Mechanism-of-Action Illustrations *(cont'd)*

Drugs with illustrated mechanisms of action	Drugs with similar mechanisms of action
enoxacin	alatrofloxacin mesylate, cinoxacin, ciprofloxacin, gatifloxacin, levofloxacin, lomefloxacin hydrochloride, moxifloxacin hydrochloride, nalidixic acid, norfloxacin, ofloxacin, sparfloxacin, trovafloxacin mesylate
etanercept	infliximab
exenatide	none
ezetimibe	none
famotidine	cimetidine, nizatidine, ranitidine hydrochloride
hydrochlorothiazide	chlorothiazide, chlorothiazide sodium, chlorthalidone, indapamide, metolazone
ipratropium bromide	none
isosorbide dinitrate, isosorbide mononitrate	nitroglycerin
lanthanum carbonate	sevelamer hydrochloride
levodopa	none
linezolid	none
memantine hydrochloride	none
milrinone lactate	inamrinone (formerly amrinone lactate)
nateglinide	repaglinide
olmesartan medoxomil	irbesartan, losartan potassium, valsartan
omeprazole	esomeprazole magnesium, lansoprazole, pantoprazole sodium, rabeprazole sodium
orlistat	none
palonosetron hydrochloride	alosetron, dolasetron, granisetron, ondansetron
pegvisomant	none
phenelzine sulfate	isocarboxazid, tranylcypromine sulfate

(continued)

Mechanism-of-Action Illustrations *(cont'd)*

Drugs with illustrated mechanisms of action	Drugs with similar mechanisms of action
remifentanil hydrochloride	codeine phosphate, codeine sulfate, fentanyl citrate, fentanyl transdermal, fentanyl transmucosal, hydrocodone bitartrate and acetaminophen, hydrocodone and ibuprofen, hydromorphone hydrochloride, levomethadyl acetate hydrochloride, levorphanol tartrate, meperidine hydrochloride, methadone hydrochloride, morphine sulfate, oxycodone and acetaminophen, oxycodone hydrochloride, oxymorphone hydrochloride, propoxyphene hydrochloride
reserpine	guanadrel sulfate, guanethidine monosulfate
spironolactone	none
tacrine hydrochloride	donepezil hydrochloride, galantamine hydrobromide, rivastigmine tartrate
teriparatide	none
ticlopidine hydrochloride	clopidogrel bisulfate
tubocurarine chloride	atracurium besylate
vasopressin	desmopressin acetate, lypressin
ziconotide	none

2016
Nurse's
Drug
Handbook

Jones & Bartlett Learning

2016 Nurse's Drug Handbook

Fifteenth Edition

JONES & BARTLETT
L E A R N I N G

World Headquarters
Jones & Bartlett Learning
5 Wall Street
Burlington, MA 01803
978-443-5000
info@jblearning.com
www.jblearning.com

Jones & Bartlett Learning books and products are available through most bookstores and online booksellers. To contact Jones & Bartlett Learning directly, call 800-832-0034, fax 978-443-8000, or visit our website, www. jblearning.com.

Substantial discounts on bulk quantities of Jones & Bartlett Learning publications are available to corporations, professional associations, and other qualified organizations. For details and specific discount information, contact the special sales department at Jones & Bartlett Learning via the above contact information or send an email to specialsales@jblearning.com.

Copyright © 2016 by Jones & Bartlett Learning, LLC, an Ascend Learning Company

ISBN: 978-1-284-08067-4

Production Credits

VP, Executive Publisher: David Cella
Executive Editor: Amanda Martin
Acquisitions Editor: Teresa Reilly
Editorial Assistant: Danielle Bessette
Senior Production Editor: Amanda Clerkin
Marketing Communications Manager: Katie Hennessy
VP, Manufacturing and Inventory Control: Therese Connell

Clinical Reviewer: Marlene Ciranowicz-Steenburg, MSN, RN
Composition: Integra Software Services Pvt. Ltd.
Cover Design: Kristin E. Parker
Rights & Media Specialist: Wes DeShano
Cover Image: © ajt/ShutterStock
Printing and Binding: Edwards Brothers Malloy
Cover Printing: Edwards Brothers Malloy

6048

Printed in the United States of America
19 18 17 16   10 9 8 7 6 5 4 3 2

Contents

Reviewers and Clinical Consultants.................................... ix
How to Use This Book xiii
Foreword xviii
Overview of Pharmacology......................... xx
Principles of Drug Administration.................... xxvii
Drug Therapy and the Nursing Process xxxi

Individual Drugs (organized alphabetically)
A... 1
B.. 121
C... 163
D.................................. 295
E F 389
G H I... 525
J K L.. 625
M 697
N O.. 803
P................................. 893
Q R S.. 1005
T 1103
U V W 1211
X Y Z.. 1247

Appendices
Parenteral Insulin Preparations 1267
Oral Allergen Extracts.................................. 1270
Antihistamines 1271
Selected Ophthalmic Drugs 1273
Selected Topical Drugs................................ 1283
Selected Antivirals 1299
Selected Antineoplastic Drugs 1308
Selected Antihypertensive Combinations 1326
Selected Obstetrical Drugs 1334
Vitamins 1336
Interferons... 1348

Compatible Drugs in a Syringe.. 1354
Drug Formulas and Calculations... 1356
Weights and Equivalents.. 1361
Equianalgesic Doses for Opioid Agonists 1363
Abbreviations.. 1364

Index 1367

Reviewers

Peter J. Ambrose, PharmD
Clinical Professor
Los Angeles–Orange County Area
Clerkships
University of California, San Francisco
San Francisco, CA

Michael C. Barros, PharmD, BCPS, CACP
Clinical Assistant Professor of Pharmacy
Practice
Temple University School of Pharmacy
Clinical Pharmacist, Heart Failure/
Transplant
Temple University Hospital
Philadelphia, PA

Edward M. Bednarczyk, PharmD
Clinical Assistant Professor
Pharmacy Practice and Nuclear Medicine
State University of New York at Buffalo
Buffalo, NY

Cristina E. Bello, PharmD
Assistant Professor of Pharmacy Practice
College of Pharmacy
Nova Southeastern University
Fort Lauderdale, FL

Scott M. Bonnema, PharmD
Consultant Pharmacist
Emissary Pharmacy and Infusion
Casper, WY

Felesia R. Bowen, RN, MS, PNP-C
Clinical Nurse Specialist
Children's Hospital at Robert Wood
Johnson University Hospital
New Brunswick, NJ

Cynthia Burman, PharmD
Clinical Assistant Professor
School of Pharmacy
Temple University
Philadelphia, PA

Jason M. Cota, PharmD, MS, BCPS
Assistant Professor, Department of
Pharmacy Practice
University of the Incarnate Word
Feik School of Pharmacy
Infectious Diseases, Clinical Pharmacist
Brooke Army Medical Center (BAMC)
San Antonio, TX

Kimberly A. Couch, PharmD
Clinical Pharmacy Specialist, Infectious
Diseases
Department of Pharmacy
Christiana Care Health System
Newark, DE

Brenda S. Frymoyer, RN, MSN
Clinical Nurse Specialist
Berks Cardiologists, Inc.
Reading, PA

Jason Gallagher, PharmD, BCPS
Associate Professor
Clinical Specialist, Infectious Diseases
Director, Infectious Diseases
Pharmacotherapy Residency
Temple University
Philadelphia, PA

Kimberly A. Galt, PharmD, FASHP
Associate Professor of Pharmacy
Practice
Director
Drug Information Services
Co-Director
Center for Practice Improvement and
Outcomes Research
Creighton University
Omaha, NE

John Gatto, RPh
Clinical Pharmacist
Eckerd Pharmacy
Owego, NY

Deborah L. Green, RN, MSN
Director
Medical Telemetry-CHF Program
Moses H. Cone Health System
Greensboro, NC

Reviewers and Clinical Consultants (cont'd)

Reviewers (cont'd)

Ronald L. Greenberg, PharmD, CPS
Clinical Pharmacy Coordinator
Fairview Ridges Hospital
Burnsville, MN

Jan K. Hastings, PharmD
Assistant Professor
College of Pharmacy
University of Arkansas for Medical Science
Little Rock, AR

Michael D. Hogue, PharmD
Assistant Professor of Pharmacy Practice
McWhorter School of Pharmacy
Samford University
Clinical Coordinator
Walgreens Drug Store
Birmingham, AL

Kimberly A. Hunter, PharmD
Assistant Professor of Pharmacy Practice
Albany College of Pharmacy
Albany, NY

William A. Kehoe, Jr., PharmD, CPS, FCCP
Professor of Clinical Pharmacy and Psychology
School of Pharmacy and Health Sciences
University of the Pacific
Stockton, CA

Julienne K. Kirk, PharmD, CPS, CDE
Assistant Professor
Department of Family Medicine
School of Medicine
Wake Forest University
Winston-Salem, NC

Peter G. Koval, PharmD, BCPS
Clinical Pharmacist
Moses H. Cone Family Practice
Greensboro, NC

Lisa M. Krupa, RN-C, CEN, FNP
Nurse Practitioner
Medical Specialists
Munster, IN

Amista A. Lone, PharmD
Clinical Assistant Professor
College of Pharmacy
University of Arizona
Tucson, AZ

Jennifer L. Lutz, PharmD
Pharmacy Resident
Samuel S. Stratton Veterans Affairs Medical Center
Albany, NY

T. Donald Marsh, PharmD, FASCP, ASHP
Director
Department of Pharmacotherapy
Mountain Area Health Education Center
Asheville, NC

Patrick McDonnell, PharmD
Assistant Professor of Clinical Pharmacy
School of Pharmacy
Temple University
Philadelphia, PA

Kenyetta N. Nesbitt, PharmD
Assistant Professor
Wayne State University
Detroit, MI

Catherine M. Oliphant, PharmD
Assistant Professor of Pharmacy Practice
School of Pharmacy
University of Wyoming
Laramie, WY

Vinita B. Pai, PharmD
Assistant Professor of Clinical Pharmacy
College of Pharmacy
Ohio State University
Columbus, OH

David J. Quan, PharmD
Clinical Pharmacist
University of California, San Francisco
San Francisco, CA

Brenda M. Reap-Thompson, RN, MSN
Assistant Clinical Professor
Drexel University
Philadelphia, PA

Nancy Jex Sabin, RN, MSN, APRN
Clinical Assistant Professor
University of San Diego
San Diego, CA

Elizabeth Sloand, PhD, RN, PNP-BC
Assistant Professor
School of Nursing
Johns Hopkins University
Baltimore, MD

Craig Williams, PharmD
Clinical Specialist
Wishard Memorial Hospital
Assistant Professor of Clinical Pharmacy
School of Pharmacy
Purdue University
Indianapolis, IN

Clinical Consultants

Madeline Albanese, RN, MSN
Nurse Educator
Hospital of the University of Pennsylvania
Philadelphia, PA

Marlene Ciranowicz-Steenburg,
 MSN, RN
Independent Consultant
Binghamton, New York

Sheree M. Fitzgerald, RN-C, MSN,
 CNA
Program Coordinator
Ancora Psychiatric Hospital
Hammonton, NJ

Maryann Foley, RN, BSN
Independent Consultant
Flourtown, PA

Grace Hukushi, RN, BSN, LNC
Critical Care Nurse
Nursing Enterprises, Inc.
Brick, NJ

Sammie Justesen, RN, BSN
Independent Nurse Consultant
Providence, UT

Catherine T. Kelly, RN, PhD, CCRN,
 CEN, ANP
Faculty
School of Nursing
Mount Saint Mary College
Newburgh, NY

Sharon Kumm, RN, MN, CCRN
Assistant Professor
School of Nursing
University of Kansas
Kansas City, KS

Leanne McQuade, RN, BSN, CEN
Staff Nurse
Emergency Department
Doylestown Hospital
Case Manager
CAB Medical Consultant
Doylestown, PA

Pamela S. Ronning, RN, MPA
Program Coordinator
Kirkhof College of Nursing
Grand Valley State University
Allendale, MI

Maureen Ryan, RN, CS, MSN, FNP
Assistant Professor
Grand Valley State University
Allendale, MI
Nurse Practitioner
Emergency Dept.
St. Mary's Hospital
Grand Rapids, MI

Julie M. Smith, RN, BA
Staff Nurse
Radiology-Heart Station
Rancocas Hospital
Willingboro, NJ

Aaron J. Strehlow, RN, PhD, FNP
Administrator and Director of Clinical
 Services
UCLA School of Nursing
Health Center at the Rescue Mission
Los Angeles, CA

Maria Wilson, RN, MSN, CCRN
Staff Nurse
Emergency Department
Chestnut Hill Hospital
Philadelphia, PA

Jones & Bartlett Learning *2016 Nurse's Drug Handbook* gives you what today's nurses and nursing students need: accurate, concise, and reliable drug facts. This book emphasizes the vital information you need to know before, during, and after drug administration. The information is presented in easy-to-understand language and organized alphabetically, so you can find what you need quickly.

What's Special

In addition to the drug information you expect to find in each entry (see "Drug Entries" for details), the *2016 Nurse's Drug Handbook* boasts these special features:

- **A new design** makes it easy to find the most need-to-know drug information, such as indications, dosages, dosage adjustments, and warnings.
- **A new size** makes the *2016 Nurse's Drug Handbook* easier and more convenient to carry and use. But even though the book is now smaller and more convenient to carry, this new edition contains more drug information than ever. We made the book smaller and better without taking anything out.
- **Practical trim size** allows the book to open flat so you can find the information you need without wrestling with a book that wants to close. You can hold the book in one hand, see complete pages at a glance, and use your other hand to document or perform other activities.
- **Introductory material** reviews essential general information you need to know to administer drugs safely and effectively, including an overview of pharmacology and the principles of drug administration. In addition, the five steps of the nursing process are explained and related specifically to drug therapy.
- **Highly useful illustrations** throughout the text help you visualize selected mechanisms of action by showing how drugs work at the cellular, tissue, and organ levels. In addition, the inside

front cover features a table listing all the drugs whose mechanisms of action are illustrated, as well as other drugs with the same mechanisms of action.

- **No-nonsense writing style** speaks in everyday language and uses the terms and abbreviations you typically encounter in your practice and your studies. To avoid sexist language, we alternate between male and female pronouns throughout the book.
- **Up-to-date drug information** includes the latest FDA-approved drugs, new and changed indications, new warnings, and newly reported adverse reactions.
- **Dosage adjustment,** headlined in color, alerts you to expected dosage changes for a patient with a specific condition or disorder, such as advanced age or renal impairment.
- **Warning,** displayed in color, calls attention to important facts that you need to know before, during, and after drug administration. For example, in the alatrofloxacin entry, this feature informs you that the drug is usually reserved for hospitalized patients and is given for no more than 2 weeks because of the high risk of severe liver damage.
- **Easy-to-use tables** showing route, onset, peak, and duration (see page *xv* for more details), and other tables in the appendices provide a time-saving way to track and check information. The appendices give you an overview of the most important facts and nursing considerations for important drug groups, including insulin preparations and selected antihistamines, topical drugs, antivirals, antineoplastic drugs, interferons, and antihypertensive combination drugs. You'll also find handy instructions for calculating drug dosages and I.V. flow rates.

Drug Entries

The *2016 Nurse's Drug Handbook* clearly and concisely presents all the vital facts on the drugs that you'll typically administer. To help you find the information you need quickly, drug entries are organized alphabetically by generic drug name—from abatacept to zonisamide. For ease of use, every drug entry follows a consistent format. However, if specific details are unknown or don't apply, the heading isn't included so you can go right to the next section.

GENERIC AND TRADE NAMES

First, each entry identifies the drug's main generic name, as well as alternate generic names. (For drugs prescribed by trade name, you can quickly check the comprehensive index, which refers you to the appropriate generic name and page.)

Next, the entry lists the most common U.S. trade names for each drug. It also includes common trade names available only in Canada, marked (CAN).

CLASS, CATEGORY, AND SCHEDULE

Each entry lists the drug's chemical and therapeutic classes. With this information, you can compare drugs in the same chemical class but in different therapeutic classes, and vice versa.

The entry also lists the FDA's pregnancy risk category, which categorizes drugs based on their potential to cause birth defects. (For details, see *FDA pregnancy risk categories.*)

However, after June 30, 2015, new prescription drugs submitted to the FDA for approval will no longer be allowed to use the lettering system to categorize drugs based on their potential to cause birth defects. Instead, new, more comprehensive text will be required in the label to explain the risks. Prescription drugs currently using the lettering system to identify potential for a drug to cause birth defects will be gradually phased into the new labeling requirement. Labeling of over-the-counter drugs will remain unchanged and is not affected by the FDA-mandated change.

Where appropriate, the entry also includes the drug's controlled substance schedule. (For details, see *Controlled substance schedules,* page *xv.*)

FDA pregnancy risk categories

Each currently prescribed drug may be placed in a pregnancy risk category based on the FDA's estimate of risk to the fetus. If the FDA hasn't provided a category, the *Drug Handbook* notes that the drug is "Not rated." The categories range from A to X, signifying least to greatest fetal risk. Note that pregnancy risk categories will no longer be used in drug labeling for drugs approved after June 30, 2015, and existing drug labels that use the category will be gradually phased into the new labeling requirements.

A   Controlled studies show no risk

Adequate, well-controlled studies with pregnant women have failed to demonstrate a risk to the fetus in any trimester of pregnancy.

B   No evidence of risk in humans

Adequate, well-controlled studies with pregnant women haven't shown increased risk of fetal abnormalities, despite adverse findings in animals, or, in the absence of adequate human studies, animal studies show no fetal risk. The chance of fetal harm is remote, but remains possible.

C   Risk can't be ruled out

Adequate, well-controlled human studies are lacking, and animal studies have shown a risk to the fetus or are lacking as well. A chance of fetal harm exists if the drug is given during pregnancy, but the potential benefits may outweigh the risk.

D   Positive evidence of risk

Studies in humans, or investigational or postmarketing data, have shown fetal risk. Nevertheless, potential benefits from the drug's use may outweigh risks. For example, the drug may be acceptable if needed in a life-threatening situation or to treat a serious disease for which safer drugs can't be used or are ineffective.

X   Contraindicated in pregnancy

Studies in animals or humans, or investigational or postmarketing reports, have shown positive evidence of fetal abnormalities or risks that clearly outweigh any possible benefit to the patient.

Controlled substance schedules

The Controlled Substances Act of 1970 mandated that certain prescription drugs be categorized in schedules based on their potential for abuse. The greater their potential for abuse, the greater the restrictions on their prescription. The controlled substance schedules range from I to V, signifying highest to lowest abuse potential.

I High potential for abuse
No accepted medical use exists for Schedule I drugs, which include heroin and lysergic acid diethylamide (LSD).

II High potential for abuse
Use may lead to severe physical or psychological dependence. Prescriptions must be written in ink or typewritten and must be signed by the prescriber. Oral prescriptions must be confirmed in writing within 72 hours and may be given only in a genuine emergency. No renewals are permitted.

III Some potential for abuse
Use may lead to low-to-moderate physical dependence or high psychological dependence. Prescriptions may be oral or written. Up to five renewals are permitted within 6 months.

IV Low potential for abuse
Use may lead to limited physical or psychological dependence. Prescriptions may be oral or written. Up to five renewals are allowed within 6 months.

V Subject to state and local regulation
Abuse potential is low; a prescription may not be required.

INDICATIONS AND DOSAGES
This section lists FDA-approved therapeutic indications. For each indication, you'll find the applicable drug form or route, age group (adults, adolescents, or children), and dosage (which includes amount per dose, timing, and duration, when known and appropriate).

ROUTE, ONSET, PEAK, AND DURATION
Quick-reference tables show the drug's onset, peak, and duration (when known) for each administration route. The onset of action is the time a drug takes to be absorbed, reach a therapeutic blood level, and elicit an initial therapeutic response. The peak therapeutic effect occurs when a drug reaches its highest blood concentration and the greatest amount of drug reaches the site of action to produce the maximum therapeutic response. The duration of action is the amount of time the drug remains at a blood level that produces a therapeutic response.

MECHANISM OF ACTION
This section concisely describes how a drug achieves its therapeutic effects at cellular, tissue, and organ levels, as appropriate. Illustrations of selected mechanisms of action lend exceptional clarity to sometimes complex processes.

INCOMPATIBILITIES
In this section, you'll be alerted to drugs or solutions that are incompatible with the topic drug when mixed in a syringe or solution, or when infused through the same I.V. line.

CONTRAINDICATIONS
An alphabetical list details the conditions and disorders that preclude administration of the topic drug.

INTERACTIONS
This section includes drugs, foods, and activities (such as alcohol use and smoking) that can cause important, problematic, or life-threatening interactions with the topic drug. For each interacting drug, food, or activity, you'll learn the effects of the interaction.

ADVERSE REACTIONS
Organized by body system, this section highlights common, serious, and life-threatening adverse reactions.

NURSING CONSIDERATIONS
Warnings, general precautions, and key information that you must know before, during, and after drug administration are

Teaching your patient about drug therapy

Your teaching about drug therapy will vary with your patient's needs and your practice setting. To help guide your teaching, each drug entry provides key information that you must teach your patient about that drug. For all patients, however, you also should:

✓ Teach the generic and trade name for each prescribed drug that he'll take after discharge—even if he took the drug before admission.

✓ Clearly explain why each drug was prescribed, how it works, and what it's supposed to do. To help your patient understand the drug's therapeutic effects, relate its action to her disorder or condition.

✓ Review the drug form, dosage, and route with the patient. Tell him whether the drug is a tablet, suppository, spray, aerosol, or other form, and explain how to take it correctly. Also, tell him how often to take the drug and for what length of time. Emphasize that he should take the drug exactly as prescribed.

✓ Describe the drug's appearance, and explain that scored tablets can be broken in half for safe, accurate dosing. Warn the patient not to break unscored tablets, because doing so may alter the drug dosage. If your patient has trouble swallowing capsules, explain that she can open ones that contain sprinkles and take them with food or a drink but that she shouldn't do this with capsules that contain powder. Also, warn her not to crush or chew enteric-coated, extended-release, sustained-release, or similar drug forms.

✓ Teach the patient about common adverse reactions that may occur. Advise him to notify the prescriber at once if a dangerous adverse reaction, such as syncope, occurs.

✓ Warn her not to suddenly stop taking a drug if she's bothered by unpleasant adverse reactions, such as a rash and mild itching. Instead, encourage her to discuss the reactions with her prescriber, who may adjust the dosage or substitute a drug that causes fewer adverse reactions.

✓ Because drugs may cause adverse reactions (such as dizziness and drowsiness) that can impair the patient's ability to perform activities that require alertness, help him develop a dosing schedule that prevents these adverse reactions.

✓ Inform the patient which adverse reactions resolve with time.

✓ Teach the patient how to store the drug properly. Let him know if the drug is sensitive to light or temperature and how to protect it from these elements.

✓ Instruct the patient to store the drug in its original container, if possible, with the drug's name and dosage clearly printed on the label.

✓ Inform the patient which devices to use—and which to avoid—for drug storage or administration. For example, warn him not to take liquid cyclosporine with a plastic cup or utensils.

✓ Teach the patient what to do if she misses a dose. Generally, she should take a once-daily drug as soon as she remembers—provided that she remembers within the first 24 hours. If 24 hours have elapsed, she should take the next scheduled dose, but she should not double the dose. If she has questions or concerns about missed doses, tell her to contact the prescriber.

✓ Provide information specific to the prescribed drug. For example, if a patient takes a diuretic to manage heart failure, instruct him to weigh himself daily at the same time of day, using the same scale, and wearing the same amount of clothing. Or, if the patient takes digoxin or an antihypertensive drug, teach him how to measure his pulse and blood pressure and how to record the measurements. Then instruct him to bring the diary to his regular appointments so the prescriber can monitor his response to the drug.

✓ Advise the patient to refill prescriptions promptly, unless she no longer needs the drug. Also instruct her to discard expired drugs because they may become ineffective or even dangerous over time.

✓ Warn the patient to keep all drugs out of the reach of children at all times.

detailed in this section. Examples include whether a pill can be crushed and how to properly reconstitute, dilute, store, handle, or dispose of a drug.

Patient teaching information is also included here. You'll find important guidelines for patients, such as how and when to take each prescribed drug, how to spot and manage adverse reactions, which cautions to observe, when to call the prescriber, and more. To save you time, however, this section doesn't repeat basic patient-teaching points. (For a summary of those, see *Teaching your patient about drug therapy*, page *xvi*, and *Federal guidelines for drug disposal*, page *xvii*.)

In short, Jones & Bartlett Learning *2016 Nurse's Drug Handbook* is designed expressly to give you more of what you need. It puts vital drug information at your fingertips and helps you always stay current in this critical part of your practice or studies.

Federal guidelines for drug disposal

Give patients these important instructions for properly disposing of their unwanted prescription drugs:

✓ Take unused, unneeded, or outdated prescription drugs out of their original containers and throw them in the trash.

✓ Consider mixing discarded prescription drugs with a substance like coffee grounds or used cat litter and putting them in impermeable, nondescript containers, such as empty cans or sealable bags.

✓ Flush prescription drugs down the toilet only if the label or accompanying patient information specifically tells you to do so.

✓ See if your community has a pharmaceutical take-back program that allows citizens to bring unused drugs to a central location for proper disposal.

Safe, effective drug therapy is one of your most important responsibilities. Not infrequently, a patient's life will depend on your ability to give drugs accurately and safely. In addition, you must keep up with the latest drug information, including newly approved drugs and recently reported life-threatening adverse reactions, as well as those drugs withdrawn from the market after widespread use.

Despite all the drug information available, medication errors remain one of the greatest threats to patients' well-being and a leading cause of lawsuits against nurses, physicians, and hospitals.

Your Responsibilities in Drug Therapy

Your basic responsibilities in drug therapy include the following:

- Administer the right drug in the right dose by the right route at the right time to the right patient.
- Know the therapeutic use, dosage, interactions, adverse reactions, and warnings of each administered drug.
- Be aware of newly approved drugs that may be prescribed.
- Know about changes to existing drugs, such as new indications and dosages and recently discovered adverse reactions and interactions.
- Concentrate fully when preparing and administering drugs.
- Respond promptly and appropriately to serious or life-threatening adverse reactions, interactions, and complications.
- Instruct each patient about the drug, how it's administered, which effects it causes or may cause, and which reactions to watch for and report.

Several factors may reduce your ability to meet these basic responsibilities—and contribute to medication errors. First, hospitals and other healthcare facilities have budget constraints that may result in elimination of professional nursing positions or the hiring of less qualified technicians to fill them. This forces the remaining nurses to care for more patients. Second, hospital patients are older and more acutely ill, and they typically receive more complex drug therapy than ever. Together, these factors place greater demands on you—increasing your stress level, reducing the time you have to concentrate on drug administration, and increasing your risk of making medication errors or overlooking serious adverse reactions or interactions.

The same factors reduce your time and energy for learning the latest drug facts—which you need to have at your command. You must have this information at your fingertips because your next patient may need a recently approved drug or a complex and unfamiliar drug regimen.

How can you balance your limited time with your need to know the latest developments?

Meeting Your Needs

Nurses and students need a reliable, accurate, easy-to-use, quick-reference drug book. They need a book clearly written by and for nurses that has been reviewed by experts in nursing and pharmacology. You hold such a book in your hands: Jones & Bartlett Learning 2016 Nurse's Drug Handbook, with features that are always current.

The content of 2016 Nurse's Drug Handbook was developed, written, and edited by experienced practicing nurses. Expert consultants, reviewers, and advisors—both nurses and pharmacists—help ensure the accuracy and reliability of the information covered in each entry and help target that information to your needs. What's more, every drug fact is checked against the most prominent drug references today, including the American Hospital Formulary Service Drug Information, Drug Facts and Comparisons, The Physicians' Desk Reference, the FDA's website of new drug approvals, and the

USP DI's *Drug Information for the Health Care Professional*. In addition, to help you quickly access much-needed information, the book is organized alphabetically by generic drug name, follows a consistent format, and is concise.

To ensure that you're always current, Jones & Bartlett Learning *Nurse's Drug Handbook* is updated every year. This newest edition contains:

• Important new drug entries in the main part of the book and in the appendices.
• New drug facts on hundreds of existing entries, including updated information on new indications and dosages, new incompatibilities and interactions, new adverse reactions, and new nursing considerations.
• Hundreds of patient-teaching guidelines and suggestions.
• Thoroughly updated appendices on insulin preparations, antiviral drugs, topical drugs, antihistamines, combination antihypertensive drugs, interferons, ophthalmic drugs, and antineoplastic drugs.
• A comprehensive new index.

And as always, you'll find the same color-coded, highly readable type that reduces eyestrain as you speed to the information you need.

Getting More from Your Drug Reference Handbook

Whether you currently work in or are preparing to work in acute care, home care, long-term care, or another healthcare setting, you'll want your own copy of the *2016 Nurse's Drug Handbook*. That's because this book can help you:

• Reduce your risk of medication errors because you'll have easy access to accurate, reliable drug information that's relevant to your practice.
• Stay current on the most up-to-date drug developments of the year.

• Improve your drug administration skills and patient care before, during, and after drug therapy.
• Quickly detect and manage serious or life-threatening adverse reactions and complications or prevent them from occurring.
• Save time because you won't have to sift through volumes of information to find what you need, search for a book that's up-to-date, or look through several drug handbooks to get enough information.
• Increase your confidence about drug administration and enhance your professional interactions with other healthcare team members.
• Ensure the delivery of safe, effective care.
• Improve the depth and quality of your patient teaching.

Reaping the Rewards

Your patients deserve the best and safest care possible—and you deserve to have the tools to deliver that care. Whether you're a student or an experienced clinician, Jones & Bartlett Learning *2016 Nurse's Drug Handbook* will help you provide safe, effective drug therapy because of its practical, easy-to-understand, accurate, and reliable information on virtually all the drugs you're likely to administer.

This handbook has aided thousands of nurses in their patient care. Take it with you to the clinical setting, share it with your peers, and use it to enhance your present and future position in the nursing profession.

Kathleen Dracup, RN, FNP, DNSc, FAAN
Dean and Professor
School of Nursing
University of California, San Francisco
San Francisco, CA

Overview of Pharmacology

Understanding the basics of pharmacology is an essential nursing responsibility. Pharmacology is the science that deals with the physical and chemical properties, and biochemical and physiologic effects, of drugs. It includes the areas of pharmacokinetics, pharmacodynamics, pharmacotherapeutics, pharmacognosy, and toxicodynamics.

The *2016 Nurse's Drug Handbook* deals primarily with pharmacokinetics, pharmacodynamics, and pharmacotherapeutics—the information you need to administer safe and effective drug therapy (discussed as follows). Pharmacognosy is the branch of pharmacology that deals with the biological, biochemical, and economic features of naturally occurring drugs. Toxicodynamics is the study of the harmful effects that excessive amounts of a drug produce in the body; in a drug overdose or drug poisoning, large drug doses may saturate or overwhelm normal mechanisms that control absorption, distribution, metabolism, and excretion.

Drug Nomenclature

Most drugs are known by several names—chemical, generic, trade, and official—each of which serves a specific function. (See *How drugs are named.*) However, multiple drug names can also contribute to medication errors. You may find a familiar drug packaged with an unfamiliar name if your institution changes suppliers or if a familiar drug is newly approved in a different dose or for a new indication.

Drug Classification

Drugs can be classified in various ways. Most pharmacology textbooks group drugs by their functional classification, such as psychotherapeutics, which is based on common characteristics. Drugs can also be classified according to their therapeutic use, such as antipanic or

How drugs are named

A drug's chemical, generic, trade, and official names are determined at different phases of the drug development process and serve different functions. For example, the various names of the commonly prescribed anticonvulsant divalproex sodium are:

- Chemical name: Pentanoic acid, 2-propyl-, sodium salt (2:1), or ($C_{16}H_{31}O_4Na$)
- Generic name: divalproex sodium
- Trade name: Depakote
- Official name: Divalproex Sodium Delayed-Release Tablets, USP

A drug's chemical name describes its atomic and molecular structure. The chemical name of divalproex sodium—pentanoic acid, 2-propyl-, sodium salt (2:1), or $C_{16}H_{31}O_4Na$ (pronounced valproate semisodium)—indicates that the drug is a combination of two valproic acid compounds with a sodium molecule attached to only one side.

Once a drug successfully completes several clinical trials, it receives a generic name, also known as the nonproprietary name. The generic name is usually derived from, but shorter than, the chemical name. The United States Adopted Names Council is responsible for selecting generic names, which are intended for unrestricted public use.

Before submitting the drug for FDA approval, the manufacturer creates and registers a trade name (or brand name) when the drug appears ready to be marketed. Trade names are copyrighted and followed by the symbol ® to indicate that they're registered and that their use is restricted to the drug manufacturer. Once the original patent on a drug has expired, any manufacturer may produce the drug under its own trade name.

A drug's official name is the name under which it's listed in the United States Pharmacopoeia (USP) and the National Formulary (NF).

antiobsessional drugs. Drugs within a certain therapeutic class may be further divided into subgroups based on their mechanisms of action. For example, the therapeutic class antineoplastics can be further classified as alkylating agents, antibiotic antineoplastics, antimetabolites, antimitotics, biological response modifiers, antineoplastic enzymes, and hormonal antineoplastics.

Pharmacokinetics

Pharmacokinetics is the study of a drug's actions—or fate—as it passes through the body during absorption, distribution, metabolism, and excretion.

ABSORPTION

Before a drug can begin working, it must be transformed from its pharmaceutical dosage form to a biologically available (bioavailable) substance that can pass through various biological cell membranes to reach its site of action. This process is known as absorption. A drug's absorption rate depends on its route of administration, its circulation through the tissue into which it's administered, and its solubility—that is, whether it's more water soluble (*hydrophilic*) or fat soluble (*lipophilic*).

Although drugs may penetrate cellular membranes either actively or passively, most drugs do so by *passive diffusion*, moving inertly from an area of higher concentration to an area of lower concentration. Passive diffusion may occur through water or fat. Passive diffusion through water—*aqueous diffusion*—occurs within large water-filled compartments, such as interstitial spaces, and across epithelial membrane tight junctions and pores in the epithelial lining of blood vessels. Aqueous diffusion is driven by concentration gradients. Drug molecules that are bound to large plasma proteins, such as albumin, are too large to pass through aqueous pores in this way. Passive diffusion through fat—*lipid diffusion*—plays an important role in drug metabolism because of the large number of lipid barriers that separate the aqueous compartments of the body. The tendency of a drug to move through lipid layers between aqueous compartments often depends on the pH of the medium—that is, the ability of the water-soluble or fat-soluble drug to form weak acid or weak base.

Drugs with molecules that are too large to readily diffuse may rely on active *diffusion*, in which special carriers on molecules, including peptides, amino acids, and glucose, transport the drug through the membranes. However, some molecules with selective membrane carriers can expel foreign drug molecules; this is why many drugs can't cross the blood-brain barrier.

Drug absorption begins at the administration route. The three main administration route categories are enteral, parenteral, and transcutaneous. Depending on its nature or chemical makeup, a drug may be better absorbed from one site than from another.

Enteral Administration

Enteral administration consists of the oral, nasogastric, and rectal routes.

Oral: Drugs administered orally are absorbed in the GI tract and then proceed by the hepatic portal vein to the liver and into the systemic circulation. Although generally considered the preferred route, oral drug administration has a number of disadvantages:

• The oral route doesn't always yield sufficiently high blood concentrations to be effective.

• Bioavailability may be less than optimal because of incomplete absorption and first-pass elimination (the part of metabolism that occurs during transit through the liver before the drug reaches the general circulation).

• Drug absorption may be incomplete if the drug is degraded by digestive enzymes or the acidic pH in the stomach or if it's excreted from the liver into the bile.

• Food in the GI tract, gastric emptying time, and intestinal motility may also impede drug absorption.

Nasogastric: Drugs administered through a nasogastric tube enter the stomach directly and are absorbed in the GI tract.

xxii   Overview of Pharmacology

Rectal: Rectal drugs and suppositories also enter the GI tract directly after being inserted in the rectum and absorbed through the rectal mucosa. After being absorbed into the lower GI tract, rectal drugs enter the circulation through the inferior vena cava, bypassing the liver and thus avoiding first-pass metabolism. Suppositories, however, tend to travel upward into the rectum, where veins, such as the superior hemorrhoidal vein, lead to the liver. As a result, drug absorption by this route is often unreliable and difficult to predict.

Parenteral Administration

Parenteral routes may be used whenever enteral routes are contraindicated or inadequate. These routes include intramuscular (I.M.), intravenous (I.V.), subcutaneous, and intradermal administration. Drug absorption is much faster and more predictable after parenteral administration than after enteral administration.

I.M.: Drugs administered by the I.M. route are injected deep into the muscle, where they're absorbed relatively quickly. The rate of drug absorption depends on the vascularity of the injection site, the physiochemical properties of the drug, and the solution in which the drug is contained.

I.V.: I.V. drug administration involves injecting or infusing the drug directly into the blood circulation, allowing for rapid distribution throughout the body. This route usually provides the greatest bioavailability.

Subcutaneous: Drugs administered by the subcutaneous route are injected into the connective tissue just below the skin and are absorbed by simple diffusion from the injection site. The factors that affect I.M. absorption also affect subcutaneous absorption. Absorption by the subcutaneous route may be slower than by the I.M. route.

Intradermal: Drugs administered intradermally, such as purified protein derivative (PPD), are injected into the dermis, from which they diffuse slowly into the local microcapillary system.

Transcutaneous Administration

Transcutaneous drug administration allows drug absorption through the skin or soft-tissue surface. Drugs may be inhaled, inserted sublingually, applied topically, or administered by the eyes, ears, nose, or vagina.

Inhalation: Inhaled drugs may be given as a powder and aerosolized or mixed in solution and nebulized directly into the respiratory tract, where they're absorbed through the alveoli. Inhaled drugs are usually absorbed quickly because of the abundant blood flow in the lungs, though some inhaled drugs have low systemic absorption.

Sublingual: Sublingual drug administration involves placing a tablet, troche, or lozenge under the tongue. The drug is absorbed across the epithelial lining of the mouth, usually quickly. This route avoids first-pass metabolism.

Topical: Topical drugs—creams, ointments, lotions, and patches—are placed on the skin and then cross the epidermis into the capillary circulation. They may also be absorbed through sweat glands, hair follicles, and other skin structures. Absorption by the skin is enhanced if the drug is in a solution.

Ophthalmic: Ophthalmic drugs include solutions and ointments that are instilled or applied directly to the cornea or conjunctiva as well as small, elliptical disks that are placed directly on the eyeball behind the lower eyelid. The movements of the eyeball promote distribution of these drugs over the surface of the eye. Although ophthalmic drugs produce a local effect on the conjunctiva or anterior chamber, some preparations may be absorbed systemically and therefore produce systemic effects.

Otic: Drops administered into the external auditory canal, otic drugs are used to treat infection or inflammation and to soften and remove ear wax. Otic solutions exert a local effect and may result in minimal systemic absorption with no adverse effects.

Nasal: Nasal solutions and suspensions are applied directly to the nasal mucosa by instillation or inhalation to produce local effects, such as vasoconstriction to reduce nasal congestion. Some nasal solutions, such as vasopressin, are administered by this route specifically to produce systemic effects.

Vaginal: Vaginal drugs include creams, suppositories, and troches that are inserted into the vagina, sometimes using a special applicator. These drugs are administered locally to treat such conditions as bacterial and fungal infections.

DISTRIBUTION
Distribution is the process by which a drug is transported by the circulating fluids to various sites, including its sites of action. To ensure maximum therapeutic effectiveness, the drug must permeate all membranes that separate it from its intended site of action. Drug distribution is influenced by blood flow, tissue availability, and protein binding. Drugs that cannot distribute to the tissues in which they are needed are not effective.

METABOLISM
Drug metabolism is the enzymatic conversion of a drug's structure into substrate molecules or polar compounds that are either less active or inactive and are readily excreted. Drugs can also be synthesized to larger molecules. Metabolism may also convert a drug to a more toxic compound. Because the primary site of drug metabolism is the liver, children, the elderly, and patients with impaired hepatic function are at risk for altered therapeutic effects.

Biotransformation is the process of changing a drug into its active metabolite. Compounds that require metabolic biotransformation for activation are known as *prodrugs*. During phase I of biotransformation, the parent drug is converted into an inactive or partially active metabolite. Much of the original drug may be eliminated during this phase. During phase II, the inactive or partially active metabolite binds with available substrates, such as acetic acid, glucuronic acid, sulfuric acid, or water, to form its active metabolite. When biotransformation leads to synthesis, larger molecules are produced to create a pharmacologic effect.

EXCRETION
The body eliminates drugs by both metabolism and excretion. Drug metabolites—and, in some cases, the active drug itself—are eventually excreted from the body, usually through bile, feces, and urine. The primary organ for drug elimination is the kidney. Impaired renal function may alter drug elimination, thereby altering the drug's therapeutic effect. Other excretion routes include evaporation through the skin, exhalation from the lungs, and secretion into saliva and breastmilk.

A drug's elimination half-life is the amount of time required for half of the drug to be eliminated from the body. The half-life roughly correlates with the drug's duration of action and is based on normal renal and hepatic function. Typically, the longer the half-life, the less often the drug has to be given and the longer it remains in the body.

Pharmacodynamics
Pharmacodynamics is the study of the biochemical and physiologic effects of drugs and their mechanisms of action. A drug's actions may be structurally specific or nonspecific. Structurally specific drugs combine with cell receptors, such as proteins or glycoproteins, to enhance or inhibit cellular enzyme actions. Drug receptors are the cellular components affected at the site of action. Many drugs form chemical bonds with drug receptors, but a drug can bond with a receptor only if it has a similar shape— much the same way that a key fits into a lock. When a drug combines with a receptor, channels are either opened or closed and cellular biochemical messengers, such as cyclic adenosine monophosphate or calcium ions, are activated. Once activated, cellular functions can be turned either on or off by these messengers.

Structurally nonspecific drugs, such as biological response modifiers, don't combine with cell receptors; rather, they produce changes within the cell membrane or interior.

The mechanisms by which drugs interact with the body are not always known. Drugs may work by physical action (such as the protective effects of a topical ointment) or chemical reaction (such as an antacid's effect on the gastric mucosa), or by modifying the metabolic activity of invading pathogens (such as an antibiotic) or replacing a missing biochemical substance (such as insulin).

AGONISTS

Agonists are drugs that interact with a receptor to stimulate a response. They alter cell physiology by binding to plasma membranes or intracellular structures. *Partial agonists* can't achieve maximal effects even though they may occupy all available receptor sites on a cell. *Strong agonists* can cause maximal effects while occupying only a small number of receptor sites on a cell. *Weak agonists* must occupy many more receptor sites than strong agonists to produce the same effect.

ANTAGONISTS

Antagonists are drugs that attach to a receptor but don't stimulate a response; instead, they inhibit or block responses that would normally be caused by agonists. *Competitive antagonists* bind to receptor sites that are also compatible with an agonist, thus preventing the agonist from binding to the site. *Noncompetitive antagonists* bind to receptor sites that aren't occupied by an agonist; this changes the receptor site so that it's no longer recognized by the agonist. *Irreversible antagonists* work in much the same way that noncompetitive ones do, except that they permanently bind with the receptor.

Antagonism plays an important role in drug interactions. When two agonists that cause opposite therapeutic effects, such as a vasodilator and a vasoconstrictor, are combined, the effects cancel each other out. When two

antagonists, such as morphine and naloxone, are combined, both drugs may become inactive.

Pharmacotherapeutics

Pharmacotherapeutics is the study of how drugs are used to prevent or treat disease. Understanding why a drug is prescribed for a certain disease can assist you in prioritizing drug administration with other patient care activities. Knowing a drug's desired and unwanted effects may help you uncover problems not readily apparent from the admitting diagnosis. This information may also help you prevent such problems as adverse reactions and drug interactions.

A drug's *desired effect* is the intended or expected clinical response to the drug. This is the response you start to evaluate as soon as a drug is given. Dosage adjustments and the continuation of therapy often depend on your accurate evaluation and documentation of the patient's response.

An *adverse reaction* is any noxious and unintended response to a drug that occurs at therapeutic doses used for prophylaxis, diagnosis, or therapy. Adverse reactions associated with excessive amounts of a drug are considered drug overdoses. Be prepared to follow your institution's policy for reporting adverse drug reactions.

An *idiosyncratic response* is a genetically determined abnormal or excessive response to a drug that occurs in a particular patient. The unusual response may indicate that the drug has saturated or overwhelmed mechanisms that normally control absorption, distribution, metabolism, or excretion, thus altering the expected response. You may be unsure whether a reaction is adverse or idiosyncratic. Once you report the reaction, the pharmacist usually determines the appropriate course of action.

An *allergic reaction* is an adverse response that results from previous exposure to the same drug or to one that's chemically similar to it. The patient's immune system reacts to the drug as if it were a foreign invader and may produce a mild hypersensitivity reaction, characterized by localized dermatitis, urticaria, angioedema, or photosensitivity. Allergic reactions should be reported to the prescriber immediately and the drug should be discontinued. Follow-up care may include giving drugs, including antihistamines and corticosteroids, to counteract the allergic response.

An *anaphylactic reaction* involves an immediate hypersensitivity response characterized by urticaria, pruritus, and angioedema. Left untreated, an anaphylactic reaction can lead to systemic involvement, resulting in shock. It's often associated with life-threatening hypotension and respiratory distress. Be prepared to assist with emergency life-support measures, especially if the reaction occurs in response to I.V. drugs, which have the fastest rate of absorption.

A *drug interaction* occurs when one drug alters the pharmacokinetics of another drug—for example, when two or more drugs are given concurrently. Such concurrent administration can increase or decrease the therapeutic or adverse effects of either drug. Some drug interactions are beneficial. For example, when taken with penicillin, probenecid decreases the excretion rate of penicillin, resulting in higher blood levels of penicillin. Drug interactions also may occur when a drug's metabolism is altered, often owing to the induction of or competition for metabolizing enzymes. For example, H_2-receptor agonists, which reduce secretion of the enzyme gastrin, may alter the breakdown of enteric coatings on other drugs. Drug interactions due to carrier protein competition typically occur when a drug inhibits the kidneys' ability to reduce excretion of other drugs. For example, probenecid is completely reabsorbed by the renal tubules and is metabolized very slowly. It competes with the same carrier protein as sulfonamides for active tubular

secretion and so decreases the renal excretion of sulfonamides. This particular competition can lead to an increased risk of sulfonamide toxicity.

Special Considerations

Although every drug has a usual dosage range, certain factors—such as a patient's age, weight, culture and ethnicity, gender, pregnancy status, and renal and hepatic function—may contribute to the need for dosage adjustments. When you encounter special considerations such as these, be prepared to reassess the prescribed dosage to make sure that it's safe and effective for your patient.

CULTURE AND ETHNICITY

Certain drugs are more effective or more likely to produce adverse effects in particular ethnic groups or races. For example, blacks with hypertension respond better to thiazide diuretics than do patients of other races; on the other hand, blacks also have an increased risk of developing angioedema with angiotensin-converting enzyme (ACE) inhibitors. A patient's religious or cultural background also may call for special consideration. For example, a drug made from porcine products may be unacceptable to a Jewish or Muslim patient.

ELDERLY PATIENTS

Because aging produces certain changes in body composition and organ function, elderly patients present unique therapeutic and dosing problems that require special attention. For example, the weight of the liver, the number of functioning hepatic cells, and hepatic blood flow all decrease as a person ages, resulting in slower drug metabolism. Renal function may also decrease with aging. These processes can lead to the accumulation of active drugs and metabolites as well as increased sensitivity to the effects of some drugs in elderly patients. Because they're also more likely to have multiple chronic illnesses, many elderly patients take multiple prescription drugs each day, thus increasing the risk of drug interactions.

CHILDREN

Because their bodily functions aren't fully developed, children—particularly those under age 12—may metabolize drugs differently than adults. In infants, immature renal and hepatic function delay metabolism and excretion of drugs. As a result, pediatric drug dosages are very different from adult dosages.

The FDA has provided drug manufacturers with guidelines that define pediatric age categories. Unless the manufacturer provides a specific age range, use these categories as a guide when administering drugs:

• neonates—birth up to age 1 month
• infants—ages 1 month to 2 years
• children—ages 2 to 12
• adolescents—ages 12 to 16.

PREGNANCY

The many physiologic changes that take place in the body during pregnancy may affect a drug's pharmacokinetics and alter its effectiveness. Additionally, exposure to drugs may pose risks for the developing fetus. Before administering a drug to a pregnant patient, be sure to check its assigned FDA pregnancy risk category and intervene appropriately.

Principles of Drug Administration

Because there are thousands of drugs and hundreds of facts about each one, taking responsibility for drug administration can seem overwhelming. One way that you can enhance your understanding of the principles of drug administration is to *associate*, *ask*, and *predict* during the critical thinking process. For example, associate each drug with general information you may already know about the drug or drug class. *Ask* yourself why a drug is administered by a certain route and why it's given multiple times throughout the day rather than only once. Learn to *predict* a drug's actions, uses, adverse effects, and possible drug interactions based on your knowledge of the drug's mechanism of action. As you apply these principles to drug administration, you'll begin to intuitively know which facts you need to make rational clinical decisions.

Prescriptions for patients in hospitals and other institutions typically are written by a physician on a form called the *physicians order sheet* or they're directly input into a computerized system with an electronic signature. Drugs are prescribed based not only on their specific mechanisms of action but also on the patient's profile, which commonly includes age, ethnicity, gender, pregnancy status, smoking and drinking habits, and use of other drugs.

"Rights" of Drug Administration

Always keep in mind the following "rights" of drug administration: the right drug, right time, right dose, right patient, right route, and right preparation and administration.

RIGHT DRUG

Many drugs have similar spellings, different concentrations, and several generic forms. Before administering any drug, compare the exact spelling and concentration of the prescribed drug that appears on the label with the information contained in the medication administration record or drug profile.

Regardless of which drug distribution system your facility uses, you should read the drug label and compare it to the medication administration record at least three times:
- before removing the drug from the dispensing unit or unit dose cart
- before preparing or measuring the prescribed dose
- before opening a unit dose package (just before administering the drug to the patient).

RIGHT TIME

Various factors can affect the time that a drug is administered, such as the timing of meals and other drugs, scheduled diagnostic tests, standardized times used by the institution, and factors that may alter the consistency of blood levels and drug absorption. Before administering any p.r.n. drug, check the patient's chart to ensure that no one else has already administered it and that the specified time interval has passed. Also, document administration of a p.r.n. drug immediately.

RIGHT DOSE

Whenever you're dispensing an unfamiliar drug or in doubt about a dosage, check the prescribed dose against the range specified in a reliable reference. Be sure to consider any reasons for a dosage adjustment that may apply to your particular patient. Also, make sure you're familiar with the standard abbreviations your institution uses for writing prescriptions.

RIGHT PATIENT

Always compare the name of the patient on the medication record with the name on the patient's identification bracelet. When using a unit dose system, compare the name on the drug profile with that on the identification bracelet.

RIGHT ROUTE

Each drug prescription should specify the administration route. If the administration route is missing from the prescription, consult the prescriber before giving the drug. Never substitute one route for another unless you obtain a prescription for the change.

RIGHT PREPARATION AND ADMINISTRATION

For drugs that need to be mixed, poured, or measured, be sure to maintain aseptic technique. Follow any specific directions included by the manufacturer regarding diluent type and amount and the use of filters, if needed. Clearly label any drug that you've reconstituted with the patient's name, the strength or dose, the date and time that you prepared the drug, the amount and type of diluent that you used, the expiration date, and your initials.

Administration Routes

Drugs may be administered by a variety of routes and dosage forms. A particular route may be chosen for convenience or to maximize drug concentration at the site of action, to minimize drug absorption elsewhere, to prolong drug absorption, or to avoid first-pass metabolism.

Different dosage forms of the same drug may have different drug absorption rates, times of onset, and durations of action. For example, nitroglycerin is a coronary vasodilator that may be administered by the I.V., sublingual, oral, or buccal route, or as a topical ointment or disk. The I.V., sublingual, and buccal forms of nitroglycerin provide a rapid onset of action, whereas the oral, ointment, and disk forms have a slower onset and a prolonged duration of action.

Drug administration routes include the enteral, parenteral, and transcutaneous routes.

ENTERAL

The enteral route consists of oral, nasogastric, and rectal administration. Drugs administered enterally enter the blood circulation by way of the GI tract. This route is considered the most natural and convenient route as well as the safest. As a result, most drugs are taken enterally, usually to provide systemic effects.

Oral

• *Tablets:* Tablets, the most commonly used dosage form, come in a variety of colors, sizes, and shapes. Some tablets are specially coated for various purposes. Enteric coatings permit safe passage of a tablet through the stomach, where some drugs may be degraded or may produce unwanted effects, to the environment of the intestine. Some coatings protect the drug from the destructive influences of moisture, light, or air during storage; some coatings actually contain the drug, such as procainamide; still others conceal a bad taste. Coatings are also used to ensure appropriate drug release and absorption. Some tablets shouldn't be crushed or broken because doing so may alter drug release.

• *Capsules:* Capsules are solid dosage forms in which the drug and other ingredients are enclosed in a hard or soft shell of varying size and shape. Drugs typically are released faster from capsules than from tablets.

• *Solutions:* Drugs administered in solution are absorbed more rapidly than many of those administered in solid form; however, they don't always produce predictable drug levels in the blood. Some drugs in solution should be administered with meals or snacks to minimize their irritating effect on the gastric mucosa.

• *Suspensions:* Suspensions are preparations consisting of finely divided drugs in a suitable vehicle, usually water. Suspensions should be shaken before administration to ensure the uniformity of the preparation and administration of the proper dosage.

Nasogastric

Drugs administered through a nasogastric or gastrostomy tube enter the stomach directly, bypassing the mouth and esophagus. They're usually administered in liquid form because an intact tablet or capsule could cause an obstruction in a gastric tube. Sometimes a tablet may be crushed or a capsule opened for nasogastric administration; however, doing so will affect the drug's release. You may need to consult a pharmacist to determine which tablets can be crushed or capsules opened.

Rectal

Some enteral drugs are administered rectally—as suppositories, solutions, or ointments—to provide either local or systemic effects. When inserted into the rectum, suppositories soften, melt, or dissolve, releasing the drug contained inside them. The rectal route may be preferred for drugs that are destroyed or inactivated by the gastric or intestinal environment or that irritate the stomach. It also may be indicated when the oral route is contraindicated because of vomiting or difficulty swallowing. The drawbacks of rectal administration include inconvenience, noncompliance, and incomplete or irregular drug absorption.

PARENTERAL

In parenteral drug administration, a drug enters the circulatory system through an injection rather than through GI absorption. This administration route is chosen when rapid drug action is desired; when the patient is uncooperative, unconscious, or unable to accept medication by the oral route; or when a drug is ineffective by other routes. Drugs may be injected into the joints, spinal column, arteries, veins, and muscles. However, the most common parenteral routes are the intramuscular (I.M.), intravenous (I.V.), subcutaneous (SubQ), and intradermal (I.D.) routes. Drugs administered parenterally may be mixed in either a solution or a suspension; those mixed in a solution typically act more rapidly than those mixed in a suspension. Parenteral administration has several disadvantages: The drug can't be removed or the dosage reduced once it has been injected, and injections typically are more expensive to administer than other dosage forms because they require strict sterility.

Intramuscular

I.M. injections are administered deep into the anterolateral aspect of the thigh (vastis lateralis), the dorsogluteal muscle (gluteus maximus), the upper arm (deltoid), or the ventrogluteal muscle (gluteus medius). I.M. injections typically provide sustained drug action. This route is commonly chosen for drugs that irritate the subcutaneous tissue. The drug should be injected as far as possible from major nerves and blood vessels.

Intravenous

In I.V. drug administration, an aqueous solution is injected directly into the vein—typically of the forearm. Drugs may be administered as a single, small-volume injection or as a slow, large-volume infusion. Because drugs injected I.V. don't encounter absorption barriers, this route produces the most rapid drug action, making it vital in emergency situations. Except for I.V. fat emulsions used as nutritional supplements, oleaginous preparations aren't usually administered by this route because of the risk of fat embolism.

Subcutaneous

The subcutaneous route may be used to inject small volumes of medication, usually 1 ml or less. Subcutaneous injections typically are given below the skin in the abdominal area, lateral area of the anterior thigh, posterior surface of the upper arm, or lateral lumbar area. Injection sites should be rotated to minimize tissue irritation if the patient receives frequent subcutaneous injections—as, for example, in a patient who takes insulin.

Intradermal

Common sites for intradermal injection are the arm and the back. Because only about 0.1 ml may be administered intradermally, this route is rarely used except in diagnostic and test procedures, such as screening for allergic reactions.

TRANSCUTANEOUS

In transcutaneous administration, a drug crosses the skin layers from either the outside (dermal) or the inside (muco-cutaneous). This route includes sublingual, inhalation, ophthalmic, otic, nasal, topical, and vaginal administration.

Sublingual

In sublingual administration, tablets are placed under the tongue and allowed to dissolve. Nitroglycerin is commonly administered by this route, which allows rapid drug absorption and action. The sublingual route also avoids first-pass metabolism.

Inhalation

Some drugs may be inhaled orally or nasally to produce a local effect on the respiratory tract or a systemic effect. Although drugs given by inhalation avoid first-pass hepatic metabolism, the lungs can also serve as an area of first-pass metabolism by providing respiratory conversion to more water-soluble compounds.

Ophthalmic

Ophthalmic solutions and ointments are applied directly to the cornea or conjunctiva for enhanced local penetration and decreased systemic absorption. These drugs usually are used in eye examinations and to treat glaucoma. Ophthalmic solutions pose a greater risk of drug loss through the nasolacrimal duct into the nasopharynx than ophthalmic ointments do.

Otic

Otic solutions are instilled directly into the external auditory canal for local

penetration and decreased systemic absorption. These drugs, which include anesthetics, antibiotics, and anti-inflammatory drugs, usually require occlusion of the ear canal with cotton after instillation.

Nasal

Nasal solutions and suspensions are applied directly to the nasal mucosa for enhanced local penetration and decreased systemic absorption. These drugs are usually used to reduce the inflammation typically associated with seasonal or perennial rhinitis.

Topical

Topical drugs—including creams, ointments, lotions, and pastes—are applied directly to the skin. Transdermal delivery systems, usually in the form of an adhesive patch or a disk, are among the latest developments in topical drug administration. Because they provide slow drug release, these systems are typically used to avoid first-pass metabolism and ensure prolonged duration of action.

Vaginal

Vaginal troches, suppositories, and creams are inserted into the vagina for slow, localized absorption. Body pH that differs from blood pH causes drug trapping or reabsorption, which delays drug excretion through the renal tubules. Vaginal secretions are alkaline, with a pH of 3.4 to 4.2, whereas blood has a pH of 7.35 to 7.45.

Drug Therapy and the Nursing Process

A systematic approach to nursing care, the nursing process helps guide you as you develop, implement, and evaluate your care and ensures that you'll deliver safe, consistent, and effective drug therapy to your patients. The nursing process consists of five steps, including assessment, nursing diagnosis, planning, implementation, and evaluation. Even though documentation is not a step in the nursing process, you're legally and professionally responsible for documenting all aspects of your care before, during, and after drug administration.

Assessment

The first step in the nursing process, assessment involves gathering information that's essential to guide your patient's drug therapy. This information includes the patient's drug history, present drug use, allergies, medical history, and physical examination findings. Assessment is an ongoing process that serves as a baseline against which to compare any changes in your patient's condition; it's also the basis for developing and individualizing your patient's plan of care.

DRUG HISTORY

The patient's drug history is critical in your planning of drug-related care. Ask about his previous use of over-the-counter and prescription drugs, as well as herbal remedies. For each drug, determine:

• the reason the patient took it
• the prescribed dosage
• the administration route
• the frequency of administration
• the duration of the drug therapy
• any adverse reactions the patient may have experienced and how he handled them.

Also determine if the patient has a history of drug abuse or addiction. Depending on his physical and emotional state, you may need to obtain the drug history from other sources, such as family members, friends, other caregivers, and the medical record.

PRESENT DRUG USE

Ask about the patient's current use of over-the-counter and prescription drugs, as well as herbal remedies. As you did in the drug history, find out the specific details for each drug (dosage, route, frequency, and reason for taking). Also ask the patient if he thinks the drug has been effective and when he took the last dose.

If the patient uses herbal remedies, similarly explore the use of these products because herbs may interact with certain drugs. Also ask about the patient's use of recreational drugs, such as alcohol and tobacco, as well as illegal drugs, such as marijuana and heroin. If the patient acknowledges use of these drugs, be alert for possible drug interactions. This information also may provide you with insight about the patient's response—or lack of response—to his current drug treatment plan.

Try to find out if the patient has any other problems that might affect his compliance with the drug treatment plan, and intervene appropriately. For instance, a patient who is unemployed and has no health insurance may fail to fill a needed prescription. In such a case, contact an appropriate individual in your facility who may be able to help the patient obtain financial assistance.

Be sure to ask the patient if his drug treatment plan requires special monitoring or follow-up laboratory tests. For example, patients who take antihypertensives need to have their blood pressure checked routinely, and those who take warfarin must have their prothrombin time tested regularly. Other patients must undergo periodic blood tests to assess their hepatic and renal function. Determine whether the patient has complied with this part of his treatment plan, and ask him if he knows the results of the latest monitoring or laboratory tests.

ALLERGIES

Find out if the patient is allergic to any drugs or foods. If he has an allergy, explore it further by determining the type of drug or food that triggers a reaction, the first time he experienced a reaction, the characteristics of the reaction, and other related information. Keep in mind that some patients consider annoying symptoms, such as indigestion, an allergic reaction. However, be sure to document a true allergy according to your facility's policy to ensure that the patient doesn't receive that drug or any related drug that may cause a similar reaction. Also, document allergies to foods because they may lead to drug interactions or adverse drug reactions. For example, sulfite is a food additive as well as a drug additive, so a patient with a known allergy to sulfite-containing foods is likely to react to sulfite-containing drugs.

MEDICAL HISTORY

While reviewing your patient's medical history, determine if he has any acute or chronic conditions that may interfere with his drug therapy. Certain disorders involving major body systems, such as the cardiovascular, GI, hepatic, and renal systems, may affect a drug's absorption, transport, metabolism, or excretion and interfere with its action; they also may increase the incidence of adverse reactions and lead to toxicity. For each disorder identified, try to determine when the condition was diagnosed, what drugs were prescribed, and who prescribed them. This information can help you determine whether the patient is receiving incompatible drugs and whether more than one prescriber is managing his drug therapy.

Ask a female patient if she is or may be pregnant or if she's breastfeeding. Many drugs are safe to use during pregnancy, but others may harm the fetus. Also, some drugs are distributed into breastmilk. If your patient is or might be pregnant, check the FDA's pregnancy risk category for the prescribed drug and notify the prescriber if the drug may pose a risk to the fetus. If the patient is breastfeeding, find out if the drug is distributed in breastmilk and intervene appropriately.

PHYSICAL EXAMINATION FINDINGS

As part of the physical examination, note the patient's age and weight. Be aware that age determines the dosage of certain drugs, such as sedatives and hypnotics, whereas weight determines the dosage of others, including some I.V. antibiotics and anticoagulants. As you perform the physical examination, note any abnormal findings that may point to body organ or system dysfunction. For example, if you detect liver enlargement and ascites, the patient may have impaired hepatic function, which can affect the metabolism of a drug he's taking and lead to harmful adverse or toxic effects. Also note whether a body organ or system appears to be responding to drug treatment. For example, if a patient has been taking an antibiotic to treat chronic bronchitis, thoroughly evaluate his respiratory status to measure his progress. And be sure to assess the patient for possible adverse reactions to the drugs he's taking.

Assess the patient's neurologic function to make sure that he can understand his drug regimen and carry out required tasks, such as performing a fingerstick to obtain blood for glucose measurement. If the patient can't understand essential drug information, you'll need to identify a family member or another person who is willing to become involved in the teaching process.

Nursing Diagnosis

Based on information derived from the assessment and physical examination findings, the nursing diagnoses are statements of actual or potential problems that a nurse is licensed to treat or manage alone or in collaboration with other members of the healthcare team. They're worded according to guidelines established by NANDA International.

One of the most common nursing diagnoses related to drug therapy is *knowledge deficit*, which indicates that the patient doesn't have sufficient understanding of his drug regimen. However, adverse reactions are the basis for most nursing diagnoses related to drug administration. For example, a patient receiving an opioid analgesic might have a nursing diagnosis of *constipation* related to decreased intestinal motility or *ineffective breathing* pattern related to respiratory depression. A patient receiving longterm, high-dose corticosteroids may have a risk for *impaired skin integrity* related to cortisone acetate or *self-concept disturbance* related to physical changes from prednisone therapy. Many antiarrhythmics cause orthostatic hypotension and thus may place an elderly patient at *high risk for injury* related to possible syncope. Broad-spectrum antibiotics, especially penicillin, may lead to the overgrowth of *Clostridium difficile*, a bacterium that normally is present in the intestine. This overgrowth in turn may lead to pseudomembranous colitis, characterized by abdominal pain and severe diarrhea. The nursing diagnoses in such a case might include *potential for infection* related to bacterial overgrowth, *alteration in comfort* related to abdominal pain, and *fluid balance deficit* related to diarrhea.

Planning

During the planning phase, you'll establish expected outcomes—or goals—for the patient and then develop specific nursing interventions to achieve them. Expected outcomes are observable or measurable goals that should occur as a result of nursing interventions and sometimes in conjunction with medical interventions. Developed in collaboration with the patient, the outcomes should be realistic and objective and should clearly communicate the direction of the plan of care to other nurses. They should be written as behaviors or responses for the patient, not the nurse, to achieve and should include a time frame for measuring the patient's progress. An example of a typical expected outcome is, *The patient will accurately demonstrate self-administration of insulin*

before discharge. Based on each outcome statement you establish, you'd then develop appropriate nursing interventions, which might include drug administration techniques, patient teaching, monitoring of vital signs, calculation of drug dosages based on weight, and recording of intake and output.

Implementation

As you implement the nursing interventions, be sure to stringently follow the classic rule of drug administration: administer the right dose of the right drug by the right route to the right patient at the right time. Also, keep in mind that you have a legal and professional responsibility to follow institutional policy regarding standing orders, prescription renewal, and the use of nursing judgment. During the implementation phase, you'll also begin to evaluate the patient's expected outcomes and nursing interventions and make necessary changes to the plan of care.

Evaluation

Evaluation is an ongoing process rather than a single step in the nursing process. During this phase, you evaluate each expected outcome to determine whether or not it has been achieved and whether the original plan of care is working or needs to be modified. In evaluating a patient's drug treatment plan, you should determine whether or not the drug is controlling the signs and symptoms for which it was prescribed. You also should evaluate the patient for psychological or physiologic responses to the drug, especially adverse reactions. This constant monitoring allows you to make appropriate and timely suggestions for changes to the plan of care, such as dosage adjustments or changes in delivery routes, until each expected outcome has been achieved.

Documentation

You're responsible for documenting all your actions related to the patient's drug therapy, from the assessment phase to evaluation. Each time you administer a drug, document the drug name, dose, time given, and your evaluation of its effect. When you administer drugs that require additional nursing judgment, such as those prescribed on an as-needed basis, document the rationale for administering the drug and follow-up assessment or interventions for each dose administered.

If you decide to withhold a prescribed drug based on your nursing judgment, document your action and the rationale for it, and notify the prescriber of your action in a timely manner. Whenever you notify a prescriber about a significant finding related to drug therapy, such as an adverse reaction, document the date and time, the person you contacted, what you discussed, and how you intervened.

A

abatacept
Orencia

Class and Category
Chemical class: Soluble fusion protein, human recombinant fusion protein
Therapeutic class: Antirheumatic
Pregnancy category: C

Indications and Dosages
➤ *To reduce signs and symptoms, induce major clinical response, inhibit progression of structural damage, and improve physical function in patients with moderate to severe active rheumatoid arthritis and an inadequate response to methotrexate or a tumor necrosis factor antagonist*
I.V. INFUSION
Adults weighing more than 100 kg (220 lb). *Initial:* 1,000 mg infused over 30 min, repeated in 2 to 4 wk. *Maintenance:* 1,000 mg infused over 30 min every 4 wk starting at wk 8.
Adults weighing 60 to 100 kg (132 to 220 lb). *Initial:* 750 mg infused over 30 min, repeated in 2 to 4 wk. *Maintenance:* 750 mg infused over 30 min every 4 wk starting at wk 8.
Adults weighing less than 60 kg. *Initial:* 500 mg infused over 30 min, repeated in 2 to 4 wk. *Maintenance:* 500 mg infused over 30 min every 4 wk starting at wk 8.
SUBCUTANEOUS INJECTION
Adults. Following a single I.V. loading dose as per body weight categories listed above, 125 mg given within a day, followed by 125 mg once wk. Alternate if unable to receive I.V. loading dose: 125 mg once wk.
DOSAGE ADJUSTMENT For patient transitioning from I.V. therapy to SubQ injection, first subQ dose should be administered instead of the next scheduled I.V. dose.
➤ *To reduce signs and symptoms of moderate to severe active polyarticular juvenile idiopathic arthritis*

I.V. INFUSION
Children ages 6 to 17 weighing more than 100 kg. *Initial:* 1,000 mg infused over 30 min, repeated in 2 to 4 wk. *Maintenance:* 1,000 mg infused over 30 min every 4 wk starting at wk 8.
Children ages 6 to 17 weighing 75 to 100 kg. *Initial:* 750 mg infused over 30 min, repeated in 2 to 4 wk. *Maintenance:* 750 mg infused over 30 min every 4 wk starting at wk 8.
Children ages 6 to 17 weighing less than 75 kg. *Initial:* 10 mg/kg infused over 30 min, repeated in 2 to 4 wk. *Maintenance:* 10 mg/kg infused over 30 min every 4 wk starting at wk 8.

Mechanism of Action
Inhibits T-cell activation by binding to CD80 and CD86 to block interaction with CD28. CD28 is part of the co-stimulatory signal needed for full activation of T cells. Activated T cells have been implicated in the pathogenesis of rheumatoid arthritis. With decreased proliferation of T cells, inflammation and other evidence of rheumatoid arthritis decrease.

Incompatibilities
Don't infuse abatacept solution with other drugs in the same intravenous line concurrently because it is not known whether the drugs may interact.

Contraindications
Hypersensitivity to abatacept or its components

Interaction
DRUGS
immunosuppressants: Possibly increased risk of serious infection
live-virus vaccines: Possibly decreased response to vaccine, and risk of infection with live virus
tumor necrosis factor antagonists: Increased risk of serious infection

Adverse Reactions
CNS: Dizziness, fever, headache
CV: Hypertension, hypotension
EENT: Nasopharyngitis, rhinitis, sinusitis
GI: Abdominal pain, diarrhea, diverticulitis, dyspepsia, nausea
GU: Acute pyelonephritis, UTI
MS: Back or limb pain

RESP: Bronchitis, COPD worsening, cough, dyspnea, pneumonia, upper respiratory tract infection, wheezing
SKIN: Cellulitis, flushing, pruritus, rash, urticaria
Other: Anaphylaxis, antibody formation, herpes simplex, herpes zoster infection, influenza, malignancies, serious infections such as sepsis, varicella infection

Nursing Considerations

• Screen patient for latent tuberculosis with a tuberculin skin test before starting abatacept. If test is positive, expect to provide treatment, as ordered, before starting abatacept. Also screen patient for hepatitis B. If present, expect abatacept to be withdrawn because antirheumatic therapies such as abatacept may reactivate hepatitis B.
• Review patient's immunization record, and make sure all immunizations are current before therapy starts. Drug may blunt effectiveness of some vaccines and increase the risk of infection with live viruses.
• Use cautiously in patients with a history of recurrent infections, underlying conditions that may predispose them to infection, or existing chronic, latent, or localized infection. They have an increased risk of infection with abatacept therapy.
• Use cautiously in patients with COPD and monitor respiratory status closely because abatacept may worsen COPD and increase the risk of adverse respiratory reactions.
• Tumor necrosis factor antagonists shouldn't be given with abatacept because of an increased risk of serious infection.
• For I.V. injection, reconstitute each vial with 10 ml of sterile water for injection. Use only the silicone-free disposable syringe provided with each vial because a siliconized syringe may cause translucent particles to form in solution. After injecting sterile water into vial, gently swirl vial until contents are completely dissolved. To minimize foaming, don't shake. Vent the vial with a needle to dissipate any foam that may be present.

• For I.V. injection, further dilute reconstituted solution with 0.9% sodium chloride injection to achieve a final solution of 100 ml. Slowly add solution into infusion bag or bottle using the same silicone-free disposable syringe provided with each vial. Mix gently. Do not shake the bag or bottle.
• Give entire I.V. dose of fully diluted drug over 30 minutes using an infusion set and a sterile, nonpyrogenic, low protein-binding filter with a pore size of 0.2 μm.
• Once fully diluted, I.V. solution may be kept for 24 hours at room temperature or refrigerated. If reconstituted solution isn't used within 24 hours, discard.
• Administer subcutaneous injection using only the supplied 125 mg/ml single-dose prefilled glass syringe. Know that the 125 mg/syringe is never to be used for intravenous infusion.
• When administering abatacept sub-cutaneously, rotate sites and never give in areas where the skin is tender, bruised, red, or hard.
• After giving abatacept, monitor patient closely for evidence of hypersensitivity reaction such as rash, pruritus, urticaria, dyspnea, or wheezing. If present, stop drug immediately, notify prescriber, and provide emergency care, as ordered.
• Monitor patient closely for evidence of infection or malignancy because abatacept inhibits T-cell activation, increasing the risk of both.

PATIENT TEACHING
• Instruct patient receiving abatacept subcutaneously on how to administer the drug. Inform patient that injection sites should be rotated and should never be administered in an area where the skin is tender, bruised, red, or hard.
• Instruct patient not to receive immunizations with live vaccines during abatacept therapy and for 3 months afterward.
• Emphasize need to report any evidence of infection or hypersensitivity to prescriber.
• Alert patient that abatacept may increase the risk of malignancy.
• Warn patient to avoid crowds and people with infections.

abciximab

Reopro

Class and Category

Chemical class: Fab fragment of chimeric 7E3 antibody
Therapeutic class: Platelet aggregation inhibitor
Pregnancy category: C

Indications and Dosages

➤ *To prevent acute myocardial ischemic complications after percutaneous transluminal coronary angioplasty (PTCA) in patients at high risk for abrupt closure of treated coronary artery*

I.V. INFUSION OR INJECTION
Adults. 250-mcg/kg bolus 10 to 60 min before PTCA. *Maintenance:* 0.125 mcg/kg/min by continuous infusion for 12 hr. *Maximum:* 10 mcg/min.

➤ *To treat unstable angina in patients who haven't responded to conventional therapy and are scheduled for PTCA within 24 hr*

I.V. INFUSION OR INJECTION
Adults. 250-mcg/kg by bolus; then 10 mcg/min by continuous infusion over 18 to 24 hr, concluding 1 hr after PTCA.

Route	Onset	Peak	Duration
I.V.	Unknown	Unknown	48 hr

Mechanism of Action

Binds to glycoprotein IIb/IIIa receptor sites on the surface of activated platelets. Circulating fibrinogen can bind to these receptor sites and link platelets together, forming a clot that eventually blocks a coronary artery. By binding to receptor sites, abciximab prevents normal binding of fibrinogen and other factors and inhibits platelet aggregation.

Incompatibilities

Don't mix abciximab with other drugs. Give through separate I.V. line when possible.

Contraindications

Active internal bleeding, arteriovenous malformation or aneurysm, bleeding disorders, stroke in past 2 years or that caused significant neurologic deficit at any time, GI or GU bleeding in past 6 weeks, hypersensitivity to abciximab, intracranial neoplasm, I.V. dextran use before or during PTCA, oral anticoagulant therapy in past 7 days unless PT is less than 1.2 times control, severe uncontrolled hypertension, surgery in past 6 weeks, thrombocytopenia, vasculitis

Interaction

DRUGS
dipyridamole, heparin, NSAIDs, oral anticoagulants, thrombolytic drugs, ticlopidine: Increased risk of bleeding

Adverse Reactions

CNS: Confusion, dizziness, hyperesthesia
CV: Atrial fibrillation or flutter, bradycardia, embolism, hypotension, peripheral edema, pseudoaneurysm, supraventricular tachycardia, third-degree AV block, thrombophlebitis, weak pulse
GI: Dysphagia, hematemesis, nausea, vomiting
GU: Dysuria, hematuria, renal dysfunction, urinary frequency, urinary incontinence, urine retention
HEME: Anemia, bleeding, leukocytosis, thrombocytopenia
RESP: Bronchitis, bronchospasm, crackles, dyspnea, pleural effusion, pneumonia, pulmonary edema, pulmonary embolism, wheezing
SKIN: Pruritus, rash, urticaria
Other: Development of human antichimeric antibodies

Nursing Considerations

• Know that abciximab may be used with heparin and aspirin therapy.
• Inspect abciximab for particles; don't use if opaque particles are present.
• For continuous I.V. infusion, withdraw 4.5 ml from 2-mg/ml solution and inject prescribed amount into 250-ml bag of normal saline solution or D_5W using an in-line sterile, nonpyrogenic, low–protein-binding 0.2- to 0.22-micron filter. Discard unused portion.
• Give I.V. bolus with sterile, nonpyrogenic, low–protein-binding 0.2- to 0.22-micron filter.
• Avoid I.M. injections, venipunctures, and use of indwelling urinary catheters, NG tubes, and automatic blood pressure cuffs

during therapy to prevent bleeding. If appropriate, insert an intermittent I.V. access device to obtain blood samples.
• Watch for GI, GU, and retroperitoneal bleeding and bleeding at puncture sites.
WARNING If hemorrhage occurs, prepare to stop infusion immediately. Expect to treat severe thrombocytopenia with platelet transfusions if needed.
• Monitor patient for hypersensitivity reactions, such as rash, pruritus, wheezing, and dysphagia from laryngeal edema. If such reactions occur, stop infusion and notify prescriber immediately. If anaphylaxis occurs, give epinephrine, antihistamines, and corticosteroids, as prescribed.
• Obtain platelet count 2 to 4 hours after initial bolus and every 24 hours during therapy as ordered. Expect platelet function to return to normal within 48 hours after therapy ends.
• Monitor vital signs and continuous ECG tracings during treatment.
PATIENT TEACHING
• Teach about possible adverse reactions, including bleeding and hypersensitivity reactions, which may cause rash, urticaria, and dyspnea.
• Tell patient to prevent injury from falls by maintaining bed rest, and injury from bleeding by keeping limb immobile while catheter sheath is in place.

acamprosate calcium

Campral

Class and Category
Chemical class: Synthetic endogenous amino acid homotaurine, gamma-aminobutyric acid (GABA) analogue
Therapeutic class: Antialcoholic
Pregnancy category: C

Indications and Dosages
➤ *To maintain abstinence from alcohol for alcohol-dependent patients who are abstinent at the start of treatment*
E.R. TABLETS
Adults. 666 mg three times daily.

DOSAGE ADJUSTMENT For patients with moderate renal impairment (creatinine clearance of 30 to 50 ml/min), 333 mg three times daily.

Route	Onset	Peak	Duration
P.O.	Unknown	3–8 hr	Unknown

Contraindications
Hypersensitivity to acamprosate or its components, severe hepatic (Child-Pugh class C) or renal impairment

Interaction
DRUGS
antidepressants: Increased weight gain
tetracyclines: Decreased absorption of tetracyclines

Adverse Reactions
CNS: Abnormal thinking, amnesia, anxiety, asthenia, chills, depression, dizziness, headache, insomnia, paresthesia, somnolence, suicidal ideation, syncope, tremor
CV: Chest pain, hypertension, palpitations, peripheral edema, vasodilation
EENT: Abnormal vision, dry mouth, pharyngitis, rhinitis, taste perversion
GI: Abdominal pain, anorexia, constipation, diarrhea, flatulence, increased appetite, indigestion, nausea, vomiting
GU: Acute renal failure, decreased libido, impotence
HEME: Leukopenia, lymphocytosis, thrombocytopenia
MS: Arthralgia, back pain, myalgia
RESP: Bronchitis, cough, dyspnea
SKIN: Diaphoresis, pruritus, rash
Other: Flulike symptoms, infection, weight gain

Nursing Considerations
• Acamprosate should start as soon as possible after patient has undergone alcohol withdrawal and achieved abstinence.
• Continue to give acamprosate even during periods of alcohol relapse.
PATIENT TEACHING
• Instruct patient to take acamprosate exactly as prescribed, even if a relapse occurs, and to seek help for a relapse.
• Warn patient that acamprosate won't reduce symptoms of alcohol withdrawal if relapse occurs followed by cessation.

Mechanism of Action

Chronic alcoholism may alter the balance between excitation and inhibition in neurons in the brain; acamprosate restores it.

When the neurotransmitter gammaaminobutyric acid (GABA) binds to its receptors in the CNS, it opens the chloride ion channel and releases chloride (Cl-) into the cell (below left), thereby reducing neuronal excitability by inhibiting depolarization. By interacting with GABA receptor sites, acamprosate prevents GABA from binding (below right).

When glutamate binds to its receptors, it closes the chloride ion channel, increasing neuronal excitability by promoting depolarization (below left). This imbalance fosters a craving for alcohol. By interacting with glutamate receptor sites, acamprosate prevents glutamate from binding (below right).

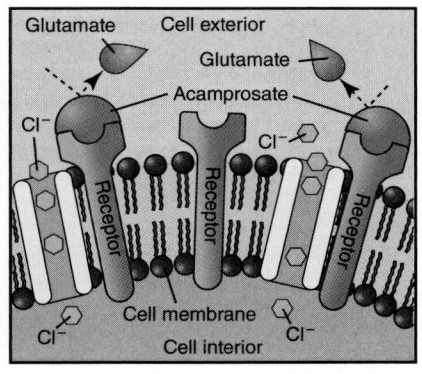

• Urge caregivers to monitor patient for evidence of depression (lack of appetite or interest in life, fatigue, excessive sleeping, difficulty concentrating) or suicidal tendencies because a small number of patients taking acamprosate have attempted suicide.

• Advise patient to use caution when performing hazardous activities until adverse CNS effects of drug are known.
• Tell female patient to notify prescriber if she is or intends to become pregnant while taking acamprosate; the drug may need to be stopped because fetal risks are unknown.

acarbose

Precose

Class and Category

Chemical class: Alpha-glucosidase inhibitor, oligosaccharide
Therapeutic class: Antidiabetic drug
Pregnancy category: B

Indications and Dosages

➤ *To control blood glucose level in patients with type 2 (non–insulin-dependent) diabetes mellitus when the level can't be controlled by diet alone*

TABLETS

Adults. *Initial:* 25 mg three times daily with first bite of each meal. *Maintenance:* Increased to maximum at 4- to 8-wk intervals p.r.n. *Maximum:* 50 mg three times daily for patients weighing 65 kg (143 lb) or less; 100 mg three times daily for patients weighing more than 65 kg.

Mechanism of Action

Inhibits action of alpha-amylase and alpha-glucoside enzymes. Normally, alpha-amylase hydrolyzes complex starches to oligosaccharides in the small intestine and alpha-glucoside hydrolyzes oligosaccharides, trisaccharides, and disaccharides to glucose and other monosaccharides in the brush border of the small intestine. In diabetic patients, acarbose inhibits these actions and delays glucose absorption, reducing blood glucose level after meals.

Contraindications

Chronic intestinal disease, cirrhosis, colonic ulceration, conditions that may deteriorate because of increased gas formation in intestines, diabetic ketoacidosis, digestive or absorption disorders, history of bowel obstruction, hypersensitivity to acarbose, inflammatory bowel disease

Interaction

DRUGS

calcium channel blockers, digestive enzymes (such as pancreatin), diuretics, estrogen, intestinal adsorbents (such as activated charcoal), isoniazid, nicotinic acid, oral contraceptives, phenothiazines, phenytoin, sympathomimetics, thyroid hormones: Possibly decreased therapeutic effects of acarbose

digoxin: Decreased serum level and therapeutic effects of digoxin
insulin, sulfonylureas: Decreased insulin action, possibly increased risk of hypoglycemia

Adverse Reactions

CV: Edema
GI: Abdominal distention and pain, diarrhea, flatulence, fulminant hepatitis, hepatotoxicity, ileus, intestinal wall gas-filled cysts, jaundice
HEME: Thrombocytopenia
SKIN: Erythema, exanthema, rash, urticaria

Nursing Considerations

WARNING Be aware that acarbose isn't recommended for patients with significant renal dysfunction and a serum creatinine level above 2 mg/dl.

- If patient is receiving acarbose and a sulfonylurea or insulin to enhance glucose control, check blood glucose level often, as appropriate.
- Store drug in sealed container in cool environment.
- Expect to decrease dosage to control GI upset.
- Monitor glycosylated hemoglobin level as ordered every 3 months for first year to evaluate glucose control and patient compliance.
- Monitor hematocrit and serum AST level every 3 months during first year of therapy and periodically thereafter, as ordered, because acarbose may decrease hematocrit and increase serum AST level.

PATIENT TEACHING

- Explain importance of self-monitoring glucose level during acarbose therapy.
- Teach patient to recognize hypoglycemia and hyperglycemia.
- Warn patient that noncompliance with treatment can increase risk of diabetic complications, including neuropathy, retinopathy, and renal insufficiency.
- Explain that temporary insulin therapy may be needed if fever, trauma, infection, illness, surgery, or other stress alters blood glucose control.
- Warn patient not to take other drugs within 2 hours of acarbose unless specifically instructed by prescriber.
- Tell him to consult prescriber before taking OTC drugs during acarbose therapy.
- Advise patient who also takes another antidiabetic to carry glucose with him at all times in case hypoglycemia occurs.

acebutolol hydrochloride

Monitan (can), Sectral

Class and Category
Chemical class: Beta$_1$-selective (cardio-selective) adrenergic receptor blocker
Therapeutic class: Antihypertensive, class II antiarrhythmic
Pregnancy category: B

Indications and Dosages
➤ *To treat hypertension*
TABLETS
Adults. *Initial:* 400 mg daily or 200 mg twice daily. *Usual:* 200 to 800 mg daily. Increased to 1,200 mg daily in divided doses twice daily for severe hypertension or hypertension that isn't well controlled with usual dosage.
➤ *To treat premature ventricular arrhythmias*
TABLETS
Adults. *Initial:* 200 mg twice daily. *Usual:* 600 to 1,200 mg daily.
DOSAGE ADJUSTMENT Maximum of 800 mg daily for elderly patients. Dosage reduced by 50% for patients with creatinine clearance less than 50 ml/min/1.73 m^2. Dosage reduced by 75% for patients with creatinine clearance less than 25 ml/min/1.73 m^2.

Route	Onset	Peak	Duration
P.O.	1–1.5 hr	2–8 hr	24 hr or longer

Mechanism of Action
Inhibits stimulation of beta$_1$ receptors in the heart, decreasing cardiac excitability, heart rate, cardiac output, and myocardial oxygen demand. Acebutolol also decreases kidneys' release of renin, which helps reduce blood pressure. Drug suppresses SA node automaticity and AV node conductivity, which suppresses atrial and ventricular ectopy. By decreasing myocardial oxygen demand, acebutolol decreases myocardial ischemia. At high doses, it inhibits stimulation of beta$_2$ receptors in the lungs and may cause bronchoconstriction.

Contraindications
Cardiogenic shock, heart failure unless from tachyarrhythmia, hypersensitivity to acebutolol, overt heart failure, second- and third-degree heart block, severe bradycardia

Interaction
DRUGS
alpha agonists, nasal decongestants: Increased risk of hypertension
aluminum salts, barbiturates, calcium salts, cholestyramine, colestipol, indomethacin, NSAIDs, penicillins, rifampin, salicylates, sulfinpyrazone: Decreased antihypertensive effects
anticholinergics, hydralazine, methyldopa, prazosin, reserpine: Increased risk of bradycardia and hypotension
beta$_2$ agonists, theophylline: Decreased bronchodilation
epinephrine: Increased risk of blocked sympathomimetic effects
ergot alkaloids: Increased risk of peripheral ischemia and gangrene
flecainide: Possibly increased effects of both drugs
lidocaine: Possibly increased serum lidocaine level, causing toxicity
oral contraceptives, quinidine: Possibly increased serum acebutolol level
sulfonylureas: Possibly decreased hypoglycemic effects
verapamil: Increased cardiac effects, leading to bradycardia and hypotension

Adverse Reactions
CNS: Abnormal dreams, anxiety, confusion, depression, dizziness, fatigue, fever, headache, insomnia
CV: Bradycardia, chest pain, edema, heart block, heart failure, hypotension
EENT: Abnormal vision, conjunctivitis, dry eyes, eye pain, pharyngitis, rhinitis
GI: Constipation, diarrhea, flatulence, hepatotoxicity, indigestion, nausea
GU: Dysuria, impotence, polyuria
MS: Arthralgia, myalgia
RESP: Bronchospasm, cough, dyspnea, wheezing
SKIN: Rash

Nursing Considerations
• Before therapy begins, obtain baseline renal function tests, as ordered.
• Check apical and radial pulses before giving acebutolol. Also, frequently monitor blood pressure and pulse rate, rhythm, and quality during treatment.

- Give drug with food to prevent GI upset.
- Acebutolol may elevate uric acid, potassium, triglyceride, lipoprotein, and antinuclear antibody levels; it also may interfere with accuracy of glucose tolerance tests.
- Monitor diabetic patient's blood glucose level to spot alterations.
- Notify prescriber if you detect a heart rate below 50 beats/min or signs of heart failure, such as dyspnea, crackles, unexplained weight gain, and jugular vein distention.
- Monitor patient for peripheral edema, and evaluate fluid intake and output.
- Be aware that chronic beta-blocker therapy, such as acebutolol, is not routinely withheld prior to major surgery because the benefits outweigh the risks associated with its use with general anesthesia and surgical procedures.

PATIENT TEACHING
- Tell patient that tablets may be crushed or swallowed whole.
- Warn against stopping acebutolol abruptly because doing so could cause angina or dangerously high blood pressure.
- Instruct patient to take a missed dose as soon as possible, up to 6 hours before next scheduled dose, but not to double the next dose.
- Advise patient to consult prescriber before taking OTC drugs that contain alpha agonists, such as nasal decongestants and cold preparations.
- Instruct patient to report dizziness, confusion, and fever immediately.
- Urge patient to maintain diet and lifestyle changes to help control blood pressure.

acetaminophen

Abenol (CAN), Acephen, Aceta Elixir, Acetaminophen Uniserts, Aceta Tablets, Apacet Capsules, Apacet Elixir, Apacet Extra Strength Tablets, Apacet Regular Strength Tablets, Aspirin-Free Pain Relief, Exdol (CAN), Feverall, Feverall Sprinkle Caps, Genapap Infants' Drops, Genebs Extra Strength, Halenol Children's Junior Strength, Liquiprin Elixir, Liquiprin Infants' Drops, Meda Cap, Neopap, Oraphen-PD, Panadol, Panadol Infants' Drops, Pediaphen, Redutemp, Robigesic (CAN), St. Joseph Aspirin-Free

Infant Drops, Tapanol Extra Strength, Tempra, Tempra Drops, Tylenol, Tylenol Caplets, Tylenol Children's Chewable Tablets, Tylenol Extra Strength, Tylenol Gelcaps, Tylenol Infants' Drops, Parenteral: Ofirmev.

Class and Category
Chemical class: Nonsalicylate, para-aminophenol derivative
Therapeutic class: Antipyretic, nonopioid analgesic
Pregnancy category: B

Indications and Dosages
➤ *To relieve mild to moderate pain from headache, muscle ache, backache, minor arthritis, common cold, toothache, or menstrual cramps; to reduce fever*
REGULAR STRENGTH (325 MG): CAPLETS, CAPSULES, CHEWABLE TABLETS, ELIXIR, GELCAPS, LIQUID SOLUTION, SPRINKLES, SUSPENSION, TABLETS
Adults and children 12 yrs and over.
650 mg (2 tablets) every 4 to 6 hr, as needed. *Maximum:* 3,250 mg (5 doses) in 24 hr.
Children ages 6 to 11 yr. 325 mg (1 tablet) every 4 to 6 hr, as needed. *Maximum:* 1,625 mg (5 doses) in 24 hr.
JUNIOR CHEWABLE TABLETS (160 MG/TABLET), JUNIOR MELTAWAYS (160 MG/TABLET)
Children age 11. 480 mg (3 tablets) every 4 hr, as needed. *Maximum:* 2,400 mg (5 doses) in 24 hr.
Children ages 9 and 10. 400 mg (2.5 tablets) every 4 hr, as needed. *Maximum:* 2,000 mg (5 doses) in 24 hr.
Children ages 6 to 8. 320 mg (2 tablets) every 4 hr, as needed. *Maximum:* 1,600 mg (5 doses) in 24 hr.
CHILDREN'S SUSPENSION (160 MG/5 ML), CHILDREN'S CHEWABLE TABLETS (80 MG/TABLET), CHILDREN'S MELTAWAYS (80 MG/TABLET)
Children age 11. 480 mg (15 ml or 6 tablets) every 4 hr, as needed. *Maximum:* 2,400 mg (5 doses) in 24 hr.
Children ages 9 and 10. 400 mg (12.5 ml or 5 tablets) every 4 hr, as needed. *Maximum:* 2,000 mg (5 doses) in 24 hr.
Children ages 6 to 8. 320 mg (10 ml or 4 tablets) every 4 hr, as needed. *Maximum:* 1,600 mg (5 doses) in 24 hr.

Children ages 4 and 5. 240 mg (7.5 mg or 3 tablets) every 4 hr, as needed. *Maximum:* 1,200 mg (5 doses) in 24 hr.
Children ages 2 and 3. 160 mg (5 ml or 2 tablets) every 4 hr, as needed. *Maximum:* 800 mg (5 doses) in 24 hr.
Children under age 2: Individualized.
8 HR E.R. CAPLETS (650 MG/CAPLET)
Adults and children age 12 and over. 1,300 mg (2 caplets) q 8 hr, as needed. *Maximum:* 3,900 mg (3 doses) in 24 hr.
EXTRA-STRENGTH (500 MG): CAPLETS, RAPID-RELEASE GELCAPS, EZ TABS
Adults and children age 12 and over. 500 mg (2 caplets, gelcaps, tabs) q 6 hr, as needed. *Maximum:* 3,000 mg (3 doses) in 24 hr.
EXTRA-STRENGTH RAPID-RELEASE LIQUID (1,000 MG PER 30 ML)
Adults and children age 12 and over. 1,000 mg (30 ml) q 6 hr, as needed. *Maximum:* 3,000 mg (3 doses) in 24 hr.
SUPPOSITORIES
Adults and adolescents. 650 mg every 4 to 6 hr, as needed. *Maximum:* 3,000 mg in 24 hr.
Children ages 6 to 12. 325 mg every 4 to 6 hr, as needed. *Maximum:* 1,950 mg in 24 hr.
Children ages 3 to 6. 120 to 125 mg every 4 to 6 hr, as needed. *Maximum:* 750 mg in 24 hr.
Children ages 1 to 3. 80 mg every 4 hr, as needed. *Maximum:* 480 mg in 24 hr.
Children ages 3 months to 11 months. 80 mg every 6 hr, as needed. *Maximum:* 320 mg in 24 hr.
➤ *To relieve mild to moderate pain; to manage moderate to severe pain with adjunctive opioid analgesics; to reduce fever*
I.V. INFUSION (OFIRMEV)
Adults and adolescents age 13 and over weighing 50 kg (110 lb) or more. 650 mg administered over 15 min every 4 hr, as needed, or 1,000 mg administered over 15 min every 6 hr, as needed. *Maximum:* 4,000 mg in 24 hr.
Adults and adolescents age 13 and over, and children age 2 and over weighing less than 50 kg (110 lb). 12.5 mg/kg administered over 15 min every 4 hr, as needed, or 15 mg/kg (up to 750 mg) administered over 15 min every 6 hr, as needed. *Maximum:* 75 mg/kg in 24 hr.

Mechanism of Action
Inhibits the enzyme cyclooxygenase, blocking prostaglandin production and interfering with pain impulse generation in the peripheral nervous system. Acetaminophen also acts directly on temperature-regulating center in the hypothalamus by inhibiting synthesis of prostaglandin E_2.

Incompatibilities
Don't mix parenteral acetaminophen with any other medication. Diazepam and chlorpromazine are physically incompatible with parenteral acetaminophen.

Route	Onset	Peak	Duration
P.O., P.R., I.V.	Varies	1–3 hr	3–4 hr

Contraindications
Hypersensitivity to acetaminophen or its components, severe hepatic impairment, severe active liver disease

Interaction
DRUGS
anticholinergics: Decreased onset of acetaminophen action
barbiturates, carbamazepine, hydantoins, isoniazid, rifampin, sulfinpyrazone: Decreased therapeutic effects and increased hepatotoxic effects of acetaminophen
lamotrigine, loop diuretics: Possibly decreased therapeutic effects of these drugs
oral contraceptives: Decreased effectiveness of acetaminophen
probenecid: Possibly increased therapeutic effects of acetaminophen
propranolol: Possibly increased action of acetaminophen
warfarin: Possibly increased international normalized ratio
zidovudine: Possibly decreased zidovudine effects
ACTIVITIES
alcohol use: Increased risk of hepatotoxicity

Adverse Reactions
GI: Abdominal pain, hepatotoxicity (possibly severe), nausea, vomiting
HEME: Hemolytic anemia (with long-term use), leukopenia, neutropenia, pancytopenia, thrombocytopenia
SKIN: Acute generalized exanthematous pustulosis, blisters, jaundice, pruritus, rash, reddening, Stevens-Johnson syndrome, toxic epidermal necrolysis, urticaria
Other: Anaphylaxis, angioedema, hypersensitivity reaction, hypoglycemic coma

Nursing Considerations

• Use acetaminophen cautiously in patients with hepatic impairment or active hepatic disease, alcoholism, chronic malnutrition, severe hypovolemia, or severe renal impairment.

• Before and during long-term therapy including parenteral therapy, monitor liver function test results, including AST, ALT, bilirubin, and creatinine levels, as ordered because acetaminophen may cause hepatotoxicity. Ensure that the daily dose of acetaminophen from all sources does not exceed maximum daily limits.

• Monitor renal function in patient on long-term therapy. Keep in mind that blood or albumin in urine may indicate nephritis; decreased urine output may indicate renal failure; and dark brown urine may indicate presence of the metabolite phenacetin.

• Expect to reduce dosage for patients with renal dysfunction.

• Store suppositories under 80° F (26.6° C).

WARNING When preparing and administering the parenteral form of acetaminophen, do not confuse a dose in milligrams with a dose in milliliters. Also, make sure the dose is based on the patient's weight if the patient weighs less than 50 kg (110 lbs) and infusion pumps are properly programmed.

• Be aware that patients weighing 50 kg (110 lb) or more and requiring 1,000-mg doses of parenteral acetaminophen (Ofirmev) can have the dose administered by inserting a vented intravenous set through the septum of the 100-ml vial. Further dilution is not required. For doses less than 1,000 mg, the appropriate dose must be withdrawn from the vial and placed into a separate container prior to administration to prevent inadvertent overdose. Place small-volume pediatric doses up to 60 ml in a syringe and administer over 15 minutes using a syringe pump.

• Monitor the end of a parenteral infusion to prevent possibility of air embolism.

• Use parenteral drug within 6 hours once vacuum seal of glass vial has been penetrated or contents transferred to another container.

WARNING Be aware that Pediaphen is a concentrated form of acetaminophen containing 80 mg/0.8 ml (standard liquid forms contain 32 mg/ml). Make sure to use correct concentration and dosage of liquid acetaminophen because serious adverse reactions can result from confusing concentrated form with regular liquid form.

PATIENT TEACHING

• Tell patient that tablets may be crushed or swallowed whole.

• Concentrated infant drops are being phased out and are no longer manufactured, but may still be available.

• Instruct patient to read manufacturer's label and follow dosage guidelines precisely. Explain that infants' and children's acetaminophen liquid aren't equal in drug concentration and aren't interchangeable. Until concentrated infant drops are completely phased out, parents should use extra caution to ensure the correct dose is given with strength being used. Tell them to use only the measuring device that comes with the bottle to help ensure accurate dosage.

• Caution patient not to exceed recommended dosage or take other drugs containing acetaminophen at the same time because of risk of liver damage. Advise him to contact prescriber before taking other prescription or OTC products because they may contain acetaminophen.

• Teach patient to recognize signs of hepatotoxicity, such as bleeding, easy bruising, and malaise, which commonly occurs with chronic overdose.

WARNING Caution patient that serious skin reactions, although rare, may occur even with first-time use and any time acetaminophen is used, even if no skin reactions occurred with a previous use of drug. Tell patient that if a skin rash, redness, or blisters occur, he should stop using drug and seek emergency treatment immediately.

acetazolamide

Acetazolam (CAN), Ak-Zol, Apo-Acetazolamide (CAN), Dazamide, Diamox, Diamox Sequels, Storzolamide

Class and Category
Chemical class: Sulfonamide derivative
Therapeutic class: Anticonvulsant,
antiglaucoma, diuretic
Pregnancy category: C

Indications and Dosages
➤ *To treat chronic simple (open-angle) glaucoma*
S.R. CAPSULES, TABLETS, I.V. OR I.M. INJECTION
Adults. 250 to 1,000 mg daily (divided for doses exceeding 250 mg).
➤ *As short-term therapy to treat secondary glaucoma and preoperatively to treat acute congestive (closed-angle) glaucoma*
S.R. CAPSULES, TABLETS, I.V. OR I.M. INJECTION
Adults. 250 mg twice daily or every 4 hr; or 1 S.R. capsule (500 mg) twice daily; or 500 mg initially, followed by 125 to 250 mg every 4 to 6 hr for severe acute glaucoma. To initially lower intraocular pressure rapidly, 500 mg I.V.; may repeat in 2 to 4 hr in acute cases, depending on patient response. Oral therapy usually started after initial I.V. dose.
S.R. CAPSULES, TABLETS
Children. 10 to 15 mg/kg daily in divided doses every 6 to 8 hr.
I.V. OR I.M. INJECTION
Children. 5 to 10 mg/kg/dose every 6 hr.
➤ *To induce diuresis in heart failure*
TABLETS, I.V. OR I.M. INJECTION
Adults. *Initial:* 250 to 375 mg or 5 mg/kg daily in morning. *Maintenance:* 250 to 375 mg or 5 mg/kg on alternate days or for 2 days followed by a drug-free day.
➤ *To treat drug-induced edema*
TABLETS, I.V. OR I.M. INJECTION
Adults. 250 to 375 mg daily for 1 to 2 days.
TABLETS, I.V. INJECTION
Children. 5 mg/kg/dose daily in morning.
➤ *To treat seizures, including generalized tonic-clonic, absence, and mixed seizures, and myoclonic jerk patterns*
TABLETS, I.V. OR I.M. INJECTION
Adults and children. 8 to 30 mg/kg daily in divided doses. *Optimal:* 375 to 1,000 mg daily. When used with other anticonvulsants, 250 mg daily.
➤ *To prevent or relieve symptoms of acute mountain sickness*

S.R. CAPSULES, TABLETS
Adults. 500 to 1,000 mg daily in divided doses, given 24 to 48 hr before ascent and continued for 48 hr or longer while at high altitude p.r.n. to control symptoms.

Route	Onset	Peak	Duration
P.O.	1–1.5 hr	2–4 hr	8–12 hr
P.O. (S.R.)	2 hr	8–12 hr	18–24 hr
I.V.	2 min	15 min	4–5 hr

Mechanism of Action
Inhibits the enzyme carbonic anhydrase, which normally appears in the eyes' ciliary processes, brain's choroid plexes, and kidneys' proximal tubule cells. In the eyes, enzyme inhibition decreases aqueous humor secretion, which lowers intraocular pressure. In the brain, inhibition may delay abnormal, intermittent, and excessive discharge from neurons that cause seizures. In the kidneys, it increases bicarbonate excretion, which carries out water, potassium, and sodium, thus inducing diuresis and metabolic acidosis. This acidosis counteracts respiratory alkalosis and reduces symptoms of mountain sickness, including headache, dizziness, nausea, and dyspnea.

Contraindications
Chronic noncongestive closed-angle glaucoma; cirrhosis; hyperchloremic acidosis; hypersensitivity to acetazolamide; hypokalemia; hyponatremia; severe pulmonary obstruction; severe renal, hepatic, or adrenocortical impairment

Interaction
DRUGS
amphetamines, methenamine, phenobarbital, procainamide, quinidine: Decreased excretion and possibly toxicity of these drugs
corticosteroids: Increased risk of hypokalemia
cyclosporine: Increased cyclosporine level, possibly nephrotoxicity or neurotoxicity
diflunisal: Possibly significantly decreased intraocular pressure
lithium: Increased excretion and decreased effectiveness of lithium
primidone: Decreased serum and urine primidone levels
salicylates: Increased risk of salicylate toxicity

A

Adverse Reactions

CNS: Ataxia, confusion, depression, disorientation, dizziness, drowsiness, fatigue, fever, flaccid paralysis, headache, lassitude, malaise, nervousness, paresthesia, seizures, tremor, weakness
EENT: Altered taste, tinnitus, transient myopia
GI: Anorexia, constipation, diarrhea, hepatic dysfunction, melena, nausea, vomiting
GU: Crystalluria, decreased libido, glycosuria, hematuria, impotence, nephrotoxicity, phosphaturia, polyuria, renal calculi, renal colic, urinary frequency
HEME: Agranulocytosis, hemolytic anemia, leukopenia, pancytopenia, thrombocytopenia, thrombocytopenic purpura
SKIN: Photosensitivity, pruritus, rash, Stevens-Johnson syndrome, urticaria
Other: Acidosis, hyperuricemia, hypokalemia, weight loss

Nursing Considerations

• Use acetazolamide cautiously in patients with calcium-based renal calculi, diabetes mellitus, gout, or respiratory impairment.
• Know that acetazolamide may increase risk of hepatic encephalopathy in patients with hepatic cirrhosis.
• To avoid painful I.M. injections (caused by alkaline solution), give acetazolamide by mouth or I.V. injection if possible.
• Reconstitute each 500-mg vial with at least 5 ml sterile water for injection. Use within 24 hours because drug has no preservative.
• Monitor blood tests during acetazolamide therapy to detect electrolyte imbalances.
• Monitor fluid intake and output every 8 hours and body weight daily to detect excessive fluid and weight loss.

PATIENT TEACHING
• Inform patient that acetazolamide tablets may be crushed and suspended in chocolate or another sweet syrup. Or, one tablet may be dissolved in 10 ml hot water and added to 10 ml honey or syrup.
• Advise patient to avoid hazardous activities if dizziness or drowsiness occurs.
• Instruct patient who takes high doses of salicylates to notify prescriber immediately about evidence of salicylate toxicity, such as anorexia, tachypnea, and lethargy.

• If patient plans to mountain climb, urge her to descend mountain gradually and to seek immediate medical care if symptoms of mountain sickness occur.

acetohexamide

Dimelor (CAN), Dymelor

Class and Category

Chemical class: Sulfonylurea
Therapeutic class: Antidiabetic
Pregnancy category: C

Indications and Dosages

➤ *To treat stable type 2 (non–insulin-dependent) diabetes mellitus*

TABLETS
Adults. *Initial:* 250 to 1,500 mg daily. Dosages of 1,000 mg or more daily may be divided and given twice daily before morning and evening meals.

DOSAGE ADJUSTMENT For patient being switched from another antidiabetic, acetohexamide dosage reduced to half the usual tolbutamide dosage or twice the usual chlorpropamide dosage. For patient being switched from insulin to acetohexamide monotherapy, dosages adjusted as follows: if insulin dosage is less than 20 units daily, acetohexamide starts at 250 mg daily and insulin is discontinued; if insulin dosage exceeds 20 units daily, acetohexamide starts at 250 mg daily and insulin is tapered by 25% to 30% before being reduced further according to patient response.

Route	Onset	Peak	Duration
P.O.	1 hr	Unknown	12–24 hr

Mechanism of Action

Stimulates insulin release from active beta cells in the pancreas, resulting in decreased blood glucose level. Improves insulin binding to insulin receptors. Increases the number of insulin receptors (with long-term administration). May reduce basal hepatic glucose secretion.

Contraindications

Diabetes mellitus complicated by keto-acidosis or pregnancy, hypersensitivity to acetohexamide, renal failure, sole therapy for type 1 (insulin-dependent) diabetes mellitus

Interaction

DRUGS

activated charcoal: Possibly reduced absorption and effectiveness of acetohexamide
androgens, anticoagulants, azole antifungals, chloramphenicol, clofibrate, fluconazole, gemfibrozil, H$_2$-receptor antagonists, magnesium salts, MAO inhibitors, methyldopa, probenecid, salicylates, sulfinpyrazone, sulfonamides, tricyclic antidepressants, urinary acidifiers: Enhanced hypoglycemic effect of acetohexamide
beta blockers, calcium channel blockers,cholestyramine, corticosteroids, diazoxide, estrogens, hydantoins, isoniazid, nicotinic acid, oral contraceptives, phenothiazines, rifampin, sympathomimetics, thiazide diuretics, thyroid drugs, urinary alkalizers: Decreased hypoglycemic effect
digitalis glycosides: Possibly increased serum digitalis level

Adverse Reactions

CNS: Anxiety, chills, confusion, depression, dizziness, drowsiness, fatigue, headache, hyperesthesia, insomnia, malaise, nervousness, paresthesia, somnolence, syncope, tremor, vertigo, weakness
CV: Arrhythmias, edema, hypertension, vasculitis
EENT: Blurred vision, conjunctivitis, eye pain, pharyngitis, retinal hemorrhage, rhinitis, tinnitus
ENDO: Hypoglycemia
GI: Abdominal pain, anorexia, constipation, diarrhea, epigastric fullness, flatulence, heartburn, hepatitis, hepatotoxicity, indigestion, nausea, proctocolitis, vomiting
GU: Decreased libido, dysuria, polyuria
HEME: Agranulocytosis, aplastic anemia, eosinophilia, hemolytic anemia, leukopenia, pancytopenia, thrombocytopenia
MS: Abnormal gait, arthralgia, hypertonia, leg cramps
RESP: Dyspnea
SKIN: Diaphoresis, eczema, erythema multiforme, exfoliative dermatitis, flushing, jaundice, lichenoid reaction (skin thickening, accentuated lesions), maculopapular rash, photosensitivity, pruritus, rash, urticaria
Other: Disulfiram-like reaction (flushing, head throbbing, hypotension, nausea, tachycardia, vomiting), hyponatremia

Nursing Considerations

• Use acetohexamide cautiously in elderly patients and in those with cardiac, hepatic, or renal disease or thyroid dysfunction. Drug's duration of action is prolonged in patients with renal disease.
• Give acetohexamide 30 minutes before meals, crushing tablets if desired. If GI upset occurs, give in divided doses, as prescribed.
• Watch for evidence of hypoglycemia and hyperglycemia, especially after meals.
• Check blood glucose level often, as ordered. Provide additional insulin if needed during stressful periods, as prescribed.
• Monitor liver enzyme levels during therapy; acetohexamide may increase AST, ALT, and alkaline phosphatase levels.
• Store acetohexamide in tightly sealed container in a cool environment.

PATIENT TEACHING

• Emphasize need to adhere to prescribed drug regimen, diet, and exercise program.
• Advise patient to take acetohexamide with food to avoid GI upset.
• Teach patient how to self-monitor blood glucose level and check urine for glucose and ketones, as appropriate.
• Teach patient to recognize and report signs of hypoglycemia and hyperglycemia.

acetohydroxamic acid
Lithostat

Class and Category

Chemical class: Synthetic hydroxylamine and ethylacetate derivative
Therapeutic class: Urease inhibitor
Pregnancy category: X

Indications and Dosages

➤ *As an adjunct to antimicrobial therapy to treat chronic UTI caused by urea-splitting bacteria*

TABLETS

Adults. *Initial:* 12 mg/kg daily in divided doses every 6 to 8 hr. *Usual:* 250 mg three or four times daily for a total of 10 to 15 mg/kg daily. *Maximum:* 1,500 mg daily.
Children. 10 mg/kg daily.

DOSAGE ADJUSTMENT Maximum dosage reduced to 1,000 mg daily or 500 mg every 12 hr for patients with serum creatinine level that exceeds 1.8 mg/dl.

Mechanism of Action

Inhibits urease, the enzyme that catalyzes urea's hydrolysis to carbon dioxide and ammonia in urine infected with urea-splitting bacteria. This action reduces the urine ammonia level and pH, enhancing antimicrobial drug effectiveness.

Contraindications

Contributing disorder that's treatable by surgery or appropriate antimicrobial therapy, hypersensitivity to ace-tohydroxamic acid, inadequate renal function (serum creatinine level above 2.5 mg/dl or creatinine clearance below 20 ml/min/1.73 m²), risk of pregnancy, UTI caused by non–urease-producing organisms, UTI that could be controlled by appropriate antimicrobial therapy

Interaction

DRUGS

iron: Decreased intestinal absorption of iron, decreased effects of iron and acetohydroxamic acid

ACTIVITIES

alcohol use: Increased risk of severe rash 30 to 45 minutes after drinking alcohol

Adverse Reactions

CNS: Anxiety, depression, fever, lack of coordination, malaise, headache, nervousness, slurred speech, tiredness, tremor
CV: Calf pain (deep vein blood clot), palpitations, sudden chest pain
EENT: Pharyngitis, sudden change in vision
GI: Anorexia, nausea, vomiting
HEME: Reticulocytosis, unusual bleeding
RESP: Dyspnea
SKIN: Ecchymosis, hair loss, nonpruritic macular rash

Nursing Considerations

• Use acetohydroxamic acid cautiously in patients with severe chronic renal disease or anemia and those who've had phlebitis or thrombophlebitis.
• Be aware that risk of adverse psychomotor effects increases if patient drinks alcohol or

takes drugs that affect alertness and reflexes, such as antihistamines, tranquilizers, sedatives, analgesics, and narcotics.
• Administer tablets with food or liquid, crushing them if needed.
WARNING Acetohydroxamic acid chelates with dietary iron. If patient has iron deficiency anemia, expect to administer I.M. iron as needed during acetohydroxamic acid therapy.
• Monitor follow-up laboratory tests to check renal and hepatic function and urine pH, as ordered.

PATIENT TEACHING

• Instruct patient to take drug at same time each day, as prescribed.
• Tell patient to take a missed dose up to 2 hours after scheduled time. If more than 2 hours have passed, he should wait for next scheduled dose and shouldn't double that dose.
• Warn patient not to take drug with alcohol or iron and to consult prescriber before taking it with any other drug.
• Instruct patient to avoid hazardous activities during therapy.

acetylcysteine

Acetadote, Mucomyst, Mucosil

Class and Category

Chemical class: N-acetyl derivative of cysteine
Therapeutic class: Antidote (for acetaminophen overdose), mucolytic
Pregnancy category: B

Indications and Dosages

➤ *To liquefy abnormal, viscid, or thickened mucus secretions in chronic pulmonary disorders (including emphysema, bronchitis, tuberculosis, bronchiectasis, and cystic fibrosis) and in pneumonia, pulmonary complications of thoracic or cardiovascular surgery, and tracheostomy care*

SOLUTION BY DIRECT INSTILLATION INTO TRACHEOSTOMY (MUCOMYST, MUCOSIL)

Adults and children. 1 to 2 ml of 10% or 20% solution instilled every 1 to 4 hr, as needed.

A

SOLUTION BY INHALATION
Adults and children. 1 to 10 ml of 20% solution or 2 to 20 ml of 10% solution nebulized through face mask, mouthpiece, or tracheostomy every 2 to 6 hr. *Usual:* 3 to 5 ml of 20% solution or 6 to 10 ml of 10% solution three or four times daily.
➤ *To treat acetaminophen overdose*
SOLUTION P.O. (MUCOMYST, MUCOSIL)
Adults and children. *Loading dose:* 140 mg/kg. *Maintenance:* 70 mg/kg 4 hr after loading dose and then every 4 hr to a total of 17 doses.
I.V. INFUSION (ACETADOTE)
Adults and children weighing 40 kg (88 lb) or more. 150 mg/kg in 200 ml of diluent infused over 60 min, followed by 50 mg/kg in 500 ml of diluent infused over 4 hr, followed by 100 mg/kg in 1,000 ml of diluent infused over 16 hr.
Adults and children weighing more than 20 kg (44 lb) but less than 40 kg. 150 mg/kg in 100 ml of diluent infused over 60 min, followed by 50 mg/kg in 250 ml of diluent infused over 4 hr, followed by 100 mg/kg in 500 ml of diluent infused over 16 hr.
Children weighing 20 kg or less. 150 mg/kg in 3 ml/kg of diluent infused over 60 min, followed by 50 mg/kg in 7 ml/kg of diluent infused over 4 hr, followed by 100 mg/kg in 14 ml/kg of diluent infused over 16 hr.

Mechanism of Action

Decreases viscosity of pulmonary secretions by breaking disulfide links that bind glycoproteins in mucus. Reduces liver damage from acetaminophen overdose. Usually, acetaminophen's toxic metabolites bind with glutathione in the liver, which detoxifies them. When acetaminophen overdose depletes glutathione stores, toxic metabolites bind with protein in liver cells, killing them. Acetylcysteine maintains or restores levels of glutathione or acts as its substitute, which reduces liver damage from acetaminophen overdose.

Incompatibilities

Don't give acetylcysteine with nebulization equipment if drug can contact iron, copper, or rubber. Don't give drug with amphotericin B, ampicillin sodium, chlortetracycline, chymotrypsin, ery-thromycin, hydrogen peroxide, iodized oil, oxytetracycline, tetracycline, or trypsin.

Contraindications

Hypersensitivity to acetylcysteine, no contraindications when used as antidote

Interaction

DRUGS
activated charcoal: Possibly adsorption and decreased effectiveness of oral acetylcysteine
nitroglycerin: Increased effects of nitroglycerin and possibly significant hypotension and headache

Adverse Reactions

CNS: Chills, dizziness, drowsiness, fever, headache
CV: Edema, hypertension, hypotension, tachycardia
EENT: Rhinorrhea, stomatitis, tooth damage
GI: Anorexia, constipation, hepatotoxicity, nausea, vomiting
RESP: Bronchospasm, chest tightness, cough, hemoptysis, respiratory distress, shortness of breath, stridor, wheezing
SKIN: Clammy skin, facial flushing, pruritus, rash, urticaria
Other: Anaphylaxis, angioedema

Nursing Considerations

• Acetylcysteine should be used cautiously in patients with asthma or a history of bronchospasm because drug may adversely affect respiratory function.
WARNING To avoid fluid overload and possibly fatal hyponatremia or seizures, adjust total administered volume, as ordered, for patients weighing less than 40 kg (88 lb) and for those who need fluid restriction.
• If needed, dilute 20% instillation or inhalation solution with normal saline solution or sterile water. The 10% solution may be used undiluted.
• When treating acetaminophen overdose, dilute 20% oral solution with cola or other soft drink to a concentration of 5%, and use within 1 hour. Dilute parenteral solution with D_5W or half-normal saline (0.45% sodium chloride) solution for injection following manufacturer guidelines because dilution is based on dosage. Acetadote may turn from colorless to slight pink or purple once the stopper is punctured, but color change has no effect on product quality.

• Acetylcysteine is most effective if given within 24 hours of acetaminophen ingestion. For specific instructions, contact a regional poison center at 1-800-222-1222 or a special health professional assistance hotline at 1-800-525-6115.
• If patient vomits loading dose or any maintenance dose within 1 hour of administration, repeat dose as prescribed.
• Keep in mind that suicidal patient may not provide reliable information about vomiting. Watch such a patient to ensure that he ingests all of prescribed dosage.
• During treatment for acetaminophen overdose, watch for signs of hepatotoxicity, such as prolonged bleeding time, altered coagulation, and easy bruising.
• Be aware that acetylcysteine may have a disagreeable odor, which disappears as treatment progresses.
• Because nebulization causes sticky residue on face and in mouth, have patient wash his face and rinse his mouth at the end of each treatment.
• Be aware that an open vial of solution may turn light purple but that this doesn't alter its effectiveness.
• Refrigerate opened vials and discard after 96 hours.
• Assess type, frequency, and characteristics of patient's cough. Particularly note sputum. If cough doesn't clear secretions, prepare to perform mechanical suctioning.
• Monitor patient for tachycardia.

PATIENT TEACHING
• Instruct patient to notify prescriber immediately about nausea, rash, or vomiting.
• Warn patient about acetylcysteine's unpleasant smell; reassure him that it subsides as treatment progresses.
• To decrease mucus viscosity, urge patient to consume 2 to 3 L of fluid daily unless contraindicated by another condition.

acitretin
Soriatane

Class and Category
Chemical class: Synthetic retinoid
Therapeutic class: Antipsoriatic
Pregnancy category: X

Indications and Dosages
➤ *To treat severe psoriasis*
CAPSULES
Adults. 25 to 50 mg once daily with a meal.

Route	Onset	Peak	Duration
P.O.	Unknown	2–5 hr	Unknown

Mechanism of Action
Binds to several retinoid receptors to regulate gene transcription. Exactly how the action of this second-generation retinoid allows normal growth and development of skin is unknown.

Contraindications
Alcohol consumption; blood donation; breastfeeding; chronic hyperlipidemia; concurrent use of etretinate, methotrexate, or tetracycline; hypersensitivity to acitretin, other retinoids, or their components; pregnancy; severe hepatic or renal impairment

Interaction
DRUGS
methotrexate: Increased risk of hepatitis
oral contraceptives containing only progestin: Possibly decreased effectiveness of oral contraceptive
phenytoin: Possibly decreased protein binding of phenytoin
sulfonylureas: Possibly increased risk of hypoglycemia
tetracyclines: Increased intracranial pressure
vitamin A and other oral retinoids: Increased risk of hypervitaminosis A
ACTIVITIES
alcohol use: Increased risk of adverse reactions and acitretin toxicity

Adverse Reactions
CNS: Aggression, depression, fatigue, headache, hyperesthesia, hypotonia, insomnia, intracranial hypertension, paresthesia, peripheral neuropathy, rigors, somnolence, stroke, suicidal ideation, thirst
CV: Chest pain, decreased high-density lipoproteins, edema, elevated cholesterol or triglyceride levels, MI, thromboembolism
EENT: Abnormal or blurred vision, blepharitis, conjunctivitis, corneal epithelial abnormality, decreased night vision, deafness, dry eyes or mouth, earache, epistaxis, eye pain, gingival bleeding,

gingivitis, increased saliva, photophobia, sinusitis, stomatitis, taste perversion, tinnitus, ulcerative stomatitis
ENDO: Hot flashes, hyperglycemia
GI: Anorexia, abdominal pain, diarrhea, elevated liver enzymes, hepatitis, hepatotoxicity, nausea, pancreatitis
GU: Vulvovaginitis
HEME: Capillary leak syndrome, hemorrhage, increased bleeding time
MS: Arthralgia, arthrosis, back pain, hyperostosis, myalgia, myopathy
SKIN: Abnormal skin or hair texture, alopecia, bullous eruption, cold or clammy skin, dermatitis, diaphoresis, dry or peeling skin, erythematous rash, exfoliative dermatitis/erythroderma, flushing, fragility or thinning of skin, loss of eyelashes or eyebrows, photosensitivity, pruritus, purpura, pyogenic granuloma, rash, scaling, seborrhea, skin fissure or ulceration
Other: Hypervitaminosis A, increased appetite

Nursing Considerations

WARNING Don't give acitretin to a pregnant woman, a woman contemplating pregnancy, or a woman who may not use reliable contraception during drug therapy and for at least 3 years afterward because acitretin causes major fetal abnormalities.

• Make sure patient has had two negative urine or serum pregnancy tests with a sensitivity of at least 25 mIU/ml before receiving acitretin. First test should be obtained when decision is made to use acitretin and second test during first 5 days of the menstrual period just before acitretin therapy starts. For patients with amenorrhea, second test should be done at least 11 days after the last act of unprotected sexual intercourse (which means without using two effective forms of contraception simultaneously).

• Check to make sure female patient of childbearing age has signed the patient agreement and informed consent form before starting acitretin therapy.

• Obtain a lipid profile, as ordered, before acitretin therapy starts and every 1 to 2 weeks for up to 8 weeks or until lipid effects are known. In high-risk patients, such as those with diabetes, obesity, or a history of alcohol abuse and those taking acitretin long-term, check lipid profile periodically throughout therapy.

• Monitor liver function test results, as ordered. If hepatotoxicity is suspected, expect to stop drug and investigate cause.

• Monitor patient closely for capillary leak syndrome demonstrated by localized or generalized edema, weight gain, fever, hypotension, and myalgias. If present, notify prescriber and expect to obtain laboratory studies for evidence of neutrophilia, hypoalbuminemia, and an elevated hematocrit. If confirmed, discontinue acitretin therapy, as ordered.

• If patient takes acitretin long-term or she develops a skeletal disorder, prepare her for periodic bone radiography because ossification abnormalities can occur, especially of the vertebral column, knees, and ankles.

• Monitor patient's eyes for abnormalities throughout therapy. Expect patient to stop drug and have an ophthalmologic examination if eye abnormalities occur.

• Monitor patient for evidence of increased intracranial pressure, such as papilledema, headache, nausea, vomiting, and visual disturbances. If papilledema occurs, stop drug therapy immediately and obtain a neurologic evaluation, as ordered. Patient should never receive a tetracycline while taking acitretin because combined use can increase intracranial pressure.

• Assess patient for suicidal ideation because depression and other psychiatric symptoms, including thoughts of self-harm, may occur with acitretin use. Expect drug to be discontinued if psychiatric symptoms develop.

• Significantly lower doses of phototherapy are needed during acitretin therapy because drug increases the risk of erythema. If patient develops serious skin reactions, notify prescriber and expect acitretin therapy to be discontinued.

PATIENT TEACHING

WARNING Warn women of childbearing age that acitretin causes major fetal abnormalities.

• Inform woman of childbearing age that she must have a pregnancy test before acitretin therapy starts, every month during acitretin therapy, and every 3 months for 3 years after therapy stops.

• Emphasize to woman of childbearing age that she must use two effective forms of contraception simultaneously unless she has chosen absolute abstinence or has had a hysterectomy. This must begin at least 1 month before acitretin therapy starts and continue throughout therapy and for at least 3 years after therapy ends.

• Caution women taking oral contraceptives that some prescribed and OTC drugs, including herbal supplements such as St. John's wort, may interfere with oral contraceptives. Urge her to tell prescriber about all drugs she takes.

• Caution patient not to consume alcohol or products that contain alcohol during acitretin therapy and for 2 months after therapy ends.

• Inform patient that regular blood tests will be needed to monitor liver function. Tell him to notify prescriber if any of the following develops: nausea and vomiting, loss of appetite, dark urine, or whites of eyes or skin turns yellow.

• Warn patient, male or female of any age, not to donate blood during acitretin therapy and for at least 3 years after it ends.

• Review acitretin medication guide with patient, and answer the patient's questions.

• Inform patient that psoriasis may worsen during initial treatment and that full effects of drug may not be seen for up to 3 months.

• Caution patient to avoid hazardous activities until drug's CNS and ophthalmic effects are known.

• Inform patient that tolerance to contact lenses may decrease during acitretin therapy and for a period of time after treatment ends.

• Advise patient not to take more than the minimum recommended daily allowance of vitamin A during acitretin therapy because of the risk of vitamin A toxicity.

• Caution patient not to use sun lamps and to avoid excessive exposure to sunlight because the effects of UV light are enhanced by retinoids such as acitretin.

• Tell patient to notify prescriber of any new skin changes that become serious or prolonged, as acitretin therapy may need to be discontinued, if present.

aclidinium bromide

Tudorza Pressair

Class and Category
Chemical class: Anticholinergic
Therapeutic class: Bronchodilator
Pregnancy category: C

Indications and Dosages
➤ *To provide long-term maintenance treatment of bronchospasm associated with chronic obstructive pulmonary disease (COPD), including chronic bronchitis and emphysema*
INHALATION AEROSOL
Adults. 1 inhalation (400 mcg) twice daily.

Mechanism of Action
Inhibits muscarinic receptor, M3, in smooth muscle in the airways to produce bronchodilation.

Contraindications
Hypersensitivity to aclidinium or its components

Interaction
DRUGS
other anticholinergics: Potential additive effect

Adverse Reactions
CNS: Headache
CV: Cardiac failure (rare), cardio-respiratory arrest (rare), first degree AV block
EENT: Dry mouth, nasopharyngitis, rhinitis, sinusitis, worsening of glaucoma
ENDO: Hyperglycemia
GI: Diarrhea, vomiting
GU: Worsening of urinary retention
RESP: Cough, paradoxical bronchospasm
Other: Immediate hypersensitivity reaction

Nursing Considerations
• Use aclidinium with extreme caution in patients with known hypersensitivity reactions to atropine or severe hypersensitivity to milk proteins as aclidinium may produce a similiar reaction.
• Use aclidinium cautiously in patients with narrow-angle glaucoma or urinary retention because drug can make these conditions worse.

• Monitor patient closely, especially after first dose, for signs and symptoms of hypersensitivity such as bronchospasms and shortness of breath because aclidinium may cause an immediate hypersensitivity reaction. Be prepared to treat such a reaction, as ordered and expect drug to be discontinued.

PATIENT TEACHING

• Caution patient that aclidinium is not intended to be used as a rescue inhaler for the treatment of acute episodes of bronchospasms. Instruct patient that if bronchospasms occur while using aclidinium, he or she should stop using aclidinium and immediately notify the prescriber.

• Teach patient how to get the inhaler ready by pressing the green button all the way down and then releasing it. Next, patient should check the control window on the inhaler to make sure it has turned green. If it is still red, tell patient to press the green button again. Then instruct how to use the inhaler by first breathing out completely, then putting lips tightly around the mouthpiece and breathing in quickly but deeply through the mouth. Patient should hear a click but should keep breathing in to be sure the full dose is received. After removing mouthpiece, patient should check the control window again to be sure it has now turned to red.

• Inform patient that some people may taste the medicine during their inhalation but that an extra dose should not be taken if the patient is not able to taste the medication

• Emphasize importance of not allowing the powder to get into eyes when using the inhaler because this may cause blurring of vision and pupil dilation.

• Advise patient with narrow-angle glaucoma to notify prescriber if eye pain or discomfort, blurred vision, visual halos or colored images in association with red eyes from conjunctival congestion and corneal edema occurs at any time with aclidinium therapy and to stop using the drug until seen by prescriber.

adalimumab
Humira

Class and Category
Chemical class: Recombinant human IgG1 monoclonal antibody
Therapeutic class: Disease-modifying antirheumatic
Pregnancy category: B

Indications and Dosages
➤ *To reduce signs and symptoms, induce major clinical response, inhibit progression of structural damage, and improve physical function in patients with moderately to severely active rheumatoid arthritis; to reduce signs and symptoms, inhibit progression of structural damage, and improve physical function in patients with psoriatic arthritis; to reduce signs and symptoms in patients with active ankylosing spondylitis*

SUBCUTANEOUS INJECTION

Adults. 40 mg every other wk.

DOSAGE ADJUSTMENT Dosage may be adjusted to 40 mg every wk, as needed and prescribed, for patients not taking methotrexate.

➤ *To reduce signs and symptoms and induce and maintain clinical remission in patients with moderately to severely active Crohn's disease who have had an inadequate response to conventional therapy or who have stopped responding to or have become intolerant of infliximab (adults) or who have had an inadequate response to corticosteroids or immunomodulators such as azathioprine, 6-mercaptopurine, or methotrexate (children)*

SUBCUTANEOUS INJECTION

Adults. *Initial:* 40 mg four times daily for 1 day or 40 mg twice daily for 2 consecutive days, followed by 80 mg 2 wk later. *Maintenance:* 40 mg every other wk starting at week 4.

Children age 6 and older who weigh 40 kg (88 lb) or more. *Initial:* 40 mg four times daily on 1 day or 40 mg twice daily for 2 days, followed by 80 mg on day 15 given in 2 divided doses of 40 mg each. *Maintenance:* 40 mg every other wk starting on day 29.

Children age 6 and older who weigh less than 40 kg (88 lb) but at least 17 kg (37 lb). *Initial*: 40 mg twice daily on day 1, followed by 40 mg on day 15. *Maintenance*: 20 mg every other week starting on day 29.

➤ *To reduce signs and symptoms of moderately to severely active polyarticular juvenile idiopathic arthritis*

SUBCUTANEOUS INJECTION

Children age 2 and over who weigh 30 kg (66 lb) or more. 40 mg every other wk.

Children age 2 and over who weigh less than 30 kg but at least 15 kg (33 lb). 20 mg every other wk.

Children age 2 and over who weigh less than 15 kg (33 lb) but at least 10 kg (22 lb). 10 mg every other wk.

➤ *To treat moderate to severe chronic plaque psoriasis in patients who are candidates for systemic therapy or phototherapy, and when other systemic therapies are less appropriate*

SUBCUTANEOUS INJECTION

Adults. *Initial*: 80 mg followed 1 wk later with 40 mg.

Maintenance: 40 mg every other wk.

➤ *To induce and sustain a remission in patients with moderate to severe active ulcerative colitis who have had an inadequate response to immunosuppressants such as corticosteroids, azathioprine, or 6-mercaptopurine*

SUBCUTANEOUS INJECTION

Adults. *Initial*: 160 mg given as four 40-mg injections on day 1 or given as two 40-mg injections on day 1 and repeated on day 2, followed by 80 mg on day 15 and 40 mg on day 29. *Maintenance*: 40 mg every other wk.

Mechanism of Action

Binds to tumor necrosis factor (TNF) to block interaction with p55 and p75 cell-surface TNF receptors, and lyses surface TNF-expressing cells in the presence of complement. TNF may be a major component of rheumatoid arthritis inflammation and joint destruction. Reduced TNF level in synovial fluid improves signs and symptoms and prevents further structural damage in rheumatoid arthritis.

Contraindications

Active infection, breastfeeding, hypersensitivity to adalimumab or its components

Interaction

DRUGS

abatacept, anakinra, rituximab: Possibly increased risk of serious infection and neutropenia in patients with rheumatoid arthritis

azathioprine, 6-mercaptopurine: Increased risk of hepatosplenic T-cell lymphoma

live vaccines: Increased risk of adverse vaccine effects

Adverse Reactions

CNS: Confusion, CVA, demyelinating disorders such as Guillain-Barré syndrome or multiple sclerosis, fever, headache, hypertensive encephalopathy, paresthesia, subdural hematoma, syncope, tremor

CV: Arrhythmias, atrial fibrillation, cardiac arrest, chest pain, coronary artery disease, congestive heart failure, deep vein thrombosis, hypercholesterolemia, hyperlipidemia, hypertension, MI, palpitations, pericardial effusion, pericarditis, peripheral edema, systemic vasculitis, tachycardia

EENT: Cataracts, optic neuritis, sinusitis

ENDO: Ketosis, parathyroid disorder

GI: Abdominal pain, cholecystitis, cholelithiasis, diverticulitis, elevated alkaline phosphatase level, elevated liver enzyme levels, esophagitis, gastroenteritis, hemorrhage, hepatic failure or necrosis, hepatitis, large bowel perforation, nausea, pancreatitis, vomiting

GU: Hematuria, paraproteinemia, pyelonephritis, UTI

HEME: Agranulocytosis, aplastic anemia, granulocytopenia, leukopenia, lymphocytosis, pancytopenia, polycythemia, thrombocytopenia

MS: Arthritis (including pyogenic or septic arthritis); back, extremity, pelvic, or thorax pain; bone disorder, fracture, or necrosis; muscle spasms; myasthenia; prosthetic infections; synovitis

RESP: Asthma, bronchitis, bronchospasm, decreased pulmonary function, dyspnea, pleural effusion, pneumonia, pulmonary embolism, pulmonary fibrosis or tuberculosis, upper respiratory tract infection

SKIN: Alopecia, cellulitis, cutaneous vasculitis, erysipelas, erythema multiforme, herpes zoster, Merkel cell carcinoma, new

or worsening psoriasis, rash, Stevens-Johnson syndrome, urticaria
Other: Anaphylaxis; angioedema; antibody formation against adalimumab; bacterial, mycobacterial, fungal, viral, parasitic, and other opportunistic infections; benign or unspecified cysts or polyps; dehydration; flare-up of disease process; flulike symptoms; healing abnormalities; injection-site erythema, hemorrhage, itching, pain, or swelling; lupus-like symptoms; lymphomas and other malignancies such as breast, colon, lung, melanoma, and prostate; postsurgical infection; sarcoidosis, sepsis; new onset or reactivation of tuberculosis

Nursing Considerations

• Use adalimumab cautiously in patients with recurrent infection or increased risk of infection and in patients who live in regions where tuberculosis and certain mycoses, such as *Histoplasma*, are endemic. Be aware that *Legionella* and *Listeria*, two bacterial infections, also have occurred with tumor necrosis factor–alpha blockers such as adalimumab. Monitor patient closely because infections associated with tumor necrosis factor–alpha blocker therapy may involve multiple organ systems and become life-threatening.

WARNING If patient has evidence of an active infection when drug is prescribed, therapy shouldn't start until the infection has been treated. Monitor all patients for infection during therapy, especially those receiving concomitant immunosuppressants. If a serious infection develops, the drug should be stopped.

• Ensure that children with juvenile idiopathic arthritis are up to date with current immunization guidelines prior to adalimumab therapy being started. However, know that they may receive vaccinations, except for live vaccines, while taking adalimumab if needed.

• Use cautiously in a patient with a preexisting or recent onset of a central or peripheral nervous system demyelinating disorder such as multiple sclerosis, optic neuritis, or Guillain-Barré because, although rare, new onset or exacerbation of demyelinating disorders have occurred with adalimumab therapy.

• Make sure patient has a tuberculin skin test before therapy starts. If skin test is positive, treatment of latent tuberculosis will start before adalimumab, as prescribed. Also, ensure that patient previously treated for tuberculosis, including prophylactic treatment, has a tuberculin skin test periodically throughout therapy, as adalimumab may induce new onset or reactivate tuberculosis.

• Be aware that the needle cover of the syringe contains dry rubber. Don't handle if you're allergic to latex.

• To activate the protection device on needles of prefilled syringes delivered to institutions, hold the syringe in one hand and, with the other hand, slide outer protective shield over exposed needle until it locks into place.

• Know that adalimumab may come in a single-use glass vial containing 40 mg (0.8 ml) of adalimumab referred to as an "institutional use vial" because the drug should only be given in a medical institution. Withdraw only one dose when using the "institutional use vial" and administer promptly. Since the vial does not contain preservatives, discard any unused portions.

WARNING Stop adalimumab immediately and tell prescriber if patient has an allergic reaction. Expect to provide supportive care.

• Watch closely for evidence of congestive heart failure (sudden, unexplained weight gain; dyspnea; crackles; anxiety), and notify prescriber if they occur.

• Monitor patient's CBC, as ordered, because adalimumab may have adverse hematologic effects. Notify prescriber about persistent fever, bruising, bleeding, or pallor.

• Although rare, malignancies, especially lymphomas and leukemias, have occurred in patients receiving TNF blockers such as adalimumab. These malignancies have also occurred in children. Patients with rheumatoid arthritis, especially those with very active disease, and patients with Crohn's disease, ankylosing spondylitis, psoriatic arthritis, or plaque psoriasis are at greatest risk. Monitor patients closely.

PATIENT TEACHING
- Inform patient that the first injection of adalimumab must take place with a healthcare professional present.
- Teach patient or caregiver how to give adalimumab as a subcutaneous injection at home, if applicable. Emphasize importance of injecting the full amount in the syringe to obtain the correct dose.
- If patient is allergic to latex, explain that the needle cover contains rubber.
- Caution patient against reusing needles and syringes. Provide patient or caregiver with a puncture-resistant container for disposal of needles and syringes at home.
- Instruct patient or caregiver to rotate injection sites in the thigh and abdomen and to avoid injecting in any area that's tender, bruised, red, or hard.
- Inform patient that prefilled syringes must be refrigerated (not frozen) but may be left at room temperature for 15 to 30 minutes before injecting to decrease injection discomfort. Keep the cap or cover on while allowing it to reach room temperature. Also keep syringe protected from light and stored in the original container.
- Urge patient to check expiration dates and not to use outdated drug.
- Review signs and symptoms of an allergic reaction (rash, swollen face, difficulty breathing), and tell patient to seek emergency care immediately if these occur.
- Inform patient that injection-site reactions (such as redness, rash, swelling, itching, and bruising) may occur but are usually mild and transient. Instruct him to apply a towel soaked with cold water on the injection site if it hurts or remains swollen. If reaction does not disappear or seems to worsen, tell patient to call prescriber immediately.
- Inform patient that tuberculosis may occur during adalimumab therapy. Instruct him to report persistent cough, wasting or weight loss, and low-grade fever to prescriber.
- Teach patient to recognize evidence of infection and bleeding disorders and to tell prescriber if they occur; drug may need to be stopped. Advise patient to avoid people with infections and to have all prescribed laboratory tests.
- Inform patient that the risk of certain kinds of cancer, especially lymphomas, is higher in patients taking adalimumab but still rare. Emphasize the importance of follow-up visits and reporting an unusual or sudden onset of signs or symptoms.
- Caution patient against receiving live-virus vaccines while taking adalimumab because doing so may adversely affect the immune system.
- Inform patient that blood samples may be needed periodically, but especially around week 24 of therapy, to check for autoantibody development. Explain that adalimumab therapy will need to be stopped if it's detected.
- Instruct patient to report lupus-like signs and symptoms that, although rare, may occur during therapy, such as chest pain that doesn't go away, shortness of breath, joint pain, or a rash on cheeks or arms that's sensitive to the sun. Explain that drug may be stopped if these occur.
- Advise patient to inform all healthcare providers about adalimumab use and to inform prescriber about any OTC medications being taken, including herbal remedies and vitamin and mineral supplements.
- Instruct women of childbearing age to notify prescriber immediately if pregnancy is suspected or known, as adalimumab may affect the immune response of an uteroexposed newborn or infant.

adenosine
Adenocard, Adenoscan

Class and Category
Chemical class: Monophosphorylated adenine riboside
Therapeutic class: Antiarrhythmic
Pregnancy category: C

Indications and Dosages
➤ *To convert paroxysmal supraventricular tachycardia (PSVT) to normal sinus rhythm*
I.V. INJECTION (ADENOCARD)
Adults and children weighing 50 kg (110 lb) or more. *Initial:* 6 mg by rapid peripheral I.V. bolus over 1 to 2 sec. If

A

PSVT continues after 1 to 2 min, 12 mg given as rapid bolus and repeated in 1 to 2 min if needed. Don't give single doses of more than 12 mg.
Children weighing less than 50 kg. *Initial:* 0.05 to 0.1 mg/kg as rapid central or peripheral I.V. bolus followed by saline flush. If PSVT continues after 1 to 2 min, additional bolus injections are given, incrementally increasing dose by 0.05 to 0.1 mg/kg. Follow each bolus with saline flush. Injections continue until PSVT converts to normal sinus rhythm or until patient reaches maximum single dose of 0.3 mg/kg.
➤ *Adjunct to thallium-201 myocardial perfusion scintigraphy in patients unable to exercise adequately during testing*
I.V. INJECTION (ADENOSCAN)
Adults. 140 mcg/kg/min infused continuously for 6 minutes (total infused dose of 0.84 mg/kg).

Route	Onset	Peak	Duration
I.V.	Immediate	Immediate	Unknown

Mechanism of Action
Slows conduction time through the AV node and can interrupt AV node reentry pathways to restore normal sinus rhythm.

Incompatibilities
Don't mix adenosine with other drugs.

Contraindications
Atrial fibrillation or flutter; bronchoconstrictive or bronchospastic lung disease; hypersensitivity to adenosine; second- or third-degree heart block or sick sinus syndrome, except in patients with a functioning artificial pacemaker; ventricular tachycardia

Interaction
DRUGS
aminophylline: Increased risk of seizures
carbamazepine: Increased heart block
digoxin, verapamil: Possibly increased depressant effect on SA or AV node
dipyridamole: Increased adenosine effects
methylxanthines, such as theophylline: Antagonized adenosine effects
FOODS
caffeine: Antagonized adenosine effects

Adverse Reactions
CNS: Apprehension, CVA, dizziness, headache, heaviness in arms, lightheadedness, nervousness, paresthesia, seizures
CV: Atrial fibrillation, bradycardia, cardiac failure, fatal and nonfatal cardiac arrest, chest pain or pressure, heart block, hypertension, hypotension, MI, palpitations, prolonged asystole, tachycardia, sinus exit block or pause, sustained ventricular tachycardia, torsades de pointes, transient hypertension, ventricular fibrillation
EENT: Blurred vision, metallic taste, throat tightness
GI: Nausea, vomiting
MS: Jaw, neck, and back pain
RESP: Bronchoconstriction, bronchospasm, dyspnea, hyperventilation, respiratory arrest
SKIN: Diaphoresis, erythema, facial flushing, rash
Other: Injection-site reactions including pain, sensitivity reactions

Nursing Considerations
• Know that Adenoscan should not be given to patients with signs and symptoms of acute myocardial ischemia, as these patients may be at greater risk for serious cardiovascular reactions, including a myocardial infarction during a medical stress test.
• Before use, inspect adenosine for crystals. If solution isn't clear, don't give it.
• Give Adenocard used to convert PSVT to normal sinus rhythm by rapid I.V. bolus over 1 to 2 seconds. Slower delivery can cause systemic vasodilation and reflex tachycardia. Give Adenoscan used as an adjunct to thallium-201 myocardial perfusion scintigraphy as a continuous peripheral intravenous infusion over 6 minutes. Know that the required dose of thallium-201 should be injected at the midpoint of the Adenoscan infusion. It is compatible with Adenoscan and may be injected directly into the Adenoscan infusion set.
• Expect prescriber to inject adenosine directly into a vein to make sure drug reaches systemic circulation. If given into an I.V. line, give drug as close to insertion site as possible and follow with rapid saline flush.

WARNING Don't give single doses of Adenocard more than 12 mg.
• Monitor heart rate and rhythm, blood pressure, and respiratory status often during adenosine therapy.
• Be aware that at the time of conversion to normal sinus rhythm, arrhythmias (such as PVCs, premature atrial contractions, sinus bradycardia, sinus tachycardia, and AV block) may occur for a few seconds, but they don't usually require intervention.

WARNING Stop drug use and notify prescriber immediately if severe respiratory difficulties develop or patient develops other signs of hypersensitivity such as chest discomfort, erythema, flushing, or rash.
• Store adenosine at room temperature. Discard unused portion.

PATIENT TEACHING
• Inform patient of increased risk for serious adverse effects. Instruct patient to report chest pain, palpitations, difficulty breathing, or severe headache during adenosine therapy.
• Warn patient that mild, temporary reactions may occur, such as flushing, nausea, and dizziness.

alatrofloxacin mesylate
Trovan I.V.
trovafloxacin mesylate
Trovan

Class and Category
Chemical class: Fluoroquinolone
Therapeutic class: Antibacterial
Pregnancy category: C

Indications and Dosages
➤ *To treat life-threatening nosocomial pneumonia*
TABLETS, I.V. INFUSION
Adults. 300 mg I.V. every 24 hr followed by 200 mg P.O. every 24 hr when patient is stabilized for total of 10 to 14 days.

➤ *To treat life-threatening community-acquired pneumonia*
TABLETS, I.V. INFUSION
Adults. 200 mg I.V. every 24 hr followed by 200 mg P.O. every 24 hr when patient is stabilized for total of 7 to 14 days; or 200 mg P.O. every 24 hr for total of 7 to 14 days.
➤ *To treat complicated, life-threatening intra-abdominal infections, including post-surgical, gynecologic, and pelvic infections*
TABLETS, I.V. INFUSION
Adults. 300 mg I.V. every 24 hr followed by 200 mg P.O. every 24 hr when patient is stabilized for total of 7 to 14 days.
➤ *To treat complicated, life-threatening or limb-threatening skin and soft-tissue infections, including diabetic foot infections*
TABLETS, I.V. INFUSION
Adults. 200 mg P.O. every 24 hr—or 200 mg I.V. every 24 hr followed by 200 mg P.O. every 24 hr when patient is stabilized—for total of 10 to 14 days.
DOSAGE ADJUSTMENT For patients with mild to moderate cirrhosis, 300-mg I.V. dosage reduced to 200 mg and 200-mg I.V. and P.O. dosage reduced to 100 mg.

Mechanism of Action
Interferes with DNA gyrase, the enzyme needed for DNA replication in aerobic and anaerobic bacteria. May be active against pathogens resistant to such antibiotics as penicillins, cephalosporins, aminoglycosides, macrolides, and tetracyclines.

Incompatibilities
Don't mix alatrofloxacin with or infuse it simultaneously through same I.V. line as other drugs. Don't dilute it with normal saline solution or lactated Ringer's solution.

Contraindications
Hypersensitivity to alatrofloxacin, quinolone antimicrobials, trovafloxacin, or their components

Interaction
DRUGS
antacids that contain aluminum, citric acid, magnesium, or sodium citrate; iron; morphine sulfate; sucralfate: Reduced absorption of trovafloxacin

Adverse Reactions
CNS: Dizziness, headache, light-headedness, seizures

A

CV: Hypotension
EENT: Hoarseness, throat tightness
GI: Abdominal pain, acute hepatic failure (anorexia, dark urine, dysphagia, fatigue, jaundice, pale stool, and vomiting)
GU: Vaginitis
RESP: Dyspnea
SKIN: Photosensitivity, rash, urticaria, or other skin reactions
Other: Angioedema

Nursing Considerations
• Infuse alatrofloxacin over 60 minutes; rapid or bolus I.V. delivery may cause hypotension.
• Periodically assess patient's liver function test results. Results may be elevated for up to 21 days after alatrofloxacin use.
WARNING Be aware that alatrofloxacin may cause severe liver damage, requiring liver transplantation or leading to death. Expect therapy to last no longer than 2 weeks to reduce risk of liver damage. Alatrofloxacin is reserved for hospitalized patients with life- or limb-threatening infections.
PATIENT TEACHING
• Instruct patient to report rash; urticaria; trouble swallowing; swelling of the lips, face, or tongue; hoarseness; or throat tightness.

albiglutide
Tanzeum

Class and Category
Chemical class: Recombinant fusion protein
Therapeutic class: Antidiabetic
Pregnancy category: C

Indications and Dosages
➤ *Adjunct to diet and exercise to improve glycemic control in patients with type 2 diabetes mellitus*
SUBCUTANEOUS INJECTION
Adults. 30 mg once weekly, increased to 50 mg once weekly, as needed.

Mechanism of Action
Lowers fasting glucose levels and reduces postprandial glucose elevations by augmenting glucose-dependent insulin secretion and slowing gastric emptying.

Contraindications
Diabetic ketoacidosis, hypersensitivity to albiglutide or its components, personal or family history of medullary thyroid carcinoma or multiple endocrine neoplasia syndrome, preexisting severe gastrointestinal disease

Interaction
DRUGS
insulin, insulin secretagogues: Increased risk of hypoglycemia
orally administered drugs: Possibly decreased absorption of orally administered drugs

Adverse Reactions
CV: Atrial fibrillation or flutter
EENT: Sinusitis
ENDO: Hypoglycemia
GI: Acute pancreatitis, constipation, diarrhea, dyspepsia, elevated liver enzymes, gastroesophageal reflux disease, nausea, vomiting
GU: Acute renal failure, worsening renal failure
MS: Arthralgia, back pain
RESP: Cough, dyspnea, pneumonia, upper respiratory infection
SKIN: Pruritus, rash
Other: Flu-like syndrome; injection site reactions such as erythema, hematoma, hemorrhage, pruritus, rash

Nursing Considerations
• Know that albiglutide should not be used as first-line therapy for patients who have inadequately controlled their blood glucose levels on diet and exercise alone.
• Use caution when beginning albiglutide therapy or titrating dose in patients with renal impairment. Monitor renal function in these patients if they experience severe adverse gastrointestinal reactions.
• Reconstitute the powder found in the pen prior to administration. First, hold the pen body with the clear cartridge pointing up to see the number 1 in the number window. Twist the clear cartridge on the pen in the direction of the arrow until the pen is felt or heard to "click" into place and the number 2 is seen in the number window. Slowly and

gently rock the pen side-to-side five times to mix the reconstituted solution. Do not shake the pen hard to avoid mixture foaming. Wait 15 minutes for the 30-mg pen and 30 minutes for the 50-mg pen to ensure that the reconstituted solution is mixed. Look in the viewing window to be sure there are no particles present and the solution is clear yellow. The reconstituted solution may be administered up to 8 hours after mixing. Alternatively, as a healthcare professional but not for the patient, after the number 2 is seen in the number window, hold the pen with the clear cartridge pointing up and maintain this orientation throughout the rest of the reconstitution process. Gently swirl the pen in small circular motions for at least 1 minute while avoiding shaking the pen to prevent foaming, which may affect the dose. A small amount of foam, on top of the solution at the end of reconstitution, is normal. Look in the view window to be sure no particles are present and the solution is clear yellow. Know that complete dissolution usually occurs within 2 to 5 minutes for the 30-mg pen using this method and 7 to 10 minutes for the 50-mg pen using this method.

• Prepare to administer albiglutide by first slowly and gently rocking the pen side-to-side five additional times to mix the reconstituted solution if the drug was not administered immediately after mixing. Holding the pen upright, attach the needle to the pen by first peeling the tab from the outer needle cap. Then hold the pen with the clear cartridge pointing up and push the needle straight down onto the clear cartridge until a "click" is heard and the needle feels as if it has "snapped" into place. With the needle pointing up, gently tap the clear cartridge two or three times to bring large bubbles to the top (small bubbles do not need to rise to the top). Remove air bubbles by slowly twisting the pen until the number 3 is seen in the number window. Know that at the same time, the injection button will be automatically released from the bottom of the pen. Administer immediately after the needle is attached and primed because the drug

can clog the needle if allowed to dry in the primed needle.

• Remove the outer needle cap and the inner needle cap immediately before administrating. A few drops of liquid may come out of the needle but will not affect the dose. Administer by inserting the needle subcutaneously into the skin in the abdomen, thigh, or upper arm region and then pressing the injection button. Hold the injection button until a "click" is heard and then hold the button for 5 additional seconds to deliver the full dose.

• There is a possibility that albiglutide may be linked to the development of thyroid C-cell tumors. While elevated serum calcitonin is a biological marker, its value in routine monitoring is unclear. If an elevated serum calcitonin level is found at any time during therapy, expect the patient to be referred to an endocrinologist for further evaluation.

• Monitor patient for signs and symptoms of pancreatitis, such as persistent severe abdominal pain, sometimes radiating to the back, which may or may not be accompanied by vomiting. If confirmed, expect albiglutide to be discontinued.

• Monitor patient also receiving insulin or insulin secretagogue therapy concomitantly for hypoglycemia. The dosage of insulin or insulin secretagogue may need to be lowered to reduce the risk of hypoglycemia. If hypoglycemia occurs, treat it according to the standard of care and notify prescriber.

• Monitor patient for signs of hypersensitivity such as dyspnea, pruritus, or rash. If present, withhold drug, notify prescriber, and expect drug to be discontinued.

• Monitor patient for signs of diarrhea, dehydration, nausea, or vomiting, which may suggest renal impairment. If present, notify prescriber because the frequency of these gastrointestinal symptoms may increase as renal function declines.

PATIENT TEACHING

• Inform patient that the drug may be administered at any time of day without regard to meals but that it should be

administered on the same day each week. However, if the day of the week needs to be changed, the change may be made as long as the last dose was administered 4 or more days earlier.
• Instruct patient that if a dose is missed, he should administer the drug as soon as possible within 3 days after the missed dose. If more than 3 days has elapsed since the last injection, he should wait to administer albiglutide until the next scheduled weekly dose.
• Teach patient how to reconstitute the powder in the pen, how to operate the pen during administration, and how to administer the drug as a subcutaneous injection.
• Remind patient that the reconstituted solution must be used within 8 hours after mixing.
• Tell patient to administer the injection into the abdomen, thigh, or upper arm region. Instruct patient that if the same body region is being used each week, the sites of injection should be rotated within that region. Tell patient how to safely dispose of the used pen and needle.
• Warn patient also receiving insulin to use separate injections for the two drugs and to never mix the drugs. However, let patient know that it is acceptable to inject both injections in the same body region but not adjacent to each other.
• Ensure that patient has been informed of the potential risk for developing thyroid tumors before starting albiglutide therapy. Tell patient to report any symptoms of thyroid tumors such as a mass in the neck, difficulty swallowing or breathing, or persistent hoarseness.
• Instruct patient on the signs and symptoms of hypoglycemia and how to treat it. Inform patient who is also receiving a sulfonylurea or insulin that the risk of hypoglycemia is greater. Tell patient to notify prescriber if hypoglycemia occurs frequently or is severe.
• Tell patient to notify prescriber if any orally administered drugs appear to be losing their effectiveness, as albiglutide causes a delay of gastric emptying and has the potential to impact the absorption of drugs taken by mouth.

albuterol

A

(salbutamol)

Proventil

albuterol sulfate

(salbutamol sulphate)

Accuneb, Airet, Gen-Salbutamol (CAN), Novo-Salmol (CAN), Proair HFA, Proventil, Proventil HFA, Proventil Repetabs, Proventil Syrup, Ventolin HFA, Ventolin Syrup, Volmax

Class and Category
Chemical class: Selective beta$_2$-adrenergic agonist, sympathomimetic
Therapeutic class: Bronchodilator
Pregnancy category: C

Indications and Dosages
➤ *To prevent exercise-induced asthma*
INHALATION AEROSOL
Adults and children over age 4. Two inhalations 15 to 30 min before exercise.
➤ *To treat bronchospasm in patients with reversible obstructive airway disease or acute bronchospastic attack*
E.R. TABLETS
Adults and children over age 12.
Initial: 4 or 8 mg every 12 hr. *Maximum:* 32 mg daily in divided doses every 12 hr.
Children ages 6 to 12.
Initial: 4 mg every 12 hr. *Maximum:* 24 mg daily in divided doses every 12 hr.
REPETABS
Adults and children over age 12.
Initial: 4 to 8 mg every 12 hr. *Maximum:* 32 mg daily in divided doses every 12 hr.
Children ages 6 to 11.
Initial: 4 mg every 12 hr. *Maximum:* 24 mg daily in divided doses every 12 hr.
SYRUP
Adults and children over age 14.
Initial: 2 to 4 mg (1 to 2 tsp) t.i.d. or q.i.d. *Maximum:* 32 mg daily in divided doses.
Children ages 6 to 14.
Initial: 2 mg (1 tsp) three or four times daily. *Maximum:* 24 mg daily in divided doses.
Children ages 2 to 6.
Initial: 0.1 mg/kg three times daily (not to exceed 2 mg three times daily), increased to

0.2 mg/kg three times daily (not to exceed 4 mg three times daily).
TABLETS
Adults and children over age 12.
Initial: 2 or 4 mg three or four times daily. *Maximum:* 32 mg daily in divided doses.
Children ages 6 to 12.
Initial: 2 mg three or four times daily. *Maximum:* 24 mg daily in divided doses.
DOSAGE ADJUSTMENT For elderly patients, initial dosage reduced to 2 mg (1 tsp) of syrup three or four times daily or 2 mg of tablets three or four times daily (up to 32 mg daily).
INHALATION AEROSOL
Adults and children age 4 and over.
1 inhalation every 4 hr to 2 inhalations every 4 to 6 hr.
INHALATION CAPSULES (ROTOCAPS)
Adults and children age 4 and over.
200 mcg inhaled every 4 to 6 hr using inhalation device. *Maximum:* 400 mcg every 4 to 6 hr.

INHALATION SOLUTION
Adults and children age 12 and over.
2.5 mg three or four times daily by nebulization over 5 to 15 min.
Children ages 2 to 12.
Initial: 0.1 to 0.15 mg/kg three or four times daily. *Maximum:* 2.5 mg three or four times daily.

Route	Onset	Peak	Duration
P.O. (E.R. tab)	30 min	2–3 hr	12 hr
P.O. (syrup)	Rapid	2 hr	Unknown
P.O. (tab)	30 min	2–3 hr	4–8 hr

Route	Onset	Peak	Duration
Inhalation (aerosol)	5–15 min	50–55 min	3–6 hr
Inhalation (rotocap)	5–15 min	0.5–3 min	2–6 hr
Inhalation (solution)	5–15 min	1–2 hr	3–6 hr

Contraindications
Hypersensitivity to albuterol or its components

Interaction
DRUGS
beta blockers: Inhibited effects of albuterol
bronchodilators (sympathomimetics), such as theophylline: Possibly adverse CV effects
digoxin: Decreased serum digoxin level
MAO inhibitors, tricyclic antidepressants: Increased vascular effects of albuterol
methyldopa: Increased vasopressor effect of methyldopa
potassium-lowering drugs: Possibly hypokalemia
potassium-wasting diuretics: Possibly increased hypokalemia

Adverse Reactions
CNS: Anxiety, dizziness, drowsiness, headache, hyperkinesia, insomnia, irritability, nervousness, tremor, vertigo, weakness
CV: Angina; arrhythmias, including atrial fibrillation, extrasystoles, supraventricular tachycardia, and tachycardia; chest pain; hypertension; hypotension; palpitations
EENT: Altered taste, dry mouth and throat, ear pain, glossitis, hoarseness,

Mechanism of Action
Albuterol attaches to $beta_2$ receptors on bronchial cell membranes, which stimulatesthe intracellular enzyme adenylate cyclase to convert adenosine triphosphate (ATP) to cyclic adenosine monophosphate (cAMP). This reaction decreases intracellular calcium levels. It also increases intracellular levels of cAMP, as shown. Together, these effects relax bronchial smooth-muscle cells and inhibit histamine release.

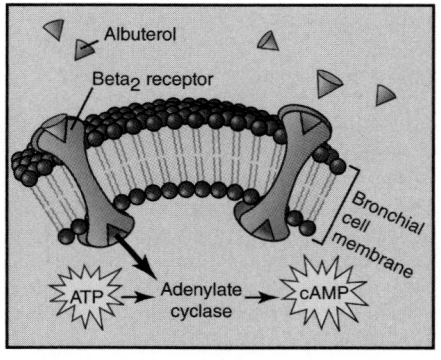

oropharyngeal edema, pharyngitis, rhinitis, taste perversion
ENDO: Hyperglycemia
GI: Anorexia, diarrhea, dysphagia, heartburn, nausea, vomiting
GU: UTI
MS: Muscle cramps
RESP: Bronchospasm, cough, dyspnea, paradoxical bronchospasm, pulmonary edema
SKIN: Diaphoresis, flushing, pallor, pruritus, rash, urticaria
Other: Angioedema, hypokalemia, infection, metabolic acidosis

Nursing Considerations
• Administer pressurized inhalations of albuterol during second half of inspiration, when airways are open wider and aerosol distribution is more effective.
WARNING Use cautiously in patients with cardiac disorders, diabetes mellitus, digitalis intoxication, hypertension, hyperthyroidism, or history of seizures. Albuterol can worsen these conditions.
• Monitor serum potassium level because albuterol may cause transient hypokalemia.
• Be aware that drug tolerance can develop with prolonged use.
PATIENT TEACHING
• Teach patient to use inhaler. Tell him to shake canister before use and to check that a new canister is working by spraying it the appropriate number of times (once to four times based on manufacturer instructions) into the air while looking for a fine mist.
• Instruct patient to wash mouthpiece with water once a week and let it air-dry.
• Advise patient to wait at least 1 minute between inhalations.
• Tell patient to check with his prescriber before using other inhaled drugs.
• Warn patient not to exceed prescribed dose or frequency. If doses become less effective, tell patient to contact his prescriber.
• Tell patient to immediately report signs and symptoms of allergic reaction, such as difficulty swallowing, itching, and rash.

alefacept
Amevive

Class and Category
Chemical class: Recombinant leukocyte function-associated antigen-3 immunoglobulin GI fusion protein
Therapeutic class: Immunosuppressant
Pregnancy category: B

Indications and Dosages
➤ *To treat moderate to severe chronic plaque psoriasis in patients who are candidates for systemic therapy or phototherapy*
I.V. INJECTION
Adults. *Initial:* 7.5 mg every wk for 12 wk. After at least 12 wk in which drug isn't given, a second 12-wk course may be given, if needed and if patient's CD4 and T-lymphocyte counts are within normal ranges.
I.M. INJECTION
Adults. 15 mg every week for 12 wk. After at least 12 wk in which drug isn't given, a second 12-wk course may be given, if needed and if patient's CD4 and T-lymphocyte counts are within normal ranges.

Mechanism of Action
Interferes with T-lymphocyte activation by binding to lymphocyte antigen and CD2, inhibiting LFA-3/CD2 interaction, and reducing the subsets of CD2+ T lymphocytes. This interference helps prevent plaque formation in chronic plaque psoriasis.

Incompatibilities
Don't add other drugs to solutions containing alefacept.

Contraindications
Breastfeeding, hypersensitivity to alefacept or its components

Adverse Reactions
CNS: Chills, dizziness, headache
CV: Coronary artery disease, MI
EENT: Pharyngitis
GI: Cholecystitis, gastroenteritis, nausea
HEME: Lymphopenia
MS: Myalgia
RESP: Increased cough, pneumonia
SKIN: Cellulitis, pruritus, urticaria
Other: Abscesses; angioedema; herpes infections; injection-site pain or inflammation; serious infections; toxic

shock syndrome; malignancies such as skin cancer, solid organ malignancies, and lymphomas; wound infections

Nursing Considerations
• Use alefacept cautiously in patients at high risk for malignancy because the drug increases risk of malignancy development. Know that drug isn't recommended for use in patients with a history of a systemic malignancy.
• Also use alefacept cautiously in patients with chronic infections or history of recurrent infection. Drug may increase risk of infection because of its immunosuppressive action.
• Obtain a CD4+ and T-lymphocyte count before starting alefacept therapy, as ordered. If counts are below normal, be aware that therapy shouldn't be started. After therapy starts, monitor patient's CD4+ and T-lymphocyte counts weekly throughout therapy. If levels drop below 250 cells/microliter, notify prescriber because drug will need to be withheld. If counts remain below 250 cells/microliter for 1 month, expect that drug will be discontinued.
• Reconstitute drug with 0.6 ml using only the supplied diluent (sterile water for injection) before administration. With the needle pointed at sidewall of vial, slowly inject diluent into vial of alefacept. Be aware that some foaming will occur. To prevent excessive foaming, don't shake or vigorously agitate vial. Instead, gently swirl vial during dissolution, which usually takes less than 2 minutes.
• Administer drug as soon as possible after reconstitution. Discard solution if not used within 4 hours.
• Don't filter reconstituted solution during preparation or administration.
• For I.M. administration, inject the full 0.5 ml of solution. Use a different injection site for each subsequent injection, injecting at least 1 inch away from previous sites. Never inject the drug into tender, bruised, red, or hard areas.
• For I.V. administration, prepare two syringes with 3 ml normal saline solution for preadministration and postadministration flush. Then prime the winged infusion set

with 3 ml normal saline solution and insert into vein. Attach filled syringe to infusion set, and administer solution over no more than 5 seconds. Finish by flushing set with 3 ml of normal saline solution.
• Be aware that drug shouldn't be started in a patient with a concurrent serious infection. Monitor patient closely during and after therapy for signs and symptoms of infection. If these occur, report them to the prescriber immediately and begin treatment, as prescribed, to reduce risk of serious infection. If infection becomes serious, expect drug to be discontinued.
• Monitor patient for allergic reactions. If these occur, discontinue drug and notify prescriber immediately.

PATIENT TEACHING
• Advise patient that weekly blood tests will be required to monitor his WBC count during alefacept therapy.
• Teach patient signs and symptoms of infection and common warning signs of malignancy. Emphasize importance of complying with follow-up visits and promptly reporting any unusual or sudden signs or symptoms suggesting malignancy or infection.
• Instruct female patient to notify prescriber if she becomes pregnant while taking alefacept or within 8 weeks after stopping it.

alendronate sodium
Binosto, Fosamax

Class and Category
Chemical class: Aminobisphosphonate
Therapeutic class: Bone resorption inhibitor
Pregnancy category: C

Indications and Dosages
➤ *To prevent postmenopausal osteoporosis*
TABLETS
Adults. 5 mg daily or 35 mg once/wk in the morning with a full glass of water at least 30 min before first food, drink, or other drugs.
➤ *To treat postmenopausal osteoporosis*
ORAL SOLUTION, TABLETS
Adults. 10 mg daily or 70 mg once/wk in the morning with a full glass of water at

least 30 min before first food, drink, or other drugs.

EFFERVESCENT TABLETS

Adults. 70 mg once/wk in the morning dissolved in 4 oz of room temperature water at least 30 min before first food, drink, or other drugs.

➤ *To treat Paget's disease of the bone in patients whose alkaline phosphatase level is twice the upper limit of normal or higher and who are symptomatic and at risk for further complications*

TABLETS

Adults. 40 mg daily with a full glass of water for 6 mo.

➤ *To increase bone mass in men with osteoporosis*

ORAL SOLUTION, TABLETS

Adults. 10 mg daily or 70 mg once/wk in the morning with a full glass of water at least 30 min before first food, drink, or other drugs.

EFFERVESCENT TABLETS

Adults. 70 mg once/wk in the morning dissolved in 4 oz of room temperature water at least 30 min before first food, drink, or other drugs.

➤ *To treat glucocorticoid-induced osteoporosis in men and women who receive a daily glucocorticoid dosage of 7.5 mg or greater of prednisone and who have low bone-mineral density*

TABLETS

Adults. 5 mg daily in the morning with a full glass of water at least 30 min before first food, drink, or other drugs.

DOSAGE ADJUSTMENT Dosage increased to 10 mg daily for postmenopausal women not receiving estrogen.

Route	Onset	Peak	Duration
P.O.	Unknown	Unknown	6 wk*

Mechanism of Action

Reduces activity of cells that cause bone loss, slows rate of bone loss after menopause, and increases amount of bone mass. May act by inhibiting osteoclast activity on newly formed bone resorption

---

* After single 5-mg dose for osteoporosis; 6 mo after single 5-mg dose for Paget's disease.

surfaces, which reduces the number of sites where bone is remodeled. Bone formation then exceeds bone resorption at these remodeling sites, which gradually increases bone mass. May also inhibit bone dissolution by binding to hydroxyapatite crystals, which are composed of calcium, phosphate, and hydroxide and give bone its rigid structure.

Contraindications

Esophageal abnormalities that delay esophageal emptying, such as stricture or achalasia; hypersensitivity to alendronate or its components; hypocalcemia; inability to stand or sit upright for at least 30 minutes

Interaction

DRUGS

antacids, calcium, iron, multivalent cations: Decreased absorption of alendronate
aspirin: Increased risk of GI distress

FOODS

any food: Delayed absorption and decreased serum level of alendronate

Adverse Reactions

CNS: Asthenia, dizziness, headache, vertigo
CV: Peripheral edema
GI: Abdominal distention and pain, constipation, diarrhea, dysphagia, esophageal perforation or ulceration, esophagitis, flatulence, gastritis, gastroesophageal reflux disease, heartburn, indigestion, melena, nausea, vomiting
MS: Arthralgia; femoral shaft or subtrochanteric fractures; focal osteomalacia; jaw osteonecrosis; joint swelling; muscle spasms; myalgia severe bone, joint, and/or muscle pain
RESP: Asthma exacerbation
SKIN: Photosensitivity, pruritus, rash, Stevens-Johnson syndrome, toxic epidermal necrolysis
Other: Anaphylaxis, hypocalcemia

Nursing Considerations

• Prepare to administer effervescent form of alendronate by dissolving one tablet in 4 ounces of plain water (do not use mineral water or flavored water) that is at room temperature. Wait 5 minutes after effervescence stops and then stir the solution for about 10 seconds before handing to patient to ingest.

• Monitor patient's serum calcium level before, during, and after treatment. Expect hypocalcemia to be treated before alendronate therapy. If hypocalcemia occurs during therapy, expect prescriber to order a calcium supplement.

• Ensure adequate dietary intake of calcium and vitamin D before, during, and after treatment.

• Be aware that oral osteoporosis drugs such as alendronate may have the potential to increase the risk of esophageal cancer. While studies are underway to determine this potential, assess patient regularly for painful or difficulty swallowing, chest pain, or new or worsening heartburn; notify prescriber if present.

WARNING Alendronate may irritate upper GI mucosa, causing adverse reactions such as esophageal ulceration. To help minimize these reactions, have patient take drug with a full glass of water and remain upright for at least 30 min.

• Monitor patient for jaw pain because alendronate may cause osteonecrosis of the jaw, with risk increasing as therapy duration becomes longer. Patients at increased risk include those who have poor oral hygiene, preexisting dental or periodontal disease, wear ill-fitting dentures, or require an invasive dental procedure. Patients are also at increased risk if they have a cancer diagnosis, concomitant therapy such as chemotherapy or corticosteroid therapy, or other illnesses, such as pre-existing dental or periodontal disease, anemia, coagulopathy, or infection.

PATIENT TEACHING

• Advise patient to take alendronate in the morning with a full glass of water. Explain that beverages such as orange juice, coffee, and mineral water reduce alendronate's effects.

• Instruct patient who is prescribed the effervescent tablet form to dissolve the tablet in 4 ounces of room temperature water (mineral water or flavored water should not be used). After the effervescence stops, tell the patient to wait 5 minutes and then stir the solution for about 10 seconds and ingest.

• To help reduce esophageal irritation, tell patient not to chew or suck on tablet.

• Instruct patient to wait at least 30 minutes after taking alendronate before eating, drinking, or taking other drugs. Teach patient to remain upright for 30 minutes after taking alendronate and until she has eaten the first food of the day.

• Encourage patient to consume adequate daily amounts of calcium and vitamin D.

• Instruct patient to report to prescriber any new or unusual pain in hip or thigh.

• Tell patient to inform dentist of alendronate therapy prior to dental work and to notify dentist of any signs of infection or delayed healing after an extraction.

• Instruct patient to report any difficulty swallowing or pain when swallowing, chest pain, or new or worsening heartburn to prescriber.

• Inform patient receiving the effervescent tablet form to be aware that each tablet contains 650 mg sodium, which is equivalent to approximately 1650 mg of sodium chloride per tablet.

alfuzosin hydrochloride
Uroxatral

Class and Category
Chemical class: Tetrahydro-2-furancarboxamide hydrochloride
Therapeutic class: Selective alpha$_1$-adrenergic antagonist
Pregnancy category: B

Indications and Dosages
➤ *To treat signs and symptoms of benign prostatic hyperplasia*
E.R. TABLETS
Adults. 10 mg daily taken immediately after same meal each day.

Mechanism of Action
Selectively blocks alpha$_1$-adrenergic receptors in smooth muscle of the bladder neck and prostate, causing relaxation, and blocks postsynaptic alpha$_1$ adrenoreceptors in bladder base and neck, prostate, prostatic capsule, and urethra, preventing further action at these sites. These actions improve urine flow and bladder emptying and reduce urinary hesitancy, frequency, and nocturia.

Contraindications

Hypersensitivity to alfuzosin or its components, moderate or severe hepatic insufficiency, use with CYP3A4 inhibitors, such as itraconazole, ketoconazole, and ritonavir

Interaction

DRUGS

alpha blockers, PDE5 inhibitors: May potentiate alfuzosin action
antihypertensives, nitrates: Possibly synergistic lowering of blood pressure and syncope
CYP3A4 inhibitors (such as itraconazole, ketoconazole, ritonavir): Increased alfuzosin effects

Adverse Reactions

CNS: Dizziness, fatigue, headache
CV: Angina (preexisting coronary artery disease), atrial fibrillation, chest pain, edema, orthostatic hypotension, QT-interval prolongation, tachycardia
EENT: Intraoperative floppy iris syndrome, pharyngitis, rhinitis, sinusitis
GI: Abdominal pain, constipation, diarrhea, indigestion, jaundice, hepatotoxicity, nausea
GU: Impotence, priapism
HEME: Thrombocytopenia
RESP: Bronchitis, upper respiratory tract infection
SKIN: Flushing, pruritus, rash, toxic epidermal necrolysis, urticaria
Other: Angioedema, generalized pain

Nursing Considerations

• Use alfuzosin cautiously in patients who have symptomatic hypotension or who have had a hypotensive response to other drugs. Orthostatic hypotension (with or without symptoms such as dizziness) may occur within hours after alfuzosin administration.
• Use cautiously in patients with severe renal insufficiency; decreased drug clearance may increase risk of adverse reactions.
• Be aware that alfuzosin shouldn't be used to treat bladder symptoms in women.
• Know that alpha$_1$ blockers such as alfuzosin may predispose patients to intraoperative floppy iris syndrome during cataract surgery that may require surgical repair.
• Monitor patient for chest pain. If symptoms of angina pectoris occur or worsen, notify prescriber immediately and expect drug to be discontinued.

PATIENT TEACHING

• Emphasize need to take alfuzosin immediately after a meal because absorption is decreased by 50% if taken on an empty stomach.
• Tell patient not to crush or chew tablets but to swallow them whole.
• Caution patient to avoid hazardous activities until drug's CNS effects are known and also for several hours after taking dose; blood pressure may drop suddenly after use.
• Advise patient to change position slowly to minimize drop in blood pressure.

alglucerase

Ceredase

Class and Category

Chemical class: Glucocerebrosidase beta-glucosidase
Therapeutic class: Enzyme replacement
Pregnancy category: C

Indications and Dosages

➤ *To treat chronic nonneuropathic Gaucher's disease in patients with moderate to severe anemia, thrombocytopenia with bleeding tendencies, bone disease, or significant hepatomegaly or splenomegaly*

I.V. INFUSION

Adults and children age 2 and over. Individualized. 2.5 units/kg to 60 units/kg infused over 1 to 2 hr, usually every 2 wk.
DOSAGE ADJUSTMENT Highly individualized based on body size and disease severity. Some patients may need infusion once every other day; others may need it once every 4 wk. Maintenance dosage progressively reduced every 3 to 6 mo to as low as 1 unit/kg.

Route	Onset	Peak	Duration
I.V.	Up to 60 min	Unknown	Variable

Mechanism of Action

Catalyzes hydrolysis of glucocerebroside to glucose and ceramide in membrane lipids. Gaucher's disease results from deficiency of the enzyme beta-glucocerebrosidase and causes the lipid glucocerebroside to accumulate in tissue macrophages.

Contraindications

Hypersensitivity to alglucerase

Adverse Reactions

CNS: Chills, dizziness, fatigue, fever, headache
CV: Transient peripheral edema, vasomotor irritability
EENT: Oral ulcerations
GI: Abdominal discomfort or pain, diarrhea, nausea, vomiting
GU: Nephrotic syndrome, proteinuria
MS: Backache
Other: I.V. site burning, itching, or swelling

Nursing Considerations

• Before starting alglucerase therapy, expect to give antihistamines if patient is hypersensitive to drug.
• On day of dose, use aseptic technique to dilute alglucerase with normal saline solution to final volume of no more than 200 ml.
• Don't shake drug because doing so could inactivate it.
• Don't use alglucerase if it's discolored or contains precipitate.
• Be aware that drug doesn't contain preservatives. Discard unused portion.
• Infuse drug with in-line I.V. particle filter.

PATIENT TEACHING

• Tell patient that he may experience flulike symptoms with each dose of alglucerase.
• Instruct patient to report headache, hot flashes, nausea, and other adverse reactions.
• Inform patient that alglucerase is derived from pooled human placental tissue and poses a slight risk of viral contamination.
• Advise patient to keep appointments for scheduled doses of alglucerase.

---

aliskiren

Tekturna

Class and Category

Chemical class: Hemifumarate salt
Therapeutic class: Antihypertensive (direct renin inhibitor)
Pregnancy category: D

Indications and Dosages

➤ *To treat hypertension*

TABLETS

Adults. 150 mg once daily, increased to 300 mg once daily, as needed.

Route	Onset	Peak	Duration
P.O.	Unknown	1–3 hr	Unknown

Mechanism of Action

Inhibits renin secreted by the kidneys in response to decreased blood volume and renal perfusion. Renin cleaves angiotensinogen to form angiotensin I, which is converted to angiotensin II by ACE and non-ACE pathways. Angiotensin II is a powerful vasoconstrictor that induces release of catecholamines from the adrenal medulla and prejunctional nerve endings. It also promotes aldosterone secretion and sodium reabsorption. Together, these actions increase blood pressure. By inhibiting renin release, aliskiren impairs the renin-angiotensin-aldosterone system. Without the vasoconstrictive effect of angiotension II, blood pressure decreases.

Contraindications

Hypersensitivity to aliskiren or its components; presence of diabetes and concurrent angiotensin converting enzyme inhibitor (ACEI) or angiotensin receptor blocker (ARB) therapy; pregnancy; renal impairment, disease, or failure

Interaction

DRUGS

ACE inhibitors, ARBs, NSAIDs, potassium-sparing diuretics, potassium supplements: Increased risk of hyperkalemia
ACE inhibitors, ARBs, NSAIDs: Possible increased risk of renal dysfunction, especially in the elderly and patients who are volume-depleted or already have renal impairment
atorvastatin, cyclosporine, itraconazole, ketoconazole, verapamil: Increased aliskiren blood level
furosemide: Decreased blood furosemide levels
irbesartan: Decreased blood aliskiren level
P-glycoprotein: Possible alteration in absorption and disposition of aliskiren at Pgp site

Adverse Reactions

CNS: Dizziness, fatigue, headache, seizures
CV: Hypotension, peripheral edema

EENT: Nasopharyngitis
GI: Abdominal pain, diarrhea, dyspepsia, gastroesophageal reflux
GU: Elevated blood creatinine, renal calculi
HEME: Decreased hemoglobin and hematocrit
MS: Back pain
RESP: Increased cough, upper respiratory tract infection
SKIN: Rash, Stevens-Johnson syndrome, toxic epidermal necrolysis
Other: Anaphylaxis, angioedema of head and neck, elevated creatine kinase or uric acid level, gout, hyperkalemia

Nursing Considerations
• Be aware that aliskiren should not be used in patients with diabetes who are concurrently taking ARBs or ACEIs because of the increased risk of serious adverse effects such as renal dysfunction, hyperkalemia, and hypotension. Also know that aliskiren should not be given to patients with moderate renal impairment (glomerular filtration rate of less than 60 ml/min) who are also receiving ARB or ACEI therapy because renal impairment may worsen.
• Monitor patient's renal function closely, especially in patients receiving drugs such as ARBs, ACEIs, NSAIDs, potassium supplements or potassium-sparing diuretics that affect the renin-angiotensin system. Use aliskiren cautiously in patients whose renal function may depend in part on the activity of this system such as those with renal artery stenosis, severe heart failure, post-myocardial infarction, or who are elderly or experiencing volume depletion because aliskiren therapy increases the risk of renal dysfunction in these patients that could lead to acute renal failure.
• To prevent hypotension, take measures to correct volume or salt depletion from high-dose diuretic therapy before starting aliskiren. If hypotension occurs during aliskiren therapy, place patient in a supine position and give normal saline solution intravenously, as needed and prescribed.
WARNING Watch closely for angioedema of the head or neck. if angioedema occurs, discontinue aliskiren, notify prescriber,

and provide supportive therapy until swelling has ceased. if swelling of the tongue, glottis, or larynx is involved, be prepared to give epinephrine solution 1:1,000 (0.3 to 0.5 ml), as prescribed, and provide measures to ensure a patent airway. Be aware that patient shouldn't receive aliskiren again.
• Monitor serum electrolytes, especially potassium levels, as ordered in patients who already are experiencing renal insufficiency or who have diabetes because of increased risk for hyperkalemia in the presence of aliskiren therapy. Also monitor patients who are taking ARBs, ACEIs, or NSAIDs along with aliskiren because of increased risk of hyperkalemia.

PATIENT TEACHING
• Advise patient to avoid high-fat meals while taking aliskiren because fat decreases drug absorption significantly.
• Instruct patient how to monitor blood pressure to determine effectiveness of aliskiren therapy.
• Explain that decreased blood pressure could lead to light-headedness, especially in the first few days of therapy. Advise patient to change positions slowly and, if light-headedness develops, to notify prescriber. Tell patient to stop taking aliskiren and to notify prescriber if she faints.
• Explain that light-headedness and fainting could also result from dehydration caused by inadequate fluid intake, excessive perspiration, diarrhea, or vomiting.
• Instruct patient to avoid using potassium supplements or potassium salt substitutes and to inform all prescribers about her aliskiren and ACE inhibitor or ARD therapy.
• Emphasize importance of stopping aliskiren and seeking immediate medical attention if patient has swelling of face, extremities, eyes, lips, or tongue, or if patient has trouble swallowing or breathing.
• Instruct female patient to notify prescriber immediately if she is or could be pregnant because drug will need to be discontinued and another antihypertensive chosen.

allopurinol

Apo-Allopurinol (CAN), Lopurin,
Purinol (CAN), Zyloprim

allopurinol sodium

Aloprim

Class and Category
Chemical class: Hypoxanthine derivative,
xanthine oxidase inhibitor
Therapeutic class: Antigout
Pregnancy category: C

Indications and Dosages
➤ *To treat gout and hyperuricemia*
TABLETS
Adults. 200 to 600 mg daily in divided
doses, depending on disease severity. *Usual:*
200 to 300 mg daily. *Maximum:* 800 mg
daily.
➤ *To treat secondary hyperuricemia
caused by neoplastic disease*
TABLETS
Children ages 6 to 10. 300 mg daily,
adjusted after 48 hr, depending on response
to treatment.
Children under age 6. 150 mg daily,
adjusted after 48 hr, depending on response
to treatment.
➤ *To prevent gout attack*
TABLETS
Adults. 100 mg daily increased by 100 mg/
wk until serum uric acid level is 6 mg/dl or
less.
➤ *To prevent uric acid nephropathy
during vigorous treatment of neoplastic
disease*
TABLETS
Adults. 600 to 800 mg daily for 2 to 3 days,
then adjusted to keep serum uric acid level
within normal limits.
➤ *To treat recurrent calcium oxalate
calculi*
TABLETS
Adults. 200 to 300 mg daily as a single dose
or in divided doses, adjusted based on
24-hr urine urate level.
DOSAGE ADJUSTMENT For patient with
impaired renal function, dosage adjusted to
200 mg daily if creatinine clearance is 10 to
20 ml/min/1.73 m^2, 100 mg daily if
creatinine clearance is 3 to 10 ml/min/1.73

m^2, or 100 mg every other day if creatinine
clearance falls below 3 ml/min/1.73 m^2.
➤ *To treat increased serum and urine uric
acid levels in patients with leukemia,
lymphoma, and solid tumors whose
cancer chemotherapy has increased
those levels and who can't tolerate oral
therapy*
I.V. INFUSION
Adults. 200 to 400 mg/m^2 daily as a single
infusion or in equally divided infusions
every 6, 8, or 12 hr. *Maximum:* 600 mg
daily.
Children. 200 mg/m^2 daily as a single
infusion or in equally divided infusions
every 6, 8, or 12 hr.

Route	Onset	Peak	Duration
P.O.	2–3 days	1–3 wk*	1–2 wk

Mechanism of Action
Inhibits uric acid production by inhibiting
xanthine oxidase, the enzyme that converts
hypoxanthine and xanthine to uric acid.
Allopurinol is metabolized to oxipurinol,
which also inhibits xanthine oxidase.

Incompatibilities
Don't combine I.V. allopurinol in solution
with amikacin, amphotericin B, carmustine,
cefotaxime sodium, chlorpromazine
hydrochloride, cimetidine hydrochloride,
clindamycin phosphate, cytarabine,
dacarbazine, daunorubicin hydrochloride,
diphenhydramine hydrochloride, doxorubicin
hydrochloride, doxycycline hyclate,
droperidol, floxuridine, gentamicin sulfate,
haloperidol lactate, hydroxyzine
hydrochloride, idarubicin hydrochloride,
imipenem-cilastatin sodium,
mechlorethamine hydrochloride, meperidine
hydrochloride, metoclopramide
hydrochloride, methylprednisolone sodium
succinate, minocycline hydrochloride,
nalbuphine hydrochloride, netilmicin sulfate,
ondansetron hydrochloride, prochlorperazine
edisylate, promethazine hydrochloride,
sodium bicarbonate, streptozocin, tobramycin
sulfate, vinorelbine tartrate.

Contraindications
Hypersensitivity to allopurinol

---

* For hyperuricemia; several months for
gout attack prevention.

Interaction
DRUGS
ACE inhibitors: Increased risk of hypersensitivity reactions
amoxicillin, ampicillin: Increased risk of rash
azathioprine, mercaptopurine: Inactivation of these drugs
chlorpropamide: Increased risk of hypoglycemia in patients with renal insufficiency
cyclophosphamide, other cytotoxic drugs: Enhanced bone marrow suppression
dicumarol: Increased half-life and anticoagulant action of dicumarol
thiazide diuretics: Possibly increased risk of allopurinol toxicity
uricosuric agents: Increased urinary excretion of uric acid
vitamin C (large doses): Possibly urine acidification and increased risk of renal calculus formation

Adverse Reactions
CNS: Chills, drowsiness, fever, headache, neuritis, paresthesia, peripheral neuropathy, somnolence
CV: Vasculitis
EENT: Epistaxis, loss of taste
GI: Abdominal pain, diarrhea, dysphagia, elevated liver function test results, gastritis, granulomatous hepatitis, hepatic necrosis, hepatomegaly, nausea, vomiting
GU: Exacerbated renal calculi, renal failure
HEME: Agranulocytosis, aplastic anemia, bone marrow depression, eosinophilia, leukocytosis, leukopenia, thrombocytopenia
MS: Arthralgia, exacerbation of gout, myopathy
SKIN: Alopecia; ecchymosis; jaundice; maculopapular, scaly, or exfoliative rash (sometimes fatal); pruritus; urticaria

Nursing Considerations
• As ordered, obtain baseline CBC and uric acid level, and review results of renal and liver function tests before and during allopurinol therapy.
• Reconstitute and dilute I.V. preparation to a concentration of 6 mg/ml or less.
WARNING Discontinue allopurinol and notify prescriber immediately at first sign of hypersensitivity reaction, such as rash, which may precede more severe reactions.

• To decrease risk of calculus formation, maintain fluid intake of up to 3 L daily and monitor patient for output of 2 L daily. Also, don't give vitamin C.
PATIENT TEACHING
• Advise patient to take allopurinol after meals and to drink at least 10 large glasses of water daily.
• Instruct patient to report unusual bleeding or bruising, fever, chills, gout attack, numbness, and tingling.
• Inform patient that acute gout attacks may occur more often early in allopurinol treatment and that results may not be noticeable for 2 weeks or longer.
• Instruct patient not to drive or perform hazardous tasks if drug causes drowsiness.

almotriptan malate
Axert

Class and Category
Chemical class: Selective 5-hydroxytryptamine$_1$ (5-HT$_1$) receptor agonist
Therapeutic class: Antimigraine drug
Pregnancy category: C

Indications and Dosages
➤ *To treat acute migraine*
TABLETS
Adults and adolescents ages 12 to 17.
Initial: 6.25 to 12.5 mg as a single dose, repeated in 2 hr as needed. *Maximum:* 2 doses/24 hr or 4 migraine treatments/mo.
DOSAGE ADJUSTMENT For patient with impaired renal or hepatic function, initial dose reduced to 6.25 mg with maximum daily dose of 12.5 mg.

Mechanism of Action
May stimulate 5-HT$_1$ receptors on intracranial blood vessels and sensory nerves in trigeminal vascular system. By activating these receptors, almotriptan selectively constricts inflamed and dilated cranial blood vessels and inhibits production of proinflammatory neuropeptides. It also interrupts transmission of pain signals to the brain.

Contraindications

Basilar or hemiplegic migraine; cerebrovascular, peripheral vascular, or ischemic or vasospastic coronary artery disease (CAD); hypersensitivity to almotriptan or its components; hypertension (uncontrolled); use within 24 hours of other serotonin-receptor agonists or ergotamine-containing or ergot-type drugs

Interaction

DRUGS

ergotamine-containing drugs: Prolonged vasospastic reactions
erythromycin, itraconazole, ketoconazole, ritonavir: Possibly increased blood almotriptan level
MAO inhibitors, verapamil: Increased blood almotriptan level
selective serotonin reuptake inhibitors, such as citalopram, escitalopram, fluoxetine, fluvoxamine, paroxetine, sertraline: Increased risk of serotonin syndrome
serotonin norepinephrine reuptake inhibitors, such as duloxetine, venlafaxine: Increased risk of serotonin syndrome

Adverse Reactions

CNS: Confusion, dizziness, headache, hemiplegia, hypoesthesia, malaise, paresthesia, restlessness, seizures, somnolence, syncope, vertigo
CV: Angina pectoris, coronary artery vasospasm, hypertension, ischemia, MI, palpitations, tachycardia, vasodilation, ventricular fibrillation, ventricular tachycardia
EENT: Blepharospasm, dry mouth, oral hypoesthesia, swollen tongue, visual impairment
GI: Abdominal pain or discomfort, colitis, nausea
MS: Arthralgia, extremity coldness or pain, myalgia
SKIN: cold sweat, diaphoresis, erythema
Other: Anaphylaxis, angioedema, serotonin syndrome

Nursing Considerations

WARNING Because almotriptan can cause coronary artery vasospasm, monitor patient with CAD for angina. Because it may cause peripheral vasospastic reactions, such as ischemic bowel disease, watch for abdominal pain and bloody diarrhea.

• For patient with risk factors for CAD but no known cardiovascular abnormalities, expect to give first dose of almotriptan in a medical facility.
• In patient with risk factors for CAD, obtain an ECG immediately after first dose of almotriptan, as ordered, because cardiac ischemia can occur without causing clinical symptoms.
• Expect to give a lower dosage to patients with hepatic or renal dysfunction because of impaired drug metabolism or excretion.
• Monitor blood pressure regularly during therapy in patients with hypertension because almotriptan may produce a transient increase in blood pressure.
WARNING Monitor patient for evidence of serotonin syndrome, such as agitation, chills, confusion, diaphoresis, diarrhea, fever, hyperactive reflexes, poor coordination, restlessness, shaking, talking or acting with uncontrolled excitement, tremor, and twitching. In its most severe form, serotonin syndrome can resemble neuroleptic malignant syndrome, which includes a high fever, muscle rigidity, autonomic instability with possible fluctuations in vital signs, and mental status changes.
• Monitor patients hypersensitive to sulfonamides for hypersensitivity to almotriptan because cross-sensitivity may occur.
PATIENT TEACHING
• Inform patient that almotriptan is used to treat acute migraine and that he shouldn't take it to treat nonmigraine headaches.
• Advise patient to consult prescriber before taking any OTC or prescription drugs.
• Advise patient not to take more than maximum prescribed, as medication overuse can cause migraine-like daily headaches or a marked increase in frequency of migraine attacks requiring detoxification to treat, which could lead to withdrawal symptoms.
• Caution patient that drug may cause adverse CNS reactions, and advise him to avoid hazardous activities until he knows how drug affects him.
• Instruct patient to seek emergency care immediately for signs of hypersensitivity such as breathing difficulties, itching, or a rash; cardiac symptoms (such as heaviness, pain, pressure, or tightness in chest, jaw,

neck, or throat); or if multiple new symptoms develop (such as mental changes, high fever, incoordination, nausea, vomiting, diarrhea) after taking drug.

alogliptin
Nesina

Class and Category
Chemical class: Beta amino acid derivative
Therapeutic class: Antidiabetic
Pregnancy category: B

Indications and Dosages
➤ *To achieve control of glucose level in type 2 diabetes mellitus as monotherapy or in conjunction with combination therapy*
TABLETS
Adults. 25 mg once daily.
DOSAGE ADJUSTMENT For patients with moderate renal impairment (creatinine clearance less than 60 ml/min but equal to or greater than 30 ml/min), dosage decreased to 12.5 mg once daily. For patients with severe renal impairment (creatinine clearance is less than 30 ml/min but equal to or greater than 15 ml/min), dosage decreased to 6.25 mg once daily.

Mechanism of Action
Inhibits the dipeptidyl peptidase-4 enzyme to slow inactivation of incretin hormones. These hormones are released by the intestine in response to a meal. When blood glucose level is increased, incretin hormones increase insulin synthesis and release from pancreatic beta cells. One type of incretin hormone, glucagon-like peptide (GLP-1), also lowers glucagon secretion from pancreatic alpha cells, which reduces hepatic glucose production. These combined actions decrease blood glucose level in type 2 diabetes.

Contraindications
Diabetic ketoacidosis, hypersensitivity to alogliptin or its components including anaphylaxis, angioedema, or severe cutaneous adverse reactions, type 1 diabetes

Interaction
DRUGS
insulin, sulfonylureas: Possibly increased risk of hypoglycemia

Adverse Reactions
CNS: Headache
EENT: Nasopharyngitis
ENDO: Hypoglycemia
GI: Acute pancreatitis, elevated hepatic enzymes, fulminant hepatic failure
RESP: Upper respiratory tract infection
SKIN: Rash, Stevens-Johnson syndrome, urticaria
Other: Anaphylaxis, angioedema, serum sickness

Nursing Considerations
• Use alogliptin cautiously in patients with a history of angioedema to another drug in the same class because it is not known if patient will be predisposed to angioedema with alogliptin therapy.
• Assess patient's renal function before starting alogliptin therapy. Know that in moderate to severe renal dysfunction, dosage will need to be reduced.
• Assess patient's liver function before starting alogliptin therapy. If abnormalities are present, monitor patient closely for signs and symptoms of liver dysfunction. If patient develops fatigue, anorexia, right upper abdominal discomfort, dark urine, or becomes jaundiced during therapy, notify prescriber and expect liver enzymes to be assessed. If elevated, expect drug to be discontinued.
• Monitor patient for serious hypersensitivity reactions, including severe cutaneous adverse reactions. If present, notify prescriber, expect alogliptin to be discontinued, and provide supportive care, as ordered.
• Monitor patient's blood glucose level, as ordered, to determine effectiveness of alogliptin therapy.
WARNING Monitor patient for signs and symptoms of acute pancreatitis, such as acute upper abdominal pain, fever, nausea, and vomiting. If suspected, notify prescriber and expect alogliptin to be discontinued, if confirmed.
PATIENT TEACHING
• Emphasize the need to follow an exercise program and a diet control program during alogliptin therapy.
• Advise patient to notify prescriber immediately if he has trouble breathing, develops swelling or skin reactions such as hives, rash, or other cutaneous abnormalities.

• Inform patient that periodic blood tests will be done to determine effectiveness of drug.
• Teach patient how to monitor blood glucose level and when to report changes.
• Caution patient that taking other drugs used to decrease blood glucose level may lead to hypoglycemia. Review signs, symptoms, and appropriate prescribed treatment with him.
• Instruct patient to contract prescriber if he develops other illnesses, such as infection, or experiences trauma or surgery, because his diabetes medication may need adjustment.
• Advise patient to carry identification indicating that he has diabetes.
• Instruct patient to stop taking alogliptin and to report persistent severe abdominal pain, possibly radiating to the back, that may or may not be accompanied by vomiting.

alosetron hydrochloride

Lotronex

Class and Category

Chemical class: Selective serotonin 5-HT$_3$ receptor antagonist
Therapeutic class: Antidiarrheal
Pregnancy category: B

Indications and Dosages

➤ *To treat women with severe diarrhea-predominant irritable bowel syndrome (IBS) who haven't responded to conventional therapy*

TABLETS
Adults. *Initial:* 1 mg daily for 4 wk, increased to 1 mg twice daily, if needed. Discontinued if no response in first 4 wk of therapy, or if drug doesn't adequately control symptoms after 4 wk of twice daily regimen.

Mechanism of Action

Inhibits activation of 5-HT$_3$ nonselective cation channels found in enteric neurons in the GI tract, thereby decreasing visceral sensations, colonic transit, and secretions in the GI tract. These changes reduce GI pain and

hyperactivity, symptoms that are prominent in diarrhea-predominant IBS.

Contraindications

Administration with fluvoxamine, history of chronic or severe constipation or sequelae from constipation, Crohn's disease, diverticulitis, GI perforation or adhesions, hypercoagulable state, impaired intestinal circulation, intestinal obstruction or stricture, ischemic colitis, thrombophlebitis, toxic megacolon, or ulcerative colitis; hypersensitivity to alosetron or its components; severe hepatic impairment

Interaction

DRUGS
fluvoxamine, ketoconazole: Increased blood alosetron level
cimetidine, clarithromycin, itraconazole, protease inhibitors, quinolones, telithromycin, voriconazole: Possibly increased alosetron level

Adverse Reactions

CNS: Anxiety, fatigue, headache, hypnagogic effects, malaise, temperature regulation disturbances
CV: Tachyarrhythmias
GI: Abdominal or GI discomfort and pain, abdominal distention, constipation (may be severe), diarrhea, dyspepsia, flatulence, GI spasms or lesions, hemorrhoids, hemorrhoidal hemorrhage, hyposalivation, ileus, impaction, ischemic colitis, nausea, obstruction, perforation, regurgitation and reflux, small-bowel mesenteric ischemia, ulceration
GU: Urinary frequency
RESP: Breathing disorders
SKIN: Diaphoresis, rash, urticaria
Other: Nonspecific cramps or pain

Nursing Considerations

• Be aware that only physicians enrolled in GlaxoSmithKline's prescribing program for alosetron should prescribe the drug and only patients who have read and signed the patient–physician agreement can receive the drug. Confirm that the agreement has been signed before therapy starts.
• Use alosetron cautiously in patients with mild to moderate liver dysfunction because alosetron is extensively metabolized in the liver.

• Report all adverse reactions to alosetron to the prescriber and to Prometheus at 1-888-423-5227.
WARNING Monitor patient for constipation, especially if she's elderly or debilitated or takes drugs that decrease GI motility. Also watch for evidence of ischemic colitis, such as rectal bleeding, bloody diarrhea, or new or worsening abdominal pain. Serious adverse GI reactions may occur without warning. If they do, be prepared to stop alosetron therapy immediately. If discontinued for ischemic colitis, drug shouldn't be resumed later; however, a patient who no longer has constipation can resume it, if needed.
• Make sure program stickers required by drug maker are affixed to all prescriptions, including refills, before giving to patient.
PATIENT TEACHING
• Explain that alosetron therapy can't begin until patient has read the medication guide that outlines drug's risks and benefits and has signed the permission form.
• Instruct patient not to start alosetron if constipated and to notify prescriber.
• Advise patient that serious adverse GI effects may occur without warning. Tell her to stop taking alosetron immediately and to notify prescriber if evidence of ischemic colitis or constipation arises. Tell her to notify prescriber if constipation doesn't resolve after stopping drug.
• Inform patient that alosetron will be stopped after 4 weeks of 1 mg b.i.d. if it dosen't control IBS symptoms.

alpha₁-proteinase inhibitor (human)

Aralast NP, Glassia, Prolastin, Prolastin-C, Zemaira

Class and Category
Chemical class: Plasma protein
Therapeutic class: Enzyme replacement
Pregnancy category: C

Indications and Dosages
➤ *To treat congenital alpha₁-antitrypsin deficiency in patients with signs of*

panacinar emphysema (Prolastin); to augment and maintain patients with emphysema who are deficient in alpha₁-proteinase inhibitor
I.V. INFUSION
Adults. 60 mg/kg infused over 30 min (Prolastin) at a rate of at least 0.08 ml/kg/min once weekly; 60 mg/kg infused over 15 min (Prolastin-C, Zemaira) at a rate of at least 0.08 ml/kg/min once weekly; 60 mg/kg infused (Aralast NP) at a rate of at least 0.08 ml/kg/min once weekly; or 60 mg/kg infused over 60 to 80 min (Glassia) at a rate not to exceed 0.04 ml/kg/min once weekly.

Mechanism of Action
Replaces the enzyme alpha₁-antitrypsin, which normally inhibits the proteolytic enzyme elastase in patients with alpha₁-antitrypsin deficiency. Without alpha₁-proteinase inhibitor, elastase attacks and destroys alveolar membranes and causes emphysema.

Contraindications
Hypersensitivity to alpha₁-proteinase inhibitor, its components, or other alpha₁-proteinase products; selective immunoglobulin A (IgA) deficiency in patients with anti-IgA antibodies
Interactions
ACTIVITIES
smoking: Inactivation of alpha₁-proteinase inhibitor

Adverse Reactions
CNS: Asthenia, chills, dizziness, fever, headache, light-headedness, malaise, paresthesia
EENT: Nasopharyngitis, pharyngolaryngeal pain, sinusitis
ENDO: Hot flashes
GI: Cholangitis, elevated liver enzymes
HEME: Mild, transient leukocytosis
RESP: Cough, upper respiratory tract infection, worsening of existing COPD
SKIN: Pruritus, rash
Other: Anaphylactic reactions, flulike symptoms, infusion-site pain

Nursing Considerations
• Use alpha₁-proteinase inhibitor cautiously in patients at risk for circulatory overload because drug is a colloid solution that increases plasma volume.

• Remove drug and diluent (if required) from refrigerator and let it warm to room temperature.

• To reconstitute (except for Glassia, which comes in a ready-to-use solution), remove caps from vials and clean rubber stoppers with antiseptic. After stoppers are dry, remove protective cover from diluent end of transfer device and insert into center of upright diluent vial. Then remove protective cover from drug end of transfer device, invert diluent vial with attached transfer device, and using minimal force, insert drug end of transfer device into center of rubber stopper of upright drug vial. Make sure flange of transfer device rests on stopper surface so that diluent flows into drug vial.

• During diluent transfer, wet lyophilized cake completely by gently tilting drug vial. Don't let air inlet filter face downward. (Take care not to lose the vacuum because this will prolong drug reconstitution.) Once diluent transfer is complete, pull transfer device along with attached diluent vial out of drug vial and discard. Gently swirl drug vial until powder is completely dissolved. Avoid shaking because this may cause drug to foam and degrade.

• If more than one vial of alpha₁-proteinase inhibitor is required, use aseptic technique to transfer reconstituted solution from each vial into a sterile I.V. administration container.

• Administer at room temperature within 3 hr of reconstitution as an I.V. infusion, using the large-volume 5-micron conical filter provided. Plce filter between distal end of I.V. administration set and infusion set, and infuse at 0.08 ml/kg/min, except for Glassia, which should be infused at a rate not to exceed 0.04 ml/kg/min. If adverse reactions occur, slow infusion rate or stop infusion until symptoms subside. Then, resume infusion at a rate determined by patient response and comfort.

WARNING Alpha₁-proteinase inhibitor is made from human plasma and may contain infectious agents, such as viruses. Make sure patient is immunized against hepatitis B before giving drug. If time doesn't allow for antibody formation, give a single dose of hepatitis B immune globulin with hepatitis B vaccine, as prescribed.

• Monitor patient for delayed fever, which may occur up to 12 hours after therapy. Fever usually resolves within 24 hours.

PATIENT TEACHING

• Tell patient to report immediately early evidence of allergic reaction, such as chest tightness, trouble breathing, faintness, hives, wheezing, and any other unusual symptoms.

• Advise patient to notify prescriber about signs or symptoms of viral infection (chills, drowsiness, fever, and runny nose, followed 2 weeks later by joint pain and a rash) after receiving drug.

• Emphasize importance of receiving weekly doses to maintain an adequate antielastase barrier in the lungs. Explain that treatment must continue for life.

• Warn patient not to smoke.

alprazolam

Apo-Alpraz (CAN), Niravam, Novo-Alprazol (CAN), Nu-Alpraz, Xanax, Xanax XR

Class and Category

Class, Category, and Schedule
Chemical class: Benzodiazepine
Therapeutic class: Antianxiety drug
Pregnancy category: D
Controlled substance schedule: IV

Indications and Dosages

➤ *To control anxiety disorders, relieve anxiety (short-term therapy), or treat anxiety associated with depression*

ORALLY DISINTEGRATING TABLETS, TABLETS
Adults. *Initial:* 0.25 to 0.5 mg three times daily, adjusted to patient's needs. *Maximum:* 4 mg daily in divided doses.

DOSAGE ADJUSTMENT In elderly or debilitated patients or patients with advanced hepatic disease, initial dosage 0.25 mg twice daily or three times daily and increased gradually, as needed and tolerated.

➤ *To treat panic attack*

ORALLY DISINTEGRATING TABLETS, TABLETS
Adults. *Initial:* 0.5 mg three times daily, increased every 3 to 4 days by no more than 1 mg daily, based on patient response. *Maximum:* 10 mg daily in divided doses.
E.R. TABLETS
Adults. *Initial:* 0.5 to 1 mg daily in morning, increased every 3 to 4 days by no more than 1 mg daily, based on patient response. *Maximum:* 10 mg daily as single dose in morning.

Mechanism of Action
May increase effects of gamma-aminobutyric acid (GABA) and other inhibitory neurotransmitters by binding to specific benzodiazepine receptors in limbic and cortical areas of the CNS. GABA inhibits excitatory stimulation, which helps control emotional behavior. The limbic system contains many benzodiazepine receptors, which may help explain drug's antianxiety effects.

Contraindications
Acute angle-closure glaucoma; hypersensitivity to alprazolam, its components, or other benzodiazepines; itraconazole or ketoconazole therapy

Interaction
DRUGS
antacids: Altered alprazolam absorption rate
cimetidine, disulfiram, fluoxetine, isoniazid, metoprolol, oral contraceptives, propoxyphene, propranolol, valproic acid: Decreased alprazolam elimination and increased effects
CNS depressants: Possibly increased CNS effects of both drugs
digoxin: Possibly increased serum digoxin level, causing digitalis toxicity
itraconazole, ketoconazole: Possibly profoundly inhibited alprazolam metabolism
levodopa: Decreased effects of levodopa
neuromuscular blockers: Possibly potentiated or antagonized effects of these drugs
phenytoin: Possibly increased serum phenytoin level, causing phenytoin toxicity
probenecid: Possibly faster onset or prolonged effects of alprazolam
ranitidine: Possibly reduced absorption of alprazolam
ACTIVITIES
alcohol use: Enhanced adverse CNS effects of alprazolam

Adverse Reactions
CNS: Agitation, akathisia, confusion, depression, dizziness, drowsiness, fatigue, hallucinations, headache, insomnia, irritability, lack of coordination, light-headedness, memory loss, nervousness, paresthesia, rigidity, speech problems, syncope, tremor, weakness
CV: Chest pain, edema, hypotension, nonspecific ECG changes, palpitations, peripheral edema, tachycardia
EENT: Blurred vision, altered salivation, dry mouth, nasal congestion, tinnitus
ENDO: Galactorrhea, gynecomastia, hyperprolactinemia
GI: Abdominal discomfort, anorexia, constipation, diarrhea, elevated liver function test results, hepatitis, hepatic failure, nausea, vomiting
GU: Altered libido, urinary hesitancy
MS: Dysarthria, muscle rigidity and spasms
RESP: Hyperventilation, upper respiratory tract infection
SKIN: Dermatitis, diaphoresis, pruritus, rash, Stevens-Johnson syndrome
Other: Angioedema, weight gain or loss

Nursing Considerations
• Expect to give a higher dosage if patient's panic attacks occur unexpectedly or during such activities as driving.
• Because use can lead to dependency, expect to reduce dosage gradually when stopping drug. To prevent withdrawal symptoms, don't stop drug abruptly.
PATIENT TEACHING
• Warn against stopping drug abruptly because withdrawal symptoms may occur.
• Instruct patient never to increase prescribed dose because of risk of dependency.
• Tell patient prescribed orally disintegrating tablets to use dry hands to remove tablet from bottle just prior to administration. Then she should immediately place the tablet on top of her tongue to dissolve. Inform patient that drinking a liquid beverage is not necessary after taking this form of alprazolam.
• Urge patient to avoid drinking alcohol during alprazolam therapy.
• Advise patient to avoid driving and activities that require alertness until alprazolam's effects are known.

• Instruct female patient of childbearing age to notify prescriber immediately if she becomes or might be pregnant. Drug isn't recommended during pregnancy.

apremilast

Otezla

Class and Category
Chemical class: Phosphodiesterase 4 inhibitor
Therapeutic class: Antirheumatic
Pregnancy category: C

Indications and Dosages
➤ *To treat active psoriatic arthritis*
TABLETS
Adults. *Initial:* 10 mg in a.m. on day 1; 10 mg in a.m. and p.m. on day 2; 10 mg in a.m. and 20 mg in p.m. on day 3; 20 mg in a.m. and p.m. on day 4; 20 mg in a.m. and 30 mg in p.m. on day 5; and 30 mg in a.m. and p.m. on day 6 and thereafter. *Maintenance:* 30 mg in a.m. and p.m.
DOSAGE ADJUSTMENT For patients with severe renal impairment, dosage titration decreased to once daily using only the a.m. titration schedule and maintenance dosage kept at 30 mg once daily in a.m.

Mechanism of Action
Inhibits phosphodiesterase 4, which is specific for cyclic adenosine monophosphate (cAMP). This action results in increased intracellular cAMP levels, which are thought to help relieve symptoms of psoriatic arthritis.

Contraindications
Hypersensitivity to apremilast or its components

Interaction
DRUGS
carbamazepine, phenobarbital, phenytoin, rifampin: Decreased apremilast exposure with loss of effectiveness

Adverse Reactions
CNS: Depression, fatigue, headache, insomnia, migraine, suicidal ideation
EENT: Nasopharyngitis
GI: Anorexia, diarrhea, dyspepsia, gastroesophageal reflux disease, nausea, upper abdominal pain, vomiting
MS: Back pain

RESP: Bronchitis, cough, upper respiratory infection
SKIN: Rash
Other: Weight loss

Nursing Considerations
• Watch patient closely for evidence of depression, especially when apremilast therapy begins, because apremilast therapy may increase risk of depression and possibly lead to suicidal thinking or behavior.
• Monitor patient's weight regularly because apremilast may cause weight loss. Notify prescriber if weight loss occurs that is unexplained or is significant.
PATIENT TEACHING
• Tell patient to follow titration schedule exactly, as this will help reduce the incidence and severity of gastrointestinal symptoms associated with initial therapy.
• Instruct patient to swallow the tablets whole and not to crush, split, or chew the tablets.
• Instruct caregivers to watch patient closely for evidence of suicidal tendencies, especially when therapy starts, and to report concerns to prescriber immediately.

alprostadil

Caverject, Edex, Muse

Class and Category
Chemical class: Prostaglandin E_1
Therapeutic class: Anti-impotence drug
Pregnancy category: C

Indications and Dosages
➤ *To treat erectile dysfunction caused by vascular or psychogenic causes or both*
INTRACAVERNOUS INJECTION (CAVERJECT, EDEX)
Adults. *Initial:* 2.5 mcg. Increased to 5 mcg if partial response or 7.5 mcg if no response, followed by incremental increases of 5 to 10 mcg until erection suitable for intercourse (not exceeding 1-hr duration) is achieved. No more than 2 doses, separated by 1 hr, should be given on a single day during initial titration phase. *Maximum:* 3 doses/wk, separated by 24 hr.
URETHRAL SUPPOSITORY (MUSE)
Adults. *Initial:* 125 to 250 mcg. If no response, dosage increased in increments to

500 or 1,000 mcg until erection suitable for intercourse (not exceeding 1-hr duration) is achieved. *Maximum:* 2 doses/24 hr.
➤ *To treat erectile dysfunction caused by spinal cord injury*
INTRACAVERNOUS INJECTION (CAVERJECT, EDEX)
Adults. *Initial:* 1.25 mcg. Increased to 2.5 mcg if partial response, then to 5 mcg, and increased in 5-mcg increments until erection suitable for intercourse (not exceeding 1-hr duration) is achieved. No more than 2 doses, separated by 1 hr, should be given on a single day during initial titration phase. *Maximum:* 3 doses/wk, separated by 24 hr.

Route	Onset	Peak	Duration
Intra-cavernous	5–20 min	Unknown	60 min
Intra-urethral	5–10 min	Unknown	30–60 min

Contraindications
Anuria, balanitis (inflammation of head of penis), cavernosal fibrosis, hypersensitivity to alprostadil or its components, hyperviscosity syndrome, indwelling urethral catheter, leukemia, men for whom sexual activity is contraindicated, multiple myeloma, penile angulation, penile implants, Peyronie's disease, polycythemia, severe hypospadius (urethral opening on underside of penis), sickle cell anemia or trait, tendency to develop venous thrombosis, thrombocythemia, urethral obstruction or stricture, urethritis

Interaction
DRUGS
anticoagulants: Possibly increased risk of bleeding
cyclosporine: Possibly decreased blood cyclosporine level

Adverse Reactions
CNS: Dizziness, headache, syncope

Mechanism of Action
Alprostadil causes penile erection by increasing blood flow to the penis through relaxation of trabecular smooth muscles and dilation of cavernosal arteries (*upper right*). A naturally occurring prostaglandin, alprostadil interacts with specific membrane-bound receptors in the corpora cavernosa cells of the penis. This action activates intracellular adenyl cyclase (*lower right*), which in turn converts adenosine triphosphate (ATP) into cyclic adenosine monophosphate (cAMP). Increased intracellular levels of cAMP activate protein kinase, an enzyme that activates other enzymes to initiate a cascade of chemical reactions.

These chemical reactions cause the trabecular smooth muscles to relax and the cavernosal arteries to dilate. Blood flow to the penis is then increased, which distends the penile lacunar spaces and compresses the veins, trapping blood in the penis and causing it to become enlarged and rigid.

Transverse section of penis

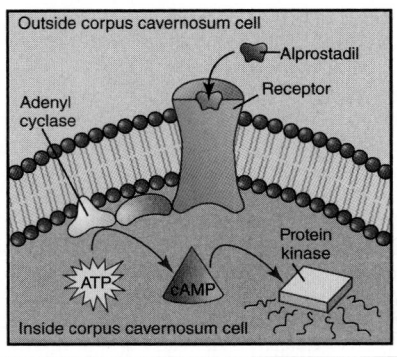

CV: Hypertension, hypotension, tachycardia, vasodilation
EENT: Nasal congestion, sinusitis
GU: Pelvic pain; penile disorders, including edema, fibrosis, pain, and rash; priapism; prolonged erection; prostatic pain or enlargement; urethral abrasions; urethral bleeding
MS: Back pain
RESP: Cough, upper respiratory tract infection
Other: Device malfunction or failure (Caverject Impulse device), flulike symptoms, injection-site bruising or hematoma, needle breakage

Nursing Considerations

• Reconstitute solution with 1 ml diluent, for a concentration of 5, 10, 20, or 40 mcg/ml, depending on vial strength. Gently swirl contents of reconstituted vial. Use reconstituted solution within 24 hours when stored at room temperature. Don't use vials that contain precipitate or discolored solution. Discard unused reconstituted solution.

• Using a 1/2-inch 27G to 30G needle, inject drug at a 90-degree angle into proximal third of spongy tissue that runs the length of the dorsolateral aspect of penis, avoiding any visible veins. Rotate injection sites by alternating sides of the penis.

• Know that alprostadil is also available as a disposable, single-dose, dual-chamber syringe for one use only under the trade name of Caverject Impulse. Be aware that this device uses a superfine 29 gauge needle, so care must be taken to prevent needle breakage. In addition, patient must be assessed closely for drug effectiveness, as device malfunction or failure has occurred with this product.

• Carefully examine penis for evidence of penile fibrosis. Expect to discontinue treatment if patient develops cavernosal fibrosis, penile angulation, or Peyronie's disease (hardening of the corpora cavernosa, which causes penis to become distorted when erect) during therapy.

WARNING Watch for prolonged erection after giving drug. Notify prescriber, and be prepared to treat patient for priapism if erection lasts longer than 4 hours.

• If patient is receiving an anticoagulant, such as warfarin or heparin, watch for bleeding at injection site because drug may inhibit platelet aggregation.

PATIENT TEACHING

• Inform patient that initial therapy must be performed in the office setting. Teach him how to correctly administer intracavernous injections or urethral suppositories. Inform him that the goal of treatment is to produce an erection that lasts no longer than 1 hour.

• Advise patient to use alprostadil for injection no more than three times/week and to separate doses by 24 hours. Inform patient using urethral suppositories not to exceed two doses in a 24-hour period.

• Alert patient using the Caverject Impulse device that needle on syringe is very fine and prone to break if not handle carefully. Also inform him that if the desired effect is not achieved, he should have the device checked, as device malfunction or failure has been reported.

• Tell patient to inform prescriber immediately about nodules or hard tissue in the penis; an erection that persists for more than 4 hours; new or worsened penile pain; or persistent curvature, redness, swelling, or tenderness of the erect penis.

• Inform patient that common adverse reactions include mild to moderate pain immediately after injection and burning after suppository insertion. Also, needle may break. Advise patient to prevent breakage by following prescriber's instructions exactly and by handling injection device properly. If needle breaks during injection and he can see and grasp broken end, he should remove it and contact prescriber. If he can't see or grasp broken end, he should seek medical care.

• Instruct patient using suppository form to urinate just before inserting suppository and to insert it with applicator supplied with drug. Tell patient to hold penis upright after insertion and to roll it firmly between his hands to distribute drug.

• Tell patient to sit, stand, or walk for 10 minutes after inserting suppository to increase blood flow and enhance erection.

• Tell patient to expect an erection 5 to 20 minutes after injecting drug or about 10 minutes after inserting suppository.

• Advise patient not to change dosage without consulting prescriber and to keep scheduled follow-up appointments.
• Warn patient that alprostadil offers no protection from sexually transmitted diseases. Urge him to use a condom to decrease risk of blood-borne disease, because injection can cause minor bleeding at injection site.
• Instruct patient not to reuse or share needles or syringes. Inform him of proper procedure for sharps disposal.
• Warn patient using suppository form not to have sexual intercourse with a pregnant woman unless a condom is used because drug's effect on pregnancy is unknown.
• Advise patient who plans to travel not to check drug with airline baggage or store it in a closed car.

alteplase
(tissue plasminogen activator, recombinant)

Activase, Activase rt-PA (CAN)

Class and Category
Chemical class: Purified glycoprotein
Therapeutic class: Thrombolytic
Pregnancy category: C

Indications and Dosages
➤ *To treat acute MI*
ACCELERATED I.V. INFUSION
Adults weighing more than 67 kg (148 lb). 15-mg bolus followed by 50 mg infused over next 30 min and then by 35 mg infused over next 60 min.
Adults weighing 67 kg or less. 15-mg bolus followed by 0.75 mg/kg (up to 50 mg) infused over next 30 min and then 0.5 mg/ kg (up to 35 mg) infused over next 60 min.
I.V. INFUSION
Adults weighing more than 65 kg (143 lb). 100 mg infused over 3 hr as follows: 6 to 10 mg by bolus over first 1 to 2 min, 50 to 54 mg over remainder of first hr, 20 mg over second hr, and 20 mg over third hr.
Adults weighing 65 kg or less. 1.25 mg/kg infused over 3 hr on similar schedule as those weighing more than 65 kg.
➤ *To treat acute ischemic stroke*

To avoid acute bleeding complications, treatment for acute ischemic stroke must begin within 3 hr after onset of stroke symptoms and only after computed tomography or other diagnostic imaging method excludes intracranial hemorrhage.
I.V. INFUSION
Adults. 0.9 mg/kg infused over 60 min, with 10% of total dose given as bolus over first min. *Maximum:* 90 mg.
➤ *To treat pulmonary embolism*
I.V. INFUSION
Adults. 100 mg infused over 2 hr.

Route	Onset	Peak	Duration
I.V.	Immediate	20–120 min	4 hr

Mechanism of Action
Binds to fibrin in a thrombus and converts trapped plasminogen to plasmin. Plasmin breaks down fibrin, fibrinogen, and other clotting factors, which dissolves the thrombus.

Incompatibilities
Don't add other drugs to solution that contains alteplase.

Contraindications
For all indications: Active internal bleeding, arteriovenous malformation or aneurysm, bleeding diathesis, intracranial neoplasm, severe uncontrolled hypertension
For acute MI and pulmonary embolism only: History of stroke, intracranial or intraspinal surgery or trauma in past 2 months
For acute ischemic stroke only: Recent head trauma, recent intracranial surgery, recent stroke, seizure activity at onset of stroke, subarachnoid hemorrhage, suspicion or history of intracranial hemorrhage

Interaction
DRUGS
drugs that alter platelet function, such as abciximab, acetylsalicylic acid, and dipyridamole; heparin; vitamin K antagonists: Increased risk of bleeding

Adverse Reactions
CNS: Cerebral edema, cerebral herniation, fever, seizure, stroke
CV: Arrhythmias (including bradycardia and electromechanical dissociation), cardiac

arrest, cardiac tamponade, cardiogenic shock, cholesterol embolism, coronary thrombolysis, heart failure, hypotension, mitral insufficiency, myocardial reinfarction or rupture, pericardial effusion, pericarditis, venous thrombosis and embolism
EENT: Epistaxis, gingival bleeding, laryngeal edema
GI: GI bleeding, nausea, retroperitoneal bleeding, vomiting
GU: GU bleeding
RESP: Pleural effusion, pulmonary edema, pulmonary reembolization
SKIN: Bleeding at puncture sites, ecchymosis, rash, urticaria
Other: Anaphylaxis

Nursing Considerations
WARNING To avoid acute bleeding complications, treatment for acute ischemic stroke must begin within 3 hr after onset of stroke symptoms and only after computed tomography or other diagnostic imaging method excludes intracranial hemorrhage.
• Immediately before use, reconstitute alteplase with sterile water for injection only. Swirl gently to dissolve powder; don't shake.
• Monitor patient for bleeding, especially at arterial puncture sites.
• Monitor blood pressure and heart rate and rhythm frequently during and after therapy.
WARNING Alteplase therapy may cause arrhythmias from sudden reperfusion of the myocardium. Monitor continuous ECG for arrhythmias during drug therapy.
• Minimize bleeding from noncompressible sites by avoiding internal jugular and subclavian venous puncture sites.
• Discontinue alteplase immediately if serious bleeding occurs.
• After administering alteplase, apply pressure for at least 30 minutes, followed by a pressure dressing.
• Store reconstituted solution at room temperature (about 86° F [30° C]) or refrigerated (36° to 46° F [2.2° to 7.7° C]).
PATIENT TEACHING
• Tell patient to immediately report bleeding, including from the nose or gums.
• Advise patient to limit physical activity during alteplase administration to reduce risk of injury and bleeding.

aluminum carbonate
Basaljel

aluminum hydroxide
AlternaGEL, Alu-Cap, Alugel (CAN), Alu-Tab, Amphojel, Dialume

Class and Category
Chemical: Aluminum salt
Therapeutic: Antacid, phosphate binder
Pregnancy category: Not rated

Indications and Dosages
➤ *To treat hyperacidity associated with gastric hyperacidity, gastritis, hiatal hernia, peptic esophagitis, and peptic ulcers; to prevent phosphate renal calculus formation; to reduce hyperphosphatemia in chronic renal failure*
ALUMINUM CARBONATE CAPSULES, SUSPENSION, TABLETS
Adults. 2 capsules or tablets or 10 ml suspension every 2 hr up to 12 times daily, as needed.
ALUMINUM HYDROXIDE CAPSULES, SUSPENSION, TABLETS
Adults. 500 to 1,500 mg as capsules or tablets in divided doses 3 to 6 times daily, taken between meals and at bedtime; 5 to 30 ml as suspension, as needed, taken between meals and at bedtime.

Route	Onset	Peak	Duration
P.O.	Varies	Unknown	20–40 min*

Mechanism of Action
Neutralizes or reduces gastric acidity, increasing stomach and duodenal alkalinity. Protects stomach and duodenum lining by inhibiting pepsin's proteolytic activity. Binds with phosphate ions in intestine to form insoluble aluminum-phosphate compounds, which lower blood phosphate level.

---

* If fasting; at least 3 hr if given 1 hr after meals.

A

Contraindications
Hypersensitivity to aluminum

Interaction
DRUGS
allopurinol, chloroquine, corticosteroids, diflunisal, digoxin, ethambutol, H_2-receptor blockers, iron, isoniazid, penicillamine, phenothiazines, ranitidine, tetracyclines, thyroid hormones, ticlopidine: Decreased effects of these drugs
benzodiazepines: Increased benzodiazepine effects

Adverse Reactions
CNS: Encephalopathy
GI: Constipation, intestinal obstruction, white-speckled stool
MS: Osteomalacia, osteoporosis
Other: Aluminum accumulation in serum, bone, and CNS; aluminum intoxication; electrolyte imbalances

Nursing Considerations
• Don't give aluminum hydroxide within 1 to 2 hours of other oral drugs.
• Know that two 0.6-g aluminum hydroxide tablets can neutralize 16 mEq of acid.
• Monitor patient's serum levels of sodium, phosphate, and other electrolytes, as appropriate.
PATIENT TEACHING
• Instruct patient to chew tablets thoroughly before swallowing and then to drink a full glass of water.
• Warn patient not to take maximum dosage for more than 2 weeks unless prescribed because doing so may cause stomach to secrete excess hydrochloric acid.
• Teach patient to prevent constipation with a high-fiber diet and increased fluid intake (2 to 3 L daily), if appropriate.
• If patient takes other prescription drugs, advise him to notify prescriber about them before taking aluminum because of risk of interactions.
• Advise patient to notify prescriber if symptoms worsen or don't subside.

alvimopan
Entereg

Class and Category
Chemical class: Single stereoisomer
Therapeutic class: Mu opioid receptor antagonist
Pregnancy category: B

Indications and Dosages
➤ *To accelerate GI recovery in hospitalized patients after partial large- or small-bowel resection with primary anastomosis*
CAPSULES
Adults. *Initial:* 12 mg 30 min to 5 hr before surgery, followed by 12 mg twice daily, starting the day after surgery for up to 7 days or until discharge. *Maximum:* 24 mg/day with a maximum of 15 doses total.

Route	Onset	Peak	Duration
P.O.	Unknown	2 hr	Unknown

Mechanism of Action
Competitively binds to selective mu opioid receptors in GI tract, antagonizing peripheral effects of opioids on GI motility and secretion without reversing the central analgesic effects of opioid agonists. This action alleviates postoperative ileus by causing bowel function to return more quickly after part of bowel has been removed and an end-to-end anastomosis performed.

Contraindications
Complete gastrointestinal obstruction, hypersensitivity to alvimopan or its components, presence of gastric or pancreatic anastomosis, severe hepatic or renal impairment, use of opioids for more than 7 consecutive days immediately before alvimopan starts

Interaction
DRUGS
opioids given within previous 7 days at therapeutic doses: Increased sensitivity to alvimopan

Adverse Reactions
GI: Abdominal pain, constipation, diarrhea, dyspepsia, flatulence
GU: Urine retention
HEME: Anemia

MS: Back pain
Other: Hypokalemia

Nursing Considerations

• Don't give alvimopan to patients with severe hepatic or renal impairment or to patients having surgery to correct a complete bowel obstruction.
• Know that alvimopan is prescribed only for short-term use with maximum of 15 doses and is only dispensed in hospitals enrolled in Entereg Access Support and Education (E.A.S.E.) program. Closely monitor number of doses given, and expect to stop drug when patient has received 15 doses or is discharged from hospital, because there is a potential risk for patient to experience a myocardial infarction if drug is used beyond 15 doses.
• Monitor patient's serum potassium level closely, as ordered, because drug may cause hypokalemia. Also check patient's hemoglobin level and hematocrit because drug has been associated with anemia.
• Monitor patient with mild to moderate hepatic or renal failure for evidence of high alvimopan levels, such as abdominal pain or cramping, diarrhea, nausea, and vomiting. Also monitor patients recently exposed to opioids, as they may be more sensitive to the effects of alvimopan and experience greater gastrointestinal effects. If present, alert prescriber.
• Monitor Japanese patients closely for possible adverse effects because alvimopan level may be higher in this population.

PATIENT TEACHING
• Explain the need to accurately describe long-term or intermittent use of opioid pain therapy, including any use of opioids in the week before receiving alvimopan. Taking alvimopan after such use may cause serious adverse GI reactions.
• Inform patient that the most common adverse effects of alvimopan are constipation, dyspepsia, and flatulence.
• Tell patient that drug is for in-hospital use only and will not be taken at home.

amantadine hydrochloride
(adamantanamine hydrochloride)

Endantadine (CAN), Gen-Amantadine (CAN), Symmetrel

Class and Category

Chemical class: Adamantane derivative
Therapeutic class: Antidyskinetic, antiviral
Pregnancy category: C

Indications and Dosages

➤ *To manage symptoms of primary Parkinson's disease, postencephalitic parkinsonism, arteriosclerotic parkinsonism, and parkinsonism caused by CNS injury from carbon monoxide intoxication*

CAPSULES, SYRUP, TABLETS
Adults. *Initial:* 100 mg twice daily.
Maximum: 400 mg daily in divided doses.

➤ *To treat drug-induced extrapyramidal reactions*

CAPSULES, SYRUP, TABLETS
Adults. *Initial:* 100 mg twice daily.
Maximum: 300 mg daily in divided doses.

DOSAGE ADJUSTMENT For elderly patients, patients taking high doses of other antidyskinetics, and patients who have a serious medical condition (such as heart failure, epilepsy, or psychosis), initial dosage reduced to 100 mg daily, with gradual titration to 100 mg twice daily after 1 to several wk. For patients with impaired renal function, dosage adjusted to 200 mg on day 1 and then to 100 mg daily if creatinine clearance is 30 to 50 ml/min/1.73 m^2; to 200 mg on day 1 and then to 100 mg every other day if creatinine clearance is 15 to 29 ml/min/1.73 m^2; and to 200 mg every wk if creatinine clearance is less than 15 ml/min/1.73 m^2 or if patient is receiving hemodialysis.

➤ *To prevent and treat respiratory tract infection caused by influenza A*

CAPSULES, SYRUP, TABLETS
Adults and children age 12 and over.
Initial: 200 mg daily or 100 mg twice daily.
Maximum: 200 mg daily.

DOSAGE ADJUSTMENT In impaired renal function, if creatinine clearance is 30 to 50 ml/min/1.73 m², 200 mg on day 1 and then 100 mg daily. If clearance is 15 to 29 ml/min/1.73 m², 200 mg on day 1 and then 100 mg every other day. If clearance is less than 15 ml/min/1.73 m² or patient is having hemodialysis, 200 mg every wk. **Children ages 9 to 12.** 100 mg every 12 hr. *Maximum:* 200 mg daily. **Children ages 1 to 9.** 1.5 to 3 mg/kg every 8 hr or 2.2 to 4.4 mg/kg every 12 hr. *Maximum:* 150 mg/day.

Route	Onset	Peak	Duration
P.O.	In 48 hr*	Unknown	Unknown

Mechanism of Action

Affects dopamine, a neurotransmitter that is synthesized and released by neurons leading from substantia nigra to basal ganglia and is essential for normal motor function. In Parkinson's disease, progressive degeneration of these neurons reduces intrasynaptic dopamine. Amantadine may cause dopamine to accumulate in the basal ganglia by increasing dopamine release or by blocking dopamine reuptake into the presynaptic neurons of the CNS. Amantadine also may stimulate dopamine receptors or make postsynaptic receptors more sensitive to dopamine. These actions help control alterations in involuntary muscle movements, such as tremors and rigidity, that are associated with Parkinson's disease.

Amantadine may inhibit influenza A viral replication by blocking uncoating of virus and release of viral nucleic acid into respiratory epithelial cells. It also may interfere with early replication of viruses that have already penetrated cells.

Contraindications

Angle-closure glaucoma, hypersensitivity to amantadine or its components

Interaction

DRUGS
anticholinergics or other drugs with anticholinergic activity, other antidyskinetics, antihistamines, phenothiazines, tricyclic antidepressants:

* Antidyskinetic action; antiviral action unknown.

Possibly increased anticholinergic effects and risk of paralytic ileus
carbidopa-levodopa, levodopa: Increased effectiveness of these drugs
CNS stimulants: Excessive CNS stimulation, possibly causing arrhythmias, insomnia, irritability, nervousness, or seizures
hydrochlorothiazide, triamterene: Possibly decreased amantadine clearance and increased risk of toxicity
live-virus vaccines: Possibly interference with vaccine effectiveness
quinidine, quinine, trimethoprim-sulfamethoxazole: Increased blood amantadine level
ACTIVITIES
alcohol use: Possibly increased risk of CNS effects—including confusion, dizziness, and light-headedness—and orthostatic hypotension

Adverse Reactions

CNS: Agitation, anxiety, confusion, dizziness, drowsiness, fatigue, fever, hallucinations, insomnia, irritability, light-headedness, mental impairment, nervousness, neuroleptic malignant syndrome, nightmares, suicidal ideation, syncope
CV: Arrhythmias, cardiac arrest, orthostatic hypotension, peripheral edema, tachycardia
EENT: Blurred vision; dry mouth, nose, or throat; keratitis; mydriasis
GI: Constipation, diarrhea, dysphagia, nausea
GU: Dysuria, increased libido
HEME: Agranulocytosis, leukopenia, neutropenia
RESP: Acute respiratory failure, pulmonary edema, tachypnea
SKIN: Diaphoresis, livedo reticularis (purplish, netlike rash), pruritus
Other: Anaphylaxis; intense urges to perform certain activities, such as gambling or sexual acts

Nursing Considerations

• Be aware that prophylactic therapy with amantadine should begin as soon as possible after exposure to persons infected with influenza A virus and should continue for 10 days. During an influenza epidemic, expect drug to be given daily throughout the epidemic, which typically lasts 6 to 8 weeks. If patient has previously received inactivated influenza A vaccine, prescriber may discontinue it when sure that patient has developed active immunity against the virus. If patient receives inactivated influenza A vaccine at the same time amantadine therapy starts, expect amantadine to be given for 2 to 3 weeks.

• Expect amantadine therapy to start 24 to 48 hours after the onset of influenza A symptoms and to continue 48 hours after they resolve.

• Monitor patients who have a history of psychiatric illness or substance abuse because amantadine may worsen these conditions. Some patients taking amantadine have attempted suicide or had suicidal ideation.

• If patient has a history of heart failure or peripheral edema, monitor for weight gain and edema because drug may cause redistribution of body fluid.

• Amantadine may increase seizure activity in patients with a history of seizures.

WARNING Monitor patient for evidence of neuroleptic malignant syndrome during dosage reduction or discontinuation of therapy. These include fever, hypertension or hypotension, involuntary motor activity, mental changes, muscle rigidity, tachycardia, and tachypnea. Be prepared to provide supportive treatment and additional drug therapy, as prescribed.

• Be aware that patients receiving more than 200 mg daily are more likely to experience adverse or toxic reactions.

• Monitor patient for decreased drug effectiveness over time. If therapeutic response declines, expect to increase dosage or discontinue drug temporarily, as ordered.

• Assess patient regularly for skin changes because melanoma risk is higher in those with Parkinson's disease. It isn't clear whether the risk is increased by the disease or by its treatment.

PATIENT TEACHING
• Instruct patient to take amantadine exactly as prescribed and not to stop abruptly. Advise patient to notify prescriber if drug becomes less effective.

• Tell patient to notify prescriber if influenza symptoms don't improve after 2 to 3 days.

WARNING Advise patient or family member to notify prescriber immediately if patient reveals thoughts of suicide.

• Encourage patient to avoid consuming alcohol during amantadine therapy because alcohol may increase the risk of confusion, dizziness, light-headedness, or orthostatic hypotension.

• Advise patient to avoid driving and other activities that require a high level of alertness until he knows how the drug affects him because it may cause blurred vision and mental impairment.

• Advise patient to change positions slowly to minimize effects of orthostatic hypotension.

• Tell patient to use ice chips or sugarless candy or gum to relieve dry mouth.

• Caution patient to resume physical activities gradually as signs and symptoms improve.

• Urge patient to have regular skin examinations by a dermatologist or other qualified health professional.

• Instruct patient to notify prescriber about intense urges, such as for gambling or sex, because dosage may need to be reduced or drug discontinued.

amikacin sulfate
Amikin

Class and Category
Chemical class: Aminoglycoside
Therapeutic class: Antibiotic
Pregnancy category: D

Indications and Dosages
➤ *To treat serious gram-negative bacterial infections (including septicemia; neonatal sepsis; respiratory tract, bone, joint, CNS, skin, soft-tissue, intra-abdominal, burn, and postoperative infections; and serious, complicated, and recurrent UTI) caused by* Acinetobacter, Enterobacter, Escherichia coli, Klebsiella, Proteus, Providencia, Pseudomonas, *and* Serratia; *and staphylococcal infections when penicillin is contraindicated*

I.V. INFUSION, I.M. INJECTION
Adults and children. 15 mg/kg daily in equal doses at equally spaced intervals (7.5 mg/kg

every 12 hr or 5 mg/kg every 8 hr) for 7 to 10 days. *Maximum:* 1,500 mg daily.
DOSAGE ADJUSTMENT For patients with impaired renal function, loading dose of 7.5 mg/kg daily; then maintenance dosage based on creatinine clearance and serum creatinine level and given every 12 hr. For morbidly obese patients, dosage not to exceed 1.5 g daily.
Neonates. Loading dose: 10 mg/kg. *Maintenance:* 7.5 mg/kg every 12 hr for 7 to 10 days.
➤ *To treat uncomplicated UTI*
I.V. INFUSION, I.M. INJECTION
Adults. 250 mg three times daily for 7 to 10 days.

Route	Onset	Peak	Duration
I.V.	Immediate	Unknown	Unknown
I.M.	Rapid	Unknown	Unknown

Mechanism of Action
Binds to negatively charged sites on bacteria's outer cell membrane, disrupting cell integrity. Also binds to bacterial ribosomal subunits and inhibits protein synthesis. Both actions lead to cell death.

Incompatibilities
Don't mix or infuse amikacin with other drugs.

Contraindications
Hypersensitivity to amikacin or other aminoglycosides

Interaction
DRUGS
cephalosporins, enflurane, methoxyflurane, vancomycin: Increased nephrotoxic effects
general anesthetics: Increased risk of neuromuscular blockade
loop diuretics: Increased risk of ototoxicity
neuromuscular blockers: Possibly increased neuromuscular blockade and prolonged respiratory depression
penicillins: Possibly inactivation of or synergistic effects with amikacin

Adverse Reactions
CNS: Drowsiness, headache, loss of balance, neuromuscular blockade, tremor, vertigo
EENT: Hearing loss, ototoxicity, tinnitus
GI: Nausea, vomiting

GU: Azotemia, dysuria, nephrotoxicity, oliguria or polyuria, proteinuria
MS: Acute muscle paralysis; arthralgia; muscle fatigue, spasms, and weakness
RESP: Apnea
Other: Hyperkalemia

Nursing Considerations
• Expect to obtain results of culture and sensitivity testing before therapy begins.
• Prepare amikacin I.V. solution by adding contents of 500-mg vial to 100 to 200 ml of sterile diluent. Then infuse drug over 30 to 60 minutes.
• Give I.M. injection in large muscle mass.
• Watch for signs of ototoxicity, such as tinnitus and vertigo, especially during high-dosage or prolonged amikacin therapy.
WARNING Because amikacin may produce nephrotoxic effects, assess renal function before and daily during therapy, as ordered. To minimize renal tubule irritation, maintain hydration during therapy.
• Be aware that amikacin may exacerbate muscle weakness in such conditions as myasthenia gravis and Parkinson's disease.
• Measure serum amikacin concentrations as ordered, usually 30 to 90 minutes after injection (for peak concentration) and just before administering next dose (for trough concentration).
PATIENT TEACHING
• Tell patient that daily laboratory tests are necessary during treatment.
• Instruct patient to report ringing in ears, hearing changes, headache, nausea, vomiting, and changes in urination.

amiloride hydrochloride
Midamor

Class and Category
Chemical class: Pyrazine-carbonyl-guanidine
Therapeutic class: Potassium-sparing diuretic
Pregnancy category: B

Indications and Dosages
➤ *As adjunct to thiazide or loop diuretic in patient with heart failure or hypertension*

to correct diuretic-induced hypokalemia or to prevent diuretic-induced hypokalemia that increases the risk of arrhythmias or other complications

TABLETS

Adults. 5 to 10 mg daily as single dose; if hypokalemia persists, increased to 15 mg daily and then 20 mg daily.

Route	Onset	Peak	Duration
P.O.	2 hr	6–10 hr	24 hr

Mechanism of Action
Inhibits sodium reabsorption in distal convoluted tubules and cortical collecting ducts, causing sodium and water loss and enhancing potassium retention.

Contraindications
Hypersensitivity to amiloride; impaired renal function; serum potassium level above 5.5 mEq/L; therapy with another potassium-sparing diuretic, such as spironolactone or triamterene, or a potassium supplement

Interaction
DRUGS

angiotensin II receptor antagonists, captopril, enalapril, lisinopril, potassium products, spironolactone: Increased risk of hyperkalemia
digoxin: Decreased effectiveness of digoxin
lithium: Reduced renal clearance of lithium and increased risk of lithium toxicity
NSAIDs: Reduced diuretic effect of amiloride
sympathomimetics: Possibly reduced antihypertensive effects of amiloride

FOODS

high-potassium food: Increased risk of hyperkalemia

Adverse Reactions
CNS: Confusion, depression, dizziness, drowsiness, encephalopathy, fatigue, headache, insomnia, nervousness, paresthesia, somnolence, tremor, vertigo
CV: Angina, arrhythmias, orthostatic hypotension, palpitations
EENT: Dry mouth, increased intraocular pressure, nasal congestion, tinnitus, vision disturbances
GI: Abdominal pain or fullness, anorexia, appetite changes, constipation, diarrhea, GI bleeding, heartburn, indigestion, nausea, thirst, vomiting
GU: Bladder spasms, dysuria, impotence, loss of libido, polyuria
HEME: Aplastic anemia, neutropenia
MS: Arthralgia, muscle spasms or weakness
RESP: Cough, dyspnea
SKIN: Alopecia, jaundice, pruritus, rash
Other: Dehydration, hyperchloremia, hyperkalemia, hypernatremia, metabolic acidosis

Nursing Considerations
- Administer amiloride with food to reduce GI upset and early in the day to minimize sleep interference from polyuria.
- Monitor renal function test results, fluid intake and output, and weight. Also monitor serum potassium level to detect hyperkalemia.

WARNING Don't administer amiloride with other potassium-sparing diuretics.

PATIENT TEACHING

- Warn patient to avoid high-potassium food and salt substitutes that contain potassium.
- Advise patient to consult prescriber before taking other drugs, including OTC remedies, especially sympathomimetics.
- Tell patient to report dizziness, trembling, numbness, and muscle weakness or spasms.
- Advise patient to increase fluid and fiber intake to prevent constipation.
- Warn patient to expect reversible hair loss and impotence.

aminocaproic acid
Amicar

Class and Category
Chemical class: Aminohexanoic acid
Therapeutic class: Antifibrinolytic, antihemorrhagic
Pregnancy category: C

Indications and Dosages
➤ *To treat excessive bleeding caused by fibrinolysis*

SYRUP, TABLETS

Adults. *Initial:* 5 g in first hour, followed by 1 to 1.25 g/hr to sustain drug plasma level of 0.13 mg/ml. *Maximum:* 30 g daily.

I.V. INJECTION
Adults. 4 to 5 g in 250 ml of diluent over 1 hr followed by continuous infusion of 1 g/hr in 50 ml of diluent. Continue for 8 hr or until bleeding stops.

Route	Onset	Peak	Duration
P.O.	Rapid	Unknown	Unknown
I.V.	Immediate	Unknown	Under 3 hr

Mechanism of Action
Inhibits breakdown of blood clots by interfering with plasminogen activator substances and producing antiplasmin activity.

Contraindications
Hypersensitivity to aminocaproic acid; signs of active intravascular clotting, as in disseminated intravascular coagulation; upper urinary tract bleeding

Interaction
DRUGS
activated prothrombin, prothrombin complex concentrates: Increased risk of thrombosis
estrogens, oral contraceptives: Increased risk of hypercoagulation

Adverse Reactions
CNS: Delirium, dizziness, hallucinations, headache, malaise, stroke, weakness
CV: Bradycardia, cardiomyopathy, elevated serum CK level, hypotension, ischemia, thrombophlebitis
EENT: Nasal congestion, tinnitus
GI: Abdominal cramps and pain, diarrhea, elevated AST level, nausea, vomiting
GU: Elevated BUN level, intrarenal obstruction, renal failure
HEME: Agranulocytosis, leukopenia, thrombocytopenia
MS: Myopathy
RESP: Dyspnea, pulmonary embolism
SKIN: Pruritus, rash
Other: Elevated serum aldolase and potassium levels

Nursing Considerations
• Be aware that patients on oral therapy may need up to 10 tablets during the first hour of treatment and tablets around the clock during continued treatment.

• Mix aminocaproic acid solution with sterile water for injection, normal saline solution, D_5W, or Ringer's solution.
WARNING Avoid rapid I.V. delivery because it increases risk of hypotension and bradycardia.
• Monitor neurologic status for drug-induced changes. Note that increased clotting may lead to stroke.
PATIENT TEACHING
• Tell patient that he'll be closely monitored during I.V. therapy and will have blood drawn for laboratory tests before, during, and after treatment.
• Advise patient who takes aminocaproic acid at home to report adverse reactions, take drug exactly as prescribed, and keep follow-up appointments with prescriber.

aminoglutethimide
Cytadren

Class and Category
Chemical class: Hormone
Therapeutic class: Adrenal steroid inhibitor
Pregnancy category: D

Indications and Dosages
➤ *To suppress adrenal function in patients with Cushing's syndrome who are waiting for surgery or for whom other treatment can't be used*
TABLETS
Adults. *Initial:* 250 mg every 6 hr. Increased as needed by 250 mg daily every 1 to 2 wk. *Maximum:* 2,000 mg daily.

Route	Onset	Peak	Duration
P.O.	3–5 days	Unknown	72 hr

Mechanism of Action
Inhibits the conversion of cholesterol to delta-5-pregnenolone, which is needed to produce certain hormones, including adrenal glucocorticoids, mineralocorticoids, estrogens, and androgens.

Contraindications
Hypersensitivity to aminoglutethimide or glutethimide

Interaction
DRUGS
antidiabetics, dexamethasone, digoxin, medroxyprogesterone, synthetic glucocorticoids, theophylline, warfarin and other oral anticoagulants: Decreased effects of these drugs

Adverse Reactions
CNS: Dizziness, drowsiness, fever, headache
CV: Hypotension, orthostatic hypotension, tachycardia
ENDO: Adrenal insufficiency, hypothyroidism, masculinization
GI: Anorexia, nausea
SKIN: Hair growth, morbilliform rash, pruritus, urticaria

Nursing Considerations
• Expect to reduce aminoglutethimide dosage or discontinue treatment if extreme drowsiness, severe rash, or excessively low cortisol level occurs.
WARNING Monitor for signs of hypothyroidism, including lethargy, dry skin, and slow pulse. If prescribed, administer thyroid hormone supplement.
• Monitor blood pressure for orthostatic or persistent hypotension.
PATIENT TEACHING
• Teach patient to recognize orthostatic hypotension (dizziness, weakness when moving from sitting to standing position) and to minimize it (as by rising slowly from a supine to an upright position).
• Tell patient to report dizziness, appetite loss, nausea, headache, or severe drowsiness. Warn him to avoid driving if drowsy.
• Instruct patient to take a missed dose as soon as remembered and to space out the day's remaining doses evenly.
• Advise patient that rash, sometimes accompanied by fever, may appear on day 10 of treatment and should subside by day 15 or 16. Tell him to report severe rash or one that doesn't disappear.

aminophylline
(theophylline ethylenediamine)
Phyllocontin, Truphylline

Class and Category
Chemical class: Xanthine
Therapeutic class: Bronchodilator
Pregnancy category: C

Indications and Dosages
➤ *To relieve acute bronchospasm*
I.V. INFUSION
Adults and children not currently receiving theophylline products. *Initial:* 6 mg/kg (equal to 4.7 mg/kg anhydrous theophylline), not to exceed 25 mg/min. *Maintenance:* For adults (nonsmokers), 0.7 mg/kg/hr for first 12 hr, then 0.5 mg/kg/hr. For children ages 9 to 16, 1 mg/kg/hr for first 12 hr, then 0.8 mg/kg/hr. For children ages 6 months to 9 years and young adult smokers, 1.2 mg/kg/hr for first 12 hr, then 1 mg/kg/hr.
Adults and children currently receiving theophylline products. *Initial:* If possible, determine the time, amount, administration route, and form of last dose. Loading dose is based on the principle that each 0.63 mg/kg (0.5 mg/kg anhydrous theophylline) given raises serum theophylline level by 1 mcg/ml. Defer loading dose if serum theophylline level can be readily obtained. If this isn't possible and patient has no obvious signs of theophylline toxicity, prescriber may order 3.1 mg/kg (2.5 mg/kg anhydrous theophylline), which may increase serum theophylline level by about 5 mcg/ml. *Maintenance:* For adults (nonsmokers), 0.7 mg/kg/hr for first 12 hr, then 0.5 mg/kg/hr. For children ages 9 to 16, 1 mg/kg/hr for first 12 hr, then 0.8 mg/kg/hr. For children ages 6 months to 9 years and young adult smokers, 1.2 mg/kg/hr for first 12 hr, then 1 mg/kg/hr.
DOSAGE ADJUSTMENT For elderly patients and those with cor pulmonale, dosage reduced to 0.6 mg/kg for 12 hr, then 0.3 mg/kg. For patients with heart failure and hepatic disease, dosage reduced to 0.5 mg/kg for 12 hr, then 0.1 to 0.2 mg/kg.
➤ *To prevent or treat reversible bronchospasm from asthma, chronic bronchitis, and emphysema and to maintain patent airways*
E.R. TABLETS, ORAL LIQUID, TABLETS, SUPPOSITORIES
Adults and children. *Initial (rapidly absorbed forms):* 16 mg/kg daily or 400 mg daily (whichever is less) in divided doses

every 6 to 8 hr. *Maintenance:* Daily dosage increased in increments of 25% every 3 days, as tolerated, until response achieved or maximum dose reached. When maximum dose is reached, dosage adjusted according to peak serum theophylline level. *Initial (E.R. forms):* 12 mg/kg daily or 400 mg daily (whichever is less) in divided doses every 8 to 12 hr. *Maintenance:* Daily dosage increased in increments of 2 to 3 mg/kg every 3 days. When maximum dose is reached, dosage adjusted according to peak serum theophylline level.

Route	Onset	Peak	Duration
P.O. (E.R.)	Unknown	Unknown	8–12 hr
P.O. (tab)	Unknown	Unknown	6–8 hr
I.V.	Immediate	Unknown	4–8 hr

Mechanism of Action

Inhibits phosphodiesterase enzymes, causing bronchodilation. Normally, these enzymes inactivate cyclic adenosine monophosphate (cAMP) and cyclic guanosine monophosphate (cGMP), which are responsible for bronchial smooth-muscle relaxation. Other mechanisms of action may include translocation of calcium, prostaglandin antagonism, stimulation of catecholamines, inhibition of cGMP metabolism, and adenosine receptor antagonism.

Incompatibilities

Don't add other drugs to prepared bag or bottle of aminophylline. Don't mix aminophylline in same syringe with doxapram. Also avoid administering amiodarone, ciprofloxacin, diltiazem, dobutamine, hydralazine, or ondansetron into the Y-port of a continuous infusion of aminophylline.

Contraindications

Active peptic ulcer disease, hypersensitivity to aminophylline, rectal or lower intestine irritation or infection (suppository form), underlying seizure disorder

Interaction

DRUGS

activated charcoal, aminoglutethimide, barbiturates, ketoconazole, rifampin, sulfinpyrazone, sympathomimetics: Decreased serum theophylline level

allopurinol, calcium channel blockers, cimetidine, corticosteroids, disulfiram, ephedrine, influenza virus vaccine, interferon, macrolides, mexiletine, nonselective beta blockers, oral contraceptives, quinolones, thiabendazole: Increased serum theophylline level
benzodiazepines: Antagonized sedative effects of benzodiazepines
beta agonists: Increased effects of aminophylline and beta agonist
carbamazepine, isoniazid, loop diuretics: Altered serum theophylline level
halothane: Increased risk of cardiotoxicity
hydantoins: Decreased hydantoin level
ketamine: Increased risk of seizures
lithium: Decreased serum lithium level
nondepolarizing muscle relaxants: Reversed neuromuscular blockade
propofol: Antagonized sedative effects of propofol
tetracyclines: Enhanced adverse effects of theophylline

FOODS

all foods: Altered bioavailability and absorption of E.R. form, leading to toxicity
high-carbohydrate, low-protein diet: Decreased theophylline elimination and prolonged aminophylline half-life
low-carbohydrate, high-protein diet; charbroiled beef: Increased theophylline elimination and shortened aminophylline half-life

ACTIVITIES

alcohol abuse: Increased aminophylline effects
smoking (1 or more packs daily): Decreased effects of aminophylline

Adverse Reactions

CNS: Dizziness, fever, headache, insomnia, irritability, restlessness, seizures
CV: Arrhythmias (including sinus tachycardia and life-threatening ventricular arrhythmias), hypotension, palpitations
EENT: Bitter aftertaste
ENDO: Hyperglycemia, syndrome of inappropriate ADH secretion
GI: Anorexia, diarrhea, epigastric pain, heavy feeling in stomach, hematemesis, indigestion, nausea, rectal bleeding or irritation (suppositories), vomiting
GU: Diuresis, proteinuria, urine retention in men with prostate enlargement
MS: Muscle twitching

RESP: Respiratory arrest, tachypnea
SKIN: Alopecia, exfoliative dermatitis, flushing, rash, urticaria

Nursing Considerations

WARNING Because aminophylline has a narrow therapeutic window (10 to 20 mcg/ml), closely monitor serum theophylline level and watch for evidence of toxicity (tachycardia, tachypnea, nausea, vomiting, restlessness, seizures). Keep in mind that acetaminophen, furosemide, phenyl-butazone, probenecid, theobromine, coffee, tea, soft drinks, and chocolate can alter serum theophylline result.

• To determine peak serum theophylline level, draw blood sample 15 to 30 minutes after administering I.V. loading dose.
• Give immediate-release and liquid forms with food to reduce GI upset. Give E.R. form 1 hour before or 2 hours after meals because food can alter drug absorption.

PATIENT TEACHING

• Advise patient to avoid excessive caffeine (in coffee, tea, soft drinks, and chocolate); it can falsely elevate theophylline level.
• Explain that blood tests may be needed to monitor drug's therapeutic effect.

aminosalicylate sodium

(para-aminosalicylate, PAS)

Nemasol Sodium (CAN), PAS

Class and Category

Chemical class: Para-aminobenzoic acid analogue
Therapeutic class: Antitubercular
Pregnancy category: C

Indications and Dosages

➤ *To treat tuberculosis as adjunct to isoniazid, streptomycin, or both and in patients with multidrug-resistant tuberculosis or when therapy with rifampin and isoniazid isn't possible because of resistance or intolerance*

TABLETS

Adults. 14 to 16 g daily in 2 or 3 divided doses.

Children. 275 to 420 mg/kg daily in 3 or 4 divided doses.

Mechanism of Action

Inhibits incorporation of para-aminobenzoic acid into folic acid and prevents synthesis of folic acid, a compound needed for bacterial growth. Aminosalicylate sodium is bacteriostatic against *Mycobacterium tuberculosis,* and it delays bacterial resistance to streptomycin and isoniazid.

Contraindications

Hypersensitivity to aminosalicylate sodium, severe renal disease

Interaction

DRUGS

digoxin: Decreased serum digoxin level
probenecid: Increased serum aminosalicylate level
rifampin: Decreased serum rifampin level

Adverse Reactions

CNS: Encephalopathy, fever
CV: Vasculitis
ENDO: Goiter with or without myxedema
GI: Abdominal pain, diarrhea, hepatitis, nausea, vomiting
HEME: Agranulocytosis, hemolytic anemia, leukopenia, thrombocytopenia
SKIN: Jaundice, various types of eruptions
Other: Infectious mononucleosis-like syndrome, Loeffler's syndrome (anorexia, breathlessness, fever, and weight loss)

Nursing Considerations

• Administer aminosalicylate with food to reduce GI upset.
WARNING Protect drug from water, heat, and sunlight to prevent rapid deterioration. Don't give tablets with brown or purple discoloration—a sign of deterioration.

PATIENT TEACHING

• Teach patient to discard aminosalicylate that appears brown or purple.
• Instruct patient to take drug with food.

amiodarone hydrochloride

Cordarone, Nexterone, Pacerone

Class and Category

Chemical class: Iodinated benzofuran derivative
Therapeutic class: Class III antiarrhythmic
Pregnancy category: D

Indications and Dosages

➤ *To treat life-threatening, recurrent ventricular fibrillation and hemodynamically unstable ventricular tachycardia when these arrhythmias don't respond to other drugs or when patient can't tolerate other drugs*

TABLETS

Adults. *Loading:* 800 to 1,600 mg daily in divided doses for 1 to 3 wk. *Maintenance:* 600 to 800 mg daily in divided doses for 1 mo; then if cardiac rhythm is stable, 400 mg daily in 1 or 2 doses. Use lowest possible dose.

I.V. INFUSION

Adults. *Loading:* 150 mg over 10 min (15 mg/min) followed by 360 mg infused over 6 hr (1 mg/min). *Maintenance:* 540 mg infused over 18 hr (0.5 mg/min); then after the first 24 hr, 720 mg infused over 24 hr (0.5 mg/min), continued up to 2 to 3 wk, as needed. Rate may be increased in first 24 hr, if needed, but initial infusion rate shouldn't exceed 30 mg/min. Change to oral form as soon as possible.

➤ *To treat life-threatening, recurrent ventricular fibrillation and hemodynamically unstable ventricular tachycardia when these arrhythmias don't respond to other drugs, when patient can't tolerate other drugs, or when oral amiodarone is indicated but patient is unable to take oral medication*

I.V. INFUSION (NEXTERONE)

Adults. *Loading:* 150 mg/100 ml premixed in dextrose over 10 min (15 mg/min) followed by 360 mg/200 ml premixed in dextrose infused over 6 hr (1 mg/min). *Maintenance:* 540 mg infused over 18 hr (0.5 mg/min) using 360 mg/200 ml premixed in dextrose; then after the first 24 hr, 720 mg infused over 24 hr (0.5 mg/min) using 360 mg/200 ml premixed in dextrose, continued up to 2 to 3 wk, as needed. Rate may be increased in first 24 hr, if needed, but initial infusion rate shouldn't exceed 30 mg/min. Change to oral form as soon as possible.

➤ *To treat breakthrough episodes of ventricular fibrillation or hemodynamically unstable ventricular tachycardia*

I.V. INFUSION (NEXTERONE)

Adults. 150 mg/100 ml premixed in dextrose and infused over 10 min (15 mg/min).

Route	Onset	Peak	Duration
P.O.	2 days– 3 wk	1–5 mo	Weeks– months
I.V.	Hours– 3 days	1–3 wk	Weeks– months

Mechanism of Action

Acts on cardiac cell membranes, prolonging repolarization and the refractory period and raising ventricular fibrillation threshold. Drug relaxes vascular smooth muscles, mainly in coronary circulation, and improves myocardial blood flow. It relaxes peripheral vascular smooth muscles, decreasing peripheral vascular resistance and myocardial oxygen consumption.

Incompatibilities

Amiodarone is incompatible with heparin. To prevent precipitation, don't add amiodarone admixed with D_5W to aminophylline 4 mg/ml, cefamandole nafate, cefazolin sodium, or mezlocillin sodium, and don't mix amiodarone 3 mg/ml with sodium bicarbonate. Also, don't use evacuated glass containers for admixing because precipitation may occur.

Contraindications

Bradycardia that causes syncope (unless pacemaker present), cardiogenic shock, hypersensitivity to amiodarone or its components, hypokalemia, hypomagnesemia, SA node dysfunction, second- and third-degree AV block (unless pacemaker present)

Interaction

DRUGS

anticoagulants: Increased anticoagulant response and possibly serious bleeding
azole antifungals, fluoroquinolones, macrolide antibiotics: Increased risk of prolonged QT interval and life-threatening arrhythmias

beta blockers: Increased serum levels of beta blockers with increased risk of AV block, hypotension, and bradycardia

calcium channel blockers: Increased serum levels of these drugs and increased risk of AV block, bradycardia, and hypotension

cholestyramine, phenytoin, rifampin, St. John's wort: Decreased amiodarone level

cimetidine: Increased amiodarone level

clopidogrel: Increased risk of ineffective inhibition of platelet aggregation

cyclosporine: Increased cyclosporine level

dextromethorphan, methotrexate, phenytoin: Increased serum levels of these drugs and increased risk of toxicity if amiodarone is taken orally for more than 2 weeks

digoxin: Increased serum digoxin level and risk of digitalis toxicity

diltiazem, propranolol, verapamil: Increased risk of hemodynamic and electrophysiologic abnormalities

disopyramide: Increased serum disopyramide level with QT prolongation and increased risk of arrhythmias

fentanyl: Increased serum fentanyl level with increased risk of bradycardia, decreased cardiac output, and hypotension

flecainide: Increased serum flecainide level

HMG-CoA reductase inhibitors such as atorvastatin and simvastatin: Increased risk of myopathy and rhabdomyolysis

hydantoins: Increased serum hydantoin level with long-term use and reduced serum amiodarone level

lidocaine: Increased serum lidocaine level and risk of seizures and bradycardia

loratadine, trazodone: Increased risk of QT-interval prolongation and torsades de pointes

potassium- and magnesium-depleting drugs: Increased risk of hypokalemia and hypomagnesemia

procainamide: Increased serum procainamide or N-acetylprocainamide level

quinidine: Increased serum quinidine level with risk of life-threatening arrhythmias

ritonavir: Increased serum amiodarone level with increased risk of cardiotoxicity

theophylline: Increased serum theophylline level; increased risk of theophylline toxicity

warfarin: Increased PT and risk of bleeding

FOODS

grapefruit juice: Increased amiodarone level

Adverse Reactions

CNS: Abnormal gait, ataxia, confusion, delirium, demyelinating polyneuropathy, disorientation, dizziness, fatigue, fever, hallucinations, headache, insomnia, involuntary motor activity, lack of coordination, malaise, paresthesia, parkinsonian symptoms, peripheral neuropathy, pseudotumor cerebri, sleep disturbances, tremor

CV: Arrhythmias (including bradycardia, electromechanical dissociation, torsades de pointes, and ventricular tachycardia or fibrillation), cardiac arrest, cardiogenic shock, edema, heart failure, hypotension, vasculitis

EENT: Abnormal salivation, abnormal taste and smell, blurred vision, corneal microdeposits, dry eyes or mouth, halo vision, lens opacities, macular degeneration, optic neuritis, optic neuropathy, papilledema, permanent blindness, photophobia, scotoma

ENDO: Hyperthyroidism, hypothyroidism, syndrome of inappropriate ADH secretion, thyroid nodules or cancer

GI: Abdominal pain, anorexia, cirrhosis, constipation, diarrhea, elevated liver function test results, hepatitis, nausea, pancreatitis, vomiting

GU: Acute renal failure, decreased libido, epididymitis, impotence

HEME: Agranulocytosis, aplastic or hemolytic anemia, coagulation abnormalities, neutropenia, pancytopenia, spontaneous bruising, thrombocytopenia

MS: Muscle weakness, myopathy, rhabdomyolysis

RESP: Acute respiratory distress syndrome; bronchiolitis obliterans organizing pneumonia; bronchospasm; eosinophilic pneumonia; infiltrates that lead to dyspnea, cough, hemoptysis, hypoxia, pulmonary fibrosis, pulmonary alveolar hemorrhage, pulmonary interstitial pneumonitis, crackles, and wheezing; pleural effusion; pleuritis; pneumonia; respiratory arrest or failure

SKIN: Alopecia, bluish gray pigmentation, bullous dermatitis, eczema, erythema multiforme, exfoliative dermatitis, flushing, photosensitivity, pruritus, rash with eosinophilia and systemic symptoms (DRESS), skin cancer, solar dermatitis, Stevens-Johnson syndrome, toxic epidermal necrolysis, urticaria

Other: Anaphylaxis including shock, angioedema

Nursing Considerations

- If patient has an implantable cardiac device, have it checked, as ordered, at the start of and during amiodarone therapy because drug may affect pacing or defibrillating thresholds.
- Parenteral amiodarone may be diluted in D_5W or normal saline solution and given in polyvinyl chloride (PVC), polyolefin, or glass containers except for Nexterone, which is already premixed.
- Use an in-line filter during I.V. administration of amiodarone. Also use a central venous catheter whenever possible. A central venous catheter is required when infusion rate exceeds 2 mg/ml because drug may cause peripheral vein phlebitis at higher rates. Amiodarone I.V. must be given by volumetric infusion pump.
- Monitor amiodarone I.V. infusion closely because loading doses at higher concentrations and rates may cause hepatocellular necrosis, acute renal failure, and death.
- Although maintenance therapy is usually only needed for up to 96 hours, infusion of up to 0.5 mg/minute may be continued for 2 to 3 weeks, regardless of patient's age, renal function, or left ventricular function.

WARNING Amiodarone may cause or worsen pulmonary disorders that may develop days to weeks after therapy and progress to respiratory failure or even death. Expect to obtain chest x-ray and pulmonary function tests before therapy starts and then chest x-ray and follow-up exams every 3 to 6 months during therapy.

- Monitor vital signs and oxygen level often during and after giving amiodarone. Keep emergency equipment and drugs nearby.

WARNING Monitor continuous ECG; check for increased PR and QRS intervals, arrhythmias, and heart rate below 60 beats/min because amiodarone toxicity may cause or worsen arrhythmias.

- Monitor serum amiodarone level, which normally ranges from 1.0 to 2.5 mcg/ml.
- Assess liver enzyme and thyroid hormone levels; drug inhibits conversion of T_4 to T_3 and may cause drug-induced hyperthyroidism, thyrotoxicosis, and new or worsened arrhythmias. If new signs of arrhythmia occur, notify prescriber at once.

PATIENT TEACHING

- Explain that patient will need frequent monitoring and laboratory tests during treatment.
- Advise patient to report swollen hands and feet, wheezing, dyspnea, cough, nausea, vomiting, dark urine, fatigue, yellow skin or sclerae, stomach pain, light-headedness, fainting, or a rapid, slow, pounding, or irregular heartbeat.
- Instruct patient to report abnormal bleeding or bruising.
- Advise patient to avoid corneal refractive laser surgery while taking drug.

amitriptyline hydrochloride

Apo-amitriptyline (CAN), Endep, Levate (CAN), Novotriptyn (CAN)

Class and Category

Chemical class: Tertiary amine
Therapeutic class: Tricyclic antidepressant
Pregnancy category: D

Mechanism of Action

Normally, when an impulse reaches adrenergic nerves, the nerves release serotonin and norepinephrine from their storage sites. Some serotonin and norepinephrine reaches receptor sites on target tissues. Most is taken back into the nerves and stored by the reuptake mechanism, as shown below on the left.

Amitriptyline blocks serotonin and norepinephrine reuptake by adrenergic nerves. By doing so, it raises serotonin and norepinephrine levels at nerve synapses. This action may elevate mood and reduce depression.

Indications and Dosages

➤ *To relieve depression, especially when accompanied by anxiety and insomnia*

TABLETS

Adults and children over age 12. *Outpatient:* 75 mg daily in divided doses, increased to 150 mg daily, if needed. *In-patient:* 100 mg daily, gradually increased to 300 mg daily, if needed. *Maintenance:* 40 to 100 mg daily at bedtime.

DOSAGE ADJUSTMENT Maintenance dosage reduced to 10 mg three times day plus 20 mg at bedtime for adolescent and elderly patients.

Route	Onset	Peak	Duration
P.O.	14–21 days	Unknown	Unknown

Contraindications

Acute recovery phase after MI, hypersensitivity to amitriptyline, MAO inhibitor therapy within 14 days

Interaction

DRUGS

anticholinergics, epinephrine, norepinephrine: Increased effects of these drugs
barbiturates: Decreased amitriptyline level
carbamazepine: Decreased serum amitriptyline level and increased serum carbamazepine level, which increases therapeutic and toxic effects of carbamazepine
cimetidine, disulfiram, fluoxetine, fluvoxamine, haloperidol, H$_2$-receptor antagonists, methylphenidate, oral contraceptives, paroxetine, phenothiazines, sertraline: Increased serum amitriptyline level
cisapride: Possibly prolonged QT interval and increased risk of arrhythmias

clonidine, guanethidine, and other antihypertensives: Decreased antihypertensive effects
dicumarol: Increased anticoagulant effect
levodopa: Decreased levodopa absorption; sympathetic hyperactivity, sinus tachycardia, hypertension, agitation
MAO inhibitors: Possibly seizures and death
thyroid replacement drugs: Arrhythmias and increased antidepressant effects

ACTIVITIES

alcohol use: Enhanced CNS depression
smoking: Decreased amitriptyline effects

Adverse Reactions

CNS: Anxiety, ataxia, coma, chills, delusions, disorientation, drowsiness, extrapyramidal reactions, fatigue, fever, headache, insomnia, nightmares, peripheral neuropathy, suicidal ideation, tremor
CV: Arrhythmias (including prolonged AV conduction, heart block, and tachycardia), cardiomyopathy, hypertension, MI, nonspecific ECG changes, orthostatic hypotension, palpitations
EENT: Abnormal taste, black tongue, blurred vision, dry mouth, increased salivation, nasal congestion, tinnitus

Mechanism of Action

Normally, when an impulse reaches adrenergic nerves, the nerves release serotonin and norepinephrine from their storage sites. Some serotonin and norepinephrinereach receptor sites on target tissues. Most of this is taken back into the nerves and stored by the reuptake mechanism, as shown below on the left.

Amitriptyline blocks serotonin and norepinephrine reuptake by adrenergic nerves. By doing so, it raises serotonin and norepinephrine levels at nerve synapses. This action may elevate mood and reduce depression.

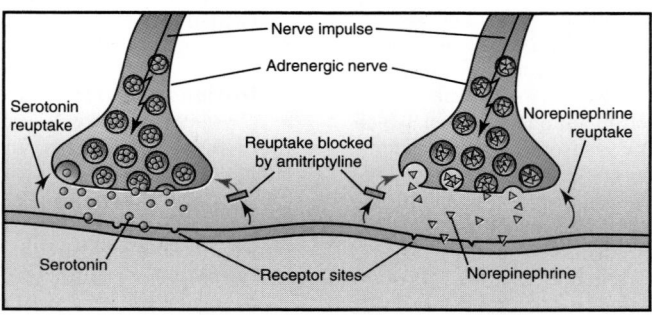

ENDO: Gynecomastia, increased or decreased blood glucose level, increased prolactin level, syndrome of inappropriate ADH secretion
GI: Abdominal cramps, constipation, diarrhea, flatulence, ileus, increased appetite, nausea, vomiting
GU: Impotence, libido changes, menstrual irregularities, testicular swelling, urinary hesitancy, urine retention
HEME: Agranulocytosis, bone marrow depression, eosinophilia, leukopenia, thrombocytopenia
SKIN: Alopecia, flushing, purpura
Other: Weight gain

Nursing Considerations

• Because of amitriptyline's atropine-like effects, use caution if patient has a history of seizures, urine retention, or angle-closure glaucoma.
WARNING Don't give an MAO inhibitor within 14 days of amitriptyline because of the risk of seizures and death.
• Closely monitor patient with CV disorder because amitriptyline may cause arrhythmias, such as sinus tachycardia.
• Watch patients closely (especially children, adolescents, and young adults), for suicidal tendencies, particularly when therapy starts and dosage changes. Depression may worsen temporarily during these times.
• Monitor blood pressure for hypotension or hypertension.
• Stay alert for behavior changes, such as hallucinations and decreased interest in personal appearance. Be aware that psychosis may develop in schizophrenic patients, and symptoms may increase in paranoid patients.
• Abrupt withdrawal after long use may cause nausea, headache, vertigo, and nightmares.
PATIENT TEACHING
• Instruct patient to take amitriptyline at bedtime to avoid daytime drowsiness.
• Instruct patient to avoid using alcohol or OTC drugs that contain alcohol during amitriptyline therapy because alcohol enhances CNS depressant effects.
• Urge family or caregiver to watch patient closely for suicidal tendencies, especially when therapy starts or dosage changes and particularly if patient is a child, teenager, or young adult.

amlodipine besylate   A
Norvasc

Class and Category

Chemical class: Dihydropyridine
Therapeutic class: Antianginal, antihypertensive
Pregnancy category: C

Indications and Dosages

➤ *To control hypertension*
TABLETS
Adults. *Initial:* 5 mg daily, increased gradually over 10 to 14 days, as needed. *Maximum:* 10 mg daily.
Children age 6 to 17 years. 2.5 mg to 5 mg once daily. Maximum: 5 mg once daily.
DOSAGE ADJUSTMENT Initially 2.5 mg daily for elderly patients or patients with impaired hepatic function. Increased gradually over 7 to 14 days based on response.
➤ *To treat chronic stable angina and Prinzmetal's (variant) angina*
TABLETS
Adults. 5 to 10 mg daily.
DOSAGE ADJUSTMENT 2.5 to 5 mg daily for elderly patients and those with impaired hepatic function.

Route	Onset	Peak	Duration
P.O.	Unknown	6–12 hr	24 hr

Mechanism of Action

Binds to dihydropyridine and nondihydropyridine cell membrane receptor sites on myocardial and vascular smooth-muscle cells and inhibits influx of extracellular calcium ions across slow calcium channels. This decreases intracellular calcium level, inhibiting smooth-muscle cell contractions and relaxing coronary and vascular smooth muscles, decreasing peripheral vascular resistance, and reducing systolic and diastolic blood pressure. Decreased peripheral vascular resistance also decreases myocardial workload, oxygen demand, and possibly angina. Also, by inhibiting coronary artery muscle cell contractions and restoring blood flow, drug may relieve Prinzmetal's angina.

Contraindications

Aliskiren therapy in patients with diabetes or renal impairment (GRF less than 60 ml/min), hypersensitivity to amlodipine or its components

Interaction

DRUGS

ACE inhibitors, aliskiren (in patients with diabetes or renal impairment): Increased risk of hyperkalemia, hypotension, and renal dysfunction
beta blockers: Possibly excessive hypotension
cyclosporine: Possibly increased blood cyclosporine levels
CYP3A4 inhibitors such as diltiazem, ketoconazole, itraconazole, and ritonavir: Possible increased blood amlodipine level
fentanyl: Increased risk of severe hypotension and increased fluid volume requirements during surgery
simvastatin: Increased exposure to simvastatin

Adverse Reactions

CNS: Anxiety, dizziness, fatigue, headache, lethargy, light-headedness, paresthesia, somnolence, syncope, tremor
CV: Arrhythmias, chest pain, hypotension, palpitations, peripheral edema
EENT: Dry mouth, gingival hyperplasia, pharyngitis
ENDO: Hot flashes
GI: Abdominal cramps, abdominal pain, anorexia, constipation, diarrhea, dysphagia, elevated hepatic enzymes, esophagitis, flatulence, indigestion, jaundice, nausea, pancreatitis, vomiting
GU: Decreased libido, impotence, urinary frequency
MS: Myalgia
RESP: Dyspnea
SKIN: Dermatitis, flushing, rash
Other: Weight loss

Nursing Considerations

• Use amlodipine cautiously in patients with heart block, heart failure, impaired renal function, hepatic disorder, or severe aortic stenosis.
• Monitor patient with impaired hepatic function closely because amlodipine is extensively metabolized by the liver, and expect to titrate dosage slowly when

administering drug to patients with severe hepatic impairment.
• Monitor blood pressure while adjusting dosage, especially in patients with heart failure or severe aortic stenosis because symptomatic hypotension may occur.
• Assess patient frequently for chest pain when starting or increasing the dose of amlodipine, because worsening of angina or an acute myocardial infarction can occur, especially in patients with severe obstructive coronary artery disease.

PATIENT TEACHING

• Tell patient to take missed dose as soon as remembered and next dose in 24 hours.
• Tell patient to immediately notify prescriber of dizziness, arm or leg swelling, difficulty breathing, hives, or rash.
• Suggest taking amlodipine with food to reduce GI upset.
• Advise patient to have blood pressure checked routinely for possible hypotension.

ammonium chloride

Class and Category

Chemical class: Ammonium ion
Therapeutic class: Acidifier
Pregnancy category: C

Indications and Dosages

➤ *To treat hypochloremia and metabolic alkalosis*

I.V. INFUSION

Adults. Individualized based on serum bicarbonate level. *Usual:* 100 to 200 mEq added to 500 or 1,000 ml of normal saline solution, infused at 5 ml/min or less (about 3 hr for an infusion of 1,000 ml).

Route	Onset	Peak	Duration
I.V.	1–3 min	3–6 hr	Unknown

Mechanism of Action

Drug is converted to urea and hydrochloric acid in the liver. During conversion, drug breaks into ammonium and chloride ions, and hydrogen ions are released. They enter the blood and extracellular fluid, where hydrogen reacts with bicarbonate ions to form water and carbon dioxide. This process decreases bicarbonate ions and increases chloride ions in blood and extracellular fluid, which decreases blood and urine pH and corrects alkalosis.

Incompatibilities
Don't mix I.V. ammonium chloride with codeine, levorphanol, or methadone.

Contraindications
Hypersensitivity to ammonium chloride or its components, markedly impaired renal or hepatic function, metabolic alkalosis caused by vomiting of hydrochloric acid and accompanied by sodium loss caused by sodium bicarbonate excretion in urine

Interaction
DRUGS
amphetamines, salicylates, sulfonylureas, tricyclic antidepressants: Decreased therapeutic blood level of ammonium
chlorpropamide: Increased ammonium effects

Adverse Reactions
CNS: Fever, headache
CV: Phlebitis or thrombosis extending from injection site
GI: Indigestion, nausea, severe hepatic dysfunction, vomiting
RESP: Hyperventilation
SKIN: Extravasation
Other: Injection-site infection, irritation, or pain; hypovolemia; severe metabolic acidosis (with large doses)

Nursing Considerations
• Before use, warm ammonium chloride solution to room temperature to dissolve crystals by placing infusion in warm water.
• During I.V. use, keep sodium bicarbonate or sodium lactate nearby to treat overdose.
• Infuse ammonium chloride slowly to avoid I.V. site pain and irritation.
WARNING Monitor patient for ammonia toxicity (arrhythmias, such as bradycardia; coma; irregular breathing; pallor; retching; seizures; diaphoresis; and twitching).
• Watch for signs of metabolic acidosis, such as increased respirations, increased serum pH, restlessness, and diaphoresis.
• Monitor serum bicarbonate level, urinalysis results, and renal and liver function test results as appropriate.

PATIENT TEACHING
• Tell patient to eat potassium-rich foods, such as bananas, oranges, cantaloupe, spinach, dried fruit, and potatoes, during therapy.

amobarbital sodium
Amytal, Novamobarb (CAN)

Class, Category, and Schedule
Chemical class: Barbiturate
Therapeutic class: Anticonvulsant, sedative-hypnotic
Pregnancy category: D
Controlled substance schedule: II

Indications and Dosages
➤ *To produce preanesthesia sedation*
CAPSULES, ELIXIR, TABLETS
Adults. 200 mg 1 to 2 hr before surgery.
Children. 2 to 6 mg/kg up to a maximum of 100 mg/dose.
➤ *To produce sedation*
CAPSULES, ELIXIR, TABLETS, I.V. OR I.M. INJECTION
Adults. 30 to 50 mg (may range from 15 to 120 mg) twice daily or three times daily. *Maximum I.V.:* 1,000 mg/dose. *Maximum I.M.:* 500 mg/dose.
Children over age 6. 2 mg/kg daily in four divided doses.
➤ *To treat insomnia*
CAPSULES, ELIXIR, TABLETS
Adults. 65 to 200 mg at bedtime for up to 2 wk.
➤ *To induce a hypnotic state*
CAPSULES, ELIXIR, TABLETS, I.V. OR I.M. INJECTION
Adults. 65 to 200 mg/dose. *Maximum I.V.:* 1,000 mg/dose. *Maximum I.M.:* 500 mg/dose
Children up to age 6. 2 to 3 mg/kg I.M. per dose.
➤ *To manage seizures*
I.V. OR I.M. INJECTION
Use I.V. route only when other routes aren't appropriate. For I.V. injection, use I.M. dose and inject slowly at 50 mg/min or less to prevent sudden respiratory depression, apnea, laryngospasm, or hypotension.
Adults. *Usual:* 65 to 500 mg to a maximum of 1,000 mg. Dosage for acute seizures is

determined by response; 200- to 500-mg doses are typically needed to control seizures. **Children age 6 and over.** 65 to 500 mg I.V. **Children up to age 6.** 3 to 5 mg/kg/dose.

Route	Onset	Peak	Duration
P.O.*	60 min	Unknown	10–12 hr
I.V.	Unknown	Unknown	10–12 hr
I.M.	Unknown	Unknown	10–12 hr

Mechanism of Action

Nonselectively acts on the CNS to depress the sensory cortex, decrease motor activity, alter cerebellar function, and produce drowsiness, sedation, and hypnosis. Appears to reduce wakefulness and alertness by acting in the thalamus, where it depresses the reticular activating system and interferes with impulse transmission from the periphery to the cortex. Produces CNS depressant effects ranging from mild sedation and anxiety reduction to anesthesia and coma, depending on the dose, route, and individual patient's response.

Incompatibilities

Don't mix amobarbital in solution with other drugs.

Contraindications

Alcoholism, history of porphyria, history of sedative or barbiturate addiction, hypersensitivity to barbiturates, renal or hepatic disease, severe respiratory disease, sleep apnea, suicidal tendency, uncontrolled pain

Interaction

DRUGS

acetaminophen: Increased blood acetaminophen level and risk of hepatotoxicity
antihistamines, CNS depressants, phenothiazines, tranquilizers: Increased CNS depression
beta blockers, carbamazepine, clonazepam, corticosteroids, digitoxin, doxycycline, estrogens, griseofulvin, metronidazole, oral anticoagulants, oral contraceptives, phenylbutazones, quinidine, theophyllines, tricyclic antidepressants: Decreased blood levels and effects of these drugs

* For capsules, elixir, and tablets.

chloramphenicol: Inhibited amobarbital metabolism; enhanced chloramphenicol metabolism
MAO inhibitors: Increased serum level and sedative effects of amobarbital
methoxyflurane: Increased nephrotoxicity
phenytoin: Altered effects of phenytoin
rifampin: Decreased serum level and effects of amobarbital
valproic acid: Increased amobarbital effects
ACTIVITIES
alcohol use: Increased serum level of amobarbital and additive CNS depressant effects

Adverse Reactions

CNS: Agitation, anxiety, ataxia, CNS depression, confusion, dizziness, hallucinations, hangover, headache, hyperkinesia, insomnia, nightmares, nervousness, paradoxical stimulation, permanent neurologic deficit (with injection near nerve), psychiatric disturbance, somnolence, syncope, vertigo
CV: Bradycardia, hypotension, shock
EENT: Laryngospasm
GI: Constipation, diarrhea, epigastric pain, nausea, vomiting
RESP: Apnea, bronchospasm, hypoventilation, respiratory depression
SKIN: Exfoliative dermatitis, rash, Stevens-Johnson syndrome, urticaria
Other: Angioedema, gangrene of arm or leg from accidental injection into artery, injection-site tissue damage and necrosis, physical and psychological dependence, potentially fatal withdrawal syndrome, tolerance

Nursing Considerations

• Use amobarbital cautiously in patients with cardiac disease, debilitation, diabetes mellitus, fever, hyperthyroidism, severe anemia, shock, status asthmaticus, or uremia.
• Administer by deep I.M. injection, preferably in large muscle.
WARNING To prevent tissue damage and necrosis at I.M. injection site, don't give more than 5 ml of this highly alkaline drug at any one site. Know that accidental arterial injection may cause gangrene of the arm or leg.
• During I.V. administration, closely monitor blood pressure, pulse, and respiration. Keep emergency equipment

and drugs nearby in case respiratory depression occurs.

WARNING Use I.V. route only when other routes aren't appropriate.

WARNING Don't administer solution after 30 minutes of exposure to air. Solution quickly becomes unstable because amobarbital sodium hydrolyzes in solution.

• To prevent withdrawal symptoms, such as diaphoresis, insomnia, irritability, nightmares, and tremors, expect to taper amobarbital dosage gradually after long-term use, especially for epileptic patients.

PATIENT TEACHING

• Advise patient to use caution when driving or doing tasks that require alertness.

• Instruct patient not to use alcohol or other CNS depressants (unless prescribed) because they increase amobarbital's effects.

• Warn patient not to stop taking drug abruptly; withdrawal symptoms can occur.

• Instruct patient to report severe dizziness, persistent drowsiness, rash, or skin lesions.

• Explain that drug effects, such as drowsiness, may be less pronounced after a few days and when drug is taken with food.

amoxapine

Asendin

Class and Category

Chemical class: Dibenzoxazepine derivative
Therapeutic class: Tricyclic antidepressant
Pregnancy category: C

Indications and Dosages

➤ *To relieve depression, including endogenous (long-term) depression and depression associated with anxiety and agitation*

TABLETS

Adults and children age 16 and over. *Initial:* 50 mg twice daily or three times daily, increased to 100 mg twice daily or three times daily by end of first wk, if tolerated. *Maintenance:* If 300-mg daily dose is ineffective after 2-wk trial period, dosage increased to a maximum of 400 mg daily in divided doses. Inpatients may receive up to a maximum of 600 mg daily in divided doses. When effective dose is achieved, a single dose may be given at bedtime, not to exceed 300 mg.

DOSAGE ADJUSTMENT For elderly patients. *Initial:* 25 mg twice daily or three times daily, increased to 50 mg twice daily or three times daily by end of first wk. *Maintenance:* 100 to 150 mg daily in divided doses, carefully increased to 300 mg daily as tolerated. When effective dose is achieved, a single dose may be given at bedtime, not to exceed 300 mg.

Route	Onset	Peak	Duration
P.O.	2–3 wk	Unknown	Unknown

Mechanism of Action

Blocks serotonin and norepinephrine reuptake by adrenergic nerves, thus raising serotonin and norepinephrine levels at nerve synapses. This action may elevate mood and reduce depression.

Normally, when an impulse reaches adrenergic nerves, they release serotonin and norepinephrine from their storage sites. Some serotonin and norepinephrine reach receptor sites on target tissues. The majority is taken back into the nerves and stored by the reuptake mechanism.

Contraindications

Acute recovery phase after MI, hypersensitivity to amoxapine or its components, MAO inhibitor therapy within 14 days

Interaction

DRUGS

anticholinergics, epinephrine, norepinephrine: Increased effects of these drugs
barbiturates: Decreased amoxapine level
carbamazepine: Decreased serum amoxapine level; increased serum carbamazepine level, increasing its therapeutic and toxic effects
cimetidine, disulfiram, fluoxetine, fluvoxamine, haloperidol, H₂-receptor antagonists, methylphenidate, oral contraceptives, paroxetine, phenothiazines, sertraline: Increased blood amoxapine level
clonidine, guanethidine, other antihypertensives: Decreased antihypertensive effects
dicumarol: Increased anticoagulant effect
levodopa: Decreased levodopa absorption; agitation, hypertension, sinus tachycardia, sympathetic hyperactivity
MAO inhibitors: Possibly seizures and death

thyroid replacement drugs: Arrhythmias and increased antidepressant effects
ACTIVITIES
alcohol use: Increased CNS depression
smoking: Decreased amoxapine effects

Adverse Reactions
CNS: Agitation, anxiety, ataxia, chills, confusion, dizziness, drowsiness, excitement, extrapyramidal reactions, fatigue, fever, headache, insomnia, nervousness, nightmares, paresthesia, restlessness, sedation, seizures, stroke, syncope, tremor, weakness
CV: Atrial arrhythmias, heart block, heart failure, hypertension, hypotension, MI, palpitations, tachycardia
EENT: Blurred vision, dry mouth, increased salivation, nasal congestion, taste perversion, tinnitus
ENDO: Gynecomastia, increased or decreased blood glucose level, increased prolactin level, syndrome of inappropriate ADH secretion
GI: Anorexia, constipation, diarrhea, elevated liver function test results, flatulence, increased appetite, nausea, vomiting
GU: Impotence, libido changes, menstrual irregularities, testicular swelling, urinary hesitancy, urine retention
HEME: Agranulocytosis, leukopenia
SKIN: Diaphoresis, flushing, photosensitivity, pruritus, rash
Other: Weight gain or loss; withdrawal symptoms, such as headache, nausea, nightmares, and vertigo

Nursing Considerations
WARNING Don't give an MAO inhibitor within 14 days of amoxapine.
• To avoid withdrawal, don't stop drug abruptly.
• Watch patients closely (especially children, adolescents, and young adults), for suicidal tendencies, particularly when therapy starts and dosage changes, because depression may worsen temporarily during these times.
PATIENT TEACHING
• Advise patient to take amoxapine at bedtime if daytime sedation occurs.
• Caution patient that stopping amoxapine abruptly may cause withdrawal symptoms.
• Urge patient to avoid alcohol because it can potentiate amoxapine's effects.

• Tell patient to report adverse effects of amoxapine.
• Instruct patient to take drug with food to prevent GI upset.
• Urge family or caregiver to watch patient closely for suicidal tendencies, especially when therapy starts or dosage changes and particularly if patient is a child, teenager, or young adult.

amoxicillin trihydrate (amoxycillin)
Amoxil, Apo-Amoxi (CAN), Disper Mox, Moxatag, Novamoxin (CAN), Nu-Amoxi (CAN), Polymox, Trimox, Wymox

Class and Category
Chemical class: Aminopenicillin
Therapeutic class: Antibiotic
Pregnancy category: B

Indications and Dosages
➤ *To treat ear, nose, throat, GU tract, skin, and soft-tissue infections caused by susceptible gram-positive and gram-negative organisms*
CAPSULES, CHEWABLE TABLETS, ORAL SUSPENSION, PEDIATRIC DROPS, POWDER OR TABLETS FOR ORAL SUSPENSION, TABLETS
Adults and children weighing 20 kg (44 lb) or more. 250 mg every 8 hr; for severe infections, 500 mg every 8 hr or 875 mg every 12 hr.
Children age 12 wk and over weighing less than 20 kg. 20 mg/kg daily in divided doses every 8 hr; for severe infections, 40 to 45 mg/kg/day in divided doses every 8 hr.
Children under age 12 wk. 30 mg/kg/day in divided doses every 12 hr.
➤ *To treat tonsillitis or pharyngitis caused by* Streptococcus pyogenes
E.R. TABLETS (MOXATAG)
Adults and children age 12 and over. 775 mg once daily for 10 days, taken within 1 hr of finishing a meal.
➤ *To treat lower respiratory tract infections caused by susceptible gram-positive and gram-negative organisms*

CAPSULES, CHEWABLE TABLETS, ORAL SUSPENSION, PEDIATRIC DROPS, POWDER OR TABLETS FOR ORAL SUSPENSION, TABLETS
Adults and children weighing 20 kg (44 lb) or more. 875 mg every 12 hr; for severe infections, 500 mg every 8 hr.
Children age 12 wk and over weighing less than 20 kg. 40 to 45 mg/kg daily in divided doses every 8 hr.
Children under age 12 wk. 30 mg/kg daily in divided doses every 12 hr.
➤ *To treat gonorrhea and acute uncomplicated anogenital and urethral infections caused by susceptible strains of gram-positive and gram-negative organisms*
CAPSULES, CHEWABLE TABLETS, ORAL SUSPENSION, POWDER OR TABLETS FOR ORAL SUSPENSION, TABLETS
Adults and postpubertal children. 3 g as a single dose.
Prepubertal children age 2 and over. 50 mg/kg of amoxicillin plus 25 mg/kg of probenecid as a single dose.
➤ *As adjunct to eradicate Helicobacter pylori to reduce risk of duodenal ulcer recurrence*
CAPSULES, CHEWABLE TABLETS, ORAL SUSPENSION, POWDER OR TABLETS FOR ORAL SUSPENSION, TABLETS
Adults. 1 g every 12 hr with 500 mg of clarithromycin every 12 hr and 30 mg of lansoprazole every 12 hr for 14 days, or 1 g every 8 hr with 30 mg of lansoprazole every 8 hr for 14 days.
➤ *To prevent bacterial endocarditis before dental, oral, or upper respiratory tract procedures*
CAPSULES, CHEWABLE TABLETS, ORAL SUSPENSION, POWDER OR TABLETS FOR ORAL SUSPENSION, TABLETS
Adults and children weighing 20 kg (44 lb) or more. 2 g 1 hr before procedure.
Children weighing less than 20 kg. 50 mg/kg 1 hr before procedure.

Route	Onset	Peak	Duration
P.O.	Unknown	Unknown	6–8 hr

Mechanism of Action
Kills bacteria by binding to and inactivating penicillin-binding proteins on the inner bacterial cell wall, weakening the bacterial cell wall and causing lysis.

Contraindications
History of severe hypersensitivity reactions (anaphylaxis or Stevens-Johnson syndrome) to other beta-lactam antibiotics, hypersensitivity to amoxicillin or its components,

Interaction
DRUGS
allopurinol: Increased risk of rash
chloramphenicol, erythromycins, sulfonamides, tetracyclines: Reduced bactericidal effect of amoxicillin
methotrexate: Increased risk of methotrexate toxicity
oral anticoagulants: Possible prolonged prothrombin time (increased international normalized ratio)
oral contraceptives with estrogen: Possibly reduced effectiveness of contraceptive
probenecid: Increased amoxicillin effects

Adverse Reactions
CNS: Agitation, anxiety, behavior changes, confusion, dizziness, insomnia, reversible hyperactivity, seizures
CV: Hypersensitivity vasculitis
EENT: Black, hairy tongue; mucocutaneous candidiasis; tooth discoloration
GI: Diarrhea, diarrhea related to *Clostridium difficile*, elevated liver enzymes, hemorrhagic or pseudomembranous colitis, jaundice, hepatic dysfunction, nausea, vomiting
GU: Crystalluria, vaginal mycosis
HEME: Agranulocytosis, anemia (including hemolytic anemia), eosinophilia, granulocytosis, leukopenia, thrombocytopenia, thrombocytopenic purpura
SKIN: Erythema multiforme, erythematous maculopapular rash, generalized exanthematous pustulosis, Stevens-Johnson syndrome, toxic epidermal necrolysis, urticaria
Other: Allergic reaction, anaphylaxis, serum sickness-like reaction (such as arthralgia, arthritis, fever, myalgia, rash, and urticaria)

Nursing Considerations
• Patients with mononucleosis shouldn't receive amoxicillin because this class of drugs may cause an erythematous rash.

• Use drug cautiously in patients with hepatic impairment. Monitor hepatic and renal function and CBC, as ordered, in patients on prolonged therapy. Also use cautiously in breastfeeding and elderly patients.
• Expect to start therapy before culture and sensitivity test results are known.
• Be aware that chewable tablets and tablets for oral suspension contain phenylalanine.
• Don't confuse amoxicillin tablets with amoxicillin tablets for oral suspension (DisperMox). They're not interchangeable.
WARNING If allergic reaction occurs, stop amoxicillin immediately and provide emergency care as indicated and ordered.
• Monitor patient closely for diarrhea, which may indicate pseudomembranous colitis caused by *Clostridium difficile*. If diarrhea occurs, notify prescriber, expect to withhold amoxicillin, and treat with fluids, electrolytes, protein, and an antibiotic effective against *C. difficile*.
• Expect treatment that lasts at least 10 days for hemolytic streptococci infections.
• Monitor patient for superinfection. If it occurs, expect to discontinue drug and provide treatment as ordered.
PATIENT TEACHING
• Tell patient to refrigerate reconstituted suspension and to shake well before each use.
• When amoxicillin suspension is prescribed for a child, instruct parents to place it directly on child's tongue to swallow. If this doesn't work, tell parents to mix dose of suspension with formula or cold drink (milk, fruit juice, ginger ale, water) and have child drink it immediately.
• Instruct patient using DisperMox tablets to place one tablet and about 2 teaspoonfuls of water in a glass, drink entire mixture, add more water to the glass, and drink again to ensure delivery of full dose.
• Tell patient to chew or crush chewable tablets and not to swallow them whole.
• To prevent infection from recurring, urge patient to take amoxicillin for full length of time prescribed, even if he feels better.
• Teach patient to report adverse reactions and notify prescriber if infection worsens or doesn't improve after 72 hours.

• Urge patient to tell prescriber about diarrhea that's severe or lasts longer than 3 days. Remind patient that watery or bloody stools can occur 2 or more months after antibiotic therapy and may be serious, requiring prompt treatment.

amphetamine sulfate

dexamphetamine sulfate

Dexedrine, Dextrostat, Liquadd, ProCentra

Class and Category
Chemical class: Sympathomimetic amine
Therapeutic class: CNS stimulant
Pregnancy category: C
Controlled substance schedule: II

Indications and Dosages
➤ *To treat attention deficit hyperactivity disorder (ADHD)*
ORAL SOLUTION (LIQUADD, PROCENTRA)
Children ages 3 to 6. *Initial:* 2.5 mg daily. Increased by 2.5 mg daily at 1-wk intervals until desired response occurs.
Children age 6 and over. *Initial:* 5 mg daily or twice daily. Increased by 5 mg daily at 1-wk intervals until desired response occurs.
TABLETS (DEXTROSTAT)
Children age 6 and over. *Initial:* 5 mg daily or twice daily. Increased by 5 mg daily at 1-wk intervals until desired response occurs. *Usual:* 0.1 to 0.5 mg/kg daily.
Children ages 3 to 5. *Initial:* 2.5 mg daily. Increased by 2.5 mg daily at 1-wk intervals until desired response occurs. *Usual:* 0.1 to 0.5 mg/kg daily.
ER CAPSULES (DEXEDRINE)
Children age 6 and over.
Initial: 5 mg daily or twice daily. Increased by 5 mg daily at 1-wk intervals until desired response occurs.
➤ *To treat narcolepsy*
ORAL SOLUTION (LIQUADD, PROCENTRA)
Adults and children age 12 and over.
Initial: 10 mg daily. Increased by 10 mg daily at 1-wk intervals until desired response occurs.

Children ages 6 to 12. *Initial:* 2.5 mg twice daily. Increased by 5 mg daily at 1-wk intervals until desired response occurs or adult dosage is reached to a maximum of 60 mg daily.
ER CAPSULES (DEXEDRINE)
Adults and children age 12 and over.
Initial: 10 mg daily. Increased by 10 mg daily at 1-wk intervals until desired response occurs.
Children ages 6 to 12. *Initial:* 5 mg once daily. Increased by 5 mg daily at 1-wk intervals until desired response occurs.

Mechanism of Action
May produce its CNS stimulant effects by facilitating release and blocking reuptake of norepinephrine at adrenergic nerve terminals and by direct stimulation of alpha and beta receptors in the peripheral nervous system. It also releases and blocks reuptake of dopamine in limbic regions of the brain. The drug's main action appears to be in the cerebral cortex and, possibly, the reticular activating system. These actions cause decreased motor restlessness, increased alertness, and diminished drowsiness and fatigue. Its peripheral actions include increased blood pressure and mild bronchodilation and respiratory stimulation.

Contraindications
Advanced arteriosclerosis, agitation (for narcolepsy treatment), glaucoma, history of drug abuse, hypersensitivity or idiosyncratic reaction to sympathomimetic amines, hyperthyroidism, MAO inhibitor therapy within 14 days, moderate to severe hypertension, symptomatic cardiovascular disease

Interaction
DRUGS
adrenergic blockers: Inhibited adrenergic blockade
acetazolamide, alkalinizers (such as sodium bicarbonate), some thiazides: Increased blood level and effects of amphetamine
antihistamines: Possibly reduced sedation from antihistamine
antihypertensives: Possibly decreased antihypertensive effects

chlorpromazine: Inhibited CNS stimulant effects of amphetamine
ethosuximide: Possibly delayed ethosuximide absorption
GI acidifiers (such as ascorbic acid), reserpine: Decreased amphetamine absorption
guanethidine: Decreased antihypertensive effect and decreased amphetamine absorption
haloperidol: Decreased CNS stimulation
lithium carbonate: Possibly decreased anorectic and stimulant effects of amphetamine
MAO inhibitors: Potentiated effects of amphetamine; possibly hypertensive crisis
meperidine: Increased analgesia
methenamine: Increased urine excretion and decreased effects of amphetamine
norepinephrine: Possibly increased adrenergic effect of norepinephrine
phenobarbital, phenytoin: Synergistic anticonvulsant action
propoxyphene: Increased CNS stimulation, potentially fatal seizures
tricyclic antidepressants: Possibly enhanced antidepressant effects and decreased effects of amphetamine
urinary acidifiers (such as ammonium chloride and sodium acid phosphate): Increased amphetamine excretion and decreased amphetamine blood level and effects
veratrum alkaloids: Decreased hypotensive effect
FOODS
acidic fruit juices: Decreased amphetamine absorption

Adverse Reactions
CNS: Aggression, anger, anxiety, depression, dizziness, dyskinesia, dysphoria, euphoria, exacerbation of motor and phonic tics and Tourette's syndrome, hallucinations, headache, insomnia, irritability, over-stimulation, paranoia, psychotic episodes, restlessness, tremor
CV: Cardiomyopathy, hypertension, palpitations, tachycardia
EENT: Blurred vision, dry mouth, mydriasis, unpleasant taste
GI: Anorexia, constipation, diarrhea
GU: Impotence, libido changes

SKIN: Alopecia, rash, Stevens-Johnson syndrome, toxic epidermal necrolysis, urticaria
Other: Anaphylaxis, angioedema, weight loss

Nursing Considerations
• Keep in mind that when symptoms of ADHD occur with acute stress reactions, treatment with amphetamines usually isn't indicated.

WARNING To prevent hypertensive crisis, don't give amphetamine during or for up to 14 days after MAO therapy.
• Give first dose when patient awakens and additional doses at 4- to 6-hour intervals.
• Be aware that 5 ml of oral solution contains 5 mg of dexamphetamine.
• If patient has bothersome adverse reactions, such as insomnia and anorexia, expect to decrease dosage. To minimize insomnia, administer drug earlier in day.
• Be alert for evidence of long-term amphetamine abuse, such as severe dermatoses, marked insomnia, irritability, hyperactivity, and personality changes. If patient suddenly stops drug after long-term, high-dose regimen, watch for extreme fatigue and depression.

PATIENT TEACHING
• Instruct breastfeeding patient to avoid breastfeeding during amphetamine therapy because drug is excreted in breastmilk.
• Teach patient to take first dose on awakening and subsequent doses at 4- to 6-hour intervals. Tell him not to take last dose late in evening because insomnia may occur.
• Inform patient or caregiver that each 5 ml of oral solution contains 5 mg of dexamphetamine. Advise patient to use a calibrated measuring device for accurate dose.
• Urge patient to avoid hazardous activities until drug's effects are known.
• Advise patient not to take amphetamine with acidic fruit juice because doing so decreases drug absorption.
• Explain drug's abuse potential, and caution against altering dosage unless prescribed.

amphotericin B
Amphocin, Fungizone Intravenous

amphotericin B cholesteryl sulfate complex
Amphotec

amphotericin B lipid complex
Abelcet

amphotericin B liposomal complex
AmBisome

Class and Category
Chemical class: Amphoteric polyene macrolide
Therapeutic class: Antifungal
Pregnancy category: B (I.V.); C (oral suspension)

Indications and Dosages
➤ *To treat severe fungal infections, using amphotericin B*
I.V. INFUSION
Adults and adolescents. *Initial:* 1-mg test dose in 20 ml of D_5W infused over 20 to 30 min; if test dose is tolerated, then 0.25 to 0.3 mg/kg daily prepared as a 0.1 mg/ml infusion, given over 2 to 6 hr. Increased in 5- to 10-mg increments up to 50 mg daily, based on patient tolerance and infection severity, not to exceed a total daily dose of 1.5 mg/kg. *Maximum:* 50 mg daily infused over 2 to 6 hr.
Children. *Initial:* 0.25 mg/kg daily in D_5W infused over 6 hr; then increased in 0.125- to 0.25-mg/kg increments daily or every other day as tolerated. *Maximum:* 1 mg/kg or 30 mg/m^2 of body surface daily.
➤ *To treat oral candidiasis, using amphotericin B*
ORAL SUSPENSION
Adults and children. 1 ml (100 mg) four times daily for 14 days.

➤ *To treat aspergillosis, using amphotericin B cholesteryl sulfate complex*
I.V. INFUSION
Adults and children. Test dose of 1.6 to 8.3 mg in 10 ml of D$_5$W infused over 15 to 30 min; if test dose is tolerated, then 3 to 4 mg/kg once daily infused at 1 mg/kg/hr.
➤ *To treat invasive amphotericin B-resistant fungal infections, using amphotericin B lipid complex*
I.V. INFUSION
Adults and children. 5 mg/kg daily infused at 2.5 mg/kg/hr.
➤ *To treat severe aspergillosis, candidiasis, or cryptococcosis, using amphotericin B liposomal complex*
I.V. INFUSION
Adults and children. 3 to 5 mg/kg daily infused over 2 hr. Infusion time may be decreased to 1 hr if tolerated or increased if patient experiences discomfort.
➤ *To treat leishmaniasis, using amphotericin B liposomal complex*
I.V. INFUSION
Immunocompetent adults and children. 3 mg/kg daily on days 1 through 5 and on days 14 and 21, infused over 2 hr. Infusion time may be decreased to 1 hr if tolerated or increased if patient has discomfort.
Immunocompromised adults and children. 4 mg/kg daily on days 1 through 5 and days 10, 17, 24, 31, and 38 infused over 2 hr. Infusion time may be decreased to 1 hr if tolerated or increased if patient has discomfort.
➤ *To treat presumed fungal infections in patients with febrile neutropenia, using amphotericin B lipid complex*
I.V. INFUSION
Adults and children. 3 mg/kg daily infused over 2 hr. Infusion time may be decreased to 1 hr if tolerated or increased if patient has discomfort.

Route	Onset	Peak	Duration
I.V.	Immediate	Unknown	Unknown

Mechanism of Action
Binds to sterols in fungal cell plasma membranes, which changes membrane permeability and allows loss of potassium and small molecules from cells. This action results in cell impairment or death.

Incompatibilities
Don't reconstitute amphotericin B with diluents other than those recommended because solutions with sodium chloride or bacteriostatic agents (such as benzyl alcohol) may cause drug precipitation.

Contraindications
Hypersensitivity to amphotericin B or its components

Interaction
DRUGS
antineoplastics: Increased risk of bronchospasm, hypotension, and nephrotoxicity
corticosteroids, corticotropin: Increased risk of hypokalemia and cardiac dysfunction
cyclosporine, nephrotoxic drugs: Increased risk of nephrotoxicity
digitalis glycosides: Possibly hypokalemia and more severe digitalis toxicity
flucytosine: Possibly increased flucytosine toxicity
leukocyte transfusion: Possibly dyspnea, hypoxemia, and pulmonary infiltrates
skeletal muscle relaxants: Possibly hypokalemia and increased muscle relaxation
zidovudine: Possibly myelotoxicity and nephrotoxicity

Adverse Reactions
CNS: Fever, headache, shaking chills, tiredness, weakness
CV: Chest pain, hypotension, irregular heartbeat
EENT: Difficulty swallowing, pharyngitis
GI: Abdominal pain, anorexia, diarrhea, hepatic failure, indigestion, nausea, vomiting
GU: Decreased or increased urine output, hemorrhagic cystitis, impaired renal function
HEME: Agranulocytosis, anemia, leukopenia, thrombocytopenia, unusual bleeding or bruising
MS: Arthralgia, muscle spasms, myalgia, rhabdomyolysis
RESP: Apnea, bronchospasm, cyanosis, dyspnea, hypoventilation, hypoxia, pulmonary edema, tachypnea
SKIN: Erythemia, flushing, jaundice, maculopapular rash, pruritus and redness especially around ears, urticaria

Other: Anaphylaxis, angioedema, hypocalcemia, hypokalemia, hypomagnesemia, infusion-site pain and thrombophlebitis

Nursing Considerations
• To prepare amphotericin B, add 10 ml of sterile water for injection without a bacteriostatic agent to vial containing 50 mg of amphotericin B. For I.V. infusion, dilute solution containing 5 mg/ ml to 0.1 mg/ml by adding 1 ml (5 mg) of solution to 49 ml of D_5W with a pH above 4.2.
• Before using D_5W to dilute amphotericin B solution, determine the injection's pH aseptically. If pH is below 4.2, follow manufacturer's instructions for buffering it.
• Because reconstituted amphotericin B is a colloidal suspension, avoid using in-line membrane filter or use one with a mean pore diameter of more than 1 micron to prevent significant drug removal.
• To prepare amphotericin B cholesteryl sulfate complex, reconstitute with sterile water for injection. Using a sterile syringe and 20G needle, rapidly add 10- or 20-ml sterile water for injection to a 50- or 100- mg vial, respectively, to obtain a solution containing 5 mg of amphotericin B per milliliter. Shake gently by hand, rotating vial until solids are dissolved; fluid may be clear or opalescent. For infusion, further dilute reconstituted solution to about 0.6 mg/ml. Don't filter solution or use an in-line filter. Flush existing line with D_5W or use a separate line.
• To prepare amphotericin B lipid complex, shake vial gently until you see no yellow sediment. Using an 18G needle, withdraw prescribed dose from required number of vials into one or more 20-ml syringes. Replace needle with 5-micron filter needle supplied with each vial. Empty syringe contents into bag of D_5W so that final concentration is 1 mg/ml. Expect to use a concentration of 2 mg/ml for children and patients with cardiovascular disease. Before infusion, shake bag until contents are mixed thoroughly. Flush existing line with D_5W, or use a separate line. Don't use an in-line filter. If infusion exceeds 2 hours, shake infusion bag every 2 hours.

• To prepare amphotericin B liposomal complex, add 12 ml sterile water for injection (without bacteriostatic agent) to each 50-mg vial to achieve a concentration of 4 mg amphotericin B per milliliter. Immediately shake vial vigorously for at least 30 seconds until all particles completely disperse. Withdraw prescribed dose of amphotericin B liposomal complex suspension. Then use a 5-micron filter to inject it into D_5W to provide a final concentration of 1 to 2 mg/ml. Expect to use a lower concentration (0.2 to 0.5 mg/ml) for infants and young children. Flush existing line with D_5W, or use a separate line. You may use an in-line filter with a mean pore diameter of at least 1 micron.
• To help minimize fever and shaking chills, expect to give an antipyretic, antihistamine, meperidine, or corticosteroid just before infusing amphotericin B.
• Before giving amphotericin B oral suspension, shake well. Drop suspension on tongue with calibrated dropper. Then tell patient to swish suspension in mouth for as long as possible before swallowing. If drug must be swabbed on, use a nonabsorbent swab.
• Give amphotericin B oral suspension between meals to permit prolonged contact with oral lesions.
• Assess I.V. insertion site regularly to detect extravasation of amphotericin B, which may cause severe local irritation. To minimize local thrombophlebitis, plan to add heparin to infusion or expect to administer amphotericin on alternate days, which also may help prevent anorexia. Alternate-day dose shouldn't exceed 1.5 mg/kg.
• Monitor renal function because of the risk of renal impairment. Plan to obtain serum creatinine level every other day while amphotericin B dosage is increasing and then at least twice weekly during therapy. If serum creatinine or BUN level increases significantly, expect to stop amphotericin B until renal function improves. Know that a cumulative dose of more than 4 g may cause irreversible renal dysfunction.

• Expect to monitor CBC and platelet count weekly during therapy to detect adverse hematologic effects. Also monitor serum calcium, magnesium, and potassium levels twice weekly to detect abnormalities.
• Use reconstituted amphotericin B within 24 hours if stored at room temperature, 1 week if refrigerated. Use reconstituted amphotericin B cholesteryl sulfate complex within 24 hours. Use amphotericin B lipid complex within 6 hours if stored at room temperature, 48 hours if refrigerated. Use diluted amphotericin B liposomal complex within 24 hours if refrigerated, but begin infusion within 6 hours.
• Be aware that false elevations of serum phosphate may occur when samples are analyzed using the PHOSm assay.

PATIENT TEACHING
• Instruct patient to shake bottle of oral suspension well before each dose; to drop suspension directly on his tongue using calibrated dropper; and then to swish suspension in his mouth for as long as possible before swallowing. If prescriber orders drug to be swabbed onto oral lesions, tell patient to use nonabsorbent swab. Instruct him to take drug four times a day (between meals and at bedtime).
• Tell patient to notify prescriber if he develops local irritation, if existing symptoms worsen or return, or if new symptoms arise.

---

ampicillin

Apo-Ampi (CAN), Novo-Ampicillin (CAN), Nu-Ampi (CAN), Omnipen

ampicillin sodium

Ampicin (CAN), Omnipen-N, Polycillin-N, Totacillin-N

ampicillin trihydrate

D-Amp, Omnipen, Penbritin (CAN), Polycillin, Principen-250, Principen-500, Totacillin

Class and Category
Chemical class: Semisynthetic aminopenicillin

Therapeutic class: Antibiotic
Pregnancy category: B

Indications and Dosages
➤ *To treat GI infections and genitourinary infections (other than gonorrhea) caused by susceptible strains of* Shigella, Salmonella typhi *and other species,* Escherichia coli, Proteus mirabilis, *and* enterococci

CAPSULES, ORAL SUSPENSION, I.V. INFUSION, I.M. INJECTION
Adults and children weighing 20 kg (44 lb) or more. 500 mg P.O. every 6 hr or 250 to 500 mg I.V. or I.M. every 6 hr.
Children weighing less than 20 kg. 50 to 100 mg/kg daily in divided doses P.O. every 6 hr or 12.5 mg/kg I.V. or I.M. every 6 hr.
➤ *To treat gonorrhea caused by susceptible strains of non–penicillinase-producing* Neisseria gonorrhoeae

CAPSULES, ORAL SUSPENSION
Adults and children. 3.5 g as a single dose with 1 g of probenecid.

I.V. INFUSION, I.M. INJECTION
Adults and children weighing 45 kg (99 lb) or more. 500 mg every 6 hr.
Children weighing less than 40 kg (88 lb). 50 mg/kg daily in divided doses every 6 to 8 hr.
➤ *To treat respiratory tract infections caused by susceptible strains of non-penicillinase–producing* Haemophilus influenzae, *staphylococci, and streptococci, including* Streptococcus pneumoniae

CAPSULES, ORAL SUSPENSION, I.V. INFUSION, I.M. INJECTION
Adults and children weighing 40 kg or more. 250 to 500 mg I.V. or I.M. every 6 to 8 hr.
Adults and children weighing 20 kg or more. 250 mg P.O. every 6 hr.
Children weighing less than 40 kg. 25 to 50 mg/kg daily I.V. or I.M. in divided doses every 6 to 8 hr.
Children weighing less than 20 kg. 50 mg/kg daily P.O. in divided doses every 6 or 8 hr or 12.5 mg/kg I.V. or I.M. every 6 hr.
➤ *To treat septicemia*

I.V. INFUSION, I.M. INJECTION
Adults. 8 to 14 g I.V. daily in divided doses every 3 to 4 hr for at least 3 days; then I.M.
Children. 150 to 200 mg/kg daily I.V. in divided doses every 3 to 4 hr for at least 3 days; then I.M.

➤ *To prevent bacterial endocarditis from dental, oral, or upper respiratory tract procedures*
I.V. INFUSION, I.M. INJECTION
Adults. 2 g within 30 min of procedure
Children. 50 mg/kg within 30 min of procedure
➤ *To treat bacterial meningitis caused by susceptible strains of* Neisseria meningitidis
I.V. INFUSION, I.M. INJECTION
Adults. 8 to 14 g daily or 150 to 200 mg/kg daily I.V. in equally divided doses every 3 to 4 hr for at least 3 days; then I.M. at same dosage and schedule.
Children. 100 to 200 mg/kg daily I.V. in equally divided doses every 3 to 4 hr for at least 3 days; then I.M. at same dosage and schedule.
➤ *To treat listeriosis*
I.V. INFUSION, I.M. INJECTION
Adults and children weighing 20 kg or more. 50 mg/kg every 6 hr.
Children weighing less than 20 kg. 12.5 mg/kg every 6 hr.

Route	Onset	Peak	Duration
I.V.	Immediate	Unknown	Unknown

Mechanism of Action
Inhibits bacterial cell wall synthesis. The rigid, cross-linked cell wall is assembled in several steps. Ampicillin exerts its effects on susceptible bacteria in the final stage of the cross-linking process by binding with and inactivating penicillin-binding proteins (enzymes responsible for linking the cell wall strands). This action causes bacterial cell lysis and death.

Incompatibilities
Don't mix ampicillin and any amino-glycoside in the same I.V. bag, bottle, or tubing; otherwise, both drugs will be inactivated. If patient must receive both drugs, administer them in separate sites at least 1 hour apart.

Contraindications
Hypersensitivity to any penicillin, infection caused by penicillinase-producing organism

Interaction
DRUGS
allopurinol: Increased risk of rash, particularly in hyperuricemic patient

aminoglycosides: Possibly inactivated action of aminoglycoside and ampicillin when given together
heparin, oral anticoagulants: Increased risk of bleeding
oral contraceptives: Possibly reduced contraceptive effectiveness and breakthrough bleeding
probenecid: Possibly increased serum ampicillin level and ampicillin toxicity
tetracyclines: Possibly impaired action of ampicillin

Adverse Reactions
CNS: Chills, fatigue, fever, headache, malaise
CV: Chest pain, edema, thrombophlebitis
EENT: Epistaxis, glossitis, laryngeal stridor, mucocutaneous candidiasis, stomatitis, throat tightness
GI: Abdominal distention, diarrhea, diarrhea related to *Clostridium difficile*, enterocolitis, flatulence, gastritis, nausea, pseudomembranous colitis, vomiting
GU: Dysuria, urine retention, vaginal candidiasis
HEME: Agranulocytosis, anemia, eosinophilia, leukopenia, thrombocytopenia, thrombocytopenic purpura
SKIN: Erythema multiforme; erythematous, mildly pruritic maculopapular rash or other types of rash; exfoliative dermatitis; pruritus; urticaria
Other: Anaphylaxis, facial edema, injection-site pain

Nursing Considerations
• Avoid giving ampicillin to patients with mononucleosis because of increased risk of rash.
• Expect to give ampicillin for 48 to 72 hours after patient becomes asymp-tomatic. For streptococcal infection, expect to give ampicillin for at least 10 days after cultures show streptococcal eradication to reduce risk of rheumatic fever or glomerulonephritis.
• To dilute ampicillin for I.M. use, add (depending on manufacturer) 1.2 ml of sterile water or bacteriostatic water for injection to each 125-mg vial, 1 ml of diluent to each 250-mg vial, 1.8 ml of diluent to each 500-mg vial, 3.5 ml of diluent to each 1-g vial, or 6.8 ml of diluent to each 2-g vial.

- To dilute ampicillin for intermittent infusion, add 5 ml of sterile water or bacteriostatic water for injection to each 125-, 250-, or 500-mg vial or 7.4 to 10 ml of diluent to each 1- or 2-g vial. Infuse in suitable diluent at less than 30 mg/ml.
WARNING Infuse I.V. solution for 3 to 5 minutes for each 125 or 500 mg or 10 to 15 minutes for each 1 or 2 g. More rapid infusion may cause seizures.
- Monitor patient closely for anaphylaxis, which may be life-threatening. Patients at greatest risk are those with a history of multiple allergies, hypersensitivity to cephalosporins, or a history of asthma, hay fever, or urticaria.
WARNING In an anaphylactic reaction, stop drug, notify prescriber immediately, and provide immediate treatment with epinephrine, airway management, oxygen, and I.V. corticosteroids, as needed.
- Notify prescriber if patient has evidence of superinfection; expect to stop drug and provide appropriate treatment.
- If long-term or high-dose ampicillin therapy is required, closely monitor results of renal and liver function tests and CBCs.
- Monitor patient closely for diarrhea, which may be pseudomembranous colitis caused by *Clostridium difficile.* If diarrhea occurs, notify prescriber and expect to withhold ampicillin and administer fluids, electrolytes, protein, and an antibiotic effective against *C. difficile.*

PATIENT TEACHING
- Emphasize the importance of taking the full course of ampicillin exactly as prescribed.
- Tell patient to take dose with 8 ounces of water 30 minutes before or 2 hours after meals.
- Instruct patient to shake suspension well before each use, keep bottle tightly closed between uses, and discard unused portion after 14 days if refrigerated or 7 days if stored at room temperature.
- Review signs of allergic reaction; if they occur, tell patient to hold next ampicillin dose and contact prescriber immediately.
- Urge patient to tell prescriber about diarrhea that's severe or lasts longer than 3 days. Remind patient that watery or bloody stools may occur 2 or more months after antibiotic therapy and may be serious, requiring prompt treatment.

amyl nitrite   A

Class and Category
Chemical class: Nitrite ester
Therapeutic class: Antianginal
Pregnancy category: C

Indications and Dosages
➤ *To treat acute attacks of angina pectoris*
CRUSHABLE AMPULES
Adults. 1 ampule (0.18 or 0.3 ml) inhaled and repeated in 3 to 5 min, if needed.

Route	Onset	Peak	Duration
Inhalation	10–30 sec	Unknown	3–5 min

Mechanism of Action
After inhalation is absorbed by pulmonary alveoli, which causes relaxation of vascular smooth-muscle cells, dilation of large coronary blood vessels, decreased systemic vascular resistance, decreased venous return to the heart, reduced afterload, decreased cardiac output, and subsequent relief of angina.

Contraindications
Hypersensitivity to amyl nitrite, its components, or nitrates

Interaction
DRUGS
aspirin: Increased serum level and action of amyl nitrite
calcium channel blockers: Possibly severe symptomatic hypotension
sildenafil: Increased risk of hypotension
sympathomimetics: Possibly decreased antianginal effects and severe hypotension and tachycardia
ACTIVITIES
alcohol use: Increased risk of severe hypotension and cardiovascular collapse

Adverse Reactions
CNS: Dizziness, headache, restlessness, syncope, weakness
CV: Orthostatic hypotension, tachycardia
GI: Fecal incontinence, nausea, vomiting
GU: Urinary incontinence
HEME: Hemolytic anemia, methemoglobinemia
SKIN: Face and neck flushing, pallor, rash

Nursing Considerations

• Use amyl nitrite cautiously in elderly patients and patients with cerebral hemorrhage, glaucoma, hyperthyroidism, recent head trauma or MI, or severe anemia.

• Monitor blood pressure during and after drug administration. Also monitor cardiac function periodically in patients who use amyl nitrite regularly.

WARNING Stop drug and notify prescriber if evidence of overdose, such as bluish lips, fingernails, or palms; dizziness; fainting; extreme pressure in head; dyspnea; unusual tiredness or weakness; a weak or fast heartbeat; or increased methemoglobin level. Cyanosis may occur when methemoglobin level reaches 1.5 g/dl. More pronounced signs occur at 20 to 50 g/dl.

• Expect to treat overdose with high-flow oxygen and I.V. methylene blue. If hypotension is severe, place patient's head down. If he needs a vasopressor, avoid epinephrine; it may cause severe hypotension.

PATIENT TEACHING

• Advise patient to store amyl nitrate in a tight container, protected from light.

• Tell patient to crush ampule between finger and thumb, hold it to nostrils, and inhale 1 to 6 times.

• Instruct patient to remain seated or supine during administration and to rise slowly afterward to prevent dizziness.

• Inform patient that relief usually occurs in 1 to 5 minutes. If pain continues, he should repeat dose. If pain continues after another 5 minutes, he should seek emergency help.

• Urge patient not to use any more drug than prescribed because of possible overdose.

WARNING Caution patient that drug is flammable and must be kept from flame and heat.

• Inform patient that amyl nitrite commonly causes headaches. Tell him to notify prescriber if they're severe or bothersome.

anakinra

Kineret

Class and Category

Chemical class: Recombinant human interleukin-1 receptor antagonist
Therapeutic class: Antirheumatic
Pregnancy category: B

Indications and Dosages

➤ *To reduce signs and symptoms and slow structural damage in moderate to severe active rheumatoid arthritis in patients who have not responded to disease-modifying antirheumatics*

SUBCUTANEOUS INJECTION

Adults. 100 mg daily.

➤ *To treat neonatal-onset multisystem inflammatory disease in patients with a cryopyrin-associated periodic syndrome*

SUBCUTANEOUS INJECTION

Children. *Initial:* 1 to 2 mg/kg daily or dosage split into twice daily administration followed by dosage adjustments in 0.5 to 1.0 mg/kg increments, as needed. *Maximum:* 8 mg/kg daily

DOSAGE ADJUSTMENT Interval reduced to every other day in severe renal insufficiency or end-stage renal disease (creatinine clearance less than 30 ml/min/1.73 m^2).

Mechanism of Action

Inhibits the binding of interleukin-1 (IL-1) to its type 1 receptor, blocking its activity. Inflammatory stimuli prompt T cells to release IL-1, a mediator of inflammation, pain, and stiffness in rheumatoid arthritis.

Contraindications

Active infection; hypersensitivity to anakinra, its components, or *Escherichia coli*–derived proteins

Interaction

DRUGS

etanercept, infliximab, and other drugs that block tumor necrosis factor: Increased risk of serious infection
live-virus vaccines: Possibly decreased antibody response to vaccine, potential for infection with live virus

Adverse Reactions

CNS: Headache
EENT: Sinusitis
GI: Abdominal pain, diarrhea, nausea
HEME: Neutropenia
MS: Bone and joint infections

RESP: Pneumonia, upper respiratory tract infection
SKIN: Cellulitis
Other: Flulike symptoms; hypersensitivity reaction; injection-site ecchymosis, erythema, inflammation, pain, and pruritus; malignancies; positive results for anti-anakinra antibodies; serious infections

Nursing Considerations
• Expect to obtain baseline neutrophil count before therapy and to monitor neutrophil count every month for 3 months and every 3 months for up to 1 year.
• Discard solution if it contains particles or is discolored. Use prefilled syringe and needles to administer drug. Don't shake syringe; allow time for solution to clear if it becomes foamy.
• Give drug about the same time each day.
WARNING Anakinra isn't recommended for patients with active infections. Monitor patient for evidence of infection, such as fever, chills, sore throat, and mouth sores, before and during therapy because drug increases the risk of infections, such as cellulitis, pneumonia, and bone and joint infections. Notify prescriber if signs are present. Patients with asthma and those receiving etanercept or infliximab are at increased risk for serious infections. Expect anakinra to be stopped if serious infection develops.
• Know that anakinra may possibly increase risk of reactivation of tuberculosis or development of other atypical or opportunistic infections. Follow current Center for Disease Control (CDC) guidelines to evaluate patients and, if needed, treat a possible latent tuberculosis infection, as ordered, before starting anakinra therapy.
• Be aware that live-virus vaccines shouldn't be given to patients receiving anakinra because drug decreases immune response.
• Monitor patients with impaired renal function for signs of anakinra toxicity; they're at increased risk because drug is excreted primarily by the kidneys.
• Store anakinra at 2° to 8° C (36° to 46° F). Protect from freezing and light.
PATIENT TEACHING
• Teach proper injection technique if patient will self-administer drug. Make sure

patient understands the process and can correctly prepare and inject doses.
• Instruct patient to rotate injection sites among thighs, stomach, and upper arms and to avoid areas that are tender, hard, red, or bruised. Advise him to make sure that each injection site is at least 1 inch away from the previous site.
• Urge patient to discard used needles and syringes in a puncture-resistant container and not to reuse them. Instruct him to return container to prescriber for disposal.
• Review evidence of allergic reaction, including rash and shortness of breath.
• Urge patient to immediately report signs of infection, such as cough, fever, chills, dyspnea, or headache, to prescriber.

anidulafungin
Eraxis

Class and Category
Chemical class: Semisynthetic echinocandin
Therapeutic class: Antifungal
Pregnancy category: B

Indications and Dosages
➤ *To treat Candidemia and other forms of Candida infections (intra-abdominal abscess and peritonitis)*
I.V. INFUSION
➤ *To treat candidemia, intra-abdominal, or peritoneal candidiasis*
Adults. 200 mg on day 1, followed by 100 mg daily and continued for at least 14 days following last positive culture.
➤ *To treat esophageal candidiasis*
I.V. INFUSION
Adults. 100 mg on day 1, followed by 50 mg daily and continued for at least 7 days following resolution of symptoms.

Mechanism of Action
Inhibits glucan synthase, an enzyme present in fungal cells. This results in inhibition of the formation of an essential D-glucan component of the fungal cell wall, thereby eliminating the fungal infection.

Incompatibilities
Use with other intravenous substances, additives, or medications other than 5%

Dextrose Injection and normal saline because compatibility is unknown.

Contraindications

Hypersensitivity to anidulafungin, its components, or other echinocandins

Adverse Reactions

CNS: Confusion, depression, dizziness, fever, headache, insomnia, rigors, seizures
CV: Atrial fibrillation, chest pain, deep vein thrombosis, hypertension, hypotension, peripheral edema, QT prolongation, right bundle branch block, sinus arrhythmia, superficial thrombophlebitis, ventricular extrasystoles
EENT: Blurred vision, eye pain, oral candidiasis, visual disturbance
ENDO: Hot flashes, hyperglycemia, hypoglycemia
GI: Abdominal pain, cholestasis, constipation, diarrhea, dyspepsia, elevated liver enzymes, hepatic necrosis, nausea, vomiting
GU: Elevated blood creatinine levels, UTI
HEME: Anemia, coagulopathy, leukocytosis, prolonged prothrombin time, thrombocytopenia
MS: Back pain
RESP: Bronchospasm, cough, dyspnea, pleural effusion, pneumonia, respiratory distress
SKIN: Diaphoresis, erythema, flushing, pruritus, rash, ulceration, urticaria
Other: Anaphylaxis, angioedema, bacteremia, clostridial infection, dehydration, hyperkalemia, hypokalemia, hypomagnesemia, infusion -related reactions, multi-organ failure, sepsis, systemic *Candida* infection in the arm used for infusion

Nursing Considerations

• Reconstitute each 50-mg vial with 15 ml of sterile water for injection and each 100-mg vial with 30 ml of sterile water for injection to provide a concentration of 3.33 mg/ml. The reconstituted solution can be stored for up to 24 hours at temperatures up to 77° F (25° C) prior to dilution into the infusion solution.
• Transfer the contents of the reconstituted vial(s) aseptically into the appropriately sized IV bag or bottle containing either 5% Dextrose Injection or normal saline following the manufacturer guidelines for the amount of infusion volume to use.

• Infuse at 1.4 ml/min (which is equivalent to 1.1 mg/min). Do not infuse at a higher rate because infusion-related adverse reactions that are possibly histamine-mediated may occur. If total infusion volume is 65 ml, infuse at least over 45 minutes; if total infusion volume is 130 ml, infuse over at least 90 minutes; and, if total infusion volume is 260 ml, infuse over at least 180 min. The infusion solution may be stored up to 48 hours at temperatures up to 77° F (25° C).
• Monitor patient's liver function and enzyme levels closely during anidulafungin therapy because significant hepatic dysfunction, hepatitis, or hepatic failure have been reported, although a causal relationship has not been established. If patient begins to complain of fatigue and shows signs of jaundice or the liver enzymes become abnormal, notify prescriber, as drug may be discontinued.
WARNING Monitor patient closely for hypersensitivity reactions that could lead to anaphylactic reactions, including shock. If present, withhold drug, notify prescriber, and be prepared to provide emergency treatment.

PATIENT TEACHING

• Instruct patient to promptly report any hypersensitivity reaction such as flushing, hives, itching, rash, difficulty breathing, or dizziness.
• Advise patient to comply with blood tests that may be ordered to monitor reaction to anidulafungin.
• Tell women of childbearing age that anidulafungin has not been studied in pregnant women or nursing mothers. If pregnancy is suspected or confirmed, or patient is planning to breastfeed, advise patient to alert prescriber.

anisindione
Miradon

Class and Category

Chemical class: Indanedione derivative
Therapeutic class: Anticoagulant
Pregnancy category: X

Indications and Dosages

➤ *To prevent and treat venous thrombosis, atrial fibrillation with embolization, and pulmonary embolism; as adjunct to treat coronary artery occlusion, usually in patients who can't tolerate Coumadin anticoagulant*

TABLETS

Adults. *Initial:* 300 mg on day 1; then 200 mg on day 2, and 100 mg on day 3. *Maintenance:* 25 to 250 mg daily.

Route	Onset	Peak	Duration
P.O.	In 6 hr	48–72 hr	1–3 days

Mechanism of Action

Interferes with the liver's ability to synthesize vitamin K–dependent clotting factors, which results in the depletion of clotting factors II (prothrombin), VII, IX, and X. By depleting levels of vitamin K–dependent clotting factors that are needed to form a stable fibrin clot, anisindione interferes with the clotting cascade and prevents coagulation.

Contraindications

Ascorbic acid deficiency; blood dyscrasias; continuous small-intestine drainage tube; diverticulitis; emaciation; GI, GU, or respiratory tract bleeding; hemophilia; hemorrhagic tendency; history of warfarin-induced necrosis; hypersensitivity to anisindione or its components; leukemia; major recent surgery; malnutrition; pericardial effusion; pericarditis; polyarthritis; pregnancy; prostatectomy; recent spinal puncture, percutaneous invasive procedure, diagnostic testing, or insertion of intrauterine device; recent or possible CNS or eye surgery; severe renal or hepatic disease; severe uncontrolled diabetes; severe uncontrolled malignant hypertension; subacute bacterial endocarditis; thrombocytopenic purpura; visceral carcinomas; ulcerative colitis

Interaction

DRUGS

abciximab, acetaminophen, allopurinol, alteplase, amiodarone, amitriptyline, amoxapine, androgens, aspirin, beta blockers, cephalosporins, chloral hydrate, chloramphenicol, chlorpropamide, cimetidine, cisapride, clofibrate, clomipramine, corticosteroids, co-trimoxazole, cyclophosphamide, danazol, desipramine, dextrothyroxine, diclofenac, diflunisal, disulfiram, doxepin, erythromycin, etodolac, fluconazole, fluoxymesterone, fosphenytoin, gemfibrozil, glucagon, hydantoins, ifosfamide, influenza virus vaccines, imipramine, indomethacin, isoniazid, itraconazole, ketoconazole, ketorolac, lepirudin, loop diuretics, lovastatin, low–molecular-weight heparins, meclofenamate, mefenamic acid, methyltestosterone, metronidazole, miconazole, moricizine, nabumetone, naproxen, nalidixic acid, neomycin, nortriptyline, NSAIDs, omeprazole, oxandrolone, penicillins, phenylbutazones, phenytoin, piroxicam, propafenone, propoxyphene, protriptyline, quinidine, quinine, quinolones, reteplase, salicylates, stanazolol, streptokinase, sulfamethoxazole, sulfinpyrazone, sulindac, tamoxifen, testosterone, thioamines, thyroid hormones, tomentin, urokinase: Increased anticoagulant effects

aminoglutethimide, ascorbic acid, barbiturates, carbamazepine, cholestyramine, corticosteroids, dicloxacillin, estrogen, ethanol, ethchlorvynol, etretinate, glutethimide, griseofulvin, nafcillin, oral contraceptives, rifampin, spironolactone, sucralfate, thiazide diuretics, thiopurines, trazodone, vitamin K: Decreased anticoagulant effects

aminoglycosides, mineral oil, tetracycline, vitamin E: Interference with vitamin K, leading to increased anticoagulant effects

FOODS

enteral products and foods high in vitamin K, such as dark green leafy vegetables: Interference with anticoagulant effects

ACTIVITIES

alcohol use: Possibly increased or decreased anticoagulation

Adverse Reactions

CNS: Fever, headache
EENT: Blurred vision, mouth ulcers, pharyngitis
GI: Abdominal cramps, diarrhea, hepatic dysfunction, hepatitis, nausea, steatorrhea
GU: Albuminuria, anuria, priapism, red-orange urine, renal tubular necrosis
HEME: Agranulocytosis, anemia, atypical mononuclear cells, eosinophilia,

hemorrhage, leukocytosis, leukopenia, RBC aplasia, thrombocytopenia
SKIN: Alopecia, exfoliative dermatitis, jaundice, necrosis of the skin and tissues evidenced by gangrene and purple toes, urticaria

Nursing Considerations
• Watch for PT to become prolonged 6 hours after anisindione administration, although maximum therapeutic effects may take 48 to 72 hours to appear.

WARNING Watch for signs of over-anticoagulation, such as microscopic hematuria, excessive menstrual bleeding, melena, petechiae, and bleeding from superficial trauma, such as tooth brushing or shaving.
• Monitor INR, CBC, fecal occult blood test, and urinalysis results for signs of overanticoagulation.

PATIENT TEACHING
• Advise patient to avoid alcohol, salicylates, and drastic changes in his intake of vitamin K–rich food.
• Instruct patient to promptly report pregnancy to prescriber.
• Provide patient with a list of foods rich in vitamin K. Advise him to eat consistent daily amounts of vitamin K.
• Urge patient to consult prescriber before having dental work or elective surgery.
• Tell patient to immediately report unusual bleeding, bruising, red or red-orange urine, red or tarry black stools, diarrhea, bleeding from gums or nose, or excessive bleeding from minor cuts or scratches.

---

anistreplase
(anisoylated plasminogen-streptokinase activator complex)
Eminase

Class and Category
Chemical class: p-Anisoylated derivative of the Lys-plasminogen-streptokinase activator complex
Therapeutic class: Thrombolytic enzyme
Pregnancy category: C

Indications and Dosages
➤ *To treat acute MI, lyse thrombi that are obstructing coronary arteries, reduce infarct size, improve ventricular function after acute MI, reduce mortality from acute MI*
I.V. INFUSION
Adults. 30 units injected over 2 to 5 min.

Route	Onset	Peak	Duration
I.V.	Immediate	20 min–2 hr	4–6 hr

Mechanism of Action
Indirectly promotes conversion of plasminogen to plasmin, an enzyme that breaks down fibrin clots, fibrinogen, and other plasma proteins, including procoagulant factors V and VIII.

Incompatibilities
Don't add other drugs to anistreplase solution or infuse other drugs through same I.V. line.

Contraindications
Active internal bleeding, arteriovenous malformation or aneurysm, bleeding diathesis, history of stroke, hypersensitivity to anistreplase or streptokinase, intracranial neoplasm, intracranial or intraspinal surgery or trauma within past 2 months, severe uncontrolled hypertension

Interaction
DRUGS
aspirin, dipyridamole, and other drugs that alter platelet function; heparin; vitamin K antagonists: Possibly increased risk of bleeding if administered before anistreplase

Adverse Reactions
CNS: Dizziness, fever, headache, intracranial hemorrhage
CV: Ankle edema, arrhythmias (especially accelerated idioventricular rhythm, conduction disorders, premature ventricular beats, sinus bradycardia, ventricular fibrillation, ventricular tachycardia), hypotension, vasculitis
EENT: Epistaxis
GI: Abdominal pain or swelling, constipation, GI bleeding, nausea, vomiting
GU: Hematuria, proteinuria, vaginal bleeding
HEME: Bleeding tendency, eosinophilia, mild to severe hemorrhage

MS: Arthralgia, back pain, joint stiffness, myalgia
RESP: Bronchospasm, dyspnea, hemoptysis
SKIN: Flushing, pruritus, rash, urticaria
Other: Anaphylaxis (rare), angioedema

Nursing Considerations

• Use anistreplase cautiously in patients with acute pericarditis; cerebrovascular disease; hemorrhagic ophthalmic conditions; history of major surgery, GI or GU bleeding, or trauma within past 10 days; hypertension; mitral stenosis with atrial fibrillation; pregnancy; septic thrombophlebitis; severe hepatic or renal disease; or subacute bacterial endocarditis.
• Reconstitute anistreplase by slowly directing 5 ml of sterile water for injection USP or sodium chloride for injection against side of vial. Then gently roll vial to mix dry powder and fluid and minimize foaming. Don't shake vial. The resulting solution should be colorless to pale yellow and transparent.
• Before administering, inspect solution for particles and discoloration. If present, discard and reconstitute drug from a new vial. Then withdraw entire contents of vial. Don't dilute reconstituted solution further or add it to I.V. fluid. Don't add other drugs to vial or syringe that contains anistreplase. Discard drug if not given within 30 minutes after reconstitution.
• For maximum effectiveness, expect to administer anistreplase as soon as possible after onset of MI symptoms.
• Closely monitor all puncture sites, such as catheter insertion and needle puncture sites, for bleeding.
• Don't give I.M. injections, and avoid handling patient unnecessarily during anistreplase therapy. Perform venipuncture only when necessary.
• If an arterial puncture is needed after anistreplase administration, use an arm vessel that allows easy manual compression. Apply a pressure dressing afterward, and check puncture site often for bleeding.
• Use continuous cardiac monitoring because arrhythmias may occur during reperfusion. Keep antiarrhythmics on hand during anistreplase therapy, and manage arrhythmias using facility policy.
• Keep epinephrine nearby for anaphylaxis.

• Know that anistreplase may be less effective if given more than 5 days after anistreplase or streptokinase administration. This occurs because patient may have developed antistreptokinase antibodies, which makes him more resistant to the drug and drug therapy less effective. Elevated serum antistreptokinase antibody levels and reduced drug effectiveness can persist for 5 days to 12 months.
• Closely monitor blood coagulation test results. The drug markedly decreases plasminogen and fibrinogen levels and increases thrombin time, APTT, and PT.

PATIENT TEACHING
• Instruct patient to report adverse reactions immediately, especially bleeding, dizziness, and chest pain.

apixaban
Eliquis

Class and Category
Chemical class: Factor Xa inhibitor
Therapeutic class: Antithrombolytic
Pregnancy category: B

Indications and Dosages
➤ To reduce the risk of stroke and systemic embolism in patients with nonvalvular atrial fibrillation

TABLETS
Adults. 5 mg twice daily.
DOSAGE ADJUSTMENT For patients with at least 2 of the following characteristics: 80 years or older, body weight weight of 60 kg (132 lbs) or less, or a serum creatinine of 1.5 mg/ml or greater; dosage decreased to 2.5 mg twice daily. For patients receiving strong dual inhibitors of cytochrome P450 3A4 (CYP3A4) and P-glycoprotein (P-gp) such as clarithromycin, itraconazole, ketoconazole, or ritonavir, dosage decreased to 2.5 mg twice daily.
➤ *To prevent deep vein thrombosis following hip or knee replacement surgery*
TABLETS
Adults. *Initial:* 2.5 mg 12 to 24 hours after surgery, followed by 2.5 mg twice daily for 12 days following knee replacement and for 35 days following hip replacement.

Mechanism of Action

Inhibits free and clot-bound factor Xa and prothrombinase activity. Although apixaban has no direct effect on platelet aggregation, it does indirectly inhibit platelet aggregation induced by thrombin. By inhibiting factor Xa, apixaban decreases thrombin generation and thrombus development.

Contraindications

Active pathological bleeding, severe hypersensitivity to apixaban or its components

Interaction

DRUGS

antiplatelets, aspirin, NSAIDs (chronic use), fibrinolytics, heparin: Possibly increased risk of bleeding

strong dual inducers of CYP3A4 and P-gp such as carbamazepine, phenytoin, rifampin, St. John's wort: Decreased effectiveness of apixaban

strong dual inhibitors of CYP3A4 and P-gp such as clarithromycin, itraconazole, ketoconazole, ritonavir: Increased effects of apixaban

Adverse Reactions

CNS: Syncope
HEME: Excessive bleeding, including hemorrhage
SKIN: Rash
Other: Anaphylaxis, angioedema

Nursing Considerations

• Know that apixaban should not be given to patients with severe hepatic dysfunction.
• Crush tablet and suspend in 60 ml of 5% dextrose and water and immediately administer through a nasogastric tube for patients unable to swallow whole tablets. Be aware that crushed and suspended tablets swallowed by mouth are not recommended as effects are not known.
• Expect apixaban to be discontinued 48 hours before an invasive procedure or surgery if patient has a moderate or high risk of hemorrhage and 24 hours before an invasive procedure or surgery if patient has a mild risk of hemorrhage.
• Be aware that manufacturer guidelines should be followed when patient is switching from or to other anticoagulants. For example, when patient is switching from warfarin to apixaban therapy, expect

warfarin to be discontinued and apixaban started when the International Normalized Ratio (INR) is below 2. When switching from apixaban to warfarin, expect apixaban to be discontinued and both a parenteral anticoagulant and warfarin given at the time the next dose of apixaban would have been given. Then the parenteral anticoagulant is discontinued when INR reaches an acceptable range. When switching between apixaban and anticoagulants other than warfarin, expect to discontinue the one being taken and begin the other at the next scheduled dose.
• Be aware that if apixaban is discontinued prematurely and adequate alternative anticoagulation is not present, the risk of thrombosis increases.

WARNING Monitor patient closely for bleeding, as apixaban may cause life-threatening bleeding. Expect drug to be discontinued with active pathological hemorrhage because there is no antidote for apixaban.

PATIENT TEACHING

• Emphasize the importance of taking apixaban exactly as prescribed.
• Tell patient not to stop taking apixaban without first consulting prescriber.
• Advise patient to report any unusual bleeding or bruising to the prescriber. Inform patient that it may take longer for her to stop bleeding and to take bleeding precautions, such as avoiding the use of a razor and using a soft-bristle toothbrush.
• Tell patient to alert all prescribers to use of apixaban therapy before any invasive procedure, including dental work, is scheduled.
• Advise female patient to notify prescriber immediately if pregnancy is suspected or known.

apomorphine hydrochloride

Apokyn

Class and Category

Chemical class: Nonergoline dopamine agonist

Therapeutic class: Hypomobilic antiparkinsonian
Pregnancy category: C

Indications and Dosages

➤ *To treat hypomobility "off" episodes (end-of-dose wearing off and unpredictable on/off episodes) in advanced Parkinson's disease*

SUBCUTANEOUS INJECTION

Adults. *Initial:* 0.2 ml (2 mg) as needed, adjusted as needed in 0.1-ml (1-mg) increments every few days. *Maximum:* 0.6 ml (6 mg).

DOSAGE ADJUSTMENT For patients who tolerate 0.2 ml (2 mg) but have no response, a 0.4-ml (4-mg) dose may be given under medical supervision, with standing and supine blood pressure checked every 20 min for 1 hr at the next observed "off" period, as long as it is at least 2 hr after the initial 0.2-ml (2-mg) test dose. If tolerated, a dose 0.1 ml (1 mg) lower may be given p.r.n. and increased in 0.1-ml (1-mg) increments every few days as needed to a maximum dose of 0.6 ml (6 mg). If patient doesn't tolerate a 0.4-ml (4-mg) test dose, a 0.3-ml (3-mg) test dose may be given under medical supervision, with standing and supine blood pressure checked every 20 min for 1 hr at the next observed "off" period, as long as it is at least 2 hr after the initial 0.4-ml (4-mg) test dose. If tolerated, a 0.2-ml (2-mg) dose can be started p.r.n. and increased to no more than 0.3 ml (3 mg) if needed after a few days. For patients with mild to moderate renal impairment, the initial dose should be reduced to 0.1 ml (1 mg).

Route	Onset	Peak	Duration
SubQ	10–60 min	Unknown	Unknown

Mechanism of Action

May stimulate postsynaptic dopamine D_2 receptors in the caudate-putamen of the brain. As a result, apomorphine improves motor function and activity levels in patients with Parkinson's disease.

Contraindications

Concurrent use of 5-HT_3 antagonists, such as alosetron, dolasetron, granisetron, ondansetron, and palonosetron; hypersensitivity to apomorphine or its components, including sodium metabisulfite

Interaction

DRUGS

5-HT_3 *antagonists:* Increased risk of profound hypotension and loss of consciousness
antihypertensives, vasodilators: Increased risk of serious adverse reactions, such as hypotension, MI, and bone or joint injuries
dopamine antagonists (such as butyrophenones, metoclopramide, phenothiazines, thioxanthenes): Decreased apomorphine effectiveness
drugs that prolong QT interval: Increased risk of torsades de pointes
entacapone, tolcapone: Increased risk of tachycardia, hypertension, and arrhythmias

ACTIVITIES

alcohol use: Increased risk of hypotension

Adverse Reactions

CNS: Aggravated Parkinson's disease, anxiety, confusion, depression, dizziness, drowsiness, dyskinesia, euphoria, fatigue, hallucinations, headache, insomnia, psychotic-like behavior, somnolence, weakness, yawning
CV: Angina, chest pain, congestive heart failure, edema, MI, orthostatic hypotension, prolonged QT interval
EENT: Rhinorrhea
GI: Constipation, diarrhea, nausea, vomiting
GU: UTI
MS: Arthralgia, back or limb pain
RESP: Dyspnea, pneumonia, tachypnea
SKIN: Contact dermatitis, diaphoresis, ecchymosis, flushing, pallor
Other: Dehydration; injection-site bruising, granuloma, or pruritus; intense urges to perform certain activities, such as gambling and sexual acts

Nursing Considerations

• Be aware that apomorphine therapy is usually not recommended in a patient with a major psychotic disorder because of the risk of exacerbating psychosis.
• Use apomorphine cautiously in patients with hepatic or renal insufficiency.
• An antiemetic, such as trimethobenzamide 300 mg three times daily, should be started 3 days before apomorphine starts and continue for at least the first 2 months of therapy. Apomorphine may cause severe nausea and vomiting, even with an antiemetic.

• Monitor patient's blood pressure closely because drug can cause severe orthostatic hypotension.
• Give a 0.2-ml (2-mg) test dose of apomorphine, as prescribed, and then check patient's supine and standing blood pressure 20, 40, and 60 minutes later.
• Monitor patient closely if he has an increased risk of prolonged QT interval, as from hypokalemia, hypomagnesemia, bradycardia, use of certain drugs, or genetic predisposition. QT-interval prolongation may lead to torsades de pointes.
• Monitor patient for evidence of apomorphine abuse. Although rare, drug may cause psychosexual stimulation and increased libido, which may cause patient to use apomorphine more often than needed for reducing Parkinson's disease symptoms.
• Assess patient regularly for skin changes because melanoma risk is higher in those with Parkinson's disease. It isn't clear whether the risk is increased by the disease or by its treatment.

PATIENT TEACHING
• Explain that an antiemetic will be prescribed starting 3 days before first apomorphine dose. Urge patient to take the antiemetic exactly as prescribed. Explain that it will be needed for 2 months or longer during apomorphine therapy.
• Explain that a test dose will determine response and drug's effects on blood pressure before patient goes home with drug.
• Teach patient how to use dosing pen and how to give drug subcutaneously.
• Emphasize that apomorphine doses are expressed as milliliters, not milligrams. Tell patient to draw up each dose carefully to reduce the chance of dosage error.
• Instruct patient to rotate injection sites in a systematic manner.
• Stress importance of taking apomorphine only as prescribed because serious adverse reactions may occur.
• Advise patient to avoid hazardous activities until drug's CNS effects are known. In particular, caution patient that apomorphine increases the risk of falling asleep suddenly, without feeling sleepy.

• Urge patient to have regular skin examinations by a dermatologist or other qualified health professional.
• Instruct patient to notify prescriber about intense urges, such as for gambling or sex, because dosage may need to be reduced or drug discontinued.
• Advise patient to report immediately any psychotic-like behavior, such as seeing or hearing things that are not real, confusion, excessive suspicion, aggressive behavior, agitation, believing things that are not real, or disorganized thinking.

aprepitant
Emend

fosaprepitant dimeglumine
Emend for Injection

Class and Category
Chemical class: Substance P/neurokinin 1 (NK1) receptor antagonist
Therapeutic class: Antiemetic
Pregnancy category: B

Indications and Dosages
➤ *To prevent acute and delayed nausea and vomiting associated with highly emetogenic chemotherapy, including high-dose cisplatin*
CAPSULES
Adults. 125 mg 1 hr before chemotherapy treatment, followed by 80 mg daily in morning on next 2 days.
I.V. INFUSION
Adults. 115 mg 30 min before chemotherapy begins (day 1 only).
➤ *To prevent postoperative nausea and vomiting*
CAPSULES
Adults. 40 mg within 3 hr before induction of anesthesia

Route	Onset	Peak	Duration
P.O., I.V.	Unknown	4 hr	Unknown

Mechanism of Action
Crosses the blood–brain barrier to occupy brain NK1 receptors, which prevents nerve

transmission of signals that cause nausea and vomiting.

Contraindications
Hypersensitivity to aprepitant, polysorbate 80, or their components; use of astemizole, cisapride, pimozide, or terfenadine

Interaction
DRUGS
carbamazepine, phenytoin, rifampin: Possibly decreased blood aprepitant level
corticosteroids: Increased blood corticosteroid level
CYP2C9 metabolizers (such as phenytoin, tolbutamide, and warfarin): Decreased blood level and effectiveness of CYP2C9 metabolizers
CYP3A4 inhibitors (such as clarithromycin, diltiazem, itraconazole, ketoconazole, nefazodone, nelfinavir, and troleandomycin): Increased blood aprepitant level
CYP3A4 substrates (such as astemizole, benzodiazepines, cisapride, docetaxel, etoposide, imatinib, irinotecan, paclitaxel, pimozide, terfenadine, vinblastine, vincristine, and vinorelbine): Increased level of CYP3A4 substrates, resulting in possibly serious or life-threatening adverse reactions
ifosfamide: Increased risk of neurotoxicity and possibly other serious or life-threatening adverse reactions
oral contraceptives: Possibly decreased effectiveness of oral contraceptives
paroxetine: Possibly decreased blood level of both drugs

Adverse Reactions
CNS: Anxiety, asthenia, confusion, depression, dizziness, fatigue, fever, headache, insomnia, malaise, peripheral or sensory neuropathy, rigors, somnolence, tremor
CV: Deep vein thrombosis, edema, hypertension, hypotension, myocardial infarction, palpitations, tachycardia
EENT: Conjunctivitis, dry mouth, increased salivation, mucous membrane alteration, nasal discharge, oral candidiasis, pharyngitis, stomatitis, taste perversion, tinnitus, vocal disturbance
ENDO: Hot flashes, hyperglycemia
GI: Abdominal pain, anorexia, constipation, diarrhea, dysphagia, elevated liver function test results, epigastric discomfort, flatulence, gastritis, gastroesophageal reflux, heartburn, hiccups, nausea, obstipation, vomiting
GU: Dysuria, elevated BUN and serum creatinine levels, hematuria, leukocyturia, renal insufficiency, UTI
HEME: Anemia, febrile neutropenia, leukocytosis, thrombocytopenia
MS: Arthralgia, back pain, muscle weakness, myalgia, pelvic pain
RESP: Cough, dyspnea, non–small-cell lung carcinoma, pneumonitis, pulmonary embolism, respiratory insufficiency, respiratory tract infection
SKIN: Acne, alopecia, diaphoresis, flushing, pruritus, rash, Stevens-Johnson syndrome, urticaria
Other: Anaphylaxis, angioedema, candidiasis, dehydration, herpes simplex, hypokalemia, hyponatremia, infusion-site pain or induration, malignant neoplasm, septic shock, weight loss

Nursing Considerations
• Use caution when giving aprepitant to patients with severe hepatic insufficiency because drug's effects on such patients aren't known.
• For maximum antiemetic effects, expect to administer aprepitant with dexamethasone and a 5-HT$_3$ antagonist, such as dolasetron, granisetron, or ondansetron.
• Drug is given intravenously only as the first dose 30 minutes before chemotherapy. Later doses are given orally.
• To reconstitute parental aprepitant, inject 5 ml normal saline for injection along vial wall to prevent foaming. Swirl vial gently. Withdraw contents from vial and add to an infusion bag containing 110 ml normal saline solution. Gently invert the bag two or three times. Administer over 15 minutes. Reconstituted solution may be stored at room temperature for 24 hours.
PATIENT TEACHING
• Instruct patient to take 125-mg dose of oral aprepitant 1 hour before chemo-therapy, 80-mg dose in the morning for 2 days after chemotherapy, or 40-mg dose within 3 hours before induction of anesthesia.
• Tell female patients taking oral contraceptives to use an alternative or

backup method of contraception during aprepitant therapy and for 1 month after last dose because drug reduces effectiveness of oral contraceptives.
• Tell patient taking warfarin to have clotting status monitored closely for 2 weeks after first aprepitant dose, especially every 7 to 10 days during each chemotherapy cycle in which the drug is used.
• Caution patient to inform prescriber of any drugs he's taking, including OTC drugs and herbal preparations, because they may interact with aprepitant.

arformoterol
Brovana

Class and Category
Chemical class: Selective beta2-adrenergic agonist, sympathomimetic
Therapeutic class: Bronchodilator
Pregnancy category: C

Indications and Dosages
➤ *To provide maintenance treatment of bronchoconstriction in patients with COPD, including chronic bronchitis and emphysema*
INHALATION SOLUTION
Adults. 15 mcg (contents of one 2-ml vial) twice daily (morning and evening) via nebulization. Do not exceed 30 mcg daily.

Mechanism of Action
Attaches to $beta_2$ receptors on bronchial cell membranes, stimulating the intracellular enzyme adenylate cyclase to convert adenosine triphosphate to cyclic adenosine monophosphate (cAMP). The resulting increase in intracellular cAMP level relaxes bronchial smooth-muscle cells, stabilizes mast cells, and inhibits histamine release.

Contraindications
Hypersensitivity to arformoterol, racemic formoterol, or its components; acute bronchospasm; symptoms of COPD; use to treat asthma without use of a long-term asthma control medication

Interaction
DRUGS
beta blockers: Decreased effectiveness of either drug
corticosteroids, methylxanthines such as aminophylline or theophylline, non-potassium-sparing (such as loop and thiazide) diuretics: Increased risk of hypokalemia
drugs known to prolong the QT interval, MAO inhibitors, tricyclic antidepressants: Increased risk of life-threatening ventricular arrhythmias
thyroid hormones: Increased risk of coronary insufficiency

Adverse Reactions
CNS: Agitation, asthenia, circumoral paresthesia, fatigue, fever, headache, hypokinesia, insomnia, malaise, nervousness, paralysis, somnolence, stroke, tremor
CV: Angina, arrhythmias, atrial flutter, chest pain, congestive heart failure, dizziness, heart block, hyperlipemia, hypertension, hypertension, MI, palpitations, peripheral edema, prolonged QT interval
EENT: Abnormal vision, dry mouth, glaucoma, herpes simplex or zoster, oral candidiasis, rectal hemorrhage, sinusitis, voice alteration
ENDO: Hyperglycemia, hypoglycemia
GI: Constipation, diarrhea, gastritis, melena, nausea, pelvic pain, retroperitoneal hemorrhage, vomiting
GU: Cystitis, hematuria, nocturia, PSA elevation, pyuria, renal calculi
HEME: Leukocytosis
MS: Arthralgia, arthritis, back pain, leg or muscle cramps, neck rigidity
RESP: Bronchitis, bronchospasm, COPD, dyspnea, pulmonary congestion
SKIN: Discoloration, dryness, hypertrophy, photosensitivity, rash, urticaria
Other: Anaphylaxis, angioedema, dehydration, flulike syndrome, gout, hyperkalemia, hypokalemia, metabolic acidosis

Nursing Considerations
• Know that arformoterol should not be initiated in patients with acutely deteriorating COPD, which may be a life-threatening condition because arformoterol's onset of action is too prolonged.

- Use cautiously in patients with cardiovascular disorders, especially insufficiency; cardiac arrhythmias, and hypertension; convulsive disorders; thyrotoxicosis; and unusual sensitivity to sympathomimetic amines because arformoterol may cause significant adverse effects.
- Arformoterol shouldn't be used to relieve bronchospasm quickly because of its prolonged onset of action. Patients already taking the drug twice daily shouldn't take additional doses for exercise-induced bronchospasm.
- Arformoterol shouldn't be used with other inhaled, long-acting beta$_2$-agonists or with other medications containing long-acting beta$_2$-agonists.

WARNING Asthma-related deaths have increased in patients receiving salmeterol, a drug in the same class as arformoterol. Be aware that use of long-acting beta$_2$-adrenergic agonists, such as arformoterol, is contraindicated in patients with asthma without the use of a long-term asthma control medication, such as an inhaled corticosteroid. Monitor patient closely, and notify prescriber immediately of any changes in patient's respiratory status.

- Watch for arrhythmias and changes in heart rate or blood pressure after use in patients with cardiovascular disorders because of drug's beta-adrenergic effects.

WARNING Stop arformoterol immediately and notify prescriber if patient develops paradoxical bronchospasm or an allergic reaction.

- Monitor patient's blood glucose level, especially if diabetic, and plasma potassium level, as ordered, because arformoterol may cause significant changes.

PATIENT TEACHING

- Advise patient to take doses 12 hours apart, morning and evening, for optimum effect. Caution against using drug more than every 12 hours.
- Teach patient to self-administer drug with a standard jet nebulizer connected to an air compressor and to use vial immediately after removing from foil package.
- Caution patient not to swallow solution.

- Tell patient to return unused vials to pouch and store arformoterol in the refrigerator.
- Instruct patient taking inhaled, short-acting beta$_2$-agonists on a regular basis to discontinue regular use of these drugs and to use them only for symptomatic relief of acute respiratory symptoms.
- Instruct patient to notify prescriber if he needs four or more oral inhalations of rapid-acting inhaled bronchodilator a day for 2 or more consecutive days, or if he uses more than one canister of rapid-acting bronchodilator in an 8-week period.
- Emphasize importance of seeking emergency medical attention immediately if his breathing problems worsen or if he used his rescue inhaler but it did not relieve his breathing problem.

argatroban
Acova

Class and Category
Chemical class: N2-substituted derivative of arginine
Therapeutic class: Anticoagulant
Pregnancy category: B

Indications and Dosages
➤ *To prevent or treat thrombosis in patients with heparin-induced thrombocytopenia (HIT)*

I.V. INFUSION
Adults. 2 mcg/kg/min as a continuous infusion. *Maximum:* 10 mcg/kg/min.
DOSAGE ADJUSTMENT Dosage adjusted as prescribed to maintain patient's APTT at 1.5 to 3 times the initial baseline value, not to exceed 100 sec. Initial dosage reduced to 0.5 mcg/kg/min for patients with moderate hepatic impairment.

➤ *To prevent or treat thrombosis in patients with or at risk for HIT when undergoing percutaneous coronary intervention (PCI)*

I.V. INFUSION
Adults. *Initial:* 350 mcg/kg over 3 to 5 min followed by continuous infusion of 25 mcg/kg/min.
DOSAGE ADJUSTMENT Dosage adjusted as prescribed to keep activated clotting time

(ACT) at 300 to 450 sec. If ACT is less than 300 sec, give additional I.V. bolus dose of 150 mcg/kg and increase infusion to 30 mcg/kg/min; if ACT exceeds 450 sec, reduce dosage to 15 mcg/kg/min. For dissection, impending abrupt closure, thrombus formation during PCI, or inability to reach or keep ACT above 300 sec, give additional bolus dose of 150 mcg/kg and increase infusion to 40 mcg/kg/min.

Route	Onset	Peak	Duration
I.V.	Immediate	3–4 hr	Unknown

Mechanism of Action

Forms a tight bond with thrombin, neutralizing this enzyme's actions, even when the enzyme is trapped within clots. Thrombin causes fibrinogen to convert to fibrin, which is essential for clot formation.

Contraindications

Active major bleeding, hypersensitivity to argatroban or its components

Interaction

DRUGS

alteplase, antineoplastic drugs, antiplatelets, antithymocyte globulin, heparin, NSAIDs, reteplase, salicylates, streptokinase, strontium chloride Sr 89, warfarin: Increased risk of bleeding

porfimer: Possibly decreased efficacy of porfimer photodynamic therapy

Adverse Reactions

CNS: Cerebrovascular bleeding, fever, headache
CV: Atrial fibrillation, cardiac arrest, hypotension, unstable angina, ventricular tachycardia
GI: Abdominal pain, anorexia, diarrhea, elevated liver function test results, GI bleeding, melena, nausea, vomiting
GU: Elevated BUN and serum creatinine levels, hematuria (microscopic), UTI
HEME: Hypoprothrombinemia, unusual bleeding or bruising
RESP: Cough, dyspnea, hemoptysis, pneumonia
SKIN: Bleeding at puncture site, rash
Other: Sepsis

Nursing Considerations

WARNING Argatroban isn't recommended for PCI patients with significant hepatic disease or AST/ALT levels three times or more the upper limits of normal.

• Reconstitute drug to 1 mg/ml before giving.
• Protect solution from direct sunlight.

WARNING Monitor patients with thrombocytopenia or those receiving daily doses of salicylates greater than 6 g for signs and symptoms of bleeding; these patients are at increased risk of bleeding from hypoprothrombinemia.

WARNING Expect to perform blood coagulation tests before and 2 hours after start of therapy because of the major risk of bleeding associated with argatroban. Be aware that coagulopathy must be ruled out before therapy starts. When giving drug to a patient undergoing PCI, expect to check ACT 5 to 10 minutes after each bolus and each infusion rate change and every 20 to 30 minutes during the PCI.

• Monitor the following patients for signs and symptoms of bleeding because they're at increased risk during argatroban therapy: women with active menstruation; patients with vascular or organ abnormalities, such as severe uncontrolled hypertension, advanced renal disease, infective endocarditis, dissecting aortic aneurysm, diverticulitis, hemophilia, hepatic disease (especially if associated with a deficiency of vitamin K–dependent clotting factors), inflammatory bowel disease, or peptic ulcer disease; and those who have recently had a stroke, major surgery (including eye, brain, or spinal cord surgery), large vessel puncture or organ biopsy, lumbar puncture, spinal anesthesia, or major bleeding (including intracranial, GI, intraocular, retro-peritoneal, or pulmonary bleeding).
• Whenever possible, avoid I.M. injections in patients receiving argatroban to decrease the risk of bleeding.
• Thrombin times may not be helpful for monitoring argatroban activity because the drug affects all thrombin-dependent coagulation tests.
• Expect dosage to be tapered before stopping to prevent the risk of rebound hypercoagulopathy; drug's effects last only a short time once drug is discontinued.

PATIENT TEACHING

• Inform patient that argatroban is a blood thinner that's given in the hospital by infusion into a vein. If he needs long-term anticoagulation, he'll be switched to another drug before discharge.

• Advise patient to report immediately any unusual or unexplained bleeding, such as blood in urine, easy bruising, nosebleeds, tarry stools, and vaginal bleeding.

• Instruct patient to avoid injury while receiving argatroban. For example, suggest that he brush his teeth gently, using a soft-bristled toothbrush, and take special care when flossing.

aripiprazole

Abilify, Abilify Discmelt, Abilify Maintena

Class and Category

Chemical class: Dihydrocarbostyril
Therapeutic class: Atypical antipsychotic
Pregnancy category: C

Indications and Dosages

➤ *To treat acute schizophrenia; to maintain stability in patients with schizophrenia*
SOLUTION, ORALLY DISINTEGRATING TABLETS, TABLETS
Adults. *Initial:* 10 or 15 mg daily. Increased to 30 mg daily, as needed, with dosage adjustments at 2-wk intervals. *Maintenance:* 15 mg daily.
I.M. INJECTION (ABILIFY MAINTENA)
Adults. 400 mg monthly (no sooner than 26 days after last dose).
➤ *To treat acute manic and mixed episodes in bipolar I disorder with or without psychotic features; to maintain stability in patients with bipolar I disorder; as adjunct with lithium or valproate in patients with bipolar I disorder*
ORAL SOLUTION, ORALLY DISINTEGRATING TABLETS, TABLETS
Adults. *Initial:* 15 mg daily, increased to 30 mg daily, as needed. *Maintenance:* 15 to 30 mg daily. *Maximum:* 30 mg daily.
Children ages 10 to 17. *Initial:* 2 mg daily, increased after 2 days to 5 mg daily and then after 2 days to 10 mg daily. Increased in 5-mg increments, as needed, at 2-wk intervals.

Maintenance: Lowest dose possible to maintain remission. *Maximum:* 30 mg daily.
➤ *As adjunct to treat depression in patients already taking an antidepressant*
ORAL SOLUTION, ORALLY DISINTEGRATING TABLETS, TABLETS
Adults. *Initial:* 2 to 5 mg daily, with dosage increased to 5 mg daily at 1-wk intervals.
➤ *To treat agitation in schizophrenia or bipolar mania*
I.M. INJECTION (ABILIFY)
Adults. *Initial:* Depending on severity of agitation, 5.25 to 15 mg. May be repeated 2 or more hr later, as needed. *Maximum:* 30 mg daily.
➤ *To treat irritability associated with autistic disorder*
ORAL SOLUTION, ORALLY DISINTEGRATING TABLETS, TABLETS
Children ages 10 to 17. *Initial:* 2 mg daily, with dosage increased after 1 wk to 5 mg daily and then after 1 wk to 10 mg daily and then after 1 wk to 15 mg daily, as needed.
➤ *To treat Tourette's disorder*
ORAL SOLUTION, ORALLY DISINTEGRATING TABLETS, TABLETS
Children ages 6 to 18 weighing 50 kg (110 lb) or more. *Initial:* 2 mg daily for 2 days, then 5 mg daily for 5 days, followed by dosage increased to 10 mg daily on day 8. Dosage increased 5 mg daily at weekly intervals, as needed, to control tics. *Maximum:* 20 mg daily.
Children age 6 to 18 weighing less than 50 kg (110 lb). *Initial:* 2 mg daily for 2 days, with dosage increased to 5 mg daily on day 3. Dosage increased gradually weekly, as needed, to control tics. *Maximum:* 10 mg daily
DOSAGE ADJUSTMENT Dosage reduced to half normal amount when given with clarithromycin, fluoxetine, itraconazole, ketoconazole, paroxetine, or quinidine, or in patients classified as CYP2D6 poor metabolizers. Dosage reduced to one-quarter normal amount when given along with a strong CYP3A4 inhibitor like ketoconazole or clarithromycin as well as a strong CYP2D6 such as fluoxetine, paroxetine, or quinidine, or when a strong CYP3A4 is given to a patient who is classified as a CYP3A4 poor metabolizer. Dosage doubled when given with carbamazepine.

Mechanism of Action

May produce antipsychotic effects through partial agonist and antagonist actions. Aripiprazole acts as a partial agonist at dopamine (especially D_2) receptors and serotonin (especially 5-HT_{1A}) receptors. The drug acts as an antagonist at 5-HT_{2A} serotonin receptor sites.

Contraindications

Breastfeeding, hypersensitivity to aripiprazole or its components

Interaction

DRUGS

anticholingerics: Increased risk for potentially fatal elevation of body temperature
carbamazepine and other CYP3A4 inducers: Possibly increased clearance and decreased blood level of aripiprazole
clarithromycin, fluoxetine, paroxetine, quinidine, and other CYP2D6 inhibitors; ketoconazole and other CYP3A4 inhibitors: Possibly inhibited aripiprazole elimination and increased blood level
CNS depressants: Increased CNS depression
ACTIVITIES
alcohol use: Increased CNS depression

Adverse Reactions

CNS: Abnormal gait, agitation, akathisia, anxiety, asthenia, cognitive and motor impairment, confusion, delusions, depression, dizziness, dream disturbances, dystonia, extrapyramidal reactions, fatigue, fever, hallucinations, headache, hostility, insomnia, intracranial hemorrhage, lethargy, light-headedness, mania, nervousness, neuroleptic malignant syndrome, paranoia, restlessness, schizophrenic reaction, seizures, somnolence, stroke (elderly), suicidal ideation, tardive dyskinesia, transient ischemic attack (elderly), tremor
CV: Arrhythmias, bradycardia, cardiopulmonary arrest, chest pain, circulatory collapse, deep vein thrombosis, elevated serum CK levels, heart failure, hyperlipidemia, hypertension, MI, orthostatic hypotension, peripheral edema, prolonged QT interval, tachycardia
EENT: Blurred vision, conjunctivitis, dry mouth, hepatitis, increased salivation, laryngospasm, nasopharyngitis, oropharyngeal spasm, pharyngitis, rhinitis, sinusitis
ENDO: Hyperglycemia, diabetes mellitus
GI: Abdominal discomfort, constipation, decreased appetite, diarrhea, difficulty swallowing, GI bleeding, indigestion, jaundice, nausea, vomiting
GU: Renal failure, urinary incontinence
HEME: Agranulocytosis, anemia, leukopenia, neutropenia, thrombocytopenia
MS: Arthralgia, elevated blood CK level, muscle spasms, musculoskeletal pain, myalgia, neck and limb rigidity, rhabdomyolysis
RESP: Apnea, aspiration, asthma, cough, dyspnea, pneumonia, pulmonary edema or embolism, respiratory failure
SKIN: Diaphoresis, dry skin, ecchymosis, pruritus, rash, ulceration, urticaria
Other: Anaphylaxis, angioedema, dehydration, flulike symptoms, heat stroke, weight gain

Nursing Considerations

• Aripiprazole shouldn't be used to treat dementia-related psychosis in the elderly because of an increased risk of death.
• Use cautiously in patients with CV disease, cerebrovascular disease, or conditions that would predispose them to hypotension. Also use cautiously in those with a history of seizures or with conditions that lower the seizure threshold, such as Alzheimer's disease.
• Use cautiously in elderly patients because of increased risk of serious adverse cerebrovascular effects, such as stroke and transient ischemic attack.
• Oral solution may be given on a milligram-per-milligram basis in place of tablets up to 25 mg. For example, if patient needs 30 mg of tablet and is switched to oral solution, expect to give 25 mg of solution.
• Be aware that for patients who have never taken aripiprazole, tolerability needs to be established with oral form prior to initiating Abilify Maintena therapy.
• Abilify Maintena comes in two types of kits: prefilled chamber syringe or single-use vials.
• To reconstitute Abilify Maintena lyophilized powder in prefilled dual-chamber syringe, push plunger rod

slightly to engage threads. Then rotate plunger rod until the rod stops rotating to release diluent. After plunger rod is at a complete stop, middle stopper will be at the indicator line. Vertically shake the syringe vigorously for 20 seconds until drug is uniformly milky white.

• To reconstitute Abilify Maintena using single-use vials, use the syringe with the pre-attached needle to withdraw the pre-determined volume from the vial of Sterile Water for Injection into the syringe. Slowly inject the Sterile Water for Injection into the vial containing the lyophilized powder. Withdraw air to equalize the pressure, then remove the needle from the vial. Engage the needle safety device by using the one-handed technique. Gently press the sheath against a flat surface until the needle is firmly engaged in the needle protection sheath and discard appropriately. Shake the vial vigorously for 30 seconds until the reconstituted suspension appears uniform. It should be opaque and milky-white in color. If the injection is not given immediately after reconstitution, keep the vial at room temperature and shake the vial vigorously for at least 60 seconds to re-suspend prior to administration. Do not store the reconstituted suspension in a syringe.

• To prepare Abilify Maintena prior to injection after reconstituting from a single-use vial, remove cover from the vial adapter package but do not remove the vial adapter from the package. Using the vial adapter package to handle the vial adapter, attach the prepackaged BD Luer-Lok syringe to the vial adapter. Use the syringe to remove the vial adapter from the package and discard the vial adapter package. Do not touch the spike tip of the adapter at any time. Determine the recommended volume for injection using the manufacturer chart for size vial being used and dosage prescribed. After wiping top of vial with a sterile alcohol swab, place and hold the vial of the reconstituted suspension on a hard surface. Attach the adapter-syringe assembly to the vial by holding the outside of the adapter and pushing the adapter's spike firmly through the rubber stopper until the adapter snaps

in place. Slowly withdraw the recom-mended volume from the vial into the syringe.

• Inject parenteral form slowly, deep into the gluteal muscle, and never I.V. or subcutaneously. Do not massage the injection site. Know that the parenteral form of Abilify and Abilify Maintena are NOT interchangeable. Abilify is a short-acting formulation, while Abilify Maintena is a long-acting formulation.

• Use the following guide for determining when to administer missed doses of the long-acting formulation, Abilify Maintena. If a second or third dose is missed and it's been more than 4 weeks but less than 5 weeks since the last injection, administer the injection as soon as possible. If more than 5 weeks have elapsed since the last injection, restart concomitant oral aripiprazole, as ordered, for 14 days with the next administered injection. If a fourth or subsequent doses are missed and it's been more than 4 weeks but less than 6 weeks since the last injection, administer the injection as soon as possible. If more than 6 weeks have elapsed since the last injection, restart concomitant oral aripiprazole for 14 days with the next administered injection.

• Monitor patient for difficulty swallowing or excessive somnolence, which could predispose to accidental injury or aspiration.

WARNING Aripiprazole rarely may cause neuroleptic malignant syndrome, tardive dyskinesia, and seizures. Monitor patient closely throughout therapy, and take safety precautions as needed.

• Watch patients closely (especially children, adolescents, and young adults) for suicidal tendencies, particularly when therapy starts and dosage changes, because depression may worsen temporarily during these times.

• Monitor patient's CBC, as ordered, because serious adverse hematologic reactions may occur, such as agranulocytosis, leukopenia, and neutropenia. Assess more often during first few months of therapy if patient has a history of drug-induced leukopenia or neutropenia or a significantly low WBC count. If abnormalities occur during therapy, watch for fever or other signs of

infection, notify prescriber and, if severe, expect drug to be stopped.
• Monitor patient's weight, blood glucose level, and lipid levels, as ordered, because atypical antipsychotic drugs such as aripiprazole may cause metabolic changes. If patient is already a diabetic, monitor blood glucose levels more closely.

PATIENT TEACHING
• Instruct patient prescribed orally disintegrating tablets to open the blister pack only when ready to take the tablet. Tell him to peel back the foil carefully and not to push tablet through the foil because doing so could damage the tablet. Tell him to place the tablet on his tongue without breaking it and let it dissolve. If needed, he may take a drink.
• Advise patient to get up slowly from a lying or sitting position during aripiprazole therapy to minimize orthostatic hypotension.
• Urge patient to avoid alcohol during aripiprazole therapy.
• Instruct patient to avoid hazardous activities until drug's effects are known.
• Urge patient to avoid activities that raise body temperature suddenly, such as strenuous exercise and exposure to extreme heat, and to compensate for situations that cause dehydration, such as vomiting or diarrhea.
• Instruct patient to inform all prescribers of any drugs he's taking, including OTC drugs, because of risk of interactions.
• Advise female patient of childbearing age to notify prescriber if she intends to become or suspects that she is pregnant during therapy.
• Instruct diabetic patient to monitor blood glucose levels closely, especially if taking the oral solution form because each milliliter of solution contains 400 mg of sucrose and 200 mg of fructose.
• Urge family or caregiver to watch patient closely for suicidal tendencies, especially when therapy starts or dosage changes, and particularly if patient is a child, teenager, or young adult.

armodafinil
Nuvigil

Class and Category
Chemical class: Diphenylmethyl sulfinyl-acetamide

Therapeutic class: CNS stimulant
Pregnancy category: C

Indications and Dosages
➤ *To treat narcolepsy or as adjunct to standard therapy for excessive daytime sleepiness in obstructive sleep apnea/ hypopnea syndrome*
TABLETS
Adults. 150 or 250 mg once daily in the morning.
➤ *To improve daytime wakefulness in patients with excessive sleepiness from circadian rhythm disruption (shift-work sleep disorder)*
TABLETS
Adults. 150 mg once daily about 1 hr before start of work shift.
DOSAGE ADJUSTMENT Decreased dosage recommended for patients who are elderly, have severe hepatic impairment, or take steroidal contraceptives.

Route	Onset	Peak	Duration
P.O.	Unknown	2 hr (fasting) 4–6 hr (with food)	Unknown

Mechanism of Action
May produce CNS-stimulant effects by binding to dopamine transporter in the brain and inhibiting dopamine reuptake in limbic regions. These actions increase alertness and reduce drowsiness and fatigue.

Contraindications
Hypersensitivity to armodafinil, modafinil, or their components

Interaction
DRUGS
amitriptyline, citalopram, clomipramine, diazepam, imipramine, propranolol, tolbutamide, topiramate: Possibly prolonged elimination time and increased blood levels of these drugs
barbiturates (such as phenobarbital, primidone), dexamethasone, rifabutin, rifampin: Possibly decreased blood level and effectiveness of armodafinil
carbamazepine: Possibly decreased armodafinil effectiveness and decreased blood carbamazepine level

cimetidine, clarithromycin, erythromycin, fluconazole, fluoxetine, fluvoxamine, itraconazole, ketoconazole, nefazodone, sertraline: Possibly inhibited metabolism, decreased clearance, and increased blood level of armodafinil
clozapine: Possibly increased levels of clozapine caused by decreased secondary hepatic metabolism
contraceptive-containing implants or devices: Possibly contraceptive failure
cyclosporine: Possibly decreased blood cyclosporine level and increased risk of organ transplant rejection
dextroamphetamine, methylphenidate: Possibly 1-hr delay in armodafinil absorption when these drugs are given together
fosphenytoin, mephenytoin, phenytoin: Possibly decreased effectiveness of armodafinil, increased blood phenytoin level, and increased risk of phenytoin toxicity
midazolam, triazolam: Possibly decreased effectiveness of triazolam or midazolam
oral contraceptives: Possibly decreased effectiveness of oral contraceptive
theophylline: Possibly decreased blood level and effectiveness of theophylline
warfarin: Possibly decreased warfarin metabolism and increased risk of bleeding

FOODS
alcohol use: Possibly adverse CNS effects
all foods: 2- to 4-hr delay for armodafinil to reach peak levels and possibly delayed onset of action
caffeine: Increased CNS stimulation
grapefruit juice: Possibly decreased armodafinil metabolism

Adverse Reactions

CNS: Agitation, anxiety, attention disturbance, depression, dizziness, drowsiness, excessive sleepiness, fatigue, fever, headache (including migraine), insomnia, irritability, nervousness, paresthesia, suicidal ideation, thirst, tremor
CV: Increased heart rate, palpitations
EENT: Dry mouth
GI: Abdominal pain (upper), anorexia, constipation, decreased appetite, diarrhea, dyspepsia, loose stools, nausea, vomiting
GU: Polyuria
RESP: Dyspnea

SKIN: Contact dermatitis, hyperhydrosis, rash
Other: Angioedema, flulike illness

Nursing Considerations

• Armodafinil shouldn't be given to patients with mitral valve prolapse syndrome or a history of left ventricular hypertrophy because drug may cause ischemic changes.
WARNING If patient has a history of alcoholism, stimulant abuse, or other substance abuse, ensure compliance with armodafinil therapy. Watch for signs of misuse or abuse, including frequent prescription refill requests, increased frequency of dosing, and drug-seeking behavior. Also watch for evidence of excessive armodafinil use, including agitation, anxiety, diarrhea, nausea, nervousness, palpitations, sleep disturbances, and tremor.
• Be aware that armodafinil, like other CNS stimulants, may alter mood, perception, thinking, judgment, feelings, and motor skills and may produce signs that patient needs sleep.
• If giving drug to patient with a history of psychosis, emotional instability, or psychological illness with psychotic features, be prepared for baseline behavioral assessment or frequent clinical observation.
• Stop drug at first sign of rash, and notify prescriber. Although rare, rash may indicate a potentially life-threatening event.
• Monitor patient for signs and symptoms of multisystem organ hypersensitivity, such as fever, rash, myocarditis, hepatitis, hematologic abnormalities, pruritus, asthenia, or any other serious abnormality because multi-organ hypersensitivity may vary in its presentation. While multisystem organ hypersensitivity has only occurred with modafinil, the possibility that it may occur with armodafinil cannot be ruled out because the two drugs are very closely related. Therefore, if suspected, notify prescriber immediately, expect to discontinue drug, and provide supportive care, as ordered.
• Watch closely for suicidal tendencies, especially in patients with a psychiatric history.

PATIENT TEACHING

- Inform patient that armodafinil can help, but not cure, narcolepsy and that drug's full effects may not be seen right away.
- Advise patient to avoid taking armodafinil within 2 hours of eating because food may delay time to peak drug effect and onset of action. If patient drinks grapefruit juice, encourage him to drink a consistent amount daily.
- Inform patient that drug can affect his concentration and ability to function and can hide signs of fatigue. Urge him not to drive or perform activities that require mental alertness until drug's full CNS effects are known.
- Because alcohol may decrease alertness, advise patient to avoid it with armodafinil.
- Encourage a regular sleeping pattern.
- Caution patient to avoid excessive intake of foods, beverages, and OTC drugs that contain caffeine because caffeine may lead to increased CNS stimulation.
- Advise patient to report the presence of a rash immediately to prescriber and to stop taking armodafinil. Also encourage patient to report any unusual or persistent signs and symptoms to prescriber.
- Inform woman that armodafinil can decrease effectiveness of certain contraceptives, including birth control pills and implantable hormonal contraceptives. If she uses such contraceptives, urge her to use an alternate birth control method during armodafinil therapy and for up to 1 month after it stops.
- Urge family or caregiver to watch patient closely for abnormal behaviors, including suicidal tendencies, especially if patient has a psychiatric history.
- Advise patient to keep follow-up appointments with prescriber so that her progress can be monitored.

asenapine

Saphris

Class and Category

Chemical: Dibenzo-oxepino pyrrole
Therapeutic: Second-generation antipsychotic, atypical antipsychotic
Pregnancy category: C

Indications and Dosages

➤ *To treat schizophrenia*
SUBLINGUAL TABLETS
Adults. *Initial:* 5 mg twice daily.
Maintenance: Dosage may be increased to 10 mg twice daily after 1 wk as needed and tolerated.
➤ *As adjunct therapy with lithium or valproate, to treat manic or mixed episodes associated with bipolar I disorder*
SUBLINGUAL TABLETS
Adults. *Initial:* 5 mg twice daily.
Maintenance: Dosage may be increased to 10 mg twice daily as needed and tolerated.
➤ *To treat manic or mixed episodes associated with bipolar I disorder*
SUBLINGUAL TABLETS
Adults. 10 mg twice daily.
DOSAGE ADJUSTMENT Dosage may be decreased to 5 mg twice daily if adverse reactions occur.

Route	Onset	Peak	Duration
P.O.	Unknown	30–90 min	Unknown

Mechanism of Action

May produce antipsychotic effects through antagonist actions at dopamine receptors, especially D_2, and serotonin receptors, especially $5\text{-}HT_{2A}$.

Contraindications

Hypersensitivity to asenapine or its components

Interaction

DRUGS
antihypertensives, CNS depressants: Possibly enhanced effects
class I A and III antiarrhythmics, gatifloxacin, moxifloxacin, other antipsychotic drugs: Increased risk of prolonged QT interval
paroxetine: Possibly increased paroxetine effect
ACTIVITIES
alcohol use: Possibly enhanced effect

Adverse Reactions

CNS: Akathisia, anxiety, depression, dizziness, dystonia, dyskinesia, extrapyramidal symptoms, fatigue, gait disturbance, hyperkinesias, insomnia, irritability, masked facies, parkinsonism,

seizures, somnolence, syncope, tardive dyskinesia, torticollis, tremor
CV: Hyperlipidemia, hypertension, orthostatic hypotension, prolonged QT interval
EENT: Sublingual application-site reactions such as blisters, inflammation, peeling, sloughing, or oral ulcers; blepharospasm; dry mouth; oral hypoesthesia or paraesthesia; salivary hypersecretion; toothache
ENDO: Hyperglycemia, diabetes melitus, hyperprolactinemia
GI: Constipation, dyspepsia, increased appetite, stomach discomfort, vomiting
HEME: Anemia, leukopenia, neutropenia, thrombocytopenia
MS: Arthralgia, extremity pain, muscle rigidity
Other: Anaphylaxis, angioedema, hyponatremia, weight gain

Nursing Considerations
• Asenapine should be avoided in patients with a history of cardiac arrhythmias; conditions that might prolong the QT interval, such as bradycardia, hypokalemia, or hypomagnesemia; or congenital QT-interval prolongation because of increased risk of torsades de pointes or sudden death.
• Asenapine shouldn't be used for dementia-related psychosis in elderly patients because of an increased risk of death.
• Use cautiously in patients with mild to moderate hepatic impairment. Asenapine isn't recommended in patients with severe hepatic impairment (Child-Pugh Class C).
• Use cautiously in patients with a history of seizures or who have conditions that may lower the seizure threshold, such as Alzheimer's dementia, because drug increases risk of seizures in these patients.
WARNING Monitor patient closely even with the first dose for life-threatening hypersensitivity reactions that may include anaphylaxis and angioedema.
• Monitor elderly patients with psychosis closely for adverse effects because asenapine drug exposure has been found to be higher in these patients than in younger adult patients.
• Monitor patient's weight, blood glucose level, and lipid levels, as ordered, because

atypical antipsychotic drugs such as asenapine may cause metabolic changes. If patient is already diabetic, monitor blood glucose levels more closely.
WARNING Asenapine rarely may cause neuroleptic malignant syndrome or tardive dyskinesia. Monitor patient closely throughout therapy, and take safety precautions as needed. Expect to stop drug if any of these adverse effects occur.
• Monitor patient's CBC regularly, as ordered. Notify prescriber of any change because drug may need to be stopped.
• Monitor patient for trouble swallowing or excessive somnolence, which could predispose him to injury or aspiration.
PATIENT TEACHING
• Tell patient to remove tablet from package only when ready to take it and to use dry hands. Tell him to firmly press and hold thumb button, and then pull out tablet pack from case. Then, he should peel back the colored tab, being careful not to push tablet through the tab because doing so could damage tablet. Instruct patient to place tablet under his tongue and let it dissolve completely. Tell him to then slide tablet pack back into case until it clicks.
• Caution patient not to crush, chew, or swallow tablets.
• Advise him not to eat or drink for at least 10 minutes after taking asenapine.
• Teach patient the signs and symptoms of a serious allergic reaction and to seek immediate emergency treatment if present.
• Urge patient to avoid alcohol while taking asenapine.
• Instruct diabetic patient taking asenapine to monitor blood glucose levels closely because hyperglycemia may occur.
• Advise patient to get up slowly from lying or sitting position during asenapine therapy to minimize orthostatic hypotension.
• Caution patient to avoid hazardous activities until drug's effects are known.
• Urge patient to avoid activities that raise body temperature suddenly, such as strenuous exercise and exposure to extreme heat, and to compensate for situations that cause dehydration, such as vomiting or diarrhea.
• Advise female patient of childbearing age to notify prescriber if she intends to become or suspects that she is pregnant during therapy.

aspirin
(acetylsalicylic acid, ASA)

Ancasal (CAN), Apo-As (CAN), Apo-ASEN (CAN), Arthrinol (CAN), Arthrisin (CAN), Aspergum, Aspirin, Atria S.R. (CAN), Bayer, Easprin, Ecotrin, Ecotrin Maximum Strength, Extra Strength Bayer Advanced Aspirin, 8-Hour Bayer Time Release, Empirin, Genprin, Maximum Bayer, Norwich Extra-Strength, Novasen (CAN), Sal-Adult (CAN), Sal-Infant (CAN), St. Joseph Children's, Supasa (CAN), Therapy Bayer, ZORprin

Class and Category

Chemical class: Salicylate
Therapeutic class: Anti-inflammatory, antiplatelet, antipyretic, nonopioid analgesic
Pregnancy category: D

Indications and Dosages

➤ *To relieve mild pain or fever*
CHEWABLE TABLETS, CHEWING GUM, CONTROLLED-RELEASE TABLETS, ENTERIC-COATED TABLETS, SOLUTION, TABLETS, TIMED-RELEASE TABLETS, SUPPOSITORIES
Adults and adolescents. 325 to 650 mg every 4 hr, as needed.; or 500 mg every 3 hr, as needed; or 1,000 mg every 6 hr, as needed
Children ages 2 to 14. 10 to 15 mg/kg/dose every 4 hr, as needed, up to 80 mg/kg daily.
➤ *To relieve mild to moderate pain from inflammation, as in rheumatoid arthritis and osteoarthritis*
CHEWABLE TABLETS, CHEWING GUM, CONTROLLED-RELEASE TABLETS, ENTERIC-COATED TABLETS, SOLUTION, TABLETS, TIMED-RELEASE TABLETS, SUPPOSITORIES
Adults and adolescents. 3.2 to 6 g daily in divided doses. *Maximum:* 6 g daily.
Children ages 2 to 14. 10 to 15 mg/kg, in divided doses every 4 to 6 hr. *Maximum:* 80 mg/kg daily.
➤ *To treat juvenile rheumatoid arthritis*
CHEWABLE TABLETS, CHEWING GUM, CONTROLLED-RELEASE TABLETS, ENTERIC-COATED TABLETS, SOLUTION, TABLETS, TIMED-RELEASE TABLETS, SUPPOSITORIES
Children ages 2 to 14. 60 to 110 mg/kg daily in divided doses every 6 to 8 hr.

➤ *To treat acute rheumatic fever*
CHEWABLE TABLETS, CHEWING GUM, CONTROLLED-RELEASE TABLETS, ENTERIC-COATED TABLETS, SOLUTION, TABLETS, TIMED-RELEASE TABLETS, SUPPOSITORIES
Adults and adolescents. 5 to 8 g daily in divided doses.
Children ages 2 to 14.
Initial: 100 mg/kg daily in divided doses for first 2 wk. *Maintenance:* 75 mg/kg/day in divided doses for next 4 to 6 wk.
➤ *To reduce the risk of recurrent transient ischemic attacks or stroke in men*
CHEWABLE TABLETS, CHEWING GUM, CONTROLLED-RELEASE TABLETS, ENTERIC-COATED TABLETS, SOLUTION, TABLETS, TIMED-RELEASE TABLETS, SUPPOSITORIES
Adults. 650 mg twice daily or 325 mg four times daily
➤ *To reduce the severity of or prevent acute MI*
CHEWABLE TABLETS, CHEWING GUM, CONTROLLED-RELEASE TABLETS, ENTERIC-COATED TABLETS, SOLUTION, TABLETS, TIMED-RELEASE TABLETS, SUPPOSITORIES
Adults. *Initial:* 160 to 162.5 mg (half of a 325-mg tablet or two 80- or 81-mg tablets) as soon as MI is suspected. *Maintenance:* 160 to 162.5 mg daily for 30 days.
➤ *To reduce risk of MI in patients with previous MI or unstable angina*
CHEWABLE TABLETS, CHEWING GUM, CONTROLLED-RELEASE TABLETS, ENTERIC-COATED TABLETS, SOLUTION, TABLETS, TIMED-RELEASE TABLETS, SUPPOSITORIES
Adults. 325 mg daily.

Route	Onset	Peak	Duration
P.O. (chewable tablets)	Rapid	Unknown	1–4 hr
P.O. (controlled-release)	5–30 min	1–4 hr	4–6 hr
P.O. (enteric-coated)	5–30 min	Unknown	1–4 hr
P.O. (solution)	5–30 min	15–40 min	1–4 hr

Route	Onset	Peak	Duration
P.O. (tablets)	15–30 min	1–2 hr	4–6 hr
P.O. (timed-release)	5–30 min	1–4 hr	4–6 hr
P.R.	Unknown	Unknown	4–6 hr

Mechanism of Action

Blocks the activity of cyclooxygenase, the enzyme needed for prostaglandin synthesis. Prostaglandins, important mediators in the inflammatory response, cause local vasodilation with swelling and pain. With blocking of cyclooxygenase and inhibition of prostaglandins, inflammatory symptoms subside. Pain is also relieved because prostaglandins play a role in pain transmission from the periphery to the spinal cord. Aspirin inhibits platelet aggregation by interfering with production of thromboxane A2, a substance that stimulates platelet aggregation. Aspirin acts on the heat-regulating center in the hypothalamus and causes peripheral vasodilation, diaphoresis, and heat loss.

Contraindications

Allergy to tartrazine dye, asthma, bleeding problems (such as hemophilia), hypersensitivity to aspirin or its components, peptic ulcer disease

Interaction

DRUGS

ACE inhibitors: Decreased antihypertensive effect
activated charcoal: Decreased aspirin absorption
antacids, urine alkalinizers: Decreased aspirin effectiveness
anticoagulants: Increased risk of bleeding; prolonged bleeding time
carbonic anhydrase inhibitors: Salicylism
corticosteroids: Increased excretion and decreased blood level of aspirin
heparin: Increased risk of bleeding
ibuprofen: Possibly reduced cardioprotective and stroke preventive effects of aspirin
methotrexate: Increased blood level and decreased excretion of methotrexate, causing toxicity
nizatidine: Increased blood aspirin level

NSAIDs: Possibly decreased blood NSAID level and increased risk of adverse GI effects
sulfonylureas: Possibly enhanced effect of sulfonylureas with large doses of aspirin
urine acidifiers (such as ammonium chloride, ascorbic acid): Decreased aspirin excretion
vancomycin: Increased risk of ototoxicity

ACTIVITIES

alcohol use: Increased risk of ulcers

Adverse Reactions

CNS: Confusion, CNS depression
EENT: Hearing loss, tinnitus
GI: Diarrhea, GI bleeding, heartburn, hepatotoxicity, nausea, stomach pain, vomiting
HEME: Decreased blood iron level, leukopenia, prolonged bleeding time, shortened life span of RBCs, thrombocytopenia
SKIN: Ecchymosis, rash, urticaria
Other: Angioedema, Reye's syndrome, salicylism (dizziness, tinnitus, difficulty hearing, vomiting, diarrhea, confusion, CNS depression, diaphoresis, headache, hyperventilation, and lassitude) with regular use of large doses

Nursing Considerations

• Don't crush timed-release or controlled-release aspirin tablets unless directed.
• Ask about tinnitus. This reaction usually occurs when blood aspirin level reaches or exceeds maximum for therapeutic effect.

PATIENT TEACHING

WARNING Advise parents not to give aspirin to a child or adolescent with chickenpox or flu symptoms because of risk of Reye's syndrome (rare life-threatening reaction characterized by vomiting, lethargy, belligerence, delirium, and coma). Tell them to consult prescriber for alternative drugs.
• Advise adult patient taking low-dose aspirin not to also take ibuprofen because it may reduce the cardioprotective and stroke preventive effects of aspirin.
• Instruct patient to take aspirin with food or after meals because it may cause GI upset if taken on an empty stomach.
• Instruct patient to stop taking aspirin and notify prescriber if any symptoms of stomach or intestinal bleeding occur such

A

as passage of black, bloody, or tarry stools or if patient is coughing up blood or vomit that looks like coffee grounds.

• Advise patient with tartrazine allergy not to take aspirin.

• Tell patient to consult prescriber before taking aspirin with any prescription drug for blood disorder, diabetes, gout, or arthritis.

• Tell patient not to use aspirin if it has a strong vinegar-like odor.

atenolol

Apo-Atenol (CAN), Novo-Atenol (CAN), Tenormin

Class and Category
Chemical class: Beta-adrenergic blocker (beta$_1$ and at high doses beta$_2$)
Therapeutic class: Antianginal, antihypertensive
Pregnancy category: D

Indications and Dosages
➤ *To treat angina pectoris and control hypertension*
TABLETS
Adults. 50 mg daily increased, as needed, after 1 to 2 wk to 100 mg daily.
➤ *To treat acute MI*
TABLETS, I.V. INFUSION
Adults. *Initial:* 5 mg I.V. over 5 min followed by 5 mg I.V. 10 min later. After another 10 min, 50 mg given and followed by another 50 mg in 12 hr. *Maintenance:* 50 mg P.O. twice daily or 100 mg P.O. daily for 6 to 9 days or until discharged from hospital.
DOSAGE ADJUSTMENT Dosage reduced to 50 mg daily P.O. for renally impaired patients and for elderly, renally impaired patients with creatinine clearance of 15 to 35 ml/min/1.73 m^2. Dosage reduced to 25 mg daily P.O. for renally impaired patients and for elderly, renally impaired patients with creatinine clearance less than 15 ml/min/1.73 m^2.

Route	Onset	Peak	Duration
P.O.	1 hr	2–4 hr	24 hr
I.V.	Immediate	5 min	12 hr

Mechanism of Action
Inhibits stimulation of beta$_1$-receptor sites, located mainly in the heart, decreasing cardiac excitability, cardiac output, and myocardial oxygen demand. Atenolol also acts to decrease release of renin from the kidneys, aiding in reducing blood pressure. At high doses, it inhibits stimulation of beta$_2$ receptors in the lungs, which may cause bronchoconstriction.

Contraindications
Cardiogenic shock, heart block greater than first degree, hypersensitivity to beta blockers, overt heart failure, sinus bradycardia

Interaction
DRUGS
amiodarone: Additive atenolol effects
calcium channel blockers, such as verapamil and diltiazem: Possibly symptomatic bradycardia and conduction abnormalities
catecholamine-depleting drugs, such as reserpine: Additive antihypertensive effect
clonidine: Rebound hypertension
disopyramide: Increased risk of severe bradycardia, asystole, and heart failure

Adverse Reactions
CNS: Depression, disorientation, dizziness, drowsiness, emotional lability, fatigue, fever, lethargy, light-headedness, short-term memory loss, vertigo
CV: Arrhythmias, including bradycardia and heart block; cardiogenic shock; cold arms and legs; heart failure; mesenteric artery thrombosis; mitral insufficiency; myocardial reinfarction; orthostatic hypotension; Raynaud's phenomenon
EENT: Dry eyes, laryngospasm, pharyngitis
GI: Diarrhea, ischemic colitis, nausea
GU: Renal failure
HEME: Agranulocytosis
MS: Leg pain
RESP: Bronchospasm, dyspnea, pulmonary emboli, respiratory distress, wheezing
SKIN: Erythematous rash
Other: Allergic reaction

Nursing Considerations
• Use atenolol cautiously in patients with heart failure controlled by digitalis glycosides or diuretics, patients with conduction abnormalities or left

ventricular dysfunction who take verapamil or diltiazem, patients with arterial circulatory disorders, and patients with impaired renal function.

• Use atenolol cautiously in diabetic patients because it may mask tachycardia caused by hypoglycemia. Unlike other beta-adrenergic blockers, it doesn't mask other signs of hypoglycemia, cause hypoglycemia, or delay the return of blood glucose to a normal level.

• At first sign of heart failure, expect patient to receive a digitalis glycoside, a diuretic, or both and to be monitored closely. If failure continues, expect to stop atenolol.

• Closely monitor patient with hyperthyroidism because atenolol may mask some signs of thyrotoxicosis. Abrupt withdrawal of atenolol may precipitate thyrotoxicosis.

• If patient also receives clonidine, expect to stop atenolol several days before gradually withdrawing clonidine. Then expect to restart atenolol therapy several days after clonidine has been discontinued.

• During I.V. atenolol therapy, monitor vital signs and cardiac rhythm closely.

• Discard parenteral mixture with atenolol if it isn't used within 48 hours.

• Stop atenolol and notify prescriber if patient develops bradycardia, hypotension, or other serious adverse reaction.

• Be aware that chronic beta blocker therapy such as atenolol is not routinely withheld prior to major surgery because the benefits outweigh the risks associated with its use with general anesthesia and surgical procedures.

PATIENT TEACHING

• Instruct patient not to stop taking atenolol abruptly. Otherwise, angina may worsen, and an MI or arrhythmia may occur.

• While patient is being weaned from atenolol, tell him to perform minimal physical activity to prevent chest pain.

• Instruct patient to take a missed dose as soon as possible. However, if it's within 8 hours of the next scheduled dose, tell him to skip the missed dose and return to his regular schedule.

• Explain that atenolol may alter serum glucose level and mask hypoglycemia.

• Inform the patient that he may experience fatigue and reduced tolerance to exercise and that he should notify his prescriber if this interferes with his normal lifestyle.

atomoxetine hydrochloride

Strattera

Class and Category

Chemical class: Selective norepinephrine reuptake inhibitor
Therapeutic class: Anti–ADHD agent
Pregnancy category: C

Indications and Dosages

➤ *To treat attention deficit hyperactivity disorder (ADHD)*

CAPSULES

Adults and children weighing 70 kg (154 lb) or less. *Initial:* 0.5 mg/kg daily, increased after at least 3 days to 1.2 mg/kg daily given either as a single dose in the morning or in evenly divided doses morning and late afternoon or early evening, as needed. *Maximum:* 1.4 mg/kg or 100 mg daily, whichever is less.

Adults and children weighing more than 70 kg. *Initial:* 40 mg daily, increased after at least 3 days to 80 mg daily given either as a single dose in the morning or in evenly divided doses morning and late afternoon or early evening. After 2 to 4 additional wk, dosage may be increased to 100 mg daily if optimal response hasn't been achieved. *Maximum:* 100 mg daily.

DOSAGE ADJUSTMENT For patients with moderate (Child-Pugh Class B) hepatic impairment, dosage reduced by 50%. For patients with severe (Child-Pugh Class C) hepatic impairment, dosage reduced by 75%. For patients weighing 70 kg or less and taking strong CYP2D6 inhibitors, such as paroxetine, fluoxetine, or quinidine, initial dosage of 0.5 mg/kg daily should be increased to 1.2 mg/kg daily only if symptoms fail to improve after 4 wk. For patients weighing more than 70 kg and taking strong CYP2D6 inhibitors, initial dosage of 40 mg daily should be increased to 80 mg daily only if symptoms fail to improve after 4 wk.

Mechanism of Action

Selectively inhibits presynaptic norepinephrine transport in the nervous system to increase attention span and produce a calming effect.

Contraindications

Angle-closure glaucoma, hypersensitivity to atomoxetine or its components, pheochromocytoma, severe cardiovascular disorders, use within 14 days of MAO inhibitor therapy

Interaction

DRUGS

albuterol and other beta2 agonists: May potentiate action of albuterol and other beta2 agonists on cardiovascular system
CYP2D6 inhibitors (such as fluoxetine, paroxetine, and quinidine): Increased blood atomoxetine level
MAO inhibitors: Possibly induced hypertensive crisis
pressor agents: Possibly altered blood pressure

Adverse Reactions

CNS: Aggressiveness, anxiety, chills, crying, depression, dizziness, early morning awakening, fatigue, headache, hostility, hypoaesthesia, insomnia, irritability, jittery feeling, lethargy, mood changes, paresthesia, peripheral coldness, pyrexia, rigors, sedation, seizures, sensory disturbances, sleep disturbance, somnolence, stroke, suicidal ideation (children and adolescents), syncope, tics, tremor, unusual dreams
CV: Chest pain, hypertension, orthostatic hypotension, MI, palpitations, QT-interval prolongation, Raynaud's phenomenon, tachycardia
EENT: Blurred vision, conjunctivitis, dry mouth, ear infection, mydriasis, nasal congestion, nasopharyngitis, pharyngitis, rhinorrhea, sinus congestion
ENDO: Hot flashes
GI: Abdominal pain (upper), anorexia, constipation, diarrhea, dyspepsia, elevated liver function test results, flatulence, gastroenteritis (viral), indigestion, nausea, severe hepatic dysfunction, vomiting
GU: Decreased libido, dysmenorrhea, dysuria, ejaculation disorders, erectile dysfunction, impotence, male pelvic pain, menstrual irregularities, orgasm abnormality, priapism, prostatitis, urinary hesitancy, urine retention
MS: Arthralgia, back pain, myalgia
RESP: Cough, upper respiratory tract infection
SKIN: Dermatitis, diaphoresis, hyperhidrosis, pruritus, rash, urticaria
Other: Anaphylaxis, angioedema, influenza, weight loss

Nursing Considerations

• Use atomoxetine cautiously in patients with cerebrovascular or CV disease (especially hypertension or tachycardia) because drug may increase blood pressure and heart rate. Also use cautiously in those prone to orthostatic hypotension and those with serious structural cardiac abnormalities, cardiomyopathy, serious heart rhythm abnormalities, or other serious cardiac problems because drug may increase risk of sudden death from these conditions.
WARNING Monitor children and adolescents closely for evidence of suicidal thinking and behavior as well as for psychotic or manic symptoms such as hallucinations, delusional thinking, or mania because atomoxetine increases the risk of suicidal ideation and the onset of psychotic or manic symptoms in these age groups. In addition, monitor patients, especially children and adolescents with ADHD, for the appearance or worsening of aggressive behavior or hostility. Notify prescriber if psychiatric adverse reactions are observed during atomoxetine therapy.
• Obtain baseline blood pressure and heart rate before starting therapy. Monitor patient's vital signs after dosage increases and periodically during therapy.
• Monitor patient closely for allergic reactions. If these occur, notify prescriber.
• Monitor child's or adolescent's growth and weight. Expect to interrupt therapy, as prescribed, if patient isn't growing or gaining weight appropriately.
• Monitor patient's liver function studies, as ordered. Notify prescriber immediately if

enzyme levels are elevated or patient has evidence of hepatic dysfunction (jaundice, dark urine, pruritus, right-upper-quadrant tenderness, or unexplained flulike symptoms). Expect to stop drug permanently.

PATIENT TEACHING

• Caution patient not to open capsules. If a capsule opens, urge patient to promptly wash his hands and any surface drug touches. If drug gets in his eyes, tell him to flush immediately with water and seek medical care.

• Instruct patient or parent to immediately report to prescriber any adverse reactions to atomoxetine therapy, such as facial swelling, itching, or rash.

WARNING Urge parents to watch their child or adolescent closely for evidence of abnormal thinking or behavior, or increased aggression or hostility. Emphasize need to notify prescriber about unusual changes.

• Urge patient to tell prescriber immediately about yellowing of his skin or eyes, itchiness, right upper abdominal pain, dark urine, or flulike symptoms. Also tell patient to notify prescriber immediately if he experiences exertional chest pain, unexplained syncope, or other symptoms suggestive of heart disease.

• Caution patient to assume sitting or standing position slowly because of drug's potential effect on blood pressure.

• Urge male patient to seek immediate medical attention for a penile erection that becomes prolonged or painful.

• Advise patient to report urinary hesitancy or urine retention to prescriber.

• Remind patient of the importance of alerting all prescribers to any OTC drugs, dietary supplements, or herbal remedies he's taking.

• Caution patient to avoid hazardous activities until drug's CNS effects are known.

• Reassure patient or parent that drug doesn't cause physical or psychological dependence.

• Instruct patient or parent to monitor weight during therapy.

atorvastatin calcium

Lipitor

Class and Category

Chemical class: Synthetically derived fermentation product
Therapeutic class: Antihyperlipidemic, HMG-CoA reductase inhibitor
Pregnancy category: X

Indications and Dosages

➤ *To control lipid levels as adjunct to diet in primary (heterozygous familial and nonfamilial) hypercholesterolemia and mixed dyslipidemia*

TABLETS

Adults. *Initial:* 10 or 20 mg once daily; then increased according to lipid level. *Maintenance:* 10 to 80 mg once daily.

DOSAGE ADJUSTMENT Initial dose may be increased to 40 mg once daily for patients who need cholesterol level reduced more than 45%.

➤ *To control lipid levels in homozygous familial hypercholesterolemia*

TABLETS

Adults. 10 to 80 mg daily.

➤ *To control lipid levels in pediatric heterozygous familial hyper-cholesterolemia*

TABLETS

Adolescents and children ages 10 to 17. *Initial:* 10 mg daily, adjusted at intervals of 4 wk or more, as needed. *Maximum:* 20 mg daily.

➤ *To reduce debilitating cardiovascular events such as stroke and MI in patients with multiple risk factors but without known coronary artery disease*

TABLETS

Adults. 10 mg once daily.

DOSAGE ADJUSTMENT FOR ALL INDICATIONS For patient taking lopinavir plus ritonavir, lowest dose necessary prescribed. For patient taking clarithromycin, itraconazole, saquinavir plus ritonavir, darunavir plus ritonavir, fosamprenavir, or forsamprenavir plus ritonavir, dosage should not exceed 20 mg daily. For patient taking nelfinavir or boceprevir, dosage should not exceed 40 mg daily.

Mechanism of Action

Reduces plasma cholesterol and lipoprotein levels by inhibiting HMG-CoA reductase and cholesterol synthesis in the liver and by increasing the number of LDL receptors on liver cells to enhance LDL uptake and breakdown.

Contraindications

Active hepatic disease, breastfeeding, hypersensitivity to atorvastatin or its components, pregnancy, unexplained persistent rise in serum transaminase level

Interaction

DRUGS

amlodipine, cimetidine, clarithromycin, diltiazem, erythromycin, itraconazole, ritonavir with saquinavir: Increased atorvastatin level
antacid, colestipol, efavirenz, rifampin: Possibly decreased blood atorvastatin level
azole antifungals, colchicine, clarithromycin, cyclosporine, darunavir plus ritonavir, erythromycin, fibric acid derivatives, forsamprenavir, fosamprenavir plus ritonavir, gemfibrozil, itraconazole, lopinavir with ritonavir, niacin (at dosage used for lipid modification), nicotinic acid, ritonavir with saquinavir or tipranavir, telaprevir: Increased risk of severe myopathy or rhabdomyolysis
cyclosporine: Increased atorvastatin bioavailability and risk of adverse reactions
digoxin: Possibly increased blood digoxin level, causing toxicity
oral contraceptives (such as ethinyl estradiol and norethindrone): Increased hormone level
protease inhibitors: Possible increased blood atorvastatin level; possible increased risk of myopathy and rhabdomyolysis

FOODS

grapefruit juice (more than 1.2 L daily): Increased blood atorvastatin level

Adverse Reactions

CNS: Abnormal dreams, amnesia, asthenia, cognitive impairment, depression, dizziness, emotional lability, facial paralysis, fatigue, fever, headache, hyperkinesia, lack of coordination, malaise, paresthesia, peripheral neuropathy, somnolence, syncope, weakness
CV: Arrhythmias, elevated serum CK level, orthostatic hypotension, palpitations, phlebitis, vasodilation
EENT: Amblyopia, altered refraction, dry eyes, dry mouth, epistaxis, eye hemorrhage, gingival hemorrhage, glaucoma, glossitis, hearing loss, lip swelling, loss of taste,

pharyngitis, sinusitis, stomatitis, taste perversion, tinnitus
ENDO: Hyperglycemia or hypoglycemia
GI: Abdominal or biliary pain, anorexia, colitis, constipation, diarrhea, duodenal or stomach ulcers, dysphagia, elevated liver enzymes, eructation, esophagitis, flatulence, gastroenteritis, hepatic failure, hepatitis, increased appetite, indigestion, jaundice, melena, pancreatitis, rectal hemorrhage, tenesmus, vomiting
GU: Abnormal ejaculation; cystitis; decreased libido; dysuria; epididymitis; hematuria; impotence; nephritis; nocturia; renal calculi; urinary frequency, incontinence, or urgency; urine retention; vaginal hemorrhage
HEME: Anemia, thrombocytopenia
MS: Arthralgia, back or muscle pain, bursitis, gout, immune-mediated necrotizing myopathy, leg cramps, myalgia, myasthenia gravis, myopathy, myositis, neck rigidity, rhabdomyolysis, tendon contracture or rupture, tenosynovitis, torticollis
RESP: Dyspnea, pneumonia
SKIN: Acne, alopecia, contact dermatitis, diaphoresis, dry skin, ecchymosis, eczema, erythema multiforme, petechiae, photosensitivity, pruritus, rash, seborrhea, Stevens-Johnson syndrome, toxic epidermal necrolysis, ulceration, urticaria
Other: Anaphylaxis, angioneurotic edema, flulike symptoms, infection, lymphadenopathy, weight gain

Nursing Considerations

• Atorvastatin is used in patients with homozygous familial hypercholesterolemia as an adjunct to other lipid-lowering treatments or alone only if other treatments aren't available.
• Atorvastatin may be used with colestipol or cholestyramine for additive antihyperlipidemic effects.
• Know that atorvastatin should not be used in patients taking cyclosporine, gemfibrozil, tipranavir plus ritonavir, or telaprevir because of high risk for rhabdomyolysis with acute renal failure.
• Use atorvastatin cautiously in patients who consume substantial quantities of alcohol or have a history of liver disease because atorvastatin use increases risk of liver dysfunction.

- Expect atorvastatin to be used in patients without obvious coronary artery disease (CAD) but with multiple risk factors (such as age 55 or over, smoker, history of hypertension or low HDL level, or family history of early CAD). Drug is used to reduce risk of MI, angina, and adverse effects of revascularization procedures.
- Also expect drug to be used in patients with type 2 diabetes who have no obvious CAD but multiple risk factors, such as retinopathy, albuminuria, smoking, or hypertension. Drug is used in these patients to reduce risk of MI and stroke.
- Expect liver function tests to be performed before atorvastatin therapy starts and then thereafter as clinically necessary. If clinical symptoms such as jaundice and hyper-bilirubinemia occurs, notify prescriber and expect atorvastatin therapy to be discontinued until cause of liver dysfunction has been identified. If no cause can be found, expect the drug to be discontinued permanently.
- Expect to measure lipid levels 2 to 4 weeks after therapy starts, to adjust dosage as directed, and to repeat periodically until lipid levels are within desired range.
- Monitor diabetic patient's blood glucose levels because atorvastatin therapy can affect blood glucose control.

WARNING Notify prescriber immediately and expect to withhold atorvastatin therapy if patient develops an acute condition suggestive of a myopathy (unexplained muscle pain, tenderness or weakness, especially if accompanied by malaise, fever, or elevated CPK level) or has a risk factor predisposing to the development of renal failure secondary to rhabdomyolysis, such as a severe acute infection; hypotension; major surgery; trauma; a severe metabolic, endocrine, or electrolyte disorder; or uncontrolled seizures.

PATIENT TEACHING

- Emphasize that atorvastatin is an adjunct to—not a substitute for—a low-cholesterol diet.
- Tell patient to take drug at the same time each day to maintain its effects.
- Instruct patient to take a missed dose as soon as possible. If it's almost time for his next dose, he should skip the missed dose. Tell him not to double the dose.

- Instruct patient to consult prescriber before taking OTC niacin because of increased risk of rhabdomyolysis.
- Advise patient to notify prescriber immediately if he develops unexplained muscle pain, tenderness, or weakness, especially if accompanied by fatigue or fever.
- Be aware that atorvastatin is expensive. Reinforce the benefits of therapy, and urge patient to comply if possible.
- Advise patient with diabetes to monitor blood glucose levels closely.

atovaquone
Mepron

Class and Category
Chemical class: Hydroxy-1, 4-naphthoquinone
Therapeutic class: Antiprotozoal
Pregnancy category: C

Indications and Dosages
➤ *To prevent* Pneumocystis jiroveci *(formerly* carinii*) pneumonia in patients who can't tolerate co-trimoxazole*

SUSPENSION, TABLETS
Adults and adolescents. 750 mg (5 ml) twice daily with meals for 21 days.
➤ *To treat mild to moderate* P. jiroveci *pneumonia in patients who can't tolerate co-trimoxazole*

SUSPENSION, TABLETS
Adults and adolescents. 750 mg (5 ml) twice daily with meals for 21 days. *Maximum:* 1,500 mg/day.

Mechanism of Action
May destroy *P. jiroveci* organisms by inhibiting the enzymes needed to synthesize nucleic acid and adenosine triphosphate.

Contraindications
Hypersensitivity to atovaquone or its components

Interaction
DRUGS
rifabutin, rifampin: Possibly decreased blood atovaquone level

Adverse Reactions
CNS: Fever, headache, insomnia
EENT: Rhinitis, throat tightness, vortex keratopathy
GI: Abdominal pain, diarrhea, elevated liver enzyme levels, hepatitis, hepatic failure, nausea, pancreatitis, vomiting
GU: Acute renal dysfunction
HEME: Anemia, thrombocytopenia
RESP: Bronchospasm, cough, dyspnea
SKIN: Desquamation, erythema multiforme, Stevens-Johnson syndrome, rash, urticaria
Other: Allergic reaction, angioedema, methemoglobinemia

Nursing Considerations
• Use atovaquone cautiously in patient with severe hepatic impairment because, although rare, serious adverse reactions affecting liver function may occur.
• Monitor blood test results because atovaquone may decrease serum sodium, hemoglobin levels, and neutrophil count; and may increase AST, ALT, alkaline phosphatase, and serum amylase levels.
• Crush atovaquone tablets, if needed.
• Don't use tablets and oral suspension interchangeably; they aren't bioequivalent.
PATIENT TEACHING
• Instruct patient to take atovaquone with meals for maximum effectiveness.
• Instruct patient to take a missed dose as soon as possible. If it's almost time for the next dose, tell him to skip the missed dose. Tell him not to double the next dose.
• Tell patient to notify prescriber if his condition doesn't improve in a few days or if he develops signs of an allergic reaction, such as fever or rash.

---

atracurium besylate
Tracrium

Class and Category
Chemical class: Biquaternary ammonium ester
Therapeutic class: Skeletal muscle relaxant
Pregnancy category: C

Indications and Dosages
➤ *To facilitate endotracheal intubation and induce skeletal muscle relaxation*

for surgery or mechanical ventilation as adjunct to anesthesia
I.V. INFUSION OR INJECTION
Adults and children age 2 or over. *Initial:* 0.4 to 0.5 mg/kg by I.V. bolus for nearly complete neuromuscular blockade.
Maintenance: 0.08 to 0.10 mg/kg 20 to 45 min after initial dose during prolonged surgery. Maintenance doses may be given every 15 to 25 min for patients under balanced anesthesia. For patients having extended surgical procedures, after an initial I.V. bolus, an infusion of 9 to 10 mcg/kg/min may be needed to counteract the spontaneous return of neuromuscular function and thereafter 5 to 10 mcg/kg/min as a constant infusion.
Children ages 1 month to 2 years having halothane anesthesia. *Initial:* 0.3 to 0.4 mg/kg. Frequent maintenance doses may be needed.

Route	Onset	Peak	Duration
I.V.	2–2.5 min	3–5 min	35–70 min

Mechanism of Action
Inhibits nerve impulse transmission by competing with acetylcholine for cholinergic receptors on motor end plate.

Incompatibilities
Don't mix atracurium in same syringe or give it through same I.V. needle as an alkaline solution, such as a barbiturate injection. Don't mix atracurium with lactated Ringer's injection.

Contraindications
Hypersensitivity to atracurium, its components, or benzyl alcohol

Interaction
DRUGS
aminoglycosides, enflurane, furosemide, halothane, isoflurane, lithium, magnesium salts, polymyxin antibiotics, procainamide, quinidine, thiazide diuretics: Possibly enhanced or prolonged atracurium effects
opioid analgesics: Possibly additive histamine release and increased risk and severity of bradycardia and hypotension

Adverse Reactions
CNS: Seizures
CV: Bradycardia, hypertension, hypotension, tachycardia

MS: Inadequate or prolonged neuro-muscular blockade
RESP: Apnea, bronchospasm, dyspnea, laryngospasm, wheezing
SKIN: Flushing, rash, urticaria
Other: Anaphylaxis, injection-site reaction

Nursing Considerations
• Use atracurium cautiously in patients with hypotension, and monitor blood pressure closely.
• Watch closely for adverse reactions, especially those related to histamine release. Atracurium is more likely than other neuromuscular blockers to cause skin flushing.
• Anticipate using lower doses for patients with neuromuscular disease, severe electrolyte disorders, or carcinomatosis because of risk of enhanced neuromuscular blockade and difficulties with reversal.
• Keep atropine nearby to treat atracurium-induced bradycardia.
• For I.V. infusion, dilute atracurium with normal saline solution, D_5W, or dextrose 5% in normal saline solution. To prepare a solution that yields 200 mcg/ml atracurium, add 2 ml atracurium to 98 ml diluent. To prepare a solution that yields 500 mcg/ml, add 5 ml atracurium to 95 ml diluent.
• Refrigerate solution or store at room temperature for up to 24 hours.

PATIENT TEACHING
• Explain atracurium's purpose and administration during anesthesia. Keep in mind that the patient can still hear.

atropine
AtroPen
atropine sulfate

Class and Category
Chemical class: Belladonna alkaloid
Therapeutic class: Anticholinergic, antimuscarinic
Pregnancy category: C

Indications and Dosages
➤ *To reduce respiratory tract secretions related to anesthesia*
TABLETS (ATROPINE SULFATE)
Adults. 0.4 to 0.6 mg preoperatively.

Children. 0.01 mg/kg up to total of 0.4 mg preoperatively and repeated every 4 to 6 hr, as needed.
I.V., I.M., OR SUBCUTANEOUS INJECTION
Adults. 0.4 to 0.6 mg preoperatively.
Children. 0.01 mg/kg up to total of 0.4 mg preoperatively and repeated every 4 to 6 hr, as needed.
➤ *To correct bradycardia*
I.V. INJECTION (ATROPINE SULFATE)
Adults. 0.4 to 1 mg. If no response to first dose, repeat once after 5 min.
Children. 0.01 to 0.02 mg/kg with a minimum dose of 0.1 mg and a maximum dose of 0.5 mg. If no response to first dose, repeat once after 5 min.
➤ *To treat cholinesterase inhibitor (such as neostigmine, pilocarpine, and methacholine) toxicity*
I.V. INJECTION (ATROPINE SULFATE)
Adults. 2 to 4 mg. Then 2 mg every 5 to 10 min until muscarinic signs (bradycardia, vasodilation, and pupil dilation) disappear or signs of atropine intoxication develop.
I.V. OR I.M. INJECTION (ATROPINE SULFATE)
Children. 1 mg. Then 0.5 to 1 mg every 5 to 10 min until muscarinic signs disappear or signs of atropine intoxication develop.
➤ *To treat mushroom (muscarine) toxicity*
I.V. OR I.M. INJECTION (ATROPINE SULFATE)
Adults. 1 to 2 mg every hr until respiratory signs and symptoms subside.
➤ *To treat pesticide (organophosphate) toxicity*
I.V. OR I.M. INJECTION (ATROPINE SULFATE)
Adults. 1 to 2 mg, repeated in 20 to 30 min as soon as cyanosis has cleared. Then continued until definite improvement is maintained, possibly for 2 or more days.
➤ *To treat known or suspected exposure to chemical nerve agent or insecticide*
I.M. INJECTION (ATROPEN)
Adults and children weighing over 41 kg (90 lb) with two or more mild symptoms. 2 mg. If severe symptoms develop after injection, two or more 2-mg injections given in rapid succession 10 min after initial injection.
Adults and children weighing over 41 kg who are unconscious or have other severe symptoms. 2 mg given immediately 3 times in rapid succession.
Children weighing 18 to 41 kg (40 to 90 lb) with two or more mild symptoms. 1 mg. If

severe symptoms develop after injection, two more 1-mg injections given in rapid succession 10 min after initial injection. **Children weighing 18 to 41 kg who are unconscious or exhibit any other severe symptoms.** 1 mg given immediately 3 times in rapid succession. **Children weighing 7 to 18 kg (15 to 40 lb) with two or more mild symptoms.** 0.5 mg. If severe symptoms develop after injection, two more 0.5-mg injections given in rapid succession 10 min after initial injection. **Children weighing 7 to 18 kg who are unconscious or exhibit any other severe symptoms.** 0.5 mg given immediately 3 times in rapid succession.

Mechanism of Action

Inhibits acetylcholine's muscarinic action at the neuroeffector junctions of smooth muscles, cardiac muscles, exocrine glands, SA and AV nodes, and the urinary bladder. In small doses, atropine inhibits salivary and bronchial secretions and diaphoresis. In moderate doses, it increases impulse conduction through the AV node and increases heart rate. In large doses, it decreases GI and urinary tract motility and gastric acid secretion.

Route	Onset	Peak	Duration
P.O.	30–120 min	1–2 hr	4–6 hr
I.V.	Immediate	2–4 min	Brief
I.M.	5–40 min	20–60 min	Brief
SubQ	Unknown	Unknown	Brief

Contraindications

Angle-closure glaucoma, asthma, GI obstructive disease (achalasia, pyloric obstruction, pyloroduodenal stenosis), hepatic disease, hypersensitivity to atropine or its components, ileus, intestinal atony, myasthenia gravis, myocardial ischemia, obstructive uropathy, renal disease, severe ulcerative colitis, tachycardia, toxic megacolon, unstable cardiovascular status in acute hemorrhage

Interaction

DRUGS

adsorbent antidiarrheals, antacids: Decreased atropine absorption
amantadine, anticholinergics, antidyskinetics, glutethimide, meperidine, muscle relaxants,
phenothiazines, tricyclic antidepressants and other drugs with anticholinergic properties, including antiarrhythmics (disopyramide, procainamide, quinidine), antihistamines, buclizine, meclizine: Increased atropine effects
antimyasthenics: Reduced intestinal motility
cyclopropane: Risk of ventricular arrhythmias
haloperidol: Decreased antipsychotic effect
ketoconazole: Decreased ketoconazole absorption
metoclopramide: Decreased effect on GI motility
opioid analgesics: Increased risk of ileus, severe constipation, and urine retention
potassium chloride, especially wax-matrix forms: Possibly GI ulcers
urinary alkalizers (calcium or magnesium antacids, carbonic anhydrase inhibitors, citrates, sodium bicarbonate): Delayed excretion, increased risk of adverse atropine effects

Adverse Reactions

CNS: Agitation, amnesia, anxiety, ataxia, Babinski's or Chaddock's reflex, behavioral changes, CNS stimulation (at high doses), coma, confusion, decreased concentration, decreased tendon reflexes, delirium, dizziness, drowsiness, fever, hallucinations, headache, hyperreflexia, insomnia, lethargy, mania, mental disorders, nervousness, paranoia, restlessness, seizures, somnolence, stupor, syncope, vertigo, weakness
CV: Arrhythmias, bradycardia (at low doses), cardiac dilation, chest pain, hypertension, hypotension, left ventricular failure, MI, palpitations, tachycardia (at high doses), weak or impalpable peripheral pulses
EENT: Acute angle-closure glaucoma, altered taste, blepharitis, blindness, blurred vision, conjunctivitis, cyclophoria, cycloplegia, decreased visual acuity or accommodation, dry eyes or conjunctiva, dry mucous membranes, dry mouth, eye irritation, eyelid crusting, heterophoria, increased intraocular pressure, keratoconjunctivitis, lacrimation, laryngitis, laryngospasm, mydriasis, nasal congestion, oral lesions, photophobia, pupils poorly reactive to light, strabismus, tongue chewing
GI: Abdominal distention, abdominal pain, bloating, constipation, decreased bowel

sounds or food absorption, delayed gastric emptying, dysphagia, heartburn, ileus, nausea, vomiting
GU: Bladder distention, enuresis, impotence, urinary hesitancy, urinary urgency, urine retention
MS: Dysarthria, hypertonia, muscle twitching
RESP: Bradypnea, dyspnea, inspiratory stridor, pulmonary edema, respiratory failure, shallow breathing, subcostal recession, tachypnea
SKIN: Cold skin, cyanosis, decreased sweating, dermatitis, flushing, rash, urticaria
Other: Anaphylaxis, dehydration, injection-site reaction, polydipsia, sensations of warmth

Nursing Considerations

WARNING For patient prescribed AtroPen for suspected nerve gas or insecticide exposure, dosage is determined by severity of symptoms. Mild symptoms include blurred vision, miosis, excessive unexplained teary eyes or runny nose, increased salivation, chest tightness, difficulty breathing, tremors, muscle twitching, nausea, vomiting, unexplained wheezing or coughing, acute onset of stomach cramps, tachycardia, and bradycardia. Severe symptoms include confusion or other strange behavior, severe difficulty breathing, extreme secretions from airway or lungs, severe muscle twitching and general weakness, involuntary urination and defecation, seizures, and unconsciousness.

• Avoid using high-dose atropine sulfate in patients with ulcerative colitis because of risk of toxic megacolon or in patients with hiatal hernia and reflux esophagitis because of risk of esophagitis

• AtroPen has no absolute contraindications when used to treat life-threatening nerve gas or insecticide exposure.

WARNING Assess for symptoms of toxic doses of atropine, such as excitement, agitation, drowsiness, and confusion, which are likely to affect elderly patients even with low doses. If symptoms occur, take safety precautions to prevent injury.

• Assess bowel and bladder elimination. Notify prescriber of diarrhea, constipation, urinary hesitancy, or urine retention.

PATIENT TEACHING
• For patient prescribed an AtroPen to carry because of risk of nerve gas or insecticide exposure, explain when and how to self-administer the drug.
• Instruct patient to take atropine sulfate 30 to 60 minutes before meals.
• Advise patient to notify prescriber if he has persistent or severe diarrhea, constipation, or difficulty urinating.

auranofin
Ridaura

Class and Category
Chemical class: Gold salt
Therapeutic class: Anti-inflammatory
Pregnancy category: C

Indications and Dosages
➤ *To treat active rheumatoid arthritis that's unresponsive to NSAIDs*
CAPSULES
Adults. *Initial:* 6 mg daily or 3 mg twice daily. *Maintenance:* Up to 9 mg daily after 3 mo of treatment, if needed.
Children age 6 and over. *Initial:* 0.1 mg/kg daily. *Maintenance:* 0.15 mg/kg daily. *Maximum:* 0.2 mg/kg daily.
DOSAGE ADJUSTMENT Drug discontinued if therapeutic response isn't adequate after 3 mo at 9 mg daily.

Route	Onset	Peak	Duration
P.O.	3–6 mo	1–2 hr	Up to 26 days

Mechanism of Action
Decreases rheumatoid factor and humoral antibody (immunoglobulin) levels. Although exact anti-inflammatory action is unknown, drug may suppress the increased phagocytic activity of macrophages and polymorphonuclear leukocytes that occurs with rheumatoid arthritis and thereby inhibit release of destructive enzymes that cause joint inflammation.

Contraindications
Agranulocytosis, blood dyscrasias, bone marrow aplasia, colitis, eczema, exfoliative

dermatitis, hepatic disease, history of gold or heavy metal toxicity, hypersensitivity to auranofin or its components, marked hypertension, necrotizing enterocolitis, pulmonary fibrosis, recent radiation therapy, renal disease, severe debilitation, systemic lupus erythematosus, uncontrolled diabetes mellitus, uncontrolled heart failure, urticaria, youth (under age 6)

Interaction
DRUGS
phenytoin: Possibly increased phenytoin level

Adverse Reactions
CNS: Confusion, dizziness, EEG abnormalities, hallucinations, seizures
EENT: Gingivitis, glossitis, iritis or corneal ulcers from gold deposits in ocular tissue, metallic taste, stomatitis
GI: Abdominal cramps, anorexia, constipation, diarrhea, enterocolitis, flatulence, indigestion, melena, nausea, vomiting
GU: Hematuria, elevated BUN and serum creatinine levels, proteinuria, vaginitis
HEME: Agranulocytosis, aplastic anemia, eosinophilia, leukopenia, neutropenia, thrombocytopenia
RESP: Cough, dyspnea, fibrosis, interstitial pneumonitis
SKIN: Alopecia, dermatitis, exfoliative dermatitis, jaundice, photosensitivity, pruritus, rash, urticaria

Nursing Considerations
• Monitor blood and urine tests for signs of gold toxicity during auranofin therapy.
WARNING Gold toxicity may occur during treatment or several months afterward. It usually occurs with a cumulative dose of 400 to 800 mg and may cause decreased hemoglobin level, WBC count less than 4,000/mm^3, granulocyte count less than 1,500/mm^3, platelet count less than 150,000/mm^3, severe diarrhea, stomatitis, hematuria, proteinuria, rash, and pruritus.
• Monitor fluid intake and output imbalance. If urine output decreases, assess BUN and serum creatinine levels for signs of renal impairment.
• Notify prescriber about possible allergic reaction (dermatitis, rash, pruritus). Drug may need to be discontinued.

PATIENT TEACHING
• Advise patient that diarrhea is common but that he should notify prescriber immediately if it becomes severe.
• Tell patient to take drug exactly as prescribed and to have monthly blood tests.
• Inform patient that drug may take 3 to 4 months to reach a therapeutic level.
• Urge patient to report skin problems, fatigue, or stomatitis (possible blood dyscrasias).
• Tell patient to report blood in stool or urine, easy bruising, and bleeding gums.

avanafil
Stendra

Class and Category
Chemical class: Phosphodiesterase 5 inhibitor
Therapeutic class: Anti-impotence
Pregnancy category: C

Indications and Dosages
➤ *To treat erectile dysfunction*
TABLETS
Adults. 100 mg as early as 15 min before sexual activity, as needed. *Maximum:* Once daily.
DOSAGE ADJUSTMENT Dosage may be decreased to 50 mg 30 min before sexual activity or dosage may be increased to 200 mg as early as 15 min before sexual activity, as needed. For patient who is stable on alpha-blocker therapy or who is taking a moderate CYP3A4 inhibitor such as amprenavir, aprepitant, diltiazem, erythromycin, fluconazole, fosamprenavir, or verapamil, dosage is limited to 50 mg.

Mechanism of Action
Enhances the effect of nitric oxide released in the penis through stimulation. Nitric oxide increases cGMP level, relaxes smooth muscle, and increases blood flow to the corpus cavernosum, thus producing an erection.

Contraindications
Continuous or intermittent nitrate therapy, hypersensitivity to avanafil or its components

Interaction
DRUGS
alpha blockers and other antihypertensives:
Increased risk of hypotension
CYP3A4 inhibitors: Possibly increased
plasma levels of avanafil
desipramine, omeprazole, rosiglitazone:
Possibly increased effect of these drugs
nitrates: Profound hypotension
sodium nitroprusside: Possibly potentiation
of anti-aggregatory effect of sodium
nitroprusside
ACTIVITIES
alcohol use: Increased risk of orthostatic
hypotension

Adverse Reactions
CNS: Depression, dizziness, fatigue,
headache, insomnia, somnolence,
vertigo
CV: Abnormal ECG, angina, deep vein
thrombosis, hypertension, palpitations,
peripheral edema
EENT: Epistaxis, eyelid swelling, hearing or
vision loss, nasal or sinus congestion,
nasopharyngitis, non-arteritic anterior
ischemic optic neuropathy, oropharyngeal
pain, sinusitis, tinnitus
ENDO: Alterations in blood glucose
GI: Constipation, diarrhea, dyspepsia,
elevated liver enzymes, gastric pain,
gastritis, gastroesophageal reflux disease,
nausea, vomiting
GU: Hematuria, nephrolithiasis,
pollakiuria, prolonged erection, urinary
tract infection
MS: Arthralgia, back or musculoskeletal
pain, muscle spasms, myalgia
RESP: Bronchitis, cough, exertional
dyspnea, upper respiratory infection,
wheezing
SKIN: Flushing, pruritis, rash
Other: Influenza

Nursing Considerations
• Be aware that avanafil should not be used
in a patient taking a strong CYP3A4
inhibitor (such as atanazavir,
clarithromycin, itndinavir, itraconazole,
ketoconazole, nefazadone, nelfinavir,
ritonavir, saquinavir, telithromycin)
because of increased risk of elevated
avanafil levels that could cause serious
adverse effects.

• Know that although nitrate therapy is a
contraindication to avanafil therapy, in a
life-threatening situation, at least 12 hours
should elapse after the last dose of avanafil
before nitrate administration is given. In
this situation, be prepared to
hemodynamically monitor the patient and
expect hypotension to be treated, if it
occurs.
• Use avanafil cautiously in a patient with
preexisting cardiovascular disease because
of the potential for increased cardiac
adverse effects during sexual activity.
Patient with left ventricular outflow
obstruction or severely impaired
autonomic control of blood pressure may
be especially sensitive to the vasodilatation
effect of avanafil.
• Use avanafil cautiously in the elderly and
patients with mild to moderate renal or
hepatic dysfunction. The effects of
avanafil in the presence of severe renal or
hepatic dysfunction is unknown.
• Monitor the patient's vision, especially in
patients over age 50; who have diabetes,
hypertension, coronary artery disease, or
hyperlipidemia; or who smoke, because
avanafil rarely may cause nonarteritic
anterior ischemic optic neuropathy that
may lead to decreased vision or
permanent vision loss.
PATIENT TEACHING
• Explain to patient that avanafil should
be taken about 30 minutes before
sexual activity and that sexual
stimulation is required for drug to
be effective.
• Remind patient that avanafil should not be
taken more than once a day.
WARNING Warn patient not to take avanafil
if he also takes any form of organic
nitrate, either continuously or intermittently or other PDE5 inhibitors,
because profound hypotension and death
could result.
• Tell patient to stop taking drug and
contact prescriber immediately if vision
decreases suddenly in one or both eyes, or
if he has a sudden loss of hearing, possibly
with tinnitus and dizziness.
• Advise patient taking avanafil to seek
sexual counseling to enhance the drug's
effects.

- Instruct patient to notify prescriber immediately if erection is painful or lasts longer than 4 hours.
- Warn patient that alcohol ingestion may increase risk of low blood pressure, accompanied by dizziness when changing position, increased heart rate, and headache.

azathioprine
Imuran

azathioprine sodium
Imuran

Class and Category
Chemical class: Purine analogue
Therapeutic class: Antimetabolite, immunosuppressant
Pregnancy category: D

Indications and Dosages
➤ *To prevent kidney rejection after transplantation*
TABLETS, I.V. INFUSION
Adults and children. *Initial:* 3 to 5 mg/kg daily P.O. or I.V. as a single dose on, or 1 to 3 days before, day of transplantation, followed by 3 to 5 mg/kg daily I.V. after surgery until P.O. dose is tolerated. *Maintenance:* 1 to 3 mg/kg daily P.O.
DOSAGE ADJUSTMENT Dosage reduced for patients with oliguria (as from tubular necrosis) after transplantation because drug or metabolite excretion may be delayed.
➤ *To treat refractory rheumatoid arthritis*
TABLETS
Adults. *Initial:* 1 mg/kg (50 to 100 mg) daily as a single dose or twice daily for 6 to 8 wk. *Maintenance:* If initial therapy doesn't produce therapeutic effects or serious adverse effects, dosage increased every 4 wk by 0.5 mg/kg up to 2.5 mg/kg. Optimal dosage is 2 to 2.5 mg/kg daily.
DOSAGE ADJUSTMENT Dosage reduced to 25% to 33% of usual dosage for patients who also take allopurinol.

Route	Onset	Peak	Duration
P.O., I.V.	4–8 wk	Unknown	Several days

Mechanism of Action
May prevent proliferation and differentiation of activated B and T cells by interfering with purine (protein) and nucleic acid (DNA and RNA) synthesis.

Contraindications
Hypersensitivity to azathioprine or its components

Interaction
DRUGS
ACE inhibitors and drugs that affect bone marrow and cell development in bone marrow, such as co-trimoxazole: Possibly severe leukopenia
allopurinol: Possibly increased therapeutic and adverse effects of azathioprine
anticoagulants: Possibly decreased anticoagulant action
cyclosporine: Possibly decreased plasma cyclosporine level
methotrexate: Possibly increased plasma level of azathioprine's metabolite, 6-mercaptopurine, which can lead to cell death
nondepolarizing neuromuscular blockers: Possibly decreased or reversed action of neuromuscular blocker

Adverse Reactions
CNS: Fever, malaise, progressive multifocal leukoencephalopathy
GI: Abdominal pain, diarrhea, hepatoxicity (elevated liver function test results), nausea, pancreatitis, steatorrhea, vomiting
HEME: Leukopenia, macrocytic anemia, pancytopenia, thrombocytopenia
MS: Arthralgia, myalgia
SKIN: Acute febrile neutrophilic dermatosis (Sweet's Syndrome), alopecia, cancer, rash
RESP: Reversible interstitial pneumonitis
Other: Infection, lymphomas and other neoplasms, negative nitrogen balance

Nursing Considerations
- Before I.V. use, add 20 ml sterile water for injection to azathioprine vial and swirl until clear solution forms. Resulting drug concentration is 100 mg and can be diluted further as prescribed. Calculate infusion rate based on final volume to be infused. Then give over 30 to 60 minutes or as prescribed (5 minutes to 8 hours).
- Obtain results of baseline laboratory tests, including WBC, RBC, and platelet counts. Expect to monitor results once a week

during first month of therapy, twice a month during second and third months, and once a month or more thereafter.
• Hematologic reactions typically are dose-related and may occur late in therapy, especially in patients with transplant rejection.
WARNING If WBC count decreases rapidly or remains significantly and consistently low, expect to reduce dosage or discontinue azathioprine.
WARNING Monitor patient closely for abnormal signs and symptoms suggestive of lymphomas, especially in adolescent and young adult males who have a history of inflammatory bowel disease, in patients who have received a renal transplant, or in patients with rheumatoid arthritis, because the majority of patients who develop a lymphoma fall into one of these categories.
• Periodically monitor liver function test results for early signs of hepatotoxicity.
• If patient develops thrombocytopenia, take bleeding precautions, such as avoiding I.M. injections and venipunctures, applying ice to areas of trauma, and checking I.V. infusion sites every 2 hours for bleeding.
• If patient also receives an oral anticoagulant, monitor his PT.
• Azathioprine therapy increases risk of viral, fungal, bacterial, and protozoal infections. Watch for evidence of infection, such as fever, chills, sore throat, and mouth sores. Expect to administer aggressive antibiotic, antiviral, or other drug therapy and reduce azathioprine dosage.
• Minimize the risk of infection. If patient has severe leukopenia, take neutropenic precautions, such as placing him in a private room and limiting visitors.
• Rheumatoid arthritis requires at least 12 weeks of azathioprine therapy. During this time, continue other pain-relief measures, such as rest, physical therapy, and other drugs, such as salicylates and corticosteroids.
• If oral azathioprine causes GI upset, give it in divided doses or with meals.
• Expect to use lowest possible maintenance dosage for rheumatoid arthritis, reducing it gradually in 0.5-mg/kg (about 25-mg) increments at 4-week intervals.

• Drug can be stopped abruptly, but its effects may persist several days.

PATIENT TEACHING
• Advise patient to take oral drug with food or meals to minimize GI upset.
WARNING Teach patient to recognize and report signs of infection, such as sore throat and fever and to seek medical attention for any abnormal signs and symptoms that might be suggestive of a malignancy.
• Teach patient how to reduce the risk of bleeding and falling.

azelastine hydrochloride
Astelin, Astepro 0.1%, 0.15%

Class and Category
Chemical class: Phthalazinone derivative
Therapeutic class: Antihistamine, H_1-receptor antagonist
Pregnancy category: C

Indications and Dosages
➤ *To treat symptoms of seasonal allergic rhinitis*
NASAL SPRAY (ASTELIN)
Adults and children age 12 and over. 1 or 2 sprays in each nostril twice daily.
Children age 5 to 11 years. 1 spray in each nostril twice daily.
NASAL SPRAY (ASTEPRO)
Adults and children age 12 and over. 1 or 2 sprays in each nostril twice daily. Alternatively, 0.15% solution may be administered as 2 sprays in each nostril once daily.
Children age 6 to 11 years. 1 spray in each nostril twice daily.
➤ *To treat symptoms of perennial allergic rhinitis*
NASAL SPRAY (ASTEPRO)
Adults and children age 12 and over. 2 sprays (0.15%) in each nostril twice daily.
Children age 6 to 11. 1 spray (0.1% or 0.15%) in each nostril twice daily.
➤ To treat symptoms of vasomotor rhinitis
NASAL SPRAY (ASTELIN)
Adults and children age 12 and over. 2 sprays in each nostril twice daily.

Route	Onset	Peak	Duration
Nasal	In 3 hr	Unknown	12 hr

Mechanism of Action

Binds nonselectively to central and peripheral H_1 receptors, preventing histamine from reaching its site of action, which reduces or prevents most of histamine's physiologic effects. By blocking histamine at its site of action, azelastine inhibits respiratory, vascular, and GI smooth-muscle contraction; decreases capillary permeability, which reduces wheals, flares, and itching; and decreases salivary and lacrimal gland secretions.

Contraindications

Hypersensitivity to azelastine or its components

Interaction

DRUGS

cimetidine, ketoconazole: Possibly increased blood azelastine level

CNS depressants: Possibly increased sedative effects and reduced mental alertness

ACTIVITIES

alcohol use: Possibly increased sedative effects and reduced mental alertness

Adverse Reactions

CNS: Dizziness, fatigue, headache, somnolence
CV: Atrial fibrillation, palpitations
EENT: Bitter taste, dry mouth, epistaxis, nasal burning, paroxysmal sneezing, pharyngitis, rhinitis
GI: Nausea
Other: Weight gain

Nursing Considerations

• Assess for changes in alertness, and take safety precautions, if needed.

PATIENT TEACHING

• Teach patient how to use azelastine nasal spray properly to achieve maximum therapeutic effects.
• Before patient's first use of nasal spray, instruct him to prime pump by placing his thumb on base and his index and middle fingers on shoulder area of bottle and then pressing thumb firmly and quickly against bottle four times, or until fine mist appears.
• If patient hasn't used spray in more than 3 days, instruct him to reprime pump with two sprays or until fine mist appears.

• Advise patient to clear nostrils gently, if needed, before using spray.
• Teach patient to inhale deeply after each spray and then exhale through his mouth and tilt his head back so drug can spread over nasopharynx.
• Advise patient to store bottle upright and keep it tightly closed.
WARNING Emphasize that patient must consult prescriber before taking any OTC drug, such as cough syrup or a cold remedy, because of the risk of extreme CNS depression.
• Inform patient that decreased alertness may occur. Advise him to avoid hazardous activities or those that require alertness, such as driving or operating machinery, until drug's effects are known.

azilsartan medoxomil

Edarbi

Class and Category

Chemical class: Angiotensin II receptor blocker
Therapeutic class: Antihypertensive
Pregnancy category: D

Indications and Dosages

➤ *To manage hypertension, alone or with other antihypertensives*

TABLETS

Adults. 80 mg once daily.

DOSAGE ADJUSTMENT For patients who are receiving high doses of diuretics, initial dosage is decreased to 40 mg once daily.

Mechanism of Action

Selectively blocks binding of angiotensin (AT) II to AT_1 receptor sites in many tissues, including vascular smooth muscle and adrenal glands. This inhibits vasoconstrictive and aldosterone-secreting effects of AT II, which reduces blood pressure.

Contraindications

Concurrent aliskiren use in patients with diabetes or patients with renal impairment (GFR less than 60 ml/min), hypersensitivity to azilsartan or its components

Interaction

DRUGS
ACE inhibitors, aliskiren, other angiotensin receptor blockers: Increased risk of hypotension, hyperkalemia, and renal dysfunction
diuretics, other antihypertensives: Possible increased risk of hypotension
lithium: Possibly increased risk of serum lithium concentrations resulting in lithium toxicity
NSAIDs: Possible decreased renal function in patients who are elderly, volume-depleted, or have existing compromised renal function

Adverse Reactions

CNS: Asthenia, dizziness, fatigue
CV: Hypotension, orthostatic hypotension
GI: Diarrhea, nausea
GU: Elevated BUN and serum creatinine levels
MS: Muscle spasm
RESP: Cough
SKIN: Pruritus, rash
OTHER: Angioedema

Nursing Considerations

• Expect to provide treatment for hypovolemia before starting azilsartan therapy.
• Monitor patient for hypotension. If it occurs, place patient in a supine position, and if needed, give an I.V. infusion of normal saline, as ordered. Be aware that a transient hypotensive episode does not require the drug to be discontinued.
• Watch for elevated BUN and serum creatinine levels, especially if patient has congestive heart failure, renal artery stenosis, or volume depletion. Report significant or persistent increases immediately.

PATIENT TEACHING
• Instruct patient to take azilsartan exactly as prescribed and to monitor his blood pressure for effectiveness.
• Advise female patient to report known or suspected pregnancy immediately. Explain that if she becomes pregnant, prescriber may replace azilsartan with another antihypertensive that's safe to use during pregnancy.

azithromycin

A

Zithromax, Zmax

Class and Category
Chemical class: Azalide (subclass of macrolide)
Therapeutic class: Antibiotic
Pregnancy category: B

Indications and Dosages

➤ *To treat mild community-acquired pneumonia, otitis media, pharyngitis, tonsillitis, and uncomplicated skin and soft-tissue infections*

CAPSULES, ORAL SUSPENSION, TABLETS
Adults. 500 mg as a single dose on day 1, followed by 250 mg daily on days 2 through 5.
Children age 6 months or over with acute otitis media or community-acquired pneumonia. 10 mg/kg as a single dose (not to exceed 500 mg daily) on day 1, followed by 5 mg/kg (not to exceed 250 mg daily) daily on days 2 through 5. Or, for acute otitis media, 30 mg/kg of oral suspension as a single dose or 10 mg/kg daily for 3 days.
Children age 12 or over with pharyngitis or tonsillitis. 12 mg/kg (not to exceed 500 mg daily) as single dose daily for 5 days.

➤ *To treat mild to moderate acute bacterial exacerbations of COPD*
CAPSULES, ORAL SUSPENSION, TABLETS
Adults. 500 mg daily for 3 days. Or, 500 mg as single dose on day 1, followed by 250 mg daily on days 2 through 5.

➤ *To treat community-acquired pneumonia*
CAPSULES, ORAL SUSPENSION, TABLETS, I.V. INFUSION
Adults and adolescents age 16 or over. 500 mg I.V. as a single dose daily for at least 2 days, followed by 500 mg P.O. as a single dose daily until patient completes 7 to 10 days of therapy.

➤ *To treat community-acquired pneumonia caused by* Chlamydophila pneumoniae, Haemophilus influenzae, Mycoplasma pneumoniae, *or* Streptococcus pneumoniae
E.R. ORAL SOLUTION (ZMAX)
Adults. 2 g as a single dose on an empty stomach.

➤ *To treat chancroid caused by* Haemophilus ducreyi; *gonococcal pharyngitis; urethritis, cervicitis, or other infections caused by* Chlamydia trachomatis

CAPSULES, ORAL SUSPENSION, TABLETS

Adults. 1 g as a one-time dose.

Children age 8 or over and children under age 8 weighing 45 kg (99 lb) or more (with infections caused by *C. trachomatis*). 1 g as a one-time dose.

➤ *To treat urethritis or cervicitis caused by* Neisseria gonorrhoeae

CAPSULES, ORAL SUSPENSION, TABLETS

Adults. 2 g as a one-time dose.

➤ *To prevent* mycobacterium avium complex *in patients with advanced HIV infection*

CAPSULES, ORAL SUSPENSION, TABLETS, I.V. INFUSION

Adults. 1.2 g once weekly, as indicated.

➤ *To treat pelvic inflammatory disease*

CAPSULES, ORAL SUSPENSION, TABLETS, I.V. INFUSION

Adults. 500 mg I.V. as a single dose daily for 1 to 2 days, followed by 250 mg P.O. as a single dose daily until patient completes 7 days of therapy.

➤ *To treat acute bacterial sinusitis*

ORAL SUSPENSION, TABLETS

Adults. 500 mg daily for 3 days. **Children.** 10 mg/kg daily for 3 days.

➤ *To treat acute bacterial sinusitis caused by* H. influenzae, Moraxella catarrhalis, *or* S. pneumoniae

E.R. ORAL SOLUTION (ZMAX)

Adults. 2 g as a single dose on an empty stomach.

Route	Onset	Peak	Duration
P.O.	Varies	Unknown	Unknown

Mechanism of Action

Binds to a ribosomal subunit of susceptible bacteria, blocking peptide translocation and inhibiting RNA-dependent protein synthesis. Drug concentrates in phagocytes, macrophages, and fibroblasts, which release it slowly and may help move it to infection sites.

Incompatibilities

Don't add I.V. substances, additives, or drugs to azithromycin I.V. solution, and don't infuse through the same I.V. line.

Contraindications

History of cholestatic jaundice or hepatic dysfunction associated with prior use of azithromycin; hypersensitivity to azithromycin, erythromycin, ketolide antibiotics, or other macrolide antibiotics

Interaction

DRUGS

antacids that contain aluminum or magnesium: Possibly decreased peak blood azithromycin level, but extent of absorption is unchanged

carbamazepine, cyclosporine, phenytoin, terfenadine (drugs meftabolized by P-450 cytochrome system): Possibly increased blood levels of these drugs

digoxin: Possibly increased blood digoxin level

dihydroergotamine, ergotamine: Possibly severe peripheral vasospasm and abnormal sensations (acute ergot toxicity)

HMG-CoA reductase inhibitors: Increased risk of severe myopathy or rhabdomyolysis

pimozide: Possibly sudden death

oral anticoagulants: Possibly potentiated effects of oral anticoagulants

theophylline: Possibly increased blood theophylline level

triazolam: Possibly decreased excretion and increased therapeutic effects of triazolam

warfarin: Possibly increased anticoagulation

FOODS

food: Dramatically increased absorption rate of azithromycin

Adverse Reactions

CNS: Aggressiveness, agitation, anxiety, asthenia, dizziness, fatigue, headache, hyperactivity, malaise, nervousness, paresthesia, seizures, somnolence, syncope, vertigo

CV: Arrhythmias, chest pain, edema, elevated serum CK level, hypotension, palpitations, prolonged QT interval, torsades de pointes, ventricular tachycardia

EENT: Hearing loss, mucocutaneous candidiasis, perversion or loss of taste or smell, tinnitus

ENDO: Hyperglycemia

GI: Abdominal pain, anorexia, cholestatic jaundice, constipation, diarrhea, dyspepsia, elevated liver function test results,

flatulence, hepatic necrosis or failure, hepatitis, nausea, pancreatitis, pseudomembranous colitis, vomiting
GU: Acute renal failure, elevated BUN and serum creatinine levels, nephritis, vaginal candidiasis
HEME: Leukopenia, neutropenia, thrombocytopenia
MS: Arthralgia
SKIN: Erythema multiforme, photosensitivity, pruritus, rash, Stevens-Johnson syndrome, toxic epidermal necrolysis, urticaria
Other: Allergic reaction, anaphylaxis, angioedema, elevated serum phosphorus level, hyperkalemia, infusion-site reaction (such as pain and redness), new or worsening myasthenia syndrome, superinfection

Nursing Considerations

• Be aware that azithromycin should not be used in patients with known QT prolongation, bradyarrhythmias, congenital long QT syndrome, uncompensated heart failure, or history of torsades de pointes; patients with ongoing proarrhythmic conditions such as uncorrected hypokalemia or hypomagnesemia, or significant bradycardia; or patients receiving drugs known to prolong the QT interval such as class IA (procainamide, quinidine) or class III (amiodarone, dofetilide, sotalol) antiarrhythmic agents because of increased risk of life-threatening arrhythmias such as torsades de pointes.
• Monitor elderly patients closely for arrhythmias because they are more susceptible to drug effects on the QT interval.
• Obtain culture and sensitivity test results, if possible, before starting therapy.
• Use azithromycin cautiously in patients with hepatic dysfunction not associated with prior use of azithromycin (drug is metabolized in the liver) or renal dysfunction (effects are unknown in this group).
• Give azithromycin capsules 1 hour before or 2 to 3 hours after food. Give tablets or suspension without regard to food.
WARNING Don't give azithromycin by I.V. bolus or I.M. injection because it may

cause erythema, pain, swelling, tenderness, or other reaction at the site. Infuse it over 60 minutes or longer, as prescribed (typically 1 mg/ml over 3 hours or 2 mg/ml over 1 hour.)
• If hepatic function is impaired, monitor liver function studies closely and expect to discontinue the drug immediately if signs and symptoms of hepatitis occur.
• Assess patient for bacterial or fungal superinfection, which may occur with prolonged or repeated therapy. If it occurs, expect to give another antibiotic or antifungal.
• Monitor bowel elimination; if needed, obtain stool culture to rule out pseudo-membranous colitis. If it occurs, expect to stop azithromycin and give fluid, electrolytes, and antibiotics effective with *Clostridium difficile.*

PATIENT TEACHING
• Tell patient to take azithromycin capsules 1 hour before or 2 to 3 hours after food. Instruct patient to take tablets or suspension without regard to food.
WARNING Urge patient to consult prescriber before taking OTC drugs, including antacids. If they're prescribed, tell patient to take azithromycin 1 hour before or 2 to 3 hours after taking antacids.
• Tell patient to report signs and symptoms of allergic reaction (such as rash, itching, hives, chest tightness, and trouble breathing) immediately.
• Warn patient that abdominal pain and loose, watery stools may occur. If diarrhea persists or becomes severe, urge him to contact prescriber and replace fluids.
• Because azithromycin may destroy normal flora, teach patient to watch for and immediately report signs of superinfection, such as white patches in the mouth.

aztreonam

Azactam, Cayston

Class and Category

Chemical class: Monobactam
Therapeutic class: Antibiotic
Pregnancy category: B

Indications and Dosages

➤ *To improve respiratory symptoms in cystic fibrosis patients with Pseudomonas aeruginosa*

INHALATION

Adults and children age 7 and older. 75 mg (1 vial) 3 times a day with doses at least 4 hr apart for 28 days (followed by 28 days off therapy).

➤ *To treat infections of the urinary tract, lower respiratory tract, skin, soft tissue, female reproductive tract; intra-abdominal infections; septicemia; and surgical abscesses caused by susceptible strains of gram-negative bacteria*

I.V. INFUSION, I.V. OR I.M. INJECTION

Adults. 0.5 to 2 g every 8 to 12 hr to maximum of 8 g daily. For life-threatening systemic infection, 2 g every 6 to 8 hr to maximum of 8 g daily.

Children ages 9 months to 16 years. 30 mg/kg every 6 to 8 hr up to 120 mg/kg daily; 50 mg/kg every 4 to 6 hr (for *Pseudomonas aeruginosa*).

DOSAGE ADJUSTMENT If creatinine clearance is 10 to 30 ml/min/1.73 m^2, initial dose is 1 to 2 g; then 50% of usual dose at usual interval. If creatinine clearance is less than 10 ml/min/1.73 m^2, initial dose is 500 mg to 2 g; then 25% of the usual dose every 6, 8, or 12 hr.

Route	Onset	Peak	Duration
I.V. infusion	Immediate	Immediate	Unknown
I.V. injection	Immediate	Immediate	Unknown
I.M.	Variable	60 min	Unknown
Inhalation	Variable	60 min	Unknown

Mechanism of Action

Inhibits bacterial cell wall synthesis in susceptible aerobic gram-negative bacteria. These bacteria assemble rigid, cross-linked cell walls in several steps. Aztreonam affects the final cross-linking step by inactivating penicillin-binding protein 3 (the enzyme that links cell wall strands), which causes cell lysis and death.

Incompatibilities

Don't mix aztreonam in same I.V. solution as cephradine, metronidazole, or nafcillin sodium. Don't mix it in same I.M. injection solution as local anesthetic.

Contraindications

Hypersensitivity to aztreonam or its components

Interaction

DRUGS

aminoglycosides (prolonged or high-dose therapy): Increased risk of nephrotoxicity and ototoxicity
cefoxitin, imipenem: Possibly antagonized action of aztreonam
furosemide, probenecid: Possibly increased blood aztreonam level

Adverse Reactions

CNS: Confusion, dizziness, fever, headache, insomnia, malaise, paresthesia, seizures, vertigo
CV: Chest pain, hypotension, transient ECG changes
EENT: Altered taste, diplopia, halitosis, mouth ulcers, mucocutaneous candidiasis, nasal congestion, sneezing, tinnitus, tongue numbness
GI: Abdominal cramps, diarrhea, elevated liver function test results, GI bleeding, hepatitis, nausea, pseudomembranous colitis, vomiting
GU: Breast tenderness, elevated serum creatinine level, vaginal candidiasis
HEME: Anemia, eosinophilia, leukocytosis, neutropenia, pancytopenia, positive Coombs' test, prolonged PT and APTT, thrombocytopenia, thrombocytosis
MS: Arthralgia, joint swelling, myalgia
RESP: Bronchospasm, dyspnea, wheezing
SKIN: Diaphoresis, erythema multiforme, exfoliative dermatitis, flushing, jaundice, petechiae, pruritus, purpura, rash, toxic epidermal necrolysis, urticaria
Other: Allergic reaction; injection-site pain, phlebitis, swelling, or thrombophlebitis

Nursing Considerations

• Obtain culture and sensitivity test results, if possible, before starting aztreonam therapy. If patient is acutely ill, expect to begin therapy before results are available.
• Keep in mind that other antimicrobials may be used with aztreonam in seriously ill patients at risk for gram-positive infection.

• Expect to use I.V. route for patients who need single doses over 1 g and those with life-threatening systemic infections, such as septicemia or peritonitis.

• To reconstitute aztreonam for I.V. bolus injection, use sterile water for injection. Immediately after adding diluent to vial, shake it vigorously to mix. After obtaining correct dose, discard unused solution. Reconstituted solution may turn light pink on standing at room temperature. This doesn't affect drug potency.

• Give I.V. bolus injection directly into I.V. tubing over 3 to 5 minutes.

WARNING When preparing aztreonam for I.V. infusion, use at least 50 ml of appropriate infusion solution per gram of aztreonam. Further dilute drug in I.V. solution, such as normal saline solution, D_5W, dextrose 5% in normal saline solution, lactated Ringer's solution, or Ringer's solution.

• Know that I.V. infusion may be administered over 20 to 60 minutes.

• Flush I.V. tubing with solution, such as normal saline solution, before and after administering I.V. infusion to reduce risk of incompatibilities.

• If prescribed, mix aztreonam in same I.V. solution with other antibiotics (such as ampicillin sodium, cefazolin sodium, clindamycin phosphate, gentamicin sulfate, or tobramycin sulfate), or mix it with cloxacillin sodium and vancomycin hydrochloride in peritoneal dialysis solution.

• Prepare solution for I.M. injection using sterile or bacteriostatic water or sodium chloride for injection. Administer injection deep into large muscle, such as in dorsogluteal or ventrogluteal area.

• Dilute each vial of inhalation solution with 1 ampule of diluent that comes with the drug. To do so, open the glass medication vial carefully, remove metal ring by pulling the tab, and remove the gray rubber stopper. Twist the tip off the diluent ampule and squeeze the liquid into the glass medication vial. Replace the rubber stopper, then gently swirl the vial until contents have been completely dissolved. Administer immediately.

• Administer diluted inhalation solution using only an Altera Nebulizer System.

• Be aware that patient should use a bronchodilator prior to aztreonam inhalation therapy. A short-acting bronchodilator should be used at least 15 minutes before but no longer than 4 hours prior to aztreonam inhalation therapy, or a long-acting bronchodilator at least 30 minutes before but no longer than 12 hours prior to aztreonam inhalation therapy. If patient is receiving multiple inhaled therapies, administer the bronchodilator first, followed by mucolytics, and last of all aztreonam.

• Assess for signs of bacterial or fungal superinfection, which may occur with prolonged or repeated therapy. If superinfection occurs, treat it as prescribed.

• Monitor bowel elimination; if needed, obtain stool culture to rule out pseudomembranous colitis. If it occurs, expect to discontinue aztreonam and administer fluid, electrolytes, and antibiotics effective against *Clostridium difficile.*

• Evaluate patient's renal and liver function test results, as ordered, if patient has renal or hepatic impairment.

• Monitor renal function if patient is receiving an aminoglycoside because of the increased risk of nephrotoxicity.

PATIENT TEACHING

• Emphasize the need to take full course of aztreonam exactly as prescribed, even if patient feels better before finishing it.

• Instruct patient how to dilute and administer inhalation form of drug, if ordered.

• Teach patient to recognize and immediately report signs and symptoms of allergic reactions, such as chest tightness, difficulty breathing, hives, itching, and rash.

• Warn patient that abdominal pain and loose, watery stools may occur 2 months or more after aztreonam therapy stops. If diarrhea persists or becomes severe, urge him to contact prescriber and replace fluids.

• Because aztreonam may destroy normal flora, teach patient to watch for and immediately report signs of superinfection, such as white patches in mouth.

B

bacampicillin hydrochloride

Penglobe (CAN), Spectrobid

Class and Category

Chemical class: Aminopenicillin
Therapeutic class: Antibiotic
Pregnancy category: B

Indications and Dosages

➤ *To treat upper respiratory tract infections (including otitis media) caused by streptococci, pneumococci, nonpenicillinase-producing staphylococci, and* Haemophilus influenzae; *UTI caused by* Escherichia coli, Proteus mirabilis, *or* Streptococcus faecalis; *skin and soft-tissue infections caused by streptococci and susceptible staphylococci*

TABLETS

Adults. 400 mg every 12 hr; 800 mg every 12 hr for severe infections and those caused by less susceptible organisms.
Children weighing 25 kg (55 lb) or more. 25 mg/kg daily in divided doses every 12 hr; 50 mg/kg daily in divided doses every 12 hr for severe infections and those caused by less susceptible organisms.

➤ *To treat lower respiratory tract infections caused by streptococci, pneumococci, non–penicillinase-producing staphylococci, and* H. influenzae

TABLETS

Adults. 800 mg every 12 hr.
Children weighing 25 kg or more. 50 mg/kg/day in divided doses every 12 hr.

➤ *To treat uncomplicated gonorrhea caused by* Neisseria gonorrhoeae

TABLETS

Adults. 1.6 g plus 1 g of probenecid as a single dose.

Route	Onset	Peak	Duration
P.O.	Variable	Unknown	12 hr

Mechanism of Action

Inhibits bacterial cell wall synthesis in susceptible bacteria. These bacteria assemble rigid, cross-linked cell walls in several steps. Bacampicillin, which undergoes hydrolysis to ampicillin, affects final stage of cross-linking by binding with and inactivating penicillin-binding protein (enzyme responsible for linking cell wall strands). This action inhibits bacterial cell wall synthesis and causes cell lysis and death.

Contraindications

Cholestatic jaundice and hepatic dysfunction associated with amoxicillin and clavulanate potassium; hypersensitivity to penicillins, cephalosporins, imipenem and cilastatin, or beta-lactamase inhibitors, such as piperacillin and tazobactam

Interactions

DRUGS

allopurinol: Increased risk of rash from bacampicillin use
beta-adrenergic blockers: Increased risk of anaphylaxis
disulfiram: Possibly disulfiram reaction when administered together
oral contraceptives: Possibly reduced effectiveness of oral contraceptives, contraceptive failure, and breakthrough bleeding
tetracyclines: Possibly impaired bactericidal effects of bacampicillin

Adverse Reactions

CNS: Anxiety, confusion, depression, fatigue, fever, hallucinations, lethargy, malaise, neuromuscular irritability, seizures, stroke, syncope
CV: Hypotension, palpitations, periarteritis nodosa, pulmonary hypertension, tachycardia, vascular collapse
EENT: Altered taste, black "hairy" tongue, blurred vision, glossitis, laryngospasm, mouth soreness, mucocutaneous candidiasis, stomatitis, taste disorders
GI: Abdominal cramps or pain, anorexia, diarrhea, enterocolitis, epigastric distress, elevated liver function test results, gastritis, nausea, pseudomembranous colitis, vomiting
GU: Elevated BUN and serum creatinine levels, hematuria, impotence, interstitial

nephritis, neurogenic bladder, priapism, renal failure, vaginal candidiasis
HEME: Agranulocytosis, anemia, bone marrow depression, decreased hemoglobin level and hematocrit, eosinophilia, leukopenia, neutropenia, prolonged PT, thrombocytopenia, thrombocytopenic purpura
MS: Arthralgia, arthritis exacerbation
RESP: Bronchospasm
SKIN: Exfoliative dermatitis, rash, urticaria
Other: Allergic reaction, lymphadenopathy, serum sickness

Nursing Considerations

• Obtain culture and sensitivity test results, if possible, before starting therapy. Expect to start drug before results are available.
• Expect to continue treatment for at least 48 hours after symptoms resolve or culture detects no signs of infection.
WARNING Expect to give bacampicillin for 10 days to treat infection caused by group A beta-hemolytic streptococci to prevent development of acute rheumatic fever or acute glomerulonephritis.
• Assess patient for bacterial or fungal superinfection, which may occur with prolonged or repeated therapy. If it occurs, expect to administer another antibiotic or antifungal drug.
• Monitor bowel elimination; if needed, obtain stool culture to rule out pseudo-membranous colitis. If this adverse reaction occurs, expect to discontinue bacampicillin and give fluid, electrolytes, and antibiotics effective against *Clostridium difficile.*

PATIENT TEACHING

• Teach patient to recognize and immediately report signs of allergic reaction, including rash, itching, hives, chest tightness, and difficulty breathing.
• Warn that abdominal pain and loose, watery stools may occur. If diarrhea persists or becomes severe, urge him to contact prescriber and drink plenty of fluids.
• Because bacampicillin may destroy normal flora, teach patient to watch for and immediately report signs of superinfection, such as white patches in mouth and vaginal itching and discharge.

bacitracin
Baci-IM

Class and Category
Chemical class: Bacillus subtilis derivative (polypeptide)
Therapeutic class: Antibiotic
Pregnancy category: C

Indications and Dosages
➤ *To treat pneumonia and empyema caused by susceptible staphylococci*
I.M. INJECTION
Infants weighing more than 2.5 kg (5.5 lb). 1,000 units/kg daily in 2 or 3 divided doses.
Infants weighing less than 2.5 kg. 900 units/kg daily in 2 or 3 divided doses.

Route	Onset	Peak	Duration
I.M.	Rapid	Unknown	About 6 hr

Mechanism of Action
Interferes with bacterial cell wall synthesis by binding with isoprenyl pyrophosphate (a lipid-carrying molecule that transports substances out of bacterial cells to help build new cell walls), forming an unusable complex in bacterial cells. This weakens cell walls and causes lysis and death. Bacitracin is considered bacteriostatic and bactericidal.

Incompatibilities
Don't dilute bacitracin with a solution that contains parabens.

Contraindications
Hypersensitivity or toxic reaction to bacitracin

Interactions
DRUGS
aminoglycosides: Increased risk of respiratory paralysis and renal dysfunction
nondepolarizing neuromuscular blockers: Possibly increased neuromuscular blockade

Adverse Reactions
GI: Nausea, vomiting
GU: Albuminuria, azotemia, cylindrical mucus casts in urine, nephrotoxicity
SKIN: Rash
Other: Injection-site pain, superinfection

Nursing Considerations

• Obtain culture and sensitivity test results before therapy begins, if possible. Be prepared to start bacitracin therapy before results are available.

WARNING Use parenteral bacitracin for I.M. injection only.

• For I.M. solution of 5,000 units/ml, reconstitute 50,000 units bacitracin powder with 9.8 ml sodium chloride for injection that contains 2% procaine hydrochloride.

• Administer I.M. injection into upper outer quadrant of buttocks, alternating between right and left sides. To prevent pain at injection site, avoid giving multiple injections in same site.

• During therapy, compare daily results of renal function tests with baseline results, as appropriate.

• Assess urine output often (hourly, if needed), and replace fluids orally and parenterally to maintain adequate renal function.

WARNING Because of increased risk of nephrotoxicity, avoid concurrent use of other nephrotoxic drugs, such as streptomycin, kanamycin, polymyxin B, and neomycin.

• Assess infant for signs of superinfection, especially white patches in mouth and perineum. If superinfection develops, plan to treat with appropriate antibiotics.

PATIENT TEACHING

• Advise parents that daily blood tests are needed to assess infant's renal function.

• Encourage parents to provide oral fluids to promote renal function. Teach them how to record infant's fluid intake.

• Instruct parents to report signs or symptoms of superinfection, such as white patches in mouth or perineal area and bright red diaper rash.

---

balsalazide disodium

Colazal

Class and Category

Chemical class: Prodrug of 5-aminosalicylic acid (5-ASA)
Therapeutic class: Anti-inflammatory
Pregnancy category: B

Indications and Dosages

➤ *To treat mildly to moderately active ulcerative colitis*

CAPSULES

Adults. 2.25 g three times daily for 8 wk. *Maximum:* 6.75 g daily for 12 wk.
Children ages 5 to 17. 750 mg or 2.25 g three times daily for up to 8 wk.

Mechanism of Action

After it has been metabolized to 5-ASA, balsalazide may reduce inflammation by inhibiting the enzyme cyclooxygenase and decreasing production of arachidonic acid metabolites, which may be increased in patients with inflammatory bowel disease.

Cyclooxygenase is needed to form prostaglandin from arachidonic acid. Prostaglandin mediates inflammatory activity and produces signs and symptoms of inflammation. By inhibiting prostaglandin synthesis, balsalazide may reduce signs and symptoms of inflammation in inflammatory bowel disease.

Balsalazide also interferes with leukotrine synthesis and inhibits the enzyme lipoxygenase. These substances are involved in the inflammatory response.

Contraindications

Hypersensitivity to balsalazide, salicylates, or their components

Adverse Reactions

CNS: Fatigue, fever, headache, insomnia
CV: Myocarditis, pericarditis, vasculitis
EENT: Dry mouth, nasopharyngitis, pharyngitis, rhinitis, stomatitis
GI: Abdominal cramps or pain, anorexia, cirrhosis, constipation, diarrhea, dyspepsia, elevated liver enzyme levels, exacerbation of colitis, flatulence, hepatotoxicity, jaundice, nausea, pancreatitis, vomiting
GU: Dysmenorrhea, interstitial nephritis, renal failure, UTI
MS: Arthralgia, myalgia
RESP: Alveolitis, cough, flulike syndrome, pleural effusion, pneumonia, respiratory tract infection
SKIN: Alopecia, pruritus

Nursing Considerations

WARNING Monitor patients who are sensitive to sulfasalazine or olsalazine for possible cross-sensitivity to balsalazide.

• Monitor patients with pyloric stenosis for decreased or delayed drug effects due to prolonged gastric retention of balsalazide capsules.
• Monitor patient for possible exacerbation of colitis symptoms.

PATIENT TEACHING
• Inform patient that balsalazide is used to reduce bowel inflammation and pain in ulcerative colitis and to minimize recurring inflammation.
• Instruct patient to swallow capsules whole, with a full glass of water, and not to crush or chew them.
• Advise patient to notify prescriber of any other drugs she may be taking, including OTC drugs, nutritional supplements, and herbal products, because they may interact with balsalazide.
• Instruct patient to notify prescriber immediately if colitis symptoms worsen.
• Inform patient that she can expect some improvement in symptoms in 3 to 21 days but that optimal results may take up to 6 weeks of treatment.

beclomethasone dipropionate

Beclodisk (CAN), Beclovent Rotacaps (CAN), Beconase, Beconase AQ, Qnasl, QVAR, Vancenase, Vanceril

Class and Category
Chemical class: Synthetic glucocorticoid
Therapeutic class: Antiasthmatic, anti-inflammatory
Pregnancy category: C

Indications and Dosages
➤ *To control and prevent symptoms in patients with chronic asthma and those who also require oral corticosteroids*

INHALATION AEROSOL (84 MCG)
Adults and children age 12 and over.
Initial: 2 inhalations (168 mcg) twice daily. For patients with severe asthma, 6 to 8 inhalations (504 to 672 mcg) daily with dosage reduced based on patient response. *Maximum:* 10 inhalations (840 mcg) daily.

Children ages 6 to 12. *Initial:* 2 inhalations (168 mcg) twice daily. *Maximum:* 5 inhalations (420 mcg) daily.

INHALATION AEROSOL (42 MCG)
Adults and children age 12 and over.
Initial: 2 inhalations (84 mcg) three times daily. or four times daily or 4 inhalations (168 mcg) twice daily. For patients with severe asthma, 12 to 16 inhalations (504 to 672 mcg) daily with dosage reduced based on patient response. *Maximum:* 20 inhalations (840 mcg) daily.

Children ages 6 to 12. *Initial:* 1 or 2 inhalations (42 mcg or 84 mcg) three times daily or four times daily or 4 inhalations (168 mcg) twice daily with dosage reduced based on patient response. *Maximum:* 10 inhalations (420 mcg) daily.

INHALATION AEROSOL (40 MCG, 80 MCG [QVAR])
Adults and adolescents. *Initial for patients previously taking bronchodilators alone:* 1 to 2 inhalations (40 to 80 mcg) twice daily, depending on strength used. *Maximum:* 4 to 8 inhalations (320 mcg) twice daily, depending on strength used. *Initial for patients previously taking inhaled corticosteroids:* 1 to 4 inhalations (160 mcg) twice daily, depending on strength used. *Maximum:* 4 to 8 inhalations (320 mcg) twice daily, depending on strength used.

Children ages 5 to 11. 1 inhalation (40 mcg) twice daily. *Maximum:* 1 to 2 inhalations (80 mcg) twice daily, depending on strength used.

➤ *To relieve symptoms of seasonal or perennial allergic and nonallergic (vasomotor) rhinitis and prevent nasal polyps from recurring after surgical removal*

NASAL INHALATION AEROSOL
Adults and children age 12 and over.
Initial: 1 inhalation (42 mcg) in each nostril twice daily to four times daily for total dose of 168 to 336 mcg daily. *Maintenance:* 1 inhalation (42 mcg) in each nostril three times daily for total dose of 252 mcg daily.

Children ages 6 to 12. 1 inhalation (42 mcg) in each nostril three times daily for total dose of 252 mcg daily.

NASAL SPRAY
Adults and children age 12 and over. 1 or 2 inhalations (42 or 84 mcg) in each nostril twice daily for total dose of 168 or 336 mcg daily.

➤ *To relieve symptoms of seasonal and perennial allergic rhinitis*
NASAL SPRAY (QNASL)
Adults and children age 12 and over.
2 sprays (80 mcg/spray) in each nostril once daily.
Children age 4 to 11. 1 spray (40 mcg) in each nostril once daily.

Mechanism of Action
May decrease number and activity of cells involved in the inflammatory response of asthma, allergies, and rhinitis, such as mast cells, eosinophils, basophils, lymphocytes, macrophages, and neutrophils. Also may inhibit production or secretion of chemical mediators, such as histamine, eicosanoids, leukotrienes, and cytokines. May produce direct smooth-muscle cell relaxation and decrease airway hyperresponsiveness.

Contraindications
Hypersensitivity to beclomethasone's ingredients, infrequent oral corticosteroid treatment, primary treatment of status asthmaticus or other acute asthma attack, relief of acute bronchospasm or of asthma controlled by bronchodilators or other nonsteroidal drugs, treatment of nonasthmatic bronchitis

Adverse Reactions
CNS: Aggression, depression, fatigue, fever, headache, insomnia, light-headedness, mania, psychomotor hyperactivity, suicidal ideation
CV: Chest pain, tachycardia
EENT: Cataracts, dry mouth, dysphonia, earache, epistaxis, glaucoma, hoarseness, lacrimation, nasal congestion or ulceration, nasal septal perforation, nose and throat dryness and irritation, nose and oral candidiasis, pharyngitis, rhinorrhea, sinusitis, sneezing, unpleasant smell and taste
ENDO: Adrenal insufficiency, cushingoid symptoms
GI: Diarrhea, indigestion, nausea, rectal hemorrhage
GU: Dysmenorrhea, UTI
MS: Arthralgia, growth suppression in children (nasal aerosol)
RESP: Bronchitis, bronchospasm, chest congestion, cough, pulmonary infiltrates, upper respiratory tract infection, wheezing

SKIN: Acne, eczema, pruritus, rash, skin discoloration, urticaria
Other: Angioedema, flulike symptoms, impaired wound healing, lymphadenopathy, weight gain

Nursing Considerations
• Be aware that beclomethasone should not be used with patients who have experienced recent nasal septal ulcers, nasal surgery, or nasal trauma because of corticosteroids' adverse effects on wound healing.
• If patient also takes an oral corticosteroid, expect to taper dosage slowly (by decreasing daily dosage or taking drug every other day) about 1 week after beclomethasone therapy begins. Expect dosage reductions of more than 2.5 mg daily.
WARNING When gradually switching patient from oral corticosteroid to inhaled beclomethasone, watch for signs of life-threatening adrenal insufficiency, such as fatigue, lassitude, weakness, nausea, vomiting, and hypotension, during transition period and when exposed to trauma, surgery, infection, or other stressor. If signs occur, notify prescriber immediately.
• Expect to resume oral corticosteroid during a stressful period or severe asthma attack.
• Because beclomethasone may be absorbed systemically, watch for signs of adrenal insufficiency during periods of stress.
• If patient has acute asthma attack or increased wheezing after receiving beclomethasone, give fast-acting bronchodilator, as prescribed. Expect to discontinue beclomethasone.
• Assess for signs of candidiasis, such as thick white plaques or coating on tongue and sides of mouth. If present, notify prescriber and expect to reduce dose or frequency or to stop beclomethasone. Also anticipate treatment with antifungal drug.
• When administering beclomethasone nasal spray, periodically assess nasal discharge for color or consistency changes, which may indicate infection.
• Monitor the growth of children receiving beclomethasone nasally.

B

• Monitor patient closely for altered thinking such as suicide thoughts. If present, notify prescriber because drug will need to be discontinued.

PATIENT TEACHING

• Advise patient not to abruptly stop taking beclomethasone because adrenal insufficiency may occur. Urge her to notify prescriber if she develops signs of adrenal insufficiency, such as nausea, fatigue, anorexia, dyspnea, hypotension, fever, malaise, dizziness, and fainting.

• Before patient uses nasal spray for first time, instruct her to prime pump by placing her thumb on its base, and her index and middle fingers on its shoulder area (the canister should be on top, pointing down), and then pressing her thumb firmly and quickly against the bottle four times into the air away from eyes and face. If nasal spray has not been used for 7 consecutive days, remind patient that container needs to be primed by spraying 2 times prior to use. Before patient uses nasal inhalation canister for first time, instruct her to shake it and check that it's working properly by spraying it once in the air while looking for fine mist.

• Teach patient to inhale deeply after each nasal spray or inhalation, exhaling through mouth and tilting head back to let drug spread over the nasopharynx.

• Teach patient how to properly use oral inhalation aerosol, shaking canister well before using. If patient has trouble using device and coordinating inhalation with it, suggest using a spacer device.

• If two inhalations are prescribed, advise patient to wait a minute between them.

• If patient uses an inhaled bronchodilator with beclomethasone oral inhalation, tell her to use bronchodilator first, wait 5 minutes, and then use beclomethasone.

WARNING Warn patient that beclomethasone isn't intended to relieve acute bronchospasm. Urge patient to notify prescriber if asthma symptoms don't respond.

• Advise patient to wear medical identification that states need for supplemental oral corticosteroids during stress or severe asthma attack. Inform patient that prescriber may order high-dose oral corticosteroid therapy.

• Warn patient and caretakers to report any abnormal thinking such as suicide thoughts immediately to prescriber.

WARNING Caution patient to avoid exposure to chickenpox and measles because drug may cause immunosuppression. If she's exposed to these disorders, urge her to notify prescriber immediately.

belimumab

Benlysta

Class and Category

Chemical class: B-lymphocyte stimulator (BLyS)-specific inhibitor
Therapeutic class: Biologic disease-modifying antilupus agent
Pregnancy category: C

Indications and Dosages

➤ *To treat active, autoantibody-positive systemic lupus erythematosus (SLE) in patients who are receiving standard therapy*

I.V. INFUSION

Adults. 10 mg/kg infused over 1 hour every 2 wks for first 3 doses followed by 10 mg/kg infused over 1 hour every 4 wks.

Mechanism of Action

Blocks the binding of soluble B-cell lymphocyte stimulator protein, a B-cell survival factor, to its receptors on B cells. This action causes cell death, which helps to relieve the signs and symptoms of active, autoantibody-positive, systemic lupus erythematosus.

Incompatibilities

Dextrose intravenous solutions are incompatible with belimumab.

Contraindications

Hypersensitivity to belimumab or its components, including prior history of anaphylaxis with belimumab use

Interactions

DRUGS

None

Adverse Reactions

CNS: Anxiety, depression, fatigue, headache, insomnia, myalgia, progressive multifocal leukoencephalopathy, suicidal ideation

CV: Bradycardia, hypotension
EENT: Nasopharyngitis, sinusitis
GI: Nausea
GU: UTI
RESP: Bronchitis, dyspnea, pneumonia, upper respiratory tract infection
MS: Myalgia
SKIN: Cellulitis, pruritus, rash, urticaria
Other: Anaphylaxis, angioedema, influenza, infusion reactions, malignancies

Nursing Considerations
• Know that belimumab should not be used to treat patients who are receiving drug therapy to treat a chronic infection. Monitor patient closely for signs and symptoms of infections during belimumab therapy. If present, notify prescriber. If the infection is determined to be new, belimumab therapy may need to be interrupted until infection is gone.
• Be aware that patient should be premedicated to prevent infusion and hypersensitivity reactions before each dose of belimumab. Patients with a history of multiple drug allergies or significant hypersensitivity may be at increased risk. If an infusion reaction still occurs, slow or temporarily stop the infusion, as ordered. If a serious hypersensitivity reaction occurs, discontinue drug immediately and notify prescriber. Know that a non-acute hypersensitivity reaction that may be evident as facial edema, fatigue, headache, myalgia, nausea, and rash may occur up to a week after an infusion.
• Remove vial from refrigerator and allow to stand 10 to 15 minutes prior to reconstitution. Use aseptic technique when reconstituting with 1.5 ml of sterile water for injection, USP for a 120-mg vial and 4.8 ml of sterile water for injection, USP when reconstituting a 400-mg vial. When injecting diluent solution into the vial, direct stream of sterile water toward the side of the vial to minimize foaming. Gently swirl the vial for 60 seconds every 5 minutes until the powder is dissolved. Do not shake or refrigerate during this process. It typically takes 10 to 15 minutes for powder to dissolve but may take as long as 30 minutes. Once reconstituted, protect from sunlight. When using a mechanical reconstitution device (swirler),

do not exceed 500 rpm, and swirl no longer than 30 minutes.
• Use only 0.9% sodium chloride injection, USP (normal saline) to further dilute the drug. Withdraw amount of normal saline from the infusion bag or bottle equivalent to the vial contents of reconstituted drug required for the patient's dose. Then add the required volume of the reconstituted solution of the drug into the infusion bag or bottle. Gently invert the bag or bottle to mix the solution. Discard any unused solution left in the vial(s). The solution should be stored in the refrigerator protected from direct sunlight, if not used immediately. Know that the total time from the drug being reconstituted to completion of infusion should not exceed 8 hours.
• Infuse belimumab intravenously over 1 hour separately from any other medication given concomitantly intravenously.
• Monitor patient for a hypersensitivity reaction following administration of belimumab because hypersensitivity reactions, including anaphylaxis, may occur on the same day of infusion. Notify prescriber immediately if a reaction occurs, because death has occurred with some patients experiencing hypersensitivity reactions. Expect to provide emergency medical treatment as ordered and indicated by severity of reaction.
• Be aware that other biologic therapies, such as B-cell targeted therapies or intravenous cyclophosphamide therapy, are not recommended during belimumab therapy because potential drug interactions are unknown.
PATIENT TEACHING
• Instruct patient to report any signs of a hypersensitivity reaction such as a rash, itching, hives, or difficulty breathing to prescriber, and to seek medical attention immediately.
• Caution patient to report new or worsening depression, suicidal thoughts, or other mood changes.
• Tell patient to contact the prescriber if he develops new or worsening neurologic symptoms such as confusion, difficulty talking or walking, dizziness, loss of balance, memory loss, or vision problems.

• Advise patient not to receive any immunization with live vaccines for 30 days before or concurrently with belimumab and to avoid contact with anyone who has an infection.
• Tell female patient of childbearing age to notify prescriber if pregnancy occurs and encourage her to enroll in the belimumab pregnancy registry by calling 1-877-681-6296.

belladonna alkaloids

Class and Category
Chemical class: Tertiary amine
Therapeutic class: GI anticholinergic
Pregnancy category: C

Indications and Dosages
➤ *To treat peptic ulcer disease, functional digestive disorders (including spastic, mucous, and ulcerative colitis), diarrhea, diverticulitis, pancreatitis, dysmenorrhea, nocturnal enuresis, idiopathic and postencephalitic parkinsonism, motion sickness, and nausea and vomiting of pregnancy*

TABLETS
Adults. 0.25 to 0.5 mg three times daily.
Children over age 6. 0.125 to 0.25 mg three times daily.

TINCTURE
Adults. 0.6 to 1 ml three times daily or four times daily.
Children. 0.03 ml/kg (0.8 ml/m^2) three times daily.

Route	Onset	Peak	Duration
P.O.	1–2 hr	Unknown	4 hr

Mechanism of Action
Inhibits acetylcholine's muscarinic actions at postganglionic parasympathetic receptor sites, including smooth muscles, secretory glands, and CNS. These actions relax smooth muscles and diminish GI, GU, and biliary tract secretions.

Contraindications
Hepatic disease, hypersensitivity to anticholinergic drugs or scopolamine, ileus, myasthenia gravis, myocardial ischemia, narrow-angle glaucoma, obstructive condition of GI or GU tract, renal disease, severe ulcerative colitis, tachycardia, toxic megacolon, unstable cardiovascular status in acute hemorrhage

Interactions
DRUGS
amantadine: Increased adverse anticholinergic effects
atenolol, digoxin: Possibly increased therapeutic and adverse effects of these drugs
phenothiazines: Possibly decreased phenothiazine effectiveness and increased adverse effects of belladonna alkaloids
tricyclic antidepressants: Possibly increased adverse anticholinergic effects

Adverse Reactions
CNS: CNS stimulation (with high doses), confusion, dizziness, drowsiness, headache, insomnia, nervousness, weakness
CV: Bradycardia, palpitations, tachycardia
EENT: Altered taste, blurred vision, dry mouth, increased intraocular pressure, mydriasis, nasal congestion, photophobia
GI: Bloating, constipation, dysphagia, heartburn, ileus, nausea, vomiting
GU: Impotence, urinary hesitancy, urine retention
SKIN: Decreased sweating, flushing, urticaria
Other: Anaphylaxis

Nursing Considerations
• Avoid using high doses of belladonna alkaloids in ulcerative colitis because they may inhibit intestinal motility and precipitate or aggravate toxic megacolon. Also avoid high doses in hiatal hernia and reflux esophagitis because they may aggravate esophagitis.
• Use belladonna alkaloids cautiously in patients with allergies, arrhythmias, asthma, autonomic neuropathy, coronary artery disease, debilitating chronic lung disease, heart failure, hypertension, hyperthyroidism, and prostatic hypertrophy.
• Give drug 30 to 60 minutes before a meal.
WARNING Monitor patient for excitement, agitation, drowsiness, and confusion. Elderly patients are more sensitive to the effects of the drug, even small doses, and

are more likely to develop adverse reactions. Dosage may need to be decreased.
• Take safety precautions to protect patient from injury from falling.

PATIENT TEACHING
• Instruct patient to take belladonna alkaloids 30 to 60 minutes before eating.
• Tell patient to notify prescriber if she has persistent or severe diarrhea, constipation, or difficulty urinating.
• Caution patient to avoid driving and similar activities until the effects of belladonna alkaloids are known.
WARNING Urge patient to avoid extreme heat and humidity because heatstroke could occur.

benazepril hydrochloride
Lotensin

Class and Category
Chemical class: Ethylester of benazeprilat
Therapeutic class: Antihypertensive
Pregnancy category: D

Indications and Dosages
➤ *To control hypertension alone or with a thiazide diuretic*

TABLETS
Adults who don't receive a diuretic. *Initial:* 10 mg daily. *Maintenance:* 20 to 40 mg daily as a single dose or in two divided doses.
Adults who receive a diuretic. 5 mg daily.
DOSAGE ADJUSTMENT Initial dosage of 5 mg/day for patients with impaired renal function and creatinine clearance less than 30 ml/min/1.73 m²; then increased gradually until blood pressure is controlled or dosage reaches maximum of 40 mg daily.
TABLETS, SUSPENSION
Children age 6 and over with glomerular filtration rate of 30 ml/min/1.73 m² or higher. *Initial:* 0.2 mg/kg daily. *Maximum:* 0.6 mg/kg daily or 40 mg daily.

Route	Onset	Peak	Duration
P.O.	1 hr	2–4 hr	24 hr

Mechanism of Action
May reduce blood pressure by affecting renin-angiotensin-aldosterone system. By inhibiting angiotensin-converting enzyme, benazepril:
• prevents conversion of angiotensin I to angiotensin II, a potent vasoconstrictor that also stimulates aldosterone release.
• may inhibit renal and vascular production of angiotensin II.
• decreases serum angiotensin II level and increases serum renin activity. This decreases aldosterone secretion, slightly increasing serum potassium level and fluid loss.
• decreases vascular tone and blood pressure.
• inhibits aldosterone release, which reduces sodium and water resorption, increases their excretion, and reduces blood pressure.

Contraindications
Aliskiren therapy in patients with diabetes or renal impairment (GFR less than 60 ml/min), history of angioedema, hypersensitivity to benazepril or other ACE inhibitor

Interactions
DRUGS
aliskiren (in patients with diabetes or renal impairment), angiotensin receptor blockers, other ACE inhibitors: Increased risk of hyperkalemia, hypotension, and renal dysfunction
antacids: Possibly decreased bioavailability of benazepril; separate doses by 2 hours
antidiabetics (oral): Possibly increased risk of hypoglycemia
capsaicin: Possibly induction or exacerbation of ACE cough caused by benazepril
digoxin: Increased serum digoxin level
diuretics: Possibly excessive hypotension
indomethacin: Reduced hypotensive effects of benazepril
lithium: Increased serum lithium level and risk of lithium toxicity
NSAIDs: Possible decreased renal function in patients who are elderly, volume-depleted, or have a compromised renal function

phenothiazines: Possibly increased therapeutic and adverse effects of benazepril

potassium preparations, potassium-sparing diuretics: Possibly increased serum potassium level

sodium aurothiomalate: Increased risk of nitritoid reactions, such as facial flushing, nausea, vomiting, and hypotension

Adverse Reactions

CNS: Anxiety, asthenia, dizziness, drowsiness, fatigue, headache, hypertonia, insomnia, nervousness, paresthesia, sleep disturbance, somnolence, syncope, weakness

CV: Angina, ECG changes, hypotension, orthostatic hypotension, palpitations, peripheral edema

EENT: Sinusitis

ENDO: Hyperglycemia

GI: Abdominal pain, acute liver failure, cholestatic hepatitis, constipation, elevated liver function test results, gastritis, hepatic necrosis, melena, nausea, pancreatitis, small bowel angioedema, vomiting

GU: Acute renal failure, decreased libido, elevated BUN and serum creatinine levels, impotence, nephrotic syndrome, oliguria, progressive azotemia, proteinuria, renal insufficiency, UTI

HEME: Agranulocytosis, decreased hemoglobin level, hemolytic anemia, pemphigus, leukopenia, neutropenia, thrombocytopenia

MS: Arthralgia, arthritis, myalgia

RESP: ACE cough, asthma, bronchitis, bronchospasm, dyspnea

SKIN: Dermatitis, diaphoresis, flushing, photosensitivity, pruritus, rash, Stevens-Johnson syndrome

Other: Anaphylaxis, angioedema, hyperkalemia, hyponatremia

Nursing Considerations

• Evaluate blood pressure with patient lying down, sitting, and standing before starting benazepril and then every 4 to 8 hours, as appropriate, to monitor effectiveness.

• Monitor urine output and BUN and serum creatinine levels, as needed, before therapy and then during therapy, especially in patients with renal artery stenosis, severe heart failure, post-myocardial infarction or in patients who are volume depleted.

Also monitor patients closely who are also receiving NSAID or angiotensin receptor blocker therapy because these patients may be at increased risk for developing acute renal failure.

• Monitor liver enzymes regularly, as ordered. Assess patient routinely for signs and symptoms of liver dysfunction, such as jaundice and fatigue. Notify prescriber if patient develops jaundice or exhibits elevated liver enzyme levels, as drug will need to be discontinued.

WARNING Be alert for angioedema, especially after first dose. If it extends to larynx and patient has laryngeal stridor or signs of airway obstruction, prepare to give epinephrine subcutaneously immediately, as prescribed, and discontinue benazepril. Be aware that black patients have a higher incidence of angioedema compared to nonblacks.

• Monitor WBC count periodically to detect neutropenia and agranulocytosis.

• Check serum potassium and other electrolyte levels to detect electrolyte imbalances.

• To prevent injury caused by orthostatic hypotension, take safety precautions, such as having patient change positions slowly and sit on edge of bed before arising.

PATIENT TEACHING

• Teach patient how to monitor blood pressure, if appropriate, and how to recognize signs of hypertension and hypotension.

WARNING Strongly urge patient to contact prescriber before using any OTC salt substitutes, which may contain potassium, or potassium supplements. These substances increase the risk of hyperkalemia.

• Explain that a persistent dry cough may develop and may not subside unless benazepril is stopped. If cough becomes bothersome or interferes with sleep or activities, patient should notify prescriber.

WARNING Instruct patient to contact prescriber immediately if she has signs of angioedema, such as swelling of the face, eyes, lips, or tongue.

• Caution patient to avoid sudden position changes and to rise slowly from sitting or lying to minimize orthostatic hypotension.

WARNING Advise patient to stop benazepril and notify prescriber as soon as possible if she experiences syncope.
WARNING Caution women of childbearing age to use reliable contraception and to notify prescriber immediately if pregnancy is suspected. Benazepril may cause fetal harm and should be discontinued.

benzonatate

Benzonatate Softgels, Tessalon Perles

Class and Category
Chemical class: Para-aminobenzoic acid (tetracaine-like)
Therapeutic class: Nonnarcotic antitussive
Pregnancy category: C

Indications and Dosages
To relieve cough
CAPSULES, PERLES
Adults and children over age 10. 100 mg three times daily up to 600 mg daily.

Route	Onset	Peak	Duration
P.O.	15–20 min	Unknown	3–8 hr

Mechanism of Action
Anesthetizes stretch receptors in respiratory tract, lung tissue, and pleura, interfering with their activity and reducing cough reflex at its source. In usual doses, benzonatate doesn't inhibit respiratory center.

Contraindications
Hypersensitivity to benzonatate or related compounds

Adverse Reactions
CNS: Confusion, hallucinations, headache, mild dizziness, sedation
CV: Cardiogenic shock, chest numbness
EENT: Burning eyes, laryngospasm, nasal congestion
GI: Constipation, GI upset, nausea
RESP: Bronchospasm
SKIN: Pruritus, rash

Nursing Considerations
• Assess type and frequency of cough. Don't try to suppress cough with benzonatate if cough has therapeutic benefit, such as to move secretions and improve airflow.

WARNING Don't break or crush capsules or perles or let patient chew or dissolve them in her mouth. Releasing drug in the mouth may anesthetize mouth and throat, causing risk of choking. Also don't let patient suck or chew capsule because severe local hypersensitivity reaction may occur.

PATIENT TEACHING
• Instruct patient to swallow capsules and perles whole and not to chew, suck, or open them.
• Instruct patient never to take two doses of drug at same time, as signs and symptoms of overdose may occur.
• Warn patient that mild dizziness and sedation may occur. Teach her to take safety measures, and encourage her to avoid activities that require mental alertness until benzonatate's effects are known.
• Emphasize importance of keeping drug out of the reach of children, as accidental ingestion in children may be fatal.

benzquinamide hydrochloride

Emete-Con

Class and Category
Chemical class: Benzoquinolizine amide
Therapeutic class: Antiemetic
Pregnancy category: Not rated

Indications and Dosages
➤ *To treat nausea and vomiting related to anesthesia or surgery*
I.V. OR I.M. INJECTION
Adults. 50 mg or 0.5 to 1 mg/kg I.M., repeated in 1 hr, then every 3 to 4 hr, as needed. Or, 25 mg or 0.2 to 0.4 mg/kg by slow infusion (1 ml every 0.5 to 1 min) as a single dose. Then, I.M. doses begin.
➤ *To prevent nausea and vomiting related to anesthesia and surgery*
I.M. INJECTION
Adults. 50 mg or 0.5 to 1 mg/kg 15 min before emergence from anesthesia.

Route	Onset	Peak	Duration
I.V., I.M.	15 min	Unknown	Unknown

Mechanism of Action
Exhibits antiemetic, antihistaminic, mild cholinergic, and sedative effects by unknown mechanism.

Contraindications
Hypersensitivity to benzquinamide or its components

Interactions
DRUGS
vasopressors: Increased hypertensive effects

Adverse Reactions
CNS: Chills, dizziness, drowsiness, excitement, fatigue, fever, headache, insomnia, nervousness, restlessness, tremor, weakness
CV: Atrial fibrillation, hypertension, hypotension, premature atrial or ventricular contractions
EENT: Blurred vision, dry mouth, increased salivation
GI: Anorexia, hiccups, nausea
MS: Muscle twitching
SKIN: Diaphoresis, flushing, rash, urticaria

Nursing Considerations
WARNING Avoid I.V. route in patients with cardiovascular disease because sudden blood pressure increases and transient arrhythmias may occur. Use I.V. route only for patients without cardiovascular disease who aren't receiving a preanesthetic or cardiovascular drug.
• Administer benzquinamide I.M. into large, well-developed muscle. Avoid using deltoid muscle unless it's well developed.
• Take safety precautions to reduce the risk of injury from CNS depression.
PATIENT TEACHING
• Advise patient to stay in bed and call for assistance to reduce risk of injury.
• Tell patient to report whether nausea and vomiting have been relieved.

---

benztropine mesylate

Apo-Benztropine (CAN), Cogentin, PMS Benztropine (CAN)

Class and Category
Chemical class: Tertiary amine

Therapeutic class: Antiparkinsonian, central-acting anticholinergic
Pregnancy category: C

Indications and Dosages
➤ *As adjunct, to treat all forms of Parkinson's disease*
TABLETS, I.M. OR I.V. INJECTION
Adults with Parkinson's disease. 1 to 2 mg daily (usual dose) with a range of 0.5 to 6 mg daily.
Adults with idiopathic Parkinson's disease. *Initial:* 0.5 to 1 mg at bedtime. *Maximum:* 4 to 6 mg daily.
Adults with postencephalitic Parkinson's disease. 2 mg daily in one or more doses; may begin with 0.5 mg at bedtime and increase as needed.
➤ *To control extrapyramidal symptoms (except tardive dyskinesia) caused by phenothiazines and other neuroleptics*
TABLETS, I.M. OR I.V. INJECTION
Adults. 1 to 4 mg once or twice daily.
➤ *To treat acute dystonic reactions*
TABLETS, I.M. OR I.V. INJECTION
Adults. *Initial:* 1 to 2 ml (1 to 2 mg total dose) I.V. or I.M. *Maintenance:* 1 to 2 mg P.O. twice daily to prevent recurrence.

Route	Onset	Peak	Duration
P.O.	1–2 hr	Unknown	24 hr
I.V., I.M	15 min	Unknown	24 hr

Mechanism of Action
Blocks acetylcholine's action at cholinergic receptor sites. This restores the brain's normal dopamine and acetylcholine balance, which relaxes muscle movement and decreases drooling, rigidity, and tremor. Benztropine also may inhibit dopamine reuptake and storage, which prolongs dopamine's action.

Contraindications
Achalasia, bladder neck obstruction, glaucoma, hypersensitivity to benztropine mesylate or its components, megacolon, myasthenia gravis, prostatic hypertrophy, pyloric or duodenal obstruction, stenosing peptic ulcer

Interactions
DRUGS
amantadine: Possibly increased adverse anticholinergic effects

digoxin: Possibly increased digoxin level
haloperidol: Possibly increased schizo-phrenic symptoms, decreased serum halo-peridol level, and development of tardive dyskinesia
levodopa: Possibly decreased levodopa effectiveness
phenothiazines: Possibly reduced phenothiazine effects and increased psychiatric symptoms

Adverse Reactions
CNS: Agitation, confusion, delirium, delusions, depression, disorientation, dizziness, drowsiness, euphoria, excitement, fever, hallucinations, headache, light-headedness, listlessness, memory loss, nervousness, paranoia, psychosis, weakness
CV: Hypotension, mild bradycardia, orthostatic hypotension, palpitations, tachycardia
EENT: Blurred vision, diplopia, dry mouth, increased intraocular pressure, mydriasis, narrow-angle glaucoma, suppurative parotitis
GI: Constipation, duodenal ulcer, epigastric distress, ileus, nausea, vomiting
GU: Dysuria, urinary hesitancy, urine retention
MS: Muscle spasms, muscle weakness
SKIN: Decreased sweating, dermatoses, flushing, rash, urticaria

Nursing Considerations
• Expect to administer I.V. or I.M. benztropine when patient needs more rapid response than oral drug can provide. Be aware that I.M. route is commonly used because it provides effects in about the same time as I.V. route. Watch for improvement a few minutes after administration. If Parkinsonian symptoms reappear, expect to repeat dose.
• Therapy typically begins with a low dose followed by gradual increases of 0.5 mg every 5 or 6 days because benztropine has a cumulative action.
• Assess muscle rigidity and tremor at baseline. Then monitor them often for improvement, which indicates drug's effectiveness.
• Give drug before or after meals based on patient's need and response. If patient has increased salivary secretions, expect to administer benztropine after meals.

If patient has dry mouth, plan to give drug before meals unless nausea develops.
WARNING When giving drug to patient with drug-induced extrapyramidal reactions, watch for worsening psychiatric symptoms.
• High-dose benztropine therapy may cause weakness and inability to move specific muscle groups. If this occurs, expect to reduce benztropine dosage.

PATIENT TEACHING
• Warn patient that drug has a cumulative effect, increasing risk of adverse reactions and overdose.
• Caution against driving and similar activities until benztropine's effects are known because it may cause blurred vision, dizziness, or drowsiness.
WARNING Because benztropine decreases sweating, urge patient to avoid extremely hot or humid conditions to reduce risk of heatstroke and severe hyperthermia. This is especially important for elderly patients and those who abuse alcohol or have chronic illness or CNS disease.
• Stress need for periodic eye examinations and intraocular pressure measurements because drug may cause narrow-angle glaucoma and increase intraocular pressure.

bepridil hydrochloride
Vascor

Class and Category
Chemical class: Calcium channel blocker, diarylammopropylamine derivative
Therapeutic class: Antianginal
Pregnancy category: C

Indications and Dosages
➤ *To treat chronic stable angina in patients who don't respond to or can't tolerate other antianginal drugs*

TABLETS
Adults. *Initial:* 200 mg daily for 10 days followed by dosage increases, depending on patient's response (ability to perform daily activities, length of QT interval, heart rate, and frequency and severity of angina attacks). *Maintenance:* 300 to 400 mg daily (maximum).

Route	Onset	Peak	Duration
P.O.	Unknown	8 days	Unknown

Mechanism of Action

Inhibits calcium movement into coronary and vascular smooth-muscle cells by blocking slow calcium channels in their membranes. This decreases intracellular calcium level, which inhibits smooth-muscle cell contractions and causes:
• relaxation of coronary and vascular smooth muscles, decreased peripheral vascular resistance, and reduced systolic and diastolic blood pressure, which decrease myocardial oxygen demand
• depression of impulse formation (automaticity) and conduction velocity.
• Bepridil also inhibits fast inward sodium channels, reducing speed and degree of action potential, and increasing its duration in cardiac muscle.

Contraindications

Congenital prolonged QT interval, history of serious ventricular arrhythmias, hypersensitivity to bepridil, hypotension (systolic pressure below 90 mm Hg), sick sinus syndrome and second- or third-degree AV block unless artificial pacemaker in place, uncompensated cardiac insufficiency, use of other drugs that prolong QT interval

Interactions
DRUGS
antiarrhythmics, such as quinidine and procainamide, with actions similar to bepridil's: Exaggerated and prolonged QT interval
beta blockers: Possibly increased depression of myocardial contractility and AV conduction
digoxin: Possibly increased serum digoxin level
fentanyl: Severe hypotension and increased need for fluid
nitrates: Additive hypotensive effect
tricyclic antidepressants: Exaggerated and prolonged QT interval

Adverse Reactions
CNS: Amnesia, anxiety, asthenia, depression, dizziness, drowsiness, fever, hallucinations, headache, insomnia, nervousness, paranoia, paresthesia, psychosis, syncope, tremor, vertigo
CV: Edema, hypertension, palpitations, premature ventricular contractions, prolonged QT interval, sinus bradycardia or tachycardia, torsades de pointes, vasodilation, ventricular fibrillation, ventricular tachycardia
EENT: Altered taste, blurred vision, dry mouth, pharyngitis, rhinitis, tinnitus
GI: Abdominal cramps or discomfort, anorexia, appetite increase, constipation, diarrhea, flatulence, gastritis, nausea
GU: Decreased libido, impotence
HEME: Agranulocytosis, leukopenia, neutropenia
MS: Arthritis, myalgia
RESP: Cough, dyspnea, respiratory tract infection
SKIN: Dermatitis, diaphoresis, rash
Other: Flulike symptoms

Nursing Considerations
• Use bepridil cautiously in patients with heart failure because it can induce new arrhythmias and may worsen heart failure.
• Because bepridil is metabolized by the liver and its metabolites are excreted in urine, monitor results of liver function studies as well as BUN and serum electrolyte and creatinine levels as appropriate.
• Assess patient's heart rate and rhythm to obtain baseline. Then monitor frequently during therapy. Also, monitor serial 12-lead ECG tracings. Be aware that bepridil can induce new arrhythmias, including ventricular tachycardia and fibrillation (which are more difficult to convert), torsades de pointes, and prolonged QT intervals.
WARNING Be alert for QT intervals that exceed 0.52 second. If this occurs, expect to reduce bepridil dose or discontinue drug.
• Monitor WBC count to detect agranulocytosis, which may warrant stopping bepridil therapy.
WARNING Be aware that bepridil shouldn't be discontinued abruptly. Instead, gradually taper dosage as prescribed to prevent increased frequency and duration of chest pain as increased calcium moves into cells, causing coronary artery spasm.
• Monitor blood pressure often if patient takes a nitrate or beta blocker. Assess for hypotension.

• Monitor serum electrolyte levels. Especially note decreased potassium level, which may worsen existing arrhythmias or induce new ones.

PATIENT TEACHING

• Advise patient to avoid driving and other activities that require alertness and coordination until bepridil's CNS effects are known.

betamethasone
Celestone

betamethasone acetate-betamethasone sodium phosphate
Celestone Soluspan

betamethasone sodium phosphate
Betnesol (CAN), Celestone Phosphate, Selestoject

Class and Category
Chemical class: Synthetic glucocorticoid
Therapeutic class: Anti-inflammatory
Pregnancy category: C

Indications and Dosages
➤ *To treat conditions with severe inflammation and conditions requiring immunosuppression*

SYRUP, TABLETS (BETAMETHASONE)
Adults. 0.6 to 7.2 mg daily.

I.M. INJECTION (BETAMETHASONE ACETATE-BETAMETHASONE SODIUM PHOSPHATE)
Adults. 0.5 to 9 mg I.M. daily, or one-third to one-half of P.O. dose every 12 hr.

I.M. OR I.V. INJECTION (BETAMETHASONE SODIUM PHOSPHATE)
Adults. *Initial:* Variable (given in emergency situations or when oral therapy isn't possible). *Maximum:* 9 mg daily.

➤ *To treat bursitis, gouty arthritis, osteoarthritis, periostitis of cuboid, peritendinitis, rheumatoid arthritis, skin lesions, tenosynovitis*

INTRA-ARTICULAR, INTRABURSAL, OR INTRADERMAL INJECTION (BETAMETHASONE ACETATE-BETAMETHASONE SODIUM PHOSPHATE)
Adults with bursitis, peritendinitis, or tenosynovitis. 1 ml by intrabursal or intra-articular injection. Three or four injections given every 1 to 2 wk.
Adults with osteoarthritis or rheumatoid arthritis. 0.5 to 2 ml, based on joint size.
Adults with foot bursitis. 0.25 to 0.5 ml every 3 to 7 days.
Adults with foot tenosynovitis or periostitis of cuboid. 0.5 ml every 3 to 7 days.
Adults with acute gouty arthritis. 0.5 to 1 ml every 3 to 7 days.
Adults with skin lesions. 0.2 ml/cm^2 intradermally, up to 1 ml weekly.
DOSAGE ADJUSTMENT Dosage reduced for elderly patients and accompanied by periodic monitoring of blood pressure and blood glucose and electrolyte levels.

Route	Onset	Peak	Duration
P.O.	Unknown	1–2 hr	3.25 days
I.V., I.M.*	Rapid	Unknown	Unknown
I.M.†	1–3 hr	Unknown	1 wk
Other†	Unknown	Unknown	1–2 wk‡

Mechanism of Action
Binds to intracellular glucocorticoid receptors and suppresses inflammatory and immune responses by:
• inhibiting neutrophil and monocyte accumulation at inflammation site and suppressing their phagocytic and bactericidal activity
• stabilizing lysosomal membranes
• suppressing antigen response of macrophages and helper T cells
• inhibiting synthesis of inflammatory response mediators, such as cytokines, interleukins, and prostaglandins.

Contraindications
Idiopathic thrombocytopenic purpura (I.M. injection), live virus vaccination, systemic fungal infection

---

* Sodium phosphate.
† Acetate-sodium phosphate.
‡ For intra-arterial or intrasynovial injection; 1 week for intralesional injection in soft tissue.

Interactions

DRUGS

anticholinesterase drugs: Possibly antagonized anticholinesterase effects in myasthenia gravis

barbiturates: Possibly decreased effects of betamethasone

cyclosporine: Possibly increased risk of cyclosporine toxicity

digitalis glycosides: Possibly increased risk of digitalis toxicity

estrogens: Possibly decreased excretion of betamethasone

hydantoins, rifampin: Possibly increased excretion and decreased therapeutic effects of betamethasone

isoniazid: Possibly decreased serum isoniazid level

ketoconazole: Possibly decreased excretion of betamethasone

oral anticoagulants: Possibly increased or decreased action of anticoagulants, requiring adjusted anticoagulant dosage

oral contraceptives: Possibly increased half-life and concentration and decreased excretion of betamethasone

potassium-wasting diuretics: Increased risk of hypokalemia

salicylates: Possibly decreased serum level and therapeutic effects of salicylates

somatrem: Possibly inhibition of somatrem's growth-promoting effects

theophyllines: Possibly changes in both drugs' effects

Adverse Reactions

CNS: Fatigue, headache, increased intracranial pressure with papilledema, insomnia, malaise, neuritis, paresthesia, seizures, steroid psychosis, syncope, vertigo
CV: Arrhythmias, ECG changes, fat embolism, heart failure, hypertension, thromboembolism, thrombophlebitis
EENT: Cataracts, exophthalmos, glaucoma, increased intraocular pressure
ENDO: Cushingoid symptoms (buffalo hump, central obesity, decreased carbohydrate tolerance, fat pad enlargement, moon face), fluid retention, growth suppression in children, hyperglycemia, masked signs of infection, negative nitrogen balance, secondary adrenocortical and pituitary unresponsiveness (in times of stress)

GI: Abdominal distention, increased appetite, nausea, pancreatitis, peptic ulcer possibly with perforation, ulcerative esophagitis, vomiting
GU: Amenorrhea, glycosuria, menstrual irregularities
HEME: Leukocytosis
MS: Aseptic necrosis of femoral and humeral heads, loss of muscle mass, muscle weakness, osteoporosis, spontaneous pathologic and vertebral compression fractures, tendon rupture
SKIN: Acneiform lesions, allergic dermatitis, ecchymosis, facial erythema, hirsutism, impaired wound healing, increased sweating, petechiae, lupuslike lesions, purpura, subcutaneous fat atrophy, thin and fragile skin, urticaria
Other: Angioedema, hypocalcemia, hypokalemia, sodium retention, suppressed reaction to skin tests, weight gain

Nursing Considerations

• Expect prescriber to order baseline ophthalmologic examination before starting therapy because prolonged betamethasone use may lead to increased intraocular pressure, glaucoma, and optic nerve damage. Use betamethasone cautiously in patients with ocular herpes simplex because corneal perforation may occur.

• Determine if latent or active amebiasis has been ruled out in patients who have spent time in the tropics, or who have unexplained diarrhea, before betamethasone therapy starts because drug may worsen it.

WARNING Give betamethasone with extreme care in patients with known or suspected Strongyloides (threadworm) infestation because corticosteroids such as betamethasone may result in immunosuppression, Strongyloides hyperinfection and dissemination, and widespread larval migration, resulting in severe enterocolitis and potentially life-threatening gram-negative septicemia.

• Assess for signs of infection before administering betamethasone because drug may mask those signs. Because drug may cause immunosuppression, new infection may develop during therapy. If so, expect to administer appropriate antibiotic.

- Review serum electrolyte levels, as ordered, before starting therapy. Monitor these levels often during therapy to detect imbalances. Sodium and water retention and potassium and calcium depletion may occur with high-dose betamethasone therapy. If so, expect to restrict sodium intake and provide potassium and calcium supplements.
- Because betamethasone is linked to peptic ulcer formation, expect to administer it with an antacid or H2-receptor blocker.

WARNING Monitor ECG tracings for arrhythmias, and evaluate patient for anaphylactic reactions, such as angioedema and seizures, which have been associated with rapid I.V. administration of high-dose corticosteroids.

WARNING During long-term betamethasone therapy, assess for signs of adrenal suppression and insufficiency (fatigue, hypotension, lassitude, nausea, vomiting, and weakness) when patient is exposed to stress. If she exhibits these signs, notify prescriber at once.

- Watch for signs of steroid psychosis, such as delirium, clouded sensorium, euphoria, insomnia, mood swings, personality changes, and severe depression, which may develop 15 to 30 days after therapy begins. Expect to stop therapy. If this isn't possible, expect to give psychotropic drugs.
- Rotate I.M. injection sites. To prevent muscle atrophy, avoid subcutaneous injection, injection in deltoid site, and repeated I.M. injections into same site.
- Administer oral betamethasone before 9 a.m., if appropriate, to mimic body's natural release of corticosteroids.
- After intra-articular injection, assess joint for marked increase in pain, local swelling, and more restricted movement. If patient also develops fever and malaise, suspect septic arthritis and notify prescriber immediately. Expect to assist with joint fluid aspiration to confirm septic arthritis.
- Monitor patient for cushingoid signs and symptoms, such as moon face, buffalo hump, central obesity, striae, acne, ecchymosis, and weight gain. Notify prescriber if you detect these symptoms.
- Expect to slowly taper oral betamethasone dosage to prevent adrenal insufficiency.

PATIENT TEACHING
- Instruct patient to take betamethasone with food if GI upset occurs.
- Review signs of adrenal insufficiency and possible need for dosage increases during stress. Advise patient to notify prescriber immediately if signs of insufficiency occur or if she's exposed to stress.
- Instruct patient to avoid exposure to infections because drug can cause immuno-suppression. Also teach patient to recognize and immediately report signs of infection.
- After intra-articular use, advise patient not to overuse joint and to continue other treatments such as physical therapy.

betaxolol hydrochloride
Kerlone

Class and Category
Chemical class: Selective beta$_1$-adrenergic blocker
Therapeutic class: Antihypertensive
Pregnancy category: C

Indications and Dosages
➤ *To treat hypertension alone or with other antihypertensives*

TABLETS
Adults. *Initial:* 10 mg daily. If no response in 7 to 14 days, then 20 mg daily.
DOSAGE ADJUSTMENT For elderly patients and patients who have renal failure or are undergoing hemodialysis, initial dosage reduced to 5 mg daily. If desired response isn't achieved, dosage increased by 5-mg increments every 2 wk up to 20 mg daily.

Route	Onset	Peak	Duration
P.O.	Unknown	3–4 hr	Unknown

Mechanism of Action
Inhibits stimulation of beta$_1$-adrenergic receptor sites, primarily in the heart. This decreases myocardial excitability, cardiac output, and myocardial oxygen demand. It also decreases renin release from the kidneys, which helps reduce blood pressure.

Contraindications

Cardiogenic shock, heart failure unless caused by tachyarrhythmia or overt heart failure, hypersensitivity to betaxolol, second- or third-degree heart block, sinus bradycardia

Interactions

DRUGS

aluminum salts, barbiturates, calcium salts, cholestyramine, colestipol, NSAIDs, penicillins, rifampin, salicylates, sulfinpyrazone: Decreased therapeutic and adverse effects of betaxolol

amiodarone, beta blockers, digoxin: Increased risk of additive systemic beta blockade, especially bradycardia

calcium channel blockers: Possibly increased therapeutic and adverse effects of betaxolol

ciprofloxacin, other quinolones: Possibly increased bioavailability of betaxolol, increasing the drug's pharmacologic effect

clonidine: Possibly severe hypertension when both drugs (or just clonidine) are simultaneously withdrawn

disopyramide: Possibly severe bradycardia, asystole, and heart failure

epinephrine: Possibly severe hypertension followed by bradycardia

ergot alkaloids: Possibly peripheral ischemia and gangrene

flecainide: Possibly increased therapeutic and adverse effects of both drugs

lidocaine: Possibly increased risk of lidocaine toxicity

nondepolarizing neuromuscular blockers: Possibly increased or decreased neuromuscular blockade

oral contraceptives: Possibly increased bioavailability and plasma level of betaxolol, increasing pharmacologic effect

prazosin: Possibly increased orthostatic hypotension

quinidine: Possibly increased effects of betaxolol

sulfonylureas: Possibly masking of hypoglycemic symptoms

Adverse Reactions

CNS: Amnesia, anxiety, behavior changes, confusion, depression, dizziness, emotional lability, fatigue, fever, hallucinations, headache, insomnia, lethargy, malaise, mood changes, nightmares, paresthesia, peripheral neuropathy, sedation, stroke, syncope, tremor, vertigo

CV: Arrhythmias, including asystole, bradycardia, heart block, and torsades de pointes; cardiogenic shock; chest pain; claudication; heart failure; hyper-cholesterolemia; hyperlipidemia; hypotension; mitral insufficiency; MI; orthostatic hypotension; peripheral vascular insufficiency; Raynaud's phenomenon; renal and mesenteric artery thrombosis

EENT: Altered taste, blurred vision, burning eyes, conjunctivitis, dry eyes, dry mouth, earache, eye irritation, eye pain or pressure, increased salivation, laryngo-spasm, mouth ulcers, nasal stuffiness, pharyngitis, ptosis, rhinitis, sinusitis, tinnitus

ENDO: Breast pain (women), hyper-glycemia, hypoglycemia

GI: Acute pancreatitis, anorexia, bloating, constipation, diarrhea, elevated liver function test results, epigastric pain, flatulence, gastritis, heartburn, hepatomegaly, increased appetite, indigestion, nausea, vomiting

GU: Decreased libido, dysuria, impotence, nocturia, Peyronie's disease, prostatitis, renal colic, renal failure, urinary frequency, urine retention, UTI

HEME: Agranulocytosis, eosinophilia, leukopenia, thrombocytopenia

MS: Arthralgia, arthritis, gout, muscle spasms or twitching, myalgia, neck pain, tendinitis

RESP: Bronchial obstruction, bronchitis, bronchospasm, cough, pulmonary embolus, respiratory distress, upper respiratory tract infection, wheezing

SKIN: Acne, aggravation of psoriasis, diaphoresis, dry skin, eczema, erythema, exfoliative dermatitis, flushing, increased pigmentation, pallor, photophobia, pruritus, rash

Other: Acidosis, facial edema, hyper-kalemia, hyperuricemia, lupus erythematosus, lymphadenopathy, positive ANA titer, weight gain

Nursing Considerations

- Betaxolol shouldn't be given to patients with untreated pheochromocytoma.
- Use drug cautiously in peripheral vascular disease. Assess color, temperature, and pulses in arms and legs, and ask about numbness, tingling and pain.

- Be aware that chronic beta blocker therapy such as betaxolol is not routinely withheld prior to major surgery because the benefits outweigh the risks associated with its use with general anesthesia and surgical procedures.
- Check blood pressure with patient lying, sitting, and standing before starting betaxolol therapy and periodically throughout the day to detect changes.
- Review renal function test results before and during therapy.
- Closely monitor diabetic patient for hypoglycemia because betaxolol may mask tachycardia, but not dizziness and diaphoresis. Be aware that betaxolol may mask tachycardia and blood pressure changes associated with hyperthyroidism.

WARNING Avoid abrupt withdrawal of betaxolol, which can worsen or cause thyroid storm. Expect to withdraw drug gradually and monitor patient closely.

- Expect to taper betaxolol over 2 weeks to prevent MI, ventricular arrhythmias, and possibly death from catecholamine hypersensitivity caused by beta blocker therapy.
- If systolic pressure falls below 90 mm Hg, expect to discontinue drug and prepare for hemodynamic monitoring.
- Take precautions to prevent injury from falls caused by orthostatic hypotension.

PATIENT TEACHING
- Teach patient how to check her blood pressure, if appropriate. Also discuss signs and symptoms of hypertension and hypotension.
- Advise patient to avoid sudden position changes and to rise slowly from a sitting or lying position to minimize the effects of orthostatic hypotension.
- Advise patient to avoid driving and activities that require mental alertness until drug's CNS effects are known.
- Counsel patient to consult prescriber before using an OTC product, such as a cold remedy or nasal decongestant.

bethanechol chloride

Duvoid, PMS-Bethanechol Chloride (CAN), Urabeth, Urecholine

Class and Category

Chemical class: Synthetic choline ester
Therapeutic class: Cholinergic, parasympathomimetic
Pregnancy category: C

Indications and Dosages

➤ *To treat postoperative and postpartal urine retention and retention caused by neurogenic atony of bladder*

TABLETS
Adults. 10 to 50 mg three times daily or four times daily. *To determine minimum effective dose:* 5 to 10 mg repeated every hr until response is obtained or maximum of 50 mg is reached.

SUBCUTANEOUS INJECTION
Adults. 2.5 to 5 mg three times daily or four times daily. *To determine minimum effective dose:* 2.5 mg repeated every 15 to 30 min until response is obtained or maximum of four doses is reached. Minimum effective dose may be repeated three times daily or four times daily, as needed.

Mechanism of Action

Acts directly on muscarinic receptors of the parasympathetic nervous system, increasing detrusor muscle tone in the bladder and allowing contraction strong enough to start voiding. Like natural neurotransmitter acetylcholine, bethanechol stimulates gastric motility, increases gastric tone, and enhances peristalsis.

Route	Onset	Peak	Duration
P.O.	30–90 min	60 min	6 hr
SubQ	5–15 min	15–30 min	2 hr

Contraindications

Acute inflammatory lesions of GI tract, atrioventricular conduction defects, bronchial asthma, coronary artery disease, epilepsy, hypersensitivity to bethanecol or its components, hypertension, hyperthyroidism, hypotension, marked vagotonia, mechanical obstruction of GI or GU tract, Parkinson's disease, peptic ulcer disease, peritonitis, pronounced bradycardia, questionable integrity of GI or GU mucosa, spastic GI disorders, vasomotor instability

Interactions

DRUGS

cholinergic drugs: Possibly increased effects of bethanechol
ganglionic blockers: Possibly severe hypotension, usually first manifested by severe adverse GI reactions
procainamide, quinidine: Possibly decreased effects of bethanechol

Adverse Reactions

CNS: Headache, malaise
CV: Hypotension with reflex tachycardia, vasomotor response
EENT: Excessive salivation, lacrimation, miosis
GI: Abdominal cramps, colicky pain, diarrhea, eructation, nausea, vomiting
GU: Urinary urgency
RESP: Asthma attack, bronchoconstriction

Nursing Considerations

• Assess urine elimination before starting bethanechol therapy.
WARNING Be aware that patient must have functioning urinary sphincter because a sphincter that doesn't relax when bladder contracts can push urine upward into renal pelvis and cause reflux infection.
• Give oral bethanechol 1 hour before or 2 hours after meals to reduce risk of nausea and vomiting.
WARNING Don't give bethanechol I.M. or I.V. because of risk of cholinergic overstimulation, which can cause abdominal cramps, bloody diarrhea, hypotension, shock, or sudden cardiac arrest. Always keep atropine nearby during subcutaneous administration.

PATIENT TEACHING

• Advise patient to take bethanechol on an empty stomach 1 hour before or 2 hours after meals to reduce risk of nausea and vomiting.

biperiden hydrochloride

Akineton

biperiden lactate

Akineton Lactate

Class and Category

Chemical class: Tertiary amine
Therapeutic class: Anticholinergic, antidyskinetic
Pregnancy category: C

Indications and Dosages

➤ *As adjunct to treat all forms of Parkinson's disease*

TABLETS

Adults. 2 mg three times daily or four times daily up to 16 mg daily.

➤ *To control extrapyramidal symptoms (except tardive dyskinesia) caused by phenothiazines and other neuroleptic drugs*

TABLETS

Adults. 2 mg one to three times daily.

I.V. OR I.M. INJECTION

Adults. 2 mg repeated every 30 min until symptoms resolve or maximum of four consecutive doses in 24 hr is reached.

Route	Onset	Peak	Duration
I.V.	15 min	Unknown	1–8 hr
I.M.	10–30 min	Unknown	Unknown

Mechanism of Action

Blocks acetylcholine's action at cholinergic receptor sites. This action restores the brain's normal dopamine and acetylcholine balance, which relaxes muscle movement and decreases rigidity and tremors. Biperiden also may inhibit dopamine reuptake and storage, which prolongs dopamine's action.

Contraindications

Achalasia, bladder neck obstruction, hypersensitivity to biperiden, myasthenia gravis, narrow-angle glaucoma, prostatic hypertrophy, pyloric or duodenal obstruction, stenosing peptic ulcer, toxic megacolon

Interactions

DRUGS

amantadine: Possibly increased adverse anticholinergic effects
digoxin: Possibly increased serum digoxin level
haloperidol: Possibly increased schizophrenic symptoms, decreased serum haloperidol level, and development of tardive dyskinesia

levodopa: Possibly decreased levodopa effectiveness
phenothiazines: Possibly reduced phenothiazine effects and increased psychiatric symptoms

Adverse Reactions

CNS: Agitation, confusion, delirium, delusions, depression, disorientation, dizziness, drowsiness, euphoria, excitement, fever, hallucinations, headache, light-headedness, listlessness, memory loss, nervousness, paranoia, psychosis, weakness
CV: Hypotension, mild bradycardia, orthostatic hypotension, palpitations, tachycardia
EENT: Blurred vision, diplopia, dry mouth, increased intraocular pressure, mydriasis, narrow-angle glaucoma, suppurative parotitis
GI: Constipation, duodenal ulcer, epigastric distress, ileus, nausea, vomiting
GU: Dysuria, urinary hesitancy, urine retention
MS: Muscle spasms, muscle weakness
SKIN: Decreased sweating, dermatosis, flushing, rash, urticaria

Nursing Considerations

• Expect to give I.V. or I.M. biperiden when patient needs more rapid response than oral drug can provide.
• Assess muscle rigidity and tremor as baseline. Then check them often for improvement, indicating biperiden's effectiveness.
WARNING When giving biperiden to patient with drug-induced extrapyramidal reactions, be alert for worsening of psychiatric symptoms.
PATIENT TEACHING
• Caution patient to avoid driving and other activities that require alertness until biperiden's CNS effects are known.
WARNING Because biperiden decreases sweating, urge patient to avoid extremely hot and humid conditions to reduce risk of heatstroke and severe hyperthermia. This is especially important for elderly patients and those who abuse alcohol or have chronic illness or CNS disease.
• Emphasize the need for periodic eye examinations and intraocular pressure measurement because biperiden may cause narrow-angle glaucoma and increase intraocular pressure.

bisoprolol fumarate
Zebeta

B

Class and Category
Chemical class: Selective beta$_1$-adrenergic blocker
Therapeutic class: Antihypertensive
Pregnancy category: C

Indications and Dosages
➤ *To treat hypertension, alone or with other antihypertensives*
TABLETS
Adults. 5 mg daily, increased to 10 to 20 mg daily if blood pressure doesn't respond to lower dosage.
DOSAGE ADJUSTMENT Dosage reduced to 2.5 mg daily initially and then increased gradually for patients with impaired renal function and creatinine clearance less than 40 ml/min/1.73 m^2 or who have impaired hepatic function, as from cirrhosis or hepatitis.

Mechanism of Action
Inhibits stimulation of beta$_1$-receptors primarily in the heart, which decreases cardiac excitability, cardiac output, and myocardial oxygen demand. Bisoprolol also decreases renin release from kidneys, which helps reduce blood pressure.

Contraindications
Cardiogenic shock, heart failure unless caused by tachyarrhythmia, overt heart failure, second- or third-degree heart block, sinus bradycardia

Interactions
DRUGS
aluminum salts, barbiturates, calcium salts, cholestyramine, colestipol, NSAIDs, penicillins, rifampin, salicylates, sulfinpyrazone: Possibly decreased therapeutic and adverse effects of bisoprolol
beta blockers, digoxin: Increased risk of bradycardia
calcium channel blockers: Possibly increased therapeutic and adverse effects of bisoprolol
ciprofloxacin, quinolones: Possibly increased bioavailability of bisoprolol

clonidine: Possibly severe hypertension from withdrawal of clonidine or both drugs
epinephrine: Possibly hypertension followed by bradycardia
ergot alkaloids: Possibly peripheral ischemia and gangrene
flecainide: Possibly increased therapeutic and adverse effects of either drug
lidocaine: Possibly increased risk of lidocaine toxicity
oral contraceptives: Possibly increased bioavailability and plasma level of bisoprolol
prazosin: Possibly increased orthostatic hypotension
quinidine: Possibly increased bisoprolol effects
sulfonylureas: Possibly masking of hypoglycemic symptoms

Adverse Reactions

CNS: Anxiety, confusion, depression, dizziness, emotional lability, fatigue, fever, hallucinations, headache, insomnia, malaise, nightmares, paresthesia, sleep disturbances, syncope, tremor, unsteadiness, vertigo
CV: Bradycardia, heart block, and other arrhythmias; chest pain; claudication; cold arms and legs; edema; heart failure; hypercholesterolemia; hyperlipidemia; hypotension; MI; orthostatic hypotension; palpitations; peripheral vascular insufficiency; renal and mesenteric artery thrombosis
EENT: Altered taste, blurred vision, dry mouth, eye pain or pressure, hearing loss, increased salivation, laryngospasm, pharyngitis, rhinitis, sinusitis, tinnitus
GI: Constipation, diarrhea, epigastric pain, gastritis, indigestion, ischemic colitis, nausea, vomiting
GU: Cystitis, decreased libido, impotence, Peyronie's disease, renal colic
HEME: Agranulocytosis, eosinophilia, leukopenia, thrombocytopenia, thrombocytopenic purpura
MS: Arthralgia, gout, muscle twitching, neck pain
RESP: Asthma, bronchitis, bronchospasm, cough, dyspnea, respiratory distress, upper respiratory tract infection
SKIN: Alopecia, dermatitis, diaphoresis, eczema, exfoliative dermatitis, flushing, pruritus, psoriasis, rash

Other: Angioedema, hyperkalemia, hyperuricemia, weight gain

Nursing Considerations

• Administer bisoprolol cautiously in patients with peripheral vascular disease because reduced cardiac output can cause or worsen arterial insufficiency. Assess patient's arms and legs for changes in color, temperature, and pulses; ask about numbness, tingling, and pain.
• Be aware that chronic beta blocker therapy such as bisoprolol is not routinely withheld prior to major surgery because the benefits outweigh the risks associated with its use with general anesthesia and surgical procedures.
• Measure blood pressure with patient lying, sitting, and standing before starting bisoprolol and then every 4 to 8 hours, as appropriate, to evaluate effectiveness.
• If patient has diabetes, monitor closely for signs of hypoglycemia, which drug may mask.
• If patient has hyperthyroidism, watch for tachycardia and hypertension, which may be masked by bisoprolol.
WARNING Keep in mind that abrupt withdrawal of bisoprolol may cause or worsen thyroid storm. During drug withdrawal, monitor patient closely.
• Expect to stop bisoprolol over 1 to 2 weeks to prevent MI, ventricular arrhythmias, and, possibly, death from catecholamine hypersensitivity caused by beta blocker therapy.
• If systolic blood pressure falls to less than 90 mm Hg, expect to discontinue drug. Prepare for hemodynamic monitoring, if needed.
WARNING If patient is scheduled for surgery with general anesthesia, expect to discontinue bisoprolol about 48 hours beforehand to reduce risk of excessive myocardial depression during anesthesia.
PATIENT TEACHING
• Teach patient how to monitor her blood pressure, if appropriate, and to recognize signs of hypertension and hypotension.
• Instruct patient to avoid sudden position changes and to rise slowly from a sitting or lying position to minimize the effects of orthostatic hypotension.

• Advise patient to avoid driving and other activities that require mental alertness until bisoprolol's CNS effects are known.
• Instruct patient to contact prescriber before using any OTC product, such as a cold remedy or nasal decongestant.

bitolterol mesylate

Tornalate

Class and Category

Chemical class: Acid ester of colterol
Therapeutic class: Bronchodilator, sympathomimetic
Pregnancy category: C

Indications and Dosages

➤ *To prevent and treat asthma and other conditions associated with reversible bronchospasm, such as emphysema and chronic bronchitis*

INTERMITTENT AEROSOL SOLUTION

Adults and children age 12 and over. 1 mg bitolterol diluted in 0.5 ml normal saline solution and inhaled over 10 to 15 min three times daily. *Maximum:* 8 mg daily.

CONTINUOUS AEROSOL SOLUTION

Adults and children age 12 and over. 2.5 mg bitolterol diluted in 1.25 ml normal saline solution and inhaled over 10 to 15 min three times daily. *Maximum:* 14 mg daily.

METERED-DOSE INHALER

Adults and children age 12 and over. *To treat acute bronchospasm:* 2 inhalations over 1 to 3 min and, if needed, a third inhalation.
To prevent bronchospasm: 2 inhalations every 8 hr, not to exceed 3 inhalations every 6 hr or 2 inhalations every 4 hr.

Mechanism of Action

Is hydrolyzed to active agent colterol (a long-acting agent that primarily affects $beta_2$-adrenergic receptors). Then it attaches to $beta_2$ receptors on bronchial cell membranes. This action stimulates the intracellular enzyme adenylate cyclase to convert adenosine triphosphate to cyclic adenosine monophosphate (cAMP). An increased intracellular level of cAMP relaxes bronchial smooth-muscle cells, stabilizes mast cells, and inhibits histamine release.

Route	Onset	Peak	Duration
Aerosol, inhalation	2–3 min	30–60 min	6–8 hr
Metered-dose inhalation	3–5 min	30–120 min	4–8 hr

B

Incompatibilities

Don't mix bitolterol in inhalation solution with cromolyn sodium or acetylcysteine.

Contraindications

Hypersensitivity to bitolterol or ingredients

Interactions

DRUGS

beta blockers: Possibly inhibition of bronchodilating effect of bitolterol
epinephrine, other sympathomimetic drugs: Possibly additive effects of either drug
MAO inhibitors, tricyclic antidepressants: Possibly potentiation of bitolterol's action on cardiovascular system

Adverse Reactions

CNS: Dizziness, fatigue, headache, hyperkinesia, insomnia, light-headedness, nervousness, paresthesia, somnolence, tremor, vertigo
CV: Chest pain, hypertension, irregular pulse, palpitations, tachycardia, transient ECG changes
EENT: Mouth and throat irritation, rhinitis
GI: Elevated liver function test results, nausea
HEME: Decreased hemoglobin level, hematocrit, and WBC count
RESP: Bronchospasm, cough

Nursing Considerations

• Assess respiratory rate, rhythm, and depth and breath sounds before, during, and after bitolterol therapy. Expect improved air movement and improvement in abnormal breath sounds.
• Because beta-adrenergic bronchodilators can significantly increase blood pressure and pulse rate, monitor them often.
• Expect therapy to begin with lowest effective dose because higher doses or more frequent use may reduce effectiveness and cause paradoxical reactions or overdose.

• Teach patient how to properly use and care for aerosol nebulizer or metered-dose inhaler. Before patient uses aerosol nebulizer, advise her to look for slight bubbling in solution-filled chamber and fine mist when nebulizer is turned on. Before patient uses inhaler for first time, instruct her to make sure it's working properly by spraying it once in the air and looking for fine mist.
• Teach patient to mix nebulizer solution immediately before use. Afterward, she should clean nebulizer and solution chamber according to manufacturer's recommendations.

WARNING Advise patient not to use more than the recommended dosage of bitolterol; excessive use of sympathomimetic drugs may be fatal.
• Tell patient to wait 1 to 3 minutes between metered-dose inhalations.

bivalirudin

Angiomax

Class and Category

Chemical class: Hirudin analogue
Therapeutic class: Anticoagulant
Pregnancy category: B

Indications and Dosages

➤ *As adjunct to provide anticoagulation and prevent thrombosis in patients with unstable angina who are having percutaneous transluminal coronary angioplasty or percutaneous coronary intervention*

I.V. INFUSION

Adults. *Initial:* Immediately before angioplasty, 0.75-mg/kg bolus; then 1.75 mg/kg/hr as continuous infusion for duration of procedure. Five min after bolus dose and with continuous infusion running, another 0.3-mg/kg dose may be given if needed. After procedure, 1.75 mg/kg/hr may be given for 4 hr by continuous infusion, followed by 0.2 mg/kg/hr for up to 20 hr if needed.

DOSAGE ADJUSTMENT Infusion dosage possibly reduced to 1 mg/kg/hr for patients with severe renal impairment (glomerular

filtration rate of 10 to 29 ml/min) and to 0.25 mg/kg/hr for patients having dialysis.

Route	Onset	Peak	Duration
I.V.	Immediate	Unknown	1 hr after end of infusion

Mechanism of Action

Selectively binds to thrombin, including thrombin trapped in established clots. Without thrombin, fibrinogen can't convert to fibrin and clots can't form.

Incompatibilities

Don't mix other drugs in same I.V. line before or during bivalirudin administration. Mixing with alteplase, amiodarone, amphotericin B, chlorpromazine HCL, diazepam, prochlorperazine edisylate, reteplase, streptokinase, or vancomycin HCL can result in haze, particulate formation, or precipitation.

Contraindications

Active major bleeding, hypersensitivity to bivalirudin or its components

Interactions

DRUGS

alteplase, antineoplastics, antithymocyte globulin, heparin, NSAIDs, platelet inhibitors, reteplase, streptokinase, strontium chloride Sr 89, warfarin: Risk of bleeding
porfimer: Possibly decreased efficacy of porfimer photodynamic therapy
salicylates: Increased risk of hypoprothrombinemia and bleeding

Adverse Reactions

CNS: Headache, intracranial hemorrhage
CV: Hypotension, thrombosis (with gamma brachytherapy)
EENT: Epistaxis, gingival bleeding
GI: Abdominal cramps, diarrhea, GI or retroperitoneal bleeding, nausea, vomiting
GU: Hematuria, vaginal bleeding
MS: Back pain
RESP: Hemoptysis, hemothorax
SKIN: Ecchymosis
Other: Injection-site bleeding, hematoma, or pain

Nursing Considerations

• To reconstitute bivalirudin, add 5 ml sterile water for injection to 250-mg vial and swirl gently until dissolved. For initial infusion, dilute reconstituted vial in 50 ml D$_5$W or normal saline solution to yield 5 mg/ml.

• For subsequent low-rate infusion, further dilute reconstituted drug in 500 ml D$_5$W or normal saline solution to final concentration of 0.5 mg/ml.

• Expect to give 300 to 325 mg of aspirin P.O. daily during bivalirudin therapy.

WARNING Monitor blood coagulation tests before and regularly during therapy; bleeding is a major bivalirudin risk.

WARNING Monitor patient often for bleeding because there's no antidote for bivalirudin. If life-threatening bleeding occurs, notify prescriber immediately, stop drug, and monitor APTT and other coagulation tests as ordered. Blood transfusions may be needed. Patients with increased bleeding risk include menstruating women; patients with vascular or organ abnormalities, such as severe uncontrolled hypertension, advanced renal disease, infective endo-carditis, dissecting aortic aneurysm, diverticulitis, hemophilia, hepatic disease (especially from deficient vitamin K–dependent clotting factors), inflammatory bowel disease, or peptic ulcer disease; and those with recent stroke, major surgery (including eye, brain, or spinal cord), large vessel or lumbar puncture, organ biopsy, spinal anesthesia, or major bleeding (including intracranial, GI, intraocular, retroperitoneal, or pulmonary bleeding).

• If patient is receiving gamma brachy-therapy, watch closely for evidence of thrombosis (weak or absent pulse, pallor, pain); use of bivalirudin may increase the risk in these patients.

• If possible, avoid I.M. injections of any kind to decrease the risk of bleeding.

• Discard any unused portion of drug.

PATIENT TEACHING

• Inform patient that bivalirudin is a blood thinner administered only in the hospital.

• Urge patient to check her skin for bruising or red spots and to immediately report back or stomach pain, trouble breathing, dizziness, fainting, and unusual bleeding (black, tarry stool; blood in urine; coughing blood; heavy menses; nose-bleeds). Drug may need to be stopped.

• Encourage patient to reduce the risk of injury while receiving bivalirudin, such as by brushing her teeth gently with a soft-bristled toothbrush.

• Caution patient not to take anti-inflammatories, such as ibuprofen, naproxen, ketoprofen, aspirin, and aspirin-like products, or other blood thinners, such as warfarin, while receiving bivalirudin unless directed.

bretylium tosylate

Bretylate (CAN), Bretylol

Class and Category

Chemical class: Bromobenzyl quaternary ammonium compound
Therapeutic class: Class III antiarrhythmic
Pregnancy category: C

Indications and Dosages

➤ *To prevent and treat ventricular fibrillation and treat life-threatening ventricular arrhythmias that don't respond to first-line antiarrhythmics, such as lidocaine*

I.V. INFUSION, I.V. OR I.M. INJECTION

Adults with immediate life-threatening ventricular arrhythmias. *Initial:* 5 mg/kg, undiluted, by rapid I.V. injection; if ventricular fibrillation persists, 10 mg/kg repeated as often as needed. *Continuous suppression:* 1 to 2 mg/min or 5 to 10 mg/kg of diluted I.V. solution infused over at least 8 min every 6 hr.

Adults with other ventricular arrhythmias. *Initial:* 5 to 10 mg/kg of diluted I.V. solution infused over at least 8 min, repeated every 1 to 2 hr if arrhythmia continues; or 5 to 10 mg/kg undiluted I.M. injection, repeated every 1 to 2 hr if arrhythmia continues. *Maintenance:* 5 to 10 mg/kg diluted I.V. solution infused over at least 8 min every 6 hours, 1 to 2 mg/min infused continuously, or 5 to 10 mg/kg undiluted I.M. injection every 6 to 8 hr.

DOSAGE ADJUSTMENT Interval between dosages increased for patients with impaired renal function because bretylium is excreted mainly by kidneys.

Children with acute ventricular fibrillation. 5 mg/kg I.V. given over 8 to

10 min, followed by 10 mg/kg every 15 to 30 min up to total dose of 30 mg/kg.
Maintenance: 5 to 10 mg/kg every 6 hr.
Children with other ventricular arrhythmias. 5 to 10 mg/kg every 6 hr.

Route	Onset	Peak	Duration
I.V.	5–10 min*	6–9 hr	6–24 hr
I.M.	20–60 min*	6–9 hr	6–24 hr

* For suppression of ventricular fibrillation; 20 to 120 min for suppression of ventricular tachycardia.

Contraindications
Digitalis toxicity, hypersensitivity to bretylium

Interactions
DRUGS
catecholamines (such as dopamine and norepinephrine): Increased vasopressor effects of catecholamines
digoxin: Possibly worsened digitalis toxicity

Adverse Reactions
CNS: Anxiety, confusion, dizziness, emotional lability, fever, lethargy, light-headedness, paranoia, psychosis, syncope, vertigo
CV: Angina, arrhythmias (including bradycardia and more frequent PVCs), hypotension, orthostatic hypotension, transient hypertension
EENT: Mild conjunctivitis, nasal stuffiness
GI: Abdominal pain, diarrhea, hiccups, nausea, vomiting
GU: Renal impairment
RESP: Dyspnea
SKIN: Diaphoresis, erythematous macular rash, flushing
Other: Injection-site pain

Nursing Considerations
WARNING Use bretylium cautiously in patients with severe aortic stenosis or pulmonary hypertension because hypotension may occur.
• For I.V. infusion, dilute bretylium and administer at 1 to 2 mg/min.
• Dilute bretylium in compatible I.V. solution, such as D_5W, dextrose 5% in normal saline solution, dextrose 5% in lactated Ringer's solution, normal saline solution, 5% sodium bicarbonate, 20%

mannitol, 1/6 molar sodium lactate, lactated Ringer's solution, calcium chloride in D_5W, and potassium chloride in D_5W.
WARNING Patient may experience hypotension while supine. Have her remain supine until tolerance develops. If supine systolic blood pressure falls below 75 mm Hg, expect to give dopamine or norepinephrine and monitor blood pressure closely because vasopressor effects are increased when these drugs are given together.
• Be alert for transient hypertension and increased frequency of arrhythmias because bretylium initially triggers release of norepinephrine. Monitor patient's ECG tracings and blood pressure continuously, and notify prescriber of changes.
• Monitor blood bretylium level. Notify prescriber if level falls outside therapeutic range of 0.5 to 1.5 mcg/ml.
PATIENT TEACHING
• Advise patient to immediately report chest pain or pressure, pain at I.V. site, or rash.
• Warn patient that she may feel dizzy or light-headed even when lying down. Tell her to stay supine and ask for help when trying to move or sit up. Tell her that this sensation usually subsides in a few days.

bromocriptine mesylate
Alti-Bromocriptine (CAN), Apo-Bromocriptine (CAN), Cycloset, Parlodel, Parlodel SnapTabs

Class and Category
Chemical class: Ergot alkaloid derivative
Therapeutic class: Antidiabetic, anti-dyskinetic, antihyperprolactinemic, dopamine-receptor agonist, growth hormone suppressant, infertility therapy adjunct
Pregnancy category: B

Indications and Dosages
➤ *To treat amenorrhea, galactorrhea, male hypogonadism, and infertility from hyperprolactinemia*

Mechanism of Action
Bretylium prolongs the repolarization phase of the action potential and lengthens the effective refractory period, which helps terminate reentry arrhythmias. The drug also acts on adrenergic nerve terminals initially causing early release of norepinephrine, which increases heart rate and blood pressure. Then it blocks release of norepinephrine, as shown here. This reduces heart rate and blood pressure. Bretylium also increases the ventricular threshold, making the ventricular myocardium less responsive to ectopic impulses and preventing ventricular fibrillation.

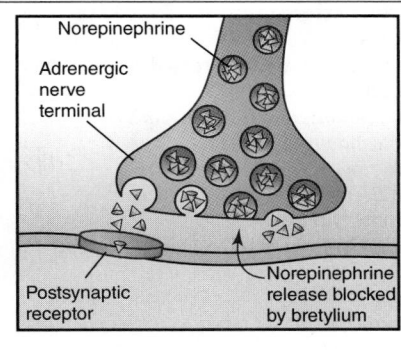

CAPSULES, TABLETS
Adults. *Initial:* 1.25 to 2.5 mg at bedtime with snack. Increased by 2.5 mg every 3 to 7 days as needed to a total daily dose of 5 to 7.5 mg, given in divided doses with snacks. *Maintenance:* 2.5 mg twice daily or three times daily with meals.
➤ *To treat prolactin-secreting adenoma*
CAPSULES, TABLETS
Adults and adolescents age 15 and over. *Initial:* 1.25 mg twice daily or three times daily with meals. Increased gradually over several weeks, if needed, to 10 to 20 mg daily in divided doses with meals. Some patients may need higher doses. *Maintenance:* 2.5 to 20 mg daily in divided doses with meals.
➤ *To treat Parkinson's disease*
CAPSULES, TABLETS
Adults. *Initial:* 1.25 mg at bedtime with snack or twice daily with meals. Increased by 2.5 mg every 14 to 28 days, if needed. *Maintenance:* 2.5 to 40 mg daily in divided doses with meals.
➤ *To treat acromegaly*
CAPSULES, TABLETS
Adults and children age 15 and over. *Initial:* 1.25 to 2.5 mg at bedtime with snack for 3 days. Then increased by 1.25 to 2.5 mg every 3 to 7 days, if needed, up to 30 mg daily. *Maintenance:* Usually 10 to 30 mg daily at bedtime with snack or in divided doses with meals.
➤ *To control blood glucose level in type 2 diabetes mellitus, with diet and exercise*

TABLETS
Adults. *Initial:* 0.8 mg once daily within 2 hr after waking up in morning. Increased weekly in increments of 0.8 mg, as needed. *Maximum:* 4.8 mg daily.

Route	Onset	Peak	Duration
P.O.*	2 hr	8 hr	24 hr
P.O.†	30–90 min	2 hr	Unknown
P.O.‡	1–2 hr	4–8 wk	4–8 hr

Mechanism of Action
Inhibits release of prolactin and growth hormone from the anterior pituitary gland, thus restoring testicular or ovarian function and suppressing lactation. Bromocriptine decreases dopamine turnover in the CNS, depleting dopamine or blocking its receptors in the brain, alleviating dyskinesia.

Contraindications
Breastfeeding; hypersensitivity to bromocriptine, other ergot alkaloids, or their components; ketoacidosis; severe ischemic heart disease or peripheral vascular disease; syncopal migraine; type 1 diabetes mellitus

---

* For amenorrhea, galactorrhea, male hypogonadism, infertility from hyperprolactinemia, and prolactin-secreting adenoma.
† For Parkinson's disease.
‡ For acromegaly.

Interactions
DRUGS
antihypertensives: Increased hypotensive effects
clarithromycin, erythromycin, troleandomycin: Increased risk of bromocriptine toxicity
CYP3A4 inhibitors: Increased bromocriptine level
CYP3A4 inducers: Decreased bromocriptine level
dopamine receptor antagonists, including neuroleptic drugs (such as butyrophenones, phenothiazines, or thioxanthenes), metoclopramide: Possibly decreased effectiveness of both drugs
ergot alkaloids or derivatives: Increased risk of hypertension
haloperidol, loxapine, MAO inhibitors, methyldopa, metoclopramide, molindone, phenothiazines, pimozide, reserpine, risperidone, thioxanthenes: Increased serum prolactin level, decreased bromocriptine effectiveness
levodopa: Additive effects requiring reduced levodopa dose
ritonavir: Increased bromocriptine level
sympathomimetic drugs: Possibly increased risk of hypertension and tachycardia
ACTIVITIES
alcohol use: Possibly disulfiram-like reaction

Adverse Reactions
CNS: Asthenia; confusion; dizziness; drowsiness; fatigue; hallucinations; headache; intense urges to gamble, engage in sexual activity, or spend money uncontrollably; light-headedness; syncope
CV: Hypertension, hypotension, orthostatic hypotension, pericarditis, pericardial effusion, Raynaud's phenomenon
EENT: Amblyopia, dry mouth, nasal congestion, rhinitis, sinusitis
ENDO: Hypoglycemia
GI: Abdominal cramps, anorexia, constipation, diarrhea, GI bleeding, indigestion, nausea, vomiting
RESP: Pleural effusion or thickening, pulmonary fibrosis
Other: Intense impulse to gamble

Nursing Considerations
• Use bromocriptine cautiously if patient has a history of psychosis or cardiovascular disease, especially after MI with residual arrhythmia. In severe psychotic disorder, bromocriptine isn't recommended because it may worsen the disorder or reduce the effects of drugs used to treat it.
• Use bromocriptine cautiously in patients with Parkinson's disease because high doses of the drug may cause confusion and mental disturbances in these patients. Drug should not be discontinued abruptly, as a symptom complex resembling the neuroleptic malignant syndrome has occurred with rapid dose reduction, withdrawal, or changes in antiparkinsonian therapy.
• Expect to perform a pregnancy test every 4 weeks during the amenorrheic period. Once menses resume, test whenever a period is missed, as ordered.
• Plan to withhold bromocriptine if patient becomes pregnant.
• If rapidly expanding adenoma needs continued therapy, watch closely for hypertensive crisis.
• Bromocriptine shouldn't be given postpartum if patient has a history of coronary artery disease or other severe cardiovascular problem unless risk of withdrawing drug is greater than risk of use. If so, monitor closely for signs and symptoms of CV dysfunction, such as chest pain.
• Expect to give drug with levodopa if patient is being treated for Parkinson's disease.
• Assess for hypotension when bromocriptine therapy starts and hypertension (typically during second week). Monitor blood pressure often if patient takes other antihypertensives.
• If patient has a history of peptic ulcer or GI bleeding, watch for new bleeding.
• Take safety precautions, such as keeping bed in low position with side rails up, because drug can cause dizziness, drowsiness, light-headedness, and syncope.
PATIENT TEACHING
• Tell patient to take each dose with a meal, milk, or a snack to minimize nausea.
• Caution patient about possible dizziness, drowsiness, and light-headedness. Urge patient to avoid hazardous activities until drug effects are known.

- Advise against sudden position changes to minimize orthostatic hypotension.
- Warn patient to avoid alcohol while taking bromocriptine because it may cause disulfiram-like reactions, such as chest pain, confusion, a fast or pounding heartbeat, facial flushing, diaphoresis, nausea, vomiting, a throbbing headache, blurred vision, and severe weakness.
- Tell patient to take a missed dose as soon as she remembers it, unless it's almost time for the next dose. In that case, tell her to wait until the next scheduled dose. Warn her not to double the dose. Advise her to contact prescriber if she misses more than one dose.
- Urge patient to report adverse reactions, such as an unremitting headache, nausea, vomiting, or other signs of CNS toxicity.
- Tell patient who takes large doses of bromocriptine to schedule regular dental checkups because the drug can decrease saliva flow, which may encourage dental caries, periodontal disease, oral candidiasis, and discomfort.
- Tell patient with acromegaly to keep her fingers warm to prevent cold-sensitive digital vasospasm.
- If patient has type 2 diabetes, provide instruction about diet, exercise, effects of hyperglycemia and hypoglycemia, hygiene, foot care, and ways to avoid infection.
- Warn patient to report intense urges to gamble, engage in sexual activity, or spend money uncontrollably.

budesonide

Entocort EC, Pulmicort Flexhaler, Pulmicort Respules, Pulmicort Turbuhaler, Rhinocort, Rhinocort Aqua, Rhinocort Turbuhaler (CAN), Uceris

Class and Category
Chemical class: Glucocorticoid
Therapeutic class: Antiasthmatic, anti-inflammatory
Pregnancy category: B

Indications and Dosages
➤ *To manage symptoms of seasonal or perennial allergic rhinitis*

NASAL AEROSOL
Adults and children over age 6. 64 mcg in each nostril twice daily or 128 mcg in each nostril daily. *Maximum:* 256 mcg daily. *Maintenance:* Lowest dosage that controls symptoms.
NASAL POWDER
Adults and children over age 6. 200 mcg in each nostril daily. *Maximum:* 800 mcg daily (adults and adolescents); 400 mcg daily (children). *Maintenance:* Lowest dosage that controls symptoms.
NASAL SUSPENSION
Adults and children over age 6. 32 mcg in each nostril daily. *Maximum:* 256 mcg daily (adults and adolescents); 128 mcg daily (children). *Maintenance:* Lowest dosage that controls symptoms.
➤ *To manage symptoms of perennial nonallergic rhinitis*
NASAL AEROSOL
Adults and adolescents. 64 mcg in each nostril twice daily or 128 mcg in each nostril daily. *Maximum:* 256 mcg daily. *Maintenance:* Lowest dosage that controls symptoms.
NASAL POWDER
Adults and adolescents. 200 mcg in each nostril daily. *Maximum:* 800 mcg daily. *Maintenance:* Lowest dosage that controls symptoms.
➤ *To provide maintenance therapy in chronic bronchial asthma*
ORAL INHALATION
Adults previously on bronchodilators alone. 1 or 2 inhalations (200 to 400 mcg) twice daily. *Maximum:* 800 mcg daily.
Adults previously on inhaled corticosteroids. 1 or 2 inhalations (200 to 400 mcg) twice daily. *Maximum:* 800 mcg twice daily, as needed and tolerated.
Adults previously on systemic corticosteroids. 2 to 4 inhalations (400 to 800 mcg) twice daily. *Maximum:* 1,600 mcg daily.
Children age 6 and over. 1 inhalation (200 mcg) twice daily. *Maximum:* 400 mcg twice daily, as needed and tolerated.
ORAL INHALATION (PULMICORT FLEXHALER)
Adults and adolescents age 18 and over.
Initial: 180 or 360 mcg twice daily, increased as needed. *Maximum:* 720 mcg twice daily.
Children ages 6 to 17.
Initial: 180 or 360 mcg twice daily. *Maximum:* 360 mcg twice daily.

B

➤ *To prevent or provide maintenance therapy in chronic bronchial asthma*

NEBULIZED INHALATION (PULMICORT RESPULES)
Children ages 1 to 8 previously on bronchodilators alone. 0.25 mg twice daily. or 0.5 mg daily by jet nebulizer. *Maximum:* 0.5 mg/day.
Children ages 1 to 8 previously on inhaled steroids. 0.25 mg twice daily or 0.5 mg daily inhaled by jet nebulizer. *Maximum:* 1 mg/day.
Children ages 1 to 8 previously on systemic corticosteroids. 0.5 mg twice daily or 1 mg daily inhaled by jet nebulizer. *Maximum:* 1 mg/day.

➤ *To treat mild to moderate active Crohn's disease involving the ileum, the ascending colon, or both*

CAPSULES
Adults. 9 mg daily in the morning for 8 wk.

➤ *To maintain clinical remission of mild to moderate Crohn's disease involving the ileum, the ascending colon, or both*

CAPSULES
Adults. 6 mg daily in the morning for up to 3 months.

➤ *To induce remission in patients with active, mild to moderate ulcerative colitis*

E.R. TABLETS (UCERIS)
Adults. 9 mg daily in the morning for up to 8 wks.

DOSAGE ADJUSTMENT Dosage reduced for patients with hepatic insufficiency and those taking ketoconazole or other CYP3A4 inhibitor.

➤ *To induce remission in patients with active, mild to moderate distal ulcerative colitis extending up to 40 cm from the anal verge*

RECTAL FOAM (UCERIS)
Adults. 1 metered dose (2 mg) twice daily for 2 wks followed by 1 metered dose (2 mg) once daily for 4 wks.

Route	Onset	Peak	Duration
Nasal aerosol	10 hr–3 days	3 days–3 wk	Unknown
Nasal powder or suspension	In 4 wk	Unknown	Unknown
Oral inhalation	In 4 wk	Unknown	Unknown

Route	Onset	Peak	Duration
Nebulized inhalation	2–8 days	4–6 wk	Unknown
P.O. (capsules)	Unknown	30 min–10 hr	Unknown

Mechanism of Action

Inhibits inflammatory cells and mediators, possibly by decreasing influx into nasal passages or bronchial walls. As a result, nasal or airway inflammation decreases. Oral inhalation form also inhibits mucus secretion in airways, decreasing the amount and viscosity of sputum.

Contraindications

Hypersensitivity to budesonide or its components, recent septal ulcers or nasal surgery or trauma (nasal spray); status asthmaticus or other acute asthma episodes (oral inhalation)

Interactions
DRUGS
clarithromycin, erythromycin, itraconazole, ketoconazole, other CYP3A4 inhibitors: Possibly increased blood budesonide level
FOOD
grapefruit juice: Possibly increased blood budesonide level

Adverse Reactions

CNS: Amnesia, asthenia, benign intra-cranial hypertension, changes in mood, dizziness, fatigue, fever, headache
CV: Hypertension, peripheral edema
EENT: Bad taste, cataracts, dry mouth, epistaxis, glaucoma, nasal irritation, oral or pharyngeal candidiasis, pharyngitis, rhinitis, sinusitis
ENDO: Adrenal insufficiency, decreased blood cortisol level, growth suppression in children, hypercorticism
GI: Abdominal pain, diarrhea, dyspepsia, flatulence, indigestion, nausea, pancreatitis, vomiting
GU: UTI
MS: Arthralgia, back pain
RESP: Bronchospasm, increased cough, respiratory tract infection
SKIN: Allergic or contact dermatitis, maculo-papular rash, pruritus, purpura, rash, urticaria
Other: Anaphylaxis, angioedema, increased risk of infection

Nursing Considerations

• Use budesonide cautiously if patient has tubercular infection; untreated fungal, bacterial, or systemic viral infection; or ocular herpes simplex.

• Closely monitor a child's growth pattern; budesonide may stunt growth.

WARNING Assess patient who switches from a systemic corticosteroid to inhaled budesonide for adrenal insufficiency (fatigue, hypotension, lassitude, nausea, vomiting, weakness), which may be life-threatening. Hypothalamic-pituitary-adrenal axis function may take several months to recover after stopping systemic corticosteroids. Stopping budesonide abruptly may cause adrenal insufficiency.

• Administer Respules by jet nebulizer connected to an air compressor.

• Patient exposed to chickenpox may receive varicella zoster immune globulin or pooled I.V. immunoglobulin. If chickenpox develops, give antiviral as ordered. A patient exposed to measles may need pooled I.M. immunoglobulin.

• Assess patient for effectiveness of budesonide therapy, especially if being weaned from a systemic corticosteroid. If patient has increased asthma or an immunologic condition previously suppressed by systemic corticosteroid—such as rhinitis, conjunctivitis, an eosinophilic condition, eczema, or arthritis—notify prescriber.

• Pulmicort Flexhaler contains small amounts of lactose, which may trigger coughing, wheezing, or bronchospasm in a patient with a severe milk-protein allergy.

• Monitor patient for evidence of hypersensitivity, such as contact dermatitis, rash, urticaria, angioedema, bronchospasm, or anaphylaxis. If present, notify prescriber immediately. Expect to stop budesonide and provide emergency supportive care.

• Monitor patients with conditions such as diabetes mellitus, glaucoma or cataracts, hypertension, osteoporosis, or peptic ulcer, as glucocorticosteroid therapy may increase adverse effects. Also monitor patients with a family history of diabetes or glaucoma.

PATIENT TEACHING

• Urge patient taking oral capsules or E.R. tablets to swallow them whole and not to chew or break them.

• Instruct patient who uses nasal spray to shake container before each use. Instruct her to blow her nose, tilt her head slightly forward, and insert tube into a nostril, pointing toward inner corner of eye, away from nasal septum. Tell her to hold the other nostril closed and spray while inhaling gently. Then have her repeat in the other nostril.

• Instruct patient to prime oral inhaler before using it for first time by holding canister upright with mouthpiece on top and twisting base of device fully to right and then fully to left until it clicks. Teach her to load each each dose just before use in the same way. After loading a dose, caution patient not to shake device or blow into it. Tell patient to turn her head away from device and exhale. Then have her hold device upright, place her lips around mouthpiece, and inhale deeply. Device will discharge a dose. Tell patient to remove her lips from mouthpiece to exhale.

• Instruct patient to empty her bowels before using rectal foam. Although product is lubricated, tell patient she may use petroleum jelly or petrolatum if more lubrication is needed. Tell her to warm the canister in her hands while shaking it vigorously for 10 to 15 seconds prior to use. Inform her that she may apply the rectal foam while standing, lying, or sitting. When applied in the evening, instruct her to do so immediately before bedtime and advise her to try not to empty her bowels again until morning. Warn patient to keep canister away from heat sources, as its contents are flammable.

• Caution patient not to use an oral inhaler with a spacer device.

• Advise patient to rinse her mouth with water after each dose and to spit the water out. Tell her to contact her prescriber if she develops a mouth or throat infection.

• Instruct patient not to use budesonide as a rescue inhaler.

• Tell patient to contact prescriber if symptoms persist or have worsened after 3 weeks. Caution against increasing the dose on her own.

• Inform parents of small children using nebulized Respules that improvement may begin within 2 to 8 days but that full effect may not be evident for 4 to 6 weeks.
• Caution patient to avoid exposure to chickenpox and measles and, if exposed, to contact prescriber immediately.
• Caution against stopping drug abruptly.
• Instruct patient on long-term therapy to have regular eye examinations.
• Urge female patient to notify prescriber if she is or could be pregnant.

bumetanide

Bumex

Class and Category

Chemical class: Sulfonamide derivative
Therapeutic class: Loop diuretic
Pregnancy category: C

Indications and Dosages

➤ *To treat edema caused by heart failure, hepatic disease, and renal disease, including nephrotic syndrome*

TABLETS
Adults. 0.5 to 2 mg daily, increased as needed, with a second or third dose every 4 to 5 hr or 0.5 to 2 mg every other day or daily for 3 or 4 days each week. *Maximum:* 10 mg daily.
I.V. INFUSION, I.V. OR I.V. INJECTION
Adults. 0.5 to 1 mg over 1 to 2 min daily, increased as needed with a second or third dose every 2 to 3 hr. *Maximum:* 10 mg daily.
DOSAGE ADJUSTMENT In patients with severe chronic renal insufficiency, continuous infusion (12 mg over 12 hr) may be more effective and less toxic than intermittent infusion.

Route	Onset	Peak	Duration
P.O.	30–60 min	1–2 hr	4–6 hr
I.V.	In min	15–30 min	3.5–4 hr

Mechanism of Action

Inhibits reabsorption of sodium, chloride, and water in the ascending limb of the loop of Henle, which promotes their excretion and reduces fluid volume.

Contraindications

Anuria, hepatic coma, hypersensitivity to bumetanide or its components, severe electrolyte depletion

Interactions

DRUGS
aminoglycosides: Increased risk of ototoxicity
antihypertensives: Increased hypotensive effect
indomethacin: Slowed increase in urine and sodium excretion, inhibited plasma renin activity
lithium: Reduced lithium renal clearance, increased risk of lithium toxicity
probenecid: Reduced sodium excretion

Adverse Reactions

CNS: Dizziness, encephalopathy, headache
CV: Hypotension
EENT: Ototoxicity
ENDO: Hyperglycemia
GI: Nausea
GU: Azotemia, elevated serum creatinine level
MS: Muscle spasms
SKIN: Stevens-Johnson syndrome, toxic epidermal necrolysis
Other: Hyperuricemia, hypocalcemia, hypochloremia, hypokalemia, hyponatremia, hypovolemia

Nursing Considerations

WARNING A patient hypersensitive to sulfonamides may be hypersensitive to bumetanide. Monitor such a patient closely when starting therapy.
• Expect to use parenteral route for patients with impaired GI absorption or in whom the oral route isn't practical. Switch to oral route, as prescribed, as soon as possible.
• Discard unused parenteral solution 24 hours after preparation.
• Assess fluid and electrolyte balance closely because bumetanide is a potent diuretic (40 to 60 times more potent than furosemide). Monitor fluid intake and output once every 8 hours, evaluate serum electrolyte levels when ordered, and assess for imbalances.
WARNING Be aware that high-dose or too-frequent administration can cause profound diuresis and water and electrolyte depletion, especially in elderly patients.

- Monitor serum potassium level regularly to check for hypokalemia, especially if patient takes a digitalis glycoside for heart failure or has hepatic cirrhosis, ascites, aldosteronism, potassium-losing nephropathy, diarrhea, or a history of ventricular arrhythmias.
- Assess for evidence of ototoxicity, such as tinnitus, daily. Rarely, drug may cause ototoxicity, especially with I.V. use, high doses, and increased frequency of dosing in a patient with renal impairment.
- Monitor results of renal function tests during therapy to detect adverse reactions.

PATIENT TEACHING
- Advise patient to avoid hazardous activities until drug's CNS effects are known.
- Stress importance of monitoring fluid intake and output and watching for evidence of electrolyte imbalance, such as dizziness, headache, and muscle spasms.
- Review adverse reactions, and tell patient to report severe or persistent reactions.
- Review potassium-rich foods, and urge patient to include them in her daily diet.
- Urge patient to return for appropriate follow-up care, especially if she's receiving bumetanide for a chronic condition.
- Tell diabetic patient to monitor blood glucose level regularly and to notify prescriber about persistent hyperglycemia.
- Advise patient to report any changes in skin that are new, unusual, persistent, or severe.

---

buprenorphine hydrochloride

Buprenex, Butrans, Subutex

Class, Category, and Schedule
Chemical class: Opioid, thebaine derivative
Therapeutic class: Opioid analgesic
Pregnancy category: C
Controlled substance schedule: III

Indications and Dosages
➤ *To control moderate to severe pain*
I.V. OR I.M. INJECTION (BUPRENEX)
Adults and children age 12 and over. 0.3 mg every 6 hr or more, as needed. A second 0.3-mg dose may be given 30 to 60 min after first dose, if needed.

DOSAGE ADJUSTMENT For patients not at high risk for opioid toxicity, I.M. dose increased to 0.6 mg or frequency increased to every 4 hr, if needed, depending on pain severity and patient response. For elderly or debilitated patients and patients who have respiratory disease or also use another CNS depressant, I.V. or I.M. dose reduced by half.

Children ages 2 to 12. 0.002 to 0.006 mg/kg every 4 to 6 hr, as needed.

➤ *To control severe chronic pain in patients requiring a continuous, around-the-clock opioid analgesic for an extended period of time for which alternative treatment options are inadequate*

TRANSDERMAL PATCH (BUTRANS)
Opioid-naive adults and adults whose daily dose of oral morphine or equivalent was less than 30 mg. *Initial:* 5 mcg/hr, increased after 72 hr, as needed, to 10 mcg/hr. *Maximum:* 20 mcg/hr.

Adults whose daily dose of oral morphine or equivalent was between 30 and 80 mg. *Initial:* Current around-the-clock opioid use tapered for up to 7 days to no more than 30 mg of morphine or equivalent per day. Then a 10 mcg/hr patch applied, increased after 72 hr, as needed, to 20 mcg/hr. *Maximum:* 20 mcg/hr.

DOSAGE ADJUSTMENT For patient with mild to moderate hepatic impairment, *initial* dosage begun at 5 mcg/hr.

➤ *To treat opioid dependence*
SUBLINGUAL TABLETS (SUBUTEX)
Adults. 12 to 16 mg daily.

Mechanism of Action
May bind with CNS receptors to alter the perception of and emotional response to pain. Buprenorphine may act by displacing narcotic agonists from their binding sites and competitively inhibiting their actions.

Incompatibilities
Don't give I.V. buprenorphine through the same I.V. line as diazepam or lorazepam.

Contraindications
Acute or severe bronchial asthma in an unmonitored setting or in the absence of

B

resuscitative equipment, hypersensitivity to buprenorphine or its components, known or suspected paralytic ileus, significant respiratory depression

Route	Onset	Peak	Duration
I.V.	Under 15 min	Under 1 hr	6–10 hr*
I.M.	15 min	1 hr	6–10 hr*
Transdermal	Unknown	17 hr	Unknown

Interactions
DRUGS
CNS depressants, MAO inhibitors: Additive hypotensive and respiratory and CNS depressant effects of these drugs that may be life threatening
opioid analgesics: Reduced therapeutic effects if buprenorphine is given before another opioid analgesic; possibly life-threatening adverse effects
Activities
alcohol use: Increased serum buprenorphine levels possibly resulting in fatal overdose owing to CNS and respiratory depression

Adverse Reactions
CNS: Dizziness, headache, sedation, seizures, vertigo
CV: Bradycardia, hypertension, hypotension, QT prolongation
EENT: Miosis
GI: Elevated serum amylase level, nausea, spasm of the sphincter of Oddi, vomiting
RESP: Bronchospasm, hypoventilation, respiratory depression
SKIN: Diaphoresis, pruritus, rash, urticaria
Other: Anaphylaxis; angioedema; application-site inflammation, burns, discharge and vesicle occurrence; injection-site pain, redness, and swelling; physical and psychological dependence

Nursing Considerations
• Know that the transdermal patch should not be used in patients whose prior total daily dose of opioid use is greater than 80 mg of oral morphine equivalents per day because the maximum 20 mcg/hour dosage may not provide adequate analgesia. An alternate analgesic should be considered.

---

* 4 to 5 hr in children ages 2 to 12.

• Be aware that opioids like buprenorphine should not be given to women during pregnancy and labor and while breast feeding, as the newborn or infant may experience neonatal opioid withdrawal syndrome (NOWS). This syndrome may exhibit as poor feeding, rapid breathing, trembling, and excessive or high-pitched crying.
• Use buprenorphine cautiously in patients with severe hepatic or renal impairment, myxedema, hypothyroidism, adrenal insufficiency, CNS depression, coma, toxic psychosis, prostatic hypertrophy, urethral stricture, acute alcoholism, alcohol withdrawal syndrome, kyphoscoliosis, orbiliary tract dysfunction. Also use cautiously in patients who take a drug that decreases hepatic clearance, are known drug abusers, or have been addicted to opioids.
• Use drug cautiously in patients with head injury, intracranial lesions, or other conditions that could increase CSF pressure. Be particularly cautious when administering drug to patients with chronic obstructive pulmonary disease or cor pulmonale and in patients who have decreased respiratory reserve, hypoxia, hypercapnia, or preexisting respiratory depression.
• To avoid causing withdrawal, drug shouldn't be given for opioid dependence until signs of withdrawal occur.
• Give I.V. form over at least 2 minutes.
• Inspect injection site for local reactions; don't use the same site twice.
• Monitor vital signs and response to drug often, especially after giving first dose and if patient develops a fever
WARNING Monitor patient closely for respiratory depression, especially in the elderly, cachectic, or debilitated patients; when initiating and titrating dosages; or when other drugs that depress respiration are given together. Report respiratory depression immediately, because respiratory arrest may occur. Be prepared to provide supportive care.
• Monitor patient with a seizure disorder, as buprenorphine may worsen seizure control.
• When buprenorphine therapy is no longer needed, drug should never be discontinued

abruptly. Instead, expect a gradual down-ward titration of the dose to prevent signs and symptoms of withdrawal.

PATIENT TEACHING
• Explain that buprenorphine may be habit forming. Urge her to notify prescriber if she develops any unusual or persistent symptoms.
• Instruct patient taking sublingual form to place tablets under her tongue until they dissolve. If patient takes more than two tablets per dose, tell her to place all tablets under her tongue at the same time. If they won't fit, tell her to place two at a time under her tongue until full dose has dissolved. Caution against swallowing tablets.
• Instruct patient prescribed the trans-dermal patch to place patch only on intact skin that is hairless and clean (washed with water only) and dry. If a hairless site is not available, instruct patient to clip, not shave, area prior to application. Emphasize importance of not applying patch to irritated skin. Inform patient patch must be applied immediately after its removal from pouch and placed on her upper outer arm, upper chest, upper back, or the side of her chest. Tell patient patch is to be worn for 7 days and that she should not cut the patch. If problems with adhesion occur, she may tape the edges of the patch with first-aid tape. If the patch should fall off during the 7-day interval, tell her to dispose of the patch and apply a new one at a different skin site. When removing the patch, tell patient to fold it over on itself and flush it down the toilet or seal it in the patch disposal unit provided and dispose of in the trash.
• Caution patient to keep patch out of the reach of others, especially children, as exposure to even one patch could be fatal.
• Inform patient wearing a buprenorphine patch not to expose it to any external heat source such as heating pads, electric blankets, heat lamps, saunas, hot tubs, or heated water beds, as absorption may be affected.
• Warn patient not to stop taking drug abruptly or to alter dosage on her own.
• Caution patient to avoid hazardous activities while receiving buprenorphine.

• Instruct patient not to drink alcohol or take sleep aids and CNS depressants without checking with prescriber first.
• Advise patient to notify prescriber if she becomes pregnant or is breastfeeding, as drug may need to be discontinued or dosage altered.

bupropion hydrochloride
Forfivo XL, Wellbutrin, Wellbutrin SR, Wellbutrin XL, Zyban

bupropion hydrobromide
Aplenzin

Class and Category
Chemical class: Aminoketone derivative
Therapeutic class: Antidepressant, smoking cessation adjunct
Pregnancy category: C

Indications and Dosages
➤ *To treat depression*
E.R. TABLETS (WELLBUTRIN SR)
Adults. *Initial:* 150 mg daily in morning for 3 days; then 150 mg twice daily and, after several wk, 200 mg twice daily, as needed and tolerated. *Maximum:* 400 mg daily or 200 mg/dose.
E.R. TABLETS (WELLBUTRIN XL)
Adults. *Initial:* 150 mg daily in morning for at least 3 days; then 300 mg daily and, after 4 wk, 450 mg daily, as needed and tolerated. *Maximum:* 450 mg daily.
E.R. TABLETS (APLENZIN)
Adults. *Initial:* 174 mg daily in the morning for 3 days. Then, if tolerated well, dosage increased to 348 mg daily in the morning. After 4 wk of therapy, dosage increased to 522 mg daily in the morning, if needed.
E.R. TABLETS (FORFIVO XL)
Adults. *Initial:* with another bupropion product and then switched to 450 mg once daily, as needed. *Maximum:* 450 mg once daily.
TABLETS (APLENZIN, WELLBUTRIN, WELLBUTRIN SR, WELLBUTRIN XL)
Adults. *Initial:* 100 mg twicedaily, increased after 3 or more days to 100 mg three times

daily, as needed. *Maximum:* 450 mg daily or 150 mg/dose.

➤ *To aid in smoking cessation*

E.R. TABLETS (ZYBAN)

Adults. *Initial:* 150 mg daily for 3 days and then 150 mg twice daily for 7 to 12 wk. *Maximum:* 300 mg daily or 150 mg/dose.

➤ *To prevent seasonal major depressive episodes in patient with seasonal affective disorder*

E.R. TABLETS (APLENZIN)

Adults. *Initial:* 150 mg once daily in morning starting in autumn, increased after 1 wk to 300 mg once daily in morning, if tolerated and needed. Decreased to 150 mg once daily 2 wk before stopping in early spring.

DOSAGE ADJUSTMENT For patients with severe hepatic cirrhosis, no more than 75 mg daily of Wellbutrin, 100 mg daily or 150 mg every other day of Wellbutrin SR, 150 mg every other day of Wellbutrin XL or Zyban, and 174 mg every other day of Aplenzin. In renal impairment, dosage or frequency decreased on an individual basis.

Route	Onset	Peak	Duration
P.O.	1–3 wk	Unknown	Unknown

Mechanism of Action

May inhibit norepinephrine, serotonin, and dopamine uptake by neurons, which significantly relieves evidence of depression.

Contraindications

Hypersensitivity to bupropion or its components, seizure disorder or conditions that increase risk of seizures (i.e., arteriovenous malformation, severe head injury, CNS tumor or infection, severe stroke, anorexia nervosa or bulimia, or abrupt discontinuation of alcohol, benzodiazepines, barbiturates, or antiepileptic drugs), use within 14 days of a MAO inhibitor (MAOI) including reversible MAOIs such as linezolid or intravenous methylene blue; use of another form of bupropion concurrently

Interactions

DRUGS

amantadine, levodopa: Increased adverse reactions to bupropion antipsychotics, concurrent use of other bupropion products, phenothiazines, systemic corticosteroids, theophylline, tricyclic antidepressants: increased risk of seizures

carbamazepine, cimetidine, phenobarbital, phenytoin: Increased bupropion metabolism

citalopram: Possibly increased citalopram effects

CYP2B6 inducers and inhibitors such as clopidogrel, cyclophosphamide, orphenadrine, thiotepa, ticlopidine: Altered bupropion effectiveness

desipramine: Possible increased effects of desipramine

efavirenz, fluvoxamine, nelfinavir, norfluoxetine, paroxetine, ritonavir, sertraline: Possibly altered effectiveness of bupropion

levodopa: Increased adverse bupropion effects

MAO inhibitors including reversible MAOIs such as linezolid and intravenous methylene blue: Increased risk of acute bupropion toxicity and serious hypertensive reactions

nicotine: Possibly increased blood pressure

ritonavir: Decreased effectiveness of bupropion

warfarin: Possibly altered PT and INR; risk of hemorrhagic or thrombotic complications

ACTIVITIES

alcohol use, recreational drug abuse: Lowered seizure threshold

Adverse Reactions

CNS: Abnormal coordination, agitation, akathisia, anxiety, asthenia, CNS stimulation, coma, confusion, decreased concentration or memory, delusions, depersonalization, depression, dizziness, emotional lability, euphoria, fever, general or migraine headache, hallucinations, hostility, hyperkinesia, hypertonia, hypersthesia, insomnia, irritability, mania, nervousness, paranoia, paresthesia, psychosis and other neuropsychiatric reactions, seizures, sleep disorder, somnolence, stroke, suicidal ideation, syncope, tremor, vertigo

CV: Arrhythmias, chest pain, complete AV block, hypertension, MI, orthostatic hypotension, palpitations, phlebitis, tachycardia, vasodilation

EENT: Acute-angle glaucoma, altered taste, amblyopia, blurred vision, dry mouth, hearing loss, increased ocular pressure,

pharyngitis, sinusitis, taste perversion, tinnitus
ENDO: Hyperglycemia, hypoglycemia, syndrome of inappropriate ADH secretion
GI: Abdominal pain, anorexia, constipation, diarrhea, dysphagia, flatulence, GI hemorrhage, GI ulceration, hepatitis, increased appetite, intestinal perforation, nausea, pancreatitis, vomiting
GU: Decreased libido, urinary frequency and urgency, UTI, vaginal hemorrhage
HEME: Anemia, leukocytosis, leukopenia, lymphadenopathy, pancytopenia, thrombocytopenia
MS: Arthralgia, arthritis, muscle twitching, myalgia, rhabdomyolysis
RESP: Bronchospasm, cough, dyspnea, pulmonary embolism
SKIN: Diaphoresis, erythema multiforme, exfoliative dermatitis, flushing, pruritus, rash, Stevens-Johnson syndrome, urticaria
Other: Anaphylaxis, angioedema, generalized pain, hot flashes, infection, serum sickness–like reaction, weight loss

Nursing Considerations

• Be aware that Forfivo XL should not be used in patients with hepatic or renal impairment because the only dosage available for Forfivo XL is 450 mg once daily, which may be too high a dose for the liver or kidneys to handle.
• Use cautiously in patients with renal impairment (all other brands); drug is excreted by kidneys.
• Know that Forfivo XL should never be used to initiate treatment of depression because the dose is too high. Only after the patient has received other bupropion products first and then requires a 450-mg dose should Forfivo XL be used.
• Assess patient's blood pressure before bupropion therapy begins and monitor periodically during therapy because bupropion may cause hypertension.
• Monitor children, adolescents, and depressed patients closely for worsened depression and increased suicide risk, especially when therapy starts or dosage changes.
• If patient takes bupropion for smoking cessation, watch for neuropsychiatric symptoms, including changes in behavior, hostility, agitation, depressed mood,

suicidal ideation, and worsening of psychiatric illness. If present, notify prescriber immediately, begin safety measures, and expect to discontinue drug.
WARNING To reduce seizure risk, allow at least 4 hours (tablets) or 8 hours (E.R. tablets) between doses. Know that maximum dosage should not be exceeded and dosage reduction should be gradual because risk of seizures is dose-related.
• Use seizure precautions, especially in patients who take OTC stimulants or anorectics; use excessive alcohol, benzodiazepines, hypnotics or sedatives; are addicted to opioids, cocaine, or stimulants; take drugs that lower the seizure threshold; have a history of seizures, head trauma, or CNS tumors; have hyponatremia, hypoxia or severe hepatic cirrhosis; or take insulin or an oral antidiabetic.
• Using transdermal nicotine with bupropion may cause hypertension. Watch closely.

PATIENT TEACHING

• Advise patient to take bupropion for 7 or more days before stopping smoking.
• Tell patient to swallow E.R. tablets whole and not to cut, crush, or chew them.
• Tell patient to take bupropion with food.
• Urge patient to avoid or minimize consuming alcohol and sedatives during therapy and not to stop drug abruptly or exceed dosage prescribed because seizures may occur.
WARNING Advise patient to seek medical help immediately and stop taking drug if signs of rash, itching, hives, chest pain, shortness of breath, or swelling, especially of face, occurs.
• Urge caregivers to monitor depressed patient closely for worsened depression, especially when therapy starts or dosage changes.
• Alert patient that drug may cause mild pupillary dilation, which can lead to an episode of acute closure glaucoma. Encourage him to have an eye exam to determine if he is susceptible to angle closure.
• If patient takes bupropion for smoking cessation, explain that it may cause serious adverse effects, including changes in behavior, hostility, agitation, depressed

B

mood, suicidal ideation, and worsening of psychiatric illness. If present, patient should notify prescriber immediately and expect to discontinue drug.
• Alert patient that bupropion therapy may produce a false-positive urine screening test for amphetamines even after drug has been discontinued. Other tests may be required to distinguish bupropion from amphetamines.

buspirone hydrochloride

BuSpar, BuSpar DIVIDOSE, Bustab (CAN)

Class and Category
Chemical class: Azaspirodecanedione
Therapeutic class: Antianxiety
Pregnancy category: B

Indications and Dosages
➤ *To manage anxiety*
TABLETS
Adults. *Initial:* 5 mg three times daily or 7.5 mg twice daily increased by 5 mg daily at 2- to 3-day intervals until desired response occurs. *Maintenance:* 20 to 30 mg daily (usual therapeutic range). *Maximum:* 60 mg daily.
DOSAGE ADJUSTMENT When used with nefazodone, dosage as little as 2.5 mg daily.

Route	Onset	Peak	Duration
P.O.	1–4 wk	3–6 wk	Unknown

Mechanism of Action
May act as a partial agonist at serotonin 5-hydroxytryptamine$_{1A}$ receptors in the brain, producing antianxiety effects.

Contraindications
Hypersensitivity to buspirone or its components, severe hepatic or renal impairment

Interactions
DRUGS
diltiazem, erythromycin, itraconazole, nefazodone, nordiazepam, verapamil:

Increased blood level and adverse effects of buspirone
haloperidol: Increased haloperidol level
hepatic enzyme CYP3A4 inducers, such as dexamethasone and certain anticonvulsants (phenytoin, phenobarbital, carbamazepine): Possibly increased rate of buspirone metabolism
hepatic enzyme CYP3A4 inhibitors, such as ketoconazole and ritonavir: Possibly inhibited buspirone metabolism and increased blood level
MAO inhibitors: Increased risk of hypertension
rifampin: Decreased blood buspirone level and pharmacodynamic effects
FOODS
food: Possibly decreased buspirone clearance
grapefruit juice: Increased blood buspirone level

Adverse Reactions
CNS: Akathisia, anger, ataxia, cogwheel rigidity, confusion, decreased concentration, depression, dizziness, dream disturbances, drowsiness, dyskinesias, dystonia, excitement, extrapyramidal symptoms, fatigue, headache, hostility, insomnia, lack of coordination, light-headedness, mood swings, nervousness, paresthesia, parkinsonism, restless leg syndrome, restlessness, serotonin syndrome, transient recall impairment, tremor, weakness
CV: Chest pain, palpitations, tachycardia
EENT: Blurred vision, dry mouth, nasal congestion, pharyngitis, tinnitus, tunnel vision
GI: Abdominal or gastric distress, constipation, diarrhea, nausea, vomiting
GU: Urine retention
MS: Myalgia
SKIN: Diaphoresis, ecchymosis, rash, urticaria
Other: Angioedema

Nursing Considerations
• Use buspirone cautiously in patients with hepatic or renal impairment.
• Institute safety precautions because of possible adverse CNS reactions.
• Follow closely if patient is being withdrawn from long-term therapy with benzodiazepines or other sedative-

hypnotic drugs while starting buspirone because buspirone won't prevent withdrawal symptoms.

PATIENT TEACHING
• Advise patient to take buspirone consistently, either always with or always without food.
• Caution patient to avoid drinking large amounts of grapefruit juice.
• Inform patient that 1 to 2 weeks of therapy may be needed before she notices drug's antianxiety effect.
• Emphasize the importance of not taking more buspirone than prescribed.
• Advise patient to avoid hazardous activities until drug's CNS effects are known.

---

butabarbital sodium

Busodium, Butalan, Butisol, Sarisol No. 2

Class, Category, and Schedule
Chemical class: Barbiturate
Therapeutic class: Sedative-hypnotic
Pregnancy category: D
Controlled substance schedule: III

Indications and Dosages
➤ *To provide daytime sedation*
ELIXIR, TABLETS
Adults. 15 to 30 mg three times daily or four times daily.
➤ *To treat insomnia*
ELIXIR, TABLETS
Adults. 50 to 100 mg every at bedtime.
➤ *To provide preoperative sedation*
ELIXIR, TABLETS
Adults. 50 to 100 mg 60 to 90 min before surgery.
Children. 2 to 6 mg/kg. *Maximum:* 100 mg/dose.
DOSAGE ADJUSTMENT Dosage reduced in patients with impaired renal or hepatic function and in elderly or debilitated patients because they may be more sensitive to drug.

Route	Onset	Peak	Duration
P.O.	45–60 min	Unknown	6–8 hr

Mechanism of Action
Inhibits the upward conduction of nerve impulses in the brain's reticular formation, which disrupts impulse transmission to the cortex. As a result, butabarbital depresses the CNS and produces drowsiness, sedation, and hypnosis.

Contraindications
History of addiction to sedative or hypnotic drug, hypersensitivity to butabarbital or its components, porphyria, severe hepatic or respiratory disease

Interactions
DRUGS
acetaminophen: Increased risk of hepato-toxicity (with large doses of or long-term therapy with butabarbital)
activated charcoal: Reduced butabarbital absorption
carbamazepine: Decreased blood carbamazepine level
chloramphenicol, corticosteroids, digitalis glycosides: Increased metabolism and decreased effects of these drugs
clonazepam: Increased clearance and reduced efficacy of clonazepam
CNS depressants, including OTC sedatives and hypnotics: Additive CNS depression
doxycycline: Shortened half-life and decreased effects of doxycycline
fenoprofen: Reduced bioavailability and effects of fenoprofen
griseofulvin: Reduced griseofulvin absorption
hydantoins, such as phenytoin: Unpredictable effects on barbiturate metabolism
MAO inhibitors: Prolonged barbiturate effects
meperidine: Prolonged CNS depressant effects of meperidine
methadone: Reduced methadone actions
methoxyflurane: Increased risk of nephrotoxicity
metronidazole: Decreased antimicrobial effect of metronidazole
oral anticoagulants: Decreased anti-coagulant effect
oral contraceptives with estrogen: Decreased contraceptive effect
phenylbutazone: Reduced elimination half-life of phenylbutazone
rifampin: Decreased butabarbital effectiveness
sodium valproate, valproic acid: Decreased butabarbital metabolism and increased adverse CNS effects

theophylline: Decreased blood level and effects of theophylline
ACTIVITIES
alcohol use: Additive CNS depression

Adverse Reactions

CNS: Agitation, anxiety, ataxia, clumsiness, CNS depression, confusion, depression, dizziness, drowsiness, fever, hallucinations, headache, hyperkinesia, insomnia, irritability, nervousness, nightmares, psychiatric disturbance, sleep driving (see Patient Teaching section), somnolence, syncope
CV: Hypertension
EENT: Laryngospasm
GI: Constipation, hepatic dysfunction, nausea, vomiting
MS: Rickets
RESP: Apnea, bronchospasm, respiratory depression
SKIN: Exfoliative dermatitis, Stevens-Johnson syndrome
Other: Anaphylaxis, angioedema, drug tolerance, physical and psychological dependence

Nursing Considerations

• Use butabarbital cautiously, if at all, in patients with depression, suicidal tendency, history of drug abuse, or hepatic dysfunction. Don't administer drug to patients with premonitory signs of hepatic coma.
WARNING Monitor patient closely following butabarbital ingestion because anaphylaxis or angioedema, although rare, may occur with first dose or later doses. Notify prescriber immediately, and provide supportive emergency care.
• Expect to give drug for no more than 2 weeks to treat insomnia because, like all barbiturates, it loses effectiveness for sleep induction and sleep maintenance after 2 weeks.
• Monitor butabarbital intake closely during long-term use because tolerance and psychological and physical dependence may develop.
• Avoid abrupt withdrawal of butabarbital to prevent withdrawal symptoms.
• Monitor elderly and debilitated patients closely because drug may cause marked excitement, depression, and confusion in these patients.

• If patient experiencing pain receives butabarbital, monitor closely for paradoxical excitement.
• If pregnant woman took butabarbital during last trimester, monitor infant for withdrawal symptoms.
• Monitor patient for worsening of insomnia or emergence of abnormal thinking or behavior during therapy. If butabarbital unmasks them, patient will need further assessment.
PATIENT TEACHING
• Emphasize the importance of taking butabarbital exactly as prescribed because it can be addictive. Warn against increasing the dose or decreasing the dosage interval without consulting prescriber.
• Advise patient to notify prescriber if insomnia persists after 7 days of butabarbital therapy.
• Tell patient to avoid alcohol and OTC sedatives and hypnotics during butabarbital therapy because of additive CNS effects.
• Advise patient to avoid hazardous activities until butabarbital's CNS effects are known.
• Advise female patient not to rely on oral contraceptives during butabarbital therapy.
• Explain that butabarbital may cause sleep driving, in which the patient drives while not fully awake and typically cannot recall doing so. Tell family members to report any episodes of sleep driving.

butorphanol tartrate

Stadol, Stadol NS

Class, Category, and Schedule
Chemical class: Opioid
Therapeutic class: Anesthesia adjunct, opioid analgesic
Pregnancy category: C
Controlled substance schedule: II

Indications and Dosages
➤ *To manage pain*

I.V. INJECTION
Adults. 0.5 to 2 mg (usually 1 mg) every 3 to 4 hr, as needed.
I.M. INJECTION
Adults. 1 to 4 mg (usually 2 mg) every 3 to 4 hr, as needed. *Maximum:* 4 mg/single dose.
NASAL INHALATION
Adults. 1 spray (1 mg) in one nostril. Dose repeated after 60 to 90 min; two-dose sequence repeated every 3 to 4 hr, as needed. For severe pain, 2 sprays (1 in each nostril) every 3 to 4 hr, as needed.
DOSAGE ADJUSTMENT Dose reduced to 1 spray in one nostril for elderly patients and those with impaired hepatic or renal function. Dose repeated after 90 to 120 min; two-dose sequence repeated every 6 hr or more, as needed.
➤ *As adjunct to provide preoperative anesthesia*
I.V. OR I.M. INJECTION
Adults. Individualized. *Average:* 2 mg 60 to 90 min before surgery.
➤ *As adjunct to provide anesthesia*
I.V. INJECTION
Adults. Individualized. *Average:* 1 to 4 mg and then supplemental doses of 0.5 to 1 mg, as needed. Total usually required during surgery is 60 to 180 mcg/kg.
DOSAGE ADJUSTMENT Parenteral doses reduced by half for elderly patients and patients with impaired hepatic or renal function.

Mechanism of Action
Binds with specific CNS receptors to alter the perception of and emotional response to pain.

Contraindications
Hypersensitivity to butorphanol or its components (including the preservative benzethonium chloride)

Route	Onset	Peak	Duration
I.V.	2–3 min	30 min	2–4 hr
I.M.	10–30 min	30–60 min	3–4 hr
Inhalation	In 15 min	1–2 hr	4–5 hr

Interactions
DRUGS
CNS depressants: Additive CNS depression
nasal vasoconstrictors, such as oxymetazoline: Decreased absorption rate and delayed onset of butorphanol

ACTIVITIES
alcohol use: Additive CNS depression

Adverse Reactions
CNS: Anxiety, confusion, difficulty making purposeful movements, difficulty speaking, dizziness, euphoria, floating feeling, headache, insomnia (with nasal form), lethargy, nervousness, paresthesia, sensation of heat, somnolence, syncope, tremor, vertigo
CV: Chest pain, hypotension, palpitations, tachycardia, vasodilation
EENT: Blurred vision, dry mouth, ear pain, epistaxis, nasal congestion or irritation (with nasal form), pharyngitis, rhinitis, sinus congestion, sinusitis, tinnitus, unpleasant taste
GI: Anorexia, constipation, epigastric pain, nausea, vomiting
RESP: Apnea, bronchitis, cough, dyspnea, respiratory depression, shallow breathing, upper respiratory tract infection
SKIN: Clammy skin, pruritus

Nursing Considerations
• Use butorphanol cautiously, if at all, in patients with depression, suicidal tendency, history of drug abuse, or hepatic or renal dysfunction.
• Because drug can raise CSF pressure, use it cautiously, if at all, in patients with head injury. Because it can increase cardiac workload, use with extreme caution in patients with acute MI, ventricular dysfunction, or coronary insufficiency.
• Be aware that butorphanol has a high potential for abuse.
• Monitor patient after first dose of nasal form; hypotension and syncope may occur.
• Take safety precautions because butorphanol causes CNS depression.
• Assess respiratory status closely because drug causes respiratory depression.
• Monitor blood pressure often after giving drug. If severe hypertension develops (rare), stop drug at once and notify prescriber. If patient isn't narcotic-dependent, expect to administer naloxone to reverse butorphanol's effects.
PATIENT TEACHING
• Emphasize the importance of taking butorphanol exactly as prescribed because it can be addictive. Warn patient not to

increase the dose or decrease the dosage interval without consulting prescriber.

• Advise patient to avoid hazardous activities until drug's CNS effects are known.

• Tell patient to avoid alcohol and other CNS depressants, including OTC drugs, while taking butorphanol because of additive adverse CNS reactions.

• Teach patient how to use nasal form properly by giving these instructions: After blowing nose to clear the nostrils, pull clear cover from the pump unit and remove protective clip from its neck. Prime pump unit by placing the nozzle between first and second fingers with thumb on the bottom of the bottle. Then pump sprayer unit firmly and quickly until a fine spray appears (7 or 8 strokes). Insert spray tip about 1 cm (one-third inch) into one nostril, pointing tip toward the back of the nose. Close other nostril with one finger and tilt head slightly forward. Then pump sprayer firmly and quickly by pushing down on the pump unit's finger grips and against the thumb at the bottom of the bottle. Sniff gently with mouth closed. After spraying, remove pump from nose, tilt head back, and sniff gently for a few more seconds. Then replace protective clip and clear cover.

➤━━━━━━━━━━━━━━━━◀

C

cabergoline
Dostinex

Class and Category
Chemical class: Ergot alkaloid derivative
Therapeutic class: Antihyperprolactinemic
Pregnancy category: B

Indications and Dosages
➤ *To treat idiopathic or adenoma-induced hyperprolactinemic disorders*
TABLETS
Adults. 0.25 mg twice/wk. Increased by 0.25 mg/wk at 4-wk intervals, if needed, up to 1 mg twice/wk.

Route	Onset	Peak	Duration
P.O.	Unknown	48 hr	Up to 14 days

Mechanism of Action
Binds with dopamine D_2 receptors to block prolactin synthesis and secretion by the anterior pituitary gland, thereby reducing the serum prolactin level.

Contraindications
History of pulmonary, pericardial, cardiac valvular, or retroperitoneal fibrotic disorders; hypersensitivity to cabergoline, ergot derivatives, or their components; uncontrolled hypertension

Interactions
DRUGS
antihypertensives: Increased risk of hypotension
dopamine antagonists (butyrophenones, metoclopramide, phenothiazines, or thioxanthenes): Decreased cabergoline effectiveness

Adverse Reactions
CNS: Aggression, asthenia, depression, fatigue, headache, nervousness, paresthesia, pathological gambling behavior, somnolence, psychotic disorder, vertigo
CV: Orthostatic hypotension, valvulopathy
EENT: Dry mouth

ENDO: Breast pain
GI: Abdominal pain, constipation, diarrhea, flatulence, indigestion, nausea, vomiting
GU: Dysmenorrhea, increased libido
RESP: Pulmonary effusion or fibrosis
SKIN: Alopecia
Other: Extracardiac fibrotic reactions

Nursing Considerations
• Ensure that patient has undergone a cardiovascular evaluation, including an echocardiogram to determine the presence of valvular disease prior to administering cabergoline because the presence of valvular disease is a contraindication to the use of cabergoline therapy.
• Obtain an erythrocyte sedimentation rate, chest x-ray, and serum creatinine measurement, as ordered, prior to initiating cabergoline therapy and repeat during therapy if the patient develops any signs and symptoms of an extracardiac fibrotic reaction.
• Before each dose increase, check serum prolactin level to assess cabergoline's effectiveness.
• If patient has moderate to severe hepatic impairment, monitor closely for adverse reactions because of decreased cabergoline metabolism.
• Expect patient who takes cabergoline long term to undergo periodic reassessment of cardiac status, including echocardiography, because valvulopathy can occur with prolonged cabergoline use.
• Monitor erythrocyte sedimentation rate, as it may increase in a patient with pleural effusion or pleural fibrosis.
WARNING If you detect evidence of overdose, such as syncope, hallucinations, light-headedness, tachycardia, and nasal congestion, notify prescriber and treat as ordered.
PATIENT TEACHING
• Urge patient to read and follow printed information that explains how to use cabergoline for best therapeutic results.
• Advise patient to take drug with meals to help decrease GI distress.
• Tell patient to take a missed dose as soon as possible within 1 to 2 days. If missed dose isn't remembered until it's time for the next dose, instruct him to double the dose if drug is generally well tolerated

and doesn't cause nausea. If drug isn't well tolerated, instruct patient to consult prescriber before taking the missed dose.
• Urge patient to change positions slowly to avoid orthostatic hypotension. Tell him to notify prescriber if it occurs.
• Urge patient to keep regular appointments to monitor drug effectiveness.
• Advise patient that drug therapy will end when serum prolactin level is normal for 6 months. Explain that he'll need periodic monitoring to determine whether therapy should resume.
• Tell female patient of childbearing age to notify prescriber if she is, could be, or plans to become pregnant during therapy; drug may need to be discontinued.
• Caution patient to avoid gambling during therapy because drug may increase the risk of pathological gambling behaviors.

calcifediol
Calderol

Class and Category
Chemical class: Sterol derivative, vitamin D analogue
Therapeutic class: Antihypocalcemic
Pregnancy category: C

Indications and Dosages
➤ *To treat metabolic bone disease or hypocalcemia in patients receiving renal dialysis*
CAPSULES
Adults and children age 10 and over. 300 to 350 mcg/wk given in divided doses daily or every other day. Increased at 4-wk intervals, p.r.n. Usual dosage 50 to 100 mcg daily or 100 to 200 mcg every other day.
Children ages 2 to 10. 0.05 mg daily.
Children up to age 2. 0.02 to 0.05 mg daily.
DOSAGE ADJUSTMENT Dosage decreased to as low as 20 mcg every other day in patients with normal serum calcium level.

Route	Onset	Peak	Duration
P.O.	Unknown	Unknown	15–20 days

Mechanism of Action
Converted to calcitriol in kidneys and then binds to specific receptors in intestinal mucosa to increase calcium absorption from intestine. Calcifediol also may regulate calcium ion transfer from bone to blood and stimulate calcium reabsorption in distal renal tubules, making more calcium available in the body.

Contraindications
Abnormal sensitivity to vitamin D effects, decreased renal function, hypercalcemia, hyperphosphatemia, hypervitaminosis, malabsorption syndrome, vitamin D toxicity

Interactions
DRUGS
aluminum-containing antacids: Increased blood aluminum level, especially in patients with chronic renal failure
barbiturates, corticosteroids, hydantoin anticonvulsants, primidone: Decreased effects of vitamin D
calcitonin, etidronate, gallium nitrate, pamidronate, plicamycin: Decreased effects of these drugs
calcium (high doses), thiazide diuretics: Increased risk of hypercalcemia
cholestyramine, colestipol, mineral oil: Decreased vitamin D absorption
digitalis glycosides: Increased risk of arrhythmias from hypercalcemia
magnesium-containing antacids: Hyper-magnesemia, especially in chronic renal failure
phosphorous-containing drugs: Increased risk of hyperphosphatemia
verapamil: Increased risk of atrial fibrillation
vitamin D derivatives, such as calcitriol, dihydrotachysterol, ergocalciferol: Increased risk of vitamin D toxicity

Nursing Considerations
• Use calcifediol cautiously in patients with sarcoidosis or other granulomatous disease because of increased sensitivity to effects of vitamin D.
• If hypercalcemia develops, expect to stop drug. Calcium level usually returns to normal in 2 to 4 weeks. To manage acute hypercalcemia, give I.V. normal saline solution and possibly a loop diuretic, as

prescribed, to enhance diuresis or prepare for dialysis with a calcium-free dialysate if needed. Chronic hypercalcemia may lead to diffuse vascular calcification, nephrocalcinosis, and other soft-tissue calcification.

- If patient receives high-dose or long-term calcifediol therapy, be alert for vitamin D toxicity. Early evidence includes bone pain, constipation, dry mouth, headache, metallic taste, myalgia, nausea, somnolence, vomiting, and weakness. Late evidence includes albuminuria, anorexia, arrhythmias, azotemia, conjunctivitis (calcific), decreased libido, elevated AST and ALT levels, elevated BUN level, generalized vascular calcification, hypercholesterolemia, hypertension, hyperthermia, irritability, mild acidosis, nephrocalcinosis, nocturia, pancreatitis, photophobia, polydipsia, polyuria, pruritus, rhinorrhea, and weight loss.

PATIENT TEACHING
- Instruct patient to swallow capsule whole and not to crush or chew it.
- Advise patient to consult prescriber before taking OTC drugs.
- Instruct patient to store drug tightly capped in a cool, dry place away from direct light.
- Encourage patient to eat a balanced diet that includes foods high in vitamin D and calcium. Calcifediol is most effective with a high-calcium diet.
- If patient takes vitamin supplements, warn him not to exceed recommended amounts.
- Tell patient to avoid calcium-, phosphate-, and magnesium-containing laxatives and antacids; mineral oil; and vitamin D preparations because they may increase the risk of calcifediol's toxic effects.
- Advise patient to immediately report possible toxicity, such as headache, irritability, nausea, photophobia, vomiting, weakness, and weight loss.
- Stress need for follow-up care, including laboratory tests to evaluate progress and identify signs of toxicity early.

calcitonin, human

Cibacalcin

calcitonin, salmon

Fortical, Miacalcin

Class and Category
Chemical class: Polypeptide hormone
Therapeutic class: Antihypercalcemic, bone resorption inhibitor, osteoporosis therapy adjunct
Pregnancy category: C

Indications and Dosages
➤ *To treat hypercalcemic emergency*
I.M. OR SUBCUTANEOUS INJECTION
Adults. *Initial:* 4 international units/kg every 12 hr. Increased after 1 or 2 days, if needed, to 8 international units/kg every 12 hr. *Maximum:* 8 international units/kg every 6 hr.
➤ *To treat postmenopausal osteoporosis in women who are at least 5 years postmenopausal*
I.M. OR SUBCUTANEOUS INJECTION (CALCITONIN, SALMON)
Adults. *Initial:* 100 international units daily, every other day, or 3 times weekly. *Maximum:* 100 international units daily.
NASAL SPRAY
Adults. 200 international units (1 spray) daily, alternating nostrils.
➤ *To treat Paget's disease of the bone*
I.M. OR SUBCUTANEOUS INJECTION (CALCITONIN, SALMON)
Adults. *Initial:* 100 international units daily. *Maintenance:* 50 to 100 international units daily or every other day. *Maximum:* 100 international units daily.
SUBCUTANEOUS INJECTION (CALCITONIN, HUMAN)
Adults. 0.5 mg daily, 0.5 mg 2 or 3 times/wk, or 0.25 mg daily.

Route	Onset	Peak	Duration
I.M., SubQ	In 15 min*	2 hr†	6–8 hr†

Mechanism of Action
Directly inhibits bone resorption. Besides reducing the serum calcium level, this action slows bone metabolism (a major factor in the development of Paget's disease) and calcium loss from the bone (a major factor in the development of osteoporosis).

* For hypercalcemia; 6 to 24 mo for paget's disease.
† For hypercalcemia; unknown for other indications.

Contraindications

Hypersensitivity to calcitonin, human; calcitonin, salmon; or their components

Interactions

DRUGS

lithium: Possibly decreased lithium level

Adverse Reactions

CNS: Agitation, anxiety, dizziness, fatigue, headache, insomnia, neuralgia, paresthesia, stroke, tremor, vertigo
CV: Bundle-branch block, hypertension, MI, palpitations, peripheral edema, tachycardia, thrombophlebitis
EENT: Blurred vision; dry mouth; earache; epistaxis; eye pain; hearing loss; nasal irritation or ulceration (nasal spray), lesions, or redness; pharyngitis; rhinitis; salty taste; sinusitis; taste perversion; tinnitus; vitreous floaters
ENDO: Goiter, hyperthyroidism, hypocalcemia
GI: Abdominal pain, anorexia, cholelithiasis, diarrhea, epigastric discomfort, flatulence, gastritis, hepatitis, increased appetite, nausea, thirst, vomiting
GU: Hematuria, nocturia, polyuria, pyelonephritis, renal calculi
HEME: Anemia
MS: Arthralgia, arthrosis, back or muscloskeletal pain, joint stiffness, polymyalgia rheumatica
RESP: Bronchitis, bronchospasm, cough, dyspnea, pneumonia, upper respiratory tract infection
SKIN: Alopecia, diaphoresis, eczema, flushing of face or hands, pruritus of earlobes, rash, ulceration
Other: Anaphylaxis, anaphylactic shock, angioedema, antibody formation, feverish sensation, influenza-like symptoms, injection-site inflammation, lymphadenopathy and other malignancies, mild tetanic symptoms

Nursing Considerations

• If sensitivity to calcitonin, human; calcitonin, salmon; or their components is suspected, expect to perform a skin test before giving drug. Prepare a mixture of 10 international units/ml by withdrawing 0.05 ml from a 200–international unit solution in a tuberculin syringe and filling the syringe to 1 ml with sodium chloride for injection. Mix well, discard 0.9 ml, and inject 0.1 ml intradermally on the inner forearm. Observe the site for 15 minutes after injection. If you detect evidence of sensitivity, such as more than mild erythema or a wheal, notify prescriber.
• If patient receives calcitonin for hypercalcemia, monitor serum calcium level. During first several doses, keep parenteral calcium available in case the calcium level is inadvertently overcorrected.
• If prescribed calcitonin dose exceeds 2 ml, expect to use I.M. route and multiple injection sites.
• For patient receiving calcitonin for postmenopausal osteoporosis, know that hypocalcemia and other mineral metabolism disorders, such as vitamin D deficiency, must be corrected before calcitonin therapy begins. These patients should also be monitored during therapy for signs and symptoms of hypocalcemia such as muscle cramps, twitching, and seizures. Also, expect to give 1.5 g supplemental calcium carbonate and at least 400 units vitamin D daily. Plan to provide a balanced diet that includes foods high in calcium and vitamin D.
• Periodically examine patient using nasal spray for nasal ulcers. If severe ulceration of the nasal mucosa occurs (ulcers greater than 1.5 mm, ulcers penetrating below the mucosa, or ulcers causing heavy bleeding), notify prescriber and expect nasal spray form to be discontinued. Also, know that nasal spray should be discontinued for smaller or less severe ulcers until healing occurs.
• Assess for nausea, especially with the first dose. Nausea tends to decrease or disappear with continued use.
• If patient with Paget's disease relapses after treatment, check for antibody formation, as ordered.

PATIENT TEACHING

• Tell patient to refrigerate injection or unopened nasal spray container.
• Teach patient to self-administer injections.
• If patient has postmenopausal osteoporosis, teach her about dietary needs, including foods rich in calcium and vitamin D.
• For nasal spray, explain how to activate nasal pump by holding the bottle upright and depressing two white side arms toward

the bottle six times. When bottle emits a faint spray, pump is activated. Tell patient to store activated nasal pump upright at room temperature and to discard it after 30 days.
• Instruct patient to place nozzle firmly into one nostril while holding head upright. Tell him to then depress the pump toward the bottle.
• Remind patient that he doesn't need to reactivate the pump before each dose.
• Instruct patient to report nasal symptoms, such as redness, lesions, sinusitis, and rhinitis, to prescriber.

calcitriol (1,25-dihydroxy-cholecalciferol)

Calcijex, Rocaltrol

Class and Category
Chemical class: Sterol derivative, vitamin D analogue
Therapeutic class: Antihypocalcemic, antihypoparathyroid
Pregnancy category: C

Indications and Dosages
➤ *To treat hypocalcemia in dialysis patients*
CAPSULES, ORAL SOLUTION
Adults. *Initial:* 0.25 mcg daily. Increased by 0.25 mcg daily every 4 to 8 wk, if needed to achieve normal serum calcium level. *Maintenance:* 0.5 to 3 mcg daily.
➤ *To treat hypocalcemia in predialysis patients*
CAPSULES, ORAL SOLUTION
Adults and children age 3 and overß. *Initial:* 0.25 mcg daily. Increased after 4 to 8 wk, if needed, to 0.5 mcg daily.
ORAL SOLUTION
Children up to age 3. 10 to 15 ng/kg daily.
➤ *To treat hypoparathyroidism*
TABLETS
Adults and children age 6 and over. *Initial:* 0.25 mcg daily in the morning. Increased every 2 to 4 wk, if needed, to achieve normal serum calcium level. *Usual:* 0.5 to 2 mcg daily.
Children ages 1 to 5. 0.25 to 0.75 mcg daily in the morning.

I.V. INJECTION
Adults. *Initial:* 1 to 2 mcg 3 times/wk given every other day. Each dose increased 0.5 to 1 mcg at 2- to 4-wk intervals, if needed.

Route	Onset	Peak	Duration
P.O.	2–6 hr	10 hr	3–5 days

Mechanism of Action
Binds to specific receptors on intestinal mucosa to increase calcium absorption from intestine. Drug also may regulate calcium ion transfer from bone to blood and stimulate calcium reabsorption in the distal renal tubules, making more calcium available in the body.

Contraindications
Hypercalcemia, vitamin D toxicity

Interactions
DRUGS
cholestyramine: Decreased calcitriol absorption
digitalis glycosides: Possibly arrhythmias
ketoconazole: Decreased calcitriol level
magnesium-containing antacids (I.V. form): Hypermagnesemia
mineral oil: Decreased blood calcitriol level (with prolonged use of mineral oil)
phenobarbital, phenytoin: Decreased synthesis and blood level of calcitriol
thiazide diuretics: Hypercalcemia

Adverse Reactions
SKIN: Erythema multiforme, lip swelling, pruritus, rash, urticaria
Other: Anaphylaxis

Nursing Considerations
• Make sure patient receives enough calcium.
• Store drug at room temperature, and protect from heat and direct light.
• In high-dose or long-term calcitriol therapy, be alert for vitamin D toxicity. Early evidence includes abdominal or bone pain, constipation, dry mouth, headache, metallic taste, myalgia, nausea, somnolence, vomiting, and weakness. Late evidence includes albuminuria, anorexia, arrhythmias, azotemia, conjunctivitis (calcific), decreased libido, elevated AST and ALT levels, elevated BUN level, vascular calcification, hypercholesterolemia, hypertension,

hyperthermia, irritability, mild acidosis, nephrocalcinosis, nocturia, pancreatitis, photophobia, polydipsia, polyuria, pruritus, rhinorrhea, and weight loss.

PATIENT TEACHING
• Warn patient not to take other forms of vitamin D while taking calcitriol.
• Instruct patient to take a missed dose as soon as possible.
• Advise patient to notify prescriber immediately about possible toxicity, such as headache, irritability, nausea, photophobia, vomiting, weakness, and weight loss.

---

calcium acetate
PhosLo

calcium carbonate
Apo-Cal (CAN), Calci-Mix, Calsan (CAN), Liqui-Cal, Liquid Cal-600, Titralac

calcium chloride
Calciject (CAN)

calcium citrate
Citracal, Citracal Liquitabs

calcium glubionate
Calcionate, Calcium-Sandoz (CAN), Neo-Calglucon

calcium gluceptate
Calcium Stanley (-)

calcium gluconate

calcium lactate

Class and Category
Chemical class: Elemental cation
Therapeutic class: Antacid, antihypermagnesemic, antihyperphosphatemic, antihypocalcemic, calcium replacement, cardiotonic
Pregnancy category: C (Not rated for calciumcarbonate, citrate, and lactate)

Indications and Dosages
➤ *To treat hyperphosphatemia*

TABLETS (CALCIUM ACETATE)
Adults. *Initial:* 2 tablets (338 mg elemental calcium, 1,334 mg calcium acetate) t.i.d. with meals. Dosage increased to reduce serum phosphorus level below 6 mg/dl as long as hypercalcemia doesn't develop. *Maintenance:* 3 or 4 tablets three times daily with each meal.
➤ *To prevent hypocalcemia*
CAPSULES, ORAL SUSPENSION, TABLETS (CALCIUM CARBONATE); EFFERVESCENT TABLETS, TABLETS (CALCIUM CITRATE); SYRUP (CALCIUM GLUBIONATE); TABLETS (CALCIUM GLUCONATE OR LACTATE)
Adults and children over age 10. 800 to 1,200 mg daily.
Pregnant and breastfeeding women. 1,200 mg daily.
Children ages 4 to 10. 800 mg daily.
Children up to age 4. 400 to 800 mg daily.
➤ *To provide antacid effects*
CHEWABLE TABLETS, ORAL SUSPENSION, TABLETS (CALCIUM CARBONATE)
Adults and children age ` 12 and over. 350 to 1,500 mg 1 hr after meals and at bedtime, as needed.
➤ *To replace calcium in hypocalcemia*
I.V. INFUSION (CALCIUM CHLORIDE)
Adults. 0.5 to 1 g every 1 to 3 days, infused at less than 1 ml/min.
Children. 25 mg/kg given over several minutes.
I.V. OR I.M. INJECTION (CALCIUM GLUCEPTATE)
Adults and children. 0.44 to 1.1 g I.M. or 1.1 to 4.4 g I.V. at a rate of no more than 2 ml (36 mg)/min.
I.V. INJECTION (CALCIUM GLUCONATE)
Adults. 970 mg given slowly, repeated if needed, until tetany is controlled.
Children. 200 to 500 mg as a single dose given slowly, repeated if needed, until tetany is controlled.
➤ *As adjunct to treat magnesium intoxication*
I.V. INJECTION (CALCIUM CHLORIDE)
Adults. 500 mg promptly and repeated as needed, based on response.
➤ *As adjunct in cardiac resuscitation*
I.V. INJECTION (CALCIUM CHLORIDE)
Adults. 0.5 to 1 g.
Children. 0.2 ml/kg.
➤ *As adjunct in exchange transfusion*
I.V. INJECTION (CALCIUM GLUCEPTATE)
Adults. 1.35 mEq with each 100 ml of citrated blood exchanged.
Neonates. 0.45 mEq after each 100 ml of citrated blood exchanged.

I.V. INJECTION (CALCIUM GLUCEPTATE)
Neonates. 110 mg after each 100 ml of
citrated blood exchanged.

Mechanism of Action
Increases levels of intracellular and
extracellular calcium, which is needed to
maintain homeostasis, especially in the
nervous and musculoskeletal systems. Also
plays a role in normal cardiac and renal
function, respiration, coagulation, and cell
membrane and capillary permeability. Helps
regulate the release and storage of
neurotransmitters and hormones. Oral
forms also neutralize or buffer stomach acid
to relieve discomfort caused by
hyperacidity.

Contraindications
Hypercalcemia, hypersensitivity to calcium
salts or their components,
hypophosphatemia, renal calculi

Incompatibilities
To avoid precipitation, don't give I.V.
calcium chloride, gluceptate, or gluconate
through same I.V. line as bicarbonates,
carbonates, phosphates, sulfates, or
tartrates.

Interactions
DRUGS
aluminum-containing antacids: Enhanced
aluminum absorption with use of calcium
citrate
atenolol: Decreased blood atenolol level and
beta blockade
calcitonin: Possibly antagonized effects of
calcitonin in hypercalcemia treatment
*calcium supplements, magnesium-containing
preparations:* Increased serum calcium or
magnesium level, especially in patients with
impaired renal function
cellulose sodium phosphate: Decreased
effectiveness of cellulose sodium phosphate
in preventing hypercalciuria
digitalis glycosides: Increased risk of
arrhythmias
*estrogens, oral contraceptives (estrogen-
containing):* Increased calcium absorption
etidronate: Decreased etidronate absorption
fluoroquinolones: Reduced fluoroquinolone
absorption by calcium carbonate
gallium nitrate: Antagonized effects of
gallium nitrate

iron salts: Decreased gastric iron absorption
magnesium sulfate (parenteral): Neutralized
effects of magnesium by parenteral calcium
*neuromuscular blockers (except
succinylcholine):* Possibly reversal of
neuromuscular blockade by parenteral
calcium salts; enhanced or prolonged
neuromuscular blockade induced by
tubocurarine
norfloxacin: Decreased norfloxacin
bioavailability
phenytoin: Decreased bioavailability of
phenytoin and calcium
*potassium phosphates, potassium and
sodium phosphates:* Increased risk of
calcium deposition in soft tissue
sodium bicarbonate: Possibly milk-alkali
syndrome
sodium fluoride: Reduced fluoride and
calcium absorption
sodium polystyrene sulfonate: Possibly
metabolic alkalosis if patient has renal
impairment
tetracyclines: Decreased tetracycline
absorption and blood level, leading to
decreased anti-infective response
thiazide diuretics: Possibly hypercalcemia
verapamil: Reversed verapamil effects
vitamin A (more than 25,000 units daily):
Possibly stimulation of bone loss, decreased
effects of calcium supplementation, and
hypercalcemia
vitamin D (high doses): Excessively
increased calcium absorption
FOODS
caffeine, high-fiber food: Possibly decreased
calcium absorption
ACTIVITIES
alcohol use (excessive), smoking: Possibly
decreased calcium absorption

Adverse Reactions
CNS: Paresthesia (parenteral form)
CV: Hypotension, irregular heartbeat
(parenteral form)
GI: Nausea or vomiting (parenteral form)
SKIN: Diaphoresis, flushing, or sensation of
warmth (parenteral form)
Other: Hypercalcemia; injection site
burning, pain, rash, or redness (parenteral
form)

Nursing Considerations
• Store at room temperature, and protect from
heat, moisture, and direct light. Don't freeze.

• Warm solution to room temperature before parenteral administration.
• Keep patient in a recumbent position for 30 minutes after parenteral administration to prevent dizziness from hypotension.
• Administer I.V. calcium through an infusing I.V. solution using a small-bore needle inserted into a large vein to minimize irritation. Give calcium slowly to prevent excess calcium from reaching the heart and causing adverse cardiovascular reactions. Adverse reactions often result from too-rapid administration. If ECG tracings are abnormal or patient reports injection site discomfort, expect to temporarily discontinue administration.
• Check regularly for infiltration because calcium causes necrosis. If infiltration occurs, stop infusion and tell prescriber immediately.
• Divide I.M. calcium gluceptate dose of 5 ml or more in half and inject in gluteal region.
• Regularly monitor serum calcium level and evaluate therapeutic response by assessing for Chvostek's and Trousseau's signs, which shouldn't appear.
• Be aware that calcium chloride injection contains three times as much calcium per milliliter as calcium gluconate injection.

PATIENT TEACHING
• For chewable tablets, urge patient to chew thoroughly before swallowing and to drink a glass of water afterward.
• If suspension is prescribed, tell patient to shake bottle well before each use.
• If calcium citrate effervescent tablets are prescribed, tell patient to dissolve them in water and drink immediately.
• Instruct patient to take calcium carbonate tablets 1 to 2 hours after meals, calcium glubionate syrup before meals (diluted in water or fruit juice, if desired, for an infant or a child), and other forms with meals.
• Advise storing calcium at room temperature away from heat, moisture, and light. Warn against freezing suspension or syrup.
• Instruct patient to avoid taking calcium within 2 hours of another oral drug because of risk of interactions.
• Urge patient to ask prescriber before taking OTC drugs because of risk of interactions.

• Tell patient to avoid excessive use of tobacco and excessive consumption of alcoholic beverages, caffeine-containing products, and high-fiber foods because these substances may decrease calcium absorption.

canagliflozin
Invokana

Class and Category
Chemical class: Hemihydrate
Therapeutic class: Antidiabetic
Pregnancy category: C

Indications and Dosages
➤ *To control blood glucose level in type 2 diabetes mellitus*
TABLETS
Adults. 100 mg once daily before first meal of the day. *Maximum:* 300 mg once daily before first meal of the day.
DOSAGE ADJUSTMENT For patients with moderate renal impairment (glomerular filtration rate less than 60 ml/min/1.73m2 but at least 45 ml/min/1.73m2), dosage limited to 100 mg once daily. For patients receiving an UDP-Glucuronosyl Transferase (UGT) enzyme inducer such as phenobarbital, phenytoin, rifampin, or ritonavir, dosage increased to 300 mg once daily before first meal of the day if renal function is normal or only mildly impaired (glomerular filtration rate greater than 60 ml/min/1.73m2).

Mechanism of Action
Inhibits sodium-glucose co-transporter 2 (SGLT2) responsible for the majority of the reabsorption of filtered glucose from the tubular lumen in the kidneys. By inhibiting SGLT2, reabsorption of filtered, glucose is reduced along with a lowering of the renal threshold for glucose, which increases urinary glucose excretion.

Contraindications
Diabetic ketoacidosis, end stage renal disease, hypersensitivity to canagliflozin or its components, severe renal impairment (glomerular filtration rate less than

30 ml/min/1.73m2), type I diabetes mellitus, use of dialysis

Interactions

DRUGS

digoxin: Possibly increased serum digoxin levels and digitalis toxicity

insulin, insulin secretagogues: Possibly increased risk of hypoglycemia

phenobarbital, phenytoin, rifampin, ritonavir: Decreased effectiveness of canaglifoxin

Adverse Reactions

CNS: Asthenia, fatigue, postural dizziness, syncope

CV: Elevation of low-density lipoprotein cholesterol (LDL-C) and non-high-density liporotein cholesterol (non-HDL-C), hypotension

ENDO: Hypoglycemia

GI: Abdominal pain, constipation, nausea, pancreatitis

GU: Acute renal failure, decreased glomerular filtration rate, elevated serum creatinine levels, genital mycotic infections, renal impairment, UTIs, vulvovaginal pruritus

HEME: Elevated hemoglobin

MS: Upper extremity fractures

SKIN: Erythema, photosensitivity, pruritus, rash, uriticaria

Other: Angioedema, dehydration, elevated phosphate levels, hyperkalemia, hypermagnesemia, thirst

Nursing Considerations

• Know that patients with volume depletion should have the condition corrected before canagliflozin therapy is begun because drug causes intravascular volume contraction. Patients especially at risk for symptomatic hypotension caused by volume depletion include patients with impaired renal function, the elderly, patients taking either diuretics or drugs that interfere with the renin-angiotensin-aldosterone system, or patients with low systolic blood pressure.

• Be aware that canagliflozin dosage should only be increased in patients who have at least a glomerular filtration rate of 60 ml/min/1.73m2 and need greater glucose control.

• Assess renal function, as ordered prior to starting canagliflozin therapy and then periodically thereafter, because canaglifozin may cause renal impairment, especially in patients with hypovolemia. Expect drug to be discontinued if the patient's glomerular filtration rate becomes persistently less than 45 ml/min/1.73m2.

• Monitor serum potassium levels regularly, as ordered, during canaglifozin therapy in patients with impaired renal function and in patients predisposed to hyperkalemia due to medications or other medical conditions.

• Monitor patient's blood glucose levels to determine effectiveness of canaglifozin therapy. Be aware that canaglifozin can increase urinary glucose excretion, leading to positive urine glucose tests, and should not be used to monitor glucose levels in patients with diabetes mellitus. Assess patient also receiving insulin or insulin secretagogues for hypoglycemia.

• Be aware that patients with a history of genital mycotic infections, as well as uncircumcised males, are at greater risk for developing genital mycotic infections.

• Assess patient for hypersensitivity reactions such as generalized urticaria , especially within hours to days after canaglifozin therapy is begun. If hypersensitivity to canaglifozin occurs, expect drug to be discontinued and provide supportive care as ordered.

• Monitor patient's lipid levels and expect to treat if an elevation occurs.

PATIENT TEACHING

• Instruct patient to take canaglifozin before the first meal of the day.

• Urge patient not to skip doses or increase dosage without consulting prescriber.

• Emphasize importance of reporting signs of hypoglycemia, such as anxiety, confusion, dizziness, excessive sweating, headache, and nausea.

• Tell patient to carry identification indicating that he has diabetes.

• Teach patient how to monitor his blood glucose level. Advise patient with diabetes mellitus to not use urine glucose tests to monitor her glycemic control.

• Inform patient that canaglifozin is not a substitute for diet and exercise management.

• Advise patient to avoid direct sunlight and to wear sunscreen when outdoors.

candesartan cilexetil

Atacand

Class and Category

Chemical class: Angiotensin II receptor antagonist
Therapeutic class: Antihypertensive
Pregnancy category: D

Indications and Dosages

➤ *To manage, or as adjunct in managing, hypertension*

TABLETS
Adults.
Initial: 16 mg daily. *Maintenance:* 8 to 32 mg daily or 4 to 16 mg every 12 hr. *Maximum:* 32 mg daily.
DOSAGE ADJUSTMENT Initial dosage decreased to 2 mg for patients with moderate to severe hepatic impairment and to 4 mg for those with renal impairment, need for hemodialysis, or possibly a risk of hypotension.

➤ *To treat heart failure in patients with an ejection fraction of 40% or less and NYHA class II–IV to reduce the risk of death from cardiovascular causes and reduce hospitalizations for heart failure*

TABLETS
Adults. *Initial:* 4 mg daily for 2 wk; then doubled every 2 wk as tolerated until reaching target dose of 32 mg daily.

Route	Onset	Peak	Duration
P.O.	In 2 wk	4–5 wk	Unknown

Mechanism of Action

Selectively blocks binding of angiotensin (AT) II to AT_1 receptor sites in many tissues, including vascular smooth muscle and adrenal glands. This inhibits vasoconstrictive and aldosterone-secreting effects of AT II, which reduces blood pressure.

Contraindications

Concurrent aliskiren therapy in presence of diabetes or renal impairment (GRF less than 60 ml/min), hypersensitivity to candesartan or its components

Interactions

DRUGS
aliskiren: Increased risk of hypotension, hyperkalemia, and renal dysfunction in presence of diabetes or existing renal dysfunction
diuretics, other antihypertensives: Possibly increased risk of hypotension
heparin, potassium-sparing diuretics, potassium supplements, potassium-containing salt substitutes: Possibly increased risk of hyperkalemia
lithium: Increased blood lithium level
NSAIDs: Possible decreased renal function in patients who are elderly, volume-depleted, or have a compromised renal function

Adverse Reactions

CNS: Dizziness, headache
CV: Hypotension
EENT: Pharyngitis, rhinitis
GI: Elevated liver enzymes, hepatitis, impaired liver function
GU: Elevated BUN and serum creatinine levels
HEME: Agranulocytosis, leukopenia, neutropenia
MS: Back pain, rhabdomyolysis
RESP: Cough, upper respiratory tract infection
SKIN: Pruritus, rash, urticaria
Other: Angioedema, hyperkalemia, hyponatremia

Nursing Considerations

• If patient has known or suspected hypovolemia and/or salt depletion such as may occur with prolonged diuretic therapy, dietary salt restriction, dialysis, diarrhea or vomiting, expect to provide treatment, such as I.V. normal saline solution, as prescribed, to correct it before starting candesartan. Continue to monitor blood pressure throughout candesartan therapy, especially after a dosage increase.
• Monitor patient closely during major surgery and anesthesia because candesartan increases risk of hypotension by blocking renin-angiotensin system.
• Watch for elevated BUN and serum creatinine levels, especially if patient has heart failure or impaired renal function; drug may cause acute renal failure. Report significant or persistent increases immediately.
• If blood pressure isn't controlled with candesartan alone, expect to give a diuretic, such as hydrochlorothiazide, as prescribed.

WARNING If patient receives a diuretic or antihypertensive with candesartan, has heart failure, or is elderly, assess blood pressure often because of added risk of hypotension.

• If patient develops hypotension, expect to stop drug temporarily. Immediately place patient in supine position and prepare to give I.V. normal saline solution, as prescribed. Expect to resume therapy after blood pressure stabilizes.

• If patient receives a diuretic, provide hydration, as ordered, to help prevent hypovolemia. Watch for evidence, such as hypotension with dizziness and fainting. If patient has heart failure and develops hypotension, dosage of diuretic, candesartan, or both may be reduced when blood pressure stabilizes and therapy resumes.

• Check CBC for decreases in hemoglobin and hematocrit. If they're significant or persistent, notify prescriber immediately.

PATIENT TEACHING

• Advise patient that full effects of candesartan may not occur for 4 to 5 weeks.

• Explain importance of lifestyle choices in controlling hypertension.

• Advise female patient of childbearing age to immediately report known or suspected pregnancy. Explain that if she becomes pregnant, candesartan will need to be discontinued as soon as possible and treatment started with another antihypertensive that's safe to use during pregnancy.

capreomycin sulfate

Capastat

Class and Category

Chemical class: Polypeptide antibiotic isolated from *Streptomyces capreolus*
Therapeutic class: Antitubercular
Pregnancy category: C

Indications and Dosages

➤ *As adjunct to treat pulmonary tuberculosis caused by* Mycobacterium tuberculosis *in which primary drugs are ineffective or can't be used because of toxicity*

I.V. INFUSION, I.M. INJECTION
Adults. 1 g daily for 60 to 120 days followed by 1 g 2 or 3 times/wk for 12 to 24 mo. *Maximum:* 20 mg/kg daily.
DOSAGE ADJUSTMENT For patient with renal impairment, dosage reduced according to patient's creatinine clearance.

Mechanism of Action

May interfere with lipid and nucleic acid biosynthesis in actively growing tubercle bacilli.

Contraindications

Hypersensitivity to capreomycin or its components

Interactions

DRUGS

aminoglycosides (parenteral): Increased risk of ototoxicity, nephrotoxicity, and neuromuscular blockade
nephrotoxic drugs, such as amphotericin B: Increased risk of nephrotoxicity
nondepolarizing neuromuscular blockers: Enhanced neuromuscular blockade
ototoxic drugs, such as quinidine: Increased risk of ototoxicity
polymyxins (parenteral): Increased risk of nephrotoxicity and neuromuscular blockade

Adverse Reactions

CNS: Dizziness, vertigo
EENT: Ototoxicity
GI: Elevated liver function test results
GU: Nephrotoxicity
HEME: Leukocytosis, leukopenia
SKIN: Maculopapular rash, sterile abscess, urticaria
Other: Hypocalcemia, hypokalemia, hypomagnesemia, injection-site pain, induration, and bleeding

Nursing Considerations

• Use capreomycin cautiously in patients with renal insufficiency, impaired hearing, or a history of hypersensitivity, especially to other drugs.

• Expect to obtain baseline renal function studies, as ordered, before starting capreomycin and weekly throughout therapy because drug may alter renal function.

• To reconstitute drug for I.V. injection, add 100 ml normal saline solution. Administer over 60 minutes.

- To reconstitute drug for I.M. injection, add 2 ml sodium chloride for injection or sterile water for injection to each 1-g vial. Allow 2 to 3 minutes for complete dissolution.
- Give I.M. injection deep into a large muscle mass, such as the gluteus maximus.
- Observe injection site for excessive bleeding or sterile abscess.
- Make sure patient receives regular audiometric and vestibular function assessment.
- Closely monitor patient for urticaria and maculopapular rash.
- Check serum electrolyte levels periodically, as ordered, because capreomycin may cause imbalances such as hypocalcemia, hypokalemia, and hypomagnesemia.

PATIENT TEACHING
- Advise patient to alert nurse or prescriber if injection site bleeds excessively.
- Warn patient to contact prescriber immediately about hearing loss or tinnitus.
- Explain the need for frequent laboratory tests to monitor renal function.
- Tell patient that tuberculosis therapy lasts for 12 to 24 months.
- Explain that noncompliance may decrease effectiveness and lengthen treatment.

captopril
Capoten

Class and Category
Chemical class: ACE inhibitor
Therapeutic class: Antihypertensive
Pregnancy category: D

Indications and Dosages
➤ *To control hypertension*
TABLETS
Adults and adolescents. *Initial:* 25 mg twice daily or three times daily. Increased to 50 mg twice daily or three times daily after 1 to 2 wk, if needed. If blood pressure isn't well-controlled at this dosage and with the addition of a diuretic, dosage increased to 100 mg twice daily or three times daily and then, if needed, to 150 mg twice daily or three times daily while continuing diuretic. *Maximum:* 450 mg daily.

➤ *To control accelerated or malignant hypertension when temporary discontinuation of current antihypertensive therapy isn't practical or when prompt titration of blood pressure is needed*
TABLETS
Adults and adolescents. *Initial:* 25 mg twice daily or three times daily while continuing diuretic but discontinuing current antihypertensive drug. Increased every 24 hr as needed until satisfactory response is obtained or maximum dosage is reached. *Maximum:* 450 mg daily.
➤ *To treat heart failure that's unresponsive to conventional therapy*
TABLETS
Adults and adolescents. *Initial:* 25 mg twice daily or three times daily. Increased to 50 mg twice daily or three times daily, as needed. After 14 days, increased to 100 mg three times daily and then to 150 mg three times daily, if needed. *Maximum:* 450 mg daily.
➤ *To treat left-sided heart failure after MI*
TABLETS
Adults and adolescents. *Initial:* 6.25 mg as single dose starting 3 days after MI and then 12.5 mg three times daily. Increased to 25 mg three times daily for several days and then again to maintenance dosage. *Maintenance:* 50 mg three times daily.
➤ *To treat diabetic nephropathy*
TABLETS
Adults and adolescents. 25 mg three times daily.
DOSAGE ADJUSTMENT Starting dosage reduced to 6.25 mg twice daily or three times daily if patient with hypertension also has heart failure, is undergoing dialysis, or is being vigorously treated with diuretics that result in hyponatremia or hypovolemia.

Route	Onset	Peak	Duration
P.O.	15–60 min	60–90 min	6–12 hr

Mechanism of Action
By inhibiting angiotensin-converting enzyme, captopril:
- prevents conversion of angiotensin I to angiotensin II, a potent vasoconstrictor that also stimulates the adrenal cortex to secrete aldosterone. Inhibiting aldosterone increases sodium and water excretion, reducing blood pressure.

- may inhibit renal and vascular production of angiotensin II.
- decreases serum angiotensin II level and increases renin activity. This decreases aldosterone secretion, slightly increasing serum potassium level and fluid loss.
- decreases vascular tone and blood pressure.

Contraindications

Concurrent aliskiren use in patients with diabetes or patients with renal impairment (GFR less than 60 ml/min), hypersensitivity to captopril, other ACE inhibitors, or their components

Interactions

DRUGS

aliskiren, other ACE inhibitors, angiotension receptor blockers: Increased risk of hypotension, hyperkalemia, and renal impairment
allopurinol: Increased risk of hypersensitivity reactions, including Stevens-Johnson syndrome, skin eruptions, fever, arthralgia
antacids: Possibly impaired captopril absorption
capsaicin: Possibly cause or worsening of cough from ACE inhibitor
cyclosporine, potassium-containing drugs, potassium-sparing diuretics, potassium supplements: Increased risk of hyperkalemia
digoxin: Increased blood digoxin level
diuretics; hypotension-producing drugs, such as hydralazine: Additive hypotensive effects
gold: Increased risk of nitritoid reaction, including facial flushing, nausea, vomiting, and hypotension
lithium: Increased risk of lithium toxicity
NSAIDs: Decreased antihypertensive response to ACE inhibition; possible decreased renal function in elderly patients or those who are volume-depleted or already have existing impaired renal function
probenecid: Increased blood level and decreased total clearance of captopril

ACTIVITIES

alcohol use: Additive hypotensive effects

Adverse Reactions

CNS: Fever
CV: Chest pain, hypotension, orthostatic hypotension, palpitations, tachycardia

EENT: Loss of taste
GU: Dysuria, impotence, nephrotic syndrome, nocturia, oliguria, polyuria, proteinuria, urinary frequency
HEME: Eosinophilia
MS: Arthralgia
RESP: Cough
SKIN: Photosensitivity, pruritus, rash
Other: Angioedema, hyperkalemia, hyponatremia, positive ANA titer

Nursing Considerations

- Closely monitor patient's blood pressure, especially when therapy starts and dosage increases. Keep patient supine if hypotension occurs.
- Monitor patient's blood pressure and electrolytes routinely if patient is receiving other drugs that also affect the renin-angiotensin system because hypotension and hyperkalemia may occur.
- Monitor renal function tests for signs of nephrotic syndrome, such as proteinuria and increased BUN and serum creatinine levels. Also watch for such renal evidence as oliguria, polyuria, and urinary frequency or other signs of impaired renal function, especially in patients who are receiving other drugs that also affect the renin-angiotensin system.
- Monitor WBC regularly, as ordered, especially if patient has collagen vascular disease or renal disease.

PATIENT TEACHING

- Instruct patient to take captopril 1 hour before meals.
- Tell patient to rise slowly from sitting or lying to minimize orthostatic hypotension.
- Tell patient to avoid sunlight or wear sunscreen in direct sunlight because photosensitivity may occur.
- Warn patient not to stop taking drug abruptly.
- Urge patient not to use salt substitutes that contain potassium and to consult prescriber before increasing potassium intake to avoid increasing risk of hyperkalemia.
- Urge patient to tell prescriber about signs and symptoms of infection, such as sore throat or fever.
- Advise female patient of childbearing age to notify prescriber immediately if pregnancy occurs.

carbamazepine

Apo-Carbamazepine (CAN),
Atretol, Carbatrol, Epitol, Equetro,
Novo-Carbamaz (CAN), Tegretol,
Tegretol-XR

Class and Category
Chemical class: Tricyclic iminostilbene
derivative
Therapeutic class: Analgesic, anticonvulsant
Pregnancy category: C

Indications and Dosages
➤ *To treat epilepsy*

E.R. CAPSULES (CARBATROL), E.R. TABLETS (TEGRETOL-XR)

Adults and children age 12 and over.
Initial: 200 mg twice daily. Increased weekly
by 200 mg daily, if needed. *Maximum:*
1,600 mg daily in adults, 1,200 mg daily in
children age 16 and over, and 1,000 mg
daily in children ages 12 to 16.
Children ages 6 to 12. *Initial:* 100 mg twice
daily. Increased weekly by 100 mg daily, if
needed. *Maximum:* 1,000 mg daily.

ORAL SUSPENSION

Adults and children age 12 and over.
Initial: 100 mg four times daily. Increased
weekly by 200 mg daily, if needed, given in
divided doses three times daily or four
times daily. *Maximum:* 1,600 mg daily in
adults, 1,200 mg daily in children age 16
and over, and 1,000 mg daily in children
ages 12 to 16.

Children ages 6 to 12. *Initial:* 50 mg four
times daily. Increased weekly by 100 mg
daily, if needed, given in divided doses
three times daily or four times daily.
Maximum: 1,000 mg daily.
Children up to age 6. *Initial:* 10 to 20 mg/
kg/day in divided doses four times daily.
Maximum: 35 mg/kg daily.

TABLETS

Adults and children age 12 and over.
Initial: 200 mg twice daily. Increased weekly
by 200 mg/day, if needed, given in divided
doses three times daily or four times daily
Maximum: 1,600 mg daily in adults,
1,200 mg daily in children age 16 and over,
and 1,000 mg daily in children ages 12 to 16.
Children ages 6 to 12. *Initial:* 100 mg twice
daily. Increased weekly by 100 mg daily, if
needed, given in divided doses three times
daily or four times daily. *Maximum:*
1,000 mg daily.
Children up to age 6. *Initial:* 10 to
20 mg/kg daily in divided doses twice daily
or three times daily. Increased weekly, if
needed, divided and given three times daily
or four times daily. *Maximum:* 35 mg/kg/
day.

➤ *To relieve pain in trigeminal neuralgia*

E.R. CAPSULES (CARBATROL), E.R. TABLETS (TEGRETOL-XR), TABLETS

Adults. *Initial:* 100 mg twice daily.
Increased by up to 200 mg daily, if needed,
in increments of 100 mg every 12 hr.
Maintenance: 400 to 800 mg/day.
Maximum: 1,200 mg daily.

Mechanism of Action
Normally, sodium moves into a neuronal
cell by passing through a gated sodium
channel in the cell membrane.
Carbamazepine may prevent or halt
seizures by closing or blocking sodium
channels, as shown here, thus preventing
sodium from entering the cell. Keeping
sodium out of the cell may slow nerve
impulse transmission, thus slowing the
rate at which neurons fire.

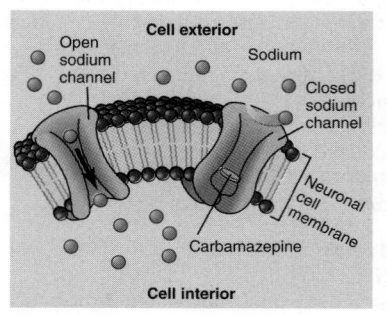

ORAL SUSPENSION (100 MG/5 ML)
Adults. 50 mg four times daily. Increased by up to 200 mg daily, if needed, in increments of 50 mg four times daily. *Maintenance:* 400 to 800 mg daily. *Maximum:* 1,200 mg daily.
➤ *To treat acute manic and mixed episodes in bipolar disorder*
E.R. CAPSULES (EQUETRO)
Adults. *Initial:* 200 mg twice daily, increased as needed in 200-mg increments. *Maximum:* 1,600 mg daily.

Contraindications
History of bone marrow depression; hypersensitivity to carbamazepine, tricyclic compounds, or their components; MAO inhibitor or nefazodone therapy

Route	Onset	Peak	Duration
P.O. (all forms)	In 1 mo*	Unknown	Unknown

Interactions
DRUGS
acetaminophen (long-term use): Increased metabolism, leading to acetaminophen-induced hepatotoxicity or decreased acetaminophen effectiveness
acetazolamide, aprepitant, cimetidine, ciprofloxacin, clarithromycin, danazol, dantrolene, diltiazem, erythromycin, fluconazole, fluoxetine, fluvoxamine, ibuprofen, isoniazid, itraconazole, ketoconazole, loratadine, loxapine, macrolides, niacinamide, nicotinamide, olanzapine, omeprazozle, oxybutynin, propoxyphene, protease inhibitors, quetiapine, terfenadine, ticlopidine, trazodone, troleandomycin, valproate, valproic acid, verapamil, voriconazozle: Increased blood carbamazepine level
albendazole, alprazolam, amitriptyline, aprepitant, buprenorphone, bupropion, buspirone, citalopram, clobazam, clonazepam, clozapine, corticosteroids, cyclosporine, delavirdine, desipramine, diazepam, dicumarol, doxycycline, ethosuximide, everolimus, felodipine, glucocorticoids, haloperidol, imatinib, imipramine, itraconazole, lamotrigine, levothyroxine, lorazepam, methadone, methsuximide,

------

* For anticonvulsant use; 8 to 72 hr for use in trigeminal neuralgia.

mianserin, midazolam, mirtazapine, nortriptyline, olanzapine, oral contraceptives, oxcarbazepine, paliperidone, phensuximide, phenytoin, praziquantel, protease inhibitors, quetiapine, risperidone, sertraline, sirolimus, tadalafil, theophylline, tiagabine, topiramate, tramadol, triazolam, trazodone, valproate, warfarin, ziprasidone, zonisamide: Decreased blood levels of these drugs
aminophylline, cisplatin, doxorubicin, felbamate, methsuximide, phenobarbital, phenytoin, primidone, rifampin, theophylline: Decreased blood carbamazepine level
clomipramine, phenytoin, primidone: Increased blood levels of these drugs
cyclophosphamide: Possibly increased cyclophosphamide toxicity
felbamate: Decreased blood level of felbamate or carbamazepine
furosemide, hydrochlorothiazide: Possibly increased risk of symptomatic hyponatremia
isoniazid: Increased risk of carbamazepine toxicity and isoniazid hepatotoxicity
lamotrigine, phenobarbital, primidone, tricyclic antidepressants, valproic acid: Decreased blood levels of these drugs, increased blood level of carbamazepine
lapatinib, temsirolimus: Altered effectiveness of these drugs
lithium: Increased risk of CNS toxicity
nefazodone: Decreased nefazodone effectiveness and increased carbamazepine level
nondepolarizing neuromuscular blockers: Possibly reduced duration or decreased effectiveness of neuromuscular blocker
oral anticoagulants: Increased metabolism and decreased effectiveness of anticoagulant
FOODS
grapefruit juice: Increased blood carbamazepine level
ACTIVITIES
alcohol use: Increased sedative effect

Adverse Reactions
CNS: Chills, confusion, dizziness, drowsiness, fatigue, fever, headache, suicidal ideation, syncope, talkativeness, unsteadiness, visual hallucinations
CV: Arrhythmias, including AV block; edema; heart failure; hypertension; hypotension; thromboembolism; thrombophlebitis; worsened coronary artery disease

EENT: Blurred vision, conjunctivitis, dry mouth, glossitis, nystagmus, oculomotor disturbances, stomatitis, tinnitus, transient diplopia
ENDO: Syndrome of inappropriate ADH secretion, water intoxication
GI: Abdominal pain, anorexia, constipation, diarrhea, dyspepsia, elevated liver enzymes, hepatitis, nausea, pancreatitis, vanishing bile duct syndrome, vomiting
GU: Acute urine retention, albuminuria, azotemia, glycosuria, impotence, oliguria, renal failure, urinary frequency
HEME: Acute intermittent porphyria, agranulocytosis, aplastic anemia, bone marrow depression, eosinophilia, leukocytosis, leukopenia, pancytopenia, thrombocytopenia
MS: Arthralgia, leg cramps, myalgia, osteoporosis
RESP: Pulmonary hypersensitivity (dyspnea, fever, pneumonia, or pneumonitis)
SKIN: Aggravation of disseminated lupus erythematosus, alopecia, altered skin pigmentation, diaphoresis, erythema multiforme, erythema nodosum, exfoliative dermatitis, jaundice, Lyell's syndrome, nail shedding (onychomadesis), photosensitivity reactions, pruritic and erythematous rash, purpura, Stevens-Johnson syndrome, toxic epidermal necrolysis, urticaria
Other: Adenopathy, drug reaction with eosinophilia and systemic symptoms (DRESS) multiorgan hypersensitivity, hypocalcemia, hyponatremia, lymphadenopathy

Nursing Considerations

• Avoid using carbamazepine in patients with a history of hepatic porphyria because it may prompt an acute attack.
WARNING If patient has Asian ancestry, make sure he has been evaluated for the genetic allelic variant HLA-B 1502 before starting carbamazepine therapy. If patient has African-American, Chinese, European, Indian including Native American, Japanese, Korean, Latin American, Taiwanese or Thai ancestry, make sure he has been evaluated for the genetic allelic variant HLA-A 3101 before starting carbamazepine therapy. Patients positive for HLA-A 3101 or HLA-B 1502 shouldn't take carbamazepine because of the risk of serious, sometimes fatal, dermatologic reactions. The risk is between 5 to 15% in patients with these variants.

• Use carbamazepine cautiously in patients with impaired hepatic function because it's mainly metabolized in the liver. Monitor liver function tests, as directed.
• Monitor patient closely for adverse reactions because many of them are serious and some can become life-threatening, such as DRESS multiorgan hypersensitivity.
• Periodically monitor blood carbamazepine level to assess for therapeutic and toxic levels; a blood level of 6 to 12 mcg/ml is optimal for anticonvulsant effects.
• Monitor patient's electrolytes, especially sodium level, as ordered. Hyponatremia may occur as an adverse reaction to carbamazepine therapy, especially in the elderly and patients treated with diuretics. Assess patient regularly for signs and symptoms of hyponatremia such as confusion, difficulty concentrating, headache, memory impairment, unsteadiness, and weakness. If present, notify prescriber and expect drug to be discontinued.
WARNING Monitor WBC and platelet counts monthly for first 2 months. Decreased counts may indicate bone marrow depression.
• Monitor patient closely for evidence of suicidal thinking or behavior, especially when therapy starts or dosage changes.
• Withdraw carbamazepine gradually to minimize risk of seizures.

PATIENT TEACHING
• Tell patient to take carbamazepine with food (except the oral suspension form, which shouldn't be taken with other liquid drugs or diluents).
• Warn patient about possible dizziness, blurred vision, and unsteadiness.
• Inform patient that coating of E.R. tablets isn't absorbed and may appear in stool.
• Advise patient not to crush or chew E.R. capsules or tablets. If he can't swallow capsules whole, have him open them and sprinkle contents on food.
• Urge patient to wear sunscreen and protective clothing to reduce photosensitivity.
• Tell patient to report unusual bleeding or bruising, fever, rash, or mouth ulcers.
• Tell female patient of childbearing age that drug decreases oral contraceptive effectiveness, and urge her to use different contraception. Because drug may cause fetal harm, tell her to notify prescriber about possible pregnancy.

• If she becomes pregnant during therapy, urge her to enroll in the antiepileptic drug pregnancy registry by calling 1-888-233-2334. Explain that the registry is collecting information about the safety of anti-epileptic drugs during pregnancy.
• Instruct caregivers to watch patient closely for evidence of suicidal tendencies, especially when therapy starts or dosage changes, and to report such tendencies to prescriber immediately.
• Advise patient to inform all prescribers of carbamazepine therapy.

carisoprodol
Soma, Vanadom

Class and Category
Chemical class: Dicarbamate
Therapeutic class: Skeletal muscle relaxant
Pregnancy category: C
Controlled substance schedule: IV

Indications and Dosages
➤ *As adjunct to relieve acute musculoskeletal pain and stiffness*
TABLETS (SOMA)
Adults and children over age 16. 250 to 350 mg three times daily and at bedtime.
TABLETS (VANADOM)
Children ages 5 to 12. 6.25 mg/kg three times daily and at bedtime.

Route	Onset	Peak	Duration
P.O.	30 min	Unknown	4–6 hr

Mechanism of Action
Blocks interneuronal activity in descending reticular formation and spinal cord, producing muscle relaxation and sedation.

Contraindications
Hypersensitivity or idiosyncratic reactions to carisoprodol, to its components, or to meprobamate-related compounds; intermittent porphyria

Interactions
DRUGS
CNS depressants, psychotropic drugs: Additive CNS depression
fluvoxamine, omeprazole: Increased blood carisoprodol level

rifampin, St. John's wort: Decreased blood carisoprodol level
ACTIVITIES
alcohol use: Additive CNS depression

Adverse Reactions
CNS: Agitation, ataxia, depression, dizziness, drowsiness, fever, headache, insomnia, irritability, seizures, somnolence, syncope, tremor, vertigo
CV: Orthostatic hypotension, tachycardia
EENT: Diplopia, transient vision loss
GI: Epigastric discomfort, hiccups, nausea, vomiting
HEME: Eosinophilia
SKIN: Erythema multiforme, facial flushing, pruritus, rash
Other: Drug dependence or withdrawal

Nursing Considerations
• Use carisoprodol cautiously in patients with history of drug addiction and in patients taking other CNS depressants, including alcohol.
• Carisoprodol therapy should last no longer than 3 weeks.
• Monitor patient closely for hypersensitivity or idiosyncratic reactions. They typically occur before the fourth dose in patients who have no previous carisoprodol exposure.
• Provide rest and other pain-relief measures.
• To avoid mild withdrawal symptoms, expect to taper therapy as prescribed, rather than stopping it abruptly.
PATIENT TEACHING
• Tell patient to take carisoprodol with meals if GI distress occurs.
• Caution patient that drug dependence and withdrawal may occur, especially if therapy lasts a long time or patient changes dosage without consulting prescriber.
• Warn patient about possible dizziness, drowsiness, syncope, and vertigo. Discourage hazardous activities, such as driving, until effects of drug are known.
• Inform patient that abruptly stopping drug can cause headache, insomnia, nausea, and other adverse reactions.
• Instruct patient to avoid alcohol and other CNS depressants while taking drug.
• Explain that saliva, urine, and sweat may appear darker (red, brown, or black). Reassure him that this discoloration is harmless but may stain garments.

• Tell patient to store drug in a tightly capped container at room temperature.
• Tell patient not to store drug in bathroom, near kitchen sink, or in other damp places to protect it from heat and moisture.

---

carteolol hydrochloride

Cartrol

Class and Category

Chemical class: Beta-adrenergic blocker
Therapeutic class: Antihypertensive
Pregnancy category: C

Indications and Dosages

➤ *To control hypertension*
TABLETS
Adults. *Initial:* 2.5 mg daily. If response is inadequate, dosage increased to 5 mg and then 10 mg daily, as needed. *Maintenance:* 2.5 or 5 mg daily.
DOSAGE ADJUSTMENT Interval increased to every 48 hr for patients with creatinine clearance of 20 to 60 ml/min/1.73 m^2 or to every 72 hr for clearance of less than 20 ml/min/1.73 m^2.

Route	Onset	Peak	Duration
P.O.	Unknown	1–3 hr	Unknown

Mechanism of Action

May reduce blood pressure by competing with beta-adrenergic receptor agonists, which helps reduce cardiac output, decrease sympathetic outflow to peripheral blood vessels, and inhibit renin.

Contraindications

Asthma, bradycardia (less than 45 beats/min), cardiogenic shock, hypersensitivity to carteolol or its components, second- or third-degree heart block

Interactions

DRUGS
allergen immunotherapy, allergenic extracts for skin testing: Increased risk of serious systemic reaction or anaphylaxis
catecholamine-depleting drugs, such as reserpine: Additive effects, increased risk of hypotension and bradycardia

clonidine: Increased risk of tachycardia and hypertension after clonidine discontinuation
diltiazem, nifedipine, verapamil: Potentiated effects of carteolol
general anesthetics: Exaggeration of hypotension
NSAIDs: Reduced antihypertensive effect of carteolol
oral antidiabetic drugs: Reduced symptomatic responses to hypoglycemia
sympathomimetics with alpha- and beta-adrenergic effects, such as pseudoephedrine: Possibly hypertension and excessive bradycardia or heart block

Adverse Reactions

CNS: Fatigue, insomnia, lassitude, paresthesia, tiredness, weakness
CV: Chest pain, heart failure, peripheral edema
EENT: Dry mouth, nasal congestion, pharyngitis
GI: Abdominal pain, diarrhea, flatulence, nausea
MS: Arthralgia, back pain, leg pain, muscle spasms
SKIN: Rash

Nursing Considerations

WARNING Be aware that stopping carteolol abruptly in patients with angina may cause worsening of angina or MI; abrupt cessation in patients with hyperthyroidism may cause thyroid storm.
• Carefully monitor blood glucose level in diabetic patient because carteolol can mask hypoglycemic symptoms. It also can interfere with endogenous insulin release in response to hyperglycemia, requiring adjustment of oral antidiabetic dosage.
PATIENT TEACHING
• Advise patient to complete dosing schedule, even if he feels better, and not to discontinue therapy abruptly.
• Instruct patient to report signs of heart failure, such as fatigue, difficulty breathing, cough, and unusually fast heartbeat.
• Tell diabetic patient to check his blood glucose level often.
• Advise patient to consult prescriber before taking OTC preparations, such as nasal decongestants and cold preparations that contain sympathomimetics, because of the risk of serious drug interactions.

carvedilol

Coreg, Coreg CR

Class and Category

Chemical class: Nonselective beta-adrenergic blocker with alpha$_1$-adrenergic blocking activity
Therapeutic class: Antihypertensive, heart failure treatment adjunct
Pregnancy category: C

Indications and Dosages

➤ *To control hypertension*

TABLETS

Adults. 6.25 mg twice daily for 7 to 14 days, if tolerated. Then dosage increased to 12.5 mg twice daily for 7 to 14 days, and up to 25 mg, if tolerated and needed. *Maximum:* 50 mg daily.

E.R. CAPSULES

Adults. *Initial:* 20 mg once daily with food. After 7 to 14 days, increased to 40 mg once daily. After another 7 to 14 days, increased to 80 mg once daily. *Maximum:* 80 mg once daily.

➤ *As adjunct to treat mild to severe heart failure of ischemic or cardiomyopathic origin*

TABLETS

Adults. 3.125 mg twice daily for 2 wk; then increased to 6.25, 12.5, and 25 mg twice daily at successive 2-wk intervals, as tolerated. *Maximum (for patients with mild to moderate heart failure):* 50 mg twice daily if patient weighs more than 85 kg (187 lb).

E.R. CAPSULES

Adults. *Initial:* 10 mg once daily with food for 2 wk. Then increased to 20 mg once daily, as needed. Subsequent dosage increased by 20 mg every 2 wk, as needed. *Maximum:* 80 mg once daily.

➤ *To reduce CV mortality after acute phase of MI in patients with left ventricular ejection fraction of 40% or less*

TABLETS

Adults. 6.25 mg twice daily for 3 to 10 days, if tolerated. Then dosage increased to 12.5 mg twice daily for 3 to 10 days and up to 25 mg twice daily, if needed and tolerated.

E.R. CAPSULES

Adults. *Initial:* 10 to 20 mg once daily. After 3 to 10 days, increased to 20 to 40 mg once daily. Increased again as needed every 3 to 10 days until reaching tolerance or target dose of 80 mg once daily. *Maximum:* 80 mg once daily.

DOSAGE ADJUSTMENT For patient with fluid retention or low blood pressure or heart rate, starting dosage may be decreased to 3.125 mg twice daily, increase may be slowed, or both for tablet form. For patient with heart rate below 55 beats/min, extended-release dosage decreased as clinical condition indicates.

Route	Onset	Peak	Duration
P.O.	In 30 min	1.5–7 hr	Unknown

Mechanism of Action

Reduces cardiac output and tachycardia, causes vasodilation, and decreases peripheral vascular resistance, which reduces blood pressure and cardiac workload. When given for at least 4 weeks, carvedilol reduces plasma renin activity.

Contraindications

Asthma or related bronchospastic conditions; cardiogenic shock; decompensated heart failure that requires I.V. inotropics; history of serious hypersensitivity reactions, such as anaphylaxis, angioedema, or Stevens-Johnson syndrome; hypersensitivity to carvedilol or its components; second- or third-degree AV block, severe bradycardia or hepatic impairment, or sick sinus syndrome unless pacemaker is in place

Interactions

DRUGS

amiodarone; other CYP2C9 drugs, such as fluconazole: Increased risk of bradycardia or heart block
beta blockers, digoxin: Increased risk of bradycardia
calcium channel blockers (especially diltiazem and verapamil): Abnormal cardiac conduction and, possibly, increased adverse effects of calcium channel blockers
catecholamine-depleting drugs (such as reserpine, MAO inhibitors): Additive effects, increased risk of hypotension and bradycardia

cimetidine: Increased blood carvedilol level
clonidine: Risk of tachycardia and hypertension when clonidine is discontinued
cyclosporine, digoxin: Increased blood levels of these drugs
digoxin: Possibly increased digoxin level
oral antidiabetics: Increased risk of hypoglycemia
rifampin: Decreased blood carvedilol level

Adverse Reactions
CNS: Asthenia, depression, dizziness, fatigue, fever, headache, hypesthesia, hypotonia, insomnia, light-headedness, malaise, paresthesia, somnolence, stroke, syncope, vertigo
CV: Angina, AV block, bradycardia, edema, heart failure, hypertension, hypertriglyceridemia, orthostatic hypotension, palpitations, peripheral vascular disorder
EENT: Blurred vision, dry eyes, periodontitis, pharyngitis, rhinitis
ENDO: Hyperglycemia, hypoglycemia
GI: Abdominal pain, diarrhea, elevated liver function test results, melena, nausea, vomiting
GU: Albuminuria, hematuria, elevated BUN and creatinine levels, impotence, incontinence, renal insufficiency, UTI
HEME: Aplastic anemia, decreased PT, thrombocytopenia, unusual bleeding or bruising
MS: Arthralgia, arthritis, back pain, muscle cramps
RESP: Dyspnea, increased cough, interstitial pneumonitis
SKIN: Erythema multiforme, jaundice, pruritus, purpura, Stevens-Johnson syndrome, toxic epidermal necrolysis, urticaria
Other: Anaphylaxis, angioedema, fluid overload, gout, hyperkalemia, hyperuricemia, hyponatremia, hypovolemia, viral infection, weight gain or loss

Nursing Considerations
• Use carvedilol cautiously in patients with peripheral vascular disease because it may aggravate symptoms of arterial insufficiency. In patients with diabetes mellitus it may mask signs of hypoglycemia, such as tachycardia, and may delay recovery.
• Monitor patient's blood glucose level, as ordered, during carvedilol therapy because drug may alter blood glucose level.

WARNING Avoid stopping drug abruptly in patients with hyperthyroidism because thyroid storm may occur, and in patients with angina because it may worsen or MI may occur.
• If patient has heart failure, expect to also give digoxin, a diuretic, and an ACE inhibitor.
• Be aware that chronic beta blocker therapy such as carvedilol is not routinely withheld prior to major surgery because the benefits outweigh the risks associated with its use with general anesthesia and surgical procedures.
PATIENT TEACHING
• Instruct patient prescribed extended-release capsules to swallow them whole. If swallowing capsules is difficult, tell patient he may open capsule and sprinkle beads on a spoonful of cold applesauce and then eat the applesauce immediately without chewing.
• Warn patient that drug may cause orthostatic hypotension, light-headedness, and dizziness; advise him to take precautions.
• Tell patient with heart failure to notify prescriber if he gains 5 lb or more in 2 days or if shortness of breath increases, which may signal worsening heart failure.
• Alert patient with diabetes to monitor his glycemic control closely because drug may increase blood glucose level or mask symptoms of hypoglycemia.
• Emphasize the need to seek emergency care if patient develops hives or swelling of the face, lips, tongue, or throat that causes trouble swallowing or breathing.
• Advise patient to notify ophthalmologist of carvedilol therapy because if cataract surgery is required, modifications of the surgical technique may be necessary.

caspofungin acetate
Cancidas

Class and Category
Chemical class: Echinocandins
Therapeutic class: Antifungal
Pregnancy category: C

Indications and Dosages

➤ *To treat invasive aspergillosis in patients refractory to or intolerant of other therapies; to treat candidemia and candidal infections in intra-abdominal abscesses, peritonitis, and pleural space infections*

I.V. INFUSION

Adults. *Initial:* 70 mg on day 1, followed by 50 mg daily. *Maximum:* 70 mg daily.

Children ages 3 months to 17 years. *Initial:* 70 mg/m² on day 1, followed by 50 mg/m² daily. *Maximum:* 70 mg daily

regardless of dose calculated based on patient's body surface area.

➤ *To treat presumed fungal infections in febrile, neutropenic patients*

I.V. INFUSION

Adults. *Initial:* 70 mg on day 1, followed by 50 mg daily for at least 14 days, including at least 7 days after neutropenia and symptoms have resolved. Increased to 70 mg daily as needed. *Maximum:* 70 mg daily.

Children ages 3 months to 17 years. *Initial:* 70 mg/m² on day 1, followed by 50 mg/m² daily for at least 14 days,

---

Mechanism of Action

Caspofungin acetate interferes with fungal cell membrane synthesis by inhibiting the synthesis of β (1, 3)-D-glucan. A polypeptide, β (1, 3)-D-glucan is the essential component of the fungal cell membrane that makes it rigid and protective. Without it, fungal cells rupture and die. This mechanism of action is most effective against susceptible filamentous fungi, such as Aspergillus.

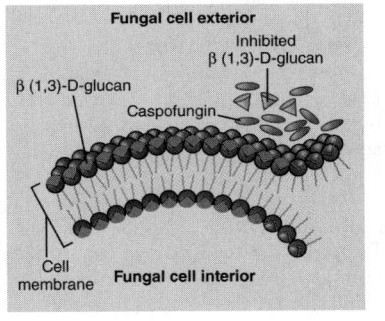

---

including at least 7 days after neutropenia and symptoms have resolved. *Maximum:* 70 mg daily regardless of dose calculated based on patient's body surface area.

DOSAGE ADJUSTMENT Dosage reduced to 35 mg daily after initial 70-mg loading dose in moderate hepatic insufficiency.

➤ *To treat esophageal candidiasis*

I.V. INFUSION

Adults. 50 mg daily.

Children ages 3 months to 17 years. *Initial:* 70 mg/m² on day 1, followed by 50 mg/m² daily. *Maximum:* 70 mg daily regardless of dose calculated based on patient's body surface area.

DOSAGE ADJUSTMENT Dosage reduced to 35 mg daily in moderate hepatic insufficiency.

Incompatibilities

Don't mix or infuse with other drugs. Don't admix with diluents that contain dextrose.

Contraindications

Hypersensitivity to caspofungin acetate or its components

Interactions

DRUGS

carbamazepine, dexamethasone, efavirenz, nelfinavir, nevirapine, phenytoin, rifampin: Possibly decreased blood caspofungin level

cyclosporine: Transient increases in ALT and AST levels

tacrolimus: Possibly decreased blood tacrolimus level

Adverse Reactions

CNS: Chills, dizziness, fever, headache, insomnia, paresthesia, tremor, warmth sensation

CV: Edema, hypertension, hypotension, phlebitis, tachycardia, thrombophlebitis

EENT: Mucosal inflammation

GI: Abdominal pain, diarrhea, elevated liver function test results, hepatic dysfunction or necrosis, jaundice, nausea, pancreatitis, vomiting

GU: Elevated BUN or serum creatinine level, proteinuria, renal insufficiency

HEME: Decreased hemoglobin and hematocrit

MS: Back pain, myalgia
RESP: Bronchospasm, cough, crackles, dyspnea, pleural effusion, pneumonia, respiratory failure, stridor, tachypnea
SKIN: Diaphoresis, erythema including multiforme, flushing, pruritus, rash, sensation of warmth, skin exfoliation, Stevens-Johnson syndrome
Other: Anaphylaxis, angioedema, decreased serum bicarbonate level, elevated gamma-glutamyltransferase level, facial edema, hypercalcemia, hyperkalemia, hyperphosphatemia, hypokalemia, hypomagnesemia, infusion-site reaction, sepsis, septic shock

Nursing Considerations
• To prepare 70-mg loading dose, let vial reach room temperature. Reconstitute by adding 10.5 ml normal saline solution to vial. Dilute for admin-istration by transferring 10 ml of reconstituted drug to 250 ml normal saline solution.
• To prepare 70-mg loading dose from two 50-mg vials, add 10.5 ml normal saline solution to each vial; then transfer 14 ml of prepared solution to 250 ml normal saline solution.
• To prepare daily 50-mg infusion, let vial reach room temperature. Reconstitute by adding 10.5 ml normal saline solution to vial. Dilute for admin-istration by transferring only 10 ml of reconstituted drug to 250 ml normal saline solution.
• To prepare daily 50-mg infusion at reduced volume, add 10 ml of reconstituted drug to 100 ml normal saline solution.
• To prepare 35-mg daily dose for patient with moderate hepatic insufficiency, recon-stitute 50-mg vial with 10.5 ml normal saline solution. To dilute, transfer only 7 ml of reconstituted drug to 250 ml normal saline solution or, if needed, to 100 ml normal saline solution.
• When preparing powder for recon-stitution, mix gently to obtain clear solution. Don't use if solution is cloudy or contains precipitate. Discard unused solution after 24 hours.
• Infuse drug slowly over about 1 hour.
• Expect to increase daily dose to 70 mg for adults and 70 mg/m² for children

(not to exceed the adult dose of 70 mg regardless of calculated dose), as prescribed, for patients also receiving carbamazepine, dexamethasone, efavirenz, nelfinavir, nevirapine, phenytoin, or rifampin.
• Watch for flushed skin, and assess patient often for unexplained temperature elevation.
• Monitor patient for possible histamine-mediated adverse reactions such as angioedema, bronchospasm, facial swelling, pruritus, rash, or warmth sensation. Report these symptoms immediately and expect caspofungin therapy to be discontinued.
WARNING Assess for airway patency if patient develops excessive facial edema or respiratory stridor. Provide emergency airway management if complete obstruction occurs.
• Monitor patient's liver function test results, as ordered, and report abnormalities.
PATIENT TEACHING
• Urge patient to notify prescriber immediately if he has difficulty talking, swallowing, or breathing during drug administration.

cefaclor

Apo-Cefaclor (CAN), Ceclor, Ceclor CD, Raniclor

Class and Category
Chemical class: Second-generation cephalosporin, 7-aminocephalosporanic acid
Therapeutic class: Antibiotic
Pregnancy category: B

Indications and Dosages
➤ *To treat otitis media caused by* Haemophilus influenzae, *staphylococci,* Streptococcus pneumoniae, *and* Streptococcus pyogenes; *lower respiratory tract infections, including pneumonia caused by* H. influenzae, S. pneumoniae, *and* S. pyogenes; *pharyngitis and tonsillitis caused by* S. pyogenes; *UTI, including cystitis and pyelonephritis, caused by* Escherichia coli, Klebsiella *species,* Proteus mirabilis, *and coagulase-negative*

staphylococci; and skin and soft-tissue infections caused by S. pyogenes *and* Staphylococcus aureus

CAPSULES

Adults and adolescents. 250 mg every 8 hr. For severe infections, such as pneumonia, or those caused by less susceptible organisms, 500 mg every 8 hr. *Maximum:* 4 g daily.

CHEWABLE TABLETS, ORAL SUSPENSION

Adults and adolescents. 250 mg every 8 hr. For severe infections, such as pneumonia, or those caused by less susceptible organisms, 500 mg every 8 hr. *Maximum:* 4 g daily.

Children. 20 mg/kg daily in divided doses every 8 hr. For serious infections, such as otitis media, and infections caused by less susceptible organisms, 40 mg/kg daily in divided doses every 8 hr. For otitis media and pharyngitis, total daily dosage divided and given every 12 hr, if needed. *Maximum:* 1 g daily.

➤ *To treat acute bacterial infection in chronic bronchitis or secondary bacterial infection in acute bronchitis (not caused by* H. influenzae*)*

E.R. TABLETS

Adults and adolescents age 16 and over. 500 mg every 12 hr for 7 days.

➤ *To treat pharyngitis and tonsillitis (not caused by* H. influenzae*)*

E.R. TABLETS

Adults and adolescents age 16 and over. 375 mg every 12 hr for 10 days.

➤ *To treat uncomplicated skin and soft-tissue infections caused by* S. aureus

E.R. TABLETS

Adults and adolescents age 16 and over. 375 mg every 12 hr for 7 to 10 days.

Mechanism of Action

Interferes with bacterial cell wall synthesis by inhibiting cross-linking of peptidoglycan strands, which stiffen cell membranes. As a result, bacterial cells rupture.

Contraindications

Hypersensitivity to cephalosporins or their components

Interactions

DRUGS

aminoglycosides, loop diuretics: Increased risk of nephrotoxicity

antacids: Decreased blood cefaclor level (E.R. tablets)

oral anticoagulants: Increased anticoagulation

Adverse Reactions

CNS: Chills, fever, headache, seizures
CV: Edema
EENT: Hearing loss
GI: Abdominal cramps, diarrhea, elevated liver function test results, hepatic failure, hepatomegaly, nausea, oral candidiasis, pseudomembranous colitis, vomiting
GU: Elevated BUN level, nephrotoxicity, renal failure, vaginal candidiasis
HEME: Eosinophilia, hemolytic anemia, hypoprothrombinemia, neutropenia, thrombocytopenia, unusual bleeding
MS: Arthralgia
RESP: Dyspnea
SKIN: Ecchymosis, erythema, erythema multiforme, pruritus, rash, Stevens-Johnson syndrome
Other: Anaphylaxis, superinfection

Nursing Considerations

• Use cefaclor cautiously in patients with impaired renal function or a history of GI disease, particularly colitis, and in patients who are hypersensitive to penicillin; about 10% of them have cross-sensitivity.
• If possible, obtain culture and sensitivity test results, as ordered, before giving drug.
• Monitor BUN and serum creatinine levels for early signs of nephrotoxicity. Also monitor fluid intake and output; decreasing urine output may indicate nephrotoxicity.
• Be aware that an allergic reaction may occur a few days after therapy starts.
• Assess bowel pattern daily; severe diarrhea may indicate pseudomembranous colitis.
• Assess patient for superinfection: perineal itching, fever, malaise, redness, pain, swelling, rash, drainage, diarrhea, cough, sputum changes.

PATIENT TEACHING

• Instruct patient to complete the prescribed course of therapy, even if he feels better.
• Tell patient to swallow E.R. tablets whole and not to crush, break, or chew them.
• Advise patient to take E.R. tablets with food to enhance absorption.
• Instruct patient to take capsules or E.R. tablets with a full glass of water.
• Tell patient to shake oral suspension well before measuring and to use a calibrated measuring device to ensure accurate dose.

• Tell patient to refrigerate oral suspension and to discard unused portion after 14 days.
• Instruct patient to report severe diarrhea to prescriber immediately.
• Explain that yogurt and buttermilk protect intestinal flora and decrease diarrhea.
• Urge patient to report evidence of superinfection.

cefadroxil
Duricef

Class and Category
Chemical class: First-generation cephalosporin, 7-aminocephalosporanic acid
Therapeutic class: Antibiotic
Pregnancy category: B

Indications and Dosages
➤ *To treat UTI caused by* Escherichia coli, Klebsiella *species, or* Proteus mirabilis
CAPSULES, TABLETS
Adults. For uncomplicated lower UTI, 1 to 2 g daily or in divided doses every 12 hr. For all other UTIs, 2 g every 12 hr.
ORAL SUSPENSION
Adults. For uncomplicated lower UTI, 1 to 2 g daily or in divided doses every 12 hr. For all other UTIs, 2 g every 12 hr.
Children. 30 mg/kg daily in divided doses every 12 hr. *Maximum:* Adult dosage.
➤ *To treat skin and soft-tissue infections caused by staphylococci or streptococci*
CAPSULES, TABLETS
Adults. 1 g daily or 500 mg every 12 hr.
ORAL SUSPENSION
Adults. 1 g daily or 500 mg every 12 hr.
Children. 30 mg/kg daily in divided doses every 12 hr. *Maximum:* Adult dosage.
➤ *To treat pharyngitis and tonsillitis caused by group A beta-hemolytic streptococci*
CAPSULES, TABLETS
Adults. 1 g daily or 500 mg twice daily for 10 days.
ORAL SUSPENSION
Adults. 1 g daily or 500 mg twice daily for 10 days.
Children. 30 mg/kg daily in divided doses every 12 hr for 10 days. *Maximum:* 1 g daily or 500 mg twice daily for 10 days.

DOSAGE ADJUSTMENT Initial dose of 1 g; then maintenance of 0.5 g every 12 hr if creatinine clearance is 25 to 50 ml/min/1.73 m^2; 0.5 g every 24 hr if creatinine clearance is 10 to 25 ml/min/1.73 m^2; and 0.5 g every 36 hr if creatinine clearance is 0 to 10 ml/min/1.73 m^2.

Mechanism of Action
Interferes with bacterial cell wall synthesis by inhibiting the final step in the cross-linking of peptidoglycan strands. Peptidoglycan makes cell membranes rigid and protective. Without it, bacterial cells rupture and die.

Contraindications
Hypersensitivity to cephalosporins or their components

Interactions
DRUGS
aminoglycosides, loop diuretics: Increased toxicity of these drugs

Adverse Reactions
CNS: Chills, fever, headache, seizures
CV: Edema
EENT: Hearing loss
GI: Abdominal cramps, diarrhea, elevated liver function test results, hepatic failure, hepatomegaly, nausea, oral candidiasis, pseudomembranous colitis, vomiting
GU: Elevated BUN level, nephrotoxicity, renal failure, vaginal candidiasis
HEME: Eosinophilia, hemolytic anemia, hypoprothrombinemia, neutropenia, thrombocytopenia, unusual bleeding
MS: Arthralgia
RESP: Dyspnea
SKIN: Ecchymosis, erythema, erythema multiforme, pruritus, rash, Stevens-Johnson syndrome
Other: Anaphylaxis, superinfection

Nursing Considerations
• Use cefadroxil cautiously in patients with impaired renal function or a history of GI disease, particularly colitis. Also use drug cautiously in patients who are hyper-sensitive to penicillin because cross-sensitivity has occurred in about 10% of such patients.
• If possible, obtain culture and sensitivity test results, as ordered, before giving drug.

- Be aware that an allergic reaction may occur a few days after therapy starts.
- Monitor BUN and serum creatinine levels for early signs of nephrotoxicity. Also monitor fluid intake and output; decreasing urine output may indicate nephrotoxicity.
- Assess bowel pattern daily; severe diarrhea may indicate pseudomembranous colitis.
- Assess for signs of superinfection, such as perineal itching, fever, malaise, redness, pain, swelling, drainage, rash, diarrhea, and cough or sputum changes.

PATIENT TEACHING
- Instruct patient to complete the prescribed course of therapy.
- Tell patient to shake oral suspension before measuring and to use a liquid-measuring device to ensure accurate doses.
- Tell patient to refrigerate oral suspension and to discard the unused portion after 14 days.
- Urge patient to report watery, bloody stools to prescriber immediately, even up to 2 months after drug therapy has ended.
- Inform patient that yogurt and buttermilk can help maintain intestinal flora and decrease diarrhea.
- Teach patient to recognize and report evidence of superinfection, such as furry tongue, perineal itching, and loose, foul-smelling stools.

cefazolin sodium

Ancef

Class and Category

Chemical class: First-generation cephalosporin, 7-aminocephalosporanic acid
Therapeutic class: Antibiotic
Pregnancy category: B

Indications and Dosages

➤ *To treat respiratory tract infections caused by group A beta-hemolytic streptococci,* Haemophilus influenzae, Klebsiella *species,* Staphylococcus aureus, *and* Streptococcus pneumoniae; *skin and soft-tissue infections*

caused by S. aureus, *group A beta-hemolytic and other strains of streptococci; biliary tract infections caused by* Escherichia coli, Klebsiella *species,* Proteus mirabilis, S. aureus, *and various strains of streptococci; bone and joint infections caused by* S. aureus; *genital infections, such as epididymitis and prostatitis, caused by* E. coli, Klebsiella *species,* P. mirabilis, *and some strains of enterococci; septicemia caused by* E. coli, Klebsiella *species,* P. mirabilis, S. aureus, *and* S. pneumoniae; *and endocarditis caused by group A beta-hemolytic streptococci and* S. aureus

I.V. INFUSION, I.V. OR I.M. INJECTION
Adults. For mild infections, 250 to 500 mg every 8 hr; for moderate to severe infections, 500 to 1,000 mg every 6 to 8 hr; and for severe life-threatening infections, 1,000 to 1,500 mg every 6 hr. *Maximum:* 6 g daily.
Children. For mild to moderate infections, 25 to 50 mg/kg daily divided equally and given three times daily or four times daily; for severe infections, 100 mg/kg daily divided equally and given three times daily or four times daily.

➤ *To treat pneumococcal pneumonia*
I.V. INFUSION, I.V. OR I.M. INJECTION
Adults. 500 mg every 12 hr.

➤ *To treat acute uncomplicated UTI caused by* E. coli, Klebsiella *species,* P. mirabilis, *and some strains of* Enterobacter *and* Enterococcus
I.V. INFUSION, I.V. OR I.M. INJECTION
Adults. 1 g every 12 hr.

➤ *To provide surgical prophylaxis*
I.V. INFUSION, I.V. OR I.M. INJECTION
Adults. 1 g 30 to 60 min before surgery; 0.5 to 1 g during surgery if it lasts 2 hr or longer; 0.5 to 1 g every 6 to 8 hr for 24 hr after surgery.

DOSAGE ADJUSTMENT After initial loading dose appropriate to infection's severity, dosage interval restricted to at least 8 hr for adults with creatinine clearance of 35 to 54 ml/min/1.73 m^2; dosage reduced by 50% and given every 12 hr for adults with creatinine clearance of 11 to 34 ml/min/1.73 m^2; and dosage reduced by 50% and given every 18 to 24 hr for adults with creatinine clearance of 10 ml/min/1.73 m^2 or less. Dosage reduced to 60% and given every

12 hr for children with creatinine clearance of 40 to 70 ml/min/1.73 m^2; dosage reduced to 25% and given every 12 hr for children with creatinine clearance of 20 to 40 ml/min/1.73 m^2; and dosage reduced to 10% and given every 24 hr for children with creatinine clearance of 5 to 20 ml/min/1.73 m^2.

Mechanism of Action

Interferes with bacterial cell wall synthesis by inhibiting the final step in the cross-linking of peptidoglycan strands. Peptidoglycan makes cell membranes rigid and protective. Without it, bacterial cells rupture and die.

Incompatibilities

To prevent mutual inactivation, don't mix cefazolin with aminoglycosides. Also avoid mixing cefazolin with other drugs, including pentamidine isethionate.

Contraindications

Hypersensitivity to cephalosporins or their components

Interactions

DRUGS

aminoglycosides, loop diuretics: Additive nephrotoxicity
probenecid: Increased and prolonged blood cefazolin level

Adverse Reactions

CNS: Chills, fever, headache, seizures
CV: Edema
EENT: Hearing loss
GI: Abdominal cramps, diarrhea, elevated liver function test results, hepatic failure, hepatitis, hepatomegaly, nausea, oral candidiasis, pseudomembranous colitis, vomiting
GU: Elevated BUN and serum creatinine levels, nephrotoxicity, renal failure, vaginal candidiasis
HEME: Eosinophilia, hemolytic anemia, hypoprothrombinemia, neutropenia, thrombocytopenia, unusual bleeding
MS: Arthralgia
RESP: Dyspnea
SKIN: Ecchymosis, erythema, erythema multiforme, pruritus, rash, Stevens-Johnson syndrome
Other: Anaphylaxis; injection-site pain, redness, and swelling; superinfection

Nursing Considerations

• Use cefazolin cautiously in patients with impaired renal function or a history of GI disease, particularly colitis. Also use cautiously in patients hypersensitive to penicillin because cross-sensitivity has occurred in about 10% of such patients.
• If possible, obtain culture and sensitivity test results, as ordered, before giving drug.
WARNING To prevent unintentional overdose, cefazolin for injection USP and dextrose injection USP shouldn't be used in children who require less than the full adult dose.
• Reconstitute 500-mg drug vial with 2 ml of sterile water for injection (or 1-g vial with 2.5 ml). Shake well until dissolved.
• For direct I.V. injection, further dilute reconstituted solution with at least 5 ml sterile water for injection. Inject slowly over 3 to 5 minutes through tubing of a flowing compatible I.V. solution.
• For intermittent I.V. infusion, reconstitute 500 to 1,000 mg in 50 to 100 ml normal saline solution, D$_5$W, D$_{10}$W, dextrose 5% in lactated Ringer's solution, dextrose 5% in quarter-normal (0.2) saline solution, dextrose 5% in half-normal (0.45) saline solution, dextrose 5% in normal saline solution, lactated Ringer's injection, 5% or 10% invert sugar in sterile water for injection, 5% sodium bicarbonate (Ancef), or Ringer's injection.
• Administer I.M injection deep into large muscle mass, such as the gluteus maximus.
• Store reconstituted drug up to 24 hours at room temperature or 10 days refrigerated.
• Monitor I.V. site for irritation, phlebitis, and extravasation.
• Monitor BUN and serum creatinine for early signs of nephrotoxicity. Also monitor fluid intake and output; decreasing urine output may indicate nephrotoxicity.
• Be aware that an allergic reaction may occur a few days after therapy starts.
• Assess bowel pattern daily; severe diarrhea may indicate pseudo-membranous colitis.
• Watch for evidence of superinfection: cough, diarrhea, drainage, fever, malaise, pain, perineal itching, rash, redness, swelling.

- Assess for pharyngitis, ecchymosis, bleeding, and arthralgia; they may indicate a blood dyscrasia.

PATIENT TEACHING
- Instruct patient to complete the prescribed course of therapy.
- Reassure patient that I.M. injection doesn't typically cause pain.
- Tell patient to report watery, bloody stools to prescriber immediately, even up to 2 months after drug therapy has ended.

cefdinir
Omnicef

Class and Category
Chemical class: Cephalosporin
Therapeutic class: Antibiotic
Pregnancy category: B

Indications and Dosages
➤ *To treat community-acquired pneumonia caused by* Haemophilus influenzae *(including beta-lactamase–producing strains),* Haemophilus parainfluenzae *(including beta-lactamase–producing strains),* Streptococcus pneumoniae *(penicillin-susceptible strains only), and* Moraxella catarrhalis *(including beta-lactamase–producing strains)*

CAPSULES
Adults and adolescents. 300 mg every 12 hr for 10 days. *Maximum:* 600 mg daily.
➤ *To treat pharyngitis or tonsillitis caused by* Streptococcus pyogenes *and acute exacerbations of chronic bronchitis caused by* H. influenzae *(including beta-lactamase–producing strains),* H. parainfluenzae *(including beta-lactamase–producing strains),* S. pneumoniae *(penicillin-susceptible strains only), and* M. catarrhalis *(including beta-lactamase–producing strains)*

CAPSULES
Adults and adolescents. 300 mg every 12 hr for 5 to 10 days or 600 mg every 24 hr for 10 days. *Maximum:* 600 mg daily.
ORAL SUSPENSION
Children ages 6 months to 12 years. 7 mg/kg every 12 hr for 5 to 10 days or 14 mg/kg every 24 hr for 10 days (for pharyngitis or tonsillitis).

➤ *To treat acute maxillary sinusitis caused by* H. influenzae *(including beta-lactamase–producing strains),* S. pneumoniae *(penicillin-susceptible strains only), and* M. catarrhalis *(including beta-lactamase–producing strains)*

CAPSULES
Adults and adolescents. 300 mg every 12 hr or 600 mg every 24 hr for 10 days. *Maximum:* 600 mg daily.
ORAL SUSPENSION
Children ages 6 months to 12 years. 7 mg/kg every 12 hr or 14 mg/kg every 24 hr for 10 days.
➤ *To treat uncomplicated skin and soft-tissue infections caused by* Staphylococcus aureus *(including beta-lactamase–producing strains) and* Streptococcus pyogenes

CAPSULES
Adults and adolescents. 300 mg every 12 hr for 10 days. *Maximum:* 600 mg daily.
ORAL SUSPENSION
Children ages 6 months to 12 years. 7 mg/kg every 12 hr for 10 days.
➤ *To treat acute bacterial otitis media caused by* H. influenzae *(including beta-lactamase–producing strains),* S. pneumoniae *(penicillin-susceptible strains only), and* M. catarrhalis *(including beta-lactamase–producing strains)*

ORAL SUSPENSION
Children ages 6 months to 12 years. 7 mg/kg every 12 hr for 5 to 10 days or 14 mg/kg every 24 hr for 10 days.
DOSAGE ADJUSTMENT For adults with creatinine clearance less than 30 ml/min/1.73 m^2, expect to reduce cefdinir dosage to 300 mg daily; for children with creatinine clearance less than 30 ml/min/1.73 m^2, dosage is 7 mg/kg (up to 300 mg) daily. For patients undergoing intermittent hemodialysis, dosage is 300 mg or 7 mg/kg every other day, beginning at the end of each hemodialysis session, as prescribed.

Mechanism of Action
Interferes with bacterial cell wall synthesis by inhibiting the final step in the cross-linking of peptidoglycan strands. Peptido-glycan makes cell membranes rigid and protective. Without it, bacterial cells

rupture and die. Because cefdinir is not degraded by some bacterial beta-lactamase enzymes, it's effective against many organisms that are resistant to both penicillins and some cephalosporins.

Contraindications

Hypersensitivity to cefdinir, other cephalosporins, or their components

Interactions

DRUGS

antacids that contain aluminum or magnesium: Decreased cefdinir absorption if given within 2 hours of antacid
iron salts: Reduced cefdinir absorption if given within 2 hours of iron
probenecid: Increased blood level and prolonged half-life of cefdinir

Adverse Reactions

CNS: Asthenia, dizziness, drowsiness, headache, insomnia, somnolence
EENT: Dry mouth, pharyngitis, rhinitis
GI: Abdominal pain, anorexia, constipation, diarrhea, flatulence, indigestion, nausea, pseudomembranous colitis, stool discoloration, vomiting
GU: Leukorrhea, vaginal candidiasis, vaginitis
HEME: Leukopenia
SKIN: Pruritus, rash
Other: Anaphylaxis, serum sickness–like reaction

Nursing Considerations

• To reconstitute cefdinir powder for oral suspension, tap bottle to loosen powder, and then dilute with water to 125 mg/5 ml. Shake well before each use. Discard any unused portion after 10 days. Keep suspension bottle tightly closed, and store it at room temperature.
• Give antacids that contain aluminum or magnesium and iron salts at least 2 hours before or after cefdinir because they may interfere with cefdinir absorption.
• Monitor patient allergic to penicillin for evidence of hypersensitivity reaction, from a mild rash to fatal anaphylaxis, because cross-sensitivity can occur.
• Monitor patient with a chronic GI condition, such as colitis, for signs

and symptoms of a drug-related exacerbation.
• Because all cephalosporins have the potential to cause bleeding, monitor elderly patients and patients with a preexisting coagulopathy, including vitamin K deficiency, for elevated PT or APTT.
• Monitor patient closely for diarrhea, which may indicate pseudomembranous colitis caused by *Clostridium difficile.* If diarrhea occurs, notify prescriber and expect to withhold cefdinir and treat with fluids, electrolytes, protein, and an antibiotic effective against *C. difficile.*
• Assess for other evidence of superinfection, including perineal itching; loose, foul-smelling stools; and vaginal drainage.

PATIENT TEACHING
• Advise patient taking cefdinir oral suspension to shake bottle well before use and to use a liquid-measuring device to ensure accurate dose.
• Inform patient that tablet coating may cause stools to become a reddish color.
• Instruct patient to complete entire course of therapy, even if he feels better.
• Advise patient to take iron salts and aluminum- or magnesium-containing antacids at least 2 hours before or after taking cefdinir.
• Inform patient with history of colitis that cefdinir may worsen it; urge him to notify prescriber promptly if symptoms develop.
• Inform patient with diabetes mellitus that oral suspension contains 2.86 g of sucrose per teaspoon; advise him to monitor his blood glucose levels as appropriate.
• Teach patient to recognize and report evidence of superinfection, such as perineal itching; loose, foul-smelling stools; and vaginal drainage.
• Inform patient that yogurt and buttermilk can help prevent superinfection and may decrease diarrhea.
• Urge patient to tell prescriber about diarrhea that's severe or lasts longer than 3 days. Remind patient that watery or bloody stools can occur 2 or more months after antibiotic therapy and can be serious, requiring prompt treatment.

cefditoren pivoxil
Spectracef

Class and Category
Chemical class: Cephalosporin
Therapeutic class: Antibiotic
Pregnancy category: B

Indications and Dosages
➤ *To treat mild to moderate acute bacterial exacerbation of chronic bronchitis or community-acquired pneumonia caused by* Haemophilus influenzae *(including beta-lactamase–producing strains),* Haemophilus parainfluenzae *(including beta-lactamase–producing strains),* Streptococcus pneumoniae *(penicillin-susceptible strains), or* Moraxella catarrhalis *(including beta-lactamase–producing strains)*

TABLETS
Adults and children age 12 and over. 400 mg twice daily for 10 days or for 14 days for community-acquired pneumonia.

➤ *To treat mild to moderate pharyngitis and tonsillitis caused by* Streptococcus pyogenes

TABLETS
Adults and children age 12 and over. 200 mg twice daily for 10 days.

➤ *To treat mild to moderate uncomplicated skin and soft-tissue infections caused by* Staphylococcus aureus *(including beta-lactamase–producing strains) or* S. pyogenes

TABLETS
Adults and children age 12 and over. 200 mg twice daily for 10 days.

DOSAGE ADJUSTMENT In moderate renal impairment (creatinine clearance 30 to 49 ml/min/1.73 m^2), maximum dosage reduced to 200 mg twice daily In severe renal impairment (creatinine clearance less than 30 ml/min/1.73 m^2), maximum dosage reduced to 200 mg daily.

Mechanism of Action
Interferes with bacterial cell wall synthesis by inhibiting the final step in the cross-linking of peptidoglycan strands. Peptidoglycan makes the cell membrane rigid and protective. Without it, bacterial cells rupture and die. This mechanism of action is most effective against bacteria that divide rapidly, including many gram-positive and gram-negative bacteria. Cefditoren isn't inactivated by beta lactamase produced by some bacteria.

Contraindications
Carnitine deficiency or inborn metabolic disorder that causes it; hypersensitivity to cephalosporins or their components

Interactions
DRUGS
aluminum- and magnesium-containing antacids, H$_2$-receptor antagonists: Reduced cefditoren absorption
probenecid: Increased and prolonged blood cefditoren level
FOODS
food: Increased cefditoren absorption

Adverse Reactions
CNS: Headache, hyperactivity, hypertonia, seizures
GI: Abdominal pain, diarrhea, dyspepsia, hepatic dysfunction, nausea, pseudomembranous colitis, vomiting
GU: Acute renal failure, renal dysfunction, toxic nephropathy
HEME: Aplastic anemia, hemolytic anemia, hemorrhage, thrombocytopenia
MS: Arthralgia
RESP: Pneumonia
SKIN: Erythema multiforme, Stevens-Johnson syndrome, toxic epidermal necrolysis
Other: Allergic reaction, anaphylaxis, carnitine deficiency, drug fever, serum sickness–like reaction, superinfection

Nursing Considerations
WARNING Before starting cefditoren therapy, determine if patient is hypersensitive to milk protein because cefditoren contains sodium caseinate, a milk protein. Drug should not be given to patient with this hypersensitivity. Also determine if patient has had a hypersensitivity reaction to cefditoren or other cephalosporins (because drug is contraindicated in these patients) or to penicillin (because cross-sensitivity has occurred in about 10% of such patients).

• Cefditoren shouldn't be used for prolonged treatment because of the risk of carnitine deficiency.
• If possible, obtain culture and sensitivity test results before giving cefditoren.
• Assess patient for evidence of *Clostridium difficile* infection and pseudomembranous colitis, such as profuse, watery diarrhea. For mild cases, expect to discontinue cefditoren. For moderate to severe cases, expect to also give fluids and electrolytes, protein supplementation, and an antibacterial drug effective against *C. difficile*.
• If an allergic reaction occurs, expect to discontinue drug, as prescribed. For serious acute hypersensitivity reactions, expect to also give epinephrine, oxygen, and I.V. fluids, antihistamines, corticosteroids, and vasopressors, as prescribed.
• Monitor BUN and serum creatinine levels to detect early signs of renal dysfunction. Also monitor fluid intake and output.
• Watch for a decreased PT, as ordered, in at-risk patients, such as those with renal or hepatic impairment, those with a poor nutritional state, and those receiving anticoagulant or prolonged antibiotic therapy. Notify prescriber if a decrease occurs, and give vitamin K as ordered.

PATIENT TEACHING
• Urge patient to complete prescribed course of therapy.
• Instruct patient to take cefditoren with meals to enhance drug absorption.
• Advise patient not to take cefditoren with aluminum- or magnesium-containing antacids or other drugs used to reduce stomach acids because these drugs may interfere with cefditoren absorption.
• Explain that yogurt and buttermilk help maintain normal intestinal flora and can decrease diarrhea during therapy.
• Instruct patient to report severe diarrhea to prescriber immediately.

cefepime
hydrochloride

Maxipime

Class and Category
Chemical class: Fourth-generation cephalosporin, 7-aminocephalosporanic acid
Therapeutic class: Antibiotic
Pregnancy category: B

Indications and Dosages
➤ *To treat mild to moderate UTI caused by* Escherichia coli, Klebsiella pneumoniae, *or* Proteus mirabilis
I.V. INFUSION, I.M. INJECTION (ONLY FOR UTI CAUSED BY *E. COLI*)
Adults and children age 12 and over. 500 to 1,000 mg every 12 hr for 7 to 10 days.
➤ *To treat severe UTI caused by* E. coli *or* K. pneumoniae, *moderate to severe skin and soft-tissue infections caused by* Staphylococcus aureus *or* Streptococcus pyogenes
I.V. INFUSION
Adults and children age 12 and over. 2 g every 12 hr for 10 days.
➤ *To treat moderate to severe pneumonia caused by* Enterobacter *species,* K. pneumoniae, Pseudomonas aeruginosa, *or* Streptococcus pneumoniae
I.V. INFUSION
Adults and children age 12 and over. 1 to 2 g every 12 hr for 10 days.
➤ *To treat febrile neutropenia*
I.V. INFUSION
Adults and children age 12 and over. 2 g every 8 hr for 7 days or until neutropenia resolves.
➤ *To treat complicated intra-abdominal infections (together with metronidazole) caused by alpha-hemolytic streptococci,* Bacteroides fragilis, E. coli, Enterobacter *species,* K. pneumoniae, *or* P. aeruginosa
I.V. INFUSION
Adults and children age 12 and over. 2 g every 12 hr for 7 to 10 days.
DOSAGE ADJUSTMENT For patient with creatinine clearance between 30 and 60 ml/min/1.73 m^2, dosing interval increased to every 24 hr if dosing interval had been every 12 hr, and dosing interval increased to every 12 hr if dosing interval had been every 8 hr. For patient with creatinine clearance between 11 and 29 ml/min/1.73 m^2, dosage decreased to 500 mg every 24 hr if dosage had been 1 gram every 24 hr; dosage decreased to 1 gram every 24 hr if dosage

had been 2 grams every 24 hr; and dosing interval decreased to 24 hr if dosing interval had been every 12 hour while maintaining a dosage of 2 grams. For patient with creatinine clearance less than 11 ml/min/1.73 m^2, dosage decreased to 250 mg every 24 hr if dosage had been 500 mg every 24 hr; dosage decreased to 500 mg every 24 hr if dosage had been 1 gram every 24 hr; and dosage decreased to 1 gram every 24 hr if dosage had been 2 grams every 24 hr. For patient on continuous abdominal peritoneal dialysis or hemodialysis, dosage interval and dosage further altered.

Mechanism of Action

Interferes with bacterial cell wall synthesis by inhibiting the final step in the cross-linking of peptidoglycan strands. Peptidoglycan makes cell membranes rigid and protective. Without it, bacterial cells rupture and die.

Incompatibilities

Don't add cefepime to solutions that contain ampicillin in a concentration of more than 40 mg/ml. Don't add drug to solutions that contain aminophylline, gentamycin, metronidazole, netilmicin sulfate, tobramycin, or vancomycin.

Contraindications

Hypersensitivity to cephalosporins, their components, other beta-lactam antibiotics, or penicillins

Interactions

DRUGS

aminoglycosides, loop diuretics: Increased risk of renal failure in renal disease

Adverse Reactions

CNS: Chills, coma, confusion, encephalopathy, fever, hallucinations, headache, myoclonus, neurotoxicity, nonconvulsive status epilepticus, seizures, stupor
CV: Edema
EENT: Hearing loss
GI: Abdominal cramps, diarrhea, elevated liver function test results, hepatic failure, hepatomegaly, nausea, oral candidiasis, pseudomembranous colitis, vomiting
GU: Elevated BUN level, nephrotoxicity, renal failure, vaginal candidiasis

HEME: Agranulocytosis, eosinophilia, hemolytic anemia, hypoprothrombinemia, leukopenia, neutropenia, thrombocytopenia, unusual bleeding
MS: Arthralgia
RESP: Dyspnea
SKIN: Ecchymosis, erythema, erythema multiforme, pruritus, rash, Stevens-Johnson syndrome
Other: Anaphylaxis; injection-site pain, redness, and swelling; superinfection

Nursing Considerations

• Use cefepime cautiously in patients with impaired renal function or a history of GI disease, particularly colitis. Also use cautiously in patients hypersensitive to other cephalosporins, other drugs, or penicillins because cross-sensitivity has occurred.
• If possible, obtain culture and sensitivity test results, as ordered, before giving drug.
• For I.V. infusion, reconstitute using manufacturer's guidelines. Give over 30 minutes.
• For I.M. injection, reconstitute 500-mg vial of drug with 1.3 ml of diluent, such as sterile water for injection (or 1-g vial with 2.4 ml of diluent). See drug guidelines for complete list of appropriate diluents.
WARNING Monitor patient closely for hypersensitivity reactions. Be aware that an allergic reaction may occur even up to a few days after therapy starts. Notify prescriber immediately and expect cefepime to be discontinued. Be prepared to administer treatment with epinephrine, oxygen, corticosteroids, intravenous fluids, intravenous antihistamines, pressor amines and airway management, if reaction is severe.
• Monitor BUN and serum creatinine levels for early signs of nephrotoxicity. Also monitor fluid intake and output; decreasing urine output may indicate nephrotoxicity. Be aware that unadjusted dosages of cefepime in renally impaired patients may cause neurotoxicity. If neurotoxicity occurs, notify prescriber and expect dosage to be modified or drug discontinued.
• Assess bowel pattern daily; severe diarrhea may indicate pseudomembranous colitis.
• Assess for signs of superinfection, such as perineal itching, fever, malaise, redness,

pain, swelling, drainage, rash, diarrhea, and cough or sputum changes.
• Assess for pharyngitis, ecchymosis, bleeding, and arthralgia; they may indicate a blood dyscrasia.
• Monitor patient for evidence of encephalopathy, such as changes in level of consciousness, myoclonus, and seizures. Patient will need immediate treatment, and the cefepime dosage will need to be adjusted or the drug discontinued.

PATIENT TEACHING
• Tell patient to immediately report severe diarrhea to prescriber.
• Instruct patient and caregiver to immediately seek emergency care for any change in mental status, such as coma, hallucinations, decreased responsiveness, abnormal movements, or seizures. Cefepime should be stopped until patient is evaluated.

cefixime
Suprax

Class and Category
Chemical class: Third-generation cephalosporin, 7-aminocephalosporanic acid
Therapeutic class: Antibiotic
Pregnancy category: B

Indications and Dosages
➤ *To treat uncomplicated UTI caused by* Escherichia coli *and* Proteus mirabilis; *otitis media caused by* Haemophilus influenzae, Moraxella catarrhalis, *or* Streptococcus pyogenes; *pharyngitis and tonsillitis caused by* S. pyogenes; *acute bronchitis and acute exacerbations of chronic bronchitis caused by* h. influenzae *and* Streptococcus pneumoniae

ORAL SUSPENSION
Children. 8 mg/kg daily or 4 mg/kg every 12 hr.

TABLETS
Adults and children over 50 kg (110 lb) or age 12. 400 mg daily or 200 mg every 12 hr.
➤ *To treat uncomplicated gonorrhea caused by* Neisseria gonorrhoeae

TABLETS
Adults and children over 50 kg or age 12. 400 mg daily.

DOSAGE ADJUSTMENT Dosage reduced to 75% for patients who have creatinine clearance of 21 to 60 ml/min/1.73 m² or receive hemodialysis. Dosage reduced to 50% for patients who have creatinine clearance of 20 ml/min/1.73 m² or less.

Mechanism of Action
Interferes with bacterial cell wall synthesis by inhibiting the final step in the cross-linking of peptidoglycan strands. Peptidoglycan makes cell membranes rigid and protective. Without it, bacterial cells rupture and die.

Contraindications
Hypersensitivity to cephalosporins or their components

Interactions
DRUGS
aminoglycosides, loop diuretics: Increased risk of nephrotoxicity
carbamazepine: Increased blood carbamazepine level

Adverse Reactions
CNS: Chills, fever, headache, seizures
CV: Edema
EENT: Hearing loss
GI: Abdominal cramps, diarrhea, elevated liver function test results, hepatic failure, hepatitis, hepatomegaly, jaundice, nausea, oral candidiasis, pseudomembranous colitis, vomiting
GU: Elevated BUN level, nephrotoxicity, renal failure, vaginal candidiasis
HEME: Eosinophilia, hemolytic anemia, hypoprothrombinemia, neutropenia, thrombocytopenia, unusual bleeding
MS: Arthralgia
RESP: Dyspnea
SKIN: Ecchymosis, erythema, erythema multiforme, pruritus, rash, Stevens-Johnson syndrome, toxic epidermal necrolysis
Other: Anaphylaxis, angioedema, facial edema, superinfection

Nursing Considerations
• Use cefixime cautiously in patients with impaired renal function or a history of GI disease, especially colitis. Also use cautiously in patients hypersensitive to penicillin because cross-sensitivity has occurred in about 10% of such patients.

- If possible, obtain culture and sensitivity test results, as ordered, before giving drug.
- Tablets shouldn't be substituted for oral suspension to treat otitis media because cefixime suspension produces a higher peak blood level than do tablets when administered at the same dose.
- Monitor BUN and serum creatinine for early signs of nephrotoxicity. Also monitor fluid intake and output; decreasing urine output may indicate nephrotoxicity.
- Be aware that an allergic reaction may occur a few days after therapy starts.
- Assess bowel pattern daily; severe diarrhea may indicate pseudomembranous colitis.
- Assess for signs of superinfection, such as perineal itching, fever, malaise, redness, pain, swelling, drainage, rash, diarrhea, and cough or sputum changes.
- Assess for pharyngitis, ecchymosis, bleeding, and arthralgia; they may indicate a blood dyscrasia.

PATIENT TEACHING

- Instruct patient to complete the prescribed course of therapy.
- Advise patient to shake oral suspension well before pouring dose and to use a calibrated device to obtain an accurate dose.
- Instruct patient to store oral suspension at room temperature and to discard unused portion after 14 days.
- Tell patient to report severe diarrhea to prescriber immediately.
- Inform patient that yogurt and buttermilk can help maintain intestinal flora and decrease diarrhea.
- Teach patient to recognize and report signs of superinfection, such as furry tongue, perineal itching, and loose, foul-smelling stools.

cefmetazole sodium

Zefazone

Class and Category

Chemical class: Second-generation cephalosporin, 7-aminocephalosporanic acid
Therapeutic class: Antibiotic
Pregnancy category: B

Indications and Dosages

➤ *To treat UTI caused by* Escherichia coli; *lower respiratory tract infections, such as bronchitis and pneumonia, caused by* E. coli, Haemophilus influenzae, Staphylococcus aureus, *and* Streptococcus pneumoniae; *skin and soft-tissue infections caused by* Bacteroides fragilis, Bacteroides melaninogenicus, E. coli, Klebsiella oxytoca, Klebsiella pneumoniae, Morganella morganii, Proteus mirabilis, Proteus vulgaris, S. aureus, Staphylococcus epidermidis, Streptococcus agalactiae, *and* Streptococcus pyogenes; *intra-abdominal infections caused by* B. fragilis, Clostridium perfringens, E. coli, K. oxytoca, *and* K. pneumoniae

I.V. INFUSION

Adults. 2 g every 6 to 12 hr for 5 to 14 days.

DOSAGE ADJUSTMENT Dosage reduced to 1 to 2 g every 12 hr if creatinine clearance is 50 to 90 ml/min/1.73 m²; 1 to 2 g every 16 hr if creatinine clearance is 30 to 49 ml/min/1.73 m²; 1 to 2 g every 24 hr if creatinine clearance is 10 to 29 ml/min/1.73 m²; and 1 to 2 g every 48 hr if creatinine clearance is less than 10 ml/min/1.73 m².

➤ *To provide surgical prophylaxis for vaginal hysterectomy*

I.V. INFUSION

Adults. 2 g as a single dose 30 to 90 min before surgery or 1 g 30 to 90 min before surgery and repeated 8 and 16 hr later.

➤ *To provide surgical prophylaxis for abdominal hysterectomy and for high-risk cholecystectomy*

I.V. INFUSION

Adults. 1 g 30 to 90 min before surgery and repeated 8 and 16 hr later.

➤ *To provide surgical prophylaxis for cesarean section*

I.V. INFUSION

Adults. 2 g as a single dose after cord is clamped or 1 g after cord is clamped and then repeated 8 and 16 hr later.

➤ *To provide surgical prophylaxis for colorectal surgery*

I.V. INFUSION

Adults. 2 g as a single dose 30 to 90 min before surgery or 2 g 30 to 90 min before surgery and repeated 8 and 16 hr later.

Mechanism of Action

Interferes with bacterial cell wall synthesis by inhibiting the final step in the cross-linking of peptidoglycan strands. Peptidoglycan makes cell membranes rigid and protective. Without it, bacterial cells rupture and die.

Contraindications

Hypersensitivity to cephalosporins or their components

Interactions

DRUGS
aminoglycosides, loop diuretics: Increased risk of nephrotoxicity
anticoagulants: Possibly increased anticoagulant effect
probenecid: Increased and prolonged blood cefmetazole level
ACTIVITIES
alcohol use: Possibly disulfiram-like reaction

Adverse Reactions

CNS: Chills, fever, headache, seizures
CV: Edema
EENT: Hearing loss
GI: Abdominal cramps, diarrhea, elevated liver function test results, hepatic failure, hepatomegaly, nausea, oral candidiasis, pseudomembranous colitis, vomiting
GU: Elevated BUN level, nephrotoxicity, renal failure, vaginal candidiasis
HEME: Eosinophilia, hemolytic anemia, hypoprothrombinemia, neutropenia, thrombocytopenia, unusual bleeding
MS: Arthralgia
RESP: Dyspnea
SKIN: Ecchymosis, erythema, erythema multiforme, pruritus, rash, Stevens-Johnson syndrome
Other: Anaphylaxis; injection site pain, redness, and swelling; superinfection

Nursing Considerations

• Use cefmetazole cautiously in patients hypersensitive to penicillin; cross-sensitivity has occurred in about 10% of such patients.
• If possible, obtain culture and sensitivity test results, as ordered, before giving drug.
• Reconstitute drug with sterile or bacteriostatic water for injection or sodium chloride for injection.

• Dilute primary solution as needed to 1 to 20 mg/ml in D_5W, normal saline solution, lactated Ringer's solution, or 1% lidocaine solution without epinephrine.
• Store reconstituted solution for up to 24 hours at room temperature or 7 days refrigerated.
• Monitor BUN and serum creatinine levels and fluid intake and output to detect early signs of nephrotoxicity.
• Assess bowel pattern daily; severe diarrhea may indicate pseudomembranous colitis.
• Assess for signs of superinfection, such as perineal itching, fever, malaise, redness, rash, diarrhea, and cough or sputum changes.
• Assess for pharyngitis, bleeding, and arthralgia, which may indicate blood dyscrasia. Monitor PT and bleeding time, as ordered.

PATIENT TEACHING
• Advise patient to report severe diarrhea to prescriber immediately.
• Instruct patient to avoid alcohol during therapy and for at least 3 days after last dose.

cefonicid sodium

Monocid

Class and Category

Chemical class: Second-generation cephalosporin, 7-aminocephalosporanic acid
Therapeutic class: Antibiotic
Pregnancy category: B

Indications and Dosages

➤ *To treat lower respiratory tract infections caused by* Escherichia coli, Haemophilus influenzae, Klebsiella pneumoniae, *and* Streptococcus pneumoniae; *UTI caused by* E. coli, K. pneumoniae, Morganella morganii, Proteus mirabilis, Proteus vulgaris, *and* Providencia rettgeri; *skin and soft-tissue infections caused by* Staphylococcus aureus, Staphylococcus epidermidis, Streptococcus agalactiae, *and* Streptococcus pyogenes; *septicemia caused by* E. coli *and* S. pneumoniae; *and bone and joint infections caused by* S. aureus

I.V. INFUSION, I.V. OR I.M. INJECTION

Adults. For mild to moderate infections, 1 g every 24 hr. For severe or life-threatening infections, 2 g every 24 hr.

➤ *To treat uncomplicated UTI*

I.V. INFUSION, I.V. OR I.M. INJECTION

Adults. 500 mg every 24 hr.

DOSAGE ADJUSTMENT Initial dose reduced to 75 mg/kg I.V. or I.M. in patients with impaired renal function. Then reduced to 10 to 25 mg/kg every 24 hr if creatinine clearance is 60 to 79 ml/min/1.73 m^2; 8 to 20 mg/kg every 24 hr if creatinine clearance is 40 to 59 ml/min/1.73 m^2; 4 to 15 mg/kg every 24 hr if creatinine clearance is 20 to 39 ml/min/1.73 m^2; 4 to 15 mg/kg every 48 hr if creatinine clearance is 10 to 19 ml/min/1.73 m^2; 4 to 15 mg/kg every 3 to 5 days if creatinine clearance is 5 to 9 ml/min/1.73 m^2; and 3 to 4 mg/kg every 3 to 5 days if creatinine clearance is less than 5 ml/min/1.73 m^2.

➤ *To provide surgical prophylaxis*

I.V. INFUSION, I.V. OR I.M. INJECTION

Adults. 1 g 60 min before surgery. Dose repeated once daily, if needed, for 2 days after prosthetic arthroplasty or open-heart surgery.

Mechanism of Action

Interferes with bacterial cell wall synthesis by inhibiting the final step in the cross-linking of peptidoglycan strands. Peptidoglycan makes cell membranes rigid and protective. Without it, bacterial cells rupture and die.

Incompatibilities

To prevent mutual inactivation, don't mix cefonicid with aminoglycosides.

Contraindications

Hypersensitivity to cephalosporins or their components

Interactions

DRUGS

aminoglycosides, loop diuretics: Increased risk of nephrotoxicity

Adverse Reactions

CNS: Chills, fever, headache, seizures
CV: Edema
EENT: Hearing loss
GI: Abdominal cramps, diarrhea, elevated liver function test results, hepatic failure, hepatomegaly, nausea, oral candidiasis, pseudomembranous colitis, vomiting
GU: Elevated BUN level, nephrotoxicity, renal failure, vaginal candidiasis
HEME: Eosinophilia, hemolytic anemia, hypoprothrombinemia, neutropenia, thrombocytopenia, unusual bleeding
MS: Arthralgia
RESP: Dyspnea
SKIN: Ecchymosis, erythema, erythema multiforme, pruritus, rash, Stevens-Johnson syndrome
Other: Anaphylaxis; injection-site pain, redness, and swelling; superinfection

Nursing Considerations

• Use cefonicid cautiously in patients with impaired renal function. Also use cautiously in patients hypersensitive to penicillin because cross-sensitivity has occurred in about 10% of such patients.

• If possible, obtain culture and sensitivity test results, as ordered, before giving drug.

• Reconstitute each 500-mg vial of drug with 2 ml sterile water for injection (or each 1-g vial with 2.5 ml).

• For I.V. infusion, dilute further in 50 to 100 ml compatible solution, such as D$_5$W, D$_{10}$W, dextrose 5% in quarter-normal (0.2) saline solution, dextrose 5% in half-normal (0.45) saline solution, or dextrose 5% in normal saline solution.

• Give I.V. injection slowly over 3 to 5 minutes through tubing of a flowing compatible I.V. solution.

• For I.M. dose larger than 1 g, divide dose in half and give into large muscle mass, such as the gluteus maximus, at two different sites.

• Reconstituted solution may be stored 24 hours at room temperature, 72 hours refrigerated.

• Monitor patient's BUN and serum creatinine levels to detect early signs of nephrotoxicity. Also monitor fluid intake and output; decreasing urine output may indicate nephrotoxicity.

• Assess patient's bowel pattern daily; severe diarrhea may indicate pseudomembranous colitis.

• Watch for evidence of superinfection, such as perineal itching, fever, malaise, redness, pain, swelling, drainage, rash, diarrhea, and cough or sputum changes.

C

• Assess patient for pharyngitis, ecchymosis, bleeding, and arthralgia; they may indicate a blood dyscrasia.

PATIENT TEACHING
• Warn patient that I.M. injection may be painful.
• Tell patient to report severe diarrhea to prescriber immediately.

cefoperazone sodium
Cefobid

Class and Category
Chemical class: Third-generation cephalosporin, 7-aminocephalosporanic acid
Therapeutic class: Antibiotic
Pregnancy category: B

Indications and Dosages
➤ *To treat respiratory tract infections caused by* Enterobacter *species,* Escherichia coli, Haemophilus influenzae, Klebsiella pneumoniae, Proteus mirabilis, Pseudomonas aeruginosa, Staphylococcus aureus, Streptococcus pneumoniae, Streptococcus pyogenes, *and other streptococci (excluding enterococci); UTI caused by* E. coli *and* P. aeruginosa; *uncomplicated gonorrhea caused by* Neisseria gonorrhoeae; *gynecologic infections caused by anaerobic grampositive cocci,* Bacteroides *species,* Clostridium *species,* E. coli, Staphylococcus epidermidis, *and* Streptococcus agalactiae; *bacterial septicemia caused by* E. coli, Klebsiella *species,* S. aureus, Serratia marcescens, *and streptococci; skin and soft-tissue infections caused by* P. aeruginosa, S. aureus, *and* S. pyogenes; *and intraabdominal infections caused by anaerobic gram-negative bacilli,* E. coli, *and* P. aeruginosa

I.V. INFUSION, I.M. INJECTION
Adults. 1 to 2 g every 12 hr. For severe infections or those caused by less sensitive organisms, 6 to 12 g daily divided into equal doses and given twice daily, three times daily, or four times daily. *Maximum:* 12 g daily.

Mechanism of Action
Interferes with bacterial cell wall synthesis by inhibiting the final step in the crosslinking of peptidoglycan strands. Peptidoglycan makes cell membranes rigid and protective. Without it, bacterial cells rupture and die.

Incompatibilities
To prevent mutual inactivation, don't mix cefoperazone with aminoglycosides. Also avoid mixing cefoperazone with other drugs, including pentamidine isethionate.

Contraindications
Hypersensitivity to cephalosporins or their components

Interactions
DRUGS
aminoglycosides, loop diuretics: Increased risk of nephrotoxicity
oral anticoagulants, other drugs that affect blood clotting: Increased anticoagulant effect
ACTIVITIES
alcohol use: Disulfiram-like reaction

Adverse Reactions
CNS: Chills, fever, headache, seizures
CV: Edema
EENT: Hearing loss
GI: Abdominal cramps, diarrhea, elevated liver function test results, hepatic failure, hepatomegaly, nausea, oral candidiasis, pseudomembranous colitis, vomiting
GU: Elevated BUN level, nephrotoxicity, renal failure, vaginal candidiasis
HEME: Eosinophilia, hemolytic anemia, hypoprothrombinemia, neutropenia, thrombocytopenia, unusual bleeding
MS: Arthralgia
RESP: Dyspnea
SKIN: Ecchymosis, erythema, erythema multiforme, pruritus, rash, Stevens-Johnson syndrome
Other: Anaphylaxis; injection-site pain, redness, and swelling; superinfection

Nursing Considerations
• Use cefoperazone cautiously in patients with a history of bleeding problems, GI disease (especially colitis), or severely impaired hepatic or renal function. Also use cautiously in patients hypersensitive to penicillin because cross-sensitivity has occurred in about 10% of such patients.

- If possible, obtain culture and sensitivity test results, as ordered, before giving drug.
- For I.V. use, reconstitute with required amount of diluent. Then further dilute in compatible solution, such as D_5W, $D_{10}W$, dextrose 5% in lactated Ringer's solution, dextrose 5% in quarter-normal (0.2) saline solution, dextrose 5% in normal saline solution, lactated Ringer's injection, normal saline solution, Normosol M and D_5W, or Normosol R. (See manufacturer's guidelines for details.)
- Give I.V. drug as intermittent infusion over 15 to 30 minutes or as continuous infusion. Direct bolus injection isn't recommended.
- For I.M. injection, reconstitute drug with bacteriostatic water for injection (that contains benzyl alcohol or parabens) or sterile water for injection.
- After reconstitution, let foam dissipate, and inspect the solution to ensure complete dissolution.
- Store reconstituted solution at room temperature for 24 hours.
- Monitor BUN and serum creatinine levels to detect early signs of nephrotoxicity. Also monitor fluid intake and output; decreasing urine output may indicate nephrotoxicity.
- Assess bowel pattern daily; severe diarrhea may indicate pseudomembranous colitis.
- Assess for pharyngitis, ecchymosis, bleeding, and arthralgia; they may indicate a blood dyscrasia.
- Assess for evidence of superinfection, such as perineal itching, fever, malaise, redness, pain, swelling, drainage, rash, diarrhea, and cough or sputum changes.

PATIENT TEACHING
- Advise patient to avoid alcohol during therapy and for at least 3 days after last dose.
- Explain that I.M. injection may hurt.
- Tell patient to immediately report severe diarrhea to prescriber.

cefotaxime sodium

Claforan

Class and Category
Chemical class: Third-generation cephalosporin, 7-aminocephalosporanic acid
Therapeutic class: Antibiotic
Pregnancy category: B

Indications and Dosages
➤ *To provide perioperative prophylaxis*
I.V. INFUSION, I.V. OR I.M. INJECTION
Adults and children weighing more than 50 kg (110 lb). 1 g 30 to 90 min before surgery.
➤ *To provide perioperative prophylaxis related to cesarean section*
I.V. INFUSION, I.V. OR I.M. INJECTION
Adults. 1 g as soon as cord is clamped, then 1 g every 6 hr for up to two doses.
➤ *To treat gonococcal urethritis and cervicitis in men and women*
I.M. INJECTION
Adults weighing more than 50 kg. 500 mg as a single dose.
➤ *To treat rectal gonorrhea in women*
I.M. INJECTION
Adults weighing more than 50 kg. 500 mg as a single dose.
➤ *To treat rectal gonorrhea in men*
I.M. INJECTION
Adults weighing more than 50 kg. 1 g as a single dose.
➤ *To treat disseminated gonorrhea*
I.V. INFUSION OR INJECTION
Adults and children weighing more than 50 kg. 1 g every 8 hr.
➤ *To treat uncomplicated infections caused by susceptible organisms*
I.V. INFUSION, I.V. OR I.M. INJECTION
Adults and children weighing more than 50 kg. 1 g every 12 hr.
Children ages 1 month to 12 years weighing less than 50 kg. 50 to 180 mg/kg daily in four to six divided doses.
Children ages 1 to 4 weeks. 50 mg/kg I.V. every 8 hr.
Children age 1 week and under. 50 mg/kg I.V. every 12 hr.
➤ *To treat moderate to severe infections caused by susceptible organisms*
I.V. INFUSION, I.V. OR I.M. INJECTION
Adults and children weighing more than 50 kg. 1 to 2 g every 8 hr.
Children ages 1 month to 12 years weighing less than 50 kg. 50 to 180 mg/kg daily in four to six divided doses. For more

serious infections, including meningitis, higher dosages are used.

Children ages 1 to 4 weeks. 50 mg/kg I.V. every 8 hr.

Children age 1 week and younger. 50 mg/kg I.V. every 12 hr.

➤ *To treat septicemia and other infections that commonly require antibiotics in higher doses than those used to treat moderate to severe infections*

I.V. INFUSION OR INJECTION

Adults and children weighing more than 50 kg. 2 g every 6 to 8 hr.

➤ *To treat life-threatening infections caused by susceptible organisms*

I.V. INFUSION OR INJECTION

Adults and children weighing more than 50 kg. 2 g every 4 hr. *Maximum:* 12 g daily.

Children ages 1 month to 12 years weighing less than 50 kg. 50 to 180 mg/kg daily in four to six divided doses.

Children ages 1 to 4 weeks. 50 mg/kg every 8 hr.

Children age 1 week and younger. 50 mg/kg every 12 hr.

DOSAGE ADJUSTMENT Dosage reduced by 50% for patients with estimated creatinine clearance below 20 ml/min/1.73 m².

Mechanism of Action

Interferes with bacterial cell wall synthesis by inhibiting cross-linking of peptidoglycan strands. Peptidoglycan makes cell membranes rigid and protective. Without it, bacterial cells rupture and die.

Incompatibilities

To prevent mutual inactivation, don't mix cefotaxime with aminoglycosides. Also avoid mixing cefotaxime with other drugs, including pentamidine isethionate.

Contraindications

Hypersensitivity to cephalosporins or their components

Interactions

DRUGS

aminoglycosides, loop diuretics: Increased risk of nephrotoxicity

probenecid: Increased and prolonged blood cefotaxime level

Adverse Reactions

CNS: Chills, fever, headache, seizures

CV: Edema

EENT: Hearing loss

GI: Abdominal cramps, cholestasis, diarrhea, elevated liver function test results, hepatic failure, hepatitis, hepatomegaly, jaundice, nausea, oral candidiasis, pseudomembranous colitis, vomiting

GU: Elevated BUN level, nephrotoxicity, renal failure, vaginal candidiasis

HEME: Eosinophilia, hemolytic anemia, hypoprothrombinemia, neutropenia, thrombocytopenia, unusual bleeding

MS: Arthralgia

RESP: Dyspnea

SKIN: Ecchymosis, erythema, erythema multiforme, pruritus, rash, Stevens-Johnson syndrome, toxic epidermal necrolysis

Other: Anaphylaxis; injection-site pain, redness, and swelling; superinfection

Nursing Considerations

• Use cefotaxime cautiously in patients with impaired renal function, a history of GI disease (especially colitis), or hypersensitivity to penicillin because crosssensitivity has occurred in about 10% of such patients.

• If possible, obtain culture and sensitivity test results, as ordered, before giving drug.

• For I.V. use, reconstitute each 0.5-, 1-, or 2-g vial with 10 ml of sterile water for injection. Shake to dissolve.

• For intermittent I.V. infusion, further dilute in 50 to 100 ml of D₅W or normal saline solution.

• For I.M. use, reconstitute each 500-mg vial with 2 ml sterile water for injection or bacteriostatic water for injection; each 1-g vial with 3 ml diluent; and each 2-g vial with 5 ml diluent. Shake to dissolve.

WARNING When preparing drug for a neonate, don't use diluent that contains benzyl alcohol; it could cause a fatal toxic syndrome.

• Give cefotaxime by I.V. injection over 3 to 5 minutes through tubing of a free-flowing compatible I.V. solution. Temporarily stop other solutions being given through same I.V. site.

• Discard unused drug after 24 hours if stored at room temperature, 5 days if refrigerated.

• Protect cefotaxime powder and solution from light and heat.
• Monitor I.V. sites for signs of phlebitis or extravasation. Rotate I.V. sites every 72 hours.
• Monitor BUN and serum creatinine levels and fluid intake and output for signs of nephrotoxicity.
• Be aware that allergic reaction may occur a few days after cefotaxime therapy starts.
• Assess bowel pattern daily; severe diarrhea may indicate pseudomembranous colitis caused by *Clostridium difficile*. If diarrhea occurs, notify prescriber and expect to withhold cefotaxime and treat with fluids, electrolytes, protein, and an antibiotic effective against *C. difficile*.
• Assess patient for pharyngitis, ecchymosis, bleeding, and arthralgia, which may indicate a blood dyscrasia. Monitor CBC, PT, and bleeding time, as ordered.
• Monitor patient closely for superinfection. If evidence appears, notify prescriber and expect to stop drug and provide care.
• Be aware that cephalosporins, such as cefotaxime, may produce a positive direct Coombs' test.

PATIENT TEACHING
• Explain that I.M. injection may be painful.
• Instruct patient to report watery, bloody stools to prescriber immediately, even up to 2 months after drug therapy has ended.

cefotetan disodium
Cefotan

Class and Category
Chemical class: Second-generation cephalosporin, 7-aminocephalosporanic acid
Therapeutic class: Antibiotic
Pregnancy category: B

Indications and Dosages
➤ *To provide surgical prophylaxis*
I.V. INJECTION
Adults. 1 to 2 g 30 to 60 min before surgery or, in cesarean section, as soon as cord is clamped.

➤ *To treat lower respiratory tract infections caused by* Escherichia coli, Haemophilus influenzae, Klebsiella *species,* Proteus mirabilis, Serratia marcescens, Staphylococcus aureus, *and* Streptococcus pneumoniae; *gynecologic infections caused by* Bacteroides *species (excluding* B. distasonis, B. ovatus, *and* B. thetaiotaomicron)*,* E. coli, Fusobacterium *species, gram-positive anaerobic cocci,* Neisseria gonorrhoeae, P. mirabilis, S. aureus, Staphylococcus epidermidis, *and* Streptococcus *species (excluding enterococci); intra-abdominal infections caused by* Bacteroides *species (excluding* B. distasonis, B. ovatus, *and* B. thetaiotaomicron)*,* Clostridium *species,* E. coli, Klebsiella *species, and* Streptococcus *species (excluding enterococci); and bone and joint infections caused by* S. aureus
I.V. INFUSION, I.V. OR I.M. INJECTION
Adults. For mild to moderate infections, 1 to 2 g every 12 hr.
I.V. INFUSION OR INJECTION
Adults. For severe infections, 2 g every 12 hr; for life-threatening infections, 3 g every 12 hr.

➤ *To treat UTI caused by* E. coli, Klebsiella *species, or* Proteus *species*
I.V. INFUSION, I.V. OR I.M. INJECTION
Adults. 0.5 to 2 g every 12 hr or 1 to 2 g every 24 hr.

➤ *To treat skin and soft-tissue infections caused by* E. coli, Klebsiella pneumoniae, Peptostreptococcus *species,* S. aureus, S. epidermidis, Streptococcus pyogenes, *and* Streptococcus *species (excluding enterococci)*
I.V. INFUSION, I.V. OR I.M. INJECTION
Adults. For mild to moderate infections due to *K. pneumoniae*, 1 or 2 g every 12 hr. For mild to moderate infections caused by other organisms, 1 g I.M. or I.V. every 12 hr or 2 g I.V. every 24 hr; for severe infections, 2 g I.V. every 12 hr.
DOSAGE ADJUSTMENT Dosing interval reduced to 24 hr if creatinine clearance is 10 to 30 ml/min/1.73 m^2 and to 48 hr if creatinine clearance is less than 10 ml/min/1.73 m^2.

Mechanism of Action
Interferes with bacterial cell wall synthesis by inhibiting the final step in the cross-

linking of peptidoglycan strands. Peptidoglycan makes cell membranes rigid and protective. Without it, bacterial cells rupture and die.

Incompatibilities
To prevent mutual inactivation, don't mix cefotetan with aminoglycosides.

Contraindications
Hypersensitivity to cephalosporins or their components

Interactions
DRUGS
aminoglycosides, loop diuretics: Increased risk of nephrotoxicity
oral anticoagulants, other drugs that affect blood clotting: Enhanced anticoagulant effect
probenecid: Increased and prolonged blood cefotetan level
ACTIVITIES
alcohol use: Disulfiram-like reaction

Adverse Reactions
CNS: Chills, fever, headache, seizures
CV: Edema
EENT: Hearing loss
GI: Abdominal cramps, diarrhea, elevated liver function test results, hepatic failure, hepatomegaly, nausea, oral candidiasis, pseudomembranous colitis, vomiting
GU: Elevated BUN level, nephrotoxicity, renal failure, vaginal candidiasis
HEME: Eosinophilia, hemolytic anemia, hypoprothrombinemia, neutropenia, thrombocytopenia, unusual bleeding
MS: Arthralgia
RESP: Dyspnea
SKIN: Ecchymosis, erythema, erythema multiforme, pruritus, rash, Stevens-Johnson syndrome
Other: Anaphylaxis; injection-site pain, redness, and swelling; superinfection

Nursing Considerations
• Use cefotetan cautiously in patients with impaired renal function or a history of GI disease, especially colitis. Also use cautiously in patients hypersensitive to penicillin because cross-sensitivity has occurred in about 10% of such patients.
• If possible, obtain culture and sensitivity test results, as ordered, before giving drug.

• For I.V. use, reconstitute each 1-g vial of drug with 10 ml sterile water for injection. For each 2-g vial, use 10 to 20 ml diluent. For I.V. infusion, further dilute solution in 50 to 100 ml D_5W or normal saline solution.
• For direct I.V. injection, give drug slowly over 3 to 5 minutes through tubing of a flowing compatible I.V. solution.
• For I.M. use, reconstitute each 1-g vial of drug with 2 ml of sterile or bacteriostatic water for injection, or sodium chloride for injection. For a 2-g vial, use 3 ml diluent.
• Monitor I.V. site for signs and symptoms of phlebitis and extravasation; rotate sites every 72 hours.
• Protect reconstituted solution from light, and store for up to 24 hours at room temperature or 96 hours under refrigeration.
• Be aware than an allergic reaction may occur a few days after therapy starts.
• Monitor BUN and serum creatinine levels and fluid intake and output for signs of nephrotoxicity.
• Monitor patient receiving even short-term cefotetan therapy for signs and symptoms of hemolytic anemia, such as marked pallor and fatigue.
• If patient receives long-term therapy, monitor CBC and serum AST, ALT, bilirubin, LD, and alkaline phosphatase levels.
• Assess patient's bowel pattern daily; severe diarrhea may indicate pseudomembranous colitis.
• Watch for pharyngitis, ecchymosis, bleeding, and arthralgia, which may indicate a blood dyscrasia. Monitor PT and bleeding time, as ordered. Be prepared to give vitamin K, if ordered, to treat hypoprothrombinemia.
PATIENT TEACHING
• Explain that I.M. injection may be painful.
• Tell patient to immediately report severe diarrhea to prescriber.
• Urge patient to avoid alcohol during and for at least 3 days after cefotetan therapy.

cefoxitin sodium
Mefoxin

Class and Category

Chemical class: Second-generation cephalosporin, 7-aminocephalosporanic acid
Therapeutic class: Antibiotic
Pregnancy category: B

Indications and Dosages

➤ *To provide surgical prophylaxis*

I.V. INFUSION OR INJECTION

Adults. 2 g 30 to 60 min before surgery and then 2 g every 6 hr after first dose for up to 24 hr.

Children age 3 months or over. 30 to 40 mg/kg 30 to 60 min before surgery and every 6 hr after first dose for up to 24 hr.

➤ *To provide surgical prophylaxis for cesarean section*

I.V. INFUSION OR INJECTION

Adults. 2 g as a single dose as soon as cord is clamped; or 2 g as soon as cord is clamped, followed by 2 g 4 and 8 hr after initial dose.

➤ *To provide surgical prophylaxis for transurethral prostatectomy*

I.V. INFUSION OR INJECTION

Adults. 1 g 30 to 60 min before surgery and then 1 g every 8 hr for up to 5 days.

➤ *To treat infections, including septicemia, gynecologic infections, intra-abdominal infections, UTI, and infections of the lower respiratory tract, skin, soft tissue, bones, and joints caused by anaerobes (including* Bacteroides *species,* Clostridium *species,* Fusobacterium *species,* Peptococcus niger, *and* Peptostreptococcus *species), gram-negative organisms (including* Escherichia coli, Haemophilus influenzae *[also ampicillin-resistant strains],* Klebsiella, *and* Proteus *species), and gram-positive organisms (including* Staphylococcus aureus *[penicillinase- and non–penicillinase-producing strains],* Staphylococcus epidermidis, Streptococcus agalactiae, Streptococcus pneumoniae, *and* Streptococcus pyogenes)*

I.V. INFUSION OR INJECTION

Adults. For uncomplicated infections, 1 g every 6 to 8 hr; for moderate to severe infections, 1 g every 4 hr or 2 g every 6 to 8 hr. For infections that commonly require high-dose antibiotics (such as gas gangrene), 2 g every 4 hr, or 3 g every 6 hr.

Children age 3 months or over. 80 to 160 mg/kg daily in equal doses given every 4 to 6 hr (higher dosages used for more severe infections). *Maximum:* 12 g daily.

➤ *To treat uncomplicated gonorrhea*

I.M. INJECTION

Adults. 2 g as a single dose along with 1 g oral probenecid concurrently or within 30 min of cefoxitin.

DOSAGE ADJUSTMENT Dosage reduced to 1 to 2 g every 8 to 12 hr if creatinine clearance is 30 to 50 ml/min/1.73 m^2; 1 to 2 g every 12 to 24 hr if clearance is 10 to 29 ml/min/1.73 m^2; 0.5 to 1 g every 12 to 24 hr if clearance is 5 to 9 ml/min/1.73 m^2; and 0.5 to 1 g every 24 to 48 hr if clearance is less than 5 ml/min/1.73 m^2.

Mechanism of Action

Interferes with bacterial cell wall synthesis by inhibiting the final step in the cross-linking of peptidoglycan strands. Peptidoglycan makes cell membranes rigid and protective. Without it, bacterial cells rupture and die.

Incompatibilities

To prevent mutual inactivation, don't mix cefoxitin with aminoglycosides. Also avoid mixing cefoxitin with other drugs, including pentamidine isethionate.

Contraindications

Hypersensitivity to cephalosporins or their components

Interactions

DRUGS

aminoglycosides, loop diuretics: Increased risk of nephrotoxicity

Adverse Reactions

CNS: Chills, fever, headache, seizures
CV: Edema
EENT: Hearing loss
GI: Abdominal cramps, diarrhea, elevated liver function test results, hepatic failure, hepatomegaly, nausea, oral candidiasis, pseudomembranous colitis, vomiting
GU: Elevated BUN level, nephrotoxicity, renal failure, vaginal candidiasis
HEME: Eosinophilia, hemolytic anemia, hypoprothrombinemia, neutropenia, thrombocytopenia, unusual bleeding
MS: Arthralgia
RESP: Dyspnea

SKIN: Ecchymosis, erythema, erythema multiforme, flushing, pruritus, rash, Stevens-Johnson syndrome, urticaria
Other: Anaphylaxis; injection-site pain, redness, and swelling; superinfection

Nursing Considerations

• Use cefoxitin cautiously in patients hypersensitive to penicillin; cross-sensitivity has occurred in about 10% of such patients.
• Also use cautiously in patients with a history of GI disease, particularly colitis, because of an increased risk of pseudomembranous colitis.
• If possible, obtain culture and sensitivity test results, as ordered, before giving drug.
• For I.V. use, reconstitute 1 g with 10 ml sterile water for injection, or 2 g with 10 to 20 ml diluent.
• For I.V. injection, give slowly over 3 to 5 minutes through tubing of a flowing compatible I.V. solution.
• For intermittent infusion, further dilute with 50 to 100 ml D₅W or normal saline solution.
• For continuous high-dose infusion, add cefoxitin to I.V. solutions of D₅W, normal saline solution, or dextrose 5% in normal saline solution.
• For I.M. use, reconstitute each 1 g with 2 ml sterile water for injection.
• Discard unused drug after 24 hours if stored at room temperature, or after 1 week if refrigerated.
• Be aware that powder or solution may darken during storage, which doesn't reflect altered potency.
• Be aware that an allergic reaction may occur a few days after therapy starts.
• Monitor BUN and serum creatinine for early signs of nephrotoxicity. Also monitor fluid intake and output; decreasing urine output may indicate nephrotoxicity.
• Assess patient's bowel pattern daily; severe diarrhea may indicate pseudomembranous colitis.
• Assess for pharyngitis, ecchymosis, bleeding, and arthralgia; they may indicate a blood dyscrasia.

PATIENT TEACHING
• Tell patient to report severe diarrhea to prescriber immediately.
• Instruct patient to complete the course of therapy as prescribed.

cefpodoxime proxetil

Vantin

Class and Category

Chemical class: Third-generation cephalosporin, 7-aminocephalosporanic acid
Therapeutic class: Antibiotic
Pregnancy category: B

Indications and Dosages

➤ *To treat acute community-acquired pneumonia caused by* Haemophilus influenzae *or* Streptococcus pneumoniae

ORAL SUSPENSION, TABLETS
Adults and adolescents over age 13.
200 mg every 12 hr for 14 days.

➤ *To treat acute bacterial exacerbation of chronic bronchitis caused by* H. influenzae, Moraxella catarrhalis, *or* S. pneumoniae

TABLETS
Adults and adolescents over age 13.
200 mg every 12 hr for 10 days.

➤ *To treat uncomplicated gonorrhea in men and women and rectal gonococcal infections in women caused by* Neisseria gonorrhoeae

ORAL SUSPENSION, TABLETS
Adults. 200 mg as a single dose.

➤ *To treat uncomplicated UTI caused by* Escherichia coli, Klebsiella pneumoniae, Proteus mirabilis, *or* Staphylococcus saprophyticus

ORAL SUSPENSION, TABLETS
Adults. 100 mg every 12 hr for 7 days.

➤ *To treat skin and soft-tissue infections caused by* Staphylococcus aureus *or* Staphylococcus pyogenes

ORAL SUSPENSION, TABLETS
Adults and adolescents over age 13.
400 mg every 12 hr for 7 to 14 days.

➤ *To treat acute otitis media caused by* H. influenzae, M. catarrhalis, *or* S. pneumoniae

ORAL SUSPENSION, TABLETS
Children ages 5 months through 12 years.
5 mg/kg every 12 hr (*maximum:* 200 mg/ dose) or 10 mg/kg every 24 hr (*maximum:* 400 mg/dose) for 10 days.

➤ *To treat pharyngitis and tonsillitis caused by* S. pyogenes

ORAL SUSPENSION, TABLETS
Adults and adolescents over age 13.
100 mg every 12 hr for 5 to 10 days.
Children ages 2 months through 12 years.
5 mg/kg every 12 hr for 5 to 10 days.
Maximum: 100 mg/dose.
DOSAGE ADJUSTMENT Dosing interval
increased to 24 hr in patients with
creatinine clearance less than 30 ml/
min/1.73 m².

Mechanism of Action

Interferes with bacterial cell wall synthesis
by inhibiting the final step in the cross-
linking of peptidoglycan strands.
Peptidoglycan makes cell membranes rigid
and protective. Without it, bacterial cells
rupture and die.

Contraindications

Hypersensitivity to cephalosporins or their
components

Interactions
DRUGS
aminoglycosides, loop diuretics: Increased
risk of nephrotoxicity
antacids, H₂-receptor antagonists: Reduced
bioavailability and blood level of
cefpodoxime
oral anticholinergics: Delayed peak blood
level of cefpodoxime
probenecid: Possibly increased and
prolonged blood cefpodoxime level

Adverse Reactions

CNS: Chills, fever, headache, seizures
CV: Edema
EENT: Hearing loss
GI: Abdominal cramps, diarrhea,
elevated liver function test results, hepatic
failure, hepatomegaly, nausea, oral
candidiasis, pseudomembranous colitis,
vomiting
GU: Elevated BUN level, nephrotoxicity,
renal failure, vaginal candidiasis
HEME: Eosinophilia, hemolytic anemia,
hypoprothrombinemia, neutropenia,
thrombocytopenia, unusual bleeding
MS: Arthralgia
RESP: Dyspnea
SKIN: Ecchymosis, erythema, erythema
multiforme, pruritus, rash, Stevens-Johnson
syndrome
Other: Anaphylaxis, superinfection

Nursing Considerations

• Use cefpodoxime cautiously in patients
who have impaired renal function or
are receiving potent diuretics. Also use
drug cautiously in patients hypersensitive
to penicillin because cross-sensitivity
has occurred in about 10% of such patients.
• If possible, obtain culture and sensitivity
test results, as ordered, before giving
cefpodoxime.
• Assess patient's bowel pattern daily; severe
diarrhea may indicate pseudomembranous
colitis.
• Be aware that an allergic reaction may
occur a few days after therapy starts.
PATIENT TEACHING
• Urge patient to complete the prescribed
course of therapy.
• Tell patient to take tablets with food to
enhance absorption.
• Advise patient to refrigerate oral
suspension and discard after 14 days.
• Instruct patient to shake oral suspension
bottle well before pouring dose and to use
a calibrated liquid-measuring device to
ensure accurate doses.
• Inform patient that yogurt and buttermilk
can help maintain intestinal flora and
decrease diarrhea.
• Warn patient not to take an antacid within
2 hours before or after taking
cefpodoxime.
• Tell patient to report watery, bloody stools
to prescriber immediately, even up to
2 months after drug therapy has ended.

cefprozil
Cefzil

Class and Category

Chemical class: Second-generation
cephalosporin, 7-aminocephalosporanic acid
Therapeutic class: Antibiotic
Pregnancy category: B

Indications and Dosages

➤ *To treat secondary bacterial infections
in patients with acute bronchitis and
acute bacterial exacerbations of acute
bronchitis caused by* Haemophilus
influenzae, Moraxella catarrhalis, *and*
Streptococcus pneumoniae

ORAL SUSPENSION, TABLETS
Adults and adolescents. 500 mg every 12 hr for 10 days.
➤ *To treat uncomplicated skin and soft-tissue infections caused by* Staphylococcus aureus *and* Streptococcus pyogenes
ORAL SUSPENSION, TABLETS
Adults and adolescents. 250 mg every 12 hr or 500 mg every 12 to 24 hr for 10 days.
Children ages 2 to 12. 20 mg/kg every 24 hr for 10 days.
➤ *To treat pharyngitis and tonsillitis caused by* S. pyogenes
ORAL SUSPENSION, TABLETS
Adults and adolescents. 500 mg every 24 hr for 10 days.
Children ages 2 to 12. 7.5 mg/kg every 12 hr for 10 days.
➤ *To treat otitis media caused by* H. influenzae, M. catarrhalis, *and* S. pneumoniae
ORAL SUSPENSION, TABLETS
Children ages 6 months to 12 years. 15 mg/kg every 12 hr for 10 days.
➤ *To treat acute sinusitis caused by* H. influenzae, M. catarrhalis, *and* S. pneumoniae
ORAL SUSPENSION, TABLETS
Adults and adolescents. 250 to 500 mg every 12 hr for 10 days.
Children ages 6 months to 12 years. 7.5 or 15 mg/kg every 12 hr for 10 days.
DOSAGE ADJUSTMENT Dosage reduced by half and given at usual intervals in patients with creatinine clearance less than 30 ml/min/1.73 m².

Mechanism of Action

Interferes with bacterial cell wall synthesis by inhibiting the final step in the cross-linking of peptidoglycan strands. Peptidoglycan makes the cell membrane rigid and protective. Without it, bacterial cells rupture and die.

Contraindications

Hypersensitivity to cephalosporins or their components

Interactions

DRUGS
aminoglycosides, loop diuretics: Increased risk of nephrotoxicity
probenecid: Increased blood cefprozil level

Adverse Reactions

CNS: Chills, fever, headache, seizures
CV: Edema
EENT: Hearing loss
GI: Abdominal cramps, diarrhea, elevated liver function test results, hepatic failure, hepatomegaly, nausea, oral candidiasis, pseudomembranous colitis, vomiting
GU: Elevated BUN level, nephrotoxicity, renal failure, vaginal candidiasis
HEME: Eosinophilia, hemolytic anemia, hypoprothrombinemia, neutropenia, thrombocytopenia, unusual bleeding
MS: Arthralgia
RESP: Dyspnea
SKIN: Ecchymosis, erythema, erythema multiforme, pruritus, rash, Stevens-Johnson syndrome
Other: Anaphylaxis, superinfection

Nursing Considerations

• Use cefprozil cautiously in patients who have impaired renal function or a history of GI disease, especially colitis. Also use drug cautiously in patients who are hypersensitive to penicillin because cross-sensitivity has occurred in about 10% of such patients.
• If possible, obtain culture and sensitivity test results, as ordered, before giving drug.
WARNING Don't administer oral suspension to patients with phenylketonuria because it contains phenylalanine 28 mg/5 ml.
• Monitor BUN and serum creatinine levels to detect early signs of nephrotoxicity. Also monitor fluid intake and output; decreasing urine output may indicate nephrotoxicity.
• Be aware that an allergic reaction may occur a few days after therapy starts.
• Assess patient's bowel pattern daily; severe diarrhea may indicate pseudomembranous colitis.

PATIENT TEACHING
• Urge patient to complete the prescribed course of therapy.
• Tell patient to refrigerate oral suspension and discard after 14 days.
• Instruct patient to shake oral suspension well before pouring and to use a

calibrated measuring device to ensure accurate doses.
- Inform patient that yogurt and buttermilk can help maintain intestinal flora and decrease diarrhea.
- Tell patient to report watery, bloody stools to prescriber immediately, even up to 2 months after drug therapy has ended.

ceftaroline fosamil
Teflaro

Class and Category
Chemical class: Fifth-generation cephalosporin, 7-aminocephalosporanic acid
Therapeutic class: Antibiotic
Pregnancy category: B

Indications and Dosages
➤ *To treat acute bacterial skin and skin structure infection caused by* Staphylococcus aureus, Streptococcus pyogenes, Streptococcus agalactiae, Escherichia coli, Klebsiella pneumoniae, *and* Klebsiella oxytoca

I.V. INFUSION
Adults. 600 mg administered over 1 hr every 12 hr for 5 to 14 days.

➤ *To treat community-acquired bacterial pneumonia caused by* Streptococcus pneumoniae, Staphylococcus aureus, Haemophilus influenzae, Klebsiella pneumoniae, Klebsiella oxytoca, *and* Escherichia coli

I.V. INFUSION
Adults. 600 mg administered over 1 hr every 12 hr for 5 to 7 days.

DOSAGE ADJUSTMENT For patients with a creatinine clearance above 30 ml/min but no higher than 50 ml/min, dosage reduced to 400 mg every 12 hr; for patients with a creatinine clearance above 15 ml/min but no higher than 30 ml/min, dosage reduced to 300 mg every 12 hr; for patients with a creatinine clearance of less than 15 ml/min including those on hemodialysis, dosage reduced to 200 mg every 12 hr.

Mechanism of Action
Interferes with bacterial cell wall synthesis by inhibiting the final step in the cross-linking of peptidoglycan strands. Peptidoglycan makes the cell membrane rigid and protective. Without it, bacterial cells rupture and die. Ceftaroline is unique in that it is effective against methicillin-resistant *Staphylococcus aureus,* unlike other cephalosporins.

Incompatibilities
Don't mix parenteral ceftaroline with any other drug because compatibility is not known.

Contraindications
Hypersensitivity to cephalosporins or their components

Adverse Reactions
CNS: Dizziness, fever, seizures
CV: Bradycardia, palpitations, phlebitis
ENDO: Hyperglycemia
GI: Abdominal pain, *Clostridium difficile*–associated diarrhea, constipation, diarrhea, elevated liver enzymes, hepatitis, nausea, vomiting
GU: Renal failure
HEME: Anemia (including hemolytic anemia), eosinophilia, neutropenia, thrombocytopenia
SKIN: Rash, urticaria
Other: Anaphylaxis, direct Coombs' test seroconversion, hyperkalemia, hypokalemia, hypersensitivity reactions

Nursing Considerations
- Use ceftaroline cautiously in patients hypersensitive to penicillins or carbapenems because cross-sensitivity may occur.
- If possible, obtain culture and sensitivity results, as ordered, before giving drug.
- Reconstitute each drug vial with 20 ml of sterile water for injection. Mix gently to ensure drug is completely dissolved. Color may range from clear to light to dark yellow, depending on the concentration and storage conditions. Then further dilute in 250 ml of appropriate solution such as normal saline solution, dextrose in water, half normal saline, or lactated Ringer's solution.
- Infuse reconstituted solution within 6 hours of mixing if stored at room temperature or within 24 hours if refrigerated.
- Administer as an I.V. infusion over 1 hour.

• Monitor patient for hypersensitivity to ceftaroline. If present, discontinue ceftaroline, as ordered, and prepare to provide emergency supportive care.
• Assess bowel pattern daily; severe diarrhea may indicate pseudomembranous colitis caused by *Clostridium difficile*. If diarrhea occurs, notify prescriber and expect to withhold drug and treat with fluids, electrolytes, protein, and an antibiotic effective against *C. difficile*.
• Be aware that seroconversion from a negative to a positive direct Coombs' test result may occur. If anemia develops during or after ceftaroline therapy, expect a direct Coombs' test to be ordered. If drug-induced hemolytic anemia is suspected, expect to discontinue the drug and provide supportive care, as indicated.

PATIENT TEACHING
• Urge patient to report hypersensitivity reactions, such as a rash, immediately.
• Instruct patient to report watery, bloody stools to prescriber immediately, even up to 2 months after drug therapy has ended.

ceftazidime

Ceptaz, Fortaz, Tazicef, Tazidime

Class and Category
Chemical class: Third-generation cephalosporin, 7-aminocephalosporanic acid
Therapeutic class: Antibiotic
Pregnancy category: B

Indications and Dosages
➤ *To treat infections caused by gram-negative organisms (including* Acinetobacter, Citrobacter, Enterobacter, Escherichia coli, Haemophilus influenzae, Klebsiella, Neisseria, Proteus mirabilis, Proteus vulgaris, Pseudomonas aeruginosa, Salmonella, Serratia, *and* Shigella*), gram-positive organisms (including* Streptococcus agalactiae, Streptococcus pneumoniae, *and* Streptococcus pyogenes *[group B streptococci]), as well as* Staphylococcus aureus *(penicillinase-and non–penicillinase-producing strains)*

I.V. INFUSION, I.M. INJECTION
Adults and children age 12 and over. 1 g every 8 to 12 hr.
I.V. INFUSION
Children ages 1 month to 12 years. 30 to 50 mg/kg every 8 hr.
Neonates up to age 1 month. 30 mg/kg every 12 hr. *Maximum:* 6 g daily.
➤ *To treat uncomplicated UTI*
I.V. INFUSION, I.M. INJECTION
Adults and children age 12 and over. 250 mg every 12 hr.
➤ *To treat complicated UTI*
I.V. INFUSION, I.M. INJECTION
Adults and children age 12 and over. 500 mg every 8 to 12 hr.
➤ *To treat uncomplicated pneumonia and mild skin and soft-tissue infections*
I.V. INFUSION, I.M. INJECTION
Adults and children age 12 and over. 0.5 to 1 g every 8 hr.
➤ *To treat bone and joint infections*
I.V. INFUSION
Adults and children age 12 and over. 2 g every 12 hr.
➤ *To treat serious gynecologic and intra-abdominal infections, meningitis, and life-threatening infections, especially in immunocompromised patients*
I.V. INFUSION
Adults and children age 12 and over. 2 g every 8 hr.
➤ *To treat pseudomonal lung infection in patients with cystic fibrosis and normal renal function*
I.V. INFUSION
Adults and children age 1 month and over. 30 to 50 mg/kg every 8 hr. *Maximum:* 6 g daily.
Neonates up to age 1 month. 30 mg/kg every 12 hr.
DOSAGE ADJUSTMENT Dosage reduced to 1 g every 12 hr if creatinine clearance is 31 to 50 ml/min/1.73 m^2; to 1 g every 24 hr if 16 to 30 ml/min/1.73 m^2; to 0.5 g every 24 hr if 6 to 15 ml/min/1.73 m^2; and to 0.5 g every 48 hr if less than 6 ml/min/1.73 m^2.

Mechanism of Action
Interferes with bacterial cell wall synthesis by inhibiting the cross-linking of peptidoglycan strands. Peptidoglycan makes the cell membrane rigid and protective. Without it, bacterial cells rupture and die.

Incompatibilities

Don't mix ceftazidime with aminoglycosides to prevent mutual inactivation. Vancomycin is physically incompatible with ceftazidime (precipitate may form); flush I.V. line between these drugs if given through same tubing. Avoid mixing ceftazidime with other drugs, including pentamidine isethionate.

Contraindications

Hypersensitivity to cephalosporins or their components

Interactions

DRUGS

aminoglycosides, loop diuretics: Increased risk of nephrotoxicity
oral combined estrogen-progesterone contraceptives: Decreased effectiveness of oral contraceptive

Adverse Reactions

CNS: Chills, fever, headache, seizures
CV: Edema
EENT: Hearing loss
GI: Abdominal cramps, diarrhea, elevated liver function test results, hepatic failure, hepatomegaly, nausea, oral candidiasis, pseudomembranous colitis, vomiting
GU: Elevated BUN level, nephrotoxicity, renal failure, vaginal candidiasis
HEME: Eosinophilia, hemolytic anemia, hypoprothrombinemia, neutropenia, thrombocytopenia, unusual bleeding
MS: Arthralgia
RESP: Dyspnea
SKIN: Ecchymosis, erythema, erythema multiforme, pruritus, rash, Stevens-Johnson syndrome
Other: Anaphylaxis; injection site pain, redness, and swelling; superinfection

Nursing Considerations

• Use ceftazidime cautiously in patients hypersensitive to penicillin because cross-sensitivity occurs in about 10% of such patients. Watch for allergic reactions a few days after therapy starts.
• Use cautiously in patients with a history of GI disease, particularly colitis, because risk of pseudomembranous colitis is increased.
• Ceftazidime l-arginine (Ceptaz) is not recommended for children under age 12.

• If possible, obtain culture and sensitivity test results, as ordered, before giving drug.
• Protect ceftazidime powder and reconstituted drug from heat and light; both tend to darken during storage.
• If pharmacy delivers frozen solution, thaw it at room temperature, not in water bath or microwave. Store thawed solution for up to 12 hours at room temperature or 7 days in refrigerator; don't refreeze.
WARNING When preparing drug for neonates or immature infants, don't use diluents containing benzyl alcohol because they are linked to a fatal toxic syndrome.
• For I.V. bolus, reconstitute 1 to 2 g with 10 ml sterile water for injection, D_5W, or sodium chloride for injection. Shake to dissolve. Administer I.V. injection slowly over 3 to 5 minutes through tubing of a flowing compatible I.V. fluid.
• For intermittent infusion, further dilute in 50 to 100 ml D_5W or normal saline solution. Avoid using sodium bicarbonate injection as a diluent because drug is least stable in it. During ceftazidime administration, temporarily stop other solutions being given at the same I.V. site.
• For I.M. use, reconstitute each gram with 3 ml sterile water for injection or bacteriostatic water for injection.
• Give I.M. injection deep into large muscle mass, such as gluteus maximus.
• Rotate I.V. sites every 72 hours. Assess for phlebitis and extravasation.
• Assess patient's bowel pattern daily; severe diarrhea may indicate pseudomembranous colitis.
• Monitor CBC, hematocrit, and serum AST, ALT, bilirubin, LD, and alkaline phosphatase levels during long-term therapy.
• Monitor PT, as ordered, in at-risk patients, such as those with renal or hepatic impairment or poor nutritional state and those receiving anticoagulant or prolonged antibiotic therapy. Notify prescriber if PT decreases, and expect to give vitamin K.
• Assess patient for perineal itching, fever, malaise, redness, swelling, rash, and change in cough or sputum; they may indicate a superinfection.

C

• Watch for pharyngitis, ecchymosis, bleeding, and arthralgia (possible blood dyscrasia). Monitor PT and bleeding time.

PATIENT TEACHING
• Tell patient to take ceftazidime exactly as prescribed.
• Tell patient to report evidence of blood dyscrasia or superinfection to prescriber immediately.
• Urge patient to report watery, bloody stools to prescriber immediately, even up to 2 months after drug therapy has ended.

ceftibuten
Cedax

Class and Category
Chemical class: Third-generation cephalo-sporin, 7-aminocephalosporanic acid
Therapeutic class: Antibiotic
Pregnancy category: B

Indications and Dosages
➤ *To treat acute bacterial exacerbations of chronic bronchitis caused by* Haemophilus influenzae, Moraxella catarrhalis, *or* Streptococcus pneumoniae; *pharyngitis and tonsillitis caused by* Streptococcus pyogenes; *and acute bacterial otitis media caused by* H. influenzae, M. catarrhalis, *or* S. pneumoniae

CAPSULES, ORAL SUSPENSION
Adults and children age 12 and over.
400 mg daily for 10 days.
➤ *To treat pharyngitis and tonsillitis caused by* S. pyogenes *and acute bacterial otitis media caused by* H. influenzae, M. catarrhalis, *or* S. pneumoniae

ORAL SUSPENSION
Children under age 12. 9 mg/kg daily for 10 days. *Maximum:* 400 mg daily.
DOSAGE ADJUSTMENT Dosage reduced to 4.5 mg/kg or 200 mg every 24 hr if creatinine clearance is 30 to 49 ml/min/1.73 m²; to 2.25 mg/kg or 100 mg every 24 hr if it's 5 to 29 ml/min/1.73 m².

Mechanism of Action
Interferes with bacterial cell wall synthesis by inhibiting the cross-linking of

peptidoglycan strands. Peptidoglycan makes the cell membrane rigid and protective. Without it, bacterial cells rupture and die.

Contraindications
Hypersensitivity to cephalosporins or their components

Interactions
DRUGS
aminoglycosides, loop diuretics: Increased risk of nephrotoxicity

Adverse Reactions
CNS: Aphasia, chills, fever, headache, psychosis, seizures
CV: Edema
EENT: Hearing loss
GI: Abdominal cramps, diarrhea, elevated liver function test results, hepatic failure, hepatomegaly, jaundice, melena, nausea, oral candidiasis, pseudomembranous colitis, vomiting
GU: Elevated BUN level, nephrotoxicity, renal failure, vaginal candidiasis
HEME: Eosinophilia, hemolytic anemia, hypoprothrombinemia, neutropenia, thrombocytopenia, unusual bleeding
MS: Arthralgia
RESP: Dyspnea
SKIN: Ecchymosis, erythema, erythema multiforme, pruritus, rash, Stevens-Johnson syndrome, toxic epidermal necrolysis
Other: Anaphylaxis, serum sickness, superinfection

Nursing Considerations
• Use ceftibuten cautiously in patients hypersensitive to penicillins because cross-sensitivity occurs in up to 10% of such patients.
• If possible, obtain culture and sensitivity test results, as ordered, before giving drug.
• Refrigerate oral suspension; shake well before using. Discard after 14 days.
• Monitor BUN and serum creatinine levels to detect early signs of nephrotoxicity. Also monitor fluid intake and output; decreasing urine output may indicate nephrotoxicity.
• Be aware that an allergic reaction may occur a few days after therapy starts.
• Assess bowel pattern daily; severe diarrhea may indicate pseudomembranous colitis.
• Assess patient for perineal itching, fever, malaise, redness, swelling, rash, and

change in cough or sputum; they may indicate a superinfection.
• Assess for pharyngitis, ecchymosis, bleeding, and arthralgia; they may indicate a blood dyscrasia.

PATIENT TEACHING
• Urge patient to complete the drug therapy as prescribed.
• Instruct patient to take drug on an empty stomach at least 2 hours before or 1 hour after meals.
• Inform patient that unflavored oral suspension has a bitter taste. Suggest having a flavor added when prescription is filled.
• Advise patient that yogurt and buttermilk can help maintain intestinal flora and decrease diarrhea during therapy.
• Tell patient to immediately report hypersensitivity reactions, severe diarrhea, and evidence of blood dyscrasia or superinfection.

ceftizoxime sodium

Cefizox

Class and Category
Chemical class: Third-generation cephalosporin, 7-aminocephalosporanic acid
Therapeutic class: Antibiotic
Pregnancy category: B

Indications and Dosages
➤ *To treat mild to moderate infections of the lower respiratory tract, skin, soft tissue, bones, and joints; septicemia; meningitis; and intra-abdominal infections caused by anaerobes (such as* Bacteroides *species,* Peptococcus, *and* Peptostreptococcus*), gram-negative organisms (including* Escherichia coli, Haemophilus influenzae, Klebsiella, *and* Proteus mirabilis*), and gram-positive organisms (including* Enterobacter *species,* Serratia *species,* Staphylococcus aureus, Staphylococcus epidermidis, Streptococcus agalactiae, Streptococcus pneumoniae, *and* Streptococcus pyogenes*)*
I.V. INFUSION, I.V. OR I.M. INJECTION
Adults and children age 12 and over. 1 to 2 g every 8 to 12 hr.

➤ *To treat severe or refractory infections of the type listed above*
I.V. INFUSION OR INJECTION
Adults and children age 12 and over. 1 g every 8 hr, or 2 g every 8 to 12 hr.
➤ *To treat life-threatening infections of the type listed above*
I.V. INFUSION OR INJECTION
Adults and children age 12 and over. 3 to 4 g every 8 hr or, if required, up to 2 g every 4 hr.
➤ *To treat bacterial infections in children*
I.V. INFUSION, I.V. OR I.M. INJECTION
Children age 6 months and over. 50 mg/kg every 6 to 8 hr.
➤ *To treat uncomplicated UTI*
I.V. INFUSION, I.V. OR I.M. INJECTION
Adults. 500 mg every 12 hr.
➤ *To treat pelvic inflammatory disease*
I.V. INFUSION OR INJECTION
Adults. 2 g every 8 hr.
➤ *To treat uncomplicated gonococcal infections*
I.M. INJECTION
Adults. 1 g as a single dose.
DOSAGE ADJUSTMENT Dosage reduced to 0.5 g every 8 hr for less severe infections, and 0.75 to 1.5 g every 8 hr for life-threatening infections if creatinine clearance is 50 to 79 ml/min/1.73 m^2; to 0.25 to 0.5 g every 12 hr for less severe infections, and 0.5 to 1 g every 12 hr for life-threatening infections if creatinine clearance is 5 to 49 ml/min/1.73 m^2; and to 0.5 g every 48 hr or 0.25 g every 24 hr for less severe infections, and 0.5 to 1 g every 48 hr or 0.5 g every 24 hr for life-threatening infections if creatinine clearance is 4 ml/min/1.73 m^2 or less.

Mechanism of Action
Interferes with bacterial cell wall synthesis by inhibiting the final step in the cross-linking of peptidoglycan strands. Peptidoglycan makes the cell membrane rigid and protective. Without it, bacterial cells rupture and die.

Contraindications
Hypersensitivity to cephalosporins or their components

Interactions
DRUGS
aminoglycosides, loop diuretics: Increased risk of nephrotoxicity

Adverse Reactions

CNS: Chills, fever, headache, seizures
CV: Edema
EENT: Hearing loss
GI: Abdominal cramps, diarrhea, elevated liver function test results, hepatic failure, hepatomegaly, nausea, oral candidiasis, pseudomembranous colitis, vomiting
GU: Elevated BUN level, nephrotoxicity, renal failure, vaginal candidiasis
HEME: Eosinophilia, hemolytic anemia, hypoprothrombinemia, neutropenia, thrombocytopenia, unusual bleeding
MS: Arthralgia
RESP: Dyspnea
SKIN: Ecchymosis, erythema, erythema multiforme, pruritus, rash, Stevens-Johnson syndrome
Other: Anaphylaxis; injection-site pain, redness, and swelling; superinfection

Nursing Considerations

• Use ceftizoxime cautiously in patients hypersensitive to penicillin because cross-sensitivity has occurred in about 10% of such patients.
• If possible, obtain culture and sensitivity test results, as ordered, before giving drug.
• For I.V. administration, reconstitute with sterile water for injection as follows: for 500-mg vial, add 5 ml; for 1-g vial, add 10 ml; and for 2-g vial, add 20 ml. Shake well. Dilute reconstituted solution further with 50 to 100 ml of a compatible solution, such as normal saline solution or D₅W, before administration. Give I.V. injection slowly over 3 to 5 minutes through tubing of a flowing compatible I.V. fluid.
• For I.M. administration, reconstitute with sterile water for injection as follows: for 500-mg vial, add 1.5 ml; for 1-g vial, add 3 ml; and for 2-g vial, add 6 ml. Shake well. Divide 2-g doses and administer in different sites. Inject deep in large muscle mass, such as the gluteus maximus.
• Reconstituted drug may be stored 24 hours at room temperature or 96 hours if refrigerated.
• Assess I.V. site for extravasation and phlebitis.
• Monitor BUN and serum creatinine levels to detect early signs of nephrotoxicity.

Also monitor fluid intake and output; decreasing urine output may indicate nephrotoxicity.
• Assess patient's bowel pattern daily; severe diarrhea may indicate pseudomembranous colitis.
• Monitor patient for allergic reactions a few days after therapy starts.
• Assess CBC, hematocrit, and serum AST, ALT, bilirubin, LD, and alkaline phosphatase levels during long-term therapy.
• Assess patient for pharyngitis, ecchymosis, bleeding, and arthralgia; they may indicate a blood dyscrasia.

PATIENT TEACHING

• Advise patient to immediately report severe or persistent diarrhea or evidence of blood dyscrasia to prescriber.

ceftriaxone sodium

Rocephin

Class and Category

Chemical class: Third-generation cephalosporin, 7-aminocephalosporanic acid
Therapeutic class: Antibiotic
Pregnancy category: B

Indications and Dosages

➤ *To treat infections of the lower respiratory tract, skin, soft tissue, urinary tract, bones, and joints; sinusitis; intra-abdominal infections; and septicemia caused by anaerobes (including* Bacteroides bivius, Bacteroides fragilis, Bacteroides melaninogenicus, *and* Peptostreptococcus *species), gram-negative organisms (including* Citrobacter species, Enterobacter aerogenes, Escherichia coli, Haemophilus influenzae, Klebsiella *species,* Neisseria *species,* Proteus mirabilis, Proteus vulgaris, Providencia *species,* Salmonella *species,* Serratia marcescens, Shigella, *and some strains of* Pseudomonas aeruginosa*), and gram-positive organisms (including* Staphylococcus aureus, Streptococcus pneumoniae, *and* Streptococcus pyogenes*)*

I.V. INFUSION, I.M. INJECTION
Adults. 1 to 2 g daily or in equally divided doses twice daily. *Maximum:* 4 g daily.
Children. 50 to 75 mg/kg daily in divided doses every 12 hr. *Maximum:* 2 g daily.
➤ *To treat meningitis*
I.V. INFUSION
Children. *Initial:* 100 mg/kg on first day, then 100 mg/kg daily or in divided doses every 12 hr for 7 to 14 days. *Maximum:* 4 g daily.
➤ *To treat acute bacterial otitis media*
I.M. INJECTION
Children. 50 mg/kg as a single dose. *Maximum:* 1 g.
➤ *To treat chancroid* (Haemophilus ducreyi *infection) and uncomplicated gonorrhea*
I.M. INJECTION
Adults. 250 mg as a single dose.
➤ *To treat gonococcal conjunctivitis*
I.M. INJECTION
Adults. 1 g as a single dose.
➤ *To treat disseminated gonoccocal infection and pelvic inflammatory disease*
I.V. INFUSION, I.M. INJECTION
Adults. 1 g every 24 hr.
➤ *To treat gonococcal meningitis and endocarditis*
I.V. INFUSION
Adults. 1 to 2 g every 12 hr for 10 to 14 days (meningitis), or for 4 wk or longer (endocarditis).
➤ *To provide surgical prophylaxis*
I.V. INFUSION
Adults. 1 g 30 min to 2 hr before surgery.

Mechanism of Action
Interferes with bacterial cell wall synthesis by inhibiting cross-linking of peptidoglycan strands. Peptidoglycan makes the cell membrane rigid and protective. Without it, bacterial cells rupture and die.

Incompatibilities
Don't admix ceftriaxone with pentamidine isethionate, labetalol, or other antibiotics, such as aminoglycosides, because of potential for incompatibility, such as substantial mutual inactivation. Also don't mix with calcium-containing solutions or products because a ceftriaxone-calcium salt may precipitate in the lungs and kidneys and may be fatal, especially in newborns.

Contraindications
Calcium-containing I.V. solutions; hyperbilirubinemic neonates; hypersensitivity to ceftriaxone, other cephalosporins, or their components; neonates who are 28 days old or less if they're expected to need calcium-containing solutions, including parenteral nutrition. Cefotaxime is a better choice of therapy for neonates.

Interactions
DRUGS
aminoglycosides, loop diuretics: Increased risk of nephrotoxicity

Adverse Reactions
CNS: Chills, fever, headache, hypertonia, reversible hyperactivity, seizures
CV: Edema
EENT: Glossitis, hearing loss, stomatitis
GI: Abdominal cramps, cholestasis, diarrhea, elevated liver function test results, gallbladder dysfunction, hepatic failure, hepatomegaly, nausea, oral candidiasis, pancreatitis, pseudolithiasis, pseudo-membranous colitis, vomiting
GU: Elevated BUN level, nephrotoxicity, oliguria, renal failure, vaginal candidiasis
HEME: Aplastic anemia, eosinophilia, hemolytic anemia, hemorrhage, hypoprothrombinemia, neutropenia, thrombocytopenia, unusual bleeding
MS: Arthralgia
RESP: Allergic pneumonitis, dyspnea
SKIN: Allergic dermatitis, ecchymosis, erythema, erythema multiforme, exanthema, pruritus, rash, Stevens-Johnson syndrome, toxic epidermal necrolysis, urticaria
Other: Anaphylaxis; drug fever; injection-site pain, redness, and swelling; serum sickness; superinfection

Nursing Considerations
WARNING Calcium-containing products must not be given I.V. within 48 hours of ceftriaxone, including solutions given through a different I.V. line and at a different site, because a ceftriaxone-calcium salt may precipitate in the lungs and kidneys and could be fatal.
• Use ceftriaxone cautiously in patients who are hypersensitive to penicillins because cross-sensitivity has occurred in about 1% to 3% of such patients.

• If possible, obtain culture and sensitivity results, as ordered, before giving drug.
• Protect powder from light.
• For I.V. use, reconstitute with an appropriate diluent, such as sterile water for injection or sodium chloride for injection, as follows: for 250-mg vial, add 2.4 ml; for 500-mg vial, add 4.8 ml; for 1-g vial, add 9.6 ml; and for 2-g vial, add 19.2 ml to yield 100 mg/ml. For piggyback bottles, reconstitute with 10 ml of diluent indicated above for 1-g bottle and 20 ml for 2-g bottle. After reconstitution, further dilute to 50 to 100 ml with diluent indicated above and infuse over 30 minutes. Never use a diluent that contains calcium, such as Ringer's solution or Hartmann's solution, because a precipitate can form and may be fatal if injected.

WARNING Never give ceftriaxone by I.V. infusion and calcium-containing IV solutions at the same time, including such continuous calcium-containing infusions as parenteral nutrition via Y-site. For patients other than neonates, ceftriaxone and calcium-containing solutions may be given sequentially if infusion lines are thoroughly flushed with a compatible fluid between infusions.

• For I.M. administration, reconstitute with an appropriate diluent, such as sterile water for injection or sodium chloride for injection, as follows: for 250-mg vial, add 0.9 ml; for 500-mg vial, add 1.8 ml; for 1-g vial, add 3.6 ml; and for 2-g vial, add 7.2 ml to make a 250-mg/ml concentration. Shake well. Inject deep into large muscle mass, such as the gluteus maximus.

• Monitor BUN and serum creatinine levels to detect early signs of nephrotoxicity. Also monitor fluid intake and output; decreasing urine output may indicate nephrotoxicity.
• Monitor patient for allergic reactions throughout ceftriaxone therapy and after drug is discontinued. Notify prescriber and stop drug, as ordered, at first sign of an allergic reaction. Be prepared to provide supportive care, including epinephrine administration and other emergency measures, as indicated and ordered.
• Assess CBC, hematocrit, and serum AST, ALT, bilirubin, LD, and alkaline phosphatase levels during long-term therapy. If abnormalities occur, notify prescriber. Drug may need to be discontinued.

• Assess bowel pattern daily; severe diarrhea may indicate pseudomembranous colitis caused by *Clostridium difficile*. If diarrhea occurs, notify prescriber and expect to treat with fluids, electrolytes, protein, and an antibiotic effective against *C. difficile*. Ceftriaxone therapy may be withheld also.
• Monitor patient for evidence of gallbladder disease (abdominal pain, nausea, vomiting) because drug may cause ceftriaxone-calcium salt to deposit in the gallbladder, which may mimic gallstones. Expect drug to be discontinued if gallbladder disorders arise.
• Assess for perineal itching, fever, malaise, redness, swelling, rash, and change in cough or sputum; they may indicate a superinfection.
• Assess for pharyngitis, ecchymosis, bleeding, and arthralgia; they may indicate a blood dyscrasia.

PATIENT TEACHING
• Tell patient to report evidence of blood dyscrasia or superinfection to prescriber immediately.
• Urge patient to report watery, bloody stools to prescriber immediately, even up to 2 months after drug therapy has ended.
• Advise patient to report any hypersensitivity reactions, such as a rash, itching skin, or hives, to prescriber immediately and to stop taking the drug.

cefuroxime axetil
Ceftin

cefuroxime sodium
Zinacef

Class and Category
Chemical class: Second-generation cephalosporin, 7-aminocephalosporanic acid
Therapeutic class: Antibiotic
Pregnancy category: B

Indications and Dosages
➤ *To treat pharyngitis and tonsillitis*

ORAL SUSPENSION
Children ages 3 months to 12 years. 10 mg/ kg daily in equally divided doses twice daily for 10 days. *Maximum:* 500 mg daily.
TABLETS
Adults and children age 13 and over. 250 mg twice daily for 10 days.
Children under age 13 who can swallow tablets. 125 mg twice daily for 10 days.
➤ *To treat acute otitis media*
ORAL SUSPENSION
Children ages 3 months to 12 years. 30 mg/kg daily in equally divided doses twice daily for 10 days. *Maximum:* 1,000 mg daily.
TABLETS
Children under age 13 who can swallow tablets. 250 mg twice daily for 10 days.
➤ *To treat impetigo*
ORAL SUSPENSION
Children ages 3 months to 12 years. 30 mg/ kg daily in equally divided doses twice daily for 10 days. *Maximum:* 1,000 mg daily.
➤ *To treat acute bacterial maxillary sinusitis*
ORAL SUSPENSION
Children ages 3 months to 12 years. 30 mg/kg daily in equally divided doses twice daily for 10 days. *Maximum:* 1,000 mg daily.
TABLETS
Adults and children age 13 and over and children under age 13 who can swallow tablets. 250 mg twice daily for 10 days.
➤ *To treat acute bacterial exacerbations of chronic bronchitis and uncomplicated skin and soft-tissue infections*
TABLETS
Adults and children age 13 and over. 250 to 500 mg twice daily for 10 days.
I.V. INFUSION, I.V. OR I.M. INJECTION
Adults. 750 mg every 8 hr.
➤ *To treat secondary bacterial infection in patients with acute bronchitis*
Adults and children age 13 and over. 250 to 500 mg twice daily for 5 to 10 days.
➤ *To treat early Lyme disease*
TABLETS
Adults and children age 13 and over. 500 mg twice daily for 20 days.
➤ *To treat uncomplicated UTI*
TABLETS
Adults. 125 to 250 mg twice daily for 7 to 10 days.

I.V. INFUSION, I.V. OR I.M. INJECTION
Adults. 750 mg every 8 hr.
➤ *To treat uncomplicated gonorrhea*
TABLETS
Adults. 1 g as a single dose.
I.V. INJECTION
Adults. 1.5 g as a single dose divided equally and injected into two different sites; given with oral probenecid 1 g.
➤ *To treat disseminated gonococcal infection and uncomplicated pneumonia*
I.V. INFUSION, I.V. OR I.M. INJECTION
Adults. 750 mg every 8 hr.
➤ *To treat bone and joint infections*
I.V. INFUSION, I.V. OR I.M. INJECTION
Adults. 1.5 g every 8 hr.
Children over age 3 months. 50 to 150 mg/ kg daily in divided doses every 8 hr. *Maximum:* Adult dose.
➤ *To treat bacterial meningitis*
I.V. INFUSION
Adults. 1.5 to 3 g every 8 hr.
Children over age 1 month. 50 to 80 mg/ kg every 6 to 8 hr.
Neonates up to age 1 month. 33.3 to 50 mg/kg every 8 to 12 hr.
➤ *To treat moderate infections other than those listed above*
I.V. INFUSION, I.V. OR I.M. INJECTION
Adults. 750 mg every 8 hr for 5 to 10 days.
I.V. INFUSION OR INJECTION
Children over age 3 months. 50 mg/kg daily in equally divided doses every 6 to 8 hr.
➤ *To treat severe or complicated infections other than those listed above*
I.V. INFUSION OR INJECTION
Adults. 1.5 g every 8 hr.
Children over age 3 months. 100 mg/kg daily in equally divided doses every 6 to 8 hr.
➤ *To treat life-threatening infections other than those listed above*
I.V. INFUSION OR INJECTION
Adults. 1.5 g every 6 hr.
➤ *To provide perioperative prophylaxis*
I.V. INFUSION OR INJECTION
Adults. 1.5 g 30 to 60 min before surgery (at induction of anesthesia for open-heart surgery), and then 0.75 g every 8 hr thereafter (1.5 g every 12 hr for total of 6 g with open-heart surgery).
DOSAGE ADJUSTMENT Parenteral dosage reduced to 0.75 g every 12 hr if creatinine

C

clearance is 10 to 20 ml/min/1.73 m^2 or to 0.75 g every 24 hr if creatinine clearance less than 10 ml/min/1.73 m^2.

Mechanism of Action

Interferes with bacterial cell wall synthesis by inhibiting the final step in the cross-linking of peptidoglycan strands. Peptidoglycan makes the cell membrane rigid and protective. Without it, bacterial cells rupture and die.

Incompatibilities

Don't admix parenteral cefuroxime with other antibiotics, such as aminogly-cosides, because of potential for incompatibility, such as substantial mutual inactivation. If they're administered concurrently, don't mix them in the same I.V. bag or bottle.

Contraindications

Hypersensitivity to cephalosporins or their components

Interactions

DRUGS

aminoglycosides, loop diuretics: Increased risk of nephrotoxicity
antacids, H$_2$-receptor antagonists, omeprazole: Decreased cefuroxime axetil absorption
probenecid: Increased and prolonged blood cefuroxime level

Adverse Reactions

CNS: Chills, fever, headache, seizures
CV: Edema
EENT: Hearing loss, oral candidiasis
GI: Abdominal cramps, diarrhea, elevated liver function test results, hepatic failure, hepatomegaly, nausea, pseudomembranous colitis, vomiting
GU: Elevated BUN level, nephrotoxicity, renal failure, vaginal candidiasis
HEME: Eosinophilia, hemolytic anemia, hypoprothrombinemia, neutropenia, thrombocytopenia, unusual bleeding
MS: Arthralgia
RESP: Dyspnea
SKIN: Ecchymosis, erythema, erythema multiforme, pruritus, rash, Stevens-Johnson syndrome
Other: Anaphylaxis; injection-site edema, pain, and redness; superinfection

Nursing Considerations

• Use cefuroxime cautiously in patients hypersensitive to penicillin because cross-sensitivity has occurred in about 10% of such patients.
• If possible, obtain culture and sensitivity results, as ordered, before giving drug.
• Give oral form with food to decrease GI distress, as needed.
• Remember that oral forms—tablets and suspension—aren't bioequivalent.
• For I.V. use, reconstitute using manufacturer's instructions according to type of preparation available. Solution ranges in color from light yellow to amber.
• For I.M. use, add 3 or 3.6 ml sterile water for injection to each 750-mg vial to yield 220 mg/ml.
• If using a container of frozen parenteral solution, thaw at room temperature or under refrigeration before administration; make sure all ice crystals have melted. Don't force thawing by microwaving.
• Store reconstituted parenteral drug for up to 24 hours at room temperature or 96 hours in refrigerator. (Thawed solutions may be stable 24 hours at room temperature or 28 days if refrigerated.) Store reconstituted oral suspension in refrigerator or at room temperature up to 10 days.
• Give I.V. injection over 3 to 5 minutes through tubing of a flowing compatible I.V. fluid.
• Monitor I.V. site for extravasation and phlebitis.
• Monitor BUN and serum creatinine levels and fluid intake and output to detect signs of nephrotoxicity. Monitor patients with renal impairment closely because they may have greater toxic reactions to cefuroxime.
• Monitor patient for allergic reactions continuing up to a few days after therapy starts. Patients with a history of some form of allergy, especially to drugs, are at increased risk for an allergic reaction.
• Assess bowel pattern daily; severe diarrhea may indicate pseudomembranous colitis. If it's suspected, stop drug, as ordered, and provide treatment as prescribed.
• Assess patient for pharyngitis, ecchymosis, bleeding, and arthralgia, which may indicate a blood dyscrasia.

- Monitor PT and bleeding time, as ordered. Be prepared to administer vitamin K, if ordered, to treat hypothrombinemia.

PATIENT TEACHING
- Instruct patient to shake oral suspension well before measuring each dose and to use a calibrated liquid-measuring device.
- Advise patient using single-dose packets of oral suspension to empty contents of one packet into a glass and add at least 10 ml (2 tsp) of cold water; apple, grape, or orange juice; or lemonade. Tell him to stir well and consume entire mixture at once.
- Inform patient that yogurt and buttermilk help maintain intestinal flora and can decrease diarrhea during therapy.
- Instruct patient to report evidence of blood dyscrasia to prescriber immediately.
- Urge patient to report watery, bloody stools to prescriber immediately, even up to 2 months after drug therapy has ended.

celecoxib
Celebrex

Class and Category
Chemical class: Diaryl-substituted pyrazole derivative
Therapeutic class: Anti-inflammatory, antirheumatic
Pregnancy category: C

Indications and Dosages
➤ *To relieve signs and symptoms of osteoarthritis*
CAPSULES
Adults. 200 mg daily or 100 mg twice daily.
➤ *To relieve signs and symptoms of rheumatoid arthritis*
CAPSULES
Adults. 100 to 200 mg twice daily.
➤ *To relieve signs and symptoms of juvenile rheumatoid arthritis*
CAPSULES
Children age 2 and older weighing 10 to 25 kg (22 to 55 lb). 50 mg twice daily.
Children age 2 and older weighing more than 25 kg. 100 mg twice daily.
➤ *To relieve pain from ankylosing spondylitis*

CAPSULES
Adults. 200 mg daily or 100 mg twice daily. Dosage increased to 400 mg daily or 200 mg twice daily after 6 weeks if needed.
➤ *As adjunct to reduce adenomatous colorectal polyps in patients with familial adenomatous polyposis*
CAPSULES
Adults. 400 mg twice daily.
➤ *To manage acute pain, to treat primary dysmenorrhea*
CAPSULES
Adults. 400 mg, followed by 200 mg if needed, on 1st day. On subsequent days, 200 mg twice daily as needed.
DOSAGE ADJUSTMENT Daily dosage reduced for patients with hepatic impairment. For those weighing less than 50 kg (110 lb), expect to start with lowest recommended dose. For patients who are poor CYP2C9 metabolizers, starting dosage should be half the lowest recommended dose.

Mechanism of Action
Selectively inhibits the enzymatic activity of cyclooxygenase-2 (COX-2), the enzyme needed to convert arachidonic acid to prostaglandin. Prostaglandins are responsible for mediating the inflammatory response and causing local vasodilation, swelling, and pain. Prostaglandins also play a role in peripheral pain transmission to the spinal cord. By inhibiting COX-2 activity and prostaglandin production, this NSAID reduces inflammatory symptoms and relieves pain. Celecoxib's mechanism of action in reducing the number of colorectal polyps is unknown.

Contraindications
Allergic reaction (such as anaphylaxis or angioedema) to aspirin, other NSAIDs, or sulfonamide derivatives or history of aspirin-induced nasal polyps with bronchospasm; hypersensitivity to celecoxib or its components; treatment of perioperative pain after coronary artery bypass graft surgery

Interactions
DRUGS
ACE inhibitors, angiotensin II receptor antagonists: Decreased antihypertensive effect of ACE inhibitors and angiotensin II receptor antagonists, increased risk of renal failure

C

aspirin: Increased risk of GI ulceration and other GI complications
fluconazole: Increased blood celecoxib level
furosemide, thiazide diuretics: Reduced diuretic effects of these drugs, increased risk of renal failure
lithium: Possibly elevated blood lithium level
warfarin: Possibly increased PT and risk of bleeding

Adverse Reactions

CNS: Aseptic meningitis, cerebral hemorrhage, depression, dizziness, fever, headache, insomnia, ischemic stroke, stroke, suicidal ideation, syncope, transient ischemic attacks, vertigo
CV: Aortic valve incompetence, chest pain, congestive heart failure, deep vein thrombosis, fluid retention, hypertension, MI, palpitations, peripheral edema or gangrene, sinus bradycardia, tachycardia, thrombosis, unstable angina, vasculitis, ventricular fibrillation, ventricular hypertrophy
EENT: Conjunctival hemorrhage, deafness, labyrinthitis, nasopharyngitis, pharyngitis, rhinitis, sinusitis, vitreous floaters
ENDO: Hyperglycemia, hypoglycemia
GI: Abdominal pain, diarrhea, elevated liver function test results, esophageal perforation, flatulence, GI bleeding or ulceration, hepatic failure, ileus, indigestion, jaundice, nausea, pancreatitis, perforation of stomach or intestine, vomiting
GU: Acute renal failure, interstitial nephritis, ovarian cyst, proteinuria, UTI, urinary incontinence
HEME: Agranulocytosis, aplastic anemia, decreased hematocrit and hemoglobin, leukopenia, pancytopenia, prolonged APTT, thrombocytopenia
MS: Arthralgia, back pain, elevated serum CK level, epicondylitis, tendon rupture
RESP: Bronchospasm, cough, dyspnea, pneumonia, pulmonary embolism, upper respiratory tract infection
SKIN: Erythema multiforme, exfoliative dermatitis, phototoxicity, rash, Stevens-Johnson syndrome, toxic epidermal necrolysis, urticaria
Other: Anaphylaxis, angioedema, hyperkalemia, hypernatremia, hyponatremia, sepsis

Nursing Considerations

• Use celecoxib with extreme caution in patients who have a history of ulcer disease or GI bleeding because NSAIDs, such as celecoxib, increase the risk of GI bleeding and ulceration. In these patients, drug should be used for shortest time possible.
• Be aware that serious GI tract ulceration and bleeding, as well as perforation of stomach or intestine, can occur without warning or symptoms. Elderly patients are at greatest risk. To minimize risk, give celecoxib with food. If patient develops GI distress, withhold celecoxib and notify prescriber immediately.
• Use celecoxib cautiously in patients with hypertension, and monitor blood pressure closely throughout therapy because drug can start or worsen hypertension.
• Use celecoxib cautiously in children with systemic onset juvenile rheumatoid arthritis because serious adverse reactions can occur, including disseminated intravascular coagulation.
• Use celecoxib cautiously in patients known to be poor CYP2C9 metabolizers based on history or experience with other CYP2C9 substrates, such as warfarin or phenytoin. Dosage should start at half the lowest recommended amount. For patients with juvenile rheumatoid arthritis who are also poor CYP2C9 metabolizers, alternative management should be considered.
WARNING Monitor patient closely for thrombotic events, including MI and stroke, because use (especially long-term use) of NSAIDs such as celecoxib increases the risk.
WARNING In patient who has bone marrow suppression or is receiving antineoplastic therapy, monitor laboratory results (including WBC) and assess for infection because celecoxib's anti-inflammatory and antipyretic actions may mask signs and symptoms, such as fever and pain.
• Monitor patient—especially if elderly or receiving long-term celecoxib therapy—for less common but serious adverse GI reactions, including anorexia, constipation, diverticulitis, dysphagia, esophagitis, gastritis, gastroenteritis, gastroesophageal reflux disease,

hemorrhoids, hiatal hernia, melena, stomatitis, and vomiting.
• Monitor liver function test results because, in rare cases, elevation may progress to severe hepatic reaction, including fatal hepatitis, hepatic necrosis, and hepatic failure.
• Monitor BUN and serum creatinine levels in elderly patients; patients taking diuretics, ACE inhibitors, or angiotensin II receptor antagonists; and patients with heart failure, impaired renal function, or hepatic dysfunction because drug may cause renal failure.
• Monitor CBC for decreased hemoglobin level and hematocrit because drug may worsen anemia.
• Assess patient's skin regularly for signs of rash or other hypersensitivity reaction because celecoxib is a sulfur drug and may cause serious skin reactions without warning, even in patients with no history of sensitivity to sulfur. At first sign of reaction, stop drug and notify prescriber.
• Avoid using celecoxib with a non-aspirin NSAID, regardless of the dose, because celecoxib reduces inflammation and fever, which may mask signs of infection.

PATIENT TEACHING
• Instruct patient to swallow celecoxib capsules whole with a full glass of water and with food or milk to prevent stomach upset.
• Tell patient to take celecoxib exactly as prescribed and not to increase dosage or take drug longer than prescribed because serious adverse reactions can occur.
• Advise patient to notify prescriber if pain continues or is poorly controlled.
• Explain that celecoxib may increase the risk of serious adverse CV events; urge patient to seek immediate medical attention if signs or symptoms arise, such as chest pain, shortness of breath, slurred speech, and weakness.
• Tell patient that celecoxib may increase the risk of serious adverse GI reactions. Stress the need to seek immediate medical attention if signs or symptoms develop, such as epigastric or abdominal pain, indigestion, black or tarry stools, and vomiting blood or material that resembles coffee grounds.
• Alert patient that celecoxib may cause serious skin reactions. Advise immediate

medical attention if signs or symptoms develop, such as rash, blisters, fever, itching, or other evidence of hypersensitivity.
• Urge patient to avoid smoking and alcohol consumption during celecoxib therapy because they may increase the risk of adverse GI reactions.

cephalexin hydrochloride
Keftab

cephalexin monohydrate
Apo-Cephalex (CAN), Keflex, Novo-Lexin (CAN), Nu-Cephalex (CAN), PMS-Cephalexin (CAN)

Class and Category
Chemical class: First-generation cephalosporin, 7-aminocephalosporanic acid
Therapeutic class: Antibiotic
Pregnancy category: B

Indications and Dosages
➤ *To treat streptococcal tonsillitis, pharyngitis, and skin and soft-tissue infections*
CAPSULES, ORAL SUSPENSION, TABLETS
Adults and adolescents age 15 and over. 500 mg every 12 hr. *Maximum:* 4 g daily.
Children and adolescents ages 2 to 15. 25 to 50 mg/kg daily divided into two equal doses and given every 12 hr. If infection is severe, dose may be doubled.
➤ *To treat mild to moderate respiratory tract, skin, soft-tissue, bone, and GU infections caused by susceptible organisms other than streptococci*
CAPSULES, ORAL SUSPENSION, TABLETS
Adults. 250 mg every 6 hr.
ORAL SUSPENSION
Children. 25 to 50 mg/kg daily in equally divided doses twice daily or four times daily.
➤ *To treat severe respiratory tract, skin, soft-tissue, bone, and GU infections*

Mechanism of Action

Like all cephalosporins, cephalexin interferes with bacterial cell wall synthesis by inhibiting the final step in the cross-linking of peptidoglycan strands. Peptidoglycan makes the cell membrane rigid and protective. Without it, bacterial cells rupture and die. This mechanism of action is most effective against bacteria that divide rapidly, including many grampositive and gram-negative bacteria.

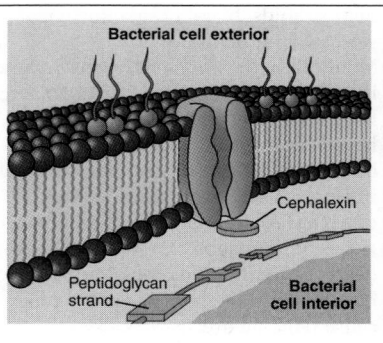

CAPSULES, ORAL SUSPENSION, TABLETS
Adults. 0.5 to 1 g every 6 hr. *Maximum:* 4 g daily.
Children. 50 to 100 mg/kg daily in equally divided doses four times daily.
➤ *To treat otitis media*
ORAL SUSPENSION
Children. 75 to 100 mg/kg daily in equally divided doses four times daily.
➤ *To treat uncomplicated cystitis*
CAPSULES, ORAL SUSPENSION, TABLETS
Adults and adolescents age 15 and over. 500 mg every 12 hr.

Contraindications

Hypersensitivity to cephalosporins or their components

Interactions

DRUGS
aminoglycosides, loop diuretics: Increased risk of nephrotoxicity
probenecid: Increased and prolonged blood cephalexin level

Adverse Reactions

CNS: Chills, fever, headache, seizures
CV: Edema
EENT: Hearing loss
GI: Abdominal cramps, diarrhea, elevated liver function test results, hepatic failure, hepatomegaly, nausea, oral candidiasis, pseudomembranous colitis, vomiting
GU: Elevated BUN level, nephrotoxicity, renal failure, vaginal candidiasis
HEME: Eosinophilia, hemolytic anemia, hypoprothrombinemia, neutropenia, thrombocytopenia, unusual bleeding
MS: Arthralgia

RESP: Dyspnea
SKIN: Ecchymosis, erythema, erythema multiforme, pruritus, rash, Stevens-Johnson syndrome
Other: Anaphylaxis, superinfection

Nursing Considerations

• Use cephalexin cautiously in patients hypersensitive to penicillin because cross-sensitivity occurs in about 10% of them.
• If possible, obtain culture and sensitivity test results, as ordered, before giving drug.
• Monitor patient's BUN and serum creatinine levels to detect early signs of nephrotoxicity. Also monitor fluid intake and output; decreasing urine output may indicate nephrotoxicity.
• Monitor for allergic reactions a few days after therapy starts.
• Assess CBC, hematocrit, and serum AST, ALT, bilirubin, LD, and alkaline phosphatase levels during long-term therapy.
• Assess patient's bowel pattern daily; severe diarrhea may indicate pseudomembranous colitis caused by *Clostridium difficile.* If diarrhea occurs, notify prescriber and expect to withhold cefotaxime and treat with fluids, electrolytes, protein, and an antibiotic effective against *C. difficile.*
• Assess patient for pharyngitis, ecchymosis, bleeding, and arthralgia; they may indicate a blood dyscrasia.
PATIENT TEACHING
• Advise patient to complete prescribed course of therapy.

- Instruct patient to shake oral suspension well before measuring each dose and to use a calibrated liquid-measuring device to ensure an accurate dose.
- Tell patient that yogurt and buttermilk can help maintain intestinal flora and decrease diarrhea during therapy.
- Urge patient to report watery, bloody stools to prescriber immediately, even if they occur up to 2 months after cephalexin therapy has ended.

cephapirin sodium

Cefadyl

Class and Category

Chemical class: First-generation cephalosporin, 7-aminocephalosporanic acid
Therapeutic class: Antibiotic
Pregnancy category: B

Indications and Dosages

➤ *To treat respiratory tract infection, skin and soft-tissue infections, UTI, septicemia, endocarditis, and osteomyelitis caused by gram-negative organisms (including* Escherichia coli, Haemophilus influenzae, Klebsiella *species, and* Proteus mirabilis*) and gram-positive organisms (including* group A beta-hemolytic streptococci, Streptococcus pneumoniae, *and* staphylococci, including coagulase-positive, coagulase-negative, and penicillinase-producing strains but not methicillin-resistant* Staphylococcus aureus*)*

I.V. INFUSION, I.V. OR I.M. INJECTION
Adults. 0.5 to 1 g every 4 to 6 hr.
Maximum: 12 g daily. For serious infections, higher doses are given by I.V. route.
Children over age 3 months. 40 to 80 mg/kg daily divided into four equal doses and given every 6 hr. *Maximum:* 12 g daily.
➤ *To provide surgical prophylaxis*
I.V. INFUSION, I.V. OR I.M. INJECTION
Adults. 1 to 2 g 30 to 60 min before surgery, 1 to 2 g during long procedure, and 1 to 2 g every 6 hr after surgery for 24 hr.

DOSAGE ADJUSTMENT For open-heart surgery or prosthetic arthroplasty, prophylaxis continued 3 to 5 days after procedure, if needed.

Mechanism of Action

Interferes with bacterial cell wall synthesis by inhibiting the final step in the cross-linking of peptidoglycan strands. Peptidoglycan makes the cell membrane rigid and protective. Without it, bacterial cells rupture and die.

Contraindications

Hypersensitivity to cephalosporins or their components

Interactions

DRUGS
aminoglycosides, loop diuretics: Increased risk of nephrotoxicity
probenecid: Increased and prolonged blood cephapirin level

Adverse Reactions

CNS: Chills, fever, headache, seizures
CV: Edema
EENT: Hearing loss
GI: Abdominal cramps, diarrhea, elevated liver function test results, hepatic failure, hepatomegaly, nausea, oral candidiasis, pseudomembranous colitis, vomiting
GU: Elevated BUN level, nephrotoxicity, renal failure, vaginal candidiasis
HEME: Eosinophilia, hemolytic anemia, hypoprothrombinemia, neutropenia, thrombocytopenia, unusual bleeding
MS: Arthralgia
RESP: Dyspnea
SKIN: Ecchymosis, erythema, erythema multiforme, pruritus, rash, Stevens-Johnson syndrome
Other: Anaphylaxis; injection site pain, redness, and swelling; superinfection

Nursing Considerations

- Use cephapirin cautiously in patients hypersensitive to penicillins because cross-sensitivity has occurred in about 10% of such patients.
- If possible, obtain culture and sensitivity test results, as ordered, before giving drug.
- For I.V. injection, reconstitute 1 g with 10 ml or more of appropriate diluent, such as sterile water for injection. Administer I.V. injection slowly over 3 to 5 minutes through tubing of a flowing compatible I.V. fluid.

• For I.V. infusion, dilute further in 50 ml of D₅W or normal saline solution and infuse over 15 to 30 minutes. Stop primary I.V. solution during cephapirin delivery.

• For I.M. injection, reconstitute 1-g vial with 2 ml sterile water for injection or bacteriostatic water for injection. Inject deep into large muscle mass, such as the gluteus maximus.

• Store reconstituted drug up to 24 hours at room temperature or 10 days refrigerated.

• Don't give cloudy solution.

• Assess I.V. site for extravasation and phlebitis.

• Monitor BUN and serum creatinine levels to detect early signs of nephrotoxicity. Also, monitor fluid intake and output; decreasing urine output may indicate nephrotoxicity.

• Monitor patient for allergic reactions a few days after therapy starts.

• Assess CBC, hematocrit, and serum AST, ALT, bilirubin, LD, and alkaline phospha-tase levels during long-term therapy.

• Assess patient's bowel pattern daily; severe diarrhea may indicate pseudomembranous colitis.

• Assess patient for pharyngitis, ecchymosis, bleeding, and arthralgia; they may indicate a blood dyscrasia.

• Assess patient for furry tongue, perineal itching, and loose, foul-smelling stool; they may indicate superinfection.

PATIENT TEACHING

• Instruct patient to report severe diarrhea or evidence of blood dyscrasia or super-infection to prescriber immediately.

cephradine
Velosef

Class and Category
Chemical class: First-generation cephalosporin, 7-aminocephalosporanic acid
Therapeutic class: Antibiotic
Pregnancy category: B

Indications and Dosages
➤ *To treat respiratory tract infections (other than lobar pneumonia) and skin and soft-tissue infections*

CAPSULES, ORAL SUSPENSION
Adults. 250 mg every 6 hr or 500 mg every 12 hr. *Maximum:* 4 g daily.
ORAL SUSPENSION
Children age 9 months and over. 25 to 50 mg/kg daily in equally divided doses every 6 or 12 hr. *Maximum:* 4 g daily.
➤ *To treat lobar pneumonia*
CAPSULES, ORAL SUSPENSION
Adults. 0.5 g every 6 hr or 1 g every 12 hr. *Maximum:* 4 g daily.
ORAL SUSPENSION
Children age 9 months and over. 25 to 50 mg/kg daily in equally divided doses every 6 or 12 hr. *Maximum:* 4 g daily.
➤ *To treat uncomplicated UTI*
CAPSULES, ORAL SUSPENSION
Adults. 500 mg every 12 hr. For more serious infections, 500 mg every 6 hr or 1,000 mg every 12 hr. *Maximum:* 4 g daily.
➤ *To treat otitis media caused by* Haemophilus influenzae
ORAL SUSPENSION
Children. 75 to 100 mg/kg daily in equally divided doses every 6 to 12 hr. *Maximum:* 4 g daily.
DOSAGE ADJUSTMENT Dosage reduced to 500 mg every 6 hr if creatinine clearance exceeds 20 ml/min/1.73 m²; 250 mg every 6 hr if clearance is 5 to 20 ml/min/1.73 m²; and 250 mg every 12 hr if clearance is less than 5 ml/min/1.73 m².

Mechanism of Action
Interferes with bacterial cell wall synthesis by inhibiting the final step in the cross-linking of peptidoglycan strands. Peptidoglycan makes the cell membrane rigid and protective. Without it, bacterial cells rupture and die.

Contraindications
Hypersensitivity to cephalosporins or their components

Interactions
DRUGS
aminoglycosides, loop diuretics: Increased risk of nephrotoxicity
probenecid: Increased and prolonged blood cephradine level

Adverse Reactions
CNS: Chills, fever, headache, seizures
CV: Edema

EENT: Hearing loss, oral candidiasis
GI: Abdominal cramps, diarrhea, elevated liver function test results, hepatic failure, hepatomegaly, nausea, pseudomembranous colitis, vomiting
GU: Elevated BUN level, nephrotoxicity, renal failure, vaginal candidiasis
HEME: Eosinophilia, hemolytic anemia, hypoprothrombinemia, neutropenia, thrombocytopenia, unusual bleeding
MS: Arthralgia
RESP: Dyspnea
SKIN: Ecchymosis, erythema, erythema multiforme, pruritus, rash, Stevens-Johnson syndrome
Other: Anaphylaxis, superinfection

Nursing Considerations

• If possible, obtain culture and sensitivity test results, as ordered, before giving drug.
• Monitor patients hypersensitive to penicillin for evidence of hypersensitivity reaction because cross-sensitivity has occurred in about 10% of such patients.
• Store oral suspension for 7 days at room temperature or for 14 days if refrigerated.
• Monitor BUN and serum creatinine levels to detect early signs of nephrotoxicity. Also monitor fluid intake and output; decreasing urine output may indicate nephrotoxicity.
• Monitor patient for allergic reactions a few days after therapy starts. If hypersensitivity develops, be prepared to stop drug and administer antihistamines, corticosteroids, and vasopressors, as ordered. Also prepare to administer oxygen, maintain an open airway, and assist with endotracheal intubation, as appropriate.
• Assess CBC, hematocrit, and serum AST, ALT, bilirubin, LD, and alkaline phosphatase levels during long-term therapy.
• Assess patient's bowel pattern daily; severe diarrhea may indicate pseudomembranous colitis. Obtain a stool specimen to test for *Clostridium difficile*. Keep in mind that this serious adverse reaction can occur during therapy or up to several weeks after therapy ends. Also avoid giving anti-peristaltic antidiarrheals, such as atropine and diphenoxylate or loperamide, because they may delay elimination of toxins from

the bowel and damage the colon from toxin retention. Mild cases may respond after cephradine is discontinued. For moderate or severe cases, be prepared to administer fluids, electrolytes, and protein replacement as ordered.
• If patient has a history of GI disease, especially ulcerative colitis, regional enteritis, or antibiotic-associated colitis, assess him often for diarrhea because he is at risk for pseudomembranous colitis.
• Assess patient for pharyngitis, ecchymosis, bleeding, and arthralgia; these may indicate a blood dyscrasia.
• If patient has a seizure, notify prescriber immediately and expect to discontinue drug. Institute seizure precautions according to facility policy.

PATIENT TEACHING
• If patient develops GI distress, advise him to take cephradine with food.
• Advise patient to complete prescribed course of therapy.
• Urge patient to avoid missing doses and to take the drug at evenly spaced intervals. If patient misses a dose, instruct him to take it as soon as possible unless it's almost time for the next dose. Emphasize that he shouldn't double the dose.
• Tell patient that yogurt and buttermilk help maintain intestinal flora and can decrease diarrhea during therapy.
• Instruct patient to report to prescriber severe diarrhea or evidence of blood dyscrasia or superinfection immediately. Warn patient not to take any OTC antidiarrheals before consulting prescriber.
• Tell patient to notify prescriber if symptoms don't improve within a few days.

certolizumab pegol
Cimzia

Class and Category

Chemical class: Recombinant, humanized antibody Fab fragment
Therapeutic class: Disease modifying anti-inflammatory
Pregnancy category: B

Indications and Dosages

➤ *To reduce signs and symptoms of Crohn's disease and maintain clinical response in patients with moderately to severely active disease who have had an inadequate response to conventional therapy*

SUBCUTANEOUS INJECTION

Adults. *Initial:* 400 mg (given as two 200-mg injections) and repeated at wk 2 and 4. *Maintenance:* 400 mg (given as two 200-mg injections) every 4 wk if clinical response occurs.

➤ *To treat active ankylosing spondylitis, active psoriatic arthritis, or moderate to severe active rheumatoid arthritis*

SUBCUTANEOUS INJECTION

Adults. *Initial:* 400 mg (given as two 200-mg injections) and repeated at wk 2 and 4. *Maintenance:* 200 mg every other wk, or 400 mg (given as two 200-mg injections) every 4 wk if clinical response occurs.

Route	Onset	Peak	Duration
SubQ	Unknown	54–171 hr	Unknown

Mechanism of Action

Binds to human tumor necrosis factor (TNF) alpha, inhibiting it. TNF alpha stimulates production of inflammatory mediators, including interleukin-1, prostaglandins, platelet activating factor, and nitric oxide. TNF alpha level is increased in patients with Crohn's disease. Inhibition of TNF alpha causes C-reactive protein level to decline in patients with Crohn's disease, and the disease improves.

Contraindications

Active infection, concurrent therapy with disease modifying anti-rheumatic drugs or other tumor necrosis factor blocker therapy, hypersensitivity to cetolizumab or its components, I.V. administration

Interactions

DRUGS

anakinra: Possibly increased risk of serious infection and neutropenia
immunosuppressants: Possibly increased risk of infection
live-virus vaccines: Increased risk of adverse vaccine effects

Adverse Reactions

CNS: Anxiety, bipolar disorder, dizziness, fever, malaise, suicidal ideation, syncope
CV: Angina, arrhythmias, heart failure, hypertension, hypotension, MI, pericardial effusion, pericarditis, peripheral edema, vasculitis
EENT: Optic neuritis, retinal hemorrhage, uveitis
ENDO: Hot flashes
GI: Abdominal pain, diarrhea, elevated liver enzymes, hepatitis, intestinal obstruction
GU: Menstrual dysfunction, nephrotic syndrome, pyelonephritis, renal failure, UTI
HEME: Anemia, leukopenia, lymphadenopathy, pancytopenia, thrombophilia
MS: Arthralgia, extremity pain
RESP: Dyspnea, pneumonia, upper respiratory infection
SKIN: Allergic dermatitis, alopecia, erythema multiforme, erythema nodosum, new or worsening psoriasis, rash, Stevens-Johnson syndrome, toxic epidermal necrolysis, urticaria
Other: Angioedema; bacterial, invasive fungal, mycobacterial, parasitic, viral or other opportunistic infections including aspergillosis, blastomycosis, candidiasis, coccidioidomycosis, histoplasmosis, legionellosis, listeriosis, pneumocytosis, and tuberculosis; injection-site reactions (redness, pain); leukemia, lymphomas, and other malignancies; lupus-like syndrome; sarcoidosis, serum sickness

Nursing Considerations

• Be aware that certolizumab should not be initiated in a patient with an active infection, including serious localized infections.

• Use certolizumab cautiously in patients with recurrent or increased risk of infection, patients who live in regions where tuberculosis and histoplasmosis are endemic, and patients with a history of CNS demyelinating disorders because any of these disorders can occur, rarely, during certolizumab therapy. Be aware that a falsely negative antigen and antibody test for histoplasmosis may occur in some patients during certolizumab therapy, even when an active infection is present. Patient should be monitored closely throughout therapy.

• Use cautiously in patients who are chronic carriers of hepatitis B virus because drug may reactivate the virus. Assess patient for evidence of hepatitis B viral infection before starting and periodically throughout certolizumab therapy. If HBV reactivation occurs, notify prescriber, stop drug, and start appropriate therapy, as ordered.

• Make sure patient has a tuberculin skin test before therapy starts. If skin test is positive (induration 5 mm or greater), treatment of latent tuberculosis must start before certolizumab is given, as prescribed. In addition, expect anti-tuberculosis therapy to be given to a patient with a past history of latent or active tuberculosis in whom an adequate course of treatment cannot be confirmed, and for patients with a negative test for latent tuberculosis but having risk factors for tuberculosis infection. Be aware that a falsely negative test for latent tuberculosis may occur during certolizumab therapy, so any signs and symptoms suggestive of tuberculosis should be carefully evaluated.

WARNING Monitor all patients for infection during therapy, especially those who are at higher risk for infection, such as patients receiving immunosuppressants, those who are over 65 years of age, or who have co-morbid conditions. If serious infection develops, expect prescriber to stop drug.

• Reconstitute two 200-mg certolizumab vials for each dose after drug has reached room temperature. Inject 1 ml sterile water for injection using a 20G needle into each vial. Gently swirl each vial without shaking. Then leave vials undisturbed for up to 30 minutes to allow time for powder to completely dissolve. Do not leave at room temperature, once reconstituted, for more than 2 hours before administration. If administration will be delayed, reconstituted drug can be refrigerated up to 24 hours. Do not let drug freeze.

• Administer drug only when solution has reached room temperature. Using a 20G needle, withdraw drug from vial using a separate syringe and needle for each vial. Switch to a 23G needle and administer subcutaneously into two separate areas on patient's abdomen or thigh.

WARNING Stop drug immediately and notify prescriber if patient has an allergic reaction. Expect to provide supportive care.

• Monitor patient closely for evidence of congestive heart failure (sudden, unexplained weight gain; dyspnea; crackles; anxiety), and notify prescriber if they occur.

• Monitor patient's CBC, as ordered, because certolizumab may have adverse hematologic effects. Notify prescriber about persistent fever, bruising, bleeding, or pallor.

• Certolizumab is a TNF inhibitor. Although rare, malignancies (especially lymphomas and leukemias) have been reported in patients receiving these drugs, including children. Patients with rheumatoid arthritis, especially those with very active disease, and patients with Crohn's disease, ankylosing spondylitis, psoriatic arthritis, and plaque psoriasis are at greatest risk. Monitor these patients closely.

PATIENT TEACHING

• Know that the patient may receive vaccinations, except for live or live attenuated vaccines.

• Review signs and symptoms of allergic reaction (rash, swollen face, trouble breathing), and tell patient to seek emergency care immediately if these occur.

• Inform patient that injection-site reactions such as redness or pain may occur and usually are mild and transient. Instruct him to apply a towel soaked in cold water to the site if it hurts. Tell patient to call prescriber if reaction persists or worsens.

• Inform patient that tuberculosis may occur during therapy. Instruct him to report persistent cough, wasting or weight loss, and low-grade fever to prescriber.

• Tell patient to report evidence of infections and bleeding disorders to prescriber; drug may need to be stopped. Advise patient to avoid people with infections and to comply with all prescribed tests.

• Inform patient that certain kinds of cancer, especially lymphomas and leukemias, are more likely in patients taking certolizumab but still rare. Emphasize need to keep follow-up visits and to report unusual or sudden signs or symptoms. Also advise patient to have periodic skin examinations, especially if they are at risk for skin cancer.

• Caution against receiving live-virus vaccines while taking certolizumab; doing so may adversely affect the immune system.
• Instruct patient to report lupus-like signs and symptoms that, although rare, may occur during therapy, such as chest pain that doesn't go away, shortness of breath, joint pain, or rash on cheeks or arms that's sensitive to the sun. Explain that drug may need to be discontinued if these occur.
• Advise patient to inform all healthcare providers about certolizumab use and to inform prescriber about any OTC medications, herbal remedies, and vitamin and mineral supplements being taken.

cevimeline hydrochloride

Evoxac

Class and Category

Chemical class: Quinuclidine derivative of acetylcholine
Therapeutic class: Cholinergic enhancer, dry mouth reliever
Pregnancy category: C

Indications and Dosages

➤ *To treat dry mouth associated with Sjögren's syndrome*
CAPSULES
Adults. 30 mg three times daily. *Maximum:* 90 mg daily.

Mechanism of Action

As a cholinergic agonist, binds to and activates muscarinic receptors of the parasympathetic nervous system and increases secretions of the exocrine glands, such as salivary glands.

Contraindications

Acute iritis, angle-closure glaucoma, hypersensitivity to cevimeline or its components, uncontrolled asthma

Interactions

DRUGS
amiodarone, cimetidine, clarithromycin, diltiazem, erythromycin, fluconazole, haloperidol, itraconazole, ketoconazole, metoclopramide, mibefradil, nefazodone, propafenone, quinidine, ritonavir, selective

serotonin reuptake inhibitors, thioridazine, tricyclic antidepressants, troleandomycin, verapamil: Possibly inhibited metabolism and increased blood level of cevimeline
anticholinergics: Decreased effectiveness of anticholinergics
antimuscarinics: Altered effects of antimuscarinics and decreased therapeutic action of cevimeline
beta blockers: Possibly cardiac conduction disturbances
parasympathomimetics: Additive effects of either drug

Adverse Reactions

CNS: Depression, fatigue, fever, hypoesthesia, insomnia, migraine headache, tremor
CV: Edema, palpitations
EENT: Abnormal vision, conjunctivitis, dry mouth, earache, epistaxis, excessive salivation, eye pain, rhinitis, salivary gland pain
GI: Abdominal pain, anorexia, cholecystitis, constipation, eructation, heartburn, hiccups, nausea, vomiting
HEME: Anemia
MS: Arthralgia, leg cramps, myalgia
RESP: Cough, dyspnea
SKIN: Diaphoresis, pruritus
Other: Flulike symptoms, hot flashes

Nursing Considerations

• Give cevimeline on an empty stomach because food may decrease rate and extent of absorption, delaying peak concentration.
• Assess patient with a pulmonary disorder for wheezing and increased respiratory secretions because drug may cause increased bronchiolar smooth-muscle contractions, airway resistance, and respiratory secretions.
• Monitor patient with known or suspected gallbladder disease for abdominal pain and other warnings of biliary obstruction, cholecystitis, or cholangitis; each of these conditions may be precipitated by cevimeline.
PATIENT TEACHING
• Instruct patient to take cevimeline on an empty stomach.
• Inform patient that cevimeline may cause vision changes; advise him to avoid driving at night or performing hazardous activities until drug's adverse effects are known.

• Urge patient to drink plenty of fluids during hot weather and while exercising because drug may cause excessive sweating and dehydration.

chloral hydrate

Aquachloral Supprettes, Novo-Chlorhydrate (CAN), PMS-Chloral Hydrate (CAN)

Class, Category, and Schedule
Chemical class: Chloral derivative
Therapeutic class: Sedative-hypnotic
Pregnancy category: C
Controlled substance schedule: IV

Indications and Dosages
➤ *To prevent or suppress alcohol withdrawal symptoms, act as an adjunct to opioids and analgesics to control postoperative pain*
CAPSULES, SYRUP, SUPPOSITORIES
Adults. 250 mg three times daily after meals. *Maximum:* 2,000 mg.
➤ *To produce nocturnal sedation*
CAPSULES, SYRUP, SUPPOSITORIES
Adults. 0.5 to 1 g 30 min before bedtime. *Maximum:* 2 g.
➤ *To produce preoperative sedation*
CAPSULES, SYRUP, SUPPOSITORIES
Adults. 0.5 to 1 g 30 min before surgery.
➤ *To provide sedation before dental or medical procedure*
SYRUP, SUPPOSITORIES
Children. 25 mg/kg up to 500 mg/single dose; up to 75 mg/kg for dental procedure supplemented by nitrous oxide.

Route	Onset	Peak	Duration
P.O.	30–60 min	Unknown	4–8 hr
P.R.	Unknown	Unknown	4–8 hr

Mechanism of Action
Produces CNS depression by an unknown mechanism involving trichloroethanol, the drug's active metabolite.

Contraindications
Gastritis; hypersensitivity or idiosyncrasy to chloral hydrate or its components; severe cardiac, hepatic, or renal disease

Interactions
DRUGS
CNS depressants: Increased CNS effects of chloral hydrate
furosemide (I.V.): Increased adverse effects when given after chloral hydrate
phenytoin: Increased excretion and decreased effectiveness of phenytoin
warfarin: Transient increase in anticoagulant effect
ACTIVITIES
alcohol use: Increased CNS effects of chloral hydrate

Adverse Reactions
CNS: Ataxia, disorientation, hangover, incoherence, paranoia, somnolence
GI: Gastric irritation, nausea, vomiting
SKIN: Rash, urticaria
Other: Drug dependence

Nursing Considerations
• Administer with full glass of water or juice to minimize GI distress from chloral hydrate capsules. Dilute syrup in a half-glass of water, ginger ale, or fruit juice.
WARNING Monitor carefully for hypersensitivity reaction in patients with a history of tartrazine sensitivity.
• Suspect physical or psychological dependence if withdrawal of chloral hydrate produces confusion, hallucinations, nausea, nervousness, restlessness, stomach pain, tremor, unusual excitement, or vomiting.
PATIENT TEACHING
• Instruct patient to take capsules with a full glass of water or juice or to mix syrup in a half-glass of water, ginger ale, or fruit juice.
• Advise patient to avoid hazardous activities until CNS effects of chloral hydrate are known.
• Caution patient that drug may be habit-forming. Advise taking it exactly as prescribed and not to stop taking it abruptly because withdrawal symptoms could occur.
• Instruct patient to notify prescriber right away about stomach pains or tarry stools.

C

chloramphenicol
Chloromycetin, Novochlorocap (CAN)

chloramphenicol palmitate
Chloromycetin

chloramphenicol sodium succinate
Chloromycetin

Class and Category
Chemical class: Dichloroacetic acid derivative
Therapeutic class: Antibiotic
Pregnancy category: Not rated

Indications and Dosages
➤ *To treat serious infections for which less potentially dangerous drugs are ineffective or contraindicated*
I.V. INFUSION
Adults. 12.5 mg/kg every 6 hr. *Maximum:* 4 g daily.
Children. 50 to 75 mg/kg daily in divided doses every 6 hr.
Full-term infants age 2 weeks and over. 12.5 mg/kg every 6 hr or 25 mg/kg every 12 hr.
Preterm and full-term infants up to age 2 weeks. 6.25 mg/kg every 6 hr.
➤ *To treat bacteremia or meningitis*
I.V. INFUSION
Children. 50 to 100 mg/kg daily in divided doses every 6 hr.
DOSAGE ADJUSTMENT Dosage limited to 25 mg/kg daily for infants and children with immature metabolic processes.

Mechanism of Action
Produces a bacteriostatic effect on susceptible organisms by inhibiting protein synthesis, thus preventing amino acids from being transferred to growing polypeptide chains.

Contraindications
Hypersensitivity to chloramphenicol or its components

Interactions
DRUGS
alfentanil: Prolonged alfentanil effect
barbiturates: Increased blood barbiturate level; decreased chloramphenicol level

blood-dyscrasia–causing drugs (such as captopril and cephalosporins), bone marrow depressants (including colchicine and methotrexate): Increased bone marrow depression
chlorpropamide, tolbutamide: Increased hypoglycemic effects
clindamycin, erythromycin, lincomycin: Decreased antibacterial effects of these drugs
cyclophosphamide: Decreased or delayed activation of cyclophosphamide, increased bone marrow depression
hepatic enzyme inducers (including rifampin): Decreased chloramphenicol level
hydantoins: Increased blood hydantoin level, possibly resulting in toxicity; increased or decreased blood chloramphenicol level
iron salts: Increased serum iron level
oral anticoagulants: Enhanced anticoagulant action
oral contraceptives containing estrogen: Decreased contraceptive effect with prolonged chloramphenicol use
penicillins: Decreased penicillin activity; synergistic effects with treatment of certain microorganisms
vitamin B_{12}: Antagonized hematopoietic response to vitamin B_{12}

Adverse Reactions
CNS: Confusion, delirium, depression, fever, headache, peripheral neuropathy
CV: Gray syndrome in neonates
EENT: Optic neuritis
GI: Diarrhea, nausea, vomiting
HEME: Aplastic anemia, bone marrow depression, granulocytopenia, hypoplastic anemia, leukopenia, reticulocytopenia, thrombocytopenia
SKIN: Rash
Other: Anaphylaxis, angioedema

Nursing Considerations
• As appropriate and ordered, obtain specimen for culture and sensitivity testing before starting chloramphenicol therapy.
• Keep in mind that chloramphenicol should never be used to treat minor infections or as prophylaxis because of its many serious toxicities.
• Repeated courses of therapy should be avoided because of the risk of serious adverse reactions.
• For I.V. use, prepare a 10% solution by adding 10 ml sterile water for injection or

D₅W to each 1-g vial. Administer over at least 1 minute.
• Know that diluted I.V. solution is stable for 24 to 48 hours when stored at room temperature or refrigerated. Don't use if cloudy.
• Assess patient for fever, sore throat, tiredness, unusual bleeding, or ecchymosis; these may indicate a blood dyscrasia.
• Perform neurologic assessments regularly, looking for signs of peripheral neuropathy.
WARNING If early signs of gray syndrome appear (failure to eat, pallor, cyanosis, abdominal distention, irregular respirations, and vasomotor collapse), notify prescriber and be prepared to stop drug immediately.
• Monitor blood chloramphenicol level as appropriate. Keep in mind that therapeutic peak levels are 10 to 20 mcg/ml and trough levels are 5 to 10 mcg/ml.
• Monitor CBC and platelet and reticulocyte counts as ordered to detect signs of blood dyscrasia. Notify prescriber immediately about abnormal results.

PATIENT TEACHING
• Instruct patient to immediately report to prescriber signs of blood dyscrasia.
WARNING Tell patient to stay alert for signs of potentially fatal, irreversible bone marrow depression that leads to aplastic anemia and is characterized by fever, pallor, pharyngitis, severe fatigue and weakness, and unusual bleeding or bruising. Bone marrow depression may occur weeks to months after therapy stops. Emphasize the need for follow-up care.

---

chlordiazepoxide hydrochloride

Apo-Chlordiazepoxide (CAN), Librium, Novo-Poxide (CAN)

Class, Category, and Schedule
Chemical class: Benzodiazepine
Therapeutic class: Antianxiety
Pregnancy category: Not rated
Controlled substance schedule: IV

Indications and Dosages
➤ *To provide short-term management of mild anxiety*

CAPSULES, TABLETS
Adults. 5 to 10 mg three or four times daily.
Children over age 6. 5 mg two to four times daily increased as needed to 10 mg two or three times daily, or 0.5 mg/kg daily in equally divided doses every 6 to 8 hr.
➤ *To provide short-term management of severe anxiety*
CAPSULES, TABLETS
Adults. 20 to 25 mg three or four times daily.
I.V. OR I.M. INJECTION
Adults. *Initial:* 50 to 100 mg. Then, 25 to 50 mg three or four times daily, as needed. *Maximum:* 300 mg daily.
I.M. INJECTION
Children age 12 and over. 0.5 mg/kg daily in equally divided doses every 6 to 8 hr.
➤ *To provide short-term treatment of acute alcohol withdrawal*
CAPSULES, TABLETS, I.V. OR I.M. INJECTION
Adults. *Initial:* 50 to 100 mg, usually given I.V. or I.M. Repeated in 2 to 4 hr followed by individualized oral dosage if needed to control symptoms. *Maximum:* 300 mg daily.
➤ *To provide perioperative relaxation and reduce apprehension and anxiety*
CAPSULES, TABLETS, I.M. INJECTION
Adults. 5 to 10 mg P.O. three or four times daily several days before surgery; 50 to 100 mg I.M. 1 hr before surgery.
DOSAGE ADJUSTMENT Dosage reduced to 5 mg P.O. two to four times daily, as needed, for elderly or debilitated patients.

Mechanism of Action
May potentiate the effects of gamma-aminobutyric acid (GABA) and other inhibitory neurotransmitters by binding to specific benzodiazepine receptors in limbic and cortical areas of the CNS. By binding to these receptors, chlordiazepoxide increases GABA's inhibitory effects and blocks cortical and limbic arousal, which helps control emotional behavior. It also helps relieve symptoms of alcohol withdrawal by causing CNS depression.

Contraindications
Hypersensitivity to chlordiazepoxide or its components

Interactions
DRUGS
antacids: Altered rate of chlordiazepoxide absorption

cimetidine, disulfiram, fluoxetine, isoniazid, ketoconazole, metoprolol, oral contraceptives, propoxyphene, propranolol, valproic acid: Increased blood chlordiazepoxide level
CNS depressants: Increased CNS effects
digoxin: Increased blood digoxin level and risk of digitalis toxicity
levodopa: Decreased efficacy of levodopa's antiparkinsonian effects
neuromuscular blockers: Potentiated, counteracted, or diminished effects of neuromuscular blockers
phenytoin: Possibly increased phenytoin toxicity
probenecid: Shortened onset of action or prolonged effect of chlordiazepoxide
rifampin: Decreased chlordiazepoxide effect
theophyllines: Antagonized sedative effects of chlordiazepoxide
ACTIVITIES
alcohol use: Increased CNS effects

Adverse Reactions

CNS: Ataxia, confusion, depression, drowsiness, suicidal ideation
CV: ECG changes, hypotension, tachycardia
GI: Hepatic dysfunction
HEME: Agranulocytosis
SKIN: Jaundice
Other: Injection-site pain, redness, and swelling

Nursing Considerations

• Use chlordiazepoxide cautiously in patients with renal or hepatic impairment or porphyria.
WARNING Be aware that prolonged use of chlordiazepoxide at therapeutic doses can lead to dependence.
• For I.V. use, reconstitute ampule contents with 5 ml sterile water for injection or sodium chloride for injection. Agitate gently until completely dissolved. Give slowly over 1 minute.
• For I.M. use, reconstitute only with diluent provided by manufacturer.
WARNING Don't use supplied diluent to prepare drug for I.V. use because air bubbles form on the surface.
• Don't give opalescent or hazy solution.
• Monitor patient for evidence of phlebitis or thrombophlebitis after I.V. chlordiazepoxide administration.
• Monitor liver function test results during therapy.

• If patient is a hyperactive, aggressive child or has a history of psychiatric disorders, watch for paradoxical reactions, such as excitement, stimulation, and acute rage, during first 2 weeks of therapy.
• Watch patients closely (especially children, adolescents, and young adults) for suicidal tendencies, particularly when chlordiazepoxide therapy starts and dosage changes.
PATIENT TEACHING
• Warn that drug may cause drowsiness.
• Advise patient to avoid other CNS depressants during therapy.
• Warn patient not to take antacids with chlordiazepoxide.
• Urge family or caregiver to watch patient closely for suicidal tendencies, especially when therapy starts or dosage changes and particularly if patient is a child, teenager, or young adult.

chlorothiazide
Diuril

chlorothiazide sodium
Diuril

Class and Category

Chemical class: Sulfonamide derivative
Therapeutic class: Antihypertensive, diuretic
Pregnancy category: B

Indications and Dosages

➤ *To treat hypertension*
ORAL SUSPENSION, TABLETS
Adults. 250 to 1,000 mg daily in a single dose or divided doses twice daily. *Maximum:* 2,000 mg daily in divided doses.
Children age 6 months and over. 10 to 20 mg/kg daily in a single dose or divided doses twice daily. *Maximum:* 1,000 mg daily for ages 2 to 12; 375 mg daily for ages 6 months to 2 years.
Children under age 6 months. Up to 30 mg/kg daily in divided doses given twice daily.
➤ *To produce diuresis*

ORAL SUSPENSION, TABLETS
Adults. 250 mg every 6 to 12 hr. Administered on an intermittent schedule, if needed, such as alternate days or 3 to 5 days/wk.
Children age 6 months and over. 10 to 20 mg/kg daily in a single dose or divided doses twice daily. *Maximum:* 1,000 mg daily for children ages 2 to 12; 375 mg daily for children ages 6 months to 2 years.
Children under age 6 months. Up to 33 mg/kg daily in divided doses twice daily.
I.V. INFUSION OR INJECTION
Adults. 250 mg every 6 to 12 hr.

Route	Onset	Peak	Duration
P.O.	2 hr	4 hr	6–12 hr
I.V.	15 min	4 hr	6–12 hr

Mechanism of Action

May promote sodium, chloride, and water excretion by inhibiting sodium reabsorption in the kidneys' distal tubules. Initially, chlorothiazide may reduce blood pressure by decreasing extracellular fluid volume, plasma volume, and cardiac output. It also may dilate arteries directly, reducing peripheral vascular resistance. After several weeks, extracellular fluid and plasma volume and cardiac output return to normal, but peripheral vascular resistance remains decreased.

Contraindications

Anuria; hepatic coma; hypersensitivity to chlorothiazide or its components, sulfonamides, or related thiazide diuretics; renal failure

Interactions
DRUGS

allopurinol: Increased risk of allopurinol hypersensitivity
amiodarone: Increased risk of arrhythmias from hypokalemia
amphotericin B, glucocorticoids: Intensified electrolyte depletion
anesthetics: Potentiated effects of anesthetics
anticholinergics: Increased chlorothiazide absorption
anticoagulants, methenamines, sulfonylureas: Decreased effects of these drugs

antihypertensives: Increased antihypertensive effect
antineoplastics: Prolonged antineoplastic-induced leukopenia
calcium: Possibly increased blood calcium level
cholestyramine, colestipol: Decreased chlorothiazide absorption
diazoxide: Hyperglycemia, hypotension
digitalis glycosides: Increased risk of digitalis-induced arrhythmias
dopamine: Increased diuretic effect
lithium: Increased risk of lithium toxicity
loop diuretics: Synergistic effects, resulting in profound diuresis and serious electrolyte imbalances
methyldopa: Potential development of hemolytic anemia
neuromuscular blockers: Increased neuromuscular blockade
NSAIDs: Possibly reduced diuretic effect of chlorothiazide; increased risk of renal failure if patient has compromised renal function
sympathomimetics: Possibly inhibited antihypertensive effect of chlorothiazide
vitamin D: Enhanced vitamin D action

Adverse Reactions

CNS: Dizziness, headache, paresthesia, restlessness, vertigo, weakness
CV: Orthostatic hypotension
ENDO: Hyperglycemia
GI: Abdominal cramps, anorexia, constipation, diarrhea, gastric irritation, nausea, pancreatitis, vomiting
GU: Glycosuria, hematuria (I.V. form), impotence, interstitial nephritis, renal dysfunction or failure
HEME: Agranulocytosis, aplastic anemia, hemolytic anemia, leukopenia, thrombocytopenia
MS: Muscle spasms
SKIN: Jaundice, photosensitivity, purpura, rash, urticaria
Other: Anaphylactic reactions, hypercalcemia, hyperuricemia, hypochloremic alkalosis, hypokalemia, hypomagnesemia, hyponatremia, hypovolemia

Nursing Considerations

• Don't give parenteral form of chlorothiazide by I.M. or subcutaneous route.
• For I.V. use, reconstitute with at least 18 ml of sterile water for injection.

Discard unused solution after 24 hours. Reconstituted solution is compatible with dextrose solution or normal saline solution for infusion.

• Watch I.V. site closely. If extravasation occurs, stop infusion and tell prescriber at once.

• Weigh patient daily to assess fluid loss and drug effectiveness. If used to treat hypertension, check blood pressure often; antihypertensive effect may not appear for days.

• Assess patient for electrolyte imbalances.

• Monitor renal function closely, especially in elderly patients, because risk of toxicity increases with renal impairment.

PATIENT TEACHING

• Tell patient to take chlorothiazide early in the day to avoid nocturia and to take it with food or milk if GI distress occurs.

• Urge patient to eat a high-potassium diet.

• Instruct patient to rise slowly to minimize effects of orthostatic hypotension.

• Urge patient to weigh himself at least weekly and to notify prescriber if weight rises or falls by 5 lb (2.25 kg) or more in 2 days.

• Tell patient to immediately notify prescriber if he develops weakness, cramps, nausea, vomiting, restlessness, excessive thirst, drowsiness, tiredness, increased heart rate, diarrhea, sudden joint pain, or dizziness.

• If patient has diabetes mellitus, tell him to check blood glucose level often. Oral antidiabetic dosage may need to be increased.

• Tell patient to avoid prolonged exposure to sun, use sunscreen, and wear protective clothing.

• Advise patient to consult prescriber or pharmacist before using alcohol and such OTC drugs as those used for appetite control, colds, cough, hay fever, and sinus problems.

chlorphenesin carbamate

Maolate

Class and Category

Chemical class: Chemically related to mephenesin
Therapeutic class: Skeletal muscle relaxant
Pregnancy category: Not rated

Indications and Dosages

➤ *As adjunct to relieve pain in acute musculoskeletal conditions*

TABLETS

Adults. 800 mg three times daily until desired effect occurs. *Maintenance:* 400 mg four times daily or less, as needed.

Mechanism of Action

May act on the CNS, rather than directly on skeletal muscle, producing a sedative effect that aids in muscle relaxation.

Contraindications

Hypersensitivity to chlorphenesin or its components

Interactions

DRUGS

CNS depressants: Increased adverse CNS effects

ACTIVITIES

alcohol use: Increased adverse CNS effects

Adverse Reactions

CNS: Confusion, dizziness, drowsiness, headache, insomnia, nervousness, paradoxical stimulation
EENT: Diplopia, transient vision loss
GI: Epigastric discomfort, nausea
Other: Anaphylaxis, drug-induced fever

Nursing Considerations

WARNING Use chlorphenesin cautiously in patients hypersensitive to aspirin; it contains tartrazine, which may cause hypersensitivity.

• Expect drug therapy to last for no more than 8 weeks because safety beyond this point is unknown.

• Provide rest and other pain-relief measures.

PATIENT TEACHING

• Because of possible reduced alertness, advise patient to avoid potentially hazardous activities until drug's CNS effects are known.

• Instruct patient to notify prescriber if these symptoms occur: confusion, dizziness, drowsiness, insomnia, nervousness, or paradoxical stimulation.

• Tell patient to immediately notify prescriber if he develops a fever or any signs or symptoms of an allergic reaction, such as rash, hives, itching, facial swelling, or difficulty breathing.

chlorpromazine

Largactil (CAN), Thorazine

chlorpromazine hydrochloride

Chlorpromanyl (CAN), Novo-Chlorpromazine (CAN), Thorazine, Thorazine Spansule

Class and Category

Chemical class: Propylamine derivative of phenothiazine
Therapeutic class: Antiemetic, antipsychotic, tranquilizer
Pregnancy category: No

Indications and Dosages

➤ *To manage symptoms of psychotic disorders or control manic manifestations of manic-depression in outpatients*

E.R. CAPSULES

Adults. 30 to 300 mg 1 to 3 times daily, with dosage adjusted as needed. *Maximum:* 1 g daily.

ORAL CONCENTRATE, SYRUP, TABLETS

Adults. 10 mg three times daily or four times daily, or 25 mg twice daily or three times daily. After 1 or 2 days, dose increased by 20 to 50 mg semiweekly until patient is calm. After 2 wk of calmness, dosage gradually reduced to maintenance level of 200 to 800 mg daily in equally divided doses.

➤ *To control acutely disturbed or manic hospitalized patients*

I.M. INJECTION

Adults. 25 mg. Repeated 25 to 50 mg in 1 hr, if needed. Increased gradually over several days up to 400 mg every 4 to 6 hr for severe cases until behavior is controlled. Then, regimen switched to oral form and outpatient dosage.

➤ *To treat severe behavioral problems in children*

ORAL CONCENTRATE, SYRUP, TABLETS

Children ages 6 months to 12 years. 0.55 mg/kg every 4 to 6 hr, as needed.

SUPPOSITORIES

Children ages 6 months to 12 years. 1 mg/kg every 6 to 8 hr, as needed.

I.M. INJECTION

Children ages 6 months to 12 years. 0.55 mg/kg every 6 to 8 hr. *Maximum:* 75 mg daily for children ages 5 to 12 years or weighing 50 to 100 lb (23 to 45 kg), except in unmanageable cases; 40 mg daily for children up to age 5 or weighing up to 50 lb.

➤ *To treat nausea and vomiting*

ORAL CONCENTRATE, SYRUP, TABLETS

Adults and adolescents. 10 to 25 mg every 4 to 6 hr, as needed.

Children ages 6 months to 12 years. 0.55 mg/kg every 4 to 6 hr, as needed.

I.M. INJECTION

Adults. 25 mg. If no hypotension occurs, 25 to 50 mg every 3 to 4 hr, as needed, until vomiting stops; then drug switched to oral form.

Children age 6 months and over. 0.55 mg/kg every 6 to 8 hr, as needed. *Maximum:* 75 mg daily for children ages 5 to 12 or weighing 50 to 100 lb; 40 mg daily for children up to age 5 or weighing up to 50 lb.

SUPPOSITORIES

Adults and adolescents. 50 to 100 mg every 6 to 8 hr, as needed.

Children ages 6 months to 12 years. 1 mg/kg every 6 to 8 hr, as needed.

➤ *To provide intraoperative control of nausea and vomiting*

I.V. INJECTION

Adults. 25 mg diluted to 1 mg/ml with sodium chloride for injection and given at no more than 2 mg every 2 min. *Maximum:* 25 mg.

Children age 6 months and over. 0.275 mg/kg diluted to at least 1 mg/ml with sodium chloride for injection and given at no more than 1 mg every 2 min. *Maximum:* 75 mg/day for children ages 5 to 12 or weighing 50 to 100 lb; 40 mg daily for children up to age 5 years or weighing up to 50 lb.

I.M. INJECTION

Adults. 12.5 mg. Repeated in 30 min if needed and no hypotension occurs.

Children age 6 months and over. 0.275 mg/kg. Repeated in 30 min if needed and tolerated.

➤ *To treat intractable hiccups*

TABLETS

Adults. 25 to 50 mg three times daily or four times daily. If hiccups last longer than 2 days, route switched to I.M., as prescribed.

I.V. INFUSION
Adults. 25 to 50 mg diluted in 500 to 1,000 ml of normal saline solution and given at 1 mg/min with patient supine.
I.M. INJECTION
Adults. 25 to 50 mg given only if oral route is ineffective. If symptoms persist, route switched to I.V., as prescribed.
➤ *To provide preoperative relaxation*
ORAL CONCENTRATE, SYRUP, TABLETS
Adults and adolescents. 25 to 50 mg 2 to 3 hr before surgery.
Children ages 6 months to 12 years. 0.55 mg/kg 2 to 3 hr before surgery.
I.M. INJECTION
Adults. 12.5 to 25 mg 1 to 2 hr before surgery.
Children age 6 months and over. 0.55 mg/ kg 1 to 2 hr before surgery.
➤ *To treat acute intermittent porphyria*
ORAL CONCENTRATE, SYRUP, TABLETS
Adults and adolescents. 25 to 50 mg three times daily or four times daily.
I.M. INJECTION
Adults. 25 mg three times daily or four times daily until oral route is possible.
➤ *To treat tetanus (usually as adjunct with barbiturates)*
I.V. INFUSION
Adults. 25 to 50 mg diluted to at least 1 mg/ ml and given at no more than 1 mg/min.
Children age 6 months and over. 0.55 mg/kg every 6 to 8 hr, diluted to at least 1 mg/ml and given at no more than 1 mg/2 min. *Maximum:* 75 mg daily for children ages 5 to 12 years or weighing 50 to 100 lb; 40 mg daily for children up to age 5 years or weighing up to 50 lb.
I.M. INJECTION
Adults. 25 to 50 mg three times daily or four times daily.
Children age 6 months and over. 0.55 mg/ kg every 6 to 8 hr. *Maximum:* 75 mg daily for children ages 5 to 12 or weighing 50 to 100 lb; 40 mg daily for children up to age 5 years or weighing up to 50 lb.
DOSAGE ADJUSTMENT Dosage possibly reduced for patients with hepatic dys-function. Dosage reduced to one-third to one-half the normal adult dosage for elderly or debilitated patients.

Mechanism of Action

Depresses brain areas that control activity and aggression, including the cerebral cortex, hypothalamus, and limbic system, by an unknown mechanism. Prevents nausea and vomiting by inhibiting or blocking dopamine receptors in the medullary chemoreceptor trigger zone and peripherally by blocking the vagus nerve in the GI tract. May relieve anxiety by indirect reduction in arousal and increased filtering of internal stimuli to the reticular activating system in the brain stem.

Incompatibilities

Don't mix chlorpromazine with thiopental, atropine, or solutions that don't have a pH of 4 to 5 because a precipitate will form. Don't mix chlorpromazine injection with other drugs in a syringe.

Contraindications

Comatose states; hypersensitivity to chlorpromazine, phenothiazines, or their com-ponents; use of large amounts of CNS depressants

Interactions
DRUGS
amphetamines: Decreased amphetamine effectiveness, decreased antipsychotic effectiveness of chlorpromazine
antacids (aluminum hydroxide or magnesium trisilicate gel): Decreased chlorpromazine absorption and effectiveness
barbiturates: Decreased plasma level and, possibly, effectiveness of chlorpromazine
CNS depressants: Prolonged and intensified CNS depression
metrizamide: Possibly lowered seizure threshold
oral anticoagulants: Decreased anti-coagulation
phenytoin: Interference with phenytoin metabolism, increased risk of phenytoin toxicity
propranolol: Increased plasma levels of both drugs
thiazide diuretics: Possibly increased orthostatic hypotension
ACTIVITIES
alcohol use: Prolonged and intensified CNS depression

Adverse Reactions
CNS: Drowsiness, extrapyramidal reactions (such as dystonia, fever, motor restlessness, pseudoparkinsonism, and tardive dyskinesia), neuroleptic malignant syndrome, seizures

CV: ECG changes, such as nonspecific, usually reversible Q- and T-wave changes; orthostatic hypotension; tachycardia
EENT: Blurred vision, dry mouth, nasal congestion, ocular changes (fine particle deposits in lens and cornea) with long-term therapy
ENDO: Gynecomastia, hyperglycemia, hypoglycemia, lactation, moderate breast engorgement
GI: Constipation, ileus, nausea
GU: Amenorrhea, ejaculation disorders, impotence, priapism, urine retention
HEME: Agranulocytosis, aplastic anemia, eosinophilia, hemolytic anemia, leukopenia, pancytopenia, thrombocytopenic purpura
SKIN: Exfoliative dermatitis, jaundice, photosensitivity, tissue necrosis, urticaria

Nursing Considerations
• Don't open or crush E.R. capsules.
• Chlorpromazine shouldn't be used to treat dementia-related psychosis in the elderly because of an increased risk of death.
• Use chlorpromazine cautiously in patients (especially children) with chronic respiratory disorders (such as severe asthma or emphysema) or acute respiratory tract infections because drug has CNS depressant effect. Also use cautiously in patients with cardiovascular, hepatic, or renal disease because of increased risk of developing hypotension, heart failure, and arrhythmias.
• Because of chlorpromazine's anticholinergic effects, use it cautiously in patients with glaucoma. Also use it cautiously in those who are exposed to extreme heat or organophosphate insecticides and those receiving atropine or related drugs.
• Protect concentrate from light. Refrigeration isn't required.
• Dilute concentrate in at least 60 ml of diluent just before administering it. Use tomato or fruit juice, milk, simple syrup, orange syrup, a carbonated beverage, coffee, tea, water, or semisolid food, such as pudding and soup.
• Protect parenteral solution from light. Solution should be clear and colorless to pale yellow. Discard markedly discolored solution.
• Don't inject drug by subcutaneous route because it can cause severe tissue necrosis.

• Wear gloves when working with liquid or injectable form because parenteral solution may cause contact dermatitis.
• For I.V. injection, dilute chlorpromazine with sodium chloride to a concentration of 1 mg/ml.
• Give I.M. injection slowly and deep into upper outer quadrant of buttocks, such as in the gluteus maximus. To minimize hypotensive effects, keep patient lying flat and monitor blood pressure for 30 minutes after injection.
WARNING Stay alert for possible suppressed cough reflex, which increases the risk of the patient's aspirating vomitus.
• Monitor patient for increased sensitivity to drug's CNS effects if patient has a history of hepatic encephalopathy from cirrhosis.
WARNING If neuroleptic malignant syndrome (hyperpyrexia, muscle rigidity, altered mental status, autonomic instability) develops, notify prescriber immediately and expect to stop drug and start intensive treatment. Watch for recurrence if patient resumes antipsychotic therapy.
PATIENT TEACHING
• Instruct patient to swallow E.R. capsules whole and not to crush, break, or chew them.
• Tell patient not to take drug within 2 hours of an antacid. Allow him to take drug with food or a full glass of milk or water.
• If patient uses suppository form, tell him to chill the suppository, moisten it with cold water, and insert it well into rectum.
• Tell patient to store oral concentrate at room temperature, away from light, to measure it with the dropper provided, and to dilute it in 4 oz of fluid just before use.
• Because of possible drowsiness, dizziness, and blurred vision (especially during the first few days of therapy), advise patient to avoid hazardous activities until drug's CNS effects are known.
• Tell patient to avoid alcohol because of possible additive effects and hypotension.
• Advise patient, especially if elderly, to rise slowly from a supine or seated position to avoid dizziness, light-headedness, and fainting.
• Tell patient to inform doctors and dentists that he's taking chlorpromazine

C

before he has surgery, medical tests, or dental work.
• Explain that drug may reduce the body's response to heat and cold; tell patient to avoid temperature extremes, as in a sauna, hot tub, or very cold or hot shower. Remind patient to dress warmly in cold weather.
• Warn patient not to take OTC drugs for a cold or an allergy because they can increase the risk of heatstroke and other unwanted effects.
• Inform patient that drug increases sensitivity to sunlight; tell him to stay out of the sun as much as possible and to protect his skin.
• If patient has dry mouth, suggest sugarless chewing gum, hard candy, and fluids.
• Urge patient to report sudden sore throat or other signs of infection.
• Advise female patient of childbearing age to notify prescriber if she intends to become or suspects that she is pregnant during therapy.

chlorpropamide

Apo-Chlorpropamide (CAN), Diabinese, Novo-Propamide (CAN)

Class and Category
Chemical class: Sulfonylurea
Therapeutic class: Antidiabetic
Pregnancy category: C

Indications and Dosages
➤ *As adjunct to manage non–insulin-dependent diabetes when diet alone fails to lower blood glucose level*
TABLETS
Adults. *Initial:* 250 mg daily for 5 to 7 days. After therapy begins, dosage may be adjusted up or down in increments of 50 to 125 mg at intervals of 3 to 5 days to obtain optimal control. *Maintenance:* 100 to 500 mg daily. *Maximum:* 750 mg daily.
DOSAGE ADJUSTMENT If patient takes more than 40 units of insulin daily, dosage reduced to half usual insulin dose for first few days of chlorpropamide therapy. Insulin dose can be reduced, depending on response. If patient takes oral antidiabetic drug or less than 40 units of insulin daily, it may be stopped abruptly when chlor-propamide starts.

Dosage reduced to half usual dose if patient has mild renal failure because metabolites and unchanged drug are excreted in urine. To avoid hypoglycemic reactions, initial dosage reduced to 100 to 125 mg daily for elderly, debilitated, or malnourished patients and patients with impaired hepatic function.

Mechanism of Action
Lowers blood glucose level by stimulating release of insulin from the pancreas in patients who have functioning beta cells. It also may increase insulin sensitivity in target tissues, which may result in a decrease in liver breakdown of glycogen to glucose or the liver's production of new glucose.

Route	Onset	Peak	Duration
P.O.	1 hr	3–6 hr	24–72 hr

Contraindications
Diabetic ketoacidosis (with or without coma), hypersensitivity to chlorpropamide or its components, type I diabetes mellitus

Interactions
DRUGS
androgens, anticoagulants, azole antifungals, chloramphenicol, clofibrate, fenfluramine, fluconazole, gemfibrozil, H₂-receptor antagonists, magnesium salts, MAO inhibitors, methyldopa, probenecid, salicylates, sulfinpyrazone, sulfonamides, tricyclic antidepressants, urinary acidifiers: Increased hypoglycemic effect
barbiturates: Prolonged barbiturate action
beta blockers, calcium channel blockers, cholestyramine, corticosteroids, diazoxide, estrogens, hydantoins, isoniazid, nicotinic acid, oral contraceptives, phenothiazines, rifampin, sympathomimetics, thiazide diuretics, thyroid drugs, urinary alkalinizers: Decreased hypoglycemic effect
digitalis glycosides: Increased blood digitalis level
oral miconazole: Risk of severe hypoglycemia
ACTIVITIES
alcohol use: Disulfiram-like reaction

Adverse Reactions
ENDO: Hypoglycemia
GI: Anorexia, cholestatic jaundice, diarrhea, hepatitis, hunger, nausea, vomiting
HEME: Hemolytic anemia

SKIN: Maculopapular eruptions, photosensitivity, pruritus, urticaria
Other: Disulfiram-like reaction

Nursing Considerations

- Use chlorpropamide cautiously in patients with renal or hepatic dysfunction; in elderly, debilitated, or malnourished patients; and in those with adrenal or pituitary insufficiency because of increased susceptibility to drug's hypoglycemic action. Also know that, although rare, drug may cause cholestatic jaundice and hepatitis that may progress to liver failure. If patient shows signs and symptoms of hepatic dysfunction, notify prescriber and expect drug to be discontinued.
- Use chlorpropamide cautiously in patients with glucose 6-phosphate dehydrogenase deficiency because sulfonylureas, such as chlorpropamide, can cause hemolytic anemia.
- Monitor patient's blood glucose level often at start of therapy and during dosage adjustments or changes in patient's life, such as during stress and illness. Hypoglycemia may be difficult to recognize in elderly patients and those who take beta-adrenergic blockers.
- Assess patient for hypoglycemia—the most common adverse reaction to chlorpropamide—especially in patients whose caloric intake is deficient, who have just engaged in strenuous or prolonged exercise, who have ingested alcohol, or who take more than one glucose-lowering drug.
- Treat hypoglycemia promptly by giving 15 g of simple carbohydrate, such as 4 oz of orange juice or soda or 8 oz of milk. Repeat in 15 minutes, if needed. Because of drug's long half-life, careful monitoring and frequent feedings are required for 3 to 5 days after a hypoglycemic episode. Hospitalization and I.V. glucose may be needed.
- Monitor patients receiving long-term chlorpropamide therapy for secondary failure, which causes loss of blood glucose control despite adherence to prescribed drug therapy and diet and exercise guidelines. If secondary failure occurs, therapy should be discontinued and a different antidiabetic drug substituted.

PATIENT TEACHING
- Instruct patient to store chlorpropamide in a sealed container, protected from heat and light.
- Tell patient to take chlorpropamide with breakfast.
- Emphasize that drug works with diet and exercise to help control blood glucose level and isn't a substitute for them.
- Tell patient to monitor blood glucose level as instructed.
- Instruct patient not to skip meals or exercise excessively.
- Teach patient how to recognize and treat hypoglycemia. Tell him to report frequent or severe hypoglycemia to prescriber.
- Caution patient with confirmed or suspected hypoglycemia not to drive or operate machinery until blood glucose levels return to normal.
- Tell patient to take a missed dose as soon as he remembers it unless it's almost time for the next scheduled dose.
- Urge patient to wear or carry medical identification showing that he has diabetes and listing his drugs.
- Advise the patient to protect his skin from the sun.
- Instruct patient to report about fever, sore throat, dark yellow or brown urine, yellow skin and eyes, bleeding, and bruising.

chlorthalidone

Apo-Chlorthalidone (CAN), Hygroton, Novo-Thalidone (CAN), Thalitone, Uridon (CAN)

Class and Category

Chemical class: Phthalimidine derivative of benzenesulfonamide (thiazide-like diuretic)
Therapeutic class: Antihypertensive, diuretic
Pregnancy category: B

Indications and Dosages

➤ *To reduce edema caused by heart failure, hepatic cirrhosis, corticosteroid or estrogen therapy, or renal dysfunction*
TABLETS
Adults. *Initial:* 50 to 100 mg (Thalitone, 30 to 60 mg) daily, 100 mg (Thalitone, 60 mg) every other day, or 150 to 200 mg (Thalitone, 90 to 120 mg) daily or every

other day. *Maintenance:* Individualized; may be lower than initial dosage.

➤ *To treat hypertension*

TABLETS

Adults. *Initial:* 25 mg daily (Thalitone, 15 mg daily). If response is insufficient, dosage increased to 50 mg daily (Thalitone, 30 to 50 mg daily). If additional control is required, dosage increased to 100 mg daily (except Thalitone) or a second antihypertensive added. *Maintenance:* Individualized; may be lower than initial dosage.

Mechanism of Action

May promote sodium, chloride, and water excretion by inhibiting sodium reabsorption in the distal tubules of the kidneys. Initially, chlorthalidone may decrease extracellular fluid volume, plasma volume, and cardiac output, which helps explain how it reduces blood pressure. It also may dilate arteries directly, which helps reduce peripheral vascular resistance and blood pressure. After several weeks, extracellular fluid and plasma volume and cardiac output return to normal, but peripheral vascular resistance remains decreased.

Route	Onset	Peak	Duration
P.O.	2–3 hr	2–6 hr	24–72 hr

Contraindications

Anuria; hypersensitivity to chlorthalidone, other sulfonamides, or their components; renal decompensation

Interactions

DRUGS

allopurinol: Increased risk of allopurinol hypersensitivity

amphotericin B, glucocorticoids: Intensified electrolyte depletion

anesthetics: Potentiated effects of anesthetics

anticholinergics: Increased chlorthalidone absorption

antidiabetics, methenamines, oral anticoagulants, sulfonylureas: Decreased effects of these drugs

antihypertensives: Potentiated action of antihypertensives and chlorthalidone

antineoplastics: Prolonged antineoplastic-induced leukopenia

cholestyramine, colestipol: Decreased chlorthalidone absorption

diazoxide: Increased risk of hyperglycemia and hypotension

digitalis glycosides: Increased risk of digitalis-induced arrhythmias

lithium: Decreased renal lithium clearance and increased risk of lithium toxicity

loop diuretics: Increased synergistic effects, resulting in profound diuresis and serious electrolyte imbalances

methyldopa: Potential development of hemolytic anemia

neuromuscular blockers: Increased neuromuscular blockade

NSAIDs: Possibly reduced diuretic effect of chlorthalidone

vitamin D: Enhanced vitamin D action

Adverse Reactions

CNS: Dizziness, headache, insomnia, light-headedness, paresthesia, restlessness, vertigo, weakness

CV: Orthostatic hypotension, vasculitis

EENT: Yellow vision

ENDO: Hyperglycemia

GI: Abdominal cramps or pain, anorexia, bloating, constipation, diarrhea, gastric irritation, nausea, pancreatitis, vomiting

GU: Decreased libido, impotence

HEME: Agranulocytosis, aplastic anemia, hypoplastic anemia, leukopenia, thrombocytopenia

MS: Gout attacks, muscle spasms

SKIN: Cutaneous vasculitis, exfoliative dermatitis, jaundice, necrotizing vasculitis, photosensitivity, purpura, rash, urticaria

Other: Hyperuricemia

Nursing Considerations

• Use chlorthalidone cautiously in patients with impaired hepatic function or progressive hepatic disease because minor changes in fluid and electrolyte balance may cause hepatic coma.

• Assess BUN, serum electrolyte, uric acid, and blood glucose levels before therapy and periodically throughout therapy. Monitor patient for signs of fluid and electrolyte imbalance.

WARNING Monitor renal function periodically to detect cumulative drug effects, which may cause azotemia in patients with impaired renal function.

PATIENT TEACHING
• Stress the importance of taking chlorthalidone even when feeling well.
• Tell patient to store drug at room temperature in tightly closed container.
• Tell patient to take drug in the morning with food or milk.
• To minimize effects of orthostatic hypotension, instruct patient to rise slowly from a seated or lying position.
• Advise patient to check blood pressure regularly.
• Instruct patient to report signs of low potassium level, such as muscle weakness and fatigue.
• Advise patient to protect his skin from the sun.
• Urge patient to immediately report sudden joint pain to prescriber because drug can cause sudden gout attacks.
• Instruct patient to take a missed dose as soon as he remembers it. If he misses one day in an every-other-day schedule, tell him to take the dose on the off day and then resume usual dosing schedule. Warn against taking double or extra doses.

chlorzoxazone
EZE-DS, Paraflex, Parafon Forte DSC, Relaxazone, Remular, Remular-S, Strifon Forte DSC

Class and Category
Chemical class: Benzoxazole derivative
Therapeutic class: Skeletal muscle relaxant
Pregnancy category: C (Parafon Forte DSC, not rated)

Indications and Dosages
➤ *As adjunct to relieve acute musculoskeletal pain and stiffness*
TABLETS
Adults. 250 to 750 mg three times daily or four times daily, usually 500 mg three times daily or four times daily, increased or decreased according to patient response.

Route	Onset	Peak	Duration
P.O.	In 1 hr	Unknown	3–4 hr

Mechanism of Action
Reduces muscle spasm by inhibiting multisynaptic reflex arcs at the level of the spinal cord and subcortical areas of the brain that are active in producing and maintaining skeletal muscle spasm.

Contraindications
Hypersensitivity or known intolerance to chlorzoxazone or any of its components

Interactions
DRUGS
CNS depressants: Additive CNS depression
ACTIVITIES
alcohol use: Additive CNS depression

Adverse Reactions
CNS: Dizziness, drowsiness, headache, lightheadedness, malaise, paradoxical stimulation
GI: Abdominal cramps or pain, constipation, diarrhea, GI bleeding, heartburn, hepatotoxicity, nausea, vomiting
GU: Urine discoloration
HEME: Agranulocytosis, anemia
SKIN: Allergic dermatitis, ecchymosis, petechiae
Other: Anaphylaxis, angioedema

Nursing Considerations
• If needed, crush chlorzoxazone tablets and mix with food or liquid for easier swallowing.
• Assess patients, especially those who have a history of allergies, for evidence of hypersensitivity, such as rash, hives, and itching.
WARNING Monitor patient for signs of hepatotoxicity, including fever, rash, jaundice, and darkened urine. Notify prescriber immediately and expect to discontinue drug if any of these signs or symptoms occur. Monitor patient for abnormal liver function test results, such as elevated AST, ALT, alkaline phosphatase, and bilirubin levels, and expect to discontinue drug, as ordered, if any of these occurs.
• Ensure adequate rest, and provide other pain-relief measures as needed.
• Institute safety measures to prevent falls or injury (such as raising bed rails and assisting with ambulation) until drug's full CNS effects are known.
PATIENT TEACHING
• Advise patient to take a missed dose of chlorzoxazone as soon as possible unless it's almost time for the next dose.

• Advise patient to avoid hazardous activities until drug's CNS effects are known.
• Instruct patient to avoid alcohol and other CNS depressants during therapy.
• Inform patient that, in rare instances, urine may turn orange or reddish purple during therapy.
• Advise patient to store drug in a tightly capped container at room temperature.

cholestyramine

Questran, Questran Light

Class and Category

Chemical class: Quaternary ammonium anion exchange resin
Therapeutic class: Antihyperlipidemic, antipruritic (cholestasis)
Pregnancy category: Not rated

Indications and Dosages

➤ *As adjunct to reduce serum cholesterol level in patients with primary hyper-cholesterolemia, to relieve pruritus associated with partial biliary obstruction*

ORAL SUSPENSION

Adults. *Initial:* 4 g once or twice daily before meals. *Maintenance:* 8 to 24 g equally divided and given 2 to 6 times a day. *Maximum:* 24 g daily when used as antihyperlipidemic and 16 g daily when used as antipruritic.

Route	Onset	Peak	Duration
P.O.	In 1–2 wk*	Unknown	2–4 wk†

Mechanism of Action

Increases bile acid excretion in feces. The resulting decreased bile acid level increases the activity of the enzyme that regulates cholesterol synthesis in the liver. As a result, the liver increases its cholesterol synthesis to produce more bile acids. However, the liver's synthesis of cholesterol typically can't match the amount needed to synthesize bile acids, which reduces the cholesterol level. Also, a decreased cholesterol level causes liver cells to increase their uptake of LDLs,

---

*For hypercholesterolemia; in 1 to 3 wk for pruritus.
† For hypercholesterolemia; 1 to 2 wk for pruritus.

which further reduces the cholesterol level. Cholestyramine may relieve pruritus by decreasing the body's bile acid level. This reduces the amount of excess bile acids that are deposited in the dermis and that typically cause pruritus in patients with cholestasis.

Contraindications

Complete biliary obstruction (when bile isn't excreted into intestine), hyper-sensitivity to cholestyramine or its components

Interactions

DRUGS

chenodiol, digitalis glycosides, fat-soluble vitamins, folic acid, gemfibrozil, penicillin G (oral), phenylbutazone, propranolol (oral), tetracyclines (oral), thiazide diuretics (oral), thyroid hormones, ursodiol, vancomycin (oral): Decreased absorption and effects of these drugs
oral anticoagulants: Decreased or increased anticoagulant effect

Adverse Reactions

CNS: Headache, dizziness
GI: Bloating, constipation, diarrhea, epigastric pain, eructation, fecal impaction, flatulence, indigestion, nausea, vomiting

Nursing Considerations

• Store cholestyramine at room temperature.
• Don't give dry powder because it may cause esophageal distress; mix it in a beverage.
WARNING Be aware that long-term use may increase bleeding tendency from hyper-prothrombinemia caused by vitamin K deficiency. If this occurs, patient will require treatment with vitamin K_1.
• Monitor for deficiencies of fat-soluble vitamins, such as A and D. If long-term therapy prevents absorption of these vitamins, expect to provide supplementation.

PATIENT TEACHING

• Urge patient to follow a low-cholesterol, low-fat diet and regular exercise program.
• Tell patient to take drug before meals.
• Instruct patient to mix dry powder as follows: Place amount of powder needed for dose in any beverage and stir vigorously. Then, vigorously stir in another 2 to 4 oz of beverage. After

drinking mixture, rinse glass with more liquid, and swallow it to make sure full dose is taken. Patient also may mix drug in thin soups or moist, pulpy fruits, such as applesauce or crushed pineapple.
• Tell patient to drink plenty of fluids and increase bulk in his diet to minimize constipation; remind him to notify prescriber if constipation, nausea, or other adverse GI reactions develop.
• Explain that serum cholesterol level will need to be measured often for first few months of therapy and periodically thereafter.
• Advise patient to take other drugs at least 1 hour before or 4 to 6 hours after cholestyramine to avoid interference with their absorption.
• Tell patient to take a missed dose as soon as he remembers but not to take double or extra doses.

choline salicylate
Arthropan

Class and Category
Chemical class: Salicylate
Therapeutic class: Analgesic, anti-inflammatory, antipyretic
Pregnancy category: C (first trimester), Not rated (later trimesters)

Indications and Dosages
➤ *To treat mild to moderate pain, reduce fever*
LIQUID
Adults and adolescents. 435 to 870 mg every 4 hr, as needed. *Maximum:* 5,325 mg daily.
Children ages 11 to 12. 435 to 652.5 mg every 4 hr, as needed. *Maximum:* Five doses daily.
Children ages 9 to 11. 435 to 543.8 mg every 4 hr, as needed. *Maximum:* Five doses daily.
Children ages 6 to 9. 435 mg every 4 hr, as needed. *Maximum:* Five doses daily.
Children ages 4 to 6. 326.5 mg every 4 hr, as needed. *Maximum:* Five doses daily.
Children ages 2 to 4. 217.5 mg every 4 hr, as needed. *Maximum:* Five doses daily.
Children up to age 2. Individualized dosage. *Maximum:* Five doses daily.

➤ *To treat rheumatoid arthritis*
LIQUID
Adults and adolescents. 870 to 1,740 mg up to four times daily.
Children age 12 and younger. 107 to 133 mg/kg daily in divided doses.

Route	Onset	Peak	Duration
P.O.	Unknown	Several wk*	Unknown

Mechanism of Action
Blocks cyclooxygenase, an enzyme needed for prostaglandin synthesis. As mediators in the inflammatory process, prostaglandins cause local vasodilation, swelling, and pain. They also influence pain transmission from the periphery to the spinal cord. By blocking cyclo-oxygenase and inhibiting prostaglandins, this NSAID decreases inflammatory symptoms and relieves pain. It also acts on the heat-regulating center in the hypothalamus and causes peripheral vasodilation, sweating, and heat loss.

Contraindications
Hypersensitivity to nonacetylated salicylates

Interactions
DRUGS
antacids: Increased clearance and decreased blood level of salicylate
carbonic anhydrase inhibitors, phenytoin, valproic acid: Decreased blood levels and therapeutic effects of these drugs
corticosteroids: Decreased blood salicylate level, increased salicylate dosage requirements
insulin, sulfonylureas: Increased hypoglycemic response
methotrexate: Increased therapeutic and toxic effects of methotrexate, especially when given in chemotherapeutic doses
oral anticoagulants: Increased blood level of unbound anticoagulant and risk of bleeding
salicylate-containing products: Increased plasma salicylate level, possibly to toxic level
uricosuric drugs: Decreased uricosuric drug efficacy

---
*For rheumatoid arthritis.

Adverse Reactions

CNS: Confusion, dizziness, drowsiness, hallucinations, headache, light-headedness
CV: Tachycardia
EENT: Hearing loss, tinnitus
GI: Constipation, diarrhea, epigastric pain, GI bleeding, heartburn, indigestion, nausea, vomiting
HEME: Easy bruising, unusual bleeding

Nursing Considerations

• Use choline salicylate cautiously in patients with renal impairment.
• Don't give salicylates to children and adolescents with chickenpox or influenza symptoms because of the risk of Reye's syndrome.
WARNING During high-dose or long-term therapy, watch for salicylate intoxication, (headache, dizziness, tinnitus, hearing loss, confusion, drowsiness, diaphoresis, vomiting, diarrhea, hyperventilation, and possibly CNS disturbance, electrolyte imbalance, respiratory acidosis, hyperthermia, and dehydration). Prepare for induced vomiting, gastric lavage, activated charcoal, and peritoneal dialysis or hemodialysis, as ordered.

PATIENT TEACHING
• Tell patient to store drug at room temperature, away from heat, light, and moisture.
• Instruct patient to take drug with full glass of water or with food.
• Tell patient to take a missed dose as soon as he remembers but to avoid doubling the dose.
• If patient has arthritis, explain that optimal drug effects may not occur for 2 to 3 weeks.
• Teach patient to recognize and immediately report signs of salicylate toxicity.
• Because drug is closely related to aspirin, advise against taking aspirin-containing OTC products during therapy.
• Instruct patient to stop taking drug and notify prescriber immediately if he experiences any symptoms of bleeding in his stomach or intestines such as passing black, bloody, or tarry stool or coughing up blood or vomit that looks like coffee grounds.

ciclesonide

Alvesco, Omnaris, Zetonna

Class and Category

Chemical class: Nonhalogenated glucocorticoid
Therapeutic class: Antiasthmatic, anti-inflammatory
Pregnancy category: C

Indications and Dosages

➤ *To prevent asthma attacks as part of maintenance therapy*
INHALATION AEROSOL (ALVESCO)
Adults and children age 12 and over using bronchodilator therapy. *Initial:* 80 mcg twice daily. *Maximum:* 160 mcg twice daily.
Adults and children age 12 and over switching from another inhaled corticosteroid. *Initial:* 80 mcg twice daily, adjusted to lowest effective dose when stabilized. *Maximum:* 320 mg twice daily.
Adults and children age 12 and older using oral corticosteroid therapy. *Initial and maximum:* 320 mcg twice daily, adjusted to lowest effective dose when stabilized.
➤ *To treat nasal congestion in seasonal allergic rhinitis*
NASAL AEROSOL (OMNARIS)
Adults and children age 6 and over. 200 mcg daily as 2 sprays in each nostril.
NASAL AEROSOL (ZETONNA)
Adults and children age 12 and over. 74 mcg daily as 1 spray in each nostril.
➤ *To treat nasal congestion in perennial allergic rhinitis*
NASAL AEROSOL (OMNARIS)
Adults and children age 12 and over. 200 mcg daily as 2 sprays in each nostril.
NASAL AEROSOL (ZETONNA)
Adults and children age 12 and over. 74 mcg daily as 1 spray in each nostril.

Mechanism of Action

Inhibits cells involved in the asthma inflammatory response, such as mast cells, eosinophils, basophils, lymphocytes, macrophages, and neutrophils. Ciclesonide also inhibits production or secretion of chemical mediators, such as histamine, eicosanoids, leukotrienes, and cytokines.

Route	Onset	Peak	Duration
Inhalation	Unknown	4 wk or longer	Several days
Nasal aerosol	Unknown	Unknown	Unknown

Contraindications

Hypersensitivity to ciclesonide or its components, primary treatment of status asthmaticus or other acute asthma episodes that require intensive measures

Interactions
DRUGS
ketoconazole: Increased exposure time of ciclesonide

Adverse Reactions

CNS: Dizziness, fatigue, headache
EENT: Cataracts, conjunctivitis, dry mouth or throat, dysphonia, epistaxis, glaucoma, hoarseness, nasal congestion or ulceration, nasal septal perforation, nasopharyngitis, oral candidiasis, pharyngolaryngeal pain, sinusitis
ENDO: Adrenal insufficiency, cushingoid symptoms, decreased bone mineral density, hyperglycemia, slower growth in children
GI: Nausea
MS: Arthralgia, back or limb pain, musculoskeletal chest pain
RESP: Bronchospasm, cough, pneumonia, upper respiratory tract infection
SKIN: Facial edema, urticaria
Other: Angioedema, infections, influenza

Nursing Considerations

• Ciclesonide should not be used in patients with recent nasal septal ulcers, nasal surgery, or nasal trauma until healing has occurred.
• Use cautiously in patients with tuberculosis; fungal, bacterial, viral, or parasitic infection; ocular herpes simplex; or measles or chickenpox because these conditions may worsen with ciclesonide therapy.
• Also use cautiously in patients with a history of increased intraocular pressure, glaucoma, or cataracts because ciclesonide may increase intraocular pressure or cause cataract formation; and in patients with major risk factors for decreased bone mineral content, such as prolonged immobilization, family history of osteoporosis, or long-term use of drugs that can reduce bone mass, such as anticonvulsants and oral corticosteroids.
• Inspect patient's oral cavity if using inhaler form, or nasal cavity if using nasal spray regularly for abnormalities. Have patient rinse mouth following inhalation of ciclesonide to reduce risk of oral candidiasis. If nasal or oral candidiasis occurs, expect to continue ciclesonide therapy, unless severe. If nasal erosion, ulceration, or perforation occurs, notify prescriber and expect nasal spray to be discontinued.
• If patient takes a systemic corticosteroid, expect to taper dosage by no more than 2.5 mg/day at weekly intervals, starting 1 week after ciclesonide therapy begins.
WARNING If patient is switched from systemic corticosteroid to ciclesonide, assess for adrenal insufficiency (fatigue, hypotension, lassitude, nausea, vomiting, weakness) early in therapy and whenever patient has infection, stress, trauma, surgery, or other steroid-depleting conditions or procedures. Notify prescriber immediately if signs or symptoms develop.
• As prescribed, administer a fast-acting inhaled bronchodilator if an acute asthma attack occurs. Ciclesonide inhalation is not a bronchodilator and its action takes longer than needed to abort acute asthma symptoms. If bronchospasm occurs immediately after ciclesonide use, expect to stop drug and start another drug regimen.
• Monitor growth in children because ciclesonide may suppress growth.
PATIENT TEACHING
• Urge patient to use ciclesonide regularly, as prescribed, but not for acute bronchospasm. Also tell her never to increase or decrease the dosage without consulting prescriber.
• Tell patient to use inhalation form only with the actuator supplied with the product. Explain that when the dose indicator shows a red zone in the window, about 20 inhalations are left, indicating a need for a refill. When the indicator shows zero, she should discard the inhaler.

Advise against relying solely on the dose indicator, especially if inhaler has been dropped, but to keep track of number of inhalations used.
• Instruct patient to use inhaler form according to package instructions. Emphasize need to make sure canister is firmly seated in the plastic mouthpiece adapter before each use and to press inhaler slowly but firmly until it can go no further in the adapter for each spray. Inform patient that she doesn't need to shake inhaler before use.
• On first use, advise her to spray three times into the air (away from her eyes), looking for a fine mist. If inhaler or spray hasn't been used for more than 4 days (Omnaris) or 10 days (Alvesco, Zetonna), it should be primed again.
• Advise patient using nasal spray form to avoid spraying the drug directly onto the nasal septum.
• Instruct patient to gargle and rinse her mouth after each dose of inhaler to help prevent dry mouth and throat, relieve throat irritation, and prevent oral yeast infection.
• Tell patient to always replace cap on inhaler after use, to keep mouthpiece clean, and to clean mouthpiece once a week with a clean, dry tissue or cloth.
• Explain that the full effect of drug may not occur for 4 weeks or more.
• Stress importance of notifying prescriber if symptoms continue or worsen.
• Instruct patient to notify prescriber immediately if asthma attacks don't respond to bronchodilators during ciclesonide inhaler use.
• If patient is switching from an oral corticosteroid to inhaled ciclesonide, urge her to carry medical identification indicating the need for supplemental systemic corticosteroids during stress or severe asthma attack.
• Caution patient to avoid contact with people who have infections because drug suppresses the immune system, increasing the risk of infection. Instruct patient to notify prescriber about exposure to chickenpox, measles, or other infections because additional treatment may be needed.

cilostazol
Pletal

Class and Category
Chemical class: Quinolinone derivative
Therapeutic class: Phosphodiesterase III inhibitor, platelet aggregation inhibitor
Pregnancy category: C

Indications and Dosages
➤ *To reduce symptoms of intermittent claudication*
TABLETS
Adults. 100 mg twice daily taken at least 30 min before or 2 hr after breakfast and dinner.

Mechanism of Action
May inhibit phosphodiesterase, decreasing phosphodiesterase activity and suppressing cyclic adenosine monophosphate (cAMP) degradation. This action increases cAMP in platelets and blood vessels, which inhibits platelet aggregation and causes vasodilation. This in turn relieves symptoms of claudication.

Contraindications
Heart failure, hypersensitivity to cilostazol or its components

Interactions
DRUGS
diltiazem, erythromycin, itraconazole, ketoconazole, omeprazole: Increased plasma cilostazol level
FOODS
grapefruit: Increased risk of adverse reactions
high-fat foods: Faster cilostazol absorption and increased risk of adverse reactions
ACTIVITIES
smoking: Decreased cilostazol effects by about 20%

Adverse Reactions
CNS: Cerebral hemorrhage, dizziness, headache, paresthesia
CV: Angina, chest pain, hypertension, hypotension, palpitations, peripheral edema, prolonged QT interval, subacute thrombosis, tachycardia, torsades de pointes
EENT: Pharyngitis, rhinitis

ENDO: Diabetes mellitus, hot flashes, hyperglycemia
GI: Abdominal pain, abnormal stool, diarrhea, elevated liver function test results, flatulence, GI hemorrhage, hepatic dysfunction, indigestion, jaundice, vomiting
GU: Elevated BUN level, hematuria
HEME: Agranulocytosis, aplastic anemia, bleeding tendency, decreased platelet count, granulocytopenia, leukopenia, thrombocytopenia
MS: Back pain, myalgia
RESP: Cough, interstitial pneumonia, pulmonary hemorrhage
SKIN: Eruptions, pruritus, rash, Stevens-Johnson syndrome
Other: Infection, increased blood uric acid level

Nursing Considerations
• Monitor patient's vital signs and cardiovascular status closely because cilostazol may cause cardiovascular lesions, which could lead to problems, such as endocardial hemorrhage.
• Monitor blood glucose level to detect hyperglycemia. Also assess for signs of type 2 diabetes mellitus, such as polyuria, polydipsia, polyphagia, and fatigue.
PATIENT TEACHING
• Instruct patient to take cilostazol on an empty stomach because high-fat foods can increase the risk of adverse reactions.
• Warn patent to avoid grapefruit juice during therapy because it can increase the risk of adverse reactions.
• Urge patient not to smoke because it decreases drug's effects.
• Explain that assessment of drug effectiveness is based on ability to walk increased distances. Stress that drug effects won't appear until 2 to 4 weeks after therapy starts and that full effects may take up to 12 weeks.

---

cimetidine

Apo-Cimetidine (CAN), Gen-Cimetidine (CAN), Novo-Cimetine (CAN), Nu-Cimet (CAN), PMS-Cimetidine (CAN), Tagamet, Tagamet HB

cimetidine hydrochloride

Novo-Cimetine (CAN), Tagamet

Class and Category
Chemical class: Imidazole derivative
Therapeutic class: Antiulcer agent, gastric acid secretion inhibitor, H_2-receptor antagonist
Pregnancy category: B

Indications and Dosages
➤ *To treat and prevent recurrence of duodenal ulcer*
ORAL SOLUTION, TABLETS
Adults and adolescents. *Initial:* 800 mg at bedtime, 300 mg four times daily with meals and at bedtime, or 400 to 600 mg in morning and at bedtime for 4 to 6 wk. *Maintenance:* 400 mg at bedtime.
Children. 20 to 40 mg/kg daily in divided doses four times daily with meals and at bedtime.
I.V. OR I.M. INJECTION
Adults. *Initial:* 300 mg every 6 to 8 hr. Dosage increased, if needed, by increasing frequency. *Maximum:* 2,400 mg daily.
➤ *To treat active, benign gastric ulcer*
ORAL SOLUTION, TABLETS
Adults and adolescents. 800 mg at bedtime, 300 mg four times daily with meals and at bedtime, or 600 mg twice daily in morning and at bedtime, or 800 mg at bedtime for up to 8 wk.
Children. 20 to 40 mg/kg daily in divided doses four times daily with meals and at bedtime.
I.V. OR I.M. INJECTION
Adults and adolescents. *Initial:* 300 mg every 6 to 8 hr. Dosage increased, if needed, by increasing frequency. *Maximum:* 2,400 mg daily.
➤ *To manage gastroesophageal reflux disease*
ORAL SOLUTION, TABLETS
Adults and adolescents. 1,600 mg daily in divided doses (800 mg twice daily or 400 mg four times daily) for up to 12 wk.
Children. 40 to 80 mg/kg daily in divided doses four times daily.
➤ *To treat pathological hypersecretory conditions, such as Zollinger-Ellison syndrome*

ORAL SOLUTION, TABLETS
Adults and adolescents. 300 mg four times daily with meals and at bedtime. Given more often, if needed. *Maximum:* 2,400 mg daily.
I.V. OR I.M. INJECTION
Adults and adolescents. *Initial:* 300 mg every 6 to 8 hr. Dosage increased, if needed, by increasing frequency. *Maximum:* 2,400 mg daily.
➤ *To treat heartburn and acid indigestion*
ORAL SOLUTION, TABLETS
Adults and adolescents. *Initial:* 200 mg with water at onset of symptoms. *Maximum:* 400 mg every 24 hr for no more than 2 wk unless prescribed.
DOSAGE ADJUSTMENT Oral dosage for all indications reduced to 300 mg every 12 hr (and increased to every 8 hr with caution, if needed) for patients with renal impairment.
➤ *To prevent stress-related upper GI bleeding during hospitalization*
I.V. INFUSION
Adults. 50 mg/hr by continuous infusion for 7 days.

Mechanism of Action
Blocks histamine's action at H_2-receptor sites on stomach's parietal cells. This action reduces gastric fluid volume and acidity. Cimetidine also decreases the amount of gastric acid secreted in response to food, caffeine, insulin, betazole, or pentagastrin.

Route	Onset	Peak	Duration
P.O.	Unknown	1–2 hr	4–5 hr
I.V., I.M.	Unknown	Unknown	4–5 hr

Incompatibilities
Don't mix cimetidine with aminophylline or barbiturates in I.V. solution. Don't mix drug with pentobarbital sodium in the same syringe.

Contraindications
Hypersensitivity to cimetidine or its components

Interactions
DRUGS
antacids, anticholinergics, metoclopramide: Decreased cimetidine absorption
benzodiazepines, calcium channel blockers, carbamazepine, chloroquine, labetalol,
lidocaine, metoprolol, metronidazole, moricizine, pentoxifylline, phenytoin, propafenone, propranolol, quinidine, quinine, sulfonylureas, tacrine, theophyllines, triamterene, tricyclic antidepressants, valproic acid, warfarin: Reduced metabolism and increased blood levels and effects of these drugs, possibly toxicity from these drugs
carmustine: Increased carmustine myelotoxicity
digoxin, fluconazole: Possibly decreased blood levels of these drugs
ferrous salts, indomethacin, ketoconazole, tetracyclines: Decreased effects of these drugs
flecainide: Increased flecainide effects
fluorouracil: Increased blood fluorouracil level after long-term cimetidine use
ketoconazole: Decreased blood ketoconazole level
opioid analgesics: Increased toxic effects of opioid analgesics
oral anticoagulants: Increased anticoagulant effect
procainamide: Increased blood procainamide level
succinylcholine: Increased neuromuscular blockade
tocainide: Decreased tocainide effects
FOODS
caffeine: Reduced metabolism and increased blood level and effects of caffeine
ACTIVITIES
alcohol use: Possibly increased blood alcohol level

Adverse Reactions
CNS: Confusion, dizziness, hallucinations, headache, peripheral neuropathy, somnolence
ENDO: Mild gynecomastia if used longer than 1 month
GI: Mild and transient diarrhea
GU: Impotence, transiently elevated serum creatinine level
SKIN: Rash
Other: Pain at I.M. injection site

Nursing Considerations
WARNING Be aware that rapid administration of cimetidine can increase risk of arrhythmias and hypotension.
• For I.V. injection, dilute cimetidine in normal saline solution to a total volume of 20 ml. Inject over 5 minutes or more.

- For intermittent I.V. infusion, dilute cimetidine in at least 50 ml of D_5W or other compatible I.V. solution. Infuse over 15 to 20 minutes.
- For I.M. injection, don't dilute cimetidine before administering it.
- Be alert for confusion in elderly or debilitated patients who receive cimetidine.

PATIENT TEACHING
- Tell patient to use a liquid-measuring device to ensure accurate dose of solution.
- Advise patient to avoid alcohol while taking cimetidine to prevent inter-actions.
- Instruct patient to avoid taking antacids within 1 hour of taking cimetidine.
- Warn patient that cigarette smoking increases gastric acid secretion and can worsen gastric disease.
- Caution patient not to take drug for more than 14 days, unless prescribed.

cinacalcet hydrochloride
Sensipar

Class and Category
Chemical class: Calcimimetic
Therapeutic class: Calcium reducer
Pregnancy category: C

Indications and Dosages
➤ *To treat secondary hyperparathyroidism in patients with chronic renal disease who are on dialysis*
TABLETS
Adults. *Initial:* 30 mg daily, increased by 30 mg every 2 to 4 wk daily, as needed. *Maximum:* 180 mg daily.
➤ *To treat hypercalcemia in patients with parathyroid carcinoma; to treat primary hyperparathyroidism in patients who are unable to undergo parathy-roidectomy*
TABLETS
Adults. *Initial:* 30 mg twice daily, increased in 2 to 4 wk to 60 mg twice daily., then in 2 to 4 wk to 90 mg twice daily, and then in 2 to 4 wk to 90 mg three

times daily or four times daily, as needed to normalize serum calcium level.

Route	Onset	Peak	Duration
P.O.	Unknown	2–6 hr	Unknown

Mechanism of Action
Increases sensitivity of calcium-sensing receptors on the surface of parathyroid cells to extracellular calcium. This sensitivity directly reduces parathyroid hormone (PTH) level, which in turn decreases serum calcium level.

Contraindications
Hypersensitivity to cinacalcet or its components, hypocalcemia

Interactions
DRUGS
amitriptyline, carvedilol, desipramine, flecainide, metoprolol, thioridazine, tricyclic antidepressants (most), vinblastine: Possibly increased blood level of these drugs
erythromycin, itraconazole, ketoconazole: Possibly increased blood cinacalcet level

Adverse Reactions
CNS: Asthenia, dizziness, seizures
CV: Arrhythmia, hypertension, hypotension (in the presence of impaired cardiac function), worsening heart failure (in the presence of impaired cardiac function)
ENDO: Hypocalcemia
GI: Anorexia, diarrhea, nausea, vomiting
MS: Myalgia
SKIN: Rash, urticaria
Other: Allergic reaction, angioedema, noncardiac chest pain

Nursing Considerations
- Cinacalcet is not recommended for use in patients with chronic kidney disease who are not on dialysis because of an increased risk of hypocalcemia.
- Use cinacalcet cautiously in patients with a history of seizures because reduced blood calcium level may lower seizure threshold. Also use cautiously in patients with hepatic insufficiency because cinacalcet metabolism may be reduced.
- ***WARNING*** Monitor patient for hypocalcemia exhibited by cramping, myalgia, paresthesia, prolonged QT interval that may cause ventricular arrhythmias, seizures, and tetany. Also monitor patient's

blood calcium and phosphorus levels within 1 week after starting therapy or adjusting dosage, and every month or two once maintenance dose is established, as ordered. If hypocalcemia develops, notify prescriber immediately because treatment to raise calcium level will be needed. Treatment may include giving supplemental calcium, starting or increasing dosage of calcium-based phosphate binder or vitamin D sterols, or temporarily withholding cinacalcet.

• Be aware that if patient starts or stops therapy with a strong CYP3A4 inhibitor, such as erythromycin, itraconazole, or ketoconazole, cinacalcet dosage may need to be adjusted.

• Monitor dialysis patient's intact PTH levels 1 to 4 weeks after therapy starts or dose is adjusted and then every 1 to 3 months thereafter, as ordered. Expect to reduce dosage or discontinue cinacalcet, as ordered, in a patient whose intact PTH level falls below the target range of 150 to 300 pg/ml.

PATIENT TEACHING
• Instruct patient to take cinacalcet with food or shortly after a meal.
• Caution patient to take tablet whole and not divide it or crush it.
• Review signs and symptoms of hypocalcemia with patient and urge him to notify prescriber of changes.

ciprofloxacin
Cipro, Cipro I.V., Cipro XR, Proquin XR

Class and Category
Chemical class: Fluoroquinolone derivative
Therapeutic class: Antibiotic
Pregnancy category: C

Indications and Dosages
➤ *To prevent inhalation anthrax after exposure or to treat inhalation anthrax*
ORAL SUSPENSION, TABLETS
Adults and adolescents. 500 mg every 12 hr for 60 days.
Children. 15 mg/kg every 12 hr for 60 days. *Maximum:* 500 mg/dose.

I.V. INFUSION
Adults and adolescents. 400 mg every 12 hr for 60 days.
Children. 10 mg/kg every 12 hr for 60 days. *Maximum:* 400 mg/dose or 800 mg daily.

➤ *To treat acute sinusitis caused by gram-negative organisms (including* Campylobacter jejuni, Citrobacter diversus, Citrobacter freundii, Enterobacter cloacae, Escherichia coli, Haemophilus influenzae, Haemophilus parainfluenzae, Klebsiella pneumoniae, Morganella morganii, Neisseria gonorrhoeae, Proteus mirabilis, Proteus vulgaris, Providencia rettgeri, Providencia stuartii, Pseudomonas aeruginosa, Serratia marcescens, Shigella flexneri, *and* Shigella sonnei) *and gram-positive organisms (including* Enterococcus faecalis, Staphylococcus aureus, Staphylococcus epidermidis, *and* Streptococcus pneumoniae)

ORAL SUSPENSION, TABLETS
Adults. 500 mg every 12 hr for 10 days.
I.V. INFUSION
Adults. For mild to moderate infections, 400 mg every 12 hr.

➤ *To treat bone and joint infections caused by susceptible organisms listed above*
ORAL SUSPENSION, TABLETS
Adults. For mild to moderate infections, 500 mg every 12 hr for 4 to 6 wk. For severe or complicated infections, 750 mg every 12 hr for 4 to 6 wk.
I.V. INFUSION
Adults. For mild to moderate infections, 400 mg every 12 hr for 4 to 6 wk. For severe or complicated infections, 400 mg every 8 hr.

➤ *To treat skin and soft-tissue infections caused by susceptible organisms listed above*
ORAL SUSPENSION, TABLETS
Adults. For mild to moderate infections, 500 mg every 12 hr for 7 to 14 days. For severe or complicated infections, 750 mg every 12 hr for 7 to 14 days.
I.V. INFUSION
Adults. For mild to moderate infections, 400 mg every 12 hr. For severe or complicated infections, 400 mg every 8 hr.

➤ *To treat chronic bacterial prostatitis caused by susceptible organisms listed above*

ORAL SUSPENSION, TABLETS
Adults. 500 mg every 12 hr for 28 days.

I.V. INFUSION
Adults. 400 mg every 12 hr.

➤ *To treat infectious diarrhea caused by susceptible organisms listed above*

ORAL SUSPENSION, TABLETS
Adults. 500 mg every 12 hr for 5 to 7 days.

➤ *To treat UTI caused by susceptible organisms listed above*

ORAL SUSPENSION, TABLETS
Adults. For acute uncomplicated infections, 100 mg every 12 hr for 3 days. For mild to moderate infections, 250 mg every 12 hr for 7 to 14 days. For severe or complicated infections, 500 mg every 12 hr for 7 to 14 days.

I.V. INFUSION
Adults. For mild to moderate infections, 200 mg every 12 hr. For severe or complicated infections, 400 mg every 12 hr.

➤ *To treat complicated UTI caused by* E. coli, K. pneumoniae, Enterococcus faecalis, P. mirabilis, *or* P. aeruginosa *or acute uncomplicated pyelonephritis caused by* E. coli

E.R. TABLETS
Adults. 1,000 mg daily for 7 to 14 days.

➤ *To treat acute cystitis caused by* E. coli, P. mirabilis, E. faecalis, *or* Staphylococcus saprophyticus

E.R. TABLETS
Adults. 500 mg daily for 3 days.

➤ *To treat lower respiratory tract infections caused by susceptible organisms listed above*

ORAL SUSPENSION, TABLETS
Adults. For mild to moderate infections, 500 mg every 12 hr for 7 to 14 days. For severe or complicated infections, 750 mg every 12 hr for 7 to 14 days.

I.V. INFUSION
Adults. For mild to moderate infections, 400 mg every 12 hr. For severe or complicated infections, 400 mg every 8 hr.

➤ *To treat intra-abdominal infections caused by susceptible organisms listed above*

I.V. INFUSION
Adults. 400 mg every 8 hr along with parenteral metronidazole.

➤ *To treat mild to severe nosocomial pneumonia caused by susceptible organisms listed above*

I.V. INFUSION
Adults. 400 mg every 8 hr.

➤ *To treat typhoid fever caused by* Salmonella typhi *or infectious diarrhea caused by* C. jejuni, E. coli, S. flexneri, *or* S. sonnei

ORAL SUSPENSION, TABLETS
Adults. 500 mg every 12 hr for 10 days.

➤ *To treat uncomplicated urethral or cervical gonococcal infections caused by* N. gonorrhoeae

ORAL SUSPENSION, TABLETS
Adults. 250 mg as a single dose.

DOSAGE ADJUSTMENT Dosage reduced to 250 to 500 mg every 12 hr if creatinine clearance is 30 to 50 ml/min/1.73 m^2; and to 250 to 500 mg P.O. or 200 to 400 mg I.V. every 18 hr if creatinine clearance is 5 to 29 ml/min/1.73 m^2.

➤ *To treat acute cystitis caused by* E. coli *or* K. pneumoniae

E.R. TABLETS (PROQUIN XR)
Adults. 500 mg daily for 3 days with evening meal.

Mechanism of Action
Inhibits the enzyme DNA gyrase, which is responsible for the unwinding and supercoiling of bacterial DNA before it replicates. By inhibiting this enzyme, ciprofloxacin causes bacterial cells to die.

Incompatibilities
Don't administer parenteral ciprofloxacin with aminophylline, amoxicillin, cefepime, clindamycin, dexamethasone, floxacillin, furosemide, heparin, or phenytoin.

Contraindications
Hypersensitivity to ciprofloxacin, quinolones, or their components, myasthenia gravis

Interactions
DRUGS
antacids, didanosine, iron supplements, sucralfate, multivitamins that contain iron or zinc: Decreased ciprofloxacin absorption
clozapine, methotrexate, methylxanthines, olanzapine, ropinirole, theophyllin, tizanidine: Increased plasma levels of these

drugs and increased risk of serious adverse reactions including toxicity
cyclosporine: Elevated serum creatinine and blood cyclosporine levels
NSAIDs (except acetylsalicylic acid): Increased risk of seizures with high doses of ciprofloxacin
oral anticoagulants: Enhanced anticoagulant effects
oral hypoglycemics: Possibly increased risk of hypoglycemia that may be severe (especially with glyburide)
phenytoin: Increased or decreased blood phenytoin level
probenecid: Increased blood ciprofloxacin level and, possibly, toxicity
FOODS
caffeine: Increased caffeine effects
dairy products: Delayed drug absorption

Adverse Reactions

CNS: Abnormal gait, agitation, anxiety, ataxia, cerebral thrombosis, confusion, depersonalization, depression, dizziness, drowsiness, fever, hallucinations, headache, increased intracranial pressure including pseudotumor cerebri, insomnia, irritability, lethargy, light-headedness, malaise, manic reaction, migraine, nervousness, nightmares, paranoia, paresthesia, peripheral neuropathy, phobia, restlessness, seizures, status epilepticus, suicidal ideation, syncope, tremor, toxic psychosis, unresponsiveness, weakness
CV: Angina, atrial flutter, cardiopulmonary arrest, cardiovascular collapse, hypertension, MI, orthostatic hypotension, palpitations, phlebitis, tachycardia, torsades de pointes, vasculitis, ventricular ectopy
EENT: Oral candidiasis
GI: Abdominal pain, anorexia, constipation, diarrhea, dysphagia, elevated liver enzymes, flatulence, GI bleeding, hepatic failure or necrosis, hepatitis, indigestion, intestinal perforation, jaundice, nausea, pancreatitis, pseudomembranous colitis, vomiting
GU: Acute renal failure or insufficiency, crystalluria, hematuria, increased serum creatinine level, interstitial nephritis, nephrotoxicity, renal calculi, renal failure, urine retention, vaginal candidiasis
HEME: Agranulocytosis, aplasitc or hemolytic anemia, bone marrow depression, leukopenia, lymphadenopathy, pancytopenia, thrombocytopenia

MS: Arthralgia, myalgia, tendinitis, tendon rupture
RESP: Allergic pneumonitis
SKIN: Acute generalized exanthematous pustulosis (AGEP), erythema multiforme, exfoliative dermatitis, photosensitivity, rash, Stevens-Johnson syndrome, toxic epidermal necrolysis, urticaria
RESP: Bronchospasm, pulmonary embolism, respiratory arrest
Other: Acidosis, anaphylaxis, angioedema, serum sickness-like reaction

Nursing Considerations

• Obtain culture and sensitivity test results, as ordered, before giving ciprofloxacin.
• Use drug cautiously in patients with CNS disorders and disorders that may predispose patient to seizures, such as history of epilepsy or conditions that may lower the seizure threshold, such as history of severe cerebral arteriosclerosis, reduced cerebral blood flow, altered brain structure, or stroke. Take seizure precautions. If a seizure occurs, expect ciprofloxacin to be discontinued immediately.
• Use drug cautiously in patients who may be more susceptible to drug's effect on QT interval, such as those taking Class IA or III antiarrhythmics; those with uncorrected hypokalemia or hypomagnesemia; or in the presence of a history of QT-interval prolongation, torsades de pointes or cardiac disease such as heart failure.
• are that E.R. and immediate-release tablets aren't interchangeable and that Proquin XR and Cipro XR aren't interchangeable.
• Patient should be well hydrated during therapy to help prevent alkaline urine, which may lead to crystalluria and nephrotoxicity.
• Assess patient's hepatic, renal, and hematologic functions periodically, as ordered. Report any abnormalities, including signs and symptoms of dysfunction, to prescriber. For example, severe liver toxicity has occurred with ciprofloxacin use (within 1 to 39 days of therapy) and has been associated more frequently with hypersensitivity reactions. If dysfunction occurs, expect drug to be discontinued and provide supportive care, as ordered and needed.

• Assess patient routinely for signs of rash or other hypersensitivity reactions, even after patient has received multiple doses. Stop drug at first sign of rash, jaundice, or other sign of hypersensitivity, and notify prescriber immediately. Be prepared to provide supportive emergency care.
• Monitor patient closely for diarrhea, which may reflect pseudomembranous colitis. If it occurs, notify prescriber and expect to withhold drug and treat diarrhea.
• Assess patient for evidence of peripheral neuropathy. Notify prescriber and expect to stop drug if patient complains of burning, numbness, pain, tingling, or weakness in extremities or if physical examination reveals deficits in light touch, pain, temperature, position sense, vibratory sensation, or motor strength.
• Monitor patients (especially children, elderly patients, patients receiving corticosteroids, and patients who have renal failure or who have had a kidney, heart, or lung transplant) for evidence of tendon rupture, such as inflammation, pain, and swelling at the site. Be aware that tendon rupture may occur within the first 48 hours of therapy, throughout therapy, or months after ciprofloxacin therapy. Notify prescriber about suspected tendon rupture, and have patient rest and refrain from exercise until tendon rupture has been ruled out. If present, expect to provide supportive care as ordered.
• Monitor patient closely for changes in mood or behavior that may be caused by ciprofloxacin-induced depression or worsening psychotic reactions potentially resulting in self-injurious behavior, such as suicide. Be aware these reactions may occur even after just one dose. Notify prescriber immediately and expect to discontinue ciprofloxacin therapy, if present, and institute precautions to keep patient safe until adverse effects have disappeared.

PATIENT TEACHING
• Urge patient to complete the prescribed course of therapy, even if he feels better before it's finished.
• Tell patient not to take drug with dairy products or calcium-fortified juices alone.
• Advise patient to take ciprofloxacin 2 hours before or 6 hours after antacids,

iron supplements, or multivitamins that contain iron or zinc. Tell him to shake oral suspension for 15 seconds, not to chew microcapsules, and not to split, crush, or chew E.R. tablets.
• Encourage patient to drink plenty of fluids during therapy to help prevent crystalluria.
• Urge patient to avoid caffeinated products because caffeine may accumulate in the body during ciprofloxacin therapy and cause excessive stimulation.
• Caution patient to avoid excessive exposure to sunlight or artificial ultraviolet light because severe sunburn may result. Tell patient to notify prescriber if sunburn develops; drug will need to be stopped.
• Urge patient to avoid hazardous activities until CNS effects of drug are known.
• Advise patient to notify prescriber about changes in limb sensation or movement and about inflammation, pain, or swelling over a joint. Urge patient to rest the affected limb at the first sign of discomfort.
• Tell patient to stop taking drug and to notify prescriber at first sign of rash or other hypersensitivity reaction.
• Urge patient to report watery, bloody stools to prescriber immediately, even up to 2 months after drug therapy has ended.
• If patient develops depression or worsening of psychotic behavior, urge caregivers to monitor him closely for suicidal tendencies and to notify prescriber,

citalopram hydrobromide
Celexa

Class and Category
Chemical class: Racemic, bicyclic phthalate derivative
Therapeutic class: Antidepressant
Pregnancy category: C

Indications and Dosages
➤ *To treat depression*

ORAL SOLUTION, TABLETS
Adults. *Initial:* 20 mg daily. Increased to 40 mg daily, as needed. *Maximum:* 40 mg daily.

DOSAGE ADJUSTMENT Dosage should not exceed 20 mg daily in patients taking concomitant cimetidine or CYP2C19 inhibitors, who are poor CYP2C19 metabolizers, who have hepatic impairment, or who are older than 60 years of age.

Route	Onset	Peak	Duration
P.O.	1–wk	Unknown	Unknown

Mechanism of Action

Blocks serotonin reuptake by adrenergic nerves, which normally release this neurotransmitter from their storage sites when activated by a nerve impulse. This blocked reuptake increases serotonin levels at nerve synapses, which may elevate mood and reduce depression.

Contraindications

Congenital long QT syndrome, hypersensitivity to citalopram or its components, pimozide therapy, use within 14 days of MAO inhibitor therapy

Interactions

DRUGS
antipsycotics, Class IA and Class III antiarrhythmics, CYP2C19 inhibitors, gatifloxacin, moxifloxacin: Increased risk of QT prolongation and torsades de pointes
amitriptyline, bromocriptine, buspirone, clomipramine, dextromethorphan, fluoxetine, fluvoxamine, furazolidone, imipramine, levodopa, lithium, meperidine, naratriptan, nefazodone, paroxetine, pentazocine, phenelzine, procarbazine, selegiline, sertraline, sibutramine, sumatriptan, tramadol, tranylcypromine, trazodone, venlafaxine, zolmitriptan: Possibly enhanced serotonergic effects of citalopram, resulting in agitation, chills, confusion, diaphoresis, diarrhea, fever, hyperreflexia, hypomania, incoordination, myoclonus, or tremor *aspirin, NSAIDs, warfarin:* Increased risk of bleeding ranging from ecchymoses to life-threatening hemorrhage
carbamazepine: Possibly increased clearance of citalopram

cimetidine: Possibly increased blood citalopram level
desipramine, metoprolol: Increased blood levels of these drugs
furazolidone, procarbazine, selegiline: Possibly hyperthermia, rigidity, myoclonus, and extreme agitation progressing to delirium and coma
itraconazole, ketoconazole, macrolide antibiotics, omeprazole: Possibly decreased clearance of citalopram
MAO inhibitors: Increased risk of life-threatening serotonin syndrome or neuroleptic malignant syndrome
warfarin: Possibly increased PT

Adverse Reactions

CNS: Agitation, akathisia, amnesia, anxiety, apathy, asthenia, confusion, CVA, delirium, depression, dizziness, drowsiness, dyskinesia, fatigue, fever, impaired concentration, insomnia, migraine, myoclonus, neuroleptic malignant syndrome, paresthesia, seizures, serotonin syndrome, suicidal ideation, tremor
CV: Angina, bundle branch block, chest pain, heart failure, MI, orthostatic hypotension, prolonged QT interval, tachycardia, thrombosis, ventricular arrhythmias
EENT: Abnormal accommodation, acute-angle glaucoma, blurred vision, dry mouth, rhinitis, sinusitis, taste perversion
GI: Abdominal pain, anorexia, diarrhea, flatulence, GI bleeding, hepatic necrosis, indigestion, nausea, pancreatitis, vomiting
GU: Acute renal failure, amenorrhea, anorgasmia, decreased libido, dysmenorrhea, ejaculation disorders, impotence, polyuria, priapism
HEME: Abnormal bleeding, decreased PT, hemolytic anemia, thrombocytopenia
MS: Arthralgia, myalgia, rhabdomyolysis
RESP: Cough, upper respiratory tract infection
SKIN: Diaphoresis, ecchymosis, erythema multiforme, pruritus, rash
Other: Anaphylaxis, angioedema, hyponatremia, weight gain or loss

Nursing Considerations

WARNING When citalopram dosage increases, monitor patient for possible serotonin syndrome, which may include agitation, chills, confusion, diaphoresis, diarrhea, fever, hyperactive reflexes, poor coordination, restlessness, shaking, talking or acting with uncontrolled excitement, tremor, and twitching. In its most severe form, serotonin syndrome can resemble neuroleptic malignant syndrome, which includes a high fever, muscle rigidity, autonomic instability with possible changes in vital signs, and mental status changes.

• Be aware that citalopram should not be given to patients with congenital long QT syndrome, bradycardia, hypokalemia or hypomagnesemia, recent acute myocardial infarction, or uncompensated heart failure because of increased risk of prolonged QT interval and torsades de pointes. It should also not be given to patients who are taking other drugs that prolong the QT interval. Expect hypokalemia and hypomagnesemia to be corrected before citalopram therapy is begun.

• Also use citalopram cautiously in patients with other cardiac conditions. ECG monitoring may be ordered to monitor the patient's QT interval and detect the development of serious arrhythmias.

• Use citalopram cautiously in patients with hepatic impairment because citalopram clearance is affected and can lead to increased plasma citalopram levels.

• Be aware that effective antidepressant therapy may convert depression into mania in predisposed people. If patient develops symptoms of mania, notify prescriber immediately and expect to discontinue citalopram.

• Assess elderly patients and those taking diuretics for signs suggesting syndrome of inappropriate secretion of antidiuretic hormone, including hyponatremia and increased serum and urine osmolarity.

• If patient (especially a child or adolescent) takes citalopram for depression, monitor him closely for suicidal tendencies, especially when therapy starts or dosage changes, because depression may worsen at these times.

• To stop therapy, expect to reduce dosage gradually to avoid serious adverse reactions.

PATIENT TEACHING
• Inform patient that citalopram's full effects may take up to 4 weeks.

• Advise patient not to self-medicate for coughs, colds, or allergies without consulting prescriber because these preparations can increase the risk of adverse reactions.

• Caution patient not to stop citalopram abruptly because doing so may lead to serious adverse reactions.

• If patient (especially a child or adolescent) takes citalopram for depression, urge caregivers to monitor him closely for suicidal tendencies, especially when therapy starts or dosage changes.

• Caution against taking OTC NSAIDs, aspirin, or other remedies (including herbal products, such as St. John's wort) while taking citalopram because they may increase the risk of bleeding.

• Advise patient that drug may cause mild pupillary dilation, which may lead to an episode of acute closure glaucoma. Encourage patient to have an eye exam before starting therapy to see if he is at risk.

• Urge patient to report sudden, severe, or unusual adverse reactions promptly to prescriber. Although uncommon, life-threatening adverse effects may occur.

clarithromycin
Biaxin, Biaxin XL, Biaxin XL-PAK

Class and Category
Chemical class: Macrolide derivative
Therapeutic class: Antibiotic
Pregnancy category: C

Indications and Dosages
➤ *To treat pharyngitis and tonsillitis caused by* Streptococcus pyogenes
ORAL SUSPENSION, TABLETS
Adults and adolescents. 250 mg every 12 hr for 10 days.
Children. 15 mg/kg daily in divided doses every 12 hr for 10 days.
➤ *To treat acute maxillary sinusitis caused by* Haemophilus influenzae, Moraxella catarrhalis, *or* Streptococcus pneumoniae

ORAL SUSPENSION, TABLETS
Adults and adolescents. 500 mg every 12 hr for 14 days.
Children. 15 mg/kg daily in divided doses every 12 hr for 10 days.
E.R. TABLETS
Adults and adolescents. 1,000 mg every 24 hr for 14 days.
➤ *To treat acute exacerbations of chronic bronchitis caused by* H. influenzae, M. catarrhalis, *or* S. pneumoniae
ORAL SUSPENSION, TABLETS
Adults and adolescents. 250 to 500 mg every 12 hr for 7 to 14 days.
Children. 15 mg/kg daily in divided doses every 12 hr for 10 days.
E.R. TABLETS
Adults and adolescents. 1,000 mg every 24 hr for 7 days.
➤ *To treat uncomplicated skin and soft-tissue infections caused by* Staphylococcus aureus *or* S. pyogenes
ORAL SUSPENSION, TABLETS
Adults and adolescents. 250 mg every 12 hr for 7 to 14 days.
Children. 15 mg/kg daily in divided doses every 12 hr for 10 days.
➤ *To treat pneumonia caused by* Chlamydia pneumoniae, Mycoplasma pneumoniae, *or* S. pneumoniae
ORAL SUSPENSION, TABLETS
Adults and adolescents. 250 mg every 12 hr for 7 to 14 days.
Children. 15 mg/kg daily in divided doses every 12 hr for 10 days.
➤ *To treat pneumonia caused by* H. influenzae
ORAL SUSPENSION, TABLETS
Adults and adolescents. 250 mg every 12 hr for 7 days.
Children. 15 mg/kg daily in divided doses every 12 hr for 10 days.
➤ *To treat acute otitis media caused by* H. influenzae, M. catarrhalis, *or* S. pneumoniae
ORAL SUSPENSION, TABLETS
Children. 15 mg/kg daily in divided doses every 12 hr for 10 days.
➤ *To treat active duodenal ulcer caused by* Helicobacter pylori
ORAL SUSPENSION, TABLETS
Adults and adolescents. 500 mg every 8 hr for 14 days with omeprazole 40 mg daily in the morning. Then, omeprazole

continued at 20 mg daily in the morning days 15 through 28. Or, 500 mg every 12 hr for 14 days with lansoprazole 30 mg and amoxicillin 1 g every 12 hr for 14 days.
➤ *To prevent or treat* Mycobacterium avium *complex in patients with HIV infection*
ORAL SUSPENSION, TABLETS
Adults and adolescents. 500 mg every 12 hr for 7 to 14 days.
Children. 7.5 mg/kg every 12 hr.
Maximum: 500 mg twice daily.
DOSAGE ADJUSTMENT For patient with severe renal impairment (creatinine clearance less than 30 ml/min), dosage reduced by 50%. For patient with moderate renal impairment (creatinine clearance 30 to 60 ml/min) who is also taking atazanavir or ritonavir, dosage reduced by 50%. For patient with severe renal impairment (creatinine clearance less than 30 ml/min) who is also taking atazanavir or ritonavir, dosage reduced by 75%.

Mechanism of Action
Inhibits RNA-dependent protein synthesis in many types of aerobic, anaerobic, gram-positive, and gram-negative bacteria. By binding with the 50S ribosomal subunit of the bacterial 70S ribosome, clarithromycin causes bacterial cells to die.

Contraindications
Concurrent therapy with astemizole, cisapride, colchicine (in patients with renal or hepatic impairment), dihydroergotamine, ergotamine, lovastatin, pimozide, simvastatin, or terfenadine; history of cholestatic jaundice, hepatic dysfunction, QT prolongation or ventricular cardiac arrhythmias, including torsades de pointes; hypersensitivity to clarithromycin, erythromycin, or any macrolide antibiotic

Interactions
DRUGS
allopurinol, atorvastatin,fibrates, lovastatin, pravastatin, simvastatin: Risk of rhabdomyolysis
alprazolam, midazolam, triazolam: Possibly increased effects of these triazolo-benzodiazepines, including increased and/ or prolonged sedation

amlodipine, diltiazem, verapamil: Increased risk of hypotension
astemizole, cisapride, Class IA or Class III antiarrhythmias, disopyramide, pimozide, quinidine, terfenadine: Possibly prolonged QT interval, torsades de pointes or other serious arrhythmias
carbamazepine, other drugs metabolized by cytochrome P450 enzyme system, tolterodine: Increased blood levels of these drugs
colchicine: Increased risk of colchicine toxicity
digoxin: Increased serum digoxin level
dihydroergotamine, ergotamine: Risk of acute ergot toxicity
efavirenz, etravirine, nevirapine, rifabutin, rifampicin, rifapentine: Decreased blood clarithromycin levels
oral anticoagulants: Potentiated anticoagulant effects
oral hypoglycemics, insulin: Increased risk of serious hypoglycemia
sildenafi, tadalafil, vardenafil: Possibly increased exposure of these phosphodiesterase inhibitors
terfenadine: Possibly increased blood clarithromycin levels
theophylline: Increased blood theophylline level
zidovudine: Decreased blood zidovudine level

Adverse Reactions

CNS: Anxiety, confusion, dizziness, fatigue, hallucinations, headache, insomnia, mania, nightmares, seizures, somnolence, tremor, vertigo
CV: Prolonged QT interval, ventricular arrhythmias
EENT: Altered smell, altered taste, glossitis, hearing loss, oral moniliasis, stomatitis, tinnitus, tongue or tooth discoloration
ENDO: Hypoglycemia
GI: Abdominal pain, anorexia, cholestatic hepatitis, diarrhea, elevated liver enzymes, hepatitis, hepatotoxicity, indigestion, jaundice, nausea, pancreatitis, pseudomembranous colitis
GU: Elevated BUN level, hepatic dysfunction, vomiting
HEME: Leukopenia, neutropenia, increased prothrombin time, thrombocytopenia
MS: Rhabdomyolysis
SKIN: Drug rash with eosinophilia and systemic symptoms (DRESS), Henoch-Schonlein purpura, pruritus, rash, Stevens-Johnson syndrome, toxic epidermal necrolysis, urticaria
Other: Anaphylaxis, angioedema, new or worsening myasthenia gravis symptoms, superinfection

Nursing Considerations

• Expect to obtain a specimen for culture and sensitivity tests before giving first dose.
• Know that clarithromycin therapy should be avoided in patients at risk for QT prolongation such as uncorrected hypokalemia or hypomagnesemia or significant bradycardia, and in patients receiving Class IA or Class III antiarrhythmics. Elderly patients are more susceptible to clarithromycin's effect on the QT interval, as well.
• Use clarithromycin cautiously in patients with renal impairment. Be aware that patients with severe renal impairment may need decreased dosage or prolonged dosage interval and that clarithromycin is not recommended in combination with ranitidine bismuth citrate therapy if patient has a creatinine clearance less than 2.5 ml/min/1.73 m² or a history of acute porphyria.
• Monitor patient closely for acute hypersensitivity reactions such as anaphylaxis and serious skin disorders. If present, expect clarithromycin therapy to be discontinued immediately and appropriate emergency treatment initiated.
• Monitor patient for signs and symptoms of liver dysfunction, especially hepatitis (anorexia, dark urine, jaundice, pruritus, or tender abdomen). Notify prescriber immediately if present, and expect clarithromycin to be discontinued.
• Monitor patients with diabetes who are also receiving oral hypoglycemics or insulin closely for hypoglycemia, which could be severe.
• Be watchful for an elevated INR and prothrombin time in patients who are also taking warfarin, as serious bleeding may occur.
• Assess patient's bowel pattern daily; severe diarrhea may indicate pseudomembranous colitis caused by *Clostridium difficile.* If diarrhea occurs, notify prescriber and expect to withhold clarithromycin and

treat with fluids, electrolytes, protein, and an antibiotic effective against *C. difficile.*

PATIENT TEACHING
• Emphasize importance of taking the full course of clarithromycin exactly as prescribed, even after feeling better.
• Caution patient not to crush or chew E.R. tablets.
• Advise patient to take drug with food if he takes E.R. tablets or has GI distress.
• If patient takes suspension form, instruct him not to refrigerate it.
• Tell patient to report severe nausea, rash, or itching.
• Instruct patient not to take OTC or prescription drugs without consulting prescriber of clarithromycin.
• Urge patient to report watery, bloody stools to prescriber immediately, even if they occur up to 2 months after therapy has ended.
• Advise patient to report signs and symptoms of liver dysfunction immediately to prescriber.
• Instruct patient with diabetes who is also taking an oral hypoglycemic agent or insulin, to monitor his blood glucose level closely.

clidinium bromide

Quarzan

Class and Category

Chemical class: Synthetic quaternary ammonium derivative
Therapeutic class: Anticholinergic
Pregnancy category: Not rated

Indications and Dosages

➤ *As adjunct to treat peptic ulcer*

CAPSULES
Adults. 2.5 to 5 mg three times daily or four times daily 30 to 60 min before meals and at bedtime.

DOSAGE ADJUSTMENT Dosage limited to 2.5 mg t.i.d. before meals for elderly or debilitated patients.

Route	Onset	Peak	Duration
P.O.	1 hr	Unknown	Up to 3 hr

Mechanism of Action

Inhibits acetylcholine's muscarinic actions at postganglionic parasympathetic receptor sites, including smooth muscles, secretory glands, and the CNS. These actions relax smooth muscles and diminish GI, GU, and biliary tract secretions.

Contraindications

Angle-closure glaucoma, benign bladder neck obstruction, hypersensitivity to clidinium bromide or its components, ileus, intestinal atony (elderly or debilitated patients), intestinal obstruction, myasthenia gravis, myocardial ischemia, ocular adhesions between lens and iris, prostatic hypertrophy, renal disease, severe ulcerative colitis, tachycardia, toxic megacolon, unstable cardiovascular status in acute hemorrhage

Interactions

DRUGS
amantadine: Increased risk of clidinium adverse effects
atenolol: Increased atenolol effects
CNS depressants: Increased clidinium effects
phenothiazines: Decreased antipsychotic effectiveness
tricyclic antidepressants: Increased clidinium adverse effects

ACTIVITIES
alcohol use: Increased clidinium effects

Adverse Reactions

CNS: Confusion, dizziness, drowsiness, excitement, fever, headache, insomnia, memory loss, nervousness, weakness
CV: Palpitations, tachycardia
EENT: Blurred vision, cycloplegia, dry mouth, increased intraocular pressure, loss of taste, mydriasis, nasal congestion, pharyngitis, photophobia
GI: Bloating, constipation, dysphagia, heartburn, ileus, nausea, vomiting
GU: Impotence, urinary hesitancy, urine retention
SKIN: Decreased sweating, flushing, rash, urticaria

Nursing Considerations

• Avoid high doses in patients with ulcerative colitis because clidinium may inhibit intestinal motility and cause or worsen toxic megacolon. Also avoid high doses in patients with hiatal hernia or reflux esophagitis because drug may aggravate esophagitis.

• Use drug cautiously in patients with heart failure, arrhythmias, hypertension, autonomic neuropathy, hyperthyroidism, allergies, asthma, or debilitating chronic lung disease.

WARNING Monitor elderly patients for excitement, agitation, drowsiness, and confusion, even with small doses, because these patients are more sensitive to clidinium's effects. If these reactions occur, notify prescriber and expect to decrease dosage.

• Take safety precautions to protect patient from injury from falling.

PATIENT TEACHING

• Instruct patient to take clidinium exactly as prescribed and not to stop taking it suddenly because it can cause withdrawal symptoms, such as vomiting, diaphoresis, and dizziness.

• Advise patient to take drug 30 to 60 minutes before meals.

• Tell patient not to store capsules in damp places, such as the bathroom.

• Teach patient how to prevent or relieve constipation and dry mouth.

• Instruct patient to avoid alcohol and other CNS depressants because they increase the drug's effects.

• Instruct patient to report constipation, vision changes, sore throat, difficulty urinating, and palpitations.

clindamycin hydrochloride

Cleocin, Dalacin C

clindamycin palmitate hydrochloride

Cleocin Pediatric, Dalacin C Flavored Granules (CAN)

clindamycin phosphate

Cleocin, Clindesse, Dalacin C Phosphate (CAN), Evoclin

Class and Category

Chemical class: Lincosamide
Therapeutic class: Antibacterial and antiprotozoal antibiotic
Pregnancy category: B

Indications and Dosages

➤ *To treat serious respiratory tract infections caused by anaerobes such as occur with anaerobic pneumonitis, empyema, and lung abscess and those caused by pneumococci, staphylococci, and streptococci; serious skin and soft-tissue infections caused by anaerobes, staphylococci, and streptococci; septicemia caused by anaerobes; intra-abdominal infections caused by anaerobes such as occur with intra-abdominal abscess and peritonitis; infections of the female pelvis and genital tract caused by anaerobes such as occur with endometritis, nongonococcal tubo-ovarian abscess, pelvic cellulitis, and postsurgical vaginal cuff infection; bone and joint infections caused by* Staphylococcus aureus; *as adjunct therapy in chronic bone and joint infections*

CAPSULES, ORAL SOLUTION

Adults and adolescents. For serious infections, 150 to 300 mg every 6 hr; for severe infections, 300 to 450 mg every 6 hr.

Children. For serious infections, 8 to 16 mg/kg daily in equally divided doses three times daily or four times daily; for severe infections, 16 to 20 mg/kg/day in equally divided doses three times daily or four times daily.

I.V. INFUSION, I.M. INJECTION

Adults and adolescents age 16 and over. For serious infections, 600 to 1,200 mg daily in equally divided doses twice daily to four times daily; for severe infections, 1,200 to 2,700 mg daily in equally divided doses twice daily to four times daily; for life-threatening infections, 4,800 mg daily in equally divided doses twice daily to four times daily.

Children ages 1 month to 16 years. 20 to 40 mg/kg daily in equally divided doses three times daily or four times daily, depending on severity of infection. **Neonates less than age 1 month.** 15 to 20 mg/kg daily in equally divided doses three times daily or four times daily, depending on severity of infection.

➤ *To treat vaginal infections caused by* Gardnerella *or* Haemophilus

VAGINAL CREAM

Nonpregnant adults. 100 mg (1 applicatorful) into vagina daily, preferably at bedtime, for 3 to 7 consecutive days.

Pregnant adults in second or third trimester. 100 mg (1 applicatorful) into vagina daily, preferably at bedtime, for 7 consecutive days.

➤ *To treat acne vulgaris*

FOAM

Adults and adolescents. Apply to affected area daily.

Mechanism of Action

Inhibits protein synthesis in susceptible bacteria by binding to the 50S subunits of bacterial ribosomes and preventing peptide bond formation, which causes bacterial cells to die.

Incompatibilities

To prevent physical incompatibility, don't administer with aminophylline, ampicillin, barbiturates, calcium gluconate, magnesium sulfate, or phenytoin.

Contraindications

History of regional enteritis, ulcerative colitis, or antibiotic-associated colitis; hypersensitivity to clindamycin or lincomycin

Interactions

DRUGS

erythromycin: Possibly blocked access of clindamycin to its site of action
kaolin-pectin antidiarrheals: Decreased absorption of oral clindamycin
neuromuscular blockers: Increased neuromuscular blockade
serotonin norepinephrine reuptake inhibitors, serotonin reuptake inhibitors: Increased risk of bleeding

Adverse Reactions

CNS: Fatigue, headache
CV: Hypotension, thrombophlebitis (after I.V. injection)

EENT: Glossitis, metallic or unpleasant taste (with high I.V. doses), stomatitis
GI: Abdominal pain, diarrhea, esophagitis, nausea, pseudomembranous colitis, vomiting
GU: Cervicitis, vaginitis, and vulvar irritation (with vaginal form)
HEME: Agranulocytosis, eosinophilia, leukopenia, neutropenia, thrombocytopenic purpura
SKIN: Acute generalized exanthematous pustulosis, erythema multiforme, irritation, maculopapular rash, pruritus, rash, Stevens-Johnson syndrome, toxic epidermal necrolysis, urticaria
Other: Anaphylaxis; drug rash with eosinophilia and systemic symptoms (DRESS); induration, pain, or sterile abscess after injection; superinfection

Nursing Considerations

• Expect to obtain a specimen for culture and sensitivity testing before giving first dose.
• Use clindamycin cautiously in patients who have a history of asthma, significant allergies, or GI disease; in those with renal or hepatic dysfunction; and in elderly or atopic patients.
WARNING Don't give 75- and 150-mg capsules to tartrazine-sensitive patients.
• Store oral solution for up to 2 weeks at room temperature or reconstituted parenteral solution for up to 24 hours at room temperature.
• Give I.V. dose by infusion only; don't give bolus dose. Dilute 300 mg of clindamycin in 50 ml of diluent and give over 10 minutes. Dilute 600 mg of clindamycin in 50 ml of diluent and give over 20 minutes. Dilute 900 mg of clindamycin in 50 to 100 ml of diluent and give over 30 minutes. Dilute 1,200 mg of clindamycin in 100 ml of diluent and give over 40 minutes.
WARNING Don't use diluents that contain benzyl alcohol when clindamycin is to be administered to neonates because a fatal toxic syndrome may occur.
• Do not dilute clindamycin phosphate prior to administering I.M. Give I.M. injection deep into large muscle mass, such as the gluteus maximus. Rotate injection sites, and avoid giving more than 600 mg by I.M. injection.
• Check I.V. site often for phlebitis and irritation.

- For topical foam, wash the affected area with mild soap, let it dry fully, and then apply foam to entire affected area. Be aware that if irritation or dermatitis develops, notify prescriber as foam will need to be discontinued.
- Monitor results of liver function tests, CBC, and platelet counts during prolonged therapy.
- Observe patient for signs and symptoms of superinfection, such as vaginal itching and sore mouth, which may occur 2 to 9 days after therapy begins.
- Assess patient's bowel pattern daily; severe diarrhea may indicate pseudomembranous colitis caused by *Clostridium difficile*. If diarrhea occurs, notify prescriber and expect to withhold clindamycin and treat with fluids, electrolytes, protein, and an antibiotic effective against *C. difficile*.

PATIENT TEACHING
- Tell patient to complete the prescribed course of therapy, even if he feels better before it's finished.
- Instruct patient to take oral clindamycin with at least 8 oz of water to prevent esophageal irritation.
- Advise patient to take oral drug with food, if needed, to reduce GI distress.
- Tell patient not to refrigerate reconstituted oral solution because it may become thick and difficult to pour and to discard unused drug after 14 days.
- If patient will use topical foam, tell him to wash affected area with mild soap, let it dry fully, and then apply foam to entire area. Caution against dispensing foam directly onto hands or face because foam will melt when it contacts warm skin. Instead, patient should dispense amount to be used into the cap or onto a cool surface. Tell patient to pick up a small amount with fingertips and gently massage into affected area until foam disappears. If foam feels warm or looks runny, tell patient to run the can under cold water before dispensing.
- Advise patient using topical foam to avoid contact with eyes, mouth, lips, other mucous membranes or areas of broken skin. If contact occurs, tell patient to rinse area thoroughly with water.

- Warn patient not to rely on latex or rubber condoms and diaphragms for 72 hours after vaginal treatment because mineral oil in vaginal cream may weaken these items.
- Explain that having sexual intercourse after using vaginal cream can increase irritation.
- Inform patient that I.M. injection may be painful.
- Tell patient to immediately report an inflamed mouth or vagina, and rash or lesions.
- Urge patient to report watery, bloody stools to prescriber immediately, even up to 2 months after drug therapy has ended.

clobazam
Onfi

Class and Category
Chemical class: Benzodiazepine
Therapeutic class: Anticonvulsant
Pregnancy category: C
Controlled substance schedule: IV

Indications and Dosages
➤ *Adjunct treatment of seizures associated with Lennox-Gastaut syndrome*
ORAL SUSPENSION, TABLETS
Adults and children age 2 and older weighing less than or equal to 30 kg (66 lbs). *Initial:* 5 mg once daily increased to 5 mg twice daily on day 7 and further increased to 10 mg twice daily on day 14. *Maximum:* 20 mg daily.
Adults and children age 2 and older weighing more than 30 kg (66 lbs). *Initial:* 5 mg twice daily increased to 10 mg twice daily on day 7 and further increased to 20 mg twice daily on day 14. *Maximum:* 40 mg daily.
DOSAGE ADJUSTMENT For elderly patients and patients who are CYP2C19 poor metabolizers or those with hepatic dysfunction, initial dose begun at 5 mg once daily regardless of weight and then titrated according to weight, but only to half the dose normally given for weight category. If needed, an additional titration to the maximum dose for the patient's weight may be started on day 21.

Mechanism of Action

May possibly involve potentiation of GABAergic neurotransmission, which causes binding at the benzodiazepine site of the $GABA_A$ receptor to stop seizure activity.

Contraindications

Hypersensitivity to clobazam or its components

Interactions

DRUGS

CNS depressants: Possible potentiated action of CNS depressants

dextromethorphan: Increased effect of dextromethorphan

fluconazole, fluvoxamine, ketoconazole, ticlopidine and other strong inhibitors of CYP2C19 and omeprazole, a moderate inhibitor of CYP2C19: Increased action of clobazam and adverse effects

midazolam: Decreased effect of midazolam

oral contraceptives: Possible diminished effectiveness of oral contraceptive

ACTIVITIES

alcohol use: Additive CNS effect; increased effect of clobazam

Adverse Reactions

CNS: Aggression, agitation, anxiety, apathy, ataxia, confusion, depression, delirium, delusion, fatigue, hallucination, insomnia, irritability, lethargy, psychomotor hyperactivity, pyrexia, sedation, somnolence, suicidal ideation

EENT: Blurred vision, diplopia, drooling

GI: Abdominal distention, change in appetite, constipation, dysphagia, elevated liver enzymes, vomiting

GU: UTI

HEME: Anemia, eosinophilia, leukopenia, thrombocytopenia

MS: Dysarthria, muscle spasms

RESP: Bronchitis, cough, pneumonia, respiratory depression, upper respiratory infection

SKIN: Rash, Stevens-Johnson syndrome, toxic epidermal necrolysis, urticaria

Other: Physical and psychological dependence

Nursing Considerations

• Watch for signs of physical and psychological dependence (strong desire or need to increase dose to maintain drug effects), especially in patients with a history of substance abuse. Alert prescriber, if present.

• Monitor patient closely for skin reactions, especially during the first 8 weeks of therapy or when re-introducing clobazam therapy. If the patient develops a rash, notify prescriber immediately and expect drug to be discontinued, as serious dermatological adverse reactions have occurred with clobazam therapy.

• Monitor patient for suicidal tendencies, particularly when therapy starts and dosage changes.

• Expect to withdraw clobazam therapy gradually when the drug is discontinued by decreasing total daily dose by 5 to 10 mg/day on a weekly basis until discontinued, as ordered, to avoid withdrawal symptoms such as anxiety, dysphoria, and insomnia.

PATIENT TEACHING

• Advise patient or parents that clobazam may be given as a whole tablet or crushed and mixed in applesauce.

• Instruct patient prescribed oral suspension form to shake container well before every administration. The oral dosing syringe provided with the product should be the only device used to measure dosage. Tell patient to firmly insert adapter into the neck of the bottle before the first use and keep it there. To withdraw the dose, she should pull back on dosing syringe to dosage amount that will be withdrawn from bottle, insert the dosing syringe into the adapter, invert bottle, slowly push the air from the syringe into the bottle and then slowly pull back the plunger to the prescribed dose. After removing the syringe from the bottle adapter, the patient should be told to slowly squirt the suspension into the corner of her mouth. Then she should replace the cap over the adapter until next dose is due and rinse syringe well with warm water.

• Tell patient not to take more drug or more often, or for a longer time than prescribed. Warn her that physical and psychological dependence can occur and teach her to recognize the signs.

• Warn patient to stop taking drug at the first sign of a rash and to notify prescriber immediately.

- Instruct patient to avoid performing hazardous activities such as driving until the effects of clobazam are known.
- Tell patient not to stop taking clobazam abruptly, as withdrawal symptoms may occur.
- Urge family or caregiver to watch patient closely for suicidal tendencies, especially when therapy starts or dosage changes.
- Inform female patient of childbearing age to discuss clobazam therapy with her prescriber because drug could interfere with the effectiveness of oral contraceptives. Additional nonhormonal forms of contraception should be used during clobazam therapy if pregnancy is not desired.

clofibrate
Abitrate, Atromid-S, Claripex (CAN), Novofibrate (CAN)

Class and Category
Chemical class: Aryloxyisobutyric acid derivative
Therapeutic class: Antihyperlipidemic
Pregnancy category: C

Indications and Dosages
➤ *To treat primary hyperlipidemia (type III) that doesn't respond to diet, and type IV and type V hyperlipidemia that don't respond to diet in patients at risk for abdominal pain and pancreatitis*
CAPSULES
Adults. 1.5 to 2 g daily in divided doses twice daily to four times daily.

Route	Onset	Peak	Duration
P.O.	2–5 days	3 wk	3 wk

Mechanism of Action
Increases the amount of cholesterol that's secreted into bile and of bile that's excreted in the feces. Clofibrate also may increase the activity of lipoprotein lipase, which degrades VLDLs.

Contraindications
Hepatic dysfunction, hypersensitivity to clofibrate, lactation, peptic ulcer, pregnancy, primary biliary cirrhosis, renal dysfunction

Interactions
DRUGS
chenodiol, ursodiol: Counteracted effectiveness of these drugs
dantrolene: Decreased plasma protein binding of dantrolene
furosemide: Increased furosemide and clofibrate effects
insulin, sulfonylureas: Increased antidiabetic effect
oral anticoagulants: Increased bleeding tendency
oral contraceptives: Decreased effectiveness of clofibrate
phenytoin: Displacement of phenytoin from binding site
probenecid: Increased clofibrate effects
rifampin: Decreased clofibrate effects

Adverse Reactions
CNS: Dizziness, drowsiness, fatigue, headache, weakness
CV: Angina, edema, phlebitis
EENT: Stomatitis
GI: Abdominal pain, bloating, diarrhea, flatulence, nausea, vomiting
GU: Decreased libido, decreased urine output, impotence, proteinuria
HEME: Eosinophilia
MS: Arthralgia, myalgia
SKIN: Alopecia, dry skin and hair, pruritus, rash, urticaria
Other: Weight gain

Nursing Considerations
- Obtain baseline CBC, liver and renal function studies, and cholesterol profile, as ordered.
- Use clofibrate cautiously in patients with a history of hepatic disease or jaundice and in those with peptic ulcer disease.
PATIENT TEACHING
- Tell patient to take clofibrate with milk or food to reduce GI distress.
- Tell patient that repeated laboratory tests will be needed to evaluate serum cholesterol and triglyceride levels.
- Stress the importance of diet, exercise, and weight loss to control cholesterol.
- Tell patient to report ankle or leg swelling, chest pain, decreased urine output, severe GI reactions, and unusual weight gain.

• If patient takes an anticoagulant, tell him to watch carefully for signs and symptoms of abnormal bleeding.
• If patient takes antidiabetic drugs, instruct him to stay alert for signs of hypoglycemia from interactions with these drugs.
• Advise women of childbearing age to use contraception during and for several months after clofibrate therapy because of teratogenic effects.

clomipramine hydrochloride

Anafranil

Class and Category
Chemical class: Dibenzazepine derivative
Therapeutic class: Antiobsessional tricyclic antidepressant
Pregnancy category: C

Indications and Dosages
➤ *To treat obsessive-compulsive disorder*
CAPSULES, TABLETS
Adults. *Initial:* 25 mg daily. Gradually increased to 100 mg daily in divided doses over 2 wk, then to maximum of 250 mg daily in divided doses over next few weeks. At maximum dose, total daily amount may be given at bedtime.
Children age 10 and over. *Initial:* 25 mg daily. Gradually increased to the lesser of 3 mg/kg daily or 100 mg daily in divided doses over 2 wk, then to maximum of 3 mg/kg daily or 200 mg daily, whichever is less. At maximum dose, total daily amount may be given at bedtime.

Route	Onset	Peak	Duration
P.O.	Unknown	2–4 wk	Unknown

Mechanism of Action
May inhibit neuronal reuptake of norepinephrine and serotonin, which may be a factor in normalizing neurotransmission in obsessive-compulsive behavior.

Contraindications
Acute recovery period after MI, hypersensitivity to clomipramine or its components, linezolid or I.V. methylene blue administration, use of an MAO inhibitor within 14 days

Interactions
DRUGS
anticholinergics: Increased anticholinergic effects
barbiturates: Decreased level and effects of clomipramine; additive CNS depression
bupropion, cimetidine, haloperidol, H_2-receptor antagonists, selective serotonin reuptake inhibitors, valproic acid: Increased blood level and therapeutic and adverse effects of clomipramine
carbamazepine: Decreased blood clomipramine level; increased carbamazepine level
clonidine: Severely increased blood pressure and risk of hypertensive crisis
CNS depressants: Increased CNS depression dicumarol: Increased anticoagulant effect
grepafloxacin, quinolones, sparfloxacin: Increased risk of life-threatening arrhythmias
guanethidine: Antagonized antihypertensive effect of guanethidine
levodopa: Delayed absorption and decreased bioavailability of levodopa
MAO inhibitors: Increased risk of seizures, coma, or death
rifamycins: Decreased clomipramine level
sympathomimetics: Possibly potentiated cardiovascular effects
thyroid drugs: Increased effects of thyroid drugs and clomipramine
ACTIVITIES
alcohol use: Increased CNS depression

Adverse Reactions
CNS: Anxiety, confusion, depersonalization, depression, dizziness, drowsiness, emotional lability, fatigue, headache, insomnia, panic reaction, paresthesia, serotonin syndrome, somnolence, suicidal ideation (children and teens), syncope, tremor, unusual dreams, yawning
CV: Orthostatic hypotension, palpitations, tachycardia
EENT: Acute-angle glaucoma, blurred vision, dry mouth, epistaxis, pharyngitis, rhinitis, sinusitis, unpleasant taste
GI: Abdominal pain, anorexia, constipation, diarrhea, flatulence, increased appetite, indigestion, nausea, vomiting

GU: Dysmenorrhea, ejaculation failure, impotence, urinary hesitancy, urine retention
RESP: Bronchospasm
SKIN: Abnormal skin odor, acne, dermatitis, dry skin, photosensitivity, rash, urticaria
Other: Weight gain

Nursing Considerations
• Be aware that stopping clomipramine abruptly may cause withdrawal symptoms and worsen disorder.
WARNING Don't give drug within 14 days of an MAO inhibitor to avoid possible seizures, coma, or death.
WARNING Monitor children and teens closely for evidence of suicidal ideation; clomipramine increases the risk in these groups.
WARNING Monitor patient closely for evidence of serotonin syndrome, such as agitation, hallucinations, coma, tachycardia, labile blood pressure, hyperthermia, hyperreflexia, incoordination, nausea, vomiting, or diarrhea. Notify prescriber at once because serotonin syndrome maybe life-threatening. Be prepared to discontinue drug and provide supportive care.

PATIENT TEACHING
• Tell patient not to use alcohol, barbiturates, or other CNS depressants; clomipramine increases their effects.
WARNING Urge parents to watch their child or teen closely for abnormal thinking or behavior, or increased aggression or hostility. Emphasize the need to notify prescriber if they occur.
• Inform male patients about risk of sexual dysfunction while taking drug.
• Caution patient that drug may cause drowsiness, especially during initial dosage adjustment.
• Warn patient not to stop taking drug abruptly.
• Instruct patient to take a missed dose as soon as he remembers unless it's almost time for the next scheduled dose, in which case he should skip the missed dose. Warn against doubling the next dose.
• Teach patient how to prevent photo-sensitivity reactions.
• Tell patient to report difficulty urinating, dizziness, dry mouth, sedation, and mental changes.

• Advise patient that drug may cause mild pupillary dilation, which may lead to an episode of acute-angle glaucoma. Encourage patient to have an eye exam before starting therapy to see if he is at risk.
• Caution patient to avoid hazardous activities until CNS effects of drug are known.

clonazepam
Apo-Clonazepam (CAN), Clonapam (CAN), Gen-Clonazepam (CAN), Klonopin, Rivotril (CAN)

Class, Category, and Schedule
Chemical class: Benzodiazepine
Therapeutic class: Anticonvulsant
Pregnancy category: D
Controlled substance schedule: IV

Indications and Dosages
➤ *To treat Lennox-Gastaut syndrome (type of absence seizure disorder) and akinetic and myoclonic seizures*
TABLETS
Adults and children over age 10. 1.5 mg daily in divided doses three times daily. Increased by 0.5 to 1 mg every 3 days, if needed, until seizures are controlled. *Maximum:* 20 mg daily.
Children age 10 and under or weighing less than 30 kg (66 lb). 0.01 to 0.03 mg/kg daily in divided doses twice daily or three times daily. Increased by 0.25 to 0.5 mg every third day up to maintenance dosage. *Maintenance:* 0.1 to 0.2 mg/kg daily, preferably in three equal doses, or if unequal, with largest dose given at bedtime. *Maximum:* 0.05 mg/kg daily.
➤ *To treat panic disorder*
TABLETS
Adults. *Initial:* 0.25 mg twice daily. Increased, if needed, to 1 mg daily after 3 days. If more than 1 mg daily is required, dosage increased in increments of 0.125 to 0.25 mg twice daily every 3 days until panic disorder is controlled or adverse reactions make further increases undesirable. This maintenance dosage may be given as a single dose at bedtime. *Maximum:* 4 mg daily.

Mechanism of Action

Prevents seizures by potentiating the effects of gamma-aminobutyric acid (GABA), which is an inhibitory neurotransmitter. Suppresses the spread of seizure activity caused by seizure-producing foci in the cortex, thalamus, and limbic structures.

Contraindications

Acute angle-closure glaucoma, hepatic disease, hypersensitivity to benzodiazepines or their components

Interactions

DRUGS

antianxiety drugs, barbiturates, MAO inhibitors, opioids, phenothiazines, tricyclic antidepressants: Increased CNS depression

ACTIVITIES

alcohol use: Increased CNS depression

Adverse Reactions

CNS: Ataxia, confusion, depression, dizziness, drowsiness, emotional lability, fatigue, headache, memory loss, nervousness, reduced intellectual ability, suicidal ideation
CV: Palpitations
EENT: Blurred vision, eyelid spasm, increased salivation, loss of taste, pharyngitis, rhinitis, sinusitis
GI: Abdominal pain, anorexia, constipation
GU: Difficult ejaculation, dysmenorrhea, dysuria, enuresis, impotence, nocturia, urine retention, UTI
HEME: Anemia, eosinophilia, leukopenia, thrombocytopenia
MS: Dysarthria, myalgia
RESP: Bronchitis, cough
Other: Allergic reaction

Nursing Considerations

• Use clonazepam cautiously in patients with renal failure, mixed seizure disorder (because drug can increase the risk of generalized tonic-clonic seizures), or respiratory disease and troublesome secretions (because clonazepam increases salivation) and in elderly patients (because they're more sensitive to drug's CNS effects).
• Monitor blood drug level, CBC, and liver function test results during long-term or high-dose therapy, as ordered.

WARNING Don't stop drug abruptly; expect to taper dosage gradually to avoid withdrawal symptoms and seizures.
• Monitor patient closely for evidence of suicidal thinking or behavior, especially when therapy starts or dosage changes.

PATIENT TEACHING

• Tell patient to take drug exactly as prescribed. Explain that stopping abruptly can cause seizures and withdrawal symptoms.
• Advise patient to avoid alcohol and sleep-inducing drugs during therapy. Instruct him to consult prescriber before taking any OTC drugs.
• Urge patient to carry medical identification of his seizure disorder and drug therapy.
• Warn patient about possible drowsiness.
• Instruct patient to report severe dizziness, persistent drowsiness, palpitations, difficulty urinating, seizure activity, and other disruptive adverse reactions.
• Suggest that parents monitor child's performance in school because clonazepam can cause drowsiness or inattentiveness.
• Urge caregivers to watch patient closely for evidence of suicidal tendencies, especially when therapy starts or dosage changes, and to report concerns to prescriber immediately.
• Urge female patient who becomes pregnant while taking clonazepam to enroll in the Antiepileptic Drug Pregnancy Registry by calling 1-888-233-2334. Explain that the registry is studying the safety of antiepileptic drugs during pregnancy.

clonidine

Catapres-TTS

clonidine hydrochloride

Catapres, Dixarit (CAN), Duraclon, Jenloga, Kapvay

Class and Category

Chemical class: Imidazoline derivative

Therapeutic class: Analgesic, antihypertensive
Pregnancy category: C

Indications and Dosages

➤ *To manage hypertension*

TABLETS

Adults. *Initial:* 0.1 mg twicedaily, increased by 0.1 mg/wk to produce desired response. *Maintenance:* 0.2 to 0.6 mg daily in divided doses twice daily or three times daily. *Maximum:* 2.4 mg daily.

E.R. TABLETS (JENLOGA)

Adults. *Initial:* 0.1 mg at bedtime, increased by 0.1 mg/wk to produce desired response. With dosage increase, total daily dosage should be equally divided and administered twice daily.

TRANSDERMAL PATCH

Adults. *Initial:* 0.1-mg patch applied to hairless area of intact skin on upper arm or torso every 7 days. After 1 to 2 wk, if blood pressure isn't controlled, two 0.1-mg patches or one 0.2-mg patch applied to skin. Dosage adjusted, as needed, every 7 days. *Maximum:* Two 0.3-mg patches worn at same time.

➤ *To treat severe hypertension*

TABLETS

Adults. 0.2 mg, then 0.1 mg every 1 hr until diastolic blood pressure reaches acceptable range or 0.8 mg has been administered. *DOSAGE ADJUSTMENT* Dosage individualized for patients with renal failure.

➤ *To treat attention deficit hyperactivity disorder (ADHD) alone or as adjunct therapy with stimulant drugs*

E.R. TABLETS (KAPVAY)

Adolescents up to age 17 and children age 6 and over. *Initial:* 0.1 mg at bedtime, increased in increments of 0.1 mg daily at weekly intervals, as needed, with total daily dosage equally divided and given twice a day as soon as dosage begins to be increased. *Maximum:* 0.4 mg/day.

➤ *As adjunct to relieve severe pain (in cancer patients) that isn't adequately relieved by opioid analgesics alone*

CONTINUOUS EPIDURAL INFUSION

Adults. *Initial:* 30 mcg/hr. Titrated up or down, if needed, depending on comfort. *Maximum:* 40 mcg/hr.

Children old enough to tolerate placement and management of epidural catheter. *Initial:* 0.5 mcg/kg/hr. Then, titrated to achieve comfort.

Route	Onset	Peak	Duration
P.O.	30–60 min	2–4 hr	8 hr
Trans-dermal	2–3 days	Unknown	7 days

Mechanism of Action

Stimulates peripheral alpha-adrenergic receptors in the CNS to produce transient vasoconstriction and then stimulates central alpha-adrenergic receptors in the brain stem to reduce peripheral vascular resistance, heart rate, and systolic and diastolic blood pressure. May produce analgesia by preventing transmission of pain signals to the brain at presynaptic and postjunctional alpha$_2$-adrenoreceptors in the spinal cord. With epidural administration, clonidine produces analgesia in body areas innervated by the spinal cord segments in which the drug concentrates.

Contraindications

Anticoagulant therapy (epidural infusion); bleeding diathesis; hypersensitivity to clonidine or its components, including adhesive used in transdermal patch; injection-site infection (epidural infusion)

Interactions

DRUGS

barbiturates, other CNS depressants: Increased depressant effects of these drugs
beta blockers, calcium channel blockers, digoxin: Additive effects, such as bradycardia and AV block; increased risk of worsened hypertensive response when clonidine is withdrawn (beta blockers only)
diuretics, other antihypertensive drugs: Increased hypotensive effect
epidural local anesthetics: Prolonged effects of epidural local anesthetics when used with epidural clonidine
levodopa: Decreased levodopa effectiveness
neuroleptics: Increased risk of orthostatic hypotension, dizziness, and fatigue

prazosin, tricyclic antidepressants: Decreased antihypertensive effect of clonidine

sympatholytics: Increased risk of worsening sinus node dysfunction and AV block, if present

ACTIVITIES

alcohol use: Enhanced CNS depressant effects of alcohol

Adverse Reactions

CNS: Agitation, delusional perception, depression, dizziness, drowsiness, fatigue, hallucinations, headache, malaise, nervousness, paresthesia, sedation, syncope, weakness, tremor

CV: Arrhythmias, AV block, bradycardia (severe), chest pain, congestive heart failure, orthostatic hypotension, Raynaud's phenomenon

EENT: Accommodation disorder, blurred vision, burning eyes, decreased lacrimation, dry eyes and mouth, salivary gland pain

GI: Constipation, hepatitis, mildly elevated liver function test results, nausea, vomiting

GU: Decreased libido, erectile dysfunction, nocturia

HEME: Thrombocytopenia

SKIN: Angioneurotic edema, pruritus, rash, urticaria

Other: Weight gain, withdrawal symptoms

Nursing Considerations

• Be aware that clonidine should not be used in most patients with severe cardiovascular disease or in those who are not hemodynamically stable because of the potential for severe hypotension.

• Use clonidine cautiously in elderly patients, who may be more sensitive to its hypotensive effect.

• Monitor blood pressure and heart rate often during clonidine therapy because clonidine may worsen sinus node dysfunction and AV block, especially if patient is taking another sympatholytic drug. If severe bradycardia occurs, be prepared to administer IV atropine or isoproterneol and assist with insertion of temporary cardiac pacing.

• Be aware that extended-release tablets are not interchangeable with immediate-release tablets.

• Expect transdermal clonidine to take 2 to 3 days to lower blood pressure.

• Remove patch before patient has an MRI to avoid possible burns at the patch site.

• Be aware that stopping drug abruptly can elevate serum catecholamine levels and cause such withdrawal symptoms as nervousness, agitation, headache, confusion, tremor, and rebound hypertension. When drug has been used to treat ADHD, be aware that dosage should be decreased by 0.1 mg every 3 to 7 days when it is being discontinued.

• Monitor patient with sinus node dysfunction and AV block closely if patient is taking sympatholytics concurrently with clonidine because these conditions may worsen, causing severe bradycardia, requiring treatment with IV atropine or isoproternol therapy and temporary cardiac pacing.

• Expect hypertension to return within 48 hours after drug is discontinued.

PATIENT TEACHING

• Advise patient to take drug exactly as prescribed and not to stop abruptly because withdrawal symptoms and severe hypertension may occur.

• Instruct patient to consult prescriber if dry mouth or drowsiness becomes a problem during oral clonidine therapy. To minimize these effects, prescriber may suggest taking most of dosage at bedtime.

• If a transdermal patch loosens during 7-day application period, tell patient to place adhesive overlay directly over patch to ensure adhesion.

• Tell patient to rotate transdermal sites.

• Instruct patient to remove patch and place a fresh one on another site if skin irritation, redness, or rash develops at patch site.

• Advise patient to fold used transdermal patch in half with adhesive sides together and discard it out of the reach of children.

• Instruct patient to swallow E.R. tablets whole and never crush, cut, or chew the tablets.

• Because of possible sedation, advise patient to avoid hazardous activities until

drug's CNS effects are known. Caution patient that these effects are increased by concomitant use of alcohol, barbiturates, or other sedating drugs.
- Advise men that libido may decrease.
- Instruct patient to report chest pain, dizziness with position changes, excessive drowsiness, rash, urine retention, and vision changes. As needed, tell patient to rise slowly to avoid hypotensive effects.
- Inform patient who wears contact lenses that clonidine may cause dry eyes.

clopidogrel bisulfate

Plavix

Class and Category

Chemical class: Thienopyridine derivative
Therapeutic class: Platelet aggregation inhibitor
Pregnancy category: B

Indications and Dosages

➤ *To reduce atherosclerotic events, such as stroke and MI, in patients with atherosclerosis documented by recent stroke, MI, or peripheral artery disease*

TABLETS

Adults. 75 mg daily.

➤ *To reduce atherosclerotic events, such as stroke and MI, in patients with acute coronary syndrome (unstable angina or non–Q-wave MI)*

TABLETS

Adults. *Loading dose:* 300 mg. *Maintenance:* 75 mg daily.

➤ *To reduce rate of death, reinfarction, or stroke in patients with ST-segment elevation acute MI*

TABLETS

Adults. 75 mg once daily. Or, loading dose of 300 mg followed by 75 mg once daily.

Mechanism of Action

Binds to adenosine diphosphate (ADP) receptors on the surface of activated platelets. This action blocks ADP, which deactivates nearby glycoprotein IIb/IIIa receptors and prevents fibrinogen from attaching to receptors. Without fibrinogen, platelets can't aggregate and form thrombi.

Route	Onset	Peak	Duration
P.O.	2 hr	3–7 days*	5 days

Contraindications

Active pathological bleeding, including peptic ulcer and intracranial hemorrhage; hypersensitivity to clopidogrel or its components

Interactions

DRUGS

aspirin: Increased risk of bleeding
CYP2C19 inhibitors, such as cimetidine, esomeprazole, etravirine, felbamate, fluconazole, fluoxetine, fluvoxamine, ketoconazole, omeprazole, ticlopidine, voriconazole: Decreased plasma clopidogrel level, decreased platelet inhibition
fluvastatin, phenytoin, tamoxifen, tolbutamide, torsemide: Interference with metabolism of these drugs
NSAIDs: Increased risk of GI bleeding, interference with NSAID metabolism
warfarin: Prolonged bleeding time, interference with warfarin metabolism

Adverse Reactions

CNS: Confusion, depression, dizziness, fatal intracranial bleeding, fatigue, fever, hallucinations, headache
CV: Chest pain, edema, hyper-cholesterolemia, hypertension, hypotension, vasculitis
EENT: Altered taste; conjunctival, ocular, or retinal bleeding; epistaxis; rhinitis; stomatitis; taste disorders
GI: Abdominal pain; acute liver failure; colitis; diarrhea; duodenal, gastric, or peptic ulcer; elevated liver function test results; gastritis; gastrointestinal and retroperitoneal hemorrhage, indigestion; nausea; noninfectious hepatitis; pancreatitis
GU: Elevated serum creatinine level, glomerulopathy, UTI
HEME: Acquired hemophilia A, agranulocytosis, aplastic anemia, neutropenia, pancytopenia, prolonged bleeding time, thrombocytopenic purpura, thrombotic thrombocytopenic purpura, unusual bleeding or bruising
MS: Arthralgia, back pain, musculoskeletal bleeding, myalgia

*With repeated doses.

C

RESP: Bronchitis, bronchospasm, cough, dyspnea, eosinophilic pneumonia, interstitial pneumonitis, respiratory tract bleeding, upper respiratory tract infection
SKIN: Bullous dermatitis, drug rash with eosinophilia and systemic symptoms (DRESS), eczema, erythema multiforme, exfoliative rash, lichen planus, pruritus, purpura, rash, skin bleeding, Stevens-Johnson syndrome, toxic epidermal necrolysis, urticaria
Other: Anaphylaxis, angioedema, flulike symptoms, serum sickness

Nursing Considerations
• Avoid clopidogrel in patients who have a genetic variation in CYP2C19 or are receiving CYP2C19 inhibitors. Platelet inhibition may decline, increasing the risk of adverse cardiovascular effects after MI.
• Determine if patient has a history of hypersensitivity that may have included a hematologic reaction to any other thieno-pyridine drug, such as prasugrel or ticlopidine, because allergic cross-reactivity has been reported.
• Use clopidogrel cautiously in patients with severe hepatic or renal disease, risk of bleeding from trauma or surgery, or conditions that predispose to bleeding (such as peptic ulcer disease or thrombotic thrombocytopenic purpura).
• Expect to give aspirin with clopidogrel in patient with acute coronary syndrome,.
WARNING Clopidogrel prolongs bleeding time; expect to stop it 5 days before elective surgery.
• Obtain blood cell count, as ordered, whenever signs and symptoms suggest a hematologic problem.
• Monitor patient who takes aspirin closely because risk of bleeding is increased.
PATIENT TEACHING
• Discourage use of NSAIDs, including OTC preparations, during clopidogrel therapy because of potential for bleeding.
• Caution patient that bleeding may continue longer than usual. Instruct him to report unusual bleeding or bruising.
• Urge patient to inform all other healthcare providers, including dentists, that he takes clopidogrel before having surgery or other procedures or taking a new drug because he has an increased risk of bleeding.
• Advise patient to notify prescriber promptly if he experiences fever, weakness, extreme skin paleness, purple skin patches, yellowing of his skin or eyes, or neurologic changes.
• Instruct patient not to discontinue clopidogrel abruptly or without first consulting prescriber.

clorazepate dipotassium

Apo-Clorazepate (CAN), Novo-Clopate (CAN), Tranxene (CAN), Tranxene-SD, Tranxene-SD Half Strength

Class, Category, and Schedule
Chemical class: Benzodiazepine
Therapeutic class: Alcohol withdrawal adjunct, antianxiety drug, anticonvulsant
Pregnancy category: Not rated
Controlled substance schedule: IV

Indications and Dosages
➤ *To relieve anxiety*
CAPSULES, TABLETS
Adults and adolescents. *Initial:* 15 mg at bedtime or 7.5 to 15 mg twice daily. Dosage adjusted, as needed, to 15 to 60 mg daily in divided doses twice daily to four times daily. *Maximum:* 90 mg daily.
E.R. TABLETS
Adults and adolescents. 11.25 mg daily as substitute for capsules or tablets in patients who were stabilized on 3.75 mg three times daily of those forms; 22.5 mg daily as substitute for capsules or tablets in patients who were stabilized on 7.5 mg three times daily of those forms.
➤ *To relieve symptoms of acute alcohol withdrawal*
CAPSULES, TABLETS
Adults. *Initial:* 30 mg followed by 15 mg twice daily to four times daily on day 1 of therapy; 15 mg three to six times on day 2; 7.5 to 15 mg three times daily on day 3; 7.5 mg twice daily to four times daily on day 4; and thereafter, 3.75 mg twice daily to four times daily. *Maximum:* 90 mg daily.

➤ *As adjunct to treat partial seizure disorder*
CAPSULES, TABLETS
Adults and adolescents. *Initial:* Up to
7.5 mg three times daily. Increased, if
needed, by up to 7.5 mg/wk. *Maximum:*
90 mg daily.
Children ages 9 to 12.
Initial: 7.5 mg twice daily. Increased, if
needed, by up to 7.5 mg/wk. *Maximum:*
60 mg daily.
E.R. TABLETS
Adults and adolescents. 11.25 mg daily as
substitute for capsules or tablets in patients
who were stabilized on 3.75 mg three times
daily of those forms; 22.5 mg daily as
substitute for capsules or tablets in patients
who were stabilized on 7.5 mg three times
daily of those forms.
DOSAGE ADJUSTMENT Initial dosage reduced
to 3.75 to 15 mg daily to treat anxiety in
elderly patients.

Mechanism of Action
Potentiates action of gamma-aminobutyric
acid (GABA) and other inhibitory neurotransmitters by binding to specific
benzodiazepine receptor sites in limbic and
cortical areas of CNS, which helps control
emotional behavior and suppresses spread
of seizure activity. Drug also helps relieve
symptoms of alcohol withdrawal by
depressing CNS.

Contraindications
Angle-closure glaucoma, hypersensitivity to
chlorazepate or its components

Interactions
DRUGS
*barbiturates, MAO inhibitors, opioids, other
antidepressants, phenothiazines:* Potentiated
effects of clorazepate
*cimetidine, disulfiram, fluoxetine, isoniazid,
ketoconazole, metoprolol, oral contraceptives,
propoxyphene, propranolol, valproic acid:*
Increased blood clorazepate level
clozapine: Possibly increased risk of shock
ACTIVITIES
alcohol use: Potentiated clorazepate effects

Adverse Reactions
CNS: Anxiety, ataxia, confusion,
depression, dizziness, drowsiness, fatigue,
headache, insomnia, irritability,
nervousness, psychosis, slurred speech,
suicidal ideation, tremor

CV: Hypotension
EENT: Blurred vision, diplopia, dry
mouth
GI: Anorexia, constipation, diarrhea,
elevated liver function test results, nausea,
vomiting
GU: Elevated BUN and serum creatinine
levels, incontinence, libido changes,
menstrual irregularities, urine retention
HEME: Decreased hematocrit
SKIN: Rash
Other: Drug dependence

Nursing Considerations
WARNING Be aware that prolonged use of
therapeutic doses can lead to
dependence.
• Monitor liver function test results during
therapy.
• Watch closely for evidence of suicidal
thinking or behavior, especially when
therapy starts or dosage changes.
PATIENT TEACHING
• Tell patient to take clorazepate with food if
GI distress occurs.
• Advise patient to avoid alcohol and other
CNS depressants while taking drug.
• Urge patient to avoid hazardous activities
until CNS effects of drug are known.
• Urge caregivers to watch patient closely for
evidence of suicidal tendencies, especially
when therapy starts or dosage changes,
and to report concerns to prescriber
immediately.
• Urge female patient who becomes
pregnant while taking clorazepate to
enroll in the antiepileptic drug pregnancy
registry by calling 1-888-233-2334.
Explain that the registry is studying the
safety of antiepileptic drugs during
pregnancy.

cloxacillin sodium
Apo-Cloxi (CAN), Cloxapen, Novo-
Cloxin (CAN), Nu-Cloxi (CAN),
Orbenin (CAN), Tegopen

Class and Category
Chemical class: Penicillinase-resistant
isoxazolyl penicillin derivative
Therapeutic class: Antibiotic
Pregnancy category: B

Indications and Dosages

➤ *To treat mild to moderate upper respiratory tract infections or localized skin and soft-tissue infections caused by penicillinase-producing staphylococci*

CAPSULES, ORAL SOLUTION, I.V. INFUSION, I.V. OR I.M. INJECTION

Adults and children weighing 20 kg (44 lb) or more. 250 mg every 6 hr. *Maximum:* 6 g daily.

Children and infants weighing less than 20 kg. 50 mg/kg daily in equally divided doses every 6 hr.

➤ *To treat severe lower respiratory tract infections or disseminated infections caused by penicillinase-producing staphylococci*

CAPSULES, ORAL SOLUTION, I.V. INFUSION, I.V. OR I.M. INJECTION

Adults and children weighing 20 kg or more. 500 mg every 6 hr. *Maximum:* 6 g daily.

Infants and children weighing less than 20 kg. 100 mg/kg daily in divided doses every 6 hr.

Mechanism of Action

Inhibits cell wall synthesis and causes cell lysis and death in bacteria that make rigid, cross-linked cell walls in several steps. Cloxacillin affects the final stage of cross-linking by binding with and inactivating penicillin-binding protein, the enzyme that causes linkage in cell wall strands.

Incompatibilities

Don't mix cloxacillin with aminoglycosides because of risk of mutual inactivation.

Contraindications

Hypersensitivity to cloxacillin, penicillin, or their components

Interactions

DRUGS

chloramphenicol, erythromycins, sulfonamides, tetracyclines: Decreased cloxacillin effects
hepatotoxic drugs, such as fluconazole: Increased risk of hepatotoxicity
methotrexate: Increased blood methotrexate level and risk of toxicity
probenecid: Increased and prolonged blood cloxacillin level

Adverse Reactions

CNS: Headache
EENT: Glossitis, oral candidiasis
GI: Abdominal pain, diarrhea, elevated liver function test results, nausea, pseudomembranous colitis, vomiting
GU: Hematuria, vaginal candidiasis
MS: Muscle twitching
SKIN: Pruritus, rash, urticaria
Other: Anaphylaxis

Nursing Considerations

• Use cloxacillin cautiously in patients hypersensitive to cephalosporins (allergic reaction may be delayed) and those with hypertension (drug is relatively high in sodium).
• For I.V. injection, reconstitute 250-mg vial with 4.9 ml of sterile water for injection, 500-mg vial with 4.8 ml, and 2,000-mg vial with 6.8 ml. Shake to dissolve.
• For direct I.V. injection, give over 2 to 4 minutes through tubing of a compatible infusing I.V. solution. If giving by intermittent I.V. infusion, further dilute with a suitable diluent (see package insert) and administer over 30 to 40 minutes.
• For I.M. injection, reconstitute 250-mg vial with 1.9 ml of sterile water for injection and 500-mg vial with 1.7 ml of sterile water. Shake to dissolve.
• Be aware that parenteral solutions are stable 24 hours at room temperature and 72 hours if refrigerated.

PATIENT TEACHING

• Tell patient to finish full course of therapy, even if he feels better before drug is gone.
• Instruct patient to take oral cloxacillin 1 to 2 hours before meals.
• Tell patient to take oral form of cloxacillin with a full glass of water (not fruit juice or soda).
• Instruct patient taking oral solution to refrigerate container and to discard unused portion after 14 days. Also instruct him to use a calibrated measuring device to ensure accurate doses.
• Advise patient to report signs or symptoms of allergic reaction.

clozapine

Clozaril, Fazaclo, Versacloz

Class and Category
Chemical class: Dibenzodiazepine derivative
Therapeutic class: Antipsychotic
Pregnancy category: B

Indications and Dosages
➤ *To treat severe schizophrenia unresponsive to standard drugs; to reduce risk of recurrent suicidal behavior in schizophrenia or schizoaffective disorders*
ORALLY DISINTEGRATING TABLETS, ORAL SUSPENSION, TABLETS
Adults. *Initial:* 12.5 mg once or twice daily. Increased by 25 to 50 mg daily to 300 to 450 mg daily in divided doses by the end of 2 wk. Dosage titration shouldn't exceed 100 mg twice per wk. *Maximum:* 900 mg daily.
DOSAGE ADJUSTMENT If patient is receiving a strong CYP1A2 inhibitor such as ciprofloxacin, enoxacin, or fluvoxamine concurrently, dosage decreased by two-thirds and then adjusted according to clinical response. If a patient is receiving a strong CYP1A2 inducer such as carbamazepine, phenytoin, rifampin, or St. John's wort concurrently, clozapine dosage may need to be increased if clinical response is ineffective. If patient has significant renal or hepatic impairment or is a CYP2D6 poor metabolizer, clozapine dosage may be decreased if patient develops significant adverse reactions.

Route	Onset	Peak	Duration
P.O.	1–6 hr	Unknown	4–12 hr

Mechanism of Action
May produce antipsychotic effects by interfering with dopamine binding to dopamine—especially D_4—receptors in the limbic region of the brain and by antagonizing adrenergic, cholinergic, histaminic, and serotoninergic receptors.

Contraindications
Angle-closure glaucoma, coma, history of clozapine-induced agranulocytosis or severe granulocytopenia, hypersensitivity to clozapine or its components, myelo-proliferative disorders, severe CNS depression, uncontrolled epilepsy, WBC count below 3,500/mm³

Interactions
DRUGS
anticholinergics: Potentiated anticholinergic effects
benzodiazepines, psychotropics: Additive hypotensive effects; increased risk of cardiopulmonary collapse
bone marrow depressants: Potentiated myelosuppressive effects
bupropion, cimetidine, citalopram, ciprofloxacin, duloxetine, enoxacin, erythromycin, escitalopram, fluoxetine, fluvoxamine, oral contraceptives, paroxetine, quinidine, sertraline, terbinafine: Possibly increased blood clozapine level and increased risk of adverse reactions
carbamazepine, phenytoin, rifampin, St. John's wort: Decreased blood clozapine level
chlorpromazine, class 1Aa antiarrhythmias such as quinidine or procainamide, class III antiarrhythmias such as amiodarone or sotalol, dolasetron, droperidol, erythromycin, gatifloxacin, halofantrine, iloperidone, levomethadyl, mesoridazine, mefloquine, methadone, moxifloxacin, pentamidine, pimozide, probucol, sparfloxacin, tacrolimus, thioridazine: Possible increased risk of prolonged QT interval
CNS depressants: Increased CNS depression
digoxin, warfarin: Increased blood level of digoxin and warfarin; displacement of clozapine from its binding site
lithium: Increased risk of confusion, dyskinesia, neuroleptic malignant syndrome, and seizures
selective serotonin reuptake inhibitors: Markedly increased blood clozapine level; increased risk of adverse effects and leukocytosis
ACTIVITIES
alcohol use: Increased CNS depression
caffeine: Increased blood clozapine level
smoking: Decreased blood clozapine level

Adverse Reactions
CNS: Agitation, akinesia, anxiety, ataxia, confusion, depression, dizziness, drowsiness, dystonia, fatigue, fever, headache, hyperkinesia, hypokinesia, insomnia, lethargy, myoclonic jerks, neuroleptic malignant syndrome, nightmares, obsessive compulsive symptoms, restlessness, rigidity, sedation, seizures, sleep disturbance, slurred speech,

status epilepticus, syncope, tardive dyskinesia, tremor, vertigo, weakness
CV: Atrial or ventricular fibrillation, cardiac arrest, cardiomyopathy, chest pain, deep vein thrombosis, ECG changes, hypercholesterolemia, hypertension, hypertriglyceridemia, hypotension, myocarditis, orthostatic hypotension, QT interval prolongation, tachycardia, torsades de pointes, vasculitis, ventricular tachycardia
EENT: Blurred vision, dry mouth, increased nasal congestion, increased salivation, narrow-angle glaucoma, pharyngitis, salivary gland swelling, tongue numbness or soreness
ENDO: Ketoacidosis, severe hyperglycemia
GI: Abdominal discomfort, acute pancreatitis, anorexia, cholestasis, constipation, diarrhea, dysphagia, elevated liver function test results, heartburn, hepatitis, jaundice, nausea, vomiting
GU: Abnormal ejaculation; acute interstitial nephritis; nocturnal enuresis; priapism; renal failure; urinary frequency, urgency, and incontinence; urine retention
HEME: Agranulocytosis; elevated hemoglobin, hematocrit and erythrocyte sedimentation rate; eosinophilia; leucopenia; neutropenia; thrombocytopenia; thrombocytosis
MS: Back or leg pain, muscle spasm or weakness, myalgia, myasthenic syndrome, rhabdomyolysis
RESP: Dyspnea, lower respiratory tract infection, pleural effusion, pneumonia, pulmonary embolism, respiratory arrest
SKIN: Erythema multiforme, photosensitivity, pruritus, rash, Stevens-Johnson syndrome, urticaria
Other: Hypersensitivity reactions, hyperuricemia, hyponatremia, sepsis, weight gain

Nursing Considerations
• Use clozapine cautiously in patients with hepatic, renal, or cardiovascular disease and in elderly patients with dementia-related psychosis because they have increased risk of serious or fatal adverse reactions. Also use cautiously in patients with risk factors for a stroke because drug use may increase risk of cerebrovascular adverse events.

• Use cautiously in patients with a history of prolonged QT syndrome or who have existing conditions that might prolong the QT interval such as a recent MI, uncompensated heart failure, or serious cardiac arrhythmia. Drug should also be used cautiously in patients with cardiovascular disease or a family history of prolonged QT syndrome because clozapine therapy may increase the QT interval enough to cause life-threatening arrhythmias such as torsades de pointes, especially in patients who are hypokalemic. Know that hypokalemia should be corrected, if present, before clozapine therapy begins and the serum potassium level monitored closely throughout therapy. If QT prolongation occurs, notify prescriber and expect drug to be discontinued if the QT interval exceeds 500 msec.

WARNING Rarely, clozapine causes severe or life-threatening adverse reactions, such as agranulocytosis, cardiac or respiratory arrest, deep vein thrombosis, myocarditis (especially in first month), neuroleptic malignant syndrome, and severe hyperglycemia with ketoacidosis in nondiabetic patients. It also may cause seizures and tardive dyskinesia. Monitor patient closely.

WARNING Check patient's baseline WBC count and absolute neutrophil count (ANC) before therapy and weekly for first 6 months, as ordered. If WBC count is at least 3,500/mm^3 and ANC at least 2,000/mm^3, check every 2 weeks for next 6 months, as ordered. If counts remain stable, expect to continue checking every 4 weeks thereafter.

• If patient develops mild leukopenia (WBCs 3,000 to 3,500/mm^3) or granulocytopenia (ANC 1,500 to 2,000/mm^3), expect to check counts twice weekly until normal. In moderate leukopenia (WBCs 2,000 to 3,000/mm^3) or granulocytopenia (ANC 1,000 to 1,500/mm^3), expect to stop drug temporarily and check counts daily until improved. Follow manufacturer's direction for resuming drug and monitoring. In severe leukopenia (WBCs less than 2,000/mm^3) or granulocytopenia (ANC less than 1,000/mm^3), expect to stop drug permanently and monitor counts daily, then as specified by manufacturer.

- Monitor temperature. A transient increase above 100.4° F (38° C) may occur, most often within the first 3 weeks of therapy.
- When therapy ends, expect to check WBC count and ANC weekly for at least 4 weeks or until WBC count is 3,500/mm³ or more and ANC is 2,000/mm³ or more.
- Monitor patients, especially male patients and younger patients, for dystonia, particularly during the first few days of treatment. Be alert for complaints of neck spasms, which sometimes may progress to throat tightness, trouble swallowing or breathing, and tongue protrusion.

PATIENT TEACHING

- Tell patient that he'll receive only a 1-week supply at a time.
- Instruct patient taking orally disintegrating tablets (Fazaclo) to leave tablet in blister pack until ready to take it. Tell him to peel foil back to remove tablet (rather than pushing tablet through foil) and then to immediately place tablet in mouth and let it dissolve before swallowing. Explain that no water is needed.
- Instruct patient prescribed oral suspension form to shake container for 10 seconds before every administration. The oral dosing syringe provided with the product should be the only device used to measure dosage. Tell patient to firmly insert adapter into the neck of the bottle before the first use and keep it there. Instruct patient to first fill the syringe with air equivalent to the dose being withdrawn from the bottle. To withdraw the dose, he should insert the dosing syringe into the adapter and push air from syringe into bottle. Then he should invert bottle and slowly pull back the plunger to the prescribed dose. After removing the syringe from the bottle adapter, the patient should be told to slowly squirt the suspension into his mouth. Then he should replace the cap over the adapter until next dose is due and rinse syringe well with warm water and dry.
- Inform patient that he'll need weekly blood tests. Review evidence of dyscrasias (fatigue, fever, sore throat, weakness); urge patient to report them to prescriber if they occur.
- Instruct patient to avoid hazardous activities until drug's CNS effects are known.

- Advise patient to rise slowly from lying or sitting position to minimize orthostatic hypotension.
- If patient stops drug for more than 2 days, emphasize need to contact prescriber for instructions; dosage will need to be changed.
- Tell patient to consult prescriber before using alcohol or taking OTC drugs.
- Advise female patients of childbearing age to notify prescriber if pregnancy occurs or is suspected.

codeine phosphate
codeine sulfate

Class, Category, and Schedule

Chemical class: Phenanthrene derivative
Therapeutic class: Antitussive, opioid analgesic
Pregnancy category: C
Controlled substance schedule: II

Indications and Dosages

➤ *To treat mild to moderate pain*

ORAL SOLUTION, TABLETS, I.M. OR SUBCUTANEOUS INJECTION

Adults. 15 to 60 mg (usual, 30 mg) every 4 hr, as needed.
Children age 1 year or over. 0.5 mg/kg every 4 to 6 hr, as needed.

I.V. INJECTION

Adults. 15 to 60 mg (usual, 30 mg) every 4 hr.

➤ *To treat cough from chemical or mechanical irritation of respiratory system*

ORAL SOLUTION, TABLETS

Adults and adolescents. 10 to 20 mg every 4 to 6 hr. *Maximum:* 120 mg daily.
Children ages 6 to 12. 5 to 10 mg every 4 to 6 hr. *Maximum:* 60 mg daily.
Children ages 2 to 6. 2.5 to 5 mg every 4 to 6 hr. *Maximum:* 30 mg daily.

Route	Onset	Peak	Duration
P.O.	30–45 min	1–2 hr	4 hr*
I.M.	10–30 min	30–60 min	4 hr*
SubQ	10–30 min	Unknown	4 hr*

*For pain; 4 to 6 hr for cough.

Mechanism of Action

May produce analgesia through partial metabolism to morphine. Drug binds with mu, delta, and kappa receptors in the spinal cord and with mu_1 and $kappa_3$ receptors higher in the CNS, decreasing intracellular cAMP, which inhibits adenylate cyclase activity and prevents release of pain neurotransmitters, such as substance P and dopamine, and altering perception of and emotional response to pain. Drug also suppresses cough by acting on opiate receptors in the cough center.

Contraindications

Hypersensitivity to codeine, other opioids, or their components; significant respiratory depression; use for postoperative pain management in children who have undergone tonsillectomy and/or adenoidectomy

Interactions

DRUGS

anticholinergics, paregoric: Increased risk of severe constipation
antihypertensives, diuretics: Potentiated hypotensive effects
buprenorphine: Decreased codeine effectiveness
CNS depressants: Additive CNS effects
hydroxyzine: Increased analgesia; increased CNS depressant and hypotensive effects
MAO inhibitors: Increased risk of unpredictable, severe, and sometimes fatal reactions
metoclopramide: Antagonized effect of metoclopramide on GI motility
naloxone: Antagonized codeine effect
naltrexone: Precipitated withdrawal symptoms in codeine-dependent patients
neuromuscular blockers: Additive respiratory depressant effects
other opioids: Additive CNS, respiratory depressant, and hypotensive effects

ACTIVITIES

alcohol use: Additive CNS effects

Adverse Reactions

CNS: Coma, delirium, depression, disorientation, dizziness, drowsiness, euphoria, hallucinations, headache, lack of coordination, lethargy, light-headedness, mental and physical impairment, mood changes, restlessness, sedation, seizures, tremor

CV: Bradycardia, heart block, hypertension, orthostatic hypotension, palpitations, tachycardia
EENT: Altered taste, blurred vision, diplopia, dry mouth, laryngeal edema, laryngospasm, miosis
GI: Abdominal cramps and pain, anorexia, constipation, flatulence, gastroesophageal reflux, ileus, indigestion, nausea, vomiting
GU: Decreased libido, difficult ejaculation, dysuria, impotence, oliguria, ureteral spasm, urinary incontinence, urine retention
MS: Muscle rigidity
RESP: Apnea, bronchoconstriction, bronchospasm, depressed cough reflex, respiratory depression
SKIN: Diaphoresis, flushing, pallor, pruritus, rash, urticaria
Other: Anaphylaxis, facial edema, physical and psychological dependence

Nursing Considerations

WARNING Know that codeine should not be given to children following tonsillectomy and/or adenoidectomy and patients who are known ultra-rapid metabolizers of codeine, including mothers who are breastfeeding, as breast-fed infants have died when exposed to high levels of morphine (codeine converts to morphine) in breastmilk. Monitor any patient receiving codeine closely, especially the patient who has never received a narcotic like codeine or morphine, for signs of overdose such as extreme sleepiness, confusion, or shallow breathing because patient may not know he is an ultra-rapid metabolizer. Some patients are ultra-rapid metabolizers because of a CYP2D6 polymorphism. How prevalent this phenotype is varies widely. It is estimated that 0.5 to 1% Chinese, Japanese, and Hispanics; 1 to 10% Caucasians; 3% African Americans; and 16 to 28% of North Africans, Ethiopians, and Arabs may carry the CYP2D6 genotype.

• Evaluate patient for therapeutic response, including decreased pain, cough, and facial grimacing.
• Take safety precautions, if needed.
• Monitor respiratory depth, effort, and rate. Notify prescriber immediately if respiratory rate drops below 10 breaths/min.

WARNING Monitor pediatric patients receiving codeine after a tonsillectomy and/or adenoidectomy for obstructive sleep apnea syndrome closely because, although rare, life-threatening respiratory depression has occurred.
• Assess urine output to detect retention.
WARNING Assess patient for evidence of physical and psychological dependence.
• Rotate sites for subcutaneous delivery. Repeated injection in same site may cause tissue irritation, pain, and induration.

PATIENT TEACHING
• Advise patient to avoid alcohol or other CNS depressants while taking codeine.
• To minimize nausea, suggest that patient take drug with food.
• Advise patient to avoid hazardous activities until drug's CNS effects are known.
• Caution patient to get up slowly from a sitting or lying position.
• To prevent constipation, urge patient to consume plenty of fluids and high-fiber foods, if not contraindicated.
• Instruct patient to take codeine exactly as prescribed and not to adjust dose or frequency without consulting prescriber.
• Advise patient to report shortness of breath or difficulty breathing.
WARNING Advise parents who have a child with obstructive sleep apnea who is being treated with codeine for pain management to give codeine on an "as needed" basis and not to give more than 6 doses in a 24-hour period. They should also observe their child for unusual sleepiness, confusion, or difficult or noisy breathing. If any of these symptoms occur, they should stop giving the codeine and seek emergency care for their child immediately, as these are signs of an overdose.
• Urge breastfeeding women to notify prescriber before taking codeine because drug appears in breastmilk and could lead to overdose in infant.

---

colchicine
Colcrys, Mitigare

Class and Category
Chemical class: Colchicum alkaloid derivative
Therapeutic class: Antigout, anti-inflammatory
Pregnancy category: C (oral form), D (parenteral forms)

Indications and Dosages
➤ *To prevent gouty arthritis attacks*
TABLETS
Adults and adolescents age 16 and over. 0.5 to 0.6 mg once or twice daily. *Maximum:* 1.2 mg daily.
➤ *To treat acute gouty arthritis*
TABLETS
Adults. *Initial:* 1.2 mg at first sign of flare; then 0.6 mg 1 hr later. *Maximum:* 1.8 mg over a 1-hr period.
DOSAGE ADJUSTMENT For elderly patients, maximum dosage reduced to 2 mg/24 hr. If treatment of a gout flare occurs during prophylactic treatment, dosage shouldn't exceed 1.2 mg at the first sign of flare, followed by 0.6 mg 1 hour later, and then prophylactic dose resumed 12 hr later. For patient taking strong CYP3A4 inhibitor (atazanavir, clarithromycin, indinavir, itraconazole, ketoconazole, nefazodone, nelfinavir, ritonavir, saquinavir, telithromycin), moderate CYP3A4 inhibitor (amprenavir, aprepitant, diltiazem, erythromycin, fluconazole, fosamprenavir, grapefruit juice, verapamil), or P-gp inhibitor (cyclosporine, ranolazine), dosage usually halved and not repeated for 3 days. For patient with moderate to severe renal impairment, dosage adjusted on individual basis. For patient with severe hepatic impairment receiving colchicine prophylactically, dosage decreased on individual basis. For patient with severe hepatic impairment receiving colchicine treatment for acute gout flare but not prophylaxis, dosage not adjusted but treatment course shouldn't be repeated more than once very 2 weeks.
➤ *To treat familial Mediterranean fever (FMF)*
TABLETS
Adults and adolescents ages 12 and over. 1.2 mg to 2.4 mg daily, with daily total divided into two doses, if desired.

Children ages 6 to 12. 0.9 mg to 1.8 mg daily, with daily total divided into two doses, if desired.

Children ages 4 to 6. 0.3 mg to 1.8 mg daily, with daily total divided into two doses, if desired.

DOSAGE ADJUSTMENT For adults needing control of FMF, dosage increased in increments of 0.3 mg daily to a maximum of 2.4 mg daily.

For adults with intolerable adverse effects, dosage decreased in increments of 0.3 mg daily to tolerable level.

For patients taking strong CYP3A4 inhibitor (atazanavir, clarithromycin, indinavir, itraconazole, ketoconazole, nefazodone, nelfinavir, ritonavir, saquinavir, telithromycin), moderate CYP3A4 inhibitor (amprenavir, aprepitant, diltiazem, erythromycin, fluconazole, fosamprenavir, grapefruit juice, verapamil), or P-gp inhibitor (cyclosporine, ranolazine), dosage usually halved and not repeated for 3 days. For patient with moderate to severe renal impairment or severe hepatic impairment, dosage adjusted on individual basis.

Route	Onset	Peak	Duration
P.O.	In 12 hr	In 24–48 hr	Unknown

Contraindications
Blood dyscrasias; hypersensitivity to colchicine or its components; serious cardiac, GI, hepatic, or renal disorders

Incompatibilities
Don't combine colchicine with bacterio-static agents, any solution or injection that contains D_5W, and any other solution that may change colchicine's pH because precipitation may occur.

Mechanism of Action
In gouty arthritis, leukocytes phagocytose urate crystals in affected joints, a process that releases chemotactic factors, degradation enzymes, and other inflammatory substances. Colchicine helps stop this process, probably by disrupting microtubules in leukocytes. Normally, microtubules contribute to cell structure and movement. When colchicine binds to tubulin (protein from which microtubules are made), the microtubule falls apart, as shown. This process disrupts cell function and prevents leukocytes from invading joints and causing inflammation.

Interactions
DRUGS
anticoagulants, such as heparin; platelet aggregation inhibitors, such as aspirin; thrombolytics, such as alteplase: Increased risk of GI ulcers or hemorrhage
antineoplastics: Possibly increased serum uric acid level and decreased therapeutic effectiveness of colchicine
cyclosporine: Increased cyclosporine level
moderate CYP3A4 inhibitors, such as amprenavir, aprepitant, diltiazem, erythromycin, fluconazole, fosamprenavir, grapefruit juice, verapamil: Increased risk of colchicine toxicity
NSAIDs, such as phenylbutazone: Possibly increased risk of bone marrow depression, GI bleeding, leukopenia, thrombo-cytopenia
strong CYP3A4 inhibitors, such as atazanavir, clarithromycin, indinavir, itraconazole, ketoconazole, nefazodone, nelfinavir, ritonavir, saquinavir, telithromycin: Increased risk of colchicine toxicity
P-gp inhibitors, such as cyclosporine, ranolazine: Increased risk of colchicine toxicity
vitamin B_{12} : Possibly impaired absorption of and increased dosage requirements for vitamin B_{12}

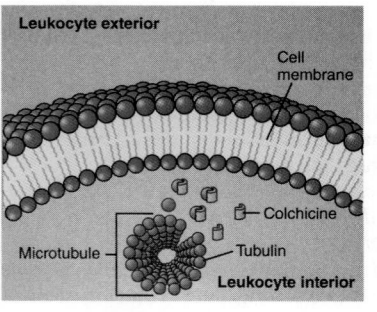

Leukocyte exterior
Cell membrane
Colchicine
Microtubule
Tubulin
Leukocyte interior

ACTIVITIES
alcohol use: Increased risk of adverse GI effects

Adverse Reactions
CNS: Peripheral neuropathy
GI: Abdominal pain, anorexia, diarrhea, nausea, vomiting
HEME: Agranulocytosis, aplastic anemia, thrombocytopenia
MS: Myopathy
SKIN: Alopecia, rash

Nursing Considerations
• Patients receiving prophylactic treatment for gout and who have hepatic impairment or are being treated with CYP3A4 inhibitors shouldn't receive colchicine for acute gout flares.
• Know that elderly or debilitated patients and those with a history of cardiac disease or impaired renal or hepatic function are at increased risk for cumulative toxicity.
• Expect to monitor CBC and platelet and reticulocyte counts at baseline and every 3 months after therapy starts.
• Notify prescriber immediately and expect to stop colchicine if patient develops evidence of toxicity, such as abdominal pain, diarrhea, nausea, or vomiting.

PATIENT TEACHING
• Instruct patient to have blood tests every 3 months, as ordered, during therapy.
• Explain that gouty arthritis pain and swelling typically subside in 24 to 48 hours after therapy begins.
• Advise patient to notify prescriber immediately if abdominal pain, diarrhea, nausea, or vomiting occurs.
• Tell patient to inform all prescribers of colchicine therapy, especially if patient has kidney or liver dysfunction because of potential drug interactions.

colesevelam hydrochloride
Welchol

Class and Category
Chemical class: Nonabsorbed hydrogel polymer

Therapeutic class: Bile acid sequestrant
Pregnancy category: B

Indications and Dosages
➤ *As adjunct to diet and exercise to improve glycemic control in type 2 diabetes mellitus*
ORAL SUSPENSION, TABLETS
Adults. 3.75 g once daily or 1.875 g twice daily with a meal and a beverage.
➤ *As adjunct to diet and exercise to reduce elevated LDL cholesterol levels in patients with primary hypercholesterolemia*
ORAL SUSPENSION, TABLETS
Adults and children age 10 to 17: 3.75 g once daily or 1.875 g twice daily with a meal and a beverage.

Mechanism of Action
Binds with bile acids in intestine, preventing their absorption and forming an insoluble complex that's excreted in feces. This action decreases amount of bile acids returning through enterohepatic circulation to the liver. As a result, the liver must convert more cholesterol to bile acids, which increases liver's demand for cholesterol. This, in turn, causes increase in production and activity of the hepatic enzyme hydroxymethyl-glutaryl-coenzyme A (HMG-CoA) reductase, which is needed for cholesterol production. However, synthesis of cholesterol in the liver typically can't match the amount needed to synthesize bile acids. Because cholesterol levels can't be sustained, LDLs, lipoproteins composed mostly of cholesterol, are increasingly removed from the blood, thereby decreasing the LDL level in the blood.

Contraindications
History of bowel obstruction or pancreatitis induced by hypertriglyceridemia, hypersensitivity to colesevelam or its components, serum triglyceride level greater than 500 mg/dl

Interactions
DRUGS
cyclosporine, drugs with narrow therapeutic index, glimepiride, glipizide, glyburide, olmesartan, oral contraceptives containing ethinyl estradiol and norethindrone, thyroid hormone replacement: Possibly altered effectiveness of these drugs

metformin E.R.: Increased blood metformin level, increasing risk of hypoglycemia
phenytoin: Decreased plasma phenytoin levels increasing risk of seizures
warfarin: Reduced INR, increasing risk of clotting

Adverse Reactions
CNS: Asthenia
CV: Hypertension, hypertriglyceridemia
EENT: Oral blistering, pharyngitis, rhinitis
ENDO: Hypoglycemia, hypertriglyceridemia
GI: Abdominal distention or pain, bowel or esophageal obstruction, constipation, dyspepsia, dysphagia, elevated liver enzymes, fecal impaction, indigestion, nausea, pancreatitis, worsening of hemorrhoids
MS: Myalgia
SKIN: Rash
Other: Flu syndrome

Nursing Considerations
• Colesevelam shouldn't be given to patients with gastroparesis or other GI motility disorders or to patients who had major GI tract surgery and are at risk for bowel obstruction from constipating effects.
• Use cautiously in patients with dysphagia or esophageal obstruction because size of tablet can cause dysphagia or esophageal obstruction.
• Use colesevelam cautiously in patients whose total triglycerides exceed 300 mg/dl; bile acid sequestrants can increase it.
• Evaluate patient's lipid levels before starting therapy for primary hyperlipidemia, again in 4 to 6 weeks, and then periodically, as ordered, during therapy. Expect drug to be discontinued if patient develops hypertriglyceridemia-induced pancreatitis or triglyceride level exceeds 500 mg/dl.
• Monitor diabetic patient's blood glucose level regularly, as ordered, to assess effectiveness of colesevelam therapy.
• Mix one packet of oral suspension with 4 to 8 ounces of water, fruit juice, or diet soft drinks. Stir well and have patient drink immediately.

• When giving colesevelam with a drug that has a narrow therapeutic index, expect to give that drug at least 4 hours before colesevelam to prevent reduced effectiveness.
• Because colesevelam may decrease or delay absorption of other drugs, administer it separately if possible.
• Make sure that patient drinks enough fluid when taking drug.
WARNING Monitor patients with preexisting constipation, who are at increased risk for developing fecal impaction.
• Monitor frequency of bowel movements and consistency of stools in patients with coronary artery disease or hemorrhoids because constipation may aggravate these conditions.
PATIENT TEACHING
• Instruct patient to take drug with meals and drink plenty of liquids when taking it.
• Tell patient to protect tablets from moisture.
WARNING Alert patient or caregiver prescribed oral suspension form that it contains phenylatanine and should not be taken by anyone who has a PKU diagnosis. If PKU is present, instruct patient not to take oral suspension and notify prescriber to get a different form of the drug.
• Instruct patient prescribed the oral suspension form to mix 1 packet with 4 to 8 ounces of water, fruit juice, or diet soft drinks; stir well; and then drink immediately. Caution patient never to ingest the contents of the packet dry.
• Caution patient against changing prescribed dosage or stopping colesevelam abruptly because serum lipid level may increase significantly.
• Remind patient that drug therapy doesn't reduce the need for dietary changes.
• Urge patient to keep regularly scheduled appointments for follow-up blood tests.
• Instruct patient to take vitamin supplements at least 4 hours before colesevelam.

colestipol hydrochloride
Colestid

Class and Category
Chemical class: Diethylenetriamine and 1-chloro-2,3-epoxypropane copolymer, high-molecular-weight anion exchange resin
Therapeutic class: Antihyperlipidemic
Pregnancy category: Not rated

Indications and Dosages
➤ *To treat primary hypercholesterolemia*
GRANULES
Adults. 15 to 30 g daily in divided doses twice daily to four times daily, before meals and at bedtime.
TABLETS
Adults.
Initial: 2 g once daily or in divided doses twice daily, increased every 1 to 2 mo in 2-g increments once or twice daily. *Maximum:* 16 g daily.

Mechanism of Action
Combines with bile acids in the intestine, preventing their absorption and forming an insoluble complex that's excreted in feces. Loss of bile acids increases hepatic production of cholesterol to form new bile acids and increases oxidation of cholesterol to bile acids. Depletion of cholesterol increases hepatic LDL receptor activity, which removes LDLs from the blood.

Contraindications
Complete biliary obstruction, hypersensitivity to colestipol or its components

Interactions
DRUGS
chenodiol, ursodiol: Possibly reduced therapeutic effects of colestipol
digitalis glycosides: Possibly increased risk of digitalis toxicity when colestipol is stopped
furosemide, sulfonylureas, thyroid hormones: Decreased absorption and therapeutic effects of these drugs
mycophenolic acid: Possibly reduced effectiveness of mycophenolic acid
oral anticoagulants: Possibly increased or decreased anticoagulant effect
penicillin G, propranolol, tetracyclines (oral), thiazide diuretics: Decreased absorption of these drugs
vancomycin (oral): Possibly marked decrease in vancomycin antibacterial action

vitamins (fat-soluble): Possibly interference with vitamin absorption

Adverse Reactions
CNS: Headache
GI: Abdominal distention and pain, constipation, diarrhea, eructation, esophageal reaction, fecal impaction, heartburn, nausea, vomiting

Nursing Considerations
• Mix colestipol granules with at least 90 ml of fluid before giving it to prevent accidental inhalation or esophageal distress.
• Because colestipol may interact with various drugs, give it on a separate schedule from other drugs when possible.
• Make sure patient has adequate fluid intake, and obtain an order for a stool softener or laxative to prevent constipation. To prevent impaction, expect to decrease dosage or discontinue drug if constipation occurs or worsens.
• Expect to discontinue drug if no response occurs after 3 months.
• Monitor patient's serum cholesterol level as appropriate, usually at baseline, 4 to 6 weeks after starting therapy, and then every 3 months. Expect to reduce monitoring frequency to every 4 months if response is adequate.
• Be aware that HDL and serum triglyceride levels may increase or remain unchanged during colestipol therapy.
• Keep in mind that adverse GI reactions are more common in patients over age 60.
PATIENT TEACHING
• To help minimize adverse GI reactions, advise patient to mix granules thoroughly in fluid so they're completely wet before drinking.
• Remind patient that colestipol doesn't reduce the importance of dietary changes.
• Caution patient not to increase or decrease prescribed dosage or to stop taking drug suddenly. Explain that stopping drug abruptly may significantly increase serum lipid levels.
• Instruct patient to keep appointments for follow-up blood tests.

• Teach patient how to prevent constipation, and advise him to contact prescriber if constipation occurs or worsens.

colistimethate sodium

Coly-Mycin M

Class and Category

Chemical class: Polypeptide
Therapeutic class: Antibiotic
Pregnancy category: C

Indications and Dosages

➤ *To treat acute or chronic gram-negative infections caused by* Enterobacter aerogenes, Escherichia coli, Klebsiella pneumoniae, *and* Pseudomonas aeruginosa

I.M. INJECTION, I.V. INJECTION, I.V. INFUSION
Adults. 2.5 to 5 mg/kg daily in 2 to 4 divided doses. *Maximum:* 5 mg/kg/day.
DOSAGE ADJUSTMENT For obese patients, dosage should be based on ideal body weight. For patients with severe renal impairment, dosage reduced to 1.5 mg/kg daily and interval reduced to every 36 hr. For patients with moderate renal impairment, interval shouldn't exceed twice daily and may need to be once daily or every 36 hr. For patients with mild renal impairment, interval shouldn't exceed twice daily.

Mechanism of Action

Penetrates into and disrupts bacterial cell membrane, resulting in cell death. Colistimethate is an inactive prodrug of the bioactive form colistin. Colistin binds to gram-negative bacterial cell membrane phospholipids, increasing cell membrane permeability and causing loss of metabolites essential to bacterial existence.

Contraindications

Hypersensitivity to colistimethate or its components, renal disease

Interactions

DRUGS
aminoglycosides, vancomycin: Increased risk of developing nephrotoxicity

curaniform muscle relaxants, such as tubocurarine, decamethonium, ether, gallamine, succinylcholine: Potentiated neuromuscular blocking effect of these drugs
sodium cephalothin: Possibly enhanced nephrotoxicity

Adverse Reactions

CNS: Dizziness, fever, paresthesia, slurred speech, tingling of extremities, vertigo
GI: Nausea, pseudomembranous colitis, vomiting
GU: Decreased creatinine clearance and urine output, increased BUN and serum creatinine, nephrotoxicity
MS: Muscle weakness
RESP: Apnea, respiratory distress
SKIN: Pruritus, rash, urticaria

Nursing Considerations

• Use colistimethate cautiously in patients with impaired renal function.
• Reconstitute each 150-mg vial with 2 ml sterile water for injection to yield 75 mg/ml. During reconstitution, swirl vial gently to avoid frothing.
• When giving by I.V. injection, slowly inject half of total daily dose over 3 to 5 minutes and repeat dose 12 hours later, as ordered.
• When giving by I.V. infusion, slowly inject half of total daily dose over 3 to 5 minutes. Then add remaining half of total daily dose to an appropriate solution, such as normal saline solution or D_5W, with type and amount of solution dictated by patient's fluid and electrolyte needs. Starting 1 to 2 hours after first dose, slowly infuse remaining drug over 22 to 23 hours. If patient has renal impairment, use a reduced infusion rate. Once the infusion is prepared, use within 24 hours.
• Notify prescriber if patient develops neurologic changes (paresthesia, tingling of limbs, pruritus, vertigo, dizziness, slurred speech). Dosage may need to be reduced.
WARNING Monitor patient's BUN and serum creatinine levels, as ordered. If elevated, notify prescriber because drug may cause nephrotoxicity (usually reversible if drug is stopped) with possible renal shutdown.

Toxic levels interfere with nerve transmission at neuromuscular junctions, resulting in apnea and muscle weakness.
• Monitor patient receiving drug I.M. because apnea and neuromuscular blockade may occur with this route, especially in patients with impaired renal function. Before giving drug I.M., make sure dose is appropriate for degree of renal function.
• Monitor patient's bowel elimination. If diarrhea develops, obtain stool culture to check for pseudomembranous colitis. If confirmed, expect to stop drug and give fluid, electrolytes, and antibiotics effective against *Clostridium difficile.*

PATIENT TEACHING
• Caution patient to avoid performing hazardous activities, including driving, during colistimethate therapy.
• Tell patient to immediately report tingling in her extremities, vertigo, dizziness, generalized pruritus, or slurred speech because dosage may need to be decreased.
• Explain need for frequent blood tests during therapy to check kidney function.
• Urge patient to tell prescriber about diarrhea that's severe or lasts longer than 3 days. Remind patient that watery or bloody stools can occur 2 or more months after antibiotic therapy and can be serious, requiring prompt treatment.

conivaptan hydrochloride

Vaprisol

Class and Category
Chemical class: Arginine vasopressin antagonist (antidiuretic hormone)
Therapeutic class: Aquaretic (sodium/water stabilizer)
Pregnancy category: C

Indications and Dosages
➤ *To treat euvolemic and hypervolemic hyponatremia in hospitalized patients such as may occur in the syndrome of inappropriate antidiuretic hormone, hypothyroidism, adrenal insufficiency, or pulmonary disorders*

I.V. INFUSION
Adults. *Loading dose:* 20 mg over 30 minutes followed by 20 mg as a continuous infusion over 24 hours. Additional 20 mg daily may be given by continuous infusion for 1 to 3 days, as needed. *Maximum:* 40 mg daily with total duration of therapy, including loading dose, not to exceed 4 days.
DOSAGE ADJUSTMENT For patient with moderate hepatic impairment, loading dose decreased to 10 mg over 30 minutes followed by a decrease in daily dose to 10 mg per day as a continuous infusion for 2 to 4 days. If serum sodium level does not rise, dosage may be titrated up to 20 mg per day.

Route	Onset	Peak	Duration
I.V.	Unknown	24 hr	Unknown

Mechanism of Action
Binds with arginine vasopressin V2 receptor sites in collecting ducts of kidneys. By doing so, drug blocks action of arginine vasopressin on V2 receptor, decreases water resorption in collecting ducts, increases excretion of free water (urine output), and increases serum sodium concentration, thus correcting water and sodium imbalance.

Incompatibilities
Don't mix with lactated Ringer's solution, normal saline solution, or other drugs.

Contraindications
Anuria; hypersensitivity to conivaptan or its components or to corn or corn products; patients with hypovolemic hyponatremia; use with potent CYP3A4 inhibitors such as clarithromycin, indinavir, itraconazole, ketoconazole, and ritonavir

Interactions
DRUGS
amphotericin B, cisplatin, corticosteroids: Possibly additive hypokalemic effects
clarithromycin, indinavir, itraconazole, ketoconazole, ritonavir, and other strong CYP3A inhibitors: Increased blood conivaptan level
digoxin: Possibly increased digoxin level and risk of digoxin toxicity
drugs metabolized by CYP3A, such as HMG-CoA reductase inhibitors: Possibly increased risk of rhabdomyolysis

warfarin: Possibly increased blood warfarin level

Adverse Reactions
CNS: Confusion, fever, headache, insomnia
CV: Atrial fibrillation, hypertension, hypotension, orthostatic hypotension, peripheral edema
EENT: Dry mouth, oral candidiasis, pharyngeal pain
ENDO: Hyperglycemia, hypoglycemia
GI: Constipation, diarrhea, nausea, thirst, vomiting
GU: Hematuria, pollakiuria, polyuria, UTI
HEME: Anemia
RESP: Pneumonia
SKIN: Erythema, pruritus
Other: Dehydration, hypokalemia, hypomagnesemia, hyponatremia, infusion-site reactions (erythema, pain, phlebitis, swelling)

Nursing Considerations
• Conivaptan shouldn't be used to treat patients with heart failure nor is it recommended in patients with severe renal impairment because of a high incidence of infusion-site phlebitis, which can reduce potential vascular access sites.
• Use cautiously in patients with hepatic or mild to moderate renal dysfunction because levels remain elevated longer in these patients.
• Give drug only through large veins, and change infusion site every 24 hours. Drug may cause serious infusion-site reactions even when diluted and infused correctly. Inspect site regularly; change immediately if reactions occur.
• Dilute 20-mg (4-ml) loading dose with 100 ml of 5% dextrose injection before administration. Gently invert bag several times to mix thoroughly. Use mixture within 24 hours, infusing over 30 minutes.
• Dilute 20-mg (4-ml) or 40-mg (8-ml) continuous infusion dose with 250 ml of D$_5$W before use. Gently invert the bag several times to mix thoroughly. Infuse immediately over 24 hours. If infusion is interrupted for any reason, discard any remaining solution 24 hours after mixing.
• Monitor neurologic status and serum sodium level closely during therapy because rapid increase in serum sodium level (more than 12 mEq/L/24 hr) may result in serious

neurologic impairment. If serum sodium level rises faster than expected, stop infusion temporarily and notify prescriber. If it keeps rising, expect conivaptan to be discontinued. If hyponatremia persists or recurs and patient has no neurologic abnormalities, drug may be resumed at a reduced rate.
• Monitor vital signs, and assess patient regularly for hypovolemia. If patient develops hypovolemia or hypotension while receiving conivaptan, stop infusion, notify prescriber, and provide supportive care, as prescribed. After hypovolemia and hypotension have been corrected, drug may be resumed at a reduced rate.
• Store ampules in cardboard container, protected from light, until ready for use.
PATIENT TEACHING
• Instruct patient to report any infusion-site discomfort immediately.
• Tell patient that frequent laboratory tests will be performed to monitor his serum sodium level and volume status.

cortisone acetate

Cortisone Acetate-ICN (CAN), Cortone (CAN), Cortone Acetate

Class and Category
Chemical class: Glucocorticoid
Therapeutic class: Anti-inflammatory, corticosteroid replacement, immunosuppressant
Pregnancy category: Not rated

Indications and Dosages
➤ *To treat allergic and inflammatory disorders, collagen disorders, congenital adrenal hyperplasia, dermatologic disorders, edema (from systemic lupus erythematosus or nephrotic syndrome), GI disorders, hematologic disorders, multiple sclerosis (acute exacerbations), neoplastic diseases, primary or secondary adrenocortical insufficiency, respiratory disorders, rheumatic disorders, trichinosis with myocardial or neurologic involvement, and tuberculous meningitis*

TABLETS
Adults and adolescents. *Initial:* 25 to 300 mg before 9 a.m. daily. *Maintenance:* Dosage adjusted based on patient response. **Children.** 2.5 to 10 mg/kg daily before 9 a.m. For adrenocortical insufficiency, 0.7 mg/kg/day before 9 a.m.

I.M. INJECTION
Adults and adolescents. *Initial:* 25 to 300 mg daily. *Maintenance:* Dosage adjusted based on patient response. **Children.** 0.83 to 5 mg/kg every 12 to 24 hr. For adrenocortical insufficiency, 0.7 mg/kg daily or every third day, or 0.23 to 0.35 mg/kg daily.

Route	Onset	Peak	Duration
P.O.	Rapid	2 hr	1.25–1.5 days
I.M.	Slow	20–48 hr	1.25–1.5 days

Mechanism of Action
Binds to intracellular glucocorticoid receptors and suppresses inflammatory and immune responses by:
• inhibiting neutrophil and monocyte accumulation at the inflammation site and suppressing their phagocytic and bactericidal activity
• stabilizing lysosomal membranes
• suppressing the antigen response of macrophages and helper T cells
• inhibiting synthesis of cellular mediators of inflammatory response, such as cytokines, interleukins, and prostaglandins.

Contraindications
Hypersensitivity to cortisone or its components, idiopathic thrombocytopenic purpura (parenteral form), live-virus vaccine administration, systemic fungal infection

Interactions
DRUGS
anticholinesterases: Possibly antagonized anticholinesterase effects in myasthenia gravis
barbiturates: Decreased cortisone effectiveness, increased cortisol clearance
digitalis glycosides: Possibly digitalis toxicity
estrogens, oral contraceptives: Increased cortisone effects and risk of toxicity
hydantoins, rifampin: Increased metabolism and decreased effects of cortisone

isoniazid: Decreased blood isoniazid level
neuromuscular blockers: Possibly enhanced blockade of neuromuscular blockers, leading to increased or prolonged respiratory depression or apnea
oral anticoagulants: Possibly obstructed anticoagulant effects
potassium-wasting diuretics: Possibly hypokalemia
salicylates: Decreased effectiveness and blood level of salicylates
somatrem: Decreased growth-promoting effect

Adverse Reactions
CNS: Ataxia, behavior changes, depression, dizziness, euphoria, fatigue, headache, increased ICP with papilledema, insomnia, lassitude, malaise, mood swings, paresthesia, seizures, steroid psychosis, syncope, vertigo
CV: Arrhythmias (from hypokalemia), fat embolism, heart failure, hypertension, hypotension, thromboembolism, thrombophlebitis
EENT: Exophthalmos, glaucoma, increased intraocular pressure, nystagmus, posterior subcapsular cataracts
ENDO: Adrenal insufficiency during stress, Cushing's syndrome, diabetes mellitus, growth suppression in children, hyperglycemia, negative nitrogen balance from protein catabolism
GI: Abdominal distention, hiccups, increased appetite, nausea, pancreatitis, peptic ulcer, ulcerative esophagitis, vomiting
GU: Glycosuria, menstrual irregularities, perineal burning or tingling
HEME: Leukocytosis
MS: Arthralgia; aseptic necrosis of femoral and humeral heads; compression fractures; muscle atrophy, weakness, and twitching; myalgia; osteoporosis; spontaneous fractures; steroid myopathy; tendon rupture
SKIN: Acne; diaphoresis; ecchymosis; erythema; hirsutism; hyperpigmentation; hypopigmentation; necrotizing vasculitis; petechiae; purpura; rash; scarring; sterile abscesses; striae; subcutaneous fat atrophy; thin, fragile skin; urticaria
Other: Anaphylaxis, hypocalcemia, hypokalemia, hypokalemic alkalosis, impaired wound healing, masking of infection,

metabolic alkalosis, suppressed skin test reaction, weight gain

Nursing Considerations

- Use cortisone cautiously in patients with ocular herpes simplex because corneal perforation may occur.
- Expect prescriber to order baseline ophthalmologic examination before therapy starts because prolonged use of cortisone may result in glaucoma, increased intraocular pressure, and damage to optic nerve.
- Assess patient for signs and symptoms of infection before giving cortisone because drug may mask them. Be aware that new infections may develop during therapy because of risk of immunosuppression. If a new infection develops, expect to administer appropriate antibiotics.
- Obtain serum electrolyte levels before therapy, as ordered, and monitor results often during therapy to detect electrolyte imbalances. Increased calcium excretion, potassium depletion, and sodium and water retention may occur with large doses of cortisone. Anticipate the need for potassium and calcium supplementation and sodium restriction, if indicated.
- Keep in mind that prescriber will order lowest effective dose.
- To avoid peptic ulcer formation from cortisone, expect patient to receive concurrent antacid or antihistamine therapy.

WARNING Be aware that live-virus vaccines shouldn't be given during cortisone therapy because patient may become immunosuppressed and develop the viral infection.

WARNING Assess for adrenal suppression or insufficiency (fatigue, hypotension, lassitude, nausea, vomiting, and weakness) in patient exposed to stress or receiving prolonged cortisone therapy. Notify prescriber immediately if patient has evidence of this life-threatening adverse reaction.

- Watch for signs and symptoms of steroid psychosis (confusion, delirium, euphoria, insomnia, mood swings, personality changes, severe depression), which may develop 15 to 30 days after starting drug. Be prepared to stop drug if such signs

occur. If stopping isn't possible, expect to administer a psychotropic drug.
- Watch for cushingoid signs, such as acne, buffalo hump, central obesity, ecchymosis, moon face, striae, and weight gain. Notify prescriber at once if they occur.
- Expect to taper oral cortisone dosage slowly to prevent withdrawal syndrome (abdominal or back pain, anorexia, dizziness, fever, headache, and syncope).

PATIENT TEACHING
- Instruct patient to take oral cortisone exactly as prescribed, every morning before 9 a.m. Advise him to take it with food if GI distress occurs.
- Caution patient not to stop drug abruptly because doing so may lead to adrenal insufficiency, withdrawal symptoms, or both.
- Inform patient about adrenal insufficiency and need for possible dosage increases during stress. Advise him to notify prescriber immediately if signs or symptoms develop or if he's exposed to stress.
- Caution patient to avoid exposure to people with infections because cortisone can cause immunosuppression. Also, teach him to recognize and immediately report signs and symptoms of infection.
- Teach patient to recognize and report adverse reactions, including Cushing's syndrome.
- Urge patient receiving long-term cortisone therapy to carry medical identification.
- Recommend regular eye examinations.
- Urge patient to keep follow-up appointments with prescriber, which may include laboratory tests, to evaluate effects of therapy.

crofelemer
Fulyza

Class and Category
Chemical class: Oligomeric proanthocyanidin mixture
Therapeutic class: Anti-diarrheal
Pregnancy category: C

Indications and Dosages
➤ *To provide symptomatic relief of non-infectious diarrhea in patients with HIV/AIDS on anti-retroviral therapy*

E.R. TABLETS
Adults.125 mg twice daily.

Mechanism of Action
Inhibits both the cyclic adenosine monophosphate (cAMP)-stimulated cystic fibrosis transmembrane conductance regulator (CFTR) chloride ion channel, and the calcium-activated chloride channel (CaCC) at the luminal membrane of enterocytes. By blocking chloride secretion and accompanying high-volume water loss in diarrhea, the flow of chloride and water in the GI tract becomes normalized.

Contraindications
Hypersensitivity to crofelemer or its components

Adverse Reactions
CNS: Anxiety, depression, dizziness
EENT: Dry mouth, nasopharyngitis, sinusitis
GI: Abdominal distention or pain, constipation, dyspepsia, elevated bilirubin or liver enzymes, flatulence, gastroenteritis, giardiasis (intestinal parasitic infection), nausea
GU: Frequent daytime urination syndrome, nephrolithiasis, UTI
HEME: Decreased white blood cell count
MS: Arthralgia: back, extremity, or musculoskeletal pain
RESP: Bronchitis, cough, upper respiratory infection
SKIN: Acne, dermatitis
Other: Herpes zoster

Nursing Considerations
• Be aware that crofelemer is used only to treat non-infectious diarrhea in patients with HIV/AIDS on anti-retroviral. Infectious etiologies should be ruled out before drug is started because crofelemer is not effective against infectious causes of diarrhea.
• Know that no dosage adjustment is needed related to the patient's CD4 cell count and HIV viral load.
PATIENT TEACHING
• Instruct patient to swallow tablet whole, avoiding crushing or chewing tablet.
• Inform patient that crofelemer may be taken with or without food.

• Advise patient to inform prescriber if no improvement in diarrhea is noted.

cromolyn sodium
(disodium cromoglycate, sodium cromoglycate)
Apo-Cromolyn (CAN), Gastrocrom, Intal Syncroner (CAN), Nalcrom (CAN), Nasalcrom, Novo-cromolyn (CAN)

Class and Category
Chemical class: Disodium chromoglycate
Therapeutic class: Antiasthmatic, anti-inflammatory
Pregnancy category: B

Indications and Dosages
➤ *To prevent bronchial asthma attacks*
AEROSOL (METERED-DOSE INHALER)
Adults and children over age 5. 2 metered sprays (1.6 to 2 mg) every 4 to 6 hr. *Maximum:* 16 sprays (12.8 to 16 mg) daily.
CAPSULES FOR INHALATION
Adults and children over age 2. 1 capsule (20 mg) every 4 to 6 hr. *Maximum:* 8 capsules (160 mg) daily.
SOLUTION FOR NEBULIZATION
Adults and children over age 2. 20 mg every 4 to 6 hr. *Maximum:* 160 mg daily.
➤ *To prevent bronchospasm caused by environmental exposure or exercise*
AEROSOL (METERED-DOSE INHALER)
Adults and children over age 5. 2 metered sprays (1.6 to 2 mg) as a single dose at least 10 to 15 min (no longer than 1 hr) before exposure or exercise. *Maximum:* 16 sprays (12.8 to 16 mg) daily.
CAPSULES FOR INHALATION
Adults and children over age 2. 1 capsule (20 mg) as single dose inhaled at least10 to 15 min (no longer than 1 hr) before exposure or exercise. *Maximum:* 8 capsules (160 mg) daily.
SOLUTION FOR NEBULIZATION
Adults and children over age 2. *Initial:* 20 mg inhaled 10 to 15 min (no longer than 1 hr) before exposure or exercise. Repeated as needed during prolonged exercise. *Maximum:* 160 mg daily.
➤ *To treat allergic rhinitis*

C

Mechanism of Action
In asthma, inflammation results when antigen reexposure causes mast cells todegranulate and release histamine and chemical mediators. Cromolyn helps reduce inflammation by preventing degranulation. After exposure to an antigen, mast cells become sensitized to it and immunoglobulin E (IgE) antibodies appear on their surfaces. When the antigen returns, it attaches to IgE (1 in the illustration) and triggers events that lead to degranulation (2). By preventing granules from opening on the cells' surfaces (3), cromolyn blocks release of histamine and chemical mediators.

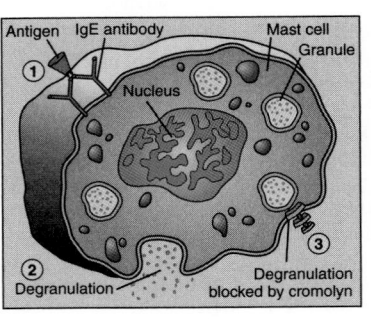

NASAL SOLUTION
Adults and children over age 2. 1 spray (5.2 mg) in each nostril at regular intervals three times daily or four times daily. *Maximum:* 1 spray (5.2 mg) in each nostril 6 times daily.
➤ *To prevent systemic mastocytosis*
CAPSULES, ORAL CONCENTRATE
Adults and adolescents. 200 mg four times daily, 30 min before meals and at bedtime.
Children ages 2 to 12. 100 mg four times daily, 30 min before meals and at bedtime. *Maximum:* 40 mg/kg/day.
Children under age 2. 5 mg/kg four times daily. *Maximum:* 40 mg/kg daily.

Contraindications
Arrhythmias, coronary artery disease (aerosol); hypersensitivity to cromolyn or its components, status asthmaticus (all forms); nasal polyps (nasal solution)

Route	Onset	Peak	Duration
Aerosol	Minutes	Unknown	Up to 2 hr
Nasal solution	1 wk	1–4 wk	Unknown
Nebulizer solution	Minutes	Unknown	3–6 hr

Adverse Reactions
CNS: Dizziness, headache, neuritis
EENT: Burning eyes, hoarseness, laryngeal edema, nasal congestion, and swollen parotid glands (all forms); increased sneezing, nasal stinging, and throat irritation (nasal solution); taste perversion (aerosol)
GI: Anorexia, diarrhea (capsules and oral concentrate), nausea, vomiting
GU: Dysuria, urinary frequency
MS: Arthralgia, joint swelling
RESP: Cough, wheezing
SKIN: Rash, urticaria

Nursing Considerations
WARNING Be aware that cromolyn sodium shouldn't be used to relieve acute asthma attack or severe bronchospasm; it should be used only for prevention.
• Don't give cromolyn sodium through handheld nebulizer. Instead, administer via power-operated nebulizer with a face mask or mouthpiece.
• Evaluate patient for effective inhalation; patient must be able to inhale adequately for nebulizer solution to be effective.
• Thoroughly mix oral concentrate or capsule contents into half a glass of hot water (not fruit juice, milk, or food), and let cool before administering.
• Give drug at regular intervals to maximize effectiveness.
PATIENT TEACHING
• Teach patient how to use power-operated nebulizer; warn against using handheld nebulizer.
• Advise patient to use cromolyn sodium 10 to 15 minutes before exercising or exposure to other precipitating factors.

• Instruct patient to thoroughly mix oral concentrate with hot water (not fruit juice, milk, or food) and let it cool before drinking.
• Inform patient that nasal spray may cause minor nasal irritation.
• Explain that cromolyn sodium may take up to 1 month to reach full therapeutic effects.

crotamiton

Eurax

Class and Category
Chemical class: Synthetic chloroformate salt
Therapeutic class: Antipruritic, scabicide
Pregnancy category: C

Indications and Dosages
➤ *To treat scabies*
CREAM, LOTION
Adults. 30 to 60 g (thin layer) massaged into skin from chin down and repeated in 24 hr. Applied as needed to skin folds, creases, and areas of intense pruritus for up to 48 hr.
➤ *To relieve pruritus caused by scabies*
CREAM, LOTION
Adults. 30 to 60 g (thin layer) massaged gently into affected areas until drug is completely absorbed. Repeated as needed.

Mechanism of Action
Exerts a toxic effect on *Sarcoptes scabiei* by an unknown mechanism.

Contraindications
Abrasions, application to mucous membranes, breaks in skin, hypersensitivity to crotamiton or its components, inflammation

Adverse Reactions
SKIN: Contact dermatitis, irritation, pruritus, rash

Nursing Considerations
• Expect pruritus to continue for 4 to 6 weeks after treatment.
PATIENT TEACHING
• Advise patient to shake lotion bottle well before applying.
• Warn him to keep drug away from eyes, nose, mouth, and inflamed skin.

• Advise patient to use a topical corticosteroid for dermatitis and an antihistamine for pruritus, as prescribed.
• Instruct patient to change clothing and bed linens the morning after final application and to take a cleansing bath 48 hours after final application.
• Inform patient that pruritus may continue for 4 to 6 weeks after treatment.
• Advise patient to notify prescriber if skin irritation or rash occurs.

cyclizine hydrochloride

Marezine

cyclizine lactate

Marzine (CAN)

Class and Category
Chemical class: Piperazine derivative
Therapeutic class: Anticholinergic, antiemetic
Pregnancy category: B

Indications and Dosages
➤ *To prevent postoperative vomiting*
I.M. INJECTION
Adults and adolescents. 50 mg 15 to 30 min before surgery ends; then every 4 to 6 hr, as needed, for first few postoperative days.
Children ages 6 to 12. 25 mg 15 to 30 min before surgery ends; then three times daily, as needed, for first few postoperative days.
Children up to age 6. 12.5 mg 15 to 30 min before surgery ends; then three times daily, as needed, for first few postoperative days.
➤ *To prevent and treat motion sickness*
TABLETS
Adults and adolescents. 50 mg 30 min before travel; then every 4 to 6 hr, as needed. *Maximum:* 200 mg daily.
Children ages 6 to 12. 25 mg 30 min before travel; then every 6 to 8 hr, as needed. *Maximum:* 75 mg daily.
I.M. INJECTION
Adults and adolescents. 50 mg every 4 to 6 hr, as needed.
Children. 1 mg/kg three times daily, as needed.

Route	Onset	Peak	Duration
P.O., I.M.	30–60 min	Unknown	4–6 hr

Mechanism of Action

May act centrally on the vomiting center by blocking chemoreceptor trigger zones. Cyclizine also may reduce the sensitivity of the labyrinthine apparatus in the inner ear.

Contraindications

Hypersensitivity to cyclizine or its components, shock

Interactions

DRUGS

anticholinergics: Possibly potentiated anticholinergic effects
apomorphine: Possibly decreased emetic response of apomorphine
CNS depressants: Possibly potentiated CNS depression

ACTIVITIES

alcohol use: Possibly potentiated CNS depression

Adverse Reactions

CNS: Dizziness, drowsiness, euphoria, excitation, hallucinations, insomnia, nervousness, restlessness, seizures (in children), vertigo
CV: Hypotension, palpitations, tachycardia
EENT: Blurred vision; diplopia; dry mouth, nose, and throat; tinnitus
GI: Anorexia, constipation, diarrhea, nausea, vomiting
GU: Urinary frequency and hesitancy, urine retention
SKIN: Jaundice, rash, urticaria

Nursing Considerations

• Help patient with ambulation, and take safety precautions to prevent injury from falls if drowsiness or dizziness occurs.
• Don't schedule allergen skin tests until at least 5 days after stopping cyclizine; drug may interfere with test results.

PATIENT TEACHING

• Urge patient to avoid alcohol and other CNS depressants during cyclizine therapy.
• Advise patient to ask for help with ambulation if he feels drowsy or dizzy.

cyclobenzaprine hydrochloride

Amrix, Flexeril

Class and Category

Chemical class: Tricyclic amine salt
Therapeutic class: Skeletal muscle relaxant
Pregnancy category: B

Indications and Dosages

➤ *As adjunct to rest and physical therapy for relief of muscle spasm associated with acute, painful musculoskeletal conditions*

TABLETS (FLEXERIL)

Adults and adolescents. 5 mg three times daily, increased as needed to 10 mg three times daily. *Maximum:* 30 mg daily for 3 wk.

DOSAGE ADJUSTMENT Dosage frequency reduced in elderly patients and those with hepatic impairment.

➤ *As adjunct to rest and physical therapy for relief of muscle spasm associated with acute, painful musculoskeletal conditions*

E.R. CAPSULES (AMRIX)

Adults. 15 mg once daily, increased to 30 mg once daily, as needed. *Maximum:* 30 mg once daily for no longer than 3 weeks.

Route	Onset	Peak	Duration
P.O.	1 hr	1–2 wk	12–24 hr

Mechanism of Action

Acts in the brain stem to reduce or abolish tonic muscle hyperactivity. Because cyclobenzaprine doesn't act at the neuromuscular junction or directly on skeletal muscle, it relieves muscle spasm without disrupting muscle function.

Contraindications

Acute recovery phase of MI; age less than 12; arrhythmias, including heart block and other conduction disturbances; heart failure; hypersensitivity to cyclobenzaprine or its components; hyperthyroidism; MAO inhibitor use within 14 days

Interactions

DRUGS

anticholinergics, antidyskinetics: Possibly potentiated anticholinergic effects of these drugs

bupropion, meperidine, MAO inhibitors, selective serotonin reuptake inhibitors (SSRIs), serotonin norepinephrine reuptake inhibitors (SNRIs), tramadol, tricyclic antiepressants: Possibly increased risk of serotonin syndrome

CNS depressants, tricyclic antidepressants: Possibly additive CNS depressant effects of these drugs, increased risk of adverse effects of antidepressants and cyclo-benzaprine

guanadrel, guanethidine: Possibly decreased or blocked antihypertensive effects of these drugs

MAO inhibitors: Possibly hyperpyretic crisis, severe seizures, and death

tricyclic antidepressants: Increased risk of MI or stroke

ACTIVITIES

alcohol use: Possibly additive CNS depression

Adverse Reactions

CNS: Asthenia, confusion, depression, dizziness, drowsiness, fatigue, fever, headache, insomnia, irritability, nervousness, paresthesia, seizures, tremor, weakness
CV: Arrhythmias, including tachycardia; orthostatic hypotension; palpitations; vasodilation
EENT: Blurred vision, diplopia, dry mouth, transient vision loss, unpleasant taste
GI: Constipation, hiccups, indigestion, nausea, vomiting
GU: Libido changes, urinary frequency, urine retention
SKIN: Diaphoresis, facial flushing, pruritus, rash

Nursing Considerations

• Use cyclobenzaprine cautiously in patients with history of low seizure threshold.
• If possible, avoid giving drug to elderly patients because of its anticholinergic effects. Know that extended-release capsules should not be given to the elderly or to patients with any degree of hepatic dysfunction.
WARNING Monitor patient closely if cyclobenzaprine is being given with other serotonergic drug, especially when treatment is started and during dosage increases, because of the potential for life-threatening serotonin syndrome to develop. Assess patient for autonomic instability, mental status changes, and nervous system abnormalities. If present, stop both cyclobenzaprine and other serotonergic drugs immediately and notify prescriber. Provide supportive care, as ordered.
• To prevent falls, take safety precautions if patient is confused, dizzy, or weak.

PATIENT TEACHING

• Urge patient to avoid alcohol and other CNS depressants during therapy.
• Inform patient about possible lack of alertness and dexterity.
• Advise patient to ask for assistance with walking, driving, or hazardous activities if he experiences dizziness or weakness.

cycloserine
Seromycin

Class and Category

Chemical class: D-alanine analogue, *Streptomyces garyphalus* or *Streptomyces orchidaceus* derivative
Therapeutic class: Antitubercular
Pregnancy category: C

Indications and Dosages

➤ *To treat tuberculosis with other antit-uberculotics after failure of primary drugs, including ethambutol, isoniazid, pyrazinamide, rifampin, streptomycin*

CAPSULES

Adults and adolescents. 250 mg every 12 hr for 2 wk; then every 6 to 8 hr for 2 wk. Dosage increased gradually to maintain blood cycloserine level below 30 mcg/ml. *Maximum:* 1 g daily.
Children. 10 to 20 mg/kg daily in divided doses every 12 hr. *Maximum:* 1 g daily.

Mechanism of Action

Inhibits bacterial cell wall synthesis in gram-positive organisms, including *Mycobacterium tuberculosis*. In early stages of bacterial cell wall synthesis, cycloserine inhibits two enzymes that help form peptidoglycan, which is needed to make the cell membrane rigid and protective.

Contraindications
Chronic alcoholism, depression, hypersensitivity to cycloserine or its components, psychosis, renal disease, seizure disorder, severe anxiety

Interactions
DRUGS
ethionamide: Possibly increased risk of seizures
isoniazid: Possibly increased risk of adverse CNS effects
phenytoin: Possibly increased blood phenytoin level
pyridoxine: Possibly anemia or peripheral neuritis
ACTIVITIES
alcohol use: Possibly increased risk of seizures

Adverse Reactions
CNS: Aggression, anxiety, coma, confusion, depression, dizziness, drowsiness, headache, irritability, lethargy, memory loss, nervousness, nightmares, psychosis, restlessness, seizures, suicidal tendencies, tremor, vertigo
CV: Heart failure
HEME: Leukocytosis, megaloblastic anemia
MS: Dysarthria, hyperreflexia
SKIN: Dermatitis, photosensitivity
Other: Folic acid deficiency, vitamin B$_{12}$ deficiency

Nursing Considerations
• Monitor blood cycloserine level, as appropriate. Blood level should be maintained at 25 to 30 mcg/ml.
• Monitor mental status, mood, and affect for aggression or depression.
• Monitor CBC to detect blood dyscrasias.
• To prevent injury from falls, take safety precautions if adverse CNS reactions, such as dizziness or drowsiness, develop.
PATIENT TEACHING
• Urge patient to avoid alcohol while taking cycloserine.
• Instruct patient to seek help immediately if he has suicidal thoughts.
• Advise patient to avoid driving and to ask for assistance with walking or hazardous activities if he develops adverse CNS reactions, such as dizziness and drowsiness.

• Tell patient to contact prescriber if symptoms haven't improved after 2 to 3 weeks.
• Emphasize the importance of complying with drug therapy because effective treatment may take years to complete.

cyclosporine
(cyclosporin A)
Neoral, Sandimmune, SangCya

Class and Category
Chemical class: Tolypocladium inflatum Gams– or Cylindrocarpon lucidum Booth–derived polypeptide
Therapeutic class: Antipsoriatic, antirheumatic, immunosuppressant
Pregnancy category: C

Indications and Dosages
➤ *To prevent or treat organ rejection in kidney, liver, and heart allogenic transplantation*
CAPSULES, MODIFIED CAPSULES, MODIFIED ORAL SOLUTION, ORAL SOLUTION
Adults and children. *Initial:* 12 to 15 mg/kg daily in divided doses every 12 hr starting 4 to 12 hr before surgery and continuing 1 to 2 wk afterward. Then, dosage reduced by 5% every wk to maintenance dose. *Maintenance:* 5 to 10 mg/kg daily in divided doses every 12 hr.
I.V. INFUSION
Adults. 2 to 6 mg/kg daily starting 4 to 12 hr before surgery and continuing afterward until patient can tolerate oral form of drug.
➤ *To treat severe rheumatoid arthritis*
MODIFIED CAPSULES, MODIFIED ORAL SOLUTION
Adults. 2.5 mg/kg daily in divided doses every 12 hr, increased by 0.5 to 0.75 mg/kg daily after 8 wk and again after 12 wk. *Maximum:* 4 mg/kg daily.
➤ *To treat psoriasis*
MODIFIED CAPSULES, MODIFIED ORAL SOLUTION
Adults. *Initial:* 2.5 mg/kg daily in divided doses twice daily, increased by 0.5 mg/kg daily after 4 wk. Then dosage increased every 2 wk, if needed. *Maximum:* 4 mg/kg daily.

Mechanism of Action

Causes immunosuppression by inhibiting the proliferation of T lymphocytes, the production and release of lymphokines, and the release of interleukin-2.

Contraindications

Abnormal renal function, neoplastic diseases, and uncontrolled hypertension in patients with psoriasis or rheumatoid arthritis (modified capsules and oral solution); hypersensitivity to cyclosporine, its components, or polyoxyethylated castor oil (I.V. infusion)

Interactions

DRUGS

ACE inhibitors, angiotensin II receptor antagonists, potassium-sparing diuretics, potassium supplements: Increased risk of hyperkalemia
aliskiren, ambrisentan, bosentan, colchicine, digoxin, daunorubicin, doxorubicin, etoposide, HMG-CoA reductase inhibitors (statins), methotrexate, mitoxantrone, NSAIDs, prednisolone, repaglinide, sirolimus: Increased blood concentrations of these drugs and possible toxicity
allopurinol, amiodarone, azithromycin, bromocriptine, clarithromycin, colchicine, danazol, diltiazem, erythromycin, fluconazole, HIV protease inhibitors, hormonal contraceptives, imatinib, itraconazole, ketoconazole, methyl-prednisolone, metoclopramide, nefazodone, nicardipine, oral contraceptives, quinupristin and dalfopristin, verapamil, voriconazole: Increased cyclosporine level
amphotericin B, azapropazon, cimetidine, ciprofloxacin, colchicine, co-trimoxazole, diclofenac, fibric acid derivatives (bezafibrate, fenofibrate), gentamicin, ketoconazole, melphalan, naproxen, NSAIDs, ranitidine, sulindac, tacrolimus, tobramycin, vancomycin: Increased risk of nephrotoxicity
atorvastatin, fluvastatin, lovastatin, pravastatin, simvastatin: Risk of myotoxicity
bosentan, carbamazepine, nafcillin, octreotide, orlistat, oxcarbazepine, phenobarbital, phenytoin, rifampin, St. John's wort, sulfinpyrazone, terbinafine, ticlopidine: Decreased blood cyclosporine level and therapeutic response

methotrexate: Increased blood methotrexate level and risk of renal dysfunction
methylprednisolone (high dose): Increased risk of seizures
nifedipine: Increased risk of gingival hyperplasia
other immunosuppressants: Possibly excessive immunosuppression
repaglinide: Possibly increased repaglinide level and risk of hypoglycemia
vaccines (killed or live virus): Possibly suppressed immune response and increased adverse effects of vaccine

FOODS

grapefruit, grapefruit juice: Increased risk of nephrotoxicity
potassium-rich foods: Increased risk of hyperkalemia

Adverse Reactions

CNS: Altered level of consciousness, confusion, encephalopathy, headache, intracranial hypertension, lethargy, loss of motor function, migraine, neurotoxicity, paresthesia, progressive multifocal leukoencephalopathy, posterior reversible encephalopathy syndrome (PRES), psychiatric disturbances, seizures, tremor
CV: Chest pain, hypertension, MI
EENT: Gingival hyperplasia, optic disc edema, oral candidiasis, sinusitis, visual impairment including blindness
ENDO: Gynecomastia
GI: Cholestasis, diarrhea, hepatitis, hepatotoxicity, jaundice, liver failure, nausea, pancreatitis, vomiting
GU: Albuminuria, elevated serum creatinine and blood urea nitrogen levels, glomerular capillary thrombosis, hematuria, nephropathy associated with BK virus, nephrotoxicity, proteinuria, renal failure
HEME: Anemia, leukopenia, thrombo-cytopenia
SKIN: Acne, cancer, flushing, hirsutism, pruritus, rash
Other: Anaphylaxis; bacterial, fungal, protozoal, and viral infections including opportunistic infections such as poly-omavirus infections that may become life-threatening; hyperkalemia; hyperuricemia; hypomagnesemia,; lymphoma and other malignancies

C

Nursing Considerations

• Be aware that capsules and oral solution aren't interchangeable with modified capsules and modified oral solution. Modified forms have greater bioavailability. Also know that Neoral is not bioequivalent to Sandimmune and requires close monitoring of blood concentration to avoid the potential of underdosing if a conversion from Neoral to Sandimmune is ordered.

• Prepare I.V. infusion by diluting each milliliter of concentrate in 20 to 100 ml of normal saline solution or D_5W. Use glass containers because of possible leaching of diethylhexyphthalate from polyvinyl chloride bags into cyclosporine solution.

• Administer I.V. infusion over 2 to 6 hr. If needed, drug may be infused over 24 hr.

WARNING Closely monitor patient for anaphylaxis, at least during first 30 minutes of I.V. administration. Make sure emergency equipment and drugs are immediately available.

WARNING Be aware that rapid I.V. infusion may cause acute nephrotoxicity.

• Don't draw blood to measure cyclosporine level through same I.V. tubing used to administer drug, even if line was flushed after administration. Blood level may be falsely elevated.

• Discard diluted solution after 24 hours.

• Be aware that oral and intravenous solutions contains alcohol and shouldn't be administered to patient who drinks heavily or has a history of alcohol dependence. In addition, these forms of cyclosporine should not used in patients in whom alcohol intake should be avoided or minimized, such as pregnant or breastfeeding women, patients with epilepsy or liver disease, and children. Be aware that for an adult weighing 70 kg or 150 pounds, the maximum daily oral dose would deliver about 6% and a daily intravenous dose would deliver about 15% of the amount of alcohol contained in a standard drink.

• Don't add water to oral solution because it will alter drug's effectiveness.

• Avoid giving oral cyclosporine with grapefruit juice, which may raise trough level, increasing risk of nephrotoxicity.

WARNING Monitor patient closely for hypersensitivity reactions, especially at the beginning of cyclosporine therapy and for at least the first 30 minutes following the start of an intravenous dose and then frequently thereafter. Know that while anaphylaxis may rarely occur, anaphylactic reactions have not occurred with the use of soft gelatin capsules or oral solution that did not contain Cremophor EL (polyoxyethylated castor oil). If anaphylaxis occurs, stop drug immediately and be prepared to administer epinephrine and oxygen, as ordered.

• Monitor blood pressure, especially in patients with a history of hypertension, because drug can worsen this condition. Expect to decrease dosage if hypertension develops.

• Monitor liver and renal function tests, as ordered, to detect decreased function. Be aware that it is not unusual for serum creatinine and BUN levels to be elevated during cyclosporine therapy. These elevations warrant investigation but do not always reflect kidney transplant rejection. If not related to rejection, a dosage reduction of cyclosporine often helps to decrease these levels.

• Be aware that an association between the development of interstitial fibrosis and higher cumulative doses or persistently high circulating trough concentrations of cyclosporine, especially during first 6 months post transplant, may increase the risk of chronic nephrotoxicity.

• Although uncommon, cyclosporine may cause neurotoxicity, especially after liver transplantation. Watch for evidence of encephalopathy (impaired consciousness, loss of motor function, psychiatric disturbance, seizures, visual disturbance). Notify prescriber immediately if present, and expect cyclosporine dosage to be decreased or the drug discontinued to increase possibility of a reversible or improvement of encephalopathy. Also monitor patients closely for seizures, especially if they are also receiving high-dose methylprednisolone therapy.

• Be aware that cyclosporine use may result in increased serum cholesterol levels.

• Be aware that St. John's Wort may decrease blood cyclosporine level.

• Store capsules at 77° F (25° C) in prepackaged foil wrap to protect them from light.
• Expect about 50% of patients treated for psoriasis to relapse about 4 months after therapy stops. Know that patients with chronic plaque psoriasis may develop erythrodermic psoriasis or generalized pustular psoriasis when cyclosporine dose is reduced or drug is discontinued.
WARNING Watch for evidence of infection (such as fever, pain, cough, malaise) because patients receiving immuno-suppressants such as cyclosporine are at increased risk for viral, bacterial, fungal, and parasitic infection. Watch for both generalized and localized infections, including worsening of preexisting infections, and be aware that these infections may become life-threatening. Activation of latent viral infections may also occur and include BK virus–associated nephropathy that can lead to decreased renal function and renal graft loss.

PATIENT TEACHING
• Instruct patient to take drug at same time each day and in same relation to type and timing of food intake to help increase compliance and maintain steady blood level.
• Advise patient to mix oral solution in a glass—not plastic—container with room-temperature orange or apple juice to improve flavor. Caution him to avoid grapefruit juice because it alters drug metabolism.
• Instruct patient to use syringe supplied by manufacturer to ensure accurate measure-ment of oral solution dose and to wipe—not rinse—syringe after use to prevent cloudiness.
• Advise patient not to stop taking drug without consulting prescriber.
• Instruct patient to avoid virus vaccines during therapy and people who have received such vaccines. Or, suggest wearing a protective mask when he's around them.
• Caution patient to avoid people who have infections during therapy because cyclosporine causes immunosuppression.
• Advise good dental hygiene because of risk of gingival hyperplasia.
• Advise patient to discard oral solution after it has been opened for 2 months.
• Inform patient with rheumatoid arthritis that drug effects may not appear for 4 to 6 weeks.
• Caution patient to avoid excessive exposure to ultraviolet light.

D

dabigatran etexilate
Pradaxa

Class and Category
Chemical class: Methanesulfonate
Therapeutic class: Direct thrombin inhibitor
Pregnancy category: C

Indications and Dosages
➤ *To reduce the risk of stroke and systemic embolism in patients with nonvalvular atrial fibrillation*
CAPSULES
Adults with creatinine clearance greater than 30 ml/min. 150 mg twice daily.
Adults with creatinine clearance between 15 and 30 ml/min. 75 mg twice daily.
DOSAGE ADJUSTMENT For patient with a creatinine level between 30 and 50 ml/min and taking dronedarone or systemic ketoconazole concomitantly, dosage decreased to 75 mg twice daily.
➤ *To reduce risk of recurrence of deep venous thrombosis or pulmonary embolism; to treat deep venous thrombosis or pulmonary embolism*
Adults with creatinine clearance greater than 30 ml/min. 150 mg twice daily.
DOSAGE ADJUSTMENT For patient with a creatinine clearance less than 50 ml/min, be aware that co-administration with P-gp inhibitors such as dronedarone or ketoconazole should be avoided.

Route	Onset	Peak	Duration
P.O.	Unknown	1 hr (fasting) 2 hr (after high-fat meal)	Unknown

Mechanism of Action
Directly inhibits thrombin from converting fibrinogen into fibrin during the coagulation cascade. Inhibition of this activity prevents the development of a blood clot.

Contraindications
Active pathologic bleeding, hypersensitivity to dabigatran or its components, presence of mechanical prosthetic heart valve

Interactions
DRUGS
dronedarone, ketoconazole: Increased dabigatran exposure
rifampin: Reduced effectiveness of rifampin
warfarin: Increased INR, increasing risk of bleeding

Adverse Reactions
CNS: Intracranial or intraspinal hemorrhage
CV: Intra-articular or pericardial bleeding
EENT: Intraocular bleeding
GI: Diarrhea, dyspepsia, esophageal ulcer, gastritis-like symptoms, gastrointestinal hemorrhage, nausea, retroperitoneal bleeding, upper abdominal pain
HEME: Bleeding (serious), thrombo-cytopenia
MS: Intramuscular bleeding with compartment syndrome
SKIN: Pruritus, rash, urticaria
Other: Anaphylactic reaction or shock, angioedema

Nursing Considerations
• Assess renal function, as ordered, prior to beginning dabigatran therapy because dose is based on the patient's creatinine level. Continue to monitor the patient's serum creatinine level throughout therapy, as ordered, and expect frequency of serum creatinine tests to increase if patient develops a condition that affects renal function because a dosing adjustment may be required. Know that the drug should be discontinued if the patient develops acute renal failure.
• Be aware that patients converting from warfarin to dabigatran therapy should begin dabigatran therapy when their international normalized ratio (INR) is below 2.0.
• Expect patients converting from dabigatran to warfarin therapy to do so based on their creatinine clearance level. For patients who have a creatinine clearance level greater than 50 ml/min, expect warfarin to be started 3 days before dabigatran is discontinued. For patients

who have a creatinine clearance level of 31 ml/min to 50 ml/min, expect warfarin to be started 2 days before dabigatran is discontinued. For patients who have a creatinine clearance level of 15 ml/min to 30 ml/min, expect warfarin to be started 1 day before dabigatran is discontinued. No recommendations are available for patients who have a creatinine clearance level of less than 15 ml/min.

• Be aware that degree of anticoagulation does not need to be assessed by routine laboratory testing with dabigatran use. However, when necessary, expect the prescriber to use aPTT or ECT, and not INR, to assess for anticoagulant activity for the patient receiving dabigatran therapy.

• Know that dabigatran can elevate the patient's INR. Therefore, when patients are transitioned, dabigatran must be stopped for at least 2 days before the most accurate effects of warfarin can be known.

• Begin dabigatran therapy, as ordered, for a patient currently receiving a parenteral anticoagulant, such as heparin, within 2 hours before the next dose of the parenteral drug was to have been administered. If the parenteral anti-coagulant being used is continuous in nature, expect to begin dabigatran therapy upon discontinuation of the continuously administered parenteral anticoagulant.

• Expect to begin treatment with a parenteral anticoagulant, if ordered, 12 hours after the patient's final dabigatran dose if the patient has a creatinine clearance of 30 ml/min or greater, and 24 hours after the patient's final dabigatran dose if the patient's creatinine clearance is less than 30 ml/min.

• Know that dabigatran therapy should be discontinued, if possible, 1 to 2 days before invasive or surgical procedures for patients with a creatinine clearance of 50 ml/min or more, and 3 to 5 days for patients whose creatinine clearance is less than 50 ml/min because of the increased risk for bleeding. Longer times may be required for patients undergoing major surgery, spinal puncture, or placement of a spinal or epidural catheter or port, in whom complete hemostasis is required. If surgery cannot be postponed, monitor

patient closely for bleeding and assess bleeding risk with the ecarin clotting time (ECT). If an ECT measurement is not possible, know that the activated partial thromboplastin time (aPTT) can provide an approximation of dabigatran's anticoagulant activity.

WARNING Monitor patient closely for bleeding because dabigatran increases risk for bleeding, which can become severe. Bleeding risk increases in patients taking concurrent antiplatelet drugs, heparin, or fibrinolytic therapy, or with chronic use of NSAIDs. It also increases during labor and delivery. **Monitor patient very closely.** Promptly report any signs or symptoms of bleeding such as a drop in hemoglobin and/or hematocrit or the development of hypotension or overt bleeding. Expect to discontinue drug if active bleeding occurs and is serious or persistent. Know that protamine sulfate and vitamin K will not affect the anticoagulant activity of dabigatran. Instead, the prescriber may prescribe platelet concentrates if thrombocytopenia is present or the patient has been exposed to long-acting antiplatelet drugs.

• Be aware that patients receiving spinal/epidural anesthesia or a spinal puncture are at risk of developing an epidural or spinal hematoma, which can result in long-term or permanent paralysis. Monitor patient frequently for signs or symptoms of neurologic impairment. Notify prescriber immediately if patient complains of bladder or bowel dysfunction, midline back pain, or numbness, tingling, or weakness in the lower extremities.

• Assess patient closely for stroke if dabigatran therapy must be discontinued temporarily because of an active bleed, elective surgery, or an invasive procedure. Know that therapy should be restarted as soon as possible. If the drug must be discontinued for reasons other than pathological bleeding, expect patient to receive coverage with another anti-coagulant to decrease the risk of thrombotic events, such as stroke.

PATIENT TEACHING

• Many of the same bleeding precautions that apply to patients who receive warfarin also apply to dabigatran.

- Tell patient to take dabigatran exactly as prescribed.
- Instruct patient to swallow capsule whole without breaking, chewing, or emptying the contents of the capsule prior to ingestion.
- Tell patient that if she misses a dose, she should take it as soon as she remembers on the same day she missed the dose, unless it is within 6 hours of the next dose. She should never double a dose to make up for a missed dose.
- Instruct patient to keep bottle tightly closed when not in use and store in the original package to protect from moisture. Have patient date bottle when opened and tell her to discard any remaining drug if not used within 4 months of initially opening the bottle.
- Urge patient to take precautions against bleeding, such as using an electric shaver and a soft-bristled toothbrush.
- Caution patient to avoid activities that could cause traumatic injury and bleeding.
- Urge patient to notify prescriber immediately about unusual bleeding and any unexplained symptoms, such as abnormal vaginal bleeding; dizziness; easy bruising; gum bleeding; black or tarry stool; red or dark brown urine; vomiting blood or vomit that looks like coffee grounds; and weakness.
- Caution patient not to stop taking dabigatran abruptly.
- Urge patient to carry medical identification that reveals she is taking dabigatran.
- Tell patient to inform all healthcare providers that she is taking dabigatran and not to take any medication, including OTC drugs, without first consulting the prescriber.

dalbavancin

Dalvance

Class and Category
Chemical class: Synthetic lipoglycopeptide
Therapeutic class: Antibacterial
Pregnancy category: C

Indications and Dosages
➤ *To treat acute bacterial skin and skin structure infections caused by* Staphylococcus aureus *(including* methicillin-susceptible and methicillin-resistant strains),* Streptococcus pyogenes, Streptococcus agalactiae, *and* Streptococcus anginosus *group (including* S. anginosus, S. intermedius, *and* S. constellatus)

I.V. INFUSION
Adults. 1,000 mg over 30 min, followed by 500 mg over 30 min 1 wk later.
DOSAGE ADJUSTMENT For patients with renal impairment (creatinine clearance less than 30 ml/min) and who are not receiving hemodialysis, initial dosage reduced to 750 mg, followed by 375 mg 1 wk later.

Mechanism of Action
Interferes with bacterial cell wall synthesis, which leads to impaired bacterial cell growth or cell death.

Incompatibilities
Do not co-infuse with other medications or electrolytes. Also, do not mix or infuse with saline-based infusion solutions because a precipitation may occur.

Contraindications
Hypersensitivity to dalbavancin or its components

Adverse Reactions
CNS: Dizziness, headache
EENT: Oral candidiasis
ENDO: Hypoglycemia
GI: Abdominal pain, *Clostridium difficile*–associated colitis, diarrhea, elevated liver enzymes, gastrointestinal hemorrhage, hepatotoxicity, melena, nausea, passage of bright red blood through anus
GU: Vulvovaginal mycotic infection
HEME: Anemia, elevated international normalized ratio, eosinophilia, hemorrhagic anemia, leukopenia, neutropenia, spontaneous hematoma, thrombocytosis, thrombocytopenia
RESP: Bronchospasm
SKIN: Flushing of upper body, petechiae, pruritus, rash, urticaria
Other: Anaphylaxis, phlebitis, red man syndrome (with rapid infusion), wound hemorrhage

Nursing Considerations
- Use cautiously in patients with a history of glycopeptides allergy because of a possibility of cross-sensitivity.

• Use cautiously in patients with a history of hepatic impairment because dosing adjustments for dalbavancin in patients with moderate to severe hepatic impairment are not known. Dosage adjustment is not required for patients with mild hepatic impairment.

• Reconstitute with 25 ml of sterile water for injection, USP for each 500-mg vial. Avoid foaming by alternating between gently swirling and inverting the vial until contents are completely dissolved. Do not shake. Solution should appear clear and colorless to yellow. Once reconstituted, the vial may be refrigerated for up to 48 hours. Do not freeze. Prior to administration, further dilute reconstituted vial by aseptically transferring the required dose from the vial to an intravenous bag or bottle containing enough solution of 5% dextrose injection, USP to provide a final dalbavancin concentration of 1 to 5 mg/ml. Discard any unused portion of the reconstituted solution. Once diluted, the intravenous bag or bottle may be refrigerated until administration as long as the total time from the vial being reconstituted until administration does not exceed 48 hours. Never freeze the diluted solution.

• Administer as an intravenous infusion over 30 minutes to minimize the risk of infusion-related reactions that resemble red man syndrome, such as flushing of the upper body, pruritus, rash, or urticaria. If present, stopping or slowing the infusion may cause these reactions to disappear. Always flush intravenous line with 5% dextrose injection, USP before and after administration if the line is used to administer other drugs.

• Assess patient for signs of secondary infection, such as profuse, watery diarrhea. If such diarrhea develops, contact prescriber and expect to obtain a stool specimen to rule out pseudomembranous colitis caused by *Clostridium difficile*. If diarrhea occurs, notify prescriber and expect to withhold dalbavancin and treat patient with fluids, electrolytes, protein, and an antibiotic effective against *C. difficile*.

PATIENT TEACHING
• Emphasize importance of obtaining second dose of dalbavancin.
• Tell patient to immediately report any signs and symptoms of an allergic reaction.
• Advise patient to report severe diarrhea to prescriber immediately.

dalteparin sodium
(tedelparin)
Fragmin

Class and Category
Chemical class: Low-molecular-weight heparin
Therapeutic class: Anticoagulant, antithrombotic
Pregnancy category: B

Indications and Dosages
➤ *To prevent ischemic complications in patients who receive aspirin as part of treatment for unstable angina and non–Q-wave MI*
SUBCUTANEOUS INJECTION
Adults. 120 international units/kg every 12 hr with aspirin (75 to 165 mg daily) until patient is stable, usually 5 to 8 days. *Maximum:* 10,000 international units/dose.
➤ *To prevent blood clots in patients undergoing hip replacement surgery*
SUBCUTANEOUS INJECTION
Adults. *Initial:* 2,500 international units 1 to 2 hr before surgery, repeated in 8 to 12 hr and again 8 to 12 hr later. *Maintenance:* 5,000 international units every morning for 5 to 10 days postoperatively or until patient is fully ambulatory. *Alternate:* 5,000 international units the evening before surgery; then 5,000 international units daily (starting the next evening) for 5 to 10 days or until patient is fully ambulatory.
➤ *To prevent blood clots in patients undergoing abdominal surgery who are at risk for thromboembolic complications*
SUBCUTANEOUS INJECTION
Adults. 2,500 international units daily, starting 1 to 2 hr before surgery and repeated for 5 to 10 days. For patients at high risk (those with cancer), 5,000 international units the evening before surgery,

repeated daily for 5 to 10 days; or 2,500 international units 1 to 2 hr before surgery followed by 2,500 international units 12 hr later and then 5,000 international units daily for 5 to 10 days.

➤ *To prevent blood clots in patients with severe mobility restrictions during acute illness*
SUBCUTANEOUS INJECTION
Adults. 5,000 international units daily.

➤ *To treat symptomatic venous thromboembolism and prevent recurrence in patients with cancer*
SUBCUTANEOUS INJECTION
Adults. 200 international units/kg (not to exceed 18,000 international units) once daily for 30 days. Then 150 international units/kg once daily for 5 more mo.

Mechanism of Action
Binds to and accelerates the activity of antithrombin III, thus inhibiting thrombin and blocking the formation of fibrin clots.

Incompatibilities
Don't mix dalteparin with other drugs.

Contraindications
Active major bleeding; hypersensitivity to low-molecular-weight heparins, heparin, or pork products; thrombocytopenia associated with positive tests for antiplatelet antibodies in the presence of dalteparin

Interactions
DRUGS
NSAIDs, oral anticoagulants, platelet aggregation inhibitors, thrombolytics: Possibly increased risk of hemorrhage and spinalor epidural hematoma

Adverse Reactions
GI: Elevated liver enzymes
HEME: Hemorrhage, thrombocytopenia
SKIN: Alopecia, bullous eruption, necrosis, pruritus, rash
Other: Anaphylaxis, injection-site hematoma and pain

Nursing Considerations
• Use dalteparin with extreme caution in patients with a history of heparin-induced thrombocytopenia; those at increased risk for hemorrhage (such as those who use a platelet inhibitor or have bacterial endocarditis, bleeding disorders,

active ulcerative GI disease, uncontrolled hypertension, or hemorrhagic stroke); and those with recent brain, eye, or spinal surgery.
• Use drug cautiously in patients with bleeding diathesis, diabetic retinopathy, platelet defects, recent GI bleeding, severe hepatic or renal insufficiency, or thrombocytopenia.
• Before giving first dose, tell Jewish or Islamic patients that drug comes from porcine intestine.
WARNING Question patient regarding use of aspirin and other NSAIDs, platelet inhibitors or other anticoagulants prior to dalteparin therapy, especially if the patient is to receive neuraxial anesthesia or spinal puncture, because unusually prolonged or severe bleeding may occur at the puncture site. Hematoma formation may be severe enough to produce paralysis that may not be reversible.
• Risk factors for thromboembolic events include age over 40, cancer, history of deep vein thrombosis or pulmonary embolism, obesity, and planned use of anesthesia for more than 30 minutes.
• Don't give drug by I.M. or I.V. injection.
• With patient seated or supine, administer drug deep into subcutaneous tissue in U-shaped area around navel, upper outer thigh, or upper outer quadrant of buttocks. If using area around navel or on thigh, lift skin fold with thumb and forefinger while giving injection. Insert entire length of needle at a 45- to 90-degree angle. Rotate sites daily.
• Routine coagulation tests and dosage adjustments usually aren't required.
WARNING Monitor patient receiving dalteparin and epidural or spinal anesthesia or spinal puncture because spinal hematomas can occur, causing long-term or permanent paralysis. Watch for evidence of neurologic impairment, such as changes in sensory or motor function. If present, notify prescriber immediately; patient needs urgent care to minimize effect of hematoma. Use of indwelling epidural catheters; concurrent use of other drugs that affect hemostasis such as nonsteroidal anti-inflammatory drugs, platelet inhibitors, and other anticoagulants; a history of traumatic or repeated epidural

D

or spinal punctures; or a history of spinal deformity or spinal surgery increases the risk of spinal or epidural hematoma in patients receiving dalteparin.

PATIENT TEACHING
• If therapy will continue at home, teach patient or caregiver to select injection sites, give subcutaneous injections, and rotate sites daily. Tell patient to discard drug if it's discolored or contains particles. Review safe handling and disposal of syringes and needles.
• Teach patient to store drug at room temperature, away from moisture and heat.
• Urge patient to report adverse reactions, especially bleeding, and to seek help immediately if signs of blood clots develop, such as severe difficulty breathing or changes in mental status or motor or sensory abnormalities.
• Emphasize the importance of follow-up visits.

danaparoid sodium

Organon

Class and Category

Chemical class: Glycosaminoglycan heparinoid, low-molecular-weight heparin
Therapeutic class: Anticoagulant, antithrombotic
Pregnancy category: B

Indications and Dosages

➤ *To prevent deep vein thrombosis after hip replacement surgery*

SUBCUTANEOUS INJECTION
Adults. 750 anti-factor Xa units b.i.d. (first dose 1 to 4 hr preoperatively; second dose no sooner than 2 hr after surgery) for 7 to 14 days, as indicated.

Mechanism of Action

Inhibits thrombin generation in coagulation pathway, thus preventing fibrin formation and clotting.

Contraindications

Active major bleeding (including hemorrhagic stroke); hypersensitivity to low-molecular-weight heparins, heparin, or pork products; severe hemorrhagic

disorders, such as hemophilia and thrombocytopenic purpura; sulfite sensitivity; type II thrombocytopenia associated with positive laboratory tests for antiplatelet antibodies in the presence of danaparoid

Interactions

DRUGS
NSAIDs, oral anticoagulants, platelet aggregation inhibitors: Possibly increased risk of bleeding

Adverse Reactions

CNS: Asthenia, dizziness, fever, headache, insomnia
CV: Chest pain, edema
GI: Abdominal pain, constipation, nausea, vomiting
GU: Urine retention, UTI
HEME: Anemia, excessive bleeding
MS: Arthralgia, myalgia
SKIN: Pruritus, rash
Other: Anaphylaxis, injection-site pain

Nursing Considerations

• Use danaparoid with extreme caution in patients at increased risk for hemorrhage (such as those with severe uncontrolled hypertension, acute bacterial endocarditis, bleeding disorders, active ulcerative GI disease, severe renal dysfunction, or nonhemorrhagic stroke); those with a postoperative indwelling epidural catheter; and those with recent had brain, eye, or spinal surgery.
• Before administering first dose, inform Jewish and Islamic patients that drug comes from porcine intestinal mucosa.
• Don't give drug by I.M. or I.V. injection.
• Administer drug with patient lying down. Use a 25G or 26G needle to minimize tissue trauma. Select site on left or right anterolateral or posterolateral abdominal wall. Hold skin fold gently between thumb and forefinger, and insert entire length of needle deep into subcutaneous tissue at a 45- to 90-degree angle. Don't pinch or rub site afterward. Rotate sites.
• Expect to monitor results of CBC and fecal occult blood tests during therapy. Typical coagulation tests, such as PT, APTT, clotting time, whole blood clotting time, and thrombin time, aren't useful for monitoring drug's anticoagulant effect.

PATIENT TEACHING
• If therapy must continue at home, teach patient or caregiver how to give subcutaneous injections. Review injection sites, and instruct her to rotate them daily. Tell her to discard drug if it's discolored or contains particles. Review safe handling and disposal of syringes and needles.
• Teach patient to store drug at room temperature, away from moisture and heat.
• Instruct patient to consult prescriber before using aspirin, ibuprofen, indomethacin, ketoprofen, naproxen, and other NSAIDs because they may increase the risk of bleeding.
• Advise patient to stop taking drug and seek help immediately if she experiences severe dizziness, fever, rash, wheezing, or prolonged or unexplained bleeding and pain at the injection site.

---

dantrolene sodium
Dantrium, Dantrium Intravenous

Class and Category
Chemical class: Hydantoin derivative, imidazolidinedione sodium salt
Therapeutic class: Antispastic, malignant hyperthermia therapy adjunct
Pregnancy category: C (parenteral), Not rated (oral)

Indications and Dosages
➤ *To treat chronic spastic conditions caused by severe chronic disorders, such as cerebral palsy, stroke, multiple sclerosis, and spinal cord injury*
CAPSULES
Adults and adolescents. *Initial:* 25 mg daily for 7 days. Then dosage increased to 25 mg/day every 4 to 7 days until desired response occurs or dosage reaches 100 mg four times daily. *Maximum:* 400 mg daily.
Children. *Initial:* 0.5 mg/kg twice daily for 7 days. Then increased by 0.5 mg/kg daily every 4 to 7 days until desired response occurs or dosage reaches 3 mg/kg four times daily. *Maximum:* 400 mg daily.
➤ *To prevent malignant hyperthermia before surgery*

CAPSULES
Adults and children. 4 to 8 mg/kg daily in divided doses three times daily or four times daily 1 or 2 days before surgery, with last dose given 3 to 4 hr before surgery.
I.V. INFUSION
Adults and children. *Initial:* 2.5 mg/kg 60 to 75 min before anesthesia and infused over 1 hr. Additional individualized doses given as needed during surgery.
➤ *To treat malignant hyperthermic crisis*
I.V. INFUSION
Adults and adolescents. *Initial:* 1 mg/kg by rapid bolus; repeated, as needed, until symptoms subside or cumulative dose of 10 mg/kg has been reached and if symptoms reappear.
➤ *To treat postmalignant hyperthermic crisis*
CAPSULES
Adults and children. 4 to 8 mg/kg daily in divided doses four times daily for 1 to 3 days.
I.V. INFUSION
Adults and children. *Initial:* Individualized dosage beginning with 1 mg/kg or more as needed if oral therapy can't be used. *Maximum:* 10 mg/kg total dose.

Route	Onset	Peak	Duration
P.O.	1 wk*	Unknown	Unknown

Mechanism of Action
Acts directly on skeletal muscle to reduce the force of reflex muscle contraction. This in turn reduces hyperreflexia, spasticity, involuntary movements, and clonus, probably by preventing calcium release from the sarcoplasmic reticulum of skeletal muscle cells. Blocked calcium release also inhibits the activation of acute catabolism associated with malignant hyperthermic crisis syndrome.

Incompatibilities
Don't administer parenteral dantrolene with acidic solutions, including D_5W and normal saline solution.

Contraindications
For oral drug only: Active hepatic disease (such as cirrhosis and hepatitis), conditions in which spasticity helps maintain upright posture and improve balance or function, skeletal muscle spasms caused by rheumatic disorders

---
* For spasticity; unknown for malignant hyperthermia.

Interactions

DRUGS
calcium channel blockers (especially verapamil): Possibly hyperkalemia, shock, life-threatening arrhythmias
CNS depressants: Possibly profound sedation
estrogens: Possibly increased risk of hepatotoxicity
hepatotoxic drugs: Increased risk of hepatotoxicity with long-term oral dantrolene use
vecuronium: Possibly potentiated vecuronium-induced neuromuscular block
ACTIVITIES
alcohol use: Possibly increased CNS depression

Adverse Reactions

CNS: Chills, confusion, depression, dizziness, drowsiness, fatigue, fever, headache, insomnia, light-headedness, malaise, nervousness, seizures, slurred speech or other speech problems, weakness
CV: Heart failure (I.V.), labile blood pressure, pericarditis, phlebitis, tachycardia
EENT: Abnormal vision, altered taste, diplopia, drooling, excessive tearing, lacrimation
GI: Abdominal cramps, anorexia, constipation, diarrhea, dysphagia, gastric irritation, GI bleeding, hepatitis, hepatotoxicity, intestinal obstruction, nausea, vomiting
GU: Crystalluria, dysuria, erectile dysfunction, hematuria, nocturia, urinary frequency, urinary incontinence, urine retention
HEME: Aplastic anemia, anemia, leukopenia, lymphocytic lymphoma, thrombocytopenia
MS: Backache, myalgia
RESP: Feeling of suffocation, pleural effusion, respiratory depression
SKIN: Acne, diaphoresis, eczematoid eruption, erythema (I.V.), extravasation with tissue damage, hirsutism, pruritus, rash, urticaria
Other: Anaphylaxis

Nursing Considerations

• Use dantrolene cautiously in patients with impaired pulmonary function, especially those with COPD, and in those with severe cardiac or hepatic dysfunction.

• Reconstitute drug with 60 ml sterile water for injection. Shake vial until clear. Store reconstituted solution at room temperature, protected from direct sunlight. Discard after 6 hours.
• To prevent precipitation, transfer reconstituted drug to a plastic I.V. bag, rather than a glass bottle, for infusion.
• Because drug has a high pH, infuse into a central vein, if possible, to avoid tissue damage from extravasation.
• Monitor blood pressure and heart rate often during administration to detect tachycardia and blood pressure changes.
• Notify prescriber about persistent diarrhea with oral therapy; drug may need to be stopped.
• Monitor results of liver function tests—especially ALT, AST, alkaline phosphatase, and total bilirubin levels—to detect hepatotoxicity. Expect to stop drug after 45 days if benefits aren't sufficient because risk of hepatotoxicity increases with dose and time, especially for women and patients over age 35.

PATIENT TEACHING
• Advise patient to take dantrolene with food if gastric irritation develops.
• Tell patient that drug may weaken muscles used for walking and climbing stairs.
• Explain drug's sedating effects. Caution patient to avoid sedatives (unless prescribed), including alcohol.
• Advise patient to report yellow skin or sclerae, itching, anorexia, and fatigue.
• If patient misses a dose, tell her to wait until the next scheduled dose if more than 2 hours have passed since the missed dose. Instruct her not to double the dose.
• Caution patient not to stop taking drug without consulting prescriber. Gradual dosage reduction may be required, especially after long-term use.

dapagliflozin

Farxiga

Class and Category

Chemical class: Sodium glucose co-transporter 2 inhibitor
Therapeutic class: Antidiabetic
Pregnancy category: C

Indications and Dosages
➤ *Adjunct to diet and exercise to improve glycemic control in patients with type 2 diabetes mellitus*

TABLETS
Adults. 5 mg once daily in morning, increased to 10 mg once daily in morning as needed.

Mechanism of Action
Inhibits sodium glucose co-transporter 2 in the kidneys, which prevents glucose reabsorption. This decreases blood glucose levels.

Contraindications
Diabetic ketoacidosis, dialysis therapy, end-stage renal disease, hypersensitivity to dapagliflozin or its components, severe renal impairment

Interaction
DRUGS
insulin, insulin secretagogues: Increased risk of hypoglycemia

Adverse Reactions
CNS: Syncope
CV: Dyslipidemia, elevated low-density lipoprotein cholesterol, hypotension
EENT: Nasopharyngitis
ENDO: Hypoglycemia
GI: Constipation, nausea
GU: Decreased glomerular filtration rate, dysuria, elevated serum creatinine levels, genital mycotic infections, impaired renal function, increased urination, osmotic diuresis, potential bladder cancer, UTI
HEME: Elevated hematocrit level
MS: Back or extremity pain
SKIN: Severe cutaneous reactions, urticaria
Other: Anaphylaxis, angioedema, dehydration, elevated serum phosphorus levels

Nursing Considerations
• Know that dapagliflozin should not be given to patients with active bladder cancer, as it is not known if the drug has an effect on preexisting bladder tumors. Use cautiously in patients with a history of bladder cancer. Monitor patient throughout therapy for hematuria, as this is a potential indicator for the presence of bladder tumor.
• Assess patient's volume status and correct, if needed and as prescribed, prior to starting dapagliflozin therapy, because drug can cause intravascular volume contraction leading to symptomatic hypotension. Patients at highest risk include elderly patients, patients receiving loop diuretic therapy, and patients who have impaired renal function.
• Obtain serum creatinine level, as ordered, prior to starting dapagliflozin therapy because dapagliflozin can cause adverse renal effects. Be aware that the elderly and patients with existing impaired renal function are at higher risk for these adverse effects. Monitor renal function throughout therapy.
• Monitor patient's blood pressure and cholesterol level throughout dapagliflozin therapy.
WARNING Monitor patient for hypersensitivity reactions. Although rare, anaphylaxis, angioedema, and severe cutaneous adverse reactions have occurred. If present, stop drug immediately and notify prescriber. Provide care, as prescribed, according to the standard of care until signs and symptoms subside.
• Be aware that patients receiving insulin or insulin secretagogues may require a lower dose of these agents because dapagliflozin in combination increases risk of hypoglycemia. Monitor patient closely for hypoglycemia. If present, treat according to standard of care and notify prescriber.
• Monitor patients for genital mycotic infections, especially those with a history of such infections. If present, notify prescriber and treat, as prescribed.

PATIENT TEACHING
• Inform patient that dapagliflozin therapy is not a replacement for diet and exercise therapy.
• Instruct patient on the signs and symptoms of hypoglycemia and how to treat it. Inform patient who is also receiving a sulfonylurea or insulin that the risk of hypoglycemia is greater. Tell patient to notify prescriber if hypoglycemia occurs frequently or is severe.
• Inform patient that dapagliflozin may have an adverse effect on the bladder, increasing the risk for bladder cancer. Tell patient to report blood in the urine immediately to the prescriber.

D

• Tell patient to monitor the blood glucose level using blood tests instead of urine tests because the drug increases urinary glucose excretion and will lead to positive urine glucose tests.
• Instruct patient to stop taking drug and seek immediate medical attention if an allergic reaction such as hives or facial or throat swelling occurs while taking dapagliflozin.
• Advise female patients to notify prescriber if pregnancy occurs or is suspected because the drug may cause fetal harm if taken in the second or third trimester.
• Advise patient to maintain adequate fluid intake throughout dapagliflozin therapy.

daptomycin
Cubicin

Class and Category
Chemical class: Cyclic lipopeptide
Therapeutic class: Antibiotic
Pregnancy category: B

Indications and Dosages
➤ *To treat complicated skin and skin structure infections caused by* Staphylococcus aureus *(including methicillin-resistant isolates),* Streptococcus pyogenes, Streptococcus agalactiae, Streptococcus dysgalactiae *subspecies* Equisimilis, *and* Enterococcus faecalis *(vancomycin-susceptible isolates only)*

I.V. INFUSION, I.V. INJECTION
Adults. 4 mg/kg administered over 2 min as an I.V. injection or over 30 min as an I.V. infusion daily for 7 to 14 days. *Maximum:* 6 mg/kg I.V. every 24 hr.

DOSAGE ADJUSTMENT For patients with creatinine clearance less than 30 ml/min/ 1.73 m², 4 or 6 mg/kg (depending on infection type) once every 48 hr.
➤ *To treat* Staphylococcus aureus *bloodstream infections, including right-sided infective endocarditis, caused by methicillin-susceptible and methicillin-resistant isolates*

I.V. INFUSION, I.V. INJECTION
Adults. 6 mg/kg administered over 2 min as an I.V. injection or over 30 min as an I.V. infusion daily for 2 to 6 wk. *Maximum:* 6 mg/kg I.V. every 24 hr.

DOSAGE ADJUSTMENT For patients with creatinine clearance less than 30 ml/min/1.73 m², dosage is 4 or 6 mg/kg (depending on infection) once every 48 hr.

Mechanism of Action
Binds to bacterial membranes to cause rapid depolarization of membrane potential. This loss of membrane potential inhibits protein, DNA, and RNA synthesis, which results in bacterial cell death.

Incompatibilities
Don't mix daptomycin with dextrose-containing diluents and with other intravenously administered drugs or infusions.

Contraindications
Hypersensitivity to daptomycin or its components

Interactions
DRUGS
HMG-CoA reductase inhibitors: Possibly increased CK level and increased risk of myopathy

Adverse Reactions
CNS: Anxiety, asthenia, confusion, dizziness, fever, headache, insomnia, peripheral neuropathy
CV: Cardiac failure, chest pain, hypertension, hypotension, peripheral edema, supraventricular tachycardia
EENT: Pharyngolaryngeal pain, oral candidiasis, sore throat
ENDO: Hyperglycemia, hypoglycemia
GI: Abdominal pain, anorexia, *Clostridium difficile*-associated diarrhea, constipation, diarrhea, dyspepsia, dysphagia, elevated liver enzymes, GI hemorrhage, nausea, vomiting
GU: Renal failure, UTI, vaginal candidiasis
HEME: Anemia, eosinophilia, increased INR, leukocytosis, thrombocytopenia, thrombocytosis
MS: Arthralgia, back or limb pain, elevated myoglobin level, myopathy, rhabdomyolysis, osteomyelitis
RESP: Cough, dyspnea, pleural effusion, pneumonia including eosinophilic, shortness of breath

SKIN: Cellulitis, diaphoresis, drug rash with eosinophilia and systemic symptoms (DRESS), erythema, pruritus, rash, Stevens-Johnson syndrome, truncal erythema, urticaria, vesiculobullous rash
Other: Anaphylaxis, angioedema, elevated alkaline phosphatase level, elevated serum sodium bicarbonate level, fungal infection, hyperkalemia, hypokalemia, hypomagnesemia, injection-site reactions, sepsis

Nursing Considerations
• Use cautiously in patients with moderate to severe renal impairment and monitor drug effectiveness closely, as daptomycin may not be as effective in this patient population.
• Obtain blood samples for culture and sensitivity testing before starting daptomycin.
• Reconstitute daptomycin powder by slowly transferring 10 ml normal saline for injection into vial and pointing needle toward wall of vial to minimize foaming. Then gently rotate vial until all powder is wet. Don't agitate or shake vial. Let vial stand undisturbed for 10 minutes, and then gently rotate or swirl contents for a few minutes, as needed, to obtain a completely reconstituted solution.
• Administer as an IV injection over a period of 2 minutes. If the drug is to be administered as an IV infusion, further dilute reconstituted daptomycin solution with normal saline for injection, and administer over 30 minutes. Reconstituted drug is stable in infusion bag for 12 hours at room temperature or 48 hours refrigerated. Do not infuse with the ReadyMED elastromeric infusion pumps, as daptomycin is not as stable when stored in these pumps.
• Daptomycin may cause a significant false increase in PT and INR with some brands of laboratory assays. If this occurs during daptomycin therapy, draw blood sample just before next daptomycin dose and evaluate other causes of the increase.
• Monitor patient closely for diarrhea, which may herald pseudomembranous colitis caused by *Clostridium difficile*. If diarrhea occurs, notify prescriber. If pseudomembranous colitis develops, expect to discontinue drug and give fluids,

electrolytes, protein, and antibiotic effective against *C. difficile*.
• Monitor patient for evidence of superinfection, and inform prescriber if present. Expect to stop drug and provide care.
• Assess patient for muscle pain or weakness, especially of distal limbs. Expect to monitor CK level weekly or more often in patients recently or currently taking an HMG-CoA reductase inhibitor. Expect to stop daptomycin, as ordered, if patient has myopathy or marked rise in CK level.
• Monitor patient's BUN and serum creatinine levels closely, especially if renal insufficiency is already present.
• Expect to discontinue daptomycin therapy immediately if patient develops signs and symptoms of eosinophilic pneumonia, such as fever or dyspnea with hypoxic respiratory insufficiency and diffuse pulmonary infiltrates, and prepare to administer systemic steroids, as ordered.

PATIENT TEACHING
• Inform patient that diarrhea may occur 2 months or more after daptomycin therapy stops. If severe or prolonged, advise patient to notify prescriber as soon as possible; additional treatment may be needed.
• Urge patient to report muscle pain, tenderness, or weakness, and other symptoms of myopathy immediately.

darbepoetin alfa
Aranesp

Class and Category
Chemical class: 165-amino acid glycoprotein identical to human erythropoietin
Therapeutic class: Antianemic
Pregnancy category: C

Indications and Dosages
➤ *To treat anemia from chronic renal failure*
I.V. OR SUBCUTANEOUS INJECTION
Adults on dialysis other than hemodialysis.
Initial: 0.45 mcg/kg as a single dose every wk. Alternatively, 0.75 mcg/kg once every 2 wks. *Maintenance:* Dosage individualized

and increased monthly to maintain a hemoglobin level not to exceed 11 g/dl. **Adults not on dialysis.** *Initial:* 0.45 mcg/kg as a single dose every 4 wks., as needed. *Maintenance:* Dosage individualized and increased monthly to maintain a hemoglobin level not to exceed 10 g/dl.

I.V. INJECTION
Adults on hemodialysis. *Initial:* 0.45 mcg/kg as a single dose every wk. *Alternatively,* 0.75 mcg/kg once every 2 wks. *Maintenance:* Dosage individualized and increased monthly to maintain a hemoglobin level not to exceed 11 g/dl.

DOSAGE ADJUSTMENT Dosage reduced by about 25% if hemoglobin level increases and approaches 11 g/dl for patients on dialysis and 10 g/dl for patients not on dialysis. If it continues to increase, doses temporarily withheld until hemoglobin level begins to decrease; then therapy is restarted at a dose about 25% below previous dose. Dosage reduced by about 25% if hemoglobin level increases by more than 1 g/dl in a 2-wk period. Dosage increased by about 25% of previous dose if hemoglobin level increases less than 1 g/dl over 4 wk but only if serum ferritin level is 100 mcg/L or greater and serum transferrin saturation is 20% or greater. Further increases made at 4-wk intervals until specified hemoglobin level is obtained.

DOSAGE ADJUSTMENT For conversion from epoetin alfa to darbepoetin alfa, dosage administered every wk for patient who previously received epoetin alfa 2 to 3 times/wk and once every 2 wk for patient who previously received epoetin alfa once/wk. For conversion from epoetin alfa, 6.25 mcg/wk darbepoetin alfa given every wk for patients who received less than 2,500 units/wk of epoetin alfa; 12.5 mcg/wk darbepoetin alfa every wk for patients who received 2,500 to 4,999 units/wk of epoetin alfa; 25 mcg/wk darbepoetin alfa every wk for patients who received 5,000 to 10,999 units/wk of epoetin alfa; 40 mcg/wk darbepoetin alfa every wk for patients who received 11,000 to 17,999 units/wk of epoetin alfa; 60 mcg/wk darbepoetin alfa every wk for patients who received 18,000 to 33,999 units/wk of epoetin alfa; 100 mcg/wk darbepoetin alfa every wk for patients who received 34,000 to 89,999 units/wk of epoetin alfa; 200 mcg/wk darbepoetin

alfa every wk for patients who received 90,000 or more units/wk of epoetin alfa.

➤ *To treat chemotherapy-induced anemia in patients with nonmyeloid malignancies and hemoglobin level less than 10 g/dl*

SUBCUTANEOUS INJECTION
Adults. *Initial:* 2.25 mcg/kg as a single dose every wk until completion of a chemotherapy course. Alternatively, 500 mcg every 3 wks until completion of a chemotherapy course. *Maintenance:* Dosage individualized to maintain a target hemoglobin level.

DOSAGE ADJUSTMENT Dosage increased to 4.5 mcg/kg if hemoglobin level increases less than 1.0 g/dl after 6 wk of therapy. If it increases more than 1.0 g/dl over 2 wk, dosage reduced by about 40%. If hemoglobin level exceeds a level needed to avoid RBC transfusion, dose withheld until hemoglobin approaches level when RBC transfusion may be required. Then therapy is restarted at a dose about 40% less than last dose given.

Route	Onset	Peak	Duration
I.V., SubQ	2–6 wk	Unknown	Unknown

Mechanism of Action
Stimulates release of reticulocytes from the bone marrow into the bloodstream, where they develop into mature RBCs.

Incompatibilities
Don't mix darbepoetin alfa with any other drug.

Contraindications
Hypersensitivity to human albumin or products made from mammal cells; uncontrolled hypertension

Adverse Reactions
CNS: Asthenia, dizziness, fatigue, fever, headache, seizures, stroke, transient ischemic attack
CV: Acute MI, angina, arrhythmias, cardiac arrest or death, chest pain, congestive heart failure, hypertension, hypotension, peripheral edema, vascular access thrombosis or other thromboembolic events
GI: Abdominal pain, constipation, diarrhea, nausea, vomiting

MS: Arthralgia, back pain, limb pain, muscle spasm, myalgia
RESP: Bronchitis, cough, dyspnea, pneumonia, pulmonary embolism, upper respiratory tract infection
SKIN: Pruritus, rash, urticaria
Other: Dehydration, fluid overload, infection, flulike symptoms, injection-site pain, sepsis

Nursing Considerations
• Before starting darbepoetin alfa therapy, expect to correct folic acid or vitamin B_{12} deficiencies because these conditions may interfere with drug's effectiveness.
• Ensure that patient has received the medication guide and patient instructions for darbepoetin and that a written acknowledgment of a discussion of the risks involved with this type of therapy has been obtained before first dose is given.
• Darbepoetin alfa shouldn't be given to cancer patients when a cure is anticipated because drug may decrease survival rate and increase tumor progression in patients with certain types of cancers, such as breast, non–small cell lung, head and neck, lymphoid, and cervical cancers. Be aware that all prescribers and hospitals must enroll in and comply with the ESA APPRISE oncology program to be able to prescribe and dispense the drug.
• Use extreme caution with darbepoetin alfa therapy in patients undergoing coronary artery bypass graft surgery because of increased risk of death, and in patients undergoing orthopedic procedures because of increased risk of deep venous thrombosis.
• To ensure effective drug response, expect to monitor serum ferritin level and transferrin saturation before and during therapy, as ordered. If serum ferritin level is less than 100 mcg/L or serum transferrin saturation is less than 20%, expect to begin supplemental iron therapy.
• Don't shake vial during preparation to avoid denaturing drug and rendering it biologically inactive.
• Discard drug if you see particulate matter or discoloration.
• Don't dilute drug before giving it.

• Needle cover on prefilled syringe contains dry natural rubber and may cause allergic reaction in those with latex sensitivity.
• Discard unused portion of drug because it contains no preservatives.
• Monitor patient closely for hypertension during therapy. Expect to reduce dosage or withhold drug if blood pressure is poorly controlled with antihypertensive and dietary measures.
• Monitor hemoglobin level weekly, as ordered, until hemoglobin stabilizes and maintenance dosage has been achieved. Then monitor hemoglobin level regularly, as ordered. After each dosage adjustment, expect to check hemoglobin level weekly for 4 weeks until it stabilizes in response to dosage change.
WARNING If hemoglobin level increases more than about 1 g/dl during any 2-week period or it exceeds 11 g/d for patient on dialysis, 10 g/dl for patient not on dialysis, or target range for cancer patient, the risk of cardiac arrest, seizures, stroke, worsened hypertension, congestive heart failure, vascular thrombosis, vascular ischemia, vascular infarction, acute MI, fluid overload with peripheral edema, tumor progression, and shortened survival increases. Expect to decrease dosage if this occurs.
• Expect to discontinue darbepoetin in cancer patients if hemoglobin level hasn't increased after 8 weeks or if patient continues to need transfusions despite therapy.
• Institute seizure precautions according to facility policy.
• For patients with chronic renal failure, monitor renal function test results and fluid and electrolyte balance for signs of declining renal function. If patient starts dialysis, monitor hemoglobin and blood pressure closely and expect dosage and route of administration to be adjusted, as needed, for type of dialysis.
• Store drug at 2° to 8° C (36° to 46° F). Don't freeze, and do protect from light.
PATIENT TEACHING
• Advise patient that the risk of seizures is highest during the first 90 days of therapy. Discourage her from engaging in hazardous activities during this time.
• Emphasize the importance of complying with the dosage regimen and keeping

follow-up medical and laboratory appointments.
- Advise patient to follow up with her prescriber for blood pressure monitoring.
- Encourage patient to eat adequate quantities of iron-rich foods.
- If patient will self-administer darbepoetin, teach her and her caregiver the proper administration technique.
- Caution patient and her caregiver not to reuse needles, syringes, or drug product. Thoroughly instruct them in proper needle and syringe disposal using a puncture-resistant container.
- Explain that needle cover on prefilled syringe contains dry natural rubber and may cause allergic reaction in those with latex sensitivity.
- Review possible adverse reactions, and urge patient to notify prescriber if she experiences chest pain, headache, rash, seizures, shortness of breath, or swelling.

darifenacin
Enablex

Class and Category
Chemical class: Muscarinic receptor antagonist
Therapeutic class: Bladder antispasmodic
Pregnancy category: C

Indications and Dosages
➤ *To treat overactive urinary bladder with symptoms of urge incontinence, including urgency and frequency*
E.R. TABLETS
Adults. *Initial:* 7.5 mg daily, increased to 15 mg daily after 2 wk as needed.
DOSAGE ADJUSTMENT For patients with moderate hepatic impairment and those taking potent CYP3A4 inhibitors (such as clarithromycin, itraconazole, ketoconazole, nefazodone, nelfinavir, and ritonavir) daily dosage should not exceed 7.5 mg.

Route	Onset	Peak	Duration
P.O.	Unknown	7 hr	Unknown

Mechanism of Action
Antagonizes effect of acetylcholine on muscarinic receptors in detrusor muscle, decreasing muscle spasms that cause inappropriate bladder emptying. This action increases bladder capacity and volume, which relieves sensations of urgency and frequency and enhances bladder control.

Contraindications
Gastric retention, hypersensitivity to darifenacin or its components, uncontrolled narrow-angle glaucoma, urine retention, and patients at risk for these conditions

Interactions
DRUGS
anticholinergics: Increased frequency and severity of anticholinergic adverse reactions
flecainide, thioridazine, tricyclic antidepressants: Risk of toxicity with these drugs
potent CYP3A4 inhibitors (such as clarithromycin, itraconazole, ketoconazole, nefazodone, nelfinavir, and ritonavir): Decreased metabolism and increased effects of darifenacin, possibly increasing the risk of adverse reactions

Adverse Reactions
CNS: Asthenia, confusion, dizziness, hallucinations, headache, somnolence
CV: Hypertension, palpitations, peripheral edema
EENT: Abnormal vision, dry eyes or mouth, pharyngitis, rhinitis, sinusitis
GI: Abdominal pain, constipation, diarrhea, indigestion, nausea, vomiting
GU: Urine retention, UTI, vaginitis
MS: Arthralgia, back pain
RESP: Airway obstruction, bronchitis
SKIN: Dry skin, erythema multiforme, interstitial granuloma annulare, pruritus, rash
Other: Anaphylaxis, angioedema, flulike symptoms, hypersensitivity reactions, weight gain

Nursing Considerations
- Use darifenacin cautiously in patients with significant bladder outflow obstruction; they have increased risk of urine retention. Also use cautiously in patients with controlled narrow-angle glaucoma, as darifenacin therapy may worsen this condition.
- Use darifenacin cautiously in patients with severe constipation, ulcerative colitis, or myasthenia gravis because it may decrease

GI motility. Also use drug cautiously in obstructive GI disorders because it increases the risk of gastric retention.

• Monitor patient for signs of anticholineric CNS effects such as headache, confusion, hallucinations, and somnolence, especially at beginning of therapy and with dosage increases.

WARNING Monitor patient closely for serious adverse reactions that may become life-threatening, such as anaphylaxis and angioedema of the face, lips, tongue, and/or larynx that may occur even after just one dose. If present, withhold drug, notify prescriber immediately, and provide emergency supportive care, as indicated.

PATIENT TEACHING
• Tell patient to swallow tablets with liquid and not to crush, split, or break them.
• Advise patient to avoid exercising in hot weather because darifenacin decreases sweating, increasing the risk of heatstroke.
• Caution patient to avoid hazardous activities until drug's CNS effects are known.
• Warn patient to seek immediate medical attention if he experiences any signs of a serious drug reaction, including swelling of his face, lips, tongue, and/or throat.

deferasirox
Exjade

Class and Category
Chemical class: Benzoic acid
Therapeutic class: Iron chelator
Pregnancy category: B

Indications and Dosages
➤ *To treat chronic iron overload caused by blood transfusions*

TABLETS
Adults and children age 2 and over.
Initial: 20 mg/kg/day, increased by 5 to 10 mg/kg every 3 to 6 mo, as needed.
Maximum: 40 mg/kg/day.
➤ *To treat chronic iron overload in patients with non-transfusion-dependent Thalassemia syndromes and who have a liver iron concentration of at least 5 mg of iron per gram of liver*

dry weight and a serum ferritin greater than 300 mcg/L

TABLETS
Adults and children age 10 and over.
Initial: 10 mg/kg once daily and continued for 6 months if the liver iron concentration falls between 3 to 7 mg of iron per gram of dry liver weight. Increased to 20 mg/kg once daily after 4 wks, if baseline liver iron concentration is greater than 15 mg of iron per gram of liver dry weight or if after 6 months, the liver iron concentration remains greater than 7 mg of iron per gram of dry liver weight. *Maximum:* 20 mg/kg once daily.

DOSAGE ADJUSTMENT For adults with moderate (Child-Pugh C) hepatic or renal impairment (creatinine clearance between 40 to 60 ml/min), starting dose reduced by 50%. During deferasirox therapy to treat transfusional iron overload in adults and adolescents age 16 and older, dosage reduced by 10 mg/kg when rise in serum creatinine increases by 33% or more above the average of the pretreatment measurements seen at two consecutive visits within one week and not attributed to other causes. During deferasirox therapy to treat transfusional iron overload in children ages 2 to 15, dosage reduced by 10 mg/kg when rise in serum creatinine increases by 33% or more above the average baseline measurement and rises above the age-appropriate upper limit of normal. During deferasirox therapy to treat non-tranfusion-dependent Thalassemia syndromes in adults and adolescents age 16 years and older, dosage temporarily interrupted if current dose is 5 mg/kg or reduced by 50% if current dose is 10 or 20 mg/kg if serum creatinine increases by 33% or more above the average baseline measurement and remains elevated at 33% or more after 1 week. During deferasirox therapy to treat non-transfusion-dependent Thalasemia syndromes in children ages 10 to 15 years, current dose reduced by 5 mg/kg if serum creatinine increases to greater than 33% above the average baseline measurement and greater than the age appropriate upper limit of normal. For patients who are receiving cholestyramine, colesevelam, colestipol, or potent UGT inducers such as phenobarbital, phenytoin, rifampicin, or ritonavir, initial dosage increased by 50% with further modifications, as needed.

Mechanism of Action

Binds iron with high affinity and removes it in feces. Deferasirox is a tridentate ligan.

Route	Onset	Peak	Duration
P.O.	Unknown	1.5–4 hr	Unknown

Contraindications

Creatinine clearance of less than 40 ml/min or serum creatinine greater than 2 times the age-appropriate upper limit of normal, hypersensitivity to deferasirox or its components, hearing impairment, poor performance status, high-risk myelodysplastic syndromes or advanced malignancies, platelet counts less than 50×10^9/L, severe (Child-Pugh C) hepatic impairment

Interactions

DRUGS

aluminum-containing antacids, cholestyramine, colesevelam, colestipol, phenobarbital, phenytoin, rifampicin, ritonavir: Possibly decreased effectiveness of deferasirox

anticoagulants, corticosteroids, NSAIDs, oral bisphosphonates: Increased risk of GI ulceration or hemorrhage

cyclobenzaprine, imipramine, haloperidol, fluvoxamine, mexiletine, olanzapine, tizanidine, zileuton, zolmitriptan: Possible increased plasma levels and effects of these drugs

cyclosporine, hormonal contraceptives, midazolam, simvastatin: Possibly decreased effectiveness of these drugs

iron chelators: Possibly combined effect

paclitaxel, repaglinide, theophylline: Increased plasma levels and effects of these drugs

FOODS

food: Increased bioavailability of deferasirox

Adverse Reactions

CNS: Dizziness, fatigue, fever, headache, hyperactivity, insomnia

EENT: Acute tonsillitis, cataracts, decreased hearing, ear infection, elevated intraocular pressure, high-frequency hearing loss, lens opacities, nasopharyngitis, pharyngolaryngeal pain, pharyngitis, retinal disturbances, rhinitis

GI: Abdominal pain, diarrhea, elevated liver enzymes, gallstones, hepatic failure, hepatitis, nausea, pancreatitis, upper GI ulceration and hemorrhage, vomiting

GU: Acute renal failure, glycosuria, increased creatinine, proteinuria, renal tubulopathy, tubulointerstitial nephritis

HEME: Agranulocytosis, neutropenia, thrombocytopenia, worsening anemia

MS: Arthralgia, back pain

RESP: Bronchitis, cough, respiratory tract infection

SKIN: Erythema multiforme, leukocytoclastic vasculitis, purpura, rash, Stevens-Johnson syndrome, urticaria

Other: Anaphylaxis, angioedema, drug fever, influenza

Nursing Considerations

• Ensure that a baseline serum ferritin level has been obtained prior to initiation of deferasirox therapy when deferasirox is used to treat chronic iron overload due to blood transfusions. If drug is used to treat chronic iron overload in non-transfusion-dependent Thalassemia syndromes, ensure patient has had a liver biopsy or an FDA-approved method for identifying need for deferasirox therapy, in addition to having two serum ferritin levels done a month apart,

• Because deferasirox can cause renal failure, obtain baseline assessment of patient's renal function by collecting blood samples to measure serum creatinine level twice, as ordered, before starting deferasirox. When therapy starts, monitor serum creatinine level, as ordered, especially in elderly patients, patients taking other drugs that depress renal function, and patients with increased risk of complications, preexisting renal conditions, or comorbid conditions. For patients starting deferasirox therapy or when a dosage adjustment occurs, expect to monitor serum creatinine level weekly for first month and monthly thereafter. Report increased serum creatinine level, and expect deferasirox dosage to be decreased. Be aware that deferasirox should not be given to patients with serum creatinine levels greater than 2 times the upper limit of normal of if the creatinine clearance is less than 40 ml/min.

• Because deferasirox may cause hepatic abnormalities and failure, obtain baseline assessment of hepatic function before therapy starts by collecting blood samples to measure liver enzymes and bilirubin level. When therapy starts, monitor these levels every 2 weeks for first month and then monthly thereafter. Notify prescriber about elevations, and expect to decrease dose for severe or persistent elevations. Be aware that deferasirox should be avoided in patients with severe hepatic impairment.

• Obtain auditory and ophthalmic testing (including slit lamp examination and dilated fundoscopy) before deferasirox therapy begins and yearly thereafter, as ordered, because drug infrequently causes auditory or visual disturbances.

• Monitor patient's serum ferritin monthly and expect dosage to be adjusted, as needed. Be aware that if serum ferritin level falls consistently below 500 mcg/L in the treatment of chronic iron overload due to blood transufsions, deferasirox may be temporarily withheld.

• Monitor patient's serum ferritin monthly and the patient's liver iron concentration every 6 months, as ordered, for patients with chronic iron overload in non-transfusion-dependent Thalassemia syndromes, Expect deferasirox treatment to be temporarily withheld when serum ferritin is less than 300 mcg/L. Obtain a liver iron concentration at that time, as ordered, to determine if it has fallen to less than 3 mg of iron per gram of liver dry weight.

• Monitor patient's blood counts regularly, as ordered, because deferasirox can cause cytopenias. If cytopenia occurs, expect drug to be discontinued until blood counts return to normal. Know that deferasirox should not be given to patients with severely depressed platelet counts.

• Especially in the first month of therapy, assess patient closely for hypersensitivity reactions, such as anaphylaxis or angioedema. Notify prescriber immediately if present, and expect drug to be discontinued. Provide care, as needed.

• Inspect patient's skin regularly for rash. If it occurs and becomes severe, drug may be withheld temporarily or discontinued.

• Watch for evidence of GI ulceration and hemorrhage, especially if patient takes drugs that increase the risk of ulceration and bleeding, such as NSAIDs, corticosteroids, oral bisphosphonates, or anticoagulants, or if patient is elderly and has advanced hematologic malignancies and/or low platelet counts. Notify prescriber of suspected GI ulceration or hemorrhage, and prepare patient for further evaluation and treatment, as prescribed.

• Monitor elderly patients closely during deferasirox therapy because these patients are at an increased risk for developing deferasirox toxicity.

PATIENT TEACHING

• Instruct patient to take deferasirox 30 minutes before eating. Tell her to completely disperse the tablet in water, orange juice, or apple juice (3.5 ounces if dose is less than 1 gram and 7 ounces if dose is 1 gram or greater); drink the suspension immediately; and then add liquid to any remaining residue and drink again. Warn that she should never chew tablets or swallow them whole.

• Tell patient to avoid taking aluminum-based antacids at the same time as deferasirox and to seek prescriber advice before taking other drugs, including OTC preparations such as NSAIDs, because of potential interactions.

• Advise her to report any hearing or visual disturbances.

• If patient has diarrhea or vomiting, tell her to notify prescriber and to stay hydrated.

• Caution her to avoid hazardous activities, such as driving, if she becomes dizzy.

deferoxamine mesylate

Desferal

Class and Category

Chemical class: Monomethanesulfonate salt
Therapeutic class: Iron chelator
Pregnancy category: C

Indications and Dosages

➤ *To treat acute iron intoxication*

I.M. INJECTION
Adults and children age 3 and over who are not in shock. *Initial:* 1,000 mg, followed by 500 mg every 4 hr for 2 doses, if needed. Additional doses of 500 mg may be administered every 4 to 12 hr, as needed. *Maximum:* 6,000 mg in 24 hr.
I.V. INFUSION
Adults and children age 3 and over who are in shock. *Initial:* 1,000 mg administered at a rate not to exceed 15 mg/kg/hr, followed by 500 mg administered at a rate not to exceed 125 mg/hr every 4 hr for 2 doses, if needed. Additional doses of 500 mg may be administered at a rate not to exceed 125 mg/hr every 4 to 12 hr, as needed. *Maximum:* 6,000 mg in 24 hr.
➤ *To treat chronic iron overload*
I.M. INJECTION
Adults and children age 3 and over. 500 to 1,000 mg daily. *Maximum:* 1,000 mg daily in absence of transfusion.
I.V. INFUSION
Adults and children age 3 and over. For patients receiving daily intramuscular treatment above and requiring blood transfusion, additional 2,000 mg administered at a rate not to exceed 15 mg/kg/hr for each unit of blood transfused but infused separately from the blood. *Maximum:* 6,000 mg daily, including daily intramuscular dosage, and even if 3 or more units of blood or packed red blood cells are given.
SUBCUTANEOUS INFUSION
Adults and children age 3 and over. 20 to 40 mg/kg/day administered over 8 to 24 hr.

Mechanism of Action

Binds iron by forming a stable complex with it. This prevents iron from entering into further chemical reactions. The chelate then passes through the kidneys and out of the body in urine, thereby decreasing the iron level in the body.

Contraindications

Anuria, hypersensitivity to deferoxamine or its components, severe renal disease

Interactions
DRUGS
prochlorperazine: Possibly impaired consciousness

vitamin C: Increased availability of iron for chelation by deferoxamine

Adverse Reactions

CNS: Dizziness, exacerbation or precipitation of aluminum-related dialysis encephalopathy, fever, headache, paresthesias, peripheral neuropathy, seizures
CV: Hypotension, shock, tachycardia
EENT: Blurred vision, cataracts, decreased acuity, dyschromatopsia, high-frequency sensorineural hearing loss, loss of vision, night blindness, optic neuritis, retinopathy, scotoma, tinnitus, visual field defects
GI: Abdominal discomfort, diarrhea, hepatic dysfunction, increased liver enzymes, nausea, vomiting
GU: Acute renal failure, dysuria, increased serum creatinine, renal tubular disorder
HEME: Leukopenia, thrombocytopenia
MS: Arthralgia, growth retardation, metaphyseal dysplasia, myalgia
RESP: Acute respiratory distress syndrome, asthma
SKIN: Rash, urticaria
Other: Anaphylaxis; angioedema; infections with *Yersinia* or *Mucormycosis;* injection-site reactions such as localized irritation, pain, burning, swelling, induration, infiltration, pruritus, erythema, wheal formation, eschar, crust, vesicles, or local edema

Nursing Considerations

• Expect to administer other supportive measures, as ordered, when treating acute iron intoxication with deferoxamine because acute respiratory distress syndrome may occur. Supportive measures include induction of emesis with syrup of ipecac; gastric lavage, suction, and maintenance of a clear airway; control of shock with intravenous fluids, blood, oxygen, and vasopressors; and correction of acidosis.
• Know that patients with thalassemia inadvertently given a high dose or rapid intravenous infusion of deferoxamine may develop acute respiratory distress syndrome and other life-threatening disorders such as hypotension, CNS depression, and acute renal failure. Symptomatic treatment is required, as there is no specific antidote for deferoxamine, although the drug is readily dialyzable.

• Reconstitute drug according to how the drug will be administered. For intramuscular administration, add 2 ml of diluent (sterile water for injection) to a 500-mg vial or 8 ml of diluent to a 2-g vial. For intravenous or subcutaneous administration, add 5 ml of diluent (sterile water for injection) to a 500-mg vial or 20 ml of diluent to a 2-g vial. Make sure drug is completely dissolved before the solution is withdrawn. Discard unused portion.

• Further dilute reconstituted solution with normal or half normal saline, glucose in water, or Ringer's lactate solution if drug will be administered intravenously.

• Follow infusion rates exactly as ordered when drug is administered intravenously because flushing, urticaria, hypotension, and shock have occurred in a few patients when deferoxamine was administered by rapid intravenous injection.

• Use a portable pump capable of providing continuous mini-infusion when administering drug by subcutaneous infusion. Be aware that the duration of infusion must be individualized as some patients excrete more iron after a short infusion of 8 to 12 hours, while another patient may need a 24-hour infusion to excrete the same amount.

• Monitor patient closely for changes in hearing or vision, especially in patients receiving deferoxamine over prolonged periods of time, or at high doses, or in patients who have low ferritin levels. If present, notify prescriber immediately and expect drug to be discontinued. Expect visual acuity tests, slit-lamp examinations, fundoscopy, and audiometry to be performed periodically in patients treated for prolonged periods of time. Early detection improves the possibility of reversal of these symptoms or test abnormalities.

• Monitor patient's serum creatinine level, and assess patient for symptoms of renal dysfunction, because deferoxamine has been associated with renal dysfunction.

• Assess children regularly for growth retardation, especially if high doses of the drug are being administered in the presence of low ferritin levels. Monitor the child's body weight and growth every 3 months. If abnormalities are detected, notify the prescriber because growth velocity may partially resume to pretreatment rates after a reduction of deferoxamine dosage occurs.

• Monitor patient, especially children, closely for signs and symptoms of respiratory distress, especially following treatment with excessively high intravenous doses of deferoxamine.

• Assess patient regularly for infections because either deferoxamine therapy or iron overload may enhance susceptibility to generalized infections. Some cases of mucormycosis have been fatal. If signs and symptoms occur, notify prescriber immediately and expect drug to be discontinued and appropriate treatment instituted.

• Expect to administer vitamin C with deferoxamine therapy because iron overload usually causes a vitamin C deficiency. However, be aware that high doses (more than 500 mg daily in adults, 100 mg in children age 10 and older, and 50 mg in children under age 10) may cause cardiac dysfunction. Therefore, make sure patient is not receiving vitamin C if he has cardiac failure, expect supplemental vitamin C therapy to begin only after an initial month of regular treatment with deferoxamine, and make sure the daily dose of vitamin C does not exceed 200 mg in adults, given in divided doses. Monitor all patients receiving deferoxamine and vitamin C therapy concomitantly for cardiac dysfunction and report any dysfunction immediately to prescriber.

• Be aware that patients with aluminum-related encephalopathy who are receiving dialysis may develop seizures as a result of deferoxamine therapy. Deferoxamine therapy may also precipitate the onset of dialysis dementia in these patients, as well as cause a decrease in the patient's serum calcium levels and aggravate hyperparathyroidism, if present.

• Discontinue deferoxamine therapy, as ordered, 48 hours prior to scinitigraphy because imaging results may be distorted as a result of the rapid urinary excretion of deferoxamine-bound gallium-67.

D

PATIENT TEACHING
• Inform patient that deferoxamine therapy is an adjunct to, and not a substitute for, standard measures used to treat acute iron intoxication.
• Advise patient not to exceed the recommended dose of daily vitamin C therapy prescribed.
• Caution patient not to perform hazardous activities such as driving until CNS, visual, and auditory adverse effects are known.
• Inform patient that his urine may have a reddish discoloration because of deferoxamine therapy.

demeclocycline hydrochloride

Declomycin

Class and Category
Chemical class: Tetracycline derivative
Therapeutic class: Antibiotic
Pregnancy category: D

Indications and Dosages
➤ *To treat Rocky Mountain spotted fever, typhus infections, Q fever, and Rickettsialpox and tick fevers caused by rickettsieae; psittacosis (ornithosis), lymphogranuloma venereum, granuloma inguinale, and* Mycoplasma pneumoniae *or* Borrelia recurrentis *infections; infections caused by gram-negative organisms, such as* Bacteroides *species,* Bartonella bacilliformis, Brucella *species,* Campylobacter fetus, Francisella tularensis, Haemophilus ducreyi, Vibrio cholerae, *and* Yersinia pestis; *infections caused by susceptible strains of* Acinetobacter calcoaceticus, Enterobacter aerogenes, Escherichia coli, Haemophilus influenzae *(respiratory tract infections),* Herellea *species,* Klebsiella *species (respiratory tract infections and UTIs), and* Shigella *species; infections caused by susceptible strains of* Staphylococcus aureus *(skin and soft-tissue infections) and* Streptococcus *species; infections caused by* Actinomyces *species,* Bacillus anthracis, Clostridium *species,* Fusobacterium fusiforme, Listeria monocytogenes, Treponema pallidum, *and* Treponema pertenue; *and acute intestinal amebiasis*

CAPSULES, TABLETS
Adults and adolescents. 150 mg every 6 hr or 300 mg every 12 hr.
Children ages 8 to 12. 6 to 12 mg/kg daily in divided doses every 6 to 12 hr.
➤ *To treat gonorrhea*
CAPSULES, TABLETS
Adults and adolescents. 600 mg followed by 300 mg every 12 hr for 4 days for total dose of 3,000 mg.

Mechanism of Action
Binds with ribosomal subunits of susceptible bacteria and alters the cytoplasmic membrane, inhibiting bacterial protein synthesis and rendering organism ineffective.

Contraindications
Hypersensitivity to demeclocycline or other tetracyclines

Interactions
DRUGS
antacids, calcium supplements, cholestyramine, choline, colestipol, iron supplements, magnesium-containing laxatives, magnesium salicylate, sodium bicarbonate: Decreased demeclocycline absorption
digoxin: Possibly increased blood digoxin level and risk of digitalis toxicity
methoxyflurane: Increased nephrotoxicity
oral anticoagulants: Increased anticoagulation
oral contraceptives: Decreased contraceptive effectiveness
penicillins: Decreased bactericidal action of penicillins
vitamin A: Possibly benign intracranial hypertension
FOODS
milk, other dairy products: Decreased drug absorption

Adverse Reactions
CNS: Dizziness, headache, light-headedness, vertigo
EENT: Tinnitus, vision changes
GI: Abdominal cramps, diarrhea, nausea, pseudomembranous colitis, vomiting

GU: Elevated BUN level, nephrogenic diabetes insipidus
HEME: Eosinophilia, hemolytic anemia, neutropenia, thrombocytopenia
SKIN: Photosensitivity, pruritus, rash, urticaria
Other: Anaphylaxis, angioedema

Nursing Considerations
• Expect to monitor renal and liver function tests during demeclocycline therapy.
WARNING Watch for nephrogenic diabetes insipidus during long-term therapy.
• Assess patient's bowel pattern daily; severe diarrhea may indicate pseudomembranous colitis caused by *Clostridium difficile.* If diarrhea occurs, notify prescriber and expect to withhold demeclocycline and treat with fluids, electrolytes, protein, and an antibiotic effective against *C. difficile.*
PATIENT TEACHING
• Emphasize importance of completing therapy as prescribed, even if symptoms improve.
• Advise patient not to take demeclocycline within 3 hours of other drugs or dairy products; its absorption may decrease.
• Instruct patient to avoid taking antacids because of impaired drug absorption.
• Advise patient to avoid direct sunlight, use sunscreen, and wear protective clothing outdoors; among tetracyclines, demeclocycline causes the most photosensitivity.
• Urge patient to immediately report edema, rash, or other hypersensitivity reactions.
• Urge patient to report watery, bloody stools to prescriber immediately, even up to 2 months after drug therapy has ended.
• Tell patient to avoid hazardous activities if light-headed, dizzy, or vertigo occurs.
• Instruct female patient of childbearing age to notify prescriber if she may be pregnant; drug may need to be discontinued.

denosumab
Prolia, Xgeva

Class and Category
Chemical class: Human IgG2 monoclonal antibody
Therapeutic class: Bone resorption inhibitor

Pregnancy category: X

Indications and Dosages
➤ *To treat men and postmenopausal women with osteoporosis at high risk for fracture; to treat bone loss in men receiving androgen deprivation therapy for prostate cancer; to treat bone loss in women receiving adjuvant aromatase inhibitor therapy for breast cancer*
SUBCUTANEOUS INJECTION (PROLIA)
Adult. 60 mg once every 6 months.
➤ *To treat bone metastasis from solid tumors*
SUBCUTANEOUS INJECTION (XGEVA)
Adult. 120 mg every 4 wks.
➤ *To treat giant cell tumor of bone; to treat hypercalcemia of malignancy refractory to bisphosphonate therapy*
SUBCUTANEOUS INJECTION (XGEVA)
Adult. 120 mg every 4 wks with additional 120 mg doses on days 8 and 15 of the first month of therapy.

Route	Onset	Peak	Duration
SubQ	Unknown	10 days	Unknown

Mechanism of Action
Binds to RANKL, a transmembrane or soluble protein required for the formation, function, and survival of osteoclasts, the cells responsible for bone resorption. By preventing RANKL from activating its receptor, RANK, on the surface of osteoclasts, osteoclast formation, function, and survival are inhibited. This action decreases bone resorption and increases bone mass and strength in both cortical and trabecular bone.

Contraindications
Hypersensitivity to denosumab and its components, hypocalcemia, pregnancy

Interactions
DRUGS
other calcium lowering drugs: Augmentation of calcium-lowering effect with possible severe hypocalcemia

Adverse Reactions
CNS: Asthenia, insomnia, sciatica, vertigo
CV: Angina pectoris, atrial fibrillation, hypercholesterolemia, peripheral edema
EENT: Pharyngitis

D

ENDO: Hypocalcemia, increased serum parathyroid hormone levels (presence of severe renal impairment or dialysis)
GI: Constipation, flatulence, gastroesophageal reflux disease, pancreatitis, upper abdominal pain
GU: Cystitis
HEME: Anemia
MS: Atypical subtrochanteric and diaphyseal femoral fractures; back, bone, extremity including joint, or musculoskeletal pain; jaw osteonecrosis; myalgia; spinal osteoarthritis
RESP: Pneumonia, upper respiratory infection
SKIN: Cellulitis, dermatitis, eczema, erysipelas (infection of upper dermis and superficial lymphatics), erythema, pruritus, rash, urticaria
Other: Anaphylaxis, angioedema, herpes zoster, malignancies (breast, gastrointestinal, reproductive), serious infections

Nursing Considerations

• Know that preexisting hypocalcemia must be corrected prior to denosumab therapy.
• Be aware that the drug solution may contain trace amounts of translucent to white proteinaceous particles. However, do not use if the solution is discolored or cloudy, or if the solution contains many particles or foreign particulate matter.
• Do not handle the gray needle cap on the prefilled syringe if allergic to latex.
• Prior to administration, remove drug from refrigerator and bring to room temperature, which generally takes 15 to 30 minutes. Do not warm the drug any other way.
• When preparing to administer drug using the single prefilled syringe, do not slide the green safety guard forward over the needle, as it will lock in place and prevent injection. Do so only after the injection to prevent an accidental needle stick.
• When using the single-use vial, withdraw solution from vial using a 27-gauge needle. Also administer the drug using a 27-gauge needle.
• Administer denosumab in the upper arm, thigh, or abdomen.

WARNING Monitor patient closely for hypersensitivity reactions that may be severe such as hypotension, dyspnea, upper airway edema, lip swelling, rash, pruritis, and urticaria. If present, stop denosumab therapy immediately, notify prescriber, and provide supportive care, as needed and ordered.

WARNING Monitor patient's calcium level, as ordered, especially in patients predisposed to hypocalcemia or disturbances of mineral metabolism, such as a history of hypoparathyroidism, thyroid or parathyroid surgery, malabsorption syndromes, excision of the small intestine, or severe renal impairment. Know that severe hypocalcemia has occurred with denosumab therapy resulting, in some cases, in death. Monitor patient closely for signs and symptoms of hypocalemia such as neuromuscular irritability, and notify prescriber immediately if present. Expect drug to be discontinued, administer calcium replacement therapy, as ordered, and provide supportive care.

PATIENT TEACHING

• Instruct patient to take a calcium supplement of 1,000 mg and at least 400 international units of vitamin D daily.
• Advise patient to notify prescriber if signs and symptoms of infection occur, such as fever, pain, swelling, redness, or drainage.
• Inform patient to report bone, joint, and/or muscle pain as drug may need to be discontinued depending on the severity.
• Tell patient to notify prescriber if severe adverse skin reactions occur, as drug may need to be discontinued.
• Instruct patient on proper oral hygiene and on the need to notify dentist of denosumab therapy before invasive dental procedures are performed.
• Instruct women of childbearing age receiving drug for breast cancer to report suspected or confirmed pregnancy immediately, as drug may need to be discontinued.
• Advise patient to report new or unusual thigh, hip, or groin pain or tingling or numbness in fingers and toes.

desipramine hydrochloride

Norpramin, Pertofrane (CAN)

Class and Category

Chemical class: Dibenzazepine derivative
Therapeutic class: Antidepressant
Pregnancy category: C

Indications and Dosages

➤ *To treat depression*

TABLETS

Adults. *Initial:* 100 to 200 mg daily as single dose or divided doses. Increased gradually to 300 mg daily, if needed. *Maximum:* 300 mg daily.

Adolescents. *Initial:* 25 to 50 mg daily in divided doses. Increased gradually, if needed. *Maximum:* 100 mg daily.

Children ages 6 to 12. *Initial:* 10 to 30 mg daily, or 1 to 5 mg/kg, in divided doses.

DOSAGE ADJUSTMENT For elderly patients, initial dosage decreased to 25 to 50 mg daily in divided doses; increased gradually, if needed, to maximum of 150 mg daily.

Route	Onset	Peak	Duration
P.O.	2–3 wk	Unknown	Unknown

Mechanism of Action

Blocks serotonin and norepinephrine reuptake by adrenergic nerves, which normally release these neurotransmitters from their storage sites when activated by a nerve impulse. By blocking reuptake, this tricyclic antidepressant increases serotonin and norepinephrine levels at nerve synapses, which may elevate mood and reduce depression.

Contraindications

Acute recovery phase of MI; hypersensitivity to desipramine, other tricyclic antidepressants, or their components; linezolid or I.V. methylene blue; MAO inhibitor therapy within 14 days

Interactions

DRUGS

activated charcoal: Prevention of desipramine absorption, reduced effects

barbiturates: Decreased blood desipramine level, increased CNS depression

bupropion, haloperidol, H_2-receptor antagonists, valproic acid: Increased blood level and adverse effects of desipramine

carbamazepine: Increased blood carbamazepine level, decreased blood desipramine level

cimetidine: Increased blood desipramine level and anticholinergic effects (dry mouth, urine retention, blurred vision)

clonidine: Increased risk of hypertensive crisis

dicumarol: Increased anticoagulant effect

grepafloxacin, quinolones, sparfloxacin: Increased risk of arrhythmias, including torsades de pointes

guanethidine: Antagonized antihypertensive effect of guanethidine

levodopa: Delayed levodopa absorption, increased risk of hypotension

MAO inhibitors: Increased risk of life-threatening adverse effects, such as hyperpyretic or hypertensive crisis and severe seizures

phenothiazines: Increased desipramine level, risk of inhibited phenothiazine metabolism and neuroleptic malignant syndrome

quinidine: Increased blood quinidine level

rifamycins: Decreased desipramine effects

selective serotonin reuptake inhibitors: Increased desipramine effects

sympathomimetics: Possibly arrhythmias, possibly increased or decreased vasopressor effects of sympathomimetics

ACTIVITIES

alcohol use: Possibly increased CNS or respiratory depression, hypotension, alcohol effects

Adverse Reactions

CNS: Agitation, akathisia, anxiety, ataxia, confusion, delusions, disorientation, dizziness, drowsiness, extrapyramidal reactions, fatigue, headache, hypomania, insomnia, lack of coordination, nervousness, nightmares, paresthesia, peripheral neuropathy, psychosis exacerbation, restlessness, seizures, serotonin syndrome, sleep disturbance, stroke, suicidal ideation (children and teens), tremor, weakness

CV: Arrhythmias, including heart block; hypertension; hypotension; palpitations

EENT: Acute-angle glaucoma, black tongue, blurred vision, dry mouth, mydriasis, stomatitis, taste perversion, tinnitus

D

ENDO: Breast enlargement and galactorrhea (women), gynecomastia (men), hyperglycemia, hypoglycemia, syndrome of inappropriate ADH secretion
GI: Abdominal cramps, anorexia, constipation, diarrhea, elevated liver function test results, elevated pancreatic enzyme levels, epigastric distress, hepatitis, ileus, increased appetite, nausea, vomiting
GU: Acute renal failure, impotence, libido changes, nocturia, painful ejaculation, testicular swelling, urinary frequency and hesitancy, urine retention
HEME: Agranulocytosis, eosinophilia, thrombocytopenia
SKIN: Acne, alopecia, dermatitis, diaphoresis, dry skin, flushing, petechiae, photosensitivity, pruritus, purpura, rash, urticaria
Other: Angioedema, drug fever, weight gain

Nursing Considerations

• Use desipramine with extreme caution in patients with cardiovascular disease, glaucoma, seizure disorder, thyroid disease, or urine retention or with a family history of sudden death, cardiac arrhythmias, or conduction disturbances.
WARNING Desipramine increases risk of suicidal ideation in children and teens; monitor them closely for evidence.
WARNING Expect drug to produce sedation and possibly to lower seizure threshold. Take safety and seizure precautions. Seizures may precede arrhythmias and death in some patients. Alert prescriber immediately if seizure activity occurs.
• Monitor blood glucose level often.
• Be prepared to obtain blood sample for leukocyte and differential counts if patient develops fever during therapy.
• Expect to discontinue drug as soon as possible before elective surgery because of its possible adverse cardiovascular effects.
WARNING Monitor patient closely for evidence of serotonin syndrome, such as agitation, hallucinations, coma, tachycardia, labile blood pressure, hyperthermia, hyperreflexia, incoordination, nausea, vomiting, or diarrhea. Notify prescriber at once because serotonin syndrome maybe life-threatening. Be prepared to discontinue drug and provide supportive care.

PATIENT TEACHING
WARNING Urge parents to watch child or teen closely and to report abnormal thinking or behavior, aggression, or hostility.
• Urge patient to use sunscreen outdoors and to avoid sunlamps and tanning beds.
• Instruct patient to notify prescriber immediately about a fast and pounding heartbeat, fainting, severe agitation or restlessness, and strange behavior or thoughts.
• Caution patient not to stop drug abruptly; doing so may cause dizziness, headache, hyperthermia, irritability, malaise, nausea, sleep disturbances, and vomiting.
• Advise against drinking alcohol because of increased risk of adverse CNS reactions.
• Advise patient to avoid hazardous activities until drug's CNS effects are known.
• Advise patient that drug may cause mild pupillary dilation, which may lead to an episode of acute-angle glaucoma. Encourage patient to have an eye exam before starting therapy to see if she is at risk.
• Urge diabetic patient to monitor blood glucose level often.

desmopressin acetate

DDAVP Injection, DDAVP Nasal Spray, DDAVP Rhinal Tube, DDAVP Rhinyle Nasal Solution (CAN), DDAVP Tablets, Octostim (CAN), Stimate, Stimate Nasal Spray

Class and Category

Chemical class: Synthetic ADH analogue
Therapeutic class: Antidiuretic, antihemorrhagic
Pregnancy category: B

Indications and Dosages

➤ *To manage primary nocturnal enuresis*
TABLETS
Adults and children age 6 and over.
Initial: 0.2 mg at bedtime, increased as needed. *Maximum:* 0.6 mg daily.
➤ *To control symptoms of central diabetes insipidus*
TABLETS
Adults and children age 6 and over.

Initial: 0.05 mg twice daily, increased as needed. *Usual:* 0.1 to 0.8 mg in divided doses twice daily or three timesdaily. *Maximum:* 1.2 mg daily.

I.V. INFUSION, I.M. OR SUBCUTANEOUS INJECTION
Adults. 2 to 4 mcg daily in divided doses twice daily. Dosage adjusted as needed.

NASAL SOLUTION
Adults and adolescents. 0.1 to 0.4 ml daily (10 to 40 mcg daily) as a single dose or in divided doses twice daily or three times daily. Dosage adjusted as needed. If daily dose is divided, each dose adjusted separately.
Children ages 3 months to 12 years. 0.25 mcg/kg daily as a single dose or in divided doses twice daily. Dosage adjusted as needed. If daily dose is divided, each dose adjusted separately.

➤ *To prevent or manage bleeding episodes in hemophilia A or mild to moderate type I von Willebrand's disease*

I.V. INFUSION
Adults and children weighing more than 10 kg (22 lb). 0.3 mcg/kg diluted in 50 ml of normal saline solution and infused over 15 to 30 min. If used preoperatively, given 30 min before procedure.
Children weighing 10 kg or less. 0.3 mcg/kg diluted in 10 ml normal saline solution and infused over 15 to 30 min. If used preoperatively, given 30 min before procedure.

NASAL SOLUTION (STIMATE NASAL SPRAY)
Adults and children weighing more than 50 kg (110 lb). 150 mcg in each nostril. If used preoperatively, given 2 hr before procedure.
Adults and children weighing 50 kg or less. 150 mcg in one nostril. If used preoperatively, given 2 hr before procedure.

Route	Onset	Peak	Duration
P.O.	1 hr*	4–7 hr*	8–12 hr*
I.V.	15–30 min†	30–60 min†	3 hr‡
Nasal	In 1 hr*	1–5 hr*	8–20 hr*

Mechanism of Action

Exerts an antidiuretic effect similar to that of vasopressin by increasing cellular

---

* For antidiuretic effect.
† For antihemorrhagic effect.
‡ For von Willebrand disease; 4 to 20 hr for mild hemophilia A.

permeability of renal collecting ducts and distal tubules, thus enhancing water reabsorption, reducing urine flow, and increasing osmolality. As an antihemorrhagic, drug increases blood level of clotting factor VIII (antihemophilic factor) and activity of von Willebrand factor (factor VII_{VWF}). It also may increase platelet aggregation and adhesion at injury sites by directly affecting blood vessel walls.

Contraindications

Hypersensitivity to desmopressin or its components, moderate to severe renal impairment (creatinine clearance below 50 ml/min/1.73 m²), previous or current hyponatremia

Interactions

DRUGS
carbamazepine, chlorpromazine, lamotrigine, NSAIDs, opioid analgesics, selective serotonin reuptake inhibitors, tricyclic antidepressants: Possibly increased risk of water intoxication with hyponatremia
demeclocycline, lithium: Possibly decreased antidiuretic effect of desmopressin
imipramine, oxybutinin: Increased risk of hyponatremic seizures
vasopressor drugs: Possibly potentiated vasopressor effect of desmopressin

Adverse Reactions

CNS: Asthenia, chills, dizziness, headache, stroke
CV: Hypertension (with high doses), MI, thrombosis, transient hypotension
EENT: Conjunctivitis, epistaxis, lacrimation, nasal congestion (nasal form), ocular edema, pharyngitis, rhinitis
GI: Nausea
GU: Vulvar pain (parenteral form)
SKIN: Flushing
Other: Anaphylaxis, hyponatremia, injection-site pain and redness; water intoxication

Nursing Considerations

• Use desmopressin cautiously in patients with conditions associated with fluid and electrolyte imbalance, such as cystic fibrosis, heart failure, and renal disorders; these patients are prone to hyponatremia.
• Also use cautiously in patients with habitual or psychogenic polydipsia; they may be more likely to drink excessive water, raising the risk of hyponatremia.

• Nasal cavity scarring, edema, and other abnormalities may cause erratic absorption and require a different administration route.

• Check blood pressure often during therapy.

WARNING Monitor patient closely for evidence of hyponatremia, such as headache, nausea, vomiting, restlessness, fatigue, lethargy, depressed reflexes, and changes in mental status. If left undetected, seizures, coma, and respiratory arrest may occur. Monitor patient's serum sodium level, and notify prescriber of abnormalities.

PATIENT TEACHING

• To prevent hyponatremia and water intoxication in a child or an elderly patient, urge family to restrict patient's fluids as prescribed.

• Tell patient to refrigerate nasal solution.

• Teach patient to prime nasal spray pump (only once) and spray dose into one or both nostrils, as prescribed, while inhaling briskly. Instruct her to clean tip of sprayer with hot water and dry it with clean tissue. Advise her to keep track of doses given and to discard bottle after 50 doses.

• Instruct patient who uses Stimate Nasal Spray to prime pump before first use by pressing down four times. Advise her to discard pump after 25 or 50 doses, depending on bottle, because delivery of an accurate dose can't be assured.

• For nasal tube, teach patient to draw prescribed amount of solution into calibrated plastic tube, insert one end of tube into a nostril and the other end into her mouth, and gently blow into tube to deposit solution deep into nasal cavity. Caution her not to let drug drain into her mouth.

• Teach patient or caregiver how to administer subcutaneous injection, if appropriate.

• Urge patient to report adverse reactions.

---

dexamethasone

Decadron, Decadron Elixir, Deronil (CAN), Dexamethasone Intensol, Dexasone (CAN), Dexone, Hexadrol, Oradexon (CAN)

dexamethasone acetate

Cortastat LA, Dalalone D.P., Dalalone L.A., Decadron-LA, Decaject L.A., Dexacen LA-8, Dexacorten-LA, Dexasone L.A., Dexone LA, Solurex LA

dexamethasone sodium phosphate

Cortastat, Dalalone, Decadrol, Decadron Respihaler, Decaject, Dexacen-4, Dexacorten, Dexacort Turbinaire, Dexasone, Dexone, Hexadrol Phosphate, Primethasone, Solurex

Class and Category

Chemical class: Synthetic adrenocortical steroid
Therapeutic class: Anti-inflammatory, diagnostic aid, immunosuppressant
Pregnancy category: C

Indications and Dosages

➤ *To treat endocrine disorders, such as congenital adrenal hyperplasia, hypercalcemia associated with cancer, and nonsuppurative thyroiditis; acute episodes or exacerbations of rheumatic disorders; collagen diseases, such as systemic lupus erythematosus and acute rheumatic carditis; severe dermatologic diseases; severe allergic conditions, such as seasonal or perennial allergic rhinitis, bronchial asthma, serum sickness, and drug hypersensitivity reactions; respiratory diseases, such as symptomatic sarcoidosis, löffler's syndrome, berylliosis, fulminating or disseminated pulmonary tuberculosis, and aspiration pneumonitis; hematologic disorders, such as idiopathic thrombocytopenic purpura and secondary thrombocytopenia in adults, autoimmune hemolytic anemia, aplastic crisis, and congenital hypoplastic anemia; tuberculous meningitis and trichinosis with neurologic or myocardial involvement*
➤ *To manage leukemias and lymphomas in adults and acute leukemia in*

children; to induce diuresis or remission of proteinuria in idiopathic nephrotic syndrome without uremia or nephrotic syndrome caused by systemic lupus erythematosus

➤ *To provide palliative therapy during acute exacerbations of GI diseases, such as ulcerative colitis and regional enteritis*

ELIXIR, ORAL SOLUTION, TABLETS, I.V. OR I.M. INJECTION

Adults. Highly individualized dosage based on severity of disorder. *Usual:* 0.75 to 9 mg/day as a single dose or in divided doses.

ELIXIR, ORAL SOLUTION, TABLETS

Children. Highly individualized, based on severity of disorder. *Usual:* 83.3 to 333.3 mcg/kg daily in divided doses three times daily or four times daily.

I.M. INJECTION

Children. Highly individualized, based on severity of disorder. *Usual:* 27.76 to 166.65 mcg/kg every 12 to 24 hr.

➤ *To manage adrenocortical insufficiency*

ELIXIR, ORAL SOLUTION, TABLETS, I.V. OR I.M. INJECTION

Adults. 0.5 to 9 mg daily as a single dose or in divided doses.

ELIXIR, ORAL SOLUTION, TABLETS

Children. 23.3 mcg/kg daily in divided doses three times daily.

I.M. INJECTION

Children. 23.3 mcg/kg daily in divided doses three times daily given every third day; alternatively, 7.76 to 11.65 mcg/kg daily.

➤ *To test for Cushing's syndrome*

ELIXIR, ORAL SOLUTION, TABLETS

Adults. 0.5 mg every 6 hr for 48 hr, followed by collection of 24-hr urine specimen to determine 17-hydroxycorticosteroid level. Or, 1 mg at 11 p.m., followed by plasma cortisol test performed at 8 a.m. the next day.

➤ *To distinguish Cushing's syndrome related to pituitary corticotropin excess from Cushing's syndrome from other causes*

ELIXIR, ORAL SOLUTION, TABLETS

Adults. 2 mg every 6 hr for 48 hr, followed by collection of 24-hr urine specimen to determine 17-hydroxycorticosteroid level.

➤ *To decrease cerebral edema*

ELIXIR, ORAL SOLUTION, TABLETS

Adults. 2 mg every 8 to 12 hr as maintenance after parenteral form has controlled initial symptoms.

I.V. INFUSION AND INJECTION

Adults. 10 mg I.V. followed by 4 mg I.M. every 6 hr. Decreased after 2 to 4 days, if needed, gradually tapering off over 5 to 7 days unless inoperable or recurring brain tumor is present. If such a tumor is present, dosage gradually decreased after 2 to 4 days to maintenance dosage of 2 mg I.M. every 8 to 12 hr and switched to P.O. regimen as soon as possible.

➤ *To treat unresponsive shock*

I.V. INFUSION AND INJECTION

Adults. 20 mg as a single dose, followed by 3 mg/kg over 24 hr as a continuous infusion; 40 mg as a single dose, followed by 40 mg every 2 to 6 hr, as needed; or 1 mg/kg as a single dose. All regimens used no more than 3 days.

➤ *To decrease localized inflammation*

INTRA-ARTICULAR INJECTION

Adults. 2 to 4 mg for large joint; 0.8 to 1 mg for small joint; 2 to 3 mg for bursae; 0.4 to 1 mg for tendon sheaths.

SOFT-TISSUE INJECTION

Adults. 2 to 6 mg; 1 to 2 mg for ganglia.

INTRALESIONAL INJECTION

Adults. 0.8 to 1.6 mg/injection site.

➤ *To decrease inflammation in allergic conditions or nasal polyps (except in sinuses)*

NASAL AEROSOL

Adults and children age 12 and over. 2 sprays (0.2 mg) in each nostril twice daily or three times daily. *Maximum:* 12 sprays (1.2 mg) daily.

Children ages 6 to 12. 1 or 2 sprays (0.1 to 0.2 mg) in each nostril twice daily. *Maximum:* 8 sprays (0.8 mg) daily.

Mechanism of Action

Binds to intracellular glucocorticoid receptors and suppresses inflammatory and immune responses by:

• inhibiting neutrophil and monocyte accumulation at inflammation site and suppressing phagocytic and bactericidal action
• stabilizing lysosomal membranes
• suppressing antigen response of macrophages and helper T cells
• inhibiting synthesis of inflammatory response mediators, such as cytokines, interleukins, and prostaglandins.

Contraindications

Administration of live-virus vaccine to patient or family member, hypersensitivity to dexamethasone or its components

(including sulfites), idiopathic thrombocytopenic purpura (I.M. administration),
systemic fungal infections

Interactions

DRUGS

*aminoglutethimide, antacids, barbiturates,
carbamazepine, hydantoins, mitotane,
rifampin:* Decreased dexamethasone effects
*amphotericin B (parenteral), carbonic
anhydrase inhibitors:* Risk of hypokalemia
anticholinesterases: Decreased anticholinesterase effectiveness in myasthenia gravis
aspirin, NSAIDs: Increased risk of adverse
GI effects
cholestyramine: Increased dexamethasone
clearance
cyclosporine: Increased activity of both
drugs, possibly resulting in seizures
digoxin: Increased risk of digitalis toxicity
related to hypokalemia
ephedrine: Decreased half-life and increased
clearance of dexamethasone
erythromycin, indinavir: Increased clearance
and decreased levels of these drugs
estrogens, ketoconazole, macrolide antibiotics:
Decreased dexamethasone clearance
isoniazid: Decreased blood isoniazid level
neuromuscular blockers: Possibly potentiated
or counteracted neuromuscular blockade
oral anticoagulants: Altered coagulation times,
requiring reduced anticoagulant dosage
oral contraceptives: Increased half-life and
concentration of dexamethasone
phenytoin: Increased risk of seizures
potassium-wasting diuretics: Increased
potassium loss and risk of hypokalemia
salicylates: Decreased blood level and
effectiveness of salicylates
somatrem: Possibly inhibition of somatrem's
growth-promoting effect
thalidomide: Increased risk of toxic epidermal necrolysis
theophyllines: Altered effects of either drug
toxoids, vaccines: Decreased antibody
response

ACTIVITIES

alcohol use: Increased risk of GI bleeding

Adverse Reactions

CNS: Depression, emotional lability,
euphoria, fever, headache, increased ICP
with papilledema, insomnia, light-
headedness, malaise, neuritis, neuropathy,
paresthesia, psychosis, seizures, syncope,
tiredness, vertigo, weakness
CV: Arrhythmias, bradycardia, edema, fat
embolism, heart failure, hypercholesterolemia, hyperlipidemia, hypertension,
myocardial rupture, tachycardia, thromboembolism, thrombophlebitis, vasculitis
EENT: Cataracts, glaucoma, vision changes
(all forms); epistaxis, loss of smell and taste,
nasal burning and dryness, oral candidiasis,
perforated nasal septum, pharyngitis,
rebound nasal congestion, rhinorrhea,
sneezing (nasal aerosol)
ENDO: Cushingoid symptoms, decreased
iodine uptake, growth suppression in
children, hyperglycemia, menstrual
irregularities, secondary adrenocortical and
pituitary unresponsiveness
GI: Abdominal distention, bloody stools,
elevated liver function test results, heartburn, hepatomegaly, increased appetite,
indigestion, intestinal perforation, melena,
nausea, pancreatitis, peptic ulcer with
possible perforation, ulcerative esophagitis,
vomiting
GU: Glycosuria, increased or decreased
number and motility of spermatozoa,
perineal irritation, urinary frequency
HEME: Leukocytosis, leukopenia
MS: Aseptic necrosis of femoral and
humeral heads; muscle atrophy, spasms, or
weakness; myalgia; osteoporosis; pathologic
fracture of long bones; tendon rupture
(intra-articular injection); vertebral
compression fracture
RESP: Bronchospasm
SKIN: Acne, allergic dermatitis, diaphoresis,
ecchymosis, erythema, hirsutism, necrotizing
vasculitis, petechiae, subcutaneous fat atrophy, striae, thin and fragile skin, urticaria
Other: Aggravated or masked signs of
infection, anaphylaxis, angioedema,
hypernatremia, hypocalcemia, hypokalemia,
hypokalemic alkalosis, impaired wound
healing, metabolic acidosis, sodium and
fluid retention, suppressed skin test
reaction, weight gain

Nursing Considerations

• Use dexamethasone cautiously in patients
with congestive heart failure, hypertension,
or renal insufficiency because drug can
cause sodium retention, which may lead to
edema and hypokalemia.

- Also use cautiously in patients who have had intestinal sugery and in those with peptic ulcer, diverticulitis, or ulcerative colitis because of the risk of perforation.
- Give once-daily dose of dexamethasone in the morning to coincide with the body's natural cortisol secretion.
- Give oral drug with food to decrease GI distress.
- Be aware that dosage forms with a concentration of 24 mg/ml are for I.V. use only.
- Shake I.M. solution before injecting deep into large muscle mass.

WARNING Avoid subcutaneous injection; it may cause atrophy and sterile abscess.

- Inject undiluted I.V. dose directly into I.V. tubing of infusing compatible solution over 30 seconds or less, as prescribed.

WARNING Don't give acetate form by I.V. injection.

- Shake nasal aerosol container well, and hold it upright about 6″ (15 cm) from area being treated. Keep spray out of patient's eyes, and advise her not to inhale it.
- Expect to taper drug rather than stopping it abruptly; prolonged use can cause adrenal suppression.
- Monitor fluid intake and output and daily weight, and watch for crackles, dyspnea, peripheral edema, and steady weight gain.
- Evaluate growth if patient is a child.
- Test stool for occult blood.
- Monitor results of hematology studies and blood glucose, serum electrolyte, cholesterol, and lipid levels. Dexamethasone may cause hyperglycemia, hypernatremia, hypocalcemia, hypokalemia, or leukopenia. It also may increase serum cholesterol and lipid levels, and it may decrease iodine uptake by the thyroid.
- Assess patient for evidence of osteoporosis, Cushing's syndrome, and other systemic effects during long-term use.
- Monitor neonate for signs of hypoadrenocorticism if mother received dexamethasone during pregnancy. Be aware that some preparations contain benzyl alcohol, which may cause a fatal toxic syndrome in neonates and immature infants.
- Watch for hypersensitivity reactions after giving acetate or sodium phosphate form;

both may contain bisulfites or parabens, to which some people are allergic.

PATIENT TEACHING

- Instruct patient not to store drug in damp or hot places and to protect liquid form from freezing.
- Instruct patient to take once-daily oral dose in the morning with food to help prevent GI distress.
- Caution against consuming alcohol during dexamethasone therapy because it increases the risk of GI bleeding.
- Advise patient to follow a low-sodium, high-potassium, high-protein diet, if prescribed, to help minimize weight gain, which is common with dexamethasone therapy. Instruct her to inform prescriber if she's on a special diet.
- Instruct patient not to stop drug abruptly.
- Advise patient to notify prescriber if condition recurs or worsens after dosage is reduced or therapy stops.
- Urge patient to have regular eye examinations during long-term use.
- Advise patient on long-term therapy to carry medical identification and to notify all healthcare providers that she takes dexamethasone.
- Instruct patient (especially a child) to avoid close contact with anyone who has chickenpox or measles and to notify prescriber immediately if exposure occurs.
- Advise patient and family members to avoid live-virus vaccinations during therapy unless prescriber approves.
- Inform diabetic patient that drug may affect her blood glucose level.
- If drug is injected into a joint, instruct patient to avoid putting excessive pressure on it and to notify prescriber if it becomes red or swollen.
- Tell patient to notify prescriber about anorexia, depression, light-headedness, malaise, muscle pain, nausea, vomiting, and early hyperadrenocorticism (abdominal distention, amenorrhea, easy bruising, extreme weakness, facial hair, increased appetite, moon face, weight gain). Tell patient and family about possible changes in appearance.
- Urge patient to notify prescriber about illness, surgery, or changes in stress level.

dexchlorphenira- mine maleate

Dexchlor, Polaramine, Polaramine Repetabs

Class and Category

Chemical class: Propylamine derivative
Therapeutic class: Antihistamine
Pregnancy category: B

Indications and Dosages

➤ *To treat allergic conjunctivitis; trans- fusion reaction; dermographism; mild, uncomplicated allergic skin reactions, such as urticaria and angioedema; perennial and seasonal allergic rhinitis; and vasomotor rhinitis and as adjunct to treat anaphylaxis*

E.R. TABLETS
Adults and adolescents. 4 to 6 mg daily at bedtime or every 8 to 10 hr, as needed.
SYRUP, TABLETS
Adults and adolescents. 2 mg every 4 to 6 hr, as needed.
Children ages 6 to 12. 1 mg every 4 to 6 hr or 150 mcg/kg in divided doses four times daily, as needed.
Children ages 2 to 6. 0.5 mg every 4 to 6 hr, as needed.

Route	Onset	Peak	Duration
P.O.	15–60 min*	Unknown*	4–8 hr*

Mechanism of Action

Binds to central and peripheral H_1 receptors, competing with histamine for these sites and preventing histamine from reaching its site of action. By blocking histamine, dexchlorpheniramine:
• inhibits respiratory, vascular, and GI smooth-muscle contraction, which prevents wheezing
• decreases capillary permeability, which reduces itching, flares, and wheals
• decreases lacrimal and salivary gland secretions, reducing nasal secretions, itching, sneezing, and watery eyes.

---

* For syrup and tablets; unknown for E.R. tablets.

Contraindications

Angle-closure glaucoma; benign prostatic hyperplasia; bladder neck obstruction; hypersensitivity to dexchlorpheniramine or other antihistamines; lower respiratory tract disorders, such as asthma; MAO inhibitor use within 14 days; pyloroduodenal obstruction; stenosing peptic ulcer

Interactions

DRUGS
anticholinergics: Potentiated anticholinergic effects
CNS depressants: Increased CNS depression
MAO inhibitors: Possibly severe hypotension and prolonged and intensified anticholinergic and sedative effects of dexchlorpheniramine
ACTIVITIES
alcohol use: Increased CNS depression

Adverse Reactions

CNS: Ataxia, confusion, dizziness, drowsiness, euphoria, excitement, headache, insomnia, irritability, nervousness, neuritis, nightmares, paresthesia, restlessness, vertigo, weakness
CV: Hypotension, palpitations, tachycardia
EENT: Acute labyrinthitis, blurred vision, dry mouth, tinnitus, vision changes
GI: Anorexia, constipation, diarrhea, indigestion, nausea, vomiting
GU: Urinary hesitancy, urine retention
RESP: Tenacious bronchial secretions
SKIN: Diaphoresis, photosensitivity, rash

Nursing Considerations

• Use dexchlorpheniramine cautiously in elderly patients and those with CV disease, hyperthyroidism, increased intraocular pressure, prostatic hypertrophy, or renal disease.
• Monitor patient for adverse reactions, especially in elderly patients and children.
• Watch for evidence of overdose, including clumsiness; drowsiness; dry mouth, nose, or throat; dyspnea; flushed or red face; hallucinations; insomnia; light- headedness; seizures; and unsteadiness.
PATIENT TEACHING
• Inform patient that drug provides temporary relief of symptoms.
• Advise patient to take drug with food, water, or milk to reduce GI irritation.

Inform her that she can crush regular (not E.R.) tablets and mix with food or fluid.
- For E.R. tablets, tell patient not to break, crush, or chew them before swallowing.
- Urge patient to take missed dose as soon as possible unless it's almost time for next dose.
- Because drug may cause drowsiness, caution patient to avoid hazardous activities until its CNS effects are known.
- Instruct her to avoid prolonged sun exposure and to use a sunscreen.
- Suggest that patient use sugarless candy or gum, ice chips, or saliva substitute to relieve dry mouth. If dryness lasts longer than 2 weeks, urge her to notify prescriber.
- Caution patient to avoid alcohol and CNS depressants, such as sedatives, sleeping pills, and tranquilizers, during therapy.
- If patient takes high doses of aspirin, urge her to inform prescriber because antihistamines may mask adverse reactions to aspirin overdose, such as tinnitus.
- Inform patient that drug needs to be discontinued 3 to 4 days before skin tests for allergies are performed.

dexmethylphenidate hydrochloride

Focalin, Focalin XR

Class, and Category Schedule
Chemical class: d-threo-enantiomer of methylphenidate
Therapeutic class: CNS stimulant*Pregnancy category:* C
Controlled substance schedule: II

Indications and Dosages
➤ *To treat attention deficit hyperactivity disorder (ADHD)*
TABLETS
Adults and children age 6 and over who are new to methylphenidate. 2.5 mg twice daily at least 4 hr apart, increased weekly by 2.5 to 5 mg. *Maximum:* 10 mg twice daily.
Adults and children age 6 and over who take methylphenidate. Half of racemic methylphenidate dosage. *Maximum:* 10 mg twice daily at least 4 hr apart.

DOSAGE ADJUSTMENT Drug stopped if no improvement within 1 mo after appropriate dosage adjustments. Dosage decreased or drug stopped for paradoxical aggravation of symptoms or adverse reactions.
E.R. CAPSULES, E.R. TABLETS
Adults who are new to methylphenidate. 10 mg daily, increased after 1 wk as needed to 20 mg daily.
Children age 6 and over who are new to methylphenidate. 5 mg daily, increased weekly as needed by 5-mg increments. *Maximum:* 20 mg daily.
Adults and children age 6 and over who take methylphenidate. Half of racemic methylphenidate dosage. *Maximum:* 20 mg daily.

Mechanism of Action
May block reuptake of norepinephrine and dopamine into presynaptic neurons in cerebral cortex, which increases availability of norepinephrine and dopamine in extraneuronal space.

Contraindications
Diagnosis or family history of Tourette's syndrome; glaucoma; hypersensitivity to dexmethylphenidate, methylphenidate, or their components; marked anxiety, tension, and agitation; motor tics; use within 14 days of MAO inhibitor

Interactions
DRUGS
anticoagulants (oral), anticonvulsants, antidepressants (tricyclic and selective serotonin reuptake inhibitors): Possibly decreased metabolism of these drugs
antihypertensives: Decreased therapeutic effect of these drugs
dopamine and other vasopressors: Increased therapeutic effect of these drugs
MAO inhibitors: Increased adverse effects, risk of hypertensive crisis

Adverse Reactions
CNS: Cerebral arteritis or occlusion, dizziness, drowsiness, dyskinesia, fever, headache, insomnia, motor or vocal tics, nervousness, seizures, Tourette's syndrome, toxic psychosis
CV: Angina, arrhythmias, hypertension, hypotension, increased or decreased pulse rate, palpitations, peripheral vasculopathy including Raynaud's phenomenon, tachycardia

EENT: Accommodation abnormality, blurred vision
GI: Abdominal pain, anorexia, nausea
GU: Priapism
HEME: Thrombocytopenic purpura
MS: Arthralgia
SKIN: Erythema multiforme, exfoliative dermatitis, necrotizing vasculitis, rash, urticaria
Other: Anaphylaxis, angioedema, weight loss (prolonged therapy)

Nursing Considerations

WARNING Be aware that dexmethylphenidate may induce CNS stimulation, mania, and psychosis and may worsen behavior disturbances and thought disorders. Use drug cautiously in children with psychosis or mania. Be aware that withdrawal symptoms may occur with long-term use.
• Also know that dexmethylphenidate should be used cautiously in patients with serious structural cardiac abnormalities, cardiomyopathy, serious heart rhythm abnormalities, or other serious cardiac problems because drug may increase risk of sudden death from these conditions.
• Monitor blood pressure and pulse rate to detect hypertension and excessive stimulation. Notify prescriber if signs appear.
• Dexmethylphenidate shouldn't be used to treat severe depression or to prevent or treat normal fatigue.
WARNING Monitor patient for signs of physical or psychological dependence. Use drug cautiously in patients with a history of drug abuse, including alcoholism.
• Monitor CBC and differential and platelet counts, as ordered, during prolonged therapy.
• Expect to stop drug if seizures occur. Drug may lower seizure threshold, especially in patients with a history of seizures or EEG abnormalities.
• Assess patient for signs and symptoms of peripheral vasculopathy, including Raynaud's phenomenon. Although mild and intermittent, know that digital ulceration and/or soft tissue breakdown has occurred. Notify prescriber if present,

as drug dosage may need to be reduced or drug discontinued.
WARNING Question male patients, including male children, about prolonged and painful erections, especially after a dosage increase or during a period of drug withdrawal. Know that presence of priapism has sometimes required emergency surgical intervention, so report any findings to prescriber immediately.
• Monitor children on long-term dexmethylphenidate therapy for signs of growth suppression, which has been noted during long-term use of stimulants.
• Dosages of drugs affected by dexmethylphenidate, such as anticoagulants and antihypertensives, may need adjustment.

PATIENT TEACHING
• Tell patient that extended-release capsules should either be taken whole, without being chewed, crushed, or divided, or capsule contents should be sprinkled on a small amount of applesauce.
• Urge patient to notify prescriber if she has excessive nervousness, fever, insomnia, nausea, palpitations, or rash while taking dexmethylphenidate.
• Caution patient with seizure disorder that drug may cause seizures.
• Advise patient to protect drug from light and moisture.
• Teach patient (or arent) to watch for improvement in signs and symptoms of ADHD, such as decreased impulsiveness and increased attention. Stress the need for continued follow-up care, and suggest participation in an ADHD program.
WARNING Inform male patients and parents or caregivers of male children that dexmethylphenidate may cause abnormally sustained or frequent and painful erections, especially when a dosage increase occurs or during a period of drug withdrawal. Advise immediate emergency care if this should occur.
• Instruct patient to inspect his fingers and toes daily for changes such as ulcer formation or skin breakdown. Although usually intermittent and mild, patient should contact prescriber if abnormalities occur, as drug may need to be discontinued or dosage reduced.

dextrose
(d-glucose)

B-D Glucose, Glutose, Insta-Glucose, Insulin Reaction

glucose

2.5% Dextrose Injection, 5% Dextrose Injection, 10% Dextrose Injection, 20% Dextrose Injection, 25% Dextrose Injection, 50% Dextrose Injection, 60% Dextrose Injection, 70% Dextrose Injection

Class and Category
Chemical class: Monosaccharide
Therapeutic class: Antidiabetic, nutritional supplement*Pregnancy category:* C

Indications and Dosages
➤ *To treat insulin-induced hypoglycemia*
CHEWABLE TABLETS, ORAL GEL
Adults and children. *Initial:* 10 to 20 g. Repeated in 10 to 20 min, if needed, based on serum glucose level.
I.V. INFUSION OR INJECTION
Adults and children. *Initial:* 20 to 50 ml of 50% solution given at 3 ml/min.
Maintenance: 10% to 15% solution by continuous infusion until blood glucose level reaches therapeutic range.
Infants and neonates. 2 ml/kg of 10% to 25% solution until blood glucose level reaches therapeutic range.
➤ *To replace calories*
I.V. INFUSION
Adults and children. Individualized dosage of 2.5%, 5%, or 10% solution, based on need for fluids or calories and given by peripheral I.V. line. Or 10% to 70% solution given by central vein, if needed, typically with amino acids or other solutions.

Route	Onset	Peak	Duration
P.O.	10–20 min	40 min	Unknown
I.V.	2–3 min	Unknown	Unknown

Mechanism of Action
Prevents protein and nitrogen loss, promotes glycogen deposition, prevents or decreases ketosis, and, in large amounts,

acts as an osmotic diuretic. Dextrose is readily metabolized and undergoes oxidation to carbon dioxide and water. The oral form—glucose—is absorbed directly into the bloodstream from the intestines and is distributed, used, or stored in the liver.

Incompatibilities
Don't give dextrose through same infusion set as blood or blood products because pseudoagglutination of RBCs may occur.

Contraindications
For all solutions: Diabetic coma with excessively elevated blood glucose level
For concentrated solutions: Anuria, alcohol withdrawal syndrome in dehydrated patient, glucose-galactose malabsorption syndrome, hepatic coma, hypersensitivity to corn or corn products, intracranial or intraspinal hemorrhage, overhydration

Interactions
DRUGS
corticosteroids, corticotropin: Increased risk of fluid and electrolyte imbalance if dextrose solution contains sodium ions

Adverse Reactions
CNS: Confusion, fever
GU: Glycosuria
Other: Dehydration; hyperosmolar coma; hypervolemia; hypovolemia; injection-site extravasation with tissue necrosis, infection, phlebitis, and venous thrombosis

Nursing Considerations
• Use dextrose cautiously in patients with renal impairment because solutions contain aluminum that could be toxic in prolonged parenteral therapy.
• Give highly concentrated dextrose solution by central venous catheter—not by subcutaneous or I.M. route.
WARNING Rapid or excessive delivery of dextrose solution in a very low–birth-weight infant may increase serum osmolality and cause intracerebral hemorrhage.
• Assess infusion site regularly for signs of infiltration, such as pain or swelling.
• Assess patient for glucosuria by using a urine reagent strip or collecting a urine sample and reviewing urinalysis results.

• When discontinuing a concentrated solution, expect to give a 5% to 10% dextrose infusion to avoid rebound hypoglycemia.

• Monitor patient for signs of hypervolemia, such as jugular vein distention and crackles.

PATIENT TEACHING

• Advise patient to swallow oral dextrose; it isn't absorbed from the buccal cavity.

• Instruct patient to monitor her blood glucose level as directed.

• Emphasize importance of reporting discomfort, pain, or signs of infection at I.V. site.

dezocine
Dalgan

Class and Category
Chemical class: Aminotetralin, synthetic opioid
Therapeutic class: Analgesic
Pregnancy category: C

Indications and Dosages
➤ *To relieve pain*
I.V. INJECTION
Adult. *Initial:* 5 mg followed by 2.5 to 10 mg every 2 to 4 hr, as needed. *Maximum:* 120 mg daily.
I.M. INJECTION
Adult. *Initial:* 10 mg followed by 5 to 20 mg every 3 to 6 hr, as needed. *Maximum:* 20 mg/dose, 120 mg daily.

Route	Onset	Peak	Duration
I.V.	In 15 min	30 min	2–4 hr
I.M.	In 30 min	1–2 hr	2–4 hr

Mechanism of Action
Binds with opiate receptors at many CNS sites, affecting perception of and emotional response to pain.

Contraindications
Hypersensitivity to dezocine or its components

Interactions
DRUGS
CNS depressants, general anesthetics, hypnotics, sedatives, tranquilizers: Increased CNS depressant effects

opioids: Possibly decreased therapeutic opioid effects and withdrawal symptoms in patient receiving long-term opioid therapy
ACTIVITIES
alcohol use: Increased CNS depression

Adverse Reactions
CNS: Dizziness, sedation, vertigo
GI: Nausea, vomiting
Other: Injection-site redness and swelling

Nursing Considerations
• Use dezocine cautiously and in low doses in elderly patients and those who have common bile duct, hepatic, renal, or respiratory disease.

• Discard solution if it contains precipitate.

• Monitor blood pressure, pulse, and respiratory rate often after giving first dose, especially if given by I.V. route.

WARNING Avoid giving dezocine to opioid-dependent patient. Doing so may precipitate withdrawal symptoms because dezocine can antagonize opioid effects.

• Assess patient for pain relief often, and document findings.

PATIENT TEACHING

• Instruct patient to notify prescriber if pain isn't relieved within 1 hour.

• Advise patient to avoid hazardous activities until drug's CNS effects are known.

diazepam
Apo-Diazepam (CAN), Diastat, Diazepam Intensol, Dizac, Novo-Dipam (CAN), Valium, Vivol (CAN)

Class Category and Schedule
Chemical class: Benzodiazepine
Therapeutic class: Anticonvulsant, anxiolytic, sedative-hypnotic, skeletal muscle relaxant
Pregnancy category: DControlled substance schedule: IV

Indications and Dosages
➤ *To relieve anxiety*
ORAL SOLUTION, TABLETS
Adults. 2 to 10 mg twice daily to four times daily.
DOSAGE ADJUSTMENT Dosage reduced to 2 to 2.5 mg daily or twice daily and increased gradually as needed and tolerated for elderly or debilitated patients.

Children age 6 months and over. *Initial:* 1 to 2.5 mg three times daily or four times daily. Increased gradually as needed and tolerated.

I.V. OR I.M. INJECTION

Adults. 2 to 5 mg every 3 to 4 hr, as needed, for moderate anxiety; 5 to 10 mg every 3 to 4 hr, as needed, for severe anxiety.

Children. Individualized dosage.

Maximum: 0.25 mg/kg given over 3 min, repeated after 15 to 30 min if needed, and after another 15 to 30 min if needed.

➤ *To treat symptoms of acute alcohol withdrawal*

ORAL SOLUTION, TABLETS

Adults. 10 mg three times daily or four times daily during first 24 hr. Then 5 mg three times daily or four times daily, if needed.

I.V. OR I.M. INJECTION

Adults. 10 mg and then 5 to 10 mg in 3 to 4 hr, if needed.

➤ *To provide muscle relaxation, to provide sedation*

ORAL SOLUTION, TABLETS

Adults. 2 to 10 mg three times daily or four times daily.

DOSAGE ADJUSTMENT Dosage reduced to 2 to 2.5 mg once or twice daily and increased gradually as needed and tolerated for elderly or debilitated patients.

Children age 6 months and over. *Initial:* 1 to 2.5 mg t.i.d. or q.i.d. Increased gradually as needed and tolerated.

I.V. OR I.M. INJECTION

Adults. 2 to 5 mg every 3 to 4 hr, as needed, for moderate anxiety; 5 to 10 mg every 3 to 4 hr, as needed, for severe anxiety.

Children. Individualized dosage.

Maximum: 0.25 mg/kg given over 3 min, repeated after 15 to 30 min if needed, and after another 15 to 30 min if needed.

➤ *To treat seizures*

ORAL SOLUTION, TABLETS

Adults. 2 to 10 mg twice daily to four times daily.

DOSAGE ADJUSTMENT Dosage reduced to 2 to 2.5 mg once or twice daily and increased gradually as needed and tolerated for elderly or debilitated patients.

Children age 6 months and over. *Initial:* 1 to 2.5 mg three times daily or four times daily. Increased gradually as needed and tolerated.

➤ *To treat status epilepticus and severe recurrent seizures*

I.V. INJECTION

Adults. 5 to 10 mg repeated every 10 to 15 min, as needed, up to a cumulative dose of 30 mg. Regimen repeated, if needed, in 2 to 4 hr. (Use I.M. route if I.V. access is impossible.)

Children age 5 and over. 1 mg repeated every 2 to 5 min, as needed, up to a cumulative dose of 10 mg. Regimen repeated, if needed, in 2 to 4 hr.

Children ages 1 month to 5 years. 0.2 to 0.5 mg repeated every 2 to 5 min, as needed, up to a cumulative dose of 5 mg. Regimen repeated, if needed, in 2 to 4 hr.

RECTAL GEL

Adults and adolescents. 0.2 mg/kg rounded up to next available unit dose (or rounded down for elderly or debilitated patient). Repeated in 4 to 12 hr, if needed.

Children ages 6 to 12. 0.3 mg/kg rounded up to next available unit dose. Repeated in 4 to 12 hr, if needed.

Children ages 2 to 6. 0.5 mg/kg rounded up to next available unit dose. Repeated in 4 to 12 hr, if needed.

➤ *To provide preoperative sedation*

I.V. OR I.M. INJECTION

Adults. 5 to 10 mg 30 min before surgery.

➤ *To reduce anxiety before cardioversion*

I.V. INJECTION

Adults. 5 to 15 mg 5 to 10 min before procedure.

➤ *To reduce anxiety before endoscopic procedures*

I.V. INJECTION

Adults. Up to 20 mg titrated to desired sedation and given immediately before procedure.

I.M. INJECTION

Adults. 5 to 10 mg 30 min before procedure.

➤ *To treat tetanus*

I.V. OR I.M. INJECTION

Adults and children age 5 and over. *Initial:* 5 to 10 mg repeated every 3 to 4 hr, if needed. Sometimes larger doses for adults.

DOSAGE ADJUSTMENT Initial dose reduced to 2 to 5 mg and increased gradually as needed and tolerated for debilitated patients.

Children ages 1 month to 5 years. 1 to 2 mg repeated every 3 to 4 hr, as needed.

D

Mechanism of Action

May potentiate effects of gamma-aminobutyric acid (GABA) and other inhibitory neurotransmitters by binding to specific benzodiazepine receptors in limbic and cortical areas of CNS. GABA inhibits excitatory stimulation, which helps control emotional behavior. Limbic system contains a dense area of benzodiazepine receptors, which may explain drug's antianxiety effects. Diazepam suppresses spread of seizure activity caused by seizure-producing foci in cortex, thalamus, and limbic structures.

Incompatibilities

Don't mix diazepam injection with aqueous solutions. Don't mix diazepam emulsion for I.M. injection with morphine or glycopyrrolate or administer it through an infusion set that contains polyvinyl chloride.

Contraindications

Acute angle-closure glaucoma, hypersensitivity to diazepam or its components, untreated open-angle glaucoma

Interactions

DRUGS

antacids: Altered rate of diazepam absorption

anticonvulsants: Decreased effectiveness of these drugs

cimetidine, disulfiram, fluoxetine, fluvoxamine, isoniazid, itraconazole, ketoconazole, metoprolol, omeprazole, oral contraceptives, propoxyphene, propranolol, valproic acid: Decreased diazepam metabolism, increased blood level and risk of adverse effects

CNS depressants: Increased CNS depression and risk of falls and fractures

digoxin: Increased serum digoxin level and risk of digitalis toxicity

levodopa: Decreased antidyskinetic effect of levodopa

phenytoin: Decreased metabolic elimination of phenytoin, increased risk of adverse reactions

probenecid: Faster onset or more prolonged effects of diazepam

ranitidine: Delayed elimination and increased blood level of diazepam

rifampin: Decreased blood diazepam level

theophyllines: Antagonized sedative effect of diazepam

ACTIVITIES

alcohol use: Increased CNS depression and risk of falls and fractures

Adverse Reactions

CNS: Anterograde amnesia, anxiety, ataxia, confusion, depression, dizziness, drowsiness, fatigue, headache, insomnia, lethargy, light-headedness, paradoxical reactions, psychiatric effects, sedation, sleepiness, slurred speech, suicidal ideation, tremor, vertigo

CV: Hypotension, palpitations, tachycardia

EENT: Blurred vision, diplopia, dry mouth, increased salivation

GI: Anorexia, constipation, diarrhea, elevated liver enzymes, jaundice, nausea, vomiting

GU: Libido changes, urinary incontinence, urine retention

HEME: Neutropenia

MS: dysarthria, muscle weakness

RESP: Respiratory depression

SKIN: Dermatitis

Other: Physical and psychological dependence

Nursing Considerations

• Use diazepam with extreme caution in patients with a history of alcohol or drug abuse because it can cause physical and psychological dependence, and in patients with hepatic disorders such as hepatic fibrosis and hepatitis because of potentially significant increase in drug's half-life.

• Use diazepam cautiously in patients with hepatic or renal impairment. Severe hepatic impairment is a contraindication to use.

• Expect to give a lower diazepam dose to patient with chronic respiratory insufficiency because of the risk of respiratory depression.

• Mix concentrated oral solution (Intensol) with liquid or semisolid food. Use supplied calibrated dropper to measure doses.

• Protect diazepam injection from light. Don't use solution that's more than slightly yellow or that contains precipitate.

• Give I.M. injection into deltoid muscle for rapid, complete absorption. Using other sites may cause slow, erratic absorption.

• Before administering emulsion form, ask if patient is allergic to soybeans because this form contains soybean oil.

- For an infant or a child, administer I.V. injection slowly over 3 minutes in a dose not to exceed 0.25 mg/kg.
- Give emulsion form within 6 hours of opening ampule because it contains no preservatives and allows rapid microbial growth. Use polyethylene-lined or glass infusion sets and polyethylene or polypropylene plastic syringes for administration. Don't use a filter with a pore size less than 5 microns because a smaller size may break down the emulsion.
- Don't mix emulsion form with anything other than its emulsion base. Otherwise, it may become unstable and increase the risk of serious adverse reactions.
- Monitor patient for adverse reactions, especially if she has hypoalbuminemia, which increases the risk of sedation.

WARNING Watch for signs of physical and psychological dependence (strong desire or need to continue taking diazepam, need to increase dose to maintain drug effects, and posttherapy withdrawal symptoms, such as abdominal cramps, insomnia, irritability, nervousness, and tremor).
- Monitor patient closely for increase in frequency or severity of grand mal seizures when diazepam is used with standard anticonvulsant therapy. Dosage of other anticonvulsants may need to be increased.
- Avoid abrupt withdrawal of diazepam, as ordered, when used as part of the patient's seizure control regimen because a transient increase in frequency or severity of seizures may occur.
- Monitor severely depressed patient or one with depression-related anxiety for suicidal tendencies, particularly when therapy starts and dosage changes; depression may worsen temporarily during these times.
- Watch for psychiatric and paradoxical reactions to diazepam, especially in children and the elderly. If reactions occur, notify prescriber and expect drug to be discontinued.
- Monitor patient for decreased drug effectiveness, especially with prolonged use.
- Check patient's blood counts and liver function periodically, as ordered, because prolonged diazepam therapy rarely causes neutropenia and jaundice.

PATIENT TEACHING
- Instruct patient not to take more drug, more often, or for a longer time than prescribed. Warn her that physical and psychological dependence can occur, and teach her to recognize the signs.
- Advise patient not to take drug to relieve everyday stress.
- Instruct patient to avoid hazardous activities until drug's CNS effects are known. Warn him that risk of falls and fractures increases when diazepam is taken with other sedatives or alcohol and to avoid this combination.
- Advise patient to avoid CNS depressants and alcohol during therapy.
- Instruct patient not to stop taking drug abruptly without prescriber's supervision. If patient has a history of seizures, warn that abrupt withdrawal may trigger them.
- Instruct patient to mix Diazepam Intensol with water, soda, or a similar beverage; applesauce; or pudding just before taking it. Caution her not to save the mixture for later. Tell her to use calibrated dropper that's provided to measure each dose.
- Teach patient how to self-administer a rectal form, if prescribed.
- Instruct female patient of childbearing age to notify prescriber immediately if she is or could be pregnant because diazepam therapy will need to be discontinued.
- Urge family or caregiver to watch patient closely for suicidal tendencies, especially when therapy starts or dosage changes.

diazoxide
Hyperstat, Proglycem

Class and Category
Chemical class: Benzothiadiazine derivative
Therapeutic class: Antihypertensive, antihypoglycemic
Pregnancy category: C

Indications and Dosages
➤ *To manage hypoglycemia caused by hyperinsulinism*
CAPSULES, ORAL SUSPENSION
Adults and children. *Initial:* 1 mg/kg every 8 hr. *Maintenance:* 3 to 8 mg/kg daily in

2 or 3 equal doses given every 8 or 12 hr. *Maximum:* 15 mg/kg daily.
Infants and neonates. *Initial:* 3.3 mg/kg every 8 hr. *Maintenance:* 8 to 15 mg/kg daily in 2 or 3 equal doses given every 8 or 12 hr.

➤ *To treat severe hypertension in hospitalized patients*

I.V. INJECTION

Adults and children. *Initial:* 1 to 3 mg/kg by rapid bolus, repeated every 5 to 15 min until diastolic pressure falls below 100 mm Hg. Repeated in 4 hr and again in 24 hr, if needed, until oral antihypertensive therapy begins. *Maximum:* 150 mg/dose, 1.2 g daily.

Mechanism of Action

Directly affects smooth muscle cells of peripheral arteries and arterioles, causing them to dilate. This action decreases peripheral resistance, which helps reduce blood pressure. Diazoxide also inhibits insulin release from the pancreas, stimulates catecholamine release, and increases hepatic glucose release.

Route	Onset	Peak	Duration
P.O.	In 1 hr	Unknown	8 hr
I.V.	1 min	2–5 min	2–12 hr

Contraindications

Acute aortic dissection; hypersensitivity to diazoxide, thiazides, other sulfonamide derivatives, or their components; treatment of compensatory hypertension, as occurs with aortic coarctation

Interactions

DRUGS

allopurinol, colchicine, probenecid, sulfinpyrazone: Increased serum uric acid level
antihypertensives: Additive hypotensive effects
beta blockers: Increased hypotensive effects of diazoxide
diuretics, especially thiazides: Potentiated hyperglycemic, hyperuricemic, and antihypertensive effects of diazoxide
estrogens, NSAIDs, sympathomimetics: Antagonized diazoxide hypotensive effects
insulin, oral antidiabetics: Possibly decreased effectiveness of these drugs
oral anticoagulants: Increased anticoagulation
peripheral vasodilators, ritodrine (I.V.): Additive, possibly severe, hypotensive effects

Adverse Reactions

CNS: Anxiety, apprehension, cerebral ischemia, dizziness, euphoria, headache, insomnia, light-headedness, malaise, somnolence, weakness
CV: Bradycardia, chest pain, hypotension, palpitations, tachycardia, transient hypertension
EENT: Blurred vision, dry mouth, increased salivation, taste perversion, tinnitus, transient hearing loss
ENDO: Transient hyperglycemia
GI: Abdominal pain, anorexia, constipation, diarrhea, ileus, nausea, vomiting
MS: Gout
SKIN: Diaphoresis, flushing, pruritus, rash, sensation of warmth
Other: Extravasation with injection-site cellulitis and pain; fluid and sodium retention

Nursing Considerations

• Use diazoxide cautiously in patients with uncompensated heart failure (can cause fluid retention and heart failure) and patients with impaired cardiac or cerebral circulation in whom abrupt blood pressure drop, mild tachycardia, and decreased blood perfusion may be harmful.
• Give I.V. drug undiluted over 10 to 30 seconds. Don't give it I.M. or subcutaneously.
• Keep patient supine during I.V. injection and for 1 hour afterward.
• Monitor blood pressure throughout treatment to check for hypertension. Before monitoring ends, measure patient's standing blood pressure if she's ambulatory.
• Assess I.V. site often for extravasation; drug is alkaline and can irritate tissue.
• Expect to adjust dosage if patient switches from oral suspension to capsules; suspension causes a higher blood diazoxide level.
• If diabetic patient receives I.V. diazoxide to treat hypertension, watch for evidence of hyperglycemia because parenteral form commonly causes transient hyperglycemia.
• Monitor blood glucose level of all patients who receive oral diazoxide to see if drug has raised blood glucose level to normal.

PATIENT TEACHING

• Tell patient who receives I.V. diazoxide that she'll be on bed rest until taking oral drug.
• Advise patient to protect oral suspension from light.

• Tell patient to take oral drug on a regular schedule and not to skip or double doses.
• Urge patient to monitor blood glucose level if she takes oral drug for hypoglycemia.
• Caution patient not to take antidiabetic drugs unless prescribed.
• Advise patient to notify prescriber if she has signs of hyperglycemia, such as increased urinary frequency, increased thirst, and fruity breath.

dichlorphenamide
Daranide

Class and Category
Chemical class: Sulfonamide derivative
Therapeutic class: Antiglaucoma drug
Pregnancy category: C

Indications and Dosages
➤ *To manage chronic open-angle glaucoma, secondary glaucoma, and acute angle-closure glaucoma (preoperatively)*

TABLETS
Adults. *Initial:* 100 to 200 mg followed by 100 mg every 12 hr. *Maintenance:* 25 to 50 mg once daily to three times daily.

Mechanism of Action
Inhibits the enzyme carbonic anhydrase, which normally is in renal proximal tubule cells, choroid plexes of the brain, and ciliary processes of the eyes. In eyes, enzyme inhibition decreases aqueous humor secretion, which reduces intraocular pressure.

Route	Onset	Peak	Duration
P.O.	30–60 min	2–4 hr	6–12 hr

Contraindications
Adrenocortical insufficiency, hepatic insufficiency, hyperchloremic acidosis, hypersensitivity to dichlorphenamide or sulfa drugs or their components, hypokalemia, hyponatremia, renal failure, severe obstructive pulmonary disease

Interactions
DRUGS
diflunisal: Increased adverse effects of dichlorphenamide, significantly decreased intraocular pressure

salicylates: Increased risk of dichlorphenamide toxicity, including CNS depression and metabolic acidosis

Adverse Reactions
CNS: Depression, disorientation, dizziness, drowsiness, lassitude, paresthesia
CV: Arrhythmias
EENT: Metallic taste, pharyngitis
ENDO: Hyperglycemia
GI: Anorexia, diarrhea, hepatic dysfunction, nausea, vomiting
GU: Phosphaturia, renal calculi, renal colic, urinary frequency
HEME: Hemolytic anemia, leukopenia, pancytopenia, thrombocytopenia
SKIN: Photosensitivity
Other: Hyperchloremia, hyperuricemia, weight loss

Nursing Considerations
• Use dichlorphenamide cautiously in patients with emphysema, pulmonary obstruction, or severe respiratory acidosis.
• Monitor serum potassium level often (especially in elderly patients and those taking digoxin) because diuresis may cause hypokalemia.

PATIENT TEACHING
• Instruct patient to take dichlorphenamide with food or full glass of water to decrease GI distress.
• Advise patient to avoid hazardous activities until drug's CNS effects are known.
• *WARNING* Urge patient to immediately report evidence of blood dyscrasias, such as fever, numbness or tingling, rash, sore throat, and unusual bleeding or bruising.
• Advise patient to avoid prolonged exposure to sunlight, to apply sunscreen, and to wear protective clothing outdoors.
• Instruct patient to take a missed dose as soon as she remembers it, unless it's almost time for the next dose.
• Tell patient to store drug at room temperature and protect from moisture and heat.

diclofenac
Zorvolex

diclofenac potassium
Cataflam, Voltaren Rapide (CAN), Zipsor

diclofenac sodium

Apo-Diclo (CAN), Dyloject,
Novo-Difenac (CAN), Nu-Diclo
(CAN), Voltaren, Voltaren SR (CAN)

Class and Category
Chemical class: Phenylacetic acid derivative
Therapeutic class: Analgesic,
anti-inflammatory
Pregnancy category: C prior to 30 weeks'
gestation; D starting at 30 weeks' gestation

Indications and Dosages
➤ *To relieve pain and inflammation in
rheumatoid arthritis*
DELAYED-RELEASE TABLETS, TABLETS
Adults. *Initial:* 150 to 200 mg daily in divided
doses three times daily or four times daily.
Maintenance: 75 to 100 mg/day, divided,
three times daily. *Maximum:* 225 mg daily.
E.R. TABLETS
Adults.
Initial: 75 or 100 mg daily, morning or
evening, or 75 mg twice daily, morning and
evening.
RECTAL SUPPOSITORIES
Adults. 50 or 100 mg as substitute for last
P.O. dose of day.
➤ *To relieve pain and inflammation in
osteoarthritis*
DELAYED-RELEASE TABLETS, TABLETS
Adults. 100 to 150 mg daily in divided
doses twice daily or three times daily.
Maximum: 150 mg daily.
➤ *To relieve pain in patients with
ankylosing spondylitis*
DELAYED-RELEASE TABLETS, TABLETS
Adults. 100 to 125 mg daily in 4 or 5
divided doses.
➤ *To relieve pain and dysmenorrhea*
TABLETS
Adults. 50 mg three times daily, as needed.;
if needed, 100 mg for first dose only.
DOSAGE ADJUSTMENT Dosage reduced, if
needed, for elderly patients and those with
serious renal dysfunction.
➤ *To manage osteoarthritis pain*
CAPSULES (ZORVOLEX)
Adults. 35 mg three times daily.
➤ *To manage mild to moderate pain; to
manage moderate to severe pain alone
or in combination with opioid analgesics*

I.V. INJECTION (DYLOJECT)
Adults. 37.5 mg given over 15 seconds
every 6 hours, as needed. *Maximum:* 150
mg daily.
➤ *To relieve mild to moderate acute pain*
CAPSULES (ZIPSOR)
Adults. 25 mg four times daily.
CAPSULES (ZORVOLEX)
Adults. 18 mg or 35 mg three times daily.
DOSAGE ADJUSTMENT For patient prescribed
Zorvolex with hepatic impairment, dosage
no higher than 18 mg three times daily.

Route	Onset	Peak	Duration
P.O.*	30 min	Unknown	8 hr

Mechanism of Action
Blocks the activity of cyclooxygenase, the
enzyme needed to synthesize
prostaglandins, which mediate
inflammatory response and cause local
pain, swelling, and vasodilation. By
blocking cyclooxygenase and inhibiting
prostaglandins, diclofenac reduces
inflammatory symptoms. This mechanism
also relieves pain because prostaglandins
promote pain transmission from periphery
to spinal cord.

Contraindications
Active GI bleeding or ulcers; history of
asthma attacks, rhinitis, or urticaria from
aspirin or other NSAIDs; hypersensitivity
to diclofenac, NSAIDs, or their
components; moderate to severe renal
insufficiency in perioperative period with
patients at risk for volume depletion (I.V.
form); treatment of perioperative pain after
coronary artery bypass grafting

Interactions
DRUGS
acetaminophen: Increased risk of adverse
renal effects with long-term concurrent use
anticoagulants, thrombolytics: Prolonged PT,
increased risk of bleeding
antihypertensives: Decreased antihypertensive effectiveness
aspirin, other NSAIDs, salicylates: Increased
GI irritability and bleeding, decreased
diclofenac effectiveness
beta blockers: Impaired antihypertensive effect

---

* For tablets; unknown for delayed-release
and E.R. tablets.

cefamandole, cefoperazone, cefotetan, plicamycin, valproic acid: Increased risk of hypoprothrombinemia
cimetidine: Altered blood diclofenac level
colchicine, corticotropin (long-term use), glucocorticoids, potassium supplements: Increased GI irritability and bleeding
cyclosporine, gold compounds, nephrotoxic drugs: Increased risk of nephrotoxicity
CYP2C9 inducers such as rifampin: Decreased effectiveness of diclofenac
CYP2C9 inhibitors such as voriconazole: Increased risk of diclofenac adverse reactions and toxicity
digoxin: Increased blood digoxin level
insulin, oral antidiabetics: Decreased effects of these drugs
lithium: Increased risk of lithium toxicity
loop diuretics: Decreased diuretic effects
methotrexate: Increased risk of methotrexate toxicity
phenytoin: Increased blood phenytoin level
potassium-sparing diuretics: Increased risk of hyperkalemia
probenecid: Increased diclofenac toxicity
FOODS
food: Delayed absorption of delayed-release tablets
ACTIVITIES
alcohol use: Increased risk of GI irritability and bleeding

Adverse Reactions
CNS: Aseptic meningitis, cerebral hemorrhage, CVA, dizziness, drowsiness, headache
CV: Bradycardia and other arrhythmias, hypotension, MI, thrombotic events, vasculitis
EENT: Glaucoma, hearing loss, tinnitus
ENDO: Hypoglycemia
GI: Abdominal pain, constipation, diarrhea, dysphagia, elevated liver function test results, esophageal ulceration, flatulence, GI bleeding or ulceration, hepatic failure, hepatitis, indigestion, jaundice, nausea, perforation of stomach or intestine
GU: Acute renal failure, interstitial nephritis
HEME: Agranulocytosis, aplastic anemia, eosinophilia, leukocytosis, leukopenia, pancytopenia, porphyria, thrombocytopenia

SKIN: Erythema multiforme, exfoliative dermatitis, pruritus, rash, Stevens-Johnson syndrome, toxic epidermal necrolysis
Other: Anaphylaxis, angioedema, fluid retention, hyperkalemia, hyperuricemia, hyponatremia, lymphadenopathy

Nursing Considerations
• Use diclofenac with extreme caution and for shortest possible time in patients with a history of GI bleeding or ulcer disease because NSAIDs increase risk of GI bleeding and ulceration.
• Don't substitute one form of oral diclofenac for another. Different formulations aren't bioequivalent.
• Assess patient's hydration status before administering diclofenac intravenously because the patient must be well hydrated to reduce the risk of renal adverse reactions.
• Be aware that serious GI tract ulceration and bleeding, as well as perforation of stomach or intestine, can occur without warning or symptoms. Elderly patients are at greater risk. Monitor patient for signs of GI irritation and ulceration, especially if patient has a predisposing condition (such as a history of GI bleeding); takes an oral corticosteroid, anticoagulant, or NSAID (long-term); smokes; is an alcoholic; is over age 60; has poor general health; or tests positive for *Helicobacter pylori.* To minimize risk, give diclofenac with food. If patient develops GI distress, withhold drug and notify prescriber immediately.
• Use diclofenac cautiously in patients with hypertension, and monitor blood pressure closely; drug can cause or worsen hypertension.
• Assess patient for hypotension. If patient takes a potassium-sparing diuretic, check for elevated serum potassium level.
WARNING Monitor patient closely for thrombotic events, including MI and stroke, because NSAIDs such as diclofenac increase the risk for such events.
• Report signs of bleeding, such as bleeding gums, bloody or cloudy urine, ecchymoses, melena, and petechiae.
• Monitor BUN and serum creatinine levels in elderly patients, patients taking ACE inhibitors or diuretics, and patients with

heart failure or impaired renal or hepatic function. These patients may have an increased risk of renal failure.

• Assess patient's skin routinely for rash or other signs of hypersensitivity reaction; drug may cause serious skin reactions without warning. At first sign of reaction, stop drug and notify prescriber.

• Because severe hepatic reactions may occur during diclofenac therapy, monitor liver function test results and serum uric acid level. Liver enzyme elevations usually occur within 2 months of starting drug and should be reported promptly because dosage may need adjustment. Also monitor patient for evidence of hepatic dysfunction (diarrhea, fatigue, flulike symptoms, jaundice, lethargy, nausea, pruritus, right upper quadrant tenderness).

• Report weight gain of more than 1 kg (2 lb) in 24 hours because it suggests fluid retention.

PATIENT TEACHING

• Advise patient not to chew, crush, or dissolve tablet, but to swallow it whole.

• Instruct patient to take diclofenac with food to minimize GI distress unless he is prescribed Zorvolex, which should be taken on an empty stomach.

• To decrease risk of esophageal ulceration, instruct patient not to lie down for 15 to 30 minutes after taking drug.

• Warn patient to avoid hazardous activities until diclofenac's CNS effects are known.

• Urge patient to notify prescriber about unexplained weight gain or edema, ringing or buzzing in ears, impaired hearing, or dizziness.

• Advise patient to consult prescriber before taking aspirin or other OTC analgesics or drinking alcohol.

• Explain that diclofenac may increase risk of serious adverse cardiovascular reactions; urge patient to seek immediate medical attention for signs and symptoms such as chest pain, shortness of breath, weakness, and slurred speech.

• Tell patient that diclofenac also may increase risk of serious adverse GI reactions; stress need to seek immediate medical attention for such evidence as epigastric or abdominal pain, indigestion, black or tarry stools, and vomiting blood or material that looks like coffee grounds.

• Alert patient about possibly serious skin reactions and need to seek immediate medial attention for such as problems as blisters, fever, itching, rash, and other signs of hypersensitivity such as difficulty breathing or swelling of face or throat.

• Urge patient to promptly report adverse liver effects (nausea, fatigue, lethargy, diarrhea, pruritus, jaundice, right upper quadrant discomfort, flulike symptoms).

• Advise female patients to notify prescriber if pregnancy occurs or is suspected.

dicloxacillin sodium
Dycill, Dynapen, Pathocil

Class and Category
Chemical class: Isoxazolyl penicillin derivative
Therapeutic class: Antibiotic
Pregnancy category: B

Indications and Dosages
➤ *To treat mild to moderate upper respiratory tract and localized skin and soft-tissue infections caused by penicillinase-producing staphylococci*
CAPSULES, ORAL SOLUTION
Adults and children weighing 40 kg (88 lb) or more. 125 mg every 6 hr.
Children weighing less than 40 kg. 12.5 mg/kg daily divided into four equal doses and given every 6 hr.
➤ *To treat severe infections, such as lower respiratory tract or disseminated infections, caused by penicillinase-producing staphylococci*
CAPSULES, ORAL SOLUTION
Adults and children weighing 40 kg or more. 250 mg every 6 hr, or higher doses, if needed. *Maximum:* 6 g daily.
Children over age 1 month weighing less than 40 kg. 25 mg/kg daily divided into 4 equal doses and given every 6 hr, or higher doses if needed.

Mechanism of Action
Inhibits cell wall synthesis in susceptible bacteria, which assemble rigid, cross-linked cell walls in several steps. Dicloxacillin affects final cross-linking by inactivating penicillin-binding protein (the enzyme

needed to link cell wall strands). This action inhibits cell wall synthesis and causes cell lysis and death.

Contraindications

Hypersensitivity to dicloxacillin, other penicillins, beta-lactamase inhibitors (such as piperacillin/tazobactam), cephalosporins, imipenem, or their components

Interactions

DRUGS

hepatotoxic drugs: Increased risk of hepatotoxicity
methotrexate: Decreased methotrexate clearance and increased risk of toxicity
oral contraceptives: Decreased contraceptive action
probenecid: Increased and prolonged blood dicloxacillin level
tetracyclines: Decreased dicloxacillin effectiveness

FOODS

all foods: Possibly delayed absorption

Adverse Reactions

CNS: Dizziness, fatigue, fever, insomnia
EENT: Black "hairy" tongue, dry mouth, glossitis, laryngeal edema, laryngospasm, stomatitis, taste perversion
GI: Abdominal pain, anorexia, diarrhea, flatulence, nausea, pseudomembranous colitis, transient hepatitis, vomiting
GU: Nephropathy, vaginitis
MS: Prolonged muscle relaxation
SKIN: Dermatitis, erythema multiforme, pruritus, rash, urticaria, vesicular eruptions
Other: Anaphylaxis, serum sicknesslike reaction, superinfection

Nursing Considerations

• Before dicloxacillin therapy begins, expect to obtain body fluid and tissue samples for culture and sensitivity tests, as ordered, and review the results, if possible. Also check for history of sensitivity to cephalosporins, penicillins, and other substances.
• If diarrhea develops, notify prescriber; it could be the development of pseudo-membranous colitis.

PATIENT TEACHING

• Instruct patient to take drug 1 hour before or 2 hours after meals.

• Instruct patient to take drug around the clock, not to miss a dose, and to complete the entire prescription unless directed otherwise by prescriber.
• Advise patient to take oral solution with a cold beverage but not acidic juice, such as orange juice. Explain that solution is effective for 7 days at room temperature and for 14 days if refrigerated.
• Caution patient not to open capsules and mix contents with food or liquids because an unpleasant taste and decreased drug absorption will result.
• Instruct parent to shake oral solution thoroughly and measure doses with a calibrated device for accuracy.
• Advise patient to notify prescriber if she experiences adverse GI reactions or signs of hypersensitivity or superinfection.
• If patient takes an oral contraceptive, advise her to use an additional form of contraception during therapy.
• Instruct patient to store drug away from heat, moisture, and direct light and to refrigerate—but not freeze—oral solution.

dicumarol

Class and Category

Chemical class: Coumarin derivative
Therapeutic class: Anticoagulant
Pregnancy category: X

Indications and Dosages

➤ *To prevent and treat pulmonary embolus, thromboembolus, and venous thrombus; to prevent thromboembolism related to atrial fibrillation and mechanical heart valves*

TABLETS

Adults. *Initial:* 200 to 300 mg on the first day. *Maintenance:* 25 to 200 mg daily.
DOSAGE ADJUSTMENT Dosage reduced for elderly patients and those with hepatic or renal impairment.

Route	Onset	Peak	Duration
P.O.	1–5 days	Unknown	5–6 days

Mechanism of Action

Prevents coagulation by interfering with the liver's ability to synthesize vitamin K–

dependent clotting factors. This in turn depletes clotting factors II (prothrombin), VII, IX, and X. Normally, clots result from a cascade of proteolytic reactions that involve several clotting factors, including vitamin K–dependent factors. These clotting factors must be converted to an activated form before the clotting cascade can continue. By depleting vitamin K–dependent clotting factors, dicumarol interferes with the clotting cascade and prevents coagulation.

Contraindications

Active bleeding; aneurysm; ascorbic acid deficiency; bacterial endocarditis; blood dyscrasia; continuous tube drainage of small intestine; diverticulitis; eclampsia or preclampsia; emaciation; hemophilia; hemorrhagic tendency; history of bleeding diathesis or warfarin-induced necrosis; leukemia; major regional lumbar block anesthesia; malnutrition; pericardial effusion; pericarditis; polyarthritis; pregnancy; prostatectomy; recent surgery on brain, eye, GI tract, or prostate; recovery from spinal puncture; severe hepatic or renal impairment; stroke; surgery resulting in large, open surfaces; threatened abortion; thrombocytopenic purpura; uncontrolled or malignant hypertension; visceral cancer; vitamin K deficiency

Interactions

DRUGS

acetaminophen, androgens, beta blockers, chlorpropamide, clofibrate, corticosteroids, cyclophosphamide, dextrothyroxine, disulfiram, erythromycin, fluconazole, gemfibrozil, glucagon, hydantoins, influenza virus vaccine, isoniazid, ketoconazole, miconazole, moricizine, propoxyphene, quinolones, streptokinase, sulfonamides, tamoxifen, thioamines, thyroid drugs, urokinase: Increased effects of dicumarol and risk of bleeding

Adverse Reactions

CNS: Fever, malaise
ENDO: Adrenal hemorrhage
GI: Abdominal cramps and distention, anorexia, diarrhea, flatulence, nausea, vomiting
GU: Menorrhagia, priapism
HEME: Hemorrhage, leukopenia
SKIN: Alopecia, pruritus, rash, urticaria

Other: Allergic reaction, purple toes syndrome

Nursing Considerations

• Use dicumarol cautiously in elderly patients and those with hepatic or renal impairment.
• Monitor results of serial PT and INR tests, and expect to adjust dosage accordingly.
• If patient also receives heparin, expect heparin therapy to continue until INR reaches desired level: 2 to 3 times the control value for pulmonary embolus, thromboembolus, or venous thrombus; or 3 to 4.5 times the control value for thromboembolism related to atrial fibrillation or mechanical valves.
• If PT or INR are prolonged, withhold one dicumarol dose, as prescribed, and, to reverse anticoagulation, give vitamin K. If patient has severe bleeding, expect to give blood to offset vitamin K's delayed onset.
• Assess patient for signs of hemorrhage, such as ecchymosis, epistaxis, gingival bleeding, hematuria, and melena.
• To reduce bleeding, apply pressure to I.M. or venipuncture sites for up to 5 minutes.

PATIENT TEACHING

• Instruct patient to take dicumarol at the same time every day.
• Inform patient that drug's full effects may not occur for 2 to 7 days.
• Instruct patient to have frequent coagulation tests, as prescribed.
• Advise patient to stabilize her intake of foods high in vitamin K. Urge her to consult prescriber before starting a weight-loss diet, altering eating habits, or taking new vitamins or other nutritional supplements; these activities may alter her vitamin K intake.
• Caution patient to avoid activities that may cause bleeding. Advise the use of a soft toothbrush and an electric razor.
• Urge patient to consult prescriber before taking OTC drugs, including herbs; they may affect anticoagulant effect.
• Instruct patient to take a missed dose as soon as she remembers unless it's nearly time for the next dose. Urge her to report missed doses to prescriber.

• Caution patient to immediately notify prescriber if signs of bleeding occur, such as abdominal pain or swelling; back pain; bloody or black stools; bloody urine; coughing up blood; joint pain, swelling, or stiffness; severe or continuing headache; and vomiting blood or material that looks like coffee grounds.

• Urge patient to carry medical identification and tell all health care providers that she takes dicumarol.

• Explain that coagulation will gradually return to normal after therapy stops. Remind patient to keep watching for bleeding.

dicyclomine hydrochloride

Bentyl, Bentylol (CAN), Formulex (CAN), Spasmoban (CAN)

Class and Category
Chemical class: Tertiary amine
Therapeutic class: Anticholinergic, antispasmodic
Pregnancy category: Not rated

Indications and Dosages
➤ *To control diarrhea and GI tract spasms*
CAPSULES, TABLETS
Adults and adolescents. 10 to 20 mg three times daily or four times daily, increased as needed and tolerated. *Maximum:* 160 mg daily.
Children ages 6 to 12. 10 mg three times daily or four times daily.
E.R. TABLETS
Adults and adolescents. 30 mg twice daily.
SYRUP
Adults and adolescents. 10 to 20 mg three times daily or four times daily, increased as needed and tolerated. *Maximum:* 60 mg daily.
Children ages 2 to 13. 10 mg three times daily or four times daily
Children ages 6 months to 2 years. 5 to 10 mg three times daily or four times daily.
I.M. INJECTION
Adults. 20 mg every 4 to 6 hr. Dosage adjusted as needed and tolerated.

Mechanism of Action
Inhibits acetylcholine's muscarinic actions at postganglionic parasympathetic receptors in smooth muscles, secretory glands, and the CNS. These actions relax smooth muscles and diminish GI, GU, and biliary tract secretions.

Contraindications
Adhesions between iris and lens, angle-closure glaucoma, GI obstruction, hemorrhagic shock, hepatic disease, hiatal hernia, hypersensitivity to any anticholinergic, ileus, intestinal atony in elderly or debilitated patients, myasthenia gravis, myocardial ischemia, obstructive uropathy, renal disease, severe ulcerative colitis, tachycardia, toxic megacolon

Interactions
DRUGS
adsorbent antidiarrheals, antacids: Decreased dicyclomine absorption
amantadine, anticholinergics, phenothiazines, tricyclic antidepressants: Increased dicyclomine effects
antimyasthenics: Reduced intestinal motility
atenolol: Increased atenolol effects
cyclopropane: Risk of ventricular arrhythmias
haloperidol: Decreased antipsychotic effect of haloperidol
ketoconazole: Decreased ketoconazole absorption
metoclopramide: Decreased effect of metoclopramide on GI motility
opioid analgesics: Increased risk of ileus, severe constipation, and urine retention
potassium chloride, especially wax-matrix preparations: Possibly GI ulceration
urinary alkalinizers (antacids that contain calcium or magnesium, carbonic anhydrase inhibitors, citrates, sodium bicarbonate): Delayed excretion and increased risk of adverse effects of dicyclomine

Adverse Reactions
CNS: Agitation, delirium, dizziness, drowsiness, dyskinesia, excitement, fever, insomnia, lethargy, light-headedness (I.M. use), nervousness, paresthesia, psychosis, syncope
CV: Palpitations, tachycardia

EENT: Blurred vision, cycloplegia, dry mouth, loss of taste, mydriasis, nasal congestion, photophobia
GI: Constipation, dysphagia, heartburn, ileus, vomiting
GU: Impotence, urine retention
SKIN: Decreased sweating, flushing, pruritus
Other: Heatstroke; injection-site pain, redness, and swelling

Nursing Considerations
• Assess patient for tachycardia before giving dicyclomine; heart rate may increase.
• Don't give drug by I.V. route because thrombosis, thrombophlebitis, and injection-site reactions such as pain, edema, skin color change and reflux sympathetic dystrophy syndrome may occur.
• Watch for symptoms of hypersensitivity, such as agitation and pruritus. They usually resolve within 48 hours of stopping drug.
• During long-term use, assess patient for chronic constipation and fecal impaction, and take corrective measures, as prescribed.
• Monitor patient, especially the elderly and/or patients with mental illness, for psychosis and delirium. If present, notify prescriber and expect drug to be discontinued and symptoms to disappear within 12 to 24 hours.
PATIENT TEACHING
• Instruct patient to store dicyclomine in a tightly sealed container at room temperature, protected from moisture and direct light. Advise her not to refrigerate syrup.
• Inform patient that dicyclomine relieves symptoms but doesn't cure the disorder.
• For best results, instruct patient to take drug 30 to 60 minutes before eating.
• Advise patient not to take an antacid or an antidiarrheal within 2 hours of dicyclomine.
• Inform patient that blurred vision, dizziness, or drowsiness may occur.
• To prevent constipation, advise patient to eat high-fiber foods and drink at least eight glasses of water daily.
WARNING Urge patient to avoid getting overheated during exercise or in hot

weather because heatstroke may result. Inform patient that hot baths or saunas may cause dizziness or fainting.
• Instruct patient to change position slowly to avoid light-headedness.
• Inform patient that stopping drug abruptly may cause dizziness and vomiting.
• Tell patient to take a missed dose as soon as she remembers, unless it's nearly time for the next dose. Caution against doubling the dose.
• Urge patient and family that if psychosis or delirium occurs, stop the drug and notify the prescriber. Inform them that these symptoms usually resolve within 12 to 24 hours after drug is discontinued.

diflunisal
Apo-Diflunisal (CAN), Dolobid, Novo-Diflunisal (CAN)

Class and Category
Chemical class: Difluorophenyl, salicylic acid derivative
Therapeutic class: Analgesic, anti-inflammatory
Pregnancy category: C (first trimester), Not rated (later trimesters)

Indications and Dosages
➤ *To relieve mild to moderate pain*
TABLETS
Adults. 1 g followed by 0.5 g every 8 to 12 hr. *Maximum:* 1.5 g daily.
➤ *To reduce inflammation in osteoarthritis or rheumatoid arthritis*
TABLETS
Adults. 0.5 to 1 g daily in divided doses twice daily. *Maximum:* 1.5 g daily.
DOSAGE ADJUSTMENT Dosage reduced for elderly patients and those who use diuretics; who could be harmed by prolonged bleeding time; or who have compromised cardiac function, conditions that cause fluid retention, hepatic or renal impairment, hypertension, or upper GI disease.

Route	Onset	Peak	Duration
P.O.*	1 hr	2–3 hr	8–12 hr

Mechanism of Action
Blocks the activity of cyclooxygenase, the enzyme needed to synthesize prostaglandins, which mediate the inflammatory response and cause local vasodilation, swelling, and pain. By blocking cyclooxygenase and inhibiting prostaglandins, this NSAID reduces inflammatory symptoms. This mechanism also relieves pain because prostaglandins promote pain transmission from the periphery to the spinal cord.

Contraindications
Asthma attacks, rhinitis, or urticaria precipitated by aspirin or other NSAIDs; hypersensitivity to diflunisal; treatment of perioperative pain after coronary artery bypass graft surgery

Interactions
DRUGS
acetaminophen: Increased risk of adverse renal effects with long-term use of both drugs
antacids: Decreased blood diflunisal level
antihypertensives: Decreased antihypertensive effects
aspirin, other NSAIDs, salicylates: Increased GI irritability and bleeding, decreased diflunisal effectiveness
beta blockers: Impaired antihypertensive effects of beta blocker
cefamandole, cefoperazone, cefotetan, plicamycin, valproic acid: Increased risk of hypoprothrombinemia
colchicine, corticotropin (long-term use), glucocorticoids, potassium supplements: Increased GI irritability and bleeding
cyclosporine, gold compounds, nephrotoxic drugs: Increased risk of nephrotoxicity
digoxin: Increased blood digoxin level
heparin, oral anticoagulants, thrombolytics: Prolonged PT, increased risk of bleeding
hydrochlorothiazide: Increased blood hydrochlorothiazide level
insulin, oral antidiabetics: Increased hypoglycemic effects
loop diuretics: Decreased loop diuretic effectiveness
methotrexate: Increased risk of methotrexate toxicity
phenytoin: Increased blood phenytoin level
probenecid: Increased diflunisal toxicity

ACTIVITIES
alcohol use: Increased GI irritability and bleeding

Adverse Reactions
CNS: Aseptic meningitis, cerebral hemorrhage, dizziness, drowsiness, headache, insomnia
CV: Vasculitis
EENT: Tinnitus
ENDO: Hypoglycemia
GI: Abdominal pain, constipation, diarrhea, esophageal irritation, GI bleeding or ulceration, hepatic failure, hepatitis, indigestion, jaundice, nausea, perforation of stomach or intestine, vomiting
GU: Acute renal failure, interstitial nephritis
HEME: Agranulocytosis, aplastic anemia, leukopenia, pancytopenia, thrombocytopenia
SKIN: Erythema multiforme, exfoliative dermatitis, rash, Stevens-Johnson syndrome, toxic epidermal necrolysis
Other: Anaphylaxis, angioedema, hyponatremia

Nursing Considerations
• Use diflunisal with extreme caution and for shortest time possible in patients with a history of GI bleeding or ulcer disease because NSAIDs such as diflunisal increase the risk.
• Serious GI tract ulceration and bleeding, as well as perforation of stomach or intestine, can occur without warning or symptoms. Elderly patients are at greater risk. To minimize risk, give diflunisal with food. If patient has GI distress, withhold drug and notify prescriber immediately.
• Use diflunisal cautiously in patients with hypertension, and monitor blood pressure closely during therapy; drug can cause or worsen hypertension.
• Use drug cautiously in elderly patients, those with renal dysfunction, and those who should avoid prolonged bleeding time.
WARNING Monitor patient closely for thrombotic events, including stroke and MI, because NSAIDs such as diflunisal increase the risk of these events.
• Monitor BUN and serum creatinine levels in elderly patients, patients taking ACE inhibitors or diuretics, and patients with

heart failure or impaired hepatic or renal function. These patients may have an increased risk of renal failure.
• Assess patient's skin routinely for rash or other signs of hypersensitivity reaction; drug may cause serious skin reactions without warning. At first sign of reaction, stop drug and notify prescriber.
• Assess type, location, and intensity of pain before and 1 to 2 hours after giving drug.
• Assess patient carefully because long-term or high-dose therapy may mask fever.

PATIENT TEACHING
• Teach patient not to crush or chew diflunisal tablets.
• Instruct patient to take tablet with a full glass of water and not to lie down for 30 minutes afterward to avoid esophageal irritation.
• Inform patient that drug will start working in about 1 week but that full effects may not occur for several weeks.
• Explain that diflunisal may increase the risk of serious adverse cardiovascular reactions; urge patient to seek immediate medical attention for such signs and symptoms as chest pain, shortness of breath, slurred speech, and weakness.
• Tell patient that diflunisal also may increase risk of serious adverse GI reactions; stress need to seek immediate medical attention for signs and symptoms such as abdominal or epigastric pain, black or tarry stools, indigestion, and vomiting blood or material that resembles coffee grounds.
• Alert patient about possibly serious skin reactions and the need to seek immediate medial attention for such as problems as blisters, fever, itching, rash, and other signs of hypersensitivity.
• Caution patient to avoid acetaminophen, alcohol, aspirin, and other salicylates during diflunisal therapy, unless directed otherwise by prescriber.
• Advise patient to avoid hazardous activities until drug's CNS effects are known.
• Advise patient to tell healthcare providers about diflunisal therapy before surgery, including dental surgery. Therapy should stop for 1 week before procedure.

digoxin

Lanoxicaps, Lanoxin, Lanoxin Elixir Pediatric, Lanoxin Injection, Lanoxin Injection Pediatric, Novo-Digoxin (CAN)

Class and Category
Chemical class: Digitalis glycoside
Therapeutic class: Antiarrhythmic, cardiotonic
Pregnancy category: C

Indications and Dosages
➤ *To treat heart failure, atrial flutter, atrial fibrillation, and paroxysmal atrial tachycardia with rapid digitalization*
CAPSULES, I.V. INJECTION
Adults. *Loading:* 10 to 15 mcg/kg in 3 divided doses every 6 to 8 hr, with first dose equal to 50% of total dose. *Maintenance:* 125 to 350 mcg daily once or twice daily.
Children over age 10. *Loading:* 8 to 12 mcg/kg in 3 or more divided doses, with first dose equal to 50% of total dose. Subsequent doses given every 6 to 8 hr. *Maintenance:* 2 to 3 mcg/kg once daily.
Children ages 6 to 10. *Loading:* 15 to 30 mcg/kg in 3 or more divided doses, with first dose equal to 50% of total dose. Subsequent doses given every 6 to 8 hr. *Maintenance:* 4 to 8 mcg/kg daily in 2 divided doses.
Children ages 2 to 5. *Loading:* 25 to 35 mcg/kg in 3 or more divided doses, with first dose equal to 50% of total dose. Subsequent doses given every 6 to 8 hr. *Maintenance:* 6 to 9 mcg/kg daily in 2 divided doses.
Infants ages 1 to 24 months. *Loading:* 30 to 50 mcg/kg in 3 or more divided doses, with first dose equal to 50% of total dose. Subsequent doses every 6 to 8 hr. *Maintenance:* 7.5 to 12 mcg/kg daily in 2 divided doses.
Full-term neonates. *Loading:* 20 to 30 mcg/kg in 3 or more divided doses, with first dose equal to 50% of total dose. Subsequent doses given every 6 to 8 hr. *Maintenance:* 5 to 8 mcg/kg daily in 2 divided doses.
Premature neonates. *Loading:* 15 to 25 mcg/kg in 3 or more divided doses, with first dose equal to 50% of total dose. Subsequent doses given every 6 to 8 hr.

Maintenance: 4 to 6 mcg/kg daily in 2 divided doses.

ELIXIR, TABLETS

Adults. *Loading:* 10 to 15 mcg/kg total dose given in 3 divided doses every 6 to 8 hr, with first dose equal to 50% of total dose. *Maintenance:* 125 to 500 mcg daily.

Children over age 10. *Loading:* 10 to 15 mcg/kg total given in 3 divided doses every 6 to 8 hr, with first dose equal to 50% of total dose. *Maintenance:* 2.5 to 5 mcg/kg daily.

Children ages 5 to 10. *Loading:* 20 to 35 mcg/kg in 3 divided doses every 6 to 8 hr. *Maintenance:* 5 to 10 mcg/kg daily in 2 divided doses.

Children ages 2 to 5. *Loading:* 30 to 40 mcg/kg in 3 divided doses every 6 to 8 hr. *Maintenance:* 7.5 to 10 mcg/kg daily in 2 divided doses.

Infants ages 1 to 24 months. *Loading:* 35 to 60 mcg/kg in 3 divided doses every 6 to 8 hr. *Maintenance:* 10 to 15 mcg/kg daily in 2 divided doses.

Full-term neonates. *Loading:* 25 to 35 mcg/kg in 3 divided doses every 6 to 8 hr. *Maintenance:* 6 to 10 mcg/kg daily in 2 divided doses.

Premature neonates. *Loading:* 20 to 30 mcg/kg in 3 divided doses every 6 to 8 hr. *Maintenance:* 5 to 7.5 mcg/kg daily in 2 divided doses.

DOSAGE ADJUSTMENT Dosage carefully adjusted for patients who are elderly or debilitated or have implanted pacemakers because toxicity may develop at doses tolerated by most patients.

Route	Onset	Peak	Duration
P.O.	30–120 min	6–8 hr	3–4 days
I.V.	5–30 min	1–5 hr	3–4 days

Mechanism of Action

Increases the force and velocity of myocardial contraction, resulting in positive inotropic effects. Digoxin produces antiarrhythmic effects by decreasing the conduction rate and increasing the effective refractory period of the AV node.

Contraindications

Hypersensitive carotid sinus syndrome, hypersensitivity to digoxin, presence or history of digitalis toxicity or idiosyncratic reaction to digoxin, ventricular fibrillation, ventricular tachycardia unless heart failure occurs unrelated to digoxin therapy

Interactions

DRUGS

adsorbent antidiarrheals, such as kaolin and pectin; bulk laxatives; cholestyramine; colestipol; oral neomycin; sulfasalazine: Inhibited digoxin absorption

amiodarone, propafenone: Elevated blood digoxin level, possibly to toxic level

antacids: Inhibited digoxin absorption

antiarrhythmics, pancuronium, parenteral calcium salts, rauwolfia alkaloids, sympathomimetics: Increased risk of arrhythmias

beta blockers: Increased additive effects of slowing heart rate, possibly producing bradycardia

carvedilol: Increased digoxin level

diltiazem, verapamil: Increased blood digoxin level, possibly excessive bradycardia

edrophonium: Excessive slowing of heart rate

erythromycin, neomycin, tetracycline: Possibly increased blood digoxin level

hypokalemia-causing drugs, potassium-wasting diuretics: Increased risk of digitalis toxicity from hypokalemia

indomethacin: Decreased renal clearance and increased blood level of digoxin

magnesium sulfate (parenteral): Possibly cardiac conduction changes and heart block

quinidine, quinine: Increased blood digoxin level

spironolactone: Increased half-life and risk of adverse effects of digoxin

succinylcholine: Increased risk of digoxin-induced arrhythmias

sucralfate: Decreased digoxin absorption

FOODS

high-fiber food: Inhibited digoxin absorption

Adverse Reactions

CNS: Confusion, depression, drowsiness, extreme weakness, headache, syncope
CV: Arrhythmias, heart block
EENT: Blurred vision, colored halos around objects
GI: Abdominal discomfort or pain, anorexia, diarrhea, nausea, vomiting
Other: Electrolyte imbalances

Nursing Considerations

• Be aware that digoxin therapy is not recommended in patients with restrictive cardiomyopathy, constrictive pericarditis, amyloid heart disease, or acute cor pulmonale involving heart failure associated with preserved left ventricular ejection fraction because of increased susceptibility to digoxin toxicity. The drug is also not recommended in patients with idiopathic hypertrophic subaortic stenosis because outflow obstruction may worsen because of the inotropic effects of digoxin.

• Expect to treat underlying thiamine deficiency in patients with beri beri heart disease because if left untreated, digoxin therapy may be ineffective.

• Give parenteral digoxin undiluted, or dilute with a fourfold or greater volume of sterile water for injection, normal saline solution, or D_5W for I.V. administration. Once diluted, give immediately. Discard if solution is markedly discolored or contains precipitate.

• Before giving each dose, take patient's apical pulse and notify prescriber if it's below 60 beats/minute (or other specified level).

• Monitor patient closely for signs of digitalis toxicity, such as altered mental status, arrhythmias, heart block, nausea, vision disturbances, and vomiting. If they appear, notify prescriber, check serum digoxin level as ordered, and expect to withhold drug until level is known. Monitor ECG tracing continuously.

• If patient has acute or unstable chronic atrial fibrillation, assess for drug effectiveness. Ventricular rate may not normalize even when serum drug level falls within therapeutic range; raising the dosage probably won't produce a therapeutic effect and may lead to toxicity.

• Frequently obtain ECG tracings as ordered in elderly patients because of their smaller body mass and reduced renal clearance. Elderly patients, especially those with coronary insufficiency, are more susceptible to arrhythmias—particularly ventricular fibrillation—if digitalis toxicity occurs.

• Monitor patient's serum potassium level regularly because hypokalemia predisposes to digitalis toxicity and serious arrhythmias. Also monitor potassium level often when giving potassium salts because hyperkalemia in patients receiving digoxin can be fatal.

PATIENT TEACHING

• Emphasize importance of taking digoxin exactly as prescribed. Warn about possible toxicity from taking too much and decreased effectiveness from taking too little.

• Instruct patient to take digoxin at same time each day to help increase compliance.

• Teach patient how to take her pulse, and instruct her to do so before each dose. Urge her to notify prescriber if pulse falls below 60 beats/minute or suddenly increases.

• Inform patient that small, white 0.25-mg tablets can easily be confused with other drugs. Caution against carrying digoxin in anything other than its original labeled container.

• Emphasize need to use special dropper supplied with elixir to ensure accurate dose measurement.

• Instruct patient to take a missed dose as soon as she remembers if within 12 hours of scheduled dose. If not, urge her to notify prescriber immediately.

• Urge patient to notify prescriber if she experiences adverse reactions, such as GI distress or pulse changes.

• Instruct patient to carry medical identification that indicates her need for digoxin.

• Advise patient to consult prescriber before using other drugs, including OTC products.

digoxin immuneFab (ovine)

Digibind

Class and Category

Chemical class: Digoxin-specific antigen-binding fragments
Therapeutic class: Digitalis glycoside antidote
Pregnancy category: C

Indications and Dosages

➤ *To treat acute toxicity from a known amount of digoxin elixir or tablets*

I.V. INJECTION

Adults and children. Individualized dosage based on amount ingested. Dose (mg) = dose ingested (mg) multiplied by 0.8 and then divided by 0.5, multiplied by 38, and rounded up to next whole vial.

➤ *To treat acute toxicity from a known amount of digoxin capsules, digitoxin tablets, or I.V. injection of digoxin or digitoxin*

I.V. INJECTION

Adults and children. Individualized dosage based on amount ingested. Dose (mg) 5 dose ingested (mg) divided by 0.5, then multiplied by 38 and rounded up to next whole vial.

➤ *To treat acute toxicity from an unknown amount of digoxin or digitoxin during long-term therapy*

I.V. INJECTION

Adults and children. Individualized dosage for digoxin toxicity: dose (mg) 5 serum digoxin level (ng/ml) multiplied by body weight (kg), then divided by 100, and then multiplied by 38. Individualized dosage for digitoxin toxicity: dose (mg) 5 serum digitoxin level (ng/ml) multiplied by body weight (kg) and then divided by 1,000, multiplied by 38, and rounded up to next whole vial.

DOSAGE ADJUSTMENT Higher dose administered, as prescribed, if the dose based on ingested amount differs substantially from the dose based on serum digoxin or digitoxin level. Dose repeated after several hours, if needed.

Route	Onset	Peak	Duration
I.V.	15–30 min	Unknown	8–12 hr

Mechanism of Action

Binds with digoxin or digitoxin molecules. The resulting complex is excreted through the kidneys. As the free serum digoxin level declines, tissue-bound digoxin enters the serum and also is bound and excreted.

Contraindications

Hypersensitivity to digoxin immune Fab

Adverse Reactions

CV: Increased ventricular rate (in atrial fibrillation), worsening of heart failure or low cardiac output

Other: Allergic reaction (difficulty breathing, urticaria), febrile reaction, hypokalemia

Nursing Considerations

• Expect each 38-mg vial of purified digoxin immune Fab to bind about 0.5 mg of digoxin or digitoxin.

• To reconstitute for I.V. use, dissolve 38 mg in 4 ml of sterile water for injection to yield 9.5 mg/ml. Mix gently. Further dilute with normal saline solution to proper volume for I.V. infusion. For very small doses, reconstituted 38-mg vial may be diluted with 34 ml of normal saline solution to yield 1 mg/ml.

WARNING Before giving digoxin immune Fab to high-risk patient, test for allergic reaction as prescribed by diluting 0.1 ml of reconstituted drug in 9.9 ml sodium chloride for injection and then injecting 0.1 ml (9.5 mcg/0.1 ml) intradermally. After 20 minutes, observe for an urticarial wheal surrounded by erythema. Alternatively, perform a scratch test by placing one drop of 9.5 mcg/0.1 ml dilution on patient's skin and making a 1/40 scratch through the drop with a sterile needle. Inspect site in 20 minutes. Test is considered positive if it produces a wheal surrounded by erythema. If test causes a systemic reaction, apply tourniquet above test site, notify prescriber, and prepare to respond to anaphylaxis. Be aware that if a skin or systemic reaction occurs, additional drug shouldn't be given unless essential; if more of the drug must be given, expect prescriber to pretreat patient with corticosteroids and diphenhydramine. Prescriber should be on standby to treat anaphylaxis.

• For an infant, reconstitute digoxin immune Fab as ordered and administer with a tuberculin syringe.

• When administering to a child, watch for fluid volume overload.

• When giving a large dose, expect a faster onset but watch closely for febrile reaction.

• Give I.V. infusion through a 0.22-micron membrane filter over 30 minutes. Keep in mind that drug may be given by rapid I.V. injection if cardiac arrest is imminent.

• Monitor serum potassium level often, especially during first few hours of therapy. Potassium level may drop rapidly.

D

dihydroergotamine mesylate

D.H.E. 45, Dihydroergotamine-Sandoz (CAN), Migranal

Class and Category
Chemical class: Semisynthetic ergot alkaloid
Therapeutic class: Antimigraine
Pregnancy category: X

Indications and Dosages
➤ *To treat acute migraine with or without aura*
I.V. INJECTION
Adults. 1 mg, repeated in 1 hr, if needed.
Maximum: 6 mg/wk.
I.M. INJECTION
Adults. 1 mg at first sign of headache, repeated every hr up to 3 mg, if needed.
Maximum: 3 mg/24 hr, 6 mg/wk.
NASAL SPRAY
Adults. 1 spray (0.5 mg) in each nostril, repeated in 15 min for a total dose of 2 sprays in each nostril or 2 mg. *Maximum:* 3 mg/24 hr, 4 mg/wk.

Route	Onset	Peak	Duration
I.V.	In 5 min	15 min–2 hr	About 8 hr
I.M.	15–30 min	15 min–2 hr	3–4 hr
Nasal	In 30 min	30–60 min	Unknown

Mechanism of Action
Produces intracranial and peripheral vasoconstriction by binding to all known 5-hydroxytryptamine$_1$ (5-HT$_1$) receptors, alpha$_1$- and alpha$_2$-adrenergic receptors, and dopaminergic receptors. Activation of 5-HT$_1$ receptors on intracranial blood vessels probably constricts large intracranial arteries and closes arteriovenous anastomoses to relieve migraine headache. Activation of 5-HT$_1$ receptors on sensory nerves in the trigeminal system also may inhibit the release of pro-inflammatory neuropeptides.

Peripherally, dihydroergotamine causes vasoconstriction by stimulating alpha-adrenergic receptors. At therapeutic doses, it inhibits norepinephrine reuptake, increasing vasoconstriction. Drug constricts veins more than arteries, increasing venous return while decreasing venous stasis and pooling.

Contraindications
Coronary artery disease, including vasospasm; hemiplegic or basilar migraine; hypersensitivity to dihydroergotamine or other ergot alkaloids; malnutrition; peripheral vascular disease or after vascular surgery; pregnancy; sepsis; severe hepatic or renal impairment; severe pruritus; uncontrolled hypertension; use of macrolide antibiotics or protease inhibitors; use within 24 hours of 5-HT$_1$ agonist, ergotamine-containing or ergot-type drug, or methysergide

Interactions
DRUGS
beta blockers: Possibly peripheral vasoconstriction and peripheral ischemia, increased risk of gangrene
macrolides, protease inhibitors: Possibly increased risk of vasospasm, acute ergotism with peripheral ischemia
nitrates: Decreased antianginal effects of nitrates
other ergot drugs, including ergoloid mesylates, ergonovine, methylergonovine, methysergide, and sumatriptan: Increased risk of serious adverse effects from nasal dihydroergotamine
systemic vasoconstrictors: Risk of severe hypertension
ACTIVITIES
smoking: Possibly increased ischemic response to ergot therapy

Adverse Reactions
CNS: Anxiety, confusion, dizziness, fatigue, headache, paresthesia, somnolence, weakness
CV: Bradycardia, chest pain, peripheral vasospasm (calf or heel pain with exertion, cool and cyanotic hands and feet, leg weakness, weak or absent pulses), tachycardia
EENT: Abnormal vision; dry mouth; epistaxis, nasal congestion or rhinitis, and sore nose (nasal spray); miosis; pharyngitis; sinusitis; taste perversion

GI: Diarrhea, nausea, vomiting
MS: Muscle stiffness
SKIN: Localized edema of face, feet, fingers, and lower legs; sensation of heat or warmth; sudden diaphoresis

Nursing Considerations

WARNING Monitor patient for signs of dihydroergotamine overdose, such as abdominal pain, confusion, delirium, dizziness, dyspnea, headache, nausea, pain in legs or arms, paresthesia, seizures, and vomiting.
• Assess patient's peripheral pulses, skin sensation, warmth, and capillary refill. After giving nasal dihydroergotamine, monitor patient for signs of widespread blood vessel constriction and adverse reactions caused by decreased circulation to many body areas.

PATIENT TEACHING
• Instruct patient to use nasal spray when headache pain—not aura—begins.
• Teach her to prime spray pump by squeezing it four times.
• Advise patient to wait 15 minutes between each set of nasal sprays.
• Encourage patient to lie down in a quiet, dark room after using drug.
• Instruct patient to use more dihydro-ergotamine if headache returns or worsens but not to exceed maximum prescribed amount or frequency.
• Remind patient to take drug only as needed, not on a daily basis.
• Instruct patient to discard residual nasal spray in an open ampule after 8 hours.
• If patient has a headache different from her usual migraines, caution her not to use dihydroergotamine and to notify prescriber.
• Inform patient that nasal drug won't relieve pain other than throbbing headaches.
• Advise patient to avoid alcohol, which can cause or worsen headaches, and to avoid smoking, which may cause an ischemic response.
• Warn patient about possible dizziness during or after a migraine for which she took dihydroergotamine.

dihydrotachysterol
DHT, DHT Intensol, Hytakerol

Class and Category
Chemical class: Sterol derivative, vitamin D analogue
Therapeutic class: Antihypocalcemic, antihypoparathyroid
Pregnancy category: C

Indications and Dosages
➤ *To treat hypocalcemic and idiopathic tetany*
CAPSULES, ORAL SOLUTION, TABLETS
Adults and adolescents. *Initial:* 0.75 to 2.5 mg daily for 3 days for acute cases; 0.25 to 0.5 mg daily for 3 days for less acute cases. *Maintenance:* 0.25 mg/wk to 1 mg daily, as needed to maintain normal serum calcium level.
➤ *To treat hypoparathyroidism*
CAPSULES, ORAL SOLUTION, TABLETS
Adults and adolescents. *Initial:* 0.75 to 2.5 mg daily for several days. *Maintenance:* 0.2 to 1 mg daily.
Children. *Initial:* 1 to 5 mg daily for 4 days; then continued or decreased to one-quarter the dose. *Maintenance:* 0.5 to 1.5 mg daily.

Route	Onset	Peak	Duration
P.O.	Several hr	Unknown	Up to 9 wk

Mechanism of Action
Stimulates intestinal calcium absorption and mobilizes bone calcium when parathyroid hormone and renal tissue fail to raise the serum calcium level.

Contraindications
Hypercalcemia, hypersensitivity to vitamin D, hypervitaminosis D, malabsorption syndrome, renal dysfunction

Interactions
DRUGS
aluminum-containing antacids: Possibly increased serum aluminum level, leading to toxicity
barbiturates, phenytoin: Decreased half-life and therapeutic effects of vitamin D
calcium-containing drugs, thiazide diuretics: Risk of hypercalcemia in patients with hypoparathyroidism
cholestyramine, colestipol, mineral oil: Decreased vitamin D absorption
digitalis glycosides: Possibly hypercalcemia; possibly potentiated effects of digitalis glycosides, resulting in arrhythmias

magnesium-containing antacids: Risk of hypermagnesemia, especially in patients with chronic renal failure
phosphorus-containing drugs: Increased risk of hyperphosphatemia
vitamin D analogues: Increased risk of vitamin D toxicity

Adverse Reactions
Other: Vitamin D toxicity (long-term, high-dose therapy)

Nursing Considerations
• After thyroid surgery, expect to give 0.25 mg once daily with 6 g of oral calcium lactate until danger of tetany has passed.
• Monitor serum calcium level regularly to determine dosage schedule and detect or prevent hypercalcemia. The difference between therapeutic and toxic doses may be small.
• Watch closely for signs of vitamin D toxicity: abdominal cramps, amnesia, anorexia, ataxia, coma, constipation, depression, diarrhea, disorientation, hallucinations, headache, hypotonia, lethargy, nausea, syncope, tinnitus, vertigo, vomiting, and weakness. Renal impairment may cause albuminuria, polydipsia, and polyuria. Delayed treatment can result in death from cardiac and renal failure caused by widespread calcification of soft tissues, including the heart, blood vessels, kidneys, and lungs.
• If toxicity occurs, notify prescriber and expect to stop dihydrotachysterol immediately. Place patient on bed rest, administer fluids and a laxative, and give low-calcium diet as ordered. For hypercalcemic crisis with dehydration, prepare to give I.V. normal saline solution and a loop diuretic (such as furosemide or ethacrynic acid) to increase urinary calcium excretion.

PATIENT TEACHING
• Emphasize importance of not exceeding prescribed dihydrotachysterol dosage because of the risk of vitamin D toxicity.
• If patient detects signs of toxicity, caution her not to take the next dose and to notify prescriber immediately.
• Advise patient to drop solution directly into her mouth or to mix it with fruit juice, cereal, or other food.

• Tell patient to take a missed dose as soon as she remembers unless it's nearly time for next dose. Warn her not to double it.
• Advise patient to avoid OTC drugs and dietary supplements that contain aluminum, calcium, phosphorus, or vitamin D, unless directed by prescriber. Also advise her to avoid antacids that contain magnesium.
• Urge patient to keep follow-up appointments and to have her serum calcium level measured periodically.

diltiazem hydrochloride
Apo-Diltiaz (CAN), Cardizem, Cardizem CD, Cardizem LA, Cardizem SR, Dilacor XR, Novo-Diltiazem (CAN), Nu-Diltiaz (CAN), Tiazac ER

Class and Category
Chemical class: Benzothiazepine derivative
Therapeutic class: Antianginal, antiarrhythmic, antihypertensive
Pregnancy category: C

Indications and Dosages
➤ *To treat prinzmetal's (variant) angina and chronic stable angina*
TABLETS
Adults and adolescents. *Initial:* 30 mg three times daily or four times daily before meals and at bedtime, increased every 1 or 2 days as appropriate. *Maximum:* 360 mg daily in divided doses three times daily or four times daily.
E.R. TABLETS
Adults and adolescents. *Initial:* 180 mg daily, increased every 7 to 14 days as needed. *Maximum:* 360 mg daily.
➤ *To control hypertension*
E.R. CAPSULES
Adults and adolescents. *Initial:* 180 to 240 mg daily, adjusted after 14 days as appropriate. *Maximum:* 360 mg daily.
E.R. CAPSULES
Adults and adolescents. *Initial:* 60 to 120 mg twice daily., adjusted after 14 days as appropriate. *Maximum:* 360 mg daily.

TABLETS

Adults and adolescents. *Initial:* 30 mg three times daily or four times daily before meals and at bedtime, increased every 1 or 2 days as appropriate. *Maximum:* 360 mg daily in divided doses three times daily or four times daily.

E.R. TABLETS

Adults. *Initial:* 180 to 240 mg daily, adjusted after 14 days, as needed. *Maximum:* 540 mg daily.

➤ *To treat atrial fibrillation, atrial flutter, and paroxysmal supraventricular tachycardia*

I.V. INFUSION OR INJECTION

Adults and adolescents. 0.25 mg/kg given by bolus over 2 min. If response is inadequate after 15 min, 0.35 mg/kg given by bolus over 2 min. Then 10 mg/hr for continued reduction of heart rate after bolus, increased by 5 mg/hr, as needed. *Maximum:* 15 mg/hr for up to 24 hr.

Route	Onset	Peak	Duration
P.O.	30–60 min	In 2 wk	Unknown
P.O. (E.R.)	2–3 hr	In 2 wk	Unknown
P.O. (S.R.)	Unknown	In 2 wk	Unknown
I.V.	In 3 min	2– 7 min	30 min–10 hr*

Incompatibilities

Don't give diltiazem through same I.V. line as acetazolamide, acyclovir, aminophylline, ampicillin sodium/ sulbactam sodium, cefamandole, cefoperazone, diazepam, furosemide, heparin, hydrocortisone sodium succinate, methylprednisolone sodium succinate, mezlocillin, nafcillin, phenytoin, rifampin, or sodium bicarbonate.

Contraindications

Acute MI; cardiogenic shock; Lown-Ganong-Levine or Wolff-Parkinson-White syndrome, second- or third-degree AV block, and sick sinus syndrome, unless artificial pacemaker is in place; pulmonary edema; systolic blood pressure below 90 mm Hg; ventricular tachycardia (wide complex)

---

* For infusion; 1 to 3 hr for injection.

Interactions

DRUGS

anesthetic: Additive hypotension; possibly decreased cardiac contractility, conductivity, and automaticity

benzodiazepines: Increased risk of prolonged sedation

beta blockers: Possibly increased risk of adverse cardiovascular effects

buspirone: Increased effects and risk of buspirone toxicity

carbamazepine, cyclosporine, lovastatin, quinidine, theophyllines: Decreased hepatic clearance and increased serum levels of these drugs, leading to toxicity

cimetidine: Decreased diltiazem metabolism, increased blood diltiazem level

clonidine: Increased risk of serious sinus bradycardia

digoxin: Increased blood digoxin level

lithium: Possibly neurotoxicity

NSAIDs: Possibly antagonized antihypertensive effect of diltiazem

prazocin: Possibly increased risk of hypotension

procainamide: Possibly increased risk of prolonged QT interval

quinidine: Increased risk of adverse quinidine effects

rifampin: Decreased blood diltiazem level to undetectable amounts

statins: Increased blood statin level

Adverse Reactions

CNS: Abnormal gait, amnesia, asthenia, depression, dizziness, dream disturbances, extrapyramidal reactions, fatigue, hallucinations, headache, insomnia, nervousness, paresthesia, personality change, somnolence, syncope, tremor, weakness

CV: Angina, atrial flutter, AV block (first-, second-, and third-degree), bradycardia, bundle-branch block, heart failure, hypotension, palpitations, peripheral edema, PVCs, sinus arrest, sinus tachycardia, 12-lead ECG abnormalities, ventricular fibrillation, ventricular tachycardia

EENT: Amblyopia, dry mouth, epistaxis, eye irritation, gingival bleeding and hyperplasia, gingivitis, nasal congestion, retinopathy, taste perversion, tinnitus

ENDO: Hyperglycemia

D

Mechanism of Action

Diltiazem inhibits calcium movement into coronary and vascular smooth-muscle cells by blocking slow calcium channels in cell membranes, as shown. This action decreases intracellular calcium, which:
• inhibits smooth-muscle cell contractions
• decreases myocardial oxygen demand by relaxing coronary and vascular smooth
• muscle, reducing peripheral vascular resistance and systolic and diastolic blood pressures
• slows AV conduction time and prolongs AV nodal refractoriness
• interrupts the reentry circuit in AV nodal reentrant tachycardias.

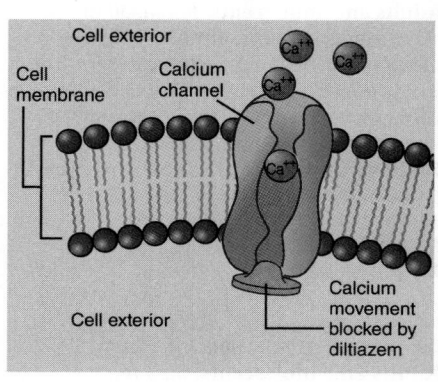

GI: Anorexia, constipation, diarrhea, elevated liver function test results, indigestion, nausea, thirst, vomiting
GU: Acute renal failure, impotence, nocturia, polyuria, sexual dysfunction
HEME: Hemolytic anemia, leukopenia, prolonged bleeding time, thrombocytopenia
MS: Arthralgia, muscle spasms, myalgia
RESP: Cough, dyspnea
SKIN: Acute generalized exanthematous pustulosis, alopecia, diaphoresis, erythema multiforme, exfoliative dermatitis, flushing, leukocytoclastic vasculitis, petechiae, photosensitivity, pruritus, purpura, rash, Stevens-Johnson syndrome, toxic epidermal necrolysis, urticaria
Other: Angioedema, hyperuricemia, weight gain

Nursing Considerations

• Use diltiazem cautiously in patients with impaired hepatic or renal function, and monitor liver and renal function, as appropriate; drug is metabolized mainly in the liver and excreted by the kidneys.
WARNING Monitor patient's blood pressure, pulse rate, and heart rate and rhythm by continuous ECG as appropriate during therapy. Keep emergency equipment and drugs available.
• Assess patient for signs and symptoms of heart failure.
• If patient takes digoxin, watch for digitalis toxicity (nausea, vomiting, halo vision, elevated serum digoxin level).

• Administer sublingual nitroglycerin, as prescribed, during diltiazem therapy.
• Expect to discontinue drug if adverse skin reactions, usually transient, persist.
PATIENT TEACHING
• Explain that capsules and E.R. tablets must be swallowed whole.
WARNING Tell patient that stopping drug suddenly may have life-threatening effects.
• Advise patient to monitor blood pressure and pulse rate regularly and to report significant changes to prescriber.
• Urge patient to report chest pain, difficulty breathing, dizziness, fainting, irregular heartbeat, rash, or swollen ankles.
• Instruct patient to maintain good oral hygiene, perform gum massage, and see a dentist every 6 months to prevent gingival bleeding and hyperplasia and gingivitis.

dimenhydrinate

Dinate, Dramanate, Gravol (CAN), Hydrate

Class and Category

Chemical class: Ethanolamine derivative
Therapeutic class: Antiemetic, antivertigo
Pregnancy category: B

Indications and Dosages

➤ *To treat nausea, vomiting, dizziness, or vertigo associated with motion sickness*

CHEWABLE TABLETS, ORAL SOLUTION, SYRUP, TABLETS

Adults and adolescents. 50 to 100 mg every 4 to 6 hr, as needed. *Maximum:* 400 mg/24 hr.

Children ages 6 to 12. 25 to 50 mg every 6 to 8 hr, as needed. *Maximum:* 150 mg/24 hr.

Children ages 2 to 6. 12.5 to 25 mg every 6 to 8 hr, as needed. *Maximum:* 75 mg/24 hr.

I.M. INJECTION

Adults and adolescents. 50 mg every 4 hr, as needed.

Children. 1.25 mg/kg or 37.5 mg/m^2 every 6 hr, as needed. *Maximum:* 300 mg daily.

I.V. INFUSION OR INJECTION

Adults and adolescents. 50 mg in 10 ml of normal saline solution administered slowly, over at least 2 min, every 4 hr, as needed.

Children. 1.25 mg/kg or 37.5 mg/m^2 in 10 ml of normal saline solution administered slowly, over at least 2 min, every 6 hr, as needed. *Maximum:* 300 mg daily.

Route	Onset	Peak	Duration
P.O.	Unknown	Unknown	3–6 hr
I.M.	20–30 min	Unknown	3–6 hr
I.V.	Immediate	Unknown	3–6 hr

Mechanism of Action

May inhibit vestibular stimulation and labyrinthine stimulation and function by acting on the otolith system and, with larger doses, on the semicircular canals.

Contraindications

Age less than 1 month, hypersensitivity to dimenhydrinate or its components

Interactions

DRUGS

aminoglycosides, other ototoxic drugs: Masked symptoms of ototoxicity
anticholinergics, drugs with anticholinergic activity: Potentiated anticholinergic effects of dimenhydrinate
apomorphine: Possibly decreased emetic response to apomorphine in treatment of poisoning
barbiturates, other CNS depressants: Possibly increased CNS depression
MAO inhibitors: Increased anticholinergic and CNS depressant effects of dimenhydrinate

alcohol use: Possibly increased CNS depression
MAO inhibitors: Increased anticholinergic and CNS depressant effects of dimen-hydrinate

ACTIVITIES

alcohol use: Possibly increased CNS depression

Adverse Reactions

CNS: Confusion, drowsiness, hallucinations, nervousness, paradoxical stimulation
CV: Hypotension, palpitations, tachycardia
EENT: Blurred vision, diplopia, dry eyes, dry mouth, nasal congestion
GI: Anorexia, constipation, diarrhea, epigastric discomfort, nausea, vomiting
GU: Dysuria
HEME: Hemolytic anemia
RESP: Thickening of bronchial secretions, wheezing
SKIN: Photosensitivity, rash, urticaria
Other: Anaphylaxis

Nursing Considerations

WARNING Be aware that I.V. dimenhydrinate shouldn't be administered to premature or full-term neonates. Some I.V. preparations may contain benzyl alcohol, which can cause a fatal toxic syndrome characterized by CNS, respiratory, circulatory, and renal impairment and metabolic acidosis.

WARNING Be aware that the 50-mg/ml concentration of dimenhydrinate is intended for I.M. use. For I.V. use, the solution must be diluted further with at least 10 ml of diluent, such as D$_5$W or normal saline solution, for each milliliter of dimenhydrinate.

• Monitor patients with prostatic hyperplasia, stenosing peptic ulcer, pyloroduodenal obstruction, bladder neck obstruction, angle-closure glaucoma, bronchial asthma, or cardiac arrhythmias for worsening of these conditions caused by anticholinergic effects.

• Monitor elderly patients for increased sensitivity to dimenhydrinate, such as excessive drowsiness, confusion, and restlessness.

• Assess patients, especially children and elderly patients, for evidence of paradoxical stimulation, such as nightmares, unusual excitement, nervousness, restlessness, or irritability.

• Store parenteral drug at 15° to 30° C (59° to 86° F); don't freeze.

D

PATIENT TEACHING
• Because dimenhydrinate may cause drowsiness, instruct patient to avoid hazardous activities until drug's CNS effects are known.
• Advise patient to inform health care providers about dimenhydrinate therapy, especially if she's being evaluated for medical conditions that are affected by this drug, such as appendicitis.
• Instruct patient to avoid alcohol, sedatives, and tranquilizers while taking dimenhydrinate.
• Encourage patient to use sunscreen to prevent photosensitivity reactions.

dimethyl fumarate
Tecfidera

Class and Category
Chemical class: Butenedioate
Therapeutic class: Antimultiple sclerotic
Pregnancy category: C

Indications and Dosages
➤ To treat relapsing forms of multiple sclerosis
DELAYED RELEASE CAPSULES
Adults. *Initial:* 120 mg twice daily for 7 days; then increased to 240 mg twice daily. *Maintenance:* 240 mg twice daily.
DOSAGE ADJUSTMENT Dosage decreased to 120 mg twice daily for up to 4 weeks for patients who cannot initially tolerate maintenance dose.

Mechanism of Action
Possibly activates the Nuclear factor (erythroid-derived 2)-like 2 (Nrf2) pathway, which is involved in the cellular response to oxidative stress thought to be a factor in multiple sclerosis.

Contraindications
Hypersensitivity to dimethyl fumarate or its components

Adverse Reactions
CNS: Progressive multifocal leukoencephalopathy
GI: Abdominal pain, diarrhea, dyspepsia, elevated liver enzymes, nausea, vomiting
GU: Albuminuria

HEME: Eosinophilia, lymphopenia
SKIN: Erythema, flushing, pruritus, rash
Other: Anaphylaxis, angioedema

Nursing Considerations
• Check to be sure patient has had a complete blood cell count (CBC) within the past 6 months prior to starting dimethyl fumarate therapy to identify patients with preexisting low lymphocyte counts. Know that a CBC should be obtained 6 months after therapy begins and then repeated every 6 to 12 months thereafter, and as needed.
• Know that dimethyl fumarate may decrease patient's lymphocyte counts as much as 30% during the first year of treatment but then stabilizes.
• Notify prescriber if patient is suspected of having an infection, as dimethyl fumarate may need to be withheld if confirmed until it is resolved.
PATIENT TEACHING
• Instruct patient to swallow capsule whole, avoiding crushing or chewing it.
• Remind patient that drug should not be sprinkled on food.
• Warn patient that dimethyl fumarate may cause flushing but that it is generally not severe, nor is it life-threatening. Advise patient that taking dimethyl fumarate with food or taking up to 325 mg of non-enteric-coated aspirin 30 minutes prior to taking drug may reduce flushing. Tell her that it generally begins soon after drug therapy has begun and usually improves or resolves over time.
WARNING Instruct patient to seek immediate emergency medical attention if a severe allergic reaction occurs, such as difficulty breathing, swelling of throat and tongue, or hives. Tell patient that an allergic reaction can occur after the first dose or at any time during treatment.
• Advise patient to report any signs and symptoms of infection such as fever, chills, redness, swelling, or drainage to prescriber immediately. Also, advise patient to report severe or persistent abdominal pain, diarrhea, and nausea.
• Inform women of childbearing age to alert prescriber if pregnancy is suspected or known, as effects of drug on the fetus is unknown and drug may need to be

discontinued. Also, if pregnancy occurs while taking drug, encourage patient to enroll in the pregnancy registry by calling 1-866-810-1462 or visiting the online site: www.tecfiderapregnancyregistry.com.
• Warn patient to protect capsules from light and to discard any unused capsules if container has been opened for 90 days.

diphenhydramine hydrochloride

Allerdryl (CAN), Banophen, Benadryl, Benadryl Allergy, Diphenhist CapTabs, Genahist, Hyrexin, Nytol QuickCaps, Siladryl, Sleep-Eze D Extra Strength, Unisom SleepGels Maximum Strength

Class and Category
Chemical class: Ethanolamine derivative
Therapeutic class: Antianaphylactic adjunct, antidyskinetic, antiemetic, antihistamine, antitussive (syrup), antivertigo, sedative-hypnotic
Pregnancy category: B

Indications and Dosages
➤ *To treat hypersensitivity reactions, such as perennial and seasonal allergic rhinitis, vasomotor rhinitis, allergic conjunctivitis, uncomplicated allergic skin eruptions, and transfusion reactions*
CAPSULES, TABLETS
Adults and adolescents. 25 to 50 mg every 4 to 6 hr, as needed. *Maximum:* 300 mg daily.
Children ages 6 to 12. 12.5 to 25 mg every 4 to 6 hr. *Maximum:* 150 mg daily.
Children up to age 6. 6.25 to 12.5 mg every 4 to 6 hr.
ELIXIR
Adults and adolescents. 25 to 50 mg every 4 to 6 hr, as needed. *Maximum:* 300 mg daily.
Children. 1.25 mg/kg every 4 to 6 hr. *Maximum:* 300 mg daily.
I.V. OR I.M. INJECTION
Adults and adolescents. 10 to 50 mg every 4 to 6 hr up to 100 mg/dose, as needed. *Maximum:* 400 mg daily.

Children. 1.25 mg/kg every 4 to 6 hr. *Maximum:* 300 mg daily.
➤ *To treat sleep disorders*
CAPSULES, TABLETS
Adults and adolescents. 50 mg 20 to 30 min before bedtime.
➤ *To provide antitussive effects*
ELIXIR
Adults and adolescents. 25 mg every 4 hr. *Maximum:* 100 mg/24 hr.
Children ages 6 to 12. 12.5 mg every 4 to 6 hr. *Maximum:* 75 mg daily.
Children ages 2 to 6. 6.25 mg every 4 to 6 hr. *Maximum:* 25 mg daily.
➤ *To prevent motion sickness or treat vertigo*
CAPSULES, ELIXIR, TABLETS
Adults and adolescents. 25 to 50 mg every 4 to 6 hr, as needed. *Maximum:* 300 mg daily.
Children. 1 to 1.5 mg/kg every 4 to 6 hr, as needed. *Maximum:* 300 mg daily.
I.V. OR I.M. INJECTION
Adults and adolescents.
Initial: 10 mg. Increased to 20 to 50 mg every 2 to 3 hr, if needed. *Maximum:* 100 mg/dose, 400 mg daily.
Children. 1 to 1.5 mg/kg I.M. every 4 to 6 hr, as needed. *Maximum:* 300 mg daily.
➤ *To treat symptoms of Parkinson's disease and drug-induced extrapyramidal reactions in elderly patients who can't tolerate more potent antidyskinetic drugs*
CAPSULES, ELIXIR, TABLETS
Adults. 25 mg three times daily, increased gradually to 50 mg four times daily, as needed. *Maximum:* 300 mg daily.
I.V. OR I.M. INJECTION
Adults and adolescents. 10 to 50 mg four times daily, as needed. *Maximum:* 100 mg/ dose, 400 mg daily.

Route	Onset	Peak	Duration
P.O.	15–60 min	1–3 hr	6–8 hr
I.V.	Immediate	1–3 hr	6–8 hr
I.M.	30 min	1–3 hr	6–8 hr

Mechanism of Action
Binds to central and peripheral H_1 receptors, competing with histamine for these sites and preventing it from reaching its site of action. By blocking histamine,

Children. 1.25 mg/kg every 4 to 6 hr. *Maximum:* 300 mg daily.

diphenhydramine produces antihistamine effects, inhibiting respiratory, vascular, and GI smooth-muscle contraction; decreasing capillary permeability, which reduces wheals, flares, and itching; and decreasing salivary and lacrimal gland secretions.

Diphenhydramine produces antidyskinetic effects, possibly by inhibiting acetylcholine in the CNS. It also produces antitussive effects by directly suppressing the cough center in the medulla oblongata in the brain. Diphenhydramine's antiemetic and antivertigo effects may be related to its ability to bind to CNS muscarinic receptors and depress vestibular stimulation and labyrinthine function. Its sedative effects are related to its CNS depressant action.

Contraindications

Bladder neck obstruction, hypersensitivity to diphenhydramine or its components, lower respiratory tract symptoms (including asthma), MAO inhibitor therapy, narrow-angle glaucoma, pyloroduodenal obstruction, stenosing peptic ulcer, symptomatic benign prostatic hyperplasia

Interactions

DRUGS

apomorphine: Possibly decreased emetic response in treatment of poisoning
barbiturates, other CNS depressants: Possibly increased CNS depression
MAO inhibitors: Increased anticholinergic and CNS depressant effects of diphenhydramine

ACTIVITIES

alcohol use: Possibly increased CNS depression

Adverse Reactions

CNS: Confusion, dizziness, drowsiness
CV: Arrhythmias, palpitations, tachycardia
EENT: Blurred vision, diplopia
GI: Epigastric distress, nausea
HEME: Agranulocytosis, hemolytic anemia, thrombocytopenia
RESP: Thickened bronchial secretions
SKIN: Photosensitivity

Nursing Considerations

• Expect to give parenteral form of diphenhydramine only when oral ingestion isn't possible.
• Keep elixir container tightly closed. Protect elixir and parenteral forms from light.

• Expect to discontinue drug at least 72 hours before skin tests for allergies because drug may inhibit cutaneous histamine response, thus producing false-negative results.

PATIENT TEACHING

• Instruct patient to take diphenhydramine at least 30 minutes before exposure to situations that may cause motion sickness.
• Advise her to take drug with food to minimize GI distress.
• Urge patient to avoid alcohol while taking diphenhydramine.
• Instruct her to use sunscreen to prevent photosensitivity reactions.
• Advise patient to avoid taking other OTC drugs that contain diphenhydramine to prevent additive effects.

dipyridamole

Apo-Dipyridamole FC (CAN), Apo-Dipyridamole SC (CAN), Novo-Dipiradol (CAN), Persantine

Class and Category

Chemical class: Pyrimidine
Therapeutic class: Coronary vasodilator, diagnostic aid, platelet aggregation inhibitor
Pregnancy category: B

Indications and Dosages

➤ *To prevent thromboembolic complications of cardiac valve replacement*

TABLETS

Adults. 75 to 100 mg four times daily with coumarin or indanedione derivative anticoagulant.

➤ *To aid diagnosis during thallium perfusion imaging of myocardium*

I.V. INFUSION

Adults. 0.57 mg/kg in 50 ml of D_5W infused over 4 min. *Maximum:* 60 mg.

Route	Onset	Peak	Duration
I.V.	Unknown	3.8–Unknown	8.7 min*

Mechanism of Action

May increase the intraplatelet level of adenosine, which causes coronary vasodilation and inhibits platelet

---

* After start of infusion, for increased velocity of coronary artery blood flow.

aggregation. Dipyridamole also may increase the intraplatelet level of cyclic adenosine monophosphate (cAMP) and may inhibit formation of the potent platelet activator stimulant thromboxane A$_2$, which decreases platelet activation. Vasodilation and increased blood flow occur preferentially in nondiseased coronary vessels, which results in redistribution of blood away from significantly diseased vessels. These changes in perfusion are observed during thallium imaging studies.

Contraindications
Asthma (I.V.), hypersensitivity to dipyridamole or its components, hypotension, unstable angina pectoris

Interactions
DRUGS
adenosine: Potentiated effects of adenosine
cefamandole, cefoperazone, cefotetan, plicamycin, valproic acid: Possibly hypoprothrombinemia and increased risk of bleeding
heparin, NSAIDs, thrombolytics: Possibly increased risk of bleeding
theophylline: Reversal of coronary vasodilation caused by dipyridamole, possibly false-negative thallium imaging result

Adverse Reactions
CNS: Dizziness, headache
CV: Angina, arrhythmias, ECG changes (specifically, ST-segment and T-wave changes)
GI: Abdominal pain, diarrhea, nausea, vomiting
RESP: Dyspnea
SKIN: Flushing, pruritus, rash

Nursing Considerations
• Protect I.V. form of dipyridamole from direct light and freezing.
• Monitor blood pressure, pulse rate and rhythm, and breath sounds every 10 to 15 minutes during I.V. infusion.
• Keep parenteral aminophylline available to relieve adverse reactions to dipyridamole infusion.
• At therapeutic doses, expect adverse reactions to be minimal and transient. They typically resolve with long-term use.
PATIENT TEACHING
• Urge patient to take dipyridamole at least 1 hour before or 2 hours after meals for faster absorption. If she experiences GI distress, advise her to take drug with meals or milk.
• Advise patient to take drug at evenly spaced intervals.
• Inform patient that drug commonly is taken with other anticoagulants.
• Urge her to keep appointments for coagulation tests.
• Instruct patient to seek immediate emergency treatment if chest pain occurs.
• Caution patient to consult prescriber before taking aspirin and other OTC NSAIDs because of the possible increased risk of bleeding.
• Advise patient to notify all healthcare providers about dipyridamole use.

dirithromycin
Dynabac

Class and Category
Chemical: Semisynthetic macrolide
Therapeutic: Antibiotic
Pregnancy category: C

Indications and Dosages
➤ *To treat acute bacterial exacerbations and secondary bacterial infections in patients with bronchitis caused by* Moraxella catarrhalis *or* Streptococcus pneumoniae, *and uncomplicated skin and soft-tissue infections caused by methicillin-susceptible* Staphylococcus aureus
TABLETS
Adults and adolescents. 500 mg daily for 7 days.
➤ *To treat streptococcal pharyngitis*
TABLETS
Adults and adolescents. 500 mg daily for 10 days.
➤ *To treat community-acquired pneumonia caused by* Legionella pneumophila, Mycoplasma pneumoniae, *or* S. Pneumoniae
TABLETS
Adults and adolescents. 500 mg daily for 14 days.

Mechanism of Action
Binds with the 50S ribosomal subunit of the 70S ribosome in susceptible bacteria.

This action inhibits RNA-dependent protein synthesis in bacterial cells, causing them to die.

Contraindications

Concurrent use of astemizole, cisapride, or pimozide; hypersensitivity to dirithromycin, erythromycin, other macrolide antibiotics, or their components; known, potential, or suspected bacteremia

Interactions

DRUGS

antacids, H_2-receptor antagonists: Increased dirithromycin absorption
astemizol, terfenadine: Possibly life-threatening arrhythmias
theophylline: Possibly increased serum theophylline level

Adverse Reactions

CNS: Dizziness, headache, weakness
GI: Abdominal pain, diarrhea, nausea, pseudomembranous colitis, vomiting
SKIN: Pruritus, rash, urticaria

Nursing Considerations

• Use dirithromycin cautiously in patients with impaired hepatic function. Monitor liver function test results as indicated because drug is metabolized in liver.

PATIENT TEACHING

• Instruct patient to take dirithromycin at the same time each day with food or within 1 hour of eating.
• Caution patient not to cut, chew, or crush tablets.
• Advise patient to store drug at room temperature in a dry place.
• Instruct patient to complete the full course of prescribed therapy, even if she feels better before drug is gone.
• Advise patient to notify prescriber immediately if GI problems persist.

disopyramide

Rythmodan (CAN)

disopyramide phosphate

Norpace, Norpace CR, Rythmodan-LA (CAN)

Class and Category

Chemical class: Substituted pyramide derivative
Therapeutic class: Class IA antiarrhythmic
Pregnancy category: C

Indications and Dosages

➤ *To rapidly control ventricular arrhythmias*

CAPSULES

Adults. *Loading:* 300 mg (200 mg if patient weighs less than 50 kg [110 lb]). If no response within 6 hr, 200 mg given every 6 hr. If no response within 48 hr, drug discontinued or dosage carefully increased to 250 to 300 mg every 6 hr.

➤ *To treat ventricular arrhythmias*

CAPSULES

Adults. 400 to 800 mg daily in divided doses every 6 hr, limited to 400 mg daily if patient weighs less than 50 kg. *Maximum:* 800 mg daily.
Children ages 12 to 18. 6 to 15 mg/kg daily in divided doses every 6 hr.
Children ages 4 to 12. 10 to 15 mg/kg daily in divided doses every 6 hr.
Children ages 1 to 4. 10 to 20 mg/kg daily in divided doses every 6 hr.
Children under age 1. 10 to 30 mg/kg daily in divided doses every 6 hr.
DOSAGE ADJUSTMENT Initial dosage reduced to 100 mg every 6 to 8 hr for adults with cardiomyopathy or possible cardiac decompensation. In renal insufficiency, dosage reduced to 100 mg every 6 hr if creatinine clearance exceeds 40 ml/min/1.73 m^2 or hepatic function is impaired; to 100 mg every 8 hr if clearance is 30 to 40 ml/min/1.73 m^2; to 100 mg every 12 hr if clearance is 15 to 29 ml/min/1.73 m^2; and to 100 mg every 24 hr if clearance is less than 15 ml/min/1.73 m^2.

E.R. CAPSULES, E.R. TABLETS

Adults. 400 to 800 mg daily in divided doses every 12 hr, limited to 200 mg every 12 hr if patient weighs less than 50 kg. *Maximum:* 800 mg daily.

Mechanism of Action

Inhibits sodium influx through fast channels of myocardial cell membranes, thus increasing recovery period after repolarization. Disopyramide decreases automaticity in the His-Purkinje system and conduction velocity in atria, ventricles, and accessory pathways. It prolongs QRS and QT intervals in normal sinus rhythm and atrial arrhythmias. Drug has a potent negative inotropic effect. It also acts as an anticholinergic and increases peripheral vascular resistance.

Contraindications

Cardiogenic shock, congenital QT-interval prolongation, hypersensitivity to disopyramide or its components, second- or third-degree AV block (without pacemaker), sick sinus syndrome

Interactions

DRUGS

antiarrhythmics: Widened QRS complex, prolonged QT interval, risk of arrhythmias, serious negative inotropic effects
anticholinergics: Possibly additive anticholinergic effects
cisapride: Possibly increased risk of prolonged QT interval
clarithromycin, erythromycin: Increased blood disopyramide level
digoxin: Increased serum digoxin level
hydantoins, rifampin: Decreased blood disopyramide level
insulin, oral antidiabetic drugs: Possibly intensified antidiabetic effects
quinidine: Increased blood disopyramide level, decreased quinidine level, or both
verapamil: Widened QRS complex, prolonged QT interval, possibly death

Adverse Reactions

CNS: Depression, dizziness, fatigue, fever, headache, insomnia, nervousness, syncope
CV: Chest pain; conduction disturbances; edema; heart failure (new or worsened); hypercholesterolemia; hypertriglyceridemia; hypotension; palpitations; proarrhythmias, including torsades de pointes; ventricular fibrillation; ventricular tachycardia
EENT: Blurred vision; dry eyes, mouth, nose, and throat
ENDO: Gynecomastia, hypoglycemia
GI: Abdominal distention, anorexia, constipation, diarrhea, vomiting
GU: Impotence, urinary frequency and urgency, urine retention
HEME: Reversible agranulocytosis (rare), thrombocytopenia
MS: Muscle weakness

RESP: Dyspnea
SKIN: Decreased sweating, pruritus, rash, reversible cholestatic jaundice
Other: Hypokalemia, lupus erythematosus–like symptoms

Nursing Considerations

WARNING Because of disopyramide's anticholinergic activity, avoid using drug in patients with glaucoma, myasthenia gravis, or urine retention.
• Use disopyramide cautiously and expect to reduce dosage in patients with impaired hepatic or renal function. Monitor hepatic and renal function, as ordered. Be aware that E.R. form shouldn't be given to patients with severe renal insufficiency.
• When changing from immediate-release to E.R. form, expect to start maintenance schedule 6 hours after last immediate-release dose.
• At therapeutic doses in hemodynamically uncompromised patients, expect drug to reduce cardiac output without decreasing resting sinus rate or affecting blood pressure. Keep in mind, however, that 2 mg/kg given I.V. over 3 minutes can increase heart rate and total peripheral resistance.
• Monitor heart rate and rhythm by continuous ECG.
• Assess serum electrolyte levels, especially potassium level, because drug may be ineffective in hypokalemia and its toxic effects enhanced in hyperkalemia.
• If patient takes quinidine, expect to start disopyramide 6 to 12 hours after last dose of quinidine. If patient takes procainamide, expect to start disopyramide 3 to 6 hours after the last dose of procainamide. A loading dose may not be required in either case.

PATIENT TEACHING

• Warn patient not to stop taking disopyramide abruptly; doing so may cause life-threatening cardiac problems.
• Advise patient to take a missed dose as soon as possible after she remembers, unless it's nearly time for the next dose. Caution her against doubling the dose. Urge her to notify prescriber if she misses more than one dose.
• Instruct patient to store drug at room temperature in a dry place.

D

• Instruct patient to check her pulse rate regularly and report significant changes.
• Urge patient to report blurred vision, constipation, difficulty urinating, dizziness, dry mouth, and trouble breathing.
• Advise patient to avoid hazardous activities until drug's CNS effects are known.
• Instruct patient to rise slowly from a lying or sitting position to reduce dizziness.
• Urge patient to avoid becoming overheated during hot weather or exercise because of risk of heatstroke.

disulfiram

Antabuse

Class and Category
Chemical class: Thiuram derivative
Therapeutic class: Alcohol abuse deterrent
Pregnancy category: Not rated

Indications and Dosages
➤ *As adjunct to maintain sobriety in treatment of chronic alcoholism*
TABLETS
Adults. *Initial:* Up to 500 mg daily for 1 to 2 wk. *Maintenance:* 125 to 500 mg daily. *Maximum:* 500 mg daily.

Route	Onset	Peak	Duration
P.O.	1–2 hr	Unknown	Up to 14 days

Mechanism of Action
Interferes with the enzyme responsible for hepatic oxidation of acetaldehyde to acetate, which occurs during alcohol catabolism. Ingestion of even a small amount of alcohol after taking disulfiram raises the blood acetaldehyde level to 5 to 10 times normal. Disulfiram doesn't alter the rate of alcohol elimination. Its major metabolite, diethyl-dithiocarbamate, inhibits norepinephrine synthesis and may be responsible for the drug's hypotensive effect.

Contraindications
Alcohol intoxication; coronary artery occlusion; hypersensitivity to disulfiram, its components, rubber, pesticides, or fungicides; psychosis; recent use of alcohol, alcohol-containing preparations, metronidazole, or paraldehyde; severe myocardial disease

Interactions
DRUGS
alfentanil: Decreased plasma clearance and prolonged duration of action of alfentanil
amoxicillin-clavulanate, bacampicillin: Possibly disulfiram-alcohol reaction
ascorbic acid: Possibly interference with disulfiram-alcohol reaction
CNS depressants: Possibly increased CNS depressant effects of either drug
isoniazid: Increased risk of additive neurotoxic effect of disulfiram; possibly increased adverse CNS effects
metronidazole: Risk of CNS toxicity, resulting in confusion and psychosis
oral anticoagulants: Possibly increased anticoagulant effects
paraldehyde: Decreased paraldehyde metabolism, increased blood paraldehyde level
phenytoin: Possibly increased blood phenytoin level and risk of phenytoin toxicity
tricyclic antidepressants: Possibly temporary delirium
FOODS
caffeine: Possibly increased cardiovascular and CNS effects of caffeine
ACTIVITIES
alcohol use: Disulfiram-alcohol reaction (if within 14 days of disulfiram therapy)

Adverse Reactions
CNS: Drowsiness, headache, peripheral neuropathy, psychotic reaction, tiredness
EENT: Blurred vision, garlic or metallic taste, optic atrophy, optic neuritis
GU: Impotence
SKIN: Rash

Nursing Considerations
• Disulfiram is given only to patients who are highly motivated to stop drinking and who are receiving psychotherapy or substance abuse counseling.
• Alcohol content of patient's other drugs should be checked before starting therapy.
WARNING Never give drug to patient without her knowledge or if she is intoxicated.

• If needed, crush tablet and mix with fluids before administration.
• Don't give drug within 14 days of patient's ingestion of alcohol-containing substance.
• Expect alcohol ingestion during disulfiram therapy to produce a severe reaction that lasts from 30 minutes to several hours. Symptoms may include angina, anxiety, blurred vision, confusion, diaphoresis, dyspnea, heart failure, hypotension, nausea, palpitations, sinus tachycardia, syncope, thirst, throbbing headache, throbbing in neck, vertigo, vomiting, and weakness. A deep sleep usually follows.

WARNING Ingestion of three or more alcoholic beverages with a disulfiram dose greater than 500 mg daily may cause respiratory depression, arrhythmias, and cardiac arrest.
• If patient takes phenytoin, monitor blood phenytoin level before and during disulfiram therapy, and adjust dosage of either drug as prescribed. Interactions may not occur if disulfiram therapy starts before phenytoin therapy. A subtherapeutic phenytoin level may result if disulfiram therapy stops.
• If patient takes an oral anticoagulant, monitor PT before and during disulfiram therapy, and adjust anticoagulant dosage as prescribed. Drug interactions may not occur if disulfiram therapy starts before warfarin therapy. If disulfiram therapy stops, be prepared to adjust warfarin dosage to avoid loss of hypoprothrombinemic effects.
• Expect some adverse reactions, such as drowsiness, headache, and impotence, to subside over time or with a brief dosage reduction.
• Because one-fifth of a disulfiram dose may stay in the body for 1 week or longer, alcohol ingestion may continue to produce unpleasant symptoms for up to 2 weeks after therapy stops.
• Expect therapy to last months to years, depending on patient's ability to abstain from alcohol.

PATIENT TEACHING
• Teach patient's household and family members about precautions needed and risks associated with disulfiram therapy.
• Explain that drug doesn't cure alcoholism but does help deter alcohol consumption.

• If patient reports daytime drowsiness, advise her to take drug in the evening.
• Warn patient to avoid alcohol-containing substances, such as vinegar, cough syrup, and sauces, during therapy because a disulfiram-alcohol reaction may occur after ingesting as little as 15 ml of 100-proof alcohol. Urge her to avoid alcohol-containing liniments and lotions as well.
• Teach patient what to expect if disulfiram-alcohol reaction occurs. Inform her that a deep sleep usually follows the reaction.
• Advise patient that a reaction can occur up to 14 days after therapy stops and that a severe reaction may cause respiratory depression, arrhythmias, and cardiac arrest.
• Instruct patient to carry medical identification that indicates drug, describes possible reactions, and lists someone to notify in case of emergency.

D

dobutamine hydrochloride
Dobutrex

Class and Category
Chemical class: Synthetic catecholamine
Therapeutic class: Cardiac stimulant
Pregnancy category: Not rated

Indications and Dosages
➤ *To treat low cardiac output and heart failure*
I.V. INFUSION
Adults. 2.5 to 10 mcg/kg/min as continuous infusion adjusted according to hemodynamic response.
Children. 5 to 20 mcg/kg/min as continuous infusion adjusted according to hemodynamic response.

Route	Onset	Peak	Duration
I.V.	1–2 min	Unknown	Under 5 min

Mechanism of Action
Mainly stimulates beta$_1$-adrenergic receptors, and mildly stimulates beta$_2$- and alpha$_1$-adrenergic receptors. Beta$_1$-receptor stimulation produces a positive inotropic effect on the myocardium, increasing cardiac output by boosting myocardial contractility

and stroke volume. Increased myocardial contractility raises coronary blood flow and myocardial oxygen consumption. Systolic blood pressure typically rises as a result of increased stroke volume. Other hemodynamic effects include decreased systemic vascular resistance, which reduces afterload, and decreased ventricular filling pressure, which reduces preload.

Incompatibilities

Don't combine dobutamine with cefamandole, cefazolin, hydrocortisone sodium succinate, cephalothin, penicillin, sodium ethycrynate, and sodium heparin because of incompatibility. Don't mix dobutamine with alkaline solutions, such as sodium bicarbonate, because of possible physical incompatibility. Don't use diluents that contain sodium bisulfite or ethanol.

Contraindications

Hypersensitivity to dobutamine or its components, idiopathic hypertrophic subaortic stenosis

Interactions

DRUGS

beta blockers: Possibly increased alpha-adrenergic activity and peripheral resistance
bretylium: Potentiated vasopressor activity, possibly arrhythmias
cyclopropane, halothane: Possibly serious arrhythmias
guanethidine: Decreased hypotensive effect of guanethidine, possibly resulting in severe hypertension
thyroid hormones: Increased cardiovascular effects of thyroid hormones or dobutamine
tricyclic antidepressants: Possibly potentiated cardiovascular and vasopressor effects of dobutamine, resulting in arrhythmias, hyperpyrexia, or severe hypertension

Adverse Reactions

CNS: Fever, headache, nervousness, restlessness
CV: Angina, bradycardia, hypertension, hypotension, palpitations, PVCs, tachycardia
GI: Nausea, vomiting
RESP: Dyspnea
SKIN: Extravasation with tissue necrosis and sloughing, rash
Other: Hypokalemia

Nursing Considerations

• Avoid giving dobutamine to patients with uncorrected hypovolemia. Expect prescriber to order whole blood or plasma volume expanders to correct hypovolemia. Also avoid giving dobutamine to patients with acute MI because it can intensify or extend myocardial ischemia.

• Use drug cautiously in patients allergic to sulfites because drug may cause anaphylactic-like signs and symptoms; commercially available dobutamine injections contain sodium bisulfite. Also use drug cautiously in patients with atrial fibrillation because drug increases AV conduction. Keep in mind that patient should be adequately digitalized before administration.

• Dilute concentrate with at least 50 ml compatible I.V. solution. A common dilution is 500 mg (40 ml from 250-ml bag) in 210 ml D_5W or normal saline solution to yield 2,000 mcg/ml. Or dilute 1,000 mg (80 ml from 250-ml bag) in 170 ml D_5W or normal saline solution to yield 4,000 mcg/ml. Adjust maximum concentration according to patient's fluid requirements as prescribed. Don't exceed 5,000 mcg/ml. Discard solution after 24 hours.

• Inspect parenteral solution for particles and discoloration before administering it.

• Give I.V. drug using an infusion pump.

• Monitor blood pressure often during therapy, preferably by continuous intra-arterial monitoring; systolic increase of 10 to 20 mm Hg may indicate dobutamine-induced increase in cardiac output.

• If hypotension develops, expect to reduce dosage or discontinue drug.

• Monitor heart rate and rhythm continuously for PVCs, which may result from drug's stimulatory effect on heart's conduction system, and sinus tachycardia, which results from positive chronotropic effect of beta stimulation and may increase heart rate by 5 to 15 beats/minute.

• Monitor hemodynamic parameters, such as central venous pressure, pulmonary artery wedge pressure, and cardiac output, as indicated, to assess drug's effectiveness.

WARNING Monitor serum potassium level to check for hypokalemia, a rare result of $beta_2$ stimulation that causes electrolyte imbalance.

- Monitor urine output hourly, as appropriate, to check for improved renal blood flow.
- Dobutamine isn't indicated for long-term treatment of heart failure because it may not be effective and may increase the risk of hospitalization and death.

PATIENT TEACHING
- Explain the need for frequent hemo-dynamic monitoring.

docusate calcium
(dioctyl calcium sulfosuccinate)
Albert Docusate (CAN), DC Softgels, Docucal-P, Doxidan (CAN), Pro-Cal-Sof, Sulfolax, Surfak

docusate potassium
(dioctyl potassium sulfosuccinate)
Diocto-K, Kasof

docusate sodium
(dioctyl sodium sulfosuccinate)
Afko-Lube, Afko-Lube Lax, Bilax, Colace, Colax, Correctol Stool Softener Soft Gels, Dialose, Diocto, Dioeze, DOK, D.O.S. Softgels, Ex-Lax Light Formula (CAN), Modane Soft, Regulax SS, Silace

Class and Category
Chemical class: Anionic surfactant
Therapeutic class: Laxative, stool softener
Pregnancy category: C

Indications and Dosages
➤ *To treat constipation*
CAPSULES (DOCUSATE CALCIUM)
Adults and adolescents. 240 mg at bedtime until bowel movements are normal.
Children age 6 and over. 50 to 150 mg at bedtime.
CAPSULES, LIQUID, SYRUP, TABLETS (DOCUSATE SODIUM)
Adults and adolescents. 50 to 500 mg at bedtime.
Children ages 6 to 12. 40 to 120 mg at bedtime.

Children ages 3 to 6. 20 to 60 mg at bedtime.
Children under age 3. 10 to 40 mg at bedtime.
CAPSULES, TABLETS (DOCUSATE POTASSIUM)
Adults and adolescents. 100 mg three times daily until bowel movements are normal.
Children age 6 and over. 100 mg at bedtime.

Route	Onset	Peak	Duration
P.O.	24–72 hr	Unknown	Unknown

Mechanism of Action
Acts as a surfactant that softens stool by decreasing surface tension between oil and water in feces. This action lets more fluid penetrate stool, forming a softer fecal mass.

Contraindications
Fecal impaction; hypersensitivity to docusate salts or their components; intestinal obstruction; nausea, vomiting, or other symptoms of appendicitis; undiagnosed abdominal pain

Interactions
DRUGS
mineral oil: Increased mineral oil absorption, increased risk of toxicity
tetracycline: Decreased tetracycline absorption

Adverse Reactions
CNS: Dizziness, syncope
CV: Palpitations
GI: Abdominal cramps and distention, diarrhea, nausea, perianal irritation, vomiting
MS: Muscle weakness

Nursing Considerations
WARNING Expect long-term or excessive use of docusate to cause dependence on laxatives for bowel movements, electrolyte imbalances, osteomalacia, steatorrhea, and vitamin and mineral deficiencies.
- Assess for laxative abuse syndrome, especially in women with depression, personality disorders, or anorexia nervosa.

PATIENT TEACHING
- Tell patient not to use docusate when she has abdominal pain, nausea, or vomiting.

- Advise patient to take docusate with a full glass of water or milk.
- To help prevent constipation, encourage patient to increase fiber intake, exercise regularly, and drink 6 to 8 glasses (240 ml/glass) of water daily.
- Instruct patient to notify prescriber about rectal bleeding; symptoms of electrolyte imbalances, such as dizziness, light-headedness, muscle cramping, and weakness; and unrelieved constipation.

dofetilide
Tikosyn

Class and Category
Chemical class: Methanesulfonanilide derivative
Therapeutic class: Class III antiarrhythmic
Pregnancy category: C

Indications and Dosages
➤ *To convert symptomatic atrial fibrillation or flutter to normal sinus rhythm or to maintain normal sinus rhythm in patients converted from symptomatic atrial fibrillation or flutter*

CAPSULES

Adults. *Initial:* 500 mcg twice daily for patients with creatinine clearance above 60 ml/min/1.73 m^2. *Maintenance:* Dosage based on QTc interval. If, 2 to 3 hr after initial dose, QTc interval increase is 15% of baseline or less, initial dose given twice daily. *Maximum:* 500 mcg twice daily.

DOSAGE ADJUSTMENT Initial dose reduced to 250 mcg twice daily if creatinine clearance is 40 to 60 ml/min/1.73 m^2 and to 125 mcg twice daily if clearance is 20 to 39 ml/min/1.73 m^2, as prescribed. If, 2 to 3 hr after initial dose, QTc interval has increased by at least 15% or is more than 500 milliseconds (msec) (550 msec in patients with ventricular conduction abnormalities), dosage decreased by 50%, as prescribed. However, for patients receiving lowest initial dose of 125 mcg twice daily, dosage reduced to 125 mcg daily, as prescribed. During next four doses (given every 2 to 3 hr, as prescribed), if QTc interval increases to more than 500 msec (550 msec in patients with ventricular conduction abnormalities), expect to discontinue drug, as prescribed.

Route	Onset	Peak	Duration
P.O.	Unknown	2 hr	4 hr

Mechanism of Action
Selectively blocks potassium channels in myocardial cell membranes involved in cardiac repolarization. By blocking potassium channels, dofetilide prolongs ventricular refractoriness (widens QT interval), effective refractory period, and action potential duration. These actions terminate or prevent reentrant tachyar-rhythmias, such as atrial fibrillation, atrial flutter, and ventricular tachycardia.

Contraindications
Cardiac conduction disturbances without an artificial pacemaker; congenital or acquired QT prolongation syndrome; concurrent therapy with cimetidine, dolutegravir, hydrochlorothiazide, ketoconazole, megestrol, prochlorperazine, trimethoprim, or verapamil; hyper-sensitivity to dofetilide or its components; severe renal impairment (creatinine clearance less than 20 ml/min/1.73 m^2)

Interactions
DRUGS

amiloride, cimetidine, cotrimoxazole, ketoconazole, megestrol, metformin, triamterene, trimethoprim: Possibly increased blood dofetilide level
azole antifungals, cannabinoids, diltiazem, nefazodone, norfloxacin, protease inhibitors, quinine, selective serotonin reuptake inhibitors, zafirlukast: Possibly increased blood dofetilide level and risk of dofetilide toxicity
bepridil, cisapride, macrolide antibiotics, phenothiazines, selected fluoroquinolones, tricyclic antidepressants: Possibly prolonged QT interval
class I and III antiarrhythmics, especially amiodarone: Possibly prolonged QT interval and increased risk of dofetilide-induced proarrhythmias
diuretics (potassium-depleting): Increased risk of torsades de pointes in patients with hypokalemia or hypomagnesemia
hydrochlorothiazide, verapamil: Possibly increased blood dofetilide level and increased risk of torsades de pointes

FOODS
grapefruit juice: Increased dofetilide level
ACTIVITIES
marijuana use: Increased dofetilide level

Adverse Reactions

CNS: Cerebral ischemia, dizziness, facial or flaccid paralysis, headache, insomnia, paresthesia, slurred speech, stroke, syncope
CV: AV block, bradycardia, cardiac arrest, chest pain, edema, MI, tachycardia, ventricular arrhythmias (including torsades de pointes and ventricular tachycardia)
GI: Abdominal pain, diarrhea, hepatic dysfunction, nausea
MS: Back pain, muscle weakness
RESP: Cough, dyspnea, respiratory tract infection
SKIN: Jaundice, rash
Other: Angioedema, flulike symptoms, weight gain

Nursing Considerations

WARNING If patient has previously received amiodarone, be aware that dofetilide shouldn't be started until blood amiodarone level is less than 0.3 mcg/ml or until amio-darone has been withdrawn for at least 3 months.
• Evaluate and document QTc interval before and during dofetilide therapy.
• Place patient on continuous ECG monitoring for at least 3 days, as ordered, during dofetilide therapy.
WARNING If patient does not convert to normal sinus rhythm within 24 hours of starting dofetilide, expect possible synchronized electrical cardioversion.
• Be prepared to reevaluate renal function and QTc interval every 3 months, as ordered, during dofetilide therapy.
• When switching to dofetilide from class I or class III antiarrhythmics, or after withdrawing antiarrhythmic treatment, monitor continuous ECG for at least 30 hours, as ordered.
• If patient requires a drug that may interact with dofetilide, expect to discontinue dofetilide, as prescribed, for 2 or more days before starting the other drug.
WARNING Monitor laboratory test results for hypokalemia or hypomagnesemia, especially in patients taking diuretics, because of the increased risk of dofetilide-induced torsades de pointes.

• Monitor women often for adverse reactions, including prolonged QTc interval and torsades de pointes; they have 12% to 18% lower renal clearance of drug than men and therefore a greater risk of adverse reactions.
PATIENT TEACHING
• Advise patient to swallow dofetilide capsules with water.
• Instruct patient to avoid drinking grapefruit juice while taking this drug.
• Inform patient that she may be hospitalized for at least 3 days if dofetilide dosage is increased.
• Teach patient to measure pulse rate and blood pressure during dofetilide therapy.
• Urge patient to report chest discomfort, fluttering, or palpitations immediately.
• Tell patient to notify prescriber immediately if she experiences severe diarrhea, unusual sweating, vomiting, loss of appetite or develops excessive thirst that may occur as a result of certain drug interactions that cause an electrolyte imbalance.
• Advise patient to consult prescriber before using any OTC drugs, nutritional supplements, or herbal products.
• Instruct patient to keep follow-up appointments to monitor heart rhythm.

dolasetron mesylate
Anzemet

Class and Category
Chemical class: Carboxylate monomethanesulfonate
Therapeutic class: Antiemetic
Pregnancy category: B

Indications and Dosages
➤ *To prevent nausea and vomiting due to chemotherapy*
ORAL SOLUTION, TABLETS
Adults and children over age 16. 100 mg within 1 hr before chemotherapy.
Children ages 2 to 16. 1.8 mg/kg within 1 hr before chemotherapy. *Maximum:* 100 mg.
➤ *To prevent postoperative nausea and vomiting*
I.V. INJECTION
Adults and children over age 16. 12.5 mg 15 min before end of anesthesia.

Children ages 2 to 16. 0.35 mg/kg 15 min before end of anesthesia. *Maximum:* 12.5 mg/dose.
➤ *To treat postoperative nausea and vomiting*
I.V. INJECTION
Adults and children over age 16. 12.5 mg as single dose as soon as symptoms develop.
Children ages 2 to 16. 0.35 mg/kg as single dose as soon as symptoms develop. *Maximum:* 12.5 mg/dose.

Mechanism of Action

With its active metabolite hydrodolasetron, prevents activation of serotonin 5-HT$_3$ receptors located peripherally on vagal nerve terminals and centrally in chemoreceptor trigger zone, thereby decreasing the vomiting reflex.

Contraindications

Congenital long-QT syndrome, hypersensitivity to dolasetron or components, hypokalemia, hypomagnesemia, intravenous administration to prevent nausea and vomiting associated with cancer chemotherapy

Interactions

DRUGS
atenolol: Possibly decreased dolasetron clearance
cimetidine: Possibly increased blood dolasetron level
fentanyl, I.V. methylene blue, lithium, mirtazapine, MAO inhibitors, selective serotonin reuptake inhibitors, serotonin and norepinehrine reuptake inhibitors: Increased risk of serotonin syndrome
rifampin: Possibly decreased blood dolasetron level

Adverse Reactions

CNS: Headache, serotonin syndrome
CV: Cardiac arrest; hypertension; hypotension; MI, prolongation of QT, PR, and QRS intervals on EKG; torsade de pointes; ventricular fibrillation and tachycardia; wide-complex tachycardia
GI: Diarrhea
SKIN: Rash
Other: injection-site pain

Nursing Considerations

• Correct hypokalemia and hypomagnesemia, if present and as ordered, prior to administering dolasetron intravenously as serious arrhythmias may result.

• Expect to give up to 100 mg of dolasetron I.V. in 30 seconds or to dilute it in normal saline solution, D$_5$W, dextrose 5% in half-normal (0.45) saline solution, or lactated Ringer's solution and infuse for up to 15 minutes, as prescribed.

• Flush I.V. line with compatible solution before and after drug administration.

• Expect to prepare an oral solution of dolasetron for patients unable to swallow tablets by diluting injection solution with apple or apple-grape juice.

WARNING Assess patient for ECG changes, including prolonged PR, QTc, and QT intervals and widened QRS complex, especially in patients with congestive heart failure, bradycardia or underlying heart disease, the elderly, and in patients with renal impairment during intravenous dolasetron therapy.

WARNING Monitor patient for serotonin syndrome, which is characterized by agitation, chills, confusion, diaphoresis, diarrhea, fever, hyperactive reflexes, poor coordination, restlessness, shaking, talking or acting with uncontrolled excitement, tremor, and twitching. In its most severe form, serotonin syndrome can resemble neuroleptic malignant syndrome, which includes a high fever, muscle rigidity, autonomic instability with possible fluctuations in vital signs, and mental status changes.

PATIENT TEACHING
• For children or patients who have trouble swallowing, explain that oral solution can be prepared by diluting injection form of drug with apple or apple-grape juice.

• Inform patient that oral solution may be refrigerated for up to 48 hours but should be discarded after 2 hours at room temperature.

• Advise patient to notify prescriber immediately if he experiences dizziness, palpitations, or an abnormally slow or irregular pulse after receiving dolasetron intravenously.

WARNING Instruct patient to seek immediate medical attention if he experiences erratic changes in his blood pressure, heart beat, or temperature; changes in his mental status; adverse gastrointestinal symptoms; or neuromuscular symptoms.

donepezil hydrochloride

Aricept

Class and Category

Chemical class: Piperidine derivative
Therapeutic class: Antidementia
Pregnancy category: C

Indications and Dosages

➤ *To treat mild to moderate Alzheimer's disease*

ORAL SOLUTION, ORALLY DISINTEGRATING TABLETS, TABLETS

Adults. *Initial:* 5 mg at bedtime. After 4 to 6 wk, dosage increased to 10 mg at bedtime, as indicated. *Maximum:* 10 mg daily.

➤ *To treat moderate to severe Alzheimer's disease*

ORAL SOLUTION, ORALLY DISINTEGRATING TABLETS, TABLETS

Adults. *Initial:* 5 mg at bedtime. After 4 to 6 wk, dosage increased to 10 mg at bedtime, as indicated. Dosage may be further increased, as needed, after 3 months to 23 mg daily at bedtime if using tablet form. *Maximum:* 23 mg daily.

Mechanism of Action

Reversibly inhibits acetylcholinesterase and improves acetylcholine's concentration at cholinergic synapses. Raising acetylcholine level in the cerebral cortex may improve cognition. Donepezil becomes less effective as Alzheimer's disease progresses and number of intact cholinergic neurons declines.

Contraindications

Hypersensitivity to donepezil, piperidine derivatives, or their components

Interactions

DRUGS

anticholinergics: Possibly interference with activity of these drugs
carbamazepine, dexamethasone, phenobarbital, phenytoin, rifampin: Increased donepezil elimination rate
cholinergic agonists, neuromuscular blockers: Possibly synergistic effects of these drugs
ketoconazole, quinidine: Inhibited donepezil metabolism

NSAIDs: Possibly increased gastric acid secretion and increased risk of GI bleeding

Adverse Reactions

CNS: Abnormal gait, agitation, anxiety, asthenia, depression, dizziness, dream disturbances, fatigue, fever, headache, hostility, insomnia, nervousness, seizures, somnolence, syncope, tremor
CV: Abnormal ECG, bradycardia, chest pain, edema, heart failure, hypertension, hypotension
EENT: Pharyngitis
ENDO: Hyperglycemia
GI: Abdominal pain, anorexia, constipation, diarrhea, dyspepsia, gastroenteritis, fecal incontinence, nausea, vomiting
GU: Cystitis, glycosuria, hematuria, urinary frequency or incontinence, UTI
HEME: Anemia, hemorrhage
MS: Arthralgia, back pain, elevated creatine kinase level, muscle spasms
RESP: Bronchitis, increased cough, pneumonia
SKIN: Ecchymosis, eczema, pruritus, rash, ulceration
Other: Angioedema, dehydration, elevated alkaline phosphatase or lactate dehydrogenase level, flu syndrome, weight loss

D

Nursing Considerations

• Use donepezil cautiously in patients with bladder obstruction because drug's weak peripheral cholinergic effect could obstruct outflow.
• Use drug cautiously in patients with asthma, COPD, or other pulmonary disorders because it has weak affinity for peripheral cholinesterase, which may increase bronchoconstriction and bronchial secretions.
• If patient has cardiac disease, monitor heart rate and rhythm for bradycardia, which may result from increased vagal tone caused by drug's inhibition of peripheral cholinesterase. Reduced heart rate may be especially significant if patient has sick sinus syndrome, bradycardia, or other supraventricular arrhythmia.
• Take safety precautions if patient is dizzy or has other adverse CNS reactions.

PATIENT TEACHING

• Advise patient to take donepezil just before going to bed.
• Inform her that drug may be taken with or without food.

• Instruct patient to avoid hazardous activities, such as driving, until drug's CNS effects are known. Urge her to take safety precautions to prevent falling if she has adverse reactions, such as dizziness.

• If patient has a history of peptic ulcer disease or gastric irritation, explain that drug may aggravate these conditions by increasing gastric acid secretion.

• Caution patient to avoid NSAIDs during therapy because of risk of GI bleeding. Urge her to notify prescriber immediately if she notices black, tarry stools.

dopamine hydrochloride

Intropin, Revimine (CAN)

Class and Category

Chemical class: Catecholamine
Therapeutic class: Cardiac stimulant, vasopressor
Pregnancy category: C

Indications and Dosages

➤ *To correct hypotension that's unresponsive to adequate fluid volume replacement or occurs as part of shock syndrome caused by bacteremia, chronic cardiac decompensation, drug overdose, MI, open-heart surgery, renal failure, trauma, or other major systemic illnesses; to improve low cardiac output*

I.V. INFUSION

Adults. 0.5 to 3 mcg/kg/min for vasodilation of renal arteries; 2 to 10 mcg/kg/min for positive inotropic effects and increased cardiac output; 10 mcg/kg/min, increased gradually according to patient's response, for increased systolic and diastolic blood pressures.

DOSAGE ADJUSTMENT Initial dosage reduced to 10% of usual amount if patient has taken MAO inhibitor in previous 2 to 3 wk.
Children. 1 to 5 mcg/kg/min increased gradually in increments of 2.5 to 5 mcg/kg/min to achieve desired results. *Maximum:* 20 mcg/kg/min.

Route	Onset	Peak	Duration
I.V.	In 5 min	Unknown	Up to 10 min

Mechanism of Action

Stimulates dopamine$_1$ (D$_1$) and dopamine$_2$ (D$_2$) postsynaptic receptors. D$_1$ receptors mediate vasodilation in renal, mesenteric, coronary, and cerebral blood vessels. D$_2$ receptors inhibit norepinephrine release. In higher doses, dopamine also stimulates alpha$_1$ and alpha$_2$ receptors, causing vascular smooth-muscle contraction.

At doses of 0.5 to 3 mcg/kg/min, this naturally occurring catecholamine mainly affects dopaminergic receptors in renal, mesenteric, coronary, and cerebral vessels, resulting in vasodilation, increased renal blood flow, improved GFR, and increased urine output. At doses of 2 to 10 mcg/kg/min, dopamine stimulates beta$_1$-adrenergic receptors, increasing cardiac output while maintaining dopaminergic-induced vasodilation. At doses of 10 mcg/kg/min or more, alpha-adrenergic agonism takes over, causing increased peripheral vascular resistance and renal vasoconstriction.

Incompatibilities

Don't add dopamine to 5% sodium bicarbonate, alkaline I.V. solutions, oxidizing agents, or iron salts.

Contraindications

Pheochromocytoma, uncorrected ventricular fibrillation, ventricular tachycardia, and other tachyarrhythmias

Interactions

DRUGS

alpha blockers, haloperidol, loxapine, phenothiazines, thioxanthenes: Antagonized peripheral vasoconstriction with high doses of dopamine
anesthetics, such as chloroform, enflurane, halothane, isoflurane, and methoxyflurane: Increased risk of severe atrial and ventricular arrhythmias
antihypertensives, diuretics used as antihypertensives: Possibly decreased antihypertensive effects of these drugs
beta blockers: Antagonized beta receptor–mediated inotropic effects of dopamine
digitalis glycosides: Possibly increased risk of arrhythmias and additive inotropic effects
diuretics: Possibly increased diuretic effects of dopamine or diuretic
doxapram: Possibly increased vasopressor effects of dopamine or doxapram

ergot alkaloids: Enhanced peripheral vasoconstriction
guanadrel, guanethidine: Possibly decreased hypotensive effects of these drugs and potentiated vasopressor response to dopamine, resulting in hypertension and arrhythmias
levodopa: Increased risk of arrhythmias
MAO inhibitors: Prolonged and intensified cardiac stimulation and vasopressor effect
maprotiline, tricyclic antidepressants: Possibly potentiated cardiovascular and vasopressor effects of dopamine, resulting in arrhythmias, hyperpyrexia, or severe hypertension
mecamylamine, methyldopa: Possibly decreased hypotensive effects of these drugs and enhanced vasopressor effect of dopamine
methylphenidate: Possibly potentiated vasopressor effect of dopamine
nitrates: Possibly decreased antianginal effects of nitrates; possibly decreased vasopressor effect of dopamine, resulting in hypotension
oxytocic drugs: Possibly severe hypertension
phenoxybenzamine: Possibly antagonized peripheral vasoconstriction of dopamine, causing hypotension and tachycardia
phenytoin: Possibly sudden bradycardia and hypotension
rauwolfia alkaloids: Possibly decreased hypotensive effects of these drugs
sympathomimetics: Possibly increased adverse cardiovascular and other effects
thyroid hormones: Increased risk of coronary insufficiency

Adverse Reactions
CNS: Anxiety, headache
CV: Angina, atrial fibrillation, bradycardia, cardiac conduction abnormalities, ectopic beats, hypertension, hypotension, palpitations, peripheral vasoconstriction, sinus tachycardia, ventricular arrhythmias, widened QRS complex
GI: Nausea, vomiting
GU: Azotemia
RESP: Dyspnea
SKIN: Extravasation with tissue necrosis, piloerection

Nursing Considerations
• If possible, avoid giving dopamine to patients with occlusive vascular disease,

such as atherosclerosis, Buerger's disease, diabetic endarteritis, or Raynaud's disease, because of risk of decreased peripheral circulation. Also, be aware that high doses of dopamine given for a prolonged period of time increase the risk of decreased peripheral circulation and could lead to gangrene in the patient's extremities.
• Use drug cautiously in patients with cardiac disease, particularly coronary artery disease, because dopamine increases myocardial oxygen demand. Also use drug cautiously in patients allergic to sulfites, which are contained in some forms of dopamine.
• Inspect parenteral solution for particles and discoloration before administration.
• Dilute dopamine concentrate with a compatible I.V. solution before administering. Typical dilution is 400 mg in 250 ml to yield 1.6 mg/ml. Don't exceed 3.2 mg/ml.
• If patient has hypovolemia, ensure adequate fluid resuscitation before giving drug.
• Give drug by I.V. infusion using an infusion pump.
WARNING When infusion rate exceeds 20 mcg/kg/min, monitor patient for excessive vasoconstriction and loss of renal vasodilating effects. Avoid using an infusion rate above 50 mcg/kg/min.
• If you must infuse more than 20 mcg/kg/min of dopamine to maintain blood pressure, expect to infuse norepinephrine as prescribed.
• To avoid extravasation and tissue necrosis, administer infusion through a central catheter. If you must give drug via peripheral line, inspect site often for signs of extravasation and necrosis. If you detect such signs, start a new I.V. line for dopamine infusion, discontinue previous I.V. line, and notify prescriber immediately.
• If drug extravasates, expect to give 5 to 10 mg phentolamine diluted in 10 to 15 ml normal saline solution, as prescribed. Phentolamine infiltrates directly into area to antagonize vasoconstriction and minimize sloughing and tissue necrosis.
• Titrate dopamine gradually to minimize hypotension, especially after a high infusion rate.
• Monitor blood pressure continuously with an intra-arterial line, as indicated.

• Place patient on continuous ECG monitoring, and assess heart rate and rhythm for arrhythmias.
• Monitor patient's hemodynamic parameters, such as central venous pressure, pulmonary artery wedge pressure, and cardiac output, as indicated, to assess effectiveness of dopamine therapy.
• Monitor urine output hourly as appropriate to assess patient for improved renal blood flow.

PATIENT TEACHING
• Explain the need for frequent hemodynamic monitoring.

doripenem
Doribax

Class and Category
Chemical class: Carbapenem
Therapeutic class: Antibiotic
Pregnancy category: B

Indications and Dosages
➤ *To treat complicated intra-abdominal infections caused by* Escherichia coli, Klebsiella pneumoniae, Pseudomonas aeruginosa, Bacteroides caccae, B. fragilis, B. thetaiotaomicron, B. uniformis, B. vulgatus, Streptococcus intermedius, S. constellatus, *and* Peptostreptococcus micros *and complicated UTIs, including pyelonephritis caused by* E. coli, K. pneumoniae, Proteus mirabilis, P. aeruginosa, *and* Acinetobacter baumannii

I.V. INFUSION
Adults. 500 mg infused over 1 hr every 8 hr for 5 to 14 days. May switch to oral therapy if improvement after 3 days.
DOSAGE ADJUSTMENT For patients with impaired renal function or creatinine clearance of 30 to 50 ml/min/1.73 m², dosage reduced to 250 mg infused over 1 hr every 8 hr. For creatinine clearance of 10 to 30 ml/min/1.73 m², dosage reduced to 250 mg infused over 1 hr every 12 hr.

Route	Onset	Peak	Duration
I.V.	Unknown	1 hr	8 hr

Mechanism of Action
Inhibits cell wall synthesis in susceptible bacteria. Doripenem inactivates multiple penicillin-binding proteins essential in cell wall synthesis to cause cell death.

Incompatibilities
Don't mix doripenem with other drugs or add to solutions containing other drugs because of potential for incompatibility.

Contraindications
History of anaphylactic reactions to beta-lactams; hypersensitivity to doripenem, its components or other carbapenems

Interactions
DRUGS
divalproex sodium, valproic acid: Decreased effectiveness of valproic acid with possible loss of seizure control
probenecid: Increased plasma concentrations of doripenem

Adverse Reactions
CNS: Headache, seizure
CV: Phlebitis
EENT: Oral candidiasis
GI: Diarrhea, liver enzyme elevation, nausea
GU: Vaginitis
HEME: Leukopenia, neutropenia, thrombocytopenia
RESP: Interstitial pneumonia
SKIN: Dermatitis, erythema, erythema multiforme, macular or papular eruptions, pruritus, rash, Stevens-Johnson Syndrome, toxic epidermal necrolysis, urticaria
Other: Anaphylaxis

Nursing Considerations
• Use cautiously in patients with a history of hypersensitivity to cephalosporins or penicillins because cross sensitivity may occur.
• Constitute vial with 10 ml sterile water for injection or normal saline solution, and gently shake to form a suspension. With-draw suspension using a syringe with a 21G needle and add it to an infusion bag containing 100 ml normal saline solution or 5% dextrose. Gently shake until clear. If administering reduced dosage of 250 mg, remove 55 ml of prepared solution from infusion bag and discard before infusion.

• Be aware that upon constitution, suspension in the vial must be diluted within 1 hour. Once drug is diluted in infusion solution, drug stored at room temperature must be used within 8 hours if mixed in normal saline solution and within 4 hours if mixed in 5% dextrose. If infusion solution is refrigerated, it must be used within 24 hours or discarded.

• Monitor patient closely for evidence of hypersensitivity, especially if patient has multiple allergies, because serious and occasionally fatal hypersensitivity reactions have occurred in patients receiving beta-lactam antibiotics. If an allergic reaction occurs, discontinue drug immediately, notify prescriber, and expect to administer emergency treatment such as epinephrine, oxygen, I.V. fluids, I.V. antihistamines, corticosteroids, and pressor amines, as ordered, and provide airway management.

• Assess patient's bowel pattern daily; severe diarrhea may be caused by *Clostridium difficile*. If suspected, expect to stop drug and provide treatment as prescribed.

PATIENT TEACHING

• Instruct patient to report any evidence such allergic reaction, such as rash, hives, itching or trouble breathing.

• Advise patient to report diarrhea if severe or persistent.

doxapram hydrochloride

Dopram

Class and Category

Chemical class: Pyrrolidinone derivative
Therapeutic class: Respiratory stimulant
Pregnancy category: B

Indications and Dosages

➤ *To stimulate respiration in COPD-related acute respiratory insufficiency*

I.V. INFUSION

Adults and adolescents. 1 to 2 mg/min titrated according to respiratory response. *Maximum:* 3 mg/min for up to 2 hr.

➤ *To treat respiratory depression after anesthesia*

I.V. INFUSION

Adults and adolescents. 5 mg/min until desired response occurs and then reduced to 1 to 3 mg/min. *Maximum:* Cumulative dose of 4 mg/kg or 300 mg.

I.V. INJECTION

Adults and adolescents. 0.5 to 1 mg/kg, repeated every 5 min, as needed. *Maximum:* 1.5 mg/kg as a single dose or 2 mg/kg every 5 min.

Route	Onset	Peak	Duration
I.V.	20–40 sec	1–2 min	5–12 min

Mechanism of Action

Activates peripheral carotid, aortic, and other chemoreceptors to stimulate respiration, resulting in increased tidal volume and respiratory rate. Doxapram also may increase respiratory rate and tidal volume by directly stimulating the respiratory center in the medulla oblongata.

Incompatibilities

To avoid precipitation and gas formation, don't mix doxapram with alkaline solutions, such as aminophylline, sodium bicarbonate, or 2.5% thiopental.

Contraindications

Age less than 1 month; cerebral edema; head injury; hypersensitivity to doxapram or its components; mechanical disorders of ventilation, including acute bronchial asthma, flail chest, muscle paresis, obstruction, pneumothorax, and pulmonary fibrosis; pulmonary embolism; seizure disorder; severe cardiovascular disorder; severe hypertension; stroke; uncompensated heart failure

Interactions

DRUGS

chloroform, cyclopropane, enflurane, halothane, isoflurane, methoxyflurane, trichloroethylene: Possibly adverse myocardial effects if doxapram given within 10 minutes of these drugs
CNS stimulants: Possibly excessive CNS stimulation, with arrhythmias, insomnia, irritability, nervousness, or seizures
MAO inhibitors, sympathomimetics: Additive vasopressor effects
skeletal muscle relaxants: Masked residual effects of muscle relaxants

Adverse Reactions

CNS: Disorientation, dizziness, headache
CV: Arrhythmias, including sinus tachycardia; hypertension
GI: Diarrhea, hiccups, nausea, vomiting
GU: Urine retention
RESP: Bronchospasm, cough, dyspnea
SKIN: Diaphoresis
Other: Injection-site pain, redness, swelling, and thrombophlebitis

Nursing Considerations

• Avoid giving doxapram to patients receiving mechanical ventilation.
• Maintain a patent airway, and assess for optimal oxygenation before giving drug.
• Monitor I.V. insertion site for extravasation and signs of thrombophlebitis or local skin irritation.
• If hypertension or dyspnea develops suddenly, stop infusion as directed.
• Assess patient for early signs and symptoms of overdose, including enhanced deep tendon reflexes, skeletal muscle hyperactivity, and tachycardia.

PATIENT TEACHING

• Explain the need for frequent pulse and blood pressure monitoring.

---

doxazosin mesylate

Cardura, Cardura-1 (CAN),
Cardura-2 (CAN), Cardura-4 (CAN)

Class and Category

Chemical class: Quinazoline derivative
Therapeutic class: Antihypertensive, benign prostatic hyperplasia therapeutic agent
Pregnancy category: C

Indications and Dosages

➤ *To manage hypertension*

TABLETS

Adults. *Initial:* 1 mg daily. Doubled every 1 to 2 wk, if needed to achieve desired blood pressure. *Maximum:* 16 mg daily.

➤ *To treat benign prostatic hyperplasia (BPH)*

TABLETS

Adults. *Initial:* 1 mg daily. Doubled every 1 to 2 wk, if needed, based on signs and symptoms. *Maximum:* 8 mg daily.

Mechanism of Action

Competitively inhibits $alpha_1$-adrenergic receptors in the sympathetic nervous system, causing peripheral vasodilation and reduced peripheral vascular resistance. This action increases heart rate and decreases blood pressure, especially when the patient stands. Doxazosin also relaxes smooth muscle of the bladder neck, prostate, and prostate capsule, which reduces urethral resistance and pressure and urinary outflow resistance.

Route	Onset	Peak	Duration
P.O.	1–2 hr*	2–6 hr†	24 hr†

Contraindications

Hypersensitivity to doxazosin, prazosin, terazosin, or their components

Interactions

DRUGS

antihypertensives, diuretics, phosphodiesterase-5 inhibitors: Enhanced hypotensive effects
cimetidine: Possibly increased blood doxazosin level
dopamine: Antagonized vasopressor effect of high-dose dopamine
ephedrine, metaraminol, methoxamine, phenylephrine: Possibly decreased vasopressor effects of these drugs
epinephrine: Possibly severe hypotension and tachycardia
NSAIDs: Possibly loss of hypotensive activity from sodium or fluid accumulation

Adverse Reactions

CNS: Dizziness, drowsiness, headache, nervousness, restlessness, vertigo
CV: Arrhythmias, including sinus tachycardia; first-dose orthostatic hypotension; palpitations; peripheral edema
EENT: Intraoperative floppy iris syndrome, rhinitis
GI: Nausea
RESP: Dyspnea

Nursing Considerations

• Don't give drug to hypotensive patients.

---

* For hypertension; in 2 wk for BPH.
† For hypertension; unknown for BPH.

• Use doxazosin cautiously in patients with hepatic disease (because normal dosage may cause exaggerated effects) and in elderly patients (because hypotensive response may be more pronounced).

WARNING Monitor patient for orthostatic hypotension (which may cause syncope) early in therapy, especially after exercise and in patients with hypovolemia.

• Monitor blood pressure for 2 to 6 hours after first dose and with each increase because orthostatic hypotension commonly occurs at this time. Adjust dose as prescribed, based on standing blood pressure.

• Carefully monitor patients with renal disease for exaggerated effects, such as first-dose orthostatic hypotension.

• Monitor urination, checking for difficulty urinating and urine retention, to assess drug's effects on BPH.

PATIENT TEACHING

• Inform patient that she may take doxazosin in the morning or evening and with food, if desired.

• Instruct patient to change position slowly to minimize orthostatic hypotension.

• Advise patient to avoid standing for long periods, exercising, using alcohol, and going outside in hot weather; these activities may worsen orthostatic hypotension.

• Advise patient to avoid hazardous activities until drug's CNS effects are known.

• Tell patient to inform surgeon that she is taking doxazosin therapy if cataract surgery is required because drug may cause intraoperative floppy iris syndrome with this procedure.

• Inform the male patient that he may become dizzy or faint if he takes an oral erectile dysfunction medicine during doxazosin therapy. Therefore, he should not use an oral erectile dysfunction medicine until he has discussed its use with the prescriber.

doxepin hydrochloride

Novo-Doxepin (CAN), Sinequan, Silenor, Triadapin (CAN)

Class and Category

Chemical class: Dibenzoxepin derivative
Therapeutic class: Antidepressant
Pregnancy category: Not rated

Indications and Dosages

➤ *To treat mild to moderate depression or anxiety*

CAPSULES, ORAL SOLUTION

Adults and adolescents. 75 to 150 mg daily at bedtime. *Maximum:* 150 mg daily.

➤ *To treat mild to moderate depression or anxiety with organic disease*

CAPSULES, ORAL SOLUTION

Adults and adolescents. 25 to 50 mg daily.

➤ *To treat severe depression or anxiety*

CAPSULES, ORAL SOLUTION

Adults and adolescents. 50 mg three times daily, gradually increased to 300 mg daily, as indicated.

➤ *To treat insomnia characterized by difficulty with sleep maintenance*

TABLET

Adults. 6 mg within 30 min of bedtime. *Maximum:* 6 mg daily.

DOSAGE ADJUSTMENT For elderly patients age 65 and over, dosage reduced to 3 mg within 30 min of bedtime but may be increased to 6 mg daily, as needed.

Mechanism of Action

May block serotonin and norepinephrine reuptake by adrenergic nerves. In this way, the tricyclic antidepressant raises serotonin and norepinephrine levels at nerve synapses, which may elevate mood and reduce depression.

Route	Onset	Peak	Duration
P.O.	2–3 wk	Unknown	Unknown

Incompatibilities

Don't mix doxepin solution with carbonated beverages or grape juice.

Contraindications

Acute recovery phase of MI; concurrent use of MAO inhibitor; glaucoma; hypersensitivity to doxepin, other tricyclic antidepressants, or their components; urine retention

Interactions

DRUGS

amantadine, anticholinergics, antidyskinetics, antihistamines: Possibly intensified anti-

cholinergic effects, causing confusion, hallucinations, and nightmares
anticonvulsants: Possibly lowered seizure threshold and decreased effects of these drugs
antithyroid drugs: Possibly increased risk of agranulocytosis
barbiturates, carbamazepine: Increased doxepin metabolism, decreased blood doxepin level, possibly lowered seizure threshold
bupropion, clozapine, cyclobenzaprine, haloperidol, loxapine, maprotiline, molindone, phenothiazines, thioxanthenes: Possibly prolonged and intensified sedative and anti-cholinergic effects of either drug, possibly increased risk of seizures
cimetidine, flecainide, phenothiazines, propafenone, quinidine, selective serotonin reuptake inhibitors, tricyclic antidepressants: Increased blood doxepin level from inhibited systemic clearance, resulting in increased risk of toxicity
clonidine, guanadrel, guanethidine: Increased risk of hypertension, especially during second week of doxepin therapy
CNS depressants: Possibly potentiated CNS depression, hypotension, and respiratory depression
corticosteroids: Possibly worsened depression
direct-acting sympathomimetics, such as epinephrine and norepinephrine: Potentiated effects of these drugs
disulfiram: Possibly transient delirium
fluoxetine: Possibly increased blood doxepin level
MAO inhibitors: Possibly hyperpyrexia, hypertension, seizures, and death
oral anticoagulants: Possibly increased anticoagulant effects of these drugs
pimozide: Increased risk of arrhythmias
probucol: Possibly prolonged QT interval, increased risk of ventricular tachycardia
thyroid hormones: Possibly increased therapeutic and toxic effects of both drugs
tolazamide: Possibly severe hypoglycemia
ACTIVITIES
alcohol use: Possibly enhanced CNS depression, hypotension, and respiratory depression

Adverse Reactions

CNS: Confusion, delirium, dream disturbances, drowsiness, fatigue, hallucinations, headache, nervousness, parkinsonism, restlessness, sedation, seizures, suicidal ideation (children and teens), tremor
CV: ECG changes, orthostatic hypotension, palpitations
EENT: Blurred vision, dry mouth, taste perversion
GI: Constipation, diarrhea, heartburn, ileus, increased appetite, nausea, vomiting,
GU: Decreased libido, ejaculation disorders
SKIN: Diaphoresis, jaundice
Other: Weight gain

Nursing Considerations

• If desired, mix oral solution in 120 ml of water; milk; or orange, grapefruit, tomato, or pineapple juice.
• Expect to observe adverse reactions within a few hours after giving drug.
• Evaluate patient for therapeutic response, such as decreased anxiety, apprehension, depression, fear, guilt, somatic symptoms, and worry; increased energy; and more restful sleep.
WARNING Monitor children and teens closely for evidence of suicidal thinking and behavior because doxepin increases the risk in these groups.
• Keep in mind that abrupt withdrawal of doxepin after prolonged therapy can cause cholinergic rebound effects, including diarrhea, nausea, and vomiting.
• Plan to discontinue drug, as prescribed, several days before elective surgery to avoid hypertension.
• Monitor elderly patients for parkinsonism, especially with high-dose therapy.
• Be alert for seizures. Patients with seizure disorder may need increased anticonvulsant dosage to maintain seizure control.
• For patients with asthma or sulfite sensitivity, doxepin tablets may aggravate asthma or cause allergic reactions because they contain sulfites.
• Follow diabetic patient's serum glucose level closely; drug may alter glucose metabolism.
• If patient takes a thyroid hormone, be alert for increased responses to both drugs and, possibly, exaggerated drug-induced effects, such as arrhythmias and CNS stimulation. Untreated hypothyroidism prevents adequate response to therapy.

PATIENT TEACHING

WARNING Alert parents to watch their child or teen closely for abnormal thinking or behavior and increased aggression or hostility. Emphasize importance of notifying prescriber about unusual changes.

• Instruct patient to avoid alcohol during doxepin therapy because mental alertness may decrease.

• Advise diabetic patient to measure serum glucose level more often than usual.

doxercalciferol
Hectorol

Class and Category

Chemical class: Fat-soluble vitamin D analogue
Therapeutic class: Antihyperparathyroid drug
Pregnancy category: B

Indications and Dosages

➤ *To reduce elevated intact parathyroid hormone (IPTH) serum level when managing secondary hyperparathyroidism in patients undergoing chronic hemodialysis*

CAPSULES

Adults. *Initial:* 10 mcg 3 times/wk (about every other day) before, during, or after dialysis. *Maintenance:* If iPTH level is decreased by 50% and above 300 picograms (pg)/ml, dosage increased by 2.5 mcg at 8-wk intervals, as needed. If iPTH level is 150 to 300 pg/ml, initial dosage maintained. If iPTH level is less than 100 pg/ml, drug stopped for 1 wk and then restarted at a dose at least 2.5 mcg less than previous dose. *Maximum:* 20 mcg 3 times/wk for a total of 60 mcg/wk.

➤ *To reduce elevated IPTH blood level when managing secondary hyperparathyroidism in patients with stage 3 or 4 chronic renal disease*

CAPSULES

Adults. 1 mcg daily. *Maintenance:* If iPTH level exceeds 70 pg/ml for stage 3 or 110 pg/ml for stage 4, dosage increased by 0.5 mcg at 2-wk intervals, as needed. If iPTH level is 35 to 70 pg/ml for stage 3 or 70 to 110 pg/ml for stage 4, dosage is maintained.

If iPTH level is less than 35 pg/ml for stage 3 or less than 70 pg/ml for stage 4, drug is stopped for 1 wk and then restarted at a dose at least 0.5 mcg lower than previous dose. *Maximum:* 3.5 mcg daily.

Mechanism of Action

Undergoes hepatic conversion to an active metabolite (1,25-dihydroxyvitamin D_2 [1,25-dihydroxyergocalciferol]), which increases intestinal absorption of dietary calcium and renal tubular reabsorption of urinary calcium. Together with parathyroid hormone, doxercalciferol also mobilizes calcium from bone. These effects serve to maintain blood calcium levels in patients with chronic renal failure, which in turn prevents hyperparathyroidism.

In patients with renal failure, decreased metabolic activation of vitamin D in the kidneys leads to chronic hypocalcemia. The parathyroid gland compensates by increasing PTH secretion, but renal failure prevents it from achieving a normal serum calcium level. Thus, secondary hyperpara-thyroidism develops. Because doxercalciferol doesn't require renal conversion to form its active metabolite, it can regulate the serum calcium level and thus suppress PTH secre-tion and reduce its serum level in patients with chronic renal failure. An elevated PTH level in these patients leads to metabolic bone disease, such as renal osteodystrophy.

Contraindications

Evidence of vitamin D toxicity, hyper-sensitivity to doxercalciferol or its components, risk or history of hypercalcemia or hyperphosphatemia

Interactions

DRUGS

antacids that contain magnesium: Possibly additive drug effects and increased risk of hypermagnesemia
cholestyramine, mineral oil, orlistat, other drugs that affect lipid absorption: Possibly decreased doxercalciferol absorption
glutethimide, phenobarbital: Possibly increased doxercalciferol metabolism and risk of adverse reactions
erythromycin, ketoconazole: Possibly inhibited doxercalciferol metabolism and decreased effectiveness

vitamin D and its analogues: Possibly additive effects, resulting in increased adverse effects, such as hypercalcemia

Adverse Reactions

CNS: Depression, dizziness, headache, insomnia, malaise, paresthesia
CV: Bradycardia, chest pain, peripheral edema
EENT: Rhinitis
ENDO: Oversuppression of iPTH
GI: Anorexia, constipation, indigestion, nausea, vomiting
HEME: Anemia
MS: Hypertonia
RESP: Cough, dyspnea
SKIN: Pruritus
Other: Dehydration, hypercalcemia, hypercalciuria, hyperphosphatemia, weight gain

Nursing Considerations

WARNING Be aware that patients who take vitamin D should not also take doxercalciferol because they may develop severe vitamin D toxicity and hyper-calcemia.
• Be alert for signs and symptoms of vitamin D toxicity and hypercalcemia in patients receiving high-dose or long-term doxercalciferol therapy. Early signs and symptoms include bone pain, consti-pation, dry mouth, headache, metallic taste, myalgia, nausea, somnolence, vomiting, and weakness. Late signs and symptoms include albuminuria, anorexia, arrhythmias, azotemia, conjunctivitis (calcific), decreased libido, elevated AST and ALT levels, elevated BUN level, generalized vascular calcification, hypercholesterolemia, hypertension, hyperthermia, irritability, mild metabolic acidosis, nephrocalcinosis, nocturia, pancreatitis, photophobia, polydipsia, polyuria, pruritus, rhinorrhea, and weight loss.
• Keep emergency equipment readily available in case patient develops toxicity.
• Expect to monitor patient's blood iPTH, calcium, and phosphorus levels before starting drug and weekly early in therapy.
• For patients with renal failure who are having hemodialysis, oral calcium-based or other non–aluminum-containing phosphate binders and a low-phosphate

diet typically are used to control serum phosphorus level. An elevated serum phosphorus level worsens secondary hyperparathyroidism and may decrease doxercalciferol's effectiveness in reducing blood iPTH level.
• After doxercalciferol therapy starts, expect to decrease dosage of phosphate binders to correct persistent mild hypercalcemia. Expect to increase dosage to correct persistent mild hyperphosphatemia.
• Avoid giving magnesium-containing antacids with doxercalciferol if patient receives long-term hemodialysis because doing so may lead to hypermagnesemia.

PATIENT TEACHING
• Urge patient who takes doxercalciferol to follow strict low-phosphorus diet and to take calcium supplement, as prescribed, to maintain serum calcium level. Stress that diet and calcium-based phosphate binder should provide 1.5 to 2 g of calcium daily.
• Explain importance of periodic follow-up blood work to measure drug effectiveness. Tell the patient that it may take several months to reach optimal PTH suppression.
• Warn patient not to take other forms of vitamin D with doxercalciferol and to ask prescriber before taking any OTC drug.
• Advise patient to contact prescriber immediately if early signs or symptoms of toxicity, such as headache or nausea, develop.

doxycycline calcium

(contains 50 mg of base per 5 ml of oral suspension)
Vibramycin

doxycycline hyclate

(contains 50 or 100 mg of base per capsule, 100 mg of base per delayed-release capsule, 100 mg of base per tablet, and 100 or 200 mg of base per injection vial)
Acticlate, Alti-Doxycycline (CAN), Apo-Doxy (CAN), Doryx, Doxycin (CAN), Vibramycin, Vibra-Tabs

doxycycline monohydrate

(contains 50 or 100 mg of base per capsule and 25 mg of base per 5 ml of oral suspension)
Monodox, Oracea, Vibramycin

Class and Category

Chemical class: Oxytetracycline derivative
Therapeutic class: Antibiotic
Pregnancy category: D

Indications and Dosages

➤ *To treat cutaneous, GI, or inhalation anthrax*

CAPSULES, DELAYED-RELEASE CAPSULES, ORAL SUSPENSION, TABLETS, I.V. INFUSION

Adults, adolescents, and children weighing more than 45 kg (99 lb). 100 mg (base) every 12 hr for 60 days.
Children weighing less than 45 kg. 2.2 mg/kg (base) every 12 hr for 60 days.

➤ *To treat inflammatory lesions (papules and pustules) of rosacea*

Adults. 40 mg once daily in morning

➤ *To treat endocervical, rectal, and urethral infections caused by* Chlamydia trachomatis

CAPSULES, DELAYED-RELEASE CAPSULES, ORAL SUSPENSION, TABLETS

Adults and children over age 8 weighing more than 45 kg. 100 mg (base) twice daily for 7 days. *Maximum:* 300 mg (base) daily.
Children weighing 45 kg or less. 2.2 mg (base)/kg twice daily on day 1 and then 2.2 to 4.4 mg (base)/kg daily or 1.1 to 2.2 mg (base)/kg twice daily.

I.V. INFUSION

Adults and children over age 8 weighing more than 45 kg. 200 mg (base) once daily or 100 mg (base) every 12 hr on day 1 and then 100 to 200 mg (base) once daily or 50 to 100 mg (base) every 12 hr. *Maximum:* 300 mg (base) daily.
Children weighing 45 kg or less. 4.4 mg (base)/kg once daily or 2.2 mg (base)/kg every 12 hr on day 1 and then 2.2 to 4.4 mg (base)/kg once daily or 1.1 to 2.2 mg (base)/kg every 12 hr.

➤ *To treat epididymoorchitis caused by* C. trachomatis *or* Neisseria gonorrhoeae

or nongonococcal urethritis caused by C. trachomatis *or* Ureaplasma urealyticum

CAPSULES, DELAYED-RELEASE CAPSULES, ORAL SUSPENSION, TABLETS

Adults and children over age 8 weighing more than 45 kg. 100 mg (base) twice daily for at least 10 days. *Maximum:* 300 mg (base)/day.
Children weighing 45 kg or less. 2.2 mg (base)/kg twice daily on day 1 and then 2.2 to 4.4 mg (base)/kg once daily or 1.1 to 2.2 mg (base)/kg twice daily.

I.V. INFUSION

Adults and children over age 8 weighing more than 45 kg. 200 mg (base) once daily or 100 mg (base) every 12 hr on day 1 and then 100 to 200 mg (base) once daily or 50 to 100 mg (base) every 12 hr. *Maximum:* 300 mg (base) daily.
Children weighing 45 kg or less. 4.4 mg (base)/kg once daily or 2.2 mg (base)/kg every 12 hr on day 1 and then 2.2 to 4.4 mg (base)/kg once daily or 1.1 to 2.2 mg (base)/kg every 12 hr.

➤ *To prevent malaria*

CAPSULES, DELAYED-RELEASE CAPSULES, ORAL SUSPENSION, TABLETS

Adults and children over age 8 weighing more than 45 kg. 100 mg (base) daily starting 1 to 2 wk before travel, continued daily during travel, and then daily for 4 wk after travel ends. *Maximum:* 300 mg (base) daily.
Children over age 8. 2 mg (base)/kg daily starting 1 to 2 days before travel, continued daily during travel, and daily for 4 wk after travel ends. *Maximum:* 100 mg (base) daily.

➤ *To treat early syphilis in penicillin-allergic patients*

CAPSULES, DELAYED-RELEASE CAPSULES, ORAL SUSPENSION, TABLETS

Adults and children over age 8 weighing more than 45 kg. 100 mg (base) twice daily for 2 wk. *Maximum:* 600 mg (base) daily.
Children weighing 45 kg or less. 2.2 mg (base)/kg twice daily on day 1 and then 2.2 to 4.4 mg (base)/kg once daily or 1.1 to 2.2 mg (base)/kg twice daily.

I.V. INFUSION

Adults and children over age 8 weighing more than 45 kg. 150 mg (base) every

D

12 hr for at least 10 days. *Maximum:* 300 mg (base) daily.
Children weighing 45 kg or less. 4.4 mg (base)/kg once daily or 2.2 mg (base)/kg every 12 hr on day 1 and then 2.2 to 4.4 mg (base)/kg once daily or 1.1 to 2.2 mg (base)/kg every 12 hr.

➤ *As adjunct to amebicides in acute intestinal amebiasis*
CAPSULES, DELAYED-RELEASE CAPSULES, I.V. INFUSION, ORAL SUSPENSION, TABLETS
Adults. 100 mg twice daily.

➤ *As adjunct therapy to treat severe acne*
CAPSULES, DELAYED-RELEASE CAPSULES, ORAL SUSPENSION, TABLETS
Adults. *Initial:* 100 mg twice daily for 3 to 6 wk or until improvement. *Maintenance:* 50 to 150 mg once daily.

➤ *To treat syphilis of more than 1 year's duration in penicillin-allergic patients*
CAPSULES, DELAYED-RELEASE CAPSULES, ORAL SUSPENSION, TABLETS
Adults and children over age 8 weighing more than 45 kg. 100 mg (base) twice daily for 4 wk. *Maximum:* 300 mg (base) daily.
I.V. INFUSION
Adults and children over age 8 weighing more than 45 kg. 150 mg (base) every 12 hr for at least 10 days. *Maximum:* 300 mg (base) daily.
Children weighing 45 kg or less. 4.4 mg (base)/kg once daily or 2.2 mg (base)/kg every 12 hr on day 1 and then 2.2 to 4.4 mg (base)/kg once daily or 1.1 to 2.2 mg (base)/kg every 12 hr.

➤ *To treat all other infections caused by susceptible organisms*
CAPSULES, DELAYED-RELEASE CAPSULES, ORAL SUSPENSION, TABLETS
Adults and children over age 8 weighing more than 45 kg. 100 mg (base) every 12 hr on day 1 and then 100 mg (base) once daily or 50 mg (base) twice daily For severe infections, 100 mg (base) continued every 12 hr. *Maximum:* 300 mg (base) daily.
Children weighing 45 kg or less. 2.2 mg (base)/kg twice daily on day 1 and then 2.2 to 4.4 mg (base)/kg once daily or 1.1 to 2.2 mg (base)/kg twice daily.
I.V. INFUSION
Adults and children over age 8 weighing more than 45 kg. 200 mg (base) once daily or 100 mg (base) every 12 hr on day 1 and

then 100 to 200 mg (base) once daily or 50 to 100 mg (base) every 12 hr. *Maximum:* 300 mg (base) daily.
Children weighing 45 kg or less. 4.4 mg (base)/kg once daily or 2.2 mg (base)/kg every 12 hr on day 1 and then 2.2 to 4.4 mg (base)/kg once daily or 1.1 to 2.2 mg (base)/kg every 12 hr.

Mechanism of Action

Exerts a bacteriostatic effect against a wide variety of gram-positive and gram-negative organisms. Doxycycline is more lipophilic than other tetracyclines, which allows it to pass more easily through the bacterial lipid bilayer, where it binds reversibly to 30S ribosomal subunits. Bound doxycycline blocks the binding of aminoacyl transfer RNA to messenger RNA, thus inhibiting bacterial protein synthesis.

Contraindications

Hypersensitivity to any tetracycline

Interactions

DRUGS
antacids that contain aluminum, calcium, magnesium, or zinc; calcium supplements; choline and magnesium salicylates; iron salts; laxatives that contain magnesium: Decreased doxycycline absorption and effects
barbiturates, carbamazepine, phenytoin: Increased clearance and decreased effects of doxycycline
cholestyramine, colestipol: Decreased doxycycline absorption
digoxin: Increased bioavailability of digoxin, possibly leading to digitalis toxicity
isotretinoin: Increased risk of intracranial hypertension
oral anticoagulants: Possibly increased hypoprothrombinemic effects of these drugs
oral contraceptives: Decreased effectiveness of estrogen-containing oral contraceptives, increased risk of breakthrough bleeding
penicillins: Inhibited bactericidal action
penthrane: Possibly increased risk of fatal renal toxicity
sodium bicarbonate: Altered doxycycline absorption from increased gastric pH
FOODS
dairy products, other foods high in calcium or iron: Decreased doxycycline absorption

Adverse Reactions

CNS: Headache, intracranial hypertension, paresthesia
CV: Phlebitis
EENT: Black "hairy" tongue, glossitis, hoarseness, oral candidiasis, pharyngitis, stomatitis, tooth discoloration, visual disturbances
GI: Anorexia; bulky, loose stools; diarrhea; dysphagia; enterocolitis; epigastric distress; esophageal ulceration; hepatotoxicity; nausea; pseudomembranous colitis; rectal candidiasis; vomiting
GU: Anogenital lesions, dark yellow or brown urine, elevated BUN level, vaginal candidiasis
HEME: Eosinophilia, hemolytic anemia, neutropenia, thrombocytopenia, thrombocytopenic purpura
SKIN: Dermatitis, drug rash with eosinophilia and systemic symptoms (DRESS), photosensitivity, rash, urticaria
Other: Anaphylaxis, angioedema, injection-site phlebitis

Nursing Considerations

• Avoid giving doxycycline to breastfeeding women because of the risk of enamel hypoplasia, inhibited linear skeletal growth, oral and vaginal candidiasis, photosensitivity reactions, and tooth discoloration in breastfeeding infant.
• Avoid giving drug to children under age 8, if possible; it may cause discoloration and enamel hypoplasia of developing teeth.
• Use oral suspension cautiously in patients allergic to sulfites because it contains sodium metabisulfite.
• Expect to adjust dosage for patients who have hepatic disease to avoid drug accumulation.
WARNING Don't give doxycycline by I.M. or subcutaneous route.
• Give doxycycline without regard to meals. Food and milk may delay absorption, but they don't significantly reduce it.
• Observe patient often for injection-site phlebitis, a common adverse reaction to I.V. administration.
• Monitor liver function test results as appropriate to detect hepatotoxicity.
• Expect oral or parenteral doxycycline to increase risk of oral, rectal, or vaginal candidiasis—especially in elderly or

debilitated patients and those on prolonged therapy—by changing the normal balance of microbial flora.
WARNING Monitor patient for signs and symptoms of intracranial hypertension, such as headache, blurred vision, diplopia, and vision loss; papilledema may be seen on fundoscopy. Patients at greater risk include women of childbearing age who are overweight or have a history of intracranial hypertension. If patient complains of visual changes, notify prescriber to obtain an immediate ophthalmologic evaluation because permanent visual loss can occur. Be aware that intracranial pressure may remain elevated for weeks after doxycycline therapy has been discontinued and warrants close follow up.
• Monitor patient closely for diarrhea, which may indicate pseudomembranous colitis. If diarrhea occurs, notify prescriber and expect to withhold doxycycline. Expect to treat pseudomembranous colitis with fluids, electrolytes, protein, and an antibiotic effective against _Clostridium difficile._

PATIENT TEACHING
• Instruct patient not to take doxycycline just before bed because it may not dissolve properly when she's recumbent and may cause esophageal burning and ulceration.
• Instruct patient taking doxycycline for rosacea to take the capsule in the morning on an empty stomach with a full glass of water.
• Advise patient to avoid dairy products; foods high in calcium or iron; antacids containing aluminum, calcium, or magnesium; bismuth subsalicylate; and iron-containing products during therapy.
• Caution patient not to take bismuth subsalicylate while taking doxycycline because doxycycline absorption will be reduced.
• Instruct patient to drink plenty of fluids while taking doxycycline to reduce the risk of esophageal burning and ulceration.
• Inform patient that her urine may become dark yellow or brown during therapy.
• Urge patient to avoid sun exposure and ultraviolet light as much as possible during therapy and to use sunscreen or sunblock as needed. If patient develops

phototoxicity, such as skin eruption, tell her to stop drug and notify prescriber.
• Advise patients who take an oral contraceptive to use an additional contraceptive method during therapy.
• If patient is being treated for a sexually transmitted disease, explain that her partner may need treatment as well.
• Tell patient to notify prescriber immediately about anorexia, epigastric distress, nausea, or vomiting as well as any visual changes during therapy.
• Urge patient to report watery, bloody stools to prescriber immediately, even up to 2 months after drug therapy has ended.
• Alert female patients that doxycycline may increase risk of vaginal candidiasis. Tell her to notify prescriber if she develops vaginal itching or discharge.
• Advise patient taking doxycycline for malaria prevention to start taking drug 1 to 2 days before traveling to the region and continue for 4 weeks after leaving the area. Note that the total length of therapy shouldn't exceed 4 months.

dronabinol
(delta-9-tetrahydro-cannabinol, THC)
Marinol

Class, Category, and Schedule
Chemical class: Synthetic tetrahydrocan-nabinol
Therapeutic class: Antiemetic, appetite stimulant
Pregnancy category: C
Controlled substance schedule: II

Indications and Dosages
➤ *To prevent nausea and vomiting caused by chemotherapy and unresponsive to other antiemetics*
CAPSULES
Adults. 5 mg/m² 1 to 3 hr before and 2 to 4 hr after chemotherapy, increased by 2.5 g/m², as needed. *Maximum:* 15 mg/m²/dose or a total of 4 to 6 doses daily.

➤ *To stimulate appetite in cancer and AIDS patients*
CAPSULES
Adults. *Initial:* 2.5 mg twice daily before lunch and supper, increased as needed. *Maximum:* 20 mg daily in divided doses.
DOSAGE ADJUSTMENT Dosage reduced to 2.5 mg before supper or at bedtime for patients who can't tolerate 5 mg daily.

Route	Onset	Peak	Duration
P.O.	Unknown	Unknown	24 hr or longer*

Mechanism of Action
May exert antiemetic effect by inhibiting the vomiting control mechanism in the medulla oblongata. As the main psychoactive substance in marijuana (*Cannabis sativa* L.), dronabinol's effects may be mediated by cannabinoid receptors in neural tissues.

Contraindications
Hypersensitivity to dronabinol, its components, sesame oil, or marijuana

Interactions
DRUGS
anticholinergics, antihistamines: Possibly increased risk of tachycardia
apomorphine: Possibly potentiated CNS depression, possibly decreased emetic response with prior use of dronabinol
CNS stimulants (such as amphetamines), and CNS depressants (such as benzodiazepines): Additive CNS effects
sympathomimetics: Possibly enhanced hypertension, tachycardia, and other adverse cardiovascular effects
ACTIVITIES
alcohol use: Additive CNS depressant effects

Adverse Reactions
CNS: Amnesia, anxiety, ataxia, confusion, delusions, depression, dizziness, drowsiness, euphoria, fatigue, hallucinations, irritability, mood changes, nervousness, seizures, sleep disturbance
CV: Orthostatic hypotension, palpitations, sinus tachycardia

---

* For appetite stimulant effects; unknown for antiemetic effects.

GI: Nausea, vomiting
Other: Physical and psychological dependence

Nursing Considerations

WARNING Dronabinol shouldn't be discontinued abruptly; if it is, withdrawal syndrome may occur.

• Use cautiously in patients with history of seizures because drug may lower seizure threshold. Notify prescriber of seizures immediately, and expect to stop drug.

• Patients under age 45 may tolerate drug better than those over age 45.

• Watch for adverse reactions that mimic psychosis, such as hallucinations and, possibly, acute anxiety, especially at high doses.

• Anticipate higher risk of cardiovascular reactions, such as increased heart rate and blood pressure changes (especially orthostatic hypotension), at higher doses.

WARNING Expect tolerance to drug to develop over time, especially if patient has smoked marijuana.

• Be aware that short-term, low-dose therapy doesn't typically lead to physical and psychological dependence, which may occur with long-term, high-dose therapy.

• Expect drug to alter REM sleep pattern, even after therapy stops.

PATIENT TEACHING

• Caution patient not to stop drug abruptly because withdrawal symptoms may occur.

• Urge patient not to use alcohol while taking dronabinol because it may enhance CNS depression.

• Instruct patient to rise slowly to sitting or standing position to minimize effects of orthostatic hypotension.

• Advise patient to avoid hazardous activities until drug's CNS effects are known.

• Inform patient that sleep pattern may be adversely affected during therapy and for sometime afterward.

---

dronedarone

Multaq

Class and Category

Chemical class: Benzofuran derivative
Therapeutic class: Antiarrhythmic
Pregnancy category: X

Indications and Dosages

➤ *To reduce risk of hospitalization for atrial fibrillation in patients in sinus rhythm with a history of paroxysmal or persistent atrial fibrillation*

TABLETS

Adults. 400 mg twice daily, with morning and evening meals

Route	Onset	Peak	Duration
P.O.	Unknown	3–6 hr	Unknown

Mechanism of Action

Although specific effect on heart rhythm is unknown, dronedarone possesses properties of all four Vaughn-Williams antiarrhythmic classes.

Contraindications

Amiodarone-induced liver toxicity; bradycardia less than 50 beats/minute; concurrent use of drugs or herbal products that prolong QT interval, such as class I and III antiarrhythmics, phenothiazine antipsychotics, oral macrolide antibiotics (selected), and tricyclic antidepressants or strong CYP3A inhibitors, such as clarithromycin, cyclosporine, ketoconazole, itraconazole, nefazodone, ritonavir, telithromycin, and voriconazole; hypersensitivity to dronedarone or its components; liver or lung toxicity related to previous use of amiodarone; nursing mothers; pregnancy; QTc Bazett interval of 500 ms or greater or a PR interval greater than 280 ms; permanent atrial fibrillation; second- or third-degree atrioventricular block or sick-sinus syndrome (except when used with a functioning pacemaker); severe hepatic impairment (Child-Pugh class C); symptomatic heart failure with recent decompensation requiring hospitalization or NYHA Class IV symptoms

Interactions

DRUGS

beta blockers: Increased risk of bradycardia
calcium channel blockers: Possibly increased dronedarone effects on conduction

calcium channel blockers, such as diltiazem, nifedipine, and verapamil; CYP3A substrates with narrow therapeutic range such as sirolimus and tacrolimus; CYP2D6 substrates, such as beta blockers, selective serotonin reuptake agents, and tricyclic antidepressant; statins, such as simvastatin: Increased effects of these drugs with possibly increased risk of adverse reactions

class I and III antiarrhythmics, macrolide antibiotics, phenothiazines, tricyclic antidepressants: Possibly increased QT interval

CYP3A inducers, such as carbamazepine, phenobarbital, phenytoin, rifampin, St. John's wort: Decreased dronedarone effects

CYP3A inhibitors, such as clarithromycin, cyclosporine, ketoconazole, itraconazole, nefazodone, ritonavir, telithromycin, and voriconazole: Increased dronedarone effects

digoxin and other P-gp substrates such as dabigatran: Increased effect of these drugs with risk of toxicity; increased risk of adverse GI reactions

diltiazem, verapamil: Increased dronedarone effect

potassium-depleting diuretics: Increased risk of hypokalemia and hypomagnesemia

warfarin: Possible increased risk of bleeding and INR

FOODS

grapefruit juice: Increased dronedarone effects

Adverse Reactions

CNS: Asthenia
CV: Bradycardia, heart failure, prolonged QT interval, vasculitis
GI: Abdominal pain, diarrhea, dyspepsia, liver injury, nausea, vomiting
GU: Increased serum creatinine levels
RESP: Dyspnea, interstitial lung disease such as pneumonitis and pulmonary fibrosis, nonproductive cough, pulmonary toxicity
SKIN: Allergic dermatitis, dermatitis, eczema, photosensitivity, pruritus, rash
Other: Anaphylaxis, angioedema, hypokalemia, hypomagnesemia

Nursing Considerations

• Check that patient has stopped taking any drug contraindicated with dronedarone, as

prescribed, before giving first dose. Also check that patient is receiving appropriate antithrombotic therapy prior to giving first dose because patients are at increased risk for stroke, especially in the first two weeks of therapy. In addition, check patient's serum potassium and magnesium levels prior to initiating therapy and throughout therapy because of increased risk of deficiency and arrhythmias, especially if patient is also taking a potassium-depleting diuretic.

• Monitor patient for evidence of heart failure, such as weight gain, dependent edema, or increasing shortness of breath. If present, notify prescriber; dronedarone may need to be discontinued.

• Monitor patient's electrocardiogram at least once every 3 months, as ordered to determine patient's rhythm. If atrial fibrillation is found, prepare patient for cardioversion, as ordered or expect dronedarone therapy to be discontinued. Monitor patient's PR and QT interval, as ordered, to see if conduction is delayed. If so, notify prescriber immediately. Dronedarone will need to be stopped.

• Monitor patient's serum creatinine levels, as ordered. Elevation may occur rapidly, plateau after 7 days, and usually is reversible after therapy stops.

• Monitor patient's liver function, as ordered, because severe liver injury may occur with dronedarone therapy. If liver enzymes become elevated or the patient develops symptoms of liver dysfunction such as anorexia, dark urine, fatigue, fever, itching, jaundice, malaise, nausea, right upper quadrant pain, or vomiting, notify prescriber and expect drug to be discontinued immediately.

• Monitor patient for dyspnea or nonproductive cough as possible development of pulmonary toxicity. If confirmed, expect drug to be discontinued.

PATIENT TEACHING

• Inform patient that dronedarone must be taken with a meal.

• Warn patient that dronedarone should not be taken with grapefruit juice.

• Urge patient to contact prescriber if he develops evidence of heart failure, such as weight gain, dependent edema, or

increasing shortness of breath, because dronedarone may need to be discontinued.
• Inform women of childbearing age of need for contraception if sexually active because drug is contraindicated during pregnancy and breastfeeding. If pregnancy occurs, she should notify prescriber immediately.
• Tell patient to inform all prescribers that he is taking dronedarone and to check with prescriber before taking any newly prescribed drug, OTC product, or herbal product with dronedarone.
• Review symptoms of liver dysfunction with patient and urge her to seek immediate medical attention, if present, and to stop taking dronedarone.

droperidol

Inapsine

Class and Category
Chemical class: Butyrophenone derivative
Therapeutic class: Antiemetic
Pregnancy category: C

Indications and Dosages
➤ *To reduce nausea and vomiting after surgery or diagnostic procedures when other treatments are ineffective*

I.V. OR I.M. INJECTION
Adults and adolescents. Dosage individualized up to a maximum initial dose of 2.5 mg I.M. or slow I.V. Additional 1.25 mg may be given to achieve desired effect if potential benefit outweighs risk.
Children ages 2 to 12. Dosage individualized to a maximum initial dose of 0.1 mg/kg. Additional dose may be given to achieve de-sired effect if potential benefit outweighs risk.
DOSAGE ADJUSTMENT Initial dosage reduced for elderly, debilitated, or critically ill patients because of the increased risk of hypotension and excessive sedation.

Route	Onset	Peak	Duration
I.V., I.M.	3–10 min	In 30 min	2–4 hr

Mechanism of Action
Produces sedation by blocking postsynaptic dopamine receptors in limbic system.

Droperidol may reduce nausea by blocking dopamine receptors in chemo-receptor trigger zone in reticular formation of the medulla oblongata. It also may produce antiemetic effects by attaching to post-synaptic gamma-amino-butyric acid (GABA) receptors in the chemoreceptor trigger zone.

Contraindications
Hypersensitivity to droperidol or its components, known or suspected prolonged QT interval (including congenital long-QT syndrome)

Interactions
DRUGS
amoxapine, haloperidol, loxapine, metoclopramide, metyrosine, molindone, olanzapine, phenothiazines, pimozide, rauwolfia alkaloids, risperidone, tacrine, thioxanthenes: Possibly increased risk of severe extrapyramidal reactions
anesthetics: Possibly hypotension and peripheral vasodilation
antiarrhythmics (class I or III), antidepressants, antimalarials, benzodiazepines, diuretics, I.V. opioids, laxatives, MAO inhibitors, volatile anesthetics, and other drugs that prolong QT interval (such as some antihistamines): Increased risk of serious adverse effects of droperidol, such as prolonged QT interval and arrhythmias
antihypertensives: Possibly orthostatic hypotension
bromocriptine, levodopa: Possibly inhibited actions of these drugs
CNS depressants: Additive CNS depression
epinephrine: Possibly paradoxical reduction of blood pressure
propofol: Possibly decreased antiemetic effect of both drugs
ACTIVITIES
alcohol use: Additive CNS depression

Adverse Reactions
CNS: Anxiety, drowsiness, dystonia, restlessness
CV: Cardiac arrest, hypertension, hypotension, potentially fatal arrhythmias (such as torsades de pointes and ventricular tachycardia), prolonged QT interval, sinus tachycardia

EENT: Fixed upward position of eyeballs, laryngospasm
MS: Spasms of tongue, face, neck, and back muscles
RESP: Bronchospasm

Nursing Considerations

WARNING Use droperidol cautiously in patients over age 65 and in patients with alcoholism, bradycardia, heart failure, hypokalemia, hypomagnesemia, parkinsonism, or preexisting QT-interval prolongation because they're at increased risk for prolonged QT interval and potentially fatal adverse reactions. Patients who take drugs that prolong the QT interval, such as some antiarrhythmics and benzodiazepines, and patients who take drugs that may cause an electrolyte imbalance, such as diuretics and laxatives, are also at increased risk.

• Expect a 12-lead ECG to be performed on all patients before droperidol administration to verify the absence of prolonged QT interval. Monitor ECG continuously for 2 to 3 hours after administering drug. Also monitor serum electrolyte levels to detect electrolyte imbalances.

• Use droperidol cautiously in patients with cardiac disease, who may not be able to compensate for drug's hypotensive effect. Monitor vital signs, including blood pressure, frequently. Be aware that hypertension and tachycardia may occur in patients with a history of pheochromocytoma.

• Expect altered level of consciousness to last up to 12 hours after drug is given. Expect dosage to be reduced if patient is taking an opioid analgesic.

• If drug causes extrapyramidal reactions, such as restlessness, dystonia, and oculogyric crisis, expect to administer an anticholinergic, such as benztropine or diphenhydramine. Be sure to maintain a patent airway and oxygenation.

• If patient develops severe hypotension, expect to give phenylephrine. If hypotension is related to hypovolemia, expect to administer fluids.

PATIENT TEACHING

• Advise patient to immediately report palpitations or faintness, which may indicate an abnormal cardiac rhythm.

• Instruct patient to ask for help with ambulation on first postoperative day because altered consciousness may last up to 12 hours.

• Caution patient to avoid drinking alcohol, taking CNS depressants, driving, and operating machinery for 24 hours after receiving droperidol.

dulaglutide
Trulicity

Class and Category
Chemical class: Fusion protein
Therapeutic class: Antidiabetic
Pregnancy category: C

Indications and Dosages
➤ *Adjunct to diet and exercise to improve glycemic control in patients with type 2 diabetes mellitus*
SUBCUTANEOUS INJECTION
Adults. 0.75 mg once weekly, increased to 1.5 mg once weekly, as needed. *Maximum*: 1.5 mg once weekly.

Mechanism of Action
Activates the GLP-1 receptor to increase intracellular cyclic AMP (cAMP) in beta cells, causing a glucose-dependent insulin release. Insulin lowers blood glucose levels. Dulaglutide also decreases glucagon secretion and slows gastric emptying to further decrease blood glucose levels.

Contraindications
Diabetic ketoacidosis, hypersensitivity to dulaglutide or its components, personal or family history of medullary thyroid carcinoma or multiple endocrine neoplasia syndrome, preexisting severe gastrointestinal disease

Interaction
DRUGS
insulin, insulin secretagogues: Increased risk of hypoglycemia
orally administered drugs: Possibly decreased absorption of the orally administered drugs

Adverse Reactions
CNS: Asthenia, fatigue, malaise

CV: First-degree AV block, prolonged PR interval, sinus tachycardia
ENDO: Hypoglycemia
GI: Abdominal distention or pain, constipation, diarrhea, dyspepsia, elevated liver enzymes, flatulence, gastroesophageal reflux disease, nausea, pancreatitis, vomiting
GU: Acute renal failure, worsening renal failure
SKIN: Pruritus, rash, urticaria
Other: Angioedema, injection site reactions such as erythema and rash

Nursing Considerations

• Know that dulaglutide should not be used as first-line therapy for patients who have inadequately controlled their blood glucose levels on diet and exercise alone.
• Use caution when beginning dulaglutide therapy or titrating dose in patients with renal impairment. Monitor renal function in these patients if they experience severe adverse gastrointestinal reactions. Also use cautiously in patients with hepatic impairment because the effect of dulaglutide therapy on the liver is unknown.
• Be aware that dulaglutide may potentially be linked to the development of thyroid C-cell tumors. While elevated serum calcitonin is a biological marker, its value in routine monitoring is unclear. If an elevated serum calcitonin level is found at any time during therapy, expect patient to be referred to an endocrinologist for further evaluation.
• Monitor patient for signs and symptoms of pancreatitis, such as persistent severe abdominal pain, sometimes radiating to the back, which may or may not be accompanied by vomiting. If confirmed, expect dulaglutide to be discontinued.
• Monitor patient also receiving insulin or insulin secretagogue therapy concomitantly for hypoglycemia. The dosage of insulin or insulin secretagogue may need to be lowered to reduce the risk of hypoglycemia. If hypoglycemia occurs, treat it according to policy and notify prescriber.
• Monitor patient for signs of hypersensitivity such as pruritus, rash, or urticaria. If present, withhold drug, notify prescriber. and expect drug to be discontinued.
• Monitor patient for signs of diarrhea, dehydration, nausea or vomiting, which may suggest renal impairment. If present, notify prescriber because the frequency of these gastrointestinal symptoms may increase as renal function declines.

PATIENT TEACHING

• Inform patient that drug may be administered at any time of day without regard to meals but that it should be administered on the same day each week. However, if the day of the week needs to be changed, that change may be made, as long as the last dose was administered 4 or more days earlier.
• Instruct patient that if a dose is missed and it is within 1 to 2 days of his next regularly scheduled dose, he should administer at the regularly scheduled time.
• Teach patient to administer the injection into the abdomen, thigh, or upper arm region. Instruct patient that if the same body region is being used each week, the sites of injection should be rotated within that region. Tell patient how to safely dispose of the used pen and needle.
• Teach female patients to alert prescriber if pregnancy occurs or is suspected.
• Ensure that patient has been informed of the potential risk for developing thyroid tumors before starting dulaglutide therapy. Tell patient to report any symptoms of thyroid tumors such as a mass in the neck, difficulty swallowing or breathing, or persistent hoarseness.
• Instruct patient on the signs and symptoms of hypoglycemia and how to treat it. Inform patient who is also receiving an insulin secretagogue or insulin that the risk of hypoglycemia is greater. Tell patient to notify prescriber if hypoglycemia occurs frequently or is severe.
• Tell patient to notify prescriber if any orally administered drugs appear to be losing their effectiveness, as dulaglutide causes a delay of gastric emptying and has the potential to impact the absorption of drugs taken by mouth.

Duloxetine hydrochloride

Cymbalta

Class and Category

Chemical: Selective serotonin and norepinephrine reuptake inhibitor
Therapeutic: Antidepressant, neuropathic and musculoskeletal pain reliever
Pregnancy category: C

Indications and Dosages

➤ *To treat major depressive disorder*
E.R. CAPSULES
Adults. 20 mg twice daily. Alternatively, 60 mg once daily or 30 mg twice daily.
➤ *To relieve neuropathic pain associated with diabetic peripheral neuropathy*
E.R. CAPSULES
Adults. 60 mg daily.
➤ *To treat generalized anxiety disorder*
E.R. CAPSULES
Adults. *Initial:* 30 or 60 mg once daily, increased in 30-mg increments weekly, as needed. *Maximum:* 120 mg once daily.
Children age 7 to 17 years of age. *Initial:* 30 mg once daily for 2 wk, then increased in 30-mg increments weekly, as needed. *Maximum:* 120 mg daily.
DOSAGE ADJUSTMENT For elderly patients, dosage initiated at 30 mg once daily for 2 weeks, before dosage increased to 60 mg once daily. Further increases in dosage made in 30-mg increments weekly, as needed, to maximum dosage of 120 mg once daily.
➤ *To treat fibromyalgia; to treat chronic musculoskeletal pain*
E.R. CAPSULES
Adults. *Initial:* 30 mg daily for 1 wk; then increased to 60 mg daily.

Mechanism of Action

Inhibits neuronal serotonin, norepine-phrine, and dopamine reuptake to potentiate serotonergic and noradrenergic activity in the CNS. These activities may elevate mood and inhibit pain signals stemming from peripheral nerves adversely affected by chronically elevated serum glucose level.

Route	Onset	Peak	Duration
P.O.	Unknown	6 hr	Unknown

Contraindications

Hepatic insufficiency, hypersensitivity to duloxetine or its components, uncontrolled angle-closure glaucoma, use within 14 days of MAO inhibitor therapy

Interactions

DRUGS
amiodarone, celecoxib, cimetidine, erythromycin, fluoxetine, fluvoxamine, haloperidol, ketoconazole, methadone, paroxetine, quinidine, quinolones, ritonavir: Increased blood duloxetine level
amiodarone, amitriptyline, desipramine, flecainide, haloperidol, imipramine, methadone, nortriptyline, phenothiazines, propafenone, ritonavir, thioridazine: Increased blood levels of these drugs
aspirin, NSAIDs, warfarin: Possibly increased risk of bleeding
CNS drugs: Increased effect of duloxetine
linezolid, methylene blue (I.V.), serotonergic drugs: Increased risk of serotonin syndrome
MAO inhibitors: Serious, sometimes fatal, autonomic instability, hyperthermia, myoclonus, rigidity
plasma protein binders (warfarin, phenytoin): Increased free concentration of these drugs and increased risk of adverse reactions
ACTIVITIES
alcohol use: Increased risk of hepatotoxicity

Adverse Reactions

CNS: Abnormal dreams, aggression, agitation, anger, anxiety, asthenia, chills, dizziness, extrapyramidal disorder, fatigue, fever, hallucinations, headache, insomnia, migraine, nervousness, neuroleptic malignant syndrome, parasthesia, restless legs syndrome, seizures, serotonin syndrome, somnolence, suicidal ideation, syncope, tremor, vertigo
CV: Hypertension, hypertensive crisis, orthostatic hypotension, palpitations, paresthesia, peripheral edema or coldness, supraventricular arrhythmia
EENT: Acute-angle glaucoma, blurred vision, dry mouth, glaucoma, nasopharyngitis, pharyngitis, taste alteration, tinnitus
ENDO: Galactorrhea, hot flashes, hyperglycemia, hyperprolactinemia

GI: Abdominal pain, anorexia, cholestatic jaundice, constipation, diarrhea, elevated liver enzymes, flatulence, hepatitis, hepatotoxicity, indigestion, jaundice, nausea, upper abdominal pain, vomiting
GU: Abnormal orgasm; decreased libido; erectile or ejaculatory dysfunction; urinary frequency, hesitancy, or retention; UTI
HEME: Bleeding episodes, leukopenia, thrombocytopenia
MS: Arthralgia, back pain, extremity pain, muscle cramp or spasm, myalgia
RESP: Cough, upper respiratory tract infection
SKIN: Diaphoresis, erythema multiforme, pruritus, rash, Stevens-Johnson syndrome, urticaria
Other: Anaphylaxis, angioedema, hyponatremia, weight loss

Nursing Considerations
• Know that duloxetine should not be given to patients with severe renal impairment or end-stage renal disease that requires hemodialysis because blood drug levels increase significantly in these patients. Also know that duloxetine should be avoided in patients with hepatic insufficiency or who use alcohol excessively because drug is metabolized by the liver.
• Use duloxetine cautiously in patients with delayed gastric emptying because drug's enteric coating resists dissolution until it reaches an area where pH exceeds 5.5.
• Give duloxetine cautiously to patients with a history of mania, which it may activate. Also give cautiously to patients with a seizure disorder because drug effects aren't known in these patients.
• Obtain patient's baseline blood pressure before duloxetine therapy starts, and assess it periodically thereafter for changes. If orthostatic hypotension occurs during therapy, notify prescriber and anticipate that drug may need to be discontinued.
• Monitor patient's serum sodium level, as ordered, especially if patient is elderly, is taking a diuretic, or has volume depletion, because drug may lower serum sodium level.
• Monitor patient's hepatic function, as ordered, because drug may increase the

risk of hepatotoxicity. Expect to discontinue duloxetine, as ordered, if patient develops jaundice or other serious liver dysfunction manifestation.
• If patient takes duloxetine for depression (especially if he's a child or an adolescent), watch closely for evidence of suicidal thinking or behavior, especially when therapy starts or dosage changes.
• Avoid stopping duloxetine therapy abruptly, if possible, because withdrawal symptoms such as dizziness, nausea, headache, fatigue, paresthesia, vomiting, irritability, nightmares, insomnia, diarrhea, anxiety, hyperhidrosis, and vertigo may occur. Taper dosage gradually, as ordered.
WARNING Monitor patient for serotonin syndrome, characterized by agitation, chills, confusion, diaphoresis, diarrhea, fever, hyperactive reflexes, poor coordination, restlessness, shaking, talking or acting with uncontrolled excitement, tremor, and twitching. In its most severe form, serotonin syndrome can resemble neuroleptic malignant syndrome, which includes a high fever, muscle rigidity, autonomic instability with possible fluctuations in vital signs, and mental status changes.
WARNING Treatment with linezolid or I.V. methylene blue is not recommended while patient is taking duloxetine because of increased risk of serotonin syndrome. However, if prescriber feels benefits outweigh the risks, expect duloxetine to be discontinued promptly. Monitor patient closely for serotonin syndrome for 5 days or until 24 hours after the last dose of linezolid or I.V. methylene blue, whichever comes first. Know that therapy with duloxetine may be resumed 24 hours after the last dose of linezolid or I.V. methylene blue.
PATIENT TEACHING
• Tell patient to take capsule whole and not to chew it, crush it, or sprinkle contents on food or liquids because doing so alters enteric coating and may affect drug absorption.
• Inform patient that full effect of duloxetine may take weeks to occur; emphasize the importance of continuing to take the drug as directed.

D

- Caution patient against excessive alcohol consumption while taking duloxetine because it may increase risk of hepatic dysfunction. Also tell him to report a yellowing of skin immediately, as drug may need to be discontinued.
- Advise patient not to stop duloxetine abruptly because adverse reactions may occur. Explain that drug will be stopped gradually.
- Instruct patient to notify prescriber if any serious or troublesome adverse effects develop.
- Advise patient to avoid hazardous activities until drug's CNS effects are known.
- Advise patient that drug may cause mild pupillary dilation, which may lead to an episode of acute-angle glaucoma. Encourage him to have an eye exam before starting therapy to see if he is at risk.
- Instruct patient to rise from a lying or sitting position slowly to minimize drug's effect on lowering blood pressure, which may possibly lead to falls or cause patient to faint.
- If patient takes duloxetine for depression, urge caregivers to watch closely for evidence of suicidal tendencies, especially if patient is a child or an adolescent and especially when therapy starts or dosage changes.
- Instruct female patients of childbearing age to notify prescriber if they are, could be, or wish to become pregnant; duloxetine therapy may cause adverse reactions in neonates exposed to it during the third trimester. If patient becomes pregnant while taking duloxetine, urge her to enroll in the Pregnancy Registry by calling 1-866-814-6975 or visiting *www.cymbaltapregnancyregistry.com*.
- Tell patient to stop taking duloxetine and notify prescriber immediately at the first sign of blisters, peeling rash, mucosal erosions, or any other sign of hypersensitivity, as drug will need to be discontinued.
- Advise patient that drug may cause mild pupillary dilation, which may lead to an episode of acute-angle glaucoma. Encourage him to have an eye exam before starting therapy to see if he is at risk.
- Instruct patient with diabetes to monitor his blood glucose levels more closely, as duloxetine therapy can alter control.

dutasteride
Avodart

Class and Category
Chemical class: Synthetic 4-azasteroid compound
Therapeutic class: Benign prostatic hyperplasia agent
Pregnancy category: X

Indications and Dosages
➤ *To treat symptomatic benign prostatic hyperplasia (BPH); as adjunct with tamsulosin therapy to treat symptomatic BPH*
CAPSULES
Adult men. 0.5 mg daily.

Contraindications
Children; women; hypersensitivity to dutasteride, its components, or other 5-alpha reductase inhibitors

Interactions
DRUGS
cimetidine, ciprofloxacin, diltiazem, ketoconazole, ritonavir, verapamil, and other CYP3A4 inhibitors: Risk of decreased dutasteride metabolism and enhanced effects

Adverse Reactions
CNS: Depression, dizziness
ENDO: Gynecomastia, increased serum testosterone and thyroid-stimulating hormone levels, male breast cancer
GU: Decreased ejaculatory volume, decreased libido, high-grade prostate cancer, impotence, testicular pain and swelling
SKIN: Localized edema, pruritus, rash, serious skin reactions, urticaria
Other: Angioedema

Nursing Considerations
WARNING Be aware that dutasteride is absorbed through the skin. If you are female and pregnant or of childbearing age, do not handle dutasteride capsule when administering it to a patient.
- Patient should be evaluated for other urologic conditions, including prostate cancer, before dutasteride therapy starts

Mechanism of Action

Dutasteride reduces prostate gland enlargement by inhibiting conversion oftestosterone to its active metabolite, 5-alpha dihydrotestosterone (DHT). DHT is the main hormone that stimulates prostate cells to grow. As men age, they may become more sensitive to DHT, resulting in excessive growth of prostatic cells and enlargement of the prostate. This condition, benign prostatic hyperplasia, may cause urinary hesitancy, urinary urgency, and nocturia.

Two forms of the intracellular enzyme 5-alpha-reductase (5α-R types 1 and 2) inliver, prostate, and skin, convert testosterone to DHT, as shown below left. Dutasteride, a dual 5α-R inhibitor, deactivates both forms. When 5α-R is inhibitedby dutasteride, production of DHT is suppressed, as shown below right. Withless circulating DHT, the prostate gland shrinks and symptoms improve.

because dutasteride therapy increases risk of patient developing high-grade prostate cancer.

• Expect patient to undergo a digital rectal examination of the prostate before and periodically during dutasteride therapy.

• Anticipate need to obtain a new baseline prostate-specific antigen (PSA) value after 3 to 6 months of dutasteride treatment because drug can decrease PSA concentration by 40% to 50%. Dutasteride also can decrease serum PSA level in the presence of prostate cancer. Any PSA reading in a patient receiving dutasteride should be doubled for comparison with normal values in untreated men. If value still falls within the normal range for men not taking a 5 alpha-reductase inhibitor, further evaluation should still be done to rule out prostate cancer.

PATIENT TEACHING

WARNING Urge patient and female partners to use reliable contraceptive method during dutasteride therapy because semen of men who take drug can harm male fetuses. Caution women and children against handling capsules.

• Advise patient to inform prescriber if he has liver disease.

• Explain how to take drug properly, and advise patient to follow instructions that accompany drug. Instruct him to swallow capsule whole and to notify pharmacist if capsules are cracked or leaking.

• Inform patient that drug may decrease ejaculatory volume and libido and may cause impotence.

• Instruct patient to postpone blood donations for 6 months after final dose to avoid transmitting dutasteride to a pregnant woman during a blood transfusion.

• Urge patient to have periodic follow-up appointments.

dyphylline

Dilor, Lufyllin

Class and Category

Chemical class: Xanthine derivative
Therapeutic class: Bronchodilator
Pregnancy category: C

Indications and Dosages

➤ *To prevent or relieve bronchospasm from acute and chronic bronchial asthma, chronic bronchitis, and emphysema*

ELIXIR, TABLETS

Adults. Up to 15 mg/kg every 6 hr.

I.M. INJECTION

Adults. *Initial:* 500 mg. *Maintenance:* 250 to 500 mg every 2 to 6 hr, as needed.

Mechanism of Action

May cause bronchodilation by inhibiting phosphodiesterase enzymes. These enzymes normally inactivate cyclic adenosine monophosphate (cAMP) and cyclic guanosine monophosphate (cGMP), which are responsible for bronchial smooth-muscle relaxation. Drug also may foster calcium translocation, prostaglandin antagonism, catecholamine stimulation, and adenosine-receptor antagonism.

Contraindications

Hypersensitivity to dyphylline, xanthines, or their components; peptic ulcer disease; seizure disorder (unless controlled by anticonvulsant therapy)

Interactions

DRUGS

beta blockers: Possibly inhibited bronchodilation by dyphylline

ephedrine: Possibly increased frequency of insomnia, nausea, and nervousness

hydrocarbon inhalation anesthetics: Possibly increased risk of ventricular arrhythmias

probenecid: Possibly decreased renal excretion of dyphylline

sucralfate: Possibly adsorption of dyphylline if drugs given within 2 hours of each other

Adverse Reactions

CNS: Headache, insomnia, irritability, nervousness, seizures, tremor
CV: Arrhythmias, hypotension, tachycardia
GI: Diarrhea, gastroesophageal reflux, nausea, vomiting
GU: Increased diuresis

Nursing Considerations

• Inspect I.M. form of dyphylline for precipitate. If present, discard drug and obtain a new ampule.
• Give oral drug at least 1 hour after meals for best absorption. However, if drug causes GI distress, give it with food if prescribed.
• Don't give parenteral drug by I.V. route.
• Evaluate for therapeutic response, including decreased respiratory rate and effort.
• Assess for signs of dyphylline toxicity, including seizures and ventricular tachycardia.

PATIENT TEACHING

• Instruct patient to take oral dyphylline with a full glass of water and on an empty stomach to promote absorption.
• Advise patient to consult prescriber about taking drug with food if she experiences GI distress.

➤━━━━━━━◄

E F

eflornithine hydrochloride
(alpha-difluoromethyl-ornithine, DFMO)
Ornidyl

Class and Category
Chemical class: Difluoromethylornithine
Therapeutic class: Antiprotozoal
Pregnancy category: C

Indications and Dosages
➤ *To treat the meningoencephalitic stage of trypanosoma brucei gambiense infection (sleeping sickness)*
I.V. INFUSION
Adults. 100 mg/kg given over at least 45 min every 6 hr for 14 days.

Route	Onset	Peak	Duration
I.V.	Unknown	4–6 hr	Unknown

Mechanism of Action
Inhibits the enzyme ornithine decarboxylase, which is needed for decarboxylation of ornithine. This process is the first step in polyamine synthesis, which is needed for protozoal cell division and differentiation.

Incompatibilities
Don't give eflornithine with any other drug.

Contraindications
Hypersensitivity to eflornithine or its components

Adverse Reactions
CNS: Asthenia, dizziness, headache, seizures
EENT: Hearing loss
GI: Abdominal pain, anorexia, diarrhea, vomiting
HEME: Anemia, eosinophilia, leukopenia, myelosuppression, thrombocytopenia
Other: Alopecia, facial edema

Nursing Considerations
• Plan to reduce eflornithine dosage as prescribed, based on renal function.

Monitor creatinine clearance in patients with renal dysfunction.
• Before infusion, dilute eflornithine concentrate with sterile water for injection. Using strict aseptic technique, withdraw the contents of a 100-ml vial and inject 25 ml into each of four I.V. diluent bags that contain 100 ml of sterile water. The resulting solution contains 40 mg/ml of eflornithine (5,000 mg of eflornithine in 125 ml total volume).
• Store bags of diluted eflornithine at 4° C (39° F) to reduce the risk of contamination. Use diluted drug within 24 hours.
• Expect to monitor the patient's CBC, including platelet count, before eflornithine treatment, twice weekly during treatment, and weekly after treatment stops until the patient's hematologic values return to baseline.
• Take infection-control and bleeding precautions because drug may cause myelosuppression. Adjust dosage or stop therapy as prescribed, based on severity.
• Take seizure precautions during eflornithine therapy.
• Consult prescriber about the need for serial audiography, if appropriate.
• Store undiluted vials of eflornithine at room temperature, and protect from freezing and light.
PATIENT TEACHING
• Emphasize need for follow-up visits because risk of relapse lasts 24 months after treatment.
• Teach patient how to follow infection-control and bleeding precautions if myelosuppression occurs.
• Warn patient about risk of seizures; advise against performing potentially hazardous activities during therapy.

eletriptan hydrobromide
Relpax

Class and Category
Chemical class: Serotonin 5-HT$_{1D}$–receptor agonist
Therapeutic class: Antimigraine agent
Pregnancy category: C

Indications and Dosages

➤ *To relieve acute migraine attacks with or without aura*

TABLETS

Adults. *Initial:* 20 or 40 mg as a single dose. Repeated in 2 hr, as needed and ordered. *Maximum:* 40 mg as single dose, 80 mg daily.

Mechanism of Action

May stimulate 5-HT$_1$ receptors, causing selective vasoconstriction of inflamed and dilated cranial blood vessels in carotid circulation, which decreases carotid arterial blood flow and relieves acute migraines.

Contraindications

Bibasilar or hemiplegic migraine, cardiovascular disease (significant), cerebrovascular syndromes (stroke, transient ischemic attack), hepatic impairment (severe), hypersensitivity to eletriptan or components, ischemic bowel disease, ischemic or vasospastic coronary artery disease (CAD), peripheral vascular disease, uncontrolled hypertension, use within 24 hours of another serotonin 5-HT$_1$–receptor agonist or ergot-type drug, use within 72 hours of a potent CYP3A4 inhibitor

Interactions

DRUGS

clarithromycin, ketoconazole, itraconazole, nefazodone, nelfinavir, ritonavir, troleandomycin and other potent CYP3A4 inhibitors: Increased metabolism of eletriptan and decreased blood eletriptan level

ergot-containing drugs, 5-HT$_1$-receptor agonists: Possibly additive or prolonged vasoconstrictive effects

fluoxetine, fluvoxamine, paroxetine, sertraline: Increased risk of weakness, hyperreflexia, and incoordination

Adverse Reactions

CNS: Asthenia, chills, dizziness, headache, hypertonia, hypesthesia, paresthesia, seizures, somnolence, tiredness, weakness, vertigo

CV: Chest tightness, pain, or pressure; coronary artery vasospasm; hypertension; MI or myocardial ischemia (transient); palpitations; shock; ventricular fibrillation or tachycardia

EENT: Dry mouth, pharyngitis, throat tightness

GI: Abdominal pain, cramps, discomfort, or pressure; dysphagia; indigestion; nausea, vomiting

MS: Back pain

SKIN: Diaphoresis, flushing

Other: Allergic reaction; angioedema; feeling of warmth, pain, or pressure

Nursing Considerations

• Ensure that patients who are at risk for CAD undergo a satisfactory CV evaluation before administering the first dose of eletriptan and that they have a periodic re-evaluation of their cardiac status during intermittent long-term therapy.

• Obtain an ECG immediately after first dose of drug in patients who have CV risk factors but who have had a satisfactory CV evaluation because of the drug's potential to cause coronary vasospasm.

• Evaluate patient for CV signs and symptoms after administration of eletriptan and notify prescriber if they occur. Expect drug to be withheld, as ordered, while patient undergoes an extensive CV workup, and discontinued if abnormalities are detected.

• Monitor patient's blood pressure during therapy because of drug's potential to increase blood pressure.

PATIENT TEACHING

• Advise patient to take eletriptan as soon as possible after onset of migraine symptoms.

• Urge patient to contact prescriber and avoid taking drug if headache symptoms aren't typical.

• Advise against exceeding prescribed dose.

• Instruct patient to seek emergency care for chest, jaw, or neck tightness after taking drug because these may indicate adverse CV reactions; subsequent doses may require ECG monitoring.

• Urge patient to report palpitations.

• Advise patient to avoid hazardous activities until drug's CNS effects are known.

• Advise yearly ophthalmic examinations during prolonged eletriptan therapy.

• Instruct patient to inform prescriber of all drugs he's taking, including OTC products and herbal remedies.

eltrombopag olamine

Promacta

Class and Category

Chemical class: Biphenyl hydrazone
Therapeutic class: Platelet formation inducer
Pregnancy category: C

Indications and Dosages

➤ *To treat thrombocytopenia in patients
with chronic immune (idiopathic)
thrombocytopenic purpura and an
insufficient response to corticosteroids,
immunoglobulins, or splenectomy*

TABLETS

Adults. *Initial:* 50 mg daily, increased as
needed to maintain a platelet count of
50 ×10^9/L. Platelet counts usually increase
in 1 to 2 wk. *Maximum:* 75 mg daily.

DOSAGE ADJUSTMENT For patients of East
Asian ancestry or patients with moderate to
severe hepatic impairment, starting dose of
25 mg daily. For patients of East Asian
ancestry who also have hepatic impairment,
starting dose of 12.5 mg daily. For patients
with a platelet count less than 50 × 10^9/L
following at least 2 weeks of therapy, dosage
increased by 25 mg daily to maximum of
75 mg/day unless patient started therapy at
12.5 mg daily, then dosage increased to 25 mg
daily before increasing the dose amount by
25 mg, as needed. For patients with a platelet
count equal to or greater than 200 × 10^9/L
but equal to or less than 400 × 10^9/L, dosage
decreased by 25 mg **daily** for at least 2 weeks
before further dosage adjustment made. For
patient with a platelet count greater than
400 × 10^9/L, drug should be withheld until
platelet count is less than 150 × 10^9/L and
then restarted at a daily dose reduced by
25 mg, unless patient had been taking 25 mg
daily, then dosage restarted at 12.5 mg daily.

➤ *To treat thrombocytopenia in patients
with chronic hepatitis C infection*

TABLETS

Adults. *Initial:* 25 mg daily, increased in
increments of 25 mg daily every 2 wk, as
needed, to achieve the target platelet count
required to initiate antiviral therapy.
Maximum: 100 mg daily.

DOSAGE ADJUSTMENT For patients with a
platelet count equal to or greater than 200 ×
10^9/L but equal to or less than 400 × 10^9/L,
dosage decreased by 25 mg for at least 2
weeks before further dosage adjustment
made. For patient with a platelet count
greater than 400 × 10^9/L, drug should be
withheld until platelet count is less than
150 × 10^9/L and then restarted at a daily dose
reduced by 25 mg, unless patient had been
taking 25 mg daily, then dosage restarted at
12.5 mg daily. For patient receiving antiviral
therapy, dosage adjusted, as needed, to avoid
dose reductions of peginterferon.

➤ *To treat severe aplastic anemia*

TABLETS

Adults. *Initial:* 50 mg once daily, increased as
needed in 50-mg increments every 2 weeks.
Maximum: 150 mg daily.

DOSAGE ADJUSTMENT For patients of East
Asian ancestry or patients with any degree of
hepatic impairment, starting dose of 25 mg
daily. For patients with a platelet count less
than 50 × 10^9/L following at least 2 weeks of
therapy, dosage increased by 50 mg daily to
maximum of 150 mg daily. For patients
taking 25 mg once daily, dosage increased to
50 mg once daily before dosage increased by
50 mg. For patients with a platelet count
equal to or greater than 200 × 10^9/L but equal
to or less than 400 × 10^9/L, dosage decreased
by 50 mg daily for at least 2 weeks before
further dosage adjustment made. For patient
with a platelet count greater than 400 × 10^9/L,
drug should be withheld for 1 week and until
platelet count is less than 150 × 10^9/L and
then drug restarted at a daily dose reduced by
50 mg.

Route	Onset	Peak	Duration
P.O.	Unknown	2–6 hr	Unknown

Mechanism of Action

Interacts with the transmembrane domain of
the thrombopoietin receptor to signal
cascades that induce proliferation and
differentiation of megakaryocytes from bone
marrow progenitor cells. This action increases
platelet production, which is abnormally low
in patients with thrombocytopenic purpura.

Contraindications

Hypersensitivity to eltrombopag or its
components

Interactions

DRUGS

acetaminophen, atorvastatin, benzyl-penicillin, fluvastatin, methotrexate, nateglinide, NSAIDs, opioids, pravastatin, repaglinide, rifampin, rosuvastatin: Possibly increased risk of adverse reactions related to excessive exposure to these drugs

antacids and mineral supplements containing aluminum, calcium, iron, magnesium, selenium, or zinc: Decreased eltrombopag absorption

ciprofloxacin, fluvoxamine, gemfibrozil, omeprazole, rifampin, trimethoprim: Increased risk of eltrombopag-induced adverse reactions

interferon, ribavirin: Increased risk of hepatotoxicity

FOODS

all foods, especially dairy: Decreased absorption of eltrombopag

ACTIVITIES

smoking: Increased risk of eltrombopag-induced adverse reactions and possibly decreased eltrombopag efficacy

Adverse Reactions

CNS: Headache, paresthesia,
CV: Portal venous system thromboses (in presence of chronic liver disease)
EENT: Cataract, conjunctival hemorrhage
GI: Abdominal pain, dyspepsia, elevated liver enzymes, hepatic decompensation (with antiviral and interferon therapy), hepatotoxicity, indirect hyperbilirubinemia (with antiviral and interferon therapy), nausea, vomiting
GU: Menorrhagia
HEME: Hemorrhage, thrombocytopenia
MS: Fatigue, myalgia
SKIN: Ecchymosis

Nursing Considerations

• Eltrombopag should be used only to treat chronic immune (idiopathic) thrombocytopenia purpura and not any other kind of thrombocytopenia because of the risk of hematologic malignancies or portal venous system thromboses in patients with chronic liver disease.

• Eltrombopag can be used only through a restricted distribution program called *Promacta Cares*. Patient, pharmacy, and prescriber must all be enrolled before therapy begins.

• Use cautiously in patients with hepatic impairment because drug may cause

hepatotoxicity and portal venous system thromboses, especially if patient with hepatic impairment also has risk factors present for thromboembolism.

• Monitor liver enzymes and bilirubin level, as ordered, before starting eltrombopag, every 2 weeks during dosage adjustment, and monthly once dose is stable. If abnormalities occur, repeat testing within 3 to 5 days and then weekly until liver enzymes return to baseline. Expect to discontinue drug if alanine aminotransferase level increases to three or more times the upper normal limit, progresses or persists for 4 or more weeks, or is accompanied by an increase in direct bilirubin or clinical symptoms of liver injury.

• Know that there is an increased risk of hepatic decomposition when eltrombopag is used in combination with interferon and ribavirin in patients with chronic hepatitis C. Monitor these patients closely for evidence of hepatic dysfunction.

• Expect to monitor platelet counts every week prior to starting antiviral therapy, as ordered, for patient with hepatitis C. Once antiviral therapy has started, expect to monitor CBCs with differentials including platelet counts weekly during antiviral therapy until a stable platelet count is achieved. Thereafter, monitor platelet counts monthly, as ordered.

• Patient should have a baseline eye examination, as ordered, before starting eltrombopag and periodically throughout therapy, because drug may cause cataracts.

• Dosage adjustments are based on platelet count response and are not used to normalize platelet counts in order to prevent or minimize thrombotic complications.

• Give eltrombopag 1 hour before or 2 hours after the patient has eaten. Separate doses of other drugs by at least 4 hours to prevent drug interactions.

• Do not administer more than one dose of eltrombopag within any 24-hour period.

• Expect to discontinue drug for patient with chronic thrombocytopenia if improvement doesn't occur within 4 weeks at maximum dose of 75 mg daily or if the platelet count remains greater than 400×10^9/L after 2 weeks of therapy at the lowest dose of eltrombopag. Expect

to discontinue drug for patient with hepatitis C if the platelet count remains greater than 400×10^9/L after 2 weeks of therapy at the lowest dose of eltrombopag or when antiviral therapy is discontinued.
• Monitor patient for hematologic malignancies because eltrombopag stimulates thrombopoietin receptor on the surface of hematopoietic cells, which increases risk of malignancies.
• Monitor patient for increased bleeding after stopping eltrombopag because thrombocytopenia may worsen, increasing bleeding risk, especially if patient is on anticoagulants or antiplatelet therapy. If bleeding occurs, obtain weekly CBC, including platelet count, for at least 4 weeks after therapy stops, and provide supportive care, as indicated and ordered.

PATIENT TEACHING
• Inform patient that before eltrombopag therapy can begin, he must be enrolled in the *Promacta Cares* program, which provides comprehensive education about the drug.
• Urge patient to tell prescriber about all health conditions and all prescribed drugs, OTC drugs, herbs, and supplements taken.
• Instruct patient to take eltrombopag on an empty stomach with a full glass of water 1 hour before or 2 hours after a meal and to separate use of other drugs by at least 4 hours because food and certain drugs (such as antacids and iron and vitamin supplements) may interfere with eltrombopag absorption.
• Instruct patient to take drug at the same time every day because no more than one dose should be taken within any 24-hour period.
• Urge patient to report any adverse reactions, especially signs and symptoms of liver problems such as yellowing of the skin or the whites of the eyes, unusual darkening of the urine, unusual tiredness, right upper stomach area pain, confusion, or swelling of the stomach area, to prescriber. In addition, tell patient to keep all appointments for blood work and follow-up.

empagliflozin

Jardiance

Class and Category

Chemical class: Sodium glucose co-transporter 2 inhibitor
Therapeutic class: Antidiabetic
Pregnancy category: C

Indications and Dosages

➤ *Adjunct to diet and exercise to improve glycemic control in patients with type 2 diabetes mellitus*

TABLETS
Adults. 10 mg once daily in morning, increased to 25 mg once daily in morning, as needed.

Mechanism of Action

Inhibits sodium glucose co-transporter 2 in the kidneys, which prevents glucose reabsorption. This decreases blood glucose levels.

Contraindications

Diabetic ketoacidosis, dialysis therapy, end-stage renal disease, hypersensitivity to empagliflozin or its components, severe renal impairment

Interaction

DRUGS
insulin, insulin secretagogues: Increased risk of hypoglycemia

Adverse Reactions

CNS: Syncope
CV: Dyslipidemia, elevated low-density lipoprotein cholesterol, hypotension
ENDO: Hypoglycemia
GI: Nausea
GU: Decreased glomerular filtration rate, dysuria, elevated serum creatinine levels, genital mycotic infections, impaired renal function, increased urination, osmotic diuresis, UTI
MS: Arthralgia
RESP: Upper respiratory tract infection
Other: Dehydration

Nursing Considerations

• Assess patient's volume status and correct, if needed and as prescribed, prior to starting empagliflozin therapy because drug can cause intravascular volume contraction leading to symptomatic hypotension. Patients at highest risk include elderly patients, patients receiving loop diuretic therapy, and patients who have impaired renal function.

E
F

• Obtain serum creatinine level, as ordered, prior to starting empagliflozin therapy because empagliflozin can cause adverse renal effects. Be aware that the elderly and patients with existing impaired renal function are at higher risk for these adverse effects. Monitor renal function throughout therapy.

• Monitor patient's blood pressure and cholesterol level throughout empagliflozin therapy.

• Be aware that patients receiving insulin or insulin secretagogues may require a lower dose of these agents because empagliflozin in combination increases risk of hypoglycemia. Monitor patient closely for hypoglycemia. If present, treat according to standard of care and notify prescriber.

• Monitor patients for genital mycotic infections or urinary tract infections, especially those with a history of such. If present, notify prescriber and treat, as prescribed.

PATIENT TEACHING

• Inform patient that empagliflozin therapy is not a replacement for diet and exercise therapy.

• Instruct patient on the signs and symptoms of hypoglycemia and how to treat it. Inform patient who is also receiving a sulfonylurea or insulin that the risk of hypoglycemia is greater. Tell patient to notify prescriber if hypoglycemia occurs frequently or is severe.

• Tell patient to monitor the blood glucose level using blood tests instead of urine tests because drug increases urinary glucose excretion and will lead to positive urine glucose tests.

• Advise female patients to notify prescriber if pregnancy occurs or is suspected because drug may cause fetal harm if taken in the second or third trimester.

• Advise patient to maintain adequate fluid intake throughout empagliflozin therapy.

enalapril maleate

Epaned, Vasotec

enalaprilat

Vasotec I.V.

Class and Category

Chemical class: Dicarbocyl-containing ACE inhibitor
Therapeutic class: Antihypertensive
Pregnancy category: D

Indications and Dosages

➤ *To control hypertension*

ORAL SOLUTION, TABLETS

Adults. *Initial:* 5 mg daily, increased after 1 to 2 wk, as needed.
Maintenance: 10 to 40 mg once daily or in divided doses twice daily.

Children. 0.08 mg/kg daily, titrated according to blood pressure response up to 5 mg daily.
Maximum: 0.58 mg/kg/dose or 40 mg/dose.

I.V. INFUSION

Adults. 1.25 mg every 6 hr.

DOSAGE ADJUSTMENT Initial dose 2.5 mg P.O. or 0.625 mg I.V. for patients who have sodium and water depletion from diuretic therapy, are receiving diuretics, or have a creatinine clearance below 30 ml/min/1.73 m^2. If response to I.V. dose is inadequate after 1 hr, I.V. dose of 0.625 mg is repeated and therapy continued at 1.25 mg every 6 hr.

➤ *To treat heart failure*

TABLETS

Adults. *Initial:* 2.5 mg once or twice daily, increased after 1 to 2 wk, as needed.
Maintenance: 5 to 40 mg daily in 2 divided doses.

➤ *To treat asymptomatic left ventricular dysfunction*

TABLETS

Adults. *Initial:* 2.5 mg twice daily, increased to 20 mg daily in 2 divided doses.

DOSAGE ADJUSTMENT Initial dosage reduced to 2.5 mg daily and, if possible, diuretic dosage reduced in patients who have a serum sodium level below 130 mEq/L or a serum creatinine level above 1.6 mg/dl.

Route	Onset	Peak	Duration
P.O.	1 hr	4–6 hr	About 24 hr
I.V.	15 min	1–4 hr	About 6 hr

Mechanism of Action

May reduce blood pressure by affecting the renin-angiotensin-aldosterone system. By inhibiting angiotensin-convering enzyme (ACE), enalapril:

• prevents conversion of angiotensin I to angiotensin II, a potent vasoconstrictor that also stimulates the adrenal cortex to secrete aldosterone
• may inhibit renal and vascular production of angiotensin II
• decreases the serum angiotensin II level and increases serum renin activity, which decreases aldosterone secretion and slightly increases serum potassium level and fluid loss
• decreases vascular tone and blood pressure
• inhibits aldosterone release, which reduces sodium and water reabsorption and increases their excretion, further reducing blood pressure.

Contraindications

Aliskiren use in patients with diabetes or renal impairment (GFR less than 60 ml/min), history of angioedema from previous ACE inhibitor; hypersensitivity to enalapril, enalaprilat, or their components

Interactions
DRUGS

aliskiren (in patients with diabetes or renal impairment), angiotensin receptor blockers, other ACE inhibitors: Increased risk of hyperkalemia, hypotension, and renal dysfunction
allopurinol, bone marrow depressants (such as amphotericin B and methotrexate), procainamide, systemic corticosteroids: Possibly increased risk of fatal neutropenia or agranulocytosis
cyclosporine, potassium-sparing diuretics, potassium supplements: Increased risk of hyperkalemia
diuretics, other antihypertensives: Additive hypotensive effects
lithium: Increased blood lithium level and lithium toxicity
NSAIDs: Possibly reduced antihypertensive effects of enalapril and enalaprilat; possibly increased risk of renal dysfunction, especially in the elderly or who are volume-depleted or already have compromised renal function
sodium aurothiomalate: Increased risk of nitritoid reactions, such as facial flushing, nausea, vomiting, and hypotension
sympathomimetics: Possibly reduced therapeutic effects of enalapril and enalaprilat

FOODS
potassium-containing salt substitutes: Increased risk of hyperkalemia
ACTIVITIES
alcohol use: Possibly additive hypotensive effect

Adverse Reactions

CNS: Ataxia, confusion, depression, dizziness, dream disturbances, fatigue, headache, insomnia, nervousness, peripheral neuropathy, somnolence, stroke, syncope, vertigo, weakness
CV: Angina, arrhythmias, cardiac arrest, hypotension, MI, orthostatic hypotension, palpitations, pulmonary embolism and infarction, Raynaud's phenomenon
EENT: Blurred vision, conjunctivitis, dry eyes and mouth, glossitis, hoarseness, lacrimation, loss of smell, pharyngitis, rhinorrhea, stomatitis, taste perversion, tinnitus
ENDO: Gynecomastia
GI: Abdominal pain, anorexia, constipation, diarrhea, hepatic failure, hepatitis, ileus, indigestion, melena, nausea, pancreatitis, vomiting
GU: Flank pain, impotence, oliguria, renal failure, UTI
MS: Muscle spasms
RESP: Asthma, bronchitis, bronchospasm, cough, dyspnea, pneumonia, pulmonary edema, pulmonary infiltrates, upper respiratory tract infection
SKIN: Alopecia, diaphoresis, erythema multiforme, exfoliative dermatitis, flushing, pemphigus, photosensitivity, pruritus, rash, Stevens-Johnson syndrome, toxic epidermal necrolysis, urticaria
Other: Anaphylaxis, angioedema, herpes zoster, hyperkalemia

Nursing Considerations
• Use enalapril and enalaprilat cautiously in patients with impaired renal function. Avoid giving drug to children with a GFR less than 30 ml/min/1.73 m².
• For children or adults who can't swallow tablets, consult with prescriber and pharmacist about preparing an oral suspension from tablets as directed by manufacturer. Alternatively, have prescriber order the oral solution form (Epaned).

• Reconstitute oral solution by tapping bottle containing the drug powder on a hard surface 5 times to loosen powder. Add about half (75 ml) of the Ora-Sweet SF diluent that comes with the drug to the powder bottle. Replace cap and shake well for 30 seconds. Reopen and add remainer diluent to the drug powder bottle. Replace cap and shake well again for 30 seconds. Calculate 60 days from the date of reconstitution and write this date as the discard date on the front of the label.

• Administer each I.V. dose over at least 5 minutes.

• Measure patient's blood pressure immediately after first dose and frequently for at least 2 hours thereafter. If hypotension requires a dosage reduction, monitor blood pressure frequently for 2 hours after reduced dosage is administered and for another hour after blood pressure has stabilized.

• Monitor blood pressure regularly during therapy. If hypotension develops, place patient in a supine position and expect to give I.V. normal saline solution or other volume expander as prescribed.

• Monitor patient's heart rate and rhythm. Expect to obtain repeated 12-lead ECG tracings.

• Monitor laboratory test results to check hepatic and renal function, leukocyte count, and serum potassium level.

• Monitor patient closely for angioedema of the face, lips, tongue, glottis, larynx, and limbs. For angioedema of the face and lips, stop drug and give an antihistamine, as prescribed. If tongue, glottis, or larynx is involved, assess patient for airway obstruction and prepare to give epinephrine 1:1,000 (0.3 to 0.5 ml) subcutaneously and maintain a patent airway.

PATIENT TEACHING

• Advise patient to take enalapril or enalaprilat at the same time each day.

• Instruct patient not to split, crush, or chew tablets.

• Teach patient how to mix oral solution, if prescribed.

• Inform patient that light-headedness and fainting may occur, especially during first few days of therapy. Advise him to change position slowly and avoid hazardous activities until drug's CNS effects are known.

• Inform patient that diarrhea, excessive sweating, vomiting, and other conditions may cause dehydration, which can lead to dizziness, fainting, and very low blood pressure during therapy. Urge sufficient fluid intake to prevent dehydration and related adverse reactions. If diarrhea or vomiting is severe or prolonged, instruct patient to notify prescriber.

• Urge patient to immediately notify prescriber if angioedema and other adverse reactions, including persistent dry cough, occur.

• Advise patient to consult prescriber before using salt substitutes, potassium supplements, or other drugs (including OTC drugs) while taking drug.

WARNING Caution women of child-bearing age that they should use a reliable form of contraception and should notify prescriber immediately if pregnancy is suspected because enalapril may cause fetal harm and should be discontinued.

enoxacin
Penetrex

Class and Category
Chemical class: Fluoroquinolone
Therapeutic class: Antibiotic
Pregnancy category: C

Indications and Dosages
➤ *To treat gonorrhea*
TABLETS
Adults. 400 mg as a single dose.
➤ *To treat uncomplicated UTI*
TABLETS
Adults. 200 mg every 12 hr for 7 days.
➤ *To treat complicated UTI*
TABLETS
Adults. 400 mg every 12 hr for 14 days.
DOSAGE ADJUSTMENT Dosage reduced by half in patients with creatinine clearance of 30 ml/min/1.73 m² or less.

Contraindications
History of tendinitis or tendon rupture, hypersensitivity to enoxacin or any quinolone antibiotic

Interactions

DRUGS

aluminum-, calcium-, or magnesium-containing antacids; didanosine (chewable or buffered tablets); ferrous sulfate; magnesium-containing laxatives; sucralfate; zinc: Interference with enoxacin absorption, decreased blood enoxacin level

bismuth: Decreased enoxacin bioavailability (by about 25% if given with or up to 60 minutes after enoxacin)

cyclosporine: Possibly increased blood cyclosporine level

digoxin: Increased serum digoxin level and risk of digitalis toxicity

NSAIDs: Possibly increased risk of CNS stimulation and seizures

theophylline: Interference with theophylline metabolism, increased risk of theophylline toxicity

warfarin: Possibly increased anti-coagulant effect and increased risk of bleeding

FOODS

caffeine: Decreased caffeine clearance, increased adverse effects of caffeine, increased blood enoxacin level

Adverse Reactions

CNS: Dizziness, drowsiness, hallucinations, headache, insomnia, nervousness, seizures, vertigo

EENT: Taste perversion

GI: Abdominal pain, diarrhea, indigestion, nausea, pseudomembranous colitis, vomiting

GU: Vaginitis

MS: Tendinitis, tendon rupture

SKIN: Photosensitivity, pruritus, rash

Other: Anaphylaxis

Nursing Considerations

• Be aware that enoxacin shouldn't be given to a patient under age 18 because it may cause arthropathy.

• Use drug cautiously in patients with a history of or susceptibility to seizures.

• Obtain a specimen for culture and sensitivity tests, as ordered, but expect to begin therapy before results are available.

• Monitor patient closely for signs and symptoms of anaphylaxis after first dose: shock, dyspnea, facial or laryngeal edema, loss of consciousness, paresthesia, pruritus, and urticaria. If they occur, stop enoxacin immediately, notify prescriber, and prepare to treat symptoms.

• Ask if patient has a history of seizures. Take seizure and safety precautions because drug may induce seizures and other adverse CNS reactions after a single dose.

E
F

Mechanism of Action

Normally, the enzyme DNA gyrase is responsible for unwinding and supercoiling bacterial DNA before replication, as shown below left. Enoxacin inhibits DNA gyrase, as shown below right, disrupting bacterial replication and causing cell death.

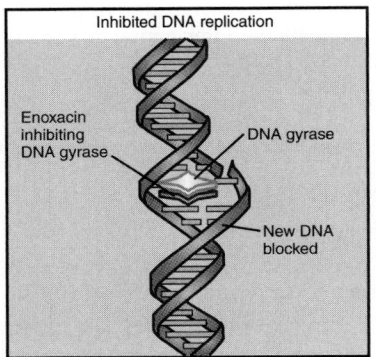

• Report severe or prolonged diarrhea, which may indicate pseudomembranous colitis.
• Watch for pain, inflammation, and tendon rupture, especially in shoulders, hands, and ankles.
• If patient has gonorrhea, expect to obtain a serologic test for syphilis at diagnosis and 3 months after enoxacin therapy ends.

PATIENT TEACHING
• Emphasize the importance of taking the full course of enoxacin exactly as prescribed, even if patient feels better before it's finished.
• Instruct patient to take drug at the same times each day—1 hour before or 2 hours after meals—with 8 oz of water.
• Urge patient to avoid potentially hazardous activities until CNS effects of enoxacin are known.
• Advise patient to notify prescriber if symptoms don't improve within a few days.
• Urge patient to drink plenty of fluids but to avoid caffeine during therapy.
• Caution patient not to take aluminum-, calcium-, or magnesium-containing antacids; bismuth; didanosine (chewable or buffered tablets), if prescribed; or products that contain iron or zinc for 8 hours before or 2 hours after taking enoxacin.
• Tell patient to avoid direct sunlight, to use sunscreen and wear protective clothing outdoors, and to report photosensitivity.
• Instruct patient to stop taking enoxacin and notify prescriber immediately if a rash or other allergic reaction develops.
• Instruct patient to take a missed dose as soon as he remembers, unless it's nearly time for the next. Warn against doubling the dose.
• Tell patient to report tendon pain or inflammation, to stop enoxacin, and to rest until tendinitis or tendon rupture is ruled out.

---

enoxaparin sodium

Lovenox

Class and Category
Chemical class: Low-molecular-weight heparin
Therapeutic class: Antithrombotic
Pregnancy category: B

Indications and Dosages
➤ *To prevent deep vein thrombosis (DVT) after hip or knee replacement and for continued prophylaxis after hospitalization for hip replacement*

SUBCUTANEOUS INJECTION
Adults. 30 mg every 12 hr, starting 12 to 24 hr after surgery for up to 14 days. Or, 40 mg daily, starting 9 to 15 hr after hip replacement surgery. *Prophylaxis:* 40 mg daily for 3 wk.

➤ *To prevent DVT after abdominal surgery for patients with thromboembolic risk factors (over age 40, obesity, general anesthesia lasting longer than 30 minutes, cancer, or a history of DVT or pulmonary embolism)*

SUBCUTANEOUS INJECTION
Adults. 40 mg daily, starting 2 hr before surgery and lasting 7 to 10 days.

➤ *To prevent ischemic complications of unstable angina and non–Q-wave MI*

SUBCUTANEOUS INJECTION
Adults. 1 mg/kg every 12 hr with 100 to 325 mg of aspirin daily for 2 to 8 days or until condition is stable.

DOSAGE ADJUSTMENT Dosage reduced to 30 mg daily if creatinine clearance is less than 30 ml/min/1.73 m² and patient is receiving drug as prophylaxis in abdominal, hip, or knee replacement surgery or is acutely ill. Reduced to 1 mg/kg daily if creatinine clearance is less than 30 ml/min/1.73 m² and drug is given with aspirin to prevent ischemic complications of unstable angina and non–Q-wave MI, with warfarin as inpatient treatment for acute DVT with or without pulmonary embolism, or with warfarin as outpatient treatment of acute DVT without pulmonary embolism.

➤ *To treat acute ST-segment–elevation MI (STEMI)*

I.V. INJECTION, THEN SUBCUTANEOUS INJECTION
Adults. 30 mg I.V. as a single dose, followed by 1 mg/kg subcutaneously (maximum, 100 mg for first two doses). Then, 1 mg/kg subcutaneously every 12 hr.

DOSAGE ADJUSTMENT If patient also receives a thrombolytic, enoxaparin should be given 15 to 30 min before and 30 min after fibrinolytic therapy starts. If patient has percutaneous coronary intervention, give 0.3-mg/kg I.V. bolus if last enoxaparin dose was given more than 8 hr before balloon inflation.

Route	Onset	Peak	Duration
SubQ	Unknown	3–5 hr	Up to 24 hr

Mechanism of Action

Potentiates the action of antithrombin III, a coagulation inhibitor. By binding with antithrombin III, enoxaparin rapidly binds with and inactivates clotting factors (primarily thrombin and factor Xa). Without thrombin, fibrinogen can't convert to fibrin and clots can't form.

Incompatibilities

Don't mix enoxaparin with other I.V. fluids or drugs.

Contraindications

Active major bleeding; hypersensitivity to benzyl alcohol (if only the multidose vial is available), enoxaparin, heparin (including low-molecular-weight heparins), or pork products; thrombocytopenia and positive antiplatelet antibody test while taking low-molecular-weight heparins

Interactions

DRUGS

cefamandole, cefoperazone, cefotetan, plicamycin, valproic acid: Possibly increased risk of hemorrhage
NSAIDs; oral anticoagulants; platelet aggregation inhibitors, such as aspirin, dipyridamole, sulfinpyrazone, and ticlopidine; thrombolytics, such as alteplase, anistreplase, streptokinase, and urokinase: Possibly increased risk of bleeding and of spinal or epidural hematoma

Adverse Reactions

CNS: Confusion, epidural or spinal hematoma, fever, headache, paralysis, stroke
CV: Atrial fibrillation, congestive heart failure, hyperlipidemia, peripheral edema, thrombosis
EENT: Epistaxis
GI: Bloody stools, cholestatic and hepatocellular liver injury, diarrhea, elevated liver function test results, hematemesis, melena, nausea, vomiting
GU: Hematuria, menstrual irregularities
HEME: Anemia, eosinophilia, hemorrhage, purpura, thrombocytopenia, thrombocytosis
MS: Osteoporosis (with long-term therapy)

RESP: Dyspnea, pneumonia, pulmonary edema or embolism
SKIN: Alopecia, cutaneous vasculitis, ecchymosis, persistent bleeding or oozing from mucous membranes or surgical wounds, pruritus, skin necrosis at injection site or distant from injection site, urticaria, vesiculobullous rash
Other: Anaphylaxis including shock; hyperkalemia; injection-site erythema, hematoma, inflammation, irritation, nodules, oozing, and pain

Nursing Considerations

• Use enoxaparin with extreme caution in patients with a history of heparin-induced thrombocytopenia or an increased risk of hemorrhage, as from bacterial endocarditis; congenital or acquired bleeding disorder; active ulcerative or angiodysplastic GI disease; hemorrhagic stroke; recent brain, spinal, or ophthalmologic surgery; or concurrent treatment with a platelet inhibitor.
• Use cautiously in those with bleeding diathesis, diabetic retinopathy, hepatic or renal impairment, recent GI ulceration or hemorrhage, or uncontrolled hypertension. Expect delayed elimination in elderly patients and those with renal insufficiency.
• Drug isn't recommended for patients with prosthetic heart valves, especially pregnant women, because of risk of prosthetic valve thrombosis. If enoxaparin is needed, monitor peak and trough anti-factor Xa levels often and adjust dosage as needed.
• Use multidose vials cautiously in pregnant women because benzyl alcohol may cross the placenta and cause fetal harm.
• Don't give drug by I.M. injection.
WARNING If patient is receiving enoxaparin with epidural or spinal anesthesia or spinal puncture, watch closely for development of spinal hematoma, which may cause long-term or permanent paralysis. If you see evidence of neurologic impairment, such as changes in sensory or motor function, notify prescriber immediately because urgent care is needed to minimize hematoma's effect. Risk of spinal or epidural hematoma during enoxaparin therapy is increased by indwelling epidural catheters, concurrent use of other drugs that affect hemostasis, a history of traumatic or

E
F

repeated epidural or spinal punctures, or a history of spinal deformity or spinal surgery. Know that placement or removal of a catheter should be delayed for at least 12 hours after administration of lower doses of enoxaparin (30 mg once or twice daily or 40 mg once daily) and at least 24 hours after the administration of higher doses. (0.75 mg/kg twice daily, 1 mg/kg twice daily, or 1.5 mg/kg once daily). However, for patients with creatinine clearance of less than 30 ml/min, timing of removal should be doubled because enoxaparin elimination is more prolonged in renal dysfunction.

• Expect to give drug with aspirin to patient with unstable angina, STEMI, and non–Q-wave MI. To minimize risk of bleeding after vascular procedures, give enoxaparin at recommended intervals.

• After percutaneous revascularization procedure, it is important to achieve hemostasis at the puncture site. A closure device may be removed right away; however, if a manual compression method is used, the sheath should be removed 6 hours after last enoxaparin dose. If enoxaparin therapy will continue, give next scheduled dose no sooner than 6 to 8 hours after sheath removal.

• Watch closely for bleeding. Notify prescriber immediately if platelet count falls below 100,000/mm^3. Expect to stop drug and start treatment if patient has a thromboembolic event, such as a stroke.

• Test stool for occult blood, as ordered.

• Keep protamine sulfate nearby in case of accidental overdose.

• Check serum potassium level for elevation, especially in patients with renal impairment or concurrent use of potassium-sparing diuretics.

PATIENT TEACHING

• Advise patient to notify prescriber about adverse reactions, especially bleeding.

• Instruct patient to seek immediate help for evidence of thromboembolism, such as neurologic changes and severe shortness of breath.

• Emphasize the importance of complying with follow-up visits with prescriber.

• Teach patient or family member how to give enoxaparin at home, if needed. Show patient how to give by deep subcutaneous injection while lying down. Instruct him not to expel air bubble from a prefilled syringe to avoid losing some of the drug. Tell him to insert the entire needle into a skin fold held between the thumb and forefinger. Remind him to alternate injection sites between the left and right anterolateral abdominal wall.

• To minimize bruising, caution patient not to rub the site after giving the injection.

• Review safe handling and disposal of syringes and needles.

entacapone
Comtan

Class and Category
Chemical class: COMT inhibitor
Therapeutic class: Antidyskinetic
Pregnancy category: C

Indications and Dosages
➤ *As adjunct to treat end-of-dose "wearing-off" in patients with Parkinson's disease*
TABLETS
Adults. 200 mg with each dose of carbidopa and levodopa. *Maximum:* 1,600 mg daily.

Mechanism of Action
Inhibits peripheral catechol-*O*-methyltransferase (COMT), the major metabolizing enzyme for levodopa. During levodopa metabolism, COMT causes the formation of a levodopa metabolite that reduces the effectiveness of levodopa. By inhibiting COMT, entacapone leads to higher sustained blood levels of levodopa and its increased availability for diffusion into the CNS, where it is converted to dopamine. By replenishing dopamine stores, entacapone increases dopaminergic stimulation in the brain and reduces the symptoms of Parkinson's disease. Carbidopa is given with levodopa because it inhibits the peripheral distribution of levodopa, making more levodopa available for transport to the brain.

Contraindications
Hypersensitivity to entacapone or its components, use within 14 days of nonselective MAO inhibitor therapy

Interactions
DRUGS
ampicillin, chloramphenicol, cholestyramine, erythromycin, probenecid, rifampin: Decreased biliary excretion of entacapone
apomorphine, bitolterol, dobutamine, dopamine, epinephrine, isoetharine, isoproterenol, methyldopa, norepinephrine: Possibly increased heart rate, arrhythmias, and excessive changes in blood pressure
MAO inhibitors (nonselective): Possibly inhibited entacapone metabolism

Adverse Reactions
CNS: Agitation, anxiety, asthenia, confusion, dizziness, dyskinesia, fatigue, falling asleep during activities of daily living, fever, hallucinations, hyperkinesia, hypokinesia, psychotic-like behavior, somnolence, syncope
CV: Orthostatic hypotension
EENT: Dry mouth, taste perversion
GI: Abdominal pain, constipation, drug-induced microscopic colitis, diarrhea, flatulence, gastritis, hepatitis, indigestion, nausea, vomiting
GU: Brown-orange urine
MS: Back pain, rhabdomyolysis
RESP: Dyspnea
SKIN: Diaphoresis, purpura
Other: Intense urges to perform certain acts, such as gambling or sex

Nursing Considerations
WARNING Be aware that entacapone should not be discontinued abruptly because doing so may precipitate signs and symptoms resembling those of neuroleptic malignant syndrome, such as fever, muscle rigidity, altered level of consciousness, confusion, and elevated creatine kinase level. Patients may also experience a rapid reemergence of parkinsonian symptoms.
- Entacapone should not be given to patients with a major psychotic disorder because the drug can exacerbate psychosis.
- Monitor patient for drug-induced diarrhea during first 4 to 12 weeks of therapy but be aware that in some patients it may appear as early as the first week of therapy and last many months after therapy is begun.
- Help patient with activities as needed because drug may increase risk of orthostatic hypotension or syncope.

- Monitor patient for daytime sleepiness or episodes of falling asleep during activities that require active participation. If present, notify prescriber and expect drug to be discontinued.
- Watch for worsening dyskinesia because entacapone potentiates dopaminergic adverse effects of levodopa.
- Drug may be taken with selective MAO inhibitors, such as selegiline.
- Assess patient for skin changes regularly because risk of melanoma is increased in those with Parkinson's disease. It isn't clear whether increased risk results from the disease or drugs used to treat it.

PATIENT TEACHING
- Instruct patient to always take entacapone with carbidopa and levodopa because it has no antidyskinetic effect of its own.
- Inform patient that dizziness and sleepiness are more common at beginning of treatment, especially in those with hypotension.
- Advise patient not to participate in potentially hazardous activities until drug's CNS effects are known, especially if he's also taking CNS depressants. Warn patient that drug has been known to cause patients to suddenly fall asleep without prior warning of sleepiness while engaged in activities of daily living.
- If patient is scheduled for surgery, instruct him to inform surgeon and anesthesiologist about entacapone use before the procedure because COMT inhibitors such as entacapone may interact with some drugs used in surgical procedures.
- Caution patient that entacapone may increase adverse effects of carbidopa and levodopa, such as nausea and uncontrolled movements. If these adverse effects do increase, advise him to contact prescriber immediately because carbidopa and levodopa dosage may need to be lowered.
- Inform patient that urine may turn brown-orange while he's taking entacapone but that this is a harmless effect.
- Urge patient to have regular skin examinations by a dermatologist or other qualified health professional.
- Advise patient to notify prescriber about intense urges, including those for

E
F

gambling or sex. Dosage may need to be reduced or drug discontinued.
• Tell patient to notify prescriber if diarrhea occurs at any time during therapy because diarrhea may become severe requiring drug to be discontinued.

epinephrine
(adrenaline)

Adrenalin, Adrenalin Chloride Solution, Ana-Guard, Bronkaid Mist, Bronkaid Mistometer (CAN), EpiPen (CAN), EpiPen Auto-Injector, EpiPen Jr. (CAN), EpiPen Jr. Auto-Injector

epinephrine bitartrate

Asthmahaler Mist, Bronkaid Suspension Mist

racepinephrine

AsthmaNefrin, MicroNefrin, Nephron, Vaponefrin

Class and Category

Chemical class: Catecholamine
Therapeutic class: Antianaphylactic, bronchodilator, cardiac stimulant, vasopressor
Pregnancy category: C

Indications and Dosages

➤ *To treat bronchospasm*
INHALED SOLUTION (EPINEPRHINE)
Adults and children age 4 and over. 1 to 3 inhalations (10 drops) by hand-bulb nebulizer no more than every 3 hr.
INHALED SOLUTION (RACEPINEPHRINE)
Adults and children age 4 and over. 3 inhalations of 0.5 ml (10 drops) by hand-bulb nebulizer, or 0.2 to 0.5 ml (4 to 10 drops) of diluted solution given over 15 min by jet nebulizer; repeated after 3 to 4 hr, if needed.
ORAL INHALED AEROSOL (EPINEPHRINE BITARTRATE)
Adults and children age 4 and over. 1 inhalation (160 mcg) repeated after 1 min, if needed; then repeated after at least 3 hr.

ORAL INHALER (EPINEPHRINE)
Adults and children age 4 and over. 1 inhalation (200 to 275 mcg) repeated after at least 1 min, if needed; then repeated after at least 3 hr.
➤ *To treat croup*
INHALED SOLUTION (RACEPINEPHRINE)
Children. 0.05 ml/kg diluted to 3 ml in normal saline solution and given over 15 min every 2 hr, as needed. *Maximum:* 0.5 ml/dose.
➤ *To treat anaphylaxis*
I.V. INFUSION
Adults and adolescents. 100 to 250 mcg given slowly.
I.M. OR SUBCUTANEOUS INJECTION
Adults and adolescents. 100 to 500 mcg repeated every 10 to 15 min, as needed. *Maximum:* 1 mg/dose; three doses.
Children. 10 mcg/kg repeated every 15 min for three doses. *Maximum:* 300 mcg/dose.
➤ *To treat severe anaphylactic shock*
I.V. INFUSION
Adults. 1 mcg/min titrated to 2 to 10 mcg/min for desired hemodynamic response.
➤ *To treat cardiac arrest*
I.V. INFUSION
Adults. 0.5 to 1 mg every 3 to 5 min during resuscitation.
Children. 10 mcg/kg followed by 100 mcg/kg every 3 to 5 min, if needed. If two doses produce no response, subsequent doses are increased to 200 mcg/kg every 5 min.
Neonates. 10 to 30 mcg/kg every 3 to 5 min.

Mechanism of Action

Acts on alpha and beta receptors. This nonselective adrenergic agonist stimulates:
• $alpha_1$ receptors, which constricts arteries and may decrease bronchial secretions
• presynaptic $alpha_2$ receptors, which inhibits norepinephrine release by way of negative feedback
• postsynaptic $alpha_2$ receptors, which constricts arteries
• $beta_1$ receptors, which induces positive chronotropic and inotropic responses
• $beta_2$ receptors, which dilates arteries, relaxes bronchial smooth muscles, increases glycogenolysis, and prevents mast cells from secreting histamine and other substances, thus reversing bronchoconstriction and edema.

Route	Onset	Peak	Duration
I.V., I.M.	Rapid	Unknown	1–2 min
SubQ	5–10 min	In 20 min	Short
Oral inhalation	1–5 min	In 5–15 min	Up to 3 hr

Incompatibilities

Don't mix epinephrine with alkalis or oxidizing agents, including bromine, chlorine, chromates, iodine, metal salts (as from iron), nitrites, oxygen, and permanganates, because these substances can destroy epinephrine.

Contraindications

Cerebral arteriosclerosis, coronary insufficiency, counteraction of phenothiazine-induced hypotension, dilated cardiomyopathy, general anesthesia with halogenated hydrocarbons or cyclopropane, hypersensitivity to epinephrine or its components, labor, angle-closure glaucoma, organic brain damage, shock (nonanaphylactic)

Interactions

DRUGS

alpha-adrenergic blockers, drugs with alpha-adrenergic action, rapid-acting vasodilators: Blockage of epinephrine's alpha-adrenergic effect, possibly causing severe hypotension and tachycardia
amyl nitrite, nitrates: Decreased antianginal effects
antihypertensives, diuretics used to treat hypertension: Decreased antihypertensive effects
beta blockers: Mutual inhibition of therapeutic effects, possibly severe hypertension and cerebral hemorrhage
chlorpheniramine, diphenhydramine, levothyroxine, MAO inhibitors, tricyclic antidepressants, tripelennamine: Possibly increased effects of epinephrine
digoxin, diuretics, quinidine: Increased risk of arrhythmias
dihydroergotamine, ergoloid mesylates, ergonovine, ergotamine, methylergonovine, methysergide, oxytocin: Increased risk of vasoconstriction, causing gangrene, peripheral vascular ischemia, or severe hypertension

ergot alkaloids: Possibly reversed pressor effects of epinephrine
hydrocarbon inhalation anesthetics: Increased risk of severe atrial and ventricular arrhythmias
insulin, oral antidiabetic drugs: Decreased effects of these drugs
MAO inhibitors: Possibly increased vasopressor effect of epinephrine and hypertensive crisis
maprotiline, tricyclic antidepressants: Potentiated cardiovascular effects of epinephrine, possibly causing arrhythmias, hyperpyrexia, severe hypertension, or tachycardia
sympathomimetics: Additive CNS stimulation, increased cardiovascular effects of either drug
thyroid hormones: Increased effects of either drug
xanthines: CNS stimulation and toxic effects

Adverse Reactions

CNS: Anxiety, apprehensiveness, chills, fever, dizziness, drowsiness, hallucinations, headache, insomnia, light-headedness, nervousness, restlessness, seizures, stroke, temporary worsening of Parkinson's disease, tremor, weakness
CV: Arrhythmias, including ventricular fibrillation; chest discomfort or pain; fast, irregular, or slow heartbeat; palpitations; severe hypertension; tachycardia
EENT: Blurred vision, dry mouth or throat, miosis
ENDO: Hyperglycemia in diabetics
GI: Anorexia, heartburn, nausea, vomiting
GU: Dysuria
MS: Muscle twitching, severe muscle spasms
RESP: Dyspnea
SKIN: Cold skin, diaphoresis, ecchymosis, flushed or red face or skin, pallor, tissue necrosis
Other: Hyperkalemia; hypokalemia; injection-site coldness, hypoaesthesia, pain, pallor, and stinging

Nursing Considerations

• Use epinephrine with extreme caution in patients with angina, arrhythmias, asthma, degenerative heart disease, or emphysema. Epinephrine's inotropic effect equals that of dopamine and dobutamine; its chronotropic effect exceeds that of both.

• Use drug cautiously in elderly patients and those with cardiovascular disease (other than listed above), diabetes mellitus, hypertension, hyperthyroidism, prostatic hypertrophy, and psychoneurologic disorders.

• Be aware that some preparations contain sulfites, which may cause allergic-type reactions. However, the presence of sulfites in epinephrine should not deter its use in a patient with anaphylaxis, even if patient is sensitive to sulfites. Monitor patient closely for adverse effects.

• Dilute the 1:1,000 (1-mg/ml) solution of parenteral epinephrine before I.V. use.

• Shake suspension thoroughly before withdrawing dose; refrigerate it between uses.

• Inspect epinephrine solution or suspension before use. If it's pink or brown, air has entered a multidose vial. If it's discolored or contains particles, discard it. Also discard unused portions of parenteral epinephrine.

• For injection, rotate sites because repeated injections in the same site may cause vasoconstriction and localized necrosis.

• Be aware that drug shouldn't be given by intra-arterial injection because marked vasoconstriction may cause gangrene.

• Avoid giving injection into buttocks because drug may be less effective when given there, especially for treating anaphylaxis.

• Monitor patient for potassium imbalances. Initially, hyperkalemia occurs when hepatocytes release potassium. Hypokalemia may quickly follow as skeletal muscles take up potassium.

• To minimize insomnia, give last dose a few hours before bedtime.

WARNING To treat cardiac arrest, at least twice the peripheral I.V. dose of epinephrine may be given by endotracheal instillation. Two dilutions are needed for this regimen; use great caution to avoid making medication errors.

PATIENT TEACHING

• Warn patient not to exceed recommended dosage or to shorten interval because of the risk of adverse reactions and tolerance.

• Advise patient to notify prescriber if symptoms don't improve or if they improve but then worsen.

• Instruct patient to take the day's last dose a few hours before bedtime to avoid insomnia.

• Caution patient not to use inhalation solution that is pink or brown or that contains particles.

• Teach patient how to use oral inhaler or inhalation solution, as needed.

• If patient also uses an oral corticosteroid inhaler, instruct him to use epinephrine inhaler first, wait 5 minutes, and then use corticosteroid inhaler to increase effectiveness.

• Teach patient and family how to administer epinephrine subcutaneously in an emergency. Tell them to inject drug into anterolateral aspect of the thigh, through the clothing if necessary. Explain that solution is light sensitive and should be stored in the carrying case and at room temperature. Tell them not to refrigerate drug and to replace solution if it discolors.

• Caution patient to avoid accidental injecting drug into his fingers, hands, toes, or feet because epinephrine is a strong vasoconstrictor and could cause loss of blood flow to the area, resulting in gangrene. If accidental injection occurs in any of these areas, instruct patient to go immediately to nearest emergency room.

• Advise patient to notify prescriber immediately if he has blurred vision, chest pain, trouble breathing, a fast or irregular heartbeat, or increased sweating.

• Inform patient with diabetes that epinephrine may cause hyperglycemia. Inform patient with Parkinson's disease that symptoms may temporarily worsen but this should not deter use of drug.

eplerenone
Inspra

Class and Category
Chemical class: Methyl ester
Therapeutic class: Antihypertensive
Pregnancy category: B

8

Indications and Dosages

➤ *To improve survival of stable patients with left ventricular systolic dysfunction and congestive heart failure after an acute MI*

TABLETS

Adults. *Initial:* 25 mg daily, increased to 50 mg daily within 4 wk, as needed.

➤ *To treat hypertension alone or with other antihypertensive drugs*

TABLETS

Adults. *Initial:* 50 mg daily, increased to 50 mg twice daily after 4 wk, if needed.

DOSAGE ADJUSTMENT For patients taking weak CYP450 3A4 inhibitors, such as erythromycin, saquinavir, verapamil, and fluconazole, initial dosage reduced to 25 mg daily.

Mechanism of Action

Blocks the binding of aldosterone at its mineralocorticoid receptor sites located in the kidneys, heart, blood vessels, and brain. This action decreases blood pressure by preventing aldosterone from inducing sodium reabsorption and possibly other mechanisms that contribute to raising blood pressure.

Contraindications

Hyperkalemia (serum potassium level greater than 5.5. mEq/L); hypersensitivity to eplerenone or its components; renal insufficiency (serum creatinine level greater than 2.0 mg/dl in men or 1.8 mg/dl in women or creatinine clearance less than 50 ml/min/1.73 m²); type 2 diabetes mellitus complicated by microalbuminuria; use of potassium supplements, potassium-sparing diuretics, or strong CYP3A4 inhibitors, such as ketoconazole or itraconazole

Interactions

DRUGS

ACE inhibitors, angiotensin II receptor antagonists: Increased risk of hyperkalemia
CYP450 3A4 inhibitors: Increased blood level and effect of eplerenone
lithium: Possibly lithium toxicity
NSAIDs: Possibly reduced antihypertensive effect of eplerenone

FOODS

grapefruit: Possibly increased blood level and effect of eplerenone

Adverse Reactions

CNS: Dizziness, fatigue, headache
CV: Angina pectoris, hypercholesterolemia, hypertriglyceridemia, MI
ENDO: Gynecomastia, mastodynia
GI: Abdominal pain, diarrhea, increased liver enzyme levels
GU: Albuminuria, elevated BUN and serum creatinine levels, vaginal bleeding
RESP: Cough
Other: Flulike symptoms, hyperkalemia, hyponatremia, increased uric acid level

Nursing Considerations

• Monitor patient's blood pressure regularly to evaluate eplerenone effectiveness.
• Monitor patient's serum potassium level every 2 weeks for the first month or two of therapy and monthly thereafter, as ordered.
• Be aware that patients who take an ACE inhibitor or an angiotensin II receptor antagonist during eplerenone therapy have an increased risk of hyperkalemia.

PATIENT TEACHING

• Caution patient not to use potassium-containing supplements or salt substitutes because increased potassium levels can lead to serious adverse reactions to eplerenone.
• Urge patient to tell all prescribers about eplerenone use because of possible interactions.

epoetin alfa
(EPO, erythropoietin alfa, recombinant erythropoietin, r-HuEPO)

Epogen, Eprex (CAN), Procrit

Class and Category

Chemical class: 165–amino acid glyco-protein identical to human erythropoietin
Therapeutic class: Antianemic
Pregnancy category: C

Indications and Dosages

➤ *To treat anemia from renal failure*
I.V. OR SUBCUTANEOUS INJECTION
Adults on dialysis but not hemodialysis.
Initial: 50 to 100 units/kg 3 times/wk, increased as needed by 25% at 4-wk

intervals or longer. *Maintenance:* Dosage gradually decreased by 25 units/kg at 4-wk intervals or longer to lowest dose that keeps hemoglobin below 11 g/dl.

Children on dialysis but not hemodialysis. 50 units/kg 3 times/wk; increased as needed by 25% at 4-wk intervals or longer. *Maintenance:* Dosage gradually decreased to lowest dose that keeps hemoglobin below 11 g/dl.

I.V. INJECTION

Adults on hemodialysis. *Initial:* 50 to 100 units/kg 3 times/wk, increased as needed by 25% at 4-wk intervals or longer. *Maintenance:* Dosage gradually decreased by 25 units/kg at 4-wk intervals or longer to lowest dose that keeps hemoglobin below 11 g/dl.

Children on hemodialysis. *Initial:* 50 units/kg 3 times/wk; increased as needed by 25% at 4-wk intervals or longer. *Maintenance:* Dosage gradually decreased to lowest dose that keeps hemoglobin below 11 g/dl.

I.V. OR SUBCUTANEOUS INJECTION

Adults not on dialysis. *Initial:* 50 to 100 units/kg 3 times/wk, increased as needed at 4-wk intervals or longer that keeps hemoglobin below 10 g/dl.

DOSAGE ADJUSTMENT For patients with anemia from renal failure on dialysis, dosage temporarily reduced or drug discontinued if hemoglobin approaches or exceeds 11 g/dl. For patients with anemia from renal failure not on dialysis, dosage temporarily reduced or drug discontinued if hemoglobin exceeds 10 g/dl. For patients with anemia from renal failure with or without dialysis, dosage reduced 25% or more if hemoglobin rises rapidly (more than 1 g/dl in any 2-week period).

➤ *To treat anemia in HIV-infected patients who take zidovudine*

I.V. OR SUBCUTANEOUS INJECTION

Adults with serum erythropoietin level of 500 mU/ml or less who receive 4,200 mg or less of zidovudine/wk. *Initial:* 100 units/kg 3 times/wk, increased by 50 to 100 units/kg every 4 to 8 wk after 8 wk of therapy. *Maintenance:* Dosage gradually titrated to maintain desired response, based on such factors as variations in zidovudine dosage and occurrence of infection or inflammation. *Maximum:* 300 units/kg 3 times/wk.

DOSAGE ADJUSTMENT For patients with anemia from zidovudine use, therapy temporarily stopped if hematocrit reaches or exceeds 40% and is resumed at a 25% lower dose when hematocrit returns to desired range.

➤ *To treat anemia from chemotherapy*

SUBCUTANEOUS INJECTION

Adults. *Initial:* 150 units/kg 3 times/wk. Dosage decreased by 25% if hemoglobin level approaches 12 g/dl or increases more than 1 g/dl in any 2-wk period. Dose withheld if hemoglobin exceeds 13 g/dl and resumed at 25% less than previous dose after hemoglobin has fallen to 12 g/dl. Dosage increased to 300 units/kg 3 times/ wk after 8 wk if response is inadequate.

Maximum: 300 units/kg 3 times/wk; or, 40,000 units weekly. Dosage decreased by 25% if hemoglobin level approaches 12 g/dl or increases more than 1 g/dl in any 2-wk period. Dose withheld if hemoglobin level exceeds 13 g/dl and resumed at 25% less than previous dose after hemoglobin has fallen to 12 g/dl. Dosage increased to 60,000 units weekly after 8 wk if hemoglobin level has not increased at least 1 g/dl without RBC transfusion.

➤ *To reduce the need for blood transfusion in anemic patients having surgery*

SUBCUTANEOUS INJECTION

Adults. 300 units/kg daily for 10 days before surgery, on day of surgery, and 4 days after surgery; or 600 units/kg/wk starting 3 wk before surgery for a total of 3 doses. Dose of 300 units/kg repeated on day of surgery.

Route	Onset	Peak	Duration
I.V., SubQ	In 2–6 wk	In 2 mo	About 2 wk

Mechanism of Action

Stimulates the release of reticulocytes from the bone marrow into the bloodstream, where they develop into mature RBCs.

Incompatibilities

Don't mix epoetin alfa with any other drug.

Contraindications

Hypersensitivity to human albumin or products made from mammal cells, uncontrolled hypertension

Interactions
DRUGS
antihypertensives: Increased blood pressure (to hypertensive level), especially when hematocrit rises rapidly
heparin: Increased heparin requirement in hemodialysis patients
iron supplements: Increased iron requirement and need for increased dose

Adverse Reactions
CNS: Anxiety, asthenia, dizziness, fatigue, fever, headache, insomnia, paresthesia, seizures, stroke
CV: Chest pain, congestive heart failure, deep vein thrombosis, edema, hypertension, MI, tachycardia, thrombosis of hemodialysis vascular access and other thromboembolic events
GI: Constipation, diarrhea, indigestion, nausea, vomiting
GU: UTI
HEME: Polycythemia
MS: Arthralgia, bone pain, muscle weakness
RESP: Cough, dyspnea, pulmonary congestion, upper respiratory tract infection
SKIN: Rash, pruritus, urticaria
Other: Flulike symptoms, hyperkalemia, injection-site reaction, trunk pain

Nursing Considerations
• Be aware that epoetin alfa shouldn't be given to cancer patients when a cure is anticipated because drug may decrease survival rate and increase tumor progression in patients with certain types of cancers, such as breast, non–small-cell lung, head and neck, lymphoid, and cervical cancers. All prescribers and hospitals must enroll and comply with the ESA APPRISE Oncology program to be able to prescribe and dispense the drug.
• Ensure that patient has received the medication guide and patient instructions for epoetin alfa and that a written acknowledgment of a discussion of the risks involved with this type of therapy has been obtained before first dose is given.
• Evaluate the patient's serum iron level before and during treatment, as ordered. Expect to give an iron supplement (I.V. iron dextran, if needed) because iron requirements rise when erythropoiesis consumes existing iron stores.

• Use epoetin alfa cautiously in patients who have conditions that could decrease or delay response to drug, such as aluminum intoxication, folic acid deficiency, hemolysis, infection, inflammation, iron deficiency, malignant neoplasm, osteitis (fibrosa cystica), or vitamin B_{12} deficiency.
• Also use drug cautiously in patients with cardiovascular disorders caused by hypertension, a history of porphyria or seizures, vascular disease, or a hematologic disorder, such as hypercoagulation, myelodysplastic syndrome, or sickle cell disease.
WARNING Multidose vial of epoetin contains benzyl alcohol, which can cause a fatal toxic syndrome in neonates and immature infants characterized by CNS, respiratory, circulatory, and renal impairment and metabolic acidosis.
• Use lowest possible dose in cancer patients because drug has shortened survival rate and increased tumor progression in patients with certain types of cancers, such as breast, non–small-cell lung, head and neck, and lymphoid cancers. Drug should only be used to treat anemia caused by myelosuppressive chemotherapy in cancer patients.
• Don't shake vial while preparing to avoid denaturing glycoprotein, inactivating drug.
• Discard unused portion of single-dose vial because it contains no preservatives. Discard unused portion of multidose vial after 21 days.
• Baseline hemoglobin level should be above 10 but below 13 g/dl if drug is given to patient scheduled for surgery. Watch closely throughout surgical period for deep vein thrombosis, especially in patients not receiving prophylactic anticoagulation, because risk increases.
• Evaluate the patient's serum iron level before and during treatment, as ordered. Expect to give an iron supplement (I.V. iron formulation, if needed) because iron requirements rise when erythropoiesis consumes existing iron stores.
• Check hemoglobin levels, as ordered, with twice-weekly measurements recommended for chronic renal failure patients, until stable and then monthly thereafter

and weekly measurements recommended for zidovudine-treated HIV-infected and cancer patients.

WARNING Target hemoglobin shouldn't exceed 11 g/dl when treating anemia in patients with chronic renal failure on dialysis and 10 g/dl for patients not on dialysis. Exceeding these parameters increases risk of life-threatening adverse cardiovascular effects.

• Expect to increase heparin dose if patient receives hemodialysis because epoetin alfa can increase the RBC volume, which could cause clots to form in the dialyzer, hemodialysis vascular access, or both.

• Monitor patient for hypertensive or thrombotic complications, especially if hemoglobin is approaching target goal.

PATIENT TEACHING

• Before epoetin alfa therapy starts, explain its serious adverse effects.

• Teach patient how to administer drug and how to dispose of needles properly. Caution him against reusing needles.

• Emphasize the importance of complying with the dosage regimen and keeping follow-up medical appointments and appointments for laboratory tests.

• Encourage patient to eat iron-rich foods.

• Review possible adverse reactions, and urge patient to notify prescriber if he experiences chest pain, headache, hives, rapid heartbeat, rash, seizures, shortness of breath, or swelling.

• Advise women of childbearing age to use effective contraception during therapy if pregnancy isn't desired because menses may resume after epoetin alfa therapy.

---

epoprostenol sodium

(PGI$_2$, PGX, prostacyclin)

Flolan, Veletri

Class and Category

Chemical class: Natural prostaglandin
Therapeutic class: Antihypertensive, vasodilator
Pregnancy category: B

Indications and Dosages

➤ *To provide long-term treatment of primary pulmonary hypertension; to treat pulmonary hypertension associated with the scleroderma spectrum of disease in NYHA Class III and Class IV patients who do not respond adequately to conventional therapy*

I.V. INFUSION

Adults. *Initial:* 2 nanograms/kg/min, increased by 2 nanograms/kg/min every 15 min or longer until dose-limiting effects occur (abdominal, chest, or musculoskeletal pain; anxiety; bradycardia; dizziness; dyspnea; flushing; headache; hypotension; nausea; tachycardia; vomiting; or other adverse reactions).

DOSAGE ADJUSTMENT Infusion rate adjusted based on persistence, recurrence, or worsening of primary pulmonary hypertension and dose-related adverse reactions, with dosage reduction done gradually in decrements of 2 nanograms/kg/min every 15 min or longer until the dose-limiting effects resolve; or if symptoms of pulmonary hypertension persist or reoccur after improving, dosage increased by 1 to 2 nanograms/kg/min every 15 min or longer to obtain new effective dose but absence of dose-limiting effects.

Mechanism of Action

Directly relaxes vascular smooth muscles through its action as a natural prostaglandin. This results in arterial dilation and inhibition of platelet aggregation. These actions decrease pulmonary vascular resistance, increase cardiac index and oxygen delivery, and limit thrombus formation.

Incompatibilities

Don't mix epoprostenol with other parenteral solutions or drugs.

Contraindications

Hypersensitivity to epoprostenol or its components; long-term use in patients with heart failure caused by severe left ventricular systolic dysfunction; pulmonary edema that developed while establishing epoprostenol dosage

Interactions

DRUGS

anticoagulants, antiplatelet drugs, NSAIDs:
Increased risk of bleeding
antihypertensives, diuretics, vasodilators:
Decreased blood pressure

Adverse Reactions

CNS: Agitation, anxiety, chills, confusion, dizziness, fever, headache, nervousness, paresthesia, syncope, weakness
CV: Bradycardia, chest pain, hypotension, tachycardia
ENDO: Hyperthyroidism
GI: Abdominal pain, diarrhea, nausea, vomiting
HEME: Anemia, bleeding events, hypersplenism, pancytopenia, splenomegaly, thrombocytopenia
MS: Arthralgia, jaw pain, myalgia
RESP: Dyspnea, hypoxia, pulmonary edema
SKIN: Diaphoresis, flushing, rash
Other: Flulike symptoms, injection-site infection and pain, sepsis, weight loss or gain

Nursing Considerations

• Use epoprostenol cautiously in elderly patients because they may have decreased hepatic, renal, or cardiac function, or other diseases or may receive other drugs that can interact with epoprostenol.

• Reconstitute drug only with sterile diluent that comes with package for Flolan or use sterile water for injection or normal saline for injection for Veletri. Don't dilute reconstituted epoprostenol.

• To make 100 ml of Flolan reconstituted solution at 3,000 nanograms/ml, dissolve contents of 0.5-mg Flolan vial with 5 ml of diluent; withdraw 3 ml and add diluent to make 100 ml. To make 100 ml of Flolan solution at 5,000 nanograms/ml, dissolve contents of 0.5-mg Flolan vial with 5 ml of diluent; withdraw contents and add diluent to make 100 ml. To make 100 ml of Flolan solution at 10,000 nanograms/ml, dissolve contents of two 0.5-mg Flolan vials each with 5 ml of diluent; withdraw contents and add diluent to make 100 ml. To make 100 ml of Flolan solution at 15,000 nanograms/ml, dissolve contents of 1.5-mg Flolan vial with 5 ml of diluent; withdraw contents and add diluent to make 100 ml Flolan.

• To make 100 ml of Veletri reconstituted solution, dissolve contents of 1.5-mg Veletri vial with 5 ml of diluent (sterile water for injection or normal saline for injection) and withdraw amount needed to make final concentration. For example, to make a 3,000-nanograms/ml concentration after dissolving contents, withdraw 1 ml of the Veletri vial contents and add to a sufficient volume of the identical diluent to make a total of 100 ml; to make a 6,000-nanograms/ml concentration after dissolving contents, withdraw 2 ml of the Veletri vial contents and add to a sufficient volume of the identical diluent to make a total of 100 ml; to make a 9,000-nanograms/ml concentration after dissolving contents, withdraw 3 ml of the Veletri vial contents and add to a sufficient volume of the identical diluent to make a total of 100 ml; to make a 12,000-nanograms/ml concentration after dissolving contents, withdraw 4 ml of the Veletri vial contents and add to a sufficient volume of the identical diluent to make a total of 100 ml; to make a 15,000-nanograms/ml concentration after dissolving contents, withdraw entire Veletri vial contents and add to a sufficient volume of the identical diluent to make a total of 100 ml; and to make a 30,000-nanograms/ml concentration, dissolve contents of two 1.5-mg Veletri vials each with 5 ml of diluent and withdraw entire vial contents and add to a sufficient volume of the identical diluent to make a total of 100 ml.

• Give continuous infusion through central venous catheter. Use peripheral I.V. infusion only until central access established.

• Use a small, lightweight, ambulatory infusion pump able to deliver 2 nanograms/kg/min. It should have alarms for occlusion, end of infusion, and low battery. It should also be positive pressure driven (continuous or pulsatile) with intervals between pulses not exceeding 3 minutes. Use a polyvinyl chloride, polypropylene, or glass reservoir. Keep a backup pump and infusion set nearby to minimize disruptions in delivery.

• At room temperature, administer a single container of reconstituted Flolan solution

E
F

over 8 hours. For extended use at temperatures above 77° F (25° C), use a cold pouch with frozen gel packs to keep Flolan at 36° to 46° F (2° to 8° C) for 12 hours. Check manufacturer guidelines for administration of Veletri reconstituted solutions because variation occurs depending on if the drug was stored prior to administration and for how long.

• After a new infusion rate has been established, monitor patient closely for adverse reactions. Measure blood pressure with patient standing and supine. Also, monitor heart rate for several hours after dosage adjustment.

• During prolonged infusion, watch for dose-related adverse reactions. If they develop, expect to decrease infusion by 2 nanograms/kg/min every 15 minutes, as prescribed, until reactions resolve.

• Avoid abrupt withdrawal or a sudden large reduction in infusion rate, which could cause rebound pulmonary hypertension (asthenia, dizziness, dyspnea) or death.

• Protect reconstituted drug from light, and refrigerate for no more than 48 hours if using Flolan and for no more than 5 days if using Veletri. Discard solution that has been frozen or refrigerated for more time than is allowed.

• Watch for evidence of bleeding, especially if patient has other risk factors for bleeding, because epoprostenol is a potent inhibitor of platelet aggregation.

PATIENT TEACHING

• Explain that epoprostenol is infused continuously through permanent indwelling central venous catheter by infusion pump.

• Emphasize that patient must commit to long-term therapy, possibly for years.

• Teach patient or caregiver how to reconstitute drug, administer it, and care for the permanent central venous catheter.

• Urge patient to maintain prescribed infusion rate and to consult prescriber before altering it.

• Caution patient that even brief interruptions in drug delivery may cause rapid worsening of symptoms.

• Instruct patient to notify prescriber if adverse reactions occur.

• Make sure patient or caregiver has ready access to emergency phone numbers.

eprosartan mesylate
Teveten

Class and Category
Chemical class: Monomethanesulfonate, nonbiphenyl nontetrazole angiotensin II receptor antagonist
Therapeutic class: Antihypertensive
Pregnancy category: D

Indications and Dosages
➤ *To control blood pressure in patients with essential hypertension*
TABLETS
Adults. *Initial:* 600 mg daily. *Maximum:* 800 mg once daily or in divided doses twice daily.

Mechanism of Action
Blocks the effects of angiotensin II (a potent vasoconstrictor that's part of the renin-angiotensin-aldosterone system) by blocking its binding to angiotensin I receptors in vascular smooth muscles, adrenal glands, and other tissues. This action halts angiotensin II's negative feedback on renin secretion. Thus, circulating renin and angiotensin II levels rise and vascular resistance declines.

Contraindications
Aliskirein use in patients with diabetes or renal impairment (GRF less than 60 ml/min); hypersensitivity to eprosartan or components

Interactions
DRUGS
aliskiren (in patients with diabetes or renal impairment), angiotensin receptor blockers, other ACE inhibitors: Increased risk of hyperkalemia, hypotension, and renal dysfunction
lithium: Possibly increased serum lithium level and lithium toxicity
NSAIDs: Possible decreased renal function in patients who are elderly, volume-depleted, or have a compromised renal function

Adverse Reactions
CNS: Depression, dizziness, drowsiness, fatigue
CV: Angina pectoris, atrial fibrillation, bradycardia, extrasystole,

hypertriglyceridemia, hypotension, palpitations, tachycardia
EENT: Pharyngitis, rhinitis
GI: Abdominal pain
GU: Oliguria, UTI
MS: Myalgia, rhabdomyolysis
RESP: Cough, upper respiratory tract infection

Nursing Considerations
• Watch for excessive hypotension if patient receives other cardiac drugs.
• Expect maximum blood pressure response after about 3 weeks.
• Be aware that, unlike ACE inhibitors, eprosartan doesn't affect bradykinin breakdown and cause the characteristic ACE cough.

PATIENT TEACHING
• Explain that maximum blood pressure response may not occur for 3 to 4 weeks.
• Tell patient that drug may cause dizziness, drowsiness, or very low blood pressure. Urge him to rise slowly to upright position.

WARNING Caution women of childbearing age to use reliable contraception and to notify prescriber immediately if pregnancy is suspected. Eprosartan may cause fetal harm and should be discontinued.

eptifibatide
Integrilin

Class and Category
Chemical class: Cyclic heptapeptide
Therapeutic class: Platelet aggregation inhibitor
Pregnancy category: B

Indications and Dosages
➤ *To treat unstable angina and non–Q-wave MI*
I.V. INFUSION
Adults. *Initial:* 180 mcg/kg over 1 to 2 min as soon as possible after diagnosis. *Maintenance:* 2 mcg/kg/min by continuous infusion starting immediately after initial dose and continuing until discharge or coronary artery bypass grafting, up to 72 hr.

DOSAGE ADJUSTMENT For non-dialysis-dependent patient with serum creatinine level less than 50 ml/min, initial bolus remains unchanged at 180 mcg/kg over 1 to 2 min so soon as possible after diagnosis but maintenance dosage decreased to 1.0 mcg/kg/min by continuous infusion.
➤ *To treat patients undergoing percutaneous transluminal coronary angioplasty (PTCA), including intracoronary stenting*
I.V. INFUSION
Adults. *Initial:* 180 mcg/kg over 1 to 2 min immediately before procedure followed by second bolus of 180 mcg/kg over 1 to 2 minutes 10 minutes after the first bolus. *Maintenance:* 2 mcg/kg/min by continuous infusion beginning just after initial bolus and continued for at least 12 hr but could be infused up to 24 hr.
DOSAGE ADJUSTMENT For non-dialysis-dependent patient with serum creatinine level less than 50 ml/min, initial bolus remains unchanged at 180 mcg/kg over 1 to 2 minutes immediately before procedure, immediately followed by a continuous infusion of 1.0 mcg/kg/min, and a second 180 mcg/kg bolus administered 10 minutes after the first.

Route	Onset	Peak	Duration
I.V.	Immediate	In 15 min	4–8 hr

Mechanism of Action
Reversibly inhibits platelet aggregation by preventing fibrinogen, von Willebrand factor, and other adhesive ligands from binding to glycoprotein IIb/IIIa receptors on activated platelets. As a result, eptifibatide disrupts final cross-linking stage of platelet aggregation—and thrombus formation.

Incompatibilities
Don't administer eptifibatide through the same I.V. line as furosemide.

Contraindications
Active bleeding or stroke during prior 30 days, bleeding diathesis, dependency on dialysis, history of hemorrhagic stroke, hypersensitivity to eptifibatide, major surgery during previous 4 weeks, serum creatinine level of 2 mg/dl or higher (for

E
F

180-mcg/kg dose or 2-mcg/kg/min infusion) or 4 mg/dl or higher (for 135-mcg/kg dose or 0.5-mcg/kg/min infusion), severe uncontrolled hypertension (systolic pressure above 200 mm Hg, diastolic pressure above 110 mm Hg), thrombocytopenia (platelet count below 100,000/mm³)

Interactions
DRUGS
anticoagulants, clopidogrel, dipyridamole, NSAIDs, thrombolytics, ticlopidine: Additive pharmacologic effects, increased risk of bleeding
other platelet aggregation inhibitors (especially inhibitors of platelet receptor glycoprotein IIb/IIIa, such as abciximab): Increased risk of additive pharmacologic effects

Adverse Reactions
CNS: Intracranial hemorrhage
CV: Hypotension
GI: GI hemorrhage, hematemesis
GU: Hematuria
HEME: Bleeding, decreased hemoglobin level, immune-mediated thrombocytopenia, thrombocytopenia
RESP: Pulmonary hemorrhage
Other: Anaphylaxis

Nursing Considerations
• Expect to obtain APTT and PT as a baseline and hematocrit, platelet count, and hemoglobin and serum creatinine levels before therapy.
• Withdraw bolus dose of eptifibatide from a 10-ml (2 mg/ml) vial into a syringe.
• Using vented I.V. infusion set, give continuous infusion directly from the 100-ml (0.75 mg/ml) vial. Be sure to center the spike in the circle on top of vial stopper.
• Expect to keep APTT between 50 and 70 seconds or per facility protocol during therapy unless patient has PTCA.
• If patient has PTCA, expect to maintain activated clotting time between 200 and 250 seconds during the procedure.
• During therapy, avoid arterial and venous punctures, I.M. injections, urinary catheters, nasotracheal or nasogastric intubation, and use of noncompressible

I.V. sites, such as subclavian and jugular veins.
• Expect to discontinue eptifibatide and heparin and monitor patient closely if platelet count falls below 100,000/mm³.
• Plan to stop drug, as prescribed, if patient undergoes coronary artery bypass surgery.
PATIENT TEACHING
• Instruct patient to immediately report bleeding during eptifibatide therapy.
• Reassure patient that he'll be monitored closely throughout therapy.
• Advise patient to avoid activities that may lead to bruising and bleeding.

ergoloid mesylates
(dihydrogenated ergot alkaloids)
Gerimal, Hydergine, Hydergine LC

Class and Category
Chemical class: Dihydrogenated ergot alkaloid derivative
Therapeutic class: Antidementia adjunct, cerebral metabolic enhancer
Pregnancy category: Not rated

Indications and Dosages
➤ *To treat age-related decline in mental capacity*
CAPSULES, ORAL SOLUTION, S.L. TABLETS, TABLETS
Adults. 1 to 2 mg three times daily.

Route	Onset	Peak	Duration
P.O.	3 wk or more	Unknown	Unknown

Mechanism of Action
May increase cerebral metabolism, blood flow, and oxygen uptake. These actions may increase neurotransmitter levels.

Contraindications
Acute or chronic psychosis, hypersensitivity to ergoloid mesylates or their components

Interactions
DRUGS
delavirdine, efavirenz, indinavir, nelfinavir, saquinavir: Increased risk of ergotism (blurred vision, dizziness, and headache)
dopamine: Increased risk of gangrene

Adverse Reactions

CNS: Dizziness, headache, light-headedness, syncope
CV: Bradycardia, orthostatic hypotension
EENT: Blurred vision, nasal congestion, tongue soreness (with S.L. tablets)
GI: Abdominal cramps, anorexia, nausea, vomiting
SKIN: Flushing, rash

Nursing Considerations

• Expect ergoloid mesylates to be prescribed only after a pathophysiologic cause for mental decline has been ruled out.
• Measure blood pressure and pulse rate and rhythm before therapy begins and monitor them frequently during therapy.
• If bradycardia or hypotension develops, expect to discontinue drug permanently.

PATIENT TEACHING

• Stress the importance of adhering to prescribed dosage and schedule.
• Teach caregiver to place S.L. tablet under patient's tongue and withhold food, fluids, and cigarettes until tablet dissolves.
• Instruct patient not to swallow S.L. tablets.
• Advise caregiver to skip a missed dose and resume the regular dosing schedule. Warn against doubling the dose, and urge caregiver to notify prescriber if patient misses two or more doses in a row.
• Instruct caregiver to store drug in a tightly closed, light-resistant container.
• Inform caregiver and family that drug may take 3 to 4 weeks to produce its effects.
• Emphasize the importance of follow-up care.

---

ergotamine tartrate

Ergomar (CAN), Ergostat, Gynergen (CAN), Medihaler Ergotamine (CAN)

Class and Category

Chemical class: Ergot alkaloid
Therapeutic class: Vascular headache suppressant
Pregnancy category: X

Indications and Dosages

➤ *To relieve vascular headaches, such as migraine, migraine variants, and cluster headaches*

S.L. TABLETS
Adults. *Initial:* 2 mg at first sign of attack and repeated every 30 min, as needed. *Maximum:* 6 mg/day and no more than twice/wk at least 5 days apart.
TABLETS
Adults. *Initial:* 1 to 2 mg at first sign of attack, repeated every 30 min, as needed. Increased to 3 mg for subsequent attacks as needed and if lower dose was well tolerated. *Maximum:* 6 mg daily.
ORAL INHALATION AEROSOL
Adults. 1 (360-mcg) inhalation at first sign of attack and repeated every 5 min, as needed. *Maximum:* 2.16 mg daily and no more than twice/wk at least 5 days apart.

Route	Onset	Peak	Duration
P.O., S.L.	Unknown	1–5 hr	Unknown

Mechanism of Action

Directly stimulates vascular smooth muscles, constricting arteries and veins and depressing vasomotor centers in the brain.

Contraindications

Coronary artery disease, hypersensitivity to ergot alkaloids, hypertension, impaired hepatic or renal function, malnutrition, peripheral vascular disease (Raynaud's disease, severe arteriosclerosis, syphilitic arteritis, thromboangiitis obliterans, thrombophlebitis), pregnancy or risk of pregnancy, sepsis, severe pruritus

Interactions

DRUGS
beta blockers: Increased risk of vasoconstriction and, possibly, peripheral gangrene
erythromycin, troleandomycin: Possibly increased risk of peripheral vasospasm and ischemia
nitrates: Increased ergotamine effects, decreased antianginal effects of nitrates, increased risk of hypertension
sumatriptan: Possibly additive vasoconstriction
vasoconstrictors: Increased risk of dangerous hypertension

ACTIVITIES
smoking: Possibly increased risk of peripheral vasoconstriction and ischemia

E
F

Adverse Reactions

CNS: Anxiety, confusion, dizziness, drowsiness, paresthesia, severe headache
CV: Chest pain, fast or slow heart rate, heart valve fibrosis, increased or decreased blood pressure, MI, weak pulse
EENT: Dry mouth, miosis, vision changes
GI: Nausea, vomiting
MS: Arm, back, or leg pain; muscle weakness in legs
SKIN: Cold, cyanotic, or pale feet or hands; pruritus
Other: Edema of face, feet, fingers, or lower legs; physical dependence

Nursing Considerations

• Use ergotamine cautiously in elderly patients.
• If patient receives long-term therapy, monitor pain control; he may need increasingly higher doses to obtain relief.
• Notify prescriber at the first sign of vasospasm and expect to discontinue drug.

PATIENT TEACHING
• Teach patient to take a tablet at the first sign of headache and to lie down in a quiet, dark room.
• Instruct patient not to swallow S.L. tablet but to let it dissolve under his tongue. Advise him not to drink, eat, or smoke until tablet has dissolved.
• Stress the importance of adhering to prescribed dosage and schedule because of drug's potential for dependence.
• Warn patient not to smoke while taking ergotamine (especially heavy smokers) because combining drug with nicotine, which also constricts vessels, may increase risk of peripheral vascular ischemia.
• Advise patient to notify prescriber if usual doses fail to relieve headaches or if headache frequency or severity increases.
• Urge patient to avoid alcohol because it worsens headaches. Also suggest that patient avoid excessive cold, which may increase peripheral vasoconstriction.
• Instruct patient to notify prescriber if an infection develops because severe infection may increase sensitivity to drug.
• Advise patient to notify prescriber if he experiences chest pain; numbness, pain, or tingling in fingers or toes; pulse rate changes; swelling of face, feet, fingers, or lower legs; or vision changes.

ertapenem sodium
Invanz

Class and Category

Chemical class: Synthetic 1-β methyl-carbapenem
Therapeutic class: Antibiotic
Pregnancy category: B

Indications and Dosages

➤ *To treat moderate to severe infections, such as complicated intra-abdominal infections due to* Escherichia coli, Clostridium clostridioforme, Eubacterium lentum, Peptostreptococcus *species,* Bacteroides fragilis, B.distasonis, B.ovatus, B.thetaiotaomicron, *or* B.uniformis; *complicated skin and skin-structure infections due to* staphylococcus aureus *(methicillin-susceptible strains only),* Streptococcus pyogenes, E.coli, *or* Peptostreptococcus *species; community-acquired pneumonia due to* streptococcus pneumoniae *(penicillin-susceptible strains only, including cases with concurrent bacteremia),* Haemophilus influenzae *(beta-lactamase–negative strains only), or* moraxella catarrhalis; *complicated UTI (including pyelonephritis) due to* E.coli *(including cases with concurrent bacteremia) or* Klebsiella pneumoniae; *and acute pelvic infections (including postpartum endomyometritis, septic abortion, and postsurgical gynecologic infections) due to* Streptococcus agalactiae, E.coli, B.fragilis, Porphyromonas asaccharolytica, Peptostreptococcus *species, or* Prevotella bivia

I.V. INFUSION
Adults and adolescents. 1 g daily, infused over 30 min, for up to 14 days.
Children ages 3 months to 13 years. 15 mg/kg twice daily, infused over 30 min, for up to 14 days. *Maximum:* 1 g daily.

I.M. INJECTION
Adults and adolescents. 1 g daily for up to 7 days.
Children ages 3 months to 13 years. 15 mg/kg twice daily for up to 7 days. *Maximum:* 1 g daily.

DOSAGE ADJUSTMENT Dosage decreased to 500 mg daily for patients with advanced renal insufficiency (creatinine clearance less than or equal to 30 ml/min/1.73 m²) or end-stage renal insufficiency (creatinine clearance less than or equal to 10 ml/min/1.73 m²). For patients on hemodialysis who have received 500 mg of ertapenem within 6 hr of hemodialysis, supplemental dose of 150 mg given after hemodialysis.

Mechanism of Action

Inhibits bacterial cell wall synthesis by binding to specific penicillin-binding proteins inside the cell wall. Penicillin-binding proteins are responsible for various steps in bacterial cell wall synthesis. By binding to these proteins, ertapenem leads to bacterial cell wall lysis.

Incompatibilities

Don't mix ertapenem with other drugs. Don't dilute it with solutions containing dextrose.

Contraindications

Hypersensitivity to ertapenem, its components, or other drugs in the same class; hypersensitivity to local anesthetics (I.M. form only, because lidocaine hydrochloride 1% is used as a diluent); patients who have experienced anaphylactic reactions to beta-lactam drugs

Interactions

DRUGS

probenecid: Increased ertapenem half-life, increased and prolonged blood ertapenem level

valproic acid: Possibly decreased serum valproic acid level and increased risk of breakthrough seizures

Adverse Reactions

CNS: Abnormal coordination, aggression, agitation, anxiety, asthenia, confusion, delirium, depressed level of consciousness, disorientation, dizziness, dyskinesia, fatigue, fever, gait disturbance, hallucinations, headache, hypothermia, insomnia, mental changes, myoclonus, seizures, somnolence, stupor, tremor

CV: Chest pain, edema, hypertension, hypotension, tachycardia, thrombophlebitis

EENT: Nasopharyngitis, oral candidiasis, rhinitis, rhinorrhea, teeth staining, viral pharyngitis

ENDO: Hyperglycemia

GI: Abdominal pain, acid regurgitation, anorexia, *Clostridium difficile* colitis, constipation, diarrhea, elevated liver function test results, indigestion, nausea, small-intestine obstruction, vomiting

GU: Dysuria, elevated serum creatinine level, genital rash, proteinuria, RBCs and WBCs in urine, UTI, vaginitis

HEME: Anemia, decreased hematocrit, decreased WBC count, eosinophilia, increased WBC count, neutropenia, prolonged PT, thrombocytopenia, thrombocytosis

MS: Arthralgia, leg pain, muscle weakness

RESP: Atelectasis, cough, crackles, dyspnea, pleural effusion, pneumonia, respiratory distress, upper respiratory tract infection, wheezing

SKIN: Cellulitis, dermatitis, drug rash with eosinophilia and systemic symptoms (DRESS syndrome), erythema, extravasation, pruritus, rash

Other: Anaphylaxis; death; hyperkalemia; hypokalemia; infusion-site induration, pain, phlebitis, pruritus, redness, swelling, or warmth

Nursing Considerations

• Obtain sputum, urine, or other specimens for culture and sensitivity testing, as ordered, before giving ertapenem. Expect to start therapy before results are available.

• When preparing drug for I.V. use, reconstitute 1 g with 10 ml of sterile water for injection, 0.9% sodium chloride injection, or bacteriostatic water for injection. Don't use solutions that contain dextrose. Shake well to dissolve. Immediately transfer reconstituted drug to 50 ml normal saline solution. Use within 6 hours if stored at room temperature, 24 hours if refrigerated at 5° C (41° F). Don't freeze. Give I.V. infusion over 30 minutes.

• Inspect drug for particles and discoloration after reconstitution.

• For I.M. injection, reconstitute 1 g of drug with 3.2 ml of 1% lidocaine hydrochloride injection (without epinephrine). Shake thoroughly to form solution. Use within 1 hour after

E
F

preparation. Withdraw contents of vial and inject deep into a large muscle mass such as the gluteal muscle.

WARNING Don't give reconstituted I.M. solution by I.V. route because of possible adverse reaction to lidocaine hydrochloride injection used to reconstitute drug.

• Monitor patient closely for a life-threatening anaphylactic reaction. Patients with a history of hypersensitivity to penicillin, cephalosporins, other beta-lactams, or other allergens are at increased risk.

WARNING If ertapenem triggers an anaphylactic reaction, stop drug, notify prescriber immediately, and provide appropriate therapy. Anaphylaxis requires immediate treatment with epinephrine as well as airway management and administration of oxygen and I.V. corticosteroids, as needed.

• Be aware that patients with a history of seizures, other CNS disorders that predispose them to seizures (such as brain lesions), or compromised renal function may be at increased risk for seizures. Administer anticonvulsant, as ordered.

• Monitor patient for diarrhea during and for at least 2 months after drug therapy; diarrhea may signal pseudomembranous colitis caused by *Clostridium difficile*. If diarrhea occurs, notify prescriber and expect to withhold ertapenem and treat with fluids, electrolytes, protein, and an antibiotic effective against *C. difficile*.

• Be aware that because ertapenem is excreted in breastmilk, its use by nursing mothers is carefully evaluated.

PATIENT TEACHING

• Instruct patient receiving ertapenem to immediately report signs of anaphylaxis, such as rash, itching, or shortness of breath; or signs of superinfection, such as severe diarrhea or white patches on tongue or in mouth.

• Urge patient to tell prescriber about diarrhea that's severe or lasts longer than 3 days. Remind patient that watery or bloody stools can occur 2 or more months after antibiotic therapy and can be serious, requiring prompt treatment.

• Alert patient taking valproic acid or divalproex for seizure control to notify prescriber of this type of concurrent therapy because ertapenem may interfere with these drugs' effectiveness to control seizures.

erythromycin

(contains 250, 333, or 500 mg of base per delayed-release capsule, delayed-release tablet, or tablet)
Apo-Erythro (CAN), E-Mycin, Erybid (CAN), ERYC, Ery-Tab, Ilotycin, Novo-Rythro Encap (CAN), PCE

erythromycin estolate

(contains 250 mg of base per capsule or tablet, or 125 or 250 mg of base per 5 ml of oral suspension)
Ilosone, Novo-Rythro (CAN)

erythromycin ethylsuccinate

(contains 1 g of base per 1.6 g of oral suspension or tablet)
Apo-Erythro-ES (CAN), E.E.S., EryPed, Erythro, Novo-Rythro (CAN)

erythromycin gluceptate

(contains 500 or 1,000 mg of base per vial)
Ilotycin

erythromycin lactobionate

(contains 500 or 1,000 mg of base per vial)
Erythrocin

erythromycin stearate

(contains 125 or 250 mg of base per 5 ml of oral suspension, or 250 or 500 mg of base per tablet)
Apo-Erythro-S (CAN), Erythrocin, Erythrocot, My-E, Novo-Rythro (CAN), Wintrocin

Class and Category

Chemical class: Macrolide
Therapeutic class: Antiacne agent, antibiotic
Pregnancy category: B

Indications and Dosages

➤ *To treat mild to moderate upper respiratory tract infections caused by* Haemophilus influenzae, Streptococcus pneumoniae, *or* Streptococcus pyogenes *(group A beta-hemolytic streptococcus)*

CAPSULES, CHEWABLE TABLETS, DELAYED-RELEASE CAPSULES, DELAYED-RELEASE TABLETS, ORAL SUSPENSION, TABLETS, I.V. INFUSION

Adults. 250 to 500 mg (base) every 6 hr for 10 days.

Children. 250 to 500 mg (base) four times daily or 20 to 50 mg (base)/kg daily in divided doses for 10 days. For *H. influenzae* infections, erythromycin ethylsuccinate is administered with 150 mg/kg daily of sulfisoxazole. *Maximum:* Adult dosage, or 6 g daily for erythromycin ethylsuccinate.

➤ *To treat lower respiratory tract infections caused by* S. pneumoniae *or* S. pyogenes *(group A beta-hemolytic streptococcus)*

CAPSULES, CHEWABLE TABLETS, DELAYED-RELEASE CAPSULES, DELAYED-RELEASE TABLETS, ORAL SUSPENSION, TABLETS, I.V. INFUSION

Adults. 250 to 500 mg (base) every 6 hr for 10 days.

Children. 250 to 500 mg (base) four times daily or 20 to 50 mg (base)/kg daily in divided doses for 10 days. *Maximum:* Adult dosage.

➤ *To treat respiratory tract infections caused by* Mycoplasma pneumoniae

CAPSULES, CHEWABLE TABLETS, DELAYED-RELEASE CAPSULES, DELAYED-RELEASE TABLETS, ORAL SUSPENSION, TABLETS, I.V. INFUSION

Adults. 500 mg (base) every 6 hr for 5 to 10 days or up to 3 wk for severe infections.

➤ *To treat mild to moderate skin and soft-tissue infections caused by* S. pyogenes *or* Staphylococcus aureus

CAPSULES, CHEWABLE TABLETS, DELAYED-RELEASE CAPSULES, DELAYED-RELEASE TABLETS, ORAL SUSPENSION, TABLETS, I.V. INFUSION

Adults. 250 mg (base) every 6 hr or 500 mg (base) every 12 hr for 10 days. *Maximum:* 4 g (base) daily.

Children. 250 to 500 mg (base) four times daily or 20 to 50 mg (base)/kg daily in divided doses for 10 days. *Maximum:* Adult dosage.

➤ *To treat acne vulgaris*

DELAYED-RELEASE CAPSULES, DELAYED-RELEASE TABLETS, TABLETS

Adults and adolescents. *Initial:* 250 mg (base) every 6 hr, 333 mg (base) every 8 hr, or 500 mg (base) every 12 hr for 4 wk. *Maintenance:* 333 to 500 mg (base) daily.

➤ *To treat pertussis (whooping cough) caused by* Bordetella pertussis

CAPSULES, CHEWABLE TABLETS, DELAYED-RELEASE CAPSULES, DELAYED-RELEASE TABLETS, ORAL SUSPENSION, TABLETS, I.V. INFUSION

Children. 500 mg (base) four times daily or 40 to 50 mg (base)/kg daily in divided doses for 5 to 14 days.

➤ *To treat diphtheria*

CAPSULES, CHEWABLE TABLETS, DELAYED-RELEASE CAPSULES, DELAYED-RELEASE TABLETS, ORAL SUSPENSION, TABLETS, I.V. INFUSION

Adults and children. 500 mg (base) every 6 hr for 10 days.

➤ *To treat erythrasma*

CAPSULES, CHEWABLE TABLETS, DELAYED-RELEASE CAPSULES, DELAYED-RELEASE TABLETS, ORAL SUSPENSION, TABLETS, I.V. INFUSION

Adults and children. 250 mg (base) three times daily for 21 days.

➤ *To treat intestinal amebiasis*

CAPSULES, CHEWABLE TABLETS, DELAYED-RELEASE CAPSULES, DELAYED-RELEASE TABLETS, ORAL SUSPENSION, TABLETS, I.V. INFUSION

Adults. 250 mg (base) every 6 hr for 10 to 14 days.

Children. 30 to 50 mg (base)/kg daily in divided doses for 10 to 14 days.

➤ *To treat pelvic inflammatory disease caused by* neisseria gonorrhoeae

CAPSULES, CHEWABLE TABLETS, DELAYED-RELEASE CAPSULES, DELAYED-RELEASE TABLETS, ORAL SUSPENSION, TABLETS, I.V. INFUSION

Adults. 500 mg (base) I.V. every 6 hr for 3 days and then 250 mg (base) P.O. or I.V. every 6 hr for 7 days.

➤ *To treat conjunctivitis in newborns*

I.V. INFUSION

Neonates. 50 mg (base)/kg daily in 4 divided doses for 14 days.

➤ *To treat pneumonia in neonates*

I.V. INFUSION

Neonates. 50 mg (base)/kg daily in divided doses for 21 days.

➤ *To treat urogenital infections caused by* chlamydia trachomatis *during pregnancy*

E
F

CAPSULES, CHEWABLE TABLETS, DELAYED-RELEASE CAPSULES, DELAYED-RELEASE TABLETS, ORAL SUSPENSION, TABLETS

Adults. 500 mg (base) on an empty stomach every 6 hr for 7 days; or 250 mg (base) on an empty stomach every 6 hr for at least 14 days.

➤ *To treat nongonococcal urethritis or uncomplicated urethral, endocervical, or rectal infections caused by C. trachomatis*

CAPSULES, CHEWABLE TABLETS, DELAYED-RELEASE CAPSULES, DELAYED-RELEASE TABLETS, ORAL SUSPENSION, TABLETS

Adults. 500 mg (base) every 6 hr for 7 days. If patient can't tolerate high doses, 250 mg (base) every 6 hr for 14 days.

➤ *To treat primary syphilis*

CAPSULES, CHEWABLE TABLETS, DELAYED-RELEASE CAPSULES, DELAYED-RELEASE TABLETS, ORAL SUSPENSION, TABLETS

Adults. 20 to 40 g (base) in divided doses over 10 to 15 days.

➤ *To treat Legionnaire's disease*

CAPSULES, CHEWABLE TABLETS, DELAYED-RELEASE CAPSULES, DELAYED-RELEASE TABLETS, ORAL SUSPENSION, TABLETS, I.V. INFUSION

Adults. 1 to 4 g (base) daily in divided doses for 10 to 14 days.

➤ *To treat rheumatic fever*

CAPSULES, CHEWABLE TABLETS, DELAYED-RELEASE CAPSULES, DELAYED-RELEASE TABLETS, ORAL SUSPENSION, TABLETS, I.V. INFUSION

Adults. 250 mg (base) every 12 hr.

➤ *To prevent bacterial endocarditis in patients with penicillin allergy who plan dental or upper respiratory tract surgery*

CAPSULES, CHEWABLE TABLETS, DELAYED-RELEASE CAPSULES, DELAYED-RELEASE TABLETS, ORAL SUSPENSION, TABLETS, I.V. INFUSION

Adults. 1 g (base) given 1 to 2 hr before procedure and then 500 mg (base) 6 hr after initial dose.

Children. 20 mg (base)/kg given 2 hr before procedure and then 10 mg (base)/kg 6 hr after initial dose.

➤ *To treat listeriosis*

CAPSULES, CHEWABLE TABLETS, DELAYED-RELEASE CAPSULES, DELAYED-RELEASE TABLETS, ORAL SUSPENSION, TABLETS, I.V. INFUSION

Adults. 250 mg (base) every 6 hr or 500 mg (base) every 12 hr.

Maximum: 4 g (base) daily.

Mechanism of Action

Binds with the 50S ribosomal subunit of the 70S ribosome in many types of aerobic, anaerobic, gram-positive, and gram-negative bacteria. This action inhibits RNA-dependent protein synthesis in bacterial cells, causing them to die.

Contraindications

Astemizole, cisapride, dihydroergotamine, ergotamine, pimozide, or terfenadine therapy; hypersensitivity to erythromycin, macrolide antibiotics, or their components; hepatic disease (erythromycin estolate)

Interactions

DRUGS

alfentanil: Decreased alfentanil clearance, prolonged alfentanil action

astemizole, cisapride, terfenadine: Increased risk of cardiotoxicity, torsades de pointes, ventricular tachycardia, and death

atorvastatin, lovastatin, pravastatin, simvastatin: Increased risk of rhabdomyolysis

calcium channel blockers such as amlodipine, diltiazem, verapamil: Increased risk of hypotension

carbamazepine, valproic acid: Possibly inhibited metabolism of these drugs, increasing their blood levels and risk of toxicity

chloramphenicol, lincomycins: Antagonized effects of these drugs

colchicine: Possible life-threatening colchicine toxicity

cyclosporine: Increased risk of nephrotoxicity

digoxin: Increased serum digoxin level and risk of digitalis toxicity

dihydroergotamine, ergotamine: Decreased ergotamine metabolism, increased risk of vasospasm from ergotamine use

hepatotoxic drugs: Increased risk of hepatotoxicity

midazolam, triazolam: Increased pharmacologic effects of these drugs

oral contraceptives: Failed contraception, hepatotoxicity

ototoxic drugs: Increased risk of ototoxicity if patient with impaired renal function receives high doses of erythromycin

penicillins: Interference with bactericidal effects of penicillin

sildenafil: Increased effects of sildenafil
warfarin: Prolonged PT and risk of
hemorrhage, especially in elderly patients
xanthines (except dyphylline): Increased
serum theophylline level and risk of
theophylline toxicity
ACTIVITIES
alcohol use: Increased alcohol level (by 40%)
with I.V. erythromycin

Adverse Reactions
CNS: Fatigue, fever, malaise, weakness
CV: Prolonged QT interval, torsades de
pointes, ventricular arrhythmias
EENT: Hearing loss, oral candidiasis
GI: Abdominal cramps and pain, diarrhea,
hepatotoxicity, nausea, pseudomembranous
colitis, vomiting
GU: Interstitial nephritis, vaginal candidiasis
MS: New or aggravated myasthenia gravis
syndrome
SKIN: Erythema, jaundice, pruritus, rash
Other: Fluid overload (from I.V. infusion),
injection-site inflammation and phlebitis

Nursing Considerations
• Be aware that erythromycin should not be
used in patients with history of QT
interval prolongation or in patients with
ongoing proarrhythmic conditions such as
uncorrected hypokalemia or hypomagnesemia, serious bradycardia, and in
patients receiving Class IA or Class III
antiarrhythmic agents. Monitor the elderly
closely as well because they are more
susceptible to drug effects on the QT
interval.
• Use erythromycin cautiously in patients
with impaired hepatic function because
drug is metabolized by the liver.
• Use erythromycin cautiously in elderly
patients, especially those with renal or
hepatic dysfunction, because these
patients are at increased risk of hearing
loss and torsades de pointes. They're also
at increased risk of bleeding if taking an
oral anticoagulant.
• Before giving first erythromycin dose,
expect to obtain body fluid or tissue
sample for culture and sensitivity testing.
• Reconstitute parenteral form before
administration. Add at least 10 ml of
preservative-free sterile water for injection
to each 500-mg vial or at least 20 ml of
diluent to each 1-g vial.

• For prolonged infusion, expect to infuse a
buffered solution up to 24 hours after
dilution.
• For intermittent infusion, dilute dose in
100 to 250 ml normal saline solution or
D_5W if needed; give slowly over 20 to
60 minutes.
• When giving I.V. erythromycin gluceptate,
dilute the solution if needed to 1 g/L in
normal saline solution or D_5W injection
for slow, continuous infusion. Diluted
solution remains potent for 7 days if
refrigerated.
• When giving I.V. erythromycin lactobionate, dilute the solution if needed to
1 to 5 mg/ml in normal saline solution,
lactated Ringer's solution, or other
electrolyte solution for slow, continuous
infusion. Diluted solution remains potent
for 14 days if refrigerated and for 24 hours
at room temperature.
• Be aware that infusions prepared in
piggyback infusion bottles stay potent for
30 days if frozen, 24 hours if refrigerated,
or 8 hours at room temperature. Don't
store infusions prepared in the ADD-
Vantage system.
• Don't use diluent with benzyl alcohol if
parenteral erythromycin is for a neonate.
It may cause a fatal toxic syndrome of
CNS depression, hypotension, metabolic
acidosis, renal failure, respiratory
problems, and, possibly, seizures and
intracranial hemorrhage.
• Periodically monitor liver function test
results to detect hepatotoxicity, which is
most common with erythromycin estolate.
Signs typically appear within 2 weeks after
continuous therapy starts and resolve
when it stops.
• Assess hearing regularly, especially in
elderly patients and those who receive 4 g
or more daily or have hepatic or renal
disease. Hearing impairment begins 36
hours to 8 days after treatment starts and
usually begins to improve 1 to 14 days
after it stops.
• During I.V. therapy, watch for evidence of
fluid overload, such as acute dyspnea and
crackles.
• Monitor infants for vomiting or
irritability with feeding because infantile
hypertrophic pyloric stenosis has been
reported.

E
F

- Assess myasthenia gravis patients for weakness because drug may aggravate it. Keep in mind that myasthenic syndrome may arise in patients previously undiagnosed with myasthenia gravis.
- Watch closely for signs and symptoms of superinfection. If they occur, notify prescriber and expect to stop drug and provide appropriate therapy.
- Monitor patient for diarrhea during and for at least 2 months after erythromycin therapy; diarrhea may signal pseudo-membranous colitis caused by *Clostridium difficile*. If diarrhea occurs, notify prescriber and expect to withhold drug and treat with fluids, electrolytes, protein, and an antibiotic effective against *C. difficile*.
- If patient receives an order for urine catecholamine analysis, notify prescriber because erythromycin interferes with fluorometric measurement of urine catecholamines.

PATIENT TEACHING
- Urge patient to complete prescribed therapy, even if he feels better before it's finished.
- Tell patient to notify prescriber if symptoms worsen or don't improve after a few days.
- Teach patient how to administer prescribed form of erythromycin. Instruct him to swallow capsules or tablets whole. For an oral suspension, teach him to use the calibrated measuring device provided to ensure accurate doses. Remind him to shake the suspension before measuring a dose.
- Advise patient to take oral form of erythromycin with a full glass of water on an empty stomach (except erythromycin ethylsuccinate, which is better absorbed with food).
- If GI distress occurs, instruct patient to take oral form with food.
- Instruct patient to promptly notify prescriber if he develops allergic reactions, hearing changes, or signs of hepatic dysfunction.
- Urge patient to tell prescriber about diarrhea that's severe or lasts longer than 3 days. Remind patient that watery or bloody stools can occur 2 or more months after antibiotic therapy and can be serious, requiring prompt treatment.

escitalopram oxalate
Lexapro

Class and Category
Chemical class: Pure S+ enantiomer of racemic bicyclic phthalane derivative citalopram
Therapeutic class: Antidepressant
Pregnancy category: C

Indications and Dosages
➤ *To treat generalized anxiety disorder or major depression*
ORAL SOLUTION, TABLETS
Adults. *Initial:* 10 mg daily in morning or evening, increased to 20 mg daily after 1 or more wk, as needed.
➤ *To treat major depression*
ORAL SOLUTION, TABLETS
Adults. *Initial:* 10 mg daily, morning or evening, increased to 20 mg daily after 1 wk, as needed.
Adolescents ages 12 to 17. *Initial:* 10 mg daily, morning or evening, increased to 20 mg daily after 3 wk, as needed.
DOSAGE ADJUSTMENT Dosage shouldn't exceed 10 mg daily for elderly patients and those with hepatic impairment.

Mechanism of Action
Inhibits reuptake of the neurotransmitter serotonin by CNS neurons, thereby increasing the amount of serotonin available in nerve synapses. An elevated serotonin level may result in elevated mood and reduced depression.

Contraindications
Hypersensitivity to escitalopram, citalopram or its components; use within 14 days of MAO inhibitor therapy

Interactions
DRUGS
aspirin, NSAIDs, warfarin: Possibly increased risk of bleeding
carbamazepine: Possibly increased clearance of escitalopram
cimetidine: Possibly increased plasma escitalopram level
CNS drugs: Additive CNS effects
lithium: Possible enhancement of the serotonergic effects of escitalopram

MAO inhibitors: Possibly hyperpyretic episodes, hypertensive crisis, serotonin syndrome, and severe seizures
metoprolol: Increased plasma metoprolol levels with decreased cardioselectivity of metoprolol
naratriptan, sumatriptan, zolmitriptan: Possibly weakness, hyperreflexia, and incoordination
St. John's wort: Increased risk of serotonin syndrome
sibutramine: Increased risk of serotonin syndrome
ACTIVITIES
alcohol use: Possibly increased cognitive and motor effects of alcohol

Adverse Reactions

CNS: Abnormal gait, acute psychosis, aggression, akathisia, delirium, dizziness, dyskinesia, dystonia, extrapyramidal effects, fatigue, headache, hypomania, insomnia, lethargy, mania, myoclonus, neuroleptic malignant syndrome, paresthesia, seizures, serotonin syndrome, somnolence, suicidal ideation
CV: Atrial fibrillation, cardiac failure, deep vein or phlebitis thrombosis, hypotension, MI, prolonged QT interval, thrombosis, torsades de pointes, ventricular arrhythmias
EENT: Acute-angle glaucoma, diplopia, dry mouth, nystagmus, rhinitis, sinusitis, toothache, visual hallucinations
ENDO: Diabetes mellitus, hyperpro-lactinemia, syndrome of inappropriate ADH secretion
GI: Abdominal pain, constipation, decreased appetite, diarrhea, flatulence, GI bleeding or hemorrhage, hepatic necrosis, hepatitis, indigestion, nausea, pancreatitis, rectal hemorrhage, vomiting
GU: Acute renal failure, anorgasmia, decreased libido, ejaculation disorders, impotence, priapism
HEME: Bleeding, decreased prothrombin time, hemolytic anemia, leukopenia, thrombocytopenia
MS: Neck or shoulder pain, rhabdomyolysis
RESP: Pulmonary embolism
SKIN: Ecchymosis, erythema multiforme, increased sweating, photosensitivity, Stevens-Johnson syndrome, toxic epidermal necrolysis, urticaria
Other: Anaphylaxis, angioedema, flulike symptoms, hyponatremia

Nursing Considerations

• Use escitalopram cautiously in patients with history of mania or seizures, patients with severe renal impairment, and those with diseases or conditions that produce altered metabolism or hemodynamic responses.

WARNING When escitalopram dosage increases, monitor patient for possible serotonin syndrome, which may include agitation, chills, confusion, diaphoresis, diarrhea, fever, hyperactive reflexes, poor coordination, restlessness, shaking, talking or acting with uncontrolled excitement, tremor, and twitching. In its most severe form, serotonin syndrome can resemble neuroleptic malignant syndrome, which includes a high fever, muscle rigidity, autonomic instability with possible changes in vital signs, and mental status changes.

• Be aware that escitalopram should not be given to patients with congenital long QT syndrome, bradycardia, hypokalemia or hypomagnesemia, recent acute myocardial infarction, or uncompensated heart failure because of increased risk of prolonged QT interval and torsades de pointes. It should also not be given to patients who are taking other drugs that prolong the QT interval. Expect hypokalemia and hypomagnesemia to be corrected before escitalopram therapy is begun.

• Monitor patient—especially elderly patient—for hypo-osmolarity of serum and urine and for hyponatremia (headache, trouble concentrating, impaired memory, weakness, unsteadiness) because they may may indicate escitalopram-induced syndrome of inappropriate ADH secretion.

• Watch for signs of misuse or abuse, such as development of tolerance, increasing dosage without approval, and drug-seeking behavior; drug's potential for physical and psychological dependence is unknown.

• Monitor patient for bleeding, especially if patient is also taking aspirin, an NSAID, or an anticoagulant. Bleeding can range from ecchymoses, hematomas, epistaxis and petechiae to life-threatening hemorrhages.

E
F

- Expect prescriber to reassess patient periodically to determine the continued need for therapy and evaluate dosage.
- If patient (particularly a child or an adolescent) takes escitalopram for depression, watch closely for suicidal tendencies, especially when therapy starts or dosage changes, because depression may worsen temporarily.
- If escitalopram will be stopped, expect to taper dosage to avoid serious adverse reactions.

PATIENT TEACHING
- Inform patient that alcohol use isn't recommended during escitalopram therapy because it may decrease his ability to think clearly and perform motor skills.
- Advise patient to avoid hazardous activities until drug's CNS effects are known.
- Instruct patient that drug shouldn't be taken with citalopram hydrobromide because of potentially additive effects.
- Tell patient that improvement may not be noticed for 1 to 4 weeks after therapy begins. Emphasize the importance of continuing therapy as prescribed.
- If patient (particularly a child or an adolescent) takes drug for depression, urge caregivers to watch closely for suicidal tendencies, especially when therapy starts or dosage changes.
- Warn patient not to stop taking drug abruptly. Explain that gradual tapering helps to avoid withdrawal symptoms.
- Urge patient to inform prescriber of any OTC drugs he takes because of potential for interactions.
- Review signs and symptoms of hyponatremia, and instruct patient to report them to prescriber.
- Advise patient that drug may cause mild pupillary dilation, which may lead to an episode of acute-angle glaucoma. Encourage patient to have an eye exam before starting therapy to see if he is at risk.
- Warn patient that escitalopram increases bleeding risk if taken with aspirin, an NSAID, or an anticoagulants and that bleeding events could range from mild to severe. Tell patient to seek emergency care for serious or prolonged bleeding.

eslicarbazepine acetate
Aptiom

Class and Category
Chemical class: Carboxamide derivative
Therapeutic class: Anticonvulsant
Pregnancy category: C

Indications and Dosages
➤ *Adjunct to treat of partial-onset seizures*

TABLETS
Adults. *Initial*: 400 mg once daily, increased to 800 mg once daily in 1 wk, followed by increase to 1,200 mg once daily in 1 or more wk, if needed. *Maintenance*: 800 mg once daily. *Maximum*: 1,200 mg once daily.
DOSAGE ADJUSTMENT For patients with moderate and severe renal impairment, dosage decreased by half beginning with initial dosage.

Mechanism of Action
Possibly inhibits voltage-gated sodium channels to exert anticonvulsant effect.

Contraindications
Hypersensitivity to eslicarbazepine acetate or oxcarbazepine and their components

Interaction
DRUGS
carbamazepine: Decreased plasma concentration of eslicarbazepine; increased adverse effects
clobazam, omeprazole, phenytoin: Increased plasma levels of these drugs
oral contraceptives: Decreased effectiveness of oral contraceptives
phenobarbital, phenytoin, primidone: Decreased plasma concentration of eslicarbazepine
rosuvastatin, simvastatin: Decreased plasma concentration of simvastatin
warfarin: Difficulty maintaining adequate INR level

Adverse Reactions
CNS: Amnesia, aphasia, asthenia, ataxia, attention deficits, confusion, coordination abnormality, depression, disorientation, dizziness, fatigue, gait disturbance,

headache, insomnia, lethargy, malaise, memory impairment, psychomotor disturbances, somnolence, suicidal ideation, tremor, vertigo
CV: Hypertension, peripheral edema
EENT: Blurred vision, diplopia, impaired vision, nystagmus
ENDO: Decreased serum T3 and T4 levels
GI: Abdominal pain, constipation, diarrhea, elevated liver enzymes, gastritis, liver dysfunction, nausea, vomiting
GU: UTI
MS: Dysarthria
RESP: Cough
SKIN: Rash, Stevens-Johnson syndrome, toxic epidermal necrolysis
Other: Anaphylaxis, angioedema, drug reaction with eosinophilia and systemic symptoms (DRESS), hypochloremia, hyponatremia

Nursing Considerations

• Monitor patient closely for adverse reactions because many of them are serious and some can become life threatening, such as DRESS multi-organ hypersensitivity.
• Monitor patient closely for evidence of suicidal thinking or behavior, especially when therapy starts or dosage changes.
• Monitor patient's electrolytes, especially sodium level, as ordered. Hyponatremia may occur as an adverse reaction to eslicarbazepine therapy, especially in the elderly and patients treated with diuretics. Assess patient regularly for signs and symptoms of hyponatremia such as confusion, difficulty concentrating, headache, memory impairment, unsteadiness, and weakness. If present, notify prescriber and expect drug to be discontinued.
• Withdraw eslicarbazepine slowly when discontinued and as ordered to minimize risk of seizures and status epilepticus.

PATIENT TEACHING
• Instruct patient to take eslicarbazepine exactly as prescribed and not to abruptly stop taking drug without consulting prescriber.
• Warn patient about possible dizziness and unsteadiness that may develop while taking eslicarbazepine. Discourage performing hazardous activities such as

driving until the neurologic effects of the drug are known.
WARNING Tell patient to discontinue drug immediately and seek emergency medical care if patient develops difficulty breathing, fever, or a rash or experiences facial or throat swelling.
• Instruct caregivers to watch patient closely for evidence of suicidal tendencies, especially when therapy starts or dosage changes, and to report such tendencies to prescriber immediately.
• Tell female patients taking oral contraceptives to use additional or alternative nonhormonal birth control. Encourage patient to enroll in the North American Antiepileptic Drug Pregnancy Registry if pregnancy occurs, by calling 1-888-233-2334.
• Advise patient to report symptoms of low sodium such as confusion, irritability, muscle weakness or spasms, tiredness, or more frequent or severe seizure activity.

---

esmolol hydrochloride
Brevibloc

Class and Category
Chemical class: Beta blocker
Therapeutic class: Antiarrhythmic, anti-hypertensive
Pregnancy category: C

Indications and Dosages
➤ *To treat supraventricular tachycardia*
I.V. INFUSION
Adults. *Loading:* 500 mcg/kg over 1 min. *Maintenance:* If response to loading dose is adequate after 5 min, 50 mcg/kg/min infused for 4 min. If response is inadequate after 5 min, another 500 mcg/kg may be given over 1 min followed by 100 mcg/kg/min for 4 min. Sequence repeated, as needed, until adequate response occurs, increasing maintenance dosage by 50 mcg/kg/min at each step. *Maximum:* 200 mcg/kg/min for 48 hr.
Children. 50 mcg/kg/min titrated every 10 min up to 300 mcg/kg/min.
➤ *To treat intraoperative and postoperative tachycardia and hypertension*

E
F

I.V. INFUSION
Adults. *Initial:* 250 to 500 mcg/kg over 1 min. *Maintenance:* 50 mcg/kg/min infused over 4 min. If response is inadequate after 5 min, another 250 to 500 mcg/kg may be given over 1 min followed by 100 mcg/kg/min for 4 min. Sequence repeated, as needed, up to 4 times, increasing by 50 mcg/kg/min each time. *Maximum:* 200 mcg/kg/min for 48 hr.

DOSAGE ADJUSTMENT Loading doses omitted, increments decreased to 25 mcg/kg/min, and titration intervals increased to 10 min as heart rate approaches desired level or if blood pressure decreases too much.

Route	Onset	Peak	Duration
I.V.	Immediate	Unknown	10–20 min

Mechanism of Action
Inhibits stimulation of beta$_1$ receptors mainly in the heart, which decreases cardiac excitability, cardiac output, and myocardial oxygen demand. Esmolol also decreases renin release from kidneys, which helps reduce blood pressure.

Incompatibilities
Don't mix esmolol with 5% sodium bicarbonate injection.

Contraindications
Cardiogenic shock, hypersensitivity to beta blockers, overt heart failure, second- or third-degree heart block, sinus bradycardia

Interactions
DRUGS
antihypertensives: Possibly hypotension
insulin, oral antidiabetics: Possibly masking of signs and symptoms of hypoglycemia caused by these drugs
MAO inhibitors: Possibly severe hypertension if esmolol is given within 14 days of discontinuing MAO inhibitor therapy
neuromuscular blockers: Possibly potentiated and prolonged action of these drugs
phenytoin: Possibly increased cardiac depression
reserpine: Possibly bradycardia and hypotension
sympathomimetics, xanthine derivatives: Possibly inhibited therapeutic effects of both drugs

Adverse Reactions
CNS: Anxiety, confusion, depression, dizziness, fatigue, fever, headache, syncope
CV: Bradycardia, chest pain, decreased peripheral circulation, heart block, hypotension
GI: Nausea, vomiting
RESP: Dyspnea, wheezing
SKIN: Diaphoresis, flushing, pallor
Other: Infusion site pain, redness, and swelling

Nursing Considerations
• Use esmolol cautiously if patient has supraventricular arrhythmias with decreased cardiac output, hypotension, or other hemodynamic compromise or is taking drugs that decrease peripheral resistance or myocardial filling, contractility, or impulse generation.
• Also use drug cautiously in patients with impaired renal function because drug is excreted by the kidneys. Patients with end-stage renal disease have an increased risk of adverse reactions.
• Avoid giving esmolol for intraoperative or postoperative hypertension caused by hypothermia-induced vasoconstriction.
• Expect to give lowest possible dose to patients with allergies, asthma, bronchitis, or emphysema. If patient develops broncho-spasm, expect to discontinue infusion immediately and give a beta$_2$-stimulating drug, as ordered.
• Don't give 250 mg/ml (2,500 mg/10 ml) dosage strength by direct I.V. push. Dilute it to a 10-mg/ml infusion by first removing 20 ml from 500 ml of a compatible I.V. solution, such as D$_5$W or dextrose 5% in normal saline solution, and then adding 5 g of esmolol to the solution.
• Use diluted solution within 24 hours if stored at room temperature.
• Use 100-mg vial (prediluted to 10 mg/ml) for loading dose. For 70-kg (154-lb) patient, loading dose for 500 mcg/kg/min is 3.5 ml.
• Monitor blood pressure and heart rate often during therapy. Hypotension can occur at any dose but usually is dose related. It typically reverses within 30 minutes after dose is decreased or infusion stopped.
• Inspect site often for thrombophlebitis (pain, redness, swelling at site). Infusion of 20 mg/ml is more likely to cause serious

vein irritation than 10 mg/ml.
Extravasation of 20 mg/ml may cause a
serious local reaction and skin necrosis.
Don't give more than 10 mg/ml into a
small vein or using a butterfly catheter.
PATIENT TEACHING
• Urge patient to report adverse reactions
immediately.
• Reassure patient that his blood pressure,
heart rate, and response to therapy will
be monitored throughout esmolol
therapy.

esomeprazole magnesium

Nexium, Nexium 24 HR, Nexium I.V.

esomeprazole strontium

Esomeprazole strontium

Class and Category
Chemical class: Substituted benzimidazole
Therapeutic class: Antiulcerative
Pregnancy category: C

Indications and Dosages
➤ *To treat gastroesophageal reflux disease
(GERD)*
**DELAYED-RELEASE CAPSULES, DELAYED-RELEASE
SUSPENSION (NEXIUM)**
Adults. 20 mg daily for 4 wk. *Maintenance:*
20 mg daily for up to 6 mo.
Adolescents ages 12 to 17. 20 mg once
daily for 4 wk.
Children ages 1 to 11. 10 mg once daily for
up to 8 wk.
**DELAYED-RELEASE CAPSULES (ESOMEPRAZOLE
STRONTIUM)**
Adults. 24.65 mg once daily for 4 wks.
➤ *To promote healing of erosive
esophagitis*
**DELAYED-RELEASE CAPSULES, DELAYED-RELEASE
SUSPENSION NEXIUM)**
Adults. 20 or 40 mg once daily for 4 to 8
wk, with cycle repeated once more if
healing has not taken place after first 8 wk.
Maintenance: 20 mg once daily
Adolescents ages 12 to 17. 20 or 40 mg
once daily for 4 to 8 wk.

**Children ages 1 to 11 weighing 20 kg or
more.** 10 or 20 mg once daily for 8 wk.
**Children ages 1 to 11 weighing less than
20 kg.** 10 mg once daily for 8 wk.
**Infants age 1 month to less than 1 year
weighing 7.5 to 12 kg.** 10 mg once daily for
up to 6 wk.
**Infants age 1 month to less than 1 year
weighing 5 kg to 7.5 kg.** 5 mg once daily
for up to 6 wk.
**Infants age 1 month to less than 1 year
weighing 3 to 5 kg.** 1.5 mg once daily for
up to 6 wk.
**DELAYED-RELEASE CAPSULES (ESOMEPRAZOLE
STRONTIUM)**
Adults. 24.65 mg or 49.3 mg once daily for 4
to 8 wks. *Maintenance:* 24.65 mg once daily.
➤ *To treat GERD in a patient with a
history of erosive esophagitis who can't
take the drug by mouth*
I.V. INFUSION
Adults. 20 to 40 mg daily infused over 10
to 30 min.
Children weighing 55 kg (121 lbs) or more.
20 mg daily infused over 10 to 30 min.
**Children weighing less than 55 kg (121
lbs).** 10 mg daily infused over 10 to 30 min.
Children ages 1 month to less than 1 year.
0.5 mg/kg daily infused over 10 to 30 min.
DOSAGE ADJUSTMENT For adult patient with
severe liver impairment, dosage should not
exceed 20 mg daily.
I.V. INJECTION
Adults. 20 or 40 mg daily given over no less
than 3 min.
➤ *As adjunct to treat duodenal or gastric
ulcer associated with* Helicobacter
pylori
DELAYED-RELEASE CAPSULES (NEXIUM)
Adults. 40 mg daily with amoxicillin 1,000
mg twice a day and clarithromycin 500 mg
twice a day for 10 days.
➤ *As adjunct to treat duodenal ulcer
associated with* Helicobacter pylori
**DELAYED-RELEASE CAPSULES (ESOMEPRAZOLE
STRONTIUM)**
Adults. 49.3 mg once daily with amoxicillin
1,000 mg twice daily and clarithromycin
500 mg twice daily for 10 days.
➤ *To reduce the risk of gastric ulcer
formation in patients who are receiving
continuous NSAID therapy and who
either are over age 60 or have a history
of gastric ulcer*

E
F

DELAYED-RELEASE CAPSULES (NEXIUM)
Adults. 20 or 40 mg daily for up to 6 mo.
DELAYED-RELEASE CAPSULES (ESOMEPRAZOLE STRONTIUM)
Adults. 24.65 mg or 49.3 mg once daily for up to 6 months
➤ *To treat pathological hypersecretory conditions, including Zollinger-Ellison syndrome*
DELAYED-RELEASE CAPSULES
Adults. 40 mg twice daily.
DOSAGE ADJUSTMENT For patients with severe hepatic insufficiency, maximum 20 mg daily.
DELAYED-RELEASE CAPSULES (ESOMEPRAZOLE STRONTIUM)
Adults. 49.3 mg twice daily.
➤ *To reduce risk of rebleeding of duodenal or gastric ulcers following therapeutic endoscopy for acute-bleeding duodenal or gastric ulcers*
I.V. INFUSION
Adults. 80 mg over 30 min followed by 8 mg per hour for 71.5 hr after initial 30-min dose is completed.
DOSAGE ADJUSTMENT For patients with mild to moderate liver impairment, maximum continuous infusion should not exceed 6 mg/hr; for patients with severe liver impairment, maximum continuous infusion should not exceed 4 mg/hr.

Mechanism of Action

Interferes with gastric acid secretion by inhibiting the hydrogen-potassium-adenosine triphosphatase (H^+-K^+-ATPase) enzyme system, or proton pump, in gastric parietal cells. Normally, the proton pump uses energy from hydrolysis of ATPase to drive H^+ and chloride (Cl^-) out of parietal cells and into the stomach lumen in exchange for potassium (K^+), which leaves the stomach lumen and enters parietal cells. After this exchange, H^+ and Cl^- combine in the stomach to form hydrochloric acid (HCl). Esomeprazole irreversibly inhibits the final step in gastric acid production by blocking exchange of intracellular H^+ and extracellular K^+, thus preventing H^+ from entering the stomach and additional HCl from forming.

Incompatibilities

Don't give esomeprazole with any other drug through the same I.V. site or tubing.

Contraindications

Hypersensitivity to esomeprazole, substituted benzimidazoles, or their components

Interactions

DRUGS
antimicrobials: Increased esomeprazole level
atazanavir, erlotinib, ketoconazole, iron salts, mycophenolate mofetil, nelfinavir: Decreased blood levels of these drugs
cilostazol: Possibly increased blood cilostazol levels
clopidogrel: Reduced effectiveness of clopidogrel
diazepam: Possibly increased diazepam level
digoxin: Possibly increased absorption of digoxin
digoxin, diuretics: Increased risk of hypomagnesemia
methotrexate: Increased risk of methotrexate toxicities
rifampin, St. John's Wort: Decreased blood esomeprazole level
saquinavir: Increased plasma saquinavir level with increased toxicity
tacrolimus: Increased serum tacrolimus level
voriconazole: Increased esomeprazole exposure and risk of adverse effects
warfarin: Possibly increased INR and PT, leading to abnormal bleeding
FOODS
all foods: Decreased bioavailability of esomeprazole

Adverse Reactions

CNS: Agitation, aggression, depression, dizziness, fever, headache, hallucinations, hepatic encephalopathy
EENT: Blurred vision, dry mouth, mucosal discoloration, sinusitis, stomatitis, taste disturbance
ENDO: Gynecomastia
GI: Abdominal pain; Barrett's esophagus; benign polyps or nodules; candidiasis; *Clostridium difficile*-associated diarrhea; constipation; diarrhea; duodenitis; dyspepsia; esophagitis; esophageal stricture, ulceration, or varices; flatulence; gastric ulcer; gastritis; hepatic failure; hepatitis; jaundice; microscopic colitis; nausea; pancreatitis
GU: Interstitial nephritis

HEME: Agranulocytosis, pancytopenia
MS: Bone fracture, muscle weakness, myalgia
RESP: Bronchospasm, respiratory tract infection
SKIN: Alopecia, diaphoresis, erythema multiforme, photosensitivity, pruritus, Stevens-Johnson syndrome, toxic epidermal necrolysis
Other: Anaphylaxis, cyanocobalamin deficiency (prolonged use), hypomagnesemia, infusion-site redness or pruritus

Nursing Considerations

• Give oral esomeprazole at least 1 hour before meals because food decreases bioavailability.
• Use delayed-release capsules or oral suspension specific for nasogastric tube administration and delayed-release oral suspension specific for nasogastric or gastric tube administration when administering esomeprazole to a patient with a nasogastric or gastric tube.
WARNING If patient takes drug with amoxicillin or clarithromycin for *H. pylori*–related ulcer, severe diarrhea may indicate pseudomembranous colitis. Obtain stool cultures, as ordered.
• Always flush I.V. line with normal saline solution injection, lactated Ringer's injection, or 5% dextrose injection before and after giving esomeprazole intravenously.
• For I.V. injection used to treat GERD in patients who cannot take oral esomeprazole, reconstitute powder with 5 ml of normal saline solution injection and give as a bolus dose over 3 or more minutes. Once reconstituted, drug may be stored at room temperature for up to 12 hours.
• For I.V. infusion for adults treated for GERD and unable to take esomeprazole by mouth, reconstitute powder with 5 ml of normal saline solution injection, lactated Ringer's injection, or 5% dextrose injection. Further dilute reconstituted solution to make a final volume of 50 ml, and infuse over 10 to 30 minutes. Reconstituted drug may be stored at room temperature up to 6 hours if mixed with 5% dextrose injection or up to 12 hours if

mixed with normal saline solution or lactated Ringer's injection.
• For I.V. infusion for children treated for GERD who are unable to take esomeprazole by mouth, reconstitute powder with 5 ml of 0.9% sodium chloride injection. Further dilute reconstituted solution with 0.9% sodium chloride injection to make final volume of 50 ml. Using a 40 mg vial, the final concentration will be 0.8 mg/ml. Using a 20-mg vial, the final concentration will be 0.4 mg/ml. Infuse over 10 to 30 minutes. Reconstituted drug may be stored at room temperature for up to 12 hours.
• For I.V. infusion used for adults to reduce risk of rebleeding of duodenal or gastric ulcers following therapeutic endoscopy, prepare the loading dose of 80 mg by reconstituting two 40-mg vials. Reconstitute each vial with 5 ml of 0.9% sodium chloride injection, then further dilute the contents of the two vials in 100 ml of 0.9% sodium chloride injection. Administer over 30 minutes. Prepare the continuous infusion in the same manner but administer over 71.5 hours at a rate of 8 mg/hr or decrease rate to 6 mg/hr for mild to moderate liver impairment and to 4 mg/hr for severe liver impairment, as ordered.
• Be aware that patient receiving I.V. esomeprazole should be switched to oral form as soon as possible.
• Monitor patients for bone fractures, especially in patients who are receiving multiple daily doses for a year or longer as proton pump inhibitors such as esomeprazole have been associated with an increased risk for osteoporosis-related fractures of the hip, wrist, or spine.
• Monitor patient's magnesium level, as ordered, because hypomagnesemia may occur with esomeprazole therapy that has lasted longer than 3 months, although most cases have occurred after therapy had been given for more than a year. Notify prescriber if magnesium level drops below normal as hypomagnesemia may cause tetany, arrhythmias and seizures. Expect patient to receive magnesium replacement and esomeprazole to be discontinued.

E
F

• Be aware that esomeprazole therapy may need to be temporarily halted for at least 14 days if patient is undergoing testing for neuroendocrine tumors because drug may cause false positive results in diagnostic testing.

• Monitor patient for diarrhea, especially in the hospitalized patient because esomeprazole therapy may increase the risk of *Clostridium difficile* associated diarrhea. If diarrhea occurs, expect to obtain a stool specimen to determine if diarrhea is *C. difficile* so that it may be treated appropriately.

PATIENT TEACHING

• If patient has trouble swallowing esomeprazole capsules, tell him to open capsule and sprinkle pellets into a tablespoon of cool applesauce. Tell him not to chew pellets and to discard any unused pellets.

• Remind patient that esomeprazole, including the over-the-counter preparation, is not intended for immediate relief of heartburn; the drug may take up to 4 days before the full effect is experienced.

• Urge patient to tell prescriber if he takes antacids.

• Advise patient to contact prescriber if he develops diarrhea, abdominal pain, and fever that does not improve especially if he has recently taken or is taking an antibiotic.

estazolam

Class, Category, and Schedule

Chemical class: Benzodiazepine
Therapeutic class: Sedative-hypnotic
Pregnancy category: X
Controlled substance schedule: IV

Indications and Dosages

➤ *To treat insomnia*

TABLETS

Adults. 1 to 2 mg at bedtime.

DOSAGE ADJUSTMENT Starting dose 0.5 mg for small or debilitated elderly patients.

Route	Onset	Peak	Duration
P.O.	Unknown	Unknown	6–8 hr

Mechanism of Action

May potentiate effects of gamma-amino-butyric acid (GABA) and other inhibitory neurotransmitters by binding to specific benzodiazepine receptors in limbic and cortical areas of CNS. By binding to these receptors, estazolam increases GABA's inhibitory effects and blocks cortical and limbic arousal.

Contraindications

Acute angle-closure glaucoma; hypersensitivity to estazolam, other benzodiazepines, or their components; pregnancy; psychosis

Interactions

DRUGS

barbiturates, carbamazepine, phenytoin, rifampin: Possibly decreased estazolam level
carbamazepine: Possibly increased blood carbamazepine level
cimetidine, diltiazem, disulfiram, erythromycin, fluoxetine, fluvoxamine, isoniazid, itraconazole, ketoconazole, nefazodone, oral contraceptives, propoxyphene, ranitidine, verapamil: Possibly increased blood level and impaired hepatic metabolism of estazolam
clozapine: Possibly cardiac arrest or respiratory depression
CNS depressants: Possibly potentiated CNS depression
levodopa: Possibly decreased therapeutic effects of levodopa

FOODS

grapefruit juice: Possibly increased blood level and impaired hepatic metabolism of drug

ACTIVITIES

alcohol use: Possibly potentiated CNS depression

Adverse Reactions

CNS: Amnesia, anxiety, ataxia, confusion, delusions, depression, dizziness, drowsiness, euphoria, headache, hypokinesia, irritability, malaise, nervousness, slurred speech, tremor
CV: Chest pain, palpitations, tachycardia
EENT: Blurred vision, dry mouth, increased salivation, photophobia
GI: Abdominal pain, constipation, diarrhea, nausea, thirst, vomiting
GU: Libido changes
RESP: Respiratory depression
SKIN: Diaphoresis
Other: Physical or psychological dependence

Nursing Considerations
• Use estazolam with extreme caution in patients with a history of drug or alcohol abuse because of risk of addiction. Expect to give drug for no more than 12 weeks.
• Use cautiously in elderly or debilitated patients and those with depression orimpaired hepatic, renal, or respiratory function.
• Expect to stop drug gradually to prevent withdrawal symptoms. Avoid stopping abruptly if patient has history of seizures.
• Monitor respiratory status, especially in patients with respiratory compromise, who are at increased risk for respiratory depression.
• If patient takes estazolam for depression, watch for suicidal tendencies, especially when therapy starts or dosage changes.

PATIENT TEACHING
• Warn patient not to exceed prescribed time because of risk of addiction.
• Because estazolam can reduce alertness, advise patient to avoid hazardous activities until CNS effects of the drug are known.
• Advise patient not to drink alcohol or take other CNS depressants during therapy because of the risk of additive effects.
• Warn elderly and debilitated patients and those with impaired hepatic or renal function about risk of excessive sedation or mental impairment and need to report them.
• If patient takes 2-mg dosage for a long time, warn against stopping drug abruptly.

estradiol
Estrace, Estrasorb, Estring, Estrogel, Evamist, Vagifem

estradiol acetate
Femring, Femtrace

estradiol cypionate
depGynogen, Depo-Estradiol, Depogen, Dura-Estrin, E-Cypionate, Estragyn LA 5, Estro-Cyp, Estrofem, Estro-L.A.

estradiol transdermal system
Alora, Climara, Esclim, Estraderm, Estrasorb, Estrogel, FemPatch, Menostar, Minivelle, Vivelle, Vivelle-Dot

estradiol valerate
Clinagen LA 40, Delestrogen, Dioval 40, Dioval XX, Duragen-20, Estra-L 40, Estro-Span, Femogex (CAN), Gynogen L.A. 20, Gynogen L.A. 40, Menaval-20, Valergen 10, Valergen 20, Valergen 40

ethinyl estradiol
Estinyl

E
F

Class and Category
Chemical class: Estrogen derivative, steroid hormone
Therapeutic class: Antineoplastic, antiosteoporotic agent, ovarian hormone replacement
Pregnancy category: X

Indications and Dosages
➤ *To treat menopausal symptoms*
TABLETS (ESTRADIOL)
Adult menopausal and postmenopausal women. Starting on day 5 of a cycle, 0.5 to 2 mg daily in cycles of 3 wk on, 1 wk off.
Adult postmenopausal women with intact uterus receiving progestin. 0.5 to 2 mg daily with daily progestin. Or, 0.5 to 2 mg daily on days 1 through 25 of a 28-day cycle, with progestin starting day 12 or 16 and continuing through day 25 of the cycle; then no drugs on days 26 through 28, as prescribed.
VAGINAL RING (ESTRADIOL ACETATE [FEMRING])
Adult women. One ring (0.05 mg or 0.1 mg of estradiol/24 hr) inserted into upper third of vaginal vault and replaced every 3 mo.
TABLETS (ESTRADIOL ACETATE [FEMTRACE])
Adult menopausal and postmenopausal women. *Initial:* 0.45 mg daily. May be increased to 0.9 mg daily and then 1.8 mg daily as needed.
TABLETS (ETHINYL ESTRADIOL)
Adult menopausal and postmenopausal women. 0.02 to 0.05 mg daily in cycles of 3 wk on, 1 wk off.

Adult postmenopausal women with intact uterus receiving progestin. 0.02 to 0.05 mg daily with daily progestin; or 0.02 to 0.05 mg daily on days 1 through 25 of a 28-day cycle, with progestin starting day 12 or 16 and continuing through day 25; then no drugs on days 26 through 28, as prescribed.

DOSAGE ADJUSTMENT Dosage may be reduced to less than 1 mg daily (estradiol) or 0.05 mg daily (ethinyl estradiol) for patients with only vaginal or vulvar symptoms.

I.M. INJECTION (ESTRADIOL CYPIONATE IN OIL)
Adult women. 1 to 5 mg as a single dose every 3 to 4 wk as needed.

I.M. INJECTION (ESTRADIOL VALERATE IN OIL)
Adult women. 10 to 20 mg every 4 wk as needed.

TRANSDERMAL (ALORA, ESTRADERM, VIVELLE, VIVELLE-DOT)
Adult menopausal and postmenopausal women. *Initial:* 0.025 to 0.05 mg daily in cycles of 3 wk on, 1 wk off. One patch applied to trunk or buttocks and replaced twice/wk (every 3 to 4 days). Adjust dosage to control symptoms, as prescribed.

TRANSDERMAL (CLIMARA)
Adult women. *Initial:* 0.025 mg daily. One patch applied to trunk or buttocks, replaced every wk. Titrate dosage to control symptoms, as prescribed. Schedule will be cyclic unless patient has had a hysterectomy.

TRANSDERMAL (ESCLIM)
Adult women. *Initial:* 0.025 mg daily. One patch applied to upper arm, upper thigh, or buttocks and replaced twice/wk (every 3 to 4 days). Adjust dosage to control symptoms, as prescribed. Use a cyclic schedule, as prescribed, unless patient has had a hysterectomy.

TRANSDERMAL (ESTRASORB)
Adult women. 3.48 g daily in morning. Half of dose (1 pouchful) applied to one thigh and rubbed over entire thigh and calf for 3 min, repeated on other thigh and calf.

TRANSDERMAL (ESTROGEL)
Adult women. 1.25 g daily applied in thin layer from wrist to shoulder on inside and outside of one arm.

TRANSDERMAL (FEMPATCH)
Adult women. *Initial:* 0.025 mg daily. One patch applied to buttocks and replaced every wk. If symptoms aren't relieved after 4 to 6 wk, increased to two patches every wk, as prescribed. Follow a cyclic schedule, as prescribed, unless patient has had a hysterectomy.

TRANSDERMAL MIST (EVAMIST)
Adult women. *Initial:* 1.53 mg (1 spray) once daily in the morning. Dosage may be increased to 3.06 mg (2 sprays) once daily in the morning and then to 4.59 mg (3 sprays) once daily in the morning as needed.

➤ *To treat menopausal symptoms as combination therapy in patients with an intact uterus*

TRANSDERMAL ESTRADIOL (ALORA, ESTRADERM, VIVELLE, VIVELLE-DOT), IN COMBINATION WITH ESTRADIOL AND NORETHINDRONE ACETATE (COMBIPATCH)
Adult women. 0.05 mg daily estradiol-only transdermal system applied for first 14 days of 28-day cycle and replaced twice/wk, according to product directions. Estradiol and norethindrone acetate transdermal system applied for remaining 14 days of 28-day cycle and replaced twice/wk during this period.

➤ *To treat postmenopausal vaginal and urogenital symptoms*

VAGINAL CREAM (ESTRACE)
Adult women. *Initial:* 2 to 4 g (200 to 400 mcg) daily for 1 to 2 wk. Then, dosage gradually reduced to half of initial dose, as prescribed, for 1 to 2 wk. *Maintenance:* 1 g (100 mcg) daily 1 to 3 times/wk for 3 wk, followed by 1 wk of no drugs. Repeat cyclically as needed.

VAGINAL RING (ESTRING)
Adult women. One ring (7.5 mcg of estradiol/24 hr) inserted into upper third of vaginal vault and replaced every 3 mo.

VAGINAL RING (FEMRING)
Adult women. One ring (0.05 or 0.1 mg of estradiol/24 hr) inserted into upper third of vaginal vault and replaced every 3 mo.

INTRAVAGINAL TABLETS (VAGIFEM)
Adult women. *Initial:* 10-mcg tablet daily for 2 wk, followed by 1 tablet twice weekly. Dosage increased to 25 mcg, as needed.

➤ *To treat moderate to severe vasomotor symptoms*

TRANSDERMAL (MINIVELLE)
Adult women. 0.0375 mg daily continuously. Patch replaced twice weekly.
➤ *To prevent osteoporosis secondary to estrogen deficiency due to either natural or surgical menopause*
TABLETS (ESTRADIOL)
Adult women. At least 0.5 mg daily cyclically or continuously, adjusted as needed to control concurrent menopausal symptoms, as prescribed.
TABLETS (ETHINYL ESTRADIOL)
Adult women. At least 0.02 mg daily cyclically or continuously, as prescribed.
TRANSDERMAL (ALORA, MINIVELLE, VIVELLE-DOT)
Adult women. *Initial:* 0.025 mg daily continuously. One patch applied to lower abdomen or buttocks and replaced twice/ wk. Adjust dosage to control symptoms and maintain bone density, as prescribed.
TRANSDERMAL (CLIMARA)
Adult women. *Initial:* 0.025 mg daily. One patch applied to trunk or buttocks and replaced every wk. Adjust dosage to control symptoms, as prescribed. Follow a cyclic schedule, as prescribed, unless patient has had a hysterectomy.
TRANSDERMAL (ESTRADERM)
Adult women. *Initial:* 0.05 mg daily. One patch applied to trunk or buttocks and replaced twice/wk. Adjust dosage to control symptoms, as prescribed. Follow a cyclic schedule, as prescribed, unless patient has had a hysterectomy.
TRANSDERMAL (MENOSTAR)
Adult women. *Initial:* 0.014 mg daily. One patch applied to lower abdomen and replaced every wk. Follow a cyclic schedule, as prescribed, unless patient has had a hysterectomy.
➤ *To treat estrogen deficiency due to oophorectomy, primary ovarian failure, or female hypogonadism*
TABLETS (ESTRADIOL)
Adult women. 0.5 to 2 mg daily continuously or in cycles of 3 wk on, 1 wk off.
TABLETS (ETHINYL ESTRADIOL)
Adult women. For primary ovarian failure or oophorectomy, 0.05 mg three times daily initially, then 0.05 mg daily after a few weeks, cyclically or continuously. For female hypogonadism, 0.05 mg once daily to three times daily for first 2 wk of a theoretical menstrual

cycle. A progestin may be added, as prescribed, during last half of cycle to help induce menses.
I.M. INJECTION (ESTRADIOL CYPIONATE IN OIL)
Adult women. 1.5 to 2 mg every mo (for female hypogonadism only).
I.M. INJECTION (ESTRADIOL VALERATE IN OIL)
Adult women. 10 to 20 mg every mo as needed.
TRANSDERMAL (ALORA, ESTRADERM, VIVELLE)
Adult women. *Initial:* 0.05 mg daily. One patch applied to trunk or buttocks and replaced twice/wk. Titrate dosage to control symptoms, as prescribed. Follow a cyclic schedule, as prescribed, unless patient has had a hysterectomy.
TRANSDERMAL (CLIMARA)
Adult women. *Initial:* 0.05 mg daily. One patch applied to trunk or buttocks and replaced every wk. Adjust dosage to control symptoms, as prescribed. Follow a cyclic schedule, as prescribed, unless patient has had a hysterectomy.
TRANSDERMAL (ESCLIM)
Adult women. *Initial:* 0.025 mg daily. One patch applied to upper arm, upper thigh, or buttocks and replaced twice/wk (every 3 to 4 days). Adjust dosage to control symptoms, as prescribed. Follow a cyclic schedule, as prescribed, unless patient has had a hysterectomy.
TRANSDERMAL (FEMPATCH)
Adult women. *Initial:* 0.025 mg. One patch applied to buttocks and replaced every wk. If symptoms aren't relieved after 4 to 6 wk, increased to two patches every wk, as prescribed. Follow a cyclic schedule unless patient has had a hysterectomy.
➤ *To treat dysfunctional uterine bleeding from hormonal imbalance in patients with hypoplastic or atrophic endometrium and without uterine disease*
TRANSDERMAL (CLIMARA)
Adult women. *Initial:* 0.05 mg daily. One patch applied to trunk or buttocks and replaced every wk. Adjust dosage to control symptoms, as prescribed. Follow a cyclic schedule, as prescribed.
TRANSDERMAL (FEMPATCH)
Adult women. *Initial:* 0.025 mg daily. One patch applied to buttocks and replaced every wk. If symptoms aren't relieved after

E
F

4 to 6 wk, increased to Two patches every wk, as prescribed. Follow a cyclic schedule, as prescribed.

➤ *To provide palliative treatment for inoperable, progressive breast cancer in selected men and postmenopausal women*

TABLETS (ESTRADIOL)

Adults. 10 mg three times daily for at least 3 mo.

TABLETS (ETHINYL ESTRADIOL)

Adults. 1 mg three times daily for at least 3 mo.

➤ *To treat advancing, inoperable prostate cancer*

TABLETS (ESTRADIOL)

Adult men. 1 to 2 mg twice daily or three times daily, adjusted or continued, as prescribed, according to patient response.

TABLETS (ETHINYL ESTRADIOL)

Adult men. 0.15 to 3 mg daily, adjusted or continued, as prescribed, according to patient response.

I.M. INJECTION (ESTRADIOL VALERATE)

Adult men. 30 mg every 1 to 2 wk, adjusted or continued, as prescribed, according to patient response.

Mechanism of Action

Increases the rate of DNA and RNA synthesis in cells of female reproductive organs, pituitary gland, hypothalamus, and other target organs. In the hypothalamus, estrogens reduce release of gonadotropin-releasing hormone, which decreases pituitary release of follicle-stimulating hormone and luteinizing hormone. In women, these hormones are required for normal genitourinary and other essential body functions.

At the cellular level, estrogens increase cervical secretions, cause endometrial cell proliferation, and improve uterine tone. Estrogen replacement helps maintain genitourinary function and reduces vasomotor symptoms when estrogen production declines as a result of menopause, surgical removal of ovaries, or other estrogen deficiency states. Estrogen replacement also helps prevent osteoporosis by inhibiting bone resorption.

In men, estrogens inhibit pituitary secretion of luteinizing hormone and decrease testicular secretion of testosterone. These actions may decrease prostate tumor growth and lower the level of prostate-specific antigen (PSA).

Contraindications

Active deep vein thrombosis, pulmonary embolism, or history of these conditions; active or recent (within past year) arterial thromboembolic disease, such as stroke or MI; hepatic dysfunction or disease; history of anaphylactic reaction or angioedema to estradiol; hypersensitivity to estradiol, ethinyl estradiol, or their components; hypersensitivity to tartrazine dye (contained in 0.02-mg estradiol and ethinyl estradiol tablets); known or suspected breast cancer or history of breast cancer except in appropriately selected patients being treated for metastatic disease; known or suspected estrogen-dependent cancer; known protein C, protein S, or antithrombin deficiency, or other known thrombophilic disorders; pregnancy; liver impairment or disease; undiagnosed abnormal genital bleeding

Interactions

DRUGS

aminocaproic acid: Possibly increased hypercoagulability caused by aminocaproic acid

barbiturates, carbamazepine, hydantoins, rifabutin, rifampin: Possibly reduced activity of estradiol

bromocriptine: Possibly decreased therapeutic effects of bromocriptine

calcium: Possibly increased calcium absorption

corticosteroids: Increased therapeutic and toxic effects of corticosteroids

cyclosporine: Increased risk of hepatotoxicity and nephrotoxicity

didanosine, lamivudine, zalcitabine: Possibly pancreatitis

hepatotoxic drugs, such as isoniazid: Increased risk of hepatitis and hepatotoxicity

oral antidiabetic drugs: Decreased therapeutic effects of these drugs

somatrem, somatropin: Possibly accelerated epiphyseal maturation

tamoxifen: Possibly decreased therapeutic effects of tamoxifen

thyroid hormone replacement: Decreased effectiveness

vitamin C: Decreased metabolism and possibly increased adverse effects of estradiol

warfarin: Decreased anticoagulant effect

FOODS

grapefruit juice: Decreased estradiol metabolism and possibly increased adverse effects

ACTIVITIES

smoking: Increased risk of stroke, pulmonary embolism, thrombophlebitis, and transient ischemic attack

Adverse Reactions

CNS: Affect liability, chorea, dementia, depression, dizziness, emotional lability, fatigue, headache, irritability, malaise, migraine headache, mood swings, nervousness, paresthesia, stroke

CV: Deep venous thrombosis, hypertension, MI, palpitations, peripheral edema, portal vein thrombosis, pulmonary embolism, thromboembolism, thrombophlebitis, unstable angina

EENT: Intolerance of contact lenses, oral paresthesia, pharyngeal edema, retinal vascular thrombosis, swollen lip or tongue, vision changes

ENDO: Breast enlargement, pain, tenderness, or tumors; breast cancer; fibrocystic breast changes; gynecomastia; hypercalcemia (presence of breast cancer and bone metastases); hyperglycemia; nipple discharge or nipple and areola discoloration

GI: Abdominal cramps or pain, anorexia, bloating, bowel obstruction (vaginal ring), cholelithiasis, constipation, diarrhea, elevated liver function test results, enlargement of hepatic hemangiomas, gallbladder disease or obstruction, hemorrhage, hepatitis, increased appetite, nausea, pancreatitis, vomiting

GU: Amenorrhea, breakthrough bleeding, cervical erosion, clear vaginal discharge, decreased libido (males), dysmenorrhea, endometrial cancer, impotence, increased libido (females), ovarian cancer, pelvic pain, prolonged or heavy menstrual bleeding, ring adherence, testicular atrophy, uterine leiomyomata, vaginitis, vaginal candidiasis, worsening of endometriosis

MS: Arthralgia, leg cramps, muscle spasms

RESP: Dyspnea, pulmonary embolism

SKIN: Acne, alopecia, diaphoresis, discoloration or dry skin, erythema multiforme or nodosum, facial pigmentation, hirsutism, jaundice, melasma, oily skin, prutitis, purpura, rash, seborrhea, urticaria

Other: Angioedema, application-site reactions (transdermal), folic acid deficiency, hypercalcemia (in metastatic bone disease), hypersensitivity, toxic shock syndrome (vaginal ring), weight gain or loss

Nursing Considerations

WARNING Be aware that estradiol (Estrace) and ethinyl estradiol (Estinyl) are distinct and separate products and that their dosing isn't equivalent.

• Use estradiol cautiously in patients with asthma, chorea, diabetes mellitus, epilepsy, migraine headaches, porphyria, systemic lupus erythematosus, or hepatic hemangiomas because estradiol may worsen these disorders.

• Administer oral preparations with or immediately after food to decrease nausea.

• For I.M. injection of estradiol cypionate or estradiol valerate, roll vial and syringe between palms to evenly disperse drug. Use at least a 21G needle because of viscosity of oil-based solution. Use a dry, sterile syringe. Inject deep into upper outer quadrant of gluteal muscle. Aspirate before injection to avoid injection into a blood vessel.

• Be aware that in patients who are converting from oral estrogen to transdermal system, oral estrogen should be stopped 1 week before skin patches are applied.

• Expect to begin prophylaxis treatment against osteoporosis at the start of menopause.

• Be aware that estrogen therapy should be given cyclically or combined with a progestin for 10 to 14 days per month in women with an intact uterus to minimize the risk of endometrial hyperplasia.

WARNING Be aware that severe hypercalcemia may occur in patients with bone metastasis due to breast cancer because estrogens influence the metabolism of calcium and phosphorus. Monitor for toxic effects of increased calcium absorption in patients who are predisposed to hypercalcemia or nephrolithiasis.

WARNING Assess patient for possible contact lens intolerance or changes in vision or visual acuity because estrogens can cause

E
F

keratoconus, leading to increased curvature of the cornea. Be prepared to discontinue drug immediately, as prescribed, if patient experiences sudden partial or complete loss of vision or sudden onset of diplopia, migraine, or proptosis.

• Monitor PT test results of patients receiving warfarin for loss of anticoagulant effect because estrogens increase production of clotting factors VII, VIII, IX, and X and promote platelet aggregation.

• Watch for elevated liver function test results because estrogens may worsen such conditions as acute intermittent or variegate hepatic porphyria.

• Closely monitor patient's blood pressure. A few patients may experience a substantial increase in blood pressure as an idiosyncratic reaction to estrogen. Monitor patients who already have hypertension for increases in blood pressure because estrogens may cause fluid retention. Also monitor patients with asthma, heart disease, migraines, renal disease, or seizure disorder for exacerbation of these conditions.

• Watch for peripheral edema or mild weight gain because estrogens can cause sodium and fluid retention.

• Frequently monitor serum glucose level in patients who have diabetes mellitus because estrogens may decrease insulin sensitivity and alter glucose tolerance.

WARNING Expect to stop estrogen therapy in any woman who develops signs or symptoms of cancer; cardiovascular disease, such as stroke, MI, pulmonary embolism, or venous thrombosis; or dementia.

• Be aware that exogenous estradiol and progestins may worsen mood disorders, including depression. Monitor patient for anxiety, depression, dizziness, fatigue, insomnia, or mood changes.

• Assess skin for melasma (tan or brown patches), which may develop on forehead, cheeks, temples, and upper lip. These patches may persist after drug is stopped.

• Check patient's triglyceride level routinely because, in patients with hypertriglyceridemia, estrogen therapy may increase serum triglyceride level enough to cause pancreatitis and other complications.

• Monitor serum PSA level in patients with inoperable prostate cancer to determine if patient is responding to hormone therapy. If patient responds (usually within 3 months), expect therapy to continue until disease is significantly advanced.

• Monitor thyroid function test results in patients with hypothyroidism because long-term use of ethinyl estradiol may decrease effectiveness of thyroid therapy.

• Expect to stop estrogen therapy several weeks before patient undergoes major surgery, as prescribed, because certain procedures are associated with prolonged immobilization and therefore pose a risk of thromboembolism.

• If patient takes thyroid hormone replacement therapy, monitor her for increased signs and symptoms of hypothyroidism because estradiol may increase thyroid binding globulin levels, which may make the patient's current dose of thyroid hormone insufficient.

WARNING Monitor patient closely for signs of anaphylaxis, which may occur any time during therapy and may require emergency medical treatment. Monitor patient with history of hereditary angioedema closely because estradiol may exacerbate symptoms of angioedema.

PATIENT TEACHING

• Before therapy starts, inform patient of risks involved in estrogen therapy, such as increased risk of breast, endometrial, or ovarian cancer; cardiovascular disease; dementia (if age 65 or over); gallbladder disease; and vision abnormalities.

• Advise patient to remain recumbent for at least 30 minutes after applying estradiol vaginal cream. Inform her that she may use a sanitary napkin (but not a tampon) to protect clothing after application.

• Teach patient proper application and use of transdermal patch. Instruct her not to apply patch to breasts, waistline, or other areas where it may not adhere properly. Advise her to rotate application sites at least weekly and to remove old patch before applying new one. If patch falls off, instruct her to reapply it to another area or to apply a new patch and continue the original treatment schedule. Caution her not to expose patch to sun for long periods. Explain that she may bathe while wearing the patch.

• Teach patient to apply Estrogel to clean, dry skin of one arm, using applicator. Emphasize importance of transferring all of the gel from applicator to arm. Tell patient to spread gel as thinly as possible over entire inside and outside of arm from wrist to shoulder. Advise her to wash her hands with soap and water afterward and to avoid fire and smoking until gel has dried because it's flammable. Tell patient never to apply gel to breasts. Warn that gel is alcohol-based and that patient should avoid fire, flame, or smoking until gel has dried.

• Inform patient that each pouch of Estrasorb contains half of daily dose. Instruct her to apply emulsion to clean, dry skin on top of thigh and to rub it into entire thigh and calf for 3 minutes. Tell her to rub any excess emulsion onto her buttocks. Then, advise her to repeat procedure on her other thigh and calf using the second pouch. Tell her to wash her hands with soap and water after the application and to dress only after affected areas are dry.

• Teach patient proper use of estradiol vaginal ring. Instruct her to insert ring in upper third of vagina, to keep it there for 90 days, and then to remove it and insert a new ring. Or she may remove it during the 90-day dosage period, rinse it with lukewarm (not hot or boiling) water, and reinsert it as needed for personal hygiene. Remind patient that she shouldn't be able to feel the ring when it's in place. If she does, she should use a finger to push the ring farther into her vagina. If vaginal wall ulceration or erosion occurs, suggest that patient leave ring out and not replace it until healing is complete to keep ring from adhering to healing tissue.

• Instruct patient using estradiol vaginal ring to remove ring immediately and contact prescriber if she develops fever, nausea, vomiting, diarrhea, muscle pain, dizziness, faintness, or a sunburn rash on face or body that may suggest a rare but serious bacterial infection called toxic shock syndrome. Also urge patient to seek prompt medical care if ring becomes attached to vaginal wall (rare), making removal difficult.

• Instruct patient prescribed transdermal Evamist to prime the pump of a new device before the first dose by holding the container upright with the cover in place and spraying 3 sprays. Then, to deliver a dose, she should spray the mist on the inner aspect of her forearm starting near the elbow. Instruct her to let the mist dry for 2 minutes and not to wash the area for at least 30 minutes. Warn her that secondary exposure may occur if a child or other adult comes into contact with sprayed area. To avoid this, she should cover the area with clothing after the spray dries.

• Inform patient receiving estradiol treatment that she should have an annual pelvic examination to screen for cervical dysplasia.

• Tell patient who has an intact uterus and is prescribed transdermal Menostar that she will need to receive progestin for 14 days every 6 to 12 months and have an endometrial biopsy yearly.

estrogens (conjugated)

C.E.S. (CAN), Congest (CAN), Premarin, Premarin Vaginal Cream, Synthetic Conjugated Estrogens A (SCE-A) Vaginal Cream

estrogens (conjugated) and medroxyprogesterone

Premphase, Prempro

synthetic estrogens, A (conjugated)

Cenestin

synthetic estrogens, B (conjugated)

Enjuvia

Class and Category

Chemical class: Estrogen derivative, steroid hormone

Therapeutic class: Antiosteoporotic agent, ovarian hormone replacement

Pregnancy category: X

Indications and Dosages

➤ *To treat moderate to severe vasomotor menopausal symptoms*

TABLETS (CENESTIN, PREMARIN)

Adults. 0.3 to 1.25 mg daily (Cenestin, Premarin) or cyclically 25 days on, 5 days off (Premarin only). Dosage increased as needed to control symptoms.

TABLETS (ENJUVIA)

Adults. 0.625 mg daily. Dosage increased as needed to control symptoms.

TABLETS (PREMPRO)

Adults. 0.3 mg conjugated estrogens and 1.5 mg medroxyprogesterone daily. Increased up to 0.625 mg conjugated estrogens and 5 mg medroxyprogesterone daily as needed.

TABLETS (PREMPHASE)

Adults. 0.625 mg conjugated estrogens daily on days 1 through 14 and combination product (0.625 mg conjugated estrogens and 5 mg medroxyprogesterone) on days 15 through 28.

➤ *To treat vaginal and vulvar atrophy*

TABLETS (CENESTIN, PREMARIN)

Adults. 0.3 to 1.25 mg daily (Cenestin, Premarin) or cyclically 25 days on, 5 days off (Premarin only). Dosage increased as needed to control symptoms.

TABLETS (PREMPRO)

Adults. 0.3 mg conjugated estrogens and 1.5 mg medroxyprogesterone daily. Increased up to 0.625 mg conjugated estrogens and 5 mg medroxyprogesterone daily as needed.

TABLETS (PREMPHASE)

Adults. 0.625 mg conjugated estrogens daily on days 1 through 14 and combination product (0.625 mg conjugated estrogens and 5 mg medroxyprogesterone) on days 15 through 28.

➤ *To treat atrophic vaginitis and vaginal and vulvar atrophy*

VAGINAL CREAM (PREMARIN)

Adults. 0.5 to 2 g daily in cycles of 3 wk on, 1 wk off.

➤ *To treat moderate to severe vaginal dryness and pain with intercourse and*

symptoms of vulvar and vaginal atrophy in menopause

TABLETS (ENJUVIA)

Adults. 0.3 mg daily.

VAGINAL CREAM (PREMARIN)

Adults. 0.5 g twice/wk. Or, 0.5 g daily for 21 days followed by 7 days off, with cycle repeated every 28 days.

VAGINAL CREAM (SCE-A)

Adults. 1 g daily for 1 wk, followed by 1 g twice/wk.

➤ *To prevent postmenopausal osteoporosis*

TABLETS (CENESTIN, PREMARIN)

Adults. 0.625 mg daily continuously or in cycles of 25 days on, 5 days off.

TABLETS (PREMPRO)

Adults. 0.3 mg conjugated estrogens and 1.5 mg medroxyprogesterone daily. Increased to 0.625 mg conjugated estrogens and 5 mg medroxyprogesterone daily as needed.

TABLETS (PREMPHASE)

Adults. 0.625 mg conjugated estrogens daily on days 1 through 14 and combination product (0.625 mg conjugated estrogens and 5 mg medroxyprogesterone) on days 15 through 28.

➤ *To provide palliative treatment for advanced androgen-dependent prostate cancer*

TABLETS (PREMARIN)

Adults. 1.25 to 2.5 mg three times daily

➤ *To provide palliative treatment for metastatic breast cancer*

TABLETS (PREMARIN)

Adults. 10 mg three times daily for 3 mo or longer.

➤ *To treat dysfunctional uterine bleeding*

I.V. INFUSION, I.M. INJECTION (PREMARIN)

Adults. 25 mg, repeated in 6 to 12 hr as needed.

➤ *To treat estrogen deficiency from oophorectomy or primary ovarian failure*

TABLETS (PREMARIN)

Adults. 1.25 mg daily in cycles of 3 wk on, 1 wk off.

➤ *To treat female hypogonadism*

TABLETS (PREMARIN)

Adults. 0.3 to 0.625 mg daily in cycles of 3 wk on, 1 wk off. Increased as needed every 6 to 12 mo.

Mechanism of Action

Increase the rate of DNA and RNA synthesis in the cells of female reproductive organs, hypothalamus, pituitary glands, and other target organs. In the hypothalamus, estrogens reduce the release of gonadotropin-releasing hormone, which decreases pituitary release of follicle-stimulating hormone and luteinizing hormone. In women, these hormones are required for normal genitourinary and other essential body functions. At the cellular level, estrogens increase cervical secretions, cause endometrial cell proliferation, and increase uterine tone. Estrogen replacement helps maintain genitourinary function and reduce vasomotor symptoms when estrogen production declines from menopause, surgical removal of ovaries, or other estrogen deficiency. Estrogen also helps prevent osteoporosis by keeping bone resorption from exceeding bone formation.

In men, estrogens inhibit pituitary secretion of luteinizing hormone and decrease testicular secretion of testosterone. These actions may decrease prostate tumor growth and lower the level of prostate-specific antigen.

Contraindications
Active deep vein thrombosis, pulmonary embolism, or history of these conditions; active or recent (within past year) arterial thromboembolic disease such as stroke or MI; hepatic dysfunction or disease; history of anaphylactic reaction or angioedema to estradiol; hypersensitivity to estrogens or their components; known or suspected breast cancer or history of breast cancer; known or suspected estrogen-dependent cancer; known protein C, protein S, or antithrombin deficiency or other known thrombophilic disorders; pregnancy; liver impairment or disease; undiagnosed abnormal genital bleeding

Incompatibilities
Don't combine I.V. estrogens with acid solutions, ascorbic acid, and protein hydrolysate because they're incompatible.

Interactions
DRUGS
aminocaproic acid: Possibly increased level of hypercoagulability caused by aminocaproic acid

barbiturates, carbamazepine, hydantoins, rifabutin, rifampin: Possibly reduced activity of estrogen and medroxyprogesterone
bromocriptine: Possibly interference with bromocriptine's therapeutic effects
calcium: Possibly increased calcium absorption
corticosteroids: Increased therapeutic and toxic effects of corticosteroids
cyclosporine: Increased risk of hepatotoxicity and nephrotoxicity
didanosine, lamivudine, zalcitabine: Possibly pancreatitis
hepatotoxic drugs (such as isoniazid): Increased risk of hepatitis and hepatotoxicity
oral antidiabetic drugs: Decreased therapeutic effects of these drugs
somatrem, somatropin: Possibly accelerated epiphyseal maturation
tamoxifen: Possibly interference with tamoxifen's therapeutic effects
thyroid hormone replacement: Decreased effectiveness
warfarin: Decreased anticoagulant effect
ACTIVITIES
smoking: Increased risk of stroke, pulmonary embolism, thrombophlebitis, and transient ischemic attack

Adverse Reactions
CNS: Asthenia, dementia, depression, dizziness, growth benign meningioma, headache, insomnia, migraine headache, mood disturbance, nervousness, paresthesia, stroke
CV: Hypertension, MI, peripheral edema, thromboembolism, thrombophlebitis, vasodilation
EENT: Intolerance of contact lenses, pharyngitis, retinal vascular thrombosis, rhinitis, sinusitis
ENDO: Breast enlargement, pain, tenderness, or tumors; gynecomastia (men); hot flashes; hyperglycemia
GI: Abdominal cramps or pain, anorexia, cholestatic jaundice, constipation, diarrhea, flatulence, gallbladder disease or obstruction, hepatic hemangioma enlargement, hepatitis, increased appetite, ischemic colitis, nausea, pancreatitis, vomiting
GU: Amenorrhea, breakthrough bleeding, cervical erosion, clear vaginal discharge,

decreased libido (men), dysmenorrhea, endometrial cancer or hyperplasia, impotence, increased libido (women), leukorrhea, ovarian cancer, prolonged or heavy menstrual bleeding, testicular atrophy, uterine leiomyomata enlargement, vaginal candidiasis, vaginitis, vaginal-site reactions (vaginal administration only) such as burning, irritation, and genital pruritus
MS: Arthralgias, back pain
RESP: Bronchitis, increased cough, pulmonary embolism
SKIN: Acne, alopecia, chloasma, erythema multiforme, erythema nodosum, hemorrhagic eruption, hirsutism, melasma, oily skin, pruritus, purpura, rash, seborrhea, urticaria
Other: Anaphylaxis, angioedema, flu syndrome, folic acid deficiency, hypercalcemia (in metastatic bone disease), weight gain

Nursing Considerations

• Use conjugated estrogens cautiously in patients with severe hypocalcemia because a sudden increase in serum calcium level may cause adverse reactions.
• Reconstitute conjugated estrogens with normal saline solution, dextrose, or invert sugar solution and use within a few hours. Discard solution that contains precipitate.
WARNING Monitor serum calcium level to detect severe hypercalcemia in patients with bone metastasis from breast cancer.
WARNING Monitor patient closely, especially within minutes to hours of taking first dose, as anaphylaxis may occur, requiring emergency intervention. Be aware that estrogen therapy may exacerbate symptoms of angioedema in women with hereditary angioedema. Monitor for signs of swelling of the lips, tongue, face or throat, and provide emergency care, as needed.
• Watch for elevated liver function test results because estrogen and progestins may worsen such conditions as acute inter-mittent or variegate hepatic porphyria.
• Assess hypertensive patients for increases in blood pressure because estrogens may cause fluid retention.
• Monitor patients with asthma, diabetes mellitus, endometriosis, heart disease, lupus erythematosus, migraine headaches, renal disease, or seizure disorder for worsening of these conditions.

• If patient takes warfarin, assess PT for loss of anticoagulant effects because estrogens increase production of clotting factors and promote platelet aggregation.
• Expect to stop drug during periods of immobilization, 4 weeks before elective surgery, and if jaundice develops.
WARNING Expect to stop estrogen combination therapy in any woman who develops signs or symptoms of cancer; cardiovascular disease, such as MI, pulmonary embolism, venous thrombosis, or stroke; or dementia.
• Check triglyceride level routinely because, in hypertriglyceridemia, estrogen therapy may increase triglycerides enough to cause pancreatitis and other complications.
• If patient takes thyroid hormone replacement therapy, monitor her for increased signs and symptoms of hypothyroidism because estrogen may increase thyroid-binding globulin level, which may make the patient's current dose of thyroid hormone insufficient.
• Estrogen may worsen mood disorders, including depression. Monitor patient for depression, fatigue, insomnia, or mood changes.
WARNING Monitor patient with history of hereditary angioedema closely because estrogens may exacerbate symptoms of angioedema.

PATIENT TEACHING

• Explain the risks of estrogen therapy, including increased risk of breast, endometrial, or ovarian cancer; cardiovascular disease; dementia; and gallbladder disease.
• Instruct patient how to use vaginal cream and to cleanse plunger by removing it from barrel and washing it with mild soap and warm water after each use.
• Urge patient to immediately report breakthrough bleeding to prescriber.
• Instruct patient to perform monthly breast self-examination and to comply with all prescribed follow-up examinations.
• Warn female patient that long-term use may increase risk of dementia, heart disease, stroke, gallbladder disease, and breast or endometrial cancer.
• Inform patient that estrogen vaginal cream may alter effectiveness of condoms, diaphragms, or cervical caps made of latex or rubber.

• Instruct patient to notify prescriber if she sees something that resembles a tablet in her stool.

eszopiclone
Lunesta

Class, Category, and Schedule
Chemical class: Pyrrolopyrazine derivative of cyclopyrrolone class
Therapeutic class: Sedative-hypnotic
Pregnancy category: C
Controlled substance schedule: IV

Indications and Dosages
➤ *To treat insomnia*
TABLETS
Adults. *Initial:* 1 mg immediately at bedtime. May be increased to 2 mg or 3 mg at bedtime, as needed. *Maximum:* 3 mg at bedtime.
DOSAGE ADJUSTMENT For patients with severe hepatic impairment, patients who take potent CYP3A4 inhibitors, or patients who are elderly or debilitated, dosage should not exceed 2 mg at bedtime.

Route	Onset	Peak	Duration
P.O.	Unknown	1 hr	Unknown

Mechanism of Action
May potentiate effects of the inhibitory neurotransmitter gamma-aminobutyric acid (GABA) by binding close to or with benzodiazepine receptors in limbic and cortical areas of the CNS. By binding to these receptor sites and areas, eszopiclone increases GABA's inhibitory effects and blocks cortical and limbic arousal, thereby inducing and maintaining sleep.

Contraindications
Hypersensitivity to eszopiclone or its components

Interactions
DRUGS
clarithromycin, itraconazole, ketoconazole, nefazodone, nelfinavir, ritonavir, troleandomycin: Increased eszopiclone level
other CNS depressants: Possibly additive effects
rifampin: Decreased eszopiclone level

ACTIVITIES
alcohol use: Additive effect on psychomotor performance
FOOD
Heavy, high-fat meal: Possibly reduced effectiveness of eszopiclone

Adverse Reactions
CNS: Agitation, anxiety, bizarre behavior such as sleep driving, confusion, depersonalization, depression, dizziness, hallucinations, headache (including migraine), nervousness, neuralgia, somnolence, unusual dreams
CV: Chest pain, peripheral edema
EENT: Dry mouth, smell distortion, taste perversion
ENDO: Gynecomastia
GI: Diarrhea, hepatitis, indigestion, nausea, vomiting
GU: Decreased libido, dysmenorrhea, UTI
RESP: Asthma, respiratory tract infection
SKIN: Pruritus, rash
Other: Generalized pain, heat stroke, viral infection

Nursing Considerations
• Use eszopiclone cautiously in patients with severe mental depression or reduced respiratory function; drug may intensify mental depression and lead to respiratory depression.
PATIENT TEACHING
• Instruct patient not to exceed prescribed eszopiclone dosage and not to stop drug abruptly because withdrawal symptoms may occur.
• Because eszopiclone can reduce alertness, advise patient to take drug immediately before bedtime and to avoid potentially hazardous activities until drug's CNS effects are known.
• Urge patient to avoid alcohol and CNS depressants because of additive effects.
• Advise woman of childbearing age to notify prescriber if she becomes or intends to become pregnant during therapy.
• Explain that sleep may be disturbed for the first few nights after therapy.
• Warn patient and caregiver that some patients have performed bizarre activities after taking drug, such as driving the car,

E
F

preparing and eating food, making phone calls, or having sex while not fully awake and often with no memory of the event. These episodes usually occur in patients who have taken the drug with alcohol or other CNS depressant, who have taken the drug with less than a full night of sleep remaining (7 to 8 hours), or who have exceeded the recommended dose. If such an episode occurs, the prescriber should be notified and eszopiclone therapy discontinued immediately.

etanercept

Enbrel

Class and Category
Chemical class: Dimeric recombinant human p75 tumor necrosis factor receptor
Therapeutic class: Disease-modifying antirheumatoid drug
Pregnancy category: B

Indications and Dosages
➤ *To reduce signs and symptoms of rheumatoid or psoriatic arthritis, slow structural damage in active arthritis, and improve physical function in patients with psoriatic arthritis, alone or in combination with methotrexate*
SUBCUTANEOUS INJECTION
Adults. 50 mg once/wk on same day each wk.
➤ *To reduce signs and symptoms of active ankylosing spondylitis*
SUBCUTANEOUS INJECTION
Adults. 50 mg once/wk on same day each wk.
➤ *To reduce signs and symptoms of juvenile rheumatoid arthritis*
SUBCUTANEOUS INJECTION
Children ages 4 to 17. 0.4 mg/kg twice/wk 3 to 4 days apart for 3 to 7 mo. Or, 0.8 mg/kg once/wk on same day each wk for 3 to 7 mo. *Maximum:* 25 mg twice/wk or 50 mg weekly.
➤ *To treat chronic moderate-to-severe plaque psoriasis in candidates for systemic therapy or phototherapy*
SUBCUTANEOUS INJECTION
Adults. *Initial:* 50 mg twice/wk 3 to 4 days apart for 3 mo; then reduced to 50 mg/wk.

➤ *To reduce signs and symptoms of moderately to severely active poly-articular juvenile idiopathic arthritis*
SUBCUTANEOUS INJECTION
Children ages 2 to 17. 0.8 mg/kg/wk. *Maximum:* 50 mg/wk.

Incompatibilities
Don't combine etanercept with other drugs.

Contraindications
Hypersensitivity to etanercept, hamster protein, or their components; sepsis or risk of it

Interactions
DRUGS
cyclophosphamide: Possibly increased risk of malignancy
sulfasalazine: Possibly decreased neutrophil count

Adverse Reactions
CNS: Asthenia, chills, demyelination, dizziness, fever, headache, multiple sclerosis, paresthesias, seizures
CV: Chest pain, congestive heart failure, hypertension, hypotension, peripheral edema, systemic vasculitis
EENT: Optic neuritis, pharyngitis, rhinitis, scleritis, sinusitis, uveitis
GI: Abdominal abscess, abdominal pain, autoimmune hepatitis, cholecystitis, diarrhea, elevated liver enzymes, gastroenteritis, indigestion, inflammatory bowel disease, nausea, noninfectious hepatitis, reactivation hepatitis B, vomiting
GU: Pyelonephritis
HEME: Aplastic anemia, leukopenia, lymphadenopathy, neutropenia, pancytopenia thrombocytopenia
MS: Osteomyelitis, septic arthritis, transverse myelitis
RESP: Bronchitis, cough, interstitial lung disease, pneumonia, upper respiratory tract infection
SKIN: Cellulitis, cutaneous lupus erythematosus or vasculitis, erythema multiforme, foot abscess, leg ulceration, melanoma and non-melanoma skin cancers, Merkel cell carcinoma, new or worsening psoriasis, pruritus, rash, Stevens-Johnson syndrome, toxic epidermal necrolysis, urticaria
Other: Angioedema; bacterial, fungal, mycobacterial, parasitic, and viral infections; injection-site edema, erythema,

itching, and pain; lupus-like syndromemacrophage activation syndrome, malignancy, such as leukemia or lymphoma; sarcoidosis, sepsis

Nursing Considerations

• Screen patient for latent tuberculosis with a tuberculin skin test before starting etanercept therapy. If test is positive, expect to give treatment, as ordered, before starting etanercept. Also screen patient for hepatitis B. If present, expect etanercept therapy to be withdrawn because antirheumatic therapies like etanercept may reactivate hepatitis B.
• Be aware that patients treated with tumor necrosis factor-alpha blockers such as etanercept are at increased risk for developing serious infections due to bacterial (including *Legionella* and *Listeria*), fungal, mycobacterial, parasitic, and viral pathogens. These infections can become life-threatening and involve multiple organ systems. Monitor patient closely throughout therapy.
• Tumor necrosis factor antagonists shouldn't be given with etanercept because doing so increases the risk of serious infection.
• Use cautiously in patients with a history of recurrent infection, underlying conditions that may predispose them to infections, or an existing chronic, latent, or localized infection because etanercept increases their risk of infection.
• Use cautiously in patients with COPD, and monitor respiratory status closely because etanercept therapy may increase patient's risk of adverse respiratory reactions.
• Use cautiously in patients with preexisting or recent onset CNS demyelinating disorders because drug may worsen these conditions. Also use cautiously in patients with heart failure because drug may worsen it.

E
F

Mechanism of Action

Etanercept reduces joint inflammation from rheumatoid arthritis by binding with tumor necrosis factor (TNF), a cytokine, or protein, that plays an important role in normal inflammatory and immune responses.

In rheumatoid arthritis, the immune and inflammatory process triggers release of TNF, mainly from macrophages. TNF then binds to TNF receptors on cell membranes, as shown below left. This action renders TNF biologically active and triggers a cascade of inflammatory events that results in increased inflammation of the synovial membrane, release of destructive lysosomal enzymes, and further joint destruction.

Etanercept binds to TNF and prevents it from binding with TNF receptors on the cell membranes, as shown below right. This action renders bound TNF biologically inactive, prevents TNFmediated cellular responses, and significantly reduces inflammatory activity.

WARNING Don't use the diluent provided with etanercept (bacteriostatic water for injection, USP, with 0.9% benzyl alcohol) for patients who have benzyl alcohol hypersensitivity. Instead, use sterile water for injection for these patients.

WARNING If you have a latex allergy, don't handle needle cover of diluent syringe because it contains dry natural rubber.

• When giving etanercept to children, don't use the 25-mg prefilled syringe if the child weighs less than 31 kg (68 lb). The 50-mg prefilled syringe or SureClick autoinjector may be used for children who weigh 63 kg (138 lb) or more.

WARNING Expect to stop etanercept if patient develops sepsis.

• Avoid giving live-virus vaccines to patients who are taking etanercept because drug decreases immune response and increases risk of secondary transmission of vaccine virus.

• Monitor immunosuppressed patients for evidence of acute or chronic infection, including chills, fever, and tachycardia, because etanercept decreases defenses against infection. It also increases the risk of developing malignant tumors.

• Continue giving corticosteroids, NSAIDs, and other analgesics, as prescribed, during etanercept therapy.

• Malignancies, especially lymphomas and leukemias, have been reported rarely in patients taking tumor necrosis factor blockers such as etanercept. Children, adolescents, and patients with rheumatoid arthritis, especially those with very active disease, are at greatest risk. Monitor closely.

PATIENT TEACHING

• Inform patient that etanercept is given by a small injection under the skin, and teach him proper injection technique if needed.

• If patient will take 50-mg dose, explain that a prefilled syringe is available to eliminate the need to mix or draw up drug.

• If patient will take less than 50-mg dose or prefers not to use prefilled syringe, advise him to use drug as soon as possible after dissolving powder. Dissolved powder may be kept in refrigerator for up to 6 hours after mixing and then should be discarded.

• Instruct patient to rotate injection sites among thigh, stomach, and upper arms and to avoid areas that are tender, red,

bruised, or hard. Advise him to keep each site at least 1" away from a previous site.

• Urge patient to use needles and syringes once and discard in puncture-proof container.

• Caution patient that the risk of malignancies such as leukemia and lymphoma may be higher in those who take etanercept, especially children and adolescents. Tell him to seek medical attention promptly for any suspicious signs and symptoms.

• Urge patient to consult prescriber immediately if he develops an infection because drug may decrease the body's infection-fighting ability.

• Caution patient who hasn't had chickenpox to contact prescriber right away if he's exposed because he may develop a more serious infection.

• Urge patient to seek immediate emergency care if he develops a persistent fever, bruising, bleeding, or pallor while taking drug.

ethacrynic acid
Edecrin

ethacrynate sodium
Edecrin

Class and Category
Chemical class: Ketone derivative of anyloxyacetic acid
Therapeutic class: Diuretic
Pregnancy category: B

Indications and Dosages
➤ *To promote diuresis in heart failure; hepatic cirrhosis; renal disease; ascites of short duration caused by cancer, idiopathic edema, or lymphedema; and edema in children (excluding infants with congenital heart disease or nephrotic syndrome)*

ORAL SOLUTION, TABLETS
Adults. *Initial:* 50 to 100 mg daily as a single dose or in divided doses. Dosage increased by 25 to 50 mg daily, as needed. *Maintenance:* 50 to 200 mg daily. *Maximum:* 400 mg daily.

Children (except infants). *Initial:* 25 mg daily. Dosage increased in 25-mg increments daily, as needed.

I.V. INFUSION

Adults. *Initial:* 50 mg or 0.5 to 1 mg/kg. Dose repeated in 2 to 4 hr, if needed, then every 4 to 6 hr based on patient response. In an emergency, dose repeated every 1 hr, if needed. *Maximum:* 100 mg as single dose.

Route	Onset	Peak	Duration
P.O.	30 min	2 hr	6–8 hr
I.V.	5 min	15–30 min	2 hr

Mechanism of Action

Probably inhibits the sulfhydryl-catalyzed enzyme systems that cause sodium and chloride resorption in the proximal and distal tubules and the ascending limb of the loop of Henle. These inhibitory effects increase urinary excretion of sodium, chloride, and water, causing profound diuresis. Drug also increases the excretion of potassium, hydrogen, calcium, magnesium, bicarbonate, ammonium, and phosphate.

Contraindications

Anuria; hypersensitivity to ethacrynic acid, ethacrynate sodium, sulfonylureas, or their components; infancy; severe diarrhea

Interactions

DRUGS

ACE inhibitors, antihypertensives: Possibly hypotension
aminoglycosides: Increased risk of ototoxicity
amiodarone: Increased risk of arrhythmias
amphotericin B: Increased risk of electrolyte imbalances, nephrotoxicity, and ototoxicity
anticoagulants, thrombolytics: Possibly potentiated anticoagulation and risk of hemorrhage
corticosteroids: Increased risk of gastric hemorrhage
digoxin: Increased risk of digitalis toxicity
insulin, oral antidiabetic drugs: Possibly increased serum glucose level and decreased therapeutic effects of these drugs
lithium: Increased risk of lithium toxicity
neuromuscular blockers: Possibly increased neuromuscular blockade
NSAIDs: Possibly decreased effects of ethacrynic acid

sympathomimetics: Possibly interference with hypotensive effects of ethacrynic acid and ethacrynate sodium

ACTIVITIES

alcohol use: Possibly potentiated hypotensive and diuretic effects of ethacrynic acid and ethacrynate sodium

Adverse Reactions

CNS: Confusion, fatigue, headache, malaise, nervousness
CV: Orthostatic hypotension
EENT: Blurred vision, hearing loss, ototoxicity (ringing or buzzing in ears), sensation of fullness in ears, yellow vision
ENDO: Hyperglycemia, hypoglycemia
GI: Abdominal pain, anorexia, diarrhea, dysphagia, GI bleeding (I.V. form), nausea, vomiting
GU: Hematuria (I.V. form), interstitial nephritis, polyuria
HEME: Agranulocytosis, severe neutropenia, thrombocytopenia
SKIN: Rash
Other: Hyperuricemia, hypochloremic alkalosis, hypokalemia, hypomagnesemia, hyponatremia, hypovolemia, infusion-site irritation and pain

Nursing Considerations

WARNING Give ethacrynic acid and ethacrynate sodium cautiously in patients with advanced hepatic cirrhosis, especially those with a history of electrolyte imbalance or hepatic encephalopathy; both forms of drug may lead to lethal hepatic coma.

• Dilute ethacrynate sodium with D_5W or normal saline solution for I.V. infusion. Discard unused portion after 24 hours.
• Don't use diluted ethacrynate sodium that's cloudy or opalescent.
• Infuse I.V. ethacrynate sodium slowly over 30 minutes.
• Weigh patient daily, and assess him for signs and symptoms of electrolyte imbalances and dehydration.
• Monitor blood pressure and fluid intake and output, and check laboratory test results.
• Report significant changes. Prescriber may reduce dosage or temporarily stop drug.
• If hypokalemia develops, administer replacement potassium, as ordered.
• Monitor serum glucose level frequently, especially if patient has diabetes mellitus;

E
F

both forms of drug may cause hyperglycemia or hypoglycemia.
• Notify prescriber if patient experiences hearing loss, vertigo, or ringing, buzzing, or sense of fullness in his ears. Drug may need to be discontinued.

PATIENT TEACHING
• Instruct patient to take the last dose of ethacrynic acid several hours before bedtime to avoid sleep interruption from diuresis. If patient receives once-daily dosing, advise him to take the dose in the morning to avoid sleep disturbance caused by nocturia.
• Suggest that patient take ethacrynic acid with food or milk to reduce the likelihood of GI distress.
• Advise patient to change position slowly to minimize effects of orthostatic hypotension, especially if he also takes an antihypertensive.
• Unless contraindicated, urge patient to eat more high-potassium foods and to take a potassium supplement, if prescribed, to prevent hypokalemia.
• Caution patient not to drink alcohol, stand for prolonged periods, or exercise during hot weather because these activities may exacerbate orthostatic hypotension.
• Instruct patient to notify prescriber if he has diarrhea; buzzing, fullness, or ringing in his ears; hearing loss; severe nausea; vertigo; or vomiting. Drug may need to be discontinued.
• Remind diabetic patients to check their serum glucose levels often for changes.

ethambutol hydrochloride

Etibi (CAN), Myambutol

Class and Category
Chemical class: Diisopropylethylene diamide derivative
Therapeutic class: Antitubercular
Pregnancy category: C

Indications and Dosages
➤ *As adjunct to treat tuberculosis and atypical mycobacterial infections caused by Mycobacterium tuberculosis*

TABLETS
Adults and adolescents who haven't received previous antituberculotic therapy. 15 mg/kg daily.
Adults and adolescents who have received antituberculotic therapy. 25 mg/kg daily; after 60 days, decreased to 15 mg/kg daily.

Mechanism of Action
May suppress bacterial multiplication by interfering with RNA synthesis in susceptible bacteria that are actively dividing.

Contraindications
Hypersensitivity to ethambutol or its components, inability to report changes in vision, optic neuritis

Interactions
DRUGS
antacids that contain aluminum hydroxide: Decreased absorption of ethambutol
other neurotoxic drugs: Increased risk of neurotoxicity, such as optic and peripheral neuritis

Adverse Reactions
CNS: Burning sensation or weakness in arms and legs, confusion, disorientation, dizziness, fever, headache, malaise, paresthesia, peripheral neuritis
EENT: Blurred vision, decreased visual acuity, eye pain, optic neuritis, red-green color blindness
GI: Abdominal pain, anorexia, hepatic dysfunction, nausea, vomiting
HEME: Leukopenia, neutropenia, thrombocytopenia
MS: Arthralgia, gouty arthritis, joint pain
RESP: Pulmonary infiltrates
SKIN: Dermatitis, erythema multiforme, pruritus, rash
Other: Anaphylaxis, hypersensitivity syndrome (rash or exfoliative dermatitis, eosinophilia, and one of the following: hepatitis, pneumonitis, nephritis, myocarditis, pericarditis), lymphadenopathy

Nursing Considerations
• Expect prescriber to refer patient for an ophthalmologic examination that includes tests for visual fields, acuity, and red-green color blindness before taking ethambutol and monthly thereafter. This is especially likely if therapy is prolonged or dosage exceeds 15 mg/kg daily.

WARNING Notify prescriber immediately if patient develops vision changes, and expect ethambutol to be stopped if they occur.
• Expect to give the patient at least one other antituberculotic with ethambutol, as prescribed, because bacteria may become resistant quickly to a single drug.
• Monitor laboratory test results for changes in liver function or for increased serum uric acid level if patient has gouty arthritis or impaired renal function. Notify prescriber of any abnormalities.
• Obtain a monthly sputum specimen, as ordered, to check bacteriologic response in sputum-positive patient.
• Know that successful ethambutol therapy typically takes 6 to 12 months but may take years.

PATIENT TEACHING
• Teach patient to recognize possible adverse reactions to ethambutol.
• Advise patient to take drug with food if he experiences adverse GI reactions.
• Instruct patient to take a missed dose as soon as he remembers, unless it's nearly time for the next dose, but not to double-dose.
• Explain that ethambutol therapy may last months or years and that compliance is essential.
• Advise patient to notify prescriber if no improvement occurs within 3 weeks of starting ethambutol therapy; if bothersome or severe adverse reactions occur; if his vision changes; or if a rash, fever, or joint pain (possible hypersensitivity) develops.

ethchlorvynol

Placidyl

Class, Category, and Schedule
Chemical class: Chlorinated tertiary acetylenic carbinol
Therapeutic class: Sedative-hypnotic
Pregnancy category: C
Controlled substance schedule: IV

Indications and Dosages
➤ *To provide short-term relief from insomnia*

CAPSULES
Adults. 0.5 to 1 g at bedtime for no longer than 1 wk.

Route	Onset	Peak	Duration
P.O.	15–60 min	Unknown	5 hr

Mechanism of Action
Exerts sedative-hypnotic, muscle relaxant, and anticonvulsant effects possibly by depressing the reticular activating system.

Contraindications
Hypersensitivity to ethchlorvynol or its components, porphyria

Interactions
DRUGS
CNS depressants, tricyclic antidepressants: Increased CNS depression
oral anticoagulants: Decreased anticoagulant effects
ACTIVITIES
alcohol use: Increased CNS depression

Adverse Reactions
CNS: Ataxia, dizziness, facial numbness, fatigue, light-headedness, syncope, unsteadiness, weakness
CV: Hypotension
EENT: Blurred vision, unpleasant aftertaste
GI: Epigastric pain, indigestion, nausea, vomiting
HEME: Thrombocytopenia
SKIN: Jaundice, rash, urticaria
Other: Physical and psychological dependence

Nursing Considerations
• If patient awakens too early after taking 0.5 or 0.75 g of ethchlorvynol at bedtime, ask prescriber if he may take a single supplemental dose of 200 mg.
• Assess for signs of addiction if patient has taken drug for 2 weeks or longer.
• Be aware that ethchlorvynol shouldn't be given for longer than 1 week. If patient has received prolonged therapy, expect to discontinue drug gradually to prevent withdrawal symptoms. Notify prescriber if you detect evidence of withdrawal, such as diaphoresis, hallucinations, irritability, muscle twitching, nausea, nervousness, restlessness, seizures, sleep disturbance, tremor, vomiting, and weakness.

E
F

PATIENT TEACHING
• Caution patient not to exceed prescribed dosage or dosing frequency because of ethchlorvynol's habit-forming potential. Instruct him not to use drug for more than 1 week.
• Advise patient to take ethchlorvynol with food or milk to minimize adverse GI reactions.
• If patient has taken long-term ethchlorvynol therapy, warn against stopping drug abruptly; advise him to contact prescriber for guidelines to reduce dosage.
• Direct patient to avoid alcohol and other CNS depressants during ethchlorvynol therapy because they increase the risk of adverse reactions.
• Advise patient to avoid potentially hazardous activities until drug's CNS effects are known.

ethionamide
Trecator-SC

Class and Category
Chemical class: Thiamide analogue of isonicotinic acid
Therapeutic class: Antituberculotic
Pregnancy category: Not rated

Indications and Dosages
➤ *As adjunct to treat tuberculosis*
TABLETS
Adults. 0.5 to 1 g daily in divided doses every 8 to 12 hr, together with other antituberculotics. *Maximum:* 1 g daily.
Children. 15 to 20 mg/kg daily in divided doses every 8 to 12 hr, together with other antituberculotics. *Maximum:* 750 mg daily.

Mechanism of Action
May inhibit peptide synthesis, resulting in bacteriostatic action against *Mycobacterium tuberculosis.*

Contraindications
Hypersensitivity to ethionamide or its components, severe hepatic damage

Interactions
DRUGS
cycloserine: Increased risk of adverse CNS effects, especially seizures

other neurotoxic drugs: Increased risk of neurotoxicity, such as optic and peripheral neuritis

Adverse Reactions
CNS: Burning or pain in arms and legs, clumsiness, confusion, depression, mental or mood changes, paresthesia, unsteadiness
CV: Orthostatic hypotension
EENT: Blurred vision, eye pain, increased salivation, metallic taste, optic neuritis, stomatitis, vision loss
ENDO: Goiter, hypoglycemia, hypothyroidism
GI: Anorexia, hepatitis, nausea, vomiting
SKIN: Jaundice, rash

Nursing Considerations
• Use ethionamide cautiously in patients with a history of hypersensitivity to isoniazid, niacin, pyrazinamide, or chemically related drugs; these patients also may be hypersensitive to ethionamide.
• Expect to give another antituberculotic with ethionamide to decrease the risk of development of bacterial resistance.
• Also plan to give pyridoxine to prevent or minimize peripheral neuritis (burning, numbness, pain, or tingling in hands and feet), especially if patient has already had isoniazid-induced peripheral neuritis.
• Monitor liver function test results, and assess for signs of impaired function, such as hepatitis and jaundice.
• Question patient regularly about vision changes. Notify prescriber about blurred vision, eye pain, or loss of vision or acuity.
• Monitor compliance; treatment may need to continue for 1 to 2 years or indefinitely.
PATIENT TEACHING
• Advise patient to take ethionamide with food if adverse GI reactions occur.
• Instruct patient to take a missed dose as soon as he remembers unless it's nearly time for the next dose. Caution him not to double the dose.
• Encourage patient to notify prescriber if no improvement occurs within 3 weeks; if bothersome or severe adverse reactions occur; if his vision changes; or if he has burning, numbness, pain, or tingling in his hands and feet.

• Inform patient that therapy may have to continue for months or years and that compliance is essential.

---

ethosuximide
Zarontin

Class and Category
Chemical class: Succinimide derivative
Therapeutic class: Anticonvulsant
Pregnancy category: Not rated

Indications and Dosages
➤ *To manage absence seizures in a patient who also has generalized tonic-clonic seizures*
CAPSULES, SYRUP
Adults and children age 6 and over.
Initial: 500 mg daily. *Maintenance:* Increased by 250 mg every 4 to 7 days until control is achieved with minimal adverse reactions.
Children ages 3 to 6. *Initial:* 250 mg daily. *Maintenance:* Increased by 250 mg every 4 to 7 days until control is achieved with minimal adverse reactions.

Mechanism of Action
Elevates the seizure threshold and reduces the frequency of attacks by depressing the motor cortex and elevating the threshold of CNS response to convulsive stimuli.

Contraindications
Hypersensitivity to ethosuximide, succinimides, or their components

Interactions
DRUGS
carbamazepine, phenobarbital, phenytoin, primidone: Possibly decreased blood ethosuximide level
CNS depressants: Possibly increased CNS depression
haloperidol: Possibly decreased blood haloperidol level
loxapine, MAO inhibitors, maprotiline, molindone, phenothiazines, pimozide, tricyclic antidepressants: Possibly lowered seizure threshold and reduced therapeutic effect of ethosuximide
valproic acid: Increased or decreased blood ethosuximide level

ACTIVITIES
alcohol use: Possibly increased CNS depression

Adverse Reactions
CNS: Aggressiveness, ataxia, decreased concentration, depression, dizziness, drowsiness, euphoria, fatigue, headache, hyperactivity, irritability, lethargy, nightmares, psychosis, sleep disturbance, suicidal ideation
EENT: Gingival hypertrophy, myopia, tongue swelling
GI: Abdominal and epigastric pain, abdominal cramps, anorexia, diarrhea, hiccups, indigestion, nausea, vomiting
GU: Increased libido, microscopic hematuria, vaginal bleeding
HEME: Agranulocytosis, aplastic anemia, eosinophilia, leukopenia, pancytopenia
SKIN: Erythematous and pruritic rashes, hirsutism, Stevens-Johnson syndrome, systemic lupus erythematosus, urticaria
Other: Hypersensitivity reaction, weight loss

Nursing Considerations
• Use ethosuximide with extreme caution in patients with hepatic or renal disease.
• Give other anticonvulsants concurrently, as prescribed, to control generalized tonic-clonic seizures.
• Monitor CBC and platelet count and assess for signs of infection, such as cough, fever, and pharyngitis. Also routinely evaluate liver and renal function test results.
• Take safety precautions because drug may cause adverse CNS reactions, such as dizziness and drowsiness.
• Monitor patient closely for evidence of suicidal thinking or behavior, especially when therapy starts or dosage changes.
• Assess patient regularly for signs of skin adverse effects. Stop ethosuximide immediately at first sign of rash and notify prescriber.

PATIENT TEACHING
• Emphasize the importance of complying with ethosuximide regimen.
• Advise patient to take a missed dose as soon as he remembers, unless it's nearly time for the next dose. Warn him not to double the dose.
• Instruct patient not to engage in potentially hazardous activities until drug's CNS effects are known.

E
F

• Caution patient not to stop taking drug abruptly; doing so increases the risk of absence seizures.

• Urge caregivers to watch patient closely for evidence of suicidal tendencies, especially when therapy starts or dosage changes, and to report any concerns immediately to prescriber.

• Encourage female patient who becomes pregnant while taking ethosuximide to enroll in the North American antiepileptic drug pregnancy registry by calling 1-888-233-2334. Explain that this registry is collecting information about the safety of antiepileptic drugs during pregnancy.

ethotoin
Peganone

Class and Category
Chemical class: Hydantoin derivative
Therapeutic class: Anticonvulsant
Pregnancy category: D

Indications and Dosages
➤ *To treat tonic-clonic and simple or complex partial seizures as initial or adjunct therapy, or when other drugs are ineffective*

TABLETS

Adults and adolescents. *Initial:* 0.5 to 1 g on the first day in four to six divided doses, increased over several days until desired response is reached. *Maintenance:* 2 to 3 g daily in four to six divided doses. *Maximum:* 3 g daily.

Children. *Initial:* Up to 750 mg daily, based on weight and age, in 4 to 6 divided doses, adjusted as needed and tolerated. *Maintenance:* 0.5 to 1 g daily in 4 to 6 divided doses. *Maximum:* 3 g daily.

DOSAGE ADJUSTMENT For debilitated patients, initial dosage lowered to reduce the risk of adverse reactions.

Mechanism of Action
Limits the spread of seizure activity and the start of new seizures by:
• regulating voltage-dependent sodium and calcium channels in neurons
• inhibiting calcium movement across neuronal membranes

• enhancing sodium-potassium adenosine triphosphatase activity in neurons and glial cells.

These actions may result from ethotoin's ability to slow the recovery rate of inactivated sodium channels.

Contraindications
Hematologic disorders; hepatic dysfunction; hypersensitivity to ethotoin, phenytoin, other hydantoins, or their components

Interactions
DRUGS
acetaminophen: Increased risk of hepatotoxicity with long-term acetaminophen use
amiodarone: Possibly increased blood ethotoin level and risk of toxicity
antacids: Possibly decreased ethotoin effectiveness
bupropion, clozapine, loxapine, MAO inhibitors, maprotiline, phenothiazines, pimozide, thioxanthenes: Possibly lowered seizure threshold and decreased therapeutic effects of ethotoin; possibly intensified CNS depressant effects of these drugs
chloramphenicol, cimetidine, disulfiram, fluconazole, isoniazid, methylphenidate, metronidazole, omeprazole, phenylbutazone, ranitidine, salicylates, sulfonamides, trimethoprim: Possibly impaired metabolism of these drugs and increased risk of ethotoin toxicity
corticosteroids, cyclosporine, digoxin, disopyramide, doxycycline, furosemide, levodopa, mexiletine, quinidine: Decreased therapeutic effects of these drugs
diazoxide: Possibly decreased therapeutic effects of both drugs
estrogens, progestins: Decreased effects of these drugs, increased blood ethotoin level
folic acid, leucovorin: Increased ethotoin metabolism, decreased seizure control
haloperidol: Possibly lowered seizure threshold, decreased ethotoin effects, and decreased blood haloperidol level
insulin, oral antidiabetic drugs: Possibly increased blood glucose level and decreased therapeutic effects of these drugs
lidocaine: Increased lidocaine metabolism, leading to reduced concentration
methadone: Possibly increased methadone metabolism and withdrawal symptoms

molindone: Possibly lowered seizure threshold and impaired absorption and decreased therapeutic effects of ethotoin
oral anticoagulants: Possibly impaired metabolism of these drugs and increased risk of ethotoin toxicity; possibly increased anticoagulant effect initially, but decreased effect with prolonged therapy
oral contraceptives that contain estrogen and progestin: Possibly breakthrough bleeding and decreased contraceptive effectiveness
rifampin: Possibly decreased therapeutic effects of ethotoin
streptozocin: Possibly decreased therapeutic effects of streptozocin
sucralfate: Possibly decreased ethotoin absorption
tricyclic antidepressants: Possibly lowered seizure threshold and decreased therapeutic effects of ethotoin; possibly decreased blood level of tricyclic antidepressants
valproic acid: Possibly decreased ethotoin level, increased valproic acid level
vitamin D analogues: Decreased vitamin D analogue activity; risk of anticonvulsant-induced rickets and osteomalacia
xanthines: Possibly inhibited ethotoin absorption and increased clearance of xanthines

ACTIVITIES
alcohol use: Possibly decreased ethotoin effectiveness, increased CNS depression

Adverse Reactions

CNS: Clumsiness, confusion, drowsiness, excitement, peripheral neuropathy, sedation, slurred speech, stuttering, suicidal ideation, tremor
EENT: Nystagmus
GI: Constipation, diarrhea, nausea, vomiting
HEME: Agranulocytosis, leukopenia, thrombocytopenia
SKIN: Rash, Stevens-Johnson syndrome, toxic epidermal necrolysis
Other: Lymphadenopathy, systemic lupus erythematosus

Nursing Considerations

• Obtain CBC and differential before treatment and monthly for first few months of ethotoin therapy, as ordered.
WARNING Ethotoin shouldn't be stopped abruptly because of risk of status epilepticus. Plan to reduce dosage

gradually or substitute another drug, as prescribed.
• Monitor patient for signs and symptoms of infection or unusual bleeding because ethotoin may cause hematologic toxicity.
• Because of ethotoin's potential for hepatotoxicity, monitor liver function test results and expect drug to be discontinued if test results are abnormal.
• Notify prescriber immediately and expect ethotoin to be stopped and replaced with another drug if patient has decreased blood counts, enlarged lymph nodes, or rash.
• Be aware that ethotoin may be substituted for phenytoin without loss of seizure control if patient develops severe gingival hyperplasia or other adverse reactions. Expect ethotoin dosage to be 4 to 6 times greater than phenytoin dosage.
• Institute and maintain seizure precautions according to facility protocol.
• Monitor patient closely for evidence of suicidal thinking or behavior, especially when therapy starts or dosage changes.

PATIENT TEACHING
• Instruct patient to take ethotoin exactly as prescribed and not to stop it abruptly.
• Advise patient to take drug with food to enhance absorption and reduce adverse GI effects.
• Advise patient to report easy bruising, epistaxis, fever, malaise, petechiae, or sore throat to prescriber immediately.
• Instruct patient to keep medical appointments to monitor drug effectiveness and check for adverse reactions. Explain the need for periodic laboratory tests.
• Urge patient to avoid alcohol during ethotoin therapy.
• Caution patient to avoid hazardous activities until drug's adverse effects are known.
• Encourage patient to wear or carry medical identification indicating his diagnosis and drug therapy.
• Urge caregivers to watch patient closely for evidence of suicidal tendencies, especially when therapy starts or dosage changes, and to report any concerns immediately to prescriber.
• Encourage female patient who becomes pregnant while taking ethotoin to enroll in

E
F

the North American antiepileptic drug pregnancy registry by calling 1-888-233-2334. Explain that this registry is collecting information about the safety of antiepileptic drugs during pregnancy.
• Advise patient to tell all healthcare providers about ethotoin therapy because drug may react with other medication, including over-the-counter drugs, vitamins, and herbal supplements.

etidronate disodium

Didronel

Class and Category

Chemical class: Bisphosphonate
Therapeutic class: Antihypercalcemic agent, bone resorption inhibitor
Pregnancy category: B (oral), C (parenteral)

Indications and Dosages

➤ *To treat Paget's disease of bone (osteitis deformans)*

TABLETS

Adults. 5 to 10 mg/kg daily for up to 6 mo, or 11 to 20 mg/kg daily for up to 3 mo.

➤ *To prevent and treat heterotopic ossification after total hip replacement*

TABLETS

Adults. 20 mg/kg daily for 1 mo before surgery and then 20 mg/kg daily for 3 mo after surgery for a total of 4 mo of treatment.

➤ *To prevent and treat heterotopic ossification after spinal cord injury*

TABLETS

Adults. 20 mg/kg daily for 2 wk and then 10 mg/kg daily for 10 wk for a total of 12 wk of treatment.

➤ *To treat moderate to severe hypercalcemia caused by cancer*

I.V. INFUSION

Adults. *Initial:* 7.5 mg/kg daily infused over at least 2 hr for 3 to 7 successive days. Oral etidronate may begin at 20 mg/kg/day for 30 days on the day after last infusion.

DOSAGE ADJUSTMENT Dosage reduced in renal impairment. Drug not given if serum creatinine level exceeds 5 mg/dl.

Mechanism of Action

Inhibits normal and abnormal bone resorption by reducing bone turnover and slowing the remodeling of pagetic or heterotopic bone. Etidronate also decreases the elevated cardiac output seen in Paget's disease of bone and reduces local increases in skin temperature. It also inhibits the abnormal bone resorption that may occur with cancer and reduces the amount of calcium that enters the blood from resorbed bone.

Contraindications

Esophageal abnormalities that delay gastric emptying, such as achalasia and stricture; hypersensitivity to etidronate, bisphosphonates, or their components; severe renal impairment

Interactions

DRUGS

antacids that contain aluminum, calcium, or magnesium; vitamin and mineral supplements that contain aluminum, calcium, iron, or magnesium: Decreased etidronate absorption

FOODS

high-calcium food (such as milk and other dairy products): Decreased etidronate absorption

Adverse Reactions

EENT: Altered taste, metallic taste
GI: Diarrhea, elevated liver function test results, nausea
GU: Nephrotoxicity
MS: Atypical subtrochanteric and diaphyseal femoral fractures, bone pain, osteonecrosis of jaw
Other: Hypocalcemia

Nursing Considerations

• Use etidronate cautiously in patients with upper GI problems such as Barrett's esophagus, dysphagia, other esophageal diseases, gastritis, duodenitis, or ulcers because drug may cause local irritation of the upper GI mucosa.
• Anticipate starting etidronate as soon as possible after spinal cord injury, preferably before signs of heterotopic ossification.
• Expect etidronate not to inhibit healing of spinal fractures, affect prosthesis, or disrupt trochanter attachment when used after total hip replacement.
• Give oral form 2 hours before meals to prevent decreased absorption.
• Dilute parenteral form in at least 250 ml of normal saline solution.

- Give parenteral form slowly over at least 2 hours.
- Store diluted parenteral solution at room temperature for up to 48 hours.

WARNING Watch for hypocalcemia if patient receives parenteral form for more than 3 days.

- When treating hypercalcemia, expect to continue giving drug for up to 90 days if serum calcium level remains within acceptable range.
- Monitor patient for adverse esophageal effects such as esophagitis, esophageal ulcers, and esophageal erosions that may occur with bleeding, as well as gastric and duodenal ulcers, because these adverse effects have occurred with other oral biphosphonates.
- Risk of severe adverse esophageal reactions increases in patients who lie down after taking drug, who fail to swallow it with a full glass of water, or who continue to take drug after developing symptoms of esophageal irritation.
- Make sure patient has had a dental checkup before having an invasive dental procedures during etidronate therapy, especially if he has cancer; is receiving chemotherapy, head or neck radiation, or a corticosteroid; or has poor oral hygiene because the risk of osteonecrosis is increased in these patients.

PATIENT TEACHING

- Instruct patient to take etidronate tablets on an empty stomach—2 hours before meals, antacids, or calcium supplements. Urge him to drink a full glass of water with tablets and to avoid taking drug with milk or other high-calcium foods.
- Tell patient to take a missed dose as soon as he remembers as long as 2 hours have elapsed since his last meal. Instruct him not to eat for another 2 hours. Warn against doubling the dose.
- Inform patient with Paget's disease that his response to etidronate may be slow and may continue for months after treatment.
- Instruct patient to inform prescriber if he develops difficulty swallowing or pain when swallowing, chest pain, or new or worsening heartburn.
- Advise patient to notify prescriber if he develops new or worsening groin or thigh pain.

etodolac

Lodine, Lodine XL

Class and Category

Chemical class: Pyranoindoleacetic acid derivative
Therapeutic class: Analgesic, anti-inflammatory
Pregnancy category: C

Indications and Dosages

➤ *To manage osteoarthritis*

CAPSULES, TABLETS

Adults. *Initial:* 800 to 1,200 mg daily in divided doses.
Maintenance: 600 to 1,200 mg daily in divided doses.
Maximum: 1,200 mg daily for patients weighing 60 kg (132 lb) or more; 20 mg/kg daily for those less than 60 kg.

E.R. TABLETS

Adults. 400 to 1,000 mg daily.

➤ *To relieve mild to moderate pain*

CAPSULES, TABLETS

Adults. *Initial:* 400 mg and then 200 to 400 mg every 6 to 8 hr. *Maximum:* 1,200 mg daily for patients weighing 60 kg or more; 20 mg/kg/day for patients weighing less than 60 kg.

Route	Onset	Peak	Duration
P.O.	30 min	1–2 hr	4–12 hr

Mechanism of Action

Blocks the activity of cyclooxygenase, the enzyme needed for prostaglandin synthesis. Prostaglandins, important mediators of the inflammatory response, cause local vasodilation with swelling and pain. By inhibiting cyclooxygenase and prosta-glandins, this NSAID causes inflammatory symptoms and pain to subside.

Contraindications

Angioedema, asthma, bronchospasm, nasal polyps, rhinitis, or urticaria induced by aspirin, iodides, or NSAIDs; coronary artery bypass graft surgery; hypersensitivity to etodolac or its components

Interactions

DRUGS

ACE inhibitors: Possibly decreased hypotensive effects of these drugs

acetaminophen (long-term use): Increased risk of adverse renal effects
antacids: Decreased blood etodolac level
antiplatelets, oral anticoagulants, thrombolytics: Prolonged PT (with warfarin), increased risk of bleeding
cidofovir: Possibly nephrotoxicity
corticosteroids: Increased risk of adverse GI effects
cyclosporine: Increased nephrotoxic effects, increased blood cyclosporine level
digoxin: Increased blood digoxin level and risk of digitalis toxicity
insulin, oral antidiabetic drugs: Increased risk of hypoglycemia
lithium: Increased blood lithium level and, possibly, toxicity
loop diuretics: Possibly decreased effects of loop diuretics
methotrexate: Increased risk of methotrexate toxicity
phenylbutazone: Possibly altered etodolac clearance
salicylates: Decreased blood etodolac level, increased risk of adverse GI effects
warfarin: Synergistic bleeding effects
ACTIVITIES
alcohol use, smoking: Increased risk of adverse GI effects

Adverse Reactions

CNS: Asthenia, chills, depression, dizziness, drowsiness, fatigue, fever, insomnia, irritability, malaise, nervousness, seizures, somnolence, syncope, stroke
CV: Edema, heart failure, hypertension, MI, palpitations, tachycardia, vasculitis
EENT: Blurred vision, deafness, loss of taste, photophobia, tinnitus
ENDO: Hyperglycemia in diabetics
GI: Abdominal pain or distention, anorexia, constipation, diarrhea, diverticulitis, dyspepsia, dysphagia, elevated liver function test results, esophagitis, flatulence, gastritis, gastroenteritis, gastroesophageal reflux disease, GI bleeding and ulceration, GI perforation, hemorrhoids, hepatic failure, hepatitis, hiatal hernia, indigestion, melena, nausea, pancreatitis, peptic ulcer, perforation of stomach or intestines, stomatitis, vomiting
GU: Dysuria, elevated serum creatinine level, hematuria, renal failure or insufficiency, renal papillary necrosis, urinary frequency
HEME: Agranulocytosis, aplastic anemia, easy bruising, hemolytic anemia, leukopenia, neutropenia, pancytopenia, thrombocytopenia
MS: Arthralgia, muscle pain
RESP: Asthma, bronchospasm, pulmonary infiltrate with eosinophilia, respiratory depression
SKIN: Erythema multiforme, exfoliative dermatitis, flushing, leukocytoclastic vasculitis, pruritus, Stevens-Johnson syndrome, toxic epidermal necrolysis, urticaria, vesiculobullous or other rash
Other: Anaphylaxis, angioedema, lymphadenopathy, sepsis

Nursing Considerations

• Assess patient's hydration status and rehydrate, if needed and as ordered, before starting etodolac therapy.
• Use etodolac with extreme caution in patients with a history of ulcer disease or GI bleeding because NSAIDs increase the risk of GI bleeding and ulceration. Expect to use etodolac for the shortest time possible in these patients. Also use with extreme caution in patients with advanced renal disease because etodolac is eliminated mainly by the kidneys.
• Be aware that serious GI tract ulceration, bleeding, and perforation may occur without warning symptoms. Elderly patents are at greater risk. To minimize risk, give drug with food. If GI distress occurs, withhold drug and notify prescriber immediately.
• Use etodolac cautiously in patients with hypertension, and monitor blood pressure closely throughout therapy. Drug may cause hypertension or worsen it.
WARNING Monitor patient closely for thrombotic events, including stroke and MI, because NSAIDs increase the risk.
• Especially if patient is elderly or taking etodolac long-term, watch for less common but serious adverse GI reactions, including anorexia, constipation, diverticulitis, dysphagia, esophagitis, gastritis, gastroenteritis, gastroesophageal reflux disease, hemorrhoids, hiatal hernia, melena, stomatitis, and vomiting.

• Monitor liver function test results. Rarely, elevated levels may progress to severe hepatic reactions, including fatal hepatitis, hepatic necrosis, and hepatic failure.
• Monitor BUN and serum creatinine levels in patients with heart failure, hepatic dysfunction, or impaired renal function; those taking diuretics or ACE inhibitors; and elderly patients because drug may cause renal failure.
• Monitor CBC for decreased hemoglobin level and hematocrit because drug may worsen anemia.

WARNING If patient has bone marrow suppression or is receiving antineoplastic drug therapy, monitor laboratory results (including WBC count), and watch for evidence of infection because anti-inflammatory and antipyretic actions of etodolac may mask it, such as fever and pain.

• Assess patient's skin routinely for rash or other signs of hypersensitivity reaction because etodolac and other NSAIDs may cause serious skin reactions without warning, even in patients with no history of NSAID hypersensitivity Stop drug at first sign of reaction and notify prescriber.
• If patient also takes acetaminophen, monitor fluid intake and output and BUN and serum creatinine levels for signs of adverse renal reactions.

PATIENT TEACHING

• Tell patient to take etodolac with food or after meals if adverse GI reactions occur.
• Caution him to avoid aspirin or aspirin-containing products while taking drug.
• Advise patient not to smoke or drink alcohol during therapy because these activities increase the risk of adverse GI reactions.
• Inform patient that he may experience dizziness or drowsiness.
• Instruct him to notify prescriber immediately about blood in urine, easy bruising, itching, rash, swelling, or yellow eyes or skin.
• Caution pregnant patient not to take etodolac or other NSAIDs during the third trimester because drug may cause premature closure of the ductus arteriosus.
• Explain that etodolac may increase the risk of serious adverse cardiovascular reac-

tions; urge patient to seek immediate medical attention for possible reactions, chest pain, shortness of breath, weakness, and slurring of speech.
• Tell patient that etodolac therapy also may increase the risk of serious adverse GI reactions; stress the importance of seeking immediate medical attention for such signs and symptoms as epigastric or abdominal pain, indigestion, black or tarry stools, or vomiting blood or material that looks like coffee grounds.
• Explain the possibility of rare but serious skin reactions. Urge patient to seek immediate medical attention for rash, blisters, itching, fever, or other indications of hypersensitivity.

everolimus
Zortress

Class and Category
Chemical class: Macrolide, M-TOR inhibitor
Therapeutic class: Immunosuppressant
Pregnancy category: C

Indications and Dosages
➤ *As adjunct to prevent organ rejection in renal transplantation*

TABLETS
Adults. *Initial:* 0.75 mg twice daily in combination with reduced-dose cyclosporine, administered as soon as possible after transplantation.
➤ *As adjunct to prevent organ rejection in liver transplantation*

TABLETS
Adults. *Initial:* 1 mg twice daily in combination with reduced-dose tacrolimus begun 30 days post-transplant.

DOSAGE ADJUSTMENT Dosage adjusted at 4- to 5-day intervals, as needed, according to everolimus blood concentrations, tolerability, individual response, change in concomitant medications, and the clinical situation. For patients with moderate hepatic impairment, the initial daily dose is reduced by 50% with further adjustments made according to everolimus blood concentration levels.

Mechanism of Action

Causes immunosuppression by inhibiting antigenic and interleukin (IL-2 and IL-15) stimulated activation and proliferation of T and B lymphocytes.

Contraindications

Hypersensitivity to everolimus or sirolimus or its components

Interactions

DRUGS

amprenavir, aprepitant, atazanavir, clarithromycin, cyclosporine, digoxin, diltiazem, erythromycin, fluconazole, fosamprenavir, indinavir, itraconazole, ketoconazole, macrolide antibiotics, nefazodone, nelfinavir, nicardipine, ritonavir, saquinavir, telithromycin, verapamil, voriconazle: Possible increased blood everolimus level

anticonvulsants, carbamazepine, efavirenz, nevirapine, phenobarbital, phenytoin, rifabutin, rifampin, rifapentine, St John's wort: Possibly decreased blood everolimus level

live vaccines: Possibly increased risk of contracting disease from live virus

FOODS

grapefruit, grapefruit juice: Possibly decreased metabolism of everolimus

Adverse Reactions

CNS: Progressive multiple leukoencephalopathy (PML)

CV: Hyperlipidemia, pericardial effusion, peripheral edema

ENDO: New-onset diabetes mellitus

GI: Ascites, hepatic artery thrombosis (liver transplant), pancreatitis

GU: Azospermia, BK virus-associated nephropathy, kidney graft thrombosis, nephrotoxicity, oligospermia, proteinuria

RESP: Noninfectious pneumonitis, pleural effusion, pulmonary embolism

SKIN: Skin cancer

Other: Angioedema; delayed wound healing; hypersensitivity reactions; infections such as bacterial, fungal, protozoal, and viral; lymphomas and other malignancies; opportunistic infections including polyoma virus

Nursing Considerations

• Be aware that everolimus isn't recommended in transplants other than kidney or liver transplantation. Know that everolimus therapy should not begin until 30 days after liver transplant because of patient's increased risk of developing hepatic artery thrombosis, which may lead to graft loss or death.

• Know that patients with galactose intolerance, the Lapp lactase deficiency, or glucose-galactose malabsorption should not receive everolimus therapy because this may result in diarrhea and malabsorption.

• Measure whole blood trough concentrations of both cyclosporine and everolimus in patient with kidney transplant or tacrolimus and everolimus in liver transplant because of increased risk of nephrotoxicity when either combination of drugs are used. Everolimus levels, ideally drawn 4 to 5 days after a previous dosing change, will also reveal if the therapeutic range has been achieved (3 to 8 nanograms per milliliter).

• Dosage adjustments of everolimus can then be made, as needed. In addition, everolimus levels should be obtained during concomitant administration of CYP3A4 inducers or inhibitors, when switching cyclosporine formulations, and/or when cyclosporine dosing is reduced as well as in patients with hepatic impairment. Know that there is little to no pharmacokinetic interaction of tacrolimus on everolimus. Therefore, there is no need to alter everolimus dosing if tacrolimus dosing is altered.

• Monitor patient's incision as everolimus delays wound healing and increases the occurrence of wound-related complications such as wound dehiscence, wound infection, incisional hernia, lymphocele, and seroma.

WARNING Watch for evidence of infection (such as fever, pain, cough, malaise) because patients receiving immunosuppressants such as everolimus are at increased risk for viral, bacterial, fungal, and parasitic infection. Watch for both generalized and localized infections, including worsening of preexisting infections, and be aware that these infections may become life threatening. Activation of latent viral infections may also occur and include BK virus–associated nephropathy that can lead to decreased renal function and renal graft loss.

• Monitor patient, especially within the first 30 days post transplantation, for evidence of kidney arterial and venous thrombosis (kidney transplant) or hepatic artery thrombosis (liver transplant) resulting in graft loss.
• Monitor patient's lipid levels routinely because hyperlipidemia may occur as a result of everolimus therapy. If hyperlipidemia drug therapy is required, be aware that simvastatin and lovastatin should not be used to treat it for patient with a kidney transplant because of a potential interaction with cyclosporine.
• Obtain renal function test results routinely because of increased risk of nephrotoxicity with combined everolimus and cyclosporine therapy or combined everolimus and tacrolimus therapy. Obtain liver function test results in patient with liver transplant to monitor transplanted liver function.
• Monitor patient's CBC and platelet count routinely because of increased risk of thrombotic microangiopathy, thrombotic thrombocytopenic purpura, and hemolytic uremic syndrome that may occur with combined everolimus and cyclosporine therapy used with kidney transplantation. Report abnormalities promptly to prescriber.
• Monitor patient's blood glucose levels regularly because everolimus therapy may increase the risk of new-onset diabetes mellitus after transplant.

PATIENT TEACHING
• Instruct patient to swallow tablets whole with a glass of water and not crushed before ingesting.
• Tell patient that ideally twice daily dosages should be consistently taken approximately 12 hours apart and at the same time as his cyclosporine or tacrolimus dose.
• Instruct patient to report any unusual, persistent, or severe symptoms to prescriber.
• Caution patient to avoid excessive exposure to ultraviolet light, to wear protective clothing when outdoors, and use a sunscreen with a high protection factor.
• Advise patient to avoid immunizations that use live vaccines such as intranasal influenza, measles, mumps, rubella, oral polio, BCG, yellow fever, varicella, and TY21a typhoid.

• Emphasize importance of avoiding grapefruit and grapefruit juice while receiving concomitant therapy with everolimus and cyclosporine.

exenatide
Bydureon, Byetta

Class and Category
Chemical class: Amino acid peptide amide
Therapeutic class: Antidiabetic drug
Pregnancy category: C

Indications and Dosages
➤ *Adjunct treatment to diet and exercise to improve blood glucose levels in patients with type 2 diabetes mellitus*
SUBCUTANEOUS INJECTION (BYETTA)
Adults. *Initial:* 5 mcg twice daily, given within 60 min before morning and evening meals. After 1 mo, increased, as needed, to 10 mcg twice daily, given within 60 min before morning and evening meals.
SUBCUTANEOUS INJECTION (BYDUREON)
Adults. 2 mg once every 7 days.

Route	Onset	Peak	Duration
SubQ	Immediate	2.1 hr	Unknown

Contraindications
Hypersensitivity to exenatide or its components, ketoacidosis, personal or family history of medullary thyroid carcinoma or multiple endocrine neoplasia syndrome type 2 (Bydureon), type 1 diabetes mellitus

Interactions
DRUGS
oral antidiabetics: Increased risk of hypoglycemia
oral drugs: May decrease rate and extent of absorption of these drugs
warfarin: Possibly increased INR with increased risk of bleeding

Adverse Reactions
CNS: Asthenia, dizziness, headache, jitteriness, somnolence
CV: Chest pain
EENT: Decreased taste
ENDO: Hypoglycemia

E
F

GI: Abdominal distention or pain, anorexia, constipation, diarrhea, dyspepsia, flatulence, gastroesophageal reflux, indigestion, nausea, pancreatitis (including life-threatening hemorrhagic or necrotizing), vomiting
GU: Acute renal failure, decreased renal function, elevated serum creatinine level, kidney transplant dysfunction, worsening chronic renal failure
RESP: Chronic hypersensitivity pneumonitis
SKIN: Alopecia, diaphoresis, macular or papular rash, pruritus, rash, urticaria
Other: Anaphylaxis, angioedema, anti-exenatide antibodies, dehydration, elevated anti-exenatide antibody level, injection-site reactions (abscess, cellulitis, necrosis, pruritus, subcutaneous nodules), weight loss

Nursing Considerations
• Exenatide isn't recommended for patients with severe GI disease, patients with creatinine clearance less than 30 ml/min/1.73 m^2, or patients having dialysis because of adverse GI or renal effects.
• Use exenatide cautiously in a renal transplant patient or patient with moderate renal disease when dosage is increased from 5 mcg to 10 mcg. Monitor renal function throughout therapy, and notify prescriber of abnormalities.
• If patient also takes a sulfonylurea, the sulfonylurea dosage may need to be decreased to reduce the risk of hypoglycemia. Usually, no dosage adjustment is needed for a patient taking metformin.
• Administer drug into patient's thigh, abdomen, or upper arm.
• Monitor patient's blood glucose level. If control decreases despite the patient's best efforts, drug may need to be discontinued because of the possibility that anti-exenatide antibodies have formed. Be aware that if patient is already taking the rapid release form of exenatide (Byetta) and is switching to the extended-release form of exenatide (Bydureon), Byetta needs to be discontinued first. Also know that he may experience a transient elevation in his blood glucose levels for about 2 weeks as his body adjusts to the extended release form.
• Monitor patient for evidence of acute pancreatitis, such as persistent, severe abdominal pain accompanied by vomiting, especially when drug is started or dosage increased. Notify prescriber, and expect to stop exenatide and give supportive care.

Mechanism of Action
Normally, when serum glucose level rises, insulin is secreted within 10 minutes. This first-phase insulin response is absent in patients with type 2 diabetes. Exenatide, an incretin mimetic, restores the first-phase insulin response and improves the second-phase response that immediately follows. It does so by promoting incretins that spur insulin synthesis and release from beta cells by binding and activating human GLP-1 receptors to reduce fasting and postprandial serum glucose levels.

The drug also suppresses inappropriately elevated glucagon secretion. Lower serum glucagon level leads to decreased hepatic glucose output

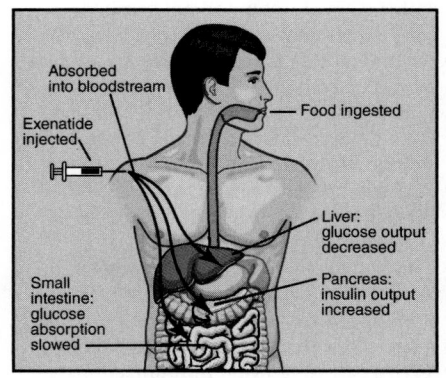

and decreased insulin demand. It also slows gastric emptying and thus the rise of serum glucose level.

• Know that the rapid release form of exenatide (Byetta) may be used concomitantly with insulin glargine (Lantus), which is along-acting insulin to help improve the patient's blood glucose control. Byetta should not be used with any other type of insulin. If the patient is susceptible to hypoglycemia, expect the insulin glargine dosage to be decreased when used with Byetta.

PATIENT TEACHING

• Teach patient how to give a subcutaneous injection and how to use pen injector if prescribed Byetta.

• Teach patient how to mix powder with diluent if prescribed Bydureon and how to give a subcutaneous injection. Remind patient to administer Bydureon immediately after the powder is suspended in the diluent and transferred to the syringe. Also tell him not to substitute needles or any other components in the tray. Alert him that a spare needle has been provided in the tray in the event he needs it.

• Inform patient that exenatide may be administered in the thigh, abdomen, or upper arm. Stress the need to rotate injection sites.

• Tell patient to inspect injection site daily and to report any adverse effects at site that are persistent or appear serious.

• Emphasize the need to use rapid release form of drug (Byetta) within 60 minutes before morning and evening meals or the two main meals of the day, about 6 hours or more apart, never after a meal.

• If patient misses a dose of Byetta, tell him to resume treatment with the next scheduled dose. If patient is prescribed Bydureon and misses a dose, tell him to administer the drug as soon as he remembers as long as his regularly scheduled dose is at least 3 days later. If the time frame is less than this, tell patient to wait until his next regularly scheduled dose. Make patient aware that he may change the day of weekly administration of Bydureon as long as the last dose was administered 3 or more days before.

• Advise patient that drug should look clear and colorless. Tell him not to use drug solution that looks cloudy or colored or contains particles.

• Instruct patient to check expiration date on the vial and not to use drug if date has passed.

• Advise patient to refrigerate rapid acting drug (Byetta) before first use and protect it from light. After first use of pen device, drug may be stored at room temperature of 77° F (25° C) or less. Advise patient to refrigerate extended-release drug (Bydureon) in refrigerator and protect from light. A single-use tray of Bydureon may be stored at room temperature for up to 4 weeks.

• Tell patient to discard pen injector 30 days after initial use, even if some drug is left.

• Alert patient that pen doesn't come with needles and that he'll need to buy them.

• Warn patient that nausea may occur at the beginning of therapy.

• Inform patient taking a sulfonylurea or insulin glargine to be alert for hypoglycemic reactions because risk increases with both drugs. Review ways to treat such reactions, and tell patient to alert prescriber if they occur often or are severe.

• Instruct female patient of childbearing potential to tell her prescriber if she is, could be, or is planning to become pregnant.

• Tell patient to seek emergency care for persistent, severe abdominal pain and vomiting.

• Caution patient that exenatide doesn't replace diet and exercise measures.

ezetimibe

Zetia

Class and Category

Chemical class: Azetidinone
Therapeutic class: Antihypercholesterolemic
Pregnancy category: C

Indications and Dosages

➤ *To treat heterozygous familial and nonfamilial hypercholesterolemia or homozygous sitosterolemia; as adjunct with HMG-CoA reductase inhibitors to treat heterozygous familial and nonfamilial hypercholesterolemia; with fenofibrate to treat mixed hyperlipidemia and with atorvastatin or simvastatin to*

E
F

treat patients with homozygous familial hypercholesterolemia

TABLETS

Adults. 10 mg daily.

Contraindications

Active hepatic dysfunction, hypersensitivity to ezetimibe or its components

Interactions
DRUGS

cholestyramine: Reduced effects of ezetimibe
cyclosporine: Increased blood cyclosporine and ezetimibe levels
fenofibrate, gemfibrozil: Increased blood ezetimibe level

Adverse Reactions

CNS: Depression, dizziness, fatigue, headache, paresthesia
CV: Chest pain
EENT: Pharyngitis, sinusitis
GI: Abdominal pain, cholelithiasis, cholecystitis, diarrhea, elevated liver function test results, hepatitis, nausea, pancreatitis

HEME: Thrombocytopenia
MS: Arthralgia, back or limb pain, elevated CK level, myalgia, myopathy, rhabdomyolysis
RESP: Cough, upper respiratory tract infection
SKIN: Erythema multiforme, rash, urticaria
Other: Anaphylaxis, angioedema, influenza, viral infection

Nursing Considerations

• Monitor liver function test results before and during ezetimibe therapy, as ordered.
• Know that you should give ezetimibe 2 hours before or 4 hours after giving bile acid sequestrant, cholestyramine, or colestipol.
PATIENT TEACHING
• Direct patient to follow a low-cholesterol diet as an adjunct to ezetimibe therapy. Recommend weight loss and exercise programs, as appropriate.
• If patient also takes a bile acid sequestrant, tell him to take ezetimibe either 2 hours

Mechanism of Action

Reduces blood cholesterol by inhibiting its absorption through the small intestine.

Normally, in the intestinal lumen, lipids break down to cholesterol and other substances that create smaller droplets called micelles, as shown below left. The micelles enter intestinal epithelial cells called enterocytes, where they combine with triglycerides, cholesterol, and other

substances to form chylomicrons. Chylomicrons then pass through to the lymphatic system to be carried to the blood.

Ezetimibe blocks cholesterol absorption into enterocytes and keeps cholesterol from moving through the intestinal wall, as shown below right. Reduced cholesterol absorption from the intestine decreases chylomicron and LDL cholesterol content.

before or at least 4 hours after it to prevent drug interactions.
• Advise patient to report unexplained muscle pain, tenderness, or weakness.

ezogabine
Potiga

Class and Category
Chemical class: Carbamic acid ethyl ester
Therapeutic class: Anticonvulsant
Pregnancy category: C
Controlled substance schedule: V

Indications and Dosages
➤ *Adjunct treatment of partial-onset seizures*

TABLETS

Adults. *Initial:* 100 mg three times daily, increased by no more than 50 mg 3 times daily on weekly basis, as needed. *Maintenance:* 200 to 400 mg 3 times daily. *Maximum:* 400 mg 3 times daily.

DOSAGE ADJUSTMENT For patients older than 65 years or for patients with moderate liver impairment, maximum dosage should not exceed 250 mg 3 times daily. For patients with a creatinine clearance less than 50 ml/min or end-stage renal disease on dialysis or in patients with severe liver impairment, maximum dosage should not exceed 200 mg 3 times daily.

Mechanism of Action
Possibly enhances transmembrane potassium currents mediated by the KCNQ family of ion channels. By activating the KCNQ channels, the resting membrane potential is stabilized, reducing brain excitability, which alters seizure activity.

Contraindications
Hypersensitivity to ezogabine and its components

Interactions
DRUGS
carbamazepine, phenytoin: Decreased effectiveness of ezogabine
digoxin: Increased blood digoxin level, resulting in possible digoxin toxicity

ACTIVITIES
alcohol use: Possibly increased CNS depression

Adverse Reactions
CNS: Abnormal coordination, amnesia, anxiety, aphasia, asthenia, attention disturbance, coma, confusion, disorientation, dizziness, dysarthria, dysphasia, encephalopathy, euphoric mood, fatigue, gait disturbance, hallucinations, hypokinesia, memory impairment, myclonus, paresthesia, psychotic symptoms, somnolence, suicidal ideation, syncope, tremor, vertigo
CV: Peripheral edema, prolonged QT interval
EENT: Blurred vision, diplopia, dry mouth, nystagmus, retinal pigment changes, visual abnormalities
GI: Constipation, dyspepsia, elevated liver enzymes, increased appetite, nausea
GU: Chromaturia, dysuria, hematuria, nephrolithiasis, renal colic, urinary hesitancy, retention
HEME: Leukopenia, enutropenia, thrombocytopenia
MS: Muscle spasms
RESP: Dyspnea
SKIN: Alopecia, blue skin discoloration, diaphoresis, rash
Other: Influenza, weight gain

Nursing Considerations
• Use ezogabine cautiously with patients who have a history of prolonged QT interval and patients who take medication known to prolong the QT interval, or those who have congestive heart failure, ventricular hypertrophy, hypokalemia or hypogmagnesemia because ezogabine may prolong the patient's QT interval.
• Use cautiously with patients who have risk factors for urinary retention (such as the presence of benign prostatic hyperplasia), patients who cannot communicate clearly, and patients who use concomitant medications that may affect voiding (such as anticholinergics) because urinary retention has occurred with ezogabine use. Know that patients at risk for urinary retention should have a urologic evaluation prior to starting ezogabine therapy.
• Ensure patient has a baseline eye exam before ezogabine therapy begins and then

E
F

at least every 6 months during therapy because drug may cause pigment changes in the retina that may lead to serious eye disease with loss of vision.
• Monitor patient for blue pigmentation of the skin, especially on or around the lips or in nail beds although more widespread involvement of the face and legs also may occur. In addition, scleral and conjunctival discoloration on the white of the eye and inside eyelids may occur. Notify prescriber immediately if present as ezogabine therapy may need to be discontinued.
• Monitor patient for urinary retention throughout drug therapy but especially during first 6 months of therapy. If present, prepare to catheterize patient, as ordered. Drug may need to be discontinued.
• Expect to reduce dosage gradually over a period of at least 3 weeks, as ordered, when drug is being discontinued to avoid withdrawal seizures.
• Monitor patient closely for evidence of psychiatric symptoms, including suicidal thinking or behavior, especially when therapy starts or dosage changes.
• Be aware that ezogabine therapy can produce falsely elevated serum and urine bilirubin readings.

PATIENT TEACHING
• Advise patient to avoid performing hazardous activities, such as driving, until the adverse effects of ezogabine are known.
• Urge caregivers to watch patient closely for evidence of psychiatric symptoms, including suicidal tendencies, especially when therapy starts or dosage changes, and to report concerns at once to prescriber.
WARNING Emphasize importance of reporting visual changes or the appearance of a blue color on her skin or white of the eye as drug may need to be discontinued and a new drug prescribed in its place.
• Encourage women who become pregnant while taking ezogabine to enroll in the North American antiepileptic drug pregnancy registry by calling 1-888-233-2334. Explain that the registry is collecting information about the safety of anti-epileptic drugs during pregnancy.

famotidine

Act (CAN), Apo-Famotidine (CAN), Dyspep HB (CAN), Gen-Famotidine (CAN), Mylanta-AR, Novo-Famotidine (CAN), Nu-Famotidine (CAN), Pepcid, Pepcid AC, Pepcid RPD

Class and Category
Chemical class: Thiazole derivative
Therapeutic class: Antiulcer agent, gastric acid secretion inhibitor
Pregnancy category: B

Indications and Dosages
➤ *To provide short-term treatment of active duodenal ulcer*
ORAL SUSPENSION, TABLETS (CHEWABLE, ORAL DISINTEGRATING, AND REGULAR)
Adults and adolescents. 40 mg daily at bedtime or 20 mg twice daily.
Children. 0.5 mg/kg daily as a single dose at bedtime or in divided doses twice daily.
I.V. INFUSION OR INJECTION
Adults and adolescents over age 16. 20 mg every 12 hr, infused over 15 to 30 min or injected over at least 2 min.
Children ages 1 to 16. *Initial:* 0.25 mg/kg every 12 hr, infused over 15 to 30 min or injected over at least 2 min. *Maximum:* 40 mg daily.
➤ *To prevent recurrence of duodenal ulcer*
ORAL SUSPENSION, TABLETS (CHEWABLE, ORAL DISINTEGRATING, AND REGULAR)
Adults and adolescents. 20 mg daily at bedtime.
➤ *To provide short-term treatment for active, benign gastric ulcer*
ORAL SUSPENSION, TABLETS (CHEWABLE, ORAL DISINTEGRATING, AND REGULAR)
Adults and adolescents. 40 mg daily at bedtime.
Children. 0.5 mg/kg daily as a single dose at bedtime or in divided doses twice daily.
I.V. INFUSION OR INJECTION
Adults and adolescents over age 16. 20 mg every 12 hr.
Children ages 1 to 16. *Initial:* 0.25 mg/kg every 12 hr. *Maximum:* 40 mg daily.
➤ *To treat gastroesophageal reflux disease (GERD)*

ORAL SUSPENSION, TABLETS (CHEWABLE, ORAL DISINTEGRATING, AND REGULAR)
Adults and adolescents. 20 mg twice daily for up to 6 wk.
Children weighing more than 10 kg (22 lb). 1 to 2 mg/kg daily in divided doses twice daily.
Children weighing less than 10 kg. 1 to 2 mg/kg daily in divided doses three times daily.
ORAL SUSPENSION
Infants age 4 months to 1 year. 0.5 mg/kg daily in divided doses twice daily for up to 8 wk.
Infants age 3 months or less. 0.5 mg/kg daily for up to 8 wk.
I.V. INFUSION OR INJECTION
Children ages 1 to 16. *Initial:* 0.25 mg/kg every 12 hr. *Maximum:* 40 mg daily.
➤ *To treat esophagitis caused by gastroesophageal reflux*
ORAL SUSPENSION, TABLETS (CHEWABLE, ORAL DISINTEGRATING, AND REGULAR)
Adults and adolescents. 20 to 40 mg twice daily for up to 12 wk.
➤ *To treat gastric hypersecretory conditions, such as Zollinger-Ellison syndrome*

ORAL SUSPENSION, TABLETS (CHEWABLE, ORAL DISINTEGRATING, AND REGULAR)
Adults and adolescents. *Initial:* 20 mg every 6 hr. Dosage adjusted, if needed, based on patient response.
I.V. INFUSION OR INJECTION
Adults and adolescents. 20 mg every 12 hr.
➤ *To prevent heartburn and indigestion*
TABLETS (CHEWABLE, ORAL DISINTEGRATING, AND REGULAR)
Adults and adolescents. 10 mg 1 hr before eating. *Maximum:* 20 mg every 24 hr.
➤ *To treat heartburn and indigestion*
TABLETS (CHEWABLE, ORAL DISINTEGRATING, AND REGULAR)
Adults and adolescents. 10 mg at onset of symptoms. *Maximum:* 20 mg every 24 hr for up to 2 wk unless prescribed otherwise.
DOSAGE ADJUSTMENT Oral or parenteral dosage reduced or dosing interval increased (to 36 to 48 hr), if needed, in patients with renal insufficiency and creatinine clearance of 49 ml/min/1.73 m^2 or less.

Route	Onset	Peak	Duration
P.O.	1 hr	1–4 hr	10–12 hr
I.V.	In 30 min	0.5–3 hr	10–12 hr

Mechanism of Action

In normal digestion, parietal cells in the gastric epithelium secrete hydrogen (H^+) ions, which combine with chloride ions (Cl^-) to form hydrochloric acid (HCl), asshown below left. However, HCl can inflame, ulcerate, and perforate gastric and intestinal mucosa normally protected by mucus. Famotidine, an H^2-receptor antagonist, reduces HCl formation by preventing histamine from binding with H^2 receptors on the surface of parietal cells, as shown below right. By doing so, the drug helps prevent peptic ulcers from forming and helps heal existing ones.

Contraindications

Hypersensitivity to famotidine, other H_2-receptor antagonists, or their components

Interactions

DRUGS

antacids, sucralfate: Possibly decreased absorption of famotidine

bone marrow depressants: Increased risk of blood dyscrasias

itraconazole, ketoconazole: Possibly decreased absorption of these drugs

ACTIVITIES

alcohol use: Possibly increased blood alcohol level

Adverse Reactions

CNS: Agitation (infants), anxiety, asthenia, confusion, depression, dizziness, fatigue, fever, hallucinations, headache, insomnia, mental or mood changes, paresthesia, seizures, somnolence

CV: Arrhythmias, AV block, palpitations, prolonged QT interval

EENT: Dry mouth, laryngeal edema, taste alteration, tinnitus

GI: Abdominal pain, anorexia, cholestatic jaundice, constipation, diarrhea, elevated liver enzymes, hepatitis, nausea, vomiting

GU: Decreased libido, impotence

HEME: Agranulocytosis, aplastic anemia, leukopenia, neutropenia, pancytopenia, thrombocytopenia

MS: Arthralgia, muscle cramps, musculoskeletal pain, rhabdomyolysis

RESP: Bronchospasm, dyspnea, interstitial pneumonia, wheezing

SKIN: Acne, alopecia, dry skin, erythema multiforme, exfoliative dermatitis, flushing, jaundice, pruritus, rash, Stevens-Johnson syndrome, toxic epidermal necrolysis, urticaria

Other: Anaphylaxis, angioedema, facial or orbital edema, hyperuricemia

Nursing Considerations

• Shake famotidine oral suspension vigorously for 5 to 10 seconds before administration.

• Dilute injection form (2 ml) with normal saline solution or other solution to 5 to 10 ml; give I.V. injection over at least 2 minutes. Or, dilute in 100 ml of D_5W and infuse over 15 to 30 minutes; or infuse premixed injection (20 mg/50 ml normal saline solution) over 15 to 30 minutes.

WARNING Be aware that Pepcid AC chewable tablets contain aspartame, which can be dangerous for patients who have phenylketonuria.

PATIENT TEACHING

• Instruct patient to store famotidine oral suspension at room temperature (below 86° F [30° C]) and to protect it from freezing. Tell her to shake the bottle vigorously, right before use, for 5 to 10 seconds after adding water.

• Advise patient who uses Pepcid RPD to store drug in unopened package. For each dose, instruct her to open blister pack with dry hands, place a tablet on her tongue, let it dissolve, and swallow it with saliva.

• If patient uses chewable tablets, instruct her to chew them thoroughly before swallowing.

• If patient also takes antacids, instruct her to wait 30 to 60 minutes after taking famotidine, if possible, before taking antacid.

• Caution patient to avoid alcohol and smoking during famotidine therapy because they irritate the stomach and can delay ulcer healing.

• Advise patient to notify prescriber if she develops pain, has trouble swallowing, or if she has bloody vomit or black stools.

• Caution patient not to take famotidine with other acid-reducing products.

febuxostat
Uloric

Class and Category

Chemical class: Non-purine xanthine oxidase inhibitor

Therapeutic class: Antigout

Pregnancy category: C

Indications and Dosages

➤ *To treat chronic hyperuricemia in patients with gout*

TABLETS

Adults. *Initial:* 40 mg once daily, increased after 2 wk to 80 mg once daily, if needed.

Route	Onset	Peak	Duration
P.O.	2–3 days	1–1.5 hr	Unknown

Mechanism of Action

Inhibits the action of xanthine oxidase, the key enzyme responsible for purine breakdown. Xanthine oxidase catalyzes conversion of xanthine to uric acid, thereby increasing uric acid levels. High uric acid levels cause gout attacks. Inhibiting xanthine oxidase causes uric acid levels to drop, decreasing the risk of gout attack.

Contraindications

Concurrent use of azathioprine or mercaptopurine, hypersensitivity to febuxostat or its components

Interactions

DRUGS

azathioprine, mercaptopurine, theophylline: Possibly increased serum levels of these drugs, leading to toxicity

Adverse Reactions

CNS: Aggression, dizziness, hemiparesis, lacunar infarction, psychotic behavior, stroke, transient ischemic attack
CV: Angina, chest pain or discomfort, ECG abnormalities, MI
EENT: Blurred vision, deafness, epistaxis, nasal dryness, paranasal sinus hypersecretion, pharyngeal edema, sneezing, taste disturbance, throat irritation, tinnitus
ENDO: Breast pain, gynecomastia, hot flashes, hypoglycemia
GI: Diarrhea, dyspepsia, elevated liver enzymes, GI discomfort, hepatic failure, hepatomegaly, jaundice, nausea, vomiting
GU: Decreased libido, erectile dysfunction, hematuria, nephrolithiasis, pollakiuria, proteinuria, renal failure or insufficiency, tubulointerstitial nephritis, urgency
HEME: Anemia, idiopathic thrombocytopenic purpura, leukocytosis, leukopenia, neutropenia, pancytopenia, splenomegaly, thrombocytopenia
MS: Arthralgia, joint stiffness or swelling, rhabdomyolysis
RESP: Upper respiratory tract infection
SKIN: Dermatitis, ecchymosis, eczema, flushing, hair color or growth changes, hyperhidrosis, peeling skin, petechiae, photosensitivity, pruritis, rash, Stevens-Johnson syndrome, urticaria
Other: Anaphylaxis, gout flares, hypersensitivity

Nursing Considerations

• Febuxostat therapy isn't recommended for patients in whom rate of urate formation is greatly increased, as in malignancy and its treatment or Lesch-Nyhan syndrome.
• Obtain a liver test panel, as ordered, prior to initiating febuxostat therapy and then periodically thereafter. Monitor patient for signs and symptoms of liver dysfunction such as fatigue, anorexia, right upper abdominal discomfort, dark urine or jaundice throughout therapy. If signs and symptoms occur or if abnormal liver tests occur, especially an elevated serum alanine aminotransferase level greater than three times the upper normal limit, notify prescriber and expect drug to be withheld until underlying cause is determined. If no other cause can be found other than febuxostat therapy, expect drug to be discontinued permanently.
• Monitor patient's serum uric acid level, as prescribed, to determine drug effectiveness. Expect it to take about 2 weeks for uric acid level to be therapeutically altered. Dose may be increased from 40 mg to 80 mg daily if target serum uric acid level fails to fall below 6 mg/dl.
• Monitor patient for gout flares, which may occur after therapy is started because of changing serum uric acid levels that result in mobilization of urate from tissue deposits. Expect prescriber to order an NSAID or colchicine when febuxostat therapy starts. If patient has a gout flare-up during treatment, notify prescriber, and expect symptoms to be managed. Know that febuxostat therapy usually isn't discontinued during this time.
• Monitor patient for evidence of cardiovascular thrombosis, such as acute MI or stroke, because drug may increase patient's risk of developing these disorders.

PATIENT TEACHING

• Inform patient that a gout attack may occur when febuxostat therapy starts and that NSAIDs or colchicine may be prescribed, usually along with febuxostat, to treat it.
• Instruct patient to seek immediate emergency care for signs or symptoms of a heart attack or stroke.

E
F

• Tell patient that periodic blood tests will be needed to determine drug's effectiveness and to detect adverse effects.

felbamate
Felbatol

Class and Category
Chemical class: Dicarbamate
Therapeutic class: Anticonvulsant
Pregnancy category: C

Indications and Dosages
➤ *To treat partial seizures in patients who don't respond to other drugs*
ORAL SUSPENSION, TABLETS
Adults and adolescents over age 14. *Initial:* 1,200 mg daily in divided doses three times daily or four times daily. Dosage increased over several weeks based on patient response. *Maximum:* 3,600 mg daily.
Children ages 2 to 14. *Initial:* 15 mg/kg daily in divided doses three times daily.or four times daily. Dosage increased over several weeks based on patient response. *Maximum:* 3,600 mg daily or 45 mg/kg daily.
➤ *As adjunct to treat generalized or partial seizures associated with Lennox-Gastaut syndrome in children*
ORAL SUSPENSION, TABLETS
Children ages 2 to 14. *Initial:* 15 mg/kg daily in divided doses three times daily or four times daily while decreasing other anticonvulsant drugs by 20% to control their blood levels. Felbamate dosage increased by 15 mg/kg daily every wk. *Maximum:* 3,600 mg daily or 45 mg/kg daily.
DOSAGE ADJUSTMENT Dosage reduced by 50% in patients with renal impairment.

Mechanism of Action
May exert anticonvulsant effects by antagonizing the amino acid glycine. When glycine binds to N-methyl-d-aspartate (NMDA) receptors in the CNS, the frequency at which receptor-gated calcium ion channels open is increased—an important factor in initiating seizures. Felbamate may raise the seizure threshold by blocking NMDA receptors so glycine can't bind to them.

Contraindications
Hepatic dysfunction; history of blood dyscrasias; hypersensitivity to felbamate, other carbamates, or their components

Interactions
DRUGS
carbamazepine: Decreased blood carbamazepine level and increased felbamate clearance, resulting in decreased blood felbamate level
fosphenytoin, phenytoin: Increased blood phenytoin level and increased felbamate clearance, resulting in decreased blood felbamate level
methsuximide: Increased adverse effects of methsuximide
oral contraceptives: Possibly decreased effectiveness of oral contraceptives
phenobarbital: Decreased blood felbamate level, increased blood phenobarbital level and risk of adverse effects
valproic acid: Increased blood valproic acid level and increased risk of adverse effects

Adverse Reactions
CNS: Abnormal gait, aggressiveness, agitation, anxiety, dizziness, drowsiness, fever, headache, insomnia, mood changes, suicidal ideation, tremor
EENT: Altered taste, diplopia, rhinitis
GI: Abdominal pain, anorexia, constipation, diarrhea, elevated liver function test results, hepatic failure, indigestion, nausea, vomiting
HEME: Aplastic anemia, leukopenia, pancytopenia, thrombocytopenia
RESP: Upper respiratory tract infection
SKIN: Photosensitivity, purpura, rash
Other: Anaphylaxis, lymphadenopathy, weight loss

Nursing Considerations
• Check liver function test results before starting felbamate, and expect to check results every 1 to 2 weeks during treatment. Notify prescriber immediately and expect to stop drug if results are abnormal.
• Plan to taper dosage by one-third every 4 to 5 days as prescribed. If patient receives adequate amounts of other anticonvulsant drugs, felbamate may be stopped without tapering, if needed.
WARNING Assess for signs of aplastic anemia and bone marrow depression. Signs may

not appear until several months after therapy begins. Expect to stop felbamate if bone marrow depression develops.

- If patient receives adjunctive therapy, expect adverse reactions to resolve as other anticonvulsant dosages decrease.
- Monitor patient closely for evidence of suicidal thinking or behavior, especially when therapy starts or dosage changes.

PATIENT TEACHING

- Direct patient to shake suspension before using and to use a calibrated spoon or container to measure each dose.
- Instruct patient to store oral suspension and tablets at room temperature.
- Because drug may cause photosensitivity, urge patient to protect skin from sun and to avoid sunlamps and tanning booths.
- Explain that dizziness and drowsiness may occur. Advise her to avoid hazardous activities until drug's CNS effects are known.
- Warn patient not to stop drug abruptly.
- Advise patient to return for ordered liver function tests and to report yellow skin or eyes and dark urine to prescriber.
- Instruct patient to tell prescriber if she experiences bleeding, infection, or fatigue.
- Advise patient to carry medical identification that indicates condition and therapy.
- Because felbamate decreases oral contraceptive effectiveness, discuss alternate contraceptive methods.
- Urge caregivers to watch patient closely for evidence of suicidal tendencies, especially when therapy starts or dosage changes, and to report any concerns immediately.
- Encourage female patient who becomes pregnant while taking felbamate to enroll in the North American antiepileptic drug pregnancy registry by calling 1-888-233-2334. Explain that this registry is collecting information about the safety of antiepileptic drugs during pregnancy.

felodipine

Plendil, Renedil (CAN)

Class and Category

Chemical class: Dihydropyridine derivative
Therapeutic class: Antihypertensive
Pregnancy category: C

Indications and Dosages

➤ *To manage essential hypertension alone or with other antihypertensives*

E.R. TABLETS

Adults. *Initial:* 5 mg daily. Dosage adjusted every 2 wk to 2.5 to 10 mg daily based on patient response.

DOSAGE ADJUSTMENT Initial or maintenance dosage reduced, if needed, in patients who are over age 65 or have impaired hepatic function.

Route	Onset	Peak	Duration
P.O.	2–5 hr	Unknown	16–24 hr

Mechanism of Action

May slow the movement of extracellular calcium into myocardial and vascular smooth-muscle cells by deforming calcium channels in cell membranes, inhibiting ion-controlled gating mechanisms, and interfering with calcium release from the sarcoplasmic reticulum. The effect of these actions is a decrease in intracellular calcium ions, which inhibits contraction of smooth-muscle cells and dilates coronary and systemic arteries. As with other calcium channel blockers, felodipine's actions result in increased oxygen to the myocardium and reduced peripheral resistance, blood pressure, and afterload.

Contraindications

Hypersensitivity to felodipine or its components

Interactions

DRUGS

anesthetics (hydrocarbon inhalation): Possibly hypotension
antihypertensives, prazocin: Increased risk of hypotension
beta blockers: Increased adverse effects of beta blockers
cimetidine: Increased felodipine bioavailability
digoxin: Transiently increased blood digoxin level and risk of digitalis toxicity
estrogens: Possibly increased fluid retention and decreased felodipine effects
lithium: Increased risk of neurotoxicity
NSAIDs, sympathomimetics: Possibly decreased therapeutic effect of felodipine

E
F

procainamide, quinidine: Increased risk of prolonged Q-T interval
tacrolimus: Possibly increased blood tacrolimus level and risk of adverse effects
FOODS
grapefruit juice: Doubled felodipine bioavailability

Adverse Reactions

CNS: Asthenia, dizziness, drowsiness, fatigue, headache, paresthesia, syncope, weakness
CV: Chest pain, hypotension, palpitations, peripheral edema, tachycardia
EENT: Gingival hyperplasia, pharyngitis, rhinitis
GI: Abdominal cramps, constipation, diarrhea, indigestion, nausea
HEME: Agranulocytosis
MS: Back pain
RESP: Cough
SKIN: Flushing, rash

Nursing Considerations

• Use felodipine cautiously in patients with heart failure or reduced ventricular function.
• Monitor blood pressure during dosage titration and throughout felodipine therapy, especially in elderly patients.
• Felodipine bioavailability increases up to twofold when taken with grapefruit juice.
WARNING Felodipine may cause severe hypotension with syncope, which may lead to reflex tachycardia. This can precipitate angina in patients with coronary artery disease or a history of angina.
• Watch for signs of overdose, such as excessive peripheral vasodilation, marked hypotension and, possibly, bradycardia. If they appear, place patient in supine position with legs elevated and give I.V. fluids, as ordered. Expect to give I.V. atropine for bradycardia.
PATIENT TEACHING
• Instruct patient to swallow tablets whole and not to crush or chew them.
• Caution patient not to alter her intake of grapefruit juice during therapy.
• Advise patient to store felodipine at room temperature and to protect it from light.
• Instruct patient to monitor her pulse rate and blood pressure.

• Teach patient how to minimize gingival hyperplasia.
• Advise patient to notify prescriber immediately if she has palpitations, pronounced dizziness, or swelling of hands or feet.

fenofibrate

Fenofibrate, Lipofen, Lofibra, Tricor, Triglide

fenofibric acid

Antara, Fibricor, Trilipix

Class and Category

Chemical class: Aryloxisobutyric acid derivative
Therapeutic class: Antihyperlipidemic
Pregnancy category: C

Indications and Dosages

➤ *To treat primary hypercholesterolemia or mixed hyperlipidemia*
CAPSULES (LIPOFEN)
Adults. 150 mg daily with food.
CAPSULES (LOFIBRA)
Adults. 200 mg daily with food.
CAPSULES (ANTARA)
Adults. 130 mg daily.
DELAYED-RELEASE CAPSULES (TRILIPIX)
Adults. 135 mg daily.
TABLETS (FENOFIBRATE)
Adults. 160 mg daily.
TABLETS (TRICOR)
Adults. 145 mg daily.
TABLETS (FIBRICOR)
Adults. 105 mg daily.
TABLETS (TRIGLIDE)
Adults. 160 mg daily.
➤ *To treat hypertriglyceridemia (fredrickson types IV and V hyperlipidemia)*
CAPSULES (LOFIBRA)
Adults. *Initial:* 67 to 200 mg daily with food, increased as needed every 4 to 8 wk.*Maximum:* 200 mg daily with meals.
TABLETS (FENOFIBRATE)
Adults. 54 to 160 mg daily, increased as needed at 4- to 8-wk intervals. *Maximum:* 160 mg daily.

➤ *As adjunct to diet to treat severe hypertriglyceridemia*

CAPSULES (ANTARA)

Adults. *Initial:* 43 to 130 mg mg daily, increased, as needed at 4-8 intervals. *Maximum:* 130 mg daily.

CAPSULES (LIPOFEN)

Adults. *Initial:* 50 to 150 mg daily with food, inceased, as needed at 4-8 wk intervals. *Maximum:* 150 mg daily with food.

DELAYED-RELEASE CAPSULES (TRILIPIX)

Adults. *Initial:* 45 to135 mg once daily, increased, as needed at 4- to 8-wk intervals. *Maximum:* 135 mg daily.

TABLETS (FIBRICOR)

Adults. *Initial:* 35 to 105 mg daily, increased, as needed at 4-8 wk intervals. *Maximum:* 105 mg daily.

TABLETS (TRICOR)

Adults. *Initial:* 48 to 145 mg daily, increased, as needed at 4-8 wk intervals. *Maximum:* 145 mg daily.

TABLETS (TRIGLIDE)

Adults. *Initial:* 50 to 160 mg daily, increased, as needed at 4-8-wk intervals. *Maximum:* 160 mg daily.

➤ *As adjunct to diet to treat primary hyperlipidemia or mixed dyslipidemia; as adjunct to diet and a HMG-CoA reductase inhibitor to treat mixed dyslipidemia*

DELAYED-RELEASE CAPSULES (TRILIPIX)

Adults. 135 mg daily.

DOSAGE ADJUSTMENT For patients with mild to moderate renal impairment or elderly patients, dosage limited for all indications to lowest dosage prescribed for treatment of severe hypertriglyceridemia once daily with increase only after drug's therapeutic and renal effects are known.

Route	Onset	Peak	Duration
P.O.	6–8 wk	Unknown	Unknown

Mechanism of Action

May increase the lipolysis of triglyceride-rich lipoproteins and decrease the synthesis of fatty acids and triglycerides by enhancing the activation of lipoprotein lipase and acyl-coenzyme A synthetase. Fenofibrate also may:

• increase hepatic elimination of cholesterol as bile salts
• promote the catabolism of larger, less dense LDLs with a high-binding affinity for cellular LDL receptors.

Contraindications

Breastfeeding; gallbladder disease; hypersensitivity to fenofibrate, fenofibric acid, choline fenofibrate, or their components; hepatic or severe renal impairment

Interactions

DRUGS

bile acid sequestrants: Decreased fenofibrate absorption
colchicine, fibrates such as gemfibrozil: Increased risk of myopathy and rhabdomyolysis
cyclosporine: Increased risk of nephro-toxicity
HMG-CoA reductase inhibitors (atorvastatin, cerivastatin, fluvastatin, lovastatin, pravastatin, simvastatin): Increased risk of myopathy, rhabdo-myolysis, and acute renal failure
oral anticoagulants: Risk of bleeding

FOODS

all foods: Increased fenofibrate bioavail-ability when given in capsule form

Adverse Reactions

CNS: Asthenia, fatigue, headache
CV: Deep vein thrombosis, severely depressed HDL cholesterol levels
EENT: Rhinitis
GI: Abdominal pain, cholelithiasis, cirrhosis, constipation, diarrhea, elevated liver function test results, hepatitis, nausea, pancreatitis, severely depressed HDL cholesterol levels
GU: Acute renal failure, increased serum creatinine level, renal failure
HEME: Agranulocytosis; anemia; decreased hematocrit, hemoglobin or white blood cell levels; thrombocytopenia
MS: Arthralgia, back pain, elevated creatinine phosphokinase, muscle spasms, myalgia, myopathy, myositis, rhabdo-myolysis
RESP: Pulmonary embolus
SKIN: Rash, Stevens-Johnson syndrome, toxic epidermal necrolysis, urticaria
Other: Flulike symptoms

E
F

Nursing Considerations
• As ordered, stop drugs that increase serum triglycerides, such as beta blockers, estrogens, and thiazides, and obtain baseline lipid levels before starting fenofibrate.
• Be aware that some brands such as Lipofen and Lofibra needed to be given with food to enhance absorption.
• Administer drug 1 hour before or 4 hours after bile acid sequestrants.
• Monitor results of liver and renal function tests. If liver enzyme levels rise to more than 3 times the upper limit of normal and persist, or if the patient develops gallstones, expect to stop drug.
• Monitor serum triglyceride and cholesterol levels at 4- to 8-week intervals. If levels don't decrease after 2 months at maximum dosage, expect to stop therapy.

WARNING Monitor patient closely for acute hypersensitivity reactions, including severe rash, and notify prescriber if they occur. Patient may need inpatient corticosteroids.
• Assess blood counts periodically, as ordered, during first 12 months of therapy to detect adverse hematologic effects.
• Watch closely for evidence of deep vein thrombosis (pain, swelling, redness in extremity) or pulmonary embolus (sudden onset of anxiety, shortness of breath, restlessness) because risk is higher in patients taking fenofibrate. Notify prescriber immediately, and start emergency treatment, as prescribed.

PATIENT TEACHING
• Emphasize that drug will be effective only if patient carefully follows prescriber's instructions about diet and exercise.
• Instruct patient prescribed Lipofen or Lofibra to take drug with food.
• Instruct patient prescribed tablet form to store the tablets in their original, desiccant-containing bottle and to avoid taking any chipped or broken tablets.
• Advise patient to have laboratory tests, as directed, to determine drug's effectiveness. They typically include liver function tests after 3 to 6 months, hematocrit and hemoglobin levels, and WBC counts periodically during first year.
• Urge patient to notify prescriber immediately about chills, fever, or sore throat. Also urge her to tell prescriber about unexplained muscle pain, tenderness, or weakness, especially if accompanied by fatigue or fever.
• Tell patient to seek emergency treatment if he develops pain, swelling, and redness in his limb or sudden shortness of breath, anxiety, and restlessness.

fenoldopam mesylate
Corlopam

Class and Category
Chemical class: Dopamine agonist
Therapeutic class: Antihypertensive
Pregnancy category: B

Indications and Dosages
➤ *To treat severe hypertension when rapid, but quickly reversible, emergency reduction of blood pressure is clinically indicated, including malignant hypertension with deteriorating end-organ function*

I.V. INFUSION
Adults. *Initial:* 0.025 to 0.3 mcg/kg/min, individualized according to patient weight and desired effect. *Usual:* 0.01 to 1.6 mcg/kg/min. *Maximum:* 1.6 mcg/kg/min for up to 48 hr.

Route	Onset	Peak	Duration
I.V.	Rapid	Unknown	Unknown

Mechanism of Action
Stimulates dopamine-1 postsynaptic receptors, which mediate renal and mesenteric vasodilation. Vasodilation lowers blood pressure and total peripheral resistance while increasing renal blood flow.

Contraindications
Hypersensitivity to fenoldopam or its components

Interactions
DRUGS
antihypertensives: Additive hypotensive effect
beta blockers: Increased risk of hypotension
dopamine antagonists, metoclopramide: Possibly decreased effects of fenoldopam

Adverse Reactions

CNS: Anxiety, headache, light-headedness
CV: Hypotension, ST- and T-wave changes, tachycardia
EENT: Increased intraocular pressure
GI: Abdominal pain, nausea
SKIN: Diaphoresis, flushing
Other: Hypokalemia, injection-site pain

Nursing Considerations

• Reconstitute by adding 40 mg fenoldopam (4 ml of concentrate) to 1,000 ml normal saline solution or D_5W, or 20 mg fenoldopam (2 ml of concentrate) to 500 ml normal saline solution or D_5W, or 10 mg fenoldopam (1 ml of concentrate) to 250 ml normal saline solution or D_5W to produce a final fenoldopam concentration of 40 mcg/ml.
• Infuse through a mechanical infusion pump for proper control of infusion rate.
• Expect to titrate fenoldopam dosage in increments of 0.05 to 0.1 mcg/kg/min, as prescribed.
• Expect to monitor heart rate and blood pressure every 15 minutes during therapy because most effect on blood pressure occurs within 15 minutes of any dosage change.
• Be aware that patient may be started on oral antihypertensive therapy, as prescribed, any time after blood pressure is stable during fenoldopam infusion.
• Discard any reconstituted solution not used within 24 hours.
• **WARNING** Assess patient for signs of increased myocardial oxygen demand, especially if patient has heart failure or a history of angina, because fenoldopam may produce a rapid decline in blood pressure, resulting in symptomatic hypotension and a dose-dependent increase in heart rate.
• Monitor serum potassium level because fenoldopam decreases serum potassium concentrations, which may result in hypokalemia, exacerbate arrhythmias, or precipitate conduction abnormalities, especially in patients with cardiac disease.
• Monitor patients with glaucoma or increased intraocular pressure for changes in vision because drug may cause a dose-dependent increase in intraocular pressure.
• Be alert for possible allergic- or anaphylactic-type reaction to sodium metabisulfite, a component of fenoldopam injection, especially in patients with asthma.

PATIENT TEACHING
• Inform patient that she'll be switched to an oral antihypertensive once her blood pressure is controlled.
• Instruct patient to expect frequent monitoring of vital signs.

---

fenoprofen calcium

Nalfon

E F

Class and Category

Chemical class: Propionic acid derivative
Therapeutic class: Analgesic, anti-inflammatory, antirheumatic
Pregnancy category: Not rated

Indications and Dosages

➤ *To manage mild to moderate pain*
CAPSULES, TABLETS
Adults. 200 mg every 4 to 6 hr, as needed.
➤ *To relieve pain, stiffness, and swelling from rheumatoid arthritis or osteoarthritis*
CAPSULES, TABLETS
Adults. 300 mg or 400 mg to 600 mg three times daily or four times daily *Maximum:* 3,200 mg daily.

Route	Onset	Peak	Duration
P.O.	15–30 min*	Unknown†	4–6 hr‡

Mechanism of Action

Blocks the activity of cyclooxygenase, the enzyme needed for prostaglandin synthesis. Prostaglandins, important mediators of the inflammatory response, cause local vaso-

---

* For analgesia; 2 days for antirheumatic effects.
† For analgesia; 2 to 3 wk for antirheumatic effects.
‡ For analgesia; unknown for antirheumatic effects.

dilation with swelling and pain. When cyclooxygenase is blocked and prostaglandins inhibited, inflammatory symptoms subside. Prostaglandin inhibition also relieves pain because prostaglandins play a role in pain transmission from the periphery to the spinal cord.

Contraindications

Angioedema, asthma, bronchospasm, nasal polyps, rhinitis, or urticaria induced by aspirin, iodides, or NSAIDs; hypersensitivity to fenoprofen or its components; renal impairment; severe hepatic impairment

Interactions

DRUGS

acetaminophen: Increased risk of renal impairment with concurrent long-term use
antacids: Decreased fenoprofen effectiveness
anticoagulants, cefamandole, cefoperazone, cefotetan, heparin, plicamycin, thrombolytics, valproic acid: Increased risk of bleeding
antineoplastics: Increased adverse hematologic effects
cyclosporine: Increased risk of nephrotoxicity
diuretics, triamterene: Decreased effectiveness of these drugs
glucocorticoids, NSAIDs, potassium supplements: Increased adverse GI effects
insulin, oral antidiabetic drugs: Increased risk of hypoglycemia
lithium: Increased risk of lithium toxicity
methotrexate: Increased risk of methotrexate toxicity
phenobarbital: Possibly decreased elimination half-life of fenoprofen
salicylates: Increased risk of GI bleeding

ACTIVITIES

alcohol use, smoking: Increased risk of GI bleeding

Adverse Reactions

CNS: Agitation, confusion, dizziness, drowsiness, headache, seizures, sleep disturbance, stroke, tremor, weakness
CV: Hypertension, MI, palpitations, peripheral edema, tachycardia, vasodilation
EENT: Blurred vision, dry or sore mouth, hearing loss, tinnitus
GI: Abdominal cramps, distention, and pain; anorexia; constipation; diarrhea;

diverticulitis; dysphagia; esophagitis; flatulence; gastritis; gastroenteritis; gastroesophageal reflux disease; GI bleeding or ulceration; hemorrhoids; hepatitis; hiatal hernia; indigestion; jaundice; liver failure; melena; nausea; perforation of stomach or intestines; vomiting
GU: Acute renal failure, dysuria, interstitial nephritis
HEME: Agranulocytosis, anemia, hemolytic anemia, leukopenia, neutropenia, pancytopenia
MS: Muscle spasms and twitching, myalgia
RESP: Dyspnea
SKIN: Diaphoresis, erythema, erythema multiforme, exfoliative dermatitis, pruritus, Stevens-Johnson syndrome, toxic epidermal necrolysis, urticaria
Other: Anaphylaxis, angioedema

Nursing Considerations

• Use fenoprofen with extreme caution in patients with a history of ulcer disease or GI bleeding because NSAIDs such as fenoprofen increase risk of GI bleeding and ulceration. Expect to use fenoprofen for the shortest time possible in these patients.

• Serious GI tract ulceration, bleeding, and perforation may occur without warning symptoms. Elderly patients are at greater risk. To minimize risk, give drug with food. If GI distress occurs, withhold drug and notify prescriber immediately.

• Use fenoprofen cautiously in patients with hypertension, and monitor blood pressure closely throughout therapy. Drug may cause hypertension or worsen it.

• Give drug with food, milk, or antacids to decrease adverse GI reactions.

• Patients with rheumatoid arthritis may need higher doses than those with osteoarthritis to control their symptoms.

WARNING If patient receives long-term therapy, watch for signs of toxicity, such as agitation; blurred vision; coma; confusion; drowsiness; elevated BUN and serum creatinine levels; indigestion; nausea; rash; seizures; severe headache; slow, labored breathing; tinnitus; and vomiting.

WARNING Monitor patient closely for thrombotic events, including MI and stroke, because NSAIDs increase the risk.

WARNING If patient has bone marrow suppression or is receiving antineoplastic drug therapy, monitor laboratory results (including WBC count), and watch for evidence of infection because anti-inflammatory and antipyretic actions of fenoprofen may mask signs and symptoms of infection, such as fever and pain.

• Monitor patient—especially if she's elderly or receiving long-term fenoprofen therapy—for less common but serious adverse GI reactions, including anorexia, constipation, diverticulitis, dysphagia, esophagitis, gastritis, gastroenteritis, gastroesophageal reflux disease, hemorrhoids, hiatal hernia, melena, stomatitis, and vomiting.

• Monitor patient's liver function test results because, in rare cases, elevations may progress to severe hepatic reactions, including fatal hepatitis, liver necrosis, and hepatic failure.

• Monitor BUN and serum creatinine levels in elderly patients, patients taking diuretics or ACE inhibitors, and patients with heart failure, impaired renal function, or hepatic dysfunction because drug may cause renal failure.

• Monitor CBC for decreased hemoglobin and hematocrit because drug may worsen anemia.

• Assess patient's skin regularly for signs of rash or other hypersensitivity reaction because fenoprofen is an NSAID and may cause serious skin reactions without warning, even in patients with no history of NSAID sensitivity. At first sign of reaction, stop drug and notify prescriber.

PATIENT TEACHING

• Advise patient to take fenoprofen with food, milk, or antacids to minimize GI distress. Also instruct her to take drug with a full glass of water and to stay upright for 30 minutes afterward to decrease the risk of drug lodging in the esophagus and causing irritation.

• Instruct patient to swallow drug whole and not to crush, break, chew, or open capsules.

• Caution patient to avoid alcohol, aspirin, and other NSAIDs, unless prescribed, while taking fenoprofen.

• If patient takes an anticoagulant, urge her to immediately report bleeding, including bloody or tarry stools and bloody vomitus.

• Caution patient to avoid hazardous activities until drug's CNS effects are known.

• Explain that NSAIDs may increase the risk of serious adverse cardiovascular reactions; urge patient to seek immediate medical attention if signs or symptoms arise, such as chest pain, shortness of breath, weakness, and slurring of speech.

• Explain that fenoprofen also may increase the risk of serious adverse GI reactions; stress the need to seek immediate medical attention for such signs and symptoms as epigastric or abdominal pain, indigestion, black or tarry stools, or vomiting blood or material that looks like coffee grounds.

• Alert patient to the possibility of rare but serious skin reactions. Urge her to seek immediate medical attention for rash, blisters, itching, fever, or other indications of hypersensitivity.

fentanyl citrate
Abstral, Actiq, Lazanda, Onsolis, Sublimaze, Subsys

fentanyl transdermal system
Duragesic

fentanyl iontophoretic transdermal
Ionsys

Class, Category, and Schedule
Chemical class: Opioid, phenylpiperidine derivative
Therapeutic class: Analgesic, anesthesia adjunct
Pregnancy category: C
Controlled substance schedule: II

Indications and Dosages
➤ *To provide surgical premedication*

E
F

I.M. INJECTION
Adults. 0.05 to 0.1 mg 30 to 60 min before surgery.

➤ *As adjunct to regional anesthesia*
I.V. OR I.M. INJECTION
Adults. 0.05 to 0.1 mg I.M. or slow I.V. over 1 to 2 min.

➤ *To manage postoperative pain in post-anesthesia care unit*
I.M. INJECTION
Adults. 0.05 to 0.1 mg. Repeated in 1 to 2 hr, if needed.

➤ *To manage acute postoperative pain in hospitalized patients requiring opioid analgesia*
IONTOPHORETIC TRANSDERMAL
Adults. 40 mg on-demand, released over 10 min. *Maximum:* Six 40-mcg doses/hour and eighty 40-mcg doses/24 hours for maximum of 72 hours.

➤ *To treat breakthrough pain in cancer patients who are receiving around-the-clock opioid therapy and have developed tolerance to it*
TRANSMUCOSAL LOZENGE (ACTIQ)
Adults. *Initial:* 200 mcg placed between cheek and gum for 15 min followed by second dose 15 min after first dose ends, if needed. Dosage increased according to patient's needs.
TRANSMUCOSAL SOLUBLE FILM (ONSOLIS)
Adults. *Initial:* 200-mcg film sheet placed against inside of cheek per episode. Increased, as needed, by 200 mcg in each subsequent episode, with doses at least 2 hours apart. *Maximum:* Four 200-mcg film sheets or one 1, 200-mcg film sheet four times daily.
SUBLINGUAL TABLETS (ABSTRAL)
Adults. *Initial:* 100 mcg followed by second dose 30 min after first dose, if needed. Dosage increased according to patient's needs and following manufacturer guidelines for titration. *Maximum:* No more than two doses per episode of breakthrough pain; dosage interval between episodes of breakthrough pain must be at least 2 hr; only four episodes of breakthrough pain can be treated per day.
NASAL SPRAY (LAZANDA)
Adults. *Initial:* 100 mcg. Increased, as needed, to 200 mcg, then 400 mcg, then 800 mcg with doses spaced at least 2 hours apart. *Maximum:* 800 mcg four times daily.

SUBLINGUAL SPRAY (SUBSYS)
Adults. *Initial:* 100 mcg followed by 100 mcg 30 minutes later, if needed. Increased, as needed, to 200 mcg, then 400 mcg, then 600 mcg, then 800 mcg, then 1,200 mcg, then 1,600 mcg with doses spaced at least 4 hours apart. A second dose of same strength may be taken 30 minutes after the first dose, as needed and counted as 1 breakthrough episode. *Maximum:* 1,600 mcg given twice 30 minutes apart four times daily.

➤ *To relieve severe chronic pain in opioid-tolerant patient who doesn't respond to less potent drugs and requires around-the-clock opioid administration for an extended time*
TRANSDERMAL SYSTEM (DURAGESIC)
Adults and children age 2 and over. *Initial:* One 25-mcg/hr patch, replaced every 72 hr (or 48 hr, if needed). Dosage increased by 12.5 mcg/hr, as needed, after first 72 hr and then every 6 days. For more than 100 mcg/hr, more than one patch is used.
DOSAGE ADJUSTMENT For elderly, cachectic, or debilitated patients, initial dosage should not exceed 25 mcg/hr, unless patient is already receiving more than 135 mg of oral morphine daily or an equivalent dose of another opioid. For patients receiving long-term opioid therapy, dosage adjusted based on previous day's drug requirement. For cancer patients who need more than 800 mcg/day for breakthrough pain, dosage altered or another long-acting opioid given, as prescribed. For patients with mild to moderate hepatic or renal failure, initial dosage decreased by 50%.

Mechanism of Action

Binds to opioid receptor sites in the CNS, altering perception of and emotional response to pain by inhibiting ascending pain pathways. Fentanyl may alter neurotransmitter release from afferent nerves responsive to painful stimuli, and it causes respiratory depression by acting directly on respiratory centers in the brain stem.

Route	Onset	Peak	Duration
I.V.	1–2 min	3–5 min	30–60 min

Route	Onset	Peak	Duration
I.M.	7–15 min	20–30 min	1–2 hr
Trans-dermal	12–24 hr	Unknown	Over 72 hr

Contraindications

I.V. or I.M. form: Under age 2, asthma, myasthenia gravis, opioid hypersensitivity or intolerance

Transmucosal form: Acute or chronic pain, including postoperative pain

Transdermal form: Acute or severe bronchial asthma; dosage that exceeds 25 mcg/hr at the start of therapy; hypersensitivity to adhesives; management of post-operative pain, mild pain, acute or intermittent pain, or in patients requiring opioid therapy for a short period of time; paralytic ileus; patients who are not opioid-tolerant; severe hepatic or renal impairment

All forms: Hypersensitivity to fentanyl (or alfentanil, sufentanil, or adhesives) or its components, intermittent pain, opioid nontolerance, significant respiratory depression, treatment of mild to moderate pain responsive to nonopioid drugs, upper airway obstruction

Interactions

DRUGS

anticholinergics, antidiarrheals (such as loperamide and paregoric): Increased risk of severe constipation

antihypertensives, diuretics: Possibly potentiated hypotension

benzodiazepines: Possibly reduced fentanyl dose required for anesthesia induction

buprenorphine: Possibly decreased therapeutic effects of buprenorphine

CNS depressants: Possibly increased CNS and respiratory depression and hypotension, possibly resulting in life-threatening effects

CYP3A4 inhibitors such as amiodarone, amprenavir, aprepitant, clarithromycin, diltiazem, erythromycin, fluconazole, fosamprenavir, itraconazole, ketoconazole, nefazodone, nelfinavir, ritonavir, troleandomycin, verapamil: Possibly increased opioid effect, leading to increased or prolonged adverse effects, including severe respiratory depression

cytochrome P-450 inducers (such as rifampin, carbamazepine, and phenytoin): Possibly induced metabolism and increased clearance of fentanyl with potential development of withdrawal syndrome in dependent patients

hydroxyzine: Possibly increased analgesic effect of fentanyl and increased CNS depression and hypotension

MAO inhibitors: Possibly unpredictable or fatal effects if taken within 14 days

metoclopramide: Possibly antagonized effect of metoclopramide on gastric motility

nalbuphine, pentazocine: Possibly antagonized analgesic, respiratory depressant, and CNS depressant effects of fentanyl; possibly additive hypotensive and CNS and respiratory depressant effects of both drugs

naloxone: Antagonized analgesic, hypotensive, serum fentanyl level, possibly resulting in fatal overdose from CNS, and respiratory depressant effects of fentanyl

naltrexone: Possibly blocked therapeutic effects of fentanyl

neuromuscular blockers: Possibly prevention or reversal of muscle rigidity by fentanyl

FOODS

grapefruit juice: Increased blood fentanyl level

ACTIVITIES

alcohol use: Increased serum fentanyl level, possibly resulting in fatal overdose from CNS and respiratory depression and hypotension

Adverse Reactions

CNS: Agitation, amnesia, anxiety, asthenia, ataxia, confusion, delusions, depression, dizziness, drowsiness, euphoria, fever, hallucinations, headache, lack of coordination, light-headedness, nervousness, paranoia, sedation, seizures, sleep disturbance, slurred speech, syncope, tremor, weakness, yawning

CV: Asystole, bradycardia, chest pain, edema, hypotension, orthostatic hypotension, tachycardia

EENT: Blurred vision, dental caries, dry mouth, gum-line erosion, laryngospasm, rhinitis, sneezing, tooth loss

GI: Anorexia, constipation, elevated serum amylase levels, ileus, indigestion, nausea, spasm of the sphincter of Oddi, vomiting

E
F

GU: Anorgasmia, decreased libido, ejaculatory difficulty, urinary hesitancy, urine retention
RESP: Apnea, depressed cough reflex, dyspnea, hypoventilation, respiratory depression
SKIN: Diaphoresis, exfoliative dermatitis, localized skin redness and swelling (with transdermal form), pruritus, rash
Other: Anaphylaxis, drug tolerance, physical or psychological dependence with long-term use, weight loss

Nursing Considerations

WARNING Fentanyl transdermal system should be used only in patients already receiving opioid therapy and with demonstrated opioid tolerance (taking for a week or longer at least 60 mg of morphine daily, 30 mg of oral oxycodone daily, 8 mg of oral hydromorphone daily, or an equianalgesic dose of another opioid), and require at least a fentanyl dosage of 25 mcg per hour to manage their pain.

• Be aware that opioids like fentanyl should not be given to women during pregnancy and labor and while breast feeding as the newborn or infant may experience neonatal opioid withdrawal syndrome (NOWS) which may be exhibited as poor feeding, rapid breathing, trembling, and excessive or high-pitched crying.

• Use with extreme caution in patients with significant chronic obstructive pulmonary disease or cor pulmonale, and in patients having a substantially decreased respiratory reserve, hypoxia, hypercapnia, or preexisting respiratory depression, because even therapeutic doses of fentanyl may decrease respiratory drive in these patients to the point of apnea.

• Use with extreme caution in patients who may be susceptible to the intracranial effects of carbon dioxide retention such as those with brain tumors, head injury, increased intracranial pressure, or impaired consciousness. Monitor these patients closely for signs of sedation and respiratory depression.

• Use caution when titrating fentanyl dosage in elderly, cachectic, and debilitated patients, especially when using intravenous route, because these patients are more sensitive to the drug's effects.

• Use cautiously in patients at risk for opioid abuse, such as those with mental illness or personal or family history of substance abuse. Monitor patient throughout therapy for fentanyl abuse or addiction.

• To reduce skin irritation, spray the allergy inhaler triamcinolone on the patient's skin, as prescribed, before applying a fentanyl patch.

• Expect the blood fentanyl level to be prolonged if patient chews or swallows the transmucosal form because drug is absorbed slowly from GI tract.

WARNING Never apply a transdermal patch if seal has been broken or patch has been cut, damaged, or changed because excessive exposure could occur, resulting in possibly fatal fentanyl overdose.

• Be aware that 100 mcg of fentanyl is equivalent in potency to 10 mg of morphine.

• To achieve optimum pain control with the lowest possible fentanyl dose, also plan to give a nonopioid analgesic, such as acetaminophen, as prescribed.

WARNING Monitor patient's respiratory status closely, especially during the first 24 to 72 hours after therapy starts or with dosage increases, because severe hypoventilation may occur without warning at any time during therapy. Patients at increased risk include the elderly, cachectic, or debilitated patients. Respiratory depression can occur in patients even if the drug is not misused or abused. Be aware that significant amounts of fentanyl can be absorbed from the skin for 24 hours or more after a transdermal patch is removed. Monitor patient for at least 72 hours after patch has been removed for respiratory depression. Have emergency equipment available including an opioid antagonist.

• Monitor cancer patients receiving sublingual spray form of fentanyl closely for oral mucositis because exposure to the drug in this form has been found to be greater than in patients without mucositis. If Grade 1 mucositis is present, the risk of respiratory or CNS depression increases, especially when therapy is initiated. Expect to avoid use of sublingual spray in cancer patients with Grade 2 mucositis or higher.

• Monitor patient closely who is receiving concurrent CYP3A4 inhibitor therapy along with fentanyl because these drugs may result in an increase in plasma fentanyl concentrations, which could increase or prolong adverse drug effects and may cause sedation and potentially fatal respiratory depression. Notify prescriber immediately, if present.

• To prevent withdrawal symptoms after long-term use, expect to taper drug dosage gradually, as prescribed. Assess patient for withdrawal symptoms after dosage reduction or conversion to another opioid analgesic.

• Monitor patient who is receiving the drug via a transdermal system and who develops a fever for opioid adverse effects because a fever may increase fentanyl release from the system and increase skin permeability. If symptoms occur, notify prescriber and anticipate dosage may be decreased.

• For patient with bradycardia, implement cardiac monitoring, as ordered, and assess heart rate and rhythm frequently during fentanyl therapy because drug may further slow heart rate.

WARNING Expect respiratory depressant effects to last longer than analgesic effects. Also be prepared for residual drug to potentiate effects of subsequent doses. Residual drug can be detected for at least 6 hours after I.V. dose and 17 hours after other forms. Monitor patient closely for at least 24 hours after therapy ends.

WARNING Assess patient for evidence of overdose, such as cardiopulmonary arrest, hypoventilation, pupil constriction, respiratory and CNS depression, seizures, and shock. Give naloxone (possibly in repeated doses), as prescribed. Be prepared to assist with endotracheal intubation and mechanical ventilation and to provide fluids.

• Monitor blood glucose level of diabetic patient receiving transdermal fentanyl because each unit contains about 2 g of sugar.

WARNING Do not substitute Actiq, Lazanda, Onsolis, or Subsys for any other fentanyl product, and do not substitute for each other. Do not convert dosage to or from other products on a mcg-per-mcg basis because doing so may result in a fatal overdose.

PATIENT TEACHING

• Instruct patient to avoid alcohol and other CNS depressants during fentanyl therapy unless prescribed.

• Advise patient not to stop taking drug unless directed by prescriber because withdrawal symptoms may occur. Warn against increasing dose or frequency without consulting prescriber because drug can cause dependency.

• For transdermal form, instruct patient to choose a site with intact (not irritated or irradiated) skin on a flat surface, such as the chest, back, flank, or upper arm, and, if appropriate, to clip, not shave, hair from the site and clean it with water (no soaps, lotions, oils, or alcohol). After site preparation, instruct patient to press patch firmly in place with palm of hand for 30 seconds, making sure edges are sealed. Tell her to wash her hands immediately after application with soap and water. If patch loosens, tell her to tape edges down but not cover the entire patch. If more than one patch is needed, the edges shouldn't touch or overlap. Instruct patient to remove patch after 72 hours, fold it in half with adhesive sides together, and flush it down the toilet. Remind her not to reuse a site for at least 3 days. Warn patient to avoid accidental secondary exposure to the drug with someone else through contact with unwashed or unclothed application sites. Examples include transfer of a patch from an adult's body to a child while hugging, sharing the same bed as the patient, accidentally sitting on a patch, and possible accidental exposure of a caregiver's skin to the medication in the patch while applying or removing the patch.

• Warn patient never to apply transdermal patch if seal has been broken or the patch has been cut, damaged, or changed in any way because drug may be released too rapidly. Also warn patient not to expose the application site and surrounding area to direct external heat sources, such as heating pads or electric blankets, heat or tanning lamps, saunas, hot tubs, and heated water beds, while wearing the

E
F

patch. She should also avoid hot baths or sunbathing because increased body temperature may increase fentanyl release, resulting in a possible overdose. If she develops a fever or becomes overheated from strenuous exercise while wearing a patch, she should contact the prescriber immediately.

• For iontophoretic transdermal form, instruct patient to press button twice firmly within 3 seconds to release a dose. An audible tone will sound when a dose is activated, and a red light will stay on throughout the 10-minute administration. Explain that no more than 6 doses can be given per hour and no more than 80 doses can be given per 24 hours. Tell the patient that the patch may be replaced once 80 doses are released or 24 hours pass, but that 72 hours is the maximum time the drug can be delivered in this way.

• For Actiq transmucosal form, instruct patient to open the package just before use and to save plastic cap for discarding the unused part of the lozenge. Tell her to place lozenge between her cheek and gum and to suck, not chew, it for 15 minutes. Show her how to move lozenge from one side of her mouth to the other using the handle provided separately.

• For Onsolis transmucosal form, instruct patient to wet inside of cheek with tongue or rinse his mouth with water. Tell him to open package just before use and place entire film sheet on the tip of a dry finger, pink side facing up. Then he should carefully place pink side of film against inside of cheek and press and hold it in place for 5 seconds. Tell him not to drink anything for 5 minutes or eat for 30 minutes. Warn patient not to cut or tear film before use. If he uses multiple film sheets, tell him to place them separately along cheek wall, not on top of each other.

• For Abstral sublingual form, instruct patient to place tablet on the floor of the mouth directly under the tongue immediately after removing tablet from the blister unit. Caution patient not to chew, suck, or swallow the tablet but to allow it to dissolve completely in the mouth. Tell him

not to eat or drink anything until the tablet is completely dissolved.

• Onsolis dosage increases must occur only in 200-mcg increments, must be done only in later pain episodes, and must be separated by at least 2 hours from previous dose. If pain isn't relieved within 30 minutes, tell him not to use another dose but to use a rescue drug instead. If dosage increase is needed and continues to be needed, tell patient to contact prescriber for new dosage strength because each episode should be treated with one film sheet of appropriate strength.

• For transmucosal form, urge patient to see a dentist regularly, to brush teeth and floss after each meal, and to avoid frequent consumption of products high in sugar because of increased risk of dental caries.

• For transmucosal form, inform diabetic patient that each unit contains 2 g of sugar. Instruct her to monitor her blood glucose levels closely.

• For nasal spray (Lazanda), tell patient to prime the device before use by spraying into the pouch 4 sprays in total. To use, insert the nozzle of the Lazanda bottle a short distance (about 1/2 inch or 1 cm) into the nose and point towards the bridge of the nose, tilting the bottle slightly. Have patient press down firmly on the finger grips until he hears a "click" and the number in the counting window advances by 1. Tell patient that the fine mist spray is not always felt on the nasal mucosal membrane and to rely on the audible click and the advancement of the dose counter to confirm a spray has been administered.

• For sublingual spray (Subsys), tell patient to open the blister package with scissors immediately prior to drug use. Tell him never to use a blister package that has been discovered to be open. Instruct him to spray the contents of the unit into his mouth carefully, underneath his tongue.

• Remind patient to keep used and unused dosage units out of reach of children and to dispose of drug properly. For buccal tablets, patient should flush leftover drug down the toilet when no longer needed. For sublingual spray, remind patient to dispose of any used or unneeded units immediately in the disposal bottle provided with every dispensed carton. For transdermal patch, patient should fold in half and flush down toilet.

• Caution patient that accidentally exposing others to transdermal fentanyl could cause serious adverse reactions that may become life threatening, especially in children, even with one dose. If accidental exposure occurs, the person should remove the patch, wash the area well with water, and seek medical attention.

• Caution patient to avoid hazardous activities until drug's CNS effects are known.

• Tell patient to increase fiber and fluid intake, unless contraindicated, because drug may cause severe constipation. If it persists or becomes severe, urge patient to notify prescriber.

• Advise patient to notify prescriber if she becomes pregnant or is breastfeeding, as drug may need to be discontinued or dosage altered.

ferric citrate
Auryxia

Class and Category
Chemical class: Iron propanetricarboxylic acid
Therapeutic class: Phosphate binder
Pregnancy category: B

Indications and Dosages
➤ *To control serum phosphorus levels in patients with chronic kidney disease on dialysis*
TABLETS
Adults. *Initial*: 2 tablets (420 mg ferric iron, equivalent to 2 g ferric citrate) three times a day with meals, increased or decreased by 1 to 2 tablets per day at 1-wk or longer intervals, as needed. *Maximum*: 12 tablets daily.

Mechanism of Action
Binds dietary phosphate in the gastrointestinal (GI) tract and precipitates as ferric phosphate, which is then excreted in the stool. By binding phosphate in the GI tract and decreasing absorption, serum phosphate levels are reduced.

Contraindications
Hypersensitivity to ferric citrate or its components, iron overload syndromes

Interaction
DRUGS
doxycycline: Decreased effectiveness of doxycycline
iron supplements: Increased iron stores

Adverse Reactions
GI: Constipation, diarrhea, nausea, vomiting
HEME: Increased serum ferritin and transferrin saturation levels
RESP: Cough

Nursing Considerations
• Be aware that ferric citrate produces dark stools because of its iron content, but this effect does not affect laboratory tests for occult bleeding.

• Know that iron absorption from ferric citrate therapy may cause an excessive elevation in iron stores. Assess patients' serum ferritin and transferrin saturation levels before initiating ferric citrate therapy, as ordered, and monitor throughout therapy.

• Expect that patients receiving iron intravenously may need a reduction in dose or discontinuation of intravenous iron therapy.

Patient teaching
• Instruct patient to take ferric citrate exactly as ordered.
WARNING Remind patient that accidental overdose of iron-containing products is a leading cause of death in children under age 6. Stress the importance of keeping ferric citrate tablets out of the reach of children. If accidental overdose occurs, the poison control center should be called and immediate emergency treatment sought for the child.

ferrous salts
ferrous fumarate
(contains 100 mg of elemental iron per capsule or per 5 ml of oral suspension, 33 mg of elemental iron per chewable tablet or per 5 ml of oral suspension, 106 mg of ele-

mental iron per E.R. capsule, 15 mg of elemental iron per 0.6 ml of oral solution, and 20 to 115 mg of elemental iron per tablet)
Femiron, Feostat, Feostat Drops, Ferretts, Fumasorb, Fumerin, Hemocyte, Ircon, Neo-Fer (CAN), Nephro-Fer, Novofumar (CAN), Palafer (CAN), Span-FF

ferrous carboxymaltose

(contains 50 mg of elemental iron per milliliter)

ferrous gluconate

(contains 10 mg of elemental iron per capsule, 34 mg of elemental iron per 5 ml of elixir, 37 mg of elemental iron per E.R. tablet, 35 mg of elemental iron per 5 ml of syrup, and 34 to 38 mg of elemental iron per tablet)
Apo-Ferrous Gluconate (CAN), Fergon, Ferralet, Ferralet Slow Release, Fertinic (CAN), Novoferrogluc (CAN), Simron

ferrous sulfate

(contains 50 mg of elemental iron per capsule, 60 mg of elemental iron per dried capsule, 30 to 50 mg of elemental iron per dried E.R. capsule, 50 mg of elemental iron per dried E.R. tablet, 65 mg of elemental iron per dried tablet, 44 mg of elemental iron per 5 ml of elixir, 60 to 65 mg of elemental iron per enteric-coated tablet, 65 to 105 mg of elemental iron per E.R. tablet, 15 mg of elemental iron per 0.6 ml of oral solution, 18 mg of elemental iron per 0.5 ml of oral solution, 25 mg of elemental iron per ml of oral solution, 30 or 60 mg of elemental iron per 5 ml of oral solution, and 39 to 65 mg of elemental iron per tablet)
Apo-Ferrous Sulfate (CAN), Feosol, Feratab, Fer-gen-sol, Fer-In-Sol Capsules, Fer-In-Sol Drops, Fer-In-Sol Syrup, Fer-Iron Drops, Fero-Grad (CAN), Fero-Gradumet, Ferospace, Ferralyn Lanacaps, Ferra-TD, Mol-Iron, Novoferrosulfa (CAN), PMS-Ferrous Sulfate (CAN), Slow-Fe

iron, carbonyl

(contains 50 mg of elemental iron per caplet)
Feosol

Class and Category

Chemical class: Trace element, mineral
Therapeutic class: Antianemic, nutritional supplement
Pregnancy category: Not rated

Indications and Dosages

➤ *To prevent iron deficiency based on U.S. and Canadian recommended daily allowances*

CAPLETS, CAPSULES, CHEWABLE TABLETS, DRIED CAPSULES, DRIED E.R. CAPSULES, DRIED E.R. TABLETS, DRIED TABLETS, ELIXIR, ENTERIC-COATED TABLETS, E.R. CAPSULES, E.R. TABLETS, ORAL SOLUTION, ORAL SUSPENSION, SYRUP, TABLETS

Adult men and children age 11 and over. 10 mg (8 to 10 mg Canadian) elemental iron daily.
Adult women and children age 11 and over. 10 to 15 mg (8 to 13 mg Canadian) elemental iron daily.
Pregnant women. 30 mg (17 to 22 mg Canadian) elemental iron daily.
Breastfeeding women. 15 mg (8 to 13 mg Canadian) elemental iron daily.
Children ages 7 to 10. 10 mg (8 to 10 mg Canadian) elemental iron daily.
Children ages 4 to 6. 10 mg (8 mg Canadian) elemental iron daily.
Children from birth to age 3. 6 to 10 mg (0.3 to 6 mg Canadian) elemental iron daily.

➤ *To replace iron in deficiency states*

CAPLETS, CAPSULES, CHEWABLE TABLETS, DRIED CAPSULES, DRIED E.R. CAPSULES, DRIED E.R. TABLETS, DRIED TABLETS, ELIXIR, ENTERIC-COATED TABLETS, E.R. CAPSULES, E.R. TABLETS, ORAL SOLUTION, ORAL SUSPENSION, SYRUP, TABLETS

Adults and adolescents. 100 to 200 mg elemental iron three times daily for 4 to 6 mo.
Children ages 2 to 12 weighing 30 to 50 kg (66 to 110 lb). 50 to 100 mg elemental iron daily in divided doses three times daily or four times daily for 4 to 6 mo.
Children ages 6 months to 2 years. Up to 6 mg/kg elemental iron daily in divided doses three times daily or four times daily for 4 to 6 mo.

Infants under age 6 months. 10 to 25 mg elemental iron daily in divided doses three times daily or four times daily for 4 to 6 mo.

➤ *To treat iron deficiency in patients who have an intolerance to oral iron, have had unsatisfactory response to oral iron, or who have non-dialysis-dependent chronic kidney disease*

I.V. INFUSION, I.V. INJECTION (INJECTAFER)

Adults weighing 50 kg (110 lbs) or more. 750 mg followed by second dose of 750 mg given no sooner than 7 days later. *Maximum:* 1500 mg per course with two doses separated by at least 7 days.

Adults weighing less than 50 kg (110 lbs). 15mg/kg followed by second dose of 15 mg/kg given no sooner than 7 days later. *Maximum:* 1500 mg per course with two doses separated by at least 7 days.

➤ *To provide iron supplementation during pregnancy*

CAPLETS, CAPSULES, CHEWABLE TABLETS, DRIED CAPSULES, DRIED E.R. CAPSULES, DRIED E.R. TABLETS, DRIED TABLETS, ELIXIR, ENTERIC-COATED TABLETS, E.R. CAPSULES, E.R. TABLETS, ORAL SOLUTION, ORAL SUSPENSION, SYRUP, TABLETS

Pregnant women. 15 to 30 mg elemental iron daily during second and third trimesters.

DOSAGE ADJUSTMENT Dosage increased if needed for elderly patients, who may not absorb iron as easily as younger adults do.

Mechanism of Action

Acts to normalize RBC production by binding with hemoglobin or by being oxidized and stored as hemosiderin or aggregated ferritin in reticuloendothelial cells of the liver, spleen, and bone marrow. Iron is an essential component of hemoglobin, myoglobin, and several enzymes, including cytochromes, catalase, and peroxidase. Iron is needed for catecholamine metabolism and normal neutrophil function.

Contraindications

Hemochromatosis, hemolytic anemias, hemosiderosis, hypersensitivity to iron salts or their components, other anemic conditions unless accompanied by iron deficiency

Interactions

DRUGS

acetohydroxamic acid: Reduced absorption of both drugs

antacids, calcium supplements: Decreased iron absorption and effectiveness

ascorbic acid (with doses of 200 mg or more): Increased iron absorption

cholestyramine, cimetidine: Decreased iron absorption

ciprofloxacin, enoxacin, etidronate, lomefloxacin, norfloxacin, ofloxacin, oral tetracyclines: Decreased effectiveness of these drugs

dimercaprol: Possibly combination with iron in body to form a harmful chemical

levodopa: Possibly chelation with iron, decreasing levodopa absorption and blood level

levothyroxine: Decreased levothyroxine effectiveness and, possibly, hypothyroidism

methyldopa: Decreased methyldopa absorption and efficacy

penicillamine: Decreased penicillamine absorption because penicillamine chelates heavy metals

vitamin E: Decreased vitamin E absorption

FOODS

coffee; eggs; foods that contain bicarbonates, carbonates, oxalates, or phosphates; milk and milk products; tea that contains tannic acid; whole-grain breads and cereals and other high-fiber foods: Decreased iron absorption and effectiveness

ACTIVITIES

alcohol abuse (acute or chronic): Increased serum iron level

Adverse Reactions

CNS: Dizziness, fever, headache, paresthesia, syncope

CV: Chest pain, hypertension, hypotension, tachycardia

EENT: Metallic taste, tooth discoloration

GI: Abdominal cramps, constipation, epigastric pain, nausea, stool discoloration, vomiting

HEME: Hemochromatosis, hemolysis, hemosiderosis

RESP: Dyspnea, wheezing

SKIN: Diaphoresis, flushing, pruritus, rash, urticaria

Other: Anaphylaxis (with I.V. administration), angioedema, injection site discoloration

Nursing Considerations

• Give iron tablets and capsules with a full glass of water or juice. Don't crush enteric-coated tablets or open capsules.
• Because iron solutions may stain teeth, dilute and administer with a straw or place drops in back of patient's throat. Mix the elixir form in water. Fer-In-Sol Drops or Syrup may be mixed with water or juice.
• To maximize absorption, give iron salts 1 hour before or 2 hours after meals. If GI irritation occurs, give with or just after meals.
• Protect liquid form from freezing.
• Administer Injectafer intravenously, either as an undiluted slow intravenous push or by infusion. When administering as a slow intravenous push, give at the rate of about 100 mg (2 ml) per minute. When administering via infusion, dilute up to 750 mg of iron in no more than 250 ml of sterile 0.9% sodium chloride injection, USP, such that the concentration of the infusion is not less than 2 mg of iron per ml, and administer over at least 15 minutes. Once diluted, solution is stable for 72 hours at room temperature.
• Avoid extravasation with intravenous administration because brown discoloration of the extravasation site may be long-lasting.
WARNING Monitor patients closely for hypersensitivity reactions such as shock, severe hypotension, loss of consciousness, and/or collapse during and for at least 30 minutes after intravenous administration. If present, discontinue drug immediately, notify prescriber, and be prepared to provide supportive care, as needed.
• Monitor patient's blood pressure after each intravenous dose for significant increases, as hypertension may occur immediately after administration but usually resolves within 30 minutes.
• Be aware that at usual dosages, serum hemoglobin level usually normalizes in about 2 months unless blood loss continues. Treatment lasts for 3 to 6 months to help replenish iron stores.

WARNING Monitor patient for signs of iron overdose, which may include abdominal pain, diarrhea (possibly bloody), nausea, severe vomiting, and sharp abdominal cramps. In case of iron toxicity or accidental iron overdose (a leading cause of fatal poisoning in children under age 6), give deferoxamine, as prescribed. As few as 3 adult iron tablets can cause serious poisoning in young children.
• Don't give antacids, coffee, tea, dairy products, eggs, or whole-grain cereals or breads within 1 hour before or 2 hours after iron.
• Remember that unabsorbed iron turns stool green or black and can mask blood in stool. Check stool for occult blood, as ordered.

PATIENT TEACHING
• Instruct patient not to chew any solid form of iron except for chewable tablets.
• Inform patient that iron deficiency may cause decreased stamina, learning problems, shortness of breath, and tiredness.
• To improve iron absorption, urge patient to eat lean red meat, chicken, turkey, and fish as well as foods rich in vitamin C (such as citrus fruits and fresh vegetables).
• Urge patient to avoid foods that impair iron absorption, including dairy products, eggs, spinach, and high-fiber foods, such as whole-grain breads and cereals and bran. Also advise her to avoid drinking coffee or tea within 1 hour of iron intake.
• Caution patient not to take antacids or calcium supplements within 1 hour before and 2 hours after taking iron supplement.
• Inform patient that stool should become dark green or black during therapy. Advise her to notify prescriber if it doesn't.
• To minimize tooth stains from liquid iron, instruct patient to mix dose with water, fruit juice, or tomato juice and to drink it with a straw. If patient must take liquid iron by dropper, direct her to place drops well back on the tongue and to follow with water or juice. Tell her that iron stains can be removed by brushing with baking soda (sodium

bicarbonate) or medicinal peroxide (hydrogen peroxide 3%).
• Advise patient to consult prescriber before taking large amounts of iron for longer than 6 months.
• Warn patient about high risk of accidental poisoning, and urge her to keep iron preparations out of the reach of children.

ferumoxytol
Feraheme

Class and Category
Chemical class: Nonstoichiometric magnetite
Therapeutic class: Iron replacement
Pregnancy category: C

Indications and Dosages
➤ *To treat iron deficiency anemia in patients with chronic kidney disease*
I.V. INJECTION
Adults. 510 mg administered at no more than 30 mg/sec followed by another 510 mg in 3 to 8 days.

Mechanism of Action
Isolates the bioactive iron from plasma components until the iron-carbohydrate complex enters the reticuloendothelial system macrophages of the liver, spleen, and bone marrow. The iron is released from the iron-carbohydrate complex within vesicles in the macrophages. Iron then either enters the intracellular storage iron pool (e.g., ferritin) or is transferred to plasma transferrin for transport to erythroid precursor cells for incorporation into hemoglobin.

Contraindications
Anemia not caused by iron deficiency, hypersensitivity to ferumoxytol or its components, iron overload

Interactions
DRUGS
oral iron preparations: Reduced absorption of these preparations

Adverse Reactions
CNS: Dizziness, fever, headache, loss of consciousness, syncope, unresponsiveness

CV: Arrhythmias, cardiac arrest, chest pain, CHF, hypertension, hypotension, myocardial ischemia, peripheral edema, tachycardia
GI: Abdominal pain, constipation, diarrhea, nausea, vomiting
GU: Chronic renal failure
HEME: Increased ferritin level
MS: Back pain, muscle spasms
RESP: Cough, cyanosis, dyspnea, respiratory arrest
SKIN: Ecchymosis, pruritus, rash, urticaria
Other: Anaphylaxis, angioedema, injection-site swelling

Nursing Considerations
• Do not dilute drug prior to administration.
• Administer drug to patient receiving hemodialysis at least 1 hour after hemodialysis has started and once the patient's blood pressure has stabilized. Monitor patient for signs and symptoms of hypotension following each injection.
• Evaluate the hematologic response by measuring the patient's hemoglobin, ferritin, iron, and transferrin saturation at least 1 month following the second injection. Expect to readminister the drug in patients with persistent or recurrent iron deficiency anemia.
• Monitor patient closely for signs and symptoms of hypersensitivity for at least 60 minutes following each injection because anaphylactoid reactions have occurred following administration. Provide supportive care, as indicated, by severity of reaction and expect drug to be discontinued.
• Monitor patient's blood pressure after administering each dose of ferumoxytol because severe hypotension has occurred with drug use.
• Monitor patient's response to ferumoxytol therapy because excessive therapy with parenteral iron can lead to excess storage of iron with the possibility of iatrogenic hemosiderosis.
• Be aware that ferumoxytol therapy may transiently affect the diagnostic ability of magnetic resonance imaging for up to3 months after the last dose.
PATIENT TEACHING
• Instruct patient to immediately report any signs and symptoms of hypersensitivity such as rash, hives, or itchiness.

E
F

• Advise patient to comply with follow-up visits and laboratory tests required to determine drug effectiveness.

fesoterodine fumarate

Toviaz

Class and Category
Chemical class: Muscarinic receptor antagonist
Therapeutic class: Antispasmodic
Pregnancy category: C

Indications and Dosages
➤ *To treat overactive bladder with symptoms of urinary incontinence, urgency, and frequency*
E.R. TABLETS
Adults. *Initial:* 4 mg daily, increased to 8 mg, as needed. *Maximum:* 8 mg daily.
DOSAGE ADJUSTMENT For patients with severe renal insufficiency or who are taking potent CYP3A4 inhibitors (such as clarithromycin, itraconazole, and ketoconazole), dosage shouldn't exceed 4 mg daily.

Route	Onset	Peak	Duration
P.O.	Unknown	5 hr	Unknown

Mechanism of Action
Exerts antimuscarinic (atropine-like) and potent direct antispasmodic (papaverine-like) actions on smooth muscle in the bladder. The result is increased bladder capacity and a decreased urge to void. Fesoterodine has an active metabolite that inhibits bladder contraction and decreases detrussor pressure.

Contraindications
Gastric retention, GI obstruction, hypersensitivity to fesoterodine or its components, ileus, pyloric stenosis, uncontrolled narrow-angle glaucoma, urine retention

Interactions
DRUGS
antimuscarinic agents: Possibly increased anticholinergic effects; possibly altered absorption of oral drugs taken concurrently

potent CYP3A4 inhibitors, such as clarithromycin, itraconazole, ketoconazole: Possibly increased serum fesoterodine level and increased risk of adverse effects
FOODS
caffeine: May aggravate bladder symptoms
ACTIVITIES
alcohol use: Increased drowsiness

Adverse Reactions
CNS: Dizziness, drowsiness, headache, insomnia, somnolence
CV: Angina, chest pain, palpitations, peripheral edema, QT-interval prolongation
EENT: Blurred vision; dry eyes, mouth, or throat
GI: Constipation, diverticulitis, dyspepsia, elevated liver enzymes, gastroenteritis, irritable bowel syndrome, nausea, upper abdominal pain
GU: Dysuria, urine retention, UTI
MS: Back pain
RESP: Cough, upper respiratory tract infection
SKIN: Decreased sweating, pruritus, rash, urticaria
Other: Angioedema

Nursing Considerations
• Use cautiously in patients with significant bladder outlet obstruction because fesoterodine can cause urine retention.
• Use cautiously in patients with myasthenia gravis, decreased GI motility, and controlled narrow-angle glaucoma because drug can make these conditions worse.
• Use cautiously in patients taking other drugs with anticholinergic effects, such as antihistamines.
• Monitor patient closely for angioedema, which may occur after the first dose. If present, discontinue fesoterodine therapy immediately, as ordered, and provide emergency supportive care, including maintaining a patent airway, as needed.
• Monitor patient for CNS anticholinergic effects, especially after beginning fesoterodine therapy or increasing the dose. If present, notify prescriber, as dosage may need to be reduced or drug discontinued.
PATIENT TEACHING
• Instruct patient to take drug exactly as prescribed.

- Tell patient to take drug with a full glass of water and not to cut, crush, or chew tablets.
- Explain that drug can cause adverse effects such as constipation and urine retention. If they occur and are severe or prolonged, patient should notify prescriber.
- Tell patient to seek immediate emergency medical attention if he experiences any swelling of his lips, tongue, face, or throat.
- Advise patient to avoid alcohol consumption during fesoterodine therapy.
- Tell patient to avoid hazardous activities until drug's CNS effects are known.
- Caution patient to avoid strenuous exercise and excessive sun exposure because of increased risk of heatstroke.
- Advise patient to limit caffeine consumption during drug therapy.
- Explain that full benefits of fesoterodine therapy may take 2 to 3 months.
- Inform patient that chewing sugarless gum or sucking hard candy (especially lemon drops) may help ease dry mouth.

---

fidaxomicin

Dificid

Class and Category
Chemical class: Macrolide
Therapeutic class: Antibiotic
Pregnancy category: B

Indications and Dosages
➤ *To treat Clostridium difficile-associated diarrhea (CDAD)*
TABLET
Adults. 200 mg twice daily for 10 days.

Mechanism of Action
Inhibits RNA synthesis in *Clostridium difficile* bacterial cells by RNA polymerases, causing the cells to die.

Contraindications
Hypersensitivity to fidaxomicin or its components

Interactions
DRUGS
cyclosporine: Possible increased blood fidaxomicin level

Adverse Reactions
ENDO: Hyperglycemia
GI: Abdominal pain or distention, dyspepsia, dysphagia, elevated liver enzymes, flatulence, GI hemorrhage, intestinal obstruction, megacolon, nausea, vomiting
HEME: Anemia, decreased platelet count, neutropenia
RESP: Dyspnea
SKIN: Drug eruption, pruritus, rash
Other: Angioedema, decreased blood bicarbonate, elevated blood alkaline phosphatase, metabolic acidosis

Nursing Considerations
- Know that fidaxomicin and other drugs for *C. difficile*-associated diarrhea are most effective when patients are not taking other antibiotics. If other antibiotics can be stopped safely, they should be.
- Monitor patient for hypersensitivity reactions that may include angioedema, dyspnea, pruritus or rash. Patients with a history of allergy to other macrolides are at increased risk. If a severe reaction occurs, discontinue fidaxomicin immediately and notify prescriber. Provide supportive care, as needed and ordered.
- Monitor patient for adverse effects and notify prescriber, if present.

PATIENT TEACHING
- Instruct patient to take fidaxomicin exactly as prescribed and for the full 10 days, regardless of how he is feeling.
- Tell patient to seek immediate emergency care if an allergic reaction occurs during fidaxomicin therapy.
- Tell patient to notify prescriber if symptoms worsen at any time or don't improve after a few days.

---

filgrastim
(granulocyte colony-stimulating factor, rG-CSF)
Neupogen

Class and Category
Chemical class: Granulocyte colony-stimulating factor

Therapeutic class: Antineutropenic,
hematopoietic stimulator
Pregnancy category: C

Indications and Dosages

➤ *To prevent infection after
myelosuppressive chemotherapy*
I.V. INFUSION
Adults and children. 5 mcg/kg daily over
15 to 30 min. Increased, as needed, by
5 mcg/kg with each chemotherapy cycle.
SUBCUTANEOUS INJECTION
Adults and children. 5 mcg/kg daily for up
to 2 wk. Increased, as needed, by 5 mcg/kg
with each chemotherapy cycle.
➤ *To reduce duration of neutropenia after
bone marrow transplantation*
I.V. INFUSION
Adults. 10 mcg/kg daily over 4 hr or as a
continuous infusion over 24 hr.
SUBCUTANEOUS INFUSION
Adults. 10 mcg/kg as a continuous infusion
over 24 hr.
➤ *To enhance peripheral blood progenitor
cell collection in autologous hemato-
poietic stem cell transplantation*
SUBCUTANEOUS INFUSION OR INJECTION
Adults. 10 mcg/kg as continuous infusion
over 24 hr or a single injection, starting 4
days before first leukapheresis and
continuing until last day of leukapheresis.
➤ *To reduce occurrence and duration of
neutropenia in congenital neutropenia*
SUBCUTANEOUS INJECTION
Adults and children. 6 mcg/kg twice
daily.
➤ *To reduce the occurrence and duration
of neutropenia in idiopathic or cyclic
neutropenia*
SUBCUTANEOUS INJECTION
Adults and children. 5 mcg/kg daily.
DOSAGE ADJUSTMENT Dosage reduced for
patients whose absolute neutrophil count
remains above 10,000/mm^3.

Route	Onset	Peak	Duration
I.V.	In 5 min	Unknown	Unknown

Mechanism of Action

Is pharmacologically identical to human
granulocyte colony-stimulating factor, an
endogenous hormone synthesized by
monocytes, endothelial cells, and fibroblasts.
Filgrastim induces formation of neutrophil
progenitor cells by binding directly to

receptors on the surface of granulocytes,
which then divide and differentiate. It also
potentiates the effects of mature neutrophils,
which reduces fever and the risk of infection
raised by severe neutropenia.

Incompatibilities

Don't mix filgrastim in vial or syringe with
normal saline solution because precipitate
will form.

Contraindications

Hypersensitivity to filgrastim, its components, or proteins from *Escherichia coli*

Interactions

DRUGS
growth hormone: Increased bone marrow
hematopoietic activity
lithium: Increased neutrophil production

Adverse Reactions

CNS: Fever, headache
CV: Transient supraventricular tachycardia
GI: Splenic rupture, splenomegaly
HEME: Leukocytosis, thrombocytopenia
MS: Arthralgia; myalgia; pain in arms, legs,
lower back, or pelvis
RESP: Acute respiratory distress syndrome
(ARDS), alveolar hemorrhage, hemoptysis
SKIN: Cutaneous vasculitis, pruritus, rash,
Sweet's syndrome (acute febrile neutrophilic
dermatosis)
Other: Anaphylaxis, injection-site pain and
redness, sickle cell crisis

Nursing Considerations

• Warm filgrastim to room temperature
  before injection. Discard drug if stored
  longer than 6 hours at room temperature
  or 24 hours in refrigerator.
• Withdraw only one dose from a vial; don't
  repuncture the vial.
• Don't shake the solution.
• For continuous infusion, dilute in D$_5$W
  (not normal saline solution) to produce
  less than 15 mcg/ml.
• For subcutaneous dose larger than 1 ml,
  divide and give in more than one site.
• After chemotherapy, give drug over 15 to
  30 minutes. Don't give within 24 hours
  before or after cytotoxic chemotherapy.
• Be aware that needle cover on single-use
  prefilled syringe contains dry natural
  rubber and may cause sensitivity reaction.
  It shouldn't be handled by allergic people.

- Expect to monitor CBC, hematocrit, and platelet count two or three times weekly.
- Inform prescriber and expect to stop drug if leukocytosis develops or absolute neutrophil count consistently exceeds 10,000/mm^3.
- Anticipate decreased response to drug if patient has received extensive radiation therapy or long-term chemotherapy.

PATIENT TEACHING
- Teach patient how to prepare, administer, and store filgrastim. Caution her not to reuse needle, syringe, or vial.
- Advise patient prescribed single-use prefilled syringe to notify prescriber if she has an allergy to latex because needle cover may cause sensitivity reaction.
- Provide patient with puncture-resistant container for needle and syringe disposal.
- Advise patient to promptly report pain in left upper quadrant of abdomen or shoulder-tip pain.
- Emphasize the importance of returning for follow-up laboratory tests.
- Advise female patient to report pregnancy to prescriber immediately and encourage her to enroll in Amgen's Pregnancy Surveillance Program by calling 1-800-77-AMGEN.

finasteride
Propecia, Proscar

Class and Category
Chemical class: 4-Azasteroid compound
Therapeutic class: Benign prostatic hyperplasia agent, hair growth stimulant
Pregnancy category: X

Indications and Dosages
➤ *To treat symptomatic benign prostatic hyperplasia; to reduce the risk of symptomatic progression of benign prostatic hyperplasia when given with doxazocin*

TABLETS
Adults. 5 mg daily.
➤ *To treat male-pattern baldness*
TABLETS
Adults. 1 mg daily.

Route	Onset	Peak	Duration
P.O.*	Unknown	8 hr	24 hr†
P.O.‡	In 3 mo	Unknown	Unknown

Mechanism of Action
Inhibits 5-alpha reductase, an intracellular enzyme that converts testosterone to its metabolite (5-alpha dihydrotestosterone) in liver, prostate, and skin. The metabolite is a potent androgen partially responsible for benign prostatic hyperplasia and hair loss.

Contraindications
Age (childhood), hypersensitivity to finasteride, sex (female)

Interactions
DRUGS
theophylline: Decreased theophylline level

Adverse Reactions
CNS: Asthenia, depression, dizziness, headache, progressive multifocal leukoencephalopathy (extremely rare)
CV: Hypotension, peripheral edema
EENT: Lip swelling, rhinitis
ENDO: Gynecomastia, male breast cancer
GI: Abdominal pain, diarrhea
GU: Altered prostate-specific antigen level, decreased ejaculatory volume, decreased libido, erectile dysfunction, high-grade prostate cancer, impotence, male infertility, testicular pain
MS: Back pain
RESP: Dyspnea
SKIN: Pruritus, rash, urticaria
Other: Angioedema

Nursing Considerations
- Be aware that patient should have a urologic evaluation prior to starting finasteride therapy and periodically throughout therapy because drug can increase the risk of prostate cancer, especially high-grade prostate cancer.
- Expect patient to have a digital rectal examination of the prostate before and periodically during finasteride therapy.

---

* For benign prostatic hyperplasia.
† With single-dose therapy; 2 wk with multiple-dose therapy.
‡ For male-pattern baldness.

E
F

• Be aware that finasteride therapy affects prostate-specific antigen (PSA) levels. For example, drug may decrease levels even in the presence of prostate cancer. Any increases, no matter how slight or even if increase is still within normal limits, warrant further evaluation because of finasteride's risk of high-grade prostate cancer.

• Pregnant female healthcare workers should not handle broken finasteride tablets because of potential adverse effect on male fetus.

PATIENT TEACHING

WARNING Urge patient and female partners to use reliable contraception during therapy because semen of men who take drug can harm male fetuses. Caution women and children not to handle broken tablets.

• Explain how to take drug, and urge patient to follow instructions that accompany it.

• Inform patient that drug may cause a variety of sexual dysfunction problems including erectile dysfunction, decreased libido, and male infertility, which may continue after drug is discontinued.

• Urge patient to have periodic follow-up to determine drug effectiveness.

• Caution patient that noncompliance with therapy may affect PSA test results.

fingolimod hydrochloride

Gilenya

Class and Category
Chemical class: Sphingosine
Therapeutic class: Antimultiple sclerotic
Pregnancy category: C

Indications and Dosages
➤ *To reduce the frequency of clinical exacerbations and to delay the accumulation of physical disability in patients with relapsing forms of multiple sclerosis (MS)*

CAPSULES
Adults. 0.5 mg once daily.

Mechanism of Action
Possibly involves reduction of lymphocyte migration into the central nervous system to produce improved physical mobility.

Contraindications
Baseline QTc interval equal to or greater than 500 ms; experience within past 6 months of class III or IV heart failure, decompensated heart failure requiring hospitalization, MI, stroke, TIA, or unstable angina; history or presence of Mobitz Type II second-degree or third-degree atrioventricular block or sick sinus syndrome unless patient has functioning pacemaker in place; hypersensitivity to fingolimod or its components; use of Class Ia or Class III anti-arrhythmic drugs

Interactions
DRUGS
antineoplastics, immunosuppressives, immunomodulators: Increased immunosuppression
beta blockers such as atenolol, calcium channel blockers such as diltiazem or verapamil, digoxin: Possibly increased severity of bradycardia or slowing of atrioventricular conduction
chlorpromazine, citalopram, Class Ia and Class III antiarrhythmics, erythromycin, haloperidol, methadone: Possibly increased risk for prolonged QT interval which may lead to torsades de pointes
ketoconazole: Increased fingolimod levels
live attenuated vaccines: Increased risk of contracting disease from live virus
vaccines: Decreased effectiveness of vaccines during and up to 2 months after fingolimod therapy

Adverse Reactions
CNS: Asthenia, depression, dizziness, headache, migraine, paresthesia, posterior reversible encephalopathy syndrome, syncope
CV: Atrioventricular blocks, bradycardia, elevated blood triglycerides, hypertension, transient asystole
EENT: Blurred vision, eye pain, macular edema, sinusitis
GI: Diarrhea, elevated liver enzymes, gastroenteritis
HEME: Leukopenia, lymphopenia

MS: Back pain
RESP: Bronchitis, cough, dyspnea
SKIN: Alopecia, eczema, pruritus, tinea infections
Other: Herpes viral infections, influenza, lymphomas, weight loss

Nursing Considerations

• Be aware that fingolimod therapy should not begin in a patient with an active acute or chronic infection until the infection is resolved.
• Immunize patient against the varicella zoster virus if he is antibody negative, as ordered. Be aware that fingolimod therapy will need to be postponed for 1 month to allow the full effect of vaccination to occur.
• Obtain an electrocardiogram on patients receiving antiarrhythmic therapy including beta-blockers and calcium channel blockers, those with cardiac risk factors, and those who have a slow or irregular heartbeat prior to beginning fingolimod therapy because drug may cause bradycardia and increased risk for atrioventricular block, especially in the first 24 hours of therapy.
• Obtain a recent complete blood count (within past 6 months) prior to starting therapy because drug increases risk of infection. Monitor patient throughout drug therapy for signs and symptoms of infection. If present, notify prescriber and expect drug to be discontinued if serious.
• Expect patient to have an ophthalmologic evaluation prior to beginning drug therapy and then again 3 to 4 months after therapy has begun to assess for macular edema. Patients with diabetes mellitus or a history of uveitis should have ongoing evaluations because they are at increased risk for macular edema. Report any visual disturbances to prescriber during drug therapy and expect additional ophthalmologic evaluation to be performed, if present, and drug discontinued. Visual acuity loss may persist even after resolution of macular edema in some patients.
• Obtain a recent liver enzyme evaluation (within past 6 months) prior to initiating fingolimod therapy because drug may cause elevation of liver enzymes. Monitor periodically throughout therapy and expect drug to be discontinued if liver enzymes exceed 5 times the upper limit of normal. Also evaluate in patient who develops symptoms suggestive of hepatic dysfunction, such as unexplained nausea, vomiting, abdominal pain, fatigue, anorexia, or jaundice and/or dark urine. Know that patients with preexisting liver disease may be at increased risk for developing elevated liver enzymes during fingolimod therapy.
• Observe patient for 24 hours after the first dose of fingolimod for signs and symptoms of bradycardia. Heart rate usually begins to decrease within an hour of the first dose. The maximal decline in heart rate usually occurs within 6 hours and recovers but not to baseline level within 10 hours after the first dose. A second decline may occur after the first within the first 24 hours after the first dose. Monitor patient closely because the second decline may be more pronounced than the first. If patient develops hypotension, dizziness, fatigue, palpitations or chest pain, notify prescriber, initiate appropriate management, as ordered, and continue observation until the symptoms have resolved. Know that with continued drug use, the heart rate returns to baseline within one month.
• Monitor patient for dyspnea throughout fingolimod therapy because drug may reduce forced expiratory volume over 1 second and diffusion lung capacity for carbon monoxide (DLCO). Expect to perform spirometric evaluations of respiratory function and evaluation of DLCO during therapy, if clinically indicated.
• Monitor patient's blood pressure regularly to detect development of hypertension.
• Be aware that it takes about 2 months for drug effects to be gone after therapy is discontinued requiring patient to be monitored for adverse effects during this time.

PATIENT TEACHING
• Inform patient that he will need to be observed for at least 6 hours after the first dose. He will need to repeat this observation period again for 6 hours if treatment is interrupted for more than 1 day within the first 2 weeks of therapy, if

treatment is interrupted for more than 7 days during week 3 and 4 of therapy, or if treatment is discontinued for more than 14 days and then treatment is reinitiated.
• Tell patient to report any adverse signs and symptoms of infection to prescriber promptly, even up to 2 months after drug has been discontinued.
• Instruct female patients to use effective contraception to avoid pregnancy during and for 2 months after fingolimod therapy is discontinued because of potential fetal harm.
• Instruct patient how to check his pulse and tell him to notify prescriber if his pulse rate drops below 60 beats per minute or becomes irregular.
• Advise patient to notify prescriber immediately if visual changes or difficulty breathing occurs.
• Tell patient to notify prescriber if he notices symptoms suggestive of liver dysfunction, such as unexplained nausea, vomiting, abdominal pain, fatigue, anorexia, or jaundice and/or dark urine.
• Alert patient of the need to have periodic blood work done during fingolimod therapy and urge him to be compliant with these evaluations.

flavoxate hydrochloride

Urispas

Class and Category
Chemical class: Flavone derivative
Therapeutic class: Urinary tract antispasmodic
Pregnancy category: B

Indications and Dosages
➤ *To relieve dysuria, nocturia, suprapubic pain, urinary frequency and urgency, and urinary incontinence caused by cystitis, prostatitis, urethrocystitis, or urethrotrigonitis*
TABLETS
Adults and adolescents. 100 to 200 mg three times daily or four times daily.

Route	Onset	Peak	Duration
P.O.	55 min	112 min	Unknown

Mechanism of Action
Relaxes muscles by cholinergic blockade and counteracts smooth-muscle spasms in the urinary tract.

Contraindications
Achalasia; GI hemorrhage; hypersensitivity to flavoxate or its components; obstruction of the duodenum, ileum, or pylorus; obstructive uropathies of the lower urinary tract

Interactions
DRUGS
bethanechol, metoclopramide: Possibly antagonized GI motility effects of these drugs

Adverse Reactions
CNS: Confusion, decreased concentration, dizziness, drowsiness, fever, headache, nervousness, vertigo
CV: Palpitations, tachycardia
EENT: Accommodation disturbances, blurred vision, dry mouth, eye pain, photophobia, worsening of glaucoma
GI: Constipation, nausea, vomiting
GU: Dysuria
HEME: Eosinophilia, leukopenia
SKIN: Decreased sweating, dermatoses, urticaria

Nursing Considerations
• Monitor for eye pain if patient has glaucoma because flavoxate's anticholinergic effects may worsen glaucoma.
PATIENT TEACHING
• Caution patient about possible dry mouth and photophobia. Advise her to wear sunglasses outdoors, and suggest sugarless candy or gum, ice chips, sips of water, or saliva substitute for dry mouth.
• Advise patient to avoid hazardous activities until CNS effects of flavoxate are known.
• Caution patient not to become overheated or to take hot baths or saunas during therapy because drug reduces sweating, which can lead to dizziness, fainting, or heatstroke.
• Instruct patient to notify prescriber immediately if she experiences confusion, drowsiness, dysuria, headache, high fever, hives, nausea, nervousness, palpitations, rash, tachycardia, vertigo, vision problems, vomiting, or worsening dry mouth.

flecainide acetate

Tambocor

Class and Category
Chemical class: Benzamide derivative
Therapeutic class: Class IC antiarrhythmic
Pregnancy category: C

Indications and Dosages
➤ *To prevent and suppress recurrent life-threatening ventricular tachycardia*
TABLETS
Adults. *Initial:* 100 mg every 12 hr (every 8 hr for some patients). Increased by 50 mg twice daily every 4 days, as needed, until response occurs. *Maintenance:* Up to 150 mg every 12 hr. *Maximum:* 400 mg daily.
DOSAGE ADJUSTMENT Initial dose reduced to 100 mg daily or 50 mg every 12 hr for patients with creatinine clearance less than 35 ml/min/1.73 m².

➤ *To prevent paroxysmal atrial fibrillation or flutter or paroxysmal supraventricular tachycardia*
TABLETS
Adults. *Initial:* 50 mg every 12 hr (every 8 hr for some patients). Increased by 50 mg twice daily every 4 days, as needed, until response occurs. *Maintenance:* Up to 150 mg every 12 hr. *Maximum:* 300 mg daily.

Mechanism of Action
Achieves antiarrhythmic effect by inhibiting fast sodium channels of myocardial cell membranes, which increase myocardial recovery after repolarization, and by depressing the upstroke of the action potential. Flecainide also produces its antiarrhythmic effect by:
• slowing intracardiac conduction, which slightly increases the duration of the action potential in atrial and ventricular muscle, thus prolonging the PR interval, QRS complex, and QT interval
• shortening the action potential of Purkinje fibers without affecting surrounding myocardial tissue
• inhibiting extracellular calcium influx (at high doses)
• stopping paroxysmal reentrant supraventricular tachycardias by acting on antegrade pathways of dysfunctional AV conduction

• decreasing conduction in accessory pathways in those with Wolff-Parkinson-White syndrome.

Contraindications
Cardiogenic shock, hypersensitivity to flecainide or its components, recent MI, right bundle-branch block associated with left hemiblock or second- or third-degree AV block unless pacemaker is present

Interactions
DRUGS
amiodarone: Increased blood flecainide level
beta blockers, disopyramide, verapamil: Possibly myocardial depression and increased blood levels of both drugs
calcium channel blockers: Increased risk of arrhythmias
digoxin: Possibly increased blood digoxin level
urinary acidifiers: Possibly increased flecainide elimination and decreased therapeutic effects
urinary alkalinizers: Possibly decreased flecainide elimination and increased therapeutic effects
FOODS
acidic juices, foods that decrease urine pH below 5.0: Increased flecainide elimination and decreased therapeutic effects
foods that increase urine pH above 7.0, strict vegetarian diet: Decreased flecainide elimination and increased therapeutic effects
ACTIVITIES
smoking: Increased flecainide clearance

Adverse Reactions
CNS: Anxiety, depression, dizziness, drowsiness, fatigue, headache, light-headedness, tremor, weakness
CV: Arrhythmias, chest pain, heart failure, hypotension
EENT: Blurred vision
GI: Abdominal pain, anorexia, constipation, hepatic dysfunction, nausea, vomiting
RESP: Dyspnea
SKIN: Rash

Nursing Considerations
• Monitor urine pH at the start of flecainide therapy.
• Check blood pressure, fluid intake and output, and weight regularly during therapy.

E
F

• Monitor trough flecainide level, as needed; therapeutic level is 0.2 to 1 mcg/ml.
• Expect drug to cause mild to moderate negative inotropic effects, minimal cardiovascular effects, and no effect on blood pressure, heart rate, and left ventricular function.

WARNING Because hypokalemia or hyperkalemia may interfere with flecainide's therapeutic effects, monitor serum potassium level before and during therapy and notify prescriber immediately if potassium imbalance develops. Also monitor for and notify prescriber about prolonged PR interval, QRS complex, or QT interval; chest pain; hypotension; and signs of heart failure. Keep in mind that drug can cause fatal proarrhythmias, which is why it isn't considered a first-line antiarrhythmic.

• Expect prolonged flecainide therapy to raise blood alkaline phosphatase level.

PATIENT TEACHING

• Instruct patient to take flecainide at regular intervals to keep a constant blood level.
• Advise patient to take a missed dose as soon as she remembers if it's within 6 hours of the scheduled time.
• Teach patient how to take her pulse, and instruct her to record it daily, along with her weight. Advise her to bring record to follow-up visits.
• Encourage family members to obtain instruction in basic cardiac life support.
• Advise patient to notify prescriber immediately about chest pain, difficulty breathing, and dizziness.
• Caution patient not to stop taking flecainide suddenly but to taper dosage gradually according to prescriber's instructions.

fluconazole
Diflucan

Class and Category
Chemical class: Triazole derivative
Therapeutic class: Antifungal
Pregnancy category: C (vaginal candidiasis indication), D (all other indications)

Indications and Dosages
➤ *To treat oral and esophageal candidiasis*
ORAL SUSPENSION, TABLETS, I.V. INJECTION
Adults and adolescents. 200 mg on day 1 followed by 100 mg daily for at least 2 (oral) or 3 (esophageal) wk after symptoms resolve.
Children. 3 mg/kg daily for at least 2 (oral) or 3 (esophageal) wk and then for 2 wk after esophageal symptoms resolve.
➤ *To treat systemic candidiasis*
ORAL SUSPENSION, TABLETS, I.V. INJECTION
Adults and adolescents. 400 mg on day 1, followed by 200 mg daily for at least 4 wk and then for additional 2 wk after symptoms resolve.
➤ *To treat cryptococcal meningitis*
ORAL SUSPENSION, TABLETS, I.V. INJECTION
Adults and adolescents. 400 mg daily until patient responds to treatment, then 200 to 400 mg daily for 10 to 12 wk after CSF culture is negative. *Maintenance:* 200 mg daily to suppress relapse.
Children. 6 to 12 mg/kg daily for 10 to 12 wk after CSF culture is negative.
➤ *To prevent candidiasis after bone marrow transplantation*
ORAL SUSPENSION, TABLETS, I.V. INJECTION
Adults and adolescents. 400 mg daily starting several days before procedure if severe neutropenia is expected and continued for 7 days after absolute neutrophil count exceeds 1,000/mm³.
➤ *To treat vaginal candidiasis*
CAPSULES, ORAL SUSPENSION, TABLETS
Adults. 150 mg as a single dose.
DOSAGE ADJUSTMENT Dosage reduced for patients with hepatic or renal impairment. Dosage reduced by 50% for patients with creatinine clearance of 11 to 50 ml/min/1.73 m².

Mechanism of Action
Damages fungal cells by interfering with a cytochrome P-450 enzyme needed to convert lanosterol to ergosterol, an essential part of the fungal cell membrane. Decreased ergosterol synthesis causes increased cell permeability, which allows cell contents to leak. Fluconazole also may inhibit endogenous respiration, interact with membrane phospholipids, inhibit transformation of yeasts to mycelial forms, inhibit purine uptake, and impair biosynthesis of triglycerides and phospholipids.

Incompatibilities
Don't add fluconazole to I.V. bag that contains any other drug.

Contraindications
Coadministration of drugs known to prolong QT interval (astemizole, cisapride, erythromycin, pimozide, or quinidine) or terfenadine (when multiple dosages reach or exceed 400 mg), hypersensitivity to fluconazole or its components

Interactions
DRUGS
alfentanil, amitriptyline, nortriptyline: Increased blood alfentanil level
astemizole, cisapride, erythromycin, pimozide, quinidine: Increased risk of QT interval prolongation possibly leading to torsades de pointes
benzodiazepines (short-acting): Possibly increased benzodiazepine level and psychomotor effects
calcium-channel blockers: Possibly increased systemic exposure of calcium-channel blockers causing adverse effects
carbamazepine: Possibly increased risk of carbamazepine toxicity
cimetidine: Decreased fluconazole level
celecoxib, cyclosporine, halofantrine, terfenadine, triazolam: Increased blood levels of these drugs
fentanyl: Possibly elevated fentanyl concentraion that may lead to respiratory depression
glipizide, glyburide, tolbutamide: Increased risk of hypoglycemia
HMG-CoA reductase inhibitors: Increased risk of myopathy and rhabdomyolysis
hydrochlorothiazide: Increased fluconazole level from decreased excretion
isoniazid, rifampin: Decreased fluconazole effects
nonsedating antihistamines: Increased blood antihistamine level, increased risk of cardiotoxicity
oral anticoagulants: Increased anticoagulant effects
phenytoin: Increased phenytoin level
rifabutin: Increased rifabutin level
theophylline: Increased theophylline level
tofacitinib: Increased systemic exposure to tofacitinib with increased risk of adverse reactions

zidovudine: Increased zidovudine level

Adverse Reactions
CNS: Chills, dizziness, drowsiness, fever, headache, seizures
CV: Prolonged QT interval, torsades de pointes
GI: Abdominal pain, anorexia, constipation, diarrhea, hepatic failure, nausea, vomiting
HEME: Agranulocytosis, leukopenia, thrombocytopenia
SKIN: Exfoliative dermatitis, photosensitivity, pruritus, rash
Other: Anaphylaxis, angioedema

Nursing Considerations
• Use fluconazole cautiously in patients with potentially proarrhythmic conditions because drug may prolong the QT interval, which can lead to life-threatening torsades de pointes.
• Expect to obtain BUN and serum creatinine levels, as well as culture, sensitivity, and liver function test results before therapy starts.
• Refrigerate, but don't freeze, fluconazole oral suspension. Shake well before administering.
• Discard I.V. solution that's cloudy or contains precipitate. Don't infuse more than 200 mg/hr or add supplemental drugs to infusion.
• Monitor hepatic and renal function periodically during therapy, and notify prescriber if you detect signs of dysfunction.
• Assess for rash every 8 hours during therapy, and notify prescriber if rash occurs.
• If patient receives an oral anticoagulant, monitor coagulation test results and assess patient for bleeding.
• Monitor patient for symptoms of overdose, such as hallucinations and paranoia. If they occur, provide supportive treatment, gastric lavage, and, possibly, hemodialysis, which can reduce blood fluconazole level by half after about 3 hours.
PATIENT TEACHING
• Instruct patient to take fluconazole tablets or oral suspension 30 minutes before or 2 hours after meals. Inform her that tablets may be crushed for easier swallowing if needed.

- Advise patient to complete entire course of therapy, even if she feels better.
- If patient takes an oral antidiabetic, urge her to monitor blood glucose level often because of increased risk of hypoglycemia.
- Alert patient that fluconazole may change the taste of food.
- Encourage patient to notify prescriber immediately about diarrhea, headache, nausea, rash, right-upper-quadrant abdominal pain, yellow skin or whites of eyes, or vomiting.
- Suggest that breastfeeding patient consult prescriber because breastfeeding may need to be stopped during therapy.
- Urge women of childbearing age to notify prescriber immediately if pregnancy is suspected or known, as drug may need to be discontinued.

fludrocortisone acetate

Florinef

Class and Category

Chemical class: Glucocorticoid
Therapeutic class: Mineralocorticoid replacement
Pregnancy category: C

Indications and Dosages

➤ *To treat primary and secondary chronic adrenocortical insufficiency*

TABLETS
Adults and adolescents. *Usual:* 100 mcg daily. Dosage may range from 100 mcg three times/wk to 200 mcg daily.
Children. 50 to 100 mcg daily.

➤ *To treat salt-losing adrenogenital syndrome*

TABLETS
Adults. 100 to 200 mcg daily.
Children. 50 to 100 mcg daily.
DOSAGE ADJUSTMENT Dosage reduced to 50 mcg daily if transient hypertension develops during therapy.

Route	Onset	Peak	Duration
P.O.	Unknown	Unknown	1–2 days

Mechanism of Action

Enhances sodium reabsorption, hydrogen and potassium excretion, and water retention by the distal renal tubules, much like aldosterone, an endogenous mineralocorticoid. In large doses, fludrocortisone can inhibit endogenous adrenocortical secretion, thymic activity, and pituitary corticotropin excretion. It also can promote glycogen deposits in the liver and induce a negative nitrogen balance when protein intake is deficient.

Contraindications

Hypersensitivity to fludrocortisone, adrenocorticoids, or their components; systemic fungal infections

Interactions
DRUGS
digoxin: Increased risk of digitalis toxicity and arrhythmias from hypokalemia
phenytoin, rifampin: Decreased fludrocortisone effects
potassium-wasting drugs, such as loop diuretics and amphotericin B: Increased risk of severe hypokalemia

Adverse Reactions
CNS: Dizziness, headache, mental changes, seizures
CV: Arrhythmias, heart failure, hypertension, peripheral edema
EENT: Cataracts (with long-term use), increased intraocular pressure
ENDO: Adrenal insufficiency, growth suppression in children, hyperglycemia
GI: Anorexia, nausea, vomiting
GU: Menstrual irregularities
HEME: Easy bruising
MS: Arthralgia, muscle weakness, myalgia, osteoporosis (with long-term use), tendon contractures
SKIN: Acne, diaphoresis, rash, urticaria
Other: Hypokalemia, hypokalemic alkalosis, impaired wound healing, weight gain

Nursing Considerations
- Monitor blood pressure, fluid status, and serum electrolyte levels periodically during fludrocortisone therapy. Watch for signs of heart failure, including adventitious breath sounds, peripheral edema, and weight gain.

• Monitor for signs and symptoms of overdose, such as cardiomegaly, edema, excessive weight gain, hypertension, and hypokalemia. These effects usually subside a few days after therapy stops. Potassium supplementation may be needed.
• Notify prescriber if patient has dizziness, headache, hypertension, hypokalemia, signs of infection, or weight gain.

PATIENT TEACHING
• Instruct patient to take a missed dose of fludrocortisone as soon as she remembers if it's within 12 hours of scheduled time. Warn against double-dosing. Advise her to notify prescriber if she misses more than one dose or if nausea or vomiting prevents her from taking drug.
• Instruct patient to reduce dietary sodium and to eat more potassium-rich foods during therapy.
• Direct patient to weigh herself each morning before breakfast in clothes of similar weight and to notify prescriber if she gains more than 2 lb (0.9 kg) per day or 5 lb (2.3 kg) per week. Instruct her to monitor how tightly her rings and shoes fit.
• Advise patient to notify prescriber about stressful events, such as dental extractions, emotional upset, illness, surgery, and trauma; dosage increase may be required.
• Instruct patient to notify prescriber about dizziness, fever, fluid retention, headache, joint pain, irregular heart rate, muscle weakness, or palpitations.
• Inform patient that drug may delay wound healing.
• Caution patient not to stop taking drug abruptly but to taper dosage gradually, as prescribed.
• Urge patient to wear or carry medical identification that documents corticosteroid use.

flumazenil

Anexate (CAN), Romazicon

Class and Category
Chemical class: Imidazobenzodiazepine derivative
Therapeutic class: Benzodiazepine antidote
Pregnancy category: C

Indications and Dosages
➤ *To reverse sedation from benzodiazepine therapy*
I.V. INJECTION
Adults. 0.2 mg, repeated after 45 to 60 sec if response is inadequate and then repeated every 1 min, if needed. If sedation recurs, regimen is repeated every 20 min or more. *Maximum:* 1 mg over 5 min or 3 mg over 1 hr.
➤ *To reverse benzodiazepine toxicity or suspected overdose*
I.V. INJECTION
Adults. 0.2 mg followed by 0.3 mg 30 to 60 sec later if response is inadequate and then 0.5 mg repeated every 1 min. If sedation recurs, regimen is repeated every 20 min. *Maximum:* 3 mg in 1-hr period.

Mechanism of Action
Antagonizes CNS effects of benzodiazepines by competing for their binding sites.

Contraindications
Evidence of tricyclic antidepressant overdose; hypersensitivity to flumazenil, benzodiazepines, or their components; use of benzodiazepine to control intracranial pressure, status epilepticus, or a potentially life-threatening condition

Route	Onset	Peak	Duration
I.V.	1–2 min	6–10 min	Variable

Interactions
DRUGS
benzodiazepines: Benzodiazepine withdrawal symptoms, including seizures
nonbenzodiazepine agonists: Loss of effectiveness of these drugs
tetracyclic or tricyclic antidepressant overdose: High risk of seizures
FOODS
all foods: Increased flumazenil clearance (by half) with food ingestion during I.V. injection

Adverse Reactions
CNS: Agitation, anxiety, ataxia, confusion, dizziness, drowsiness, emotional lability, fatigue, headache, hypoesthesia, insomnia, paresthesia, resedation, seizures, tremor, vertigo
CV: Hot flashes, hypertension, palpitations
EENT: Blurred vision, diplopia, dry mouth
GI: Nausea, vomiting

E
F

RESP: Dyspnea, hyperventilation, hypoventilation
SKIN: Diaphoresis, flushing, rash
Other: Injection-site pain and thrombophlebitis

Nursing Considerations

• Use flumazenil cautiously in patients with cardiac disease. Assess for increased stress or anxiety from benzodiazepine withdrawal because patient's blood pressure may rise.
• Give flumazenil undiluted or diluted in a syringe with D_5W, normal saline solution, or lactated Ringer's solution. Administer over 15 to 30 seconds directly into tubing of a free-flowing compatible I.V. solution. Use a large vein, if possible, to minimize pain at site. Avoid extravasation because drug may irritate tissue.
• Be aware that drug may cause signs of benzodiazepine withdrawal in drug-dependent patient. Also, abrupt awakening from benzodiazepine overdose can cause agitation, dysphoria, and increased adverse reactions.
• Be aware that benzodiazepine reversal may cause an anxiety or a panic attack for patient with a history of these episodes. Expect to adjust dosage carefully.
• Monitor patient for signs of resedation and hypoventilation for at least 2 hours after giving flumazenil because drug has a short half-life. Be aware that patient shouldn't be discharged until the risk of resedation has resolved.

PATIENT TEACHING

• Caution patient to avoid alcohol and OTC drugs for 10 to 24 hours after taking drug.
• Advise patient to avoid hazardous activities for 18 to 24 hours after discharge.
• Inform patient and family that agitation, emotional lability, fear, and panic attack (if patient has a history of them) may occur. Tell them to seek medical care if patient has depression, trouble breathing, flushing, hyperventilation, insomnia, palpitations, or tremor.
• Because drug doesn't always reverse postprocedure amnesia, provide written instructions or instructions to caregiver even if patient is alert.

flunisolide
Aerospan, Bronalide (CAN), Nasalide, Nasarel, Rhinalar (CAN)

Class and Category
Chemical class: Corticosteroid
Therapeutic class: Antiasthmatic, anti-inflammatory
Pregnancy category: C

Indications and Dosages
➤ *To provide maintenance treatment of asthma, alone or with oral corticosteroids*
INHALATION AEROSOL (BRONALIDE, NASALIDE, NASAREL, RHINALAR)
Adults and adolescents age 15 and over.
500 mcg (2 inhalations) twice daily morning and evening. *Maximum:* 2,000 mcg daily (4 inhalations twice daily).
Children ages 6 to 15. 500 mcg (2 inhalations) twice daily. *Maximum:* 1,000 mcg daily.
INHALATION AEROSOL (AEROSPAN)
Adults and adolescents age 12 and over.
Initial: 160 mcg (2 inhalations) twice daily. *Maximum:* 320 mg (4 inhalations) twice daily.
Children ages 6 to 11. *Initial:* 80 mcg (1 inhalation) twice daily. *Maximum:* 160 mcg (2 inhalations) twice daily.
➤ *To relieve symptoms of seasonal or perennial rhinitis*
NASAL SOLUTION
Adults. 50 mcg (2 sprays) twice daily in each nostril. *Maximum:* 400 mcg daily (16 sprays).
Children. 25 mcg (1 spray) three times daily in each nostril. *Maximum:* 200 mcg daily (8 sprays).

Route	Onset	Peak	Duration
Inhalation	In 4 wk	Unknown	Unknown
Nasal	3–7 days	Unknown	4–6 hr

Mechanism of Action
Inhibits cells involved in inflammatory response, such as mast cells, eosinophils, basophils, lymphocytes, macrophages, and neutrophils. Also inhibits production of chemical mediators, such as histamine, eicosanoids, leukotrienes, and cytokines.

Contraindications

Hypersensitivity to flunisolide or its components, primary treatment of status asthmaticus or other asthma episodes that require emergency care, recent nasal surgery (nasal form), untreated localized infection of nasal mucosa (nasal form)

Adverse Reactions

CNS: Anxiety, chills, depression, dizziness, headache, hyperactivity, insomnia, irritability, lethargy, mood changes, nervousness, tremor, vertigo
CV: Hypertension
EENT: Candidiasis (oral and throat), dry mouth and throat, earache, eye infection, hoarseness, loss of smell or taste, mouth irritation, pharyngitis, rhinitis, sinusitis, sneezing
GI: Abdominal pain, anorexia, constipation, diarrhea, flatulence, heartburn, increased appetite, indigestion, nausea, vomiting
GU: Menstrual irregularities
HEME: Eosinophilia
RESP: Bronchitis, dyspnea, pleurisy, pneumonia
SKIN: Acne, eczema, pruritus, rash, urticaria
Other: Growth suppression (children), lymphadenopathy

Nursing Considerations

• Use flunisolide cautiously in patients with ocular herpes simplex, pulmonary tuberculosis, or untreated systemic bacterial, fungal, parasitic, or viral infection.
• If patient receives an oral corticosteroid, expect to taper it slowly 1 week after changing to flunisolide. For patient who receives prednisone, expect to reduce it by no more than 2.5 mg daily at weekly intervals, beginning at least 1 week after flunisolide therapy starts.
WARNING Assess patient switched from systemic corticosteroid to flunisolide for adrenal insufficiency (fatigue, hypotension, lassitude, nausea, vomiting, weakness) during initial treatment and during stress, trauma, surgery, infection, or other electrolyte-depleting conditions. Notify prescriber immediately if signs or symptoms arise.
• Monitor growth in children; corticosteroids may increase risk of growth suppression.

PATIENT TEACHING

• Teach patient how to use inhaler. When starting a new canister, advise spraying once into the air (avoiding her eyes) to check for mist.
• Instruct patient to gargle or rinse after each use of flunisolide to help prevent mouth and throat dryness, relieve throat irritation, and prevent oropharyngeal infection.
• Urge patient to contact prescriber if symptoms haven't improved after 3 weeks.
WARNING Caution patient not to use flunisolide to relieve acute bronchospasm.
• If patient switches from an oral corticosteroid to flunisolide, advise her to carry medical identification indicating the need for supplemental systemic corticosteroids during stress or severe asthma attack. Advise her to ask prescriber how to respond to these problems.
• Caution patient to avoid exposure to chickenpox and measles and to contact prescriber immediately if exposure occurs.

E
F

fluoxetine hydrochloride

Prozac, Prozac Weekly, Sarafem

Class and Category

Chemical class: Phenylpropylamine derivative
Therapeutic class: Antibulimic, antidepressant, antiobsessive-compulsive
Pregnancy category: C

Indications and Dosages

➤ *To treat depression*
CAPSULES, ORAL SOLUTION, TABLETS (PROZAC)
Adults. *Initial:* 20 mg daily in the morning. Dosage increased every 4 to 8 wk as needed. Dosage greater than 20 mg daily given twice daily morning and noon. *Maximum:* 80 mg daily.
Children ages 8 and older. *Initial:* 10 mg daily. Increased after 1 wk to 20 mg daily.
DOSAGE ADJUSTMENT For lower-weight children, dosage increased to 20 mg daily only if improvement insufficient after several wk.

DELAYED-RELEASE CAPSULES (PROZAC WEEKLY)
Adults. 90 mg/wk, beginning 7 days after last 20-mg daily dose.
➤ *As adjunct to olanzapine therapy to treat acute depressive episodes associated with Bipolar I disorder*
CAPSULES, ORAL SOLUTION, TABLETS (PROZAC)
Adults. *Initial:* 20 mg once daily in evening with 5 mg olanzapine. *Maximum:* 50 mg fluoxetine and 12.5 mg olanzapine.
➤ *To treat obsessive-compulsive disorder*
CAPSULES, ORAL SOLUTION, TABLETS (PROZAC)
Adults. *Initial:* 20 mg daily in the morning. Dosage increased every 4 to 8 wk as needed. Dosage greater than 20 mg daily given twice daily morning and noon. *Maximum:* 80 mg daily.
Children and adolescents. *Initial:* 10 mg daily. Dosage increased after 2 wk to 20 mg daily. Subsequent dosage increased, as needed, at intervals of at least several wk. *Maintenance:* 20 to 60 mg daily.
DOSAGE ADJUSTMENT For lower-weight children, dosage should be increased above 10 mg daily only if clinical improvement remains insufficient after several wk. Maintenance dosage for such patients should not exceed 30 mg daily.
➤ *To treat moderate to severe bulimia nervosa*
CAPSULES, ORAL SOLUTION, TABLETS (PROZAC)
Adults. 60 mg daily in the morning. Some patients may be prescribed a lower dose, which is titrated to 60 mg daily as tolerated.
➤ *To treat panic disorder with or without agoraphobia*
CAPSULES, ORAL SOLUTION, TABLETS (PROZAC)
Adults. *Initial:* 10 mg daily. Dosage increased in 1 wk to 20 mg daily, as needed. *Maximum:* 60 mg daily.
➤ *To treat premenstrual dysmorphic disorder*
CAPSULES (SARAFEM)
Adults. 20 mg daily. Dosage increased as needed.
Maximum: 80 mg daily.
DOSAGE ADJUSTMENT Dose or frequency reduced for patients with hepatic impairment or concurrent illness, those who take multiple medications, and for elderly patients.

Route	Onset	Peak	Duration
P.O.*	1–6 wk†	Unknown	Unknown

Mechanism of Action

Selectively inhibits reuptake of the neurotransmitter serotonin by CNS neurons and increases the amount of serotonin available in nerve synapses. An elevated serotonin level may result in elevated mood and, consequently, reduced depression.

Contraindications

Concurrent therapy with pimozide or thioridazine, hypersensitivity to selective serotonin reuptake inhibitors or their components, use within 14 days of MAO inhibitor therapy, including reversible MAOIs such as linezolid or intravenous methylene blue

Interactions
DRUGS
alprazolam, diazepam: Possibly prolonged half-life of these drugs
aspirin, NSAIDs, warfarin: Increased anticoagulant activity and risk of bleeding
astemizole: Increased risk of serious arrhythmias
buspirone: Decreased buspirone effects, increased risk of serotonin syndrome
clozapine, fluphenazine, haloperidol, maprotiline, trazodone: Increased risk of adverse effects
CYP2D6-metabolized drugs, such as antiarrhythmics (especially flecainide, propafenone), selected antidepressants (tricyclics), antipsychotics (phenothiazines and most atypicals), thioridazine, and vinblastine: Increased plasma levels of these drugs and increased risk of serious adverse reactions
fentanyl, intravenous methylene blue, linezolid, lithium, serotonergics (such as amphetamines and other psychostimulants, antidepressants, and dopamine agonists), St. John's wort, tramadol, tricyclic antidepressants, triptans: Increased risk of serotonin syndrome
MAO inhibitors: Possibly severe and life-threatening adverse effects
olanzapine: Increased blood olanzapine levels with decreased clearance resulting in possible increased risk for adverse reactions
phenytoin: Increased blood phenytoin level and risk of toxicity

---

* Capsules, oral solution, and tablets.
† For depression and bulimia; 5 wk for obsessive-compulsive disorder.

pimozide, thiordazine: Increased blood levels of these drugs; possibly increased risk of prolonged QT interval

sumatriptan: Increased risk of weakness, hyperreflexia, and difficulty with coordination

tryptophan: Increased risk of central and peripheral toxicity, increased risk of serotonin syndrome

Adverse Reactions

CNS: Akathisia, anxiety, ataxia, balance disorder, chills, depersonalization, dream disturbances, drowsiness, emotional lability, euphoria, fatigue, fever, headache, hypertonia, hypomania, insomnia, mania, myoclonus, nervousness, neuroleptic malignant syndrome, paranoid reaction, restlessness, seizures, serotonin syndrome, somnolence, suicidal ideation, tremor, vertigo, weakness, yawning

CV: Arrhythmias, hypotension, palpitations, prolonged QT interval, torsades de pointes, ventricular arrhythmias

EENT: Abnormal vision, angle-closure glaucoma, dry mouth, mydriasis, pharyngitis, sinusitis, taste perversion, teeth grinding

ENDO: Galactorrhea, gynecomastia, hypoglycemia, syndrome of inappropriate antidiuretic hormone secretion (SIADH)

GI: Anorexia, diarrhea, dysphagia, gastritis, gastroenteritis, indigestion, melena, nausea, stomach ulcer

GU: Decreased or increased libido, dysuria, ejaculation disorders, gynecological bleeding, impotence, micturition disorder

HEME: Altered platelet function, unusual bleeding

MS: Arthralgia, myalgia

RESP: Dyspnea

SKIN: Alopecia, diaphoresis, ecchymosis, pruritus, rash, urticaria

Other: Flulike symptoms, hyponatremia, weight loss

Nursing Considerations

• Use fluoxetine cautiously in patients with a history of seizures.

• Use fluoxetine cautiously in patients with congenital long QT syndrome, previous history of QT prolongation, or family history of long QT syndrome or sudden cardiac death. In addition, use caution in presence of other conditions that increase risk of QT prolongation and ventricular arrhythmia, such as concurrent drug therapy with drugs known to prolong the QT interval, hypokalemia, hypomagnesemia, recent MI, significant arrhythmias, uncompensated heart failure and conditions that predispose patient to increased fluoxetine exposure, such as hepatic impairment or concurrent use of drugs known to increase blood fluoxetine levels such as CYP2D6 inhibitors, CYP2D6 poor metabolizer status, or use of other highly protein-bound drugs. Obtain an ECG recording, as ordered, before fluoxetine begins in these patients and periodically throughout therapy. Expect fluoxetine to be discontinued if the QT interval becomes prolonged or patient develops a ventricular arrhythmia.

WARNING Avoid giving fluoxetine within 14 days of an MAO inhibitor or starting MAO inhibitor therapy within 5 weeks of discontinuing fluoxetine.

• In patients taking fluoxetine for depression (especially children, adolescents, and young adults), watch closely for suicidal tendencies, particularly when therapy starts and dosage changes, because depression may worsen temporarily during those times.

• Monitor patient closely for evidence of GI bleeding, especially if patient takes another drug known to increase the risk, such as aspirin, an NSAID, or warfarin.

• Monitor patient—especially an elderly patient—for hypoosmolarity of serum and urine and for hyponatremia (headache, difficulty concentrating, memory impairment, weakness, unsteadiness), which may indicate fluoxetine-induced SIADH.

• To discontinue, expect to taper drug, as ordered, to minimize adverse reactions.

WARNING Monitor patient for possible serotonin syndrome, characterized by agitation, chills, confusion, diaphoresis, diarrhea, fever, hyperactive reflexes, poor coordination, restlessness, shaking, talking or acting with uncontrolled excitement, tremor, and twitching, especially if patient is receiving another drug that raises serotonin level (such as dopamine agonist,

E
F

MAO inhibitor, tryptophan, amphetamine, and other antidepressant or psycho-stimulant). In its most severe form, serotonin syndrome can resemble neuroleptic malignant syndrome, which includes a high fever, muscle rigidity, autonomic instability, and possible fluctuations in vital signs and mental status.

• Monitor patient with diabetes mellitus for altered blood glucose level because drug may cause hypoglycemia during therapy and hyperglycemia when it stops. Expect to adjust dosage of antidiabetic drug, as prescribed.

• Expect patient to be reevaluated period-ically to determine continued need for therapy.

• When stopping fluoxetine therapy, expect to taper drug to minimize adverse reactions.

PATIENT TEACHING

WARNING Tell patient that drug increases risk of serotonin syndrome, a rare but serious complication, especially when taken with certain other drugs. Teach patient to recognize its signs and symptoms, and advise her to notify prescriber immediately if they occur.

• Urge family or caregiver to watch patient closely for suicidal tendencies, especially when therapy starts or dosage changes, and particularly if patient is a child, teenager, or young adult.

• Caution patient to avoid hazardous activities until CNS effects of drug are known.

• Caution against stopping fluoxetine abruptly because serious adverse effects may result.

• Inform patient that drug may cause mild pupillary dilation, which may lead to an episode of acute-angle glaucoma. Encourage patient to have an eye exam prior to starting fluoxetine therapy to see if she is at risk.

• Advise patient to consult prescriber before taking OTC or prescription drugs, if a rash or hives develop, or if she becomes or intends to become pregnant during therapy.

• Inform patient that drug may take several weeks to achieve full effects.

fluphenazine decanoate

Modecate (CAN),
Modecate Concentrate (CAN),
Prolixin Decanoate

fluphenazine enanthate

Moditen Enanthate (CAN), Prolixin Enanthate

fluphenazine hydrochloride

Apo-Fluphenazine (CAN), Moditen HCl (CAN), Permitil, Permitil Concentrate, PMS Fluphenazine (CAN), Prolixin, Prolixin Concentrate

Class and Category

Chemical class: Phenothiazine, propylpiperazine derivative
Therapeutic class: Antipsychotic
Pregnancy category: Not rated

Indications and Dosages

➤ *To control psychotic disorders*

ELIXIR, ORAL SOLUTION, TABLETS (FLUPHENAZINE HYDROCHLORIDE)

Adults and adolescents. *Initial:* 2.5 to 10 mg/day in divided doses every 6 to 8 hr. When symptoms are controlled, dosage reduced to 1 to 5 mg daily. *Maximum:* 20 mg/dose with caution.

Children. 250 to 750 mcg once daily to four times daily.

I.M. INJECTION (FLUPHENAZINE HYDROCHLORIDE)

Adults and adolescents. *Initial:* 1.25 mg, increased as clinical condition tolerates up to 2.5 to 10 mg daily in divided doses every 6 to 8 hr. *Maximum:* 10 mg daily.

DOSAGE ADJUSTMENT For elderly or debilitated patients, dosage reduced to 1 to 2.5 mg daily in divided doses every 6 to 8 hr.

I.M. OR SUBCUTANEOUS INJECTION (FLUPHENAZINE DECANOATE OR ENANTHATE)

Adults. *Initial:* 12.5 to 25 mg every 1 to 4 wk, as needed (decanoate). For doses over 50 mg, next dose increased cautiously by

12.5 mg. Or 25 mg every 2 wk, with dose and dosing interval adjusted based on patient response (enanthate). *Maximum:* 100 mg/dose.
Adolescents and children age 12. *Initial:* 6.25 to 18.75 mg/wk (decanoate), increased to 12.5 to 25 mg every 1 to 3 wk, according to condition.
Children ages 5 to 12. 3.125 to 12.5 mg every 1 to 3 wk (decanoate), according to condition.

Route	Onset	Peak	Duration
P.O.	In 1 hr	Variable	6–8 hr
I.M.*	In 1 hr	Variable	6–8 hr
I.M., SubQ†	In 24–72 hr	Variable	1–6 wk‡

Mechanism of Action
May block postsynaptic dopamine receptor sites in the CNS. This action may depress areas of the brain that control activity and aggression, including the cerebral cortex, hypothalamus, and limbic system.

Incompatibilities
Don't mix fluphenazine hydrochloride oral solution with beverages that contain caffeine, such as coffee and cola; tannins, such as tea; or pectins, such as apple juice. They're physically incompatible.

Contraindications
Blood dyscrasias, bone marrow depression, cerebral arteriosclerosis, coma, concomitant use of large amounts of another CNS depressant, coronary artery disease, hepatic dysfunction, hypersensitivity to pheno-thiazines, myeloproliferative disorders, severe CNS depression, severe hypertension or hypotension, subcortical brain damage

Interactions
DRUGS
adsorbent antidiarrheals, aluminum- or magnesium-containing antacids: Possibly inhibited absorption of fluphenazine
amantadine, anticholinergics: Possibly intensified adverse effects of both drugs

---

* For hydrochloride.
† For decanoate and enanthate.
‡ For decanoate; 2 wk for enanthate.

amphetamines: Possibly decreased therapeutic effects of both drugs
antihypertensives: Possibly severe hypotension
antithyroid drugs: Increased risk of agranulocytosis
beta blockers: Possibly increased blood levels and risk of adverse effects of both drugs
bromocriptine: Decreased bromocriptine effects
CNS depressants: Possibly prolonged and intensified CNS depression
erythromycin: Possibly inhibited fluphenazine metabolism
guanethidine: Decreased hypotensive effect of guanethidine
levodopa: Possibly decreased antidyskinetic effect of levodopa
lithium: Possibly neurotoxicity (disorientation, extrapyramidal reactions, unconsciousness)
meperidine: Excessive sedation and hypotension
metrizamide: Increased risk of seizures when injected in subarachnoid area during fluphenazine therapy
oral anticoagulants: Possibly decreased anticoagulant effects
pimozide, other drugs that prolong QT interval: Prolonged QT interval and risk of arrhythmias
thiazide diuretics: Increased risk of hyponatremia, hypotension, and water intoxication
tricyclic antidepressants: Possibly prolonged and intensified sedation
ACTIVITIES
alcohol use: Possibly increased CNS depression and increased risk of heatstroke

Adverse Reactions
CNS: Ataxia, cerebral edema, dizziness, drowsiness, headache, insomnia, light-headedness, nervousness, seizures, slurred speech, syncope, worsening psychotic symptoms
CV: AV conduction disorders, bradycardia, cardiac arrest, hypercholesterolemia, hypertension, orthostatic hypotension, QT-interval prolongation, shock, ST-segment depression, tachycardia
EENT: Blurred vision, dry mouth, glaucoma, increased salivation, laryngeal edema, laryngospasm, miosis, mydriasis,

E
F

nasal congestion, papillary hypertrophy of the tongue, parotid gland enlargement, photophobia, pigmentary retinopathy, ptosis **ENDO:** Breast engorgement (females), galactorrhea, hyperglycemia, hypoglycemia, mastalgia, syndrome of inappropriate ADH secretion
GI: Anorexia, constipation, diarrhea, fecal impaction, ileus, increased appetite, nausea, vomiting
GU: Amenorrhea, bladder paralysis, decreased libido, enuresis, menstrual irregularities, polyuria, urinary frequency, urinary incontinence, urine retention
HEME: Anemia, aplastic anemia, eosinophilia, leukopenia, thrombocytopenia, thrombocytopenic or nonthrombocytopenic purpura
RESP: Bronchospasm, dyspnea, increased respiratory depth
SKIN: Contact dermatitis, dry skin, eczema, erythema, jaundice, photosensitivity, pruritus, seborrhea
Other: Heatstroke, hyponatremia, lupus-like symptoms, weight gain

Nursing Considerations
• Fluphenazine shouldn't be used to treat dementia-related psychosis in elderly patients because of an increased mortality risk.
• Use fluphenazine cautiously in patients with a history of glaucoma or renal impairment.
• For I.M. and subcutaneous injection, use at least a 21G needle.
• Monitor temperature; a significant, unexplained rise can indicate intolerance and a need to discontinue drug. Notify prescriber immediately if this occurs.
• Watch for signs of hepatic failure, such as jaundice.
• Notify prescriber about worsening psychotic symptoms: agitation, catatonic state, confusion, depression, hallucinations, lethargy, paranoid reactions.
PATIENT TEACHING
• If patient takes elixir form of fluphenazine, instruct her to keep it in an amber or opaque bottle because drug is sensitive to light.
• Advise patient not to mix oral solution with beverages that contain caffeine (coffee, cola), tannins (tea), or pectins (apple juice).

• Caution patient about possible dizziness or light-headedness.
• Teach patient how to prevent heatstroke, orthostatic hypotension, and photosensitivity reactions.
• Warn against stopping drug abruptly.

flurazepam hydrochloride
Apo-Flurazepam (CAN), Dalmane, Novo-Flupam (CAN), Somnol (CAN)

Class, Category, and Schedule
Chemical class: Benzodiazepine
Therapeutic class: Sedative-hypnotic
Pregnancy category: Not rated
Controlled substance schedule: IV

Indications and Dosages
➤ *To treat insomnia characterized by difficulty falling asleep, frequent nocturnal awakenings, or early-morning awakening*
CAPSULES
Adults. 15 to 30 mg at bedtime.
DOSAGE ADJUSTMENT Initial dose reduced to 15 mg for elderly or debilitated patients until individual response is known.

Route	Onset	Peak	Duration
P.O.	15–45 min	Unknown	7–8 hr

Mechanism of Action
May potentiate the effects of gamma-aminobutyric acid (GABA) and other inhibitory neurotransmitters by binding to specific benzodiazepine receptor sites in the limbic and cortical areas of the CNS. As a result, flurazepam increases GABA's inhibitory effects and blocks cortical and limbic arousal.

Contraindications
Acute angle-closure glaucoma, breastfeeding, hypersensitivity to other benzodiazepines, itraconazole or ketoconazole therapy, psychosis

Interactions
DRUGS
cimetidine, diltiazem, disulfiram, erythromycin, fluoxetine, fluvoxamine, itraconazole, nefazodone, estrogen-

containing oral contraceptives, propoxyphene, ranitidine, verapamil: Possibly increased blood level and impaired hepatic metabolism of flurazepam
clozapine: Possibly cardiac arrest or respiratory depression
CNS depressants: Possibly potentiated CNS depression
levodopa: Possibly decreased therapeutic effects of levodopa
FOODS
grapefruit juice: Possibly increased blood level and impaired hepatic metabolism of flurazepam
ACTIVITIES
alcohol use: Possibly potentiated CNS and respiratory depression

Adverse Reactions

CNS: Amnesia, anxiety, ataxia, bizarre behavior (such as sleep driving), confusion, delusions, depression, dizziness, drowsiness, euphoria, headache, hypokinesia, irritability, malaise, nervousness, slurred speech, tremor
CV: Chest pain, palpitations, tachycardia
EENT: Blurred vision, dry mouth, increased salivation, photophobia
GI: Abdominal pain, constipation, diarrhea, nausea, thirst, vomiting
GU: Libido changes
SKIN: Diaphoresis
Other: Anaphylaxis, angioedema, physical or psychological dependence

Nursing Considerations

• Use flurazepam cautiously in patients with severe mental depression or reduced respiratory function; drug may intensify mental depression and lead to respiratory depression.
• Expect to use lowest effective dose in elderly or debilitated patients to minimize the risk of ataxia, confusion, dizziness, and oversedation.
• Monitor liver function test results, as appropriate.
PATIENT TEACHING
• Instruct patient not to exceed prescribed dosage and not to stop drug abruptly.
WARNING Warn patient that, although rare, drug may cause swelling of the oral cavity or throat, which could cause airway obstruction. If swelling occurs, patient should seek emergency care immediately and never take flurazepam again.

• Caution patient about possible morning dizziness or drowsiness.
• Because flurazepam can reduce alertness, advise patient to avoid hazardous activities until drug's CNS effects are known.
• Caution patient to avoid alcohol and CNS depressants during therapy.
• Advise patient to notify prescriber if she becomes or intends to become pregnant during therapy.
• Inform patient that sleep may be disturbed for the first few nights after stopping drug.
• Warn patient and caregiver that some patients have performed bizarre activities after taking drug, such as driving their car, preparing and eating food, making phone calls, or having sex while not fully awake and often with no memory of the event. These episodes usually occur in patients who have taken the drug with alcohol or other CNS depressant or who have exceeded the recommended dose. If such an episode occurs, the prescriber should be notified and flurazepam therapy discontinued immediately.

flurbiprofen

Ansaid, Froben (CAN), Froben SR (CAN), Novo-Flurprofen (CAN)

Class and Category

Chemical class: Propionic acid derivative
Therapeutic class: Antiarthritis, anti-inflammatory
Pregnancy category: B (first trimester), Not rated (later trimesters)

Indications and Dosages

➤ *To treat acute or chronic rheumatoid arthritis and osteoarthritis*
E.R. CAPSULES
Adults. 200 mg daily in the evening.
TABLETS
Adults. *Initial:* 200 to 300 mg daily in divided doses twice daily to four times daily. *Maximum:* 300 mg daily (100 mg/dose).

Mechanism of Action

Blocks the activity of cyclooxygenase, the enzyme necessary for prostaglandin synthesis. Prostaglandins, important mediators in the inflammatory response, cause local vasodilation with swelling and pain. They also play a role in pain transmission from the periphery to the spinal cord. By blocking cyclooxygenase and inhibiting prostaglandins, this NSAID causes inflammatory symptoms and pain to subside.

Contraindications
Angioedema, asthma, bronchospasm, nasal polyps, rhinitis, or urticaria induced by aspirin, iodides, or NSAIDs; hypersensitivity to NSAIDs

Interactions
DRUGS
acetaminophen: Increased risk of renal impairment with long-term use of both drugs
antacids: Decreased flurbiprofen effectiveness
anticoagulants, cefamandole, cefoperazone, cefotetan, heparin, plicamycin, thrombolytics, valproic acid: Increased risk of bleeding
antineoplastics: Increased adverse hematologic effects
cyclosporine: Increased risk of nephrotoxicity
diuretics, triamterene: Decreased effectiveness of these drugs
glucocorticoids, other NSAIDs, potassium supplements: Increased adverse GI effects
insulin, oral antidiabetic drugs: Increased risk of hypoglycemia
lithium: Increased risk of lithium toxicity
methotrexate: Increased risk of methotrexate toxicity
salicylates: Increased risk of GI bleeding
ACTIVITIES
alcohol use, smoking: Increased risk of GI bleeding

Adverse Reactions
CNS: Anxiety, cerebral hemorrhage, depression, dizziness, drowsiness, forgetfulness, headache, insomnia, malaise, nervousness, stroke, tremor, weakness
CV: Arrhythmias, heart failure, hypertension, hypotension, palpitations, peripheral edema, tachycardia
EENT: Amblyopia, blurred vision, rhinitis, stomatitis, tinnitus, vision changes
GI: Abdominal cramps or distress, anorexia, constipation, diarrhea, diver-

ticulitis, dysphagia, esophagitis, flatulence, gastritis, gastroenteritis, gastroesophageal reflux disease, GI bleeding or ulceration, hemorrhoids, hiatal hernia, hepatitis, increased appetite, indigestion, jaundice, liver failure, melena, nausea, perforation of stomach or intestines, stomatitis, vomiting
GU: Hematuria, interstitial nephritis, renal failure, UTI
HEME: Agranulocytosis, aplastic anemia, eosinophilia, leukopenia, neutropenia, pancytopenia, thrombocytopenia
SKIN: Erythema multiforme, exfoliative dermatitis, flushing, rash, Stevens-Johnson syndrome, toxic epidermal necrolysis
Other: Anaphylaxis, angioedema, hyponatremia

Nursing Considerations
• Use flurbiprofen with extreme caution in patients who have a history of ulcer disease or GI bleeding because NSAIDs such as flurbiprofen increase the risk of GI bleeding and ulceration. Expect to use flurbiprofen for the shortest time possible in these patients.
• Be aware that serious GI tract ulceration, bleeding, and perforation may occur without warning signs or symptoms. Elderly patients are at greater risk. To minimize the risk, give flurbiprofen with food. If GI distress occurs, withhold drug and notify prescriber immediately.
• Use flurbiprofen cautiously in patients with hypertension, and monitor blood pressure closely throughout therapy. Drug may cause hypertension or worsen it.
WARNING Monitor patient closely for thrombotic events, including MI and stroke, because NSAIDs increase the risk.
• Monitor patient—especially if she's elderly or receiving long-term flurbiprofen therapy—for less common but serious adverse GI reactions, including anorexia, constipation, diverticulitis, dysphagia, esophagitis, gastritis, gastroenteritis, gastroesophageal reflux disease, hemorrhoids, hiatal hernia, melena, stomatitis, and vomiting.
• Monitor liver function test results because, rarely, elevations may progress to severe hepatic reactions, including fatal hepatitis, liver necrosis, and hepatic failure.

• Monitor BUN and serum creatinine levels in elderly patients, patients taking diuretics or ACE inhibitors, and patients with heart failure, impaired renal function, or hepatic dysfunction; flurbiprofen may cause renal failure.

• Monitor CBC for decreased hemoglobin and hematocrit because drug may worsen anemia.

WARNING If patient has bone marrow suppression or is receiving an antineoplastic drug, monitor laboratory results (including WBC count), and watch for evidence of infection because anti-inflammatory and antipyretic actions of flurbiprofen may mask signs and symptoms, such as fever and pain.

• Assess patient's skin regularly for signs of rash or other hypersensitivity reaction because flurbiprofen is an NSAID and may cause serious skin reactions without warning, even in patients with no history of NSAID sensitivity. At first sign of reaction, stop drug and notify prescriber.

PATIENT TEACHING

• Encourage patient to take flurbiprofen with food or milk to avoid GI distress.

• Caution patient about possible blurred vision, dizziness, and drowsiness.

• Advise patient to avoid aspirin, alcohol, and smoking during flurbiprofen therapy.

• Urge patient to notify prescriber immediately if she has blood in urine, easy bruising, itching, rash, swelling, or yellow eyes or skin.

• Caution pregnant patient not to take NSAIDs such as flurbiprofen during the last trimester because they may cause premature closure of the ductus arteriosus.

• Explain that flurbiprofen may increase the risk of serious adverse cardiovascular reactions; urge patient to seek immediate medical attention if signs or symptoms arise, such as chest pain, shortness of breath, weakness, and slurring of speech.

• Explain that flurbiprofen may increase the risk of serious adverse GI reactions; stress the importance of seeking immediate medical attention for such signs and symptoms as epigastric or abdominal pain, indigestion, black or tarry stools, or

vomiting blood or material that looks like coffee grounds.

• Alert patient to rare but serious skin reactions. Urge her to seek immediate medical attention for rash, blisters, itching, fever, or other indications of hypersensitivity.

fluticasone propionate

Flonase, Flonase Allergy Relief, Flovent

fluticasone furoate

Arnuity Ellipta, Veramyst

E
F

Class and Category

Chemical class: Trifluorinated corticosteroid
Therapeutic class: Antiasthmatic, anti-inflammatory
Pregnancy category: C

Indications and Dosages

➤ *To prevent asthma attacks, alone or with oral corticosteroids*

INHALATION AEROSOL (FLOVENT)

Adults and children age 12 and over using bronchodilator therapy. *Initial:* 88 mcg inhaled twice daily. *Maximum:* 440 mcg inhaled twice daily.

Adults and children age 12 and over switching from another inhaled corticosteroid. *Initial:* 88 to 220 mcg inhaled twice daily. *Maximum:* 440 mcg inhaled twice daily.

Adults and children age 12 and over using oral corticosteroid therapy. *Initial and maximum:* 880 mcg inhaled twice daily.

Children ages 4 to 11 regardless of previous therapy. 88 mcg twice daily. *Maximum:* 88 mcg twice daily.

INHALATION AEROSOL (ARNUITY ELLIPTA)

Adults and children age 12 and older not on oral corticosteroid therapy. 100 mcg inhaled once daily, increased after 2 wk to 200 mcg once daily, as needed.

Adults and children age 12 and older receiving other drug treatments for asthma. Highly individualized based on patient's previous asthma drug therapy and disease severity.

➤ *To prevent seasonal or perennial allergic rhinitis*
NASAL SUSPENSION (FLONASE)
Adults and children age 12 and over.
Initial: 100 mcg (2 sprays) in each nostril daily or 50 mcg (1 spray) in each nostril twice daily, as needed. *Maintenance:* 50 mcg (1 spray) in each nostril daily, as tolerated and needed. *Maximum:* 200 mcg daily (4 sprays).
Children ages 4 to 11. 50 or 100 mcg (1 or 2 sprays) in each nostril daily in the morning, as needed. *Maximum:* 200 mcg daily (4 sprays).
➤ *To treat seasonal or perennial allergic rhinitis*
NASAL SUSPENSION (FLONASE, FLONASE ALLERGY RELIEF)
Adults and children age 12 and over.
Initial: 100 mcg (2 sprays) in each nostril daily or 50 mcg (1 spray) in each nostril twice daily, as needed. *Maintenance:* 50 mcg (1 spray) in each nostril daily, as tolerated and needed. *Maximum:* 200 mcg daily (4 sprays).
NASAL SUSPENSION (FLONASE)
Children ages 4 to 11. 50 or 100 mcg (1 or 2 sprays) in each nostril daily in the morning, as needed. *Maximum:* 200 mcg daily (4 sprays).
NASAL SUSPENSION (VERAMYST)
Adults and children age 12 and over.
Initial: 110 mcg (2 sprays) in each nostril once daily, decreased to 55 mcg (1 spray) in each nostril once daily when symptoms are controlled. *Maintenance:* 55 mcg (1 spray) in each nostril once daily.
Children ages 2 to 11. *Initial:* 55 mcg (1 spray) in each nostril once daily, increased to 110 mcg (2 sprays) in each nostril once daily, as needed. *Maintenance:* 55 mcg (1 spray) in each nostril once daily.

Route	Onset	Peak	Duration
Inhalation	In 24 hr	1–2 wk	Several days
Nasal	12 hr–3 days	4–7 days	1–2 wk

Mechanism of Action

Inhibits cells involved in the inflammatory response of asthma, such as mast cells, eosinophils, basophils, lymphocytes, macrophages, and neutrophils. Fluticasone also inhibits production or secretion of chemical mediators, such as histamine, eicosanoids, leukotrienes, and cytokines.

Contraindications

Hypersensitivity to fluticasone or its components, primary treatment of status asthmaticus or other acute asthma episodes that require intensive measures, untreated nasal mucosal infection (nasal suspension)

Interactions

DRUGS
ketoconazole, ritonavir and other strong cytochrome P-450 3A4 inhibitors (long-term use): Possibly increased fluticasone level and decreased serum cortisol level

Adverse Reactions

CNS: Aggressiveness, agitation, anxiety, depression, difficulty speaking, dizziness, fatigue, fever, headache, insomnia, irritability, malaise, restlessness
EENT: Allergic rhinitis, cataracts, conjunctivitis, dental caries, dry mouth and throat, epistaxis, esophageal candidiasis, eye irritation, facial and oropharyngeal edema, glaucoma, hoarseness, impaired nasal wound healing, laryngitis, loss of voice, nasal *candida* infection, nasal congestion or discharge, nasal discomfort (burning, dryness, irritation, soreness), nasal sinus pain, nasal septal perforation or ulceration, oropharyngeal candidiasis, otitis media, pharyngitis, sinusitis, throat irritation, tonsillitis, tooth discoloration
ENDO: Adrenal insufficiency, cushingoid symptoms, hyperglycemia, slower growth in children
GI: Abdominal pain, diarrhea, indigestion, nausea, vomiting
GU: Dysmenorrhea
HEME: Churg-Strauss syndrome, easy bruising, eosinophilia
MS: Arthralgia, bone mineral density reduction (long-term use), myalgia, osteoporosis
RESP: Asthma exacerbation, bronchitis, bronchospasm, chest congestion and tightness, cough, dyspnea, pneumonia, upper respiratory tract infection, wheezing
SKIN: Dermatitis, ecchymosis, pruritus, rash, urticaria

Other: Anaphylaxis, angioedema, flulike symptoms, weight gain

Nursing Considerations

- Use fluticasone cautiously in patients with ocular herpes simplex, pulmonary tuberculosis, or untreated systemic bacterial, fungal, parasitic, or viral infection.
- Although anaphylaxis is rare, monitor patient closely at start of therapy, especially if patient has severe allergy to milk. If hypersensitivity reaction occurs, notify prescriber, expect drug to be discontinued, and provide supportive care, as prescribed.
- If patient takes a systemic corticosteroid, expect to taper dosage by no more than 2.5 mg daily at weekly intervals, starting 1 week after fluticasone therapy begins.

WARNING If patient is switched from systemic corticosteroid to fluticasone, assess for adrenal insufficiency (fatigue, hypotension, lassitude, nausea, vomiting, weakness) early in therapy and when patient has infection, stress, trauma, surgery, or other electrolyte-depleting conditions or procedures. Notify prescriber immediately if signs or symptoms develop.

- As prescribed, administer a fast-acting inhaled bronchodilator if bronchospasm occurs immediately after fluticasone use. Expect to stop fluticasone and start another drug therapy.
- Expect to titrate fluticasone to lowest effective dosage after asthma has stabilized.

PATIENT TEACHING

- Urge patient to use fluticasone regularly, as prescribed, and stress that drug is not for acute bronchospasm.
- Teach patient how to administer drug according to the form prescribed (nasal spray or oral inhaler).
- Instruct patient to shake canister and use inhaler according to package instructions. On first use, advise her to spray 4 times into the air (away from her eyes and shaking inhaler between each test spray) and look for a fine mist. If inhaler hasn't been used for more than 7 days or it's

dropped, it will need to be primed again by shaking well and then releasing 1 test spray into the air (away from her face).

- If 2 inhalations are prescribed, tell patient to wait at least 1 minute between them.
- Instruct patient to gargle and rinse her mouth after each dose to help prevent dry mouth and throat, relieve throat irritation, and prevent oropharyngeal yeast infection.
- If patient uses more than 1 inhaler, instruct her to use fluticasone last, at least 5 minutes after previous inhaler.
- Instruct patient to clean inhaler according to manufacturer guidelines at least once a week after her evening dose.
- Inform patient that, when counter reads 020, she should obtain a refill, if needed. When counter reaches 000, she should discard the inhaler.
- Instruct patient using nasal spray to shake container well before each use.
- Explain that symptoms may improve within 2 days but that full improvement may not occur for 1 to 2 weeks or longer.
- Caution patient not to increase dosage but to contact prescriber after 1 week if symptoms continue or worsen.
- Urge patient to tell prescriber immediately if asthma attacks don't respond to bronchodilators during fluticasone therapy.
- If patient is switching from an oral corticosteroid to fluticasone, urge her to carry medical identification indicating the need for supplemental systemic corticosteroids during stress or severe asthma attack.
- Caution patient to avoid people who have infections because fluticasone suppresses the immune system, increasing the risk of infection. Instruct patient to notify prescriber about exposure to chickenpox, measles, or other infections because additional treatment may be needed.

fluvastatin sodium
Lescol, Lescol XL

Class and Category
Chemical class: Heptenoic acid derivative
Therapeutic class: Antihyperlipidemic
Pregnancy category: X

Indications and Dosages

➤ *As adjunct to lower cholesterol level in primary hypercholesterolemia, to decrease progression of coronary atherosclerosis, to reduce risk in patients with coronary artery disease undergoing coronary revascularization*

CAPSULES

Adults. 20 to 40 mg daily in the evening or 40 mg twice daily. *Maximum:* 40 mg twice daily.

E.R. TABLETS

Adults. 80 mg in the evening. *Maximum:* 80 mg daily.

➤ *As adjunct to lower cholesterol level in children with heterozygous familial hypercholesterolemia*

CAPSULES

Girls ages 10 to 16 who are at least 1 year past menarche. *Initial:* 20 mg once daily, increased every 6 wk, as needed. *Maximum:* 40 mg twice daily.

DOSAGE ADJUSTMENT For pediatric patients, if maximum dose of 40 mg twice daily. is reached with immediate-release capsules, child may be switched to extended-release tablets, 80 mg once daily.

Route	Onset	Peak	Duration
P.O.	In 1–2 wk	In 4–6 wk	Unknown
P.O. (E.R.)	In 2 wk	In 4 wk	Unknown

Mechanism of Action

Interferes with the hepatic enzyme hydroxymethylglutaryl-coenzyme A reductase, reducing formation of mevalonic acid (a cholesterol precursor) and interrupting the pathway by which cholesterol is synthesized. When cholesterol level declines in hepatic cells, LDLs are consumed, which reduces circulating total cholesterol and serum triglycerides.

Contraindications

Acute hepatic disease, breastfeeding, hypersensitivity to fluvastatin or its components, pregnancy, unexplained persistently elevated liver enzyme levels

Interactions

DRUGS

bile acid sequestrants: Possibly decreased fluvastatin bioavailability

cimetidine, ketoconazole, spironolactone: Possibly decreased endogenous steroid hormonal production

cimetidine, omeprazole, ranitidine: Significantly increased blood fluvastatin level

colchicine, cyclosporine, erythromycin, gemfibrozil, niacin: Increased risk of severe myopathy and rhabdomyolysis

cyclosporine, erythromycin, gemfibrozil and other fibrates, niacin: Increased risk of acute renal failure

fluconazole: Increased fluconazole level

glyburide: Increased glyburide level

itraconazole, ketoconazole: Increased risk of myopathy

oral contraceptives: Risk of bleeding

phenytoin: Increased phenytoin levels

protease inhibitors: Possible increased blood fluvastatin level; possible increased risk of myopathy and rhabdomyolysis

rifampin: Significantly decreased blood fluvastatin level, increased plasma clearance

warfarin: Possibly increased bleeding and/or increased prothrombin times

ACTIVITIES

alcohol use: Increased bioavailability and blood level of fluvastatin

Adverse Reactions

CNS: Dizziness, fatigue, headache, hypoesthesia, insomnia, memory loss, weakness

EENT: Pharyngitis, rhinitis, sinusitis

ENDO: Decreased adrenal or gonadal steroid hormone production, elevated hemoglobin A1c levels, hyperglycemia

GI: Abdominal cramps and pain, anorexia, cirrhosis, constipation, diarrhea, elevated liver enzymes, flatuence, fulminant hepatic necrosis, hepatic failure, hepatitis, hepatoma, hyperbilirubinemia, indigestion, jaundice, nausea, pancreatitis, vomiting

GU: UTI

MS: Arthritis, back pain, immune-mediated necrotizing myopathy, muscle pain, myalgia, myopathy, myositis, rhabdomyolysis

RESP: Bronchitis, cough, upper respiratory tract infection

SKIN: Pruritus, rash

Nursing Considerations

WARNING Expect to stop drug if CK level rises sharply or myopathy is suspected.

• Expect liver function tests to be performed before fluvastatin therapy starts and then thereafter as clinically necessary.

- Assess patient for signs and symptoms of hepatic dysfunction such as fatigue, dark urine or jaundice and/or elevation in liver enzymes to more than 3 times the upper limit of normal. Also look for hyperbilirubinemia. If present, notify prescriber and expect fluvastatin to be discontinued until cause of liver dysfunction has been identified. If no cause can be found, expect the drug to be discontinued permanently.
- Monitor patient for hyperglycemia, especially diabetic patients, and for other endocrine signs and symptoms. Notify prescriber, if present.

PATIENT TEACHING

- Urge patient to comply with monthly laboratory tests early in treatment.
- Tell patient to follow prescribed low-fat diet.
- Encourage patient to notify prescriber promptly about muscle pain or unexplained weakness.
- Instruct patient with diabetes to monitor his blood glucose level more closely.

---

fluvoxamine maleate

Luvox, Luvox CR

Class and Category

Chemical class: Aralkylketone derivative
Therapeutic class: Antiobsessional
Pregnancy category: C

Indications and Dosages

➤ *To treat obsessive-compulsive disorder*

TABLETS

Adults. *Initial:* 50 mg at bedtime, increased by 50 mg every 4 to 7 days, as needed. *Maximum:* 300 mg daily.

Children ages 8 to 17. *Initial:* 25 mg at bedtime, increased by 25 mg every 4 to 7 days, as needed. *Maximum:* 200 mg daily.

DOSAGE ADJUSTMENT Doses divided for adults taking more than 100 mg daily and for children taking more than 50 mg daily; given in 2 equal doses twice daily or in 2 unequal doses with the larger dose at bedtime.

CAPSULES

Adults. *Initial:* 100 mg at bedtime, increased by 50 mg weekly, if needed. *Maximum:* 300 mg daily.

DOSAGE ADJUSTMENT For elderly patients or those with hepatic impairment, dosage increases with extended-release form are made more slowly.

➤ *To treat social anxiety disorder*

CAPSULES

Adults. *Initial:* 100 mg at bedtime, increased by 50 mg weekly, if needed. *Maximum:* 300 mg daily.

DOSAGE ADJUSTMENT For elderly patients or those with hepatic impairment, dosage increases with extended-release form are made more slowly.

Route	Onset	Peak	Duration
P.O.	3–10 wk	Unknown	Unknown

Mechanism of Action

May potentiate serotonin's action by blocking its reuptake at neuronal membranes. An elevated serotonin level may elevate mood and decrease depression and anxiety, which often accompany obsessive-compulsive disorder.

Contraindications

Alosetron, astemizole, cisapride, pimozide, terfenadine, thioridazine, or tizanidine therapy; hypersensitivity to fluvoxamine maleate or its components; use within 14 days of MAO inhibitor, including intravenous methylene blue and linezolid

Interactions

DRUGS

alosetron: Increased plasma alosetron level
alprazolam: Increased plasma alprazolam level
antihistamines: Increased risk of impaired mental and motor skills
aspirin, NSAIDs, warfarin: Risk of bleeding
astemizole, cisapride, pimozide, terfenadine: Possibly fatal QT prolongation
benzodiazepines: Decreased benzodiazepine clearance, possibly impaired memory and motor skills
buspirone: Decreased buspirone effects, increased blood fluvoxamine level, and paradoxical worsening of obsessive-compulsive disorder
carbamazepine: Increased risk of carbamazepine toxicity

clozapine: Increased blood clozapine level
diltiazem: Increased risk of bradycardia
haloperidol: Increased blood haloperidol
level, possibly delayed recall and reduced
memory and attention span
lithium: Possibly increased serotonin
reuptake action of fluvoxamine
MAO inhibitors: Possibly serious or fatal
reactions (such as agitation, autonomic
instability, coma, delirium, fluctuating vital
signs, hyperthermia, myoclonus, and rigidity)
methadone: Possibly significantly increased
blood methadone level, increased risk of
methadone toxicity
metoprolol, propranolol: Increased blood
levels of these drugs, possibly reduced
diastolic blood pressure and heart rate
induced by these drugs
*serotonergics (such as amphetamines and
other psychostimulants, antidepressants, and
dopamine agonists):* Increased risk of
serotonin syndrome
sympathomimetics: Possibly increased
effects of sympathomimetics and increased
risk of serotonin syndrome
tacrine: Increased blood level and
therapeutic and adverse effects of tacrine
theophylline: Decreased theophylline
clearance, increased risk of theophylline
toxicity
tizanidine: Increased risk of serious adverse
effects, such as hypotension and profound
sedation
tricyclic antidepressants: Increased blood
levels of antidepressants
warfarin: Increased blood warfarin level,
prolonged PT
FOODS
caffeine: Possibly decreased hepatic
clearance of caffeine
ACTIVITIES
smoking: Increased fluvoxamine metabolism

Adverse Reactions

CNS: Agitation, anxiety, apathy, chills,
confusion, depression, dizziness,
drowsiness, fatigue, headache, hypomania,
insomnia, malaise, mania, nervousness,
neuroleptic malignant syndrome, sedation,
serotonin syndrome, suicidal ideation,
tremor, vertigo, yawning
CV: Palpitations, tachycardia
EENT: Acute-angle glaucoma, altered taste,
blurred vision, dry mouth

GI: Anorexia, constipation, diarrhea,
flatulence, indigestion, nausea, upper GI
bleeding, vomiting
GU: Decreased libido, ejaculation disorders,
impotence, urinary frequency, urine
retention
HEME: Bleeding events
MS: Muscle twitching
RESP: Dyspnea, upper respiratory tract
infection
SKIN: Diaphoresis, rash
Other: Flulike symptoms, weight gain

Nursing Considerations

• Use fluvoxamine cautiously in patients
  with cardiovascular disease, impaired
  hepatic or renal function, mania, seizures,
  or suicidal tendencies.
WARNING Fluvoxamine shouldn't be given
within 14 days of an MAO inhibitor.
WARNING Monitor patient for possible
serotonin syndrome, characterized by
agitation, chills, confusion, diaphoresis,
diarrhea, fever, hyperactive reflexes, poor
coordination, restlessness, shaking, talking
or acting with uncontrolled excitement,
tremor, and twitching, especially if patient
is receiving another drug that raises
serotonin level (such as dopamine agonist,
MAO inhibitor, tryptophan, amphetamine,
or other antidepressant or psycho-
stimulant). In its most severe form,
serotonin syndrome can resemble
neuroleptic malignant syndrome, which
includes a high fever, muscle rigidity,
autonomic instability, and possible
fluctuations in vital signs and mental
status.
• Watch patient closely (especially children,
  adolescents, and young adults), for
  suicidal tendencies, particularly when
  therapy starts and dosage changes, because
  depression may worsen temporarily
  during these times and lead to suicidal
  ideation.
• Monitor patient for bleeding, especially if
  patient also takes aspirin, an NSAID, or
  an anticoagulant. Bleeding can range
  from ecchymoses, hematomas, epistaxis,
  and petechiae to life-threatening
  hemorrhage.
• Discontinue fluvoxamine therapy
  gradually, as ordered, to prevent
  unpleasant adverse reactions.

PATIENT TEACHING
• Caution patient not to drink alcohol during fluvoxamine therapy.
• Urge patient to avoid potentially hazardous activities until drug's CNS effects are known.
WARNING Inform patient that fluvoxamine increases the risk of a rare but serious problem: serotonin syndrome. Encourage her to notify prescriber immediately if symptoms develop.
• Caution patient not to stop taking drug abruptly. Explain that gradual tapering helps avoid withdrawal symptoms.
• Urge family or caregiver to watch patient closely for suicidal tendencies, especially when therapy starts or dosage changes and particularly if patient is a child, teenager, or young adult.
• Warn patient that fluvoxamine increases bleeding risk if taken with aspirin, an NSAID, or an anticoagulant and that bleeding events could range from mild to severe. Tell patient to seek emergency care for serious or prolonged bleeding.
• Advise patient that drug may cause mild pupillary dilation, which may lead to an episode of acute-angle glaucoma. Encourage patient to have an eye exam before starting therapy to see if she is at risk.
• Advise pregnant patient to consult with prescriber before her third trimester about ongoing fluvoxamine therapy because of an increased risk to her unborn child during the third trimester.

fondaparinux sodium
Arixtra

Class and Category
Chemical class: Synthetic pentasaccharide factor Xa inhibitor
Therapeutic class: Antithrombolytic
Pregnancy category: B

Indications and Dosages
➤ *To provide prophylaxis against deep vein thrombosis, which may lead to pulmonary embolism in patients undergoing hip fracture surgery, hip replacement surgery, knee replacement surgery, or abdominal surgery in patients at risk for thromboembolic complications*
SUBCUTANEOUS INJECTION
Adults. *Initial:* After hemostasis has been established, 2.5 mg subcutaneously 6 to 8 hr after surgery, followed by 2.5 mg subcutaneously daily for 5 to 9 days. *Maximum:* 2.5 mg subcutaneously daily for 11 days for hip or knee replacement and abdominal surgery and 24 days for hip fracture surgery.
➤ *To treat acute deep vein thrombosis (with warfarin); to treat acute pulmonary embolism (with warfarin) in a hospital setting*
SUBCUTANEOUS INJECTION
Adults. *Initial:* 5 mg if body weight is less than 50 kg (110 lb), 7.5 mg if body weight is 50 to 100 kg (110 to 220 lb), and 10 mg if body weight exceeds 100 kg daily for at least 5 days and until INR is between 2.0 and 3.0 (usually in 5 to 9 days)

Mechanism of Action
Selectively binds to antithrombin III, which enhances the inactivation of clotting factor Xa by antithrombin III. Inactivation of factor Xa interrupts the blood coagulation pathway, which then inhibits thrombin formation. Without thrombin, fibrinogen can't convert to fibrin and clots can't form.

Incompatibilities
Don't mix fondaparinux sodium with other injections or infusions.

Contraindications
Active major bleeding; bacterial endocarditis; body weight less than 50 kg (110 lb) if patient is having hip repair or replacement or knee replacement surgery; fondaparinux-induced thrombocytopenia associated with a positive in vitro test for antiplatelet antibodies; hypersensitivity to fondaparinux or its components; prophylactic fondaparinux therapy in patients weighing less than 50 kg (110 lb) undergoing hip repair or replacement, knee replacement, or abdominal surgery; severe renal impairment (creatinine clearance less than 30 ml/min/1.73 m²)

E
F

Interactions

DRUGS

abciximab, thrombolytics, other drugs that enhance risk of bleeding: Increased risk of hemorrhage and spinal or epidural hematoma

Adverse Reactions

CNS: Confusion, dizziness, fever, headache, insomnia
CV: Edema, elevated serum aminotransferase level, hypotension
GI: Constipation, diarrhea, elevated liver function test results, indigestion, nausea, vomiting
GU: Urine retention, UTI
HEME: Anemia, bleeding, elevated APTT, hematoma, postoperative hemorrhage, thrombocytopenia, thrombocytopenia with thrombosis
SKIN: Bullous eruption, increased wound drainage, rash, purpura
Other: Anaphylaxis, angioedema, generalized pain; hypokalemia; injection-site bleeding, pruritus, and rash

Nursing Considerations

• Fondaparinux shouldn't be given as prophylaxis for patients who have had a hip fracture, who are having hip or knee replacement or abdominal surgery, or who weigh less than 50 kg (110 lb) because of increased risk of bleeding.
• Use fondaparinux cautiously in elderly patients, especially those weighing less than 50 kg (110 lb) and are receiving the drug for pulmonary embolism or deep vein thrombosis, because the risk of drug-induced bleeding increases with age.
• Don't give initial dose of fondaparinux less than 6 hours after surgery.
• Inspect fondaparinux for particles or discoloration before administration. Be aware that needle guard on prefilled syringe contains dry natural latex rubber and shouldn't be handled by those sensitive to latex.
• Alternate injection sites using left and right anterolateral or left and right posterolateral abdominal wall. Don't expel air bubble from prefilled syringe before injection to prevent expelling drug from syringe. Don't give drug by I.M. injection.
WARNING If patient is receiving fondaparinux with epidural or spinal

anesthesia or spinal puncture, watch closely for development of spinal hematoma, which may cause long-term or permanent paralysis. If you see evidence of neurologic impairment, such as changes in sensory or motor function, notify prescriber immediately because urgent care is needed to minimize hematoma's effect. Risk of spinal or epidural hematoma during fondaparinux therapy is increased by indwelling epidural catheters, concurrent use of other drugs that affect hemostasis, a history of traumatic or repeated epidural or spinal punctures, or a history of spinal deformity or spinal surgery. **Be aware that optimal timing between the administration of fondaparinux and neuraxial procedures is unknown.**
• Closely monitor patient for bleeding (such as ecchymosis, epistaxis, hematemesis, hematuria, and melena), especially those at risk for decreased drug elimination (such as elderly patients and patients with mild to moderate renal impairment) and those at increased risk for bleeding (such as patients with congenital or acquired bleeding disorders; active ulcerative and angiodysplastic GI disease; hemorrhagic stroke; uncontrolled arterial hypertension; recent brain, spinal, or ophthalmologic surgery; diabetic retinopathy; or a history of heparin-induced thrombocytopenia; and those being treated concomitantly with platelet inhibitors).
• Perform periodic CBC, including platelet count, as ordered. Expect prescriber to discontinue drug if platelet count falls below 100,000/mm^3. Be aware that routine coagulation tests, such as PT and INR, are not used to monitor fondaparinux therapy; an anti-Xa assay may be used instead. Also, test stools for occult blood, as ordered.
• Monitor patient with thrombocytopenia for evidence of thrombosis that may appear similar to heparin-induced thrombocytopenia even when no exposure to heparin has taken place. If patient's platelet count falls below 100,000/mm^3, fondaparinux should be discontinued.
• Monitor renal function test results, as ordered. Expect to discontinue drug if severe renal impairment or labile renal function occurs during fondaparinux

therapy because the risk of hemorrhage increases as renal function decreases.
• Store drug at a controlled room temperature.
PATIENT TEACHING
• Inform patient that fondaparinux can't be taken orally.
• Instruct patient to seek immediate help if she experiences signs of thromboembolism, such as neurologic changes and severe shortness of breath.
• Inform patient about the increased risk of bleeding. Instruct her or family member to watch for and report abdominal or lower back pain, black stools, bleeding gums, bloody urine, or severe headaches.
• Teach patient or family member how to administer fondaparinux by subcutaneous injection at home, if needed. Instruct her not to expel air bubble from a prefilled syringe to avoid expelling some of the drug. Tell her to insert the entire needle into a skinfold held between thumb and forefinger, and remind her to alternate administration sites.
• To minimize bruising, caution the patient not to rub the injection site after giving the drug.
• Review safe handling and disposal of syringes and needles.
• Advise patient to have follow-up appointments and prescribed laboratory tests.

formoterol fumarate dihydrate

Foradil Aerolizer, Oxeze Turbuhaler (CAN), Perforomist

Class and Category
Chemical class: Racemic acid salt
Therapeutic class: Bronchodilator
Pregnancy category: C

Indications and Dosages
➤ *To prevent asthma-induced bronchospasm*
POWDER FOR ORAL INHALATION
Adults and children age 5 and over.
12 mcg every 12 hr through inhaler device. *Maximum:* 24 mcg daily.

➤ *To prevent exercise-induced bronchospasm*
POWDER FOR ORAL INHALATION
Adults and adolescents age 12 and over.
12 mcg at least 15 min before exercise every 12 hr as needed. *Maximum:* 24 mcg daily.
➤ *To provide long-term treatment of bronchospasm in patients with chronic bronchitis and emphysema*
POWDER FOR ORAL INHALATION
Adults. 12 mcg every 12 hr through inhaler device. *Maximum:* 24 mcg daily.
SOLUTION FOR ORAL INHALATION
Adults. 20 mcg twice daily by nebulization. *Maximum:* 40 mcg daily.

Route	Onset	Peak	Duration
Oral inhalation	1–3 min	Unknown	12 hr

Mechanism of Action
Selectively attaches to beta$_2$ receptors on bronchial membranes, stimulating the intracellular enzyme adenyl cyclase to convert adenosine triphosphate to cAMP. The resulting increase in the intracellular cAMP level relaxes bronchial smooth-muscle cells, stabilizes mast cells, and inhibits histamine release.

Contraindications
Acute asthma, hypersensitivity to formoterol fumarate or its components, treatment of asthma without use of a long-term asthma control medication

Interactions
DRUGS
adrenergics: Possibly increased sympathetic effects of formoterol
beta blockers: Decreased effects of formoterol, possibly severe bronchospasm
corticosteroids, non–potassium-sparing diuretics, xanthine derivatives: Possibly increased hypokalemic effect of formoterol
disopyramide, macrolides, MAO inhibitors, phenothiazines, procainamide, quinidine, tricyclic antidepressants: Possibly prolonged QTc interval, increasing risk of ventricular arrhythmias
halogenated hydrocarbons: Increased risk of arrhythmias

Adverse Reactions
CNS: Anxiety, dizziness, fatigue, fever, headache, insomnia, malaise, tremor

CV: Angina, arrhythmias, chest pain, hypertension, hypotension, palpitations, prolonged QT interval, tachycardia
EENT: Dry mouth; laryngeal spasm, irritation, or swelling; hoarseness; pharyngitis; rhinitis and tonsillitis (in children); sinusitis
ENDO: Hyperglycemia
GI: Abdominal pain, gastroenteritis, indigestion (in children); nausea
MS: Back pain, leg cramps, muscle spasms
RESP: Asthma exacerbation, bronchitis, bronchospasm (paradoxical or hypersensitivity-induced), cough, dyspnea, increased sputum production, upper respiratory tract infection
SKIN: Dermatitis, pruritus, rash, urticaria
Other: Anaphylaxis, angioedema, hypokalemia, metabolic acidosis, viral infection (in children)

Nursing Considerations

• Know that formoterol therapy should not be used in patients whose asthma is adequately controlled with low- or medium-dose inhaled corticosteroids. Formoterol should only be used as additional therapy for patients with asthma who are currently taking but are not adequately controlled on long-term asthma control medication, such as an inhaled corticosteroids. Once asthma is controlled and maintained, expect formoterol to be discontinued as soon as possible without loss of asthma control.
• Use caution when administering formoterol to patients with cardiovascular disorders such as coronary insufficiency, arrhythmias, hypertension, aneurysm, or pheochromocytoma; in patients with seizure disorders or thyrotoxicosis; and in patients who are unusually responsive to sympathomimetic amines.
• Be aware that children and adolescents who require the use of a long-acting beta agonist in addition to an inhaled corticosteroid should use a combination product containing both an inhaled corticosteroid and a long-acting beta agonist, to ensure compliance with both medication regimens.
• Administer formoterol capsules or solution only by oral inhalation.

• Store capsules and solution in their original packaging, and open immediately before use.
• To use delivery system for powder form, place capsule in well of inhaler device. Press and release buttons on side of device to pierce capsule. Have patient inhale rapidly and deeply through mouthpiece; drug is dispersed into airways as patient inhales.
• Give inhalation solution only by standard jet nebulizer and air compressor.
WARNING Monitor patient for worsening or deteriorating asthma because asthma-related deaths have increased in patients receiving salmeterol, a drug in the same class as formoterol. Be aware that use of long-acting beta$_2$-adrenergic agonists such as formoterol is contraindicated in patients with asthma without the use of a long-term asthma control medication, such as an inhaled corticosteroid. Monitor patient closely, and notify prescriber immediately of any changes in patient's respiratory status.
• Watch closely for paradoxical bronchospasm; if this occurs, discontinue formoterol immediately and notify prescriber.
• Monitor patients with a history of cardiovascular disorders, especially coronary insufficiency, arrhythmias, or hypertension. Notify prescriber of any significant increases in pulse rate or blood pressure or worsening of chronic conditions because formoterol may produce cardiovascular reactions, including angina, arrhythmias, hypertension or hypotension, palpitations, and tachycardia. Drug may need to be discontinued if such reactions occur.
PATIENT TEACHING
• Advise patient, especially if she has significant cardiac history, to inform prescriber of any other drugs she takes before beginning formoterol therapy to prevent harmful drug interactions.
• Instruct patient to use manufacturer's plastic device for inhaling powder form of formoterol, to always use new inhaler that comes with each refill, and not to use a spacer. Tell her never to swallow capsules.
• Teach patient how to store powdered drug and inhaler properly. Instruct her to avoid exposing capsules to moisture and to always handle them with dry hands

because powder inside capsules must be dry to be inhaled. Also advise her to keep inhaler in a dry place and not to wash it.
• Teach patient proper use of powdered formoterol delivery system. Instruct her to remove capsule from blister pack just before use, to place capsule in well of inhaler device, to press and release buttons on side of device to pierce capsule, and then to inhale rapidly and deeply through mouthpiece. Emphasize that she should only inhale, not exhale, into device.
• For solution form, teach patient how to use, clean, and store nebulizer equipment. Tell her to leave the vial in its original foil pack until just before use.
• Instruct patient who currently uses oral or inhaled corticosteroids to continue using them, as prescribed, even if she feels better after starting formoterol.
• Caution patient not to increase formoterol dosage or frequency without consulting prescriber because she may need a rapid-acting bronchodilator.
• Urge patient to notify prescriber if her symptoms worsen, if formoterol becomes less effective, or if she needs more inhalations of short-acting beta$_2$-agonist than usual. This may indicate that her asthma is worsening.
• Instruct patient to notify prescriber immediately if she experiences palpitations, chest pain, rapid heart rate, tremor, or nervousness while taking formoterol because dosage may need to be adjusted.
• Ensure that patient has been informed that long acting beta agonists, such as formoterol, increase the risk of asthma-related death and should not be used without a long-term asthma control drug prior to starting formoterol therapy.

fosfomycin tromethamine

Monurol

Class and Category
Chemical class: Phosphonic acid derivative
Therapeutic class: Antibiotic
Pregnancy category: B

Indications and Dosages
➤ *To treat uncomplicated UTI (acute cystitis) caused by* Enterococcus faecalis *or* Escherichia coli

GRANULES FOR ORAL SOLUTION
Women age 18 and over. 3 g as a single dose mixed with water.

Route	Onset	Peak	Duration
P.O.	2–3 days	48 hr	Unknown

Mechanism of Action
Disrupts the formation of bacterial cell walls by blocking cell wall precursors. Specifically, fosfomycin inactivates enolpyruvyl transferase, which irreversibly blocks the condensation of uridine diphosphate-*N*-acetylglucosamine with phosphoenolpyruvate, a preliminary step in bacterial cell wall synthesis. Fosfomycin also decreases adherence of bacteria to epithelial cells of the urinary tract.

Contraindications
Hypersensitivity to fosfomycin or its components

Interactions
DRUGS
metoclopramide: Decreased blood level and urinary excretion of fosfomycin

Adverse Reactions
CNS: Asthenia, dizziness, fever, headache, insomnia, nervousness, paresthesia, somnolence
EENT: Dry mouth, pharyngitis, rhinitis
GI: Abdominal pain, anorexia, constipation, diarrhea, flatulence, indigestion, nausea, pseudomembranous colitis, vomiting
GU: Dysmenorrhea, dysuria, hematuria, menstrual irregularities, vaginitis
MS: Back pain
SKIN: Pruritus, rash
Other: Flulike symptoms, lymph-adenopathy

Nursing Considerations
• Use fosfomycin cautiously in patients with impaired renal function because drug clearance may be decreased.
• Expect to obtain urine specimens for culture and sensitivity tests before and after fosfomycin therapy.
• To reconstitute granules, pour contents of single-dose packet into 90 to 120 ml

E
F

(3 to 4 oz) of water (not hot water) and stir. Administer immediately after dissolving.

WARNING Expect adverse reactions to increase if more than one dose is used to treat a single episode of acute cystitis.

• Monitor patient for diarrhea during and for at least 2 months after drug therapy; diarrhea may signal pseudomembranous colitis caused by *Clostridium difficile*. If diarrhea occurs, notify prescriber and expect to withhold fosfomycin and treat with fluids, electrolytes, protein, and an antibiotic effective against *C. difficile*.

PATIENT TEACHING
• Explain how to reconstitute fosfomycin, and instruct patient to take drug immediately after it dissolves. Tell her not to take dry granules or mix them with hot water.
• To treat each episode of acute cystitis, advise patient to use only a single dose, as prescribed, to avoid increasing the risk of adverse reactions.
• Urge patient to notify prescriber if symptoms don't improve in 2 to 3 days.
• Instruct patient to return to prescriber for further urine testing after taking fosfomycin.
• Urge patient to tell prescriber about diarrhea that's severe or lasts longer than 3 days. Explain that watery or bloody stools can occur 2 or more months after therapy and can be serious, requiring prompt treatment.

fosinopril sodium
Monopril

Class and Category
Chemical class: Phosphinic acid derivative
Therapeutic class: Antihypertensive, vasodilator
Pregnancy category: C (first trimester), D (later trimesters)

Indications and Dosages
➤ *To manage blood pressure, alone or with other antihypertensives*
TABLETS
Adults. *Initial:* 10 mg daily. *Maintenance:* 20 to 40 mg daily. *Maximum:* 80 mg daily.
➤ *To treat heart failure*

TABLETS
Adults. 10 mg daily.
DOSAGE ADJUSTMENT Initial dosage reduced to 5 mg daily, if needed, for patients with acute heart failure, moderate to severe renal failure, or recent aggressive diuresis. Dosage may be increased over several weeks to maximum of 40 mg daily.

Route	Onset	Peak	Duration
P.O.	1 hr	2–6 hr	24 hr

Mechanism of Action
May reduce blood pressure by affecting renin-angiotensin-aldosterone system. By inhibiting angiotensin-converting enzyme, fosinopril:
• prevents conversion of angiotensin I to angiotensin II, a potent vasoconstrictor that also stimulates the adrenal cortex to secrete aldosterone
• may inhibit renal and vascular production of angiotensin II
• decreases serum angiotensin II level and increases serum renin activity, which decreases aldosterone secretion, slightly increasing the serum potassium level and fluid loss
• decreases vascular tone and blood pressure
• inhibits aldosterone release, which reduces sodium and water reabsorption and increases their excretion, further reducing blood pressure.

Contraindications
Hypersensitivity to fosinopril, other ACE inhibitors, or their components

Interactions
DRUGS
allopurinol, bone marrow depressants, procainamide, systemic corticosteroids: Increased risk of potentially fatal neutropenia or agranulocytosis
antacids: Impaired fosinopril absorption
cyclosporine, potassium-sparing diuretics, potassium supplements: Increased risk of hyperkalemia
diuretics, other antihypertensives: Possibly additive hypotension
lithium: Increased blood lithium level and risk of lithium toxicity
NSAIDs: Possibly decreased antihypertensive effect of fosinopril

sodium aurothiomalate: Nitritoid reactions, including facial flushing, nausea, vomiting, and hypotension

FOODS

salt substitutes: Increased risk of hyperkalemia

ACTIVITIES

alcohol use: Possibly additive hypotension

Adverse Reactions

CNS: Confusion, depression, dizziness, drowsiness, fatigue, fever, headache, insomnia, mood changes, sleep disturbance, syncope, tremor, vertigo, weakness
CV: Angina, arrhythmias (including AV conduction disorders, bradycardia, and tachycardia), claudication, hypotension, MI, orthostatic hypotension, palpitations
EENT: Dry mouth, epistaxis, eye irritation, hoarseness, rhinitis, sinus problems, taste perversion, tinnitus, vision changes
GI: Abdominal distention and pain, anorexia, constipation, diarrhea, flatulence, hepatic failure, hepatitis, hepatomegaly, nausea, pancreatitis, vomiting
GU: Decreased libido, flank pain, renal insufficiency, sexual dysfunction, urinary frequency
MS: Arthralgia, gout, myalgia
RESP: Asthma; bronchitis; bronchospasm; dry, persistent, tickling cough; dyspnea; tracheobronchitis; upper respiratory tract infection
SKIN: Diaphoresis, jaundice, photosensitivity, pruritus, rash, urticaria
Other: Anaphylaxis, angioedema, hyperkalemia, weight gain

Nursing Considerations

• Monitor serum potassium level before and during fosinopril therapy, as appropriate.
• Observe patient being treated for heart failure for at least 2 hours after giving drug to detect hypotension or orthostatic hypotension. If either develops, notify prescriber and monitor patient until blood pressure stabilizes. Keep in mind that orthostatic hypotension is unlikely to develop in patients with a systolic blood pressure over 100 mm Hg who receive a 10-mg dose.
• If patient also receives an antacid, separate administration times by at least 2 hours.
• If patient also receives a diuretic or another antihypertensive, expect to reduce

its dosage over 2 to 3 days before starting fosinopril. If blood pressure isn't controlled with fosinopril alone, other antihypertensive therapy may resume, as prescribed. If so, observe for excessive hypotension.
WARNING If angioedema affects the face, glottis, larynx, limbs, lips, mucous membranes, or tongue, notify prescriber immediately. Expect to discontinue fosinopril and start appropriate therapy at once. If airway obstruction threatens, promptly give 0.3 to 0.5 ml of epinephrine solution 1:1,000 subcutaneously, as prescribed.

PATIENT TEACHING

• Instruct patient to take fosinopril at same time each day to improve compliance and maintain drug's therapeutic effect.
• Emphasize the importance of taking fosinopril as prescribed, even if patient feels well. Caution her not to stop taking drug without consulting prescriber.
• Explain that drug helps control—but doesn't cure—hypertension and that patient may need lifelong therapy.
WARNING Urge patient to seek immediate medical attention for difficulty breathing or swallowing, hoarseness, or swelling of the face, lips, tongue, or throat.
• Instruct patient to notify prescriber about persistent, severe nausea, vomiting, and diarrhea; resulting dehydration may lead to hypotension.
• Advise patient not to take other drugs or use salt substitutes without consulting prescriber.
• Encourage patient to keep scheduled appointments with prescriber to monitor blood pressure, blood test results, and effects of therapy.
• Caution patient about possible dizziness.
• To minimize effects of orthostatic hypotension, advise patient to rise slowly from a lying or sitting position and to dangle legs over bed for several minutes before standing.
• Reinforce prescriber's recommendations for lifestyle changes, such as smoking cessation, stress reduction, dietary improvements, alcohol avoidance, and regular exercise.

E
F

• If patient is a woman of childbearing age, urge her to use contraception during therapy because drug may harm fetus.

• Advise patient to use caution during exercise and hot weather because of the increased risk of dehydration from excessive sweating.

fosphenytoin sodium

Cerebyx

Class and Category

Chemical class: Hydantoin derivative
Therapeutic class: Anticonvulsant
Pregnancy category: D

Indications and Dosages

➤ *To treat status epilepticus*

I.V. INFUSION, I.M. INJECTION

Adults and adolescents. *Initial:* 15 to 20 mg of phenytoin equivalent (PE)/kg I.V. at 100 to 150 PE/min. *Maintenance:* 4 to 6 mg PE/kg daily I.V. or I.M. in divided doses twice daily to four times daily. *Maximum:* 30 mg PE/kg as total loading dose.

Children. *Initial:* 15 to 20 mg PE/kg I.V. given at up to 3 mg PE/kg/min. *Maintenance:* 4 to 6 mg PE/kg daily I.V. or I.M. in divided doses twice daily to four times daily.

➤ *To prevent or treat seizures during and after neurosurgery*

I.V. INFUSION, I.M. INJECTION

Adults and adolescents. *Initial:* 10 to 20 mg PE/kg I.V., not to exceed 150 mg PE/ min. *Maintenance:* 4 to 6 mg PE/kg daily I.V. or I.M. in divided doses twice daily to four times daily. *Maximum:* 30 mg PE/kg as total loading dose.

Mechanism of Action

Is converted from fosphenytoin (a prodrug) to phenytoin, which limits the spread of seizure activity and the start of new seizures. Phenytoin does so by regulating voltage-dependent sodium and calcium channels in neurons, inhibiting calcium movement across neuronal membranes, and enhancing the sodium-potassium-adenosine triphosphatase activity in neurons and glial cells. These actions may stem from phenytoin's ability to slow the recovery rate of inactivated sodium channels.

Contraindications

Concurrent delavirdine use, hypersensitivity to fosphenytoin, phenytoin, other hydantoins, or their components

Interactions

DRUGS

acetaminophen (long-term use): Increased risk of hepatotoxicity

acyclovir: Decreased blood phenytoin level, loss of seizure control

alfentanil: Increased clearance and decreased effectiveness of alfentanil

amiodarone, fluoxetine: Possibly increased blood phenytoin level and risk of toxicity

antacids: Possibly decreased phenytoin effectiveness

antineoplastics, diazepam, fosamprenavir, nelfinavir, reserpine, rifampin, ritonavir, St. John's wort, vigabatrin: Increased phenytoin metabolism and decreased phenytoin level

beta blockers: Increased myocardial depression

bupropion, clozapine, loxapine, MAO inhibitors, maprotiline, phenothiazines, pimozide, thioxanthenes: Possibly lowered seizure threshold and decreased therapeutic effects of phenytoin, possibly intensified CNS depressant effects of these drugs

calcium: Possibly impaired phenytoin absorption

calcium channel blockers, capecitabine, fluconazole, fluvastatin, fluvoxamine, ketoconazole, itraconazole, miconazole, omeprazole, sertraline, voriconazole: Possibly increased blood phenytoin level

carbamazepine: Decreased blood carbamazepine level, possibly decreased blood phenytoin level

chloramphenicol, cimetidine, disulfiram, isoniazid, methylphenidate, metronidazole, phenylbutazone, ranitidine, salicylates, sulfonamides, trimethoprim: Possibly impaired metabolism of these drugs, increased risk of phenytoin toxicity

CNS depressants: Possibly increased CNS depression

corticosteroids, cyclosporine, digoxin, disopyramide, doxycycline, fosamprenavir, furosemide, levodopa, mexiletine, quinidine: Decreased therapeutic effects of these drugs *delavirdine:* Possible loss of virologic response and possible resistance to delavirdine

diazoxide: Possibly decreased therapeutic effects of both drugs

dopamine: Possibly sudden hypotension or cardiac arrest after I.V. fosphenytoin administration

estrogen- and progestin-containing contraceptives: Possibly breakthrough bleeding and decreased contraceptive effectiveness

estrogens, progestins: Decreased therapeutic effects, increased blood phenytoin level

ethosuximide, felbamate, methsuximide, oxcarbazepine, topiramate: Possibly impaired metabolism and increased blood level of phenytoin

fluorouracil: Increased blood fosphenytoin level possibly causing toxicity reactions

folic acid: Increased phenytoin metabolism, decreased seizure control

fosamprenavir in combination with ritonavir: Possibly increased blood fosamprenavir level

haloperidol: Possibly lowered seizure threshold and decreased therapeutic effects of phenytoin; possibly decreased blood haloperidol level

insulin, oral antidiabetic drugs: Possibly increased blood glucose level and decreased therapeutic effects of these drugs

lamotrigine: Possibly decreased therapeutic effects of lamotrigine

lidocaine: Possibly decreased blood lidocaine level, increased myocardial depression

lithium: Increased risk of lithium toxicity

methadone: Possibly increased methadone metabolism, leading to withdrawal symptoms

molindone: Possibly lowered seizure threshold, impaired absorption, and decreased therapeutic effects of phenytoin

nondepolarizing neuromuscular blocking agents such as cisatracurium, pancuronium, rocuronium, vecuronium: Possibly more rapid recovery from neuromuscular blockade than expected

oral anticoagulants: Possibly impaired metabolism of these drugs and increased risk of phenytoin toxicity; possibly increased anticoagulant effects initially and then decreased effects with prolonged therapy

rifampin: Possibly decreased therapeutic effects of phenytoin

streptozocin: Possibly decreased therapeutic effects of streptozocin

sucralfate: Possibly decreased phenytoin absorption

tricyclic antidepressants: Possibly lowered seizure threshold and decreased therapeutic effects of phenytoin; possibly decreased blood antidepressant level

valproic acid: Decreased blood phenytoin level, increased blood valproic acid level

vitamin D analogues: Decreased vitamin D analogue activity

xanthines: Possibly inhibited phenytoin absorption and increased clearance of xanthines

zaleplon: Increased clearance and decreased effectiveness of zaleplon

ACTIVITIES

alcohol use: Possibly decreased or increased phenytoin effectiveness

Adverse Reactions

CNS: Agitation, amnesia, asthenia, ataxia, cerebral edema, chills, coma, confusion, delusions, depression, dizziness, emotional lability, encephalitis, encephalopathy, extrapyramidal reactions, fever, headache, hemiplegia, hostility, hypoesthesia, lack of coordination, malaise, meningitis, nervousness, neurosis, paralysis, personality disorder, positive Babinski's sign, seizures, somnolence, speech disorders, stroke, stupor, subdural hematoma, syncope, transient paresthesia, tremor, vertigo

CV: Atrial flutter, bradycardia, bundle-branch block, cardiac arrest, cardiomegaly, edema, heart failure, hypertension, hypotension, orthostatic hypotension, palpitations, PVCs, serious arrhythmias, shock, tachycardia, thrombophlebitis

EENT: Amblyopia, conjunctivitis, diplopia, dry mouth, earache, epistaxis, eye pain, gingival hyperplasia, hearing loss, hyper-acusis, increased salivation, loss of taste, mydriasis, nystagmus, pharyngitis, photophobia, rhinitis, sinusitis, taste perversion, tinnitus, tongue swelling, visual field defects

E
F

ENDO: Diabetes insipidus, hyperglycemia, ketosis
GI: Anorexia, constipation, diarrhea, dysphagia, elevated liver function test results, flatulence, gastritis, GI bleeding, hepatic necrosis, hepatitis, ileus, indigestion, nausea, vomiting
GU: Albuminuria, dysuria, incontinence, oliguria, polyuria, renal failure, urine retention, vaginal candidiasis
HEME: Anemia, easy bruising, leukopenia, thrombocytopenia
MS: Arthralgia, back pain, leg cramps, muscle twitching, myalgia, myasthenia, myoclonus, myopathy
RESP: Apnea, asthma, atelectasis, bronchitis, dyspnea, hemoptysis, hyperventilation, hypoxia, increased cough, increased sputum production, pneumonia, pneumothorax
SKIN: Contact dermatitis, diaphoresis, maculopapular or pustular rash, photosensitivity, skin discoloration, skin nodule, Stevens-Johnson syndrome, transient pruritus, urticaria
Other: Cachexia; cryptococcosis; dehydration; drug reaction with eosinophilia and systemic symptoms (DRESS); facial edema; flulike symptoms; hyperkalemia; hypokalemia; hypophosphatemia; infection; injection-site reaction such as Purple Glove Syndrome, edema, discoloration and pain distal to the site of injection; lymphadenopathy; sepsis

Nursing Considerations

• Express the dosage, concentration, and infusion rate of fosphenytoin in PE units. Misreading an order or a label could result in massive overdose.
• Refrigerate unopened fosphenytoin at 2° to 8° C (36° to 46° F), but don't freeze.
• Dilute drug in D_5W or normal saline solution to 1.5 to 25 mg PE/ml.
• Inspect parenteral solution before administration. Discard solution that contains particles or is discolored.
• Be aware that drug shouldn't be given I.M. for status epilepticus because I.V. route allows faster onset and peak.
• Keep in mind that I.V. fosphenytoin administration doesn't require use of a filter, as with phenytoin administration.

• Don't give fosphenytoin solution faster than 150 mg PE/minute because of the risk of severe hypotension and cardiac arrhythmias. For a 50-kg (110-lb) patient, infusion typically takes 5 to 7 minutes. Monitor patient throughout the infusion for adverse signs and symptoms of cardiovascular toxicity. If present, notify prescriber and expect infusion rate to be slowed or drug discontinued.
• Follow loading dose with maintenance dosage of oral or parenteral phenytoin or parenteral fosphenytoin, as prescribed.
• As prescribed, give I.V. benzodiazepine (such as lorazepam or diazepam) with fosphenytoin; otherwise, drug's full antiepileptic effect won't be immediate.
• Monitor ECG, blood pressure, and respiratory function for 10 to 20 minutes after infusion ends.
• Expect to obtain blood fosphenytoin (phenytoin) level 2 hours after I.V. infusion or 4 hours after I.M. injection. Therapeutic level generally ranges from 10 to 20 mcg/ml; steady-state may take several days to several weeks to reach.
• Be aware that I.V. or I.M. fosphenytoin may be substituted for oral phenytoin sodium at same total daily dose and frequency. If prescribed, give daily amount in two or more divided doses to maintain seizure control.
• When switching between phenytoin and fosphenytoin, remember that small differences in phenytoin bioavailability can lead to significant changes in blood phenytoin level and an increased risk of toxicity.
• If drug causes transient, infusion-related paresthesia and pruritus, decrease or discontinue infusion, as ordered.
• Monitor CBC for thrombocytopenia or leukopenia—signs of hematologic toxicity. Also monitor serum albumin level and results of renal and liver function tests.
• Anticipate increased frequency and severity of adverse reactions after I.V. administration in patients with hepatic or renal impairment or hypoalbuminemia.
• Discontinue drug, as ordered, if signs of hypersensitivity develop: acute hepato-toxicity (hepatic necrosis and hepatitis), fever, lymphadenopathy, and skin

reactions during first 2 months of therapy.

• Monitor phenytoin level to detect early signs of toxicity, such as diplopia, nausea, severe confusion, slurred speech, and vomiting. Expect to reduce or stop drug.

WARNING Monitor patient for seizures; at toxic levels, phenytoin is excitatory.

WARNING If patient has bradycardia or heart block rhythm, notify prescriber and expect to withhold drug; severe cardiovascular reactions and death have occurred.

• Expect to provide vitamin D supplement if patient has inadequate dietary intake and is receiving long-term anticonvulsant treatment.

• Document type, onset, and characteristics of seizures and response to treatment.

• Monitor patient for injection-site reactions such as local toxicity known as Purple Glove Syndrome, exhibited by edema, discoloration and pain distal to the site of injection. Know that this may occur without extravasation being present and up to several days after injection. If present, notify prescriber and expect drug to be discontinued.

PATIENT TEACHING

• Inform patient that fosphenytoin typically is used for short-term treatment.

• Instruct patient to notify prescriber immediately about bothersome symptoms, especially rash and swollen glands or local reaction at injection site, including pain distal to the site, swelling, and discoloration.

• Because gingival hyperplasia may develop during long-term therapy, emphasize need for good oral hygiene and gum massage.

• Urge patient to consume adequate amounts of vitamin D.

frovatriptan succinate

Frova

Class and Category

Chemical class: Selective 5-hydroxytryptamine$_1$ (5-HT$_1$) receptor agonist, triptan
Therapeutic class: Antimigraine agent

Pregnancy category: C

Indications and Dosages

➤ *To treat acute migraine with or without aura*

TABLETS

Adults. 2.5 mg, repeated in 2 hr as needed. *Maximum:* 7.5 mg daily.

Mechanism of Action

Binds to 5-HT$_{1B}$ and 5-HT$_{1D}$ receptors on extracerebral and intracranial arteries to inhibit excessive dilation of these vessels. This action may decrease carotid arterial blood flow, thus relieving acute migraines. Frovatriptan may also relieve pain by inhibiting the release of proinflammatory neuropeptides and reducing transmission of trigeminal nerve impulses from sensory nerve endings during a migraine attack.

Contraindications

Hypersensitivity to frovatriptan or its components, basilar or hemiplegic migraines, cerebrovascular or peripheral vascular disease, ischemic or vasospastic coronary artery disease (CAD), uncontrolled hypertension, use within 24 hours of other serotonin-receptor agonists or ergotamine-containing or ergot-type drugs

Interactions

DRUGS

dihydroergotamine mesylate, other ergotamine-containing drugs: Possibly prolonged vasospastic reaction
oral contraceptives, propranolol: Possibly increased blood frovatriptan level
selective serotonin reuptake inhibitors, such as citalopram, escitalopram, fluoxetine, fluvoxamine, paroxetine, sertraline; serotonin norepinephrine reuptake inhibitors, such as duloxetine, venlafaxine: Increased risk of life-threatening serotonin syndrome

Adverse Reactions

CNS: Anxiety, dizziness, dysesthesia, fatigue, headache, hypoesthesia, insomnia, paresthesia, seizures, serotonin syndrome
CV: Arrhythmias (such as bradycardia and tachycardia), chest pain, coronary artery vasospasm, ECG changes, MI, myocardial ischemia (transient), palpitations,

ventricular fibrillation, ventricular tachycardia
EENT: Abnormal vision, dry mouth, indigestion, rhinitis, sinusitis, tinnitus
GI: Abdominal pain, diarrhea, indigestion, vomiting
MS: Skeletal pain
SKIN: Diaphoresis, flushing
Other: Generalized pain

Nursing Considerations

• Use frovatriptan cautiously in patients with peripheral vascular disease because drug may cause vasospastic reactions, leading to vascular and colonic ischemia with abdominal pain and bloody diarrhea. Assess patient's peripheral circulation and bowel sounds during frovatriptan therapy.
• Don't give frovatriptan within 24 hours of another 5-HT$_1$ receptor agonist, such as sumatriptan or rizatriptan, or of an ergotamine-containing or ergot-type drug, such as dihydroergotamine or methysergide.
• Administer tablet with fluids.
• Assess patient for headache before administering second dose. Don't administer more than three 2.5-mg tablets a day.
WARNING Be aware that some patients have had serious adverse cardiac reactions— including fatal ones—after using 5-HT$_1$ receptor agonists. However, these reactions are extremely rare; most were reported in patients with risk factors for CAD.
• Assess patient's cardiovascular status and institute continuous ECG monitoring, as ordered, immediately after drug administration in patients with cardiovascular risk factors because they're at risk for asymptomatic cardiac ischemia.
• Assess patient for arrhythmias, chest pain, and other signs of heart disease in patients with risk factors for CAD. Expect to assess periodically cardiovascular status of patients on long-term therapy.
• Be aware that the safety of treating more than four migraine attacks in 30 days (on average) has not been established.
• Regularly monitor blood pressure of hypertensive patients during therapy because frovatriptan may produce a transient increase in blood pressure.
WARNING Monitor patient for possible serotonin syndrome, characterized by

agitation, chills, confusion, diaphoresis, diarrhea, fever, hyperactive reflexes, poor coordination, restlessness, shaking, talking or acting with uncontrolled excitement, tremor, and twitching, especially if patient is receiving another drug that raises serotonin level (such as selective serotonin reuptake inhibitors or serotonin norepinephrine reuptake inhibitors). In its most severe form, serotonin syndrome can resemble neuroleptic malignant syndrome, which includes a high fever, muscle rigidity, and autonomic instability with possible fluctuations in vital signs and mental status changes.

PATIENT TEACHING
• Instruct patient to read and follow manufacturer's instructions for using frovatriptan to ensure maximum therapeutic results.
• Remind patient not to exceed prescribed daily dosage.
• Encourage patient to lie down in a dark, quiet room after taking drug to help relieve migraine.
• Instruct patient to seek emergency care for chest, jaw, or neck tightness after drug use because drug may cause coronary artery vasospasm.
• Urge patient to report palpitations.
• Caution patient about possible adverse CNS effects, and advise her to avoid hazardous activities until drug's CNS effects are known.
• Emphasize need to report any unusual or severe symptoms immediately.

furazolidone

Furoxone

Class and Category

Chemical class: MAO inhibitor, nitrofuran derivative
Therapeutic class: Antibiotic, antiprotozoal
Pregnancy category: C

Indications and Dosages

➤ *To treat bacterial diarrhea and cholera*
ORAL SUSPENSION, TABLETS
Adults and adolescents. 100 mg every 6 hr for 5 to 7 days.

Infants and children age 1 month and over. 1.25 mg/kg every 6 hr for 5 to 7 days. *Maximum:* 8.8 mg/kg daily.

➤ *To treat giardiasis*

ORAL SUSPENSION, TABLETS

Adults and adolescents. 100 mg every 6 hr for 7 to 10 days.

Infants and children age 1 month and over. 1.25 to 2 mg/kg every 6 hr for 7 to 10 days. *Maximum:* 8.8 mg/kg daily.

Mechanism of Action

May interfere with several bacterial enzyme systems through DNA strand damage. Furazolidone also prevents the inactivation of tyramine by GI and hepatic MAO because it is similar in structure and actions to MAO inhibitors.

Contraindications

Age less than 1 month; hypersensitivity to furazolidone, other nitrofurans, or their components

Interactions

DRUGS

levodopa: Increased therapeutic and adverse effects (particularly hypertension) of levodopa

meperidine: Possibly agitation, apnea, coma, diaphoresis, fever, and seizures

other MAO inhibitors, sedatives, sympathomimetics, tranquilizers, tricyclic antidepressants: Possibly sudden and severe hypertensive crisis

selective serotonin reuptake inhibitors: Increased risk of serotonin syndrome

FOODS

foods and beverages with high content of tyramine or other vasopressor amines: Possibly sudden and severe hypertensive crisis

ACTIVITIES

alcohol use: Possibly disulfiram-like reaction

Adverse Reactions

CNS: Headache, malaise

ENDO: Hypoglycemia

GI: Abdominal pain, diarrhea, nausea, vomiting

GU: Darkened urine

HEME: Hemolytic anemia, leukopenia

Other: Allergic reaction (arthralgia, dyspnea, fever, hypotension, urticaria, vesicular morbilliform rash)

Nursing Considerations

• Ask patient if she has a history of blood disorders—especially glucose-6-phosphate dehydrogenase (G6PD) deficiency—before giving furazolidone.

• As ordered, check G6PD level before giving furazolidone to whites of Mediterranean and Near Eastern origin, Asians, or blacks; G6PD deficiency may worsen drug's hemolytic effect.

• If no response occurs within 7 days, expect to discontinue drug because organism is resistant. Provide therapy with other antibiotics, as prescribed.

• If giardiasis symptoms persist, expect to obtain three stool specimens for analysis several days apart, starting 3 to 4 weeks after treatment ends.

PATIENT TEACHING

• Instruct patient to take drug at evenly spaced intervals around the clock.

• Advise patient to take drug with food if GI distress occurs.

• Direct patient to take a missed dose as soon as she remembers, unless it's nearly time for the next scheduled dose. Caution against double-dosing.

• Instruct patient to take furazolidone for the full time prescribed, even if she feels better before finishing the prescription, because stopping too soon could result in reinfection.

• Advise patient to store furazolidone between 59° and 86° F (15° and 30° C), protected from moisture and light.

• Inform patient that drug may cause dizziness and usually turns urine brown.

• Instruct patient to avoid alcohol during therapy and for 4 days afterward.

• Give patient a list of products to avoid during furazolidone therapy and for at least 2 weeks afterward, such as foods and beverages that contain tyramine and other vasopressor amines (for example, ripe cheese, beer, red and white wine, and smoked or pickled meat, poultry, or fish), OTC appetite suppressants, cough and cold medicines, and other drugs, unless prescribed.

• Instruct patient to notify prescriber if she experiences difficult breathing, fever, flushing, itching, muscle aches, or rash.

E
F

furosemide

Apo-Furosemide (CAN), Furoside (CAN), Lasix, Lasix Special (CAN), Myrosemide, Novosemide (CAN), Uritol (CAN)

Class and Category
Chemical class: Sulfonamide
Therapeutic class: Antihypertensive, diuretic
Pregnancy category: C

Indications and Dosages
➤ *To reduce edema caused by cirrhosis, heart failure, and renal disease, including nephrotic syndrome*

ORAL SOLUTION, TABLETS
Adults. 20 to 80 mg as a single dose, increased by 20 to 40 mg every 6 to 8 hr until desired response occurs. *Maximum:* 600 mg daily.
Children. 2 mg/kg as a single dose, increased by 1 to 2 mg/kg every 6 to 8 hr until desired response occurs. *Maximum:* 6 mg/kg/dose.

I.V. INFUSION, I.V. OR I.M. INJECTION
Adults. 20 to 40 mg as a single dose, increased by 20 mg every 2 hr until desired response occurs.
Children. 1 mg/kg as a single dose, increased by 1 mg/kg every 2 hr until desired response occurs. *Maximum:* 6 mg/kg/dose.
DOSAGE ADJUSTMENT Initial single dose limited to 20 mg for elderly patients.

➤ *To manage mild to moderate hypertension, as adjunct to treat acute pulmonary edema and hypertensive crisis*

ORAL SOLUTION, TABLETS
Adults. *Initial:* 40 mg twice daily, adjusted until desired response occurs. *Maximum:* 600 mg daily.

I.V. INFUSION OR INJECTION
Adults with normal renal function. 40 to 80 mg as a single dose over several minutes.
Adults with acute renal failure or pulmonary edema. 100 to 200 mg as a single dose over several minutes.
DOSAGE ADJUSTMENT For patients with acute pulmonary edema without hypertensive crisis, dosage reduced to 40 mg followed by 80 mg 1 hr later if therapeutic response doesn't occur.

Route	Onset	Peak	Duration
P.O.	20–60 min	1–2 hr	6–8 hr
I.V.	5 min	In 30 min	2 hr
I.M.	30 min	Unknown	2 hr

Mechanism of Action
Inhibits sodium and water reabsorption in the loop of Henle and increases urine formation. As the body's plasma volume decreases, aldosterone production increases, which promotes sodium reabsorption and the loss of potassium and hydrogen ions. Furosemide also increases the excretion of calcium, magnesium, bicarbonate, ammonium, and phosphate. By reducing intracellular and extracellular fluid volume, the drug reduces blood pressure and decreases cardiac output. Over time, cardiac output returns to normal.

Incompatibilities
Don't mix furosemide (a milky, buffered alkaline solution) with highly acidic solutions.

Contraindications
Anuria unresponsive to furosemide; hypersensitivity to furosemide, sulfonamides, or their components

Interactions
DRUGS
ACE inhibitors, angiotensin II receptor blockers: Possibly first-dose hypotension, severe hypotension, deterioration in renal function
aminoglycosides, cisplatin, ethacrynic acid: Increased risk of ototoxicity
amiodarone: Increased risk of arrhythmias from hypokalemia
cephalosporins: Increased risk of cephalosporin-induced nephrotoxicity
chloral hydrate: Possibly diaphoresis, hot flashes, and hypertension
cyclosporine: Increased risk of gouty arthritis
digoxin: Increased risk of digitalis toxicity related to hypokalemia
ganglionic or peripheral adrenergic blocking agents: Increased furosemide effects
indomethacin: Possibly reduced natriuretic and antihypertensive effects of furosemide

insulin, oral antidiabetic drugs: Increased blood glucose level
lithium: Increased risk of lithium toxicity
methotrexate: Possibly decreased therapeutic effects of furosemide
norepinephrine: Possibly decreased arterial response to norepinephrine
NSAIDs: Possibly decreased diuresis
phenytoin, probenecid: Possibly decreased therapeutic effects of furosemide
propranolol: Possibly increased blood propranolol level
succinylcholine: Increased action of succinylcholine
sucralfate: Possibly reduced natriuretic and antihypertensive effects of furosemide
thiazide diuretics: Possibly profound diuresis and electrolyte imbalances
tubocurarine: Antagonized skeletal muscle relaxing effect of tubocurarine
ACTIVITIES
alcohol use: Possibly increased hypotensive and diuretic effects of furosemide

Adverse Reactions

CNS: Dizziness, drowsiness, fever, headache, lethargy, paresthesia, restlessness, vertigo, weakness
CV: Arrhythmias, elevated cholesterol and triglyceride levels, orthostatic hypotension, shock, tachycardia, thromboembolism, thrombophlebitis vertigo
EENT: Blurred vision, dry mouth, oral irritation, ototoxicity, stomatitis, tinnitus, transient hearing loss (rapid I.V. injection), yellow vision
ENDO: Hyperglycemia
GI: Abdominal cramps, anorexia, constipation, diarrhea, elevated liver enzymes, gastric irritation, hepatocellular insufficiency, indigestion, jaundice, nausea, pancreatitis, vomiting
GU: Azotemia, bladder spasms, glycosuria, oliguria
HEME: Agranulocytosis (rare), anemia, aplastic anemia (rare), eosinophilia, hemolytic anemia, leukopenia, thrombocytopenia
MS: Muscle pain or spasms
SKIN: Acute generalized exanthematous pustulosis, bullous pemphigoid, drug rash with eosinophilia and systemic symptoms (DRESS), erythema multiforme, exfoliative dermatitis, photosensitivity, pruritus, purpura, rash, Stevens-Johnson syndrome, toxic epidermal necrolysis, urticaria
Other: Allergic reaction (interstitial nephritis, necrotizing vasculitis, systemic vasculitis), anaphylactic reactions, dehydration, hyperuricemia, hypocalcemia, hypochloremia, hypokalemia, hypomagnesemia, hyponatremia, hypovolemia, thirst

Nursing Considerations

WARNING Use furosemide cautiously in patients with advanced hepatic cirrhosis, especially those who also have a history of electrolyte imbalance or hepatic encephalopathy; drug may lead to lethal hepatic coma.
• Be aware that patients who are allergic to sulfonamides may also be allergic to furosemide. Monitor patient closely.
• Know that furosemide may precipitate nephrocalcinosis/nephrolithiasis in premature infants. Drug may also increase the risk of persistence of patent ductus arteriosus in premature infants.
• Obtain patient's weight before and periodically during furosemide therapy to monitor fluid loss.
• For once-a-day dosing, give drug in the morning so patient's sleep won't be interrupted by increased need to urinate.
• Prepare drug for infusion with normal saline solution, lactated Ringer's solution, or D_5W.
• Administer drug slowly I.V. over 1 to 2 minutes to prevent ototoxicity.
• Expect patient to have periodic hearing tests during prolonged or high-dose I.V. therapy.
• Monitor blood pressure and hepatic and renal function as well as BUN, blood glucose, and serum creatinine, electrolyte, and uric acid levels, as appropriate.
• Be aware that elderly patients are more susceptible to hypotensive and electrolyte-altering effects and thus are at greater risk for shock and thromboembolism.
• If patient is at high risk for hypokalemia, give potassium supplements along with furosemide, as prescribed.
• Expect to discontinue furosemide at maximum dosage if oliguria persists for more than 24 hours.

• Be aware that furosemide may worsen left ventricular hypertrophy, systemic lupus erythematosus, or renal retention and adversely affect glucose tolerance and lipid metabolism as well as increase risk of decreased renal function in patients at high risk for radiocontrast nephropathy after a procedure.

• Be aware that patients with hypoproteinemia, such as occurs with nephrotic syndrome, may weaken effect of furosemide and increase its ototoxicity potential.

• Notify prescriber if patient experiences hearing loss, vertigo, or ringing, buzzing, or sense of fullness in her ears. Drug may need to be discontinued.

PATIENT TEACHING

• Instruct patient to take furosemide at the same time each day to maintain therapeutic effects. Urge her to take it as prescribed, even if she feels well.

• Instruct patient to take the last dose of furosemide several hours before bedtime to avoid sleep interruption from diuresis. If patient receives once-daily dosing, advise her to take the dose in the morning to avoid sleep disturbance caused by nocturia.

• Advise patient to change position slowly to minimize effects of orthostatic hypotension and to take furosemide with food or milk to reduce GI distress.

• Caution patient about drinking alcoholic beverages, standing for prolonged periods, and exercising in hot weather because these actions increase the hypotensive effect of furosemide.

• Emphasize the importance of weight and diet control, especially limiting sodium intake.

• Unless contraindicated, urge patient to eat more high-potassium foods and to take a potassium supplement, if prescribed, to prevent hypokalemia.

• Instruct patient to keep follow-up appointments with prescriber to monitor progress. Urge her to notify prescriber about persistent, severe nausea, vomiting, and diarrhea because they may cause dehydration.

• Inform diabetic patient that furosemide may increase blood glucose level, and advise her to check her blood glucose level frequently.

G H I

gabapentin
Gralise, Neurontin

gabapentin enacarbil
Horizant

Class and Category
Chemical class: Cyclohexane-acetic acid derivative
Therapeutic class: Anticonvulsant
Pregnancy category: C

Indications and Dosages
➤ *To manage postherpetic neuralgia*
CAPSULES, ORAL SOLUTION, TABLETS (NEURONTIN)
Adults. *Initial:* 300 mg on day 1, increased to 300 mg twice daily on day 2, increased to 300 mg three times daily on day 3, and increased gradually thereafter according to pain response, up to 600 mg three times daily. *Maximum:* 1,800 mg daily.
TABLETS (GRALISE)
Adults. *Initial:* 300 mg once daily with evening meal on day 1, 600 mg once daily with evening meal on day 2, 900 mg once daily with evening meal on days 3 through 6, 1,200 mg once daily with evening meal on days 7 through 10, 1500 mg once daily with evening meal on days 11 through 14, and 1,800 mg once daily with evening meal on day 15 and thereafter.
Extended-release tablets (Horizant)
Adults. *Initial:* 600 mg once daily in a.m. for 3 days, followed by 600 mg twice daily. *Maximum:* 600 mg twice daily.
DOSAGE ADJUSTMENT For patients taking Gralise who have a reduced creatinine clearance of 30 ml/min to 60 ml/min, dosage must be individualized and may need to be reduced. Patients with a creatinine clearance of less than 30 ml/min or who are receiving hemodialysis should not receive Gralise. For patients taking Neurontin who have a reduced creatinine clearance, including patients on hemodialysis, dosage reduced but reduction is highly individualized. For patients taking

Horizant with a creatinine clearance between 30 and 59 ml/min, dosage reduced to 300 mg once daily in a.m. for 3 days, followed by 300 mg twice daily with further increase to 600mg twice daily, as needed. For patients taking Horizant with a creatinine clearance between 15 and 29 ml/min, dosage reduced to 300 mg once daily in a.m. on day 1 and 3, followed by 300 mg once daily in a.m. with further increase to 300 mg twice daily, if needed. For patient with a creatinine clearance less than 15 ml/min and not on dialysis, dosage reduced to 300 mg once daily in a.m. every other day, followed by 300 mg once daily in a.m., if needed. For patient with a creatinine clearance less than 15 ml/min and on hemodialysis, 300 mg following every dialysis with further increase to 600 mg following every dialysis, if needed.
➤ *As adjunct to treat partial seizures*
CAPSULES, ORAL SOLUTION, TABLETS (NEURONTIN)
Adults and adolescents. *Initial:* 300 mg three times daily, increased gradually according to clinical response. *Maintenance:* 900 to 1,800 mg daily. *Maximum:* 3,600 mg daily.
DOSAGE ADJUSTMENT For patients taking Neurontin who have a reduced creatinine clearance, including patients on hemodialysis, dosage reduced but reduction is highly individualized.
➤ *To treat restless legs syndrome*
E.R. TABLETS (HORIZANT)
Adults. 600 mg once daily with food at about 5 PM.
DOSAGE ADJUSTMENT For patients taking Horizant with a creatinine clearance between 30 and 59 ml/min, dosage reduced to 300 mg daily and then increased to 600 mg, as needed. For patients taking Horizant with a creatinine clearance between 15 and 29 ml/min, dosage reduced to 300 mg daily and not increased. For patients with a creatinine clearance of less than 15 ml/min and not on hemodialysis, dosage reduced to 300 mg and given every other day. Patients taking Horizant with a creatinine clearance of less than 15 ml/min and receiving hemodialysis should not receive Horizant.

Mechanism of Action
Is structurally like gamma-aminobutyric acid (GABA), the main inhibitory

neurotransmitter in the brain. Although gabapentin's exact mechanism of action is unknown, GABA inhibits the rapid firing of neurons associated with seizures.

Contraindications
Hypersensitivity to gabapentin or its components

Interactions
DRUGS
aluminum- and magnesium-containing antacids: Decreased gabapentin bio-availability
CNS depressants: Increased CNS depression
ACTIVITIES
alcohol use: Increased CNS depression

Adverse Reactions
CNS: Agitation, altered proprioception, amnesia, anxiety, apathy, aphasia, asthenia, ataxia, cerebellar dysfunction, chills, CNS tumors, decreased or absent reflexes, delusions, depersonalization, depression, disappearance of aura, dizziness, dream disturbances, dysesthesia, dystonia, emotional lability, euphoria, facial paralysis, fatigue, fever, hallucinations, headache, hemiplegia, hostility, hyperkinesia, hyperreflexia, hypoesthesia, hypotonia, intracranial hemorrhage, lack of coordination, malaise, migraine headache, movement disorder, nervousness, occipital neuralgia, paranoia, paresis, paresthesia, positive Babinski's sign, psychosis, sedation, seizures, somnolence, stupor, subdural hematoma, suicidal ideation, syncope, tremor, vertigo
CV: Angina, hypertension, hypotension, murmur, palpitations, peripheral edema, peripheral vascular insufficiency, tachycardia, vasodilation
EENT: Abnormal vision, amblyopia, blepharospasm, cataracts, conjunctivitis, diplopia, dry eyes and mouth, earache, epistaxis, eye hemorrhage, eye pain, gingival bleeding, gingivitis, glossitis, hearing loss, hoarseness, increased salivation, inner ear infection, loss of taste, nystagmus, pharyngitis, photophobia, ptosis (bilateral or unilateral), rhinitis, sensation of fullness in ears, stomatitis, taste perversion, tinnitus, tooth discoloration, visual field defects
ENDO: Breast hypertrophy, blood glucose fluctuation

GI: Abdominal pain, anorexia, constipation, diarrhea, elevated liver function tests, fecal incontinence, flatulence, gastroenteritis, hemorrhoids, hepatitis, hepatomegaly, increased appetite, indigestion, jaundice, melena, nausea, thirst, vomiting
GU: Acute renal failure, decreased libido, impotence
HEME: Anemia, coagulation defect, decreased WBC count, leukopenia, thrombocytopenia
MS: Arthralgia, arthritis, back pain, bone fractures, dysarthria, joint stiffness or swelling, muscle twitching, myalgia, positive Romberg test, tendinitis
RESP: Apnea, cough, dyspnea, pneumonia, pseudocroup
SKIN: Abrasion, acne, alopecia, cyst, diaphoresis, drug reaction with eosinophilia and systemic symptoms (DRESS), dry skin, eczema, erythema multiforme, hirsutism, pruritus, purpura, rash, seborrhea, Stevens-Johnson syndrome, urticaria
Other: Angioedema, dehydration, elevated creatine kinase level, facial edema, hyponatremia, lymphadenopathy, viral infection, weight gain or loss

Nursing Considerations
• As needed, open gabapentin capsules and mix contents with water, fruit juice, applesauce, or pudding before administration.
• Administer initial dose for Neurontin brand at bedtime to minimize adverse reactions, especially ataxia, dizziness, fatigue, and somnolence. Administer Gralise brand with evening meal and initial dose of Horizant in the morning.
• Give drug at least 2 hours after an antacid.
• Don't exceed 12 hours between doses on a 3-times-a-day schedule.
• Be aware that routine monitoring of blood gabapentin level isn't needed.
WARNING To discontinue drug used to treat seizures or switch to a different anticonvulsant, expect to change gradually over at least 1 week, as prescribed, to avoid loss of seizure control. When gabapentin is discontinued after treating other indications, expect to reduce dosage, as ordered, over 1 week.
• Monitor renal function test results, and expect to adjust dosage, if needed.

• Monitor patient closely for evidence of suicidal thinking or behavior, especially when therapy starts or dosage changes.
• Be aware that the various brands of gabapentin are not interchangeable.
• Monitor patient for hypersensitivity, such as fever or lymphadenopathy suggestive of DRESS. Although rare, DRESS may be life-threatening. If suspected, notify prescriber immediately and expect gabapentin to be discontinued.

PATIENT TEACHING
• If patient has trouble swallowing gabapentin capsules, advise him to open them and sprinkle contents in juice or on soft food immediately before use. Tell patient taking gabapentin extended-release tablets to swallow the tablet whole and not to split, crush, or chew the tablets.
• Instruct patient not to take drug within 2 hours after taking an antacid.
• Urge patient to take a missed dose as soon as he remembers. If the next dose is in less than 2 hours, tell him to wait 1 to 2 hours before taking it and then resume his regular schedule. Caution against doubling the dose.
• Caution patient not to stop drug abruptly.
• Inform patient about possible ataxia, dizziness, drowsiness, and nystagmus. Advise him to avoid hazardous activities until drug's CNS effects are known.
• To prevent complications from adverse oral reactions (such as gingivitis), encourage patient to use good oral hygiene and to seek routine dental care.
• Explain that adverse effects usually are mild to moderate and decline with time.
• Urge patient to keep follow-up appointments with prescriber to check progress.
• Urge caregivers to watch closely for evidence of suicidal tendencies, especially when therapy starts or dosage changes, and to report concerns immediately.
• Urge woman who becomes pregnant while taking gabapentin to enroll in the North American antiepileptic drug pregnancy registry by calling 1-888-233-2334. Explain that this registry is collecting information about the safety of antiepileptic drugs during pregnancy.

galantamine hydrobromide

Razadyne, Razadyne ER

Class and Category
Chemical class: Tertiary alkaloid
Therapeutic class: Antidementia agent
Pregnancy category: B

Indications and Dosages
➤ To treat mild to moderate Alzheimer's-type dementia
ORAL SOLUTION, TABLETS
Adults. Initial: 4 mg twice daily. Dosage increased by 8 mg daily every 4 wk, if tolerated. Maximum: 12 mg twice daily.
DOSAGE ADJUSTMENT For patients with moderately impaired hepatic or renal function, maximum dosage shouldn't exceed 16 mg daily.
E.R. CAPSULES
Adults. Initial: 8 mg daily. Dosage increased by 8 mg daily every 4 wk if tolerated. Maximum: 24 mg daily.

Route	Onset	Peak	Duration
P.O.	Unknown	1 hr	Unknown

Mechanism of Action
Reduces acetylcholine metabolism by competitively and reversibly inhibiting the brain enzyme acetylcholinesterase. Acetylcholine-producing neurons degenerate in the brains of patients with Alzheimer's disease. Inhibition of acetylcholinesterase increases the amount of acetylcholine, which is needed for nerve impulse transmission.

Contraindications
Hypersensitivity to galantamine hydro-bromide or its components, severe hepatic or renal impairment (creatinine clearance less than 9 ml/min/1.73 m^2)

Interaction
DRUGS
amitriptyline, fluoxetine, fluvoxamine, quinidine: Possibly decreased galantamine clearance
anticholinergics: Possibly interference with cholinesterase activity

G
H
I

cholinergic agonists, cholinesterase inhibitors, neuromuscular blockers: Possibly exaggerated effects of these drugs and galantamine
cimetidine: Possibly increased galantamine bioavailability
ketoconazole, paroxetine: Increased galantamine bioavailability

Adverse Reactions
CNS: Aggression, asthenia, depression, dizziness, dysgeusia, fatigue, fever, headache, hypersomnia, insomnia, lethargy, malaise, somnolence, stroke, suicidal ideation, syncope, tremor
CV: AV block, bradycardia, chest pain, MI, myocardial ischemia
EENT: Blurred vision, rhinitis
GI: Abdominal pain, anorexia, diarrhea, elevated liver enzymes, flatulence, GI bleeding, hepatitis, indigestion, nausea, vomiting
GU: Hematuria, incontinence, renal failure or insufficiency, UTI
HEME: Anemia
Other: Dehydration, hypersensitivity reactions, hypokalemia, weight loss

Nursing Considerations
• Give galantamine twice daily with morning and evening meals, and ensure adequate fluid intake to prevent GI symptoms.
• If therapy is interrupted for several days, expect to restart drug at lowest dose because benefits are lost when it is discontinued.
• Monitor patient's CV status closely because cholinesterase inhibitors like galantamine may have a depressive effect on sinoatrial and AV nodes and may lead to bradycardia and AV block.
• Monitor patient for progressive deterioration of mental status because drug is less effective as Alzheimer's disease progresses and intact cholinergic neurons decrease.

PATIENT TEACHING
• Instruct patient to take or caregiver to give regular-strength drug with morning and evening meals. Extended-release capsules should be given once in the morning, preferably with food.
• Tell patient or caregiver to notify prescriber immediately if therapy stops for

several days. Prescriber may restart at lowest dose.
• Instruct patient to maintain adequate fluid intake throughout galantamine therapy.
• Advise patient not to drive or perform activities requiring alertness, especially during first weeks of treatment, because drug may cause dizziness and drowsiness.
• Inform patient and family members that drug isn't a cure for Alzheimer's disease.

gemfibrozil

Apo-Gemfibrozil (CAN), Gen-Fibro (CAN), Lopid, Novo-Gemfibrozil (CAN), Nu-Gemfibrozil (CAN)

Class and Category
Chemical class: Fibric acid derivative, phenoxypentanoic acid
Therapeutic class: Antihyperlipidemic
Pregnancy category: C

Indications and Dosages
➤ As adjunct (with diet) to treat hyper-lipidemia types IIb, IV, and V
CAPSULES, TABLETS
Adults. 600 mg before meals twice daily.

Route	Onset	Peak	Duration
P.O.	2–5 days	4 wk	Unknown

Mechanism of Action
May decrease hepatic triglyceride production by reducing VLDL synthesis, inhibiting peripheral lipolysis, and decreasing hepatic extraction of free fatty acids. Gemfibrozil also may inhibit synthesis and increase clearance of apolipoprotein B, a carrier molecule for VLDL. In addition, it may accelerate turnover and removal of total cholesterol from the liver while increasing cholesterol excretion in the feces. As a result, triglyceride, total cholesterol, and VLDL levels decrease; the HDL level increases; and the LDL level is unaffected.

Contraindications
Concurrent therapy with repaglinide or simvastatin, gallbladder disease, hepatic or severe renal dysfunction, hypersensitivity to gemfibrozil or its components

Interaction

DRUGS

chenodiol, ursodiol: Decreased effectiveness of gemfibrozil

colchicine: Increased toxicity of either drug; risk of myopathy, including rhabdomyolysis

HMG-CoA reductase inhibitors: Increased risk of rhabdomyolysis and acute renal failure

oral anticoagulants: Increased anti-coagulation

repaglinide: Increased serum repaglinide level and risk of severe hypoglycemia

resin-granule drugs such as colestipol: Decreased blood gemfibrozil levels

Adverse Reactions

CNS: Chills, fatigue, headache, hypoesthesia, paresthesia, seizures, somnolence, syncope, vertigo

CV: Vasculitis

EENT: Blurred vision, cataracts, hoarseness, retinal edema, taste perversion

GI: Abdominal or epigastric pain, cholelithiasis, colitis, diarrhea, flatulence, heartburn, hepatoma, nausea, pancreatitis, vomiting

GU: Decreased male fertility, dysuria, impotence

HEME: Anemia, bone marrow hypoplasia, eosinophilia, leukopenia, thrombocytopenia

MS: Arthralgia, back pain, myalgia, myasthenia, myopathy, myositis, rhabdomyolysis, synovitis

RESP: Cough

SKIN: Eczema, jaundice, pruritus, rash

Other: Anaphylaxis, angioedema, increased risk of bacterial and viral infections, lupus-like symptoms, weight loss

Nursing Considerations

• Monitor serum triglyceride and cholesterol levels, as appropriate.

• Periodically review CBC and liver function test results during therapy, as ordered.

• If serum triglyceride and cholesterol levels don't improve within 3 months, expect to switch to a different drug, as prescribed.

• Monitor patient's prothrombin time, as ordered, if patient is also receiving warfarin therapy because gemfibrozil therapy may cause a drug interaction with warfarin. Warfarin dosage may need to be decreased to maintain prothrombin time

at a level needed to prevent adverse bleeding effects.

PATIENT TEACHING

• Instruct patient to take gemfibrozil 30 minutes before breakfast and 30 minutes before dinner.

• Advise patient to take a missed dose as soon as he remembers, unless it's nearly time for the next dose. Caution against doubling the dose.

• Emphasize importance of a low-fat diet, regular exercise, alcohol avoidance, and smoking cessation, as appropriate.

• Caution patient to avoid hazardous activities until drug's CNS effects are known.

• Instruct patient to notify prescriber if he experiences chills; cough; fever; hoarseness; lower back, side, or muscle pain; painful or difficult urination; severe abdominal pain with nausea and vomiting; tiredness; or weakness.

• If patient also takes an oral anticoagulant, urge him to report unusual bleeding or bruising; anticoagulant dosage may need to be reduced.

• Advise patient to keep scheduled appointments with prescriber to check progress.

gemifloxacin mesylate

Factive

Class and Category

Chemical class: Fluoroquinolone
Therapeutic class: Antibiotic
Pregnancy category: C

Indications and Dosages

➤ *To treat acute bacterial exacerbation of chronic bronchitis caused by* Streptococcus pneumoniae, Haemophilus influenzae, H. parainfluenzae, *or* Moraxella catarrhalis

TABLETS

Adults. 320 mg daily for 5 days.

➤ *To treat mild to moderate community-acquired pneumonia caused by* S. pneumoniae, H. influenzae, M. catarrhalis, Mycoplasma pneumoniae, Chlamydia pneumoniae, *or* Klebsiella pneumoniae

TABLETS

Adults. 320 mg daily for 7 days.

DOSAGE ADJUSTMENT Dosage should be decreased to 160 mg daily in patients with creatinine clearance of 40 ml/min/1.73 m² or less.

Route	Onset	Peak	Duration
P.O.	0.5–2 hr	Unknown	Unknown

Mechanism of Action

Inhibits actions of the enzymes DNA gyrase and topoisomerase IV, which are required for bacterial growth, thereby causing bacterial cells to die.

Contraindications

Hypersensitivity to gemifloxacin, its components, or other fluoroquinolones; myasthenia gravis

Interaction

DRUGS

aluminum and magnesium antacids, didanosine as chewable or buffered tablets or pediatric powder for oral solution, ferrous sulfate, sucralfate, zinc, or other metal cations: Reduced blood gemifloxacin level
antipsychotics; class IA antiarrhythmics, such as procainamide and quinidine; class III antiarrhythmics, such as amiodarone and sotalol; erythromycin; tricyclic antidepressants: Possibly prolonged QT interval
probenecid: Increased blood gemifloxacin level
warfarin: Possibly enhanced warfarin anticoagulant effects

Adverse Reactions

CNS: Dizziness, fever, headache, peripheral neuropathy, syncope, transient ischemic attack
CV: Peripheral edema, prolonged QT interval, supraventricular tachycardia, vasculitis
EENT: Taste perversion
GI: Abdominal pain, acute hepatic necrosis or failure, diarrhea, elevated liver function test results, hepatitis, jaundice, nausea, pseudomembranous colitis, vomiting
GU: Acute renal insufficiency or failure, interstitial nephritis
HEME: Agranulocytosis, aplastic or hemolytic anemia, elevated platelet count,

elevated INR, hemorrhage, leukopenia, pancytopenia, thrombocytopenia
MS: Arthralgia, muscle weakness, myalgia, tendinitis, tendon rupture
RESP: Allergic pneumonitis
SKIN: Erythema multiforme, exfoliation, facial swelling, photosensitivity, rash, Stevens-Johnson syndrome, toxic epidermal necrolysis, urticaria
Other: Anaphylaxis, angioedema, serum sickness

Nursing Considerations

• Review patient's medical history before giving gemifloxacin, which shouldn't be used in patient with a history of prolonged QT interval, patient with uncorrected electrolyte disorders, or patient receiving class IA or III antiarrhythmics because of increased risk of prolonged QT interval. Monitor elderly patients closely because they may be more susceptible to prolonged QT interval.

• Use cautiously in patients with CNS disorders, such as epilepsy, or in those prone to seizures because other fluoroquinolones have caused seizures, increased intracranial pressure, and toxic psychosis. Monitor patient closely; if CNS alterations occur, notify prescriber immediately and expect drug to be discontinued.

• Monitor patient closely for hypersensitivity reaction, which may occur as soon as first dose. If patient has such evidence as angioedema, bronchospasm, dyspnea, itching, rash, jaundice, shortness of breath, and urticaria, notify prescriber immediately and expect drug to be discontinued.

• Monitor patients prone to tendinitis, such as the elderly, athletes, and those taking corticosteroids, for reports of tendon pain, inflammation, or rupture. If present, notify prescriber. Expect gemifloxacin to be discontinued, patient placed on bed rest with no exercise of affected limb, and diagnostic tests ordered to confirm rupture.

• Notify prescriber about severe or prolonged diarrhea; it may indicate pseudomembranous colitis caused by *Clostridium difficile*. If diarrhea occurs, notify prescriber and expect to withhold gemifloxacin and treat with fluids, electrolytes, protein, and an antibiotic effective against *C. difficile.*

• Monitor patients, especially women under age 40 and postmenopausal women receiving hormone replacement therapy, for rash. It may appear days after therapy stars and resolve in 7 days. Notify prescriber immediately if rash occurs because it can be severe in about 10% of patients.

• Assess patient for evidence of peripheral neuropathy. Notify prescriber and expect to stop drug if patient complains of burning, numbness, pain, tingling, or weakness in extremities or if physical examination reveals deficits in light touch, pain, temperature, position sense, vibratory sensation, or motor strength.

• If patient takes warfarin, monitor coagulation status, as ordered, because adding gemifloxacin may increase risk of bleeding.

PATIENT TEACHING

• Tell patient to swallow tablet whole and take with a full glass of liquid.

• Warn patient not to increase dose because doing so may cause life-threatening cardiac arrhythmias.

• Instruct patient to complete entire course of therapy, even if symptoms decrease before prescription is finished.

• Caution patient to avoid sun exposure as much as possible while taking gemifloxacin. Patient who can't avoid sun exposure should apply sunscreen and wear a hat, sunglasses, and long sleeves to cover as much skin as possible.

• Instruct patient to maintain adequate hydration throughout therapy to keep urine from becoming too concentrated. Tell patient to increase fluid intake if urine darkens or amount voided decreases.

• Caution patient to avoid hazardous activities until CNS effects of drug are known.

• Instruct patient to seek medical attention and notify prescriber immediately if he has tendon pain, tenderness, or rupture; evidence of hypersensitivity reaction, such as rash, urticaria, difficulty breathing, or facial swelling; or palpitations or fainting spells. The drug may need to be stopped.

• Urge patient to tell prescriber about diarrhea that's severe or lasts longer than 3 days. Explain that watery or bloody stools can occur 2 or more months after therapy and can be serious, requiring prompt treatment.

• Tell patient to consult prescriber before starting any new medications, including OTC products, because gemifloxacin may interact adversely.

• Inform patient that magnesium and/or aluminum antacids; products containing iron; multivitamins containing zinc or other metal cations; and didanosine (Videx) chewable or buffered tablets and pediatric powder for oral solution (if prescribed) shouldn't be taken within 3 hours before or 2 hours after gemifloxacin and that gemifloxacin should be taken at least 2 hours before sucralfate (if prescribed).

• Instruct patient to alert prescriber about severe diarrhea, even up to 2 months after gemifloxacin therapy has ended.

gentamicin sulfate

Cidomycin (CAN), Garamycin, G-Mycin, Jenamicin

Class and Category

Chemical class: Aminoglycoside derived from *Micromonospora purpurea*
Therapeutic class: Antibiotic
Pregnancy category: D

Indications and Dosages

➤ *To treat serious bacterial infections caused by aerobic gram-negative organisms and some gram-positive organisms, including* Citrobacter *species,* Enterobacter *species,* Escherichia coli, Klebsiella *species,* Proteus *species,* Pseudomonas aeruginosa, Serratia *species,* Staphylococcus aureus, *and many strains of* Streptococcus *species*

I.V. INFUSION, I.M. INJECTION

Adults and adolescents. 1 to 1.7 mg/kg every 8 hr or 4-7 mg/kg every 24 hours.
Children. 2 to 2.5 mg/kg every 8 hr.
Infants. 2.5 mg/kg every 8 to 16 hr.

Premature or full-term neonates up to age 1 week. 2.5 mg/kg every 12 to 24 hr.
INTRATHECAL (INTRALUMBAR OR INTRAVENTRICULAR) INJECTION
Adults and adolescents. 4 to 8 mg daily.
Infants and children age 3 months and over. 1 to 2 mg daily.
➤ *To treat uncomplicated UTI*
I.V. INFUSION, I.M. INJECTION
Adults and adolescents weighing more than 60 kg (132 lb). 160 mg once daily or 80 mg every 12 hr.
Adults and adolescents weighing less than 60 kg. 3 mg/kg once daily or 1.5 mg/kg every 12 hr.
DOSAGE ADJUSTMENT Supplemental dose of 1 to 1.7 mg/kg (2 to 2.5 mg/kg for children) given by I.M. injection or I.V. infusion after hemodialysis, based on infection severity.

Mechanism of Action

Binds to negatively charged sites on the outer cell membrane of bacteria, thereby disrupting the membrane's integrity. Gentamicin also binds to bacterial ribosomal subunits and inhibits protein synthesis. Both actions lead to cell death.

Incompatibilities

Don't administer gentamicin through same I.V. line as other drugs, especially beta-lactam antibiotics (penicillins and cephalosporins), because substantial mutual inactivation may occur. Give drugs through separate sites.

Contraindications

Hypersensitivity or serious toxic reaction to other aminoglycosides, hypersensitivity to gentamicin or its components

Interaction

DRUGS
aminoglycosides (concurrent use of two or more): Decreased bacterial uptake of each drug, increased risk of ototoxicity and nephrotoxicity
cephalosporins, enflurane, methoxyflurane, vancomycin: Increased risk of nephrotoxicity
loop diuretics: Increased risk of ototoxicity and nephrotoxicity
neuromuscular blockers: Prolonged respiratory depression, increased neuromuscular blockade

penicillins: Inactivation of gentamicin by certain penicillins, increased risk of nephrotoxicity

Adverse Reactions

CNS: Acute organic mental syndrome, confusion, depression, fever, headache, increased protein in cerebrospinal fluid, lethargy, myasthenia gravis–like syndrome, neurotoxicity (dizziness, hearing loss, tinnitus, vertigo), peripheral neuropathy or encephalopathy (muscle twitching, numbness, seizures, skin tingling), pseudotumor cerebri
CV: Hypertension, hypotension, palpitations
EENT: Blurred vision, increased salivation, laryngeal edema, ototoxicity, stomatitis, vision changes
GI: Anorexia, nausea, splenomegaly, transient hepatomegaly, vomiting
GU: Nephrotoxicity
HEME: Anemia, eosinophilia, granulocytopenia, increased or decreased reticulocyte count, leukopenia, thrombocytopenia
MS: Arthralgia, leg cramps
RESP: Pulmonary fibrosis, respiratory depression
SKIN: Alopecia, generalized burning sensation, pruritus, purpura, rash, urticaria
Other: Anaphylaxis, injection-site pain, superinfection, weight loss

Nursing Considerations

• Before gentamicin therapy begins, expect to obtain a body fluid or tissue specimen for culture and sensitivity testing, as ordered, or check test results, if available.
• Drug is best absorbed when given by I.V. route. Blood level is unpredictable after I.M. administration.
• For I.V. use, dilute each dose with 50 to 200 ml normal saline solution or D_5W to yield no more than 1 mg/ml. Administer slowly over 30 to 60 minutes.
• Don't give gentamicin through same I.V. line as other drugs without first consulting pharmacist.
• Expect to adjust dosage based on peak and trough blood drug levels drawn after third maintenance dose, as prescribed.
• Don't give gentamicin by subcutaneous route because it may be painful.

• When assisting with intrathecal injection, use only 2 mg/ml of preservative-free preparation. Drug may be injected directly or delivered by implanted reservoir.

• Don't give drug to pregnant patient because it can cause hearing loss in fetus.

• Any report of hearing loss, dizziness, or ringing in the ears should be taken very seriously. Hold drug with any report of these problems.

WARNING When giving pediatric injectable form of drug, be alert for allergic reactions—including anaphylaxis and possibly life-threatening asthmatic episodes—because drug contains sodium bisulfite.

• Assess patient for evidence of other infections because gentamicin may cause overgrowth of nonsusceptible organisms.

• Be aware that premature infants, neonates, and elderly patients have an increased risk of nephrotoxicity.

PATIENT TEACHING

• Emphasize importance of completing full course of gentamicin therapy.

• Instruct patient to report immediately adverse reactions, such as hearing loss, to avoid permanent effects.

glimepiride
Amaryl

Class and Category
Chemical class: Sulfonylurea
Therapeutic class: Antidiabetic
Pregnancy category: C

Indications and Dosages
➤ *To control blood glucose level in type 2 diabetes mellitus*

TABLETS
Adults. 1 to 2 mg daily with first meal of the day. *Maintenance:* 1 to 4 mg daily, increased by 1 to 2 mg every 1 to 2 wk as needed for blood glucose control. *Maximum:* 8 mg daily.
DOSAGE ADJUSTMENT Initial dosage reduced to 1 mg daily if needed for patients with renal impairment.

Route	Onset	Peak	Duration
P.O.	2–3 hr	Unknown	Over 24 hr

Mechanism of Action
Stimulates insulin release from beta cells in pancreas. Glimepiride also increases peripheral tissue sensitivity to insulin, either by enhancing insulin binding to cellular receptors or by increasing the number of insulin receptors.

Contraindications
Diabetes complicated by pregnancy; diabetic coma; hypersensitivity to glimepiride, sulfonamide derivatives, or their components; ketoacidosis; sole therapy for type 1 diabetes mellitus

Interaction
DRUGS
ACE inhibitors, anabolic steroids, androgens, azole antifungals, bromocriptine, chloramphenicol, clarithromycin, clonidine, cyclophosphamide, disopyramide, fibric acid derivatives, fluconazole, fluoxetine, guanethidine, H$_2$-receptor antagonists, insulin, magnesium salts, MAO inhibitors, methyldopa, NSAIDs, octreotide, oral anticoagulants, other oral hypoglycemic agents, oxyphenbutazone, pentoxifylline, phenylbutazone, phenyramidol, pramlintide, probenecid, propoxyphene, quinidine, quinolones, reserpine, salicylates, somatostatin analogs, sulfonamides, tetracyclines, theophylline, tricyclic antidepressants, urinary acidifiers: Increased risk of hypoglycemia
asparaginase, barbiturates, calcium channel blockers, cholestyramine, clonidine, clozapine, colesevelam, corticosteroids, danazol, diazoxide, estrogens, glucagon, hydantoins, isoniazid, laxatives, lithium, morphine, nicotinic acid, olanzapine, oral contraceptives, phenothiazines, phenytoin, protease inhibitors, reserpine, rifabutin, rifampin, somatropin, sympathomimetics, thiazide and other diuretics, thyroid hormones, urinary alkalinizers: Increased risk of hyperglycemia
beta blockers: Possibly hyperglycemia or masking of hypoglycemia signs
digoxin: Increased risk of digitalis toxicity
miconazole (oral): Increased risk of severe hypoglycemia
pentamidine: Initially hypoglycemia and then hyperglycemia if beta cell damage occurs

G
H
I

sympatholytic drugs such as beta blockers, clonidine, guanethidine, reserpine: Reduced or absent hypoglycemic signs and symptoms

ACTIVITIES

alcohol use: Altered blood glucose control (usually hypoglycemia)

Adverse Reactions

CNS: Abnormal gait, anxiety, asthenia, chills, depression, dizziness, fatigue, headache, hypertonia, hypoesthesia, insomnia, malaise, migraine headache, nervousness, paresthesia, somnolence, syncope, tremor, vertigo

CV: Arrhythmias, edema, hypertension, vasculitis

EENT: Blurred vision, conjunctivitis, eye pain, pharyngitis, retinal hemorrhage, rhinitis, taste perversion, tinnitus

ENDO: Hypoglycemia, increased release of antidiuretic hormone secretion (SIADH)

GI: Anorexia, cholestasis, constipation, diarrhea, elevated liver enzymes, epigastric discomfort or fullness, flatulence, heartburn, hepatic porphyria, hepatotoxicity, hunger, jaundice, liver failure, nausea, proctocolitis, trace blood in stool, vomiting

GU: Darkened urine, decreased libido, dysuria, polyuria

HEME: Agranulocytosis, aplastic anemia, eosinophilia, hemolytic anemia, leukopenia, pancytopenia, thrombocytopenia

MS: Arthralgia, leg cramps, myalgia

RESP: Dyspnea

SKIN: Allergic skin reactions, diaphoresis, eczema, erythema multiforme, exfoliative dermatitis, flushing, lichenoid reactions, maculopapular or morbilliform rash, photosensitivity, pruritus, Stevens-Johnson syndrome, urticaria

Other: Anaphylaxis, angioedema, disulfiram-like reaction, hyponatremia

Nursing Considerations

• Use cautiously in patients with glucose 6-phosphate dehyrdrogenase (G6PD) deficiency because glimepiride is a sulfonylurea, and sulfonylureas can cause hemolytic anemia in these patients.

• Monitor fasting blood glucose level to determine response to glimepiride. Expect to check glycosylated hemoglobin level every 3 to 6 months to evaluate long-term blood glucose control.

• Arrange for dietary consultation and diabetic teaching, if appropriate. Ask dietitian to discuss amount of alcohol patient can consume without risking hypoglycemia.

• Expect to switch patient to insulin therapy, as prescribed, during physical stress, such as infection, surgery, and trauma.

WARNING Expect a higher risk of hypoglycemia when giving glimepiride to a malnourished or debilitated patient or one with renal, hepatic, pituitary, or adrenal insufficiency. Also be aware that hypoglycemia may be more difficult to recognize in patients with autonomic neuropathy, the elderly, and patients taking beta blockers or other sympatholytic agents. Monitor blood glucose level closely.

• Be aware that patients taking the sulfonylurea, tobutamide, may have an increased risk of dying from cardiovascular disease. Glimepiride has not been studied for cardiovascular mortality, but because it is also a sulfonylurea, monitor patients closely.

• Monitor patient closely for allergic reactions that could become life-threatening. If allergic reaction occurs, stop drug immediately and notifiy prescriber. Provide supportive care, as ordered.

PATIENT TEACHING

• Instruct patient to take glimepiride just before first meal of the day. Caution him not to skip the meal after taking drug.

• Urge patient not to skip doses or increase dosage without consulting prescriber.

• Urge patient to report signs of hypoglycemia, such as anxiety, confusion, dizziness, excessive sweating, headache, and nausea.

• Encourage patient to carry candy or other simple sugars to treat mild hypoglycemia.

• Advise patient to consult prescriber before taking any OTC drug.

• Urge patient to carry identification indicating that he has diabetes.

• Teach patient how to monitor his blood glucose level.

• Teach patient about exercise, diet, signs of hyperglycemia and hypoglycemia, hygiene, foot care, and ways to avoid infection.

• Instruct patient to notify prescriber about darkened urine, difficulty controlling his blood glucose level, easy bruising, fever, rash, sore throat, or unusual bleeding.
• If photosensitivity is a problem, instruct patient to avoid direct sunlight and to wear sunscreen.

glipizide
Glucotrol, Glucotrol XL

Class and Category
Chemical class: Sulfonylurea
Therapeutic class: Antidiabetic
Pregnancy category: C

Indications and Dosages
➤ To control blood glucose level in type 2 diabetes mellitus

E.R. TABLETS
Adults. Initial: 5 mg daily with breakfast. Dosage increased by 5 mg daily every 3 mo, if needed. Maintenance: 5 to 10 mg daily. Maximum: 20 mg daily.

TABLETS
Adults. Initial: 5 mg 30 min before first meal of day. Dosage adjusted by 2.5 to 5 mg every 2 to 3 days. For daily dose of 15 mg or less, give as a single dose. For dose above 15 mg daily, give in 2 divided doses. Maximum: 40 mg daily.

➤ As adjunct to or replacement for insulin therapy in type 2 diabetes mellitus

CAPSULES, TABLETS
Adults who need more than 20 units insulin daily. 5 mg daily, while decreasing insulin dosage by one-half. Further insulin reductions are based on clinical response.

DOSAGE ADJUSTMENT Initial dosage reduced to 2.5 mg daily if needed for patients over age 65 and those with hepatic disease.

Route	Onset	Peak	Duration
P.O.	10–30 min	30 min–2 hr	12–24 hr
P.O. (E.R.)	Unknown	Unknown	18–24 hr

Mechanism of Action
Stimulates insulin release from beta cells in pancreas. Glipizide also increases peripheral tissue sensitivity to insulin, either by increasing insulin binding to cellular receptors or by increasing number of insulin receptors.

Contraindications
Diabetes complicated by pregnancy; diabetic coma; hypersensitivity to glipizide, sulfonylureas, or their components; ketoacidosis; sole therapy for type 1 diabetes mellitus

Interaction
DRUGS
ACE inhibitors, anabolic steroids, androgens, azole antifungals, bromocriptine, chloramphenicol, disopyramide, fibric acid derivatives, guanethidine, H_2-receptor antagonists, insulin, magnesium salts, MAO inhibitors, methyldopa, octreotide, oral anticoagulants, oxyphenbutazone, phenylbutazone, probenecid, quinidine, salicylates, sulfonamides, tetracycline, theophylline, tricyclic antidepressants, urinary acidifiers: Increased risk of hypoglycemia
asparaginase, calcium channel blockers, cholestyramine, clonidine, colesevelam, corticosteroids, danazol, diazoxide, estrogen, glucagon, hydantoins, isoniazid, lithium, morphine, nicotinic acid, oral contraceptives, phenothiazines, rifabutin, rifampin, sympathomimetics, thiazide diuretics, thyroid drugs, urinary alkalinizers: Increased risk of hyperglycemia
beta blockers: Possibly hyperglycemia or masking of hypoglycemia signs
digitalis glycosides: Increased risk of digitalis toxicity
pentamidine: Initially hypoglycemia and then hyperglycemia if beta cell damage occurs
FOODS
all foods: Possibly delayed absorption of tablets if taken within 30 minutes of meal
ACTIVITIES
alcohol use: Altered blood glucose control (usually hypoglycemia)

Adverse Reactions
CNS: Abnormal gait, anxiety, asthenia, chills, depression, dizziness, fatigue, headache, hypertonia, hypoesthesia, insomnia, malaise, migraine headache, nervousness, paresthesia, somnolence, syncope, tremor, vertigo
CV: Arrhythmias, edema, hypertension, vasculitis

EENT: Blurred vision, conjunctivitis, eye pain, pharyngitis, retinal hemorrhage, rhinitis, taste perversion, tinnitus
ENDO: Hypoglycemia
GI: Abdominal pain, anorexia, cholestatic jaundice, constipation, diarrhea, elevated liver function test results, epigastric discomfort or fullness, flatulence, heartburn, hepatitis, hunger, nausea, proctocolitis, trace blood in stool, vomiting
GU: Darkened urine, decreased libido, dysuria, polyuria
HEME: Agranulocytosis, aplastic anemia, eosinophilia, hemolytic anemia, hepatic porphyria, leukopenia, pancytopenia
MS: Arthralgia, leg cramps, myalgia
RESP: Dyspnea
SKIN: Allergic skin reactions, diaphoresis, eczema, erythema multiforme, exfoliative dermatitis, flushing, jaundice, lichenoid reactions, maculopapular or morbilliform rash, photosensitivity, urticaria
Other: Disulfiram-like reaction

Nursing Considerations

- Use cautiously in patients with glucose 6-phosphate dehydrogenase deficiency because hemolytic anemia may develop. Monitor patient's CBC closely.
- To improve blood glucose control, give drug in divided doses instead of once daily.
- Check blood glucose level at least three times daily for a patient switching from insulin to glipizide. Patients who take more than 40 units of insulin daily may need hospitalization during transition.
- If patient gradually loses responsiveness to glipizide, expect to give a second antidiabetic to maintain blood glucose control.
- Monitor fasting blood glucose level to determine response to drug. Expect to check glycosylated hemoglobin every 3 to 6 months or as ordered to evaluate long-term blood glucose control.
- Expect to switch patient to insulin therapy, as prescribed, during physical stress, such as infection, surgery, or trauma.
- *WARNING* Risk of hypoglycemia is higher when giving glipizide to a malnourished or debilitated patient or one with renal, hepatic, pituitary, or adrenal insufficiency.

PATIENT TEACHING
- Tell patient to take glipizide 30 minutes before the first meal of the day. Caution him not to skip the meal after taking the drug.
- Advise patient not to skip doses or increase the dosage without consulting prescriber.
- Urge patient to report evidence of hypoglycemia, such as anxiety, confusion, dizziness, excessive sweating, headache, and nausea.
- Encourage patient to carry candy or other simple sugars to treat mild hypoglycemia.
- Caution patient to consult prescriber before taking any OTC drugs.
- Urge patient to carry identification indicating that he has diabetes.
- Teach patient how to monitor his blood glucose level.
- Teach patient about exercise, diet, signs of hyperglycemia and hypoglycemia, hygiene, foot care, and ways to avoid infection.
- Instruct patient to notify prescriber if he experiences darkened urine, easy bruising, fever, hypoglycemia or hyperglycemia, rash, sore throat, and unusual bleeding.
- If photosensitivity is a problem, instruct patient to avoid direct sunlight and to wear sunscreen.

glucagon

GlucaGen, Glucagon Diagnostic Kit, Glucagon Emergency Kit

Class and Category

Chemical class: Synthetic hormone
Therapeutic class: Antihypoglycemic, diagnostic aid adjunct
Pregnancy category: B

Indications and Dosages

➤ *To provide emergency treatment of severe hypoglycemia*

I.V., I.M., OR SUBCUTANEOUS INJECTION
Adults and children weighing more than 20 kg (44 lb) or, with GlucaGen, more than 25 kg (55 lb). 1 mg, repeated in 15 min as needed.
Children weighing 20 kg or less or, with GlucaGen, 25 kg or less. 0.5 mg, or 0.02 to 0.03 mg/kg, repeated in 15 min, as needed.

➤ *To provide diagnostic assistance by inhibiting bowel peristalsis in radiologic examination of GI tract*

I.V. INJECTION

Adults. 0.25 to 2 mg before procedure. Dose, route, and timing vary with segment of GI tract examined and length of procedure.

Route	Onset	Peak	Duration
I.V.	5–20 min*†	Unknown	90 min*‡
I.M.	15–26 min*§	Unknown	90 min*‖
SubQ	30–45 min*	Unknown	90 min*

Mechanism of Action

Increases production of adenylate cyclase, which catalyzes conversion of adenosine triphosphate to cAMP, a process that in turn activates phosphorylase. Phosphorylase promotes breakdown of glycogen to glucose (glycogenolysis) in the liver. As a result, blood glucose level increases and GI smooth muscles relax.

Incompatibilities

Don't mix glucagon with sodium chloride or solutions that have a pH of 3.0 to 9.5; use with dextrose solutions instead.

Contraindications

Hypersensitivity to glucagon or its components, pheochromocytoma

Interaction

DRUGS

oral anticoagulants: Possibly increased anticoagulant effects

Adverse Reactions

CV: Hypertension, hypotension (with hypersensitivity reaction), tachycardia
GI: Nausea, vomiting
RESP: Bronchospasm, respiratory distress
SKIN: Urticaria

Nursing Considerations

• Rouse patient as quickly as possible because prolonged hypoglycemia can cause cerebral damage.

---

* For antihypoglycemic action.
† 45 sec to 1 min for smooth-muscle relaxation.
‡ 9 to 25 min for smooth-muscle relaxation.
§ 4 to 10 min for smooth-muscle relaxation.
‖ 12 to 32 min for smooth-muscle relaxation.

• For I.V. use, reconstitute 1-mg vial of glucagon with 1 ml of diluent or 10-mg vial with 10 ml of diluent. Don't give more than 1 mg/ml. For large doses, dilute with sterile water for injection.
• Before injecting glucagon, place unconscious patient on his side to prevent aspiration of vomitus when he regains consciousness.
• Administer by slow I.V. injection to decrease risk of adverse reactions, such as tachycardia and vomiting.
• If patient doesn't respond to glucagon, expect to give I.V. dextrose.
• When patient is conscious or diagnostic procedure is completed, give oral carbohydrates to restore hepatic glycogen stores and prevent secondary hypoglycemia.
• Keep in mind that glucagon isn't effective in patients with depleted hepatic glycogen stores caused by such conditions as adrenal insufficiency, chronic hypoglycemia, and starvation.

PATIENT TEACHING

• Instruct patient to monitor blood glucose level, especially with signs of hypoglycemia.
• Teach patient and family members how to recognize signs of hypoglycemia and when to notify prescriber.
• Advise patient to carry candy or other simple sugars to treat early hypoglycemia.
• Emphasize importance of a consistent diet, regular exercise, and proper use of insulin or oral antidiabetic drug.
• Make sure unstable diabetic patients and family members know how to give glucagon subcutaneously in case of hypoglycemia. Instruct family members to keep patient on his side and give him a carbohydrate when he awakens. Advise against giving fluids by mouth until patient is fully conscious.
• Instruct patient and family members to call for emergency medical assistance after glucagon treatment, especially if patient can't ingest oral glucose or if he's taking the sulfonylurea chlorpropamide, in case secondary hypoglycemia occurs.

G
H
I

glyburide
(glibenclamide)

Albert Glyburide (CAN), Apo-Glyburide (CAN), DiaBeta, Euglucon (CAN), Gen-Glybe (CAN), Glynase PresTab, Medi-Glybe (CAN), Micronase, Novo-Glyburide (CAN), Nu-Glyburide (CAN)

Class and Category
Chemical class: Sulfonylurea
Therapeutic class: Antidiabetic
Pregnancy category: C (B for Glynase PresTab and Micronase)

Indications and Dosages
➤ *To control blood glucose level in type 2 diabetes mellitus*
MICRONIZED TABLETS
Adults. *Initial:* 1.5 to 3 mg daily with first meal of day, increased by up to 1.5 mg at weekly intervals, if needed. *Maintenance:* 0.75 to 12 mg as a single dose or in divided doses with meals.
NONMICRONIZED TABLETS
Adults. *Initial:* 2.5 to 5 mg daily with first meal of the day, increased by up to 2.5 mg at weekly intervals, if needed. *Maintenance:* 1.25 to 20 mg daily as a single dose or in divided doses with meals.
DOSAGE ADJUSTMENT For conversion from insulin to glyburide for adults who use more than 40 units of insulin daily, initial dosage adjusted to 5 mg non-micronized or 3 mg micronized glyburide as a single dose with 50% of usual insulin dose; glyburide dosage increased gradually, as needed. For adults who use less than 40 units insulin daily, usual glyburide dosage is used when insulin is discontinued.
For elderly patients, initial dosage possibly reduced to 1.25 mg nonmicronized glyburide daily, gradually increased by 2.5 mg/wk, as needed; or 0.75 to 3 mg micronized daily, gradually increased by 1.5 mg/wk, as needed.

Route	Onset	Peak	Duration
P.O.*	1 hr	2.3–3.5 hr	12–24 hr
P.O.†	15–60 min	1–3 hr	24 hr

Mechanism of Action
Stimulates insulin release from beta cells in the pancreas. Glyburide also increases peripheral tissue sensitivity to insulin either by enhancing insulin binding to cellular receptors or by increasing the number of insulin receptors.

Contraindications
Concurrent therapy with bosentan, diabetes complicated by pregnancy; diabetic ketoacidosis; hypersensitivity to glyburide, sulfonylureas, or their components; ketoacidosis; type 1 diabetes mellitus

Interaction
DRUGS
ACE inhibitors, anabolic steroids, androgens, azole antifungals, bromocriptine, chloramphenicol, clarithromycin, disopyramide, fibric acid derivatives, fluoxetine, guanethidine, H_2-receptor antagonists, insulin, magnesium salts, MAO inhibitors, methyldopa, NSAIDs, octreotide, oral anti-coagulants, oxyphenbutazone, phenylbutazone, probenecid, quinidine, quinolones, salicylates, sulfonamides, tetracycline, theophylline, tricyclic anti-depressants, urinary acidifiers: Increased risk of hypoglycemia
asparaginase, calcium channel blockers, cholestyramine, clonidine, colesevelam, corticosteroids, danazol, diazoxide, estrogen, glucagon, hydantoins, isoniazid, lithium, morphine, nicotinic acid, oral contraceptives, phenothiazines, rifabutin, rifampin, sympathomi-metics, thiazide diuretics, thyroid drugs, urinary alkalinizers: Increased risk of hyperglycemia
beta blockers: Possibly hyperglycemia or masking of hypoglycemia signs
bosentan: Increased risk of elevated liver enzymes
cyclosporine: Increased cyclosporine plasma level and toxicity
CYP2C9 and CYP3A4 inducers or inhibitors: Possibly altered blood glucose levels
digitalis glycosides: Increased risk of digitalis toxicity
miconazole (oral): Possibly severe hypo-glycemia

---
* Micronized.
† Nonmicronized.

oral anticoagulants: Possibly potentiated or weakened anticoagulant effects
pentamidine: Initial hypoglycemia and then hyperglycemia if beta cell damage occurs
rifampin: Decreased glyburide effectiveness
FOODS
high-fat foods: Reduced bioavailability of nonmicronized glyburide
ACTIVITIES
alcohol use: Altered blood glucose control (usually hypoglycemia)

Adverse Reactions

CNS: Abnormal gait, anxiety, asthenia, chills, depression, dizziness, fatigue, headache, hypertonia, hypoesthesia, insomnia, malaise, migraine headache, nervousness, paresthesia, somnolence, syncope, tremor, vertigo
CV: Arrhythmias, edema, hypertension, vasculitis
EENT: Blurred vision, conjunctivitis, eye pain, pharyngitis, retinal hemorrhage, rhinitis, taste perversion, tinnitus
ENDO: Hypoglycemia
GI: Anorexia, constipation, cholestatic jaundice, diarrhea, elevated liver function test results, epigastric discomfort or fullness, flatulence, heartburn, hepatic failure, hepatitis, hunger, nausea, proctocolitis, trace blood in stool, vomiting
GU: Decreased libido, dysuria, polyuria
HEME: Agranulocytosis, aplastic anemia, eosinophilia, hemolytic anemia, hepatic porphyria, leukopenia, pancytopenia
MS: Arthralgia, leg cramps, myalgia
RESP: Dyspnea
SKIN: Allergic skin reactions, diaphoresis, eczema, erythema multiforme, exfoliative dermatitis, flushing, jaundice, lichenoid reactions, maculopapular or morbilliform rash, photosensitivity, urticaria
Other: Disulfiram-like reaction

Nursing Considerations

• Use cautiously in patients with glucose 6-phosphate dehydrogenase deficiency because hemolytic anemia may develop. Monitor patient's CBC closely.
• Give glyburide as single dose before first meal of the day. If patient takes more than 10 mg daily or if severe GI distress occurs, give in 2 divided doses before meals.

• Monitor fasting blood glucose level to determine patient's response to glyburide. Expect to check glycosylated hemoglobin every 3 to 6 months or as ordered to evaluate long-term blood glucose control.
• When patient switches from insulin to glyburide, check blood glucose level three times daily before meals.
• Be aware that micronized tablets aren't equal to nonmicronized tablets; they contain smaller particles, which affects drug bioavailability.
WARNING Expect a higher risk of hypoglycemia when giving drug to a malnourished or debilitated patient or one with renal, hepatic, pituitary, or adrenal insufficiency. Also be aware that hypoglycemia may be more difficult to recognize in patients with autonomic neuropathy, the elderly, and patients who are taking beta blockers or other sympatholytic agents. Monitor blood glucose level closely.
• Monitor patient with history of allergies to other sulfonamide derivatives closely because he may be allergic to glyburide. If allergic reactions persist or worsen (dyspnea, drop in blood pressure, or shock), expect drug to be discontinued.
• Administer insulin as needed and prescribed during periods of increased stress, such as infection, surgery, and trauma.
• Arrange for diabetic teaching and consultation between patient and dietitian, if appropriate.
PATIENT TEACHING
• Instruct patient to take glyburide just before first meal of the day. Caution him not to skip the meal after taking drug.
• Advise patient not to take nonmicronized glyburide with a high-fat meal because it may reduce glyburide bioavailability.
• Caution patient to avoid skipping doses, discontinuing glyburide, or taking OTC drugs without first consulting prescriber.
• Teach patient how to monitor his blood glucose level and when to notify prescriber about changes.
• Urge patient to report signs of hypoglycemia: anxiety, confusion, dizziness, excessive sweating, headache, and nausea.

G
H
I

• Suggest that patient carry candy or other simple sugars to treat mild hypoglycemia.
• Urge patient to avoid alcohol because it increases the risk of hypoglycemia.
• Advise patient to carry identification indicating that he has diabetes.
• Teach patient about exercise, diet, signs of hyperglycemia and hypoglycemia, hygiene, foot care, and ways to avoid infection.
• Instruct patient to notify prescriber if he experiences easy bruising, fever, hypoglycemia or hyperglycemia, rash, sore throat, and unusual bleeding.
• If photosensitivity is a problem, instruct patient to avoid direct sunlight and to wear sunscreen.

glycopyrrolate

Cuvposa, Robinul, Robinul Forte

Class and Category

Chemical class: Quaternary ammonium compound
Therapeutic class: Antiarrhythmic, anticholinergic, cholinergic adjunct
Pregnancy category: B

Indications and Dosages

➤ *To treat peptic ulcer disease*
TABLETS
Adults and adolescents. 1 to 2 mg twice daily or three times daily. *Maximum:* 8 mg daily.
I.V. OR I.M. INJECTION
Adults and adolescents. 0.1 to 0.2 mg every 4 hr, as needed. *Maximum:* 4 doses daily.
➤ *To reduce gastric acid and respiratory secretions before anesthesia*
I.M. INJECTION
Adults and adolescents. 0.0044 mg/kg 30 to 60 min before anesthesia or when preanesthesia sedative or opioid is given.
Children over age 2. 0.0044 to 0.0088 mg/kg 30 to 60 min before anesthesia or when preanesthesia sedative or opioid is given.
➤ *To counteract intraoperative and anesthesia-induced arrhythmias*
I.V. INJECTION
Adults and adolescents. 0.1 mg, repeated every 2 to 3 min, if needed.

Children over age 2. 0.0044 mg/kg. Dose repeated every 2 to 3 min, if needed. *Maximum:* 0.1 mg as a single dose.
➤ *As cholinergic adjunct in curariform block*
I.V. INJECTION
Adults and children over age 2. 0.2 mg glycopyrrolate for each 1 mg neostigmine or 5 mg pyridostigmine when given together.
➤ *To reduce chronic severe drooling in patients with neurologic conditions associated with problem drooling, such as cerebral palsy*
ORAL SOLUTION
Children ages 3 to 16. *Initial:* 0.02 mg/kg three times daily 1 hr before meals or 2 hr after meals, increased in increments of 0.02 mg/kg every 5 to 7 days, as needed and based on response and adverse reactions. *Maximum:* 0.1 mg/kg three times daily not to exceed 1.5 to 3 mg per dose based on weight of child.

Route	Onset	Peak	Duration
P.O.	60 min	Unknown	8–12 hr
I.V.	1 min	Unknown	2–3 hr*
I.M., SubQ	15–30 min	30–45 min	2–3 hr*

Mechanism of Action

Inhibits acetylcholine's action on postganglionic muscarinic receptors throughout the body. Depending on the receptors' location, glycopyrrolate produces various effects, such as:
• reducing the volume and acidity of gastric secretions
• controlling excessive bronchial, pharyngeal, and tracheal secretions and dilating the bronchi
• inhibiting vagal stimulation of the heart
• relaxing smooth muscle in the GI and GU tracts.

Incompatibilities

Don't mix glycopyrrolate with alkaline drugs or solutions that have a pH over 6.0 because drug stability may be affected. A pH over 6.0 may occur if glycopyrrolate is mixed with dexamethasone sodium phosphate or LR solution. Gas or precipitate may form if glycopyrrolate is mixed in same

---

* For vagal blocking effect; up to 7 hr for reduction of saliva.

syringe as chloramphenicol, diazepam, dimenhydrinate, methohexital sodium, pentobarbital sodium, secobarbital sodium, sodium bicarbonate, or thiopental sodium.

Contraindications

Angle-closure glaucoma, asthma, concomitant use of solid oral dosage forms of potassium chloride (Cuvposa), hemorrhage with unstable cardiovascular status, hepatic disease, hypersensitivity to anticholinergics, ileus, intestinal atony, myasthenia gravis, obstructive GI or urinary disorders, severe ulcerative colitis, toxic megacolon

Interaction

DRUGS

anticholinergics, antiparkinsonian drugs, phenothiazines, tricyclic antidepressants: Possibly increased anticholinergic effects
antidiarrheals (adsorbent): Decreased glycopyrrolate absorption, leading to decreased therapeutic effectiveness
antimyasthenics: Possibly reduced intestinal motility
atenolol: Possibly potentiated atenolol effects
calcium- or magnesium-containing antacids, carbonic anhydrase inhibitors, citrates, sodium bicarbonate: Possibly reduced excretion of glycopyrrolate and increased therapeutic and adverse effects
cyclopropane: Possibly ventricular arrhythmias
digoxin: Possibly potentiated digoxin effects
haloperidol, levodopa, phenothiazines: Possibly decreased effectiveness of these drugs
ketoconazole: Possibly decreased ketoconazole absorption
metformin: Possibly potentiated metformin effects
metoclopramide: Possibly antagonized effects of metoclopramide
opioids: Possibly severe constipation and urine retention, risk of ileus
potassium chloride: Possibly increased severity of potassium chloride–induced gastric lesions

Adverse Reactions

CNS: Confusion, dizziness, drowsiness, headache, insomnia, nervousness, weakness
CV: Bradycardia (low doses), heart block, palpitations, prolonged QT interval, tachycardia (high doses)

EENT: Blurred vision, cycloplegia, dilated pupils, dry mouth, increased intraocular pressure, loss of taste, mydriasis, nasal congestion, photophobia, taste perversion
GI: Abdominal distention, constipation, dysphagia, nausea, vomiting
GU: Impotence, urinary hesitancy, urine retention
RESP: Dyspnea
SKIN: Decreased sweating (heat exhaustion), dry skin, flushing, pruritus, urticaria
Other: Anaphylaxis

Nursing Considerations

• Use glycopyrrolate cautiously in patients with autonomic neuropathy, hepatic disease, mild to moderate ulcerative colitis, prostatic hypertrophy, or hiatal hernia because drug's anticholinergic effect can worsen these conditions; gastric ulcer because drug may delay gastric emptying; and renal disease because drug excretion may be altered.
• Give tablets 30 to 60 minutes before meals.
• As needed and prescribed, give 2-mg dose at bedtime to ensure overnight control of symptoms.
• For I.V. use, administer by direct injection without diluting. Or inject into tubing of flowing I.V. solution unless it contains an alkaline drug or sodium bicarbonate.
• Closure system contains dry natural rubber that may cause hypersensitivity reaction if handled by or used to inject someone with latex sensitivity.
• Use continuous cardiac monitoring, as ordered, to assess patient for arrhythmias during drug administration.
WARNING Check all doses carefully because even a slight overdose can lead to toxicity.
• To prevent overheating caused by decreased sweating, adjust the room temperature and make sure patient is well hydrated.

PATIENT TEACHING

• Advise patient to take glycopyrrolate tablets 30 to 60 minutes before meals.
• Instruct patient to consult prescriber before taking any OTC drugs.
• Caution patient about possible drowsiness and dizziness and need to avoid hazardous activities until drug's effects are known.

G
H
I

- Suggest that patient use sugarless hard candy, ice, or saliva substitute to relieve dry mouth.
- Instruct patient to avoid exertion and hot environments because he's prone to heat exhaustion while taking glycopyrrolate.
- Urge patient to drink at least 8 glasses of water daily, unless contraindicated.
- Tell patient to notify prescriber about abdominal distention, trouble breathing or urinating, eye pain, irregular heartbeat, sensitivity to light, or severe constipation.
- Advise patient to wear sunglasses in bright light.
- Inform male patient that reversible impotence may occur during therapy.
- If urinary hesitancy occurs, advise patient to void before taking each dose.

golimumab

Simponi, Simponi Aria

Class and Category

Chemical class: Human IgG$_1$ monoclonal antibody
Therapeutic class: Biologic disease-modifying anti-rheumatic drug (DMARD)
Pregnancy category: B

Indications and Dosages

➤ *To treat active psoriatic arthritis or ankylosing spondylitis with or without methotrexate or other nonbiologic Disease Modifying Antirheumatic Drugs (DMARD)s*

SUBCUTANEOUS INJECTION (SIMPONI)

Adults. 50 mg monthly.

➤ *To treat moderate to severe active rheumatoid arthritis in combination with methotrexate*

I.V. INFUSION (SIMPONI ARIA)

Adults. 2 mg/kg infused over 30 minutes at weeks 0 and 4, then every 8 wks thereafter.

SUBCUTANEOUS INJECTION (SIMPONI)

Adults. 50 mg monthly.

➤ *To treat moderate to severe active ulcerative colitis in patients who have demonstrated corticosteroid dependence or who have had an inadequate response to or failed to tolerate oral aminosalicylates, oral corticosteroids, azathioprine, or 6-mercaptopruine*

SUBCUTANEOUS INJECTION (SIMPONI)

Adults. *Initial:* 200 mg at week 0, followed by 100 mg at week 2. *Maintenance:* 100 mg every 4 wks.

Route	Onset	Peak	Duration
SubQ	Unknown	2–6 days	Unknown

Mechanism of Action

Binds to a cytokine protein, tumor necrosis factor alpha (TNFa), to block interaction with its receptors, which prevents biological activity of TNFa. Elevated TNFa levels in the blood, synovium, and joints may play an important role in pathophysiology of such inflammatory diseases as rheumatoid arthritis, psoriatic arthritis, and ankylosing spondylitis. Reduced TNFa activity in these disorders improves signs and symptoms.

Incompatibilities

Don't mix golimumab solution for intravenous infusion with other drugs, as incompatibilities are unknown.

Contraindications

Hypersensitivity to golimumab or its components

Interaction

DRUGS

abatacept, anakinra, rituximab: Possibly increased risk of serious infection
cytochrome P-450 substrates such as cyclosporine, theophylline, warfarin: Effects or blood levels of these drugs may change when golimumab therapy starts or stops
live vaccines, therapeutic infectious agents such as BCG bladder instillation for treatment of cancer: Increased risk of adverse vaccine effects

Adverse Reactions

CNS: Dizziness, fever, paresthesia
CV: Hypertension
EENT: Nasopharyngitis, oral herpes, pharyngitis, rhinitis, sinusitis
GI: Elevated liver enzyme levels
RESP: Bronchitis, interstitial lung disease, pneumonia, tuberculosis, upper respiratory tract infection
SKIN: Bullous skin reactions, cellulitis, melanoma, new or worsening psoriasis, rash, skin exfoliation
Other: Abscess; anaphylaxis; antibody formation; bacterial (including Legionella

and Listeria), fungal, mycobacterial, parasitic, or viral infections (including invasive fungal infections and reactivation of hepatitis B infection in chronic carriers); influenza; injection-site erythema; lupus-like syndrome; malignancies such as leukemia or lymphoma; sarcoidosis; sepsis

Nursing Considerations

• Make sure patient has a tuberculin skin test before therapy starts. If skin test is positive, treatment of latent tuberculosis must start before golimumab therapy starts, as prescribed. Also anti-tuberculosis therapy may be started if patient has a history of latent or active tuberculosis, if adequate therapy can't be confirmed, or if patient has a negative test for latent tuberculosis but also has risk factors for tuberculosis.

WARNING If patient has evidence of an active infection when drug is prescribed, golimumab therapy shouldn't start until infection has been treated. Monitor all patients for bacterial (including Legionella and Listeria), fungal, mycobacterial, parasitic, or viral infection during therapy, especially those receiving immunosuppressants. Know that the infection could become life-threatening and affect multiple organs. If a serious infection, an opportunistic infection, or sepsis develops, expect prescriber to stop drug and start appropriate antimicrobial therapy. Monitor patient closely for tuberculosis throughout golimumab therapy because active tuberculosis has occurred in patients during and after treatment of latent tuberculosis.

• Patients with a history of cancer, except those successfully treated for nonmelanoma skin cancer, should be thoroughly evaluated before golimumab therapy starts because treatment may pose more risks than benefits. Patients with rheumatoid arthritis may have a higher risk than the general population for developing leukemia while taking a TNF blocker such as golimumab.

• Use golimumab cautiously in patients with recurrent infection or increased risk of infection, patients who live in regions where tuberculosis and histoplasmosis are endemic, and patients with a history of

hepatitis B infection because drug increases risk of infection.

• Use golimumab cautiously in patients with congestive heart failure, demyelinating disorders such as multiple sclerosis, and hematologic cytopenias because these disorders have occurred with use of other TNF blockers.

• Be aware that needle cover of syringe used for subcutaneous injection contains dry rubber. Don't handle if you're allergic to latex.

• Take golimumab out of the refrigerator 30 minutes before giving subcutaneous injection to allow time for drug to warm up to room temperature. Never warm drug in any other way. Rotate subcutaneous injection sites. If more than one subcutaneous injection is required, administer the injections at different sites on the body.

• Know that each 4-ml vial used for intravenous infusion contains 50 mg of golimumab. Dilute the total volume of the drug solution with normal saline for intravenous infusion for a final volume of 100 ml. Gently mix. Discard any unused solution remaining in the vials. Use within 4 hours, keeping diluted solution at room temperature.

• Inspect diluted solution for intravenous infusion prior to infusion for particulate matter or discoloration. Do not use if present. Use only an infusion set with an in-line, sterile, nonpyrogenic, low protein-binding filter (pore size 0.22 micrometer or less). Do not infuse concomitantly in the same intravenous line with other drugs. Infuse the diluted solution over 30 minutes.

PATIENT TEACHING

• Explain that first injection of golimumab must be administered with a healthcare professional present.

• Teach patient or caregiver how to give golimumab as a subcutaneous injection at home, if applicable. Tell him to let prefilled syringe or autoinjector sit at room temperature outside carton for 30 minutes before injecting. Tell him not to warm drug in any other way and not to remove needle cover or cap while letting golimumab warm up.

• Teach patient using autoinjector not to pull the device away from his skin until he hears a first "click" and then a second "click" indicating the injection is finished. It may take up to 15 seconds before second click is heard and, if device is pulled away from the skin before the second click, a full dose may not have been given.
• Emphasize need to inject full amount in prefilled syringe to obtain correct dose. Instruct patient to discard any drug left in prefilled syringe or autoinjector.
• Tell patient requiring multiple injections to administer the injections at different sites on the body.
• If patient is allergic to latex, explain that needle cover contains natural dry rubber.
• Instruct patient or caregiver to use a puncture resistant container to dispose of needles and syringes at home.
• Inform patient that drug must be refrigerated (not frozen).
• Urge patient to check expiration dates and not to use outdated drug.
• Teach patient to rotate injection sites and never to give injection into an area where skin is tender, bruised, red, or hard.
• Explain that tuberculosis may occur during golimumab therapy. Instruct him to report persistent cough, wasting or weight loss, and low-grade fever to prescriber.
• Teach patient to recognize evidence of infection and bleeding disorders and to tell prescriber if they occur; drug may need to be stopped. Advise patient to avoid people with infections and to have all prescribed laboratory tests performed.
• Inform patient that golimumab therapy increases the risk of certain kinds of cancer, especially lymphomas and leukemias. Emphasize the importance of having follow-up visits and reporting unusual or sudden onset of signs or symptoms. Also, encourage patient to have regular skin examinations, as melanomas have occurred with golimumab therapy.
• Caution against receiving live-virus vaccines while taking golimumab; doing so may adversely affect the immune system.
• Tell patient to report lupus-like signs and symptoms that, although rare, may occur during therapy, such as chest pain that doesn't go away, shortness of breath, joint pain, or a rash on cheeks or arms that's

sensitive to the sun. Explain that drug may need to be discontinued if these occur.
• Advise patient to tell all healthcare providers about golimumab therapy and to tell prescriber about any OTC drugs, herbal remedies, and vitamin and mineral supplements being taken.

granisetron hydrochloride

Kytril, Sancuso

Class and Category
Chemical class: Carbazole
Therapeutic class: Antiemetic
Pregnancy category: B

Indications and Dosages
➤ *To prevent nausea and vomiting caused by chemotherapy*

ORAL SOLUTION, TABLETS
Adults and adolescents. 1 mg up to 1 hr before chemotherapy, repeated 12 hr later. Or, 2 mg up to 1 hr before chemotherapy.

I.V. INFUSION
Adults and adolescents. 10 mcg/kg diluted and infused over 5 min, starting 30 min before chemotherapy; or 10 mcg/kg undiluted and infused over 30 sec, starting 30 min before chemotherapy.

TRANSDERMAL
Adults. 3.1 mg/24 hr patch applied to upper outer arm 24 to 48 hr before chemotherapy and worn up to 7 days. Patch removed no sooner than 24 hr after chemotherapy is completed.
➤ *To prevent nausea and vomiting caused by radiation therapy*

ORAL SOLUTION, TABLETS
Adults and adolescents. 2 mg daily given 1 hr before radiation therapy.
➤ *To prevent or treat postoperative nausea and vomiting*

I.V. INJECTION
Adults and adolescents. 1 mg given over 30 sec before induction of anesthesia or immediately before reversal anesthesia for prevention. 1 mg administered over 30 sec after surgery for treatment.

Mechanism of Action

Has a high affinity for serotonin receptors along vagal nerve endings in intestines. Because of this affinity, granisetron prevents nausea and vomiting that usually result when serotonin is released by damaged enterochromaffin cells.

Incompatibilities

Don't mix granisetron in same solution as other drugs.

Contraindications

Hypersensitivity to granisetron or its components

Interaction

DRUGS

drugs that prolong the QT interval: Increased risk of QT-interval prolongation

Adverse Reactions

CNS: Asthenia, chills, CNS stimulation, drowsiness, fever, headache, insomnia, serotonin syndrome, somnolence
CV: Hypertension, prolonged QT interval
EENT: Taste perversion
GI: Abdominal pain, anorexia, constipation, diarrhea, elevated liver function test results, nausea, vomiting
HEME: Anemia, leukopenia, thrombocytopenia
SKIN: Alopecia, reactions at patch application site (pruritus, rash, redness)

Nursing Considerations

• Use cautiously in patients with arrhythmias or cardiac conduction disorders because granisetron may prolong QT interval. Patients especially at risk include those with cardiac disease or electrolyte abnormalities and those receiving cardiotoxic chemotherapy or therapy with another drug that prolongs QT interval.
• For use with chemotherapy, dilute I.V. preparation of granisetron with normal saline solution or D_5W to total volume of 20 to 50 ml. Mixture may be stored up to 24 hours. Use only on days when chemotherapy is given.
• Apply transdermal patch to patient's upper outer arm 24 to 48 hours before chemotherapy, and don't remove it until at least 24 hours after chemotherapy is completed.

WARNING Monitor patient for serotonin syndrome, characterized by agitation, chills, confusion, diaphoresis, diarrhea, fever, hyperactive reflexes, poor coordination, restlessness, shaking, talking or acting with uncontrolled excitement, tremor, and twitching.

PATIENT TEACHING

• Inform patient that granisetron is given orally or I.V. before chemotherapy to help prevent nausea.
• Instruct patient to take granisetron tablet without food to avoid reducing drug bioavailability.
• Advise patient to report constipation, fever, severe diarrhea, or severe headache. Also caution about possible drowsiness.
• Advise patient wearing granisetron patch to cover it with clothing if there's a risk of exposure to sunlight. Tell patient to continue covering application site with clothing for 10 days after removal of patch.

WARNING Instruct patient to seek immediate medical attention if the following symptoms occur: changes in mental status, autonomic instability, neuromuscular symptoms, with or without gastrointestinal symptoms.

guaifenesin

Anti-Tuss, Balminil Expectorant (CAN), Benylin-E (CAN), Breonesin, Calmylin Expectorant (CAN), Gee-Gee, Genatuss, GG-CEN, Glycotuss, Glytuss, Guaituss, Halotussin, Hytuss, Hytuss 2X, Mucinex, Organidin NR, Resyl (CAN), Robitussin, Scot-tussin Expectorant, Uni-tussin

Class and Category

Chemical class: Glyceryl guaiacolate
Therapeutic class: Expectorant
Pregnancy category: C

Indications and Dosages

➤ *To relieve cough, especially when secretions are thick*

CAPSULES, ORAL SOLUTION, SYRUP, TABLETS
Adults and adolescents. 200 to 400 mg every 4 hr. *Maximum:* 2,400 mg daily.

CAPSULES, ORAL SOLUTION, SYRUP
Children ages 6 to 12. 100 to 200 mg every 4 hr. *Maximum:* 1,200 mg daily.
➤ *To promote productive cough*
E.R. TABLETS (MUCINEX)
Adults and adolescents. 600 to 1,200 mg every 12 hr. *Maximum:* 2,400 mg daily.

Route	Onset	Peak	Duration
P.O.	30 min	Unknown	4–6 hr

Mechanism of Action
Increases fluid and mucus removal from the upper respiratory tract by increasing the volume of secretions and reducing their adhesiveness and surface tension.

Contraindications
Hypersensitivity to guaifenesin

Adverse Reactions
CNS: Dizziness, headache
GI: Nausea and vomiting (with large doses)
SKIN: Rash, urticaria

Nursing Considerations
• As prescribed and as appropriate, give liquid forms of guaifenesin to children.
• Watch for evidence of more serious condition, such as cough that lasts longer than 1 week, fever, persistent headache, and rash.
PATIENT TEACHING
• Instruct patient to take each dose with a full glass of water.
• Advise patient not to break, crush, or chew E.R. tablets but to swallow them whole.
• Tell patient to increase fluid intake (unless contraindicated) to help thin secretions.
• Advise patient not to take drug longer than 1 week and to notify prescriber about fever, persistent headache, or rash.

---

guanadrel sulfate

Hylorel

Class and Category
Chemical class: Guanidine derivative
Therapeutic class: Antihypertensive
Pregnancy category: B

Indications and Dosages
➤ *To manage hypertension*

TABLETS
Adults. 5 mg twice daily, increased to 20 to 75 mg daily in divided doses three times daily or four times daily, if needed.
DOSAGE ADJUSTMENT Initial dosage reduced to 5 mg daily if needed for patients with renal impairment or creatinine clearance of 30 to 60 ml/min/1.73 m^2. Then, adjusted after at least 7 days. Initial dosage reduced to 5 mg every other day if needed for patients with creatinine clearance less than 30 ml/min/1.73 m^2. Then, dosage adjusted after at least 2 wk.

Route	Onset	Peak	Duration
P.O.	30 min–2 hr	4–6 hr	4–14 hr

Mechanism of Action
Exerts antihypertensive effect at peripheral sympathetic nerve endings. Through an uptake mechanism, guanadrel is stored in adrenergic neurons, where it displaces norepinephrine from its storage sites. This action blocks normal release of norepinephrine in response to nerve impulses, which depletes norepinephrine stores in synapses and relaxes vessel walls, thus reducing peripheral resistance and blood pressure.

Contraindications
Heart failure not caused by hypertension, hypersensitivity to guanadrel or its components, MAO inhibitor use within 1 week of guanadrel use, pheochromocytoma

Interaction
DRUGS
alpha blockers, beta blockers, rauwolfia alkaloids: Possibly orthostatic hypotension or bradycardia
amphetamines, appetite suppressants, cyclobenzaprine, haloperidol, loxapine, maprotiline, methylphenidate, phenothiazines, thioxanthenes, tricyclic antidepressants: Decreased antihypertensive effect of guanadrel
anticholinergics: Possibly decreased inhibition of gastric acid secretion
barbiturates, opioids: Possibly increased hypotensive effect
MAO inhibitors: Possibly severe blood pressure increase
NSAIDs: Possibly sodium and water retention and decreased antihypertensive effect of guanadrel

sympathomimetics: Possibly reduced anti-hypertensive effect of guanadrel, leading to hypertension; possibly potentiated effects of sympathomimetics
vasodilators: Increased orthostatic hypotension
ACTIVITIES
alcohol use: Increased hypotensive effect

Adverse Reactions

CNS: Confusion, drowsiness, fatigue, headache, light-headedness, paresthesia, sleep disturbance
CV: Chest pain, orthostatic hypotension, palpitations, peripheral edema
EENT: Blurred vision, dry mouth and throat, glossitis
GI: Abdominal cramps or pain, anorexia, constipation, diarrhea, indigestion, nausea, vomiting
GU: Difficult ejaculation, hematuria, impotence, nocturia, urinary frequency or urgency
MS: Arthralgia, back or neck pain, joint inflammation, leg cramps, muscle weakness, myalgia
RESP: Cough, dyspnea
Other: Excessive weight gain or loss

Nursing Considerations

• Use guanadrel cautiously in patients with asthma because drug may aggravate this condition. Monitor patient for acute dyspnea, wheezing, and other evidence of asthma attack. Notify prescriber immediately if they develop.
WARNING Assess patient for evidence of overdose, such as blurred vision, dizziness, and syncope.
• Be aware that elderly patients have a greater risk of dizziness and syncope.
• Assess for signs of fluid retention and heart failure, including crackles, a new S_3 heart sound, and sudden weight gain.

PATIENT TEACHING
• Explain that guanadrel won't cure high blood pressure but will help control it.
• Instruct patient to take drug at the same time each day to improve compliance and blood pressure control.
• Caution patient about possible dizziness, light-headedness, and fainting, especially when getting up from a lying or sitting position. Advise him to rise slowly,

especially in the morning, and to sit with his feet dangling for 1 to 2 minutes before standing up.
• Instruct patient to sit or lie down immediately if he feels dizzy.
• To prevent fainting, advise patient to avoid alcohol, standing for long periods, pursuing excessive exercise, and being overly exposed to hot weather.
• Instruct patient to check with prescriber before taking OTC drugs during therapy.
• Advise patient to follow a low-sodium diet to help reduce blood pressure and prevent fluid retention.

guanethidine monosulfate

Apo-Guanethidine (CAN), Ismelin

Class and Category

Chemical class: Guanidine derivative
Therapeutic class: Antihypertensive
Pregnancy category: C

Indications and Dosages

➤ *To manage moderate to severe hypertension and renal hypertension*
TABLETS
Adults. *Initial:* 10 to 12.5 mg daily, increased as needed by 10 to 12.5 mg every wk. *Maintenance:* 25 to 50 mg daily. Some patients may need up to 300 mg daily.
Children. 0.2 mg/kg daily, increased as needed, by 0.2 mg/kg every 7 to 10 days. *Maximum:* 3 mg/kg every 24 hr.
DOSAGE ADJUSTMENT Initial dosage increased to 25 to 50 mg daily for hospitalized adults because they can be monitored more closely. Then dosage increased by 25 to 50 mg every other day, as needed.

Route	Onset	Peak	Duration
P.O.	Unknown	8 hr	Unknown

Mechanism of Action

Exerts antihypertensive effect at peripheral sympathetic nerve endings. Through an uptake mechanism, guanethidine is stored in adrenergic neurons, where it displaces norepinephrine from its storage sites. This action blocks normal release of norepinephrine in response to nerve impulses, which depletes norepinephrine stores in synapses and relaxes vessel walls, reducing peripheral resistance and blood pressure.

Contraindications

Heart failure not caused by hypertension, hypersensitivity to guanethidine or its components, MAO inhibitor use within 1 week of guanethidine use, pheochromocytoma

Interaction

DRUGS

alpha blockers, beta blockers, rauwolfia alkaloids: Possibly orthostatic hypotension or bradycardia

amphetamines, appetite suppressants, cyclobenzaprine, haloperidol, loxapine, maprotiline, methylphenidate, phenothiazines, thioxanthenes, tricyclic antidepressants: Decreased antihypertensive effect of guanethidine

anticholinergics: Possibly decreased inhibition of gastric acid secretion

barbiturates, opioids: Increased hypotensive effect

insulin, oral antidiabetic drugs: Possibly increased antidiabetic effect of these drugs

MAO inhibitors: Possibly severe blood pressure increase

NSAIDs: Possibly sodium and water retention and decreased antihypertensive effect of guanethidine

sympathomimetics: Possibly reduced antihypertensive effect of guanethidine, leading to hypertension; possibly potentiated effects of sympathomimetics

vasodilators: Increased orthostatic hypotension

ACTIVITIES

alcohol use: Increased hypotensive effect

Adverse Reactions

CNS: Depression, dizziness, fatigue, headache, lassitude, paresthesia, syncope
CV: Angina, bradycardia, orthostatic hypotension, palpitations, peripheral edema
EENT: Blurred vision, dry mouth, glossitis, nasal congestion, parotid gland tenderness, ptosis
GI: Anorexia, constipation, diarrhea (severe), indigestion, nausea, vomiting

GU: Ejaculation disorders, elevated BUN level, impotence, nocturia, priapism, urinary frequency
HEME: Anemia, leukopenia, thrombocytopenia
MS: Leg cramps, muscle twitching, myalgia
RESP: Asthma exacerbation, dyspnea
SKIN: Alopecia, dermatitis
Other: Weight gain

Nursing Considerations

• As prescribed, stop MAO inhibitor therapy at least 1 week before starting guanethidine.
• Because guanethidine has cumulative effects, give a small initial dose and increase gradually, as prescribed. When blood pressure is controlled, expect to reduce dosage to lowest effective level.
• Watch for orthostatic hypotension, which occurs most often when patient rises in the morning and is exacerbated by hot weather, exercise, and alcohol. Assess supine and standing blood pressures, especially after dosage adjustments.
• Measure daily weight to help detect fluid retention. Also observe for edema and other signs of heart failure. A thiazide diuretic may be prescribed to decrease sodium and fluid retention.
• Notify prescriber if severe diarrhea occurs. Drug may need to be discontinued.
• Monitor febrile patient for increased hypotension and adverse reactions because fever decreases drug requirements.
• As ordered, stop giving guanethidine 2 weeks before surgery to reduce risk of cardiac arrest during anesthesia.

PATIENT TEACHING

• Teach patient how to recognize orthostatic hypotension, and advise changing position slowly. Explain that symptoms are worse in the morning and worsened by exercise, hot weather, alcohol, and hot showers.
• Instruct patient to report fainting, frequent dizziness, and severe diarrhea.
• Caution patient to avoid alcohol because it may increase risk of orthostatic hypotension.
• Instruct patient to weigh himself daily at the same time, on the same scale, and wearing the same amount of clothing.

Advise him to report signs of fluid retention, such as reduced urine volume, sudden weight increase, and limb swelling.
• Urge patient to consult prescriber before taking OTC drugs during guanethidine therapy.
• If a diabetic patient takes insulin or a sulfonylurea, instruct him to monitor his blood glucose level more frequently to check for hypoglycemia.
• Advise patient to follow a low-sodium diet to help reduce blood pressure and prevent fluid retention.

guanfacine hydrochloride

Intuniv, Tenex

Class and Category
Chemical class: Dichlorobenzine derivative
Therapeutic class: Antihypertensive
Pregnancy category: B

Indications and Dosages
➤ *To manage hypertension, alone or with other antihypertensives*
TABLETS
Adults. 1 mg daily at bedtime, increased as needed to 2 mg after 3 to 4 wk. Increased to 3 mg if needed after another 3 to 4 wk. *Maintenance:* 2 or 3 mg daily.
DOSAGE ADJUSTMENT Twice-daily administration used if blood pressure tends to rise at the end of 24-hr period.
➤ *To treat attention deficit hyperactivity disorder (ADHD); adjunct therapy with stimulant medications*
E.R. TABLETS
Adults and children age 6 and over. *Initial:* 1 mg once daily, increased, as needed, by 1 mg/wk. *Maintenance:* 1 to 4 mg once daily. *Maximum:* 4 mg once daily.

Route	Onset	Peak	Duration
P.O.	Unknown*	8–12 hr†	24 hr

Mechanism of Action
Decreases sympathetic nerve impulse outflow from the vasomotor center of the brain to the heart and blood vessels by

---

* For single dose; in 1 wk for multiple doses.
† For single dose; 1 to 3 mo for multiple doses.

stimulating central alpha$_2$-adrenergic receptors. This action reduces peripheral vascular resistance, renovascular resistance, heart rate, and blood pressure. Prolonged guanfacine use may reduce total peripheral vascular resistance, slightly reducing heart rate. Guanfacine also stimulates growth hormone secretion, reduces circulating plasma catecholamine levels, and reduces left ventricular hypertrophy.

Contraindications
Hypersensitivity to guanfacine

Interaction
DRUGS
CNS depressants: Possibly increased CNS depression
ketoconazole and other strong CYP3A4/5 inhibitors: Increased plasma guanfacine level and increased risk of bradycardia, hypotension, and sedation
NSAIDs, sympathomimetics, tricyclic antidepressants: Possibly decreased antihypertensive effect of guanfacine
other antihypertensives: Possibly increased antihypertensive effect, resulting in hypotension
rifampin and other CYP3A4 inducers: Decreased plasma guanfacine level and effectiveness
valproic acid: Increased plasma valproic acid level
ACTIVITIES
alcohol use: Possibly increased CNS depression

Adverse Reactions
CNS: Anxiety, asthenia, confusion, depression, dizziness, drowsiness, fatigue, hallucinations (children), headache, irritability, lethargy, nervousness, sedation, seizures, somnolence, syncope, weakness
CV: Atrioventricular block, bradycardia, chest pain, hypertension, orthostatic hypotension, sinus arrhythmia
EENT: Conjunctivitis, dry mouth
GI: Abdominal pain, constipation, dyspepsia, elevated liver enzyme levels, nausea, vomiting
GU: Decreased libido, enuresis, impotence, urinary frequency
RESP: Asthma
SKIN: Dermatitis, diaphoresis, pallor, pruritus, purpura, rash
Other: Increased weight

G
H
I

Nursing Considerations

• Use guanfacine cautiously in patients with cerebrovascular disease, chronic renal or hepatic failure, recent MI, or severe coronary insufficiency.

• Give drug at bedtime to minimize daytime sedation.

WARNING Expect to stop hypertension treatment by decreasing dosage gradually over 2 to 4 days. Typically, if patient hasn't taken drug for 2 or more days, he may have withdrawal symptoms, including abdominal cramps, anxiety, chest pain, diaphoresis, headache, increased salivation, insomnia, irregular heart rate and rhythm, nausea, nervousness, restlessness, tremor, and vomiting.

For patients being treated for ADHD, expect to taper dosage gradually over 3 to 7 days by no more than 1 mg every 3 to 7 days to prevent rebound hypertension.

• If you suspect that patient has drug-related depression, notify prescriber immediately and expect to discontinue drug.

PATIENT TEACHING

• Instruct patient to take guanfacine at bedtime to reduce daytime drowsiness.

• Tell patient not to break, crush, or chew extended-release tablets before swallowing.

• Caution patient about possible drowsiness, and advise him to avoid hazardous activities until drug's CNS effects are known.

• Urge patient to avoid consuming alcohol and other CNS depressants while taking guanfacine.

• Advise patient to report rash.

• Inform male patient that guanfacine may cause impotence. Suggest that he discuss impotence with prescriber, if it occurs.

• Caution patient not to stop taking drug abruptly because doing so can cause a dangerous rise in blood pressure along with anxiety and nervousness.

halazepam
Paxipam

Class, Category, and Schedule

Chemical class: Benzodiazepine
Therapeutic class: Antianxiety
Pregnancy category: D
Controlled substance schedule: IV

Indications and Dosages

➤ *To manage anxiety*

TABLETS

Adults. 20 to 40 mg three times daily or four times daily. *Optimal:* 80 to 160 mg daily.

DOSAGE ADJUSTMENT Dosage reduced to 20 mg once or twice daily if needed for debilitated patients.

Route	Onset	Peak	Duration
P.O.	Slow	Unknown	6–8 hr

Mechanism of Action

May potentiate the effects of gamma-aminobutyric acid (GABA) and other inhibitory neurotransmitters by binding to specific benzodiazepine receptor sites in limbic and cortical areas of the CNS. By binding to these receptor sites, halazepam increases inhibitory effects of GABA and blocks cortical and limbic arousal.

Contraindications

Acute angle-closure glaucoma, hypersensitivity to halazepam or its components, itraconazole or ketoconazole therapy, psychosis

Interaction

DRUGS

antacids: Possibly altered rate of halazepam absorption

barbiturates, CNS depressants, opioids: Increased CNS depression, possibly sedation and impaired motor function

cimetidine, diltiazem, disulfiram, erythromycin, fluoxetine, fluvoxamine, isoniazid, itraconazole, ketoconazole, metoprolol, nefazodone, oral contraceptives, propoxyphene, propranolol, ranitidine, valproic acid, verapamil: Decreased halazepam clearance, increased blood level, and increased risk of adverse effects

clozapine: Possibly respiratory depression

digoxin: Increased blood digoxin level and risk of digitalis toxicity

levodopa: Decreased antidyskinetic effect

neuromuscular blockers: Increased or blocked neuromuscular blockade
theophyllines: Decreased sedative effect of halazepam
ACTIVITIES
alcohol use: Increased CNS depression, possibly sedation and impaired motor function
smoking: Decreased halazepam effectiveness

Adverse Reactions
CNS: Agitation, anxiety, ataxia, confusion, depression, dizziness, drowsiness, euphoria, headache, irritability, nervousness, slurred speech, tremor, weakness
CV: Angina, palpitations, sinus tachycardia
EENT: Diplopia, dry mouth, tinnitus
GI: Abdominal cramps or pain, constipation, diarrhea, increased salivation, nausea, vomiting
GU: Decreased libido, dysuria
MS: Arthralgia
SKIN: Pruritus, rash

Nursing Considerations
• Use halazepam cautiously in patients with impaired hepatic or renal function, seizure disorders, or suicidal tendencies.
• Be aware that risk of halazepam addiction and abuse is relatively high.
• Monitor renal and liver function test results, as appropriate, during long-term treatment.
• Expect to withdraw drug gradually over 2 weeks to avoid withdrawal symptoms, which include anxiety, confusion, insomnia, psychosis, and seizures.
PATIENT TEACHING
• Instruct patient to take halazepam exactly as prescribed and not to stop abruptly because withdrawal symptoms may occur.
• Caution patient to avoid alcohol and other CNS depressants during therapy. Advise patient to avoid OTC drugs, such as cough and cold remedies, because they may contain CNS depressants.
• Advise patient to avoid hazardous activities until drug's CNS effects are known.
• Instruct patient to report depression, difficulty voiding, double vision, persistent drowsiness, and rash.
• Explain that drug's full effects may not occur for 6 weeks.

haloperidol
Apo-Haloperidol (CAN), Haldol, Novo-Peridol (CAN), Peridol (CAN)

haloperidol decanoate
Haldol Decanoate, Haldol LA (CAN)

haloperidol lactate
Haldol Concentrate

Class and Category
Chemical class: Butyrophenone derivative
Therapeutic class: Antidyskinetic, antipsychotic
Pregnancy category: C (haloperidol decanoate), not rated (haloperidol, haloperidol lactate)

Indications and Dosages
➤ *To treat psychotic disorders*
ORAL SOLUTION, TABLETS
Adults and adolescents. 0.5 to 5 mg twice daily or three times daily. *Maximum:* Usually 100 mg daily.
Children ages 3 to 12. 0.05 mg/kg daily in divided doses twice daily or three times daily. Increased by 0.5 mg every 5 to 7 days, as needed. *Maximum:* 0.15 mg/kg daily.
➤ *To treat nonpsychotic behavior disorders and tourette's syndrome*
ORAL SOLUTION, TABLETS
Adults and adolescents. 0.5 to 5 mg twice daily or three times daily. *Maximum:* Usually 100 mg daily.
Children ages 3 to 12. 0.05 to 0.075 mg/kg daily in divided doses twice daily or three times daily Increased by 0.5 mg every 5 to 7 days, if needed. *Maximum:* 0.075 mg/kg daily.
DOSAGE ADJUSTMENT Initial dosage reduced to 0.5 to 2 mg twice daily or three times daily, as needed for elderly or debilitated patients.
➤ *To treat acute psychotic episodes*
I.M. INJECTION
Adults and adolescents. *Initial:* 2 to 5 mg, with subsequent doses up to every 60 min. Or, if symptoms are controlled, dose may be repeated every 4 to 8 hr. *Maximum:* Usually 100 mg daily. First oral dose may

be given 12 to 24 hr after last parenteral dose.

➤ *To provide long-term antipsychotic therapy for patients who require parenteral therapy*

LONG-ACTING I.M. (DECANOATE) INJECTION

Adults. *Initial:* 10 to 15 times the daily oral dose up to 100 mg. Repeated every 4 wk, if needed. *Maximum:* 300 mg/mo.

Mechanism of Action

May block postsynaptic dopamine receptors in the limbic system and increase brain turnover of dopamine, producing an antipsychotic effect.

Contraindications

Blood dyscrasias, bone marrow depression, cerebral arteriosclerosis, coma, concurrent use of large amounts of other CNS depressants, coronary artery disease, epilepsy, hepatic dysfunction, hypersensitivity to haloperidol or its components, Parkinson's disease, severe hypertension or hypotension, severe CNS depression, subcortical brain damage

Route	Onset	Peak	Duration
I.M.*	Unknown	3–4 days†	Unknown

Interaction

DRUGS

alprazolam, buspirone, chlorpromazine, fluoxetine, fluvoxamine, itraconazole, nefazodone, promethazine, quinidine, sertraline, venlafaxine: Increased plasma haloperidol concentrations

amphetamines: Possibly decreased stimulant effects of amphetamines and decreased antipsychotic effect of haloperidol

anticholinergics, antidyskinetics, antihistamines: Increased anticholinergic effect and risk of decreased antipsychotic effect of haloperidol

anticonvulsants: Possibly decreased effectiveness of anticonvulsants and decreased blood haloperidol level

bromocriptine: Possibly decreased effectiveness of bromocriptine

bupropion: Lowered seizure threshold, increased risk of major motor seizure

carbamazepine, rifampin: Decreased plasma haloperidol levels

CNS depressants: Increased CNS depression and risk of respiratory depression and hypotension

diazoxide: Possibly hypoglycemia

dopamine (high-dose therapy): Possibly decreased vasoconstriction

ephedrine: Possibly decreased vasopressor effect of ephedrine

epinephrine: Possibly severe hypotension and tachycardia

fluoxetine: Increased risk of severe and frequent extrapyramidal effects

guanadrel, guanethidine: Decreased hypotensive effects of these drugs

ketoconazole, paroxetine: Possible increased QT interval

levodopa, pergolide: Possibly decreased therapeutic effects of these drugs

lithium: Increased risk of neurotoxicity

MAO inhibitors, maprotiline, tricyclic antidepressants: Increased sedative and anticholinergic effects of these drugs

metaraminol: Possibly decreased vasopressor effect of metaraminol

methoxamine: Decreased vasopressor effect, shortened duration of methoxamine action

methyldopa: Possibly disorientation, slowed or difficult thought processes

phenylephrine: Decreased vasopressor response to phenylephrine

ACTIVITIES

alcohol use: Increased CNS depression and risk of respiratory depression and hypotension

Adverse Reactions

CNS: Agitation, anxiety, confusion, drowsiness, dystonia, euphoria, extrapyramidal reactions that may be irreversible (akathisia, pseudoparkinsonism, tardive dyskinesia), hallucinations, headache, insomnia, neuroleptic malignant syndrome, restlessness, slurred speech, tremor, vertigo

CV: Cardiac arrest, hypertension, orthostatic hypotension, QT-interval prolongation, ventricular arrhythmias, tachycardia, torsades de pointes

EENT: Blurred vision, dry mouth, increased salivation (all drug forms); stomatitis (oral solution)

---

* For haloperidol decanoate and lactate.

† For haloperidol decanoate only; 30 to 45 min for haloperidol lactate.

ENDO: Breast engorgement, galactorrhea
GI: Constipation, nausea, vomiting
GU: Decreased libido, difficult ejaculation, impotence, menstrual irregularities, urine retention
HEME: Agranulocytosis, anemia, leukocytosis, leukopenia
SKIN: Diaphoresis, photosensitivity, rash
Other: Heatstroke, weight gain

Nursing Considerations

• Haloperidol shouldn't be used to treat dementia-related psychosis in the elderly because of an increased mortality risk.
• Use haloperidol cautiously in patientswith a history of prolonged QT interval, patients with uncorrected electrolyte disturbances, and patients receiving Class IA or III antiarrhythmics because of an increased risk of prolonged QT interval. Monitor elderly patients closely because they may have an increased risk of prolonged QT interval.
• Dilute oral solution with a beverage, such as cola or orange, apple, or tomato juice.
• Give haloperidol decanoate (long-acting form prepared in sesame oil to produce slow, sustained release) by deep I.M. injection into gluteal muscle using Z-track technique and 21G needle. Don't give more than 3 ml per site. Expect to reach stable plasma level after third or fourth dose.
• If injection solution has a slight yellow discoloration, be aware that this change doesn't affect potency.
• Watch for tardive dyskinesia (potentially irreversible involuntary movements) in patients receiving long-term therapy, especially elderly women who take large doses.
• Monitor CBC, especially if patient has a low WBC count or history of drug-induced leukopenia or neutropenia, often during the first few months of therapy. If WBC count drops, especially if neutrophil count drops below 1,000/mm^3, expect haloperidol to be discontinued. If neutropenia is significant, also monitor patient for fever or other symptoms of infection and provide appropriate treatment, as prescribed.
• If extrapyramidal reactions occur during the first few days of treatment, reduce

dosage, as prescribed. If symptoms persist, drug may be discontinued. Dystonia also may occur during first few days of treatment, especially in patients receiving higher doses and in males and younger age-groups. Notify prescriber.
• Avoid stopping haloperidol abruptly unless severe adverse reactions occur.
• Monitor for signs of neuroleptic malignant syndrome, a rare but possibly fatal disorder linked to antipsychotic drugs. Signs include altered mental status, arrhythmias, fever, and muscle rigidity.
WARNING Sudden death, QT-interval prolongation, and torsades de pointes, although uncommon, may occur in patients receiving haloperidol despite the lack of such predisposing factors as electrolyte imbalance, concurrent therapy with drugs known to prolong the QT interval, underlying cardiac abnormalities, hypothyroidism, and familial long-QT syndrome.

PATIENT TEACHING
• Advise patient to take haloperidol exactly as prescribed and not to stop abruptly because withdrawal symptoms may occur.
• To prevent oral mucosal irritation, instruct patient to dilute liquid form with juice or cola before taking it.
• Caution patient to avoid skin contact with oral solution because it may cause a rash.
• Advise patient to take tablets with food or a full glass of milk or water to reduce GI distress.
• Instruct patient to consume adequate fluids and to take precautions against heatstroke.
• Urge patient not to drink alcohol during therapy.
• If sedation occurs, caution patient to avoid driving and other hazardous activities.
• Instruct patient to report repetitive movements, tremor, and vision changes.

heparin calcium
Calcilean (CAN), Calciparine

heparin sodium
Hepalean (CAN), Heparin Leo (CAN), Heparin Lock Flush, Liquaemin

Class and Category

Chemical class: Glycosaminoglycan
Therapeutic class: Anticoagulant
Pregnancy category: C

Indications and Dosages

➤ *To prevent and treat deep vein thrombosis and pulmonary embolism, to treat peripheral arterial embolism, and to prevent thromboembolism before and after cardioversion of chronic atrial fibrillation*

I.V. INFUSION OR INJECTION

Adults. *Loading:* 35 to 70 units/kg or 5,000 units by injection. Then 20,000 to 40,000 units infused over 24 hr.

Children. *Loading:* 50 units/kg by injection. Then 100 units/kg infused every 4 hr or 20,000 units/m² infused over 24 hr.

I.V. INJECTION

Adults. *Initial:* 10,000 units. *Maintenance:* 5,000 to 10,000 units every 4 to 6 hr.

Children. Initial: 50 units/kg. *Maintenance:* 100 units/kg/dose every 4 hr.

I.V. OR SUBCUTANEOUS INJECTION

Adults. *Loading:* 5,000 units I.V. Then 10,000 to 20,000 units subcutaneously. *Maintenance:* 8,000 to 10,000 units subcutaneously every 8 hr or 15,000 to 20,000 units subcutaneously every 12 hr.

➤ *To diagnose and treat disseminated intravascular coagulation (DIC)*

I.V. INFUSION OR INJECTION

Adults. 50 to 100 units/kg every 4 hr. Drug may be discontinued if no improvement occurs in 4 to 8 hr.

Children. 25 to 50 units/kg every 4 hr. Drug may be discontinued if no improvement occurs in 4 to 8 hr.

➤ *To prevent postoperative thromboembolism*

SUBCUTANEOUS INJECTION

Adults. 5,000 units 2 hr before surgery and then 5,000 units every 8 to 12 hr for 7 days or until patient is fully ambulatory.

➤ *To prevent clots in patients undergoing open-heart and vascular surgery*

I.V. INFUSION OR INJECTION

Adults. 300 units/kg for procedures that last less than 60 min; 400 units/kg for procedures that last longer than 60 min. *Minimum:* 150 units/kg.

Children. 300 units/kg for procedures that last less than 60 min. Then dosage based on

coagulation test results. *Minimum:* 150 units/kg.

➤ *To maintain heparin lock patency*

I.V. INJECTION

Adults. 10 to 100 units/ml heparin flush solution (enough to fill device) after each use of device.

DOSAGE ADJUSTMENT Increased dosage may be needed if patient needs aggressive anticoagulation to treat or prevent life-threatening thromboses, if heparin will be given I.V., and if heparin has been manufactured under the new standard implemented in October, 2009. (The letter "N" appears in the lot number or after the expiration date on heparin products made under the new standard. An exception is Hospira, which identifies its new-standard products using a lot number starting with "82" or higher.)

Route	Onset	Peak	Duration
I.V.	Immediate	Minutes	Unknown
SubQ	20–60 min	Unknown	Unknown

Mechanism of Action

Binds with antithrombin III, enhancing antithrombin III's inactivation of the coagulation enzymes thrombin (factor IIa) and factors Xa and XIa. At low doses, heparin inhibits factor Xa and prevents conversion of prothrombin to thrombin. Thrombin is needed for conversion of fibrinogen to fibrin; without fibrin, clots can't form. At high doses, heparin inactivates thrombin, preventing fibrin formation and existing clot extension.

Incompatibilities

Don't mix heparin with any other drug unless you have an order to do so and have checked with pharmacist. Heparin is incom-patible with many drugs and solutions, espe-cially ones that contain a phosphate buffer, sodium bicarbonate, or sodium oxalate.

Contraindications

Hypersensitivity to heparin or its components; breastfeeding; infants, neonates, or pregnant woman (Heparin Sodium Injection, USP, preserved with benzyl alcohol); severe thrombocytopenia; uncontrolled bleeding, except in DIC

Interaction

DRUGS

antihistamines, digoxin, nicotine, tetracyclines: Decreased anticoagulant effect of heparin

aspirin, NSAIDs, platelet aggregation inhibitors, sulfinpyrazone: Increased platelet inhibition and risk of bleeding

cefamandole, cefoperazone, cefotetan, methimazole, plicamycin, propylthiouracil, valproic acid: Possibly hypoprothrombinemia and increased risk of bleeding

chloroquine, hydroxychloroquine: Possibly thrombocytopenia and increased risk of hemorrhage

ethacrynic acid, glucocorticoids, salicylates: Increased risk of bleeding and GI ulceration and hemorrhage

nitroglycerin (I.V.): Possibly decreased anticoagulant effect of heparin

probenecid: Possibly increased anticoagulant effect of heparin

thrombolytics: Increased risk of hemorrhage

ACTIVITIES

smoking: Decreased anticoagulant effect

Adverse Reactions

CNS: Chills, dizziness, fever, headache, peripheral neuropathy
CV: Chest pain, thrombosis
EENT: Epistaxis, gingival bleeding, rhinitis
GI: Abdominal distention and pain, hematemesis, melena, nausea, vomiting
GU: Hematuria, hypermenorrhea
HEME: Easy bruising, excessive bleeding from wounds, thrombocytopenia
MS: Back pain, myalgia, osteoporosis
RESP: Dyspnea, wheezing
SKIN: Alopecia, cyanosis, petechiae, pruritus, urticaria
Other: Anaphylaxis; injection-site hematoma, irritation, pain, redness, and ulceration

Nursing Considerations

• Know that Heparin Sodium Injection, USP (porcine), preserved with benzyl alcohol, should not be given to neonates, infants, pregnant women, or women who are breastfeeding because benzyl alcohol has been associated with serious adverse events and death, especially in pediatric patients. Instead, a preservative-free heparin sodium solution should be used

with these patients. Various heparin products contain the preservative benzyl alcohol, which isn't recommended for children under age 1 month because it may cause gasping syndrome, which may be fatal.

• Use heparin cautiously in alcoholics; menstruating women; patients over age 60, especially women; and patients with mild hepatic or renal disease or a history of allergies, asthma, or GI ulcer.

• Read heparin label carefully. Revision has been made to state the strength of the entire container of heparin, followed by how much heparin is in 1 ml. This was done to eliminate the need to calculate the total amount of heparin in a product containing more than 1 ml, thereby reducing the risk of miscalculations that could result in medication errors.

WARNING Be aware that the new standard for manufacturing heparin in the U.S. has decreased its I.V. potency by about 10%. When using this route, determine if the heparin has been manufactured under the new standard by looking for the letter "N" in the lot number or after the expiration date (or, if made by Hospira, the number "82" or higher at the start of the lot number). If giving such heparin, be aware that more drug may be required than in the past to achieve desired level of anticoagulation in some patients. The change in potency also may require more frequent or intensive APTT or ACT monitoring. Change in potency doesn't appear problematic using subcutaneous route.

WARNING Give heparin only by subcutaneous or I.V. route; I.M. use causes hematoma, irritation, and pain.

• Avoid injecting any drugs by I.M. route during heparin therapy, to decrease risk of bleeding and hematoma.

WARNING Don't use heparin sodium injection as a catheter-lock flush because fatal errors have occurred in children when 1-ml heparin sodium injection vials were confused with 1-ml catheter-lock flush vials. Always examine vial labels closely to ensure correct product is being used.

• Administer subcutaneous heparin into anterior abdominal wall, above the iliac crest, and 5 cm (20) or more away from the umbilicus. To minimize subcutaneous tissue trauma, lift adipose tissue away from deep tissues; don't aspirate for blood before injecting drug; don't move needle while injecting drug; and don't massage injection site before or after injection. You can apply gentle pressure to the site after withdrawing needle.

• Alternate injection sites, and watch for signs of bleeding and hematoma.

• To prepare heparin for continuous infusion, invert container at least six times to prevent drug from pooling. Anticipate slight discoloration of prepared solution; this doesn't indicate a change in potency.

• During continuous I.V. therapy, expect to obtain APTT after 8 hours of therapy. Use the arm opposite the infusion site.

• For intermittent I.V. therapy, expect to adjust dose based on coagulation test results performed 30 minutes earlier. Therapeutic range is typically 1.5 to 2.5 times the control.

• Bleeding is major adverse effect of heparin therapy. Take safety precautions to prevent bleeding, such as having patient use a soft-bristled toothbrush and an electric razor. Bleeding may occur at any site and also may indicate an underlying problem, such as GI or urinary tract bleeding. Other sites of bleeding that could be fatal and require immediate attention includes adrenal, ovarian, and retroperitoneal hemorrhage.

• Monitor blood test results, and observe for signs of bleeding, such as ecchymosis, epistaxis, hematemesis, hematuria, melena, and petechiae. Thrombocytopenia of any degree should be monitored closely. If platelet count drops below 100,000/mm³ or recurrent thrombosis develops, notify prescriber and expect heparin to be discontinued. Be aware that heparin-induced thrombocytopenia and thrombosis can occur up to several weeks after heparin therapy has been discontinued.

• Make sure all healthcare providers know that patient is receiving heparin.

• Keep protamine sulfate on hand to use as an antidote for heparin. Be aware that each milligram of protamine sulfate neutralizes 100 units of heparin.

• Be aware that prescriber may order oral anticoagulants before discontinuing heparin to avoid increased coagulation caused by heparin withdrawal. Heparin may be discontinued when full therapeutic effect of oral anticoagulant is achieved.

• Know that women over age 60 have highest risk of hemorrhage during therapy.

• Watch closely if patient is receiving heparin therapy and nitroglycerin I.V. because PTT may decrease and then rebound after nitroglycerin is discontinued. Monitor PTT closely, and be prepared to adjust heparin dose, as prescribed.

WARNING Delayed-onset, heparin-induced thrombocytopenia may occur several weeks after heparin is discontinued and may progress to heparin-induced thrombocytopenia thrombosis, causing venous and arterial thromboses, including thrombus formation on a prosthetic cardiac valve.

PATIENT TEACHING

• Explain that heparin can't be taken orally.

• Inform patient about increased risk of bleeding; urge her to avoid injuries and to use a soft-bristled toothbrush and an electric razor.

• Urge patient to report any abnormal sign or symptom to prescriber, even weeks after heparin has been discontinued, because of the potential for delayed adverse reactions.

• Advise patient to avoid drugs that interact with heparin, such as aspirin and ibuprofen.

• Instruct patient and family to watch for and report abdominal or lower back pain, black stools, bleeding gums, bloody urine, excessive menstrual bleeding, nosebleeds, and severe headaches.

• Explain that temporary hair loss may occur.

• Advise patient to wear or carry appropriate medical identification.

hyaluronan (high-molecular-weight)

Euflexxa, Orthovisc

Class and Category
Chemical class: Natural complex glycosaminoglycan sugar
Therapeutic class: Analgesic
Pregnancy category: Not rated

Indications and Dosages
➤ *To relieve osteoarthritic knee pain in patients who respond inadequately to conservative nonpharmacologic therapy and to simple analgesics*
INTRA-ARTICULAR INJECTION (ORTHOVISC)
Adults. 30 mg/wk for 3 to 4 wk.
INTRA-ARTICULAR INJECTION (EUFLEXXA)
Adults. 20 mg/wk for 3 wk.

Mechanism of Action
Relieves pain associated with osteoarthritis by lubricating the joint and absorbing shock when the joint moves. Hyaluronan is a viscoelastic substance normally found in joint tissues and in the fluid that fills joints; it is instilled directly into the joint.

Contraindications
Hypersensitivity to hyaluronan avian, avian-derived products (such as eggs, feathers, or poultry) or any of their components; knee infections; skin diseases affecting the knee area

Adverse Reactions
CNS: Headache
MS: Acute arthritis, arthralgia, back pain, bursitis
Other: Injection-site bruising, edema, erythema, pain, pruritus, or rash

Nursing Considerations
• Prepare patient for removal of joint effusion, if present, before hyaluronan injection.
• Assist the trained healthcare professional who gives intra-articular injections, as needed, making sure that strict aseptic technique is followed during procedure.
• Be aware that prefilled syringe is for single use and that contents of syringe should be used immediately after opening.
PATIENT TEACHING
• Inform patient that transient knee pain, swelling, or other localized reactions, such as itchiness or bruising, may occur after hyaluronan injection.
• Instruct patient to avoid strenuous or weight-bearing activities lasting longer than 1 hour for 48 hours after injection.

• Inform patient that she may feel achy after injection but that this discomfort is typically mild and brief.
• Advise patient that pain may not be relieved until after third injection.

hydralazine hydrochloride
Apo-Hydralazine (CAN), Apresoline (CAN), Novo-Hylazin (CAN)

Class and Category
Chemical class: Phthalazine derivative
Therapeutic class: Antihypertensive, vasodilator
Pregnancy category: C

Indications and Dosages
➤ *To manage essential hypertension, alone or with other antihypertensives*
TABLETS
Adults. *Initial:* 40 mg daily in divided doses twice daily or four times daily for first 2 to 4 days and then increased to 100 mg daily in divided doses twice daily or four times daily for remainder of first wk. *Maximum:* Usually 200 mg daily, but sometimes 300 to 400 mg daily.
Children. 0.75 mg/kg daily in divided doses twice daily or four times daily. Increased gradually over 3 to 4 wk. *Maximum:* 7.5 mg/kg or 200 mg daily.
➤ *To manage severe essential hypertension when drug can't be taken orally or when need to reduce blood pressure is urgent*
I.V. OR I.M. INJECTION
Adults. 5 to 40 mg, repeated as needed.
Children. 1.7 to 3.5 mg/kg daily in divided doses every 4 to 6 hr, as needed.

Route	Onset	Peak	Duration
P.O.	20–30 min	1–2 hr	2–4 hr
I.V.	5–20 min	10–80 min	2–6 hr
I.M.	10–30 min	1 hr	2–6 hr

Mechanism of Action
May act in a manner that resembles organic nitrates and sodium nitroprusside, except that hydralazine is selective for arteries. It:
• exerts a direct vasodilating effect on vascular smooth muscle

- interferes with calcium movement in vascular smooth muscle by altering cellular calcium metabolism
- dilates arteries, not veins, which minimizes orthostatic hypotension and increases cardiac output and cerebral blood flow
- causes reflex autonomic response that increases heart rate, cardiac output, and left ventricular ejection fraction
- has a positive inotropic effect on the heart.

Incompatibilities
Don't mix hydralazine in I.V. infusion solutions.

Contraindications
Coronary artery disease, hypersensitivity to hydralazine or its components, mitral valve disease

Interaction
DRUGS
beta blockers: Increased effects of both drugs
diazoxide, MAO inhibitors, other antihypertensives: Risk of severe hypotension
epinephrine: Possibly decreased vasopressor effect of epinephrine
NSAIDs: Decreased hydralazine effects
sympathomimetics: Possibly decreased antihypertensive effect of hydralazine
FOODS
all foods: Possibly increased bioavailability of hydralazine

Adverse Reactions
CNS: Chills, fever, headache, peripheral neuritis
CV: Angina, edema, orthostatic hypotension, palpitations, tachycardia
EENT: Lacrimation, nasal congestion
GI: Anorexia, constipation, diarrhea, nausea, vomiting
RESP: Dyspnea
SKIN: Blisters, flushing, pruritus, rash, urticaria
Other: Lupus-like symptoms, especially with high doses; lymphadenopathy

Nursing Considerations
- Monitor CBC, lupus erythematosus cell preparation, and ANA titer before therapy

and periodically as appropriate during long-term treatment.
- Anticipate that drug may change color in solution. Consult pharmacist if color changes.
- Be aware that hydralazine may change color when exposed to a metal filter.
- Give tablets with food to increase bioavailability.
- Monitor blood pressure and pulse rate regularly and weigh patient daily during therapy.
- Check blood pressure with patient in lying, sitting, and standing positions, and watch for signs of orthostatic hypotension. Expect orthostatic hypotension to be most common in the morning, during hot weather, and with exercise.
WARNING Expect to discontinue drug immediately if patient has lupus-like symptoms, such as arthralgia, fever, myalgia, pharyngitis, and splenomegaly.
- Expect prescriber to withdraw hydralazine gradually to avoid a rapid increase in blood pressure.
- Expect to treat peripheral neuritis with pyridoxine.
PATIENT TEACHING
- Instruct patient to take hydralazine tablets with food.
- Advise patient to change position slowly, especially in the morning. Caution that hot showers may increase hypotension.
- Instruct patient to immediately notify prescriber about fever, muscle and joint aches, and sore throat.
- Urge patient to report numbness and tingling in limbs, which may require treatment with another drug.
- Caution patient against stopping drug abruptly because doing so may cause severe hypertension.

hydrochlorothiazide
Esidrix, Hydro-chlor, Hydro-D, HydroDIURIL, Microzide, Neo-Codema (CAN), Novo-Hydrazide (CAN), Oretic, Urozide (CAN)

Class and Category
Chemical class: Benzothiadiazide
Therapeutic class: Antihypertensive, diuretic
Pregnancy category: B

Indications and Dosages
➤ *To manage hypertension*
CAPSULES
Adults. 12.5 mg daily.
ORAL SOLUTION, TABLETS
Adults. 25 to 100 mg daily as a single dose or in divided doses twice daily.
Children age 6 months and over. 1 to 2 mg/kg daily as a single dose or in divided doses twice daily.
Infants under age 6 months. Up to 3 mg/kg daily.
➤ *As adjunct to treat edema caused by cirrhosis, corticosteroids, estrogen, heart failure, or renal disorders*
ORAL SOLUTION, TABLETS
Adults. 25 to 100 mg twice daily, once daily, or every other day for 3 to 5 days/wk.
Children age 6 months and over. 1 to 2 mg/kg daily as a single dose or in divided doses twice daily.
Infants under age 6 months. Up to 3 mg/kg daily.

Route	Onset	Peak	Duration
P.O.	2 hr	4 hr	6–12 hr

Contraindications
Anuria; hypersensitivity to hydrochlorothiazide, other thiazides, sulfonamide derivatives, or their components; renal failure

Interaction
DRUGS
ACTH, amphotericin B, corticosteroids: Increased electrolyte depletion, especially potassium
amantadine: Possibly increased blood level and risk of toxicity of amantadine
amiodarone: Increased risk of arrhythmias from hypokalemia
antihypertensives: Increased antihypertensive effects
barbiturates, opioids: Possibly orthostatic hypotension
calcium: Possibly increased serum calcium level
carbamazepine: Possibly increased risk of symptomatic hyponatremia
cholestyramine, colestipol: Reduced GI absorption of hydrochlorothiazide
cyclosporine: Possibly increased risk of hyperuricemia and gout-type complications
diazoxide: Increased antihypertensive and hyperglycemic effects of hydrochlorothiazide
diflunisal: Possibly increased blood hydrochlorothiazide level
digoxin: Increased risk of digitalis toxicity from hypokalemia
dopamine: Possibly increased diuretic effects of both drugs
insulin, oral antidiabetic drugs: Possibly increased blood glucose level
lithium: Decreased lithium clearance, increased risk of lithium toxicity
neuromuscular blockers: Possibly enhanced neuromuscular blockade from hypokalemia

G
H
I

Mechanism of Action
A thiazide diuretic, hydrochlorothiazide promotes movement of sodium (Na^+), chloride (Cl^-), and water (H_2O) from blood in peritubular capillaries into nephron's distal convoluted tubule, as shown. Initially, it may decrease extracellular fluid volume, plasma volume, and cardiac output, which helps explain blood pressure reduction. It also may reduce blood pressure by direct arterial dilation. After several weeks, extracellular fluid volume, plasma volume, and cardiac output return to normal, and peripheral vascular resistance remains decreased.

nondepolarizing skeletal muscle relaxants: Possibly increased response to muscle relaxants
NSAIDs: Decreased diuretic effect of hydrochlorothiazide, increased risk of renal failure
oral anticoagulants: Possibly decreased anticoagulant effects
sympathomimetics: Possibly decreased antihypertensive effect of hydrochlorothiazide
vitamin D: Increased risk of hypercalcemia
ACTIVITIES
alcohol use: Possibly orthostatic hypotension

Adverse Reactions

CNS: Asthenia, dizziness, fever, headache, insomnia, paresthesia, restlessness, vertigo, weakness
CV: Elevated cholesterol and triglycerides levels, hypotension, orthostatic hypotension, vasculitis
EENT: Acute myopia, acute angle-closure glaucoma, blurred vision, dry mouth
ENDO: Hyperglycemia
GI: Abdominal cramps, anorexia, constipation, diarrhea, indigestion, jaundice, nausea, pancreatitis, vomiting
GU: Decreased libido, impotence, interstitial nephritis, nocturia, polyuria, renal failure
HEME: Agranulocytosis, aplastic anemia, bone marrow failure, hemolytic anemia, leukopenia, neutropenia, thrombocytopenia
MS: Muscle spasms and weakness
RESP: Pneumonitis, pulmonary edema
SKIN: Alopecia, cutaneous vasculitis, erythema multiforme, exfoliative dermatitis, photosensitivity, purpura, rash, Stevens-Johnson syndrome, toxic epidermal necrolysis, urticaria
Other: Anaphylaxis, dehydration, hypercalcemia, hyperuricemia, hypochloremia, hypokalemia, hypomagnesemia, hyponatremia, hypovolemia, metabolic alkalosis, weight loss

Nursing Considerations
• Give hydrochlorothiazide in the morning and early evening to avoid nocturia.
• Monitor fluid intake and output, daily weight, blood pressure, and serum levels of electrolytes, especially potassium.

• Assess for evidence of hypokalemia, such as muscle spasms and weakness.
• Monitor BUN and serum creatinine levels.
• Check blood glucose level often, as ordered, in diabetic patients, and expect to increase antidiabetic dosage, as needed.
• If patient has gouty arthritis, expect increased risk of gout attacks during therapy.
• Monitor serum creatinine levels, as ordered, especially in patients with chronic kidney disease, renal artery stenosis, severe congestive heart failure, or volume depletion, because of increased risk of acute renal failure with hydrochlorothiazide therapy. Notify prescriber if serum creatinine levels become elevated, as drug may need to be withheld or discontinued.
• Monitor patient for decreased visual acuity or ocular pain, especially within hours to weeks of beginning drug therapy and in patients with a history of sulfonamide or penicillin allergy, as acute myopia and acute angle-closure glaucoma may develop. If left untreated, permanent blindness may occur. If present, notify prescriber immediately, expect to discontinue hydrochlorothiazide, and assist with prompt medical or surgical intervention, as indicated.
• **WARNING** Be aware that even minor alterations in fluid and electrolyte balance may precipitate hepatic coma in patients with impaired hepatic function.
PATIENT TEACHING
• Advise patient to take hydrochlorothiazide morning and early evening to avoid awakening during the night to urinate.
• Instruct patient to take drug with food or milk if adverse GI reactions occur.
• Tell patient to weigh herself at the same time each day wearing the same amount of clothing and to notify prescriber if she gains more than 0.9 kg (2 lb) per day or 2.3 kg (5 lb) per week.
• Instruct patient to eat a diet high in potassium-rich food, including citrus fruits, bananas, tomatoes, and dates.
• Advise patient to change position slowly to minimize effects of orthostatic hypotension.

• Urge patient to report decreased urination, muscle cramps and weakness, and unusual bleeding or bruising.

hydrocodone bitartrate

Hysingla ER, Zohydro ER

Class and Category

Chemical class: Semi-synthetic opioid agonist
Therapeutic class: Analgesic
Pregnancy category: C
Controlled substance schedule: II

Indications and Dosages

➤ To *manage severe pain in patients requiring continuous, around-the-clock opioid analgesia for an extended period of time and for which alternative treatment options are inadequate*

E.R. CAPSULES (ZOHYDRO ER)

Adults who are opioid-naïve or opioid non-tolerant. *Initial:* 10 mg every 12 hr, increased, as needed, in increments of 10 mg every 12 hr every 3 to 7 days to effective and tolerable dose. *Maximum:* 80 mg total daily dose.

Adults who are opioid tolerant and converting from another opioid. Highly individualized.

DOSAGE ADJUSTMENT For patients with renal or severe hepatic impairment, a single dose of 10 mg given, followed by close monitoring for respiratory depression and sedation. If single dose tolerated, 10 mg every 12 hr. as needed and tolerated with further titration highly individualized.

E.R. TABLETS (HYSINGLA ER)

Adults who are opioid naive or opioid nontolerant. *Initial:* 20 mg every 24 hr, increased, as needed, in increments of 10 mg to 20 mg daily every 3 to 7 days to effective and tolerable dose. *Maximum:* 80 mg every 24 hr.

Adults who are opioid tolerant and converting from another opioid. Highly individualized.

DOSAGE ADJUSTMENT For patients with severe hepatic impairment, moderate to severe renal impairment, or end-stage renal disease, initial dosage reduced to 10 mg every 24 hr.

Mechanism of Action

Binds to and activates opioid receptors at sites in the peri-aquaductal and peri-ventricular gray matter, the ventro-medial medulla, and the spinal cord to produce pain relief.

Contraindications

Acute or severe bronchial asthma or hypercarbia, hypersensitivity to hydrocodone bitartrate or any of its components, known or suspected paralytic ileus, significant respiratory depression, use within 14 days of MAO inhibitor therapy

Interaction

DRUGS

anticholinergics, other drugs with anticholinergic activity: Increased risk of urinary retention or severe constipation, which may lead to paralytic ileus
CNS depressants; nonprescription or prescription drugs containing alcohol: Increased risk of respiratory depression, profound sedation, coma, and death
CYP3A4 inducers: Increased clearance of hydrocodone with decreased effectiveness
CYP3A4 inhibitors: Decreased clearance of hydrocodone resulting in increased or prolonged opioid effects
mixed agonist/antagonist analgesics such as buprenorphine, butorphanol, nalbuphine, pentazocine: Possible reduced hydrocodone effectiveness or precipitation of withdrawal symptoms

ACTIVITIES

alcohol use: Possibly increased hydrocodone plasma levels with potentially fatal overdose

Adverse Reactions

CNS: Anxiety, depression, dizziness, fatigue, fever, headache, insomnia, lethargy, migraine, paresthesia, somnolence, syncope, tremor
CV: Hypercholesterolemia, hypotension (may be severe), peripheral edema
EENT: Dry mouth
ENDO: Hot flashes
GI: Abdominal discomfort or pain, constipation (may be severe), elevated liver enzymes, gastroesophageal reflux disease, nausea, spasm of the Sphincter of Oddi, vomiting

G
H
I

GU: UTI
MS: Arthralgia; back, extremity, musculo-skeletal, or neck pain; muscle spasms
RESP: Cough, dyspnea, respiratory depression
SKIN: Pruritis, rash, sweating including night sweats
Other: Dehydration, hypokalemia, noncardiac chest pain, physical and psychological dependence

Nursing Considerations

• Know that hydrocodone should not be given to a patient with impaired consciousness, nor should the drug be administered on an as needed basis.
• Use extreme caution when administering hydrocodone to patients with significant chronic obstructive pulmonary disease or cor pulmonale, and in patients having a substantially decreased respiratory reserve, hypoxia, hypercapnia, or preexisting respiratory depression, especially when initiating or titrating therapy. These patients may develop respiratory depression, even with usual therapeutic doses, because hydrocodone may decrease the patient's respiratory drive to the point of apnea.
• Use hydrocodone cautiously in elderly, cachectic, or debilitated patients, especially when initiating and titrating therapy, as they are at increased risk for adverse effects, especially respiratory depression.
• Be aware that patients who are considered opioid tolerant are those who have received for one week or longer, at least 60 milligrams of oral morphine daily, 25 micrograms transdermal fentanyl per hour, 30 milligrams of oral oxycodone per day, 8 mg oral hydromorphone per day, 25 milligrams of oral oxymorphone per day, or an equianalgesic dose of another opioid.
• Do not administer hydrocodone to a patient wearing a transdermal fentanyl patch until the patch has been removed for eighteen hours. Also know that close monitoring is especially important for a patient converting from methadone because methadone has a long half-life and tends to accumulate in the blood.
WARNING Be aware that hydrocodone available as an extended release formulation increases risk of overdose and death because of larger amount of drug present

in this form. Also know that crushing, chewing, snorting, or injecting the contents of the capsule dissolved in a liquid base will result in the uncontrolled delivery of hydrocodone and can result in overdose and death.
WARNING Monitor patient for respiratory depression, especially when initiating therapy or when increasing dosage, even when the drug has been used as prescribed and not misused or abused. Be aware that overestimating hydrocodone dose when converting patients from another opioid medication can result in fatal overdose with the first dose. To avoid this, know that it is recommended to underestimate a patient's 24-hour oral hydrocodone requirement and provide rescue medication, as needed, until the right dose is determined. Keep resuscitation equipment nearby.
• Monitor patients closely who may be susceptible to the intracranial effects of carbon dioxide retention from respiratory depression caused by hydrocodone therapy, such as patients with head injuries or those who have a preexisting elevation in intracranial pressure.
• Monitor patients with a seizure history or disorder because hydrocodone may cause or worsen seizures.
• Monitor effectiveness of hydrocodone in relieving pain; consult prescriber as needed.
• Assess patient for constipation.
• Monitor patient for evidence of physical dependence or abuse. Know that addiction can occur not only in those who obtain the drug illicitly but also in patients who are appropriately prescribed the drug at recommended doses.
• Notify prescriber if serious adverse reactions occur with hydrocodone therapy and expect dosage to be reduced.
• Expect to taper hydrocodone dosage gradually every two to four days when patient no longer requires therapy to prevent withdrawal symptoms in the physically dependent patient. Know that hydrocodone should not be discontinued abruptly.
• Monitor patient's vital signs closely, especially after initiating or titrating dose of hydrocodone. Know that in addition to

respiratory depression, hydrocodone may cause severe hypotension, especially in patients whose blood pressure is already compromised by a depleted blood volume or after concurrent administration of drugs that decrease blood pressure.
• Monitor patient for decreased bowel motility in post-operative patients receiving hydrocodone, as the drug may obscure the development of acute abdominal conditions.

PATIENT TEACHING
• Instruct patient to take drug exactly as ordered and not to adjust dosage without speaking to prescriber first. Warn patient of possibility of addiction even when taken as prescribed.
• Inform patient that capsules and tablets should be taken whole and never chewed, crushed, or dissolved. In addition, enough water should be taken with the tablet or capsule to ensure complete swallowing immediately after placing drug in mouth.
• Warn patient to keep hydrocodone away from the reach of children, as accidental consumption of even one capsule can cause significant respiratory depression and death.
• Caution patient to avoid ingesting alcohol, including medications containing alcohol, as the combination increases the risk of respiratory depression, overdose and death, as does taking other types of depressants together with hydrocodone therapy. Patient should notify all prescribers of hydrocodone use.
• Advise women of childbearing age to notify prescriber if pregnancy occurs or is suspected because a fetus exposed to hydrocodone during utero may require treatment for neonatal opioid withdrawal syndrome when born.
• Caution patient to avoid hazardous activities until drug's CNS effects are known.
• Instruct patient to rise slowly from a sitting or lying position and to sit or lie down if he experiences light-headedness. If effect is frequent or severe, tell him to notify prescriber.
• Urge patient to consume plenty of fluids and high-fiber foods, if not contra-indicated, to prevent constipation.

hydrocortisone (cortisol)
Cortef, Cortenema, Hydrocortone

hydrocortisone acetate
Cortifoam, Hydrocortone Acetate

hydrocortisone cypionate
Cortef

hydrocortisone sodium phosphate
Hydrocortone Phosphate

hydrocortisone sodium succinate
A-hydroCort, Solu-Cortef

Class and Category
Chemical class: Glucocorticoid
Therapeutic class: Adrenocorticoid replacement, anti-inflammatory
Pregnancy category: Not rated; C (Cortifoam)

Indications and Dosages
➤ *To treat severe inflammation or acute adrenal insufficiency*
ORAL SUSPENSION, TABLETS (HYDROCORTISONE, HYDROCORTISONE CYPIONATE)
Adults. 20 to 240 mg daily as a single dose or in divided doses.
I.V. INFUSION OR I.V., I.M., OR SUBCUTANEOUS INJECTION (HYDROCORTISONE SODIUM PHOSPHATE); I.M. INJECTION (HYDROCORTISONE)
Adults. 15 to 240 mg daily as a single dose or in divided doses. *Usual:* One-half to one-third the oral dose.
DOSAGE ADJUSTMENT Dosage increased to more than 240 mg daily if needed to treat acute disease.
I.V. INFUSION; I.V. OR I.M. INJECTION (HYDROCORTISONE SODIUM SUCCINATE)
Adults. 100 to 500 mg every 2, 4, or 6 hr.
➤ *To treat joint and tissue inflammation*

INTRA-ARTICULAR INJECTION (HYDROCORTISONE ACETATE)
Adults. 25 to 37.5 mg injected into large joints or bursae as a single dose, or 10 to 25 mg into small joints as a single dose.
INTRALESIONAL INJECTION (HYDROCORTISONE ACETATE)
Adults. 5 to 12.5 mg injected into tendon sheaths as a single dose, or 12.5 to 25 mg injected into ganglia as a single dose.
SOFT-TISSUE INJECTION (HYDROCORTISONE ACETATE)
Adults. 25 to 50 mg as a single dose. Sometimes a dose of up to 75 mg is needed.
➤ *As adjunct to treat ulcerative proctitis of the distal portion of the rectum in patients who can't retain hydrocortisone or other corticosteroid enemas*
RECTAL AEROSOL (HYDROCORTISONE ACETATE)
Adult men. Initial: 1 applicatorful once or twice daily for 2 to 3 wk; then every other day thereafter. *Maintenance:* Highly individualized.
➤ *To treat ulcerative colitis*
ENEMA (HYDROCORTISONE)
Adults. 100 mg every night for 2 to 3 wk or until condition improves.

Route	Onset	Peak	Duration
P.O.†	Unknown	1 hr	1.25–1.5 days
P.O.‖	Unknown	1–2 hr	Unknown
I.V. ‡§	Rapid	Unknown	Unknown
I.M.†	Unknown	4–8 hr	Unknown
I.M.‡	Rapid	1 hr	Unknown
I.M.§	Rapid	1 hr	Variable
Other*	Unknown	24–48 hr	3 days–4 wk

Mechanism of Action

Binds to intracellular glucocorticoid receptors and suppresses inflammatory and immune responses by:

---

† Hydrocortisone
‡ Phosphate
§ Succinate
‖ Cypionate
* Acetate; intra-articular, intralesional, and soft-tissue injection.

• inhibiting neutrophil and monocyte accumulation at inflammation site and suppressing their phagocytic and bactericidal activity
• stabilizing lysosomal membranes
• suppressing antigen response of macrophages and helper T cells
• inhibiting synthesis of cellular mediators of inflammatory response, such as cytokines, interleukins, and prostaglandins.

Contraindications

Hypersensitivity to hydrocortisone or its components, idiopathic thrombocytopenic purpura (I.M.), intestinal conditions prohibiting intrarectal steroids (P.R.), recent live-virus vaccination, systemic fungal infection

Interaction

DRUGS
acetaminophen: Increased risk of hepatotoxicity
amphotericin B, carbonic anhydrase inhibitors: Possibly severe hypokalemia
anabolic steroids, androgens: Increased risk of edema and severe acne
anticholinergics: Possibly increased intraocular pressure
anticoagulants, thrombolytics: Increased risk of GI ulceration and hemorrhage, possibly decreased therapeutic effects of these drugs
asparaginase: Increased risk of hyperglycemia and toxicity
aspirin, NSAIDs: Increased risk of GI distress and bleeding
cholestyramine: Possibly increased hydrocortisone clearance
cyclosporine: Possibly increased action of both drugs; increased risk of seizures
digoxin: Possibly hypokalemia-induced arrhythmias and digitalis toxicity
ephedrine, phenobarbital, phenytoin, rifampin: Decreased blood hydrocortisone level
estrogens, oral contraceptives: Increased therapeutic and toxic effects of hydrocortisone
insulin, oral antidiabetic drugs: Possibly increased blood glucose level
isoniazid: Possibly decreased therapeutic effects of isoniazid
macrolide antibiotics: Possibly decreased hydrocortisone clearance

mexiletine: Decreased blood mexiletine level
neuromuscular blockers: Possibly increased neuromuscular blockade, causing respiratory depression or apnea
potassium-depleting drugs, such as thiazide diuretics: Possibly severe hypokalemia
potassium supplements: Possibly decreased effects of these supplements
somatrem, somatropin: Possibly decreased therapeutic effects of these drugs
streptozocin: Increased risk of hyperglycemia
vaccines: Decreased antibody response and increased risk of neurologic complications
ACTIVITIES
alcohol use: Increased risk of GI distress and bleeding

Adverse Reactions

CNS: Ataxia, behavioral changes, depression, dizziness, euphoria, fatigue, headache, increased intracranial pressure with papilledema, insomnia, malaise, mood changes, paresthesia, seizures, steroid psychosis, syncope, vertigo
CV: Arrhythmias (from hypokalemia), fat embolism, heart failure, hypertension, hypotension, thromboembolism, thrombophlebitis
EENT: Exophthalmos, glaucoma, increased intraocular pressure, nystagmus, posterior subcapsular cataracts
ENDO: Adrenal insufficiency during stress, cushingoid symptoms (buffalo hump, central obesity, moon face, supraclavicular fat pad enlargement), diabetes mellitus, growth suppression in children, hyperglycemia, negative nitrogen balance from protein catabolism
GI: Abdominal distention; hiccups; increased appetite; nausea; pancreatitis; peptic ulcer; rectal abnormalities, such as bleeding, blistering, burning, itching, or pain (rectal form); ulcerative esophagitis; vomiting
GU: Amenorrhea, glycosuria, menstrual irregularities, perineal burning or tingling
HEME: Easy bruising, leukocytosis
MS: Arthralgia; aseptic necrosis of femoral and humeral heads; compression fractures; muscle atrophy, twitching, or weakness; myalgia; osteoporosis; spontaneous fractures; steroid myopathy; tendon rupture

SKIN: Acne; altered skin pigmentation; diaphoresis; erythema; hirsutism; necrotizing vasculitis; petechiae; purpura; rash; scarring; sterile abscess; striae; subcutaneous fat atrophy; thin, fragile skin; urticaria
Other: Anaphylaxis, hypocalcemia, hypokalemia, hypokalemic alkalosis, impaired wound healing, masking of signs of infection, metabolic alkalosis, suppressed skin test reaction, weight gain

Nursing Considerations

• Systemic hydrocortisone shouldn't be given to immunocompromised patients, such as those with fungal and other infections, including amebiasis, hepatitis B, tuberculosis, vaccinia, and varicella.
• Give daily dose of hydrocortisone in morning to mimic normal peak in adrenocortical secretion of corticosteroids.
• When possible, give oral dose with food or milk to avoid GI distress.
• Don't give acetate injectable suspension by I.V. route.
• Give hydrocortisone sodium succinate as a direct I.V. injection over 30 seconds to several minutes, or as an intermittent or a continuous infusion. For infusion, dilute to 1 mg/ml or less with D₅W, normal saline solution, or dextrose 5% in normal saline solution.
• Inject I.M. form deep into gluteal muscle, and rotate injection sites to prevent muscle atrophy. Subcutaneous injection may cause atrophy and sterile abscess.
• Shake foam container vigorously for 5 to 10 seconds before each use. Gently withdraw applicator plunger past the fill-line on the applicator barrel while container is upright on a level surface. Administer rectal foam only with provided applicator. After each use, wash applicator, container cap, and underlying tip with warm water.
• High-dose therapy shouldn't be given for longer than 48 hours. Be alert for depression and psychotic episodes.
• Monitor weight, blood pressure, and electrolyte levels regularly during therapy.
• Expect hydrocortisone to worsen infections or mask signs and symptoms.
• Monitor blood glucose level in diabetic patients, and increase insulin or oral antidiabetic drug dosage, as prescribed.

G
H
I

• Know that elderly patients are at high risk for osteoporosis during long-term therapy.
• Anticipate the possibility of acute adrenal insufficiency with stress, such as emotional upset, fever, surgery, or trauma. Increase hydrocortisone dosage, as prescribed.

WARNING Avoid withdrawing drug suddenly after long-term therapy because adrenal crisis can result. Expect to reduce dosage gradually and monitor response.

PATIENT TEACHING
• Advise patient to take daily dose of hydrocortisone at 9 a.m.
• Instruct patient to take tablets or oral suspension with milk or food.
• Teach patient how to use foam or enema form, if prescribed.
• Caution patient not to stop drug abruptly without first consulting prescriber.
• Instruct patient to report early evidence of adrenal insufficiency: anorexia, difficulty breathing, dizziness, fainting, fatigue, joint pain, muscle weakness, and nausea.
• Inform patient that he may bruise easily.
• Advise patient on long-term therapy to have periodic eye examinations.
• If patient receives long-term therapy, urge her to carry or wear medical identification.
• Caution patient to avoid people with infections because drug can suppress immune system, increasing risk of infection. If patient comes into contact with chickenpox or measles, instruct him to call prescriber because he may need prophylactic care.

---

hydromorphone hydrochloride

(dihydromorphinone)

Dilaudid, Dilaudid-HP, Exalgo, PMS-Hydromorphone (CAN), PMS-Hydromorphone Syrup (CAN)

Class, Category, and Schedule
Chemical class: Phenanthrene derivative, semisynthetic opioid derivative
Therapeutic class: Analgesic
Pregnancy category: C
Controlled substance schedule: II

Indications and Dosages
➤ *To relieve moderate to severe pain*
ORAL SOLUTION (DILAUDID, PMS-HYDROMORPHONE SYRUP)
Adults. 2.5 to 10 mg every 3 to 6 hr, as needed.
TABLETS (DILAUDID, PMS-HYDROMORPHONE)
Adults. 2 mg every 3 to 6 hr, as needed. Increased to 4 mg or more every 4 to 6 hr, if indicated.
I.V. INJECTION (DILAUDID)
Adults. 1 mg every 3 hr, as needed., given slowly over 2 to 3 minutes.
I.M. OR SUBCUTANEOUS INJECTION (DILAUDID)
Adults. 1 or 2 mg every 3 to 6 hr, as needed. Increased to 3 or 4 mg every 4 to 6 hr, as needed for severe pain.
SUPPOSITORIES (DILAUDID)
Adults. 3 mg every 4 to 8 hr, as needed.
DOSAGE ADJUSTMENT For patients with hepatic or renal impairment, initial dosage is given at 25 to 50% of normal dosage.
➤ *To treat moderate to severe pain for opioid-tolerant patients who require higher doses of opioids*
I.M., I.V. OR SUBCUTANEOUS INJECTION (DILAUDID-HP)
Adults. Highly individualized and dependent on patient's previous total daily 24-hour opioid use. If I.V. route is used, give slowly over 2 to 3 minutes.
➤ *To manage moderate to severe pain in opioid-tolerant patients requiring continuous, around-the-clock opioid analgesia for an extended period of time*
E.R. TABLETS (EXALGO)
Adults. Highly individualized and dependent on patient's previous total 24-hour opioid use. Once dosage is determined, drug is given once daily.
DOSAGE ADJUSTMENT For patients with moderate hepatic impairment, dosage started at 25% of normal dosage. For patients with moderate renal impairment, dosage started at 50% of normal dosage.

Route	Onset	Peak	Duration
P.O.	30 min	1.5–2 hr	4 hr
I.V.	10–15 min	15–30 min	2–3 hr
I.M.	15 min	30–60 min	4–5 hr
SubQ	15 min	30–90 min	4 hr
P.R.	30 min	Unknown	4 hr

Mechanism of Action

May bind with opioid receptors in the spinal cord and higher levels in the CNS. In this way, hydromorphone is believed to stimulate mu and kappa receptors, thus altering the perception of and emotional response to pain.

Contraindications

Acute asthma; history of narrowing of the GI tract or presence of blind loops in the GI tract, or GI obstruction; hypersensitivity to hydromorphone, other narcotics, or their components; increased intracranial pressure; opioid nontolerant patients (Dilaudid HP, Exalgo); paralytic ileus; severe respiratory depression; upper respiratory tract obstruction

Interaction

DRUGS

anticholinergics: Increased risk of ileus, severe constipation, or urine retention
antihypertensives, diuretics, guanadrel, guanethidine, mecamylamine: Increased risk of orthostatic hypotension
barbiturate anesthetics: Increased sedative effect of hydromorphone
belladonna alkaloids, difenoxin and atropine, diphenoxylate and atropine, kaolin pectin, loperamide, paregoric: Increased risk of CNS depression and severe constipation
buprenorphine, butorphanol, dezocine, nalbuphine, pentazocine: Possibly potentiated or suppressed symptoms of spontaneous opioid withdrawal
CNS depressants, other opioid analgesics: Additive CNS depression and hypotension, possibly resulting in life-threatening reactions
hydroxyzine: Increased analgesia, CNS depression, and hypotension
metoclopramide: Decreased effect of metoclopramide on GI motility
naloxone: Possibly withdrawal symptoms in physically dependent patients
naltrexone: Possibly prolonged respiratory depression or cardiac arrest
neuromuscular blockers: Additive CNS depression

ACTIVITIES

alcohol use: Increased CNS and respiratory depression

Adverse Reactions

CNS: Anxiety, confusion, dizziness, drowsiness, euphoria, hallucinations, headache, nervousness, restlessness, sedation, somnolence, tremor, weakness
CV: Hypertension, orthostatic hypotension, palpitations, tachycardia
EENT: Blurred vision, diplopia, dry mouth, laryngeal edema, laryngospasm, nystagmus, tinnitus
GI: Abdominal cramps, anorexia, biliary tract spasm, constipation, hepatotoxicity, nausea, vomiting
GU: Dysuria, urine retention
RESP: Dyspnea, respiratory depression, wheezing
SKIN: Diaphoresis, flushing
Other: Injection-site pain, redness, and swelling; physical and psychological dependence

Nursing Considerations

• Use extreme caution when administering hydromorphone to patients with significant chronic obstructive pulmonary disease or cor pulmonale, and in patients having a substantially decreased respiratory reserve, hypoxia, hypercapnia, or preexisting respiratory depression, especially when initiating and titrating therapy. These patients may develop respiratory depression, even with usual therapeutic doses, because hydromorphone may decrease the patient's respiratory drive to the point of apnea.
• Use hydromorphone cautiously in elderly, cachectic, or debilitated patients, especially when initiating and titrating therapy, as they are at increased risk for adverse effects, especially respiratory depression.
• Use hydromorphone cautiously in patients whose ability to maintain a normal blood pressure is already compromised by a reduced blood volume or concurrent administration of certain CNS depressant drugs; the drug may cause severe hypotension in these patients, especially when initiating or titrating the dose of hydromorphone.
• To improve analgesic action, give hydromorphone before pain becomes intense.

G
H
I

• Give I.V. form by direct injection over at least 2 minutes. For infusion, mix drug with D₅W, normal saline solution, or Ringer's solution.

• Rotate I.M. and subcutaneous injection sites.

WARNING Monitor patient for respiratory depression, especially within the first 72 hours of initiating therapy or when increasing dosage, even when the drug has been used as prescribed and not misused or abused. Patients who are especially vulnerable include the elderly and those who are cachectic or debilitated. Be aware that overestimating hydromorphone dose when converting patients from another opioid medication can result in fatal overdose with the first dose. To avoid this, know that it is recommended to underestimate a patient's 24-hour oral hydromorphone requirement and provide rescue medication (e.g., immediate-release hydromorphone), as needed, until the right dose is determined. Keep resuscitation equipment and naloxone nearby.

• Monitor patient for hypotension, profound sedation, coma, or respiratory depression when administering hydromorphone around-the-clock; these reactions can occur if alcohol or illicit drugs are being used without the prescriber's knowledge.

• Monitor patients with seizure disorders because hydromorphone therapy may induce or aggravate convulsions.

• Monitor effectiveness of hydromorphone in relieving pain; consult prescriber as needed.

• Assess patient for constipation.

• Monitor patient for evidence of physical dependence or abuse.

• Anticipate that drug may mask or worsen gallbladder pain.

• Be aware that all other around-the-clock opioid analgesics should be stopped when E.R. tablets are prescribed. Expect to give immediate-release nonopioid analgesics for exacerbation of pain and for preventing pain during certain activities. Be aware that dosage adjustments with E.R. tablets may be made every 3 to 4 days, if needed.

• Know that E.R. tablets may be visible on abdominal X-rays under certain

circumstances, especially when digital enhancing techniques are utilized, because the tablet is nondeformable and does not change much in shape in the GI tract.

• Expect to taper dosages of hydromorphone that have been administered for an extended period of time to the opioid-tolerant patient gradually by 25 to 50% every 2 to 3 days, down to a dose of 8 mg before the drug is discontinued. This will help prevent signs and symptoms of withdrawal.

PATIENT TEACHING

• Instruct patient to take drug exactly as prescribed and before pain is severe.

• Alert patient that drug is a controlled substance. She should take steps to protect drug from theft or misuse.

• Advise patient to take drug with food to avoid GI distress.

• Tell patient not to break, chew, crush, or dissolve E.R. tablets, but to swallow them whole.

• Instruct patient to refrigerate suppositories.

• Caution patient to avoid alcohol and OTC drugs during therapy, unless prescriber approves.

• Instruct patient to report constipation, difficulty breathing, severe nausea, or vomiting.

• Inform patient that drug may cause drowsiness and sedation. Advise her to avoid hazardous activities until drug's CNS effects are known.

• Tell patient to change position slowly to minimize orthostatic hypotension.

• To avoid withdrawal, instruct physically dependent patient not to stop taking hydromorphone abruptly.

• Warn patient to keep drug out of reach of children, as accidental ingestion may cause death.

• Advise women of childbearing age to notify prescriber immediately if they suspect they are pregnant or become pregnant because hydromorphone may cause fetal harm or neonatal withdrawal that could be life-threatening.

• Advise patients when hydromorphone tablets or solution are no longer needed to flush the unused tablets or solution down the toilet or remit to authorities at a certified drug take-back program.

hydroxychloroquine sulfate

Plaquenil

Class and Category

Chemical class: 4-aminoquinoline compound
Therapeutic class: Antiprotozoal, antirheumatic, lupus erythematosus suppressant
Pregnancy category: C

Indications and Dosages

➤ *To prevent malaria*

TABLETS

Adults. 400 mg the same day of each week starting 2 wk before entering endemic area and continuing until departure from endemic area. If this isn't possible, initially 800 mg in two divided doses 6 hr apart, followed 1 wk later with 400 mg, and then 400 mg on same day of each week thereafter until departure from endemic area.

Infants and children. 5 mg/kg the same day of each week, starting 2 wk before entering endemic area and continuing until departure from endemic area. If this isn't possible, initially 10 mg/kg in two divided doses 6 hr apart, followed 1 wk later with 5 mg/kg, and then 5 mg/kg on same day of each week until departure from endemic area. *Maximum:* Adult dosage.

➤ *To treat acute attacks of malaria caused by* Plasmodium vivax, P. malariae, P. ovale, *and susceptible strains of* P. falciparum

TABLETS

Adults. *Initial:* 800 mg, followed by 400 mg in 6 to 8 hr and 400 mg on next 2 consecutive days. Or, 800 mg given as a single dose or an initial dose of 10 mg base/kg (maximum, 620 mg base [800 mg]), followed by 5 mg base/kg (maximum, 310 mg base [400 mg]) 6 hr after first dose, 5 mg base/kg 18 hr after second dose, and 5 mg base/kg 24 hr after third dose.

Infants and children. Initial: 10 mg base/kg (maximum, 620 mg base [800 mg]), followed by 5 mg base/kg (maximum, 310 mg base [400 mg]) 6 hr after first dose, 5 mg base/kg 18 hr after second dose, and 5 mg base/kg 24 hr after third dose.

➤ *To treat chronic discoid and systemic lupus erythematosus*

TABLETS

Adults. *Initial:* 400 mg once or twice daily for several weeks or months. *Maintenance:* 200 to 400 mg daily.

➤ *To treat acute or chronic rheumatoid arthritis*

TABLETS

Adults. *Initial:* 400 to 600 mg daily for 4 to 12 wk. *Maintenance:* 200 mg to 400 mg daily.

DOSAGE ADJUSTMENT For patients with rheumatoid arthritis who develop troublesome adverse reactions, initial dosage decreased for 5 to 10 days and then gradually increased to optimum response level.

Mechanism of Action

May mildly suppress the immune system, inhibiting production of rheumatoid factor and acute phase reactants. Hydroxychloroquine also accumulates in WBCs, stabilizing lysosomal membranes and inhibiting enzymes such as collagenase and proteases that cause cartilage breakdown. These actions may decrease symptoms of rheumatoid arthritis and lupus erythematosus.

Hydroxychloroquine also binds to and alters DNA of malaria parasite to prevent it from reproducing. It also may increase the pH of acid vesicles, which interferes with vesicle function and may inhibit parasitic phospholipid metabolism in erythrocytes, thereby halting plasmodial activity.

Contraindications

Hypersensitivity to 4-aminoquinoline compounds (including hydroxy-chloroquine), long-term therapy in children, retinal or visual changes related to 4-aminoquinoline compounds

Interaction

DRUGS

aurothioglucose: Increased risk of blood dyscrasias
digoxin: Increased digoxin concentrations

Adverse Reactions

CNS: Abnormal nerve conduction, ataxia, dizziness, emotional lability, headache, irritability, lassitude, nervousness,

neuromuscular sensory abnormalities, nightmares, psychosis, seizures, vertigo
CV: Cardiomyopathy (prolonged high doses)
EENT: Abnormal pigmentation (bullseye appearance) or colored vision, blurred vision, central scotoma with decreased visual acuity, corneal deposits, decreased corneal sensitivity, diplopia, irreversible retinal damage (in lupus erythematosus or rheumatoid arthritis), halo vision, lassitude, macular edema or atrophy, nerve-related hearing loss, nystagmus, pericentral or paracentral scotoma, photophobia, retinal fundus changes, tinnitus, visual abnormalities
ENDO: Hypoglycemia
GI: Abdominal cramps, anorexia, diarrhea, elevated liver function test results, fulminant hepatic failure, nausea, vomiting
HEME: Agranulocytosis, aplastic anemia, hemolysis (in patients with glucose-6-phosphate dehydrogenase [G6PD] deficiency), leukopenia, thrombocytopenia
MS: Atrophy of proximal skeletal muscle groups, depressed tendon reflexes, muscle weakness
RESP: Bronchospasm
SKIN: Acute generalized exanthematous pustulosis, alopecia, altered mucosal and skin pigmentation, bleaching of hair, dermatitis (including exfoliative dermatitis), non–light-sensitive psoriasis, pruritus, psoriasis exacerbation, rash, Stevens-Johnson syndrome, urticaria
Other: Angioedema, porphyria, weight loss

Nursing Considerations

• Use hydroxychloroquine cautiously in patients with G6PD deficiency, patients with hepatic disease or alcoholism, and patients taking hepatotoxic drugs.
• Monitor children closely for adverse reactions because they're especially sensitive to 4-aminoquinoline compounds.
• Observe patients with psoriasis closely because hydroxychloroquine may lead to severe psoriasis attack. Also monitor patients with porphyria closely because hydroxychloroquine may worsen it. Expect to use hydroxychloroquine in patients with psoriasis or porphyria only after risks and benefits have been considered.

• During prolonged therapy, obtain periodic blood cell counts, as ordered, to detect adverse hematologic effects. Expect to stop drug if severe adverse effects occur.
• Monitor patient's vision when giving hydroxychloroquine for lupus erythematosus or rheumatoid arthritis because irreversible retinal damage may occur in some patients during long-term or high-dose therapy. Ask regularly about vision abnormalities, such as light flashes or streaks, that may indicate retinopathy. Expect patient to have an initial ophthalmologic examination, followed by examinations every 3 months. Report changes to prescriber immediately, and expect drug to be stopped. Retinal changes may progress even after therapy stops.
• Monitor patient on long-term therapy for muscle weakness and abnormal knee and ankle reflexes. If present, notify prescriber and expect drug to be stopped.
• Expect drug to be stopped if patient with rheumatoid arthritis shows no improvement, such as reduced joint swelling or increased mobility, in 6 months.
• If serious adverse reactions occur, notify prescriber immediately. Expect drug to be stopped. Also expect to give ammonium chloride (8 g daily in divided doses for adults) 3 or 4 days weekly for several months because acidification of urine increases renal excretion of drug.

PATIENT TEACHING
• Instruct patient to take drug with meals or milk to minimize stomach upset.
• Tell patient to take hydroxychloroquine exactly as prescribed because taking too much may cause serious adverse reactions and taking too little or skipping doses decreases effectiveness.
• Caution patient to notify prescriber about troublesome adverse reactions. Hydroxychloroquine dosage may need to be adjusted or drug stopped.
• Caution patient who takes drug for rheumatoid arthritis or lupus erythematosus about possible visual reactions and the need for periodic eye examinations. Tell patient to notify prescriber about abnormal visual changes, including blurred vision, halos around lights, and light flashes or streaks; explain that drug will need to be stopped.

• Tell patient receiving prolonged therapy about the need for periodic blood tests to detect adverse effects.
• Advise patient to notify prescriber if muscle weakness develops.

hydroxyzine hydrochloride

Apo-Hydroxyzine (CAN), Atarax, Multipax (CAN), Novo-Hydroxyzin (CAN)

hydroxyzine pamoate

Vistaril

Class and Category
Chemical class: Piperazine derivative
Therapeutic class: Antianxiety, antiemetic, antihistamine, sedative-hypnotic
Pregnancy category: C

Indications and Dosages
➤ *To relieve anxiety and induce sedation and hypnosis*
CAPSULES, ORAL SUSPENSION, SYRUP, TABLETS
Adults and adolescents. 50 to 100 mg as a single dose.
Children. 600 mcg/kg as a single dose.
I.M. INJECTION
Adults and adolescents. 50 to 100 mg every 4 to 6 hr, as needed (antianxiety); 50 mg as a single dose (sedative-hypnotic).
➤ *To treat pruritus*
CAPSULES, ORAL SUSPENSION, SYRUP, TABLETS
Adults and adolescents. 25 to 100 mg three times daily or four times daily, as needed.
Children. 500 mcg/kg every 6 hr, as needed.
➤ *To provide antiemetic effects*
CAPSULES, ORAL SUSPENSION, SYRUP, TABLETS
Adults and adolescents. 25 to 100 mg three times daily or four times daily, as needed.
Children. 500 mcg/kg every 6 hr, as needed.
I.M. INJECTION
Adults and adolescents. 25 to 100 mg, as needed.
Children. 1.1 mg/kg as a single dose.
➤ *As adjunct to permit reduction in preoperative and postoperative opioid dosage*

I.M. INJECTION
Adults and adolescents. 25 to 100 mg given with prescribed opioid.
Children. 1.1 mg/kg given with prescribed opioid.
DOSAGE ADJUSTMENT For elderly patients, treatment is started at lowest possible dosage.

Route	Onset	Peak	Duration
P.O.	15–60 min	Unknown	4–6 hr
I.M.	20–30 min	Unknown	4–6 hr

Mechanism of Action
Competes with histamine$_1$ for histamine$_1$ receptor sites on surfaces of effector cells. This suppresses results of histaminic activity, including edema, flare, and pruritus. Hydroxyzine's antiemetic effect may stem from central anticholinergic actions. Sedative actions occur at subcortical level of CNS and are dose-related.

Contraindications
Breastfeeding; early pregnancy; hypersensitivity to cetirizine, hydroxyzine, or their components

Interaction
DRUGS
CNS depressants: Increased CNS depression
ACTIVITIES
alcohol use: Increased CNS depression

Adverse Reactions
CNS: Drowsiness, hallucinations, headache, involuntary motor activity, seizures, tremor
EENT: Dry mouth
SKIN: Fixed drug eruptions, pruritus, rash, urticaria
Other: Allergic reaction, injection-site pain

Nursing Considerations
• Don't give hydroxyzine by subcutaneous or I.V. route because tissue necrosis may occur.
• Inject I.M. form deep into large muscle, using Z-track method.
• Observe for oversedation if patient takes another CNS depressant.
PATIENT TEACHING
• Urge patient to avoid alcohol.
• Caution patient about drowsiness; tell her to avoid hazardous activities until drug's CNS effects are known.

G
H
I

• Instruct woman to tell prescriber if she is or could be pregnant because drug is contraindicated in early pregnancy.

hyoscyamine sulfate

Anaspaz, A-Spas S/L, Cystospaz, Cystospaz-M, Donnamar, ED-SPAZ, Gastrosed, Levbid, Levsin, Levsin/ SL, Levsinex Timecaps, Symax SL, Symax SR

Class and Category

Chemical class: Belladonna alkaloid, tertiary amine
Therapeutic class: Antimuscarinic, antispasmodic
Pregnancy category: C

Indications and Dosages

➤ *To treat peptic ulcers and GI tract disorders caused by spasm*

ELIXIR, ORAL SOLUTION
Adults and adolescents. 0.125 to 0.25 mg every 4 to 6 hr.
Children. Dosage individualized by weight.

E.R. CAPSULES
Adults and adolescents. 0.375 mg every 12 hr.

E.R. TABLETS
Adults and adolescents. 0.375 to 0.75 mg every 12 hr. *Maximum:* 1.5 mg daily.

TABLETS
Adults and adolescents. 0.125 to 0.5 mg three times daily or four times daily.
Children. Dosage individualized by weight.

I.V., I.M., OR SUBCUTANEOUS INJECTION
Adults and adolescents. 0.25 to 0.5 mg every 4 to 6 hr.
Children. Dosage individualized by weight.

➤ *To control salivation and excessive secretions during surgical procedures*

I.V. INJECTION
Adults and adolescents. 0.5 mg 30 to 60 min before procedure.

Route	Onset	Peak	Duration
P.O.*	20–30 min	30–60 min	4 hr
P.O. (E.R.)†	20–30 min	40–90 min	12 hr
I.V., I.M., SubQ	2–3 min	15–30 min	4 hr

Mechanism of Action

Competitively inhibits acetylcholine at autonomic postganglionic cholinergic receptors. Because the most sensitive receptors are in salivary, bronchial, and sweat glands, hyoscyamine acts mainly to reduce salivary, bronchial, and sweat gland secretions. It also causes GI smooth muscle to contract and decreases gastric secretion and GI motility. It also causes bladder detrusor muscle to contract, reduces nasal and oropharyngeal secretions, and decreases airway resistance from relaxation of smooth muscle in the bronchi and bronchioles.

Contraindications

Acute hemorrhage and hemodynamic instability; angle-closure glaucoma; hepatic disease; hypersensitivity to hyoscyamine, other anticholinergics, or their components; ileus; intestinal atony; myasthenia gravis; myocardial ischemia; obstructive GI disease; obstructive uropathy; renal disease; severe ulcerative colitis; tachycardia; toxic megacolon

Interaction

DRUGS
anticholinergics: Possibly increased anticholinergic effects
antidiarrheals (adsorbent): Possibly decreased hyoscyamine effects
calcium- and magnesium-containing antacids, carbonic anhydrase inhibitors, citrates, sodium bicarbonate, urinary alkalinizers: Possibly potentiated therapeutic and adverse effects of hyoscyamine
haloperidol: Possibly decreased haloperidol effects
ketoconazole: Possibly reduced ketoconazole absorption
metoclopramide: Possibly antagonized therapeutic effects of metoclopramide
opioid analgesics: Increased risk of severe constipation and ileus

---

* For tablets only; for elixir and oral solution, onset is 5 to 20 min, and peak and duration are unknown.
† For E.R. tablets only; for E.R. capsules, onset and peak are unknown, and duration is 12 hr..

Adverse Reactions
CNS: Drowsiness, insomnia
EENT: Blurred vision; dry mouth, nose, and throat; photophobia
ENDO: Decreased lactation
GI: Constipation
GU: Impotence, urine retention
SKIN: Decreased sweating
Other: Heatstroke, injection-site redness and urticaria

Nursing Considerations
• Use hyoscyamine cautiously in patients who have arrhythmias, autonomic neuropathy, coronary artery disease, heart failure, hiatal hernia with reflux esophagitis, hypertension, hyperthyroidism, renal failure, or tachycardia.
• Give drug 30 to 60 minutes before meals and at bedtime. Give bedtime dose at least 2 hours after last meal of day.
• Anticipate that tablets may not disintegrate and may appear in stool.
WARNING Anticipate an increased risk of drug-induced heatstroke in hot or humid weather because hyoscyamine decreases sweating.
WARNING Be aware that lower doses may paradoxically decrease heart rate. Higher doses affect nicotinic receptors in autonomic ganglia, causing delirium, disorientation, hallucinations, and restlessness.
• Monitor urine output, and be alert for urine retention.
PATIENT TEACHING
• Instruct patient to void before taking each dose and to notify prescriber if she has trouble urinating during therapy.
• Advise patient to take drug 30 to 60 minutes before meals and at bedtime. Bedtime dose should be taken at least 2 hours after last meal of the day.
• Explain that drug may cause drowsiness. Advise patient to avoid hazardous activities until drug's CNS effects are known.
• If patient reports dry mouth, suggest using sugarless hard candy or gum.
• Inform male patient that drug may cause impotence. If it occurs, suggest that he discuss it with prescriber.
• Advise patient to avoid exposure to high temperatures and to increase fluid intake, unless contraindicated.

ibandronate sodium
Boniva

Class and Category
Chemical class: Bisphosphonate
Therapeutic class: Bone resorption inhibitor
Pregnancy category: C

Indications and Dosages
➤ *To prevent osteoporosis in post-menopausal women*
TABLETS
Adults. 2.5 mg daily. Alternatively, 150 mg once monthly taken same day of each month.
➤ *To treat osteoporosis in postmenopausal women*
TABLETS
Adults. 2.5 mg daily. Alternatively, 150 mg once monthly taken same day of each month.
I.V. INJECTION
Adults. 3 mg every 3 months.

Mechanism of Action
Based on its affinity for hydroxyapatite, which is part of the mineral matrix of bone, osteoclast activity is inhibited and bone resorption and turnover is reduced. In postmenopausal women, the elevated rate of bone turnover is reduced leading to, on average, a net gain in bone mass.

Incompatiblities
Do not mix with calcium-containing solutions or other intravenously administered drugs.

Contraindications
Esophageal abnormalities that delay esophageal emptying, such as stricture or achalasia (oral form); hypersensitivity to ibandronate or its components; uncorrected hypocalcemia

Interaction
DRUGS
aspirin, NSAIDs: Increased risk of GI irritation
calcium-containing preparations, including antacids: Impaired absorption of ibandronate
FOODS
all foods: Decreased ibandronate bioavailability

G
H
I

Adverse Reactions

CNS: Asthenia, depression, dizziness, fatigue, headache, insomnia, nerve root lesion, vertigo
CV: Hypercholesterolemia, hypertension
EENT: Nasopharyngitis, pharyngitis, tooth disorder
ENDO: Transient decrease in serum calcium values
GI: Abdominal pain, constipation, diarrhea, dyspepsia, gastritis, gastroenteritis, nausea, vomiting
GU: Cystitis, UTI
MS: Arthralgia; arthritis; atypical subtrochanteric and diaphyseal femoral fractures; back, bone or extremity pain; joint disorder; localized osteoarthritis; myalgia
RESP: Bronchitis, pneumonia, upper respiratory infection
SKIN: Rash
Other: Allergic reaction, infection, influenza, injection-site reactions such as redness or swelling

Nursing Considerations

• Be aware that hypocalcemia, hypovitaminosis D, and other disturbances of bone and mineral metabolism must be effectively treated before starting ibandronate therapy.
• Know that ibandronate should not be administered to patients with severe renal impairment.
• Use cautiously in patients with active upper gastrointestinal problems (such as known Barrett's esophagus, dysphagia, other esophageal diseases, gastritis, duodenitis, or ulcers because drug may cause local irritation of the upper gastrointestinal mucosa.
• Make sure patient has had a dental checkup before having invasive dental procedures during ibandronate therapy, especially if patient has cancer; is receiving chemotherapy, head or neck radiation, or a corticosteroid; or has poor oral hygiene, because the risk of jaw osteonecrosis has increased in these patients taking other bisphosphonates, a class of drugs of which ibandronate is a member.
• Obtain serum creatinine level in patients receiving injection form of ibandronate prior to administering each dose because

other bisphosphonates have been associated with serious renal toxicity. If renal deterioration occurs, expect drug to be withheld.
• Administer parenteral ibandronate intravenously over 15 to 30 seconds using the needle provided. Prefilled syringes are for single use only. Be careful not to inject drug intra-arterally or paravenously, as this could lead to tissue damage.
• If appointment is missed for parenteral ibandronate therapy, administer drug as soon as possible. Schedule next injection from the date of the last injection, as drug must not be administered more frequently than once every 3 months.

PATIENT TEACHING

• Instruct patient prescribed oral ibandronate to take the tablet at least 1 hour before first food or drink of day (except water) while in an upright position and with 6 to 8 oz of water. Caution against lying down for at least 30 minutes after taking drug to keep it from lodging in esophagus and causing irritation. Also instruct patient not to chew or suck on tablet because doing so may irritate mouth or throat.
• Inform patient of need and importance of taking supplemental calcium and vitamin D on daily basis.
• Instruct patient to take calcium supplements at least 2 hours before or after oral ibandronate.
• Advise patient to stop taking drug and to notify prescriber if GI symptoms appear or become worse.
• Alert patient that drugs in the same class as ibandronate have caused severe bone, joint, or muscle pain. If such symptoms appear while taking ibandronate, advise patient to contact prescriber. Also, tell him to report new or worsening groin or thigh pain.
• Tell patient to stop taking drug and notify prescriber if he develops dysphagia, pain while swallowing, retrosternal pain, or new or worsening heartburn.
• Urge women of childbearing age to tell prescriber about planned, suspected, or known pregnancy because of risk to fetal skeleton.
• Instruct patient on proper oral hygiene and on the need to notify prescriber about invasive dental procedures.

ibuprofen

Actiprofen Caplets (CAN), Advil, Apo-Ibuprofen (CAN), Bayer Select Ibuprofen Pain Relief Formula Caplets, Caldolor, Children's Advil, Children's Motrin, Dolgesic, Excedrin IB, Genpril, Haltran, Ibifon 600 Caplets, Ibuprin, Ibuprohm Caplets, Ibu-Tab, Medipren, Midol IB, Motrin, Motrin-IB, Novo-Profen (CAN), Nu-Ibuprofen (CAN), Nuprin, Pamprin-IB, Q-Profen, Rufen, Trendar

Class and Category
Chemical class: Propionic acid derivative
Therapeutic class: Analgesic, anti-inflammatory, antipyretic
Pregnancy category: C (before 30 weeks gestation); D (starting at 30 weeks gestation)

Indications and Dosages
➤ *To relieve pain in rheumatoid arthritis and osteoarthritis*
CAPSULES, CHEWABLE TABLETS, ORAL SUSPENSION, TABLETS
Adults. 300 mg four times daily; or 400, 600, or 800 mg three times daily; or four times daily. Range: 1.2 to 3.2 g daily.
➤ *To relieve mild to moderate pain*
CAPSULES, CHEWABLE TABLETS, ORAL SUSPENSION, TABLETS
Adults. 400 mg every 4 to 6 hr, as needed.
I.V. INFUSION
Adults. 400 to 800 mg infused over at least 30 minutes, every 6 hours, as needed.
➤ *To relieve acute migraine pain*
CAPSULES, CHEWABLE TABLETS, ORAL SUSPENSION, TABLETS
Adults. 200 to 400 mg at onset of migraine pain. *Maximum:* 400 mg daily.
➤ *To relieve pain in primary dysmenorrhea*
CAPSULES, CHEWABLE TABLETS, ORAL SUSPENSION, TABLETS
Adults. 400 mg every 4 hr, as needed.
➤ *To relieve pain in juvenile arthritis*
CAPSULES, CHEWABLE TABLETS, ORAL SUSPENSION, TABLETS
Children. 30 to 70 mg/kg daily in divided doses three times daily or four times daily; 20 mg/kg daily for mild disease.

➤ *To relieve minor aches, pains, and dysmenorrhea and to reduce fever*
CAPSULES, CHEWABLE TABLETS, ORAL SUSPENSION, TABLETS
Adults. 200 to 400 mg every 4 to 6 hr. *Maximum:* 1.2 g daily.
➤ *To relieve moderate to severe pain as an adjunct to opioid analgesics*
I.V. INFUSION
Adults. 400 mg to 800 mg infused over at least 30 minutes, every 6 hours, as needed.
➤ *To reduce fever*
CAPSULES, CHEWABLE TABLETS, ORAL SUSPENSION, TABLETS
Children ages 6 months to 12 years. 5 to 10 mg/kg every 4 to 6 hr. *Maximum:* 40 mg/kg daily.
I.V. INFUSION
Adults. 400 mg infused over at least 30 minutes, followed by 400 mg infused over at least 30 minutes, every 4 to 6 hours. Or, 100 to 200 mg infused over at least 30 minutes, every 4 hours, as needed.

Route	Onset	Peak	Duration
P.O.*	30 min	Unknown	4–6 hr
P.O.†	Up to 7 days	1–2 wk	Unknown
P.O.‡	In 1 hr	2–4 hr	6–8 hr

Mechanism of Action
Blocks activity of cyclooxygenase, the enzyme needed to synthesize prosta-glandins, which mediate inflammatory response and cause local vasodilation, swelling, and pain. By inhibiting prostaglandins, this NSAID reduces inflammatory symptoms and relieves pain. Ibuprofen's antipyretic action probably stems from its effect on the hypothalamus, which increases peripheral blood flow, causing vasodilation and encouraging heat dissipation.

Contraindications
Angioedema, asthma, bronchospasm, nasal polyps, rhinitis, or urticaria caused by hypersensitivity to aspirin, ibuprofen, iodides, or other NSAIDs; perioperative pain with coronary artery bypass graft surgery

* For analgesic effects.
† For anti-inflammatory effects.
‡ For antipyretic effects.

Interaction

DRUGS

acetaminophen: Possibly increased renal effects with long-term use of both drugs
antihypertensives: Decreased effectiveness of these drugs
aspirin: Possibly decreased cardioprotective and stroke-preventive effects of aspirin
aspirin, other NSAIDs: Increased risk of bleeding and adverse GI effects
bone marrow depressants: Possibly increased leukopenic and thrombocytopenic effects of bone marrow depressants
cefamandole, cefoperazone, cefotetan: Increased risk of hypoprothrombinemia and bleeding
colchicine, platelet aggregation inhibitors: Increased risk of GI bleeding, hemorrhage, and ulcers
corticosteroids, potassium supplements: Increased risk of adverse GI effects
cyclosporine: Increased risk of nephro-toxicity from both drugs, increased blood cyclosporine level
digoxin: Increased blood digoxin level and risk of digitalis toxicity
diuretics (loop, potassium-sparing, and thiazide): Decreased diuretic and antihypertensive effects
gold compounds, nephrotoxic drugs: Increased risk of adverse renal effects
heparin, oral anticoagulants, thrombolytics: Increased anticoagulant effects, increased risk of hemorrhage
insulin, oral antidiabetics: Possibly increased hypoglycemic effects of these drugs
lithium: Increased blood lithium level
methotrexate: Decreased methotrexate clearance and increased risk of toxicity
plicamycin, valproic acid: Increased risk of hypoprothrombinemia and GI bleeding, hemorrhage, and ulcers
probenecid: Possibly increased blood level, effectiveness, and risk of toxicity of ibuprofen

ACTIVITIES

alcohol use: Increased risk of adverse GI effects

Adverse Reactions

CNS: Aseptic meningitis, dizziness, headache, nervousness, seizures, stroke
CV: Fluid retention, heart failure, hypertension, MI, peripheral edema, tachycardia
EENT: Amblyopia, epistaxis, stomatitis, tinnitus
GI: Abdominal cramps, distention, or pain; anorexia; constipation; diarrhea; diverticulitis; dyspepsia; dysphagia; elevated liver function test results; epigastric discomfort; esophagitis; flatulence; gastritis; gastroenteritis; gastroesophageal reflux disease; GI bleeding, hemorrhage, perforation, or ulceration; heartburn; hemorrhoids; hepatic failure; hepatitis; hiatal hernia; indigestion; melena; nausea; stomatitis; vomiting
GU: Cystitis, hematuria, renal failure (acute)
HEME: Agranulocytosis, anemia, aplastic anemia, eosinophilia, hemolytic anemia, leukopenia, neutropenia, pancytopenia, prolonged bleeding time, thrombocytopenia
RESP: Bronchospasm, dyspnea, wheezing
SKIN: Blisters, erythema multiforme, photosensitivity, pruritus, rash, Stevens-Johnson syndrome, toxic epidermal necrolysis, urticaria
Other: Anaphylaxis, angioedema, flulike symptoms, hypokalemia, weight gain

Nursing Considerations

• Be aware that ibuprofen should not be used in pregnant women starting at 30 weeks gestation because premature closure of the ductus arteriosus may occur in the fetus.
• Use ibuprofen with extreme caution in patients with a history of ulcer disease or GI bleeding because NSAIDs such as ibuprofen increase risk of GI bleeding and ulceration. Expect to use ibuprofen for shortest time possible in these patients.
• Risk of serious cardiovascular thrombotic events such as a MI or stroke increases the longer ibuprofen is used. Expect to give drug for shortest time possible.
• For I.V. use, dilute Caldolor brand of ibuprofen to final concentration of 4 mg/ml or less using 0.9% sodium chloride injection, 5% dextrose injection, or lactated Ringer's solution. For an 800-mg dose, dilute 8 ml Caldolor in at least 200 ml diluent; for a 400-mg dose, dilute 4 ml Caldolor in at least 100 ml diluent. Diluted solutions may be kept at room temperature up to 24 hours. When infusing ibuprofen intravenously, infusion time must be at least 30 minutes.

- Serious GI tract ulceration, bleeding, and perforation may occur without warning symptoms. Elderly patients are at greater risk. To minimize risk, give oral drug with food. If GI distress occurs, withhold drug and notify prescriber immediately.
- Use ibuprofen cautiously in patients with hypertension, and monitor blood pressure closely throughout therapy. Drug may cause hypertension or worsen it.

WARNING Monitor patient closely for thrombotic events, including MI and stroke, because NSAIDs increase the risk.

- Monitor patient—especially if he's elderly or receiving long-term oral ibuprofen therapy—for less common but serious adverse GI reactions, including anorexia, constipation, diverticulitis, dysphagia, esophagitis, gastritis, gastroenteritis, gastroesophageal reflux disease, hemorrhoids, hiatal hernia, melena, stomatitis, and vomiting.
- Monitor liver function test results because, in rare cases, elevations may progress to severe hepatic reactions, including fatal hepatitis, liver necrosis, and hepatic failure.
- Monitor BUN and serum creatinine levels in elderly patients, patients taking diuretics or ACE inhibitors, and patients with heart failure, impaired renal function, or hepatic dysfunction; drug may cause renal failure.
- Monitor CBC for decreased hemoglobin and hematocrit. Drug may worsen anemia.

WARNING If patient has bone marrow suppression or is receiving an anti-neoplastic drug, monitor laboratory results (including WBC count), and watch for evidence of infection. Ibuprofen's anti-inflammatory and antipyretic actions may mask signs and symptoms, such as fever and pain.

- Assess patient's skin regularly for signs of rash or other hypersensitivity reaction because ibuprofen is an NSAID and may cause serious skin reactions without warning, even in patients with no history of NSAID sensitivity. At first sign of reaction, stop drug and notify prescriber.
- Although analgesic effect occurs at low doses, expect to give at least 400 mg four times daily for anti-inflammatory effect.
- Expect higher doses for rheumatoid arthritis than for osteoarthritis.
- Be aware that ibuprofen oral suspension may contain sucrose, which may affect blood glucose level in diabetic patients.

PATIENT TEACHING

- Instruct patient to take tablets with a full glass of water, and caution him not to lie down for 15 to 30 minutes to prevent esophageal irritation.
- Advise patient to take drug with food or after meals to reduce GI distress.
- Urge patient no more drug or for a longer time than prescribed because stomach bleeding may occur and risk of MI or stroke may increase.
- Instruct patient to consult prescriber if he needs to take drug for more than 3 days for fever or 10 days for pain; if stomach problems (heartburn, upset, pain) recur; if he has a history of ulcers, bleeding problems, hypertension, or heart or renal disease; if he takes a diuretic; or if he's over age 65.
- Inform patient with phenylketonuria that Motrin chewable tablets contain aspartame.
- Inform patient that full therapeutic effect for arthritis may take 2 weeks or longer.
- Urge patient to avoid taking two different NSAIDs at the same time, unless directed, and to alert prescriber before taking ibuprofen if he has ever had an allergic reaction to any other analgesic or fever-reducing drug or has a history of asthma.
- Urge patient to avoid alcohol, aspirin, and corticosteroids while taking ibuprofen, unless prescribed. If patient takes aspirin as prevention of MI or stroke, explain that ibuprofen may interfere with this effect.
- Suggest that patient wear sunscreen and protective clothing when outdoors.
- Advise patient to report flulike symptoms, rash, signs of GI bleeding, swelling, vision changes, and weight gain.
- Urge parents to tell prescriber promptly if child receiving drug develops a severe or persistent sore throat, high fever, head-ache, persistent diarrhea, nausea, or vomiting or hasn't been drinking fluids.
- Advise parents to consult prescriber before giving OTC ibuprofen to a child if the

G
H
I

child has asthma, ulcers, bleeding problems, high blood pressure, heart or kidney disease, a need for diuretic therapy, serious adverse effects from previous use of fever reducers or pain relievers, or persistent stomach problems, such as heartburn, upset stomach, or stomach pain.

• Caution pregnant patient not to take NSAIDs such as ibuprofen during last trimester because they may cause premature closure of the ductus arteriosus.

• Explain that ibuprofen may increase risk of serious adverse cardiovascular reactions; urge patient to seek immediate medical attention if signs or symptoms arise, such as chest pain, shortness of breath, weakness, and slurring of speech.

• Explain that ibuprofen may increase risk of serious adverse GI reactions; stress importance of seeking immediate medical attention for such signs and symptoms as epigastric or abdominal pain, indigestion, black or tarry stools, or vomiting blood or material that looks like coffee grounds.

• Alert patient to rare but serious skin reactions. Urge him to seek immediate medical attention for rash, blisters, itching, fever, or other indications of hypersensitivity.

ibutilide fumarate

Corvert

Class and Category

Chemical: Methanesulfonanilide derivative
Therapeutic: Class III antiarrhythmic
Pregnancy category: C

Indications and Dosages

➤ *To rapidly convert recent-onset atrial flutter or fibrillation to sinus rhythm*

I.V. INFUSION

Adults weighing 60 kg (132 lb) or more. 1 mg over 10 min. Dose repeated 10 min after first dose is finished if arrhythmia persists.

Adults weighing less than 60 kg. 0.01 mg/kg over 10 min. Dose is repeated 10 min after first dose is completed if arrhythmia persists.

DOSAGE ADJUSTMENT Infusion stopped if arrhythmia is terminated or if sustained or

nonsustained ventricular tachycardia or prolonged QT or QTc interval develops.

Mechanism of Action

May promote sodium movement through slow inward sodium channels in myocardial cell membranes. Ibutilide also may inhibit potassium channels in myocardial cell membranes involved in cardiac repolarization. These actions prolong cardiac action potential by delaying repolarization and increasing atrial and ventricular refractoriness. As a result, sinus rate slows and AV conduction is delayed.

Contraindications

Hypersensitivity to ibutilide or components

Interaction

DRUGS

amiodarone, astemizole, disopyramide, maprotiline, phenothiazines, procainamide, quinidine, sotalol, tricyclic antidepressants: Possibly prolonged QT interval, leading to increased risk of proarrhythmias

Adverse Reactions

CNS: Headache, syncope
CV: AV block, bradycardia, bundle-branch block, heart failure, hypertension, hypotension, idioventricular rhythm, orthostatic hypotension, palpitations, prolonged QT interval, sinus and supraventricular tachycardia, supraventricular arrhythmias, ventricular arrhythmias, ventricular tachycardia (sustained and nonsustained)
GI: Nausea
GU: Renal failure

Nursing Considerations

• Before giving ibutilide, check serum electrolyte levels and expect to correct abnormalities, as prescribed. Be especially alert for hypokalemia and hypomagnesemia, which can lead to arrhythmias.

• Give drug undiluted or dilute in 50 ml normal saline solution or D_5W. Add contents of 10-ml vial (0.1 mg/ml) to 50 ml solution to obtain 0.017 mg/ml. Use polyvinyl chloride plastic bags or polyolefin bags for admixtures. Give drug within 24 hours (48 hours if refrigerated).

- Infuse drug slowly over 10 minutes.
- As ordered, monitor patient's cardiac rhythm continuously during infusion and for at least 4 hours afterward—longer if arrhythmias appear or if patient has abnormal hepatic function. Observe patient for ventricular ectopy.
- Make sure defibrillator and drugs to treat sustained ventricular tachycardia are available during therapy and when monitoring patient after therapy.

PATIENT TEACHING
- Inform patient that ibutilide will be given by I.V. infusion and that his heart rhythm will be monitored continuously.
- Ask patient to report chest pain, faintness, numbness, tingling, palpitations, and shortness of breath.
- Advise patient to keep follow-up appointments to monitor heart rhythm.

icatibant
Firazyr

Class and Category
Chemical class: Synthetic decapeptide
Therapeutic class: Angioedema suppressant
Pregnancy category: C

Indications and Dosages
➤ *To treat acute attacks of hereditary angioedema (HAE)*

SUBCUTANEOUS INJECTION
Adults. *Initial:* 30 mg over at least 30 seconds, followed by 30 mg over at least 30 seconds 6 hours later, if needed. An additional 30-mg dose administered over at least 30 seconds may be given 6 hours after second dose, if needed. *Maximum:* 3 doses in a 24-hour period.

Mechanism of Action
Inhibits bradykinin, a vasodilator thought to be responsible for the characteristic HAE symptoms of localized swelling, inflammation, and pain. By inhibiting bradykinin from binding to the B2 receptor, clinical symptoms of HAE cannot develop.

Contraindications
Hypersensitivity to icatibant or its components

Interaction
DRUGS
ACE inhibitors: Increased antihypertensive effect of ACE inhibitors

Adverse Reactions
CNS: Dizziness, fever
GI: Elevated transaminase level
Other: Anti-icatibant antibody formation, injection reactions such as bruising, burning, erythema, hematoma, hypoesthesia, irritation, numbness, pain, swelling, urticaria, or warmth

Nursing Considerations
- Be aware that the only needle that should be used is the one supplied by the manufacturer. When attaching the 25-gauge needle to the syringe hub, it must be screwed on securely.
- Administer icatibant over at least 30 seconds.
- Monitor patient closely following administration of icatibant for signs of airway obstruction. Have emergency equipment nearby. Notify prescriber immediately of any signs of airway obstruction and provide emergency intervention, as indicated.

PATIENT TEACHING
- Teach patient how to attach needle to syringe hub. Caution not to use a different needle.
- Instruct patient how to administer a subcutaneous injection.
- Instruct patient to administer icatibant over at least 30 seconds immediately upon development of any signs of angioedema. Emphasize importance of seeking immediate medical attention after administering icatibant because of the potential for airway closure.

icosapent ethyl
Vascepa

Class and Category
Chemical class: Ethyl ester of eicosapentaenoic acid
Therapeutic class: Antihypertriglyceridemic
Pregnancy category: C

Indications and Dosages
➤ *Adjunct to diet to reduce triglyceride levels in patients with severe (equal to or greater than 500 mg/dl) hypertriglyceridemia*

CAPSULES

Adults. 2 grams twice daily with food.

Mechanism of Action
Reduces very low-density lipoprotein triglycerides (VLDL-TG) synthesis and/or secretion in the liver and enhances triglyceride clearance from circulating VLDL particles. Mechanisms used to accomplish this may include increased beta oxidation, inhibition of acyl-CoA:1,2-diacylglycerol acyltransferase, increased plasma lipoprotein lipase activity, and decreased lipogenesis in the liver. These mechanisms work together to lower triglyceride levels.

Contraindications
Hypersensitivity to icosapent ethyl or its components

Interaction
DRUGS

antiplatelet drugs: Possibly increased bleeding time

Adverse Reactions
EENT: Oropharyngeal pain
MS: Arthralgia

Nursing Considerations
• Use icosapent ethyl cautiously in patients with a known hypersensitivity to fish and/or shellfish because the drug contains ethyl esters of the omega-3 fatty acid obtained from the oil of fish.
• Be aware that patient should have been placed on a lipid-lowering diet and exercise regimen before starting icosapent ethyl therapy.
• Know that efforts should be made to control conditions that may increase lipid abnormalities, such as diabetes mellitus, hypothyroidism, and alcohol intake.
• Expect medications known to exacerbate hypertriglyceridemia, such as beta blockers, estrogen therapy, and immuno-suppressants.
• Obtain lipid levels prior to initiating icosapent ethyl therapy, as ordered, to determine a baseline. Monitor lipid levels

periodically throughout icosapent ethyl therapy to determine effectiveness.
• Monitor alanine aminotransferase and aspartate aminotransferase levels periodically, as ordered, in patients with hepatic impairment.

PATIENT TEACHING
• Tell patient that icosapent ethyl therapy is not a substitution for diet and exercise but that these lifestyle changes need to continue during icosapent ethyl therapy.
• Instruct patient to take capsules whole and not to break, open, crush, dissolve, or chew the capsules.
• Inform patient that periodic blood tests will be needed to monitor effectiveness of icosapent ethyl therapy.

iloperidone
Fanapt

Class and Category
Chemical class: Piperidinyl-benzisoxazole derivative
Therapeutic class: Second-generation antipsychotic; atypical antipsychotic
Pregnancy category: C

Indications and Dosages
➤ *To treat schizophrenia*

TABLETS

Adults. *Initial:* 1 mg twice daily, adjusted to target dosage range as follows: 2 mg twice daily on day 2, 4 mg twice daily on day 3, and 6 mg twice daily on day 4. Dosage may be further increased, as needed, as follows: 8 mg twice daily on day 5, 10 mg twice daily on day 6, and 12 mg twice daily on day 7. *Maximum:* 12 mg twice daily.

DOSAGE ADJUSTMENT For patients taking strong CYP2D6 or CYP3A4 inhibitors, dosage reduced by half.

Route	Onset	Peak	Duration
P.O.	1–2 wk	2–4 hr	Unknown

Mechanism of Action
Selectively blocks serotonin type 2 (5-HT$_2$) and dopamine type 2 (D$_2$) receptors in CNS, thereby suppressing psychotic symptoms.

Contraindications
Hypersensitivity to iloperidone or its components

Interaction
DRUGS
antibiotics such as fluoroquinolones or macrolides, class I A antiarrhythmics such as procainamide or quinidine, class III antiarrhythmics such as amiodarone or sotalol, other antipsychotic drugs such as chlorpromiazine or thioridazine, or any other drug that affects the QT interval, such as methadone or pentamidine: Possibly prolonged QT interval
antihypertensive drugs: Increased antihypertensive effects
CYP3A4 inhibitors such as ketoconazole, CYP2D6 inhibitors such as fluoxetine or paroxetine: Increased plasma iloperidone level
dextromethorphan: Increased blood dextromethorphan level

Adverse Reactions
CNS: Aggression, delusion, dizziness, extrapyramidal effects, fatigue, lethargy, neuroleptic malignant syndrome, seizures, somnolence, suicidal ideation, restlessness, tremor
CV: CHF, dyslipidemia, orthostatic hypotension, palpitations, QT-interval prolongation, tachycardia
EENT: Blurred vision, conjunctivitis, dry mouth, nasal congestion, nasopharyngitis, upper respiratory tract infection
ENDO: Diabetic ketoacidosis, elevated prolactin levels, hyperglycemia, hyperosmolar coma
GI: Abdominal discomfort, diarrhea, nausea
GU: Ejaculation failure, erectile dysfunction, priapism, urinary incontinence
HEME: Leukopenia
MS: Arthralgia, musculoskeletal stiffness, spasms, myalgia
RESP: Dyspnea
SKIN: Rash
Other: Weight gain

Nursing Considerations
• Iloperidone shouldn't be used in patients with a history of cardiovascular disease such as QT-interval prolongation, recent MI, uncompensated heart failure, or cardiac arrhythmias. It also shouldn't be used in patients taking other drugs known to prolong the QT interval and in patients with hepatic impairment.
WARNING Iloperidone shouldn't be used to treat patients with dementia-related psychosis, especially elderly patients, because of an increased risk of death.
• Use cautiously in patients who have a history of seizures or who have conditions that lower the seizure threshold, such as Alzheimer's dementia. Also use cautiously in patients who are at risk for aspiration pneumonia or who have moderate hepatic impairment (not recommended for use in patients with severe hepatic impairment).
• Expect to start dosage adjustment schedule in patients who have been off iloperidone therapy for more than 3 days.
• Obtain baseline serum potassium and magnesium levels in patients at risk for electrolyte imbalances, and then monitor periodically throughout therapy, as ordered, because electrolyte imbalances increase risk of prolonged QT interval or arrhythmia. If patient reports dizziness, palpitations, or syncope, notify prescriber and expect further evaluation to be done.
WARNING Neuroleptic malignant syndrome has occurred in patients taking other antipsychotic drugs. Monitor patient for hyperpyrexia, muscle rigidity, altered mental status, and autonomic instability. If present, notify prescriber immediately, expect drug to be discontinued, and start intensive treatment, as prescribed. Watch for recurrence if patient resumes antipsychotic therapy.
• Monitor patient for tardive dyskinesia, which has occurred with other antipsychotic drugs. If patient develops involuntary, dyskinetic movements, notify prescriber and expect to discontinue drug.
• Monitor blood glucose level, especially in patients with diabetes mellitus, because iloperidone may alter blood glucose enough to induce life-threatening ketoacidosis or hyperosmolar coma.
• Monitor patient's CBC periodically, as ordered, especially during first few months of therapy, because iloperidone may cause neutropenia. Also, be aware that other antipyschotic drugs have caused sometimes fatal leukopenia and agranulocytosis. If patient's WBC count decreases, expect drug to be discontinued.

• Monitor patient closely for abnormal tendencies that may suggest suicidal thinking, especially when iloperidone therapy starts or dosage is changed.

PATIENT TEACHING

• Inform patient that when iloperidone therapy starts, dosage must be adjusted for up to a week to reach target level. Also explain that adjustment process will need to be repeated if she skips drug for more than 3 days.

• Advise patient or caregiver to notify prescriber about unusual, severe, or persistent adverse reactions because drug may need to be discontinued.

• Urge patient or caregiver to report evidence of abnormal thinking, especially when therapy starts or dosage changes.

• Tell diabetic patient to monitor blood glucose levels closely and to report persistent elevations immediately to prescriber.

• Caution patient to avoid hazardous activities until CNS effects of drug are known. Patient should also avoid alcohol.

• Instruct patient to avoid activities that might raise body temperature, such as doing strenuous exercise, being exposed to extreme heat, taking other drugs with anticholinergic activity, or being subjected to dehydration.

• Emphasize the need to comply with follow-up appointments and laboratory tests.

• Tell patient to rise slowly from lying to sitting position and from sitting position to standing to avoid dizziness or light-headedness during therapy.

• Advise female patient of childbearing age to notify prescriber if she intends to become or suspects that she is pregnant during therapy.

imipramine hydrochloride

Apo-Imipramine (CAN), Impril (CAN), Norfranil, Novopramine (CAN), Tipramine, Tofranil

imipramine pamoate

Tofranil-PM

Class and Category

Chemical class: Dibenzazepine derivative
Therapeutic class: Antidepressant
Pregnancy category: Not rated

Indications and Dosages

➤ *To treat depression*

CAPSULES

Adults. *Initial:* 75 mg daily at bedtime, gradually increased as needed and tolerated. *Maximum:* 300 mg daily (hospitalized patients), 200 mg/day (outpatients).

TABLETS

Adults. *Initial:* 25 to 50 mg three times daily or four times daily, gradually increased as needed and tolerated. *Maximum:* 300 mg daily (hospitalized patients), 200 mg daily (outpatients).

DOSAGE ADJUSTMENT Initial dosage reduced to 25 mg at bedtime for depressed elderly patients; then adjusted as needed and tolerated up to 100 mg daily in divided doses.

Adolescents. *Initial:* 25 to 50 mg daily in divided doses, adjusted as needed and tolerated. *Maximum:* 100 mg daily.

Children ages 6 to 12. 10 to 30 mg daily in divided doses twice daily.

➤ *As adjunct to treat childhood enuresis*

TABLETS

Children age 6 and over. 25 mg 1 hr before bedtime. Increased to 50 mg if no response occurs within 1 wk and child is under age 12; increased to 75 mg if child is age 12 or over. *Maximum:* 2.5 mg/kg daily.

Route	Onset	Peak	Duration
P.O.	2–3 wk*	Unknown	Unknown

Mechanism of Action

May interfere with reuptake of serotonin (and possibly other neurotransmitters) at presynaptic neurons, thus enhancing serotonin's effects at postsynaptic receptors. Mood elevation may result from restoration of normal levels of neurotransmitters at nerve synapses. This tricyclic antidepressant also blocks acetylcholine receptors, which may explain how it relieves enuresis.

Contraindications

Acute recovery period after MI; hypersensitivity to imipramine, other

* For antidepressant effect.

tricyclic antidepressants, or their components; use within 14 days of MAO inhibitor therapy, including intravenous methylene blue and linezolid

Interaction
DRUGS
amantadine, anticholinergics, antidyskinetics, antihistamines: Risk of increased anticholinergic effects, including confusion, hallucinations, and nightmares
anticonvulsants: Increased risk of CNS depression, increased risk of seizures, decreased effectiveness of imipramine
antithyroid drugs: Possibly agranulocytosis
barbiturates, carbamazepine: Possibly decreased imipramine level and effects
cimetidine, fluoxetine: Possibly increased blood imipramine level
clonidine, guanadrel, guanethidine: Possibly decreased antihypertensive effects of these drugs, increased CNS depression (clonidine)
CNS depressants: Increased CNS depression, respiratory depression, and hypotension
disulfiram, ethchlorvynol: Risk of delirium, increased CNS depression (ethchlorvynol)
estramustine, estrogen-containing oral contraceptives, estrogens: Risk of increased bioavailability of imipramine, increased depression
MAO inhibitors: Increased risk of hypertensive crisis, severe seizures, and death
oral anticoagulants: Possibly increased anticoagulant activity
pimozide, probucol: Risk of arrhythmias
sympathomimetics (including ophthalmic epinephrine and vasoconstrictive local anesthetics): Increased risk of arrhythmias, hyperpyrexia, hypertension, tachycardia
thyroid hormones: Risk of increased therapeutic and adverse effects of both drugs
ACTIVITIES
alcohol use: Increased CNS depression, increased alcohol effects
sun exposure: Increased risk of photosensitivity

Adverse Reactions
CNS: Anxiety, ataxia, chills, confusion, delirium, dizziness, drowsiness, excitation, extrapyramidal reactions, fever, hallucinations, headache, insomnia, nervousness, nightmares, parkinsonism, seizures, serotonin syndrome, stroke, suicidal ideation, tremor
CV: Arrhythmias, orthostatic hypotension, palpitations
EENT: Blurred vision, dry mouth, increased intraocular pressure, pharyngitis, taste perversion, tinnitus, tongue swelling
ENDO: Gynecomastia, syndrome of inappropriate ADH secretion
GI: Constipation, diarrhea, heartburn, ileus, increased appetite, nausea, vomiting
GU: Impotence, libido changes, testicular swelling, urine retention
HEME: Agranulocytosis, bone marrow depression
RESP: Wheezing
SKIN: Alopecia, diaphoresis, jaundice, photosensitivity, pruritus, rash, urticaria
Other: Allergic reaction, facial edema, weight gain

Nursing Considerations
• Use imipramine cautiously in patients with a history of urine retention or angle-closure glaucoma because drug's anticholinergic effects may cause urine retention and increased intraocular pressure.

WARNING Don't give MAO inhibitors within 2 weeks of imipramine, including intravenous methylene blue and linezolid. Patient may experience hypertensive crisis, seizures, and death.

WARNING Monitor patient for possible serotonin syndrome, characterized by agitation, chills, confusion, diaphoresis, diarrhea, fever, hyperactive reflexes, poor coordination, restlessness, shaking, talking or acting with uncontrolled excitement, tremor, and twitching. Notify prescriber immediately if serotonin syndrome is suspected because it can become life-threatening. Expect to discontinue imipramine therapy if serotonin syndrome is confirmed.

• Frequently assess for adverse reactions during first 2 hours of therapy.
• Check supine and standing blood pressure for orthostatic hypotension before and during imipramine therapy and before dosage increases.
• Anticipate increased risk of arrhythmias in patients with a history of cardiac disease.

G
H
I

• When drug is used for depression, expect mood elevation to take 2 to 3 weeks. Watch patient closely for suicidal tendencies, especially children and adolescents and especially when therapy starts or dosage changes, because depression may worsen temporarily at these times.

• Avoid abrupt withdrawal of drug in patients on long-term therapy. Such withdrawal may cause headache, malaise, nausea, sleep disturbance, and vomiting.

• Taper drug gradually, as ordered, a few days before surgery to avoid risk of hypertension during surgery.

• Obtain CBC, as ordered, if patient experiences signs and symptoms of infection, such as fever or pharyngitis.

• Limit amount of drug given to potentially suicidal patient.

PATIENT TEACHING

• Advise patient to take imipramine exactly as prescribed. Warn that stopping drug abruptly may cause headache, malaise, nausea, trouble sleeping, and vomiting.

• Caution parents to monitor child or adolescent closely for suicidal tendencies, especially when therapy starts or dosage changes.

• Urge patient to report chills, trouble urinating, dizziness, excess sedation, fever, palpitations, signs of allergic reaction, and sore throat.

• Caution patient to avoid hazardous activities until drug's CNS effects are known.

• Urge patient to avoid alcohol during imipramine therapy because it increases CNS depression and alcohol effects.

• Suggest that patient eat small, frequent meals to help relieve nausea.

• Instruct patient to avoid prolonged exposure to sunlight because of the risk of photosensitivity.

• Inform male patient about possible impotence and increased or decreased libido.

• If patient reports dry mouth, suggest sugarless candy or gum to relieve it. Tell him to check with prescriber if dry mouth persists after 2 weeks.

immune globulin intramuscular (human)
(gamma globulin, IG)

BayGam, GamaSTAN S/D, WinRho SDF

immune globulin intravenous (human)

Bivigam 10% Liquid; Carimune NF, Nanofiltered; Gammaplex 5% Liquid, Octagam 10%

(IGIV, immune serum globulin, ISG, IVIG)

Flebogamma 5% DIF, Flebogamma 10% DIF, Gamimune N 5% S/D, Gamimune N 10% S/D, Gammagard Liquid, Gammagard S/D, Gammagard S/D 0.5 g, Gammar-P IV, Gamunex 10%, Iveegam EN, Octagam 5%, Polygam S/D, Privigen, Rhophylac, Sandoglobulin, Venoglobulin-I, Venoglobulin-S 5%, Venoglobulin-S 10%, WinRho SDF

immune globulin subcutaneous (human)

Gammagard Liquid, Gamunex-C, Hizentra 20%, Vivaglobin

Class and Category
Chemical class: Polyvalent antibody
Therapeutic class: Antibacterial, anti–Kawasaki disease agent, antipolyneuropathy agent, antiviral, immunizing agent, platelet count stimulator
Pregnancy category: C

Indications and Dosages
➤ *To treat primary immunodeficiency*

I.M. INJECTION (BAYGAM)
Adults. 0.66 ml/kg (at least 200 mg/kg) every 3 to 4 wk; initial dose may be doubled.

I.V. INFUSION (GAMIMUNE N 5% S/D OR 10% S/D)
Adults. 100 to 200 mg/kg every mo. If response is inadequate, dose may be increased to as much as 400 mg/kg, or dosing frequency may be increased.

I.V. INFUSION (GAMMAGARD S/D, POLYGAM S/D)
Adults. 200 to 400 mg/kg initially, then at least 100 mg/kg every mo thereafter. If response is inadequate, dose or frequency may be adjusted.

I.V. INFUSION (GAMMAR-P IV)
Adults. 200 to 400 mg/kg every 3 to 4 wk.
Adolescents and children. 200 mg/kg every 3 to 4 wk.

I.V. INFUSION (GAMUNEX 10%)
Adults. 300 to 600 mg/kg every 3 or 4 wk.

I.V. INFUSION (IVEEGAM EN)
Adults. 200 mg/kg every mo.

I.V. INFUSION (OCTAGAM 5%)
Adults. *Initial:* 30 mg/kg/hr for first 30 min; increased, if tolerated, to 60 mg/kg/hr for second 30 min and, if tolerated, to 120 mg/kg/hr for another 30 min; followed by maintenance infusion of up to 200 mg/kg/hr.

I.V. INFUSION (SANDOGLOBULIN)
Adults and children. 200 mg/kg every mo. If response is inadequate, dose may be increased to 300 mg/kg or dosing frequency may be increased.

I.V. INFUSION (VENOGLOBULIN-I)
Adults and children. 200 mg/kg every mo. If response is inadequate, dose may be increased to 300 to 400 mg/kg every mo or dosing frequency may be increased.

I.V. INFUSION (VENOGLOBULIN-S 5% OR 10%)
Adults and children. 200 mg/kg every mo. If response is inadequate, dose may be increased to as much as 400 mg/kg or dosing frequency may be increased.

I.V. INFUSION (CARIMUNE NF, NANOFILTERED)
Adults and children. 0.4 to 0.8 g/kg once every 3 to 4 wks initially infused at 0.5 mg/kg/min. If tolerated, after 30 min, infusion rate increased to 1 mg/kg/min for 30 min. If tolerated, infusion rate gradually increased to maximum rate of 3 mg/kg/min. For patients at risk for renal dysfunction or thrombosis

development, rate of infusion should be less than 2 mg/kg/min.

I.V. INFUSION (GAMMAPLEX 5% LIQUID)
Adults. 300 to 800 mg/kg once every 3 to 4 wks, initially infused at 0.5 mg/kg/min and then gradually rate increased every 15 minutes, if tolerated, to final infusion rate of 4 mg/kg/min.

SUBCUTANEOUS INJECTION (VIVAGLOBIN)
Adults. Highly individualized and begun 1 wk after patient's last immune globulin intravenous (IGIV) infusion with initial weekly dosage obtained by multiplying the previous IGIV dose by 1.37; this number is then divided by the number of weeks between doses during the patient's previous IGIV treatment. Average weekly dose falls in the range of 100 to 200 mg/kg.

➤ *To prevent serious infections in patients with immunoglobulin deficiencies if circulating IgG levels of about 200 mg/ml plasma are maintained*

I.M. INJECTION (GAMASTAN S/D)
Adults. 0.66 ml/kg (at least 100 mg/kg) every 3 to 4 wks with a double dose given at onset of therapy.

➤ *To treat primary immunodeficiency disorders associated with defects in humoral immunity*

I.V. INFUSION (FLEBOGAMMA 5% DIF, FLEBOGAMMA 10% DIF, GAMMAGARD LIQUID)
Adults and children. 300 to 600 mg/kg every 3 to 4 wk.

I.V. INFUSION (PRIVIGEN)
Adults and children. 200 mg/kg to 800 mg/kg every 3 to 4 wk.

I.V. INFUSION (BIVIGAM 10% LIQUID)
Adults. 300 to 800 mg/kg every 3 to 4 wk. Infuse 0.5 mg/kg/min for the first 10 min, then increase infusion rate every 20 min, if tolerated, by 0.8 mg/kg/min up to 6 mg/kg/min.

SUBCUTANEOUS INFUSION (HIZENTRA 20%)
Adults and children. Highly individualized and begun 1 wk after patient's last immune globulin intravenous (IGIV) infusion with initial weekly dosage, obtained by multiplying the previous IGIV dose in grams by the dose adjustment factor of 1.53; this number is then divided by the number of weeks between doses during the patient's previous IGIV treatment, followed by multiplying the calculated dose by 5 to convert the dose calculated in grams to milliliters.

G
H
I

SUBCUTANEOUS INFUSION (GAMMAGARD LIQUID, GAMUNEX-C)

Adults and children age 3 and over. Highly individualized and begun 1 wk after patient's last immune globulin intravenous (IGIV) infusion with initial weekly dosage obtained by multiplying the previous IGIV dose in grams by the dose adjustment factor of 1.37; this number is then divided by the number of weeks between doses during the patient's previous IGIV treatment, followed by multiplying the calculated dose by 10 to convert the dose calculated in grams to milliliters.

➤ *To treat idiopathic thrombocytopenic purpura (ITP)*

I.V. INFUSION (GAMIMUNE N 5% S/D)

Adults and children. 400 mg/kg daily for 5 days. Or, 1,000 mg/kg for 1 or 2 days for patients not at risk for increased fluid volume.

I.V. INFUSION (PRIVIGEN)

Adults and adolescents age 15 and over. 1 gram/kg (10 ml/kg) daily for 2 consecutive days for patients not at risk for increased fluid volume.

I.V. INFUSION (GAMIMUNE N 10% S/D)

Adults and children. 1,000 mg/kg for 1 or 2 days for patients not at risk for increased fluid volume.

I.V. INFUSION (OCTAGAM 10%)

Adults. 1 g/kg (10 ml/kg) daily for 2 consecutive days. Initially infuse at 0.01 ml/kg/min for 30 min. If tolerated, increase infusion rate to 0.02 ml/kg/min for next 30 min. If tolerated, further increase infusion rate to 0.04 ml/kg/min for 30 min. If tolerated, further increase infusion rate to 0.08 ml/kg/min for 30 min. If tolerated, infusion rate may be increased up to 0.12 mg/kg/min for remainder of infusion.

I.V. INFUSION (GAMUNEX 10%)

Adults. 1 g/kg daily for 2 consecutive days (second dose may be withheld if adequate increase in platelet count occurs 24 hours after first dose). Or, 0.4 g/kg daily for 5 consecutive days.

I.V. INFUSION (CARIMUNE NF, NANOFILTERED)

Adults and children. 0.4 g/kg on 2 to 5 consecutive days, initially infused at 0.5 mg/kg/min. If tolerated, after 30 min, infusion rate increased to 1 mg/kg/min for 30 min. If tolerated, infusion rate gradually increased to maximum rate of 3 mg/kg/min.

I.V. INFUSION (GAMMAPLEX 5% LIQUID)

Adults. 1 g/kg on 2 consecutive days, initially infused at 0.5 mg/kg/min and then gradually rate increased every 15 minutes, if tolerated, to final infusion rate of 4 mg/kg/min.

DOSAGE ADJUSTMENT In acute ITP of childhood, I.V. Carimune NF or Sandoglobulin therapy may be discontinued after second day of 5-day course if initial platelet count response is adequate (30,000 to 50,000/mm³). In chronic ITP, an additional I.V. infusion of 400 mg/kg (Carimune NF, Gamimune, or Sandoglobulin) may be prescribed if platelet count falls below 30,000/mm³ or if patient develops significant bleeding. If response remains inadequate, an additional I.V. infusion of 800 to 1,000 mg/kg may be given. In chronic ITP, dosage of Gammaplex 5% liquid may need to be reduced in patients at risk for thrombosis, hemolysis, acute kidney injury, or volume overload.

I.V. INFUSION (GAMMAGARD S/D)

Adults. 1 g/kg. If response is inadequate, up to three separate doses may be administered on alternate days.

I.V. INFUSION (RHOPHYLAC)

Adults. 50 mcg/kg at 2 ml/15 to 60 seconds.

I.V. INFUSION (SANDOGLOBULIN)

Adults and adolescents. 400 mg/kg daily for 2 to 5 consecutive days.

I.V. INFUSION (VENOGLOBULIN-I)

Adults and children. *Induction:* Cumulative dose up to 2 g/kg over 2 to 7 consecutive days. *Maintenance (adults):* 2 g/kg as a single dose every 2 wk as needed to maintain platelet count above 30,000/mm³ or prevent bleeding episodes. *Maintenance (children):* 1 g/kg as a single dose every 2 wk as needed to maintain platelet count above 30,000/mm³ or prevent bleeding episodes.

I.V. INFUSION (VENOGLOBULIN-S 5% OR 10%)

Adults and children. Cumulative dose up to 2,000 mg/kg over 5 consecutive days.

DOSAGE ADJUSTMENT An additional I.V. infusion of 1,000 mg/kg may be administered to maintain a platelet count of 30,000/mm³ in children, or 20,000/mm³ in adults, or to prevent bleeding episodes.

➤ *To treat acute or chronic pediatric ITP; to treat chronic adult-onset ITP; to treat pediatric- and adult-onset ITP secondary to HIV infection*

I.V. INJECTION (WINRHO SDF)

Adults and children. *Initial:* 250 iu/kg given as a single injection over 3 to 5 min. Or, 125 iu/kg given as a single injection over 3 to 5 min and repeated once on a separate day. *Maintenance:* Frequency and dosage highly individualized based on patient's hemoglobin and platelet levels.

DOSAGE ADJUSTMENT For patients with hemoglobin level less than 10 g/dl, dose reduced to 125 to 200 international units/kg.

➤ *As adjunct to treat Kawasaki disease*

I.V. INFUSION (GAMMAGARD S/D)

Adults and adolescents. 1 g/kg as a single dose; or, 400 mg/kg daily for 4 consecutive days.

I.V. INFUSION (IVEEGAM EN, VENOGLOBULIN-S 5% OR 10%)

Adults and adolescents. 2 g/kg as a single dose; or, Iveegam EN may be given at 400 mg/kg daily for 4 days.

➤ *To decrease the risk of graft-versus-host disease, interstitial pneumonia, septicemia, and other infections during first 100 days after bone marrow transplantation*

I.V. INFUSION (GAMIMUNE N 5% S/D OR 10% S/D)

Adults over age 20. 500 mg/kg on 7th and 2nd days before transplant (or at time when conditioning therapy for transplantation begins), and then weekly through 90th day after transplant.

➤ *As adjunct to treat bacterial infections secondary to B-cell chronic lymphocytic leukemia*

I.V. INFUSION (GAMMAGARD S/D, POLYGAM S/D)

Adults and adolescents. 400 mg/kg every 3 to 4 wk.

➤ *To prevent bacterial infection in children with HIV who are immunosuppressed*

I.V. INFUSION (GAMIMUNE N 5% S/D OR 10% S/D)

Children. 400 mg/kg daily every 28 days.

➤ *To prevent hepatitis A*

I.M. INJECTION (BAYGAM)

Adults with household or institutional contacts. 0.02 ml/kg (0.01 ml/lb).

Adults traveling to areas where hepatitis A is common. 0.02 ml/kg if staying less than 3 mo, 0.06 ml/kg (repeated every 4 to 6 mo) if staying 3 mo or longer.

I.M. INJECTION (GAMASTAN S/D)

Adults and children with household or institutional contacts. 0.02 ml/kg.

Adults traveling for less than 3 months to areas where hepatitis A is common. 0.02 ml/kg.

Adults traveling for 3 months or longer to areas where hepatitis A is common. 0.06 ml/kg, repeated every 4 to 6 months, as needed.

➤ *To prevent or lessen severity of measles (rubeola) in susceptible persons*

I.M. INJECTION (BAYGAM)

Adults exposed fewer than 6 days previously. 0.2 ml/kg (0.11 ml/lb).

I.M. INJECTION (GAMASTAN S/D)

Adults and children exposed fewer than 6 days previously. 0.25 ml/kg. (0.11 ml/lb).

Children exposed to rubeola and are immunocompromised. 0.5 ml/kg immediately. *Maximum:* 15 ml dose.

➤ *To provide passive immunization against varicella in immunosuppressed patients*

I.M. INJECTION (BAYGAM, GAMASTAN S/D)

Adults. 0.6 to 1.2 ml/kg if varicella-zoster immune globulin (human) is unavailable.

➤ *To improve muscle strength and disability as maintenance therapy in patients with multifocal motor neuropathy*

I.V. INFUSION (GAMMAGARD LIQUID)

Adults. *Maintenance:* 0.5 to 2.4 grams/kg/month. Initially infused at 0.5 ml/kg/hr (0.8 mg/kg/min) with rate increased, as needed, up to 5.4 ml/kg/hr (9 mg/kg/min).

➤ *To reduce the risk of infection and fetal damage in women who have been exposed to rubella in early pregnancy*

I.M. INJECTION (BAYGAM, GAMASTAN S/D)

Adults. 0.55 ml/kg.

➤ *To suppress Rh isoimmunization*

I.M. INJECTION, I.V. INFUSION (RHOPHYLAC)

Adult pregnant women. 1,500 international units as a single dose at 28- to 30-wk gestation, followed by 1,500 international units within 72 hr after delivery of an Rh-positive newborn.

I.M. INJECTION (WINRHO SDF)

Adult pregnant women. 1,500 international units as a single dose at 28-wk gestation, followed by 600 international

G
H
I

units within 72 hr after delivery of an Rh-positive newborn.

I.V. INJECTION (WINRHO SDF)

Adult pregnant women. 1,500 international units as a single dose infused over 3 to 5 min at 28-wk gestation, followed by 600 international units over 3 to 5 min within 72 hr after delivery of an Rh-positive newborn.

DOSAGE ADJUSTMENT For patients with more than 34-wk gestation and having an abortion, amniocentesis, or other manipulative procedure, 600 international units given within 72 hr but preferably immediately after procedure. For patients with 34-wk gestation or less and having amniocentesis or chorionic villus sampling, 1,500 international units given immediately after procedure and repeated every 12 wk for duration of pregnancy. For patients with threatened abortion at any stage of pregnancy, 1,500 international units given immediately.

➤ *To treat incompatible blood transfusions*

I.M. INJECTION, I.V. INFUSION (RHOPHYLAC)

Adults exposed to Rh-positive RBCs. 100 international units/2 ml transfused blood or 1 ml erythrocyte concentrate within 72 hr of exposure.

I.M. INJECTION (WINRHO SDF)

Adults exposed to Rh-positive whole blood. 6,000 international units every 12 hr until total dose (60 international units/ml of blood) is given.

Adults exposed to Rh-positive RBCs. 6,000 international units every 12 hr until total dose (120 international units/ml of cells) is given.

I.V. INJECTION (WINRHO SDF)

Adults exposed to Rh-positive whole blood. 3,000 international units infused over 3 to 5 min every 8 hr until total dose (45 international units/ml of blood) is given.

Adults exposed to Rh-positive RBCs. 3,000 international units infused over 3 to 5 min every 8 hr until total dose (90 international units/ml of cells) is given.

➤ *To treat massive fetomaternal hemorrhage*

I.M. INJECTION, I.V. INFUSION (RHOPHYLAC)

Adults exposed to Rh-positive RBCs. 1,500 international units plus 100 international units for every 1 ml of fetal RBCs exceeding 15 ml if transplacental bleeding is quantified, or an additional 1,500 international units if transplacental bleeding can't be quantified within 72 hours of hemorrhage.

I.M. INJECTION (WINRHO SDF)

Adults exposed to Rh-positive whole blood. 6,000 international units every 12 hr until total dose (60 international units/ml of blood) is given.

Adults exposed to Rh-positive RBCs. 6,000 international units every 12 hr until total dose (120 international units/ml of cells) is given.

I.V. INJECTION (WINRHO SDF)

Adults exposed to Rh-positive whole blood. 3,000 international units infused over 3 to 5 min every 8 hr until total dose (45 international units/ml of blood) is given.

Adults exposed to Rh-positive RBCs. 3,000 international units infused over 3 to 5 min every 8 hr until total dose (90 international units/ml of cells) is given.

Route	Onset	Peak	Duration
I.V.	Unknown	Unknown	21–28 day
SubQ	Unknown	Unknown	Unknown

Mechanism of Action

Releases antibody-specific globulins to produce an antibody-antigen reaction that results in bacterial lysis and facilitates bacterial phagocytosis. In treatment of ITP, immune globulin blocks iron receptors on macrophages to increase immunoglobulin action. Immune globulin also increases cytokine production and improves B-cell immune function by regulating T-cell and macrophage activity. Newly formed antigen-antibody complexes produce split complement components that cause bacterial lysis.

In Kawasaki disease and bacterial infections with B-cell chronic lymphocytic leukemia, immune globulin neutralizes bacterial and viral toxins that harm immune and inflammatory responses.

Incompatibilities

Don't mix immune globulin with any other drugs, including other immune globulins, or with any I.V. solutions other than D_5W or manufacturer's supplied diluent because effects of doing so are unknown.

Contraindications

Hypersensitivity to immune globulin (human) or its components; IgA deficiency in patients with known antibody to IgA

Interaction

DRUGS

live-virus vaccines: Possibly decreased response to vaccine

Adverse Reactions

CNS: Headache, malaise

CV: Chest discomfort, tachycardia, thrombotic events

EENT: Blurred vision, oropharyngeal pain

GI: Nausea, vomiting

GU: Hemolysis related renal dysfunction or failure

HEME: Acute hemolysis, delayed hemolytic anemia, disseminated intravascular coagulation, positive Coombs' test

MS: Arthralgia, back or extremity pain, muscle spasms or weakness, myalgia

RESP: Dyspnea, pulmonary embolism

Nursing Considerations

• Before giving immune globulin, monitor patient's fluid volume and BUN and serum creatinine levels, as ordered, to determine risk for acute renal failure. Those at increased risk include patients with renal insufficiency, diabetes mellitus, volume depletion, sepsis, or paraproteinemia; those taking nephrotoxic drugs; and those over age 65. Expect drug to be discontinued if renal function deteriorates.

• Use caution when administering immune globulin, regardless of the route of administration, because of risk for thrombosis. Monitor closely patients with increased risk of thrombosis such as a history of atherosclerosis, multiple cardiovascular risk factors, advanced age, impaired cardiac output, coagulation disorders, prolonged periods of immobilization, and/or hyperviscosity. In such patients, obtain a baseline assessment of blood viscosity, as ordered. Ensure patient is adequately hydrated prior to administration. When administering drug intravenously, expect to infuse at the lowest rate possible. Report any signs and symptoms suggestive of a thrombotic event immediately to prescriber and be prepared to administer treatment, as ordered.

• When preparing immune globulin, verify that appropriate form is being used—either immune globulin intramuscular for I.M. injection, immune globulin intravenous for I.V. infusion or immune globulin subcutaneous for subcutaneous infusion.

• To reconstitute drug if required, follow manufacturer's guidelines and use only diluent recommended by manufacturer. Don't shake solution; excessive shaking causes foaming. If drug or diluent is cold, drug may take up to 20 minutes to dissolve.

• If drug is reconstituted outside of sterile laminar airflow conditions, administer it immediately and discard unused portions.

• Be aware that an in-line filter may be required for intravenous infusion of drug. Check manufacturer's guidelines for specific product being used.

• Consult manufacturer's guidelines to determine appropriate flow rate for starting infusion. Expect to increase flow rate after 15 to 30 minutes, as specified, except for Hizentra 20%, which has a flow adjustment rate done after the first infusion is completed and Privigen, which may adjust flow rate, as needed.

• When giving drug by I.M. injection, inject it only into deltoid muscle of upper arm or anterolateral aspect of upper thigh. If giving a dose larger than 5 ml, divide it and administer at separate sites.

• When giving Hizentra by subcutaneous infusion, infuse in the abdomen, thigh, upper arm, and/or lateral hip with no more than 4 sites used simultaneously. Infusion sites should be at least 2 inches apart and sites changed with each weekly administration. For first infusion, do not infuse more than 15 ml per hour per site. The volume may be increased to 20 ml per hour per site after the fourth infusion and to a maximum of 25 ml per hour per site as tolerated. However, do not exceed a maximum flow rate of more than a total of 50 ml per hour for all sites combined at any time. Use an infusion pump to administer the drug.

• When giving Gamunex-C by subcutaneous infusion, infuse in the abdomen,

G
H
I

thigh, upper arm, and/or lateral hip with no more than 8 sites used simultaneously. Infusion sites should be at least 2 inches apart and sites changed with each weekly administration. Be aware that the average infusion rate for Gamunex-C as a subcutaneous infusion is 20 ml/hour/site. Know that if dilution is required, Gamunex-C is not compatible with saline. It may be diluted with 5% dextrose in water. Content of Gamunex-C vials may be pooled under aseptic conditions into sterile infusion bags and infused within 8 hours after pooling. Use an infusion pump to administer the drug.

• Administer Vivaglobin by subcutaneous injection into patient's abdomen, thighs, upper arms, or lateral hip. Rotate injection sites weekly. Never inject intravenously.

• Watch for an acute inflammatory reaction in patients who have never received immune globulin therapy before, in those whose last treatment was more than 8 weeks before, and in those whose initial infusion rate exceeded 1 ml/minute. Within 30 minutes to 1 hour after beginning infusion, assess for chills, fever, facial flushing, feeling of tightness in chest, dizziness, nausea, vomiting, diaphoresis, and hypotension. Notify prescriber immediately if such symptoms occur, and be prepared to stop infusion until symptoms have subsided.

• Monitor patient closely for signs and symptoms of hemolysis, especially patients with risk factors. For patients at increased risk, expect to obtain a baseline measurement of hemoglobin or hematocrit prior to infusion and within 36 to 96 hours post infusion. Notify prescriber of any abnormalities.

WARNING After immune globulin administration, monitor patient closely for aseptic meningitis. Notify prescriber if patient develops drowsiness, fever, nausea, vomiting, nuchal rigidity, photophobia, painful eye movements, or severe headache.

• Be aware that immune globulin intravenous is made from human plasma and therefore may contain infectious agents, such as viruses. Risk of transmitting a virus by infusion has been reduced by screening blood donors, testing

donated blood, and inactivating or removing certain viruses from the product.

• Monitor patient with preexisting renal insufficiency who is receiving Bivigam to be sure the patient is not volume-depleted. If renal function deteriorates, notify prescriber and expect drug to be discontinued. For the patient at risk for renal dysfunction or thrombotic events, administer Bivigam at the minimum infusion rate practicable.

• For patient receiving WinRho SDF to treat ITP, assess clinical response by monitoring patient's platelet count, RBC count, hemoglobin level, and reticulocyte level.

• For patient receiving WinRho SDF for exposure to incompatible blood transfusions or massive fetal hemorrhage, give drug within 72 hours of incident, as ordered.

PATIENT TEACHING

• Instruct patient to report immediately any symptoms he experiences after receiving immune globulin.

• Inform patient to postpone live-virus vaccinations for up to 11 months after receiving immune globulin because drug may delay or inhibit response to vaccine.

inamrinone
(amrinone)
Inocor

Class and Category
Chemical class: Bipyridine derivative
Therapeutic class: Cardiac inotrope
Pregnancy category: C

Indications and Dosages
➤ *To treat heart failure in patients who haven't responded sufficiently to digoxin, diuretics, or vasodilators*
I.V. INFUSION
Adults. *Initial:* 0.75 mg/kg by bolus over 2 to 3 min and repeated after 30 min, if needed. *Maintenance:* 5 to 10 mcg/kg/min by infusion. *Maximum:* 10 mg/kg daily.

Route	Onset	Peak	Duration
I.V.	2–5 min	In 10 min	30 min–2 hr

Mechanism of Action

Inhibits phosphodiesterase enzymes that normally degrade myocardial cAMP. This action increases intracellular levels of cAMP, which regulates intracellular and extracellular calcium balance. Increased intracellular cAMP level enhances influx of calcium into cell, thereby increasing force of myocardial contractions. Inamrinone also acts directly on peripheral vascular smooth-muscle cells, causing relaxation and dilation, which reduces preload and afterload.

Incompatibilities

Don't administer inamrinone through same I.V. line as furosemide because precipitate may form. Don't dilute inamrinone in solution that contains dextrose because a chemical interaction occurs over 24 hours.

Contraindications

Hypersensitivity to inamrinone, bisulfites, or their components; severe aortic or pulmonary valvular disease

Interaction

DRUGS
disopyramide: Possibly severe hypotension

Adverse Reactions

CNS: Fever
CV: Chest pain, hypotension, pericarditis, supraventricular tachycardia, ventricular arrhythmias
GI: Abdominal pain, anorexia, elevated liver function test results, hepatotoxicity, nausea, vomiting
HEME: Elevated erythrocyte sedimentation rate, thrombocytopenia (especially with high-dose or prolonged treatment)
MS: Myositis
RESP: Hypoxemia, pleuritis
SKIN: Jaundice
Other: Infusion-site burning

Nursing Considerations

WARNING Be aware that inamrinone may increase risk of ventricular arrhythmias in patients with atrial flutter or fibrillation. To minimize risk, expect to pretreat such patients with digoxin.

• Give drug undiluted or diluted in normal or half-normal (0.45) saline solution to a concentration of 1 to 3 mg/ml, as prescribed. Use diluted solution within 24 hours.

WARNING Monitor vital signs regularly. If blood pressure falls significantly, slow or stop infusion and notify prescriber.

• Monitor weight, cardiac index, central venous pressure, pulmonary artery wedge pressure, and fluid intake and output as appropriate to assess drug's effectiveness.

WARNING Assess often for signs of thrombocytopenia, such as bruising or bleeding and altered platelet count. If signs appear, expect to decrease inamrinone dose or discontinue drug.

PATIENT TEACHING
• Instruct patient to notify you or another nurse if he becomes dizzy, which may indicate hypotension.

---

indacaterol maleate

Arcapta Neohaler

G
H
I

Class and Category

Chemical class: Long-acting beta$_2$-adrenergic agonist
Therapeutic class: Bronchodilator
Pregnancy category: C

Indications and Dosages

➤ *To alleviate airflow obstruction in patients with chronic obstructive pulmonary disease (COPD), including chronic bronchitis and/or emphysema*
INHALATION AEROSOL
Adults. 75 mcg once daily.

Mechanism of Action

Selectively attaches to beta$_2$ receptors on bronchial membranes, stimulating the intracellular enzyme adenyl cyclase to convert adenosine triphosphate to cAMP. The resulting increase in the intracellular cAMP level relaxes bronchial smooth-muscle cells, which allows greater airflow through the airways.

Contraindications

Asthma, hypersensitivity to indacaterol or its components

Interaction

DRUGS
adrenergic drugs: potentiated sympathetic effects

beta blockers: Possible interference with the effect of beta blockers and indacaterolcytochrome P450 3A4, P-gp efflux transporter such as erythromycin *diuretics, steroids, xanthine derivatives:* Possible increased risk of hypokalemic effect
MAO inhibitors, tricyclic antidepressants: Potentiated adrenergic action on the cardiovascular system
non-potassium sparing diuretics: Increased risk of ECG changes or hypokalemia
QT prolonging drugs: Increased risk of ventricular arrhythmias

Adverse Reactions

CNS: Dizziness, headache, nervousness, tremor
CV: Angina, atrial fibrillation, peripheral edema, palpitations, tachycardia
EENT: Nasopharyngitis, oropharyngeal pain, sinusitis
ENDO: Hyperglycemia
GI: Nausea
MS: Muscle spasm, musculoskeletal pain
RESP: COPD exacerbation, cough, dyspnea, paradoxical bronchospasm, pneumonia, upper respiratory tract infection
SKIN: Pruritus, rash, urticaria
Other: Angioedema, hypokalemia, immediate hypersensitivity reactions

Nursing Considerations

• Be aware that indacaterol should not be given to patients with acutely deteriorating COPD nor should it be used for relief of acute symptoms. Instead acute symptoms should be treated with an inhaled short-acting beta$_2$-agonist.
• Use cautiously in patients with cardiovascular disorders, especially coronary insufficiency, cardiac arrhythmias, and hypertension because drug can increase pulse rate, blood pressure and cause ECG changes, such as flattening of the T wave, prolongation of the QT interval, and ST segment depression.
• Use cautiously in patients with convulsive disorders or thyrotoxicosis, or in patients who are unusually responsive to sympathomimetic amines as drug may aggravate these conditions.
• Monitor the patient's vital signs for an increase in pulse rate or blood pressure. If such effects occur, notify prescriber as indacaterol may need to be discontinued.

WARNING Monitor patient for immediate hypersensitivity reactions after administering indacaterol that may include difficulties in breathing or swallowing; swelling of tongue, lips and face; urticaria; or rash. If present, discontinue drug immediately, notify prescriber, and provide supportive care, as indicated.

PATIENT TEACHING

• Instruct patient who has been taking inhaled, short-acting beta$_2$-agonists on a regular basis to discontinue the regular use of these drugs, as directed by prescriber, and use them only for symptomatic relief of acute respiratory symptoms, as ordered.
• Tell patient indacaterol capsules are only for use in inhaler device and should never be swallowed.
• Instruct patient to store capsules in their original packaging and to open immediately before use.
• Teach patient how to use delivery system. Tell them to place capsule in well of inhaler device and then to press and release buttons on side of device only once to pierce capsule. A click-type of sound will occur. Have patient place the inhaler into his mouth with the buttons to the left and right (not up and down). Then have him inhale rapidly and deeply through mouthpiece; drug is dispersed into airways as patient inhales. A whirring noise should be heard when inhaling. If not, the capsule may be stuck in the capsule cavity. If this occurs, have the patient open the inhaler and carefully loosen the capsule by tapping the base of the device. Tell him not to press the piercing buttons to loosen the capsule. Have him repeat these steps, if needed.
• Remind patient that indacaterol is not to be used to relieve acute symptoms. Instead, he should use his short-acting beta$_2$-agonist.
• Inform patient to notify prescriber if any of the following situations occur: if indacterol no longer seems to control his symptoms, if he needs to use his short-acting beta$_2$-agonist more often than usual; or if the short-acting beta$_2$-agonist becomes less effective.

indapamide

Apo-Indapamide (CAN), Gen-Indapamide (CAN), Lozide (CAN), Lozol, Novo-Indapamide (CAN), Nu-Indapamide (CAN)

Class and Category

Chemical class: Sulfonamide
Therapeutic class: Antihypertensive, diuretic
Pregnancy category: B

Indications and Dosages

➤ *To treat edema caused by heart failure*

TABLETS

Adults. 2.5 mg daily in the morning, increased to 5 mg daily after 1 wk, if indicated.

➤ *To manage hypertension*

TABLETS

Adults. 2.5 mg daily, increased to 5 mg after 4 wk, if needed.

Route	Onset	Peak	Duration
P.O.*	1–2 hr	Unknown	36 hr
P.O.†	1–2 wk	8–12 wk	Up to 8 wk

Mechanism of Action

Acts mainly on distal convoluted tubules, where it enhances excretion of sodium, chloride, and water by inhibiting sodium ion movement across renal tubules. The resulting decrease in plasma and extracellular fluid volume decreases peripheral vascular resistance and reduces blood pressure. This thiazide diuretic also may cause arterial vasodilation by blocking calcium channels in smooth-muscle cells.

Contraindications

Anuria; hypersensitivity to thiazide or related diuretics or to sulfonamide-derived drugs

Interaction

DRUGS

amiodarone: Increased risk of arrhythmias if hypokalemia develops
cholestyramine, colestipol: Decreased indapamide absorption
diazoxide: Increased risk of hyperglycemia

---

* For edema.

† For hypertension (with multiple doses).

digoxin: Increased risk of digitalis toxicity if hypokalemia develops
hypotension-producing drugs: Increased antihypertensive or diuretic effects
lithium: Increased risk of lithium toxicity
neuromuscular blockers: Possibly increased neuromuscular blockade, risk of respiratory depression
oral anticoagulants: Possibly decreased anticoagulant effects

Adverse Reactions

CNS: Anxiety, dizziness, drowsiness, fatigue, fever, headache, mood changes, nervousness, sleep disturbance, vertigo, weakness
CV: Arrhythmias, hypercholesterolemia, orthostatic hypotension, palpitations
EENT: Dry mouth
ENDO: Hyperglycemia, hypoglycemia
GI: Anorexia, constipation, diarrhea, hepatitis, nausea, pancreatitis, thirst, vomiting
GU: Impotence, nocturia
MS: Gout, muscle spasms
SKIN: Jaundice, necrotizing vasculitis, photosensitivity, pruritus, rash, urticaria
Other: Dilutional hypochloremia and hyponatremia, hypokalemia, metabolic alkalosis, weight loss

Nursing Considerations

• Administer indapamide with food or milk to reduce adverse GI reactions.
• Give drug early in the day to avoid nocturia.
• Weigh patient daily, and monitor fluid intake and output, blood pressure, and serum electrolyte levels, especially in elderly women, because severe hyponatremia and hypokalemia may occur. Hypokalemia also commonly occurs in patients taking diuretics. Report electrolyte abnormalities, and expect to provide corrective measures, as prescribed.
• Monitor BUN and serum creatinine levels regularly, as appropriate.
• If muscle cramps and weakness develop from hypokalemia, expect prescriber to order potassium supplement or potassium-sparing diuretic.
• When managing hypertension, expect therapeutic response to indapamide to take several weeks.

G
H
I

PATIENT TEACHING

• Advise patient to take indapamide early in the day to avoid nighttime urination and to take it with food or milk to minimize GI distress.
• Encourage patient to eat high-potassium foods, such as oranges and bananas.
• Caution patient to change position slowly to minimize effects of orthostatic hypotension.
• Instruct patient to weigh himself daily at the same time and wearing similar clothing. Direct him to report a weight gain of more than 0.9 kg (2 lb) per day or 2.3 kg (5 lb) per week.
• Inform patient about possible photosensitivity.
• If patient has a dry mouth, suggest sugarless gum or hard candy to relieve it.

---

indomethacin

Apo-Indomethacin (CAN), Indocid (CAN), Indocin, Indocin SR, Novo-Methacin (CAN), Nu-Indo (CAN), Tivorbex

indomethacin sodium trihydrate

Apo-Indomethacin (CAN), Indameth, Indocid (CAN), Indocid PDA (CAN), Indocin, Indocin I.V., Novomethacin (CAN)

Class and Category

Chemical class: Indoleacetic acid derivative
Therapeutic class: Analgesic, antigout, anti-inflammatory, antirheumatic
Pregnancy category: Not rated

Indications and Dosages

➤ *To relieve symptoms of ankylosing spondylitis, osteoarthritis, and rheumatoid arthritis*
CAPSULES, ORAL SUSPENSION
Adults. 25 to 50 mg twice daily to four times daily, increased by 25 or 50 mg daily every wk, as needed. *Maximum:* 200 mg daily. After adequate response, dosage reduced as low as possible.
E.R. CAPSULES (ANTIRHEUMATIC)
Adults. 75 mg daily, increased to 75 mg twice daily, if needed.

SUPPOSITORIES
Adults. 50 mg up to four times daily.
➤ *To relieve symptoms of acute gouty arthritis*
CAPSULES, ORAL SUSPENSION
Adults. *Initial:* 100 mg. Increased up to 50 mg three times daily. *Maximum:* 200 mg daily. After pain is relieved, dosage tapered until drug is discontinued.
SUPPOSITORIES
Adults. 50 mg up to four times daily. *Maximum:* 200 mg daily.
➤ *To treat inflammation and relieve acute shoulder pain from bursitis or tendinitis*
CAPSULES, ORAL SUSPENSION
Adults. 75 to 150 mg daily in divided doses three times daily or four times daily for 7 to 14 days.
SUPPOSITORIES
Adults. 50 mg up to four times daily. *Maximum:* 200 mg daily.
➤ *To treat mild to moderate acute pain*
CAPSULES (TIVORBEX)
Adults. 20 mg three times daily or 40 mg two or three times daily.
DOSAGE ADJUSTMENT Dosage reduced for elderly patients.
➤ *To treat hemodynamically significant patent ductus arteriosus in premature infants weighing 500 to 1,750 g (1 to 3.9 lb)*
I.V. INJECTION
Infants over age 7 days. *Initial:* 200 mcg/kg (0.2 mg/kg) over 5 to 10 sec; 1 or 2 additional doses of 250 mcg/kg (0.25 mg/kg) given at 12- to 24-hr intervals, if needed.
Neonates ages 2 to 7 days. *Initial:* 200 mcg/kg (0.2 mg/kg) over 5 to 10 sec; 1 or 2 additional doses of 200 mcg/kg (0.2 mg/kg) given at 12- to 24-hr intervals, if needed.
Neonates under age 48 hours. *Initial:* 200 mcg/kg (0.2 mg/kg) over 5 to 10 sec; 1 or 2 additional doses of 100 mcg/kg (0.1 mg/kg) given at 12- to 24-hr intervals, if needed.

Route	Onset	Peak	Duration
P.O.*	2–4 hr	2–5 days	Unknown
P.O.†	30 min	Unknown	4–6 hr
P.O.‡	In 7 days	1–2 wk	Unknown

---

* For antigout effects.
† For anti-inflammatory effects.
‡ For antirheumatic effects.

Mechanism of Action

Blocks activity of cyclooxygenase, the enzyme needed to synthesize prostaglandins, which mediate inflammatory response and cause local vasodilation, swelling, and pain. By blocking cyclooxygenase and inhibiting prostaglandins, this NSAID reduces inflammatory symptoms and helps relieve pain.

Incompatibilities

Don't give indomethacin suspension with alkaline antacids or liquids. Don't mix reconstituted indomethacin sodium with I.V. infusion solutions.

Contraindications

Allergy or hypersensitivity to aspirin, indomethacin, iodides, other NSAIDs, or their components; history of proctitis or recent rectal bleeding (suppositories); perioperative pain with coronary artery bypass graft surgery (Tivorbex)

Interaction

DRUGS

Note: All effects listed are for oral forms and suppositories unless indicated.

acetaminophen: Increased risk of adverse renal effects (long-term use of both drugs)
aluminum- and magnesium-containing antacids: Possibly decreased blood indomethacin level
aminoglycosides: Increased risk of aminoglycoside toxicity
antihypertensives: Decreased effectiveness of these drugs
aspirin, other NSAIDs: Increased risk of adverse GI effects and non-GI bleeding
bone marrow depressants: Possibly increased leukopenic or thrombocytopenic effects of these drugs
cefamandole, cefoperazone, cefotetan: Increased risk of hypoprothrombinemia and bleeding
colchicine, platelet aggregation inhibitors: Increased risk of GI bleeding, hemorrhage, and ulcers
corticosteroids, potassium supplements: Increased risk of adverse GI effects
cyclosporine: Increased risk of nephrotoxicity from both drugs, increased blood cyclosporine level
diflunisal: Increased blood indomethacin level and risk of GI bleeding

digoxin: Increased blood digoxin level and risk of digitalis toxicity (all forms)
diuretics (thiazide, loop, and potassium-sparing): Decreased diuretic and anti-hypertensive effects
gold compounds, nephrotoxic drugs: Increased risk of adverse renal effects
heparin, oral anticoagulants, thrombolytics: Possibly increased anticoagulant effects and risk of hemorrhage
lithium: Increased blood lithium level and risk of toxicity
methotrexate: Increased risk of methotrexate toxicity
plicamycin, valproic acid: Increased risk of hypoprothrombinemia and GI bleeding, hemorrhage, and ulcers
probenecid: Increased blood level and effectiveness of indomethacin, increased risk of indomethacin toxicity
zidovudine: Increased blood zidovudine level and risk of toxicity, increased risk of indomethacin toxicity

ACTIVITIES

alcohol use: Increased risk of adverse GI effects

Adverse Reactions

Note: All reactions are for oral forms and suppositories unless indicated.

CNS: Confusion, depression, dizziness, drowsiness, fatigue, hallucinations, headache, intraventricular hemorrhage (I.V.), peripheral neuropathy, seizures, stroke, syncope, vertigo
CV: Arrhythmias, chest pain, edema, fluid retention (all forms), heart failure, hypertension, MI, pulmonary hypertension (I.V.), tachycardia
EENT: Blurred vision, corneal and retinal damage, epistaxis, hearing loss, tinnitus
ENDO: Hypoglycemia (I.V.)
GI: Abdominal cramps or pain, abdominal distention (I.V.), anorexia, constipation, diarrhea, diverticulitis, dyspepsia, dysphagia, epigastric discomfort, esophagitis, gastric perforation, gastritis, gastroenteritis, gastroesophageal reflux disease, GI bleeding and ulceration (all forms), hemorrhoids, hepatic dysfunction (I.V.), hepatic failure, hiatal hernia, ileus (I.V.), indigestion, melena, nausea, necrotizing enterocolitis (I.V.), pancreatitis, peptic ulcer, perforation of stomach or intestine, stomatitis, vomiting (all forms)

G
H
I

GU: Acute renal failure, hematuria, interstitial nephritis, nephrotic syndrome, oliguria (I.V.), proteinuria, renal dysfunction (I.V.), vaginal bleeding
HEME: Agranulocytosis, anemia, aplastic anemia, bone marrow depression, decreased platelet aggregation (I.V.), disseminated intravascular coagulation, hemolytic anemia, iron deficiency anemia, leukopenia, neutropenia, pancytopenia, thrombocytopenia, unusual bleeding or bruising (all forms)
RESP: Asthma, respiratory depression
SKIN: Ecchymosis, erythema multiforme, erythema nodosum, photosensitivity, pruritus, rash, Stevens-Johnson syndrome, toxic epidermal necrolysis, urticaria
Other: Anaphylaxis, angioedema, hyperkalemia (I.V.), hyponatremia (I.V.), injection-site irritation

Nursing Considerations

• Use indomethacin with extreme caution in patients with history of ulcer disease or GI bleeding because NSAIDs such as indomethacin increase risk of GI bleeding and ulceration. Expect to use drug for shortest time possible in these patients.
• Be aware that serious GI tract ulceration, bleeding, and perforation may occur without warning symptoms. Elderly patients are at greater risk. To minimize risk, give oral indomethacin with food, a full glass of water (not suspension), or an antacid to reduce GI distress.
• If GI distress occurs, withhold drug and notify prescriber immediately.
• Use indomethacin cautiously in patients with hypertension, and monitor blood pressure closely throughout therapy. Drug may cause hypertension or worsen it.
• Shake suspension well before giving it.
• For arthritis, give up to 100 mg of daily dose (not E.R. capsules) at bedtime to reduce nighttime pain and morning stiffness.
• Make sure suppository stays in rectum at least 1 hour to improve absorption.
• To reconstitute I.V. form, add 1 to 2 ml of preservative-free sodium chloride for injection or preservative-free sterile water to vial. Solution made with 1 ml diluent contains 100 mcg (0.1 mg) indomethacin/0.1 ml. Solution made with

2 ml diluent contains 50 mcg (0.05 mg) indomethacin/0.1 ml. Use solution immediately because it contains no preservatives. Discard unused portion.
• Be aware that scheduled I.V. doses may be withheld if infant or neonate has anuria or a significant decrease in urine output (less than 0.6 ml/kg/hr).
• When using I.V. form, avoid extravasation to protect surrounding tissue.
• Anticipate a second course (3 more doses) of I.V. indomethacin if patent ductus arteriosus fails to close or reopens. After two courses, surgery may be performed.
WARNING Monitor patient closely for thrombotic events, including MI and stroke, because NSAIDs increase the risk.
• Monitor patient—especially if he's elderly or receiving long-term indomethacin therapy—for less common but serious adverse GI reactions, including anorexia, constipation, diverticulitis, dysphagia, esophagitis, gastritis, gastroenteritis, gastroesophageal reflux disease, hemorrhoids, hiatal hernia, melena, stomatitis, and vomiting.
• Monitor liver function test results because, rarely, elevations may progress to severe hepatic reactions, including fatal hepatitis, liver necrosis, and hepatic failure.
• Monitor BUN and serum creatinine levels in elderly patients, those taking diuretics or ACE inhibitors, and those with heart failure, impaired renal function, or hepatic dysfunction; drug may cause renal failure.
• Monitor CBC for decreased hemoglobin and hematocrit. Drug may worsen anemia.
WARNING If patient has bone marrow suppression or is receiving an anti-neoplastic drug, monitor laboratory results (including WBC count), and watch for evidence of infection because anti-inflammatory and antipyretic actions of indomethacin may mask signs and symptoms, such as fever and pain.
• Assess patient's skin regularly for signs of rash or other hypersensitivity reaction because indomethacin is an NSAID and may cause serious skin reactions without warning, even in patients with no history of NSAID sensitivity. At first sign of reaction, stop drug and notify prescriber.

• Because indomethacin causes sodium retention, monitor weight and blood pressure, especially if patient has hypertension.
• When drug is used to treat gouty arthritis, expect its action to peak in 24 to 36 hours and significant swelling to gradually disappear over 3 to 5 days.
• Be aware that E.R. form shouldn't be used to treat gouty arthritis.
• Expect to use suppositories for patients who can't swallow oral form.
• To evaluate drug effectiveness, assess for reduced pain and inflammation and improved joint mobility.
• Expect patient to have intermittent checkups during long-term therapy and an ophthalmologic examination if vision changes.

PATIENT TEACHING
• Urge patient to take indomethacin capsules with full glass of water and to avoid lying down for 15 to 30 minutes afterward. This helps prevent drug from lodging in esophagus and causing irritation. Caution patient not to open or crush capsules.
• Instruct patient to take drug with food or an antacid to reduce GI distress.
• Instruct patient to make sure suppository stays in rectum at least 1 hour.
• Urge patient to avoid alcohol during indomethacin therapy.
• Remind patient that improvement may not occur for 2 to 4 weeks after starting indomethacin and that he should continue taking drug, as prescribed.
• Inform breastfeeding patient that indomethacin appears in breastmilk and may cause seizures in infants. Urge her to use another feeding method during therapy.
• Caution against prolonged sun exposure during therapy.
• Urge patient to notify prescriber immediately about changes in vision or hearing, fever, itching, rash, sore throat, swelling in arms or legs, and weight gain.
• Emphasize importance of having ordered laboratory tests and eye examinations during long-term therapy.
• Caution pregnant patient not to take NSAIDs such as indomethacin during last trimester because they may cause premature closure of the ductus arteriosus.

• Explain that indomethacin may increase risk of serious adverse cardiovascular reactions; urge patient to seek immediate medical attention if signs or symptoms arise, such as chest pain, shortness of breath, weakness, and slurring of speech.
• Explain that indomethacin may increase risk of serious adverse GI reactions; emphasize need to seek immediate medical attention for such signs and symptoms as epigastric or abdominal pain, indigestion, black or tarry stools, or vomiting blood or material that looks like coffee grounds.
• Alert patient to rare but serious skin reactions. Urge him to seek immediate medical attention for rash, blisters, itching, fever, or other indications of hypersensitivity.

G
H
I

infliximab
Remicade

Class and Category
Chemical class: Monoclonal antibody
Therapeutic class: Anti-inflammatory
Pregnancy category: C

Indications and Dosages
➤ *To control moderate to severe Crohn's disease long-term*
I.V. INFUSION
Adults and children. *Induction:* 5 mg/kg over 2 hr, repeated 2 and 6 wk after first infusion. *Maintenance:* 5 mg/kg over 2 hr every 8 wk.
DOSAGE ADJUSTMENT For adults who respond and then lose response, dosage may be increased to 10 mg/kg.
➤ *To reduce number of draining enterocutaneous and rectovaginal fistulas and to maintain fistula closure in fistulizing Crohn's disease*
I.V. INFUSION
Adults. *Induction:* 5 mg/kg over 2 hr, repeated 2 and 6 wk after first infusion. *Maintenance:* 5 mg/kg over 2 hr every 8 wk.
DOSAGE ADJUSTMENT For patients who respond and then lose response, dosage may be increased to 10 mg/kg.
➤ *To reduce signs and symptoms, to induce and maintain remission and*

mucosal healing, and to eliminate corticosteroid use in patients with moderate to severe active ulcerative colitis who have had an inadequate response to conventional therapy

I.V. INFUSION

Adults. 5 mg/kg over 2 hr, repeated 2 and 6 wk after infusion. *Maintenance:* 5 mg/kg over 2 hr every 8 wk.

➤ *To reduce signs and symptoms and to induce and maintain remission in pediatric patients with moderately to severely active ulcerative colitis who have had an inadequate response to conventional therapy*

I.V. INFUSION

Children age 6 and older. 5 mg/kg over 2 hr, repeated 2 and 6 wk after infusion. *Maintenance:* 5 mg/kg over 2 hr every 8 wk.

➤ *As adjunct to reduce signs and symptoms, inhibit progression of structural damage, and improve physical function in patients with moderate to severe active rheumatoid arthritis*

I.V. INFUSION

Adults. 3 mg/kg, with methotrexate, repeated 2 and 6 wk after first infusion and then every 8 wk thereafter.

➤ *To treat active ankylosing spondylitis*

I.V. INFUSION

Adults. 5 mg/kg, repeated 2 and 6 wk after first infusion and then every 6 wk thereafter.

➤ *To reduce signs and symptoms, inhibit progression of structural damage, and improve physical function in patients with psoriatic arthritis*

I.V. INFUSION

Adults. 5 mg/kg, with or without methotrexate, repeated 2 and 6 wk after first infusion and then every 8 wk thereafter.

➤ *To treat chronic severe plaque psoriasis in patients who are candidates for systemic therapy, but those therapies are medically less appropriate*

I.V. INFUSION

Adults. 5 mg/kg, repeated 2 and 6 wk after first infusion and every 8 wk thereafter.

Mechanism of Action

Binds with cytokine tumor necrosis factor-alpha (TNF-alpha), preventing it from binding with its receptors. As a result, TNF-alpha can't produce proinflammatory cytokines and endothelial permeability. Infiltration of inflammatory cells into inflamed intestine and joints declines.

Incompatibilities

Don't infuse infliximab in same I.V. line with other drugs or through plasticized polyvinyl chloride infusion equipment or devices.

Contraindications

Breast-feeding; hypersensitivity to infliximab, murine proteins, or their components; moderate or severe New York Heart Association (NYHA) Class III or IV heart failure

Interaction

DRUGS

abatacept, anakinra, etanercept, tocilizumab: Increased risk of neutropenia and serious infections

live vaccines, therapeutic infectious agents such as BCG in bladder instillation used to treat bladder cancer: Increased risk of adverse vaccine effects

Adverse Reactions

CNS: Chills, dizziness, fatigue, fever, Guillain-Barré syndrome, headache, meningitis, neuritis, numbness, paresthesia, seizures, stroke, syncope, tingling

CV: Arrhythmias, chest pain, hypertension, hypotension, MI, myocardial ischemia, myelitis, neuropathies, pericardial effusion, systemic and cutaneous vasculitis, thrombophlebitis

EENT: Laryngeal/pharyngeal edema, oral candidiasis, pharyngitis, rhinitis, sinusitis, transient vision loss, visual changes

GI: Abdominal hernia; abdominal pain; acute hepatic failure; cholecystitis; cholestasis; diarrhea; dyspepsia; elevated aminotranferases; GI hemorrhage; hepatitis; hepatotoxicity; ileus; intestinal obstruction, perforation, or stenosis; jaundice; melena; pancreatitis; nausea; splenic infarction; splenomegaly; vomiting

GU: Kidney infection, renal failure, ureteral obstruction, UTI, vaginal candidiasis, vaginitis

HEME: Anemia, leukopenia, neutropenia, pancytopenia, thrombocytopenia
MS: Ankylosing spondylitis, arthralgia, back pain, limb weakness, myalgia, psoriatic arthritis
RESP: Adult respiratory distress syndrome, bronchitis, cough, dyspnea, interstitial lung disease, pneumonia, tuberculosis, respiratory tract infection, severe bronchospasm, wheezing
SKIN: Facial flushing, melanoma, Merkel cell cancer, pruritus, psoriasis, rash, urticaria
Other: Anaphylaxis; antibody formation to infliximab; bacterial (including Legionella and Listeria), fungal, mycobacterial, parasitic, or viral infection; infusion reaction; lupuslike symptoms; lymphadenopathy; malignancies, such as leukemia and lymphomas, including hepatosplenic T-cell lymphoma; sepsis

Nursing Considerations

• Infliximab therapy shouldn't be started in a patient with an active infection, including serious localized infection.
• Use with extreme caution if patient has a history of chronic or recurrent infection, known exposure to tuberculosis, an underlying condition that predisposes to infection, or residence or travel to areas of endemic tuberculosis or mycoses, such as histoplasmosis, coccidioidomycosis, or blastomycosis.
• Use cautiously in elderly patients because they have a higher risk of infection.
• Use cautiously in patients with previous or ongoing hematologic abnormalities because infliximab may cause serious or even life-threatening adverse hematologic effects. Montior patient's CBC regularly, as ordered. If adverse effects occur, expect drug to be discontinued.
• Be aware that use of TNF-blocking therapy, including infliximab, may reactivate hepatitis B virus in patients who are chronic carriers of this virus. Ensure that patient has been tested for hepatitis B infection before infliximab therapy is begun. For patients who develop reactivation of hepatitis B, know that therapy should be stopped and antiviral therapy with appropriate supportive treatment begun.

WARNING Because drug increases risk of developing tuberculosis or reactivating latent tuberculosis, expect prescriber to evaluate patient's risk and start tuberculosis treatment, as needed, before starting infliximab.
WARNING Infliximab increases risk of serious or fatal opportunistic infections, including invasive fungal infections, as well as bacterial (including Legionella and Listeria), mycobacterial, parasitic, and viral infections. The most common ones include aspergillosis, blastomycosis, candidiasis, coccidioidomycosis, histoplasmosis, legionellosis, listeriosis, pneumocytosis, and tuberculosis.
WARNING Watch for infection, especially if patient receives immunosuppressant therapy or has a chronic infection. Upper respiratory tract infections and UTI are most common, but sepsis and fatal infections have occurred.
• To reconstitute infliximab, use 21G (or smaller) needle to add 10 ml sterile water for injection to each vial of drug. Swirl to mix; don't shake. Solution may foam and be clear or light yellow.
• Withdraw volume equal to amount of reconstituted drug from a 250-ml glass bottle or polypropylene or polyolefin infusion bag of normal saline solution. Then add reconstituted infliximab to bottle to dilute to 250 ml. Use within 3 hours.
• Infuse over at least 2 hours using polyethylene-lined infusion set and in-line, sterile, nonpyrogenic, low–protein-binding filter with pores 1.2 microns or less. Don't reuse.
• Be prepared to stop infusion if hypersensitivity or CNS reaction occurs. Keep acetaminophen, antihistamines, corticosteroids, and epinephrine on hand. A reaction may occur 2 hours to 12 days after infusion.
WARNING Avoid giving drug to patients with New York Heart Association Class III or IV congestive heart failure (CHF) because it may worsen the condition or cause death. If patient does receive infliximab, expect to stop it if CHF worsens.
• Because severe hepatic reactions may occur, monitor liver function. Expect to

G
H
I

stop drug if jaundice develops or liver enzymes are 5 times or more the upper limit of normal.
- Be aware that infliximab is a tumor necrosis factor (TNF) blocker. Malignancies, especially leukemia and such rare lymphomas as hepatosplenic T-cell lymphoma have been reported in patients, particularly children and adolescents, receiving TNF blockers. Patients at increased risk of leukemia are those with rheumatoid arthritis. Patients at increased risk of lymphomas are those with rheumatoid arthritis, Crohn's disease, ankylosing spondylitis, psoriatic arthritis, and plaque psoriasis, especially those with long-term or very active disease. Monitor them closely.

PATIENT TEACHING
- Inform patient that infliximab should take effect within 1 to 2 weeks.
- Urge patient to report evidence of infection, such as painful urination, cough, and sore throat. Infusion reaction (chest pain, chills, dyspnea, facial flushing, fever, itching, headache, rash) may occur for up to 12 days.
- Explain that infliximab increases the risk of lymphoma; urge prompt medical attention for suspicious signs or symptoms. Also, advise patient to have regular skin examinations because drug increases risk of skin cancer.
- Advise patient not to receive vaccinations using live vaccines. Also advise parents not to have their infant exposed to live vaccines for up to six months after birth if the mother was taking infliximab during the pregnancy.

insulin, inhaled

(rapid-acting)

Afrezza

Class and Category

Chemical class: Human insulin
Therapeutic class: Antidiabetic
Pregnancy category: C

Indications and Dosages

➤ *To improve glycemic control in patients with diabetes mellitus*

ORAL INHALATION

Adults who are not currently taking insulin. *Initial:* 4 units at beginning of each meal with dosage increased, as needed.
Adults converting from subcutaneous mealtime (prandial) insulin. Dosage dependent upon subcutaneous insulin dosage as follows: 4 units at beginning of each meal if up to 4 units of subcutaneous mealtime insulin was being used; 8 units at beginning of each meal if 5 to 8 units of subcutaneous mealtime insulin was used; 12 units at beginning of each meal if 13 to 16 units of subcutaneous mealtime insulin was used; 20 units at beginning of each meal if 17 to 20 units of subcutaneous mealtime insulin was used; and 24 units at beginning of each meal if 21 to 24 units of subcutaneous mealtime insulin was used. *Maintenance*: Dosage based on metabolic needs, blood glucose monitoring results, and glycemic control goal.
Adults converting from subcutaneous premixed insulin. Both basal and mealtime dosages required for conversion. *Mealtime dosage:* Beginning-of-mealtime injected dose estimated by dividing half of the total daily injected premixed insulin dose equally among the three meals of the day. Then each estimated injected mealtime dose converted as follows: 4 units if up to 4 units of subcutaneous premixed insulin was used; 8 units if 5 to 8 units of subcutaneous premixed insulin was used; 12 units if 9 to 12 units of subcutaneous premixed insulin was used; 16 units if 13 to 16 units of subcutaneous premixed insulin was used; 20 units if 17 to 20 units of subcutaneous premixed insulin was used; and 24 units if 21 to 24 units of subcutaneous premixed insulin was used. *Basal dosage:* The remaining half of the total daily injected premixed dose injected as a basal insulin dose. *Maintenance:* Mealtime and basal dosages based on metabolic needs, blood glucose monitoring results, and glycemic control goal.

DOSAGE ADJUSTMENT Dosage may need to be decreased if patient is taking any of the following drugs concurrently: ACE inhibitors, angiotensin II receptor blocking agents, disopyramide, fibrates, fluoxetine, monoamine oxidase inhibitors, other antidiabetic agents, pentoxifylline, pramlintide, propoxyphene, salicylates, somatostatin analogs, or sulfonamide antibiotics. Dosage may need to be increased if patient is taking any of the following drugs concurrently: atypical antipsychotics, corticosteroids, danazol, diuretics, estrogens, glucagon, isoniazid, niacin, oral contraceptives, phenothiazines, progestogens, protease inhibitors, somatropin, sympathomimetic agents, or thyroid hormones. Dosage may need to be increased or decreased if patient is taking any of the following concurrently: alcohol, beta blockers, clonidine, lithium, or pentamidine

Mechanism of Action
Lowers blood glucose levels by stimulating peripheral glucose uptake by skeletal muscle and fat, and by inhibiting hepatic glucose production. Also inhibits lipolysis in adipocytes, inhibits proteolysis, and enhances protein synthesis.

Contraindications
Chronic lung disease (asthma, chronic obstructive pulmonary disease), during episodes of hypoglycemia, hypersensitivity to regular human insulin or any of its components

Interaction
DRUGS
ACE inhibitors, angiotensin II receptor blocking agents, disopyramide, fibrates, fluoxetine, monoamine oxidase inhibitors, other antidiabetic agents, pentoxifylline, pramlintide, propoxyphene, salicylates, somatostatin analogs, sulfonamide antibiotics: Increased risk of hypoglycemia
atypical antipsychotics, corticosteroids, danazol, diuretics, estrogens, glucagon, isoniazid, niacin, oral contraceptives, phenothiazines, progestogens, protease inhibitors, somatropin, sympathomimetic agents, thyroid hormones: Decreased effectiveness of inhaled insulin
beta blockers, clonidine, lithium, or pentamidine: Possibly increased or decreased blood glucose levels
beta blockers, clonidine, guanethidine, reserpine: Blunted hypoglycemic signs and symptoms *thiazolidinediones:* Increased risk of fluid retention and heart failure

Activities
alcohol use: Possibly increased or decreased blood glucose levels

Adverse Reactions
CNS: Confusion, dizziness, drowsiness, fatigue, headache
CV: Tachycardia
EENT: Throat pain or irritation
ENDO: Diabetic ketoacidosis, hypoglycemia
GI: Diarrhea, nausea
GU: UTI
RESP: Acute bronchospasm, bronchitis, cough, decline in pulmonary function, dyspnea, shortness of breath
SKIN: Diaphoresis, rash
Other: Anaphylaxis, angioedema, anti-insulin antibodies, hypokalemia, weight gain

Nursing Considerations
• Be aware that inhaled insulin is not a substitute for long-acting insulin and must be used in combination with long-acting insulin in patients with type 1 diabetes mellitus.
• Know that inhaled insulin should not be used to treat diabetic ketoacidosis, nor should it be used in patients who smoke or who have recently stopped smoking.
• Ensure that patient has had a complete medical history, physical examination, and spirometry before inhaled insulin therapy is begun to identify potential lung disease, as the drug is contraindicated in patients with chronic lung disease. Spirometry should be repeated after the first 6 months of therapy and annually thereafter. Expect drug to be discontinued if patient experiences a 20% or more decline in pulmonary function.
• Administer inhaled insulin using only the Afrezza inhaler. Each cartridge provides a single inhalation.
WARNING Monitor patient closely for signs and symptoms of hypoglycemia, which could become severe, causing seizures or even death. If present, withhold inhaled insulin, treat according to standard of care, and notify prescriber.
• Monitor patient's blood glucose level closely to detect need for dosage adjustment, as ordered. Expect dosage adjustments with changes in patient's

G
H
I

physical activity, meal patterns, and renal or hepatic function, or during acute illness.

• Monitor patient for hypersensitivity reactions. If present, withhold drug, treat according to standard of care, and monitor patient closely until signs and symptoms resolve. Notify prescriber and expect drug to be discontinued and replaced with subcutaneous forms of insulin therapy.

• Monitor patient's serum potassium levels throughout inhaled insulin therapy in patients at risk for hypokalemia, such as those using potassium-lowering drugs, drugs sensitive to serum potassium concentrations, or intravenously administered insulin.

PATIENT TEACHING
• Teach patient how to use the inhaler device.

• Tell patient that doses that exceed 8 units per mealtime will require more than one cartridge.

• Instruct patient to keep the inhaler level, the white mouthpiece on the top, and the purple base on the bottom after a cartridge has been inserted into the inhaler. Remind patient that loss of drug effect can occur if the inhaler is turned upside down, held with the mouthpiece pointing down, or shaken (or dropped) after the cartridge has been inserted but before the dose has been administered. If any of these events occur, the patient should replace the cartridge before use.

WARNING Review signs and symptoms of hypoglycemia and how to treat them. If frequent or severe, tell patient to notify prescriber, as dosage may need to be adjusted. Stress importance of monitoring blood glucose levels.

• Stress importance of not smoking or ingesting alcoholic beverages while using inhaled insulin.

• Tell patient to avoid performing hazardous activities such as driving until the effects of inhaled insulin on her nervous system is known.

ipecac syrup
Ipecac Syrup

Class and Category
Chemical class: Cephaelis acuminata or Cephaelis ipecacuanha derivative
Therapeutic class: Emetic
Pregnancy category: C

Indications and Dosages
➤ *To induce vomiting after drug overdose and certain types of poisoning*
SYRUP
Adults and children over age 12. 15 to 30 ml followed by 240 ml water. Dose repeated if vomiting doesn't begin within 20 to 30 min.
Children ages 1 to 12. 15 ml preceded or followed by 120 to 240 ml water. Dose repeated if vomiting doesn't begin within 20 to 30 min.
Infants ages 6 months to 1 year. 5 to 10 ml preceded or followed by 120 to 240 ml water.

Route	Onset	Peak	Duration
P.O.	20–30 min	Unknown	20–25 min

Mechanism of Action
Induces vomiting by irritating gastric mucosa and stimulating medullary chemoreceptor trigger zone in CNS.

Contraindications
Loss of gag reflex, poisoning with strychnine or corrosives (such as alkaloid substances, petroleum distillates, and strong acids), seizures, semiconsciousness or unconsciousness, severe inebriation, shock

Interaction
DRUGS
activated charcoal: Lack of emetic effect

Adverse Reactions
CNS: Depression, drowsiness
EENT: Aspiration of vomitus, coughing
GI: Diarrhea, indigestion

Nursing Considerations
• Give ipecac syrup only to conscious patients, and follow with adequate water. Give young or frightened children water before or after ipecac.

• Expect vomiting to start in 20 to 30 minutes.

• If vomiting doesn't start within 30 minutes of second dose, prepare for gastric lavage.

• Don't give ipecac after ingestion of petroleum distillates, such as gasoline, or

caustic substances, to avoid further injury to esophagus.
• If activated charcoal will be given, expect to do so after patient vomits or 30 minutes after second ipecac dose because activated charcoal adsorbs and inhibits ipecac.
• Arrhythmias, atrial fibrillation, brady-cardia, fatal myocarditis, hypotension, myalgia, or muscle stiffness or weakness may develop if patient takes too much ipecac or doesn't vomit.

PATIENT TEACHING
• Inform patient of ipecac's effects.
• Tell adult patient to drink 8 oz (240 ml) of water after taking drug and child to drink 4 to 8 oz (120 to 240 ml) before or after taking drug.
• Inform patient or parents of child that diarrhea may occur after taking drug.
• Urge parents to keep ipecac syrup and phone number of a poison control center.

WARNING Advise parents to replace their ipecac extract or tincture with ipecac syrup. Explain that ipecac fluid extract is 14 times more concentrated than ipecac syrup and can cause serious, possibly toxic, effects if given incorrectly.

---

ipratropium bromide

Apo-Ipravent (CAN), Atrovent, Kendral-Ipratropium (CAN)

Class and Category
Chemical class: Quaternary N-methyl isopropyl derivative of noratropine
Therapeutic class: Anticholinergic, bronchodilator
Pregnancy category: B

Indications and Dosages
➤ *To treat bronchitis and COPD*
INHALATION AEROSOL
Adults and adolescents. 2 to 4 inhalations (36 to 72 mcg) three times daily or four times daily. *Maximum:* Up to 12 inhalations (216 mcg)/24 hr.
INHALATION SOLUTION FOR NEBULIZER
Adults and adolescents. 250 to 500 mcg dissolved in preservative-free sterile

normal saline solution every 6 to 8 hr. For severe COPD exacerbations, 500 mcg every 4 to 8 hr.
➤ *To treat perennial and allergic rhinitis*
NASAL SPRAY
Adults and children age 6 and over.
2 sprays of 0.03% (21 mcg/spray) per nostril twice daily or three times daily *Maximum:* 12 sprays (252 mcg)/24 hr.
➤ *To treat rhinorrhea caused by the common cold*
NASAL SPRAY
Adults and children age 5 and over.
2 sprays of 0.06% (42 mcg/spray) per nostril three times daily or four times daily for up to 4 days. *Maximum:* 16 sprays (672 mcg)/24 hr.

Route	Onset	Peak	Duration
Inhalation	5–15 min	1–2 hr	3–8 hr
Nasal	5 min	1–4 hr	4–8 hr

Contraindications
Hypersensitivity to atropine, ipratropium bromide, or their components; hypersensitivity to peanuts, soya lecithin, soybeans, or related products (with aerosol inhaler)

Interaction
DRUGS
anticholinergics: Increased anticholinergic effects
tacrine: Decreased effects of both drugs

Adverse Reactions
CNS: Dizziness, insomnia
CV: Atrial fibrillation (oral inhalation), bradycardia (nasal spray), edema, hypertension, palpitations, supraventricular tachycardia (oral inhalation), tachycardia
EENT: Acute eye pain, dry mouth or pharyngeal area, increased intraocular pressure, laryngospasm, taste perversion, oropharyngeal edema (all drug forms); blurred vision, conjunctival and corneal congestion, eye irritation and pain, mydriasis, visual halos (if nasal spray comes in contact with eyes); epistaxis, mydriasis, nasal dryness and irritation, pharyngitis, rhinitis, sinusitis, tinnitus (with nasal spray)
GI: Bowel obstruction, constipation, diarrhea, ileus, nausea, vomiting
GU: Prostatitis, urine retention
MS: Arthritis

G
H
I

Mechanism of Action

After acetylcholine is released from cholinergic fibers, ipratropium prevents it from attaching to muscarinic receptors on membranes of smooth-muscle cells, as shown at right. By blocking acetycholine's effects in bronchi and bronchioles, ipratropium relaxes smooth muscles and causes bronchodilation.

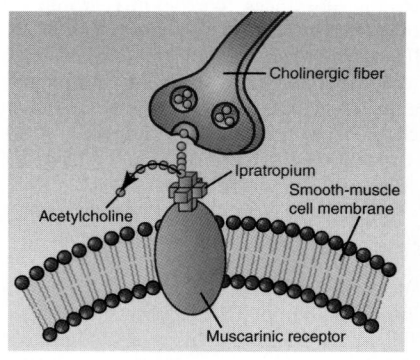

RESP: Bronchitis, bronchospasm, cough, dyspnea, increased sputum production, wheezing
SKIN: Dermatitis, pruritus, rash, urticaria
Other: Anaphylaxis, angioedema, flulike symptoms

Nursing Considerations

• Use ipratropium cautiously in patients with angle-closure glaucoma, benign prostatic hyperplasia, or bladder neck obstruction and in patients with hepatic or renal dysfunction.
• As prescribed, mix ipratropium inhalation solution with preservative-free albuterol, and preservative-free ipratropium inhalation solution with cromolyn inhalation solution. Use within 1 hour.
• When using a nebulizer, apply a mouthpiece to prevent drug from leaking out around mask and causing blurred vision or eye pain.
WARNING Monitor patient for hypersensitivity reactions that could be life-threatening. If present, stop drug use immediately, notify prescriber, and provide supportive care, as needed.
PATIENT TEACHING
• Caution patient not to use ipratropium to treat acute bronchospasm.
• Inform patient that although some people feel relief within 24 hours of drug use, maximum effect may take up to 2 weeks.
• Teach patient to use inhaler or nasal spray. Tell him to shake inhaler well at each use.
• Advise patient to keep spray out of his eyes because it may irritate them or blur his vision. If spray comes in contact with eyes, instruct him to flush them with

cool tap water for several minutes and to contact prescriber.
• Instruct patient to rinse mouth after each nebulizer or inhaler treatment to help minimize throat dryness and irritation.
• If patient is using 0.06% nasal spray for a common cold, advise against use for longer than 4 days.
• Teach patient to track canister contents by counting and recording number of doses.
• Advise patient to report decreased response to ipratropium as well as difficulty voiding, eye pain, nasal dryness, nose bleeds, palpitations, and vision changes.

irbesartan

Avapro

Class and Category

Chemical class: Nonpeptide angiotensin II antagonist
Therapeutic class: Antihypertensive
Pregnancy category: D

Indications and Dosages

➤ *To manage hypertension, alone or with other antihypertensives*
TABLETS
Adults and adolescents. *Initial:* 150 mg daily. *Maximum:* 300 mg daily.
DOSAGE ADJUSTMENT Initial dosage reduced to 75 mg daily for patients with hypovolemia or hyponatremia from such causes as hemodialysis or vigorous diuretic therapy.

Children ages 6 to 12. *Initial:* 75 mg daily. *Maximum:* 150 mg daily.

➤ *To treat nephropathy in type 2 diabetes mellitus*

TABLETS

Adults. 300 mg daily.

Route	Onset	Peak	Duration
P.O.	Unknown	In 4–6 wk	Unknown

Mechanism of Action

Selectively blocks binding of the potent vasoconstrictor angiotensin (AT) II to AT_1 receptor sites in many tissues, including vascular smooth-muscle and adrenal glands. This inhibits the vaso-constrictive and aldosterone-secreting effects of AT II, which reduces blood pressure.

Contraindications

Concurrent aliskiren use in patients with diabetes or patients with renal impairment (GFR less than 60 ml/min), hypersensitivity to irbesartan or its components

Interaction

DRUGS

ACE inhibitors, aliskiren (patients with diabetes or renal impairment), other angiotensin receptor blockers: Increased risk of hypotension, hyperkalemia, and renal dysfunction

diuretics: Possibly additive hypotensive effects

lithium: Possibly increased serum lithium level

NSAIDs: Possible decreased renal function in patients who are elderly, volume-depleted, or have a compromised renal function

potassium-sparing diuretics, potassium supplements, or salt substitutes containing potassium: Possible hyperkalemia

Adverse Reactions

CNS: Anxiety, dizziness, fatigue, headache, nervousness

CV: Chest pain, hypotension, peripheral edema, tachycardia

EENT: Pharyngitis, rhinitis

GI: Abdominal pain, diarrhea, elevated liver function tests, heartburn, hepatitis, indigestion, jaundice, nausea, vomiting

GU: Impaired renal function, renal failure, UTI

MS: Musculoskeletal pain

HEME: Thrombocytopenia

MS: Increased CPK level, rhabdomyolysis

RESP: Upper respiratory tract infection

SKIN: Rash, urticaria

Other: Angioedema, hyperkalemia

Nursing Considerations

• If patient has known or suspected hypovolemia, provide treatment, such as I.V. normal saline solution, as prescribed, to correct this condition before beginning irbesartan therapy. Or expect to begin therapy with a lower dosage.

• Check blood pressure often to evaluate drug's effectiveness.

• If blood pressure isn't controlled with irbesartan alone, expect to also give a diuretic, such as hydrochlorothiazide, as prescribed.

WARNING If patient receives a diuretic or another antihypertensive during irbesartan therapy, frequently monitor blood pressure because he's at risk for hypotension.

• If patient experiences symptomatic hypotension, expect to stop drug temporarily. Immediately place him in supine position and prepare to give I.V. normal saline solution, as prescribed. Expect to resume drug therapy after blood pressure stabilizes.

• If patient receives a diuretic, provide adequate hydration, as appropriate, to help prevent hypovolemia. Also monitor patient for signs and symptoms of hypovolemia, such as hypotension, dizziness, and fainting.

WARNING Monitor patient for increased BUN and serum creatinine levels if he has heart failure or impaired renal function because drug may cause acute renal failure. If increases are significant or persistent, notify prescriber immediately.

PATIENT TEACHING

• Advise patient to take drug at the same time each day to maintain its therapeutic effect.

• Explain importance of regular exercise, proper diet, and other lifestyle changes in controlling hypertension.

• Caution patient to avoid hazardous activities until drug's CNS effects are known.

G
H
I

• Instruct patient to consult prescriber before taking any new drug.
• To reduce risk of dehydration and hypotension, advise patient to drink adequate fluids during hot weather and exercise.
• Instruct patient to contact prescriber if severe nausea, vomiting, or diarrhea occurs and continues, because of the risk of dehydration and hypotension.
WARNING Advise female patient to notify prescriber immediately about known or suspected pregnancy. Explain that if she becomes pregnant, prescriber may replace irbesartan with another antihypertensive that's safe to use during pregnancy.
• Urge patient to keep follow-up appointments with prescriber to monitor progress.

iron dextran

(contains 50 mg of elemental iron per milliliter)
DexFerrum, DexIron (CAN), InFeD

Class and Category

Chemical class: Iron salt, mineral
Therapeutic class: Antianemic
Pregnancy category: C

Indications and Dosages

➤ *To treat iron deficiency anemia*
I.V. INFUSION
Adults and children weighing more than 15 kg (33 lb). Dose (ml) 5 0.0442 (desired hemoglobin 2 observed hemoglobin) 3 lean body weight (kg) 1 (0.26 3 lean body weight). Or, consult dosage table in package insert. *Maximum:* 2 ml (100 mg) daily.
Children over age 4 months weighing 5 to 15 kg (11 to 33 lb). Dose (ml) 5 0.0442 (desired hemoglobin 1 observed hemoglobin) 3 weight (kg) 1 (0.26 3 weight). Or, consult dosage table in package insert. *Maximum:* 1 ml (50 mg) daily.
➤ *To replace iron lost in blood loss*
I.V. INFUSION
Adults. Replacement iron (mg) 5 ml of blood loss 3 hematocrit.

Mechanism of Action

Restores hemoglobin and replenishes iron stores. Iron, an essential component of

hemoglobin, myoglobin, and several enzymes (including cytochromes, catalase, and peroxidase), is needed for catecholamine metabolism and normal neutrophil function.

In iron dextran therapy, iron binds to available protein parts after the drug has been split into iron and dextran by cells of the reticuloendothelial system. The bound iron forms hemosiderin or ferritin, physiologic forms of iron, and transferrin, which replenish hemoglobin and deplete iron stores. Dextran is metabolized or excreted.

Incompatibilities

Don't mix iron dextran with blood for transfusion, other drugs, or parenteral nutrition solutions for I.V. infusion.

Contraindications

Anemia other than iron deficiency, hypersensitivity to iron dextran or its components

Adverse Reactions

CNS: Chills, disorientation, dizziness, fever, headache, malaise, paresthesia, seizures, syncope, unconsciousness, weakness
CV: Arrhythmias, bradycardia, chest pain, hypertension, hypotension, shock, tachycardia
EENT: Altered taste
GI: Abdominal pain, diarrhea, nausea, vomiting
GU: Hematuria
HEME: Leukocytosis
MS: Arthralgia, arthritis, backache, myalgia, rhabdomyolysis
RESP: Bronchospasm, dyspnea, respiratory arrest, wheezing
SKIN: Cyanosis, diaphoresis, rash, pruritus, purpura, urticaria
Other: Anaphylaxis, infusion-site phlebitis

Nursing Considerations

• Expect oral iron therapy to stop before iron dextran therapy starts. Iron dextran is given only when oral therapy isn't feasible; it also may be given by I.M. injection.
• Expect to monitor hemoglobin level, hematocrit, serum ferritin level, and transferrin saturation, as ordered, before, during, and after iron dextran therapy.
WARNING Before starting iron dextran therapy, give a test dose of 0.5 ml iron

dextran gradually over 30 seconds, as prescribed, and monitor patient closely for anaphylactic reaction.
• Wait 1 to 2 hours before giving remainder of dose. Infuse undiluted iron dextran slowly, at no more than 1 ml/minute (50 mg/minute).
WARNING Monitor patient closely for signs and symptoms of anaphylaxis (such as severe hypotension, loss of consciousness, collapse, dyspnea, and seizures) during and after infusion. Patients with a history of asthma or allergies are at increased risk for anaphylaxis, possibly death. Institute emergency resuscitation measures as needed, including epinephrine administration, as prescribed.
WARNING Assess blood pressure often after iron dextran administration because hypotension is a common adverse effect that may be related to infusion rate; avoid rapid infusion.
• Be aware that patient may have adverse reactions, including arthralgia, backache, chills, and vomiting, 1 to 2 days after drug therapy. Symptoms should resolve within 3 to 4 days.
• Assess patients with a history of rheumatoid arthritis for exacerbation of joint pain and swelling.
• If patient has cardiovascular disease, watch for worsening from drug's adverse effects.
• Assess patient for iron overload, characterized by sedation, decreased activity, pale eyes, and bleeding in GI tract and lungs.
• Store iron dextran at 59° to 86° F (15° to 30° C).

PATIENT TEACHING
• Instruct patient to report immediately signs of adverse reaction, such as shortness of breath, wheezing, or rash, during iron dextran therapy.
• Advise patient not to take any oral iron without first consulting prescriber.
• Inform patient that symptoms of iron deficiency may include decreased stamina, learning problems, shortness of breath, and fatigue. Urge patient to plan periods of activity and rest to avoid excessive fatigue.
• Emphasize need to follow dosage regimen and keep follow-up medical and laboratory appointments.

iron sucrose
(contains 100 mg of elemental iron per 5 ml)
Venofer

Class and Category
Chemical class: Iron salt, mineral
Therapeutic class: Antianemic
Pregnancy category: B

Indications and Dosages
➤ *To treat iron deficiency anemia in hemodialysis patients receiving erythropoietin*
I.V. INJECTION
Adults. *Initial:* 100 mg elemental iron injected undiluted over 2 to 5 min during dialysis. *Usual:* 100 mg elemental iron every wk to 3 times/wk to total dose of 1,000 mg. Dosage repeated as needed to maintain target levels of hemoglobin and hematocrit and acceptable blood iron level. *Maximum:* 100 mg/dose.
I.V. INFUSION
Adults. *Initial:* 100 mg elemental iron infused diluted over 15 min during dialysis. *Usual:* 100 mg elemental iron every wk to 3 times/wk to a total dose of 1,000 mg. Dosage repeated as needed to maintain target levels of hemoglobin and hematocrit and acceptable blood iron level. *Maximum:* 100 mg/dose.
➤ *To treat iron deficiency anemia in peritoneal dialysis patients receiving erythropoietin*
I.V. INFUSION
Adults. *Initial:* 300 mg elemental iron infused diluted over 1.5 hr on days 1 and 14, followed by 400 mg elemental iron infused over 2.5 hr on day 28. Dosage repeated as needed to maintain target levels of hemoglobin and hematocrit and acceptable blood iron level. *Maximum:* 1,000 mg/28 days.
➤ *To maintain iron therapy in children with chronic kidney disease who are nondialysis-dependent receiving erythropoietin or who are peritoneal-dialysis-dependent receiving erythropoietin*
I.V. INJECTION
Children age 2 years and older. 0.5 mg/kg, not to exceed 100 mg per dose, every 4 wks

G
H
I

for 12 wks given undiluted over 5 minutes. Treatment repeated, as needed.

I.V. INFUSION

Children age 2 years and older. 0.5 mg/kg, not to exceed 100 mg per dose, every 4 wks for 12 wks diluted in 25 ml of 0.9% NaCl and given over 5 to 60 minutes. Treatment repeated, as needed.

➤ *To treat iron deficiency anemia in nondialysis patients with chronic renal disease. regardless of whether they're receiving erythropoietin*

I.V. INJECTION

Adults. *Initial:* 200 mg elemental iron injected undiluted over 2 to 5 min and repeated 4 more times over a 14-day period for a total dose of 1,000 mg. Dosage repeated as needed to maintain target levels of hemoglobin and hematocrit and acceptable blood iron level. *Maximum:* 1,000 mg/14 days.

I.V. INFUSION

Adults. 500 mg elemental iron infused diluted over 3.5 to 5 hr on days 1 and 14. Dosage repeated as needed to maintain target levels of hemoglobin and hematocrit and acceptable blood iron level. *Maximum:* 1,000 mg/14 days.

Mechanism of Action

Acts to replenish iron stores lost during dialysis because of increased erythropoiesis and insufficient absorption of iron from GI tract. Iron is an essential component of hemoglobin, myoglobin, and several enzymes, including cytochromes, catalase, and peroxidase, and is needed for catecholamine metabolism and normal neutrophil function. Iron sucrose injection also normalizes RBC production by binding with hemoglobin or being stored as ferritin in reticuloendothelial cells of the liver, spleen, and bone marrow.

Incompatibilities

Don't mix with other drugs or parenteral nutrition solutions for I.V. infusion.

Contraindications

Anemia other than iron deficiency, hypersensitivity to iron salts or their components, iron overload

Interaction

DRUGS

chloramphenicol: Possibly decreased effectiveness of iron sucrose

oral iron preparations: Possibly reduced absorption of oral iron supplements

Adverse Reactions

CNS: Asthenia, dizziness, fatigue, fever, headache, hypoesthesia, malaise

CV: Chest pain, heart failure, hypertension, hypotension, peirpheral edema

EENT: Conjunctivitis, ear pain, nasal congestion, nasopharyngitis, rhinitis, sinusitis, taste perversion

ENDO: Hyperglycemia, hypoglycemia

GI: Abdominal pain, constipation, diarrhea, elevated liver function test results, nausea, occult-positive feces, peritoneal infection, vomiting

GU: UTI

MS: Arthralgia, arthritis, back pain, leg cramps, muscle pain or weakness, myalgia

RESP: Cough, dyspnea, pneumonia, upper respiratory tract infection

SKIN: Pruritus, rash

Other: Anaphylaxis; fluid overload; gout; hypervolemia; infusion or injection-site burning, pain, or redness; sepsis

Nursing Considerations

• To reconstitute iron sucrose injection for infusion, dilute 100 mg elemental iron in maximum of 100 ml normal saline solution (for hemodialysis patients) or 250 ml (for peritoneal dialysis and nondialysis patients) immediately before infusion. Discard any unused diluted solution.

• Give drug directly into dialysis line by slow I.V. injection or by infusion.

WARNING Monitor patient closely for evidence of anaphylaxis, such as severe hypotension, loss of consciousness, collapse, dyspnea, or seizures, during and for at least 30 minutes after therapy. Institute emergency resuscitation measures as needed.

WARNING Assess blood pressure often after drug administration because hypotension is a common adverse reaction that may be related to infusion rate (avoid rapid infusion) or total cumulative dose.

• Monitor hemoglobin, hematocrit, serum ferritin, and transferrin saturation, as ordered, before, during, and after iron sucrose therapy. Test serum iron level 48 hours after last dose. Notify prescriber and

expect to stop therapy if blood iron levels are normal or elevated, to prevent iron toxicity.
• Watch for evidence of iron overload, such as sedation, decreased activity, pale eyes, and bleeding in GI tract and lungs.

PATIENT TEACHING
• Inform patient that symptoms of iron deficiency may include decreased stamina, learning problems, shortness of breath, and fatigue.

isocarboxazid
Marplan

Class and Category
Chemical class: Hydrazine derivative
Therapeutic class: Antidepressant
Pregnancy category: C

Indications and Dosages
➤ *To treat major depression*
TABLETS
Adults and adolescents over age 16. *Initial:* 10 mg twice daily, increased by 10 mg daily every 2 to 4 days, as needed and tolerated. *Maximum:* 60 mg daily.

Route	Onset	Peak	Duration
P.O.	7–10 days	Unknown	10 days

Mechanism of Action
Irreversibly binds to MAO, reducing its activity and increasing levels of neurotransmitters, including serotonin and the catecholamine neurotransmitters dopamine, epinephrine, and norepinephrine. This regulation of CNS neurotransmitters helps to ease depression. With long-term use, drug results in down-regulation (desensitization) of alpha$_2$- or beta-adrenergic and serotonin receptors after 2 to 4 weeks, which also produces an antidepressant effect.

Contraindications
Cardiovascular disease; cerebrovascular disease; heart failure; hepatic disease; history of headaches; hypersensitivity to isocarboxazid or its components; hypertension; pheochromocytoma; severe renal impairment; use of anesthetics, antihypertensives, bupropion, buspirone, carbamazepine, CNS depressants, cyclobenzaprine, dextromethorphan, meperidine, selective serotonin reuptake inhibitors, sympathomimetics, or tricyclic antidepressants; use within 14 days of another MAO inhibitor

Interaction
DRUGS
anticholinergics, antidyskinetics, antihistamines: Increased anticholinergic effect, prolonged CNS depression (with antihistamines)
anticonvulsants: Increased CNS depression, possibly altered seizure pattern
antihypertensives, diuretics: Increased hypotensive effect
bromocriptine: Possibly interference with bromocriptine effects
bupropion: Increased risk of bupropion toxicity
buspirone, guanadrel, guanethidine: Increased risk of hypertension
caffeine-containing drugs: Increased risk of dangerous arrhythmias and severe hypertension
carbamazepine, cyclobenzaprine, maprotiline, other MAO inhibitors: Increased risk of hyperpyretic crisis, hypertensive crisis, severe seizures, and death; altered pattern of seizures (with carbamazepine)
CNS depressants: Increased CNS depression
dextromethorphan: Increased risk of excitation, hypertension, and hyperpyrexia
doxapram: Increased vasopressor effects of either drug
fluoxetine, paroxetine, sertraline, trazodone, tricyclic antidepressants: Increased risk of life-threatening serotonin syndrome
haloperidol, loxapine, molindone, phenothiazines, pimozide, thioxanthenes: Prolonged and intensified anticholinergic, hypotensive, and sedative effects
insulin, oral antidiabetic drugs: Increased hypoglycemic effects
levodopa: Increased risk of sudden, moderate to severe hypertension
local anesthetics (with epinephrine or levonordefrin): Possibly severe hypertension
meperidine, other opioid analgesics: Increased risk of coma, hyperpyrexia, hypotension, immediate excitation, rigidity, seizures, severe hypertension, severe

respiratory depression, shock, sweating, and death
methyldopa: Increased risk of halluci-nations, headache, hyperexcitability, and severe hypertension
methylphenidate: Increased CNS stimulation
metrizamide: Decreased seizure threshold and increased risk of seizures
oral anticoagulants: Increased anticoagulant activity
phenylephrine (nasal or ophthalmic): Potentiated vasopressor effect of phenylephrine
rauwolfia alkaloids: Increased risk of moderate to severe hypertension, CNS depression (when isocarboxazid is added to rauwolfia alkaloid therapy), CNS excitation and hypertension (when rauwolfia alkaloid is added to isocarboxazid therapy)
spinal anesthetics: Increased risk of hypo-tension
sympathomimetics: Prolonged and intensified cardiac stimulant and vaso-pressor effects
tryptophan: Increased risk of confusion, disorientation, hyperreflexia, hyperthermia, hyperventilation, mania or hypomania, and shivering
FOODS
aged cheese; avocados; bananas; fava or broad beans; cured meat or sausage; overripe fruit; pickled or smoked fish, meats or poultry; protein extract; soy sauce; yeast extract; and other foods high in tyramine or other pressor amines: Increased risk of dangerous arrhythmias and severe hypertensive crisis
ACTIVITIES
alcohol-containing products that also may contain tyramine, such as beer (including reduced-alcohol and alcohol-free beer), hard liquor, liqueurs, sherry, and wines (red and white): Increased risk of developing hypertensive crisis

Adverse Reactions
CNS: Agitation, dizziness, drowsiness, fever, headache, insomnia, intracranial bleeding, overstimulation, restlessness, sedation, suicidal ideation, tremor, weakness
CV: Bradycardia, chest pain, edema, hyper-tensive crisis, orthostatic hypotension, palpitations, tachycardia

EENT: Blurred vision, dry mouth, mydriasis, photophobia, yellowing of sclera
GI: Abdominal pain, anorexia, constipation, diarrhea, elevated liver function test results, increased appetite, nausea
GU: Dark urine, oliguria, sexual dysfunction
HEME: Leukopenia
MS: Muscle spasms, myoclonus, neck stiffness
SKIN: Clammy skin, diaphoresis, jaundice, rash
Other: Unusual weight gain

Nursing Considerations
• Monitor patient's blood pressure during isocarboxazid therapy to detect hyper-tensive crisis and decrease risk of orthostatic hypotension.
WARNING Notify prescriber immediately if patient has evidence of hypertensive crisis (drug's most serious adverse effect), such as chest pain, headache, neck stiffness, and palpitations. Expect to stop drug imme-diately if these occur.
• Keep phentolamine readily available to treat hypertensive crisis. Give 5 mg by slow I.V. infusion, as prescribed, to reduce blood pressure without causing excessive hypotension. Use external cooling measures, as prescribed, to manage fever.
• To avoid hypertensive crisis, expect to wait 10 to 14 days when switching patient from one MAO inhibitor to another or when switching from a dibenzazepine-related drug, such as amitriptyline or perphenazine.
• Monitor patient with a history of epilepsy for seizures because isocarboxazid may alter seizure threshold. Institute seizure precautions according to facility protocol.
• Monitor liver function test results, and assess patient for abdominal pain, dark urine, and jaundice because isocarboxazid may cause hepatic dysfunction.
• Expect to observe some therapeutic effect in 7 to 10 days, but keep in mind that full effect may not occur for 4 to 8 weeks.
• Be aware that, for maintenance therapy, the smallest possible dose should be used. Once clinical effect has been achieved, expect to decrease the dosage slowly over several weeks.
• Keep dietary restrictions in place for at least 2 weeks after stopping isocarboxazid

because of slow recovery from drug's enzyme-inhibiting effects.
• Ideally, expect to stop drug 10 days before elective surgery, as prescribed, to avoid hypotension.
• Anticipate that coadministration with a selective serotonin reuptake inhibitor may cause confusion, diaphoresis, diarrhea, seizures, and other less severe symptoms.
• Monitor depressed patient for suicidal tendencies, especially when therapy starts or dosage changes, because depression may worsen temporarily. If suicidal tendencies arise, institute suicide precautions, as appropriate and according to facility policy, and notify prescriber immediately.
• Monitor patient for sudden insomnia. If it develops, notify prescriber and be prepared to give drug early in the day.

PATIENT TEACHING
• Inform patient and family members that therapeutic effects of isocarboxazid may take several weeks to appear and that he should continue taking drug as prescribed.
• Caution parents to monitor pediatric patients, including adolescents, closely for suicidal tendencies, especially when therapy starts or dosage changes.
• Caution patient to rise slowly from a lying or sitting position to minimize effects of orthostatic hypotension.
WARNING Instruct patient to avoid the following foods, beverages, and drugs during isocarboxazid therapy and for 2 weeks afterward: alcohol-free and reduced-alcohol beer and wine; appetite suppressants; beer; broad beans; cheese (except cottage and cream cheese); chocolate and caffeine in large quantities; dry sausage (including Genoa salami, hard salami, Lebanon bologna, and pepperoni); hay fever drugs; inhaled asthma drugs; liver; meat extract; OTC cold and cough medicines (including those containing dextromethorphan); nasal decongestants (tablets, drops, or spray); pickled herring; products that contain tyramine; protein-rich foods that may have undergone protein changes by aging, fermenting, pickling, or smoking; sauerkraut; sinus drugs; weight-loss products; yeast extracts (including brewer's yeast in large quantities); yogurt; and wine.

• Advise patient to notify prescriber immediately about chest pain, dizziness, headache, nausea, neck stiffness, palpitations, rapid heart rate, sweating, and vomiting.
• Advise patient to inform all healthcare providers (including dentists) that he takes an MAO inhibitor because certain drugs are contraindicated within 2 weeks of it.
• Urge patient to avoid hazardous activities until drug's adverse effects are known.
• Urge patient with diabetes mellitus who's taking insulin or an oral antidiabetic to check blood glucose level often during therapy because isocarboxazid may affect glucose control.
• Caution patient not to stop taking drug abruptly to avoid recurrence of original symptoms.

isoetharine hydrochloride

Arm-a-Med Isoetharine (0.062%, 0.125%, 0.167%, 0.2%, 0.25%), Beta-2 (1%), Bronkosol (1%), Dey-Lute Isoetharine (0.08%, 0.1%, 0.17%, 0.25%)

isoetharine mesylate

Bronkometer (0.61%)

Class and Category
Chemical class: Catecholamine
Therapeutic class: Bronchodilator
Pregnancy category: Not rated

Indications and Dosages
➤ *To prevent and treat reversible bronchospasm from chronic bronchitis or emphysema*

INHALATION AEROSOL
Adults and adolescents. 1 or 2 inhalations (340 or 680 mcg) every 4 hr.

INHALATION SOLUTION FOR HAND-BULB NEBULIZER
Adults. 3 to 7 inhalations of undiluted 0.5% or 1% solution every 4 hr.

INHALATION SOLUTION FOR NEBULIZER
Adults. 2.5 to 10 mg over 15 to 20 min. Repeated every 4 hr, as needed.

G
H
I

Route	Onset	Peak	Duration
Inhalation	5 min	5–15 min	2–3 hr

Mechanism of Action

Attaches to beta$_2$ receptors on bronchial cell membranes, which stimulates the intracellular enzyme adenylate cyclase to convert adenosine triphosphate to cyclic adenosine monophosphate (cAMP). Increased intracellular levels of cAMP help relax bronchial smooth-muscle cells, stabilize mast cells, and inhibit histamine release.

Contraindications

Hypersensitivity to isoetharine, sympathomimetic amines, or their components

Interaction

DRUGS

beta blockers: Decreased effects of both drugs
cyclopropane, halothane: Increased risk of arrhythmias
ephedrine: Increased cardiac stimulation
epinephrine: Increased epinephrine effects
guanethidine: Decreased hypotensive effects
isoproterenol: Excessive cardiac stimulation
MAO inhibitors: Increased risk of hypertensive crisis, increased vascular effects of isoetharine
methyldopa: Increased vasopressor response
nitrates: Possibly decreased effects of both drugs
oxytocic drugs: Increased risk of hypotension
rauwolfia alkaloids: Increased risk of hypertension
tricyclic antidepressants: Increased risk of arrhythmias

Adverse Reactions

CNS: Anxiety, dizziness, headache, insomnia, tremor, vertigo, weakness
CV: Angina, arrhythmias, hypertension, palpitations, tachycardia
EENT: Choking sensation, eyelid or lip swelling, laryngospasm, taste perversion
GI: Nausea, vomiting
RESP: Bronchospasm, cough, paradoxical increased airway resistance (with excessive use), wheezing
SKIN: Dermatitis, flushing, pruritus, urticaria

Other: Angioedema, facial edema

Nursing Considerations

• Dilute 1% isoetharine inhalation solution with 1 to 4 ml sterile normal saline solution; 0.062% to 0.25% solutions don't need to be diluted before use.
• Don't use a solution that's pink or darker than light yellow or one that contains precipitate.
• Wait 1 minute after initial inhaler dose to assess whether patient needs a second dose.
• Monitor blood pressure and pulse, and observe for arrhythmias during therapy.

PATIENT TEACHING

• Teach patient how to use isoetharine inhaler or nebulizer.
• Instruct patient to take drug exactly as directed and not to exceed dosage.
• Instruct patient not to take other drugs, even OTC drugs, unless prescribed.
• Teach patient how to determine when canister needs to be replaced by counting and recording number of doses.
• Instruct patient to report chest pain, difficulty breathing, failure to respond to usual isoetharine dose, irregular heartbeat, productive cough, or tremor.

isoniazid

(isonicotinic acid hydrazide, INH)

Isoniazid, Isotamine (CAN), PMS-Isoniazid (CAN)

Class and Category

Chemical class: Isonicotinic acid derivativexs
Therapeutic class: Antibiotic, antitubercular
Pregnancy category: C

Indications and Dosages

➤ *To prevent tuberculosis*
SYRUP, TABLETS, I.M. INJECTION
Adults and adolescents. 300 mg daily.
Children. 10 mg/kg daily (up to 300 mg).
➤ *As adjunct to treat active tuberculosis*
SYRUP, TABLETS
Adults and adolescents. 300 mg daily or 15 mg/kg (up to 900 mg) 2 or 3 times/wk, based on treatment regimen.

Children. 10 to 20 mg/kg (up to 300 mg) daily or 20 to 40 mg/kg (up to 900 mg) 2 or 3 times/wk, based on treatment regimen.

I.M. INJECTION

Adults and adolescents. 5 mg/kg (up to 300 mg) daily or 15 mg/kg (up to 900 mg) 2 or 3 times/wk, based on treatment regimen.
Children. 10 to 20 mg/kg (up to 300 mg) daily or 20 to 40 mg/kg (up to 900 mg) 2 or 3 times/wk, based on treatment regimen.

Mechanism of Action

Interferes with lipid and nucleic acid synthesis in actively growing tubercule bacilli cells. Isoniazid also disrupts bacterial cell wall synthesis and may interfere with mycolic acid synthesis in mycobacterial cells.

Contraindications

History of serious adverse reactions (such as hepatic injury) from isoniazid, hypersensitivity to isoniazid or its components

Interaction

DRUGS

acetaminophen: Increased risk of hepatotoxicity and possibly nephrotoxicity
alfentanil: Decreased alfentanil clearance and increased duration of effects
aluminum-containing antacids: Decreased isoniazid absorption
benzodiazepines: Decreased benzodiazepine clearance
carbamazepine: Increased blood carbamazepine level and toxicity, increased risk of isoniazid toxicity
corticosteroids: Decreased isoniazid effects
cycloserine: Increased risk of adverse CNS effects and CNS toxicity
disulfiram: Changes in behavior and coordination
enflurane: Increased risk of high-output renal failure
halothane: Increased risk of hepatotoxicity and hepatic encephalopathy
hepatotoxic drugs, rifampin: Increased risk of hepatotoxicity
ketoconazole: Possibly decreased blood ketoconazole level and resistance to antifungal treatment

---

* For treatment of bronchospasm.
† For treatment of bradycardia.

meperidine: Risk of hypotensive episodes or CNS depression
nephrotoxic drugs: Increased risk of nephrotoxicity
oral anticoagulants: Increased anticoagulation
phenytoin: Increased blood phenytoin level, increased risk of phenytoin toxicity
theophylline: Increased theophylline level

FOODS

histamine-containing foods, such as tuna, skipjack, and other tropical fish: Inhibited action of the enzyme diamine oxidase in foods, possibly resulting in headache, sweating, palpitations, flushing, and hypotension.
tyramine-containing foods, such as cheese and fish: Increased response to tyramine in foods, possibly resulting in chills; diaphoresis; headache; light-headedness; and red, itchy, clammy skin

ACTIVITIES

alcohol use: Increased risk of hepatotoxicity and increased isoniazid metabolism

Adverse Reactions

CNS: Clumsiness, confusion, dizziness, encephalopathy, fatigue, fever, hallucinations, neurotoxicity, paresthesia, peripheral neuritis, psychosis, seizures, weakness
CV: Vasculitis
EENT: Optic neuritis
ENDO: Gynecomastia, hyperglycemia
GI: Abdominal pain, anorexia, elevated liver function test results, epigastric distress, hepatitis, nausea, pancreatitis, vomiting
GU: Glycosuria
HEME: Agranulocytosis, aplastic anemia, eosinophilia, hemolytic anemia, sideroblastic anemia, thrombocytopenia
MS: Arthralgia, joint stiffness
SKIN: Jaundice, pruritus, rash, Stevens-Johnson syndrome
Other: Anaphylaxis, hypocalcemia, hypophosphatemia, injection-site irritation, lupus-like symptoms, lymphadenopathy

Nursing Considerations

• Administer isoniazid cautiously to diabetic, alcoholic, or malnourished patients and those at risk for peripheral neuritis.
• Give drug 1 hour before or 2 hours after meals to promote absorption. If GI

G
H
I

distress occurs, give drug with a small amount of food or an antacid that doesn't contain aluminum 1 hour before or 2 hours after meal.

• Monitor liver enzyme studies, which may be ordered monthly, because isoniazid can cause severe (possibly fatal) hepatitis.

• About 50% of patients metabolize isoniazid slowly, which may lead to increased toxic effects. Watch for adverse reactions, such as peripheral neuritis; if they occur, expect to decrease dosage.

• Give isoniazid with other antituberculotic drugs, as prescribed, to prevent development of resistant organisms.

• Be aware that patients with advanced HIV infection may experience more severe adverse reactions in greater numbers.

PATIENT TEACHING

• Instruct patient to take isoniazid exactly as prescribed and not to stop without first consulting prescriber. Explain that treatment may take months or years.

• Direct patient to take drug on an empty stomach 1 hour before or 2 hours after meals. If GI distress occurs, instruct him to take drug with food or an antacid that doesn't contain aluminum.

• Advise patient to report signs of hepatic dysfunction, including dark urine, decreased appetite, fatigue, and jaundice.

• Caution patient not to drink alcohol while taking isoniazid because alcohol increases the risk of hepatotoxicity.

• Give patient a list of tyramine-containing foods to avoid when taking isoniazid, such as cheese, fish, salami, red wine, and yeast extracts. Explain that consuming these foods during isoniazid therapy may cause unpleasant adverse reactions, such as chills, pounding heartbeat, and sweating.

• Tell patient to avoid histamine-containing foods such as tuna, skipjack, and other tropical fish during therapy to avoid such adverse reactions as headache, sweating, rapid heartbeat, flushing, and low blood pressure.

• Tell patient that he'll need periodic laboratory tests and physical examinations.

• Urge patient to report fever, nausea, numbness and tingling in arms or legs, rash, vision changes, vomiting, and yellowing skin.

isoproterenol (isoprenaline)

Isuprel

isoproterenol hydrochloride

Isuprel, Isuprel Mistometer

isoproterenol sulfate

Medihaler-Iso

Class and Category

Chemical class: Catecholamine
Therapeutic class: Antiarrhythmic, bronchodilator
Pregnancy category: B (inhalation), C (I.V. infusion)

Indications and Dosages

➤ *To treat bronchospasm in asthma and to prevent and treat bronchospasm in COPD*

INHALATION AEROSOL (ISOPROTERENOL HYDROCHLORIDE)

Adults and adolescents. 1 oral inhalation (120 to 131 mcg), repeated in 2 to 5 min. Inhalations repeated every 3 to 4 hr, as needed.

INHALATION AEROSOL (ISOPROTERENOL SULFATE)

Adults and adolescents. 1 oral inhalation (80 mcg), repeated in 2 to 5 min. Inhalations repeated every 4 to 6 hr, as needed.

INHALATION SOLUTION FOR NEBULIZER (ISOPROTERENOL)

Adults and adolescents. 2.5 mg diluted and administered over 10 to 20 min. Repeated every 4 hr, as needed.

Children. 0.05 to 0.1 mg/kg (up to 1.25 mg) diluted and administered over 10 to 20 min. Repeated every 4 hr, as needed.

➤ *To manage bronchospasm during anesthesia*

I.V. INJECTION (ISOPROTERENOL HYDROCHLORIDE)

Adults. 0.01 to 0.02 mg, repeated as needed.

➤ *To treat bradycardia with significant hemodynamic change, such as third-degree heart block or prolonged QT intervals*

I.V. INFUSION (ISOPROTERENOL HYDROCHLORIDE)
Adults. *Initial:* 2 mcg/min. Titrated according to heart rate, as ordered. *Maximum:* 10 mcg/min.

Route	Onset	Peak	Duration
I.V.*	Unknown	Unknown	1–2 hr
I.V.†	In 5 min	Unknown	10 min
Inhalation	In 5 min	5–15 min	In 3 hr

Mechanism of Action
Stimulates beta$_1$ receptors in the myocardium and cardiac conduction system, resulting in positive inotropic and chronotropic effects. Isoproterenol also shortens AV conduction time and refractory period in patients with AV block. This action increases ventricular rate and halts bradycardia and associated syncope.

In addition, isoproterenol attaches to beta$_2$ receptors on bronchial cell membranes. This action stimulates the intracellular enzyme adenylate cyclase to convert adenosine triphosphate to cyclic adenosine monophosphate (cAMP). An increased intracellular cAMP level relaxes bronchial smooth-muscle cells, stabilizes mast cells, and inhibits histamine release.

Contraindications
Angina pectoris, heart block or tachycardia from digitalis toxicity, ventricular arrhythmias that require inotropic therapy (I.V. form); hypersensitivity to isoproterenol or its components, such as sulfite in some preparations (inhalation form); tachyarrhythmias (I.V. and inhalation forms)

Interaction
DRUGS
Note: All interactions listed are for I.V. form unless indicated.
alpha blockers, other drugs with this action: Possibly decreased peripheral vasoconstricting and hypertensive effects of isoproterenol
anesthetics (hydrocarbon inhalation): Increased risk of atrial and ventricular arrhythmias
astemizole, cisapride, drugs that prolong QTc interval, terfenadine: Possibly prolonged QTc interval
beta blockers (ophthalmic): Decreased effects of isoproterenol, increased risk of

bronchospasm, wheezing, decreased pulmonary function, and respiratory failure
beta blockers (systemic): Increased risk of bronchospasm, decreased effects of both drugs (including inhaled isoproterenol)
digoxin: Increased risk of arrhythmias, hypokalemia, and digitalis toxicity
diuretics, other antihypertensives: Possibly decreased antihypertensive effects
ergot alkaloids: Increased vasoconstriction and vasopressor effects
MAO inhibitors: Intensified and extended cardiac stimulation and vasopressor effects
quinidine, other drugs that affect myocardial reaction to sympathomimetics: Increased risk of arrhythmias
theophylline: Increased risk of cardiotoxicity, decreased blood theophylline level
thyroid hormones: Increased effects of both drugs, increased risk of coronary insufficiency in patients with coronary artery disease
tricyclic antidepressants: Increased vasopressor response, increased risk of prolonged QTc interval and arrhythmias

Adverse Reactions
CNS: Dizziness, headache, insomnia, nervousness, syncope, tremor, weakness
CV: Angina, arrhythmias, bradycardia, hypertension, hypotension, palpitations, tachycardia, ventricular arrhythmias
EENT: Dry mouth, oropharyngeal edema, taste perversion
ENDO: Hyperglycemia
GI: Heartburn, nausea, vomiting
MS: Muscle spasms and twitching
RESP: Bronchitis, bronchospasm, cough, dyspnea, increased sputum production, pulmonary edema, wheezing
SKIN: Dermatitis, diaphoresis, erythema multiforme, flushing, pallor, pruritus, rash, Stevens-Johnson syndrome, urticaria
Other: Angioedema, hypokalemia

Nursing Considerations
• Expect to give lowest possible dose of isoproterenol for shortest possible time to minimize tolerance.
• Don't administer I.V. isoproterenol if solution is pink or brown or contains precipitate.

G
H
I

• Administer isoproterenol infusion through a large vein, and monitor patient for signs of extravasation.

• Monitor blood pressure, cardiac rhythm, central venous pressure, and urine output when giving I.V. drug. Adjust infusion rate to response, as ordered.

• Notify prescriber immediately if heart rate increases significantly or exceeds 110 beats/minute during I.V. infusion.

• Know that drug may increase pulse pressure and cause hypotension. Expect to reduce I.V. infusion slowly to decrease risk of hypotension.

WARNING Be aware that drug markedly increases risk of arrhythmias. If an arrhythmia develops, expect to give a cardioselective beta blocker, such as atenolol.

• Isoproterenol isn't used regularly to treat asthma, decreased cardiac output, hypotension, or shock because it increases the risk of arrhythmias, hypotension, and ischemia.

WARNING If drug aggravates a ventilation-perfusion problem, expect blood oxygen level to fall even as breathing seems to improve.

PATIENT TEACHING

• Instruct patient not to use isoproterenol inhaler more often than prescribed because it may cause cardiac and respiratory problems.

• Teach patient to use the inhaler. Provide a spacer, as needed.

• Instruct patient to wait 2 to 5 minutes before taking second inhalation.

• Advise patient to rinse his mouth after inhalation to remove drug residue and minimize mouth dryness.

• Inform patient that saliva may appear pink after inhalation.

• If patient uses a corticosteroid inhaler, tell him to take isoproterenol first and wait at least 2 minutes before taking corticosteroid.

• Instruct patient to notify prescriber about chest pain, dizziness, hyperglycemic symptoms (such as abdominal cramps, lethargy, nausea, and vomiting), insomnia, irregular heartbeat, palpitations, tremor, and weakness.

• Advise patient to also report reduced effectiveness of isoproterenol, increased use of inhaler, and increased symptoms after taking drug.

isosorbide dinitrate
Apo-ISDN (CAN), Cedocard-SR (CAN), Coradur (CAN), Coronex (CAN), Dilatrate-SR, Isordil Tembids, Isordil Titradose, Sorbitrate

isosorbide mononitrate
IMDUR, ISMO, Monoket

Class and Category
Chemical class: Organic nitrate
Therapeutic class: Antianginal, vasodilator
Pregnancy category: C

Indications and Dosages
➤ *To treat or prevent angina*
CHEWABLE TABLETS
Adults. 5 mg every 2 to 3 hr, as needed (dinitrate).
E.R. CAPSULES
Adults. 40 to 80 mg every 8 to 12 hr (dinitrate).
E.R. TABLETS
Adults. 20 to 80 mg every 8 to 12 hr (dinitrate); 30 to 60 mg daily, increased gradually as tolerated to 120 mg daily (mononitrate).
S.L. TABLETS
Adults. 2.5 to 5 mg every 2 to 3 hr, as needed (dinitrate).
TABLETS
Adults. 5 to 40 mg every 6 hr, adjusted as needed (dinitrate); 20 mg in 2 doses given 7 hr apart (mononitrate).

Route	Onset	Peak	Duration
P.O.*	1 hr†	Unknown	5–6 hr
P.O. (chewable)*	In 3 min	Unknown	30 min–2 hr
P.O. (E.R.)*	30 min	Unknown	6–8 hr
P.O. (S.L.)*	In 3 min	Unknown	2 hr

Contraindications
Angle-closure glaucoma; cerebral hemorrhage; concurrent use of phosphodiesterase inhibitors (sildenafil, tadalafil, vardenafil) or riociguat; head trauma; hypersensitivity to isosorbide, other nitrates, or their components; orthostatic hypotension; severe anemia

Interaction
DRUGS
acetylcholine, norepinephrine: Possibly decreased effectiveness of these drugs
antihypertensives, calcium channel blockers, opioid analgesics, other vasodilators: Increased risk of orthostatic hypotension
aspirin: Increased blood level and pharmacologic action of isosorbide
other vasodilators: Additive effects
phosphodiesterase inhibitors such as sildenafil, tadalafil, vardenafil: Increased risk of hypotension, myocardial ischemia, syncope, and possibly death
riociguat: Increased risk of hypotension
sympathomimetics: Increased risk of hypotension, possibly decreased therapeutic effects of isosorbide
ACTIVITIES
alcohol use: Increased risk of orthostatic hypotension

Adverse Reactions
CNS: Agitation, confusion, dizziness, headache, insomnia, restlessness, syncope, vertigo, weakness
CV: Arrhythmias, orthostatic hypotension, palpitations, peripheral edema, tachycardia
EENT: Blurred vision, diplopia (all forms); sublingual burning (S.L. form)
GI: Abdominal pain, diarrhea, indigestion, nausea, vomiting
GU: Dysuria, impotence, urinary frequency
HEME: Hemolytic anemia
MS: Arthralgia, muscle twitching
RESP: Bronchitis, pneumonia, upper respiratory tract infection
SKIN: Diaphoresis, flushing, rash

Nursing Considerations
• Use isosorbide cautiously in patients with hypovolemia or mild hypotension. Monitor patient for increased hypotension and reduced cardiac output.
• Give drug 1 hour before or 2 hours after meals. Give with meals if patient experiences severe headaches or adverse GI reactions.
• Know that patient may experience daily headaches from isosorbide's vasodilating effects. Give acetaminophen, as prescribed, to relieve pain.
• ***WARNING*** Be aware that stopping drug abruptly may cause angina and increase the risk of MI.
• Monitor blood pressure often during isosorbide therapy, especially in elderly patients; drug may cause severe hypotension.
• Keep isosorbide protected from heat and light.
PATIENT TEACHING
• Teach patient and family to recognize signs and symptoms of angina, including chest

G
H
I

Mechanism of Action
Isosorbide may interact with nitrate receptors in vascular smooth-muscle cell membranes. By interacting with receptors' sulfhydryl groups, drug is reduced to nitric oxide. Nitric oxide activates the enzyme guanylate cyclase, increasing intracellular formation of cyclic guanosine monophosphate (cGMP). An increased cGMP level may relax vascular smooth muscle by forcing calcium out of muscle cells, causing vasodilation. This improves cardiac output by reducing mainly preload but also afterload.

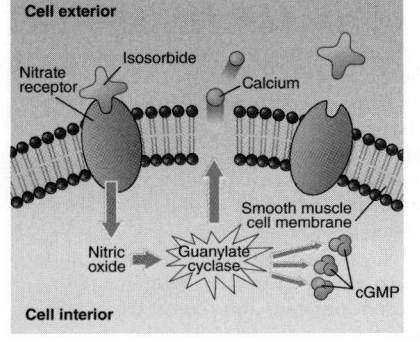

* For dinitrate.
† For mononitrate, onset also is 1 hr; peak and duration are unknown.

pain, fullness, or pressure, which commonly is accompanied by sweating and nausea. Pain may radiate down the left arm or into the neck or jaw. Inform female patients and those with diabetes mellitus or hypertension that they may experience only fatigue and shortness of breath.

• Caution patient not to crush or chew isosorbide E.R. capsules or tablets or S.L. tablets unless specifically ordered to do so by prescriber.

• Instruct patient to place S.L. tablet under tongue and not to swallow it, but to let it dissolve. Explain that moisture in mouth promotes drug absorption and that tingling or burning in the mouth indicates drug effectiveness.

• Advise patient to chew chewable tablets well and to keep them in his mouth for 1 to 2 minutes before swallowing to enhance drug absorption.

• Instruct patient to take drug before any situation or activity that might precipitate angina.

• Advise patient to carry isosorbide with him at all times.

• Caution patient that abrupt drug discontinuation may cause angina and increase the risk of MI.

• Instruct patient to notify prescriber about blurred vision, fainting, increased angina attacks, rash, and severe or persistent headaches.

• Teach patient to reduce the effects of orthostatic hypotension by changing position slowly. Advise him to lie down if he becomes dizzy.

• Inform patient that drug commonly causes headache, which typically resolves after a few days of continuous therapy. Suggest that patient take acetaminophen as needed and as prescribed.

• Advise patient to avoid potentially hazardous activities until drug's CNS effects are known.

• Urge patient to avoid alcohol consumption.

• Instruct patient to store drug in a tightly closed container and protect from light and heat.

• Advise male patient with erectile dysfunction to alert prescriber that he is taking isosorbide because sildenafil, tadalafil, and vardenafil can cause fatal reactions when taken with isosorbide.

isotretinoin

Absorica, Accutane, Claravis

Class and Category

Chemical class: Retinoid
Therapeutic class: Acne inhibitor
Pregnancy category: X

Indications and Dosages

➤ *To treat severe recalcitrant nodular acne unresponsive to conventional therapy*

CAPSULES

Adults. *Initial:* 0.5 mg to 1 mg/kg daily in 2 divided doses, increased as needed up to 2 mg/kg daily given in 2 divided doses. *Maximum:* 2 mg/kg daily. Course of therapy given for 15 to 20 wk with second course given, as needed, after a period of 2 mo or more off therapy.

Mechanism of Action

Inhibits sebaceous gland function and keratinization, which results in diminished nodular formation associated with recalcitrant nodular acne.

Contraindications

Hypersensitivity to isotretinoin or any of its components, hypersensitivity to parabens, pregnancy

Interaction

DRUGS

corticosteroids (systemic): Possibly increased risk of osteoporosis
hormonal contraceptives including microdosed progesterone preparations, medroxyprogesterone injection, levonorgestrel implants: Possibly decreased effectiveness of contraceptive
phenytoin: Possibly increased risk of osteomalacia
tetracyclines: Increased risk of benign intracranial hypertension
vitamin A supplements: Increased risk of additive toxic effects

Adverse Reactions

CNS: Aggressive or violent behavior, depression, dizziness, drowsiness, emotional instability, fatigue, headache, insomnia, lethargy, malaise, nervousness,

paresthesias, pseudotumor cerebri, psychosis, seizures, stroke, suicidal ideation, syncope, weakness
CV: Chest pain, decreased high-density lipoprotein level, edema, elevated creatinine phosphokinase level, hypercholesteremia, hypertriglyceridemia, palpitation, stroke, tachycardia, vascular thrombotic disease, vasculitis
ENDO: Abnormal menses, alterations in blood glucose levels
EENT: Bleeding and inflammation of gums, cataracts, color vision disorder, conjunctivitis, corneal opacities, decreased night vision, dry mouth or nose, dry eyes, epistaxis, eyelid inflammation, hearing impairment, keratitis, optic neuritis, photophobia, tinnitus, visual disturbances, voice alteration
GI: Colitis, hepatitis, ileitis, inflammatory bowel disease, liver enzyme elevation, nausea, pancreatitis
GU: Glomerulonephritis, hematuria, proteinuria, WBCs in urine
HEME: Anemia, agranulocytosis, neutropenia, platelet count elevation, sedimentation rate elevation, thrombo-cytopenia
MS: Arthralgia, arthritis, back pain (children), bone abnormalities, calcification of tendons and ligaments, premature epiphyseal closure, tendonitis
RESP: Bronchospasms, respiratory infection
SKIN: Alopecia, bruising, disseminated herpes simplex, dry lips or skin, eczema, eruptive xanthomas, erythema multiforme, facial erythema, flushing, fulminant acne, hair abnormalities, hirsutism, hyperpigmentation, hypopigmentation, increased sunburn susceptibility, infections, nail dystrophy, paronychia, peeling of palms and soles, photoallergic or photosensitizing reactions, pruritus, pyogenic granuloma, rash, seborrhea, skin fragility, Stevens-Johnson syndrome, sweating, toxic epidermal necrolysis, urticaria
Other: Abnormal wound healing, alkaline phosphatase increase, allergic reactions, hyperuricemia, lymphadenopathy, weight loss

Nursing Considerations

• Ensure that women of childbearing age have had two negative urine or serum

pregnancy tests with a sensitivity of at least 50 mIU/ml, joined the Accutane Survey, signed the consent form, and watched the videotape provided by manufacturer prior to beginning isotretinoin therapy.

WARNING Notify prescriber if elevated serum triglyceride levels can't be controlled or if symptoms of pancreatitis occur (abdominal pain, nausea, vomiting). Drug may need to be discontinued because fatal hemorrhagic pancreatitis has occurred with drug use.

• Obtain serum lipid level before therapy and periodically thereafter, as ordered, to detect elevated lipid levels that result from isotretinoin therapy.

• Monitor liver enzyme levels periodically, as ordered, because drug can cause hepatitis.

• Assess patient frequently for adverse reactions and report to prescriber any that occur; drug may have serious adverse effects that require discontinuation.

PATIENT TEACHING

• Instruct patient to take isotretinoin with food or milk.

• Advise women of childbearing age that two forms of contraceptives must be used simultaneously (unless absolute abstinence is the chosen method) 1 month before therapy and for 1 month after therapy has stopped because of potential for fetal harm. Inform women who use oral contraceptives that drug may lessen effectiveness of oral contraceptives. Urge patient to notify prescriber immediately if pregnancy occurs.

• Emphasize importance of picking up isotretinoin prescription within 7 days of a pregnancy test or, for male patients or women not of childbearing potential, within 30 days of prescription.

• Urge patient to report headache, nausea, vomiting and visual disturbances immediately to prescriber because drug will need to be discontinued immediately and patient referred to a neurologist.

• Caution patient and family that isotretinoin may cause aggressive or violent behavior, depression, psychosis, and suicidal ideation. Instruct patient to notify prescriber immediately if changes in mood occur.

G
H
I

• Tell patient to report hearing changes or tinnitus, visual difficulties, skin reactions, abdominal pain, rectal bleeding, or severe diarrhea to prescriber because drug may need to be discontinued.
• Advise patient to avoid hazardous activities until drug's CNS effects are known. Caution that changes in night vision may occur suddenly.
• Caution patient not to donate blood during therapy and for 1 month after therapy has stopped because blood might be given to a pregnant woman.
• Warn patient that transient exacerbation of acne may occur, especially during initial therapy and to notify prescriber if this occurs.
• Instruct patient to avoid wax epilation and skin resurfacing procedures during therapy and for at least 6 months thereafter because of scarring potential.
• Caution patient to avoid exposure to direct sunlight or UV light and to wear sunscreen when outdoors.
• Inform patient that contact lens tolerance may decrease during and after isotretinoin therapy.
• Alert patient to the potential for mild musculoskeletal adverse reactions, which usually clear rapidly after drug is discontinued. Urge patient to notify prescriber if symptoms become bothersome or serious because drug may need to be discontinued.
• Advise patient not to take vitamin A supplements while on isotretinoin therapy because of potentially additive toxic effects.
• Instruct patient to notify all prescribers of isotretinoin use because of the risk of interactions.
• Inform patient of need for frequent laboratory tests and importance of complying with scheduled appointments.

---

isradipine
DynaCirc

Class and Category
Chemical class: Dihydropyridine derivative
Therapeutic class: Antihypertensive
Pregnancy category: C

Indications and Dosages
➤ *To manage essential hypertension*
CAPSULES
Adults. *Initial:* 2.5 mg twice daily, increased by 5 mg every 2 to 4 wk, as needed. *Maximum:* 20 mg daily.

Mechanism of Action
Inhibits calcium movement into coronary vascular smooth-muscle cells by blocking the slow calcium channels in their membranes. By decreasing intracellular calcium level, isradipine inhibits smooth-muscle cell contractions. The result is relaxation of coronary and vascular smooth muscle, decreased peripheral vascular resistance, and reduced systolic and diastolic blood pressure, all of which decrease myocardial oxygen demand.

Route	Onset	Peak	Duration
P.O.	2–3 hr	2–4 wk	Unknown

Contraindications
Hypersensitivity to isradipine or its components

Interaction
DRUGS
anesthetics (hydrocarbon inhalation), antihypertensives, hydrochlorothiazide, prazocin: Increased risk of hypotension
beta blockers: Increased adverse effects of beta blockers
cimetidine: Increased blood level and bioavailability of isradipine
digoxin: Transiently increased blood digoxin level and risk of digitalis toxicity
estrogens: Possibly increased fluid retention and decreased isradipine effects
lithium: Increased risk of neurotoxicity
NSAIDs, sympathomimetics: Possibly decreased therapeutic effects of isradipine
procainamide, quinidine: Increased risk of prolonged QT interval
FOODS
grapefruit juice: Doubled isradipine bioavailability
other foods: Prolonged time to achieve peak blood level

Adverse Reactions
CNS: Asthenia, dizziness, fatigue, headache, paresthesia, somnolence, stroke, syncope, transient ischemic attack, weakness

CV: Angina, atrial fibrillation, heart failure, hypotension, MI, orthostatic hypotension, palpitations, peripheral edema, tachycardia, ventricular fibrillation
EENT: Gingival hyperplasia, pharyngitis, rhinitis
GI: Abdominal cramps, constipation, diarrhea, elevated liver function test results, indigestion, nausea, vomiting
HEME: Leukopenia
MS: Back pain
RESP: Cough
SKIN: Flushing, photosensitivity, rash, urticaria
Other: Angioedema

Nursing Considerations
• Monitor blood pressure and heart rate often during isradipine therapy.
• Monitor patient with impaired hepatic or renal function for an increased blood isradipine level.
• Avoid giving isradipine with food because doing so increases time to peak effect by about 1 hour.
• Observe for mild peripheral edema caused by vasodilation of small blood vessels. Know that this type of edema doesn't result from fluid retention or heart failure.
PATIENT TEACHING
• Inform patient that isradipine therapy will be long-term and will require laboratory tests and follow-up visits to monitor drug effects.
• Instruct patient to take drug exactly as prescribed and to swallow capsules whole, not crushing or chewing them.
• Advise patient to take drug on an empty stomach 1 hour before or 2 hours after meals.
• Instruct patient to take a missed dose as soon as he remembers it unless it's nearly time for the next dose. In that case, advise him to wait and take next scheduled dose, but not to double the dose. If more than one dose is missed, tell him to contact prescriber.
WARNING Urge patient not to stop taking drug suddenly. Doing so may lead to life-threatening problems.
• Inform patient that fragments of capsules may be visible in stool.
• Caution patient not to drink grapefruit juice during isradipine therapy.

• Urge patient to avoid potentially hazardous activities until isradipine's CNS effects are known.
• Caution patient to change position slowly to minimize orthostatic hypotension.
• Urge patient to contact prescriber if he experiences chest pain, fainting, irregular heartbeat, rash, or swollen ankles while taking isradipine.
• Instruct patient to maintain good oral hygiene, perform gum massage, and see a dentist every 6 months to prevent gum bleeding and gum disorders.
• To help prevent photosensitivity reactions, caution patient to avoid direct sunlight and to wear protective clothing and apply sunscreen when outdoors.
• Instruct patient to store drug at room temperature in a dry place.

itraconazole
Sporanox

Class and Category
Chemical class: Triazole derivative
Therapeutic class: Antifungal
Pregnancy category: C

Indications and Dosages
➤ *To treat blastomycosis caused by* Blastomyces dermatitidis *and* histoplasmosis *caused by* Histoplasma capsulatum
CAPSULES
Adults and adolescents. *Initial:* 200 mg daily, increased by 100 mg daily, as needed. *Maximum:* 400 mg daily, with dosage greater than 200 mg given in divided doses twice daily.
➤ *To treat aspergillosis unresponsive to amphotericin B*
CAPSULES
Adults and adolescents. 200 to 400 mg daily, with dosage greater than 200 mg daily given in divided doses twice daily.
➤ *To treat oropharyngeal candidiasis*
ORAL SOLUTION
Adults and adolescents. 100 mg twice daily for 7 to 14 days.
➤ *To treat esophageal candidiasis*

ORAL SOLUTION

Adults and adolescents. 100 mg daily for at least 3 wk and continued for 2 wk after symptoms resolve.

➤ *To treat onychomycosis of toenails only or of toenails and fingernails*

CAPSULES

Adults and adolescents. 200 mg daily for 12 wk.

➤ *To treat onychomycosis of fingernails only*

CAPSULES

Adults and adolescents. 200 mg twice daily for 7 days; then repeated after 3 wk.

Mechanism of Action

Inhibits the synthesis of ergosterol, an essential component of fungal cell membranes, by binding with a cytochrome P-450 enzyme needed to convert lanosterol to ergosterol. Lack of ergosterol results in increased cellular permeability and leakage of cell contents. Itraconazole also may lead to fungal cell death by inhibiting fungal respiration under aerobic conditions.

Contraindications

Concurrent therapy with cisapride, colchicine (presence of renal or hepatic impairment), disopyramide, dofetilide, dronedarone, eplerenone, ergot alkaloids, felodipine, HMG-CoA inhibitors (lovastatin and simvastatin), irinotecan, levomethadyl, lurasidone, methadone, nisoldipine, oral midazolam, pimozide, quinidine, ranolazine, or triazolam; evidence of ventricular dysfunction, as in congestive heart failure (CHF) or a history of it (onychomycosis treatment); hypersensitivity to itraconazole or its components; pregnancy or contemplating pregnancy during onychomycosis treatment

Interaction

DRUGS

alfentanil, budesonide, buspirone, busulfan, carbamazepine, cyclosporine, dexamethasone, digoxin, docetaxel, felodipine, fluticasone, indinavir, methylprednisolone, phenytoin, pimozide, rifabutin, ritonavir, saquinavir, sirolimus, tacrolimus, trimetrexate, vinca alkaloids: Possibly increased blood levels of these drugs and serious adverse effects

alprazolam, diazepam, oral midazolam, triazolam: Elevated blood levels and possibly prolonged sedative effects of these drugs

antacids, anticholinergics, H_2-receptor antagonists, proton pump inhibitors, sucralfate: Possibly decreased itraconazole absorption

atorvastatin, lovastatin, simvastatin: Increased blood levels of these drugs; possibly rhabdomyolysis

calcium channel blockers: Possibly edema and increased risk of CHF; increased blood levels of these drugs

carbamazepine, isoniazid, nevirapine, phenobarbital, phenytoin, rifabutin, rifampin: Possibly decreased blood itraconazole level

cilostazol; eletriptan; glucocorticosteroids such as budesonide, dexamethasone, fluticasone, and methylprednisolone; trimetrexate: Possibly inhibited metabolism of these drugs

cisapride, colchicine (presence of renal or hepatic impairment), dofetilide, dronedarone, eplerenone, ergot alkaloids, felodipine, halofantrine, irinotecan, levomethadyl, lovastatin, lurasidone, methadone, midazolam (oral), nisoldipine, pimozide, quinidine, ranolazine, simvastatin, triazolam: Possibly increased plasma levels of these drugs leading to potentially life-threatening cardiovascular complications such as cardiac arrest, prolonged QT interval, torsades de pointes, ventricular tachycardia, and sudden death

clarithromycin, erythromycin, indinavir, ritonavir: Possibly increased blood itraconazole level

didanosine: Possibly decreased therapeutic effects of itraconazole

ergot alkaloids: Possibly increased plasma ergot alkaloid elevation, leading to cerebral ischemia and ischemia of the extremities

fentanyl: Possibly increased plasma fentanyl level, causing potentially fatal respiratory depression

nisoldipine: Increased plasma nisoldipine levels that do not decrease after drug dosage is reduced

oral antidiabetic drugs: Possibly increased blood levels of these drugs and risk of hypoglycemia *warfarin:* Increased anticoagulant effect of warfarin

Adverse Reactions

CNS: Chills, confusion, dizziness, drowsiness, fatigue, fever, headache, hypoesthesia, paresthesia, peripheral neuropathy, vertigo
CV: Cardiac failure, chest pain, CHF, hypertriglyceridemia, hypertension, hypotension, left ventricular failure, peripheral edema, tachycardia
EENT: Altered sense of taste, blurred vision, diplopia, dysphonia, transient or permanent hearing loss, tinnitis
ENDO: Hyperglycemia
GI: Abdominal pain, anorexia, constipation, diarrhea, elevated liver function test results, flatulence, hepatic failure, hepatitis, hepatotoxicity, hyperbilirubinemia, indigestion, jaundice, nausea, pancreatitis, vomiting
GU: Erectile dysfunction, menstrual irregularities, pollakiuria, renal impairment, urinary incontinence
HEME: Leukopenia, neutropenia, thrombocytopenia
MS: Arthralgia, myalgia
RESP: Cough, dyspnea, pulmonary edema
SKIN: Acute generalized exanthematous pustulosis, alopecia, diaphoresis, erythema multiforme, exfoliative dermatitis, leukocytoclastic vasculitis, photosensitivity, pruritus, rash, Stevens-Johnson syndrome, toxic epidermal necrolysis, urticaria
Other: Anaphylaxis, angioedema, hyperkalemia, hypokalemia, hypomagnesemia, serum sickness

Nursing Considerations

• Use itraconazole with extreme caution in patients with risk factors for CHF, such as ischemic or valvular heart disease, significant COPD, and renal failure and other edematous disorders because of increased risk of developing CHF during itraconazole treatment.
• Use itraconazole cautiously in patients with hypersensitivity to other azole antifungals (because cross-hypersensitivity is unknown) and in patients with renal or hepatic impairment.
• Because itraconazole has been linked to serious adverse cardiac and hepatic effects, expect to send appropriate nail specimens

for laboratory testing to confirm onychomycosis before beginning therapy.
WARNING Keep in mind that itraconazole is a potent inhibitor of the cytochrome P-450 3A4 (CYP3A4) isoenzyme system, which may increase blood levels of drugs metabolized by this system. Patients taking such drugs as cisapride with itraconazole or other CYP3A4 inhibitors have experienced life-threatening cardiovascular complications, such as prolonged QT interval, torsades de pointes, and ventricular tachycardia, as well as sudden death.
• Administer itraconazole capsules (not oral solution) with a meal to ensure maximal absorption.
• Know that capsules and oral solution forms are not interchangeable because drug exposure is greater with oral solution.
• Keep in mind that a patient with AIDS may have hypochlorhydria, which reduces drug absorption. For such a patient, expect to administer higher doses of itraconazole.
• Monitor liver function test results in patients with impaired hepatic function and those who have experienced hepatotoxicity with other drugs.
• If patient develops signs and symptoms of peripheral neuropathy or CHF, such as fatigue, dyspnea, and peripheral edema, expect to discontinue drug.
• Assess patient for rash every 8 hours during therapy; notify prescriber if rash occurs.
• If patient also receives warfarin, monitor PT and assess patient for signs and symptoms of bleeding.
• If patient also receives digoxin, monitor blood digoxin level as appropriate to detect toxic level, and assess patient for signs and symptoms of digitalis toxicity, such as nausea and yellow vision.

PATIENT TEACHING
• Instruct patient to take itraconazole capsules with a meal and to swallow capsules whole, but oral solution without food.
• If patient also takes an oral antidiabetic drug, instruct him to check his blood glucose level often because of the increased risk of hypoglycemia.

G
H
I

- Advise patient to avoid taking antacids with oral itraconazole.
- Advise patient to notify prescriber immediately of changes in other drugs, such as new drugs and dosage changes.
- Advise patient to notify prescriber immediately about abdominal pain, diarrhea, headache, hearing loss, nausea, peripheral neuropathy, or vomiting.
- Instruct patient to stop itraconazole and notify prescriber immediately if he experiences an allergic reaction such as a skin rash, itching hives, shortness of breath or difficulty breathing, and/or swelling of his face.
- Tell him to stop itraconazole and notify prescriber immediately if he develops shortness of breath; has unusual swelling in his feet, ankles or legs; suddenly gains weight; is unusually tired; coughs up white or pink phlegm, has an unusual fast heartbeat; or begins to wake up at night.
- Instruct patient to notify prescriber if he experiences signs of liver problems, such as abdominal pain, dark urine, fatigue, loss of appetite, pale stools, weakness, or yellow eyes or skin.
- Caution patient to avoid performing hazardous activities such as driving until CNS effects such as dizziness or change in vision are not present.
- Caution breastfeeding patient to consult prescriber about continuation of breast-feeding during itraconazole therapy.

JKL

kanamycin sulfate

Kantrex

Class and Category

Chemical class: Aminoglycoside
Therapeutic class: Antibiotic
Pregnancy category: D

Indications and Dosages

➤ *To treat infections caused by gram-negative organisms (including* Acinetobacter *species,* Enterobacter aerogenes, Escherichia coli, Haemophilus influenzae, Klebsiella pneumoniae, Neisseria *species,* Proteus *species,* Providencia *species,* Salmonella *species,* Serratia marcescens, Shigella *species, and* Yersinia *species) and gram-positive organisms (including* Staphylococcus aureus *and* Staphylococcus epidermidis)

I.M. INJECTION

Adults and children. 3.75 mg/kg every 6 hr, 5 mg/kg every 8 hr, or 7.5 mg/kg every 12 hr for 7 to 10 days. *Maximum:* 1.5 g daily.

I.V. INFUSION

Adults and children. 5 mg/kg every 8 hr or 7.5 mg/kg every 12 hr for 7 to 10 days. *Maximum:* 1.5 g daily.

➤ *As adjunct to suppress intestinal bacterial growth*

CAPSULES

Adults. 1 g/hr for 4 hr and then 1 g every 6 hr for 36 to 72 hr.

➤ *To treat hepatic coma*

CAPSULES

Adults. 8 to 12 g daily in divided doses.

➤ *To treat respiratory tract infection*

INHALATION NEBULIZER

Adults. 250 mg twice daily to four times daily *Maximum:* 1.5 g daily.

DOSAGE ADJUSTMENT For elderly patients and those with renal failure, dosage reduced and blood kanamycin level and renal function test results monitored.

Mechanism of Action

Binds to negatively charged sites on bacterial outer cell membranes, which disrupts cell membrane integrity. Kanamycin also binds to bacterial ribosomal subunits and inhibits protein synthesis; these actions lead to cell death.

Route	Onset	Peak	Duration
P.O.	Slow	Unknown	Unknown
I.V.	Rapid	Unknown	Unknown
I.M.	Unknown	1–2 hr	Unknown

Incompatibilities

Don't mix kanamycin in same syringe or administer through same I.V. line as other antibiotics.

Contraindications

Hypersensitivity to kanamycin, other aminoglycosides, or their components; intestinal obstruction (oral form)

Interactions

DRUGS

cephalosporins, vancomycin: Increased risk of nephrotoxicity
digoxin, loop diuretics: Increased ototoxic and nephrotoxic effects of kanamycin
general anesthetics, neuromuscular blockers: Increased risk of neuromuscular blockade
penicillins: Inactivation of kanamycin or synergistic effects

Adverse Reactions

CNS: Ataxia, dizziness, headache
EENT: Hearing loss
GI: Diarrhea
GU: Elevated BUN and serum creatinine levels, oliguria, proteinuria
MS: Muscle paralysis
RESP: Apnea
SKIN: Injection-site irritation or pain

Nursing Considerations

• Obtain body fluid or tissue specimen for culture and sensitivity testing before kanamycin therapy begins, as indicated. Therapy may begin before test results are available.
• Administer I.M. injection deep into upper outer quadrant of gluteus maximus. Rotate injection sites.
• Be aware that oral kanamycin is minimally absorbed from intact GI mucosa but may

J
K
L

be more absorbed from mechanically irrigated areas of the GI tract.
- For I.V. use, dilute 500-mg vial with 100 to 200 ml normal saline solution or D_5W, or 1-g vial with 200 to 400 ml normal saline solution or D_5W, and infuse over 30 to 60 min. Vial contents may darken during storage but potency isn't affected.
- Keep patient well hydrated before and during therapy.
- Monitor blood kanamycin level periodically during therapy, as appropriate.
- Prolonged treatment increases risk of ototoxicity and nephrotoxicity. Monitor hearing and renal function if therapy lasts longer than 10 days.

PATIENT TEACHING
- Explain need to take kanamycin at prescribed intervals around the clock until patient completes full course of therapy.
- Advise patient to report dizziness, hearing loss, and severe diarrhea or headache.

ketoprofen
Actron, Apo-Keto (CAN), Orudis, Orudis KT, Orudis-SR (CAN), Oruvail, Rhodis

Class and Category
Chemical class: Propionic acid derivative
Therapeutic class: Analgesic, anti-inflammatory
Pregnancy category: B

Indications and Dosages
➤ *To treat symptoms of rheumatoid arthritis*
CAPSULES, TABLETS
Adults. *Initial:* 75 mg three times daily or 50 mg four times daily. *Maximum:* 300 mg daily.
E.R. CAPSULES
Adults. *Maintenance:* 150 to 200 mg daily. *Maximum:* 300 mg daily.
➤ *To relieve pain in dysmenorrhea*
TABLETS
Adults. *Initial:* 25 to 50 mg every 6 to 8 hr as needed. *Maximum:* 300 mg daily.
DOSAGE ADJUSTMENT Dosage reduced by 33% to 50% for patients with renal impairment.

Mechanism of Action
Blocks activity of cyclooxygenase, the enzyme needed for prostaglandin synthesis. Prostaglandins, important mediators of inflammatory response, cause local vasodilation with swelling and pain. By blocking cyclooxygenase and inhibiting prostaglandins, this NSAID reduces inflammatory symptoms and relieves pain.

Contraindications
Angioedema; aspirin-, iodide-, or NSAID-induced asthma, bronchospasm, nasal polyps, rhinitis, or urticaria; hypersensitivity to ketoprofen or its components

Interactions
DRUGS
ACE inhibitors: Possibly decreased hypotensive effect of ACE inhibitors
acetaminophen: Possibly increased adverse renal effects with long-term acetaminophen use
aspirin, other NSAIDs: Increased risk of bleeding and adverse GI effects, increased and prolonged blood ketoprofen levels
cefamandole, cefoperazone, cefotetan: Increased risk of hypoprothrombinemia and bleeding
colchicine, platelet aggregation inhibitors: Increased risk of GI bleeding, hemorrhage, and ulcers
corticosteroids, potassium supplements: Increased risk of adverse GI effects
cyclosporine: Increased risk of nephrotoxicity from both drugs, increased blood cyclosporine level
diuretics (loop, potassium-sparing, and thiazide): Decreased diuretic and antihypertensive effects
gold compounds, nephrotoxic drugs: Increased risk of adverse renal effects
heparin, oral anticoagulants, thrombolytics: Increased anticoagulant effects, increased risk of hemorrhage
insulin, oral antidiabetic drugs: Possibly increased hypoglycemic effects of these drugs
lithium: Increased blood lithium level and possibly toxicity
methotrexate: Decreased methotrexate clearance, increased risk of methotrexate toxicity

plicamycin, valproic acid: Increased risk of hypoprothrombinemia and GI bleeding, hemorrhage, and ulcers
probenecid: Possibly increased blood level, effectiveness, and risk of toxicity of ketoprofen
ACTIVITIES
alcohol use: Increased risk of adverse GI effects

Adverse Reactions

CNS: Headache, irritability, nervousness, seizures, stroke
CV: Edema, fluid retention, hypertension, MI, tachycardia
EENT: Tinnitus, vision changes
GI: Abdominal pain, anorexia, constipation, diarrhea, diverticulitis, dyspepsia, dysphagia, flatulence, gastritis, gastroenteritis, gastroesophageal reflux disease, GI bleeding and ulceration, hepatic failure, hiatal hernia, indigestion, melena, nausea, perforation of stomach or intestine, stomatitis, vomiting
GU: Acute renal failure, decreased urine output
HEME: Agranulocytosis, anemia, easy bruising, hemolytic anemia, leukopenia, neutropenia, pancytopenia, thrombocytopenia
RESP: Asthma, respiratory depression
SKIN: Erythema multiforme, Stevens-Johnson syndrome, toxic epidermal necrolysis, rash
Other: Anaphylaxis, angioedema, rapid weight gain

Nursing Considerations

• Use ketoprofen with extreme caution in patients with history of ulcer disease or GI bleeding because NSAIDs such as ketoprofen increase risk of GI bleeding and ulceration. Expect to use ketoprofen for shortest time possible in these patients.
• Be aware that serious GI tract ulceration, bleeding, and perforation may occur without warning symptoms. Elderly patients are at greater risk. To minimize risk, give drug with food. If GI distress occurs, withhold drug and notify prescriber immediately.
• Use ketoprofen cautiously in patients with hypertension, and monitor blood pressure closely throughout therapy. Drug may cause hypertension or worsen it.

WARNING Monitor patient closely for thrombotic events, including MI and stroke, because NSAIDs increase the risk.
• Monitor patient—especially if he's elderly or receiving long-term ketoprofen therapy—for less common but serious adverse GI reactions, including anorexia, constipation, diverticulitis, dysphagia, esophagitis, gastritis, gastroenteritis, gastroesophageal reflux disease, hemorrhoids, hiatal hernia, melena, stomatitis, and vomiting.
• Monitor liver function test results because, rarely, elevations may progress to severe hepatic reactions, including fatal hepatitis, liver necrosis, and hepatic failure.
• Monitor BUN and serum creatinine levels in elderly patients, patients taking diuretics or ACE inhibitors, and patients with heart failure, impaired renal function, or hepatic dysfunction; drug may cause renal failure.
• Monitor CBC for decreased hemoglobin level and hematocrit because drug may worsen anemia.

WARNING If patient has bone marrow suppression or is receiving an antineoplastic drug, monitor laboratory results (including WBC count), and watch for evidence of infection because antiinflammatory and antipyretic actions of ketoprofen may mask signs and symptoms, such as fever and pain.
• Assess patient's skin regularly for signs of rash or other hypersensitivity reaction because ketoprofen is an NSAID and may cause serious skin reactions without warning, even in patients with no history of NSAID sensitivity. At first sign of reaction, stop drug and notify prescriber.
• If patient takes acetaminophen, monitor fluid intake and output, BUN level, and serum creatinine level for evidence of adverse renal effects.

PATIENT TEACHING
• Instruct patient to take ketoprofen with food or after meals to prevent GI upset. Advise him to take drug with a full glass of water and to avoid lying down for 15 to 30 minutes afterward to prevent drug from lodging in esophagus and causing irritation.

J
K
L

- Advise patient to swallow drug whole and not to crush, break, chew, or open capsules.
- Instruct patient to avoid aspirin, aspirin-containing products, and alcohol while taking ketoprofen to decrease risk of adverse GI effects.
- Tell patient not to take more drug than prescribed because stomach bleeding may occur.
- If patient takes an anticoagulant, tell him to watch for and immediately report bleeding problems, such as bloody or tarry stools and bloody vomitus.
- If patient takes insulin or an oral anti-diabetic, advise him to monitor blood glucose level closely. Urge him to carry candy or other simple sugars to treat mild hypoglycemia. If he has frequent or severe episodes, instruct him to consult prescriber.
- Inform patient that he may be nervous and irritable while taking ketoprofen.
- Instruct patient to notify prescriber immediately if he develops a rash, decreased urine output, dark yellow or brown urine, or signs of fluid retention, including swelling of extremities and unexplained rapid weight gain.
- Caution pregnant patient not to take NSAIDs such as ketoprofen during last trimester because they may cause premature closure of the ductus arteriosus.
- Explain that ketoprofen may increase risk of serious adverse cardiovascular reactions; urge patient to seek immediate medical attention if signs or symptoms arise, such as chest pain, shortness of breath, weakness, and slurring of speech.
- Explain that ketoprofen may increase risk of serious adverse GI reactions; emphasize importance of seeking immediate medical attention for such signs and symptoms as epigastric or abdominal pain, indigestion, black or tarry stools, or vomiting blood or material that looks like coffee grounds.
- Alert patient to rare but serious skin reactions. Urge him to seek immediate medical attention for rash, blisters, itching, fever, or other indications of hypersensitivity.

ketorolac tromethamine

Sprix, Toradol

Class and Category
Chemical class: Acetic acid derivative
Therapeutic class: Analgesic, anti-inflammatory
Pregnancy category: C

Indications and Dosages
➤ *To treat moderate to severe pain*
TABLETS
Adults ages 16 to 64. *Initial:* 20 mg as single dose, followed by 10 mg every 4 to 6 hr as needed, up to 4 times a day. *Maximum:* 40 mg daily for no more than 5 days.
DOSAGE ADJUSTMENT For patients weighing less than 50 kg, elderly patients, and patients with impaired renal function, initial dose reduced to 10 mg.
NASAL SPRAY (SPRIX)
Adults less than 65 years of age. 15.75 mg (1 spray) in each nostril every 6 to 8 hr. *Maximum:* 126 mg (four doses) daily for no more than 5 days.
Adults 65 years of age and older, adults weighing less than 50 kg (110 lb). 15.75 mg in only one nostril every 6 to 8 hr. *Maximum:* 63 mg (four doses) daily for no more than 5 days.
I.M. INJECTION
Adults ages 16 to 64. *Initial:* 60 mg as single dose, followed by oral ketorolac if needed; or 30 mg every 6 hr as needed. *Maximum:* 120 mg daily for no more than 5 days.
DOSAGE ADJUSTMENT For patients weighing less than 50 kg, elderly patients, and patients with impaired renal function, initial dose reduced to 30 mg, followed by oral ketorolac if needed; or 15 mg every 6 hr as needed, up to maximum of 60 mg daily for no more than 5 days.
I.V. INJECTION
Adults ages 16 to 64. *Initial:* 30 mg as single dose, followed by oral ketorolac if needed; or 30 mg every 6 hr as needed. *Maximum:* 120 mg daily for no more than 5 days.
DOSAGE ADJUSTMENT For patients weighing less than 50 kg, elderly patients,

and patients with impaired renal function, initial dose reduced to 15 mg, followed by oral ketorolac if needed; or 15 mg every 6 hr as needed, up to maximum of 60 mg daily for no more than 5 days.

Route	Onset	Peak	Duration
P.O.	30–60 min	2–3 hr	5–6 hr
I.M., I.V.	30–60 min	1–2 hr	4–6 hr

Mechanism of Action

Blocks cyclooxygenase, an enzyme needed to synthesize prostaglandins. Prostaglandins mediate inflammatory response and cause local vasodilation, swelling, and pain. They also promote pain transmission from periphery to spinal cord. By blocking cyclooxygenase and inhibiting prostaglandins, this NSAID reduces inflammation and relieves pain.

Contraindications

Advanced renal impairment or risk of renal impairment due to volume depletion; before or during surgery if hemostasis is critical; breastfeeding; cerebrovascular bleeding; concurrent use of aspirin or other salicylates, other NSAIDs, or probenecid; hemorrhagic diathesis; history of GI bleeding, GI perforation, or peptic ulcer disease; hemophilia or other bleeding problems, including coagulation or platelet function disorders; hypersensitivity to ketorolac tromethamine, aspirin, other NSAIDs, or their components; incomplete hemostasis; labor and delivery; treatment of perioperative pain during coronary artery bypass graft surgery

Interactions

DRUGS

ACE inhibitors, angiotensin II receptor antagonists: Increased risk of renal impairment; decreased effectiveness of these drugs

acetaminophen, gold compounds: Increased risk of adverse renal effects

amphotericin, penicillamine, and other nephrotoxic drugs: Increased risk or severity of adverse renal reactions

antihypertensives, diuretics: Possibly reduced effects of these drugs

aspirin and other salicylates, other NSAIDs: Additive toxicity

cefamandole, cefoperazone, cefotetan: Possibly hypoprothrombinemia

corticosteroids, potassium supplements: Increased risk of gastric ulcers or hemorrhage

furosemide: Decreased effects of furosemide

heparin, oral anticoagulants, platelet aggregation inhibitors, thrombolytics: Increased risk of GI bleeding and I.M. hematoma formation

lithium: Possibly increased blood lithium level and increased risk of lithium toxicity

methotrexate: Possibly methotrexate toxicity

nondepolarizing muscle relaxants: Increased risk of apnea

pentoxifylline, selective serotonin reuptake inhibitors: Increased risk of bleeding

plicamycin, valproic acid: Possibly hypoprothrombinemia and increased risk of bleeding

probenecid: Decreased elimination of ketorolac, increased risk of adverse effects

ACTIVITIES

alcohol use: Increased risk of adverse GI effects

Adverse Reactions

CNS: Aseptic meningitis, cerebral hemorrhage, coma, dizziness, drowsiness, headache, psychosis, seizures, stroke

CV: Edema, fluid retention, hypertension

EENT: Laryngeal edema, stomatitis

ENDO: Hyperglycemia

GI: Abdominal pain; acute pancreatitis; bloating; constipation; diarrhea; diverticulitis; flatulence; GI bleeding, perforation, or ulceration; hepatitis; hepatic failure; jaundice; indigestion; nausea; perforation of stomach or intestines; vomiting; worsening of inflammatory bowel disease

GU: Interstitial nephritis, renal failure, urine retention

HEME: Agranulocytosis, anemia, aplastic or hemolytic anemia, eosinophilia, leukopenia, lymphadenopathy, pancytopenia, thrombocytopenia

RESP: Bronchospasm, pneumonia, respiratory depression

SKIN: Diaphoresis, erythema multiforme, exfoliative dermatitis, photosensitivity, pruritus, rash, Stevens-Johnson syndrome, toxic epidermal necrolysis, urticaria

Other: Anaphylaxis, angioedema, hyperkalemia, hyponatremia, injection-site pain, sepsis, unusual weight gain

Nursing Considerations

• Read ketorolac label carefully. Don't use I.M. form for I.V. route. Know that ketorolac isn't for intrathecal or epidural use.
• Inject I.M. ketorolac slowly, deep into a large muscle mass. Monitor site for bleeding, bruising, or hematoma.
• Give I.V. injection over at least 15 seconds.
• Notify prescriber if pain relief is inadequate or if breakthrough pain occurs between doses because supplemental doses of an opioid analgesic may be required.

WARNING Monitor liver function test results. If elevated levels persist or worsen, notify prescriber and expect to stop drug, as ordered, to prevent hepatic impairment.

WARNING Monitor patients with a history of peripheral edema, heart failure, or hypertension for adequate fluid balance because drug can promote fluid retention and worsen these conditions. Assess patient for dyspnea, edema, unexplained rapid weight gain, and decreased activity tolerance. Notify prescriber if such symptoms develop.
• Use ketorolac with extreme caution in patients with history of ulcer disease or GI bleeding because NSAIDs like ketorolac increase risk of GI bleeding and ulceration. Use ketorolac in these patients for shortest length of time possible.
• Serious GI tract ulceration and bleeding and perforation of stomach or intestine can occur without warning or symptoms. Elderly patients are at greater risk. To minimize risk, give drug with food. If GI distress occurs, withhold drug and notify prescriber immediately.
• Monitor patient with history of inflammatory bowel disease, such as ulcerative colitis or Crohn's disease, because ketorolac may worsen these conditions.
• Use ketorolac cautiously in patients with hypertension, and monitor blood pressure closely throughout therapy because drug can lead to onset of hypertension or worsen existing hypertension.

WARNING Monitor patient closely for thrombotic events including MI and stroke because NSAIDs such as ketorolac increase risk.
• Monitor patient—especially if elderly—for less common but serious adverse GI reactions, including anorexia, constipation, diverticulitis, dysphagia, esophagitis, gastritis, gastroenteritis, gastroesophageal reflux disease, hemorrhoids, hiatal hernia, melena, stomatitis, and vomiting.
• Monitor liver function test results because rarely, elevations may progress to severe hepatic reactions, including fatal hepatitis, liver necrosis, and hepatic failure.
• Monitor BUN and serum creatinine levels in patients with heart failure, impaired renal function, or hepatic dysfunction; those who are taking diuretics or ACE inhibitors; and the elderly because drug may cause renal failure.
• Monitor CBC for decreased hemoglobin and hematocrit because drug may worsen anemia.

WARNING In patient who has bone marrow suppression or is receiving antineoplastic drug therapy, monitor laboratory results (including WBC) and assess for evidence of infection because ketorolac has anti-inflammatory and antipyretic actions that may mask signs and symptoms, such as fever and pain.
• Assess patient's skin routinely for rash or other evidence of hypersensitivity reactions because ketorolac is an NSAID and may cause serious skin reactions without warning, even in patients with no history of NSAID hypersensitivity. Stop drug at first sign of reaction, and notify prescriber.

PATIENT TEACHING

• Instruct patient to take ketorolac tablets with a meal, a snack, or an antacid to prevent stomach upset. Advise him to take drug with a full glass of water and to stay upright for at least 15 minutes afterward.
• Teach patient how to prime bottle and administer nasal spray form, if prescribed. Remind patient nasal spray form is not to be inhaled. Tell patient not to use any single nasal spray bottle for more than

1 day, as it will not deliver the intended dose after 24 hours.

- Advise patient not to take aspirin, other salicylates, or other NSAIDs while taking ketorolac without consulting prescriber. Urge patient to limit use of acetaminophen to only a few days during ketorolac therapy and to notify prescriber of use.
- Caution patient not to use ketorolac for more than 5 days, as serious adverse effects may occur.
- Instruct him to immediately report blood in urine, easy bruising, itching, rash, swelling, or yellow eyes or skin.
- Caution pregnant patient that NSAIDs like ketorolac shouldn't be taken during last trimester because drug may cause premature closure of the ductus arteriosus.
- Explain that ketorolac may increase risk of serious adverse cardiovascular reactions; urge patient to seek immediate medical attention if signs or symptoms arise, such as chest pain, shortness of breath, weakness, and slurring of speech.
- Tell patient that ketorolac also may increase risk of serious adverse GI reactions; stress importance of seeking immediate medical attention if signs or symptoms occur, such as epigastric or abdominal pain, indigestion, black tarry stools, and vomiting blood or coffee ground material.
- Alert patient to the possibility of serious skin reactions, although rare, occurring with ketorolac therapy. Urge patient to seek immediate medical attention if signs or symptoms occur, such as a rash, blisters, fever, or other signs of hypersensitivity, such as itching.
- Caution patient to avoid hazardous activities until drug's CNS effects are known.
- Urge patient to avoid alcohol while taking ketorolac.
- Encourage patient to have dental procedures performed before starting drug therapy because of increased risk of bleeding.
- Teach patient proper oral hygiene measures, and encourage him to use a soft-bristled toothbrush while taking ketorolac.

labetalol hydrochloride

Normodyne, Trandate

Class and Category
Chemical class: Benzamine derivative
Therapeutic class: Antihypertensive
Pregnancy category: C

Indications and Dosages
➤ *To manage hypertension*
TABLETS
Adults. *Initial:* 100 mg twice daily, increased by 100 mg twice daily as needed and tolerated every 2 to 3 days. *Maintenance:* 200 to 400 mg twice daily. For severe hypertension, 1.2 to 2.4 g daily in divided doses twice daily or three times daily.
➤ *To manage severe hypertension and treat hypertensive emergencies*
I.V. INFUSION
Adults. 200 mg diluted in 160 ml of D_5W and infused at 2 mg/min until desired response occurs.
I.V. INJECTION
Adults. 20 mg given over 2 min; additional doses given in increments of 40 to 80 mg every 10 min as indicated until desired response occurs. *Maximum:* 300 mg.

Route	Onset	Peak	Duration
P.O.	20 min–2 hr	1–4 hr	8–24 hr
I.V.	2–5 min	5–15 min	2–4 hr

Mechanism of Action
Selectively blocks $alpha_1$ and $beta_2$ receptors in vascular smooth muscle and $beta_1$ receptors in heart to reduce peripheral vascular resistance and blood pressure. Potent beta blockade prevents reflex tachycardia, which commonly occurs when alpha blockers reduce resting heart rate, cardiac output, or stroke volume.

Incompatibilities
Don't dilute labetalol in sodium bicarbonate solution or give through same I.V. line as alkaline drugs, such as furosemide; doing so may cause white precipitate to form.

Contraindications

Asthma, cardiogenic shock, heart failure, hypersensitivity to labetalol or its components, second-or third-degree heart block, severe bradycardia

Interactions

DRUGS

allergen immunotherapy, allergenic extracts for skin testing: Increased risk of serious systemic reaction or anaphylaxis
beta blockers, digoxin: Increased risk of bradycardia
calcium channel blockers, clonidine, diazoxide, guanabenz, reserpine: Possibly hypotension
cimetidine: Possibly increased labetalol effects
estrogens, NSAIDs: Possibly reduced antihypertensive effect of labetalol
general anesthetics: Increased risk of hypotension and myocardial depression
insulin, oral antidiabetic drugs: Increased risk of hyperglycemia
nitroglycerin: Possibly hypertension
phenoxybenzamine, phentolamine: Possibly additive alpha$_1$-blocking effects
sympathomimetics with alpha- and beta-adrenergic effects (such as pseudoephedrine): Possibly hypertension, excessive brady-cardia, or heart block
xanthines (aminophylline and theophylline): Possibly decreased therapeutic effects of both drugs

FOODS
all food: Increased blood labetalol level
ACTIVITIES
alcohol use: Increased labetalol effects

Adverse Reactions

CNS: Anxiety, confusion, depression, dizziness, drowsiness, fatigue, paresthesia, syncope, vertigo, weakness, yawning
CV: Bradycardia, chest pain, edema, heart block, heart failure, hypotension, orthostatic hypotension, ventricular arrhythmias
EENT: Nasal congestion, taste perversion
GI: Elevated liver function test results, hepatic necrosis, hepatitis, indigestion, nausea, vomiting
GU: Ejaculation failure, impotence
RESP: Dyspnea, wheezing
SKIN: Jaundice, pruritus, rash, scalp tingling

Nursing Considerations

• During I.V. labetalol use, monitor blood pressure according to facility policy, usually every 5 minutes for 30 minutes, then every 30 minutes for 2 hours, and then every hour for 6 hours.
• Keep patient in supine position for 3 hours after I.V. administration.
WARNING Be aware that labetalol masks common signs of shock.
• Monitor blood glucose level in diabetic patient because labetalol may conceal symptoms of hypoglycemia.
• Be aware that stopping labetalol tablets abruptly after long-term therapy could result in angina, MI, or ventricular arrhythmias. Expect to taper dosage over 2 weeks while monitoring response.
PATIENT TEACHING
• Advise patient to report confusion, difficulty breathing, rash, slow pulse, and swelling in arms or legs.
• Caution patient not to stop drug abruptly because doing so could cause angina and rebound hypertension.
• Suggest that patient minimize effects of orthostatic hypotension by rising slowly, avoiding sudden position changes, and taking labetalol at bedtime, if approved by prescriber.
• Instruct diabetic patient to check blood glucose level often and to be alert for signs and symptoms of hypoglycemia.
• Inform patient that scalp tingling may occur early in treatment but is transient.
• Urge patient to avoid alcohol during labetalol therapy.
• Advise patient to inform eye healthcare provider if he needs cataract surgery because intraoperative floppy iris syndrome has occurred during cataract surgery in some patients treated with the class of drugs of which labetalol is a member.

lacosamide

Vimpat

Class and Category

Chemical class: Functionalized amino acid
Therapeutic class: Anticonvulsant
Pregnancy category: C

Indications and Dosages

➤ *To treat partial-onset seizures*
ORAL SOLUTION, TABLETS
Adults and adolescents age 17 and over.
100 mg twice daily, increased by 50 mg twice daily every week to recommended maintenance dose. Alternatively, 200 mg given as single loading dose, followed 12 hr later by 100 mg twice daily for 1 week. Dosage increased at weekly intervals by 50 mg twice daily, as needed, up to recommended maintenance dose. *Maintenance:* 300 to 400 mg daily.
I.V. INFUSION
Adults and adolescents age 17 and over.
Initial: 100 mg infused over 30 to 60 min twice daily for 1 week. Dosage increased by 50 mg/day at weekly intervals. Alternatively, 200 mg given as single loading dose infused over 30 to 60 min, followed 12 hr later by 100 mg infused over 30 to 60 min twice daily for 1 week. Dosage increased at weekly intervals by 50 mg twice daily, as needed, up to recommended maintenance dose. *Maintenance:* 300 to 400 mg daily.
➤ *As adjunct to treat partial-onset seizures in patients with epilepsy*
ORAL SOLUTION, TABLETS
Adults and adolescents age 17 and over.
Initial: 50 mg twice daily, increased by 100 mg/ day at weekly intervals based on response and tolerance. Alternatively, 200 mg given as single loading dose, followed 12 hr later by 100 mg twice daily for 1 week. Dosage increased at weekly intervals by 50 mg twice daily, as needed, up to recommended maintenance dose. *Maintenance:* 200 to 400 mg daily.
I.V. INFUSION
Adults and adolescents age 17 and over.
Initial: 50 mg infused over 30 to 60 min twice daily, increased by 100 mg/day at weekly intervals. *Maintenance:* 200 to 400 mg daily.

DOSAGE ADJUSTMENT For patients with mild to moderate hepatic impairment or severe renal impairment (creatinine clearance of 30 ml/min/1.73 m^2 or less) including end-stage renal disease, maximum dosage is 300 mg daily. Following a 4-hour hemodialysis treatment, dosage supplementation of up to 50% may be required. For patients with renal or hepatic impairment taking strong CYP3A4 or CYP2C9 inhibitors concurrently, dosage may need to be reduced.

Mechanism of Action

May selectively inactivate voltage-gated sodium channels, which prevents seizure activity by stabilizing hyperexcitable neuronal membranes and inhibiting repetitive neuronal firing in the brain.

Contraindications

Hypersensitivity to lacosamide and its components

Interactions

DRUGS
CYP3A4 inhibitors, CYP2C9 inhibitors (in presence of renal or hepatic impairment): Possibly significant increase in lacosamide exposure and adverse effects
drugs that may prolong the QT interval: Possibly further QT-interval prolongation

Adverse Reactions

CNS: Aggression, agitation, asthenia, ataxia, attention deficit, cerebellar syndrome, confusion, depression, dizziness, feeling drunk, fever, hallucinations, headache, hypoaesthesia, impaired balance, insomnia, irritability, memory impairment, mood alteration, paresthesia, psychotic disorder, somnolence, suicidal ideation, tremor, vertigo
CV: Atrial fibrillation or flutter, AV block, bradycardia, palpitations, prolonged QT interval
EENT: Blurred vision, diplopia, dry mouth, nystagmus, oral hypoaesthesia, tinnitus
GI: Constipation, diarrhea, dyspepsia, nausea, vomiting
HEME: Agranulocytosis, anemia, neutropenia
MS: Dysarthria, muscle spasms
SKIN: Pruritus, rash, Stevens-Johnson syndrome, toxic epidermal necrolysis, urticaria
Other: Angioedema, delayed multi-organ hypersensitivity reaction; injection-site pain, irritation, and erythema

Nursing Considerations

• Use cautiously in patients with conduction problems (such as AV block, sick sinus syndrome and no pacemaker in place), sodium channelopathies such as Brugada Syndrome, severe cardiac disease (such as myocardial ischemia, heart failure), or concomitant drug therapy with drugs that prolong the PR interval because lacosamide may affect conduction. For

J
K
L

these patients, ensure an ECG has been done, as ordered, prior to starting therapy and after dosage titration.

• Use cautiously in patients with diabetic neuropathy or cardiovascular disease because drug may predispose them to atrial fibrillation or flutter.

• In patients who are already taking a single antiepileptic and being converted to lacosamide monotherapy, the maintenance dose of lacosamide should be maintained for at least 3 days before beginning the withdrawal of the concomitant antiepileptic drug, as ordered. A gradual withdrawal of the concomitant antiepileptic drug over at least 6 weeks is recommended.

• Administer drug intravenously without further dilution or know that it may be mixed with diluents such as 0.9% sodium chloride injection, 5% dextrose injection, or lactated Ringer's injection. If diluted, do not store diluted solution for more than 4 hours at room temperature.

• Watch patient closely for suicidal tendencies, particularly when therapy starts and dosage changes, because depression may worsen temporarily during these times and lead to suicidal ideation.

• Be aware that lacosamide therapy should be discontinued gradually over at least 1 week to minimize seizure frequency.

• Monitor patient closely for hypersensitivity reactions to lacosamide, such as rash, pruritus, and more than one organ abnormality, such as elevated liver enzymes and myocarditis or pancreatitis.

PATIENT TEACHING
• Tell patient that lacosamide tablet or oral solution may be taken with or without food. If using oral solution, remind patient to measure and administer the dose using a calibrated measuring device because a household teaspoon or tablespoon may not deliver correct dose.

• Urge family or caregiver to watch patient closely for suicidal tendencies, especially when therapy starts or dosage changes.

• Caution patient to avoid hazardous activities until drug's CNS effects are known.

• Encourage patient to carry medical identification that indicates her diagnosis and drug therapy.

lactulose

Acilac (CAN), Cephulac, Cholac, Chronulac, Constilac, Constulose, Duphalac, Enulose, Evalose, Heptalac, Lactulax (CAN), Laxilose (CAN), PMS-Lactulose (CAN), Portalac

Class and Category
Chemical: Synthetic disaccharide sugar
Therapeutic: Ammonia reducer, laxative
Pregnancy category: B

Indications and Dosages
➤ *To treat constipation*
POWDER, SYRUP
Adults. *Initial:* 10 to 20 g daily, increased as needed. *Maximum:* 40 g daily.
➤ *To prevent and treat hepatic encephalopathy*
POWDER, SYRUP
Adults. *Initial:* 20 to 30 g three times daily or four times daily until two or three soft stools occur daily. *Usual:* 60 to 100 g daily in divided doses. For acute episodes, 20 to 30 g every 2 hr initially to achieve rapid laxative effect and then reduced to usual dosage.
RETENTION ENEMA
Adults. 200 g (300 ml) diluted in 700 ml water or normal saline solution and given every 4 to 6 hr, as needed.

Mechanism of Action
Arrives unchanged in the colon, where it breaks down into lactic acid and small amounts of formic and acetic acids, acidifying fecal contents. Acidification leads to increased osmotic pressure in the colon, which, in turn, increases stool water content and softens stool.

Also, lactulose makes intestinal contents more acidic than blood. This prevents ammonia diffusion from intestine into blood, as occurs in hepatic encephalopathy. The trapped ammonia is converted into ammonia ions and, by lactulose's cathartic effect, is expelled in feces with other nitrogenous wastes.

Route	Onset	Peak	Duration
P.O.	24–48 hr	Unknown	Unknown

Contraindications
Hypersensitivity to lactulose or its components, low-galactose diet

Interactions

DRUGS

antacids, antibiotics (especially oral neomycin), other laxatives: Decreased effectiveness of lactulose

Adverse Reactions

GI: Abdominal cramps and distention, diarrhea, flatulence
ENDO: Hyperglycemia
Other: Hypernatremia, hypokalemia, hypovolemia

Nursing Considerations

• When giving lactulose by retention enema, use a rectal tube with a balloon to help patient retain enema for 30 to 60 minutes. If not retained for at least 30 minutes, repeat dose. Be sure to deflate balloon and remove rectal tube after completing administration.
• Expect to periodically check serum electrolyte levels of elderly or debilitated patient who uses oral drug longer than 6 months.
• Monitor blood ammonia level in patient with hepatic encephalopathy. Also watch for dehydration, hypernatremia, and hypokalemia when giving higher lactulose doses to treat this condition.
• Monitor diabetic patient for hyperglycemia because lactulose contains galactose and lactose.
• Plan to replace fluids if frequent bowel movements cause hypovolemia.

PATIENT TEACHING

• Advise patient to take lactulose with food or dilute with juice to reduce sweet taste.
• Direct patient not to use other laxatives while taking lactulose.
• Instruct patient to report abdominal distention or severe diarrhea.
• Advise diabetic patient to check blood glucose level often and to report hyperglycemia.
• Instruct patient to increase fluid intake if frequent bowel movements occur.
• Teach patient with chronic constipation the importance of exercising, increasing fiber in diet, and increasing fluid intake.
• Inform patient that because oral lactulose must reach the colon to work, bowel movement may not occur for 24 to 48 hours after taking drug.

lamotrigine

Lamictal, Lamictal XR

Class and Category

Chemical class: Phenyltriazine
Therapeutic class: Anticonvulsant
Pregnancy category: C

Indications and Dosages

➤ *As adjunct to treat partial seizures; to treat generalized seizures of Lennox-Gastaut syndrome; to treat primary generalized tonic-clonic seizures*

CHEWABLE TABLETS, ORALLY DISINTEGRATING TABLETS, TABLETS

Adults and children age 12 and over taking valproate. 25 mg every other day for 2 wk, followed by 25 mg once daily for 2 wk. Increased by 25 to 50 mg every 1 to 2 wk, if needed. *Maintenance:* 100 to 400 mg daily.
Children ages 2 to 12 taking valproate. 0.15 mg/kg daily as a single dose or in divided doses twice daily for 2 wk and then 0.3 mg/kg daily as single dose or in divided doses twice daily for next 2 wk. Increased by 0.3 mg/kg every 1 to 2 wk, if needed, to reach maintenance dosage. *Maintenance:* 1 to 5 mg/kg daily as single dose or in divided doses twice daily. *Maximum:* 200 mg daily.
Adults and children age 12 and over taking an antiepileptic drug other than carbamazepine, phenytoin, phenobarbital, primidone, or valproate. 25 mg once daily for 2 wk, followed by 50 mg once daily for 2 wk. Increased by 50 mg every 1 to 2 wk, if needed. *Maintenance:* 225 to 375 mg daily in 2 divided doses. *Maximum:* 400 mg daily.
Children ages 2 to 12 taking an an antiepileptic drug other than carbamazepine, phenytoin, phenobarbital, primidone, or valproate. 0.3 mg/kg daily in 1 or 2 divided doses for 2 wk; followed by 0.6 mg/kg daily in 2 divided doses for 2 wk. Increased by 0.6 mg/kg daily every 1 to 2 wk, if needed. *Maintenance:* 4.5 to 7.5 mg/kg daily in 2 divided doses. *Maximum:* 300 mg daily.
Adults and children age 12 and over taking carbamazepine, phenytoin, phenobarbital, or primidone but NOT valproate. 50 mg once daily for 2 wk and then 100 mg daily in 2 divided doses for 2 wk. Increased by

100 mg every 1 to 2 wk, if needed. *Maintenance:* 300 to 500 mg daily in 2 divided doses *Maximum:* 700 mg daily in 2 divided doses.

Children ages 2 to 12 taking carbamazepine, phenytoin, phenobarbital, or primidone but NOT valproate. 0.6 mg/kg daily in 2 divided doses for 2 wk and then 1.2 mg/kg daily in 2 divided doses for 2 wk. Increased by 1.2 mg/kg every 1 to 2 wk, if needed to reach maintenance dosage. *Maintenance:* 5 to 15 mg/kg daily in 2 divided doses *Maximum:* 400 mg daily.

➤ *To treat partial seizures with conversion from carbamazepine, phenytoin, phenobarbital, primidone, or valproate*

CHEWABLE TABLETS, ORALLY DISINTEGRATING TABLETS, TABLETS

Adults and adolescents age 16 and over converting from carbamazepine, phenytoin, phenobarbital, or primidone. 50 mg once daily for 2 wk, followed by 50 mg twice daily for next 2 wk. Increased by 100 mg daily every 1 to 2 wk (while continuing to take carbamazepine, phenytoin, phenobarbital, or primidone), until usual maintenance dosage—300 mg to 500 mg daily in 2 divided doses is achieved. Then carbamazepine, phenytoin, phenobarbital, or primidone dosage tapered in 20% decrements weekly over 4 wk and then discontinued.

Adults and adolescents age 16 and over converting from valproate. 25 mg every other day for 2 wk followed by 25 mg once daily for 2 wk. Then increased by 25 to 50 mg daily every 1 to 2 wk until maintenance dosage of 200 mg daily is achieved. (At this time valproate dosage decreased to 500 mg daily by decrements no greater than 500 mg daily every wk and then maintained at 500 mg daily for 1 wk). After valproate dosage has been at 500 mg for one week, lamotrigine dosage increased to 300 mg daily while valproate dosage decreased to 250 mg daily for 1 wk. Then lamotrigine dosage increased by 100 mg daily every wk until maintenance dose of 500 mg daily is reached (given in two divided doses). Valproate therapy is then discontinued.

E.R. TABLETS

Adults and adolescents age 13 and over converting from carbamazepine, phenytoin, phenobarbital, or primidone. 50 mg once daily for first 2 wk, then increased as follows: 100 mg once daily for wk 3 and 4, then 200 mg once daily for wk 5, then 300 mg once daily for wk 6, then 400 mg once daily for wk 7 and 500 mg for wk 8. Once maintenance dosage of 500 mg daily has been reached, carbamazepine, phenytoin, phenobarbital, or primidone dosage tapered in 20% decrements weekly over 4 wk and then discontinued. Two weeks after carbamazepine, phenytoin, phenobarbital, or primidone has been discontinued, lamotrigine dosage decreased no faster than 100 mg/day each week until monotherapy maintenance dosage of 250 mg to 300 mg daily has been reached.

Adults and adolescents age 13 and over converting from valproate. 25 mg every other day for 2 wk, then increased as follows: 25 mg once daily for wk 3 and 4, then 50 mg once daily for wk 5, then 100 mg once daily for wk 6, then 150 mg once daily for wk 7, and 200 mg once daily for wk 8, with dosage increased to 250 mg once daily, if needed, for wk 9. Once lamotrigine dosage has reached 150 mg once daily, valproate dosage decreased by decrements no greater than 500 mg/wk to 500 mg/day and then maintained for 1 wk, followed by dosage decrease to 250 mg/day for 1 wk and then discontinued.

➤ *To treat partial seizures with conversion from a single antiepileptic drug other than carbamazepine, phenytoin, phenobarbital, primidone, or valproate*

E.R. TABLETS

Adults and adolescents age 13 and over converting from an antiepileptic drug other than carbamazepine, phenytoin, phenobarbital, primidone, or valproate. 25 mg once daily for 2 wk, followed by 50 mg once daily for next 2 wk. Increased to 100 mg once daily for wk 5 followed by 150 mg once daily for wk 6, followed by 200 mg once daily for wk 7. Further increased by 100 mg once daily at weekly intervals beginning at week 8 and onward until usual maintenance dosage—300 to 400 mg daily—is reached. Once dosage has reached 250 mg to 300 mg once daily, antiepileptic drug tapered in 20% decrements weekly over 4 wk and then discontinued.

➤ *As adjunct to treat primary generalized tonic-clonic seizures and partial-onset seizures*

E.R. TABLETS

Adults and children age 13 and over taking valproate. 25 mg every other day for 2 wk, followed by 25 mg once daily for 2 wk, followed by 50 mg once daily for 1 wk. Then 100 mg once daily for 1 wk, then 150 mg once daily. Dosage increased further, as needed, but increase not greater than 100 mg weekly. *Maintenance:* 200 to 250 mg once daily.

Adults and children age 13 and over NOT taking carbamazepine, phenytoin, phenobarbital, primidone, or valproate. 25 mg once daily for 2 wk, followed by 50 mg once daily for 2 wk, followed by 100 mg once daily for 1 wk. Then 150 mg once daily for 1 wk, followed by 200 mg once daily. Dosage increased further, as needed, but increase not greater than 100 mg weekly. *Maintenance:* 300 to 400 mg once daily.

Adults and children age 13 and over taking carbamazepine, phenytoin, phenobarbital, or primidone and NOT taking valproate. 50 mg once daily for 2 wk, followed by 100 mg once daily for 2 wk, followed by 200 mg once daily for 1 wk. Then 300 mg once daily for 1 wk, followed by 400 mg once daily. Dosage increased further, as needed, but increase not greater than 100 mg weekly. *Maintenance:* 400 to 600 mg once daily.

DOSAGE ADJUSTMENT For women taking estrogen-containing oral contraceptives, maintenance dose may need to be increased gradually by as much as twofold over recommended target maintenance dose. For women discontinuing estrogen-containing oral contraceptives who have been stabilized on lamotrigine prior to discontinuation, maintenance dose may need to be decreased gradually by as much as half. For patient with moderate to severe hepatic impairment without ascites, all dosages decreased by 25%, and for patient with severe hepatic impairment with ascites, all dosages decreased by 50%. For patient with significant renal impairment, maintenance dosage may need to be reduced on individual basis.

➤ *As maintenance therapy for bipolar 1 disorder to delay occurrence of mood episodes (depression, mania, hypomania, mixed episodes)*

CHEWABLE TABLETS, ORALLY DISINTEGRATING TABLETS, TABLETS

Adults not taking carbamazepine, phenytoin, phenobarbital, primidone, rifampin, or valproate. 25 mg once daily for 2 wk, followed by 50 mg once daily for 2 wk, followed by 100 mg once daily for 1 wk, and then increased to 200 mg once daily as maintenance dose. Maximum: 200 mg daily.

Adults taking valproate. 25 mg every other day for 2 wk, followed by 25 mg once daily for 2 wk, followed by 50 mg once daily for 1 wk, and then increased to 100 mg once daily as maintenance dose.

Adults taking carbamazepine, phenytoin, phenobarbital, primidone, or rifampin, but not valproate. 50 mg once daily for 2 wk, followed by 100 mg once daily in divided doses for 2 wk, followed by 200 mg once daily in divided doses for 1 wk, then increased to 300 mg daily in divided doses for 1 wk, and then increased to 400 mg daily in divided doses as maintenance dose.

DOSAGE ADJUSTMENT For patient starting or stopping estrogen-containing oral contraceptives, lamotrigine dosage may need to be adjusted on individual basis. For patient with moderate to severe liver impairment without ascites, dosage reduced by 25%. For patient with severe liver impairment with ascites, dosage reduced by 50%.

Mechanism of Action

May stabilize neuron membranes by blocking their sodium channels and inhibiting release of excitatory neurotransmitters, such as glutamate and aspartate, through these channels. By blocking the release of neurotransmitters, lamotrigine inhibits the spread of seizure activity in the brain and reduces seizure frequency.

Route	Onset	Peak	Duration
P.O.	Days to wks	Unknown	Unknown

Contraindications

Hypersensitivity to lamotrigine or its components

Interactions
DRUGS

acetaminophen (long-term use): Possibly decreased blood lamotrigine level
atazanavir/ritonavir, lopinavir/ritonavir, rifampin: Decreased blood lamotrigine level
carbamazepine: Decreased blood lamotrigine level; possibly increased risk of dizziness, diplopia, ataxia, and blurred vision folate inhibitors, such as cotrimoxazole and methotrexate: Increased blood lamotrigine level
oral contraceptives: Decreased blood lamotrigine level during 3 weeks of active hormonal therapy and increased blood lamotrigine level during 1 week of inactive hormonal therapy; possibly reduced effectiveness of oral contraceptives
oxcarbazepine: Possibly increased risk of headache, dizziness, nausea, and somnolence
phenobarbital, phenytoin, primidone: Decreased blood lamotrigine level, possibly increased CNS depression
topiramate: Increased topiramate level
valproic acid: Increased lamotrigine level
ACTIVITIES
alcohol use: Possibly increased CNS depression

Adverse Reactions

CNS: Amnesia, anxiety, aseptic meningitis, ataxia, confusion, depression, dizziness, drowsiness, emotional lability, exacerbation of parkinsonian symptoms, fever, headache, increased seizure activity, lack of coordination, suicidal ideation
CV: Chest pain, vasculitis
EENT: Blurred vision, diplopia, dry mouth, nystagmus
GI: Abdominal pain, anorexia, constipation, diarrhea, esophagitis, hepatic failure, pancreatitis, vomiting
HEME: Agranulocytosis, anemia, aplastic or hemolytic anemia, disseminated intravascular coagulation, eosinophilia, leukopenia, neutropenia, pancytopenia, pure red cell aplasia, thrombocytopenia
MS: Rhabdomyolysis
RESP: Apnea
SKIN: Drug reaction with eosinophilia and systemic symptoms (DRESS), petechiae, photosensitivity, pruritus, rash, Stevens-Johnson syndrome, toxic epidermal necrolysis
Other: Angioedema, flulike symptoms, lupus-like reaction, lymphadenopathy, progressive immunosuppression

Nursing Considerations

• Use cautiously in patients with illnesses that could affect metabolism or elimination of lamotrigine, such as renal, hepatic, or cardiac functional impairment.
• Be aware that the patient may be converted directly from immediate-release lamotrigine to extended-release lamotrigine with the initial dose of extended-release matching the total daily dose of immediate-release lamotrigine. However, monitor effects closely, especially for patient who is receiving an enzyme-inducing agent that may lower plasma levels of lamotrigine on conversion. If drug effectiveness appears to be altered, notify prescriber and expect a dosage adjustment.
WARNING Lamotrigine may cause potentially life-threatening rash. Notify prescriber at first sign, and expect to discontinue drug. Lamotrigine therapy shouldn't be restarted after rash subsides.
• Monitor patient for adverse reactions, especially suicidal thoughts, at start of therapy and with each dosage increase.
WARNING Monitor patient for hypersensitivity, such as fever, rash, or lymphadenopathy in association with other organ system dysfunction that may be suggestive of DRESS. Although rare, DRESS may be life-threatening. If suspected, notify prescriber immediately and expect lamotrigine to be discontinued.
WARNING Monitor patient closely for signs and symptoms of aseptic meningitis such as headache, fever, nausea, vomiting, and nuchal rigidity. Additional signs and symptoms may include rash, photophobia, myalgia, chills, altered consciousness, and somnolence. These symptoms may occur within 1 day to 1.5 months following the

initiation of lamotrigine therapy. Notify prescriber immediately, if suspected, and expect drug to be discontinued.
• Monitor patient for seizure activity during lamotrigine therapy.
• Stopping lamotrigine abruptly may increase seizure activity. Expect to taper dosage over at least 2 weeks, even for treatment of bipolar disorder.

PATIENT TEACHING
• Advise patient to take lamotrigine exactly as prescribed and not to stop abruptly because seizure activity may increase.
• Instruct patient to seek immediate emergency help or call local poison control center if too much lamotrigine is taken.
• Advise patient to notify prescriber immediately if rash or other symptoms of hypersensitivity, such as a fever or swollen glands, occur.
• Instruct patient to report increased seizure activity, vision changes, and vomiting.
• Caution patient to avoid hazardous activities until drug's CNS effects are known.
• Advise patient to avoid direct sunlight and to wear protective clothing to minimize risk of photosensitivity.
• Instruct patient to wear or carry medical identification stating that she takes an anticonvulsant.
• Caution patient or caregiver about possibility of suicidal thoughts, especially when therapy begins or dosage changes.
WARNING Advise patient to notify prescriber immediately if she develops any combination of a headache, fever, nausea, vomiting, stiff neck, rash, abnormal sensitivity to light, myalgia, chills, confusion, or drowsiness while taking lamotrigine.
• Tell female patient to notify prescriber if she becomes pregnant, is considering pregnancy, or starts or stops an oral hormonal contraceptive or other female hormonal preparation.
• Urge woman who becomes pregnant while taking lamotrigine to enroll in the North American antiepileptic drug pregnancy registry by calling 1-888-233-2334. Explain that registry is collecting information about safety of antiepileptic drugs during pregnancy.

lansoprazole
Prevacid, Prevacid I.V., Prevacid SoluTab

dexlansoprazole
Dexilant

Class and Category
Chemical class: Substituted benzimidazole
Therapeutic class: Antisecretory, antiulcer
Pregnancy category: B

Indications and Dosages
➤ *To treat duodenal ulcers and maintain healed duodenal ulcers*
DELAYED-RELEASE CAPSULES, DELAYED-RELEASE SUSPENSION, DELAYED-RELEASE ORALLY DISINTEGRATING TABLETS
Adults. 15 to 30 mg daily before morning meal for 4 wk. *Maximum:* 30 mg daily.
➤ *To treat gastric ulcers*
DELAYED-RELEASE CAPSULES, DELAYED-RELEASE SUSPENSION, DELAYED-RELEASE ORALLY DISINTEGRATING TABLETS
Adults. 15 to 30 mg daily before morning meal for up to 8 wk.
➤ *To treat gastroesophageal reflux disease*
DELAYED-RELEASE CAPSULES, DELAYED-RELEASE SUSPENSION, DELAYED-RELEASE ORALLY DISINTEGRATING TABLETS
Adults. 15 mg daily before morning meal for up to 8 wk.
➤ *To treat nonerosive gastroesophageal reflux disease*
CAPSULES (DEXLANSOPRAZOLE)
Adults. 30 mg once daily for 4 wk.
➤ *To heal all grades of erosive esophagitis*
CAPSULES (DEXLANSOPRAZOLE)
Adults. 60 mg once daily for up to 8 wk.
➤ *To maintain healed erosive esophagitis*
CAPSULES (DEXLANSOPRAZOLE)
Adults. 30 mg once daily.
➤ *To treat erosive esophagitis*
DELAYED-RELEASE CAPSULES, DELAYED-RELEASE SUSPENSION, DELAYED-RELEASE ORALLY DISINTEGRATING TABLETS
Adults. *Initial:* 30 mg daily before morning meal for up to 8 wk. Continued another 8 wk if indicated. *Maintenance:* 15 mg daily.
➤ *To treat erosive esophagitis short-term (up to 7 days) in patients unable to take oral medication*

I.V. INFUSION
Adults. 30 mg daily infused over 30 min for up to 7 days.
➤ *To treat pathological hypersecretory conditions, such as Zollinger-Ellison syndrome*
DELAYED-RELEASE CAPSULES, DELAYED-RELEASE SUSPENSION, DELAYED-RELEASE ORALLY DISINTEGRATING TABLETS
Adults. *Initial:* 60 mg daily before morning meal, increased as needed according to patient's condition. Doses exceeding 120 mg/day administered in divided doses. *Maximum:* 180 mg daily.
➤ *To eradicate* Helicobacter pylori *and reduce risk of duodenal ulcer recurrence*
DELAYED-RELEASE CAPSULES, DELAYED-RELEASE SUSPENSION, DELAYED-RELEASE ORALLY DISINTEGRATING TABLETS
Adults. 30 mg plus 1 g amoxicillin and 500 mg clarithromycin every 12 hr before meals for 10 to 14 days. Or, 30 mg plus 1 g amoxicillin t.i.d. before meals for 14 days.
➤ *To treat symptomatic pediatric gastroesophageal reflux disease*
DELAYED-RELEASE CAPSULES, DELAYED-RELEASE SUSPENSION, DELAYED-RELEASE ORALLY DISINTEGRATING TABLETS
Children ages 12 to 17. 15 mg daily for up to 8 wk.
Children ages 1 to 11 weighing 30 kg (66 lb) or less. 15 mg daily for up to 12 wk.
Children ages 1 to 11 weighing more than 30 kg. 30 mg daily for up to 12 wk.
➤ *To treat symptomatic pediatric erosive esophagitis*
DELAYED-RELEASE CAPSULES, DELAYED-RELEASE SUSPENSION, DELAYED-RELEASE ORALLY DISINTEGRATING TABLETS
Children ages 12 to 17. 30 mg daily for up to 8 wk.
Children ages 1 to 11 weighing 30 kg (66 lb) or less. 15 mg daily for up to 12 wk.
Children ages 1 to 11 weighing more than 30 kg. 30 mg daily for up to 12 wk.
➤ *To treat frequent heartburn*
E.R. CAPSULES (PREVACID 24-HR)
Adults. 1 capsule daily for 14 days. May repeat course every 4 months.

Route	Onset	Peak	Duration
P.O.	1–3 hr	Unknown	Over 24 hr

Mechanism of Action
Binds to and inactivates the hydrogen-potassium adenosine triphosphate enzyme system (also called the proton pump) in gastric parietal cells. This action blocks the final step of gastric acid production.

Incompatibilities
Don't give any other drugs with parenteral lansoprazole, and dilute only with solutions recommended by manufacturer (sterile water for initial reconstitution and normal saline solution, lactated Ringer's solution, or D_5W for further dilution).

Contraindications
Hypersensitivity to lansoprazole or its components

Interactions
DRUGS
ampicillin, digoxin, iron salts, ketoconazole, other drugs that depend on low gastric pH for bioavailability: Inhibited absorption of these drugs
atazanavir: Decreased blood level and possibly reduced effectiveness of atazanavir
methotrexate: Possibly elevated methotrexate levels, which may cause toxicity
sucralfate: Delayed lansoprazole absorption
tacrolimus: Possibly increased blood tacrolimus levels
theophylline: Slightly decreased blood theophylline level
warfarin: Increased INR and PT with possibly increased risk of serious bleeding

Adverse Reactions
CNS: Dizziness, headache
EENT: Blurred vision, oral edema
GI: Abdominal pain, anorexia, *Clostridium difficile*-associated diarrhea, diarrhea, elevated liver enzymes, hepatotoxicity, increased appetite, nausea, pancreatitis, vomiting
GU: Interstitial nephritis, urine retention
HEME: Agranulocytosis, aplastic anemia, decreased hemoglobin, hemolytic anemia, leukopenia, neutropenia, pancytopenia, thrombocytopenia, thrombotic thrombocytopenic purpura
MS: Arthralgia, bone fracture, bursitis, myositis
RESP: Upper respiratory tract infection

SKIN: Erythema multiforme, leucocyto-clastic vasculitis, pruritus, rash, Stevens-Johnson syndrome, toxic epidermal necrolysis
Other: Anaphylaxis, angioedema, hyperkalemia, hypomagnesemia, injection-site reaction

Nursing Considerations

• Give lansoprazole before meals. Antacids may be given as well, if needed.
• If patient is prescribed capsules and has trouble swallowing them, open and sprinkle granules on applesauce, Ensure, pudding, cottage cheese, yogurt, or strained pears. Don't crush granules. Have patient swallow mixture immediately. Or, empty granules into 2 ounces apple, orange, or tomato juice; mix quickly, and have patient swallow immediately. Then add 2 or more ounces of juice to glass and have patient drink immediately to ensure full dose.
• For delayed-release orally disintegrating tablets, place tablet on patient's tongue and let it dissolve, with or without water, until patient can swallow particles.
• For patient with nasogastric tube, don't use oral suspension. Instead use capsules or orally disintegrating tablets. For capsule form, open capsule, mix granules in 40 ml apple juice only, and inject through tube. Then flush tube with apple juice only. For disintegrating tablets, place tablet in syringe and draw up 4 ml (for 15-mg tablet) or 8 ml (for 30-mg tablet) of water. Shake gently, and inject through tube within 15 minutes. Then refill syringe with 5 ml of water, shake gently, and inject through tube.
• For delayed-release oral suspension, empty packet contents into a container with 2 tablespoons water (no other liquids or foods), stir well, and have patient drink immediately. If any particles remain in container, add more water, stir, and have patient drink again immediately.
• Reconstitute parenteral form by injecting 5 ml sterile water into 30-mg drug vial. Mix gently until powder dissolves. Use within 1 hour. After reconstitution, dilute with 50 ml normal saline solution, lactated Ringer's solution, or D$_5$W. Give within 12 hours if mixed with D$_5$W or 24 hours if mixed with normal saline solution or lactated Ringer's solution.

• Give parenteral drug with a filter following manufacturer's guidelines. Change filter every 24 hours. Give as I.V. infusion over 30 minutes. Flush line with normal saline solution, lactated Ringer's solution, or D$_5$W before and after giving lansoprazole.
• Expect to give lansoprazole with antibiotics because decreased gastric acid secretion helps antibiotics eradicate *H. pylori.*
• Diarrhea from *Clostridium difficile* infection can occur with or without concurrent antibiotics when lansoprazole is used. If *C. difficile*-associated diarrhea occurs, notify prescriber and expect to withhold drug and treat with fluids, electrolytes, protein, and an antibiotic effective against *C. difficile.*
• Monitor patient for bone fracture, especially in patients receiving multiple daily doses for more than a year, because proton pump inhibitors, such as lansoprazole, increase risk for osteoporosis-related fractures of the hip, wrist, or spine.
• Monitor the patient, especially the patient on long-term therapy for hypomagnesemia. If patient is to remain on lansoprazole long term, expect to monitor the patient's serum magnesium level, as ordered, and if level becomes low, anticipate that magnesium replacement therapy and lansoprazole will be discontinued.

PATIENT TEACHING

• Urge patient to take drug exactly as prescribed, usually before a meal (preferably breakfast) to decrease gastric acid output.
• If patient has trouble swallowing dexlansoprazole capsules, tell her to open them and sprinkle granules on 1 tablespoon of applesauce and swallow immediately. If patient has trouble swallowing lansoprazole capsules, tell her to open them and sprinkle granules on applesauce, Ensure, pudding, cottage cheese, yogurt, or strained pears and to swallow immediately without chewing. Or, she may empty granules into 2 ounces of apple, orange, or tomato juice, mix quickly, and swallow immediately. Tell her to refill glass with 2 or more ounces of juice and drink immediately to ensure a full dose.

J
K
L

• If patient was prescribed delayed-release orally disintegrating tablets, tell her to place tablet on tongue, let it dissolve, and then swallow particles with or without water. Also tell her not to break, cut, or chew the tablets.
• If patient was prescribed delayed-release oral suspension, tell her to empty contents of packet into a container with 2 table-spoons of water (no other liquids or foods), stir well, and drink immediately. If particles remain in container, she should add water, stir, and drink immediately.
• Inform patient that she may take antacids with lansoprazole.
• Advise patient to report severe headache, or worsening of symptoms immediately to prescriber.
• Urge patient to tell prescriber about diarrhea that's severe or lasts longer than 3 days. Remind patient that watery or bloody stools can occur 2 or more months after antibiotic therapy and can be serious, requiring prompt treatment.
• Monitor the patient, especially the patient on long-term therapy for hypomag-nesemia. If patient is to remain on lansoprazole long-term, expect to monitor the patient's serum magnesium level, as ordered, and if the level becomes low, anticipate magnesium replacement therapy and lansoprazole to be discontinued.

lanthanum carbonate

Fosrenol

Class and Category
Chemical class: Rare earth element
Therapeutic class: Phosphate binder
Pregnancy category: C

Indications and Dosages
➤ *To reduce serum phosphate levels in patients with end-stage renal disease*
ORAL POWDER, TABLETS
Adults. *Initial:* 500 mg three times daily with meals; increased, as needed, by 750 mg daily every 2 to 3 wk until acceptable serum phosphate level is reached.

Contraindications
Bowel obstruction, fecal impaction, hyper-sensitivity to lanthanum carbonate or any of its components, hypophosphatemia, ileus

Interactions
DRUGS
ACE inhibitors: antibiotics such as ampicillin, fluoroquinolones or tetracyclines; antimalarials; drugs with narrow therapeutic range; statins; thyroid hormones: Possible reduced bioavailability with these drugs
calcium channel blockers: Increased risk of adverse gastrointestinal effects

Adverse Reactions
CNS: Headache
CV: Hypotension
EENT: Rhinitis
ENDO: Hypercalcemia, hypocalcemia
GI: Abdominal pain, bowel obstruction, constipation, diarrhea, dyspepsia, fecal impaction, ileus, nausea, vomiting
GU: Dialysis graft occlusion
RESP: Bronchitis
SKIN: Pruritus, rash, urticaria
Other: Hypophosphatemia

Nursing Considerations
• Use lanthanum carbonate cautiously in patients with acute peptic ulcer, ulcerative colitis, Crohn's disease, or bowel obstruction because drug effects are unknown in these patients.
• Monitor the patient's serum phosphate levels, as ordered, especially during dosage adjustment, to determine effectiveness of lanthanum carbonate therapy. Serum phosphate levels should fall below 6.0 mg/dl.
• Monitor patient closely for signs and symptoms of bowel obstruction, fecal impaction, or ileus, especially the patient with a history of gastrointestinal surgery, colon cancer or hypomotility disorders, as well as the patient receiving calcium channel blockers. Notify prescriber, if present, because these gastrointestinal adverse effects may become serious enough to require hospitalization or surgery.
• Administer tetracyclines and drugs with a narrow therapeutic range at least one

Mechanism of Action

During digestion, phosphate is released into the upper GI tract (below left) and absorbed into the bloodstream, increasing serum phosphate levels. In patients with end-stage renal disease, however, inefficient phosphate clearance from the blood leads to abnormally elevated levels.

Lanthanum dissociates in the upper GI tract, releasing ions that attach to unbound phosphate to form an insoluble complex (below right). Unabsorbed into the bloodstream, these altered phosphate molecules can't elevate the patient's serum phosphate level.

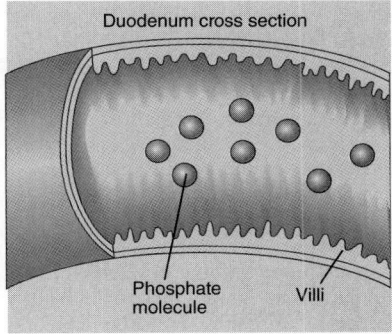

Duodenum cross section. Phosphate molecule. Villi.

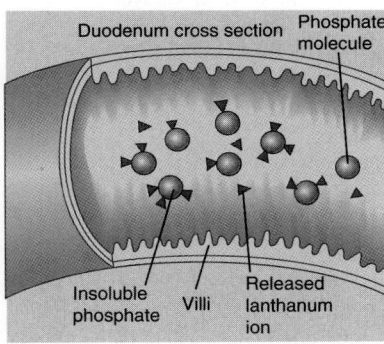

Duodenum cross section. Phosphate molecule. Insoluble phosphate. Villi. Released lanthanum ion.

hour before or three hours after lanthanum administration; quinolone antibiotics at least 1 hour before or 4 hours after lanthanum administration; and levothyroxine at least 2 hours before or 2 hours after lanthanum administration to prevent a reduction in bioavailability.

PATIENT TEACHING

• Instruct patient to take lanthanum carbonate with or immediately after meals.
• Advise patient to chew each tablet thoroughly before swallowing. If patient has trouble chewing tablets, tell her she may crush them.
• Tell patient to sprinkle the prescribed oral powder form on a small quantity of applesauce or other similar foods and consume immediately.
• Urge patient to take drug exactly as prescribed, and explain that it may take weeks to reach a desired serum phosphate level.
• Advise patient to notify prescriber if he experiences gastrointestinal discomfort that becomes severe or prolonged.

leflunomide

Arava

Class and Category

Chemical class: Malonitrilamide immunomodulator
Therapeutic class: Antirheumatic
Pregnancy category: X

Indications and Dosages

➤ *To relieve symptoms of active rheumatoid arthritis, improve physical function and slow disease progression*

TABLETS

Adults. *Loading:* 100 mg daily for 3 days. *Maintenance:* 20 mg daily, reduced to 10 mg daily if poorly tolerated. *Maximum:* 20 mg/day.

Mechanism of Action

Inhibits dihydroorotate dehydrogenase, the enzyme in autoimmune process that leads to rheumatoid arthritis. With this action, leflunomide relieves inflammation and prevents alteration of the autoimmune process.

J
K
L

Contraindications

Hypersensitivity to leflunomide, teriflunomide, or their components; pregnancy

Interactions

DRUGS

activated charcoal, cholestyramine: Decreased blood leflunomide level
live-virus vaccines: Possibly adverse reactions to vaccines caused by leflunomide-induced immunosuppression
methotrexate: Risk of hepatotoxicity
NSAIDs: Possibly impaired NSAID metabolism
rifampin, tolbutamide: Increased blood leflunomide level

Adverse Reactions

CNS: Anxiety, dizziness, drowsiness, fatigue, fever, headache, paresthesia, peripheral neuropathy
CV: Chest pain, hypertension, palpitations, tachycardia, vasculitis
EENT: Blurred vision, conjunctivitis, dry mouth, epistaxis, mouth ulcers, pharyngitis, rhinitis, sinusitis
GI: Abdominal pain, cholestasis, constipation, diarrhea, elevated liver function test results, flatulence, gastritis, gastroenteritis, hepatic injury or failure, hepatitis, jaundice, nausea, pancreatitis, vomiting
GU: Hypophosphaturia, UTI
HEME: Agranulocytosis, anemia, leukopenia, neutropenia, pancytopenia, thrombocytopenia
MS: Back pain, synovitis, tendinitis
RESP: Asthma, bronchitis, dyspnea, interstitial lung disease, pulmonary fibrosis, respiratory tract infection
SKIN: Alopecia (transient), cutaneous lupus erythematosus, cutaneous necrotizing vasculitis, erythema multiforme, erythematous rash, pruritus, pustular psoriasis, Stevens-Johnson syndrome, toxic epidermal necrolysis, urticaria, worsening psoriasis
Other: Angioedema, drug reaction with eosinophilia and systemic symptoms (DRESS), opportunistic infections, sepsis, weight loss

Nursing Considerations

• Leflunomide isn't recommended for patients with severe immunodeficiency, bone marrow dysplasia, or severe, uncontrolled infections because of its immunosuppressant effect. It is also not recommended for patients with liver disease or those with a serum alanine aminotransferase level greater than two times the upper level normal prior to initiation of therapy because drug may worsen liver dysfunction.
• Use cautiously in patients who are over 60 years of age, patients with diabetes, or in patients taking concomitant neurotoxic drugs because of an increased risk of developing peripheral neuropathy. If peripheral neuropathy occurs during leflunomide therapy, notify prescriber and expect drug to be discontinued and possibly cholestyramine washout to be ordered.
• Test patient for latent tuberculosis before starting leflunomide. If positive, expect standard medical treatment to be given before leflunomide therapy starts.
• Obtain baseline blood pressure before starting leflunomide, and monitor periodically thereafter because drug may cause hypertension.
• Assess liver enzyme (ALT and AST) levels at start of therapy, monthly during first 6 months, and if stable, every 6 to 8 weeks thereafter, as ordered. If levels become elevated greater than threefold upper level normal, notify prescriber and expect leflunomide therapy to be withheld until underlying cause is determined. If the elevation is thought to be leflunomide induced, expect to start cholestyramine washout, as ordered, and monitor liver test weekly until normalized. If another cause is found for the elevation, expect to resume leflunomide therapy.
• Obtain platelet count, WBC count, and hemoglobin or hematocrit at start of therapy and every 4 to 8 weeks thereafter, as ordered.
• Notify prescriber if patient develops serious infection because drug may need to be interrupted and cholestyramine or charcoal given to eliminate drug rapidly.
WARNING Monitor patient's respiratory function closely because drug may cause interstitial lung disease that could become

life-threatening. If patient develops a cough and dyspnea, notify prescriber; drug will need to be stopped, and patient may need cholestyramine or charcoal to eliminate drug rapidly.

WARNING Assess patient's skin regularly for evidence of serious skin reactions. If present, notify prescriber, as drug will need to be discontinued, and patient may need cholestyramine or charcoal to eliminate drug rapidly.

PATIENT TEACHING
• Advise patient that leflunomide doesn't cure arthritis but may relieve its symptoms and improve physical function.
• Inform patient that reversible hair loss may occur.
• Caution woman of childbearing potential not to become pregnant while taking drug because of the high risk of birth defects.
• Instruct patient to report signs of hepatotoxicity, such as mouth ulcers, unusual bleeding or bruising, and yellow skin or eyes.
• Tell patient to report signs of respiratory dysfunction, such as cough and dyspnea, and signs of persistent or serious skin reactions.
• Advise patient to avoid live vaccines during leflunomide therapy.
• Instruct patient to notify prescriber if she develops an infection.

leuprolide acetate

Eligard, Lupron, Lupron Depot, Lupron Depot-3 Month 11.25 mg, Lupron Depot-3 Month 22.5 mg, Lupron Depot-4 Month 30 mg, Lupron Depot-6 Month 45 mg, Lupron Depot-Ped-1 Month, Lupron Depot-Ped-3 Month

Class and Category
Chemical class: Synthetic peptide gonadotropin-releasing hormone analogue
Therapeutic class: Antianemic, antiendometrionic agent, antineoplastic, gonadotropin inhibitor
Pregnancy category: X

Indications and Dosages
➤ *To provide palliative treatment of advanced prostate cancer*
SUBCUTANEOUS INJECTION (ELIGARD)
Adults. 7.5 mg/mo., 22.5 mg every 3 mo., 30 mg every 4 mo., or 45 mg every 6 mo.
SUBCUTANEOUS INJECTION (LUPRON)
Adults. 1 mg daily.
I.M. INJECTION (LUPRON, LUPRON DEPOT-3 MONTH, LUPRON DEPOT-4 MONTH, LUPRON DEPOT-6 MONTH)
Adults. 7.5 mg/mo., 22.5 mg every 3 mo., 30 mg every 4 mo., or 45 mg every 6 mo.
➤ *To treat precocious central puberty*
I.M. INJECTION (LUPRON DEPOT-PED-1 MONTH)
Children weighing more than 37.5 kg (83 lb). *Initial:* 15 mg every 4 wk. *Maintenance:* Dosage increased as needed in increments of 3.75 mg every 4 wk. *Maximum:* 15 mg every 4 wk.
Children weighing 25 to 37.5 kg (55 to 83 lb). *Initial:* 11.25 mg every 4 wk. *Maintenance:* Dosage increased as needed in increments of 3.75 mg every 4 wk. *Maximum:* 15 mg every 4 wk.
Children weighing less than 25 kg. *Initial:* 7.5 mg every 4 wk. *Maintenance:* Dosage increased as needed in increments of 3.75 mg every 4 wk. *Maximum:* 15 mg every 4 wk.
I.M. INJECTION (LUPRON DEPOT-PED-3 MONTH)
Children age 2 and older. 11.25 mg or 30 mg once every 3 months (dose not based on weight).
SUBCUTANEOUS INJECTION (LEUPROLIDE ACETATE INJECTION)
Children. 50 mcg/kg daily. Dosage increased in increments of 10 mcg/kg daily.
➤ *To treat endometriosis*
I.M. INJECTION (LUPRON DEPOT, LUPRON DEPOT-3 MONTH)
Adults. 3.75 mg every mo or 11.25 mg every 3 mo for up to 6 mo. *Maximum:* 33.75 mg total dose.
➤ *As adjunct to treat anemia due to uterine leiomyomas*
I.M. INJECTION (LUPRON DEPOT, LUPRON DEPOT-3 MONTH)
Adults. 3.75 mg every mo up to 3 mo or 11.25 mg single dose. *Maximum:* 11.25 mg total dose.

J
K
L

Mechanism of Action

After stimulating follicle-stimulating hormone (FSH) and luteinizing hormone (LH), continuous leuprolide therapy suppresses secretion of gonadotropin-releasing hormone, decreasing testosterone and estradiol levels. In children with central precocious puberty, this stops menses and reproductive organ development.

In adult men, continuous suppression decreases testosterone levels and causes pharmacologic castration, which slows the activity of prostatic neoplastic cells. In women with endometriosis or uterine leiomyomas, leuprolide suppresses ovarian function, inactivating endometrial tissues and resulting in amenorrhea.

Route	Onset	Peak	Duration
I.M., SubQ*	1 wk	Unknown	4–12 wk after therapy
I.M., SubQ†	2–4 wk	After 1–2 mo	60–90 days after therapy

Contraindications

Women and children (leuprolide acetate injectable suspension); hypersensitivity to benzyl alcohol, gonadorelin, and gonadotropin-releasing hormone analogues, including leuprolide, and their components; pregnancy; undiagnosed abnormal vaginal bleeding

Adverse Reactions

CNS: Anxiety, depression, dizziness, fatigue, headache, insomnia, lethargy, malaise, memory loss, mood changes, nervousness (adult women), paresthesia, paralysis (from spinal fracture), peripheral neuropathy, pituitary apoplexy, rigors, seizures, stroke, syncope, transient ischemic attacks, weakness
CV: Arrhythmias, deep vein thrombosis, edema, hypertension, hypotension, palpitations, prolonged QT interval, vasodilation; angina, MI, thrombophlebitis (adult men)
EENT: Blurred vision, hearing disorder

---

* Gonadotropin inhibitor.
†Antiendometrionic, antineoplastic.

ENDO: Amenorrhea, androgenic effects in women, breast tenderness or swelling, decreased testicle size, gynecomastia, hot flashes, hyperglycemia, pituitary apoplexy
GI: Colitis, constipation in adult men, dyspepsia, gastroenteritis, hepatic dysfunction, nausea, vomiting
GU: Bladder spasm, decreased libido, decreased penis size, dysuria, endometriosis flare-up, impotence, incontinence, nocturia, prostate cancer flare-up, prostate pain, uterine bleeding, vaginal discharge in girls, vaginitis
HEME: Leukopenia
MS: Arthralgia, body pain in children, bone density loss, bone or limb pain, fibromyalgia, myalgia, spinal fracture, tenosynovitis
RESP: Asthmatic attack, dyspnea, interstitial lung disease, pulmonary embolism
SKIN: Alopecia, clamminess, night sweats, photosensitivity, rash, urticaria
Other: Anaphylaxis; elevated uric acid; injection-site abscess, burning, edema, induration, itching, pain, or redness; tumor flare; weight gain

Nursing Considerations

• Use cautiously in patients at risk for prolonged QT interval, such as in the presence of congenital long QT syndrome, congestive heart failure, or frequent electrolyte abnormalities, and in patients taking drugs that may prolong the QT interval. Know that electrolyte abnormalities should be corrected, as ordered, prior to therapy beginning. Monitor patient's electrolytes and electrocardiogram regularly throughout therapy, as ordered. Notify prescriber of any abnormalities.
• Let drug come to room temperature before using. Reconstitute leuprolide acetate depot suspension with diluent provided by manufacturer. Add diluent to powder for suspension and thoroughly shake vials to disperse particles into a uniform milky suspension. Use within 30 minutes after mixing, and discard any unused portion. If using a prefilled dual-chamber syringe, follow manufacturer's instructions to release diluent into chamber containing powder. Shake gently after diluted to disperse particles evenly in solution. No dilution or

reconstitution is needed for leuprolide acetate injection for subcutaneous administration. Rotate injection sites.
WARNING Leuprolide acetate for injectable suspension (Eligard) is approved only for use in men for palliative treatment of prostate cancer. Use provided syringes and delivery system, and read and follow instructions carefully to ensure proper mixing of product; shaking alone is inadequate to mix it.
WARNING Monitor patient for possible allergic reaction (erythema and induration) at injection site because leuprolide injections contain benzyl alcohol. Manufacturer recommends that injection be given by physician.

• During first weeks of leuprolide therapy, monitor patient being treated for prostate cancer for initial worsening of symptoms, such as increased bone pain, difficult urination, and paresthesia or paralysis (in patients with vertebral metastasis).

• During treatment for prostate cancer, monitor patient's serum testosterone and PSA levels periodically, as ordered, to determine response to leuprolide therapy.

• Monitor patient's blood glucose level, as ordered, because leuprolide therapy may elevate blood glucose levels, leading to a diagnosis of diabetes mellitus, or may adversely affect glycemic control in patients with diabetes.

• Watch patient closely for signs and symptoms of cardiovascular disease because leuprolide therapy increases risk of myocardial infarction, sudden cardiac death, and stroke.

• Expect to stop drug before age 11 in female patients and age 12 in male patients treated for precocious central puberty.

• Monitor bone density test results, as ordered, of women at risk for osteoporosis who are receiving leuprolide because of possible drug-induced estrogen loss, which may result in decreased bone density.

• Be aware that therapeutic doses of leuprolide suppress the pituitary-gonadal system and that normal function doesn't return for 4 to 12 weeks after drug is stopped.

WARNING Monitor patient for evidence of pituitary apoplexy, such as sudden headache, vomiting, visual changes, ophthalmoplegia, altered mental status, and possibly cardiovascular collapse. Although rare, it may occur within 2 weeks of first dose, sometimes within the first hour. Notify prescriber immediately and provide supportive care.

PATIENT TEACHING

• Instruct patient who is self-administering leuprolide injection to use syringe provided by manufacturer. If manufacturer's syringe is unavailable, advise her to use only a 0.5-ml disposable, low-dose, U-100 insulin syringe to ensure accurate dosage. Substitution of syringes is not recommended for leuprolide acetate for injectable suspension.

• Advise women to report monthly menses or breakthrough bleeding to prescriber immediately.

• Instruct female patient of childbearing age to use a nonhormonal form of contraception during leuprolide therapy. Advise her to stop taking drug and notify prescriber at once if she becomes pregnant. Be aware that patient should not breastfeed while receiving leuprolide.

• Inform patient with osteoporosis or at risk for developing it that drug may increase bone density loss.

• Inform parents of child being treated for central precocious puberty that they should expect normal gonadal-pituitary function to return 4 to 12 weeks after therapy ends.

• Advise patient to report symptoms of depression or memory problems.

• Caution patient being treated for prostate cancer that drug may initially worsen such symptoms as bone pain and that it may cause new signs or symptoms to occur during first few weeks of treatment. Reassure patient that this is transient.

• Instruct patient to report to prescriber any symptoms that are new, worsen, or are prolonged.

• Advise patient with diabetes to monitor his blood glucose level closely.

• Emphasize importance of seeking immediate emergency care if patient develops symptoms suggestive of a heart attack or stroke.

J
K
L

levalbuterol hydrochloride

Xopenex, Xopenex HFA

Class and Category

Chemical class: Sympathomimetic amine
Therapeutic class: Bronchodilator
Pregnancy category: C

Indications and Dosages

➤ *To prevent or treat bronchospasm in reversible obstructive airway disease*

INHALATION AEROSOL

Adults and children age 4 and over. 45 or 90 mcg (1 or 2 inhalations) every 4 to 6 hr.

INHALATION SOLUTION

Adults and children age 12 and over. 0.63 to 1.25 mg three times daily every 6 to 8 hr. *Maximum:* 1.25 mg three times daily. **Children ages 6 to 11.** 0.31 to 0.63 mg three times daily. *Maximum:* 0.63 mg three times daily.

DOSAGE ADJUSTMENT For elderly patients, dosage limited to 0.63 mg three times daily every 6 to 8 hr.

Route	Onset	Peak	Duration
Inhalation	10–17 min	1.5 hr	5–6 hr

Mechanism of Action

Attaches to beta$_2$ receptors on bronchial cell membranes, which stimulates the intracellular enzyme adenyl cyclase to convert adenosine triphosphate to cAMP. Increased intracellular cAMP level relaxes bronchial smooth muscle and inhibits histamine release from mast cells.

Contraindications

Hypersensitivity to levalbuterol, other sympathomimetic amines, or their components

Interactions

DRUGS

beta blockers: Blocked effects of both drugs
digoxin: Decreased blood digoxin level
loop or thiazide diuretics: Increased risk of hypokalemia
MAO inhibitors, sympathomimetics, tricyclic antidepressants: Increased risk of adverse cardiovascular effects

Adverse Reactions

CNS: Anxiety, chills, dizziness, dysphonia, hypertonia, insomnia, migraine headache, nervousness, paresthesia, syncope, tremor
CV: Arrhythmias, chest pain, hypertension, hypotension, tachycardia
EENT: Dry mouth and throat, rhinitis, sinusitis
GI: Diarrhea, gastroesophageal reflux disease (GERD), indigestion, nausea, vomiting
MS: Leg cramps, myalgia
RESP: Asthma exacerbation, cough, dyspnea, paradoxical bronchospasm
SKIN: Rash, urticaria
Other: Anaphylaxis, angioedema, flulike symptoms, lymphadenopathy, metabolic acidosis

Nursing Considerations

• Use levalbuterol cautiously in patients with arrhythmias, diabetes mellitus, hypertension, hyperthyroidism, or a history of seizures.
• Give oral solution form only by nebulizer.
• Monitor pulse rate and blood pressure before and after nebulizer treatment.
• Because drug may provoke paradoxical bronchospasm, observe for dyspnea, wheezing, and increased coughing.

PATIENT TEACHING

• Teach patient how to use levalbuterol nebulizer and to measure correct dose.
• Instruct patient to prime inhaler before using it for the first time or when it hasn't been used for more than 3 days by releasing 4 test sprays into the air, aiming it away from her face.
• Show patient how to clean nebulizer or inhaler, and explain the need to do so at least once weekly.
• Instruct patient to notify prescriber if drug fails to work or if she needs more treatments because asthma is worsening.
• Instruct patient not to increase dosage or frequency unless told by prescriber.
• Urge patient to stop drug and call prescriber if she has paradoxical bronchospasm.
• Instruct patient to use inhalation solution within 2 weeks of opening the foil pouch and to protect drug from light and heat.

• Urge patient to consult prescriber before using OTC or other drugs.

---

levetiracetam

Keppra, Keppra XR

Class and Category

Chemical: Pyrrolidine derivative
Therapeutic: Anticonvulsant
Pregnancy category: C

Indications and Dosages

➤ *As adjunct to treat partial seizures*

ORAL SOLUTION, TABLETS

Adults and adolescents over age 16.
Initial: 500 mg twice daily, increased by 1,000 mg daily every 2 wk if needed, and given in 2 divided doses. *Maximum:* 3,000 mg daily.

Children ages 4 to 16. *Initial:* 10 mg/kg twice daily, increased by 20 mg/kg daily every 2 wk until recommended daily dose of 60 mg/kg given in 2 divided doses is reached.

Children 6 months to 4 years. *Initial:* 10 mg/kg twice daily, increased by 20 mg/kg daily every 2 wk until the recommended daily dose of 50 mg/kg given in 2 divided doses is reached.

Infants 1 month of age to 6 months.
Initial: 7 mg/kg twice daily, increased by 14 mg/kg every two weeks until recommended daily dose of 42 mg/kg given in 2 divided doses is reached.

XR TABLETS

Adults and adolescents over age 16. 1,000 mg once daily, increased by 1,000 mg daily every 2 wk until recommended daily dose of 3,000 mg is reached given in 2 divided doses.

I.V. INFUSION

Adults and adolescents over age 16. *Initial:* 500 mg infused over 15 minutes twice daily, increased by 1,000 mg daily every 2 wk, if needed. *Maximum:* 3,000 mg daily given in 2 divided doses.

I.V. INFUSION

Children ages 4 to 16. *Initial:* 10 mg/kg infused over 15 minutes twice daily, increased by 20 mg/kg daily every 2 wk until recommended daily dose of 60 mg/kg given in 2 divided doses is reached.

Children 6 months to 4 years. *Initial:* 10 mg/kg infused over 15 minutes twice daily, increased by 20 mg/kg daily every 2 wk until the recommended daily dose of 50 mg/kg given in 2 divided doses is reached.

Infants 1 month of age to 6 months.
Initial: 7 mg/kg infused over 15 minutes twice daily, increased by 14 mg/kg every 2 wk until recommended daily dose of 42 mg/kg given in 2 divided doses is reached.

➤ *As adjunct to treat myoclonic seizures in patients with juvenile myoclonic epilepsy*

ORAL SOLUTION, TABLETS

Adults and children age 12 and over.
Initial: 500 mg twice daily, increased by 1,000 mg daily every 2 wk, if needed. *Maximum:* 3,000 mg daily.

I.V. INFUSION

Adults and children age 12 and over.
Initial: 500 mg infused over 15 minutes twice daily, increased by 1,000 mg daily every 2 wk, if needed, and given in 2 divided doses. *Maximum:* 3,000 mg daily given in 2 divided doses.

➤ *As adjunct to treat primary generalized tonic-clonic seizures in patients with idiopathic generalized epilepsy*

ORAL SOLUTION, TABLETS

Adults and children age 16 and over.
Initial: 500 mg twice daily, increased by 1,000 mg daily every 2 wk, as needed. *Maximum:* 3,000 mg daily.

I.V. INFUSION

Children ages 6 to 16. *Initial:* 10 mg/kg infused over 15 minutes twice daily, increased by 20 mg/kg daily every 2 wk, if needed, and given in 2 divided doses. *Maximum:* 60 mg/kg daily in 2 divided doses.

DOSAGE ADJUSTMENT Maximum dosage reduced to 2,000 mg daily for patients with creatinine clearance of 50 to 80 ml/min/1.73 m^2; to 1,500 mg daily for clearance of 30 to 49 ml/min/1.73 m^2; and to 1,000 mg daily for clearance less than 30 ml/min/1.73 m^2. For patients with end-stage renal disease who are having dialysis, expect to give another 250 to 500 mg, as prescribed, after each dialysis session. For children who can't tolerate 60 mg/kg daily, dosage reduced to point of tolerance.

J
K
L

Mechanism of Action
May protect against secondary generalized seizure activity by preventing coordination of epileptiform burst firing. Levetiracetam doesn't seem to involve inhibitory and excitatory neurotransmission.

Contraindications
Hypersensitivity to levetiracetam or its components

Adverse Reactions
CNS: Abnormal gait, aggression, agitation, anger, anxiety, apathy, asthenia, ataxia, behavioral difficulties (children), choreoathetosis, confusion, coordination difficulties, depersonalization, depression, dizziness, dyskinesia, emotional lability, fatigue, hallucinations, headache, hostility, increased reflexes, insomnia, irritability, involuntary movements, mental or mood changes, nervousness, neurosis, panic attacks, paresthesia, personality disorder, psychosis, seizures, somnolence, suicidal ideation, vertigo
CV: Elevated diastolic blood pressure (children up to 4 years of age)
EENT: Amblyopia, conjunctivitis, diplopia, ear pain, nasopharyngitis, pharyngitis, rhinitis, sinusitis
GI: Anorexia, constipation, diarrhea, elevated liver enzymes, gastroenteritis, hepatic failure, hepatitis, pancreatitis, vomiting
GU: Albuminuria
HEME: Decreased hemtatocrit, hemoglobin, and red and white blood cell counts; elevated eosinophil count; leukopenia; neutropenia; pancytopenia; thrombocytopenia
MS: Muscle weakness, neck pain
RESP: Asthma, cough
SKIN: Alopecia, ecchymosis, erythema multiforme, pruritus, skin discoloration, Stevens-Johnson syndrome, toxic epidermal necrolysis, vesiculobullous rash
Other: Dehydration, facial edema, hyponatremia, infection, influenza, weight loss

Nursing Considerations
• Children weighing 20 kg or less should be given only the oral solution form.
• Know that the intravenous form of levetiracetam should be used only as an alternative for patients when oral administration is temporarily not possible.
• When switching patient from oral dosing to intravenous dosing and from intravenous dosing to oral dosing, no dosage or frequency changes are needed.
• For I.V. use, dilute parenteral levetiracetam in 100 ml of compatible diluent, such as normal saline injection, lactated Ringer's injection, or dextrose 5% injection. Use within 24 hours.
• Assess compliance during first 4 weeks of therapy, when adverse reactions are most common.
• Monitor patient for seizure activity during therapy. As appropriate, implement seizure precautions according to facility policy.
• Avoid stopping drug abruptly because doing so may increase seizure activity. Expect to taper dosage gradually.
• Certain adverse effects, including somnolence, fatigue, coordination problems, and abnormal behaviors may be more likely in patients taking levetiracetam for partial seizure disorders.
• Monitor blood pressure in children because increased diastolic blood pressure may occur in patients up to 4 years old.
• Monitor patient closely for evidence of suicidal thinking or behavior, especially when therapy starts or dosage changes.
• Monitor patient for a rash and other adverse skin reactions because serious dermatological reactions have occurred with levetiracetam therapy. Although these adverse reactions usually appear within 14 to 17 days after therapy has begun, some have occurred as late as four months later. Notify prescriber at the first sign of a rash and expect drug to be discontinued.
• Monitor pregnant patient closely, especially during third trimester, because physiological changes associated with pregnancy may gradually decrease plama levetiracetam levels. Monitoring should continue through the postpartum period.
PATIENT TEACHING
• Caution patient that levetiracetam may cause dizziness and drowsiness, especially during first 4 weeks of therapy.

- Advise patient to avoid hazardous activities until drug's CNS effects are known.
- Caution patient not to stop taking levetiracetam abruptly; inform her that drug dosage should be tapered under prescriber's direction to reduce the risk of breakthrough seizures.
- Explain that levetiracetam may cause mental and behavioral changes, such as aggression, depression, irritability, and rarely psychotic symptoms. Urge her to contact prescriber about any bothersome changes.
- Advise patient to keep taking other anticonvulsants, as ordered, while taking levetiracetam.
- Encourage patient to avoid alcohol during therapy because alcohol can increase incidence of drowsiness and dizziness.
- Instruct patient to see prescriber regularly so that her progress can be monitored.
- Urge caregivers to watch patient closely for evidence of suicidal tendencies, especially when therapy starts or dosage changes, and to report concerns immediately.
- Urge woman who becomes pregnant while taking levetiracetam to enroll in the North American antiepileptic drug pregnancy registry by calling 1-888-233-2334. Explain that registry is collecting information about safety of antiepileptic drugs during pregnancy.
- Emphasize importance of notifying prescriber at the first sign of a rash.

levocetirizine

Xyzal

Class and Category
Chemical class: H_1-receptor antagonist
Therapeutic class: Antihistamine
Pregnancy category: B

Indications and Dosages
➤ *To treat chronic idiopathic urticaria; to treat allergic rhinitis*
TABLETS, ORAL SOLUTION
Adults and children age 12 and over. 2.5 to 5 mg once daily in evening. *Maximum:* 5 mg daily.
DOSAGE ADJUSTMENT For patient with mild renal impairment (creatinine clearance 50 to 80 ml/min/1.73 m²),

dosage shouldn't exceed 2.5 mg daily. For patient with moderate renal impairment (creatinine clearance 30 to 50 ml/min/1.73 m²), dosage shouldn't exceed 2.5 mg once every other day. For patient with severe renal impairment (creatinine clearance 10 to 30 ml/min/1.73 m²), dosage shouldn't exceed 2.5 mg once every 3 to 4 days.
Children ages 6 to 11. 2.5 mg once daily in evening. *Maximum:* 2.5 mg daily.

Mechanism of Action
Binds to central and peripheral H_1 receptors, competing with histamine for these sites and preventing it from reaching its site of action. By blocking histamine, levocetirizine produces antihistamine effects, inhibiting respiratory, vascular, and GI smooth-muscle contraction; decreasing capillary permeability, which reduces wheals, flares, and itching; and decreasing salivary and lacrimal gland secretions to relieve chronic urticaria and signs and symptoms of allergic rhinitis.

Contraindications
Children ages 6 to 11 with impaired renal function; creatinine clearance less than 10 ml/min/1.73 m²; end-stage renal disease in adults and children age 12 and over; hypersensitivity to levocetirizine, cetirizine or their components; renal failure

Interactions
DRUGS
CNS depressants: Possibly increased CNS depression
MAO inhibitors: Possibly prolonged and intensified anticholinergic effects
ritonavir: Possibly increased risk of adverse effects of levocetirizine
theophylline: Possibly decreased clearance of levocetirizine
ACTIVITIES
alcohol use: Possibly increased CNS depression

Adverse Reactions
CNS: Aggression, agitation, asthenia, depression, dizziness, fatigue, fever, hallucinations, insomnia, movement disorders, myoclonus and extrapyramidal

J
K
L

symptoms, paraesthesia, seizures, somnolence, suicidal ideation, syncope, tic, tremor, vertigo
CV: Edema, palpitations, tachycardia
EENT: Blurred vision, dry mouth, epistaxis, nasopharyngitis, pharyngitis, visual disturbances
GI: Hepatitis, increased appetite, nausea, vomiting
GU: Dysuria, urinary retention
MS: myalgia
RESP: Cough, dyspnea
SKIN: Fixed drug eruption, pruritus, rash, urticaria
Other: Anaphylaxis, angioedema, weight gain

Nursing Considerations

• Use levocetirizine cautiously in patients with predisposing risk factors for urinary retention, such as spinal cord lesion or prostatic hyperplasia. Monitor patient's intake and output closely. If urinary retention is suspected, notify prescriber and expect drug to be discontinued if confirmed.

• Monitor patient for abnormal thinking, such as desire to harm oneself. Notify prescriber immediately if present.

• Expect to stop drug at least 72 hours before skin tests for allergies because drug may inhibit cutaneous histamine response, thus producing false-negative results.

PATIENT TEACHING

• Instruct patient to take drug exactly as prescribed. For oral solution, patient should use appropriate measuring device.

• Urge patient to avoid alcohol while taking levocetirizine

• Advise patient to avoid hazardous activities until drug's CNS effects are known.

• Tell patient to notify prescriber if he is feeling bladder fullness or notices that his urine output is significantly less than his intake.

• Warn patient that if he develops abnormal thoughts, especially thoughts of harming himself, he should notify prescriber immediately.

Mechanism of Action

By supplementing a low level of endogenous dopamine, levodopa helps control alterations in voluntary muscle movement (such as tremors and rigidity) in Parkinson's disease. Dopamine, a neurotransmitter synthesized and released by neurons leading from substantia nigra to basal ganglia, is essential for normal motor function. By stimulating peripheral and central dopaminergic 2 (D 2) receptors on postsynaptic cells, dopamine inhibits the firing of striatal neurons (such as cholinergic neurons). In Parkinson's disease, progressive degeneration of these neurons substantially reduces the supply of intrasynaptic dopamine. Levodopa, a dopamine precursor, increases the dopamine supply in neurons, making more available to stimulate dopaminergic receptors.

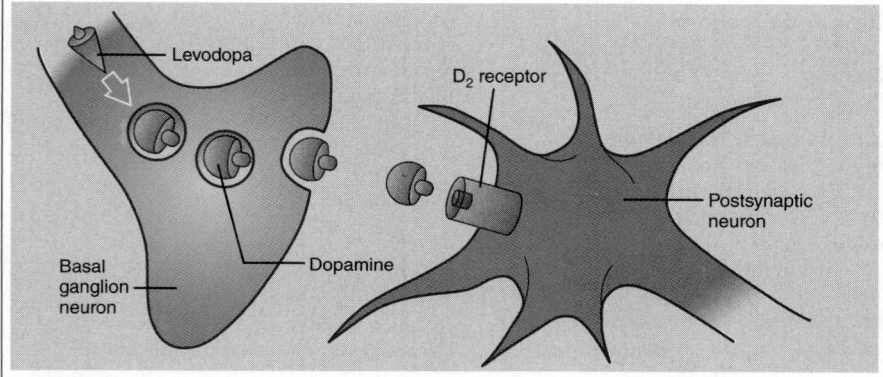

levodopa

Dopar, Larodopa

Class and Category

Chemical class: Dihydroxyphenylalanine isomer, metabolic precursor of dopamine
Therapeutic class: Antidyskinetic
Pregnancy category: Not rated

Indications and Dosages

➤ *To manage symptoms of primary Parkinson's disease, postencephalitic parkinsonism, and parkinsonism caused by CNS injury from carbon monoxide or manganese intoxication*

CAPSULES, TABLETS

Adults and children age 12 and over.
Initial: 250 mg daily in divided doses twice daily to four times daily. Increased by 100 to 750 mg every 3 to 7 days, as indicated. *Maximum:* 8 g daily.

Contraindications

Angle-closure glaucoma, history of melanoma, hypersensitivity to levodopa or its components, suspicious undiagnosed skin lesions, use within 14 days of MAO inhibitor therapy

Route	Onset	Peak	Duration
P.O.	14–21 days*	Unknown	5 hr

Interactions

DRUGS

antacids: Increased blood levodopa level
antihypertensives: Risk of orthostatic hypotension
benzodiazepines: Possibly decreased therapeutic effects of levodopa
bromocriptine: Possibly additive effects of levodopa
furazolidone, MAO inhibitors, procarbazine: Risk of severe hypertension
haloperidol, loxapine, molindone, papaverine, phenothiazines, phenytoin, rauwolfia alkaloids: Decreased effects of levodopa
inhaled anesthetics, sympathomimetics: Increased risk of arrhythmias

iron salts: Possibly decreased blood level and effectiveness of levodopa
methyldopa: Possibly toxic CNS effects
metoclopramide: Possibly worsening of Parkinson's disease and decreased therapeutic effects of metoclopramide
pyridoxine (vitamin B_6): Decreased antidyskinetic effect of levodopa

FOODS

high-protein food: Decreased levodopa absorption

ACTIVITIES

cocaine use: Increased risk of arrhythmias

Adverse Reactions

CNS: Aggressiveness, anxiety, ataxia, confusion, delusions, dizziness, dream disturbances, dyskinesia, dystonia, euphoria, hallucinations, headache, increased tremor, insomnia, malaise, mood changes, severe depression, suicidal tendencies, syncope, weakness
CV: Arrhythmias, hot flashes, orthostatic hypotension, palpitations
EENT: Bitter aftertaste, blurred vision, darkened saliva, diplopia, dry mouth, increased salivation, mydriasis, tooth clenching and grinding
GI: Abdominal pain, anorexia, constipation, diarrhea, flatulence, GI bleeding, hepatotoxicity, hiccups, indigestion, nausea, vomiting
GU: Darkened urine, priapism, urine retention
SKIN: Darkened sweat, diaphoresis, rash

Nursing Considerations

- Expect to discontinue levodopa 6 to 8 hours before surgery to avoid interactions with anesthetics.
- Observe patient for mental or behavioral changes and suicidal tendencies. Notify prescriber immediately if they occur.
- Watch for muscle twitching and blepharospasm (eyelid spasm), which are early signs of levodopa overdose. Report them at once.
- Expect patient to be tested for acromegaly and diabetes during long-term levodopa therapy. Also expect to monitor hematopoietic, hepatic, and renal function.

PATIENT TEACHING

- Advise patient to take levodopa with meals if she experiences adverse GI reactions.

---

* With multiple doses.

J
K
L

• Because protein impairs drug absorption, instruct patient to avoid high-protein meals during levodopa therapy and to distribute protein intake equally throughout the day.

• Caution patient to avoid excessive use of vitamins and fortified cereals that contain vitamin B_6 or iron, which can reduce levodopa's effects.

• Instruct patient to report fainting, increased muscle tremor, difficult urination, and severe or persistent nausea and vomiting.

• Urge patient to continue taking drug as prescribed even if results of therapy aren't evident immediately.

• Inform patient that saliva, sweat, and urine may darken but that this isn't harmful.

• Direct patient to protect drug from heat, light, and moisture and to discard darkened pills because they have lost their potency.

• Advise patient to change position slowly to minimize orthostatic hypotension.

• Caution male patient about risk of priapism (persistent, painful erection), and urge him to seek medical help immediately if it occurs.

levofloxacin

Levaquin

Class and Category

Chemical class: Fluoroquinolone
Therapeutic class: Antibiotic
Pregnancy category: C

Indications and Dosages

➤ *To reduce incidence or progression of inhalation anthrax after exposure to aerosolized Bacillus anthracis; to treat plague, including pneumonic and septicemic plague, caused by Yersinia pestis; to provide prophylaxis for plague*

TABLETS, I.V. INFUSION, ORAL SOLUTION
Adults and children weighing more than 50 kg (110 lb). 500 mg (over 60 min for I.V. infusion) daily for 60 days for treatment of inhalation anthrax and 10 to 14 days for treatment of plague.
Children weighing less than 50 kg (110 lb) and 6 months of age or older.

8 mg/kg (over 60 min for I.V. infusion) every 12 hr for 60 days for treatment of inhalation anthrax and 10 to 14 days for treatment of plague. *Maximum:* 250 mg/dose.

➤ *To treat acute maxillary sinusitis caused by* Haemophilus influenzae, Moraxella catarrhalis, *or* Streptococcus pneumoniae

TABLETS, I.V. INFUSION, ORAL SOLUTION
Adults. 500 mg daily (over 60 to 90 min for I.V. infusion) for 10 to 14 days. Or 759 mg daily for 5 days.

➤ *To treat acute exacerbation of chronic bacterial bronchitis caused by* H. influenzae, H. parainfluenzae, M. catarrhalis, S. pneumoniae, *or* Staphylococcus aureus

TABLETS, I.V. INFUSION, ORAL SOLUTION
Adults. 500 mg daily (over 60 to 90 min for I.V. infusion) for 7 days.

➤ *To treat community-acquired pneumonia caused by* Chlamydia pneumoniae, H. influenzae, H. parainfluenzae, Klebsiella pneumoniae, Legionella pneumophila, M. catarrhalis, Mycoplasma pneumoniae, S. aureus, *or* S. pneumoniae

TABLETS, I.V. INFUSION, ORAL SOLUTION
Adults. 500 mg daily (over 60 to 90 min for I.V. infusion) for 7 to 14 days. Alternatively, for infection caused by *C. pneumoniae, H. influenzae, H. parainfluenzae, M. pneumoniae,* or *S. pneumoniae,* 750 mg daily (over 60 to 90 min for I.V. infusion) for 5 days.

➤ *To treat uncomplicated UTI caused by* Escherichia coli, K. pneumoniae, *or* Staphylococcus saprophyticus

TABLETS, I.V. INFUSION, ORAL SOLUTION
Adults. 250 mg daily (over 60 to 90 min for I.V. infusion) for 3 days.

➤ *To treat complicated UTI caused by* Enterococcus faecalis, E. cloacae, E. coli, K. pneumoniae, Proteus mirabilis, *or* Pseudomonas aeruginosa *or acute pyelonephritis caused by* E. coli

TABLETS, I.V. INFUSION, ORAL SOLUTION
Adults. 250 mg daily (over 60 to 90 min for I.V. infusion) for 10 days.

➤ *To treat complicated UTI caused by* E. coli, K. pneumoniae, *or* P. mirabilis *or acute pyelonephritis caused by* E. coli

TABLETS, I.V. INFUSION, ORAL SOLUTION
Adults. 750 mg daily (over 90 min for I.V. infusion) for 5 days.
➤ *To treat mild to moderate skin and soft-tissue infections caused by* S. aureus *or* Streptococcus pyogenes
TABLETS, I.V. INFUSION, ORAL SOLUTION
Adults. 500 mg daily (over 60 to 90 min for I.V. infusion) for 7 to 10 days.
➤ *To treat complicated skin and soft-tissue infections caused by methicillin-sensitive* Enterococcus faecalis, Proteus mirabilis, S. aureus, *or* S. pyogenes; *to treat nosocomial pneumonia caused by* S. aureus, Pseudomonas aeruginosa, Serratia marcescens, E. coli, K. pneumoniae, H. influenzae, *or* S. pneumoniae
TABLETS, I.V. INFUSION, ORAL SOLUTION
Adults. 750 mg daily (over 60 to 90 min for I.V. infusion) for 7 to 14 days.
➤ *To treat chronic bacterial prostatitis caused by* E. coli, E. faecalis, *or* S. epidermidis
TABLETS, I.V. INFUSION, ORAL SOLUTION
Adults. 500 mg daily (over 60 to 90 min for I.V. infusion) for 28 days.
DOSAGE ADJUSTMENT For patients with creatinine clearance of 20 to 49 ml/min and normal dosage is 750 mg, dosage interval increased to every 48 hr; for normal dosage of 500 mg, one dose of 500 mg given, followed by 250 mg every 24 hr. For patients with creatinine clearance of 10 to 19 ml/min or who are receiving dialysis, and normal dosage is 750 mg, one dose of 750 mg given, followed by 500 mg every 48 hr; for normal dosage of 500 mg, one dose of 500 mg given, followed by 250 mg every 48 hr.; and for normal dosage of 250 mg (no information on dosing adjustment available for patient on dialysis at this dosage), dosage interval increased to every 48 hr unless the 250 mg dosage is used to treat uncomplicated UTI, then no dosage adjustment is required.

Mechanism of Action
Interferes with bacterial cell replication by inhibiting the bacterial enzyme DNA gyrase, which is essential for replication and repair of bacterial DNA.

Contraindications
Hypersensitivity to levofloxacin, other fluoroquinolones, or their components; myasthenia gravis

Interactions
DRUGS
aluminum-, calcium-, or magnesium-containing antacids; didanosine; iron; sucralfate; zinc: Reduced GI absorption of levofloxacin
antineoplastics: Decreased blood levofloxacin level
cimetidine: Increased blood levofloxacin level
cyclosporine: Increased risk of nephrotoxicity
NSAIDs: Possibly increased CNS stimulation and risk of seizures
oral anticoagulants: Increased anticoagulant effect and risk of bleeding
oral antidiabetic drugs: Possibly hyperglycemia or hypoglycemia
theophylline: Increased blood theophylline level and risk of toxicity
ACTIVITIES
sun exposure: Increased risk of photosensitivity

Adverse Reactions
CNS: Anxiety, CNS stimulation, dizziness, fever, headache, increased ICP, insomnia, light-headedness, nervousness, paranoia, peripheral neuropathy, psychosis, seizures, sleep disturbance, suicidal ideation
CV: Arrhythmias, leukocytoclastic vasculitis, prolonged QT interval, torsades de pointes, vasculitis, vasodilation
EENT: Blurred vision, decreased visual acuity, diplopia, dysphonia, scotoma, taste perversion, tinnitus, uveitis
ENDO: Hyperglycemia, hypoglycemia
GI: Abdominal pain, acute hepatic necrosis or failure, anorexia, constipation, diarrhea, flatulence, hepatitis, hepatotoxicity, indigestion, jaundice, nausea, pseudomembranous colitis, vomiting
GU: Acute renal failure or insufficiency, crystalluria, interstitial nephritis, vaginal candidiasis
HEME: Agranulocytosis, aplastic anemia, eosinophilia, hemolytic anemia, leukopenia, pancytopenia, thrombocytopenia

J
K
L

MS: Arthralgia, arthritis, back pain, gait abnormality, myalgia, rhabdomyolysis, tendon or muscle rupture, tendinopathy
RESP: Allergic pneumonitis
SKIN: Photosensitivity, pruritus, rash, Stevens-Johnson syndrome, toxic epidermal necrolysis, urticaria
Other: Anaphylaxis, angioedema, multiorgan failure, serum sickness

Nursing Considerations

• Use levofloxacin cautiously in patients with renal insufficiency. Monitor renal function as appropriate during treatment.
• Use drug cautiously in patients with CNS disorders, such as epilepsy, that may lower the seizure threshold. Also use cautiously in patients taking corticosteroids, especially elderly patients, because of increased risk of tendon rupture.
• Expect to obtain culture and sensitivity tests before levofloxacin treatment begins.
• Know that levofloxacin therapy should begin as soon as possible after suspected or confirmed exposure to *Y. pestis.*
• Avoid giving drug within 2 hours of antacids.
• Give parenteral form over 60 to 90 minutes, depending on dosage, because bolus or rapid I.V. delivery may cause hypotension.

WARNING Stop levofloxacin at first sign of hypersensitivity, including rash and jaundice, because drug may lead to anaphylaxis. Reaction may occur after first dose. Expect to give epinephrine and provide supportive care.

• Monitor blood glucose level, especially in diabetic patient who takes an oral antidiabetic or uses insulin, because levofloxacin may alter blood glucose level. If so, notify prescriber, stop drug immediately if patient has hypoglycemia, and provide prescribed treatment.
• Monitor QT interval if needed. If it lengthens, notify prescriber at once and stop drug. Patients with hypokalemia, significant bradycardia, or cardiomyopathy and those receiving a class IA or III antiarrhythmic shouldn't receive levofloxacin.
• Notify prescriber if patient has symptoms of peripheral neuropathy (pain; burning; tingling; numbness; weakness; altered

sensations of light touch, pain, temperature, position sense, or vibration sense), which could be permanent; or CNS abnormalities (seizures, psychosis, increased ICP, or CNS stimulation), which may lead to more serious adverse reactions, such as suicidal ideation. In each case, expect to discontinue levofloxacin.
• Watch for evidence of tendon rupture (inflammation, pain, swelling) during and up to several months after therapy, especially in children, elderly patients, patients receiving corticosteroids, and patients with kidney, heart, and lung transplants. Notify prescriber about suspected tendon rupture, and have patient rest and refrain from exercise until tendon rupture has been ruled out. If present, expect to provide supportive care, as ordered.
• Monitor patient's bowel elimination. If diarrhea develops, obtain stool culture to check for pseudomembranous colitis. If confirmed, expect to stop drug and give fluid, electrolytes, and antibiotics effective against *Clostridium difficile.*
• Be aware that children have a higher incidence of musculoskeletal adverse reactions, especially arthralgia, arthritis, gait abnormality, and tendinopathy. Report any complaint involving the musculoskeletal system promptly to prescriber.

PATIENT TEACHING

• If patient will take oral solution form of levofloxacin, tell him to take it 1 hour before or 2 hours after eating.
• Advise patient to increase fluid intake during therapy to prevent crystalluria.
• Direct patient to take an antacid, didanosine, iron, sucralfate, or zinc at least 2 hours before or after levofloxacin.
• Tell patient to complete the drug as prescribed, even if symptoms subside.
• Urge patient to avoid excessive sun exposure and to wear sunscreen because of increased risk of photosensitivity. Tell patient to notify prescriber at first sign.
• Caution patient to avoid hazardous activities until drug's CNS effects are known.
• Tell patient to stop drug and notify prescriber if he develops tendon pain or inflammation, or abnormal changes in motor or sensory function.

• Urge patient to stop drug and tell prescriber about rash or other allergic reaction.
• Advise diabetic patient to monitor blood glucose level and report changes.
• Urge patient to tell prescriber about severe diarrhea, even if it's more than 2 months after drug therapy ends. Additional treatment may be needed.
• Advise patient to notify prescriber about heart palpitations or loss of consciousness. An ECG may be needed to detect adverse drug effects on the patient's heart.

levomilnacipran hydrochloride

Fetzima

Class and Category

Chemical class: Selective norepinephrine and serotonin reuptake inhibitor
Therapeutic class: Antidepressant
Pregnancy category: C

Indications and Dosages

➤ *To treat major depressive disorder*
EXTENDED RELEASE CAPSULES
Adults. *Initial:* 20 mg once daily for two days then increased to 40 mg once daily. Dosage further increased in 40-mg increments at intervals of 2 or more days, as needed. *Maximum:* 120 mg once daily.
DOSAGE ADJUSTMENT For patients with moderate renal impairment (creatinine clearance of 30 to 59 ml/min), maintenance dosage should not exceed 80 mg once daily. For patients with severe renal impairment (creatinine clearance of 15 to 29 ml/min), maintenance dosage should not exceed 40 mg once daily.

Mechanism of Action

Inhibits reuptake of norepinephrine and serotonin by CNS neurons without affecting uptake of dopamine or other neurotransmitters, thereby increasing amount of norepinephrine and serotonin available in nerve synapses in the central nervous system. Elevated norepinephrine and serotonin levels may relieve symptoms of depression.

Contraindications

Hypersensitivity to levomilnacipran, milnacipran, or its components; uncontrolled narrow-angle glaucoma; use within 14 days of MAO inhibitor therapy, including reversible agents such as intravenous methylene blue or linezolid

Interactions

DRUGS
antipsychotics or other dopamine antagonists, MAO inhibitors, other serotonergic drugs (buspirone, fentanyl, lithium, St. John's Wort, tramadol, tricyclic antidepressants, triptans, tryptophan), selective serotonin reuptake inhibitors, serotonin-norepinephrine reuptake inhibitors: Possibly development of serotonin syndrome or neuroleptic malignant syndrome-like reactions
aspirin, NSAIDs, warfarin: Increased risk of bleeding
CNS-active drugs: Possibly increased CNS effects
ketoconazole: Increased exposure of levomilnacipran resulting in increased risk of adverse reactions
ACTIVITIES
alcohol use: Increased risk of adverse reactions

Adverse Reactions

CNS: Activation of hypomania or mania, aggression, agitation, anger, anxiety, delirium, depression, dizziness, extrapyramidal disorder, fatigue, fever, hallucinations, headache, hypoesthesia, insomnia, irritability, loss of consciousness, migraine, panic attack, paresthesia, seizures, serotonin syndrome, suicidal ideation, syncope, thirst, tremor
CV: Chest pain, extrasystoles, hypertension, hypertensive crisis, hypotension, increased heart rate, palpitations, peripheral edema, supraventricular tachycardia, tachycardia
EENT: Angle closure glaucoma, blurred vision, conjunctival hemorrhage, dry eye, mydriasis
ENDO: Hot flashes
GI: Abdominal distention or pain, anorexia, constipation, diarrhea, elevated liver enzymes, flatulence, nausea, vomiting
GU: Decreased libido, dysuria, ejaculation disorder, erectile dysfunction, hematuria,

J
K
L

prostatitis, proteinuria, scrotal or testicular pain, testicular swelling, urinary hesitation or retention

HEME: Ecchymosis, epitaxis, hematoma, hemorrhage, petechiae

RESP: Dyspnea,

SKIN: Dry skin, erythema multiforme, excessive sweating including night sweats, flushing, pruritus, rash, urticaria

Nursing Considerations

• Use levomilnacipran cautiously in patients with renal impairment and patients with significant hypertension or cardiac disease. Also use cautiously in patients with a history of dysuria, especially men with prostatic hypertrophy, prostatitis, and other lower urinary tract obstructive disorders.

• Know that at least 14 days should elapse between stopping an MAO inhibitor and starting levomilnacipran. At least 7 days should elapse between stopping levomilnacipran and starting an MAO inhibitor antidepressant.

• Measure patient's blood pressure and heart rate before starting and periodically during levomilnacipran therapy because drug can raise blood pressure and heart rate. If hypertension or tachycardia occurs and persists, notify prescriber and expect to reduce dosage or discontinue drug.

• Watch closely for suicidal tendencies, especially when therapy starts and after dosage changes.

WARNING Monitor patient closely for serotonin syndrome, a rare but serious adverse effect of selective serotonin reuptake inhibitors such as levomilnacipran. Signs and symptoms include agitation, confusion, diaphoresis, diarrhea, fever, hyperactive reflexes, poor coordination, restlessness, shaking, talking or acting with uncontrolled excitement, tremor, and twitching. In its most severe form, it can resemble neuroleptic malignant syndrome with muscle rigidity, autonomic instability with possible rapid fluctuation of vital signs, and mental status changes. If symptoms occur, notify prescriber immediately, expect to discontinue drug, and provide supportive care.

• Assess effectiveness of levomilnacipran periodically being aware that therapy may

be required for several months or longer. Expect to taper drug when no longer needed, as ordered, to minimize adverse reactions.

PATIENT TEACHING

• Instruct patient to take levomilnacipran capsules whole and not to open, chew or crush capsules.

• Advise patient that drug may cause mild pupillary dilation, which may lead to an episode of acute closure glaucoma. Encourage patient to have an eye exam before starting therapy to see if he is at risk.

• Urge family or caregiver to watch patient closely for suicidal tendencies, especially when therapy starts or dosage changes.

• Caution patient against stopping drug abruptly because serious adverse effects may result.

• Instruct patient to alert all prescribers of levomilnacipran therapy.

• Tell patient to have his blood pressure monitored regularly throughout levomilnacipran therapy.

• Advise patient to avoid activities, such as driving, that require alertness until the CNS effects of levomilnacipran are known.

• Monitor patient to avoid aspirin and NSAIDs, if possible, while taking levomilnacipran.

---

levorphanol tartrate

Levo-Dromoran

Class, Category, and Schedule

Chemical class: Morphinan derivative
Therapeutic class: Analgesic, anesthesia adjunct
Pregnancy category: Not rated
Controlled substance schedule: II

Indications and Dosages

➤ *To relieve moderate to severe pain*

TABLETS

Adults. 2 mg every 6 to 8 hr, as needed. Increased to 3 mg every 6 to 8 hr, if indicated.

I.V. INJECTION

Adults. Up to 1 mg every 3 to 6 hr, as needed.

Maximum: 8 mg daily for non–opioid-dependent patients.

I.M. OR SUBCUTANEOUS INJECTION
Adults. 1 to 2 mg every 6 to 8 hr, as needed.
Maximum: 8 mg daily for non–opioid-dependent patients.
➤ *To provide preoperative sedation*
I.M. OR SUBCUTANEOUS INJECTION
Adults. 1 to 2 mg 60 to 90 min before procedure.

Route	Onset	Peak	Duration
P.O.	10–60 min	90–120 min	4–5 hr
I.V.	Unknown	In 20 min	4–5 hr
I.M.	Unknown	60 min	4–5 hr
SubQ	Unknown	60–90 min	4–5 hr

Mechanism of Action
Decreases intracellular level of cyclic adenosine monophosphate by inhibiting adenylate cyclase, which regulates release of pain neurotransmitters, such as substance P, gamma-aminobutyric acid, dopamine, acetylcholine, and noradrenaline. Levorphanol also stimulates mu and kappa opioid receptors, altering perception of and emotional response to pain.

Incompatibilities
Don't mix levorphanol tartrate with solutions that contain aminophylline, ammonium chloride, amobarbital sodium, chlorothiazide sodium, heparin sodium, methicillin sodium, nitrofurantoin sodium, novobiacin sodium, pentobarbital sodium, perphenazine, phenobarbital sodium, phenytoin, secobarbital sodium, sodium bicarbonate, sodium iodide, sulfadiazine sodium, sulfisoxazole diethanolamine, or thiopental sodium.

Contraindications
Acute alcoholism, acute or severe asthma, anoxia, hypersensitivity to levorphanol tartrate or its components, increased intracranial pressure, respiratory depression, upper airway obstruction

Interactions
DRUGS
alfentanil, CNS depressants, fentanyl, sufentanil: Possibly increased CNS and respiratory depression and hypotension

anticholinergics: Increased risk of severe constipation
antidiarrheals, such as difenoxin and atropine, kaolin, and loperamide: Increased risk of severe constipation and increased CNS depression
antihypertensives: Increased risk of hypotension
buprenorphine: Possibly decreased therapeutic effects of levorphanol and increased risk of respiratory depression
hydroxyzine: Increased risk of CNS depression and hypotension
metoclopramide: Possibly antagonized effects of metoclopramide
naloxone, naltrexone: Decreased therapeutic effects of levorphanol
neuromuscular blockers: Increased risk of prolonged CNS and respiratory depression
ACTIVITIES
alcohol use: Possibly increased CNS and respiratory depression and hypotension

Adverse Reactions
CNS: Amnesia, coma, confusion, delusions, depression, dizziness, drowsiness, dyskinesia, hypokinesia, insomnia, nervousness, personality disorder, seizures
CV: Bradycardia, cardiac arrest, hypotension, orthostatic hypotension, palpitations, shock, tachycardia
EENT: Abnormal vision, diplopia, dry mouth
GI: Abdominal pain, biliary tract spasm, constipation, hepatic failure, indigestion, nausea, vomiting
GU: Dysuria, urine retention
RESP: Apnea, hyperventilation
SKIN: Cyanosis, pruritus, rash, urticaria
Other: injection-site pain, redness, and swelling; physical and psychological dependence

Nursing Considerations
WARNING Be aware that levorphanol may be habit-forming.
• Give drug with food if GI distress occurs.
• If respiratory depression occurs, expect to administer naloxone to reverse it.
• Monitor supine and standing blood pressure, and notify prescriber of orthostatic hypotension.
• Carefully assess for adverse reactions in elderly patients; they are especially sensitive to drug and are at increased risk for constipation.

J
K
L

PATIENT TEACHING
• Advise patient to avoid hazardous activities until drug's CNS effects are known.
• Instruct patient to avoid alcoholic beverages while taking levorphanol.
• Direct patient to change position slowly to minimize orthostatic hypotension.
• Advise patient to notify prescriber if constipation, nausea, or vomiting occurs.
• If patient reports dry mouth, suggest that she use sugarless candy or gum or ice chips.

levothyroxine sodium

(L-thyroxine sodium, T₄, thyroxine sodium)

Eltroxin (CAN), Levo-T, Levothroid, Levoxyl, PMS-Levothyroxine Sodium (CAN), Synthroid, Unithroid

Class and Category
Chemical class: Synthetic thyroxine (T₄)
Therapeutic class: Thyroid hormone replacement
Pregnancy category: A

Indications and Dosages
➤ *To treat mild hypothyroidism*
TABLETS
Adults. *Initial:* 50 mcg daily, increased by 25 to 50 mcg every 2 to 3 wk until desired response occurs or therapeutic blood level is reached. *Maintenance:* 75 to 125 mcg daily.
DOSAGE ADJUSTMENT For elderly patients and those with cardiovascular disease or chronic hypothyroidism, initial dosage usually reduced to 12.5 to 25 mcg daily and then increased by 12.5 to 25 mcg every 3 to 4 wk until desired response occurs. For elderly patients, maintenance dosage is limited to 75 mcg daily.
Children over age 10. 2 to 3 mcg/kg daily. *Usual:* 150 to 200 mcg daily.
Children ages 6 to 10. 4 to 5 mcg/kg daily. *Usual:* 100 to 150 mcg daily.
Children ages 1 to 5. 3 to 5 mcg/kg daily. *Usual:* 75 to 100 mcg daily.

Infants ages 6 to 12 months. 5 to 6 mcg/kg daily. *Usual:* 50 to 75 mcg daily.
Infants under age 6 months. 5 to 6 mcg/kg daily. *Usual:* 25 to 50 mcg daily.
➤ *To treat severe hypothyroidism*
TABLETS
Adults. *Initial:* 12.5 to 25 mcg daily. Increased by 25 mcg every 2 to 3 wk until desired response occurs or therapeutic blood level is reached. *Maintenance:* 75 to 125 mcg daily. *Maximum:* 200 mcg daily.
Children over age 10. 2 to 3 mcg/kg daily. *Usual:* 150 to 200 mcg daily.
Children ages 6 to 10. 4 to 5 mcg/kg daily. *Usual:* 100 to 150 mcg daily.
Children ages 1 to 5. 3 to 5 mcg/kg daily. *Usual:* 75 to 100 mcg daily.
Infants ages 6 to 12 months. 5 to 6 mcg/kg daily. *Usual:* 50 to 75 mcg daily.
Infants under age 6 months. 5 to 6 mcg/kg daily. *Usual:* 25 to 50 mcg daily.
I.V. OR I.M. INJECTION
Adults. 50 to 100 mcg daily until therapeutic blood level is reached.
Children. 75% of usual P.O. dose daily until therapeutic blood level is reached.
➤ *To treat myxedema coma*
I.V. INJECTION
Adults. 200 to 500 mcg on day 1. If no significant improvement, 100 to 300 mcg on day 2. Daily dose continued as prescribed until therapeutic blood level is reached and P.O. administration is tolerated.
Children. 75% of usual P.O. dose daily until therapeutic blood level is reached and P.O. administration is tolerated.

Route	Onset	Peak	Duration
P.O.	3–5 days	3–4 wk	1–3 wk
I.V.	6–8 hr	24 hr	Unknown
I.M.	Unknown	Unknown	1–3 wk

Mechanism of Action
Replaces endogenous thyroid hormone, which may exert its physiologic effects by controlling DNA transcription and protein synthesis. Levothyroxine has all the following actions of endogenous thyroid hormone. The drug:
• increases energy expenditure
• accelerates the rate of cellular oxidation, which stimulates body tissue growth, maturation, and metabolism

• regulates differentiation and proliferation of stem cells
• aids in myelination of nerves and development of synaptic processes in the nervous system
• regulates growth
• decreases blood and hepatic cholesterol concentrations
• enhances carbohydrate and protein metabolism, increasing gluconeogenesis and protein synthesis.

Contraindications

Acute MI (unless caused or complicated by hyperthyroidism), hypersensitivity to levothyroxine or its components, uncorrected adrenal insufficiency, untreated thyrotoxicosis

Interactions

DRUGS

adrenocorticoids: Possibly adrenocorticoid *dosage adjustments* as thyroid status changes
aluminum-and magnesium-containing antacids, bile acid sequestrants, calcium carbonate, cation exchange resins, cholestyramine, colestipol, ferrous sulfate, kayexalate, orlistat, sucralfate: Possibly reduced effects of levothyroxine
amiodarone, iodide: Possibly hyperthyroidism
beta blockers: Possibly impaired action of beta blockers and decreased conversion of T_4 to triiodothyronine (T_3)
cholestyramine, colestipol: Delayed or inhibited levothyroxine absorption
digoxin: Reduced digoxin effects
estrogen, phenylbutazone, phenytoin: Reduced binding of levothyroxine to protein, possibly requiring increased levothyroxine dosage
insulin, oral antidiabetic drugs: Possibly uncontrolled diabetes mellitus, requiring increased dosage of insulin or oral antidiabetic drug
ketamine: Possibly hypertension and tachycardia
maprotiline: Increased risk of arrhythmias
oral anticoagulants: Altered anticoagulant activity, possibly need for anticoagulant dosage adjustment
selective serotonin reuptake inhibitors, tricyclic and tetracyclic antidepressants: Increased therapeutic and toxic effects of both drugs

sympathomimetics: Increased risk of coronary insufficiency in patients with coronary artery disease
theophylline: Decreased theophylline clearance
FOODS
dietary fiber, soybean flour (infant formula), walnuts: Possibly decreased absorption of levothyroxine from GI tract

Adverse Reactions

CNS: Fatigue, headache, insomnia, somnolence
ENDO: Hyperthyroidism (with overdose)
GI: Dysphagia
MS: Muscle weakness, myalgia, slipped capital femoral epiphysis
SKIN: Alopecia (transient), rash, urticaria
Other: Weight gain

Nursing Considerations

• Administer levothyroxine tablets as a single daily dose 30 to 60 minutes before breakfast. If patient has difficulty swallowing, crush tablet and suspend in a small amount of water or food.
• To prevent decreased drug absorption, give oral levothyroxine at least 4 hours before or after aluminum-or magnesium-containing antacids, bile acid sequestrants, calcium carbonate, cation exchange resins, cholestyramine, colestipol, ferrous sulfate, kayexalate, or sucralfate.
• Expect to give drug I.V. or I.M. if patient can't take tablets. Be aware that drug shouldn't be given subcutaneously.
• For I.V. use, reconstitute drug by adding 5 ml of normal saline solution.
• Monitor PT of patient who is receiving anticoagulants; she may require a dosage adjustment.
• Monitor blood glucose level of diabetic patient. Prescriber may reduce antidiabetic drug dosage as thyroid hormone level enters therapeutic range.
• Expect patient to undergo thyroid function tests regularly during levothyroxine therapy.
PATIENT TEACHING
• Inform patient that levothyroxine replaces a hormone that is normally produced by the thyroid gland and that she'll probably need to take drug for life.
• Instruct patient to take drug at least 30 minutes before breakfast because drug absorption is increased on an empty stomach and evening doses may cause insomnia.

J
K
L

• Emphasize the need to take levothyroxine with a full glass of water to avoid choking, gagging, having tablet stick in throat, and developing heartburn afterward.

• Instruct patient to separate iron and calcium supplements and antacids by at least 4 hours from levothyroxine doses.

• Inform patient that drug may require a few weeks to take effect.

• Advise patient not to stop drug or change dosage unless instructed by prescriber.

• Instruct patient to report signs of hyperthyroidism, such as diarrhea, excessive sweating, heat intolerance, insomnia, palpitations, weight loss, chest pain, shortness of breath, leg cramps, headache, nervousness, irritability, tremors, changes in appetite, vomiting, fever, and changes in menstrual periods.

• Tell patient to notify prescriber if rash or hives develop during drug use.

• Inform patient that transient hair loss may occur during first few months of levothyroxine therapy.

• Instruct female patient of childbearing age to notify prescriber immediately if she becomes pregnant because levothyroxine dosage may need to be increased.

---

lidocaine hydrochloride

(lignocaine hydrochloride)

Alphacaine (CAN), Anestacon, DermaFlex, Dilocaine, L-Caine, Lidoderm, Xylocaine, Xylocard (CAN), Zingo

Class and Category

Chemical class: Aminoacetamide
Therapeutic class: Class IB antiarrhythmic, local anesthetic
Pregnancy category: B

Indications and Dosages

➤ *To treat ventricular tachycardia or ventricular fibrillation*

I.V. INFUSION AND INJECTION

Adults. *Loading:* 50 to 100 mg (or 1 to 1.5 mg/kg), given at 25 to 50 mg/min. If desired response isn't achieved after 5 to

10 min, second dose of 25 to 50 mg (or 0.5 to 0.75 mg/kg) given every 5 to 10 min until maximum loading dose (300 mg in 1 hr) has been given. *Maintenance:* 20 to 50 mcg/kg/ min (1 to 4 mg/min) by continuous infusion. Smaller bolus dose repeated 15 to 20 min after start of infusion if needed to maintain therapeutic blood level. *Maximum:* 300 mg (or 3 mg/kg) over 1 hr.

Children. *Loading:* 1 mg/kg. *Maintenance:* 30 mcg/kg/min by continuous infusion. *Maximum:* 3 mg/kg.

DOSAGE ADJUSTMENT For elderly patients receiving I.V. lidocaine to treat arrhythmias and for patients with acute hepatitis or decompensated cirrhosis, loading dose and continuous infusion rate reduced by 50%.

I.M. INJECTION

Adults. 300 mg, repeated after 60 to 90 min, if needed.

➤ *To provide topical anesthesia for skin or mucous membranes*

FILM-FORMING GEL, JELLY, OR OINTMENT

Adults. Thin layer applied to skin or mucous membranes as needed before procedure.

TRANSDERMAL PATCH

Adults. 1 to 3 patches applied over most painful area only once for up to 12 hr within a 24-hr period.

➤ *To provide topical anesthesia before venous access procedures*

POWDER

Children ages 3 to 18. Compressed gas application of powder to selected skin site 1 to 3 minutes before procedure.

Route	Onset	Peak	Duration
I.V.	45–90 sec	Immediate	10–20 min
I.M.	5–15 min	Unknown	60–90 min
Topical	2–5 min	Unknown	0.5–1 hr

Mechanism of Action

Combines with fast sodium channels in myocardial cell membranes, which inhibits sodium influx into cells and decreases ventricular depolarization, automaticity, and excitability during diastole. Lidocaine also blocks nerve impulses by decreasing the permeability of neuronal membranes to sodium, which produces local anesthesia.

Contraindications

Adams-Stokes syndrome; hypersensitivity to lidocaine, amide anesthetics, or their components; severe heart block (without artificial pacemaker); Wolff-Parkinson-White syndrome

Interactions

DRUGS

amiodarone, propranolol, quinidine: Additive cardiac effects possibly resulting in toxicity
beta blockers, cimetidine: Increased blood lidocaine level and risk of toxicity
MAO inhibitors, tricyclic antidepressants: Risk of severe, prolonged hypertension
mexiletine, tocainide: Additive cardiac effects
neuromuscular blockers: Possibly increased neuromuscular blockade
phenytoin, procainamide: Increased cardiac depression

Adverse Reactions

CNS: Anxiety; apprehension; confusion; difficulty speaking; dizziness; drowsiness; euphoria; hallucinations; lethargy; light-headedness; malignant hyperthermia; paresthesia; seizures; sensation of heat, cold, or numbness; tremors; twitching; unconsciousness
CV: Bradycardia, cardiac arrest, hypotension, new or worsening arrhythmias
EENT: Blurred vision, diplopia, tinnitus
GI: Nausea, vomiting
HEME: Methemoglobinemia
MS: Muscle weakness, myalgia
RESP: Respiratory arrest or depression
Other: Anaphylaxis, other less severe hypersensitivity reactions; injection-site burning, irritation, petechiae, redness, stinging, swelling, and tenderness; worsened pain

Nursing Considerations

• Use caution in patients with severe hepatic or renal disease because accumulation of lidocaine may occur and lead to toxicity. Also, use caution in patients with hypovolemia, shock, or any form of AV block, including AV block caused by digitalis toxicity.
• Use caution when administering lidocaine to patients with compromised myocardial function because of risk of fluid overload or electrolyte disturbances.

• Observe for respiratory depression after bolus injection and during I.V. infusion of lidocaine.
• Keep life-support equipment and vasopressors nearby during I.V. use in case of respiratory depression or other reactions.
• Carefully check prefilled syringes before using. Use only syringes labeled "for cardiac arrhythmias" for I.V. administration.
• As ordered, titrate I.V. dose to minimum amount needed to prevent arrhythmias. If administration is controlled by a pumping device, stop pump before container runs dry because an air embolism may result. Change intravenous administration apparatus at least once every 24 hours.
• During I.V. administration, place patient on cardiac monitor, as ordered, and closely observe her at all times. Monitor for worsening arrhythmias, widening QRS complex, and prolonged PR interval—possible signs of drug toxicity. If present, notify prescriber and expect to discontinue lidocaine therapy immediately. Although infrequent, also monitor her for hypersensitivity reactions that can be as severe as anaphylaxis following lidocaine administration. If anaphylaxis occurs, discontinue drug, notify prescriber, and provide supportive care.
• Check blood drug level, as ordered. Therapeutic level is 2 to 5 mcg/ml.
• If signs of toxicity, such as dizziness, occur, notify prescriber and expect to discontinue or slow infusion.
• Give I.M. injection in deltoid muscle only.
• Apply lidocaine jelly or ointment to gauze or bandage before applying to skin.
• Monitor vital signs as well as BUN and serum creatinine and electrolyte levels during and after therapy.

PATIENT TEACHING

• Inform patient who receives lidocaine as an anesthetic that she'll feel numbness.
• Advise patient to report difficulty speaking, dizziness, injection-site pain, nausea, numbness or tingling, and vision changes.
• Caution patient to keep lidocaine topical preparations and patches out of reach of children and pets.
• Tell patient to wash hands thoroughly after handling lidocaine topical forms or patch and to avoid getting drug in eyes.

J
K
L

• If patient uses patches, tell her to store them in their sealed envelopes until needed and to apply immediately after removing from the envelope. Tell patient to remove patch if irritation or burning occurs at the site and not to reapply until irritation is gone.
• Tell patient to fold used patches so that the adhesive side sticks to itself and discard where children or pets cannot get to them.
• Warn patient prescribed a lidocaine patch not to place external heat sources, such as a heating pad or electric blanket, on it while wearing it, because heat may cause the drug to be absorbed faster increasing the risk of adverse effects.

linaclotide

Linzess

Class and Category

Chemical class: Guanylate cyclase-C agonist
Therapeutic class: Bowel stimulator
Pregnancy category: C

Indications and Dosages

➤ *To treat irritable bowel syndrome with constipation*

CAPSULES

Adults. 290 mcg once daily on an empty stomach, at least 30 min prior to the first meal of the day.

➤ *To treat chronic, idiopathic constipation*

CAPSULES

Adults. 145 mcg once daily on an empty stomach, at least 30 min prior to the first meal of the day.

Mechanism of Action

Acts locally on the luminal surface of the intestinal epithelium through activation of guanylate cyclase-C, which increases both intracellular and extracellular concentrations of cyclic guanosine monophosphate (cGMP). Elevation in intracellular cGMP stimulates secretion of chloride and bicarbonate into the intestinal lumen, which increases intestinal fluid and accelerates GI transit to relieve constipation. Increased extracellular cGMP decreases the activity of pain-sensing nerves, resulting in a reduction of intestinal pain present with irritable bowel syndrome and constipation.

Contraindications

Hypersensitivity to linaclotide or its components, known or suspected mechanical gastrointestinal obstruction, pediatric patients under 6 years of age

Adverse Reactions

CNS: Fatigue, headache
EENT: Sinusitis
GI: Abdominal distention or pain, diarrhea, dyspepsia, fecal incontinence, flatulence, gastroesophageal reflux, melena, rectal hemorrhage, viral gastroenteritis, vomiting
RESP: Upper respiratory infection
SKIN: Urticaria
Other: Allergic reaction

Nursing Considerations

• Be aware that although linaclotide is contraindicated in children under 6 years of age, it also is not recommended to be given to children between the ages of 6 and 17 years of age.
• Monitor patient for diarrhea that may become severe. If present, withhold drug and notify prescriber.

PATIENT TEACHING

• Instruct patient to swallow the capsules whole and to avoid breaking the capsule apart or chewing it.
• Tell patient that linaclotide is to be taken on an empty stomach 30 minutes before the first meal of the day.
• Advise patient to stop taking linaclotide if severe diarrhea occurs and to contact prescriber.

linagliptin

Tradjenta

Class and Category

Chemical class: Dipeptidyl peptidase-4 enzyme inhibitor
Therapeutic class: Antidiabetic
Pregnancy category: B

Indications and Dosages

➤ *To improve glycemic control in type 2 diabetes mellitus treated with or without a supplemental oral hypoglycemic agent or insulin*

TABLETS

Adults. 5 mg once daily.

DOSAGE ADJUSTMENT For patients taking a supplemental oral hypoglycemic agent or insulin, dosage may need to be reduced.

Mechanism of Action
Inhibits the enzyme, dipeptidyl peptidase-4, that degrades incretin hormones responsible for glucose elevation. This allows levels of incretin hormones to rise, stimulating the release of insulin in a glucose-dependent manner while decreasing the glucagon level in the blood. In addition, glucagon secretion from pancreatic alpha cells is reduced, resulting in a reduction in the amount of glucose released by the liver. These combined actions reduce blood glucose levels, thereby improving glycemic control in type 2 diabetes.

Contraindications
Hypersensitivity to linagliptin or its components, ketoacidosis, sole therapy for type 1 diabetes mellitus

Interactions
DRUGS
P-gp or CYP3A4 inducers (strong) such as rifampin: Decreased linagliptin effectiveness in reducing blood glucose level
sulfonylureas, insulin: Increased risk of hypoglycemia

Adverse Reactions
CNS: Headache
CV: Hyperlipidemia, hypertriglyceridemia
EENT: Nasopharyngitis
ENDO: Hypoglycemia
GI: Acute pancreatitis, constipation, diarrhea
GU: UTI
MS: Arthralgia, back or extremity pain, myalgia
RESP: Bronchial hyperreactivity, cough
SKIN: Localized skin exfoliation, urticaria
Other: Anaphylaxis, angioedema, elevated uric acid, weight gain

Nursing Considerations
WARNING Know that linagliptin's hypersensitivity may be exhibited through serious adverse reactions such as anaphylaxis, angioedema, bronchial hyperreactivity, exfoliative skin conditions, or urticaria. Monitor patient closely for hypersensitivity reactions. If present, withhold drug immediately, notify prescriber, and be prepared to administer emergency care, as ordered.

• Monitor patient closely for hypoglycemia, especially if another antidiabetic drug, such as a sulfonylurea or insulin is used concomitantly. If signs and symptoms of hypoglycemia occur, check patient's blood glucose level. If confirmed, administer 15 grams of an oral rapid-acting carbohydrate. After 15 minutes, repeat blood glucose and, if needed, administer 15 grams of an oral rapid-acting carbohydrate again. (Administer glucagon 1 mg parenterally, as ordered; if patient is unresponsive, and repeat dose in 15 minutes, if needed.) Notify prescriber of incident, as dosage of the other antidiabetic drug may need to be reduced.
• Monitor the patient's blood glucose level routinely to determine response to drug. Expect to check the patient's glycosylated hemoglobin every 3 to 6 months or as ordered to evaluate long-term blood glucose control.
• Monitor patient for signs and symptoms of pancreatitis such as abdominal pain, fever, nausea, sweating, and vomiting. Notify prescriber if present, and expect drug to be discontinued, as acute pancreatitis may become life-threatening.
PATIENT TEACHING
• Urge patient to report evidence of hypoglycemia, such as anxiety, confusion, dizziness, excessive sweating, headache, and nausea.
• Encourage patient to carry hard candy or other simple sugars to treat mild hypoglycemia.
• Urge patient to carry identification indicating that he has diabetes.
• Teach patient how to monitor his blood glucose level.
• Instruct patient about exercise, diet, signs of hyperglycemia and hypoglycemia, hygiene, foot care, and ways to avoid infection.
• Tell patient to stop drug if he experiences signs and symptoms of an allergic reaction such as a rash, skin flaking or peeling, hives, swelling of skin or face including lips and tongue, difficulty breathing or swallowing, or signs and symptoms of acute pancreatitis such as persistent severe abdominal pain radiating to the back, which may or may not be accompanied by vomiting, and to seek medical attention immediately.

J
K
L

lincomycin hydrochloride

Lincocin

Class and Category

Chemical class: Lincosamide
Therapeutic class: Bacteriostatic or bactericidal antibiotic
Pregnancy category: C

Indications and Dosages

➤ *To treat serious respiratory, skin, and soft-tissue infections caused by susceptible strains of streptococci, pneumococci, and staphylococci*

CAPSULES

Adults and adolescents. 500 mg every 6 to 8 hr.

Children over age 1 month. 7.5 to 15 mg/kg every 6 hr; or, 10 to 20 mg/kg every 8 hr.

I.V. INFUSION

Adults. 600 mg to 1 g every 8 to 12 hr. *Maximum:* 8 g daily in divided doses for life-threatening infection.

Children over age 1 month. 10 to 20 mg/kg/day in divided doses every 8 to 12 hr, depending on severity of infection.

I.M. INJECTION

Adults and adolescents. 600 mg every 12 to 24 hr.

Children over age 1 month. 10 mg/kg every 12 to 24 hr.

DOSAGE ADJUSTMENT Dosage reduced by 25% to 30% for patients with severely impaired renal function.

Mechanism of Action

Inhibits protein synthesis in susceptible bacteria by binding to 50S subunit of bacterial ribosomes and preventing peptide bond formation, causing bacterial cells to die.

Incompatibilities

Don't give lincomycin with novobiocin or kanamycin.

Contraindications

Hypersensitivity to lincomycin, clindamycin, or their components

Interactions

DRUGS

antimyasthenic drugs: Possibly antagonized effects of these drugs

chloramphenicol, clindamycin, erythromycin: Possibly blocked access of lincomycin to its site of action
hydrocarbon inhalation anesthetics, neuromuscular blockers: Increased neuromuscular blockade, possibly severe respiratory depression
opioid analgesics: Increased risk of prolonged or increased respiratory depression

Adverse Reactions

CNS: Fever, vertigo
CV: Cardiac arrest and hypotension (with rapid administration)
EENT: Glossitis, stomatitis, tinnitus
GI: Abdominal cramps, colitis, diarrhea, nausea, pseudomembranous colitis, rectal candidiasis, vomiting
GU: Vaginal candidiasis
HEME: Agranulocytosis, eosinophilia, leukopenia, neutropenia, thrombocytopenic purpura
SKIN: Erythema multiforme, rash, Stevens-Johnson syndrome, urticaria
Other: Anaphylaxis, angioedema, superinfection

Nursing Considerations

• Expect to obtain a specimen for culture and sensitivity testing before giving first dose of lincomycin.

WARNING Be aware that some lincomycin preparations contain benzyl alcohol, which can cause a fatal toxic syndrome in neonates or premature infants characterized by CNS, respiratory, circulatory, and renal impairment and metabolic acidosis. Because drug enters breastmilk, breastfeeding patient may need to stop drug or stop breastfeeding.

• Dilute 600-mg dose in at least 100 ml D_5W, $D_{10}W$, normal saline solution, dextrose 5% in normal saline solution, or other compatible diluent recommended by manufacturer. Dilute higher doses in 100 ml of a compatible diluent for each gram being given—for example, dilute a 3-g dose in at least 300 ml of diluent. Use diluted solution within 24 hours if stored at room temperature.

WARNING Give lincomycin over at least 1 hour for each gram being administered. For example, infuse 1 g over 1 hour and 3 g over 3 hours. Too-rapid infusion may result in cardiac arrest or hypotension.

WARNING Monitor patient for hypersensitivity reaction, such as rash, pruritus, wheezing, and dysphagia from laryngeal edema. If a reaction occurs, stop infusion and notify prescriber immediately. If anaphylaxis occurs, give epinephrine, antihistamines, oxygen, and corticosteroids, as prescribed. Be aware that patients with a history of asthma or significant allergies are at increased risk of hypersensitivity.
• Observe patient for evidence of superinfection, such as vaginal itching and sore mouth.
• Monitor patient for signs of pseudomembranous colitis, such as watery, loose stools. Patients with a history of GI disease, particularly colitis or regional enteritis, are at increased risk for colitis. In elderly patients, antibiotic-related diarrhea may be more severe and less well-tolerated. Notify prescriber if severe or prolonged diarrhea develops; it may indicate pseudomembranous colitis caused by *Clostridium difficile*. Expect to withhold lincomycin and treat with fluids, electrolytes, protein, and an antibiotic effective against *C. difficile*.
• Monitor results of liver and renal function tests, CBC, and platelet counts periodically during lincomycin therapy.
• Before diluting drug, store it at a controlled room temperature of 68° to 77° F (20° to 25° C).

PATIENT TEACHING
• Advise patient to take lincomycin capsules with a full glass of water on an empty stomach 1 hour before or 2 hours after meals to maximize drug's effectiveness.
• Review with patient possibly serious adverse reactions, such as difficulty breathing, rash, and chest tightness, and tell her to report any that occur.
• Inform patient that yogurt or buttermilk can help maintain intestinal flora and may decrease the risk of diarrhea.
• Urge patient to tell prescriber about diarrhea that's severe or lasts longer than 3 days. Remind patient that watery or bloody stools can occur 2 or more months after antibiotic therapy and can be serious, requiring prompt treatment.
• Emphasize the importance of following dosage regimen and keeping follow-up medical and laboratory appointments.

lindane
Bio-Well, GBH, G-well, Hexit (CAN), Kildane, Kwell, Kwellada (CAN), Kwildane, PMS-Lindane (CAN), Scabene, Thionex

Class and Category
Chemical class: Benzene derivative
Therapeutic class: Pediculicide, scabicide
Pregnancy category: B

Indications and Dosages
➤ *To treat scabies and pediculosis*
CREAM, LOTION
Adults and children. For scabies, thin layer applied once over entire skin surface. For pediculosis, thin layer applied once to affected skin and hair.
SHAMPOO
Adults and children. 30 ml (for short hair) or 45 ml (for long hair) applied to dry hair and worked into lather for 4 to 5 min.

Mechanism of Action
Penetrates parasite skeleton and inhibits neuronal membrane function, causing seizures and death. Lindane also kills parasite eggs.

Contraindications
Hypersensitivity to lindane or its components, prematurity (in neonates), seizure disorders

Interactions
ACTIVITIES
use of oil-based hair products: Possibly increased absorption of lindane

Adverse Reactions
CNS: Dizziness, irritability, nervousness, restlessness, seizures, unsteadiness
SKIN: Erythema, pruritus, rash, urticaria

Nursing Considerations
• Use lindane cautiously in patients at risk for CNS toxicity, such as infants, elderly patients, and patients weighing less than 110 lb (50 kg).
• Wear gloves when applying drug. If another person will apply drug, supply gloves for use.
• For scabies, apply thin layer of preparation to dry skin and rub in thoroughly. Trim patient's nails, and apply under nails with

toothbrush. Apply to body from neck down, including soles. Leave drug on for 8 to 12 hours (usually overnight), and then remove with bath or shower.
- Expect to reduce application time for infants and children to 6 to 8 hours, as prescribed, because of risk of systemic absorption.
- Keep lindane away from mouth and eyes. Don't use on open wounds, cuts, or sores.
- Expect to give topical steroids or oral antihistamines to reduce pruritus, which may continue for several weeks with scabies.
- For hospitalized patients, use special linen-handling precautions until treatment is completed.

WARNING Be aware that lindane may cause seizures or other adverse CNS reactions. Use it only after other treatments have been tried.
- Monitor immunocompromised patients closely because they're at increased risk for adverse reactions.

PATIENT TEACHING
- Inform patient that lindane is for one-time use but may be reapplied after 1 week if she finds live lice or nits (eggs).
- Caution patient to avoid eyes, mucous membranes, and open areas of skin when applying drug and not to inhale vapors.
- Instruct patient (or parents of a child) to wear gloves when applying drug.
- For scabies, instruct patient to shake lotion bottle well before using and to apply lotion or cream in a thin layer all over body from neck down, avoiding face and scalp. Direct her to leave drug on for 8 to 12 hours and then wash it off in the bath or shower. Explain that itching may persist for several weeks after treatment.
- For pubic lice, instruct patient to shake lotion bottle well before using and to apply a thin layer of lotion to pubic hair and skin as well as to groin, thighs, and lower stomach if they're also affected. Direct her to leave lotion on for 12 hours and then thoroughly wash it off in the bath or shower.
- For head lice, instruct patient to shake lotion bottle well before using and to apply lotion to affected areas of head and scalp as well as nearby hairy areas and rub it in well. Tell her to leave lotion

on for 12 hours and then thoroughly wash it off.
- For head or pubic lice, instruct patient to wash and dry her hair before applying lindane shampoo, especially if she uses oil-based hair products. Instruct her to shake bottle well before using and then apply shampoo to dry hair, working it in thoroughly and adding a small amount of water if needed to form good lather. Direct her to wait 4 minutes, rinse her hair well, and then dry it with a clean towel. Instruct her to use a fine-toothed comb or tweezers to remove nits or nit shells. Direct patient not to use shampoo again for 7 days and then only if she finds live lice. Caution patient not to use shampoo in the shower to avoid getting it in her eyes and mouth.
- Advise patient to wash lindane off her skin and to contact prescriber if irritation (severe itching, hives, or redness) occurs.
- Explain that if lice come back, the problem is probably reinfestation rather than treatment failure.
- Advise patient to notify family members and sexual contacts about infestation.

linezolid
Zyvox

Class and Category
Chemical class: Oxazolidinone
Therapeutic class: Antibiotic
Pregnancy category: C

Indications and Dosages
➤ *To treat vancomycin-resistant* Enterococcus faecium *infections, including bacteremia*
ORAL SUSPENSION, TABLETS, I.V. INFUSION
Adults and adolescents. 600 mg every 12 hr for 14 to 28 days.
Infants and children. 10 mg/kg every 8 hr for 14 to 28 days.
➤ *To treat nosocomial pneumonia caused by* Staphylococcus aureus *(methicillin-susceptible and resistant strains) or* Streptococcus pneumoniae *(penicillin-*

susceptible strains only) and
community-acquired pneumonia,
including accompanying bacteremia,
caused by S. aureus (methicillin-
susceptible strains only) or
S. pneumoniae (penicillin-susceptible
strains only); to treat complicated skin
and soft-tissue infections, including
diabetic foot infections without
concomitant osteomyelitis, caused by
S. aureus (methicillin-susceptible and
resistant strains), Streptococcus
pyogenes, or Streptococcus agalactiae
ORAL SUSPENSION, TABLETS, I.V. INFUSION
Adults and adolescents. 600 mg every
12 hr for 10 to 14 days.
Infants and children. 10 mg/kg every 8 hr
for 10 to 14 days.
➤ *To treat uncomplicated skin and soft-*
tissue infections caused by S. aureus
(methicillin-susceptible strains only) or
S. pyogenes
ORAL SUSPENSION, TABLETS
Adults. 400 mg every 12 hr for 10 to 14 days.
Adolescents. 600 mg every 12 hr for 10 to
14 days.
Children age 5 to 11. 10 mg/kg every 12 hr
for 10 to 14 days.
Infants and children to age 5. 10 mg/kg
every 8 hr.

Incompatibilities
Don't add other drugs to linezolid solution.
Don't infuse linezolid in same I.V. line as
amphotericin B, chlorpromazine
hydrochloride, cotrimoxazole, diazepam,
erythromycin lactobionate, pentamidine
isethionate, or phenytoin sodium because
these drugs are physically incompatible.
Don't infuse linezolid with ceftriaxone
sodium because these drugs are chemically
incompatible.

Contraindications
Carcinoid syndrome; concurrent therapy
with buspirone, dopaminergic agents,
meperidine, sympathomimetic agents,
serotonin 5-HT$_1$ receptor agonists,
serotonin reuptake inhibitors, tricyclic
antidepressants, or vasopressive agents
without careful monitoring; hypersensitivity
to linezolid or its components;
phenylketonuria; thyrotoxicosis;
uncontrolled hypertension; use within
14 days of an MAO inhibitor

Interactions
DRUGS
*adrenergics, including pseudoephedrine and
phenylpropanolamine, dopaminergic agents,
serotonergic agents, vasopressive agents such
as epinephrine or norepinephrine:* Possibly
increased blood pressure
*buspirone, meperidine, serotonergics, tricyclic
antidepressants:* Possibly serotonin syndrome
*carbamazepine, phenytoin, phenobarbital,
rifampin:* Possibly decreased plasma
linezolid level
MAO inhibitors: Increased risk of life-
threatening adverse effects
FOODS
tyramine-containing foods and beverages:
Possibly hypertension

Adverse Reactions
CNS: Dizziness, fever, headache, insomnia,
optic and peripheral neuropathy, serotonin
syndrome
CV: Hypertension
EENT: Oral candidiasis, tooth or tongue
discoloration
ENDO: Hypoglycemia (in diabetics taking
antidiabetic agents)
GI: Abdominal pain, constipation, diarrhea,
indigestion, nausea, pseudomembranous
colitis, vomiting
GU: Vaginal candidiasis
HEME: Anemia, leukopenia, pancytopenia,
thrombocytopenia
SKIN: Pruritus, rash
Other: Lactic acidosis

Nursing Considerations
• Obtain body tissue and fluid specimens
for culture and sensitivity tests, as ordered,
before giving first dose of linezolid. Expect
to start drug before test results are known.
• Be aware that linezolid shouldn't be used to
treat catheter-related bloodstream infections,
catheter-site infections, or infections caused
by gram-negative bacteria because the risk
of death is higher in these infections.
• Infuse I.V. solution over 30 to 120 minutes
with D$_5$W, normal saline solution, or
lactated Ringer's solution.
• ***WARNING*** Monitor CBC weekly, as ordered,
to detect or track worsening myelosuppression in patients who need more
than 2 weeks of therapy, who have
preexisting myelosuppression and are

J
K
L

Mechanism of Action

Linezolid inhibits bacterial protein synthesis by interfering with translation of ribonucleic acid (RNA) to protein. In bacteria, protein synthesis begins with binding of a 30S ribosomal subunit and a 50S ribosomal subunit to a messenger RNA (mRNA) molecule to form a 70S initiation complex. The 50S ribosomal subunit consists of 23S ribosomal RNA (rRNA) and other ribosomal subunits. Then translation begins. Transfer RNA (tRNA) attaches to the 50S subunit and brings specific amino acids into place. As the tRNA and amino acids fall into place, they are joined together by peptide bonds and elongate to form a polypeptide chain, as shown below left. This chain eventually combines with other polypeptide chains to form a complete protein molecule. After translation is complete, the ribosomal subunits fall away and are ready to combine with more mRNA to start the translation process over again.

Linezolid binds to a site on the bacterial 23S rRNA of the 50S subunit. This action prevents formation of a functional 70S initiation complex, an essential component of the bacterial translation. Without proper protein production, as shown below right, susceptible bacteria are unable to multiply. Linezolid is bacteriostatic against staphylococci and enterococci, and bactericidal against most streptococci.

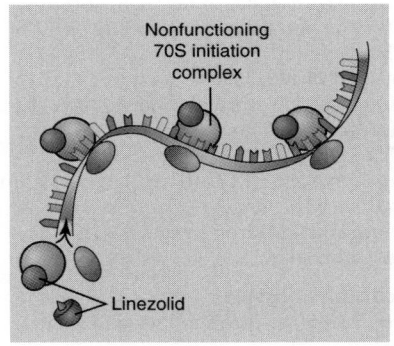

receiving drugs that produce bone marrow suppression, or who have chronic infection and are receiving or have received antibiotic therapy.

• Notify prescriber if patient develops visual impairment that suggests optic neuropathy, such as changes in visual acuity or color vision, blurred vision, lost vision, or visual field defect. If optic or peripheral neuropathy develops, the drug may need to be stopped.

• If patient takes a dopaminergic agent, sympathomimetic agent, or vasopressive agent, monitor blood pressure closely; if monitoring isn't possible, know that linezolid shouldn't be prescribed.

• Be aware that while linezolid should not be given to patients receiving serotonergic drugs, there are some conditions that may be life-threatening and require the use of linezolid, such as the presence of vancomycin-resistent *Enterococcus faecium* (VRE) or infections such as nosocomial pneumonia and complicated skin and skin structure infections, including those caused by *methicillin-resistant Staphylococcus aureus* (MRSA). If patient takes buspirone, meperidine, or a serotonergic or tricyclic antidepressant, watch closely for signs and symptoms of serotonin syndrome; if monitoring isn't possible, know that linezolid shouldn't be prescribed.

• Assess bowel pattern daily. Also watch for secondary infection, including oral candidiasis and profuse, watery diarrhea.

• Monitor patient with diabetes who is also taking antidiabetic medication for hypoglycemia because hypoglycemia has been linked to linezolid use in these patients. If hypoglycemia occurs, treat appropriately and notify prescriber, as the dosage of the antidiabetic medication may need to be decreased.

PATIENT TEACHING
• Caution patient with phenylketonuria that oral suspension contains phenylalanine and that he should receive tablets instead.
• Advise patient not to take OTC cold remedies without consulting prescriber because medications that contain pseudoephedrine or propanolamine may cause or worsen hypertension.
• Instruct patient to avoid foods and beverages that contain large amounts of tyramine, including aged cheese, fermented or air-dried meats, sauerkraut, soy sauce, tap beers, red wines, and protein-rich foods that have been stored for long periods or poorly refrigerated.
• Instruct patient to notify prescriber at once about severe diarrhea, even up to 2 months after linezolid therapy has ended, because additional treatment may be needed.
• Also tell patient to report vision changes and changes in limb sensation (such as pins and needles, numbness, or tingling) because drug may need to be stopped.
• Reassure patient with tooth discoloration that professional dental cleaning can restore tooth color.
• Advise diabetic patients prescribed antidiabetic medications to monitor their blood glucose closely and be prepared to treat hypoglycemia if it should occur. If present, tell patient to notify prescriber as a dosage adjustment may be required in his antidiabetic medication.

---

liothyronine sodium
(L-triiodothyronine, sodium L-triiodothyronine, T₃, thyronine sodium)
Cytomel, Triostat

Class and Category
Chemical class: Synthetic triiodothyronine (T_3)

Therapeutic class: Thyroid hormone replacement
Pregnancy category: A

Indications and Dosages
➤ *To treat mild hypothyroidism*
TABLETS
Adults. *Initial:* 25 mcg daily. Increased by 12.5 to 25 mcg every 1 to 2 wk until response occurs. *Maintenance:* 25 to 50 mcg daily.
DOSAGE ADJUSTMENT For elderly patients and those with cardiovascular disease, initial dose reduced to 5 mcg daily and then increased by 5 mcg every 2 wk.
➤ *To treat congenital hypothyroidism*
TABLETS
Adults and children. *Initial:* 5 mcg daily. Increased by 5 mcg every 3 to 4 days until desired response occurs. *Maintenance:* Highly individualized.
➤ *To treat simple nontoxic goiter*
TABLETS
Adults. *Initial:* 5 mcg daily. Increased by 5 to 10 mcg every 1 to 2 wk up to 25 mcg daily. Then increased by 12.5 to 25 mcg/wk, as indicated. *Maintenance:* 50 to 100 mcg daily.
➤ *To treat myxedema*
TABLETS
Adults. *Initial:* 2.5 to 5 mcg daily. Increased 5 to 10 mcg every 1 to 2 wk up to 25 mcg daily. Then increased by 12.5 to 25 mcg every 1 to 2 wk, as indicated. *Maintenance:* 25 to 50 mcg daily.
➤ *To treat myxedema coma or premyxedema coma (severe hypothyroidism)*
I.V. INJECTION
Adults. *Initial:* 25 to 50 mcg. Repeated every 4 to 12 hr according to patient's response. Then P.O. therapy is resumed as soon as possible.
DOSAGE ADJUSTMENT When treating myxedema coma in patients with known or suspected cardiovascular disease, initial dose decreased to 10 to 20 mcg.
➤ *To differentiate hyperthyroidism from euthyroidism (T_3 suppression test)*
TABLETS
Adults. 75 to 100 mcg daily for 7 days.

Route	Onset	Peak	Duration
P.O.	24–72 hr	48–72 hr	Up to 72 hr
I.V.	2–4 hr	2 days	Unknown

Mechanism of Action

Replaces endogenous thyroid hormone, which may exert its physiologic effects by controlling DNA transcription and protein synthesis. Like endogenous thyroid hormone, liothyronine:

• increases energy expenditure
• accelerates the rate of cellular oxidation, which stimulates body tissue growth, maturation, and metabolism
• regulates differentiation and proliferation of stem cells
• aids in myelination of nerves and development of synaptic processes in the nervous system
• regulates growth
• decreases blood and hepatic cholesterol concentrations
• enhances carbohydrate and protein metabolism, increasing gluconeogenesis and protein synthesis.

Contraindications

Acute MI (unless caused or complicated by hypothyroidism), hypersensitivity to liothyronine or its components, uncorrected adrenal insufficiency, untreated thyrotoxicosis

Interactions

DRUGS

adrenocorticoids: Possibly need for adrenocorticoid dosage adjustments as thyroid status changes
beta blockers: Possibly impaired action of beta blockers
cholestyramine, colestipol: Decreased liothyronine absorption
digoxin: Reduced therapeutic effects of digoxin
estrogen, phenylbutazone, phenytoin: Reduced binding of liothyronine to protein, possibly requiring increased liothyronine dosage
insulin, oral antidiabetic: Possibly uncontrolled diabetes mellitus, requiring increased dosage of insulin or oral antidiabetic
ketamine: Possibly hypertension and tachycardia
maprotiline: Increased risk of arrhythmias
oral anticoagulants: Altered anticoagulant activity, possibly need for anticoagulant dosage adjustment

sympathomimetics: Increased risk of coronary insufficiency in patients with coronary artery disease
theophylline: Decreased theophylline clearance
tricyclic antidepressants: Increased therapeutic and toxic effects of both drugs

Adverse Reactions

CNS: Insomnia
ENDO: Hyperthyroidism (with overdose)
SKIN: Alopecia (transient), rash, urticaria

Nursing Considerations

• Be aware that liothyronine is used most often for rapid onset or rapidly reversible thyroid hormone replacement.
• Administer tablet as a single daily dose before breakfast.
• Give I.V. injections more than 4 hours but less than 12 hours apart.
• Evaluate response to therapy by monitoring pulse rate and blood pressure.
• Expect patient to undergo regular tests of thyroid function during therapy.
• Monitor PT of patient receiving anticoagulants because she may require a dosage adjustment.
• Frequently monitor blood glucose level of diabetic patient. Prescriber may reduce antidiabetic drug dosage as thyroid hormone level enters therapeutic range.
• Be aware that liothyronine is used in T_3 suppression test to differentiate hyperthyroidism from euthyroidism (normal thyroid function). For this test, ^{131}I uptake test is performed before and after liothyronine administration. Suppression of ^{131}I uptake by 50% indicates normal thyroid function.

PATIENT TEACHING

• Inform patient that liothyronine usually is taken for life. Caution her not to discontinue drug or change dosage unless instructed by prescriber.
• Instruct patient to take drug before breakfast; evening doses may cause insomnia.
• Advise patient to report signs of hyperthyroidism, such as chest pain, excessive sweating, heat intolerance, increased pulse rate, nervousness, and palpitations.
• Inform patient that transient hair loss may occur during first few months of therapy.

• Instruct diabetic patient to monitor blood glucose level frequently because antidiabetic drug dosage may need to be reduced.

• Inform patient of need for periodic blood tests to monitor drug effectiveness.

liraglutide

Saxenda, Victoza

Class and Category

Chemical class: Acylated human glucagon-like peptide-1
Therapeutic class: Antidiabetic
Pregnancy category: C (Victoza), X (Saxenda)

Indications and Dosages

➤ *To improve glycemic control as an adjunct to diet and exercise in patients with type 2 diabetes mellitus*

SUBCUTANEOUS INJECTION (VICTOZA)

Adults. *Initial:* 0.6 mg daily for 1 wk, then increased to 1.2 mg daily. *Maximum:* 1.8 mg daily.

➤ *Adjunct for chronic weight management in patients with an initial body mass index of 30 kg/m² or greater, or 27 kg/ m² or greater in the presence of at least one weight-related comorbid condition such as hypertension, type 2 diabetes mellitus, or dyslipidemia*

SUBCUTANEOUS INJECTION (SAXENDA)

Adults. *Initial:* 0.6 mg daily for wk 1, increased to 1.2 mg daily for wk 2, increased to 1.8 mg daily for wk 3, increased 2.4 mg daily for wk 4, and increased to 3 mg daily for wk 5 and onward. *Maintenance:* 3 mg daily.

Route	Onset	Peak	Duration
SubQ	Unknown	8–12 hr	Unknown

Mechanism of Action

Activates the glucagon-like peptide-1 site on pancreatic beta cells, which increases intracellular cyclic AMP, which increases insulin release when blood glucose level is elevated. In addition, because insulin and glucagon levels occur in an inverse relationship to plasma glucose level, increased insulin level will decrease glucagon level, which inhibits glucagon stimulation of the liver that increases plasma glucose level. Although its exact mechanism is unclear, liraglutide also delays gastric emptying, which helps prevent a sudden rise in plasma glucose level after eating. Together these actions work to lower plasma glucose level.

Contraindications

History or presence of medullary thyroid cancer or multiple endocrine neoplasia syndrome type 2, hypersensitivity to liraglutide or its components, ketoacidosis, pregnancy (Saxenda), type 1 diabetes mellitus

Interactions
DRUGS

oral hypoglycemic agents such as sulfonylureas: Increased risk of hypoglycemia
orally administered drugs: Possibly decreased absorption of these drugs

Adverse Reactions

CNS: Anxiety, asthenia, dizziness, fatigue, headache, insomnia, suicidal ideation
CV: Hypertension
EENT: Dry mouth, nasopharyngitis, sinusitis
ENDO: Elevated calcitonin levels, hypoglycemia (type 2 diabetes), thyroid C-cell hyperplasia, thyroid cancer
GI: Abdominal distention or pain, anorexia, cholecystitis, cholelithiasis, constipation, diarrhea, dyspepsia, elevated lipase, flatulence, nausea, pancreatitis, slowed gastric emptying, vomiting
GU: Acute renal failure, elevated serum creatinine level, UTI, worsening of chronic renal failure
MS: Back pain
RESP: Upper respiratory tract infection
SKIN: Pruritus, rash, urticaria
Other: Anaphylaxis, angioedema, antiliraglutide antibodies, dehydration, influenza-like symptoms, injection-site reaction including erythema

Nursing Considerations

• Be aware that liraglutide isn't recommended as first-line therapy for patients with type 2 diabetes mellitus not well controlled with diet and exercise. It also isn't a substitute for insulin therapy.

J
K
L

• Liraglutide shouldn't be given to a patient with a history of thyroid C-cell tumors, including medullary thyroid carcinoma, or to patients with multiple endocrine neoplasia syndrome type 2 because drug may stimulate tumor growth.

• Use liraglutide cautiously in patients with a history of pancreatitis because drug can cause pancreatitis, in patients with impaired hepatic function because drug effects in these patients are unknown, and in patients with renal dysfunction because liraglutide may adversely affect renal function.

• Be aware that dosage of liraglutide given during first week of therapy isn't enough to provide glycemic control, but is given to minimize adverse effects when dosage is increased.

• Monitor patient closely for signs and symptoms of a hypersensitivity reaction that may become serious, especially in patients with a history of angioedema to other medications. If any hypersensitivity reaction occurs, discontinue liraglutide and notify the prescriber.

• Monitor patient's serum calcitonin levels, as indicated. Be aware that elevations occur more often when liraglutide dosage is 1.8 mg daily.

• Monitor patient for pancreatitis, especially when therapy starts or dosage increases. Report persistent severe abdominal pain; it may radiate to the back and may be accompanied by vomiting. If pancreatitis is confirmed, expect to stop drug and do not restart it after episode has been resolved.

• Monitor patient for hypoglycemia, especially if he takes another antidiabetic, such as a sulfonylurea. Report any episode of hypoglycemia because dosage of other antidiabetic may need adjustment. Treat hypoglycemia with a glucose-containing food or beverage, or give glucagons, as ordered, to raise blood glucose level.

• Monitor patient's blood glucose level and hemoglobin A_{1C} regularly, as ordered, to assess effectiveness of drug.

• Monitor effectiveness of all other oral drugs because liraglutide slows gastric emptying and may impair their absorption. Alert prescriber to any concerns.

• Be aware that if more than 3 days has elapsed since the last liraglutide dose, the drug should be reinitiated at the initial dose of 0.6 mg.

• Monitor patient closely for suicidal ideation such as depression, or unusual changes in mood or behavior. If patient becomes suicidal, take safety precautions immediately, discontinue liraglutide therapy, as ordered, and notify prescriber.

PATIENT TEACHING

• Teach patient how to use prefilled multi-dose pen and how to give a subcutaneous injection. Explain that he'll need to inject drug daily but that he can do it at any time of day, independent of meals. Tell patient to inject drug into his abdomen, thigh, or upper arm and to rotate sites to minimize injection-site reactions.

• Advise patient of possible risk of medullary thyroid cancer and the need to report any symptoms, such as a neck mass, dysphagia, dyspnea, or persistent hoarseness.

• Tell caregivers to monitor patient closely for depression or changes in mood or behavior. If suicidal, have them take safety precautions, stop the drug, and seek emergency medical help for patient.

• Emphasize that liraglutide therapy isn't a substitute for diet and exercise but is used to enhance the effectiveness of these measures.

• Instruct patient to discontinue drug immediately and seek emergency care if he experiences a serious hypersensitivity reaction, such as swelling of the face or throat area, difficulty breathing, or feeling acutely ill.

• Instruct female patients prescribed Saxenda to notify prescriber immediately if pregnancy is suspected or occurs, as drug will need to be discontinued.

lisdexamfetamine dimesylate
Vyvanse

Class and Category
Chemical class: Sympathomimetic amine
Therapeutic class: CNS stimulant
Pregnancy category: C

Indications and Dosages

➤ *To treat attention deficit hyperactivity disorder (ADHD)*

CAPSULES

Adults, adolescents, and children age 6 and over. *Initial:* 30 mg once daily in the morning, increased as needed in increments of 10 or 20 mg daily every wk. *Maximum:* 70 mg daily.

DOSAGE ADJUSTMENT For patients with severe renal impairment (GFR from 15 ml/min to less than 30 ml/min), maximum dose is limited to 50 mg daily. For patients with end-stage renal disease (GFR less than 15 ml/min), maximum dose is limited to 30 mg daily. For patients taking agents that alter urinary pH, dosage adjustments are individualized.

Route	Onset	Peak	Duration
P.O.	Unknown	1 hr	Unknown

Mechanism of Action

Produces CNS stimulant effects, probably by facilitating release and blocking reuptake of norepinephrine at adrenergic nerve terminals and by stimulating alpha and beta receptors in peripheral nervous system. The drug also releases and blocks reuptake of dopamine in limbic regions of brain. These actions cause decreased motor restlessness and increased alertness.

Contraindications

Advanced arteriosclerosis; agitation; glaucoma; history of drug abuse, hypersensitivity, or idiosyncratic reaction to lisdexamfetamine, other sympathomimetic amines, or their components; hyperthyroidism; MAO inhibitor therapy within 14 days; moderate to severe hypertension; symptomatic cardiovascular disease; history of seizures

Interactions

DRUGS

adrenergic blockers: Inhibited adrenergic blockade

acetazolamide, alkalinizers (such as sodium bicarbonate), some thiazides: Increased blood level and effects of lisdexamfetamine

antihistamines: Possibly reduced sedation from antihistamine

antihypertensives: Possibly decreased antihypertensive effects

chlorpromazine: Inhibited CNS stimulant effects of lisdexamfetamine

ethosuximide: Possibly delayed ethosuximide absorption

GI acidifiers (such as ascorbic acid), reserpine: Decreased amphetamine absorption

guanethine: Decreased antihypertensive effect and decreased lisdexamfetamine absorption

guanfacine: Possibly increased blood guanfacine level

haloperidol: Decreased CNS stimulation

lithium carbonate: Possibly decreased anorectic and stimulant effects of lisdexamfetamine

MAO inhibitors: Potentiated effects of lisdexamfetamine, possibly hypertensive crisis

meperidine: Increased analgesia

methenamine: Increased urine excretion and decreased effects of lisdexamfetamine

norepinephrine: Possibly increased adrenergic effect of norepinephrine

phenobarbital, phenytoin: Synergistic anticonvulsant actionphenytoin: Possible delayed absorption of phenytoin; increased synergistic anticonvulsant action

propoxyphene: Increased CNS stimulation, potentially fatal seizures

sympathomimetic drugs: Increased stimulant effect

tricyclic antidepressants: Possibly increased antidepressant effects and decreased lisdexamfetamine effects

urinary acidifiers (such as ammonium chloride and sodium acid phosphate): Increased amphetamine excretion and decreased amphetamine blood level and effects

veratrum alkaloids: Decreased hypotensive effect

Adverse Reactions

CNS: Affect lability, aggression, agitation, anxiety, compulsive skin picking, depression, dizziness, dyskinesia, dysphoria, euphoria, fever, hallucinations, headache, insomnia, irritability, jittery feeling, mania, psychomotor hyperactivity, psychotic episodes, seizures, somnolence, tics, tremor

CV: Cardiomyopathy, hypertension, palpitations, peripheral vasculopathy, including Raynaud's phenomenon, tachycardia, ventricular hypertrophy

J
K
L

EENT: Blurred vision, diplopia, dry mouth, mydriasis, teeth grinding, visual accommodation difficulties
ENDO: Long-term growth suppression
GI: Anorexia, constipation, diarrhea, eosinophilic hepatitis, nausea, vomiting, upper abdominal pain
GU: Decreased libido, erectile dysfunction, priapism
RESP: Dyspnea
SKIN: Diaphoresis, rash, Stevens-Johnson syndrome, toxic epidermal necrolysis, uncontrolled picking at skin, urticaria
Other: Anaphylaxis, angioedema, physical or psychological dependence, weight loss

Nursing Considerations

WARNING Chest pain or fainting should be reported to prescriber immediately.
WARNING Lisdexamfetamine shouldn't be given to patients with structural cardiac abnormalities, cardiomyopathy, or other serious heart problems or rhythm abnormalities because even usual CNS-stimulant dosages increase risk of sudden death in patients with these conditions.

• Use lisdexamfetamine cautiously in patients with hypertension, heart failure, recent MI, or ventricular arrhythmia because drug may increase blood pressure and worsen these conditions.
• Monitor patient's blood pressure closely; stimulant drugs such as lisdexamfetamine may increase it.
• Monitor patients with psychosis, bipolar illness, or a history of aggression or hostility; CNS stimulation may worsen symptoms.
• Assess growth pattern in pediatric patients because stimulants such as lisdexamfetamine may suppress growth. If so, notify prescriber and expect therapy to be halted.
• If patient has a history of seizures or EEG abnormality, watch for seizure activity because stimulants may lower seizure threshold. Rarely, lisdexamfetamine may cause seizures in a patient with no history of them. Take seizure precautions in all patients, and notify prescriber if a seizure occurs. Expect to discontinue lisdexamfetamine, as prescribed.
• Take safety precautions because stimulants may alter accommodation and cause blurred

vision. Although these effects haven't been reported with lisdexamfetamine, the drug is a known stimulant.
• Be aware that therapy may be stopped temporarily to assess continued need for it, as evidenced by a return of hyperactivity and attention deficit.
• Know that lisdexamfetamine can cause a significant elevation in plasma corticosteroid levels, especially in the evening, which may interfere with urinary steroid determinations.

PATIENT TEACHING

WARNING Tell patient with symptoms such as chest pain or fainting to contact prescriber immediately.
• Warn patient or caregiver that drug must be taken exactly as prescribed and dosage increased only at prescriber's instruction because drug can be abused or lead to dependence.
• Instruct patient or caregiver that capsule may be opened and contents dissolved in a glass of water or orange juice and drunk immediately. Alternatively, the contents of the capsule may be mixed with yogurt until completely dispersed; the entire mixture must be consumed immediately.
• Tell patient or caregiver that drug should only be taken in the morning because taking it later in the day may cause insomnia.
• Advise patient or caregiver to report any symptoms that suggest heart disease, such as exertional chest pain or unexplained syncope.
• Urge patient to avoid hazardous activities until drug effects are known.
• Warn male patients and parents of male children that painful or prolonged penile erections may occur while taking the drug, especially after a dose increase or during a period of drug withdrawal. In the event this happens, immediate medical attention should be sought.
• Instruct patient or parents to monitor fingers and toes for ulceration and/or soft tissue breakdown. If noticed, prescriber should be notified. Reassure patient that signs and symptoms generally improve after the dose is reduced or drug is discontinued.
• Tell female patient of childbearing age to notify prescriber if pregnancy is suspected.

lisinopril

Prinivil, Zestril

Class and Category

Chemical class: Lysine ester of enalaprilat
Therapeutic class: Antihypertensive, vasodilator
Pregnancy category: D

Indications and Dosages

➤ *To manage uncomplicated essential hypertension*

TABLETS

Adults. *Initial:* 10 mg daily. *Maintenance:* 20 to 40 mg daily. *Maximum:* 80 mg daily.

DOSAGE ADJUSTMENT For patients with renal failure, initial dosage reduced to 5 mg daily if creatinine clearance is 10 to 30 ml/min/1.73 m^2 and to 2.5 mg daily if creatinine clearance is less than 10 ml/min/1.73 m^2. For patients receiving a diuretic, initial dosage reduced to 5 mg daily.

Children age 6 and over with a GFR of at least 30 ml/min/1.73 m^2. *Initial:* 0.07 mg/kg daily, adjusted according to blood pressure response up to 5 mg daily. *Maximum:* 0.61 mg/kg or 40 mg daily.

➤ *To treat heart failure, along with digoxin and diuretics*

TABLETS

Adults. *Initial:* 5 mg daily. *Maintenance:* 5 to 20 mg daily. *Maximum:* 80 mg daily.

DOSAGE ADJUSTMENT For patients with hyponatremia or creatinine clearance of 30 ml/min/1.73 m^2 or less, initial dosage reduced to 2.5 mg daily.

➤ *To improve survival in hemodynamically stable patient after acute MI*

TABLETS

Adults. 5 mg within 24 hr after onset of symptoms, followed by 5 mg after 24 hr and 10 mg after 48 hr. *Maintenance:* 10 mg daily for 6 wk. *Maximum:* 80 mg daily.

DOSAGE ADJUSTMENT For patients with baseline systolic blood pressure of 120 mm Hg or less, initial dosage decreased to 2.5 mg daily for first 3 days after MI. If systolic blood pressure falls to 100 mm Hg or less during therapy, maintenance dosage decreased to 2.5 to 5 mg as tolerated; if

systolic blood pressure is 90 mm Hg or less for more than 1 hr, drug is discontinued.

Route	Onset	Peak	Duration
P.O.	1 hr	6–8 hr	24 hr

Mechanism of Action

May reduce blood pressure by inhibiting conversion of angiotensin I to angiotensin II. Angiotensin II is a potent vasoconstrictor that also stimulates adrenal cortex to secrete aldosterone. Lisinopril may also inhibit renal and vascular production of angiotensin II. Decreased release of aldosterone reduces sodium and water reabsorption and increases their excretion, thereby reducing blood pressure.

Contraindications

Concurrent aliskiren use in patients with diabetes or patients with renal impairment (GFR less than 60 ml/min); hypersensitivity to lisinopril, other ACE inhibitors, or their components; history of angioedema related to previous treatment with an ACE inhibitor; hereditary or idiopathic angioedema

Interactions

DRUGS

aliskiren, other ACE inhibitors, angiotension receptor blockers: Increased risk of hypotension, hyperkalemia, and renal impairment
allopurinol, bone marrow depressants (such as methotrexate), procainamide, systemic corticosteroids: Increased risk of potentially fatal neutropenia or agranulocytosis
cyclosporine, potassium-sparing diuretics, potassium supplements: Increased risk of hyperkalemia
diuretics, other antihypertensives: Increased hypotensive effect
gold: Possibly nitritoid reaction (facial flushing, hypotension, nausea, vomiting)
insulin, oral antidiabetics: Increased risk of hypoglycemia
lithium: Increased blood lithium level and risk of lithium toxicity
NSAIDs: Possibly reduced antihypertensive effect; possibly reduced renal function in patients with preexisting renal dysfunction, the elderly and patients who are volume-depleted
sympathomimetics: Possibly reduced antihypertensive effect

J
K
L

FOODS

high-potassium diet, potassium-containing salt substitutes: Increased risk of hyperkalemia

ACTIVITIES

alcohol use: Possibly increased hypotensive effect

Adverse Reactions

CNS: Ataxia, confusion, depression, dizziness, fatigue, hallucinations, headache, insomnia, irritability, memory impairment, mood alterations, nervousness, paresthesia, peripheral neuropathy, somnolence, stroke, syncope, transient ischemic attack, tremor, vertigo
CV: Arrhythmias, chest pain, fluid overload, hypotension, MI, orthostatic hypotension, palpitations, peripheral edema, vasculitis
ENDO: Hyperglycemia, hypoglycemia (patients on oral antidiabetic agents or insulin), syndrome of inappropriate ADH secretion
EENT: Blurred vision, diplopia, dry mouth, olfactory or taste disturbance, photophobia, tinnitus, visual loss
GI: Abdominal pain, anorexia, cholestatic jaundice, constipation, diarrhea, elevated liver enzyme levels, flatulence, fulminant hepatic necrosis, gastritis, hepatitis, indigestion, nausea, pancreatitis, vomiting
GU: Acute renal failure, decreased libido, impotence, pyelonephritis
HEME: Agranulocytosis, anemia, hemolytic anemia, neutropenia, thrombocytopenia
MS: Arthralgia, arthritis, bone or joint pain, muscle spasms, myalgia
RESP: Bronchospasm, cough, dyspnea, paroxysmal nocturnal dyspnea, pulmonary embolism and infarction, upper respiratory tract infection
SKIN: Alopecia, cutaneous pseudolymphoma, diaphoresis, erythema, flushing, herpes zoster, infections, pemphigus, photosensitivity, pruritus, psoriasis, rash, Stevens-Johnson syndrome, toxic epidermal necrolysis, urticaria
Other: Anaphylaxis, angioedema, dehydration, gout, hyponatremia, weight gain or loss

Nursing Considerations

• Use lisinopril cautiously in patients with fluid volume deficit, heart failure, impaired renal function, or sodium depletion.

• To prepare pediatric suspension, add 10 ml purified water to a polyethylene terephthalate (PET) bottle containing ten 20-mg tablets and shake for at least 1 minute. Add 30 ml of Bicitra diluent and 160 ml of Ora-Sweet SF to concentrate in PET bottle and shake gently for several seconds. Refrigerate up to 4 weeks. Shake suspension before each use.

• Monitor blood pressure often, especially early in treatment. If excessive hypotension develops, expect to withhold drug for several days.

WARNING If angioedema affects face, glottis, larynx, limbs, lips, mucous membranes, or tongue, notify prescriber immediately and expect to stop lisinopril and start appropriate therapy at once. If airway obstruction threatens, promptly give 0.3 to 0.5 ml of epinephrine 1:1,000 solution subcutaneously, as prescribed.

• Monitor patient for anaphylaxis, especially patient being dialyzed with high-flux membranes and treated with an ACE inhibitor such as lisinopril. If anaphylaxis occurs, stop dialysis immediately and treat aggressively (antihistamines are ineffective in this situation), as ordered. Anaphylaxis has also occurred with some patients undergoing low-density lipoprotein apheresis with dextran sulfate absorption.

• Notify prescriber if patient has persistent, nonproductive cough, a common adverse effect of ACE inhibitors such as lisinopril.

• Monitor for dehydration, which can lead to hypotension. Be aware that diarrhea and vomiting can cause dehydration.

• Monitor patient for hepatic dysfunction because lisinopril, an ACE inhibitor, may rarely cause a syndrome that starts with cholestatic jaundice or hepatitis and progresses to fulminant hepatic necrosis. If patient develops jaundice or a marked elevation in liver enzyme levels, withhold drug and notify prescriber.

• If patient takes insulin or an oral antidiabetic, monitor blood glucose level closely because risk of hypoglycemia increases, especially during first month of therapy.

PATIENT TEACHING

• Explain that lisinopril helps to control, but doesn't cure, hypertension and that patient may need lifelong therapy.

- Advise patient to take lisinopril at the same time every day.
- Emphasize need to take drug as ordered, even if patient feels well; caution her not to stop drug without consulting prescriber.
- Instruct patient to report dizziness, especially during first few days of therapy.
- Inform patient that persistent, nonproductive cough may develop during lisinopril therapy. Urge her to notify prescriber immediately if cough becomes difficult to tolerate.
- Advise patient to drink adequate fluids and avoid excessive sweating, which can lead to dehydration and hypotension. Make sure she understands that diarrhea and vomiting can also cause hypotension.
- Caution patient not to use salt substitutes that contain potassium.
- Instruct patient to report signs of infection, such as fever and sore throat, which may indicate neutropenia.
- Advise patient to change position slowly to minimize orthostatic hypotension.
- If patient has diabetes and takes insulin or an oral antidiabetic, urge her to monitor her blood glucose level closely and watch for symptoms of hypoglycemia.
- Caution female patient to notify prescriber immediately if she is or could be pregnant.
- Advise patient to inform all prescribers of lisinopril therapy.

lithium carbonate
Carbolith (CAN), Duralith (CAN), Eskalith, Eskalith CR, Lithane, Lithizine (CAN), Lithobid, Lithonate, Lithotabs

lithium citrate
Cibalith-S

Class and Category
Chemical class: Alkaline metal, monovalent cation
Therapeutic class: Antidepressant, antimanic
Pregnancy category: D

Indications and Dosages
➤ *To treat recurrent bipolar affective disorder, to prevent bipolar disorder depression*

CAPSULES, TABLETS
Adults and children age 12 and over.
Initial: 300 to 600 mg three times daily.
Maintenance: 300 mg three times daily or four times daily. *Maximum:* 2,400 g daily.
Children up to age 12. 15 to 20 mg/kg daily in divided doses twice daily or three times daily.

E.R. TABLETS
Adults and children age 12 and over.
Initial: 900 to 1,800 mg daily in divided doses twice daily or three times daily.
Maintenance: 450 mg twice daily or 300 mg three times daily. *Maximum:* 2,400 g daily.

SLOW-RELEASE CAPSULES
Adults and children age 12 and over. 600 to 900 mg on day 1, increased to 1,200 to 1,800 mg daily in divided doses three times daily.
Maintenance: 900 to 1,200 mg daily in divided doses three times daily. *Maximum:* 2,400 g daily.

SYRUP (LITHIUM CITRATE)
Adults and children age 12 and over. 8 to 16 mEq (equivalent of 300 to 600 mg of lithium carbonate) three times daily.
Maintenance: Equivalent of 300 mg of lithium carbonate three times daily or four times daily. *Maximum:* Equivalent of 2,400 g daily of lithium carbonate.
Children up to age 12. 0.4 to 0.5 mEq (equivalent of 15 to 20 mg of lithium carbonate)/kg daily in divided doses twice daily or three times daily.

Route	Onset	Peak	Duration
P.O.	1–3 wk	Unknown	Unknown

Mechanism of Action
May increase presynaptic degradation of the catecholamine neurotransmitters serotonin, dopamine, and norepinephrine; inhibit their release at neuronal synapses; and decrease postsynaptic receptor sensitivity. These actions may correct overactive catecholamine systems in patients with mania.

Antidepressant action may result from enhanced serotonergic activity.

Contraindications
Blood dyscrasias, bone marrow depression, brain damage, cerebrovascular disease, coma, coronary artery disease, excessive

intake of other CNS depressants, hypersensitivity to lithium or its components, impaired hepatic function, myeloproliferative disorders, severe depression, severe hypertension or hypotension

Interactions

DRUGS

ACE inhibitors, NSAIDs, piroxicam: Possibly increased blood lithium level and increased risk of toxicity

acetazolamide, sodium bicarbonate, urea, xanthines: Decreased blood lithium level

calcium channel blockers, molindone: Increased risk of neurotoxicity from lithium

calcium iodide, iodinated glycerol, potassium iodide: Possibly increased hypothyroid effects of both drugs

carbamazepine: Possibly increased thera-peutic effects of carbamazepine and neurotoxic effect of lithium

chlorpromazine, other phenothiazines: Possibly impaired GI absorption and decreased blood levels of these drugs; possibly masking of early signs of lithium toxicity

desmopressin, lypressin, vasopressin: Possibly impaired antidiuretic effects of these drugs

diuretics (loop and osmotic): Increased lithium reabsorption by kidneys, possibly leading to lithium toxicity

fluoxetine, methyldopa, metronidazole: Increased risk of lithium toxicity from reduced renal clearance of lithium

haloperidol and other antipyschotics: Increased risk of irreversible neurotoxicity and brain damage

neuromuscular blockers: Risk of prolonged paralysis or weakness

norepinephrine: Possibly decreased therapeutic effects of norepinephrine and severe respiratory depression

selective serotonin reuptake inhibitors: Increased risk of adverse effects, such as diarrhea, confusion, dizziness, agitation, and tremor

thyroid hormones: Possibly hypothyroidism

tricyclic antidepressants: Possibly severe mood swings from mania to depression

FOODS

high-sodium foods: Increased excretion and possibly decreased therapeutic effects of lithium

Adverse Reactions

CNS: Ataxia, coma, confusion, depression, dizziness, drowsiness, headache, lethargy, seizures, syncope, tremor (in hands), vertigo

CV: Arrhythmias (including bradycardia and tachycardia), ECG changes, edema, hypotension, palpitations, peripheral circulatory collapse, unmasking of Brugada syndrome

EENT: Dental caries, dry mouth, exophthalmos

ENDO: Diabetes insipidus, euthyroid goiter, hypothyroidism, myxedema

GI: Abdominal distention and pain, anorexia, diarrhea, nausea, thirst

GU: Stress incontinence, urinary frequency

HEME: Leukocytosis

MS: Muscle twitching and weakness

RESP: Dyspnea

SKIN: Acne; alopecia; dry, thin hair; pruritus; rash

Other: Cold sensitivity, weight gain or loss

Nursing Considerations

- Administer lithium after meals to slow absorption from GI tract and reduce adverse reactions. Dilute syrup with juice or other flavored drink before giving.
- Note that 5 ml of lithium citrate equals 8 mEq of lithium ion or 300 mg of lithium carbonate.
- Expect to monitor blood lithium level two or three times weekly during first month, and then weekly to monthly during maintenance therapy and when starting or stopping NSAID therapy. In uncomplicated cases, plan to monitor lithium level every 2 to 3 months.
- Be aware that lithium has a narrow therapeutic range. Even a slightly high blood level is dangerous, and some patients show signs of toxicity at normal levels.
- Expect prescriber to decrease dosage after acute manic episode is controlled.
- *WARNING* Be aware that lithium affects intracellular and extracellular potassium ion shift, which can cause ECG changes, such as flattened or inverted T waves; it also can increase the risk of cardiac arrest.
- Monitor ECGs, renal and thyroid function test results, and serum electrolyte levels, as appropriate, during lithium treatment.

WARNING Be aware that lithium can cause reversible leukocytosis, which usually peaks within 7 to 10 days of starting therapy; WBC count typically returns to baseline within 10 days after therapy stops.
• Weigh patient daily to detect sudden weight changes.
• Monitor blood glucose level often in diabetic patient because lithium alters glucose tolerance.
• Palpate thyroid gland to detect enlargement because drug may cause goiter.
• Ensure that patient's fluid and sodium intake is adequate during treatment.
• Monitor patient closely for unexplained syncope or palpitations after starting lithium therapy as these symptoms may be caused by the unmasking of Brugada syndrome by lithium. Know that Brugada syndrome is a disorder in which electrocardiographic abnormalities occur and can result in sudden death. Patients at risk include those with a family history of Brugada syndrome or a family history of sudden death before the age of 45 years. Notify prescriber if syncope or palpitations occur and expect to discontinue lithium therapy.

PATIENT TEACHING
• Advise patient to take lithium with or after meals to minimize adverse reactions.
• Instruct patient to swallow E.R. or slow-release form whole.
• Direct patient to mix syrup form with juice or other flavored drink before taking.
• Inform patient that frequent urination, nausea, and thirst may occur during the first few days of treatment.
• Caution patient not to stop taking lithium or adjust dosage without first consulting prescriber.
• Instruct patient to report signs of toxicity, such as diarrhea, drowsiness, muscle weakness, tremor, uncoordinated body movements, and vomiting.
• Urge patient to avoid hazardous activities until drug's CNS effects are known.
• Advise patient to maintain normal fluid and sodium intake.
• Emphasize importance of complying with scheduled checkups and laboratory tests.
• Instruct patient to see immediate emergency care if he experiences fainting, lightheadedness, abnormal heart beats, or shortness of breath.

lomefloxacin hydrochloride

Maxaquin

Class and Category
Chemical class: Fluoroquinolone
Therapeutic class: Antibiotic
Pregnancy category: C

Indications and Dosages
➤ *To treat mild to moderate lower respiratory tract infections caused by susceptible organisms, including* Haemophilus influenzae *and* Moraxella catarrhalis

TABLETS
Adults. 400 mg daily for 10 days.
➤ *To treat uncomplicated cystitis caused by* Escherichia coli; *to treat uncomplicated cystitis caused by* Klebsiella pneumoniae, Proteus mirabilis, *or* Staphylococcus saprophyticus

TABLETS
Adults. 400 mg daily for 3 days.
➤ *To treat complicated UTI caused by* Citrobacter diversus, Enterobacteriaceae, E. coli, K. pneumoniae, P. mirabilis, *or* Pseudomonas aeruginosa

TABLETS
Adults. 400 mg daily for 14 days.
➤ *To provide prophylaxis for transurethral surgery*

TABLETS
Adults. 400 mg as a single dose 2 to 6 hr before surgery.
➤ *To provide prophylaxis for transrectal biopsy*

TABLETS
Adults. 400 mg as a single dose 1 to 6 hr before surgery.
➤ *To treat gonorrhea (as alternative to ciprofloxacin or ofloxacin)*

TABLETS
Adults. 400 mg as a single dose.
DOSAGE ADJUSTMENT For patients with creatinine clearance between 11 and 39 ml/min/1.73 m^2, loading dose of 400 mg given on day 1 and followed by 200 mg daily.

Mechanism of Action
Inhibits the bacterial enzyme DNA gyrase, which normally is responsible for

J
K
L

unwinding and supercoiling of bacterial DNA before it replicates. By inhibiting this enzyme, lomefloxacin interferes with bacterial cell replication and causes cell death.

Contraindications
History of tendinitis or tendon rupture, hypersensitivity to lomefloxacin or any quinolone derivative

Interactions
DRUGS
aluminum-, calcium-, or magnesium-containing antacids; iron salts; sucralfate; zinc: Decreased absorption and blood level of lomefloxacin
cyclosporine: Possibly increased blood cyclosporine level, increased nephrotoxicity
probenecid: Decreased lomefloxacin excretion, increased risk of toxicity
warfarin: Possibly increased anticoagulant effect and risk of bleeding

Adverse Reactions
CNS: Ataxia, cerebral thrombosis, dizziness, drowsiness, hallucinations, headache, insomnia, nervousness, peripheral neuropathy, phobia, vertigo
CV: Prolonged QT interval, torsades de pointes, vasculitis
EENT: Diplopia, laryngeal edema, oral candidiasis, painful oral mucosa, taste perversion
GI: Abdominal pain, diarrhea, hepatitis, indigestion, nausea, pseudomembranous colitis, vomiting
GU: Interstitial nephritis, polyuria, renal failure, urine retention, vaginal candidiasis
HEME: Hemolytic anemia
MS: Tendinitis, tendon rupture
RESP: Pulmonary edema
SKIN: Exfoliative dermatitis, hyperpigmentation, photosensitivity, Stevens-Johnson syndrome, toxic epidermal necrolysis
Other: Anaphylaxis

Nursing Considerations
• Know that lomefloxacin shouldn't be given to patients with QT-interval prolongation or hypokalemia or to patients taking class IA antiarrhythmics (such as quinidine or procainamide) or class III antiarrhythmics

(such as amiodarone or sotalol) because of increased risk of torsades de pointes.
• Expect to obtain body fluid or tissue sample for culture and sensitivity testing and to review results, if possible, before lomefloxacin therapy begins.
• If patient's culture test results are positive for gonorrhea, expect to obtain serologic test for syphilis at diagnosis and to repeat test 3 months after lomefloxacin therapy.
• Give drug with meals and a full glass of water.
• Ensure that patient maintains adequate fluid intake during therapy.
• Monitor for evidence of secondary infections, such as sore mouth or vaginal discharge.
• Notify prescriber if patient experiences severe or prolonged diarrhea, which may indicate pseudomembranous colitis.
• Be aware that prolonged use may lead to growth of drug-resistant organisms.
• Notify prescriber and expect to stop lomefloxacin if patient develops symp-toms of peripheral neuropathy (pain, burning, tingling, numbness, weakness, or changes in sensations of light touch, pain, temperature, position, or vibration) to prevent an irreversible condition or tendon rupture that requires immediate rest and avoidance of exercise involving affected area.

PATIENT TEACHING
• Advise patient to take lomefloxacin at same time each day with meals and with a full glass of water.
• Caution patient not to take antacids, iron, sucralfate, or zinc 1 hour before or 2 hours after taking lomefloxacin because these preparations impair drug absorption.
• Urge patient to drink plenty of fluids during treatment.
• Instruct patient to complete full course of therapy, even if symptoms subside.
• Advise patient to notify prescriber if symptoms don't improve within a few days after starting lomefloxacin or if severe GI distress or diarrhea develops.
• Instruct patient to notify prescriber and stop taking drug if she has tendon inflammation or pain; advise her to rest until tendinitis and tendon rupture have been ruled out.
• Urge patient to avoid direct sunlight, to wear protective clothing, and to use

sunscreen because photosensitivity reactions can occur during therapy and for several days afterward.
• Explain that risk of photosensitivity can be decreased by taking lomefloxacin at least 12 hours before sun exposure. Urge patient to stop drug and notify prescriber at first sign of photosensitivity, such as skin burning, redness, swelling, blisters, rash, itching, or dermatitis.
• Inform patient that an allergic reaction may occur after a single dose. Tell patient to stop lomefloxacin and notify prescriber if rash or other allergic reaction develops.
• Caution patient to avoid hazardous activities until drug's CNS effects are known.

lomitapide mesylate

Juxtapid

Class and Category
Chemical class: Methanesulfonate salt
Therapeutic class: Antihyperlipidemic, Microsomal Triglyceride Transfer Protein (MTP) Inhibitor
Pregnancy category: X

Indications and Dosages
➤ *To control lipid levels as adjunct to diet and other lipid-lowering treatments in homozygous familial hypercholesterolemia*
CAPSULES
Adults. *Initial:* 5 mg once daily with full glass of water 2 hrs after evening meal with dosage increased to 10 mg once daily after 2wks, as needed. Dosage further increased in 4 wk increments to 20 mg once daily, then to 40 mgs once daily to 60 mg once daily, as needed. *Maximum:* 60 mg once daily.
DOSAGE ADJUSTMENT For patients with mild hepatic impairment or with end-stage renal impairment requiring dialysis, dosage not to exceed 40mg once daily. For patients receiving weak CYP450 3A4 inhibitors such as alprazolam, amiodarone, amlodipine, atorvastatin, bicalutamide, cilostazol, cimetidine, cyclosporine, fluoxetine, fluvoxamine, ginkgo, goldenseal, isoniazid, lapatinib, nilotinib, oral contraceptives, pazopanib, ranitidine, ranolazine, ticagrelor,

or zileuton, dosage not to exceed 30 mg once daily. For patients who develop elevated transaminases 3 times or greater but less than 5 times upper normal limits during therapy, daily dosage reduced with degree of reduction individualized.

Mechanism of Action
Binds and inhibits microsomal triglyceride transfer protein, located in the lumen of the endoplasmic reticulum of cells which in turn prevents the assembly of apo B-containing lipoproteins in enterocytes and hepatocytes. This then prevents the synthesis of chylomicrons and very low-density lipoproteins (VLDL). Lower VLDL levels leads to reduced levels of plasma low-density lipoprotein-cholesterol.

Contraindications
Active liver disease, concurrent therapy with moderate or strong CYP3A4 inhibitors, hypersensitivity to lomitapide or its components, moderate or severe hepatic impairment, pregnancy, unexplained persistent elevations of serum transaminases

Interactions
DRUGS
bile acid sequestrants: Possibly decreased absorption of lomitapide
CYP3A inhibitors: Increased lomitapide exposure with possible increased risk of adverse reactions
lovastatin, simvastatin: Increased risk of myopathy, including rhabdomyolysis
P-glycoprotein substrates such as aliskiren, colchicine, dabigatran etexilate, digoxin, everolimus, fexofenadine, imatinib, lapatinib, maraviroc, nilotinib, posaconazole, ranolazine, saxagliptin, sirolimus, sitagliptin, talinolol, tolvaptan, topotecan: Increased absorption of these drugs resulting in higher drug levels
warfarin: Increased plasma warfarin levels with possible increased risk of bleeding events
ACTIVITIES
alcohol use: Possibly increased risk of hepatic steatosis
FOODS
grapefruit juice: Increased lomitapide exposure and adverse reactions

Adverse Reactions
CNS: Dizziness, fatigue, fever, headache
CV: Chest pain, palpitations

EENT: Nasal congestion, nasopharnygitis, pharyngolaryngeal pain
GU: Abdominal distention or pain, constipation, defecation urgency, diarrhea, dyspepsia, elevated liver enzymes, flatulence, gastroenteritis, gastroesophageal reflux disease, hepatic steatosis, hepatotoxicity, nausea, rectal tenesmus, transaminase elevations, vomiting
MS: Back pain
Other: Fat soluble vitamin deficiency, flulike symptoms, serum fatty acid deficiency, weight loss

Nursing Considerations
• Be aware that lomitapide should not be given to patients with rare, hereditary problems of galactose intolerance, Lapp lactase deficiency, or glucose-galactose malabsorption because drug may cause diarrhea and malabsorption in these patients.
• Know that because lomitapide increases risk of hepatotoxicty, the drug can only be administered through the Juxtapid REMS program.
• Determine patient has had ALT, AST, alkaline phosphatase and total bilirubin measured, has had a negative pregnancy test if patient is female, and has initiated a low-fat diet supplying less than 20% of energy from fat prior to initiating lomitapide therapy.
• Be aware that ALT and AST levels should be measured prior to potential dosage increase or monthly, whichever comes first, for first year of therapy and then before each dosage increase and every three months thereafter. If transaminase values are equal to or greater than three times upper limit normal but less than five times upper limit normal, expect to confirm elevation with a repeat measurement within one week. If confirmed, expect dosage to be decreased and additional liver-related tests done, such as measurement of alkaline phosphatase, total bilirubin, and INR. Repeat tests weekly, as ordered, and expect to withhold drug if there are signs of abnormal liver function such as an elevation in patient's bilirubin or INR, If transaminase levels are above five times upper limit normal, or if transaminase levels do not fall below three times upper limit normal within about

4 weeks, expect drug to withheld or discontinued. Know that if drug therapy is resumed, dosage should be reduced and more frequent liver-related tests ordered.
• Monitor patient closely for signs and symptoms of liver impairment, such as presence of abdominal pain, fever, flulike symptoms, jaundice, or lethargy; a bilirubin result that is equal to or greater than two times upper limit normal, or active liver disease is suspected because risk of hepatotoxicity increases with lomitapide therapy.
• Monitor patient for fat-soluble vitamin and fatty acids deficiencies, especially patients with chronic bowel or pancreatic diseases that predispose to malabsorption, because lomitapide reduces the absorption of fat-soluble vitamins.
• Monitor patient for adverse reactions, especially gastrointestinal reactions, which are the most common reactions associated with lomitapide therapy. Give drug with a full glass of water two hours after evening meals. Ensure patient is adhering to a low-fat diet that supplies less than 20% of energy needs from fat to reduce the risk of adverse gastrointestinal reactions.

PATIENT TEACHING
• Advise patient to take lomitapide with a full glass of water two hours after the evening meal because taking drug with food may increase the risk of gastrointestinal adverse reactions.
• Caution patient to swallow capsule whole and not to open, crush, dissolve, or chew capsule.
• Instruct patient to take daily supplements of 400 international units of vitamin E and at least 200 milligrams linoleic acid, 210 milligrams alpha-linolenic acid, 110 milligrams eicosapentaenoic acid, and 80 milligrams of docosahexaenoic acid to prevent deficiencies.
• Remind patient of importance of adhering to the low fat diet prescribed as lomitapide therapy is not a replacement for dietary control of fat in her diet.
• Tell patient to inform all prescribers about lomitapide therapy because of potential drug interactions.
• Review signs and symptoms of liver impairment, and emphasize importance of reporting such to prescriber. Inform patient of need for blood tests to monitor

her liver function and importance of compliance with test schedule.

WARNING Instruct patient not to consume more than one alcoholic beverage daily.

WARNING Caution women of childbearing age to notify prescriber immediately if pregnancy occurs or is suspected because drug will need to be discontinued. Also, encourage them to enroll in the pregnancy exposure registry that monitors pregnancy outcomes in women exposed to the drug during pregnancy.

loracarbef
Lorabid

Class and Category
Chemical class: Carbacephem
Therapeutic class: Antibiotic
Pregnancy category: B

Indications and Dosages
➤ *To treat acute bronchitis caused by* Haemophilus influenzae, Moraxella catarrhalis, *or* Streptococcus pneumoniae
CAPSULES, ORAL SUSPENSION
Adults and adolescents. 200 to 400 mg every 12 hr for 7 days.
➤ *To treat chronic bronchitis exacerbations caused by* H. influenzae, M. catarrhalis, *or* S. pneumoniae
CAPSULES, ORAL SUSPENSION
Adults and adolescents. 400 mg every 12 hr for 7 days.
➤ *To treat pneumonia caused by* H. influenzae *or* S. pneumoniae
CAPSULES, ORAL SUSPENSION
Adults and adolescents. 400 mg every 12 hr for 14 days.
➤ *To treat pharyngitis, sinusitis, or tonsillitis caused by* Streptococcus pyogenes
CAPSULES, ORAL SUSPENSION
Adults and adolescents. 200 to 400 mg every 12 hr for 10 days.
Children. 7.5 mg/kg every 12 hr for 10 days.
➤ *To treat acute otitis media caused by* H. influenzae, M. catarrhalis, S. pneumoniae, *or* S. pyogenes
ORAL SUSPENSION
Children. 15 mg/kg every 12 hr for 10 days.
➤ *To treat uncomplicated skin and soft-tissue infections caused by* Staphylococcus aureus *or* S. pyogenes

CAPSULES, ORAL SUSPENSION
Adults and adolescents. 200 mg every 12 hr for 7 days.
ORAL SUSPENSION
Children. 7.5 mg/kg every 12 hr for 7 days.
➤ *To treat uncomplicated cystitis caused by* Escherichia coli *or* Staphylococcus saprophyticus
CAPSULES, ORAL SUSPENSION
Adults and adolescents. 200 mg daily for 7 days.
➤ *To treat uncomplicated pyelonephritis caused by* E. coli
CAPSULES, ORAL SUSPENSION
Adults and adolescents. 400 mg every 12 hr for 14 days.

DOSAGE ADJUSTMENT If creatinine clearance is 10 to 49 ml/min/1.73 m², 50% of usual dose given at normal interval or usual dose given at twice the normal interval; if clearance is less than 10 ml/min/1.73 m², usual adult dosage given every 3 to 5 days.

Mechanism of Action
Interferes with bacterial cell wall synthesis by inhibiting final step in the cross-linking of peptidoglycan strands. Peptidoglycan makes bacterial cell membrane rigid and protective. Without it, bacterial cells rupture and die.

Contraindications
Hypersensitivity to loracarbef, other cephalosporins, or their components

Interactions
DRUGS
probenecid: Inhibited renal excretion of loracarbef, resulting in increased blood level
FOODS
all foods: Inhibited drug absorption

Adverse Reactions
CNS: Dizziness, drowsiness, headache, insomnia, nervousness, seizures
EENT: Oral candidiasis
GI: Abdominal pain, anorexia, diarrhea, nausea, pseudomembranous colitis, vomiting
GU: Vaginal candidiasis
SKIN: Pruritus, rash, urticaria

Nursing Considerations
• Expect to obtain body fluid or tissue sample for culture and sensitivity testing and to review results, if possible, before giving first dose of loracarbef.

J
K
L

• Be aware that oral suspension is absorbed more rapidly and produces a higher peak plasma level than capsules.
• Monitor patient for signs of secondary infections, such as sore mouth and vaginal discharge.
• Watch for seizures, especially if patient has impaired renal function.

PATIENT TEACHING
• Advise patient to take loracarbef at least 1 hour before or 2 hours after meals.
• Tell patient to complete full course of drug as prescribed, even if symptoms decrease.
• Instruct patient to discard unused oral solution after 14 days.
• Advise patient to report diarrhea, hives, or severe rash to prescriber.

lorazepam

Apo-Lorazepam (CAN), Ativan, Lorazepam Intensol, Novo-Lorazem (CAN), Nu-Loraz (CAN)

Class, Category, and Schedule
Chemical class: Benzodiazepine
Therapeutic class: Amnestic, antianxiety, anticonvulsant, sedative
Pregnancy category: D (parenteral), Not rated (oral)
Controlled substance schedule: IV

Indications and Dosages
➤ *To treat anxiety*
ORAL CONCENTRATE, TABLETS
Adults and adolescents. 1 to 3 mg twice daily or three times daily. *Maximum:* 10 mg daily.
DOSAGE ADJUSTMENT For elderly or debilitated patients, initial dosage may be reduced to 0.5 to 2 mg daily in divided doses.
➤ *To treat insomnia caused by anxiety*
ORAL CONCENTRATE, TABLETS
Adults and adolescents. 2 to 4 mg at bedtime.
DOSAGE ADJUSTMENT Dosage possibly reduced for elderly or debilitated patients.
➤ *To provide preoperative sedation*
I.V. INJECTION
Adults and adolescents. 0.044 mg/kg or 2 mg, whichever is less, given 2 hr before procedure. *Maximum:* 0.05 mg/kg or total of 4 mg.

I.M. INJECTION
Adults and adolescents. 0.05 mg/kg 2 hr before procedure. *Maximum:* 4 mg.
➤ *To treat status epilepticus*
I.V. INJECTION
Adults and adolescents. *Initial:* 4 mg at a rate of 2 mg/min. Repeated in 10 to 15 min if seizures don't subside. *Maximum:* 8 mg/24 hr.

Route	Onset	Peak	Duration
I.V.	5 min	Unknown	12–24 hr
I.M.	15–30 min	Unknown	12–24 hr

Mechanism of Action
May potentiate the effects of gamma-aminobutyric acid (GABA) and other inhibitory neurotransmitters by binding to specific benzodiazepine receptors in limbic and cortical areas of CNS. GABA inhibits excitatory stimulation, which helps control emotional behavior. Limbic system contains a highly dense area of benzodiazepine receptors, which may explain drug's anti-anxiety effects. Also, lorazepam hyperpolarizes neuronal cells, thereby interfering with their ability to generate seizures.

Incompatibilities
Don't mix I.V. lorazepam in same syringe as buprenorphine.

Contraindications
Acute angle-closure glaucoma, hypersensitivity to lorazepam, its components, or benzodiazepines; intra-arterial delivery; psychosis

Interactions
DRUGS
aminophylline, theophylline: Possibly reduced sedative effects of lorazepam
clozapine: Increased risk of marked sedation, excessive salivation, hypotension, ataxia, delirium, and respiratory arrest
CNS depressants: Additive CNS depression, potentially fatal respiratory depression
digoxin: Possibly increased blood digoxin level and risk of digitalis toxicity
fentanyl: Possibly decreased therapeutic effects of fentanyl
probenecid: Possibly increased therapeutic and adverse effects of lorazepam
ACTIVITIES
alcohol use: Increased CNS depression

Adverse Reactions

CNS: Amnesia, anxiety, ataxia, coma, confusion, delusions, depression, dizziness, drowsiness, euphoria, extrapyramidal symptoms, fatigue, headache, hypokinesia, irritability, malaise, nervousness, seizures, slurred speech, suicidal ideation, tremor, unsteadiness, vertigo
CV: Chest pain, palpitations, tachycardia
EENT: Blurred vision, diplopia, dry mouth, increased salivation, photophobia
ENDO: Syndrome of inappropriate ADH
GI: Abdominal pain, constipation, diarrhea, increased liver enzyme levels, jaundice, nausea, thirst, vomiting
GU: Libido changes
HEME: Agranulocytosis, pancytopenia, thrombocytopenia
RESP: Apnea, respiratory depression, worsening of sleep apnea or obstructive pulmonary disease
SKIN: Diaphoresis
Other: Anaphylaxis, injection-site pain (I.M.) or phlebitis (I.V.), physical and psychological dependence, withdrawal symptoms

Nursing Considerations

• Before starting lorazepam therapy in a patient with depression, make sure he already takes an antidepressant, because of the increased risk of suicide in patients with untreated depression.
• Use extreme caution when giving lorazepam to elderly patients, especially those with compromised respiratory function, because drug can cause hypoventilation, sedation, unsteadiness, and respiratory depression.
• Use drug cautiously in patients with a history of alcohol or drug abuse or a personality disorder because of an increased risk of physical and psycho-logical dependence. Also use cautiously in patients with severe hepatic insufficiency or encephalopathy because drug may worsen hepatic encephalopathy.
• For I.M. use, inject lorazepam deep into large muscle mass, such as gluteus maximus.
• For I.V. use, dilute lorazepam with equal amount of sterile water for injection, sodium chloride for injection, or D_5W. Give diluted lorazepam slowly, at no more than 2 mg/min.

• During I.V. use, monitor patient's respirations every 5 to 15 minutes and keep emergency resuscitation equipment readily available.
WARNING Monitor patient's respiratory status closely because drug may cause life-threatening respiratory depression.
• Because stopping drug abruptly increases risk of withdrawal symptoms, expect to taper dosage gradually, especially in epileptic patients.

PATIENT TEACHING

• Instruct patient to take lorazepam exactly as prescribed and not to stop without consulting prescriber because of the risk of withdrawal symptoms.
• Advise patient to avoid hazardous activities until drug's CNS effects are known.
• Urge patient to avoid alcohol while taking lorazepam because it increases drug's CNS depressant effects.
• Instruct patient to report excessive drowsiness and nausea.
• Inform pregnant patient that lorazepam therapy will need to be discontinued early in third trimester to avoid possible withdrawal symptoms in newborn.

lorcaserin hydrochloride

Belviq

Class and Category

Chemical class: Serotonin 2C receptor agonist
Therapeutic class: Weight regulator
Pregnancy category: X

Indications and Dosages

➤ *Adjunct to reduced-calorie diet and increased physical activity for chronic weight management in patients with an initial body mass index of 30 kg/m² or greater (obese), or 27 kg/m² or greater (overweight) in the presence of at least one weight-related comorbid condition such as hypertension, dyslipidemia, or type 2 diabetes*

TABLETS

Adults. 10 mg twice daily.

Mechanism of Action

Selectively activates 5-HT$_{2C}$ receptors on anorexigenic pro-opiomelanocortin neurons located in the hypothalamus to decrease food consumption and promote satiety.

Contraindications

Hypersensitivity to lorcaserin or its components, pregnancy

Interactions

DRUGS

bupropion, dextromethorphan, linezolid, lithium, MAOIs, selective serotonin norepinephrine reuptake inhibitors (SSNRIs), selective serotonin reuptake inhibitors (SSRIs), St. John's Wort, tramadol, tricyclic antidepressants (TCAs), triptans, tryptophan: Increased risk for serotonin syndrome
cytochrome P450 (2D6) substrates: Increased exposure of these drugs
phosphodiesterase type 5 inhibitors: Possibly increased risk of priapism
serotonergic and dopaminergic drugs (e.g. cabergoline): Increased risk for cardiac valvulopathy

Adverse Reactions

CNS: Anxiety, cognitive impairment, depression, dizziness, euphoria, fatigue, headache, insomnia, neuroleptic malignant syndrome-like reaction, serotonin syndrome, stress, suicidal ideation
CV: Bradycardia, hypertension, peripheral edema, valvulopathy
EENT: Abnormal ocular sensations, blurred vision; cataracts, conjunctival infections, irritations, inflammations; dry eyes or mouth; nasopharyngitis; oropharyngeal pain; sinus congestion; toothache; visual impairment
ENDO: Elevated prolactin level, hypoglycemia, worsening of diabetes mellitus
GI: Constipation, decreased appetite, diarrhea, gastroenteritis, nausea, vomiting
GU: UTI
HEME: Anemia; decreased red blood cell count, white blood cell count, hemoglobin, or hematocrit; leukopenia; lymphopenia; neutropenia
MS: Back or musculoskeletal pain
RESP: Cough, upper respiratory infection
SKIN: Rash
Other: Seasonal allergy

Nursing Considerations

• Use extreme caution when administering lorcaserin with any drug that affects the serotonergic neurotransmitter system, especially when drug is initiated and during dosage changes, because of the risk of serotonin syndrome.
• Use caution when administering lorcaserin to patients with congestive heart failure or hemodynamically-significant valvular heart disease because lorcaserin has been linked to regurgitant cardiac valvular disease, primarily affecting the mitral and/or aortic valves. Monitor patient closely for congestive heart failure, dependent edema, dyspnea, or a new cardiac murmur. If present, notify prescriber and expect drug to be discontinued.
• Use caution when administering lorcaserin to men who have conditions that might predispose them to priapism (e.g., sickle cell anemia, multiple myeloma, or leukemia), or in men with anatomical deformation of the penis (e.g., angulation, cavernosal fibrosis, or Peyroine's disease) because priapism is a potential effect of 5-HT$_{2C}$ receptor agonism.
• Use lorcaserin cautiously in patients with bradycardia or a history of heart block greater than first degree because a decrease in heart rate may occur with lorcaserin therapy.
• Use lorcaserin cautiously in patients with moderate renal impairment or severe hepatic impairment because the effects of lorcaserin in these patients are unknown. The drug is not recommended for patients with severe renal impairment or end-stage renal disease.
• Be aware that daily dosage should not exceed 10 mg twice a day because of increased risk of psychiatric disorders such as dissociation, euphoria, or hallucinations.
• Assess patient's weight loss at the end of 12 weeks. If patient has not lost at least 5% of his baseline body weight, notify prescriber and expect lorcaserin to be discontinued, as no further benefits are likely.
WARNING Monitor patient for signs and symptoms of serotonin syndrome, which may include mental status changes (e.g., agitation, hallucinations, coma), autonomic instability (e.g., hyperthermia,

labile blood pressure, tachycardia), neuromuscular aberrations (e.g., hyperreflexia, in-coordination) and/or gastrointestinal symptoms (e.g., diarrhea, nausea, vomiting). Know that serotonin syndrome, in its most severe form, can resemble neuroleptic maligant syndrome, which includes autonomic instability with possible rapid fluctuation of vital signs, hyperthermia, mental status changes, and muscle rigidity. If present, discontinue lorcaserin immediately, notify prescriber, and provide supportive care.

• Monitor patient's blood glucose level, especially patient with type 2 diabetes mellitus who is also being treated with insulin and/or oral hypoglycemic agents. As weight is lost, the risk of hypoglycemia increases. If hypoglycemia develops, treat appropriately and notify prescriber, as a dosage reduction may be needed with the patient's antidiabetic drug regimen.

• Monitor patient's complete blood count (CBC) periodically, as ordered, as hematological changes may occur during lorcaserin therapy.

• Monitor patient for signs and symptoms of prolactin excess (e.g., galactorrhea, gynecomastia) because lorcaserin moderately elevates prolactin levels. If present, notify prescriber and expect to obtain a prolactin level to confirm.

PATIENT TEACHING
• Warn patient not to exceed prescribed dosage because serious adverse effects may occur.

• Advise patient to avoid hazardous activities until drug's CNS effects on cognition are known.

• Instruct patient with type 2 diabetes mellitus who is also taking insulin or an oral hypoglycemic agent to monitor his blood glucose level closely. If hypo-glycemia develops, tell him to notify prescriber, as a dosage adjustment of his antidiabetic agent(s) may be needed.

• Inform a male patient to seek emergency care if he develops a painful erection that lasts longer than 4 hours and to discon-tinue lorcaserin therapy immediately.

• Tell women of childbearing age to notify prescriber immediately if pregnancy is suspected or has occurred.

losartan potassium
Cozaar

Class and Category
Chemical class: Angiotensin II receptor antagonist
Therapeutic class: Antihypertensive
Pregnancy category: D

Indications and Dosages
➤ *To manage hypertension*
TABLETS
Adults. *Initial:* 50 mg daily. *Maintenance:* 25 to 100 mg as a single dose or in 2 divided doses.
➤ *To treat nephropathy in patients with type 2 diabetes and hypertension*
TABLETS
Adults. *Initial:* 50 mg daily, increased to 100 mg daily, as needed.
➤ *To reduce stroke risk in patients with hypertension and left ventricular hypertrophy*
TABLETS
Adults. *Initial:* 50 mg daily, followed by 12.5 mg hydrochlorothiazide daily. Dosage increased to 100 mg daily, as needed, followed by 25 mg hydrochlorothiazide daily, as needed.
Children age 6 and over. *Initial:* 0.7 mg/kg to a maximum of 50 mg daily. *Maximum:* 1.4 mg/kg or 100 mg daily.
DOSAGE ADJUSTMENT Initial losartan dosage reduced to 25 mg daily for patients with impaired hepatic function or volume depletion.

Route	Onset	Peak	Duration
P.O.	Unknown	6 hr	Over 24 hr

Mechanism of Action
Blocks binding of angiotensin II to receptor sites in many tissues, including vascular smooth muscle and adrenal glands. Angiotensin II is a potent vasoconstrictor that also stimulates the adrenal cortex to secrete aldosterone. The inhibiting effects of angiotensin II reduce blood pressure.

Contraindications
Concurrent aliskiren therapy (in patients with diabetes or renal impairment [GFR less than 60 ml/min]), hypersensitivity to losartan or its components

J
K
L

Interactions

DRUGS

ACE inhibitors, aliskiren (in patients with diabetes or renal impairment), other angiotensin receptor blockers: Increased risk of hyperkalemia, hypotension, and renal dysfunction

antihypertensives, diuretics: Possibly hypotension

cyclosporine, potassium-sparing diuretics, potassium supplements: Increased risk of hyperkalemia

indomethacin, sympathomimetics: Possibly decreased antihypertensive effect of losartan

lithium: Increased serum lithium levels and risk of lithium toxicity

NSAIDs: Possibly decreased renal function in elderly patients or those with renal dysfunction or volume depletion; possibly decreased effectiveness of losartan

FOODS

high-potassium diet, potassium-containing salt substitutes: Increased risk of hyperkalemia

Adverse Reactions

CNS: Dizziness, fatigue, headache, insomnia, malaise
CV: Hypotension
EENT: Nasal congestion
GI: Diarrhea, indigestion, nausea, vomiting
HEME: Thrombocytopenia
MS: Back pain, leg pain, muscle spasms
RESP: Cough, upper respiratory tract infection
SKIN: Erythroderma
Other: Angioedema, hyperkalemia, hyponatremia

Nursing Considerations

• In some patients, losartan is more effective when given in two divided doses daily; it may be used with other antihypertensives.
• Know that patients of African descent with hypertension and left ventricular hypertrophy may not benefit from losartan to reduce stroke risk.
WARNING Be aware that patients who have severe heart failure or renal artery stenosis may experience acute renal failure from losartan therapy because losartan inhibits the angiotensin-

aldosterone system, on which renal function depends.
• Monitor blood pressure and renal function studies to evaluate drug effectiveness.
• Periodically monitor patient's serum potassium level, as appropriate, to detect hyperkalemia.
• Monitor patient for muscle pain; rarely, rhabdomyolysis develops in patients taking other angiotensin II receptor blockers.

PATIENT TEACHING

• Instruct patient to avoid potassium-containing salt substitutes because they may increase risk of hyperkalemia.
• Advise patient to avoid exercising in hot weather and drinking excessive amounts of alcohol; instruct her to notify prescriber if she has prolonged diarrhea, nausea, or vomiting.
• Warn patient to tell all prescribers of losartan therapy.
• Instruct women to notify prescriber immediately if pregnancy occurs or is suspected as drug may cause fetal harm and will need to be discontinued.

lovastatin
(mevinolin)
Altoprev, Mevacor

Class and Category
Chemical class: Mevinic acid derivative
Therapeutic class: Antihyperlipidemic
Pregnancy category: X

Indications and Dosages
➤ *To reduce LDL and total cholesterol levels in patients with primary hypercholesterolemia*

TABLETS

Adults. *Initial:* 20 mg as a single dose with evening meal. *Maintenance:* 20 to 80 mg daily as a single dose or in divided doses with meals. *Maximum:* 80 mg daily.

DOSAGE ADJUSTMENT For patients who also take immunosuppressants, initial dosage decreased to 10 mg daily and maximum dosage limited to 20 mg daily.

E.R. TABLETS

Adults. *Initial:* 10 mg, 20 mg, 40 mg, or 60 mg as single dose at bedtime, increased, as needed, every 4 wk, up to maximum dose. *Maintenance:* 10 to 60 mg daily as single dose. *Maximum:* 60 mg daily.

➤ *To reduce LDL, total cholesterol, and apolipoprotein B levels in adolescents with heterozygous familial hypercholesterolemia*

TABLETS

Adolescents 1 yr postmenarche (ages 10 to 17). *Initial:* 20 mg daily for LDL reduction of 20% or more, 10 mg daily for LDL reduction of less than 20%; dosage adjusted after at least 4 wk. *Maintenance:* 10 to 40 mg daily. *Maximum:* 40 mg daily.

DOSAGE ADJUSTMENT For patients who also take amiodarone, maximum dosage limited to 40 mg daily. For patients who also take danazol, diltiazem, or verapamil, initial therapy begun at 10 mg daily and maximum dosage limited to 20 mg daily. For patients with creatinine clearance less than 30 ml/min/1.73 m², maximum dosage limited to 20 mg daily.

Route	Onset	Peak	Duration
P.O.	In 2 wk	Unknown	4–6 wk

Mechanism of Action

Interferes with the hepatic enzyme hydroxymethylglutaryl-coenzyme A reductase. By doing so, lovastatin reduces formation of mevalonic acid (a cholesterol precursor), thus interrupting the pathway by which cholesterol is synthesized. When cholesterol level declines in hepatic cells, LDLs are consumed, which also reduces amount of circulating total cholesterol and serum triglycerides. The decrease in LDLs may result in decreased level of apolipoprotein B, which is found in each LDL particle.

Contraindications

Acute hepatic disease, breastfeeding, concomitant therapy with cobicistat-containing products, cyclosporine, gemfibrozil, or strong CYP3A4 inhibitors (such as boceprevir, clarithromycin, erythromycin, HIV protease inhibitors, itraconazole, ketoconazole, nefazodone, posaconazole, telaprevir, telithromycin, voriconazole), hypersensitivity to lovastatin or its components, pregnancy, unexplained elevated liver function test results

Interactions

DRUGS

amiodarone, boceprevir, cobicistat-containing products, clarithromycin, colchicine, cyclosporine, danazol, erythromycin, fibric acid derivatives, gemfibrozil and other fibrates, HIV protease inhibitors, immunosuppressants, itraconazole, ketoconazole, nefazodone, niacin (1 g daily or more), posaconazole, ranolazine, telaprevir, telithromycin, verapamil: Increased risk of severe myopathy or rhabdomyolysis
bile acid sequestrants, cholestyramine, colestipol: Decreased bioavailability of lovastatin
cimetidine, spironolactone: Possibly decreased level or activity of endogenous steroid hormones
isradipine: Increased hepatic clearance of lovastatin
itraconazole, ketoconazole: Increased lovastatin blood level
oral anticoagulants: Increased anticoagulant effect and risk of bleeding
voriconazole: Possibly increased blood lovastatin levels

FOODS

all foods: Increased lovastatin absorption
grapefruit juice (more than 1 qt daily): Increased risk of myopathy or rhabdomyolysis

ACTIVITIES

alcohol use: Increased lovastatin blood level

Adverse Reactions

CNS: Cognitive impairment, confusion, dizziness, fatigue, headache, insomnia, memory loss
EENT: Blurred vision, cataracts, pharyngitis, rhinitis, sinusitis
ENDO: Elevated glycosylated hemoglobin levels, hyperglycemia
GI: Abdominal cramps and pain, constipation, diarrhea, elevated liver function test results, flatulence, hepatic failure (rare), hyperbilirubinemia, indigestion, nausea, vomiting
MS: Arthritis, back pain, immune-mediated necrotizing myopathy, muscle pain, myalgia, myopathy, myositis, rhabdomyolysis
RESP: Cough, upper respiratory tract infection
SKIN: Dermatomyositis, erythema multiforme, pruritus, rash, Stevens-Johnson syndrome, toxic epidermal necrolysis
Other: Anaphylaxis, angioedema

J
K
L

Nursing Considerations

• Give lovastatin cautiously in patients who have a history of liver disease and patients who consume large amounts of alcohol.

• Give drug 1 hour before or 4 hours after bile acid sequestrant, cholestyramine, or colestipol.

• Expect patient to be prescribed a standard low-cholesterol diet during therapy.

• Be aware that drug affects mainly total cholesterol and LDL levels; it has only slight effects on HDL and triglyceride levels.

• Monitor liver function test results before therapy begins. If indicated, expect to measure them during therapy, as ordered. If AST or ALT level reaches or exceeds three times upper limit of normal and persists at that level, expect to discontinue lovastatin.

• Monitor patient closely for muscle pain, tenderness, or weakness suggestive of myopathy. Also monitor creatinine kinase, as ordered. If patient becomes symptomatic or creatine kinase becomes highly elevated, withhold drug, notify prescriber and expect drug to be discontinued. Be especially alert for myopathy that could become its more severe form, rhabdomyolysis, in patients with other disorders such as diabetes complicated with renal dysfunction.

• Expect to withhold drug temporarily in patients who develop an acute or serious condition predisposing the patient to the development of renal failure secondary to rhabdomyolysis. Conditions to be watchful for include hypotension; major surgery or trauma; sepsis; uncontrolled epilepsy; or severe electrolyte, endocrine or metabolic disorders.

PATIENT TEACHING

• Tell patient who takes drug once daily to do so with evening meal to enhance absorption.

• Advise patient to report muscle aches, pains, tenderness, or weakness, being especially watchful of these symptoms when dosage is increased. If present, tell him to stop taking lovastatin immediately and notify prescriber.

• Instruct patient to report severe GI distress or vision changes, as well as the development of dark urine, fatigue, loss of appetite, right upper abdominal pain or yellowing of skin.

• Advise patient to avoid performing any hazardous activity, such as driving, if

cognitive impairment develops and to notify prescriber.

• Tell patient to alert prescriber of any prescription or over-the-counter drugs being taken because serious drug interactions could occur.

• Urge patient to avoid consuming alcohol or more than 1 quart of grapefruit juice daily while taking drug.

• Direct patient to follow a low-cholesterol diet during therapy. Recommend weight loss and exercise programs as appropriate.

• Emphasize the importance of periodic eye examinations during therapy.

• Teach female patients appropriate contraceptive methods and the need to report suspected pregnancy immediately.

loxapine hydrochloride

Loxapac (CAN), Loxitane, Loxitane C, Loxitane IM

loxapine succinate

Loxapac (CAN), Loxitane

Class and Category

Chemical class: Dibenzoxazepine derivative
Therapeutic class: Antipsychotic
Pregnancy category: C

Indications and Dosages

➤ *To treat psychotic disorders and schizophrenia*

CAPSULES, ORAL SOLUTION

Adults. *Initial:* 10 mg twice daily, increased over 7 days. *Maintenance:* 15 to 25 mg twice daily to four times daily. *Maximum:* 250 mg daily.

DOSAGE ADJUSTMENT For elderly patients, dosage reduced to 3 to 5 mg twice daily.

➤ *To treat acute exacerbations of psychotic disorders*

I.M. INJECTION

Adults. 12.5 to 50 mg every 4 to 6 hr or longer. *Maximum:* 250 mg daily.

Route	Onset	Peak	Duration
P.O.	20–30 min	1.5–3 hr	12 hr

Mechanism of Action

May treat psychotic disorders by blocking dopamine at postsynaptic receptors in the brain. With prolonged use, loxapine enhances antipsychotic effects by causing depolarization blockade of dopamine tracts, resulting in decreased dopamine neurotransmission.

Contraindications

Blood dyscrasias, bone marrow depression, cerebrovascular disease, coma, coronary artery disease, hypersensitivity to loxapine or its components, impaired hepatic function, myeloproliferative disorders, severe drug-induced CNS depression, severe hypertension or hypotension

Interactions

DRUGS

amphetamines, ephedrine: Decreased effects of these drugs

antacids, antidiarrheals (adsorbent): Possibly decreased absorption of oral loxapine

anticholinergics: Possibly increased anticholinergic effects

anticonvulsants: Lowered seizure threshold, increased risk of seizures

antidyskinetics: Possibly antagonized therapeutic effects of these drugs

bromocriptine: Possibly decreased therapeutic effects of bromocriptine

CNS depressants: Increased effects of CNS depression

dopamine: Possibly decreased alpha-adrenergic effects of dopamine

epinephrine: Possibly severe hypotension or tachycardia, decreased epinephrine effects

guanadrel, guanethidine, levodopa: Possibly decreased therapeutic effects of these drugs

MAO inhibitors, tricyclic antidepressants: Possibly increased blood levels of these drugs, increased CNS depressant and anticholinergic effects

metaraminol: Possibly decreased vasopressor effect of metaraminol

methoxamine: Possibly decreased vasopressor effect and methoxamine duration of action

ACTIVITIES

alcohol use: Increased CNS depression

Adverse Reactions

CNS: Confusion, drowsiness, dystonia, involuntary motor activity, neuroleptic malignant syndrome, pseudoparkinsonism, sleep disturbance, tardive dyskinesia

CV: Orthostatic hypotension

EENT: Blurred vision, dry mouth

ENDO: Galactorrhea, gynecomastia

GI: Constipation, ileus, nausea, vomiting

GU: Menstrual irregularities, sexual dysfunction, urine retention

SKIN: Photosensitivity (mild), rash

Other: Weight gain

Nursing Considerations

• Be aware that loxapine's full antipsychotic effect may require weeks.

• Loxapine shouldn't be given to treat dementia-related psychosis in the elderly because of an increased mortality risk.

• Assess for signs of tardive dyskinesia, including involuntary protrusion of tongue and chewing movements. These signs may appear months or years after loxapine therapy begins and may not disappear with dosage reduction.

• Observe for extrapyramidal reactions or parkinsonian symptoms, such as excessive salivation, masklike facies, rigidity, and tremor, especially in first few days of treatment. Prescriber may reduce dosage to control these symptoms.

WARNING Monitor patient for neuroleptic malignant syndrome, a rare but possibly fatal adverse reaction. Early evidence includes altered mental status, arrhythmias, fever, and muscle rigidity.

PATIENT TEACHING

• Instruct patient to dilute loxapine oral solution with orange or grapefruit juice just before taking. Advise her to use calibrated dropper that accompanies solution to ensure correct dosage.

• Tell patient not to take antacids and antidiarrheals within 2 hours of loxapine.

• Caution patient to avoid alcohol while taking loxapine.

• Advise patient to change position slowly to minimize orthostatic hypotension.

• Urge patient to avoid hazardous activities until CNS effects of loxapine are known.

• Advise patient to avoid prolonged sun exposure and to use sunscreen to minimize risk of photosensitivity.

• Urge patient to have periodic eye examinations during therapy.

J
K
L

lubiprostone

Amitiza

Class and Category

Chemical class: Chloride channel activator
Therapeutic class: Intestinal motility enhancer
Pregnancy category: C

Indications and Dosages

➤ *To treat chronic idiopathic constipation, to treat opioid-induced constipation*

CAPSULES

Adults. 24 mcg twice daily with food and water.

➤ *To treat irritable bowel syndrome with constipation*

CAPSULES

Adults. 8 mcg twice daily with food and water.

Mechanism of Action

Enhances chloride-rich intestinal fluid secretion by locally activating chloride channels. By increasing intestinal fluid secretion, lubiprostone increases intestinal motility, which aids passage of stool, alleviating constipation.

Contraindications

Diarrhea, hypersensitivity to lubiprostone or components, mechanical GI obstruction

Interactions

DRUGS

antidiarrheals: Decreased GI motility

Adverse Reactions

CNS: Asthenia, dizziness, fatigue, headache, malaise
CV: Chest discomfort or pain, edema, increased heart rate
EENT: Dry mouth, throat tightness
GI: Abdominal distention or pain, diarrhea, dyspepsia, flatulence, nausea, vomiting
MS: Muscle cramps or spasms
RESP: Dyspnea
SKIN: Rash
Other: Angioedema

Nursing Considerations

• Be aware that lubiprostone shouldn't be used in patients with severe diarrhea.

• Make sure woman has a negative pregnancy test before starting lubiprostone because safety during pregnancy is unknown.
• Watch closely for adverse reactions, particularly dyspnea, and especially after first dose.

PATIENT TEACHING

• Advise patient to take drug with food to minimize risk of nausea.
• Tell women to use effective contraception while taking lubiprostone and to notify prescriber if pregnancy is suspected. Drug may need to be discontinued.
• Instruct patient to notify prescriber if severe diarrhea occurs.

lurasidone hydrochloride

Latuda

Class and Category

Chemical class: Benzoisothiazol
Therapeutic class: Atypical antipsychotic
Pregnancy category: B

Indications and Dosages

➤ *To treat schizophrenia*

TABLETS

Adults. *Initial:* 40 mg once daily with a meal consisting of at least 350 calories, increased as needed. *Maximum:* 80 mg once daily with a meal consisting of at least 350 calories.

➤ *To treat depressive episodes associated with bipolar I disorder as monotherapy or adjunctive therapy with either lithium or valproate*

TABLETS

Adults. *Initial:* 20 mg once daily. *Maximum:* 120 mg once daily.

DOSAGE ADJUSTMENT For patients already taking a moderate CYP3A4 drug or who have moderate hepatic impairment or moderate (creatinine clearance 30 to less than 50 ml/min) or severe (creatinine clearance less than 30 ml/min) renal impairment, maximum dose should not exceed 80 mg once daily. For patient with severe hepatic impairment, maximum dose should not exceed 40 mg once daily. For patient newly prescribed a moderate

CYP3A4 inhibitor, dosage reduced to half of the original dose of lurasidone prescribed.

Mechanism of Action

Possibly mediated through a combination of central dopamine type 2 and serotonin type 2 receptor antagonism to suppress psychotic symptoms.

Contraindications

Concurrent therapy with strong CYP3A4 inhibitors such as ketoconazole and strong CYP3A4 inducers such as rifampin, hypersensitivity to lurasidone or its components

Interactions

DRUGS

CNS depressants: Additive CNS depression
CYP3A4 inducers: Possibly decreased effect of lurasidone
CYP3A4 inhibitors: Possibly increased effect of lurasidone
digoxin, midazolam: Possibly increased blood levels of these drugs

ACTIVITIES

alcohol use: Additive CNS depression

Adverse Reactions

CNS: Agitation, akathisia, anxiety, dizziness, dystonia, fatigue, impaired cognitive and motor function, insomnia, neuroleptic malignant syndrome, parkinsonism, restlessness, seizures, somnolence, stroke, suicidal ideation, syncope, tardive dyskinesia, transient ischemic attacks
CV: Orthostatic hypotension, tachycardia
EENT: Blurred vision, increased salivation
ENDO: Hyperglycemia, hyperprolactinemia
GI: Abdominal pain, anorexia, diarrhea, dyspepsia, dysphagia, nausea, vomiting
HEME: Agranulocytosis, leukopenia, neutropenia
MS: Back pain
SKIN: Pruritus, rash
Other: Elevated CPK level

Nursing Considerations

WARNING Be aware that lurasidone should not be used to treat dementia-related psychosis in the elderly because of an increased risk of death nor in patients at

risk for aspiration pneumonia because drug may cause esophageal dysmotility, resulting in dysphagia.

• Use lurasidone cautiously in patients with cardiovascular disease, cerebrovascular disease, or conditions that would predispose them to hypotension. Also, use cautiously in those with a history of seizures or with conditions that lower the seizure threshold, such as Alzheimer's disease.

• Also, use cautiously in elderly patients because of increased risk of serious adverse cerebrovascular effects, such as stroke and transient ischemic attack.

WARNING Monitor patient closely for neuroleptic malignant syndrome, tardive dyskinesia, and seizures throughout therapy, and take safety precautions, as needed. Notify prescriber immediately of any occurrence.

• Monitor patient's blood glucose level routinely; risk of hyperglycemia may increase.

• Watch patients closely for suicidal tendencies, particularly when therapy starts and dosage changes, because depression may worsen temporarily during these times.

• Monitor patient's CBC, as ordered, because serious adverse hematologic reactions may occur, such as agranulocytosis, leukopenia, and neutropenia. Assess more often during first few months of therapy if patient has a history of drug-induced leukopenia or neutropenia or a significantly low WBC count. If abnormalities occur during therapy, watch for fever or other signs of infection, notify prescriber, and, if severe, expect drug to be discontinued.

• Know that extrapyramidal symptoms and withdrawal symptoms may occur in newborns following delivery to parents taking antipsychotics.

PATIENT TEACHING

• Instruct patient or caregiver that lurasidone must be taken with a meal consisting of at least 350 calories.

• Urge patient to avoid alcohol during lurasidone therapy.

• Instruct patient to avoid hazardous activities until drug's effects are known.

J
K
L

lypressin

Diapid

Class and Category

Chemical class: Synthetic vasopressin analogue
Therapeutic class: Antidiuretic
Pregnancy category: C

Indications and Dosages

➤ *To control and prevent dehydration, polydipsia, and polyuria in patients with neurogenic diabetes insipidus that is unresponsive to other therapy*

NASAL SOLUTION

Adults and adolescents. 1 or 2 sprays four times daily. If more drug is needed, interval between doses is decreased rather than increasing number of sprays/dose.

Mechanism of Action

Increases cellular permeability of collecting ducts in kidneys, leading to increased urine osmolality and decreased urine output.

Contraindications

Hypersensitivity to lypressin or components

Route	Onset	Peak	Duration
Intranasal	In 1 hr	0.5–2 hr	3–4 hr

Interactions

DRUGS

carbamazepine, chlorpropamide, clofibrate: Possibly increased antidiuretic effect
demeclocycline, lithium, norepinephrine: Decreased antidiuretic effect of lypressin

Adverse Reactions

CNS: Headache

EENT: Conjunctivitis; nasal congestion, irritation, and itching; periorbital edema and itching; rhinorrhea

GI: Abdominal cramps, diarrhea, heartburn (if excessive intranasal use causes dripping into pharynx)

RESP: Cough, transient dyspnea (if drug is accidentally inhaled)

Other: Water intoxication

Nursing Considerations

• Assess patient for nasal congestion or upper respiratory tract infection, which can reduce lypressin absorption and require larger doses or adjunct therapy.
• Administer final spray of drug at bedtime to help control nocturia.

WARNING Inadvertent inhalation, although rare, may cause chest tightness, continuous cough, and dyspnea.

• Observe for nasal irritation during long-term therapy.
• Watch for evidence of water intoxication, including coma, confusion, drowsiness, persistent headache, seizures, urine retention, and weight gain.

PATIENT TEACHING

• Teach patient how to administer lypressin correctly by holding head upright and bottle in a vertical position and spraying 1 or 2 sprays in each nostril with each dose.
• Instruct patient to take last dose of day at bedtime to control nocturia.
• Instruct patient to use drug exactly as prescribed.
• Tell patient to report abdominal cramps, heartburn, persistent headache, severe nasal irritation, and shortness of breath.

➤━━━━━━━━━━━━━━━━━━━◄

M

magnesium chloride

(contains 64 mg of elemental magnesium per tablet, 100 mg of elemental magnesium per enteric-coated tablet, 64 mg of elemental magnesium per E.R. tablet, and 200 mg of elemental magnesium per 1 ml of injection)
Chloromag, Mag-L-100, Slow-Mag

magnesium citrate

(citrate of magnesia)

(contains 40.5 to 47 mg elemental magnesium per 5 ml oral solution)
Citroma, Citro-Mag (CAN)

magnesium gluconate

(contains 54 mg elemental magnesium per 5 ml oral solution and 27 to 29.3 mg elemental magnesium per tablet)
Almora, Maglucate (CAN), Magonate, Magtrate

magnesium hydroxide

(milk of magnesia)

(contains 135 mg elemental magnesium per tablet, 129 to 130 mg elemental magnesium per chewable tablet, and 164 to 328 mg elemental magnesium per 5 ml liquid, liquid concentrate, or oral solution)
Phillips' Chewable Tablets, Phillips' Magnesia Tablets (CAN), Phillips' Milk of Magnesia, Phillips' Milk of Magnesia Concentrate

magnesium lactate

(contains 84 mg elemental magnesium per E.R. tablet)
Mag-Tab SR Caplets

magnesium oxide

(contains 84.5 mg elemental magnesium per capsule and 50 to 302 mg elemental magnesium per tablet)
Mag-200, Mag-Ox 400, Maox, Uro-Mag

magnesium sulfate

(contains 100 to 500 mg elmenteal magnesium per 1 ml of injection, 1 to 5 g elemental magnesium per 10 ml of injection, and 40 mEq per 5 mg of crystals)

Class and Category
Chemical class: Cation, electrolyte
Therapeutic class: Antacid, antiarrhythmic, anticonvulsant, electrolyte replacement, laxative
Pregnancy category: D (parenteral magnesium sulfate), Not rated (others)

Indications and Dosages
➤ *To correct magnesium deficiency caused by alcoholism, magnesium-depleting drugs, malnutrition, or restricted diet; to prevent magnesium deficiency based on U.S. and Canadian recommended daily allowances*
CAPSULES, CHEWABLE TABLETS, CRYSTALS, ENTERIC-COATED TABLETS, E.R. TABLETS, LIQUID, LIQUID CONCENTRATE, ORAL SOLUTION, TABLETS (MAGNESIUM CHLORIDE, CITRATE, GLUCONATE, HYDROXIDE, LACTATE [EXCEPT IN CHILDREN], OXIDE, SULFATE)
Dosage individualized based on severity of deficiency and normal recommended daily allowances listed below.
Adult men and children over age 10. 270 to 400 mg daily (*Canada:* 130 to 250 mg daily).
Adult women and children over age 10. 280 to 300 mg daily (*Canada:* 135 to 210 mg daily).
Pregnant women. 320 mg daily (*Canada:* 195 to 245 mg daily).
Breastfeeding women. 340 to 355 mg daily (*Canada:* 245 to 265 mg daily).
Children ages 7 to 10. 170 mg daily (*Canada:* 100 to 135 mg daily).
Children ages 4 to 6. 120 mg daily (*Canada:* 65 mg daily).

M

Children from birth to age 3. 40 to 80 mg/ day (*Canada:* 20 to 50 mg daily).
➤ *To treat mild magnesium deficiency*
I.M. INJECTION (MAGNESIUM SULFATE)
Adults and adolescents. 1 g every 6 hr for 4 doses.
➤ *To treat severe hypomagnesemia*
I.V. INFUSION (MAGNESIUM CHLORIDE)
Adults. 4 g diluted in 250 ml D_5W and infused at no more than 3 ml/min. *Maximum:* 40 g daily.
I.V. INFUSION (MAGNESIUM SULFATE)
Adults and adolescents. 5 g diluted in 1 L I.V. solution and infused over 3 hr.
➤ *To provide supplemental magnesium in total parenteral nutrition*
I.V. INFUSION (MAGNESIUM SULFATE)
Adults. 1 to 3 g daily.
Children. 0.25 mg to 1.25 g daily.
DOSAGE ADJUSTMENT Adult dosage may be increased to 6 g daily for certain conditions, such as short-bowel syndrome.
I.M. INJECTION (MAGNESIUM SULFATE)
Adults and adolescents. Up to 250 mg/kg every 4 hr, as needed.
➤ *To prevent and control seizures in preeclampsia or eclampsia as well as seizures caused by epilepsy, glomerulonephritis, or hypothyroidism*
I.V. INFUSION OR INJECTION (MAGNESIUM SULFATE)
Adults. *Loading:* 4 g diluted in 250 ml compatible solution and infused over 30 min. *Maintenance:* 1 to 2 g/hr by continuous infusion.
I.M. INJECTION (MAGNESIUM SULFATE)
Adults. 4 to 5 g every 4 hr, as needed.
Children. 20 to 40 mg/kg, repeated as needed.
➤ *To relieve indigestion with hyperacidity*
CHEWABLE TABLETS, LIQUID, LIQUID CONCENTRATE, ORAL SOLUTION TABLETS (MAGNESIUM HYDROXIDE)
Adults and adolescents. 400 to 1,200 mg (5 to 15 ml liquid or 2.5 to 7.5 ml liquid concentrate) up to 4 times daily with water, or 622 to 1,244 mg (tablets or chewable tablets) up to 4 times daily.
CAPSULES, TABLETS (MAGNESIUM OXIDE)
Adults and adolescents. 140 mg (capsules) three times daily or four times daily with water or milk, or 400 to 800 mg daily (tablets).
➤ *To relieve constipation, to evacuate colon for rectal or bowel examination*

LIQUID, LIQUID CONCENTRATE (MAGNESIUM HYDROXIDE)
Adults and children age 12 and over. 2.4 to 4.8 g (30 to 60 ml) daily as single dose or divided doses.
Children ages 6 to 11. 1.2 to 2.4 g (15 to 30 ml)/day as a single dose or in divided doses.
Children ages 2 to 5. 0.4 to 1.2 g (5 to 15 ml) daily as single dose or divided doses.
ORAL SOLUTION (MAGNESIUM CITRATE)
Adults and children age 12 and over. 11 to 25 g daily as single dose or divided doses.
Children ages 6 to 11. 5.5 to 12.5 g daily as single dose or divided doses.
Children ages 2 to 5. 2.7 to 6.25 g daily as single dose or divided doses.
CRYSTALS (MAGNESIUM SULFATE)
Adults and children age 12 and over. 10 to 30 g daily as single dose or divided doses.
DOSAGE ADJUSTMENT Dosage limited to 20 g of magnesium sulfate every 48 hr for patients with severe renal impairment.
Children ages 6 to 11. 5 to 10 g daily as a single dose or in divided doses.
Children ages 2 to 5. 2.5 to 5 g daily as a single dose or in divided doses.
CAPSULES, TABLETS (MAGNESIUM OXIDE)
Adults. 2 to 4 g with a full glass of water or milk, usually at bedtime.

Route	Onset	Peak	Duration
P.O.*	0.5–3 hr	Unknown	Unknown
P.O.†	20 min	Unknown	20–180 min
I.M.‡	1 hr	Unknown	3–4 hr
I.V.‡	Immediate	Unknown	About 30 min

Mechanism of Action
Assists all enzymes involved in phosphate transfer reactions that use adenosine triphosphate (ATP). Magnesium is required for normal function of the ATP-dependent sodium-potassium pump in muscle membranes. It may effectively treat digitalis glycoside–induced arrhythmias because correction of hypomagnesemia improves the sodium-potassium pump's ability to distribute potassium into intracellular spaces and because magnesium decreases

---

* For laxative effect.
† For antacid effect.
‡ For anticonvulsant effect.

calcium uptake and potassium outflow through myocardial cell membranes.

As a laxative, magnesium exerts a hyperosmotic effect in the small intestine. It causes water retention that distends the bowel and causes the duodenum to secrete cholecystokinin. This substance stimulates fluid secretion and intestinal motility.

As an antacid, magnesium reacts with water, converting magnesium oxide to magnesium hydroxide. Magnesium hydroxide rapidly reacts with gastric acid to form water and magnesium chloride, which increases gastric pH.

As an anticonvulsant, magnesium depresses the CNS and blocks peripheral neuromuscular impulse transmission by decreasing available acetylcholine.

Incompatibilities

Don't combine magnesium sulfate with alkali carbonates and bicarbonates, alkali hydroxides, arsenates, calcium, clindamycin phosphate, dobutamine, fat emulsions, heavy metals, hydrocortisone sodium succinate, phosphates, polymyxin B, procaine hydrochloride, salicylates, sodium bicarbonate, strontium, and tartrates.

Contraindications

Hypersensitivity to magnesium salts or any component of magnesium-containing preparations
For magnesium chloride: Coma, heart disease, renal impairment
For magnesium sulfate: Heart block, MI, preeclampsia 2 hours or less before delivery (I.V. form)
For use as laxative: Acute abdominal problem (as indicated by abdominal pain, nausea, or vomiting), diverticulitis, fecal impaction, intestinal obstruction or perforation, colostomy or ileostomy, severe renal impairment, ulcerative colitis

Interaction

DRUGS

amphotericin B, cisplatin, cyclosporine, gentamicin: Possibly magnesium wasting and need for magnesium dosage adjustment
anticholinergics: Possibly decreased absorption and therapeutic effects of these drugs
calcium salts (I.V.): Possibly neutralization of magnesium sulfate's effects

cellulose sodium phosphate: Possibly binding with magnesium, possibly decreased therapeutic effectiveness of cellulose
CNS depressants: Increased CNS depression
digoxin (I.V.): Possibly heart block and conduction changes, especially when calcium salts are also administered
digoxin, fluoroquinolones, folic acid, H$_2$-receptor blockers, iron preparations, isoniazid, ketoconazole, penicillamine, phenothiazines, phenytoin, phosphates (oral), tetracyclines: Possibly decreased absorption and blood levels of these drugs
diuretics (loop or thiazide): Possibly hypomagnesemia
*edetate sodium, sodium polystyrene sulfonate:*Possibly binding with magnesium
enteric-coated drugs: Possibly quicker dissolution of these drugs and increased risk of adverse GI reactions
etidronate (oral): Decreased etidronate absorption
mecamylamine: Possibly prolonged effects of mecamylamine
methenamine, streptomycin, sucralfate, tetracyclines, tobramycin (oral), urinary acidifiers: Possibly decreased therapeutic effects of these drugs
misoprostol: Increased misoprostol-induced diarrhea
neuromuscular blockers: Possibly increased neuromuscular blockade
nifedipine: Possibly increased hypotensive effects when taken with magnesium sulfate
potassium-sparing diuretics: Increased risk of hypermagnesemia
salicylates: Possibly increased excretion and lower blood levels of salicylates
sodium polystyrene sulfonate resin: Possibly metabolic alkalosis

FOODS

high glucose intake: Increased urinary excretion of magnesium

ACTIVITIES

alcohol use: Increased urinary excretion of magnesium

Adverse Reactions

CNS: Confusion, decreased reflexes, dizziness, syncope
CV: Arrhythmias, hypotension
GI: Flatulence, vomiting
MS: Muscle cramps

RESP: Dyspnea, respiratory depression or paralysis
SKIN: Diaphoresis
Other: Allergic reaction, hypermagnesemia, injection-site pain or irritation (I.M. form), laxative dependence, magnesium toxicity

Nursing Considerations

• Be aware that magnesium sulfate is the elemental form of magnesium. Oral preparations aren't all equivalent.
• Be aware that drug isn't metabolized. Drug remaining in the GI tract produces watery stool within 30 minutes to 3 hours.
• Make sure patient chews chewable tablets thoroughly before swallowing.
• Avoid giving other oral drugs within 2 hours of magnesium-containing antacid.
• Before giving drug as laxative, shake oral solution, liquid, or liquid concentrate well and give with a large amount of water.
WARNING Observe for and report early evidence of hypermagnesemia: bradycardia, depressed deep tendon reflexes, diplopia, dyspnea, flushing, hypotension, nausea, slurred speech, vomiting, and weakness.
WARNING Be aware that magnesium may precipitate myasthenic crisis by decreasing patient's sensitivity to acetylcholine.
• Frequently assess cardiac status of patient taking drugs that lower heart rate, such as beta blockers, because magnesium may aggravate symptoms of heart block.
WARNING Magnesium chloride for injection contains the preservative benzyl alcohol, which may cause fatal toxic syndrome in neonates and premature infants.
• Provide adequate diet, exercise, and fluids for patient being treated for constipation.
• Monitor serum electrolyte levels in patients with renal insufficiency because they're at risk for magnesium toxicity.
• Be aware that magnesium salts aren't intended for long-term use. For example, magnesium sulfate may cause fetal abnormalities if administered for more than 5 to 7 days to pregnant women. When magnesium sulfate is administered by continuous IV infusion (especially for more than 24 hours preceding delivery) to control convulsions in a toxemic woman, monitor newborn for signs of magnesium toxicity, such as neuromuscular or respiratory depression.

PATIENT TEACHING
• Advise patient to chew magnesium chewable tablets thoroughly before swallowing, and then drink a full glass of water. Mention that tablets have a chalky taste.
• Instruct patient to take magnesium-containing antacid between meals and at bedtime. Urge him not to take other drugs within 2 hours of the antacid.
• Tell patient to notify prescriber and avoid using magnesium-containing laxative if he has abdominal pain, nausea, or vomiting.
• Instruct patient to refrigerate magnesium citrate solution.
• Caution patient about risk of dependence with long-term laxative use.
• Teach patient to prevent constipation by increasing dietary fiber and fluid intake and exercising regularly.
• Inform patient that magnesium supplements used to replace electrolytes can cause diarrhea.

mannitol
Osmitrol, Resectisol

Class and Category
Chemical class: Hexahydroxy alcohol
Therapeutic class: Antiglaucoma, diagnostic agent, osmotic diuretic, urinary irrigant
Pregnancy category: B

Indications and Dosages
➤ *To reduce intracranial or intraocular pressure*
I.V. INFUSION
Adults and adolescents. 0.25 to 2 g/kg as 15% to 25% solution given over 30 to 60 min. If used before eye surgery, 1.5 to 2 g/kg 60 to 90 min before procedure. *Maximum:* 6 g/kg daily.
DOSAGE ADJUSTMENT For small or debilitated patients, dosage reduced to 0.5 g/kg.
➤ *To diagnose oliguria or inadequate renal function*
I.V. INFUSION
Adults and adolescents. 200 mg/kg or 12.5 gas 15% to 20% solution given over 3 to 5 min. Second dose given only if patient fails to excrete 30 to 50 ml of urine in 2 to 3 hr. Drug discontinued if no response after second dose. Or, 100 ml of 20% solution

diluted in 180 ml normal saline solution (forming 280 ml of 7.2% solution) and infused at 20 ml/min; followed by measurement of urine output. *Maximum:* 6 g/kg daily.
➤ *To prevent oliguria or acute renal failure*
I.V. INFUSION
Adults and adolescents. 50 to 100 g as 5% to 25% solution. *Maximum:* 6 g/kg daily.
➤ *To treat oliguria*
I.V. INFUSION
Adults and adolescents. 50 to 100 g as 15% to 25% solution given over 90 min to several hr. *Maximum:* 6 g/kg daily.
➤ *To promote diuresis in drug toxicity*
I.V. INFUSION
Adults and adolescents. *Loading:* 25 g. *Maintenance:* Up to 200 g as 5% to 25% solution given continuously to maintain urine output of 100 to 500 ml/hr with positive fluid balance of 1 to 2 L. *Maximum:* 6 g/kg daily.
➤ *To promote diuresis in hemolytic transfusion reaction*
I.V. INFUSION
Adults. 20 g given over 5 min and repeated if needed. *Maximum:* 6 g/kg daily.
➤ *To provide irrigation during transurethral resection of prostate gland*
IRRIGATION SOLUTION
Adults. 2.5% or 5% solution, as needed.

Route	Onset	Peak	Duration
I.V.*	1–3 hr	Unknown	Up to 8 hr
I.V.†	30–60 min	Unknown	4–8 hr
I.V.‡	In 15 min	Unknown	3–8 hr

Mechanism of Action
Elevates plasma osmolality, causing water to flow from tissues, such as brain and eyes, and from CSF, into extracellular fluid, thereby decreasing intracranial and intraocular pressure.

As an osmotic diuretic, mannitol increases the osmolarity of glomerular filtrate, which decreases water reabsorption. This leads to increased excretion of water, sodium, chloride, and toxic substances.

* To produce diuresis.
† To decrease intraocular pressure.
‡ To decrease intracranial pressure.

As an irrigant, mannitol minimizes the hemolytic effects of water used as an irrigant and reduces the movement of hemolyzed blood from the urethra to the systemic circulation, which prevents hemoglobinemia and serious renal complications.

Incompatibilities
Don't administer mannitol through same I.V. line as blood or blood products.

Contraindications
Active intracranial bleeding (except during craniotomy), anuria, hepatic failure, hypersensitivity to mannitol or its components, pulmonary edema, severe dehydration, severe heart failure, severe pulmonary congestion, severe renal insufficiency

Interaction
DRUGS
digoxin: Increased risk of digitalis toxicity from hypokalemia
diuretics: Possibly increased therapeutic effects of mannitol

Adverse Reactions
CNS: Chills, dizziness, fever, headache, seizures
CV: Chest pain, heart failure, hypertension, tachycardia, thrombophlebitis
EENT: Blurred vision, dry mouth, rhinitis
GI: Diarrhea, nausea, thirst, vomiting
GU: Polyuria, urine retention
RESP: Pulmonary edema
SKIN: Extravasation with edema and tissue necrosis, rash, urticaria
Other: Dehydration, hyperkalemia, hypernatremia, hypervolemia, hypokalemia, hyponatremia (dilutional), metabolic acidosis, water intoxication

Nursing Considerations
• If crystals form in mannitol solution exposed to low temperature, place solution in hot-water bath to redissolve crystals.
• Use a 5-micron in-line filter when administering drug solution of 15% or greater.
• During I.V. infusion of mannitol, monitor vital signs, central venous pressure, and fluid intake and output every hour. Measure urine output with indwelling urinary catheter, as appropriate.

M

• Check weight and monitor BUN and serum creatinine electrolyte levels daily.
• Provide frequent mouth care to relieve thirst and dry mouth.

PATIENT TEACHING
• Inform patient that he may experience dry mouth and thirst during mannitol therapy.
• Instruct patient to report chest pain, difficulty breathing, or pain at I.V. site.

maprotiline hydrochloride

Ludiomil

Class and Category

Chemical class: Dibenzobicyclooctadiene derivative
Therapeutic class: Antidepressant, tricyclic antidepressant
Pregnancy category: B

Indications and Dosages

➤ *To treat mild to moderate depression*

TABLETS

Adults and adolescents. *Initial:* 75 mg daily in divided doses for 2 wk. Increased in 25-mg increments as needed and tolerated. *Maintenance:* 150 to 225 mg daily in divided doses; for prolonged therapy, possibly 75 to 150 mg daily in divided doses.

➤ *To treat hospitalized patients with severe depression*

TABLETS

Adults and adolescents. *Initial:* 100 to 150 mg daily in divided doses, increased as needed and tolerated. *Maintenance:* 150 to 225 mg daily in divided doses; for prolonged therapy, possibly 75 to 150 mg daily in divided doses.

DOSAGE ADJUSTMENT For patients over age 60, initial dosage reduced to 25 mg daily and then increased by 25 mg/wk up to maintenance dosage of 50 to 75 mg daily in divided doses.

Route	Onset	Peak	Duration
P.O.	1–3 wk	3–6 wk	Unknown

Mechanism of Action

Blocks norepinephrine's reuptake at adrenergic nerve fibers. Normally, when a nerve impulse reaches an adrenergic nerve fiber, norepinephrine is released from storage sites and metabolized in the nerve or at the synapse. Some norepinephrine reaches receptor sites on target organs and tissues, but most is taken back into the nerve and stored by way of reuptake mechanism. By blocking norepinephrine reuptake, maprotiline increases its level at nerve synapses. Elevated norepinephrine level may improve mood and decrease depression.

Contraindications

Hypersensitivity to maprotiline, mirtazapine, or their components; use within 14 days of MAO inhibitor therapy

Interaction

DRUGS

anticholinergics, antihistamines: Increased atropine-like adverse effects, such as blurred vision, constipation, dizziness, and dry mouth
anticonvulsants: Increased risk of CNS depression, possibly lower seizure threshold and increased risk of seizures
bupropion, clozapine, haloperidol, loxapine, molindone, other tricyclic antidepressants, phenothiazines, pimozide, thioxanthenes, trazodone: Possibly increased anticholinergic effects, possibly lowered seizure threshold and increased risk of seizures
cimetidine: Possibly increased blood maprotiline level
clonidine, guanadrel, guanethidine: Possibly decreased antihypertensive effects of these drugs, possibly increased CNS depression (with clonidine)
CNS depressants: Increased risk of CNS depression
estrogens, oral contraceptives containing estrogen: Possibly decreased therapeutic effects and increased adverse effects of maprotiline
MAO inhibitors: Increased risk of hyperpyrexia, hypertensive crisis, severe seizures, or death
sympathomimetics: Increased risk of arrhythmias, hyperpyrexia, hypertension, or tachycardia
thyroid hormones: Increased risk of arrhythmias

ACTIVITIES

alcohol use: Increased risk of CNS depression

Adverse Reactions

CNS: Agitation, dizziness, drowsiness, fatigue, headache, insomnia, seizures, suicidal ideation, tremor, weakness
EENT: Blurred vision, dry mouth, increased intraocular pressure
ENDO: Gynecomastia
GI: Constipation, diarrhea, epigastric distress, increased appetite, nausea, vomiting
GU: Impotence, libido changes, testicular swelling, urinary hesitancy, urine retention
HEME: Agranulocytosis
SKIN: Diaphoresis, photosensitivity, pruritus, rash
Other: Weight loss

Nursing Considerations

• Give largest dose of maprotiline at bedtime if daytime drowsiness occurs.
• Check CBC, as ordered, if fever, sore throat, or other evidence of agranulocytosis develops.
• Take seizure precautions according to facility policy.
• Watch patient (especially children, adolescents, and young adults) closely for suicidaltendencies, particularly when therapy startsand dosage changes, because depression may worsen temporarily during these times, possibly leading to suicidal ideation.
• Expect to taper drug gradually because stopping abruptly may produce withdrawal symptoms.

PATIENT TEACHING

• Advise patient to take maprotiline exactly as prescribed. Caution him not to stop drug abruptly because of risk of withdrawal symptoms, including headache, nausea, nightmares, and vertigo.
• Inform patient that he may not feel drug's effects for several weeks.
• Suggest that patient take drug with food if adverse GI reactions develop.
• Urge patient to report difficulty urinating, excessive drowsiness, fever, or sore throat.
• Advise patient to avoid hazardous activities until drug's CNS effects are known.
• Caution patient to avoid alcohol and other CNS depressants while taking drug.
• Urge family or caregiver to watch patient closely for suicidal tendencies, especially when therapy starts or dosage changes and particularly if patient is a child, teenager, or young adult.

meclizine hydrochloride
(meclozine hydrochloride)

Antivert, Bonamine (CAN), Bonine, Dizmiss, Dramamine II, Meclicot, Medivert, Meni-D

Class and Category

Chemical class: Piperazine derivative
Therapeutic class: Antiemetic, antivertigo
Pregnancy category: B

Indications and Dosages

➤ *To prevent and treat vertigo*
CAPSULES, CHEWABLE TABLETS, TABLETS
Adults and adolescents. 25 to 100 mg daily, as needed, in divided doses.
➤ *To treat motion sickness*
CAPSULES, TABLETS
Adults. 25 to 50 mg 1 hr before travel and then every 24 hr, as needed, for duration of trip.

Route	Onset	Peak	Duration
P.O.	1 hr	Unknown	8–24 hr

Mechanism of Action

May inhibit nausea and vomiting by reducing sensitivity of labyrinthine apparatus and blocking cholinergic synapses in the brain's vomiting center.

Contraindications

Hypersensitivity to meclizine or its components

Interaction

DRUGS
anticholinergics: Possibly potentiated anticholinergic effects
apomorphine: Possibly decreased emetic response to apomorphine
CNS depressants: Possibly potentiated CNS depression
CYP2D6 inhibitors: Possibly decreased effectiveness of meclizine
ACTIVITIES
alcohol use: Possibly potentiated CNS depression

M

Adverse Reactions

CNS: Dizziness, drowsiness, euphoria, excitement, fatigue, hallucinations, headache, insomnia, nervousness, restlessness, vertigo
CV: Hypotension, palpitations, tachycardia
EENT: Blurred vision; diplopia; dry mouth, nose, and throat; tinnitus
GI: Abdominal pain, anorexia, constipation, diarrhea, nausea, vomiting
GU: Urinary frequency and hesitancy, urine retention
RESP: Bronchospasm, thickening of respiratory secretions
SKIN: Jaundice, rash, urticaria

Nursing Considerations

• Use meclizine cautiously in patients with asthma, glaucoma, or prostate gland enlargement.
• Also, use cautiously in patients with hepatic or renal impairment and the elderly because of potential increase of drug in blood levels under these conditions.
• Be aware that drug may mask signs of brain tumor, intestinal obstruction, or ototoxicity.

PATIENT TEACHING
• Explain that meclizine works best for motion sickness when taken before travel.
• Instruct patient to chew meclizine chewable tablets thoroughly before swallowing.
• Instruct patient to report blurred vision or drowsiness.
• Urge patient to avoid alcohol while taking drug.
• Caution patient to avoid hazardous activities until drug's CNS effects are known.
• Advise patient to have regular eye examinations during long-term therapy.

meclofenamate sodium

Meclomen

Class and Category

Chemical class: Fenamate (anthranilic acid) derivative

Therapeutic class: Analgesic, antidysmenorrheal, anti-inflammatory, antirheumatic
Pregnancy category: Not rated

Indications and Dosages

➤ *To relieve pain and inflammation in rheumatoid arthritis and osteoarthritis*
CAPSULES
Adults and adolescents over age 14. 50 to 100 mg every 6 to 8 hr, as needed. *Maximum:* 400 mg/day.
➤ *To relieve mild to moderate pain*
CAPSULES
Adults and adolescents over age 14. 50 mg every 4 to 6 hr, as needed. Increased to 100 mg every 4 to 6 hr, as needed. *Maximum:* 400 mg daily.
➤ *To treat hypermenorrhea and primary dysmenorrhea*
CAPSULES
Adults and adolescents over age 14. 100 mg three times daily for up to 6 days.

Route	Onset	Peak	Duration
P.O.*	1 hr	0.5–2 hr	4–6 hr
P.O.†	Few days	2–3 wk	Unknown

Mechanism of Action

Blocks cyclooxygenase, the enzyme needed to synthesize prostaglandins, which mediate the inflammatory response and cause local vasodilation, swelling, and pain. By inhibiting prostaglandins, this NSAID reduces inflammatory symptoms. It also relieves pain because prostaglandins promote pain transmission from periphery to spinal cord.

Contraindications

Hypersensitivity to aspirin, iodides, meclofenamate, other NSAIDs, or their components

Interaction

DRUGS
acetaminophen: Increased risk of adverse renal effects with long-term use of both drugs
anticoagulants, thrombolytics: Prolonged PT and increased risk of bleeding
antihypertensives: Decreased effectiveness of antihypertensives

---

* For analgesic effect.
† For antirheumatic effect.

beta blockers: Impaired antihypertensive effect of beta blockers
cefamandole, cefoperazone, cefotetan, plicamycin, valproic acid: hypoprothrombinemia and increased risk of bleeding
cimetidine: Altered meclofenamate level
colchicine, glucocorticoids, potassium supplements: Increased GI irritability and bleeding
cyclosporine, gold compounds, nephrotoxic drugs: Increased risk of nephrotoxicity
digoxin: Increased blood digoxin level
insulin, oral antidiabetic drugs: Decreased effectiveness of these drugs
lithium: Increased risk of lithium toxicity
loop diuretics: Decreased effects of these drugs
methotrexate: Increased risk of methotrexate toxicity
NSAIDs, salicylates: Increased GI irritability and risk of bleeding, decreased meclofenamate effectiveness
phenytoin: Increased blood phenytoin level
probenecid: Increased risk of meclofenamate toxicity

ACTIVITIES
alcohol use: Increased GI irritability and bleeding

Adverse Reactions

CNS: Dizziness, drowsiness, fatigue, headache, insomnia, seizures, stroke
CV: Hypertension, MI, peripheral edema, tachycardia
EENT: Stomatitis, tinnitus
GI: Abdominal pain; anorexia; constipation; diarrhea; diverticulitis; dyspepsia; dysphagia; elevated liver function test results; esophagitis; flatulence; gastritis; gastroenteritis; gastroesophageal reflux disease; GI bleeding, perforation, and ulceration; hepatic failure; indigestion; jaundice; melena; nausea; perforation of stomach or intestines; stomatitis; vomiting
GU: Acute renal failure, dysuria, elevated BUN and serum creatinine levels
HEME: Agranulocytosis, anemia, easy bruising, hemolytic anemia, leukopenia, neutropenia, pancytopenia, thrombocytopenia
RESP: Asthma, respiratory depression
SKIN: Erythema multiforme, pruritus, rash, Stevens-Johnson syndrome, toxic epidermal necrolysis, urticaria
Other: Anaphylaxis, angioedema

Nursing Considerations

• Use meclofenamate with extreme caution in patients with a history of ulcer disease or GI bleeding because NSAIDs such as meclofenamate increase risk of GI bleeding and ulceration. Expect to use drug for shortest time possible in these patients.
• Be aware that serious GI tract ulceration, bleeding, and perforation may occur without warning symptoms. Elderly patients are at greater risk. To minimize risk, give drug with food and a full glass of water. If GI distress occurs, withhold drug and notify prescriber immediately.
• Use meclofenamate cautiously in patients with hypertension, and monitor blood pressure closely throughout therapy. Drug may cause hypertension or worsen it.
WARNING Monitor patient closely for thrombotic events, including MI and stroke, because NSAIDs increase the risk.
• Monitor patient—especially if he's elderly or taking meclofenamate long-term—for less common but serious adverse GI reactions, including anorexia, constipation, diverticulitis, dysphagia, esophagitis, gastritis, gastroenteritis, gastroesophageal reflux disease, hemorrhoids, hiatal hernia, melena, stomatitis, and vomiting.
• Monitor liver function test results because, rarely, elevations may progress to severe hepatic reactions, including fatal hepatitis, liver necrosis, and hepatic failure.
• Monitor BUN and serum creatinine levels in elderly patients, patients taking diuretics or ACE inhibitors, and patients with heart failure, impaired renal function, or hepatic dysfunction; drug may cause renal failure.
• Monitor CBC for decreased hemoglobin and hematocrit because drug may worsen anemia.
WARNING If patient has bone marrow suppression or is receiving an antineoplastic drug, monitor laboratory results (including WBC count), and watch for evidence of infection because antiinflammatory and antipyretic actions of meclofenamate may mask signs and symptoms, such as fever and pain.

M

• Assess patient's skin regularly for rash or other hypersensitivity reaction because meclofenamate is an NSAID and may cause serious skin reactions without warning, even in patients with no history of NSAID sensitivity. At first sign of reaction, stop drug and notify prescriber.

• Expect lower doses of meclofenamate to be used for long-term therapy.

PATIENT TEACHING

• Tell patient to take drug with a full glass of water to keep it from lodging in esophagus and causing irritation. Suggest taking drug with food or milk to avoid GI distress.

• Instruct patient to report itching, rash, severe diarrhea, and swelling in ankles or fingers.

• Caution patient to avoid hazardous activities until drug's CNS effects are known.

• Caution pregnant patient not to take NSAIDs such as meclofenamate during last trimester because they may cause premature closure of fetal ductus arteriosus.

• Explain that meclofenamate may increase risk of serious adverse cardio-vascular reactions; urge patient to seek immediate medical attention if signs or symptoms arise, such as chest pain, shortness of breath, weakness, or slurring of speech.

• Explain that meclofenamate may increase risk of serious adverse GI reactions; stress importance of seeking immediate medical attention for such signs and symptoms as epigastric or abdominal pain, indigestion, black or tarry stools, or vomiting blood or material that looks like coffee grounds.

• Alert patient to rare but serious skin reactions to meclofenamate. Urge him to seek immediate medical attention for rash, blisters, itching, fever, or other indications of hypersensitivity.

meloxicam

Mobic

Class and Category

Chemical class: Oxicam derivative
Therapeutic class: Anti-inflammatory
Pregnancy category: C

Indications and Dosages

➤ *To relieve signs and symptoms of osteoarthritis and rheumatoid arthritis*

ORAL SUSPENSION, TABLETS
Adults. 7.5 mg daily. *Maximum:* 15 mg daily.

➤ *To relieve pauciarticular or poly-articular signs and symptoms of juvenile rheumatoid arthritis*

ORAL SUSPENSION, TABLETS
Children age 2 and over. 0.125 mg/kg daily. *Maximum:* 7.5 mg daily.

Mechanism of Action

Blocks cyclooxygenase, the enzyme needed to synthesize prostaglandins, which mediate the inflammatory response and cause local vasodilation, swelling, and pain. By inhibiting prostaglandins, the NSAID meloxicam reduces inflammatory symptoms. It also relieves pain because prostaglandins promote pain transmission from the periphery to the spinal cord.

Contraindications

Angioedema, asthma, bronchospasm, nasal polyps, rhinitis, or urticaria induced by hypersensitivity to aspirin, meloxicam, other NSAIDs, or their components

Interaction

DRUGS
ACE inhibitors: Decreased antihypertensive effect, increased risk of renal failure
aspirin: Increased risk of GI ulceration
furosemide: Decreased diuretic effect of furosemide, possibly renal impairment
kayexalate: Increased risk of intestinal necrosis
lithium: Elevated blood lithium level, possibly lithium toxicity
oral anticoagulants, warfarin: Increased risk of bleeding

ACTIVITIES
alcohol use, smoking: Increased risk of GI bleeding

Adverse Reactions

CNS: Confusion, dizziness, fever, headache, insomnia, mood alteration, seizures, stroke
CV: Chest pain, edema, heart failure, hypertension, MI, tachycardia, vasculitis
EENT: Laryngitis, pharyngitis, sinusitis
GI: Abdominal pain, anorexia, colitis, constipation, diarrhea, diverticulitis, dyspepsia, dysphagia, elevated liver

function test results, esophagitis, flatulence, gastritis, gastroenteritis, gastroesophageal reflux disease, GI bleeding and ulceration, hepatic failure, hepatitis, indigestion, melena, nausea, pancreatitis, perforation of stomach or intestines, stomatitis, vomiting
GU: Acute renal failure, acute urine retention (children), urinary frequency, UTI
HEME: Agranulocytosis, anemia, easy bruising, hemolytic anemia, leukopenia, neutropenia, pancytopenia, thrombocytopenia
MS: Arthralgia; back pain; joint crepitation, effusion, or swelling; muscle spasms; myalgia
RESP: Asthma, bronchospasm, cough, dyspnea, respiratory depression, upper respiratory tract infection
SKIN: Erythema multiforme, exfoliative dermatitis, photosensitivity, pruritus, rash, Stevens-Johnson syndrome, toxic epidermal necrolysis
Other: Anaphylaxis, angioedema, flulike symptoms

Nursing Considerations

• Use meloxicam with extreme caution in patients with history of ulcer disease or GI bleeding because NSAIDs such as meloxicam increase risk of GI bleeding and ulceration. Expect to use drug for shortest time possible in these patients.
• Be aware that serious GI tract ulceration, bleeding, and perforation may occur without warning symptoms. Elderly patients are at greater risk. To minimize risk, give drug with food and a full glass of water. If GI distress occurs, withhold drug and notify prescriber immediately.
• Use meloxicam cautiously in patients with hypertension, and monitor blood pressure closely throughout therapy. Drug may cause hypertension or worsen it.
WARNING Monitor patient closely for thrombotic events, including MI and stroke, because NSAIDs increase the risk.
• Monitor patient—especially if elderly or taking meloxicam long-term—for less common but serious adverse GI reactions, including anorexia, constipation, diverticulitis, dysphagia, esophagitis, gastritis, gastroenteritis, gastroesophageal reflux disease, hemorrhoids, hiatal hernia, melena, stomatitis, and vomiting.
• Monitor liver function test results because, rarely, elevations may progress to severe

hepatic reactions, including fatal hepatitis, liver necrosis, and hepatic failure.
• Monitor BUN and serum creatinine levels in elderly patients; patients taking diuretics, angiotensin II receptor antagonists, or ACE inhibitors; and patients with heart failure, impaired renal function, or hepatic dysfunction. Drug may cause renal failure.
• Monitor CBC for decreased hemoglobin and hematocrit. Drug may worsen anemia.
WARNING If patient has bone marrow suppression or is receiving an antineoplastic drug, monitor laboratory results (including WBC count), and watch for evidence of infection because antiinflammatory and antipyretic actions of meloxicam may mask signs and symptoms, such as fever and pain.
• Assess patient's skin regularly for rash or other hypersensitivity reaction because meloxicam is an NSAID and may cause serious skin reactions without warning, even in patients with no history of NSAID sensitivity. At first sign of reaction, stop drug and notify prescriber.
• Monitor patient for adequate hydration before beginning meloxicam therapy to decrease risk of renal dysfunction.

PATIENT TEACHING

• Instruct patient to take meloxicam with food or after meals if she has stomach upset.
• For oral suspension, tell patient to shake container gently before use.
• Caution patient to avoid using other NSAIDs, aspirin, or products containing aspirin while taking meloxicam.
• Advise patient to refrain from smoking and alcohol use because these activities may increase risk of adverse GI reactions.
• Instruct patient to notify prescriber if she develops signs or symptoms of hepatic dysfunction, such as dark yellow or brown urine, fatigue, fever, itching, lethargy, nausea, or yellowing of eyes or skin.
• Advise patient, especially if she's taking an oral anticoagulant such as warfarin, to report immediately signs of bleeding, such as easy bruising, stomach pain, blood in urine, or black tarry stools.
• Alert women of childbearing age that meloxicam may cause a reversible delay in ovulation that may make conception more

M

difficult. If pregnancy is desired, she should consult with prescriber about discontinuing meloxicam therapy and using an alternative drug to treat her condition.
- Caution pregnant patient not to take NSAIDs such as meloxicam during the last trimester because they may cause premature closure of ductus arteriosus.
- Explain that meloxicam may increase risk of serious adverse cardiovascular reactions; urge patient to seek immediate medical attention if signs or symptoms arise, such as chest pain, shortness of breath, weakness, and slurring of speech.
- Explain that meloxicam may increase risk of serious adverse GI reactions; emphasize importance of seeking immediate medical attention for such signs and symptoms as epigastric or abdominal pain, indigestion, black or tarry stools, or vomiting blood or material that looks like coffee grounds.
- Alert patient to rare but serious skin reactions. Urge her to seek immediate medical attention for rash, blisters, itching, fever, or other indications of hypersensitivity.

memantine hydrochloride

Namenda, Namenda XR

Class and Category

Chemical class: N-methyl-D-aspartate (NMDA) receptor antagonist
Therapeutic class: Antidementia agent
Pregnancy category: B

Indications and Dosages

➤ *To treat moderate-to-severe dementia of the alzheimer's type*

TABLETS
Adults. *Initial:* 5 mg daily, increased by 5 mg/wk, as needed, to 10 mg daily in two divided doses; then 15 mg daily with one 5-mg and one 10-mg dose daily; then 20 mg daily in two divided doses.
Maintenance: 20 mg daily.

ER CAPSULES
Adults. *Initial:* 7 mg once daily, increased by 7 mg/wk, as needed, to 28 mg once daily. *Maximum:* 28 mg once daily.

DOSAGE ADJUSTMENT Maintenance dosage reduction probable for patients with severe renal impairment.

Contraindications

Hypersensitivity to memantine, amantadine, or their components

Interaction

DRUGS
amantadine, dextromethorphan, ketamine: Possibly additive effects
carbonic anhydrase inhibitors, sodium bicarbonate: Decreased memantine

Mechanism of Action

Memantine blocks the excitatory amino acid glutamate on N-methyl-D-aspartate (NMDA) receptor cells in the CNS. In Alzheimer's disease, glutamate levels areabnormally high when brain cells are both at rest and active. Normally, when certainbrain cells are resting, magnesium ions block NMDA receptors and prevent influxof sodium and calcium ions and outflow of potassium ions. When learning andmemory cells in the brain are active, glutamate engages with NMDA receptors, magnesium ions are removed from NMDA receptors, and cells are depolarized. During depolarization, sodium and calcium ions enter brain cells, and potassium ionsleave. In Alzheimer's disease, excessive circulating glutamate permanently removes magnesium ions and opens ion channels. Excessive influx of calcium may damage brain cells and play a major role in Alzheimer's disease. What's more, dying brain cells release additional glutamate, worsening the cycle of brain cell destruction.

Memantine replaces magnesium on NMDA receptors of brain cells, closing ion channels and preventing calcium influx and the resulting damage to brain cells. By preventing excessive brain cell death, memantine slows progression of Alzheimer's disease.

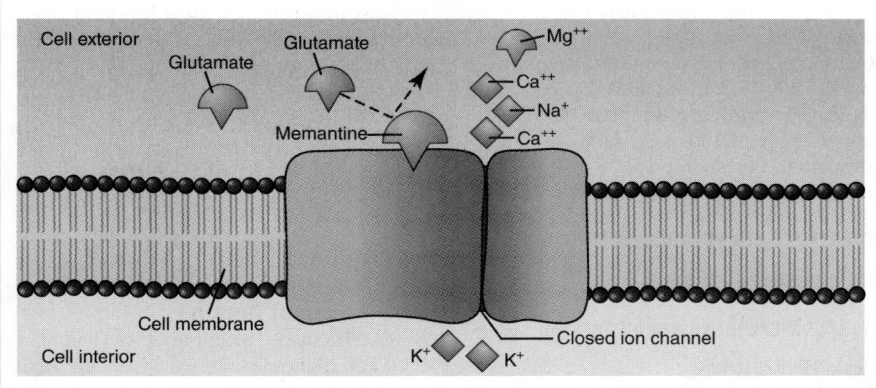

clearance, leading to increased blood drug levels and risk of adverse effects
cimetidine, hydrochlorothiazide, metformin, nicotinic acid, quinidine, ranitidine, triamterene: Possibly increased blood levels of both agents

Adverse Reactions

CNS: Abnormal gait, agitation, akathisia, anxiety, confusion, delirium, delusions, depression, dizziness, drowsiness, dyskinesia, fatigue, hallucinations, headache, hyperexcitability, insomnia, neuroleptic malignant syndrome, psychosis, restlessness, seizures, somnolence, stroke, suicidal ideation, tardive dyskinesia

CV: AV block, chest pain, congestive heart failure, hypertension, peripheral edema, prolonged QT interval, supraventricular tachycardia, tachycardia

ENDO: Hypoglycemia

GI: Acute pancreatitis, anorexia, colitis, constipation, diarrhea, hepatic failure, hepatitis, ileus, nausea, pancreatitis, vomiting

GU: Acute renal failure, elevated creatinine levels, impotence, renal insufficiency, urinary incontinence, UTI

HEME: Agranulocytosis, leukopenia, neutropenia, pancytopenia, thrombo-cytopenia, thrombotic thrombocytopenic purpura

MS: Arthralgia, back pain

RESP: Bronchitis, cough, dyspnea, upper respiratory tract infection

SKIN: Stevens-Johnson syndrome

Other: Generalized pain, flulike symptoms

Nursing Considerations

• Use memantine cautiously in patients with renal tubular acidosis or severe UTI because these conditions make urine alkaline, reducing memantine excretion and increasing the risk of adverse reactions.

• Use cautiously in patients with severe hepatic impairment because drug undergoes partial hepatic metabolism, which may increase risk of adverse reactions.

• Monitor patient's response to memantine, and notify prescriber if serious or bothersome adverse reactions occur.

• Monitor patient closely for suicidal thoughts.

PATIENT TEACHING

• Instruct patient to take memantine exactly as prescribed. Inform him to notify the prescriber if he fails to take the drug for several days, as dosage adjustments may be necessary. Caution him not to double dose if he misses a single dose. Instead, tell him to take the next dose as scheduled.

• Advise patient to avoid a diet excessively high in fruits and vegetables because these foods contribute to alkaline urine, which can alter memantine clearance and increase adverse reactions.

• Tell patient capsule should be swallowed whole and not divided, chewed, or crushed. If patient has difficulty swallowing the capsule, instruct him to open capsule, sprinkle contents on

M

applesauce, and immediately consume entire amount of applesauce.
• Caution patient to avoid hazardous activities until drug's CNS effects are known.
• Alert patient or caregiver that memantine has the potential to cause suicidal thoughts. If present, prescriber should be notified immediately.

meperidine hydrochloride (pethidine hydrochloride)
Demerol

Class, Category, and Schedule
Chemical class: Phenylpiperidine derivative opioid
Therapeutic class: Analgesic
Pregnancy category: C
Controlled substance schedule: II

Indications and Dosages
➤ *To relieve moderate to severe pain*
SYRUP, TABLETS, I.M. OR SUBCUTANEOUS INJECTION
Adults. 50 to 150 mg every 3 to 4 hr, as needed.
Children. 1.1 to 1.8 mg/kg every 3 to 4 hr, as needed.
➤ *To provide preoperative sedation*
I.V. INJECTION
Adults. 15 to 35 mg/hr, as needed.
I.M. OR SUBCUTANEOUS INJECTION
Adults. 50 to 100 mg 30 to 90 min before surgery.
Children. 1 to 2 mg/kg 30 to 90 min before surgery. *Maximum:* 100 mg every 3 to 4 hr.
➤ *As adjunct to anesthesia*
I.V. INFUSION OR INJECTION
Adults. Individualized. Repeated slow injections of 10 mg/ml solution or continuous infusion of dilute solution (1 mg/ml) titrated as needed.
➤ *To provide obstetric analgesia*
I.M. OR SUBCUTANEOUS INJECTION
Adults. 50 to 100 mg given with regular, painful contractions; repeated every 1 to 3 hr.
DOSAGE ADJUSTMENT For patients with creatinine clearance of 10 to 50 ml/min/1.73 m^2, 75% of usual dose is used;

with creatinine clearance of less than 10 ml/min/1.73 m^2, 50% of usual dose is used. For elderly patients, total daily dosage decreased.

Route	Onset	Peak	Duration
P.O.	15 min	1–1.5 hr	2–4 hr
I.V.	1 min	5–7 min	2–4 hr
I.M., SubQ	10–15 min	30–50 min	2–4 hr

Mechanism of Action
Binds with opiate receptors in the spinal cord and higher levels of the CNS. In this way, meperidine stimulates mu and kappa receptors, which alters the perception of and emotional response to pain.

Incompatibilities
Don't mix meperidine in same syringe with aminophylline, barbiturates, heparin, iodides, methicillin, morphine sulfate, phenytoin, sodium bicarbonate, sulfadiazine, or sulfisoxazole.

Contraindications
Acute asthma; hypersensitivity to meperidine, opioids, or their components; increased intracranial pressure; severe respiratory depression; upper respiratory tract obstruction; use within 14 days of MAO inhibitor therapy

Interaction
DRUGS
acyclovir, ritonavir: Possibly increased blood meperidine level
agonist or antagonist analgesics such as buprenorphine, butorphanol, nalbuphine, pentazocine: Possibly decreased therapeutic effects of meperidine and increased risk of precipitating withdrawal symptoms
alfentanil, CNS depressants, fentanyl, sufentanil: Increased risk of CNS and respiratory depression and hypotension
amphetamines, MAO inhibitors: Risk of increased CNS excitation or depression with possibly fatal reactions
anticholinergics: Increased risk of severe constipation
antidiarrheals (such as loperamide and difenoxin and atropine): Increased risk of severe constipation and increased CNS depression

antihypertensives: Increased risk of hypotension
buprenorphine: Increased risk of respiratory depression
cimetidine: Reduced clearance and volume of distribution of meperidine
hydroxyzine: Increased risk of CNS depression and hypotension
metoclopramide: Possibly decreased effects of metoclopramide
naloxone, naltrexone: Decreased pharmacologic effects of meperidine
neuromuscular blockers: Increased risk of prolonged respiratory and CNS depression
oral anticoagulants: Possibly increased anticoagulant effect and risk of bleeding
phenytoin: Possibly enhanced hepatic metabolism of meperidine

ACTIVITIES
alcohol use: Possibly increased CNS and respiratory depression and hypotension

Adverse Reactions

CNS: Agitation, confusion, delirium, depression, dizziness, drowsiness, headache, increased intracranial pressure, lack of coordination, malaise, mood changes, nervousness, nightmares, restlessness, seizures, syncope, transient hallucinations or disorientation, tremor, weakness
CV: Hypotension, orthostatic hypotension, tachycardia
EENT: Blurred vision, diplopia, dry mouth
GI: Abdominal cramps or pain, anorexia, constipation, ileus, nausea, vomiting
GU: Dysuria, urinary frequency, urine retention
MS: Involuntary muscle movements
RESP: Dyspnea, respiratory arrest or depression, wheezing
SKIN: Diaphoresis, flushing, pruritus, rash, urticaria
Other: Anaphylaxis; injection-site pain, redness, or swelling; physical and psychological dependence

Nursing Considerations
• Use meperidine with extreme caution in patients with acute abdominal conditions, hepatic or renal disorders, hypothyroidism, prostatic hyperplasia, seizures, or supraventricular tachycardia.
• Use cautiously in debilitated patients or patients with sickle cell anemia, adreno-cortical insufficiency, pheochromocytoma,

toxic psychosis and any other condition that might worsen with CNS depression, such as acute alcoholism.
• To minimize local anesthetic effect, dilute meperidine syrup with water before use.
• Give I.V. dose slowly by direct injection or as a slow continuous infusion. Mix with D₅W, normal saline solution, or Ringer's or lactated Ringer's solution.
• Keep naloxone available when giving I.V. meperidine.
• Be aware that subcutaneous injection is painful and isn't recommended.
• Be aware that oral form of meperidine is less than half as effective as parenteral meperidine. Give I.M. form when possible, and expect to increase dosage when switching patient to oral form.
• Monitor patient's respiratory and cardiovascular status during treatment. Notify prescriber immediately and expect to discontinue drug if respiratory rate falls to less than 12 breaths/minute or if respiratory depth decreases.
• Monitor patient's bowel function to detect constipation, and assess the need for stool softeners.
• Assess for signs of physical dependence and abuse. Know that prolonged use may also increase risk of toxicity exhibited by seizures from the accumulation of the meperidine metabolite, normeperidine.
• Expect withdrawal symptoms to occur if drug is abruptly withdrawn after long-term use.

PATIENT TEACHING
• Inform patient that meperidine is a controlled substance and that he'll need identification to purchase it.
• Advise patient to take drug exactly as prescribed.
• Instruct patient to report constipation, severe nausea, and shortness or breath.
• Advise patient to avoid hazardous activities until drug's CNS effects are known.
• Instruct patient to prevent postoperative atelectasis by turning, coughing, and deep breathing.
• Urge patient to avoid alcohol, sedatives, and tranquilizers during therapy.

M

mephentermine sulfate

Wyamine

Class and Category

Chemical class: Sympathomimetic amine
Therapeutic class: Vasopressor
Pregnancy category: C

Indications and Dosages

➤ To treat hypotension secondary to spinal anesthesia

I.V. INJECTION

Adults. 30 to 45 mg (15 mg for obstetric patients); may be repeated, as needed, to maintain blood pressure.

I.V. INFUSION

Adults. Dosage individualized based on patient response to therapy. Average dose is 1 to 5 mg/min.

Route	Onset	Peak	Duration
I.V.	Almost immediate	Unknown	15–30 min

Mechanism of Action

Stimulates alpha-adrenergic receptors directly and indirectly, resulting in positive inotropic and chronotropic effects. Indirect stimulation occurs by release of norepinephrine from its storage sites in the heart and other tissues. By enhancing cardiac contraction, mephentermine improves cardiac output, thereby increasing blood pressure. Increased peripheral resistance from peripheral vasoconstriction may also contribute to increased blood pressure. Drug can affect heart rate but change is variable, based on vagal tone. It also may stimulate beta-adrenergic receptors.

Contraindications

Hypersensitivity to mephentermine, phenothiazine-induced hypotension, use within 14 days of MAO inhibitor therapy

Interaction

DRUGS

alpha blockers and other drugs with alpha-blocking effects: Possibly decreased peripheral vasoconstrictive and hypertensive effects of mephentermine

beta blockers (ophthalmic): Decreased effects of mephentermine; increased risk of bronchospasm, wheezing, decreased pulmonary function, and respiratory failure
beta blockers (systemic): Increased risk of bronchospasm and decreased effects of both drugs
diuretics and other antihypertensives: Possibly reduced effectiveness of these drugs
doxapram: Possibly increased vasopressor effects of either drug
ergot alkaloids: Increased vasopressor effects
guanadrel, guanethidine, mecamylamine, methyldopa, reserpine: Possibly decreased effects of these drugs and increased risk of adverse effects
hydrocarbon inhalation anesthetics: Increased risk of atrial and ventricular arrhythmias
MAO inhibitors: Increased, lengthened cardiac stimulation and vasopressor effects, and possibly severe headache and hypertensive crisis
maprotiline, tricyclic antidepressants: Increased vasopressor response; increased risk of prolonged QTc interval, arrhythmias, hypertension, and hyperpyrexia
methylphenidate: Possibly increased vasopressor effect of mephentermine
nitrates: Possibly reduced antianginal effects of nitrates and decreased vasopressor effect
other sympathomimetics (such as dopamine): Possibly increased cardiac effects and adverse reactions
oxytocin: Possibly severe hypertension
thyroid hormones: Increased effects of both drugs, increased risk of coronary insufficiency in patients with coronary artery disease

Adverse Reactions

CNS: Anxiety, dizziness, drowsiness, euphoria, headache, incoherence, nervousness, psychosis, restlessness, seizures, weakness
CV: Angina, arrhythmias (including bradycardia, tachycardia, and ventricular arrhythmias), hypertension, hypotension, palpitations, peripheral vasoconstriction
GI: Nausea, vomiting
RESP: Dyspnea
SKIN: Peripheral necrosis

Nursing Considerations

- Before giving mephentermine, expect to intervene, as ordered, to correct hemorrhage, hypovolemia, metabolic acidosis, or hypoxia.
- Discard vial if you observe discoloration or precipitate.
- Using D$_5$W or normal saline solution, prepare a 1-mg/ml solution for infusion.
- Administer drug using an infusion pump to provide a controlled rate.
- Monitor blood pressure, cardiac rate and rhythm, central venous pressure (if appropriate), and urine output during administration. Adjust infusion rate according to patient response, as ordered. Be aware that patients with a history of cardiovascular disease (including hypertension) or hyperthyroidism and chronically ill patients are at increased risk for mephentermine's adverse cardiovascular effects.
- Assess patients with angle-closure glaucoma for signs of an exacerbation, such as eye pain or blurred vision.
- Assess circulation in patients with a history of occlusive vascular disease, such as atherosclerosis and Raynaud's disease, because mephentermine may cause decreased circulation and increase risk of necrosis or gangrene. Inspect I.V. site periodically for signs of extravasation.
- **WARNING** Be aware that weeping, excitability, seizures, and hallucinations are some of the symptoms of mephentermine overdose. Contact prescriber immediately if patient has such symptoms, and expect to provide supportive treatment.
- Be aware that mephentermine can increase contractions in pregnant women, especially during third trimester. Expect drug to be prescribed only when benefits outweigh potential adverse effects.
- Store drug at 59° to 86° F (15° to 30° C); don't freeze.

PATIENT TEACHING

- Instruct patient receiving mephentermine to report adverse reactions, including chest pain, difficulty breathing, dizziness, irregular heartbeat, headache, and weakness.

mephenytoin

Mesantoin

Class and Category

Chemical class: Hydantoin derivative
Therapeutic class: Anticonvulsant
Pregnancy category: Not rated

Indications and Dosages

➤ *To control generalized tonic-clonic, focal, and jacksonian seizures when other drugs are ineffective*

TABLETS

Adults. *Initial:* 50 to 100 mg daily during first wk. Increased by 50 to 100 mg at 1-wk intervals until desired response is reached. *Maintenance:* 200 to 600 mg daily in equally divided doses. *Maximum:* 1.2 g daily.

Children. *Initial:* 20 to 50 mg daily. Increased by 25 to 50 mg at 1-wk intervals until desired response occurs. *Maintenance:* 100 to 400 mg daily in equally divided doses. *Maximum:* 400 mg daily.

➤ *To replace other anticonvulsants*

TABLETS

Adults. 50 to 100 mg daily during first wk. Dosage gradually increased while decreasing dosage of other drug over 3 to 6 wk.

Route	Onset	Peak	Duration
P.O.	30 min	Unknown	24–48 hr

Mechanism of Action

Limits spread of seizure activity and start of new seizures by:

- regulating voltage-dependent sodium and calcium channels in neurons
- inhibiting calcium movement across neuronal membranes
- enhancing sodium-potassium adenosine triphosphatase activity in neurons and glial cells.
- These actions may reflect a slowed recovery rate of inactivated sodium channels.

Contraindications

Hypersensitivity to mephenytoin, phenytoin, other hydantoins, or their components

M

Interaction
DRUGS
acetaminophen: Increased risk of hepato-toxicity with long-term acetaminophen use
amiodarone: Possibly increased blood mephenytoin level and risk of toxicity
antacids: Possibly decreased mephenytoin effectiveness
antineoplastics: Increased mephenytoin metabolism
bupropion, clozapine, loxapine, MAO inhibitors, maprotiline, phenothiazines, pimozide, thioxanthenes: Possibly lowered seizure threshold and decreased therapeutic effects of mephenytoin, possibly intensified CNS depressant effects of these drugs
calcium channel blockers, fluconazole, itraconazole, ketoconazole, miconazole, omeprazole: Possibly increased phenytoin level
carbamazepine: Decreased blood carbamazepine level, possibly increased blood phenytoin level and risk of toxicity
chloramphenicol, cimetidine, disulfiram, isoniazid, methylphenidate, metronidazole, phenylbutazone, ranitidine, salicylates, sulfonamides, trimethoprim: Possibly impaired metabolism of these drugs and increased risk of mephenytoin toxicity
corticosteroids, cyclosporine, digoxin, disopyramide, doxycycline, furosemide, levodopa, mexiletine, quinidine: Decreased therapeutic effects of these drugs
diazoxide: Possibly decreased therapeutic effects of both drugs
estrogens, progestins: Decreased therapeutic effects of these drugs, increased blood phenytoin level
felbamate: Possibly impaired metabolism and increased blood level of phenytoin
fluoxetine: Possibly increased blood phenytoin level and risk of toxicity
folic acid: Increased mephenytoin metabolism, decreased seizure control
haloperidol: Possibly lowered seizure threshold and decreased therapeutic effects of mephenytoin; possibly decreased blood haloperidol level
insulin, oral antidiabetic drugs: Possibly increased blood glucose level and decreased therapeutic effects of these drugs
lamotrigine: Possibly decreased therapeutic effects of lamotrigine
lithium: Increased risk of lithium toxicity

methadone: Possibly increased methadone metabolism and withdrawal symptoms
molindone: Possibly lowered seizure threshold, impaired absorption, and decreased therapeutic effects of mephenytoin
oral anticoagulants: Possibly impaired metabolism of these drugs and increased risk of mephenytoin toxicity; possibly increased anticoagulant effect initially, but decreased effect with prolonged therapy
oral contraceptives containing estrogen and progestin: Possibly breakthrough bleeding and decreased contraceptive effectiveness
rifampin: Possibly decreased therapeutic effects of mephenytoin
streptozocin: Possibly decreased therapeutic effects of streptozocin
sucralfate: Possibly decreased mephenytoin absorption
tricyclic antidepressants: Possibly lowered seizure threshold and decreased therapeutic effects of mephenytoin; possibly decreased blood level of tricyclic antidepressants
valproic acid: Decreased blood phenytoin level, increased blood valproic acid level
vitamin D analogues: Decreased vitamin D analogue activity, risk of anticonvulsant-induced rickets and osteomalacia
xanthines: Possibly inhibited mephenytoin absorption and increased clearance of xanthines
zaleplon: Increased clearance and decreased effectiveness of zaleplon
ACTIVITIES
alcohol use: Possibly decreased mephenytoin effectiveness

Adverse Reactions
CNS: Ataxia, choreoathetoid movements, confusion, dizziness, drowsiness, excitement, fatigue, fever, headache, peripheral neuropathy, sedation, slurred speech, stuttering, tremor
EENT: Gingival hyperplasia, nystagmus
GI: Constipation, diarrhea, nausea, vomiting
HEME: Agranulocytosis, leukopenia, thrombocytopenia
MS: Muscle twitching
SKIN: Rash, Stevens-Johnson syndrome, toxic epidermal necrolysis
Other: Lymphadenopathy, systemic lupus erythematosus

Nursing Considerations

- Because of mephenytoin's potentially dangerous adverse effects, expect to use it only when other drugs are ineffective.
- Keep in mind that mephenytoin doesn't control absence seizures.

WARNING Be aware that drug shouldn't be discontinued abruptly because doing so may cause status epilepticus. Plan to reduce dosage gradually or substitute another drug, as prescribed.

- Obtain CBC and differential before treatment, after 2 weeks, and then monthly during first year of treatment, as ordered.
- If patient has depressed blood counts, enlarged lymph nodes, or rash, notify prescriber immediately and expect to stop mephenytoin and substitute another drug.

PATIENT TEACHING

- Urge patient to take mephenytoin exactly as prescribed and not to stop abruptly.
- Advise patient to take drug with food to enhance absorption and reduce adverse GI reactions.
- Caution patient on once-a-day therapy to be especially careful not to miss a dose.
- Advise patient to report impaired coordination, persistent headache, rash, severe GI distress, swollen gums or lymph nodes, or unusual bleeding or bruising.
- Encourage patient to maintain good oral hygiene and to have regular dental checkups to reduce risk of gum disease.
- Instruct patient to keep medical appointments to monitor drug effectiveness and check for adverse reactions. Explain the need for periodic laboratory tests.
- Advise patient to wear medical identification stating that he has epilepsy and takes mephenytoin to prevent seizures.

mephobarbital

Mebaral

Class, Category, and Schedule

Chemical class: Barbiturate derivative
Therapeutic class: Anticonvulsant, sedative
Pregnancy category: D
Controlled substance schedule: IV

Indications and Dosages

➤ *To treat seizures*

TABLETS

Adults. 400 to 600 mg daily as a single dose or in divided doses, usually beginning with low dose and increasing over 4 to 5 days until optimum dosage is determined.
Children over age 5. 32 to 64 mg three times daily or four times daily.
Children under age 5. 16 to 32 mg three times daily or four times daily.

➤ *To provide sedation*

TABLETS

Adults. 32 to 100 mg three times daily or four times daily.
Children. 16 to 32 mg three times daily or four times daily.

Route	Onset	Peak	Duration
P.O.	30–60 min	Unknown	10–16 hr

Mechanism of Action

May reduce seizure activity by reducing transmission of monosynaptic and polysynaptic nerve impulses, which decreases excitability in nerve cells. As a sedative, mephobarbital inhibits upward conduction of nerve impulses to the reticular formation of the brain, which disrupts impulse transmission to the cortex. As a result, mephobarbital depresses the CNS and produces drowsiness, hypnosis, and sedation.

Contraindications

Hepatic disease or failure; history of addiction to sedatives or hypnotics; hypersensitivity to mephobarbital, other barbiturates, or their components; nephritis; porphyria; severe respiratory disease with obstruction or dyspnea.

Interaction

DRUGS

acetaminophen: Possibly decreased effects of acetaminophen (with long-term mephobarbital use)
anesthetics (halogenated hydrocarbon): Increased risk of hepatotoxicity (with long-term mephobarbital use)
carbamazepine, chloramphenicol, corticosteroids, cyclosporine, dacarbazine, digoxin, disopyramide, doxycycline, griseofulvin, metronidazole, oral contraceptives, phenylbutazone, quinidine, theophyllines,

M

vitamin D: Decreased effectiveness of these drugs
CNS depressants: Increased CNS depression
divalproex sodium, valproic acid: Increased risk of CNS depression and neurotoxicity
guanadrel, guanethidine: Increased risk of orthostatic hypotension
haloperidol: Possibly decreased blood haloperidol level and change in seizure pattern
hydantoins: Possibly interference with hydantoin metabolism
leucovorin: Possibly decreased anti-convulsant effect of mephobarbital
maprotiline: Possibly increased CNS depression and decreased therapeutic effects of mephobarbital
mexiletine: Possibly decreased blood mexiletine level
oral anticoagulants: Possibly decreased therapeutic effects of anticoagulants, possibly increased risk of bleeding when mephobarbital is discontinued
tricyclic antidepressants: Possibly decreased therapeutic effects of tricyclic antidepressants
ACTIVITIES
alcohol use: Increased CNS depression

Adverse Reactions

CNS: Agitation, anxiety, ataxia, confusion, delusions, depression, dizziness, drowsiness, fever, hallucinations, headache, insomnia, irritability, nervousness, nightmares, para-doxical stimulation, seizures, syncope, tremor
CV: Orthostatic hypotension
EENT: Vision changes
GI: Anorexia, constipation, hepatic dysfunction, nausea, vomiting
HEME: Agranulocytosis
MS: Arthralgia, bone pain, muscle twitching or weakness
RESP: Respiratory depression
SKIN: Exfoliative dermatitis, rash, Stevens-Johnson syndrome
Other: Physical and psychological dependence, weight loss

Nursing Considerations

• Observe patient for signs of physical and psychological dependence, especially with prolonged use at high doses.
• Observe for signs of chronic barbiturate intoxication, including confusion,

insomnia, poor judgment, slurred speech, and unsteady gait.
• Assess for paradoxical stimulation in patient who receives drug for acute or chronic pain.
WARNING Expect to taper mephobarbital gradually when discontinuing. Be aware that withdrawal symptoms can be severe and may cause death. Mild signs and symptoms may include anxiety, muscle twitching, nausea, orthostatic hypo-tension, and progressive weakness and may appear 8 to 12 hours after last dose. More severe signs include delirium and seizures.
PATIENT TEACHING
• Advise patient to take mephobarbital exactly as prescribed. Caution him not to stop taking drug abruptly because of possible withdrawal symptoms and, for epileptic patients, seizures.
• Instruct patient to avoid alcohol, sleeping pills, and other sedatives while taking mephobarbital because of the risk of increased CNS depression.
• Advise patient to avoid hazardous activities until CNS effects of drug are known.
• Advise patient to change position slowly to minimize orthostatic hypotension.
• Urge patient to report confusion, fever, rash, or severe dizziness.

meprobamate
Apo-Meprobamate (CAN), Equanil, MB-Tab, Meprospan, Miltown, Neuramate

Class, Category, and Schedule
Chemical class: Carbamate derivative
Therapeutic class: Antianxiety
Pregnancy category: Not rated
Controlled substance schedule: IV

Indications and Dosages
➤ *To treat anxiety*
S.R. CAPSULES
Adults and adolescents. 400 to 800 mg every morning and bedtime. *Maximum:* 2,400 mg daily.
Children ages 6 to 12. 200 mg every morning and bedtime.

TABLETS

Adults and adolescents. 1,200 to 1,600 mg/ day in divided doses three times daily or four times daily. *Maximum:* 2,400 mg daily.
DOSAGE ADJUSTMENT For patients with creatinine clearance of 10 to 50 ml/ min/1.73 m², drug given every 12 hr; with creatinine clearance less than 10 ml/ min/1.73 m², drug given every 18 hr.
Children ages 6 to 12. 200 to 600 mg daily in divided doses twice daily or three times daily.

Route	Onset	Peak	Duration
P.O.	1 hr	Unknown	Unknown

Mechanism of Action
May act at multiple sites in CNS, including thalamus and limbic system. Meprobamate inhibits spinal reflexes, causing CNS relaxation; its sedative effects may account for its anticonvulsant action. It also has muscle relaxant properties.

Contraindications
Hypersensitivity to meprobromate or related drugs, such as carisoprodol; porphyria

Interaction
DRUGS
CNS depressants: Increased CNS depression
ACTIVITIES
alcohol use: Increased CNS depression

Adverse Reactions
CNS: Ataxia, dizziness, drowsiness, euphoria, headache, paradoxical stimulation, paresthesia, slurred speech, syncope, vertigo, weakness
CV: Arrhythmias, including tachycardia; hypotension; palpitations
EENT: Impaired visual accommodation
GI: Diarrhea, nausea, vomiting
SKIN: Erythematous maculopapular rash, pruritus, urticaria
Other: Physical dependence

Nursing Considerations
• Use meprobamate cautiously in patients with impaired hepatic or renal function, seizure disorders, or suicidal tendencies.
• Also use drug cautiously in patients with history of drug dependence or abuse because meprobamate use can lead to physical dependence and abuse.
• Observe for evidence of chronic drug intoxication, such as ataxia, slurred speech, and vertigo.
WARNING When stopping therapy, expect to taper dosage over 2 weeks because stopping abruptly can worsen previous symptoms, such as anxiety, or cause withdrawal symptoms, such as confusion, hallucinations, muscle twitching, tremor, and vomiting.

PATIENT TEACHING
• Instruct patient to take meprobamate exactly as directed and not to stop taking it abruptly.
• Advise patient not to crush or chew S.R. capsules.
• Instruct patient to avoid hazardous activities until drug's CNS effects are known.
• Direct patient to avoid alcohol, sedatives, and other CNS depressants while taking meprobamate.
• Inform patient that drug may become less effective after several months of treatment.
• Instruct patient to report rash.

meropenem
Merrem I.V.

Class and Category
Chemical class: Carbapenem
Therapeutic class: Antibiotic
Pregnancy category: B

Indications and Dosages
➤ *To treat complicated appendicitis and peritonitis caused by susceptible strains of alpha-hemolytic streptococci,* Bacteroides fragilis, Bacteroides thetaiotaomicron, Escherichia coli, Klebsiella pneumoniae, Peptostreptococcus species, *or* Pseudomonas aeruginosa
I.V. INFUSION OR INJECTION
Adults and children weighing more than 50 kg (110 lb). 1 g every 8 hr infused over 15 to 30 min or given as a bolus over 3 to 5 min.
Children over age 3 months weighing less than 50 kg. 20 mg/kg every 8 hr infused over 15 to 30 min or given as bolus over 3 to 5 min. *Maximum:* 1 g every 8 hr.

DOSAGE ADJUSTMENT For patients with creatinine clearance of 26 to 50 ml/min/1.73 m², dosage reduced to 1 g every 12 hr. For those with clearance of 10 to 25 ml/min/1.73 m², dosage reduced to 500 mg every 12 hr. For those with clearance less than 10 ml/min/1.73 m², dosage reduced to 500 mg every 24 hr.

➤ *To treat complicated skin and skin structure infections caused by* Staphylococcus aureus, Streptococcus agalactiae, Streptococcus pyogenes, *viridans group streptococci,* Enterococcus faecalis *(excluding vancomycin-resistant isolates),* Pseudomonas aeruginosa, Escherichia coli, Proteus mirabilis, Bacteroides fragilis, *and* Peptostreptococcus species

I.V. INFUSION
Adults and children weighing more than 50 kg (110 lb). 500 mg every 8 hr infused over 15 to 30 min.
Children over age 3 months weighing less than 50 kg. 10 mg/kg every 8 hr infused over 15 to 30 min. *Maximum:* 500 mg every 8 hr.
DOSAGE ADJUSTMENT For patients with creatinine clearance of 26 to 50 ml/min/1.73 m², dosage reduced to 500 mg every 12 hr. For those with clearance of 10 to 25 ml/min/1.73 m², dosage reduced to 250 mg every 12 hr. For those with clearance less than 10 ml/min/1.73 m², dosage reduced to 250 mg every 24 hr.

➤ *To treat bacterial meningitis caused by* Haemophilus influenzae, Neisseria meningitidis, *or* Streptococcus pneumoniae *in children*

I.V. INFUSION OR INJECTION
Children weighing more than 50 kg. 2 g every 8 hr infused over 15 to 30 min or given as a bolus over 3 to 5 min.
Children over age 3 months weighing less than 50 kg. 40 mg/kg every 8 hr infused over 15 to 30 min or given as bolus over 3 to 5 min. *Maximum:* 2 g every 8 hr.

Mechanism of Action
Penetrates cell walls of most gram-negative and gram-positive bacteria, inactivating penicillin-binding proteins. This action inhibits bacterial cell wall synthesis and causes cell death.

Incompatibilities
Don't mix meropenem in same solution with other drugs.

Contraindications
Hypersensitivity to meropenem, other carbapenem drugs, beta-lactams, or their components

Interaction
DRUGS
probenecid: Inhibited renal excretion of meropenem
valproic acid: Possibly reduced blood level of valproic acid to subtherapeutic level

Adverse Reactions
CNS: Headache, paresthesias, seizures
CV: Shock
EENT: Epistaxis, glossitis, oral candidiasis
GI: Anorexia, constipation, diarrhea, elevated liver function test results, nausea, pseudomembranous colitis, vomiting
GU: Elevated BUN and serum creatinine levels, hematuria, renal failure
HEME: Agranulocytosis, hemolytic anemia, leukopenia, neutropenia, positive Coombs' test
RESP: Apnea, dyspnea
SKIN: Diaper rash from candidiasis (children), erythema multiforme, pruritus, rash, Stevens-Johnson syndrome, toxic epidermal necrolysis
Other: Anaphylaxis; angioedema; injection-site inflammation, pain, phlebitis, or thrombophlebitis; sepsis

Nursing Considerations
• Obtain body fluid and tissue samples, as ordered, for culture and sensitivity testing. Expect to review test results, if possible, before giving first dose of meropenem.
• For I.V. bolus, add 10 ml sterile water for injection to 500 mg/20-ml vial, or 20 ml diluent to 1 g/30-ml vial of drug. Shake to dissolve.
WARNING Be aware that fatal hypersensitivity reactions have occurred with meropenem use. Determine whether patient has had previous reactions to antibiotics or other allergens. Monitor patient closely and stop drug immediately if signs and symptoms of anaphylaxis occur. Notify prescriber, and expect to provide supportive emergency care that may include epinephrine and I.V. steroid administration, oxygen, and airway management.

• Monitor patient closely for diarrhea, which may indicate pseudomembranous colitis caused by *Clostridium difficile.* If diarrhea occurs, notify prescriber and expect to withhold meropenem and treat with fluids, electrolytes, protein, and an antibiotic effective against *C. difficile.*
• Take seizure precautions according to facility policy, especially for patients with bacterial meningitis or CNS or renal disorders because of an increased risk of seizures with meropenem.
• Monitor patient with creatinine clearance of 10 to 26 ml/min/1.73 m^2 for signs and symptoms of seizures, heart failure, renal failure, or shock.

PATIENT TEACHING
• Tell patient to report trouble breathing, injection-site pain, and sore mouth.
• Urge patient to tell prescriber about diarrhea that's severe or lasts longer than 3 days. Remind patient that watery or bloody stools can occur 2 or more months after antibiotic therapy and can be serious, requiring prompt treatment.
• Instruct patient to avoid hazardous activities until drug's CNS effects are known.

mesalamine

Asacol, Apriso, Canasa, Delzicol, Lialda, Mesasal (CAN), Pentasa, Rowasa, Salofalk (CAN)

Class and Category
Chemical class: 5-Aminosalicylic acid derivative
Therapeutic class: Anti-inflammatory
Pregnancy category: C

Indications and Dosages
➤ *To treat and maintain remission of ulcerative colitis*
DELAYED-RELEASE TABLETS (ASACOL), DELAYED-RELEASE CAPSULES (DELZICOL)
Adults. *Initial:* 0.8 g three times daily for 6 wk. *Maintenance:* 1.6 g daily in divided doses.
DELAYED-RELEASE TABLETS (MESASAL)
Adults. 1.5 to 3 g daily in divided doses for 6 wk.

DELAYED-RELEASE TABLETS (SALOFALK)
Adults. 1 g three times daily or four times daily for 6 wk.
E.R. CAPSULES (APRISO)
Adults. 1 g four times daily for up to 8 wk.
➤ *To induce remission in patients with active mild to moderate ulcerative colitis.*
TABLETS (LIALDA)
Adults. 2.4 or 4.8 g once daily with a meal for up to 8 wk.
➤ *To maintain remission of ulcerative colitis*
TABLETS (LIALDA)
Adults. 2.4 g once daily with a meal.
➤ *To treat mild to moderate distal ulcerative colitis, proctitis, and proctosigmoiditis*
RECTAL SUSPENSION (ROWASA)
Adults. 4 g (60 ml) daily at bedtime for 3 to 6 wk.
➤ *To treat active ulcerative proctitis*
SUPPOSITORIES (CANASA)
Adults. 0.5 g twice daily or three times daily for 3 to 6 wk. Or 1 g at bedtime for 3 to 6 wk.

Mechanism of Action
May reduce inflammation by inhibiting the enzyme cyclooxygenase and decreasing production of arachidonic acid metabolites, which may be increased in patients with inflammatory bowel disease. Cyclooxygenase is needed to form prostaglandins from arachidonic acid. Prostaglandins mediate inflammatory activity and produce signs and symptoms of inflammation. Mesalamine also may reduce inflammation by interfering with leukotriene synthesis and inhibiting the enzyme lipoxygenase, both of which take part in inflammatory response.

Contraindications
Hypersensitivity to mesalamine, salicylates, or their components

Interaction
DRUGS
digoxin: Possibly decreased absorption and bioavailability of digoxin
lactulose: Possibly interference with delayed-release tablets or E.R. capsules
omeprazole: Increased mesalamine absorption

M

Adverse Reactions

CNS: Chills, confusion, depression, dizziness, emotional lability, fatigue, fever, Guillain-Barre syndrome, headache (severe), peripheral neuropathy, somnolence, transverse myelitis, tremor, vertigo, weakness
CV: Myocarditis, pericardial effusion, pericarditis
EENT: Blurred vision, dry mouth, rhinitis, taste perversion, tinnitus
GI: Abdominal cramps or pain (severe), anorexia, bloody diarrhea, cholecystitis, colitis, diarrhea, elevated liver function test results, flatulence, gastritis, gastrointestinal bleeding, hepatotoxicity, hepatitis, indigestion, jaundice, Kawasaki-like syndrome, liver failure or necrosis, nausea, pancreatitis, perforated peptic ulcer, rectal pain, vomiting
GU: Acute or chronic renal failure, interstitial nephritis, nephrotoxicity, reversible oligospermia
HEME: Agranulocytosis, anemia including aplastic anemia, eosinophilia, granulo-cytopenia, leukopenia, lymphadenopathy, thrombocytopenia
MS: Back pain, dysarthria, myalgia
RESP: Allergic alveolitis, asthma exacerbation, eosinophilic or interstitial pneumonitis, fibrosing alveolitis, pleuritis, pneumonitis
SKIN: Acne, alopecia, dryness, drug reaction with eosinophilia and systemic symptoms (DRESS), erythema nodosum, pyoderma gangrenosum, psoriasis, pruritus, rash, Stevens-Johnson syndrome, urticaria
Other: Anaphylaxis, angioedema, drug fever, drug reaction with eosinophilia and systemic symptoms (DRESS), gout, systemic lupus erythematosus

Nursing Considerations

• Use mesalamine cautiously in patients with sulfite sensitivity. Some drug formulations contain sulfites, which may cause hypersensitivity reactions in these patients.
• Use mesalamine cautiously in patients with liver disease because hepatic dysfunction may occur.
• Ensure that suppository is firm before inserting it. If it's too soft, chill in refrigerator for 30 minutes or run under cold water before removing wrapper. Moisten with water-soluble lubricant or

tap water before insertion. Have patient retain suppository for 1 to 3 hours, as directed.
• Give rectal suspension at bedtime, and have patient retain for prescribed time—about 8 hours, if possible. Retention time ranges from 3.5 to 12 hours.
• Be aware that rectal suspension may darken slightly over time but that this change doesn't affect potency. Discard rectal suspension that turns dark brown.
• Assess patient for evidence of acute intolerance similar to flare-up of inflammatory bowel disease: acute abdominal cramps and pain, bloody diarrhea, and, possibly, fever, headache, and rash.
• For patients with impaired renal function, expect to monitor renal function test results periodically during long-term therapy because drug may cause nephrotoxicity.
• Monitor patient's CBC with differential for eosinophilia, which may indicate an allergic reaction.
• Be aware that mesalamine may interfere with the measurement of urinary normetanephrine producing falsely elevated test results if the test is done by liquid chromatography with electrochemical detection.

PATIENT TEACHING
• Instruct patient taking oral drug to swallow tablets or capsules whole and not to break outer coating by cutting or chewing.
• Tell patient taking extended-release product to take it with a meal unless prescribed Delzicol which should be taken 1 hour before or 2 hours after a meal.
• Teach patient how to use rectal suspension or suppositories correctly. Emphasize shaking suspension bottle well before using.
• Advise patient to notify prescriber immediately about abdominal cramps or pain, bloody diarrhea, fever, headache, or rash.

mesoridazine besylate

Serentil

Class and Category
Chemical class: Alkylpiperidine phenothiazine derivative
Therapeutic class: Antipsychotic
Pregnancy category: Not rated

Indications and Dosages
➤ *To treat schizophrenia in patients who failed to respond to other antipsychotic drugs, either because they were ineffective or because intolerable adverse effects prevented attainment of effective dose*

ORAL SOLUTION, TABLETS
Adults and adolescents. 50 mg three times daily, increased as needed and tolerated. *Maximum:* 400 mg daily.

I.M. INJECTION
Adults and adolescents. 25 mg, repeated in 30 to 60 min, as needed. *Maximum:* 200 mg/day.

Route	Onset	Peak	Duration
P.O., I.M.	Up to several wk	6 wk–6 mo	4–8 hr

Mechanism of Action
Depresses brain areas that control activity and aggression—including cerebral cortex, hypothalamus, and limbic system—by an unknown mechanism.

Contraindications
Blood dyscrasias; bone marrow depression; cerebral arteriosclerosis; coma; concurrent use of high doses of CNS depressants; concurrent use of other drugs that prolong QTc interval, such as disopyramide, procainamide,and quinidine; congenital long-QT syndrome;coronary artery disease; hepatic dysfunction; history of arrhythmias; hypersensitivity to mesoridazine, other phenothiazines, or their components; myeloproliferative disorders; severe CNS depression; severe hypertension or hypotension; subcortical brain damage

Interaction
DRUGS
aluminum- or magnesium-containing antacids, antidiarrheals (adsorbent): Decreased mesoridazine absorption

amantadine, anticholinergics: Increased anticholinergic effects, possibly decreased therapeutic effects of mesoridazine
aminoglycosides, ototoxic drugs: Masked symptoms of ototoxicity, such as dizziness, tinnitus, and vertigo
anticonvulsants: Possibly lowered seizure threshold
antithyroid drugs: Increased risk of agranulo-cytosis
appetite suppressants: Possibly antagonized anorectic effect
astemizole, cisapride, disopyramide, erythromycin, pimozide, probucol, procainamide, quinidine: Increased risk of prolonged QT interval and life-threatening arrhythmias
beta blockers: Increased blood levels of both drugs, possibly resulting in additive hypotension, retinopathy, arrhythmias, and tardive dyskinesia
CNS depressants, general anesthetics: Increased CNS depression
dextroamphetamine: Possibly interference with action of either drug
levodopa: Possibly inhibited levodopa effects
lithium: Possibly decreased absorption of mesoridazine
opioid analgesics: Possibly decreased mesoridazine effects; increased CNS and respiratory depression and orthostatic hypotension; increased risk of severe constipation
oral anticoagulants: Possibly decreased therapeutic effects of anticoagulants
sympathomimetics: Possibly decreased therapeutic effects of these drugs and increased risk of hypotension
thiazide diuretics: Possibly orthostatic hypotension, hyponatremia, and water intoxication
tricyclic antidepressants: Increased tricyclic antidepressant levels, inhibited mesoridazine metabolism, increased risk of neuroleptic malignant syndrome
ACTIVITIES
alcohol use: Increased CNS depression

Adverse Reactions
CNS: Ataxia, dizziness, drowsiness, extrapyramidal reactions (tardive dyskinesia, pseudoparkinsonism), fever, neuroleptic malignant syndrome, restlessness, seizures, slurred speech, syncope, tremor, weakness

M

CV: Hypotension, orthostatic hypotension, prolonged QTc interval, torsades de pointes
EENT: Blurred vision, dry mouth, hypertrophic papillae of tongue, increased salivation, photophobia
ENDO: Galactorrhea, gynecomastia
GI: Constipation, hepatotoxicity, nausea, vomiting
GU: Dysuria, ejaculation disorders, impotence, menstrual irregularities, priapism
HEME: Agranulocytosis, leukopenia, thrombocytopenia
SKIN: Contact dermatitis, decreased sweating, jaundice, photosensitivity, rash
Other: Injection site pain, weight gain

Nursing Considerations

• Before starting mesoridazine, expect to obtain a 12-lead ECG to detect prolonged QTc interval. If patient's QTc interval is greater than 450 milliseconds (msec), expect to withhold drug because of risk of life-threatening torsades de pointes.
• Wear gloves when working with liquid and parenteral forms of mesoridazine, and avoid contact with clothing or skin; drug may cause contact dermatitis.
• Discard injection solution if it's frankly discolored or contains precipitate; slightly yellow color is acceptable.
• Inject I.M. drug deep into upper outer quadrant of buttocks; massage area afterward to prevent sterile abscess.
• Implement continuous ECG monitoring, as ordered, to detect arrhythmias. Expect to discontinue mesoridazine if the QTc interval exceeds 500 msec.
• Monitor serum potassium level before and during therapy, and administer potassium supplements as prescribed.
• Assess patient for hypotension and orthostatic hypotension, especially during I.M. use. Notify prescriber if either develops.
• **WARNING** Monitor patient for neuroleptic malignant syndrome, a potentially fatal reaction to antipsychotic drugs, and notify prescriber about such early signs as altered mental status, fever, hypertension or hypotension, muscle rigidity, and tachycardia.
• Assess patient for signs of blood dyscrasias, including cellulitis, fever, and pharyngitis. If they develop, expect to stop drug.

• Monitor patient for signs of tardive dyskinesia, even after treatment stops. Notify prescriber if they develop.
• Expect to taper drug dosage before discontinuation to avoid adverse reactions, such as dizziness, nausea, tremor, and vomiting.

PATIENT TEACHING
• Instruct patient to take drug exactly as prescribed and not to stop abruptly.
• Explain that I.M. injection may be painful.
• Caution patient to avoid hazardous activities until drug's CNS effects are known.
• Advise patient to change position slowly to minimize orthostatic hypotension.
• Tell patient to report fever, involuntary facial movements, sore throat, unusual bleeding or bruising, and yellowing of eyes or skin.
• Urge patient to avoid alcohol and prolonged sun exposure during therapy.
• If patient need long-term therapy, explain the risk of tardive dyskinesia. Also advise him to have regular eye examinations.

metaproterenol sulfate

Arm-a-Med Metaproterenol, Dey-Lute Metaproterenol

Class and Category

Chemical class: Sympathomimetic amine
Therapeutic class: Antiasthmatic, bronchodilator
Pregnancy category: C

Indications and Dosages

➤ *To treat bronchospasm*
SYRUP, TABLETS
Adults and children age 9 or over weighing more than 27 kg (59 lb). 20 mg every 6 to 8 hr.
Children ages 6 to 9 weighing 27 kg or less. 10 mg every 6 to 8 hr.
INHALATION AEROSOL
Adults and adolescents. 2 to 3 inhalations (1.3 to 1.95 mg) every 3 to 4 hr. *Maximum:* 12 inhalations daily.
Children ages 6 to 12. 1 to 3 inhalations (0.65 to 1.95 mg) every 3 to 4 hr. *Maximum:* 12 inhalations daily.

INHALATION NEBULIZER
Adults and adolescents. 0.2 to 0.3 ml of 5% solution diluted in 2.5 ml normal saline solution three times daily or four times daily, as needed,, but no more than every 4 hr. **Children ages 6 to 12.** 0.1 to 0.2 ml of 5% solution diluted in normal saline solution to a total volume of 3 ml three times daily or four times daily, as needed, but no more than every 4 hr.

Route	Onset	Peak	Duration
P.O.	15 min	1 hr	4 hr or longer
Inhalation (aerosol)	1 min	1 hr	4 hr or longer
Inhalation (nebulizer)	5–30 min	Unknown	4 hr or longer

Mechanism of Action
Attaches to beta$_2$ receptors on bronchial cell membranes, which stimulates intracellular enzyme adenyl cyclase to convert adenosine triphosphate to cyclic adenosine monophosphate (cAMP). Increased intracellular cAMP level relaxes bronchial smooth-muscle cells and inhibits histamine release.

Contraindications
Angina, cerebral arteriosclerosis, dilated heart failure, heart block from digitalis toxicity, hypersensitivity to metaproterenol or its components, labor, local anesthesia, organic brain damage, tachyarrhythmias

Interaction
DRUGS
beta blockers: Increased risk of broncho-spasm
MAO inhibitors, tricyclic antidepressants: Possibly potentiated cardiovascular effects of metaproterenol
other sympathomimetics: Possibly additive effects of both drugs and risk of toxicity
theophylline: Increased risk of arrhythmias

Adverse Reactions
CNS: Dizziness, fatigue, headache, insomnia, malaise, nervousness, tremor
CV: ECG changes, hypertension, palpitations, tachycardia

EENT: Dry mouth, pharyngitis, taste perversion
GI: Diarrhea, nausea, vomiting
RESP: Asthma exacerbation, cough

Nursing Considerations
• Anticipate that a single dose of nebulized metaproterenol may not completely stop an acute asthma attack.
• Monitor for adverse reactions and signs of toxicity, especially if patient uses tablets and aerosol. Notify prescriber if they develop.
• Be aware that tolerance may occur with continued use.

PATIENT TEACHING
• Caution patient not to use metaproterenol inhaler or nebulizer more often than prescribed.
• Teach patient to use metaproterenol inhaler correctly, to hold breath during second half of inhalation, and to wait 2 minutes between inhalations.
• Instruct parents to use spacer with their child's metered-dose inhaler.
• Advise patient to use metaproterenol 5 minutes before using corticosteroid inhaler, if prescribed, to maximize airway opening and drug effects.
• Instruct patient to report immediately diarrhea, increased shortness of breath, insomnia, or irregular heartbeat.
• Instruct patient to notify prescriber if drug becomes less effective.

metaxalone
Skelaxin

Class and Category
Chemical class: Oxazolidinone derivative
Therapeutic class: Skeletal muscle relaxant
Pregnancy category: Not rated

Indications and Dosages
➤ *To relieve discomfort caused by acute, painful musculoskeletal conditions*
TABLETS
Adults and children over age 12. 800 mg three times daily or four times daily.

Route	Onset	Peak	Duration
P.O.	Usually in 1 hr	Unknown	4–6 hr

M

Mechanism of Action

May depress CNS, causing sedation, which in turn may reduce skeletal muscle spasms to provide pain relief. Metaxalone doesn't directly relax tense skeletal muscles.

Contraindications

Hypersensitivity to metaxalone or its components, significant renal or hepatic disease, tendency to develop drug-induced, hemolytic, or other anemias

Interaction

DRUGS
CNS depressants: Increased CNS depression
ACTIVITIES
alcohol use: Increased CNS depression

Adverse Reactions

CNS: Dizziness, drowsiness, excitement, general CNS depression, headache, insomnia, irritability, nervousness, restlessness
GI: Abdominal cramps or pain, GI upset, jaundice, hepatotoxicity, nausea, vomiting
HEME: Hemolytic anemia, leukopenia
SKIN: Pruritus, rash

Nursing Considerations

• Metaxalone may not be prescribed for women who are or may become pregnant unless potential benefits outweigh risks because drug's effect on fetus is unknown.
• Expect to avoid giving metaxalone with food because food may increase CNS depression, especially in elderly patients.
• Monitor patient for excessive drowsiness, which may lead to respiratory depression.
• Caution patient to consult prescriber before taking other drugs, such as sleeping pills, cold or allergy preparations, opioid analgesics, and antidepressants.
• Monitor liver function test results for elevations, especially in patients with preexisting hepatic disease.
• Monitor renal function test results, as prescribed, for signs of impaired renal function because drug is excreted by kidneys.
• Provide rest and other pain-relief measures.
• Store drug at 59° to 86° F (15° to 30° C).

PATIENT TEACHING
• Advise patient to take metaxalone tablets exactly as prescribed and not to increase dosage or frequency.

• Instruct patient to take metaxalone tablets on an empty stomach.
• Caution patient to avoid hazardous activities, such as driving or operating machinery, until drug's CNS effects are known.
• Instruct patient to avoid alcohol and other CNS depressants during therapy.
• Urge patient to notify prescriber if he notices a rash or itching, which may signify a hypersensitivity reaction, or if he develops signs of hepatotoxicity, such as tiredness, nausea, yellow skin, or flulike symptoms.

metformin hydrochloride

Fortamet, Gen-Metformin (CAN), Glucophage, Glucophage XR, Glumetza, Glycon (CAN), Novo-Metformin (CAN), Riomet

Class and Category

Chemical class: Dimethylbiguanide
Therapeutic class: Antidiabetic
Pregnancy category: B

Indications and Dosages

➤ *To reduce blood glucose level in type 2 diabetes mellitus*

ORAL SOLUTION, TABLETS
Adults and children age 10 and over.
Initial: 500 mg twice daily or 850 mg daily, increased as prescribed by 500 mg/wk or by 850 mg every 2 wk until desired response occurs. *Usual:* 500 to 850 mg twice daily or three times daily. *Maximum:* 2,550 mg daily (adults and adolescents age 17 and over); 2,000 mg daily (children ages 10 to 16).
DOSAGE ADJUSTMENT If patient uses insulin, initial dosage reduced to 500 mg daily and then increased as prescribed by 500 mg weekly until blood glucose level is controlled.
E.R. TABLETS (GLUCOPHAGE XR, GLUMETZA)
Adults and adolescents age 18 and over.
Initial: 500 mg daily (Glucophage XR) or 1,000 mg daily (Glumetza) with evening meal. Increased as prescribed by 500 mg/wk. *Maximum:* 2,000 mg daily.
DOSAGE ADJUSTMENT If control isn't achieved with maximum once-daily E.R.

dosage, regimen may be changed to 1,000 mg twice daily. If control isn't achieved after 4 wk of maximum dosage, an oral sulfonylurea may be prescribed.

E.R. TABLETS (FORTAMET)
Adults and adolescents age 17 and over.
Initial: 500 to 1,000 mg once daily in evening. Increased in increments of 500 mg weekly, as needed. *Maximum:* 2,500 mg daily. If control isn't achieved after 4 wk at maximum dosage, an oral sulfonylurea may be prescribed.

➤ *As adjunct to insulin therapy in type 2 diabetes mellitus*
ORAL SOLUTION, TABLETS, E.R. TABLETS
Adults. *Initial:* 500 mg (Glucophage, Glucophage XR, Fortamet) or 1,000 mg (Glumetza) daily in addition to current dose of insulin. Increased by 500 mg/wk, as needed. *Maximum:* 2,000 mg for Glucophage XR and Glumetza; 2,500 mg for Glucophage and Fortamet.

DOSAGE ADJUSTMENT If fasting blood glucose level drops below 120 mg/dl, insulin dosage decreased by 10% to 25%. Subsequent insulin dosage decrease may be needed based upon patient's continued response.

Route	Onset	Peak	Duration
P.O. (tablets)	Unknown	Up to 2 wk	2 wk after drug discontinued

Mechanism of Action

May promote storage of excess glucose as glycogen in the liver, which reduces glucose production. Metformin also may improve glucose use by skeletal muscle and adipose tissue by increasing glucose transport across cell membranes. This drug also may increase the number of insulin receptors on cell membranes and make them more sensitive to insulin. In addition, metformin modestly decreases blood triglyceride and total cholesterol levels.

Contraindications

Hypersensitivity to metformin or its components, impaired renal function, metabolic acidosis, use of iodinated contrast media within preceding 48 hours.

Interaction

DRUGS
calcium channel blockers, corticosteroids, estrogens, isoniazid, nicotinic acid, oral contraceptives, phenothiazines, phenytoin, sympathomimetics, thiazide and other diuretics, thyroid drugs: Possibly hyperglycemia
cationic drugs (such as amiloride, cimetidine, digoxin, morphine, procainamide, quinidine, quinine, ranitidine, triamterene, trimethoprim, vancomycin), nifedipine: Increased blood metformin level
clofibrate, MAO inhibitors, probenecid, propranolol, rifabutin, rifampin, salicylates, sulfonamides, sulfonylureas: Increased risk of hypoglycemia
FOODS
all foods: Possibly delayed metformin absorption
ACTIVITIES
alcohol use: Increased risk of hypoglycemia and lactate formation

Adverse Reactions

CNS: Headache
EENT: Metallic taste
ENDO: Hypoglycemia
GI: Abdominal distention, anorexia, constipation, diarrhea, flatulence, indigestion, nausea, vomiting
HEME: Aplastic anemia, megaloblastic anemia, thrombocytopenia
SKIN: Photosensitivity, rash
Other: Lactic acidosis, weight loss

Nursing Considerations

• Give metformin tablets with food, which decreases and slightly delays absorption, thus reducing risk of adverse GI reactions. Give E.R. tablets with evening meal; don't break or crush them.
• Expect prescriber to alter dosage if patient has a condition that decreases or delays gastric emptying, such as diarrhea, gastroparesis, GI obstruction, ileus, or vomiting.
• Expect to assess BUN and serum creatinine level before and during long-term therapy in those at increased risk for lactic acidosis.
• Monitor patient's hepatic function, as ordered, because impaired hepatic function may significantly reduce the liver's ability to clear lactate, predisposing the patient to lactic acidosis.

M

- Monitor patient's blood glucose level to evaluate drug effectiveness. Assess for hyperglycemia and the need for insulin during times of increased stress, such as infection and surgery.
- Withhold drug, as ordered, if patient becomes dehydrated or develops hypoxemia or sepsis because these conditions increase the risk of lactic acidosis.
- Iodinated contrast media used in radiographic studies increases risk of renal failure and lactic acidosis during metformin therapy. Expect to withhold drug for 48 hours before and after testing.
- Be aware that women should not breastfeed while taking metformin because nursing infants may develop hypoglycemia.

PATIENT TEACHING
- Instruct patient to take metformin tablet at breakfast if taking drug once a day, or at breakfast and dinner if taking drug twice a day. Instruct him to take E.R. tablets once daily with evening meal and to swallow them whole without crushing or chewing.
- Direct patient to take drug exactly as prescribed and not to change the dosage or frequency unless instructed.
- Emphasize importance of following prescribed diet, exercising regularly, controlling weight, and checking blood glucose level.
- Teach patient how to measure blood glucose level and recognize hyperglycemia and hypoglycemia. Urge him to notify prescriber of abnormal blood glucose level.
- Caution patient to avoid alcohol, which can increase the risk of hypoglycemia.
- Instruct patient to report early signs of lactic acidosis, including drowsiness, hyperventilation, malaise, and muscle pain.
- Advise patient to expect laboratory testing of glycosylated hemoglobin every 3 months until blood glucose is controlled.

methadone hydrochloride

Dolophine, Methadose

Class, Category, and Schedule

Chemical class: Phenylheptylamine

Therapeutic class: Synthetic opiate agonist
Pregnancy category: C
Controlled substance schedule: II

Indications and Dosages

➤ *To manage opioid detoxification and then maintenance of opioid abstinence*
DISPERSIBLE TABLETS, ORAL CONCENTRATE, ORAL SOLUTION, TABLETS
Adults. *Initial on day 1:* 20 to 30 mg as a single dose, followed by 5 to 10 mg 2 to 4 hr later, if needed. *Maximum for day 1:* 40 mg. *Maintenance:* Highly individualized with dosage adjustments made until opioid withdrawal symptoms have ceased for 24 hr. *Maximum:* 120 mg daily.
I.M. OR SUBCUTANEOUS INJECTION
Hospitalized adults unable to take drug orally. Highly individualized. If oral methadone had been used prior to hospitalization, dosage initially decreased by 50%.
➤ *To manage moderate to severe pain when a continuous, around-the-clock opioid analgesic is needed for an extended period of time*
ORAL SOLUTION, TABLETS
Adults. *Initial:* 2.5 to 10 mg every 8 to 12 hr. *Maintenance:* Dosage adjustments made every 1 to 2 days, as needed. *Maximum:* 120 mg/day.
I.M. OR SUBCUTANEOUS INJECTION
Hospitalized adults unable to take drug orally. Highly individualized. If oral methadone dosage had been used prior to hospitalization, dosage initially decreased by 50%.
➤ *To treat moderate to severe pain not responsive to non-narcotic analgesics*
I.V. INJECTION
Hospitalized opioid non-tolerant adults. *Initial:* 2.5 to 10 mg every 8 to 12 hr, slowly titrated to effect with dosage interval decreased, as needed.
Hospitalized opioid tolerant adults. Highly individualized.
I.M., OR SUBCUTANEOUSINJECTION
Hospitalized adults. Highly individualized
DOSAGE ADJUSTMENT Elderly patients, debilitated patients, patients with severe hepatic or renal dysfunction, hypothyroidism, Addison's disease, prostatic hyperplasia, or urethral stricture; and patients who are taking CNS depressants

such as anxiolytics, hypnotics, neuroleptics, other opioids, or sedatives or who are suspected of alcohol or illicit drug use need individualized reduced dosages.

Route	Onset	Peak	Duration
P.O.	30–60 min	1.5–2 hr	4–6 hr
I.M.	10–20 min	1–2 hr	4–5 hr

Mechanism of Action
Binds with and activates opioid receptors (primarily mu receptors) in spinal cord and higher levels of CNS to produce analgesia and euphoric effects.

Contraindications
Acute or severe bronchial asthma in unmonitored setting or in absence of resuscitative equipment, hypersensitivity to methadone or its components, paralytic ileus, significant respiratory depression

Interaction
DRUGS
ammonium chloride, ascorbic acid, potassium, sodium phosphate: May precipitate methadone withdrawal symptoms
amitriptyline, chloripramine, nortriptyline: Increased CNS and respiratory depression
anticholinergics: Possibly severe constipation leading to ileus; urine retention
antiemetics, general anesthetics, hypnotics, phenothiazines, sedatives, tranquilizers: Possibly coma, hypotension, respiratory depression, and severe sedation
antihistamines, choral hydrate, glutethimide, MAO inhibitors, methocarbamol: Increased CNS and respiratory depressant effects of methadone
antihypertensives, hypotension-producing drugs: Increased hypotension, risk of orthostatic hypotension
azole antifungals, macrolide antibiotics: Increased or prolonged opioid effect
buprenorphine: Decreased therapeutic effect of methadone, increased respiratory depression, possibly withdrawal symptoms
calcium channel blockers, class IA and class III antiarrhythmics, diuretics, laxatives, mineralocorticoid hormones, neuroleptics, tricyclic antidepressants: Increased risk of electrolyte disturbances and prolonged QT interval

carbamazepine, phenobarbital, St. John's wort: Possibly precipitation of withdrawal symptoms
cimetidine: Increased analgesic and CNS and respiratory depressant effects of methadone
CNS depressants: Additive hypotensive, respiratory, and CNS depressant effects, possibly resulting in life-threatening reactions
desipramine: Increased plasma desipramine level
didanosine, stavudine: Decreased plasma levels of these drugs
diuretics: Decreased diuresis
efavirenz, nevirapine, ritonavir, ritonavir and lopinavir: Decreased blood methadone level
hydroxyzine: Increased analgesic, CNS depressant, and hypotensive effects of methadone
loperamide, paregoric: Increased CNS depression, possibly severe constipation
MAO inhibitors: Possibly increased risk of severe adverse reactions
metoclopramide: Possibly antagonized metoclopramide effects on GI motility
mixed agonist-antagonist analgesics: Possibly withdrawal symptoms
naloxone: Antagonized analgesic and CNS and respiratory depressant effects of methadone, and possibly withdrawal symptoms
naltrexone: Possibly induction or worsening of withdrawal symptoms if methadone given within 7 days before naltrexone
neuromuscular blockers: Increased or prolonged respiratory depression
opioid analgesics (such as alfentanil and sufentanil): Increased CNS and respiratory depression, increased hypotension
phenytoin, rifampin: May precipitate withdrawal symptoms
selective serotonin reuptake inhibitors: Possibly increased blood methadone levels and increased risk of methadone toxicity
zidovudine: Increased blood zidovudine level and risk of toxicity
ACTIVITIES
alcohol use: Increased CNS and respiratory depression, possibly hypotension

Adverse Reactions
CNS: Agitation, amnesia, anxiety, asthenia, coma, confusion, decreased concentration,

delirium, delusions, depression, dizziness, drowsiness, euphoria, fever, hallucinations, headache, insomnia, lethargy, light-headedness, malaise, psychosis, restlessness, sedation, seizures, syncope, tremor

CV: Bradycardia, cardiac arrest, cardiomyopathy, edema, heart failure, hypotension, orthostatic hypotension, palpitations, phlebitis, prolonged QT interval, shock, tachycardia, torsades de pointes, T-wave inversion on ECG, ventricular fibrillation or tachycardia

EENT: Blurred vision, diplopia, dry mouth, glossitis, laryngeal edema or laryngospasm (allergic), miosis, nystagmus, rhinitis

GI: Abdominal cramps or pain, anorexia, biliary tract spasm, constipation, diarrhea, dysphagia, elevated liver function test results, gastroesophageal reflux, hiccups, ileus and toxic megacolon (in patients with inflammatory bowel disease), indigestion, nausea, vomiting

GU: Amenorrhea, decreased ejaculate potency, decreased libido, difficult ejaculation, impotence, prolonged labor, urinary hesitancy, urine retention

HEME: Anemia, leukopenia, thrombocytopenia

MS: Arthralgia

RESP: Apnea, asthma exacerbation, atelectasis, bronchospasm, depressed cough reflex, hypoventilation, pulmonary edema, respiratory arrest and depression, wheezing

SKIN: Diaphoresis, flushing

Other: Allergic reaction; facial edema; hypokalemia; hypomagnesemia; injection-site edema, pain, rash, or redness; physical and psychological dependence; weight gain; withdrawal symptoms

Nursing Considerations

• Before giving methadone, make sure opioid antagonist and equipment for administering oxygen and controlling respiration are nearby.

• Before therapy begins, assess patient's current drug use, including all prescription and OTC drugs.

• Use extreme caution when administering methadone to patients with conditions accompanied by hypoxia, hypercapnia, or decreased respiratory reserve such as asthma, chronic obstructive pulmonary

disease or cor pulmonale, severe obesity, sleep apnea syndrome, myxedema, kyphoscoliosis, CNS depression or coma. This is because methadone, even with usual therapeutic doses, may decrease respiratory drive while simultaneously increasing airway resistance to the point of apnea.

WARNING Give drug cautiously to patients at risk for a prolonged QT interval, such as those with cardiac hypertrophy, hypokalemia, or hypomagnesemia; those with a history of cardiac conduction abnormalities; and those taking diuretics or medications that affect cardiac conduction.

• Dilute oral concentrate with water or another liquid to volume of at least 30 ml, but preferably to 90 ml or more, before administration. Dissolve dispersible tablets in 120 ml of water or another liquid before giving. Know that the dispersible tablet may not completely dissolve in water. If a residue remains in the cup after initial administration with water, add a small amount of liquid to the cup and give to patient to drink to ensure all of the drug has been ingested.

• Monitor patient for expected excessive drowsiness, unsteadiness, or confusion during first 3 to 5 days of therapy, and notify prescriber if effects continue to worsen or persist beyond this time.

WARNING Monitor respiratory and circulatory status carefully and often during methadone therapy, especially when drug therapy is initiated and when patient is being converted to methadone, because respiratory or circulatory depression, respiratory arrest, shock, hypotension, and cardiac arrest can develop. Life-threatening respiratory depression can occur even when drug is being used as prescribed and is not misused or abused. Be especially vigilant with elderly, cachectic, and debilitated patients who are at higher risk for developing respiratory depression. Assess patient for excessive or persistent sedation; dosage may need to be adjusted.

• Be aware that patients tolerant to other opioids may be incompletely tolerant to methadone. A high degree of "opioid tolerance" does not eliminate the possibility of methadone toxicity. Some patients have died during conversion from chronic high-dose therapy with other opioid agonists. Monitor patient closely during the conversion process.

• Watch for drug tolerance, especially in patients with a history of chronic drug abuse, because methadone can cause physical and psychological dependence.

• Monitor patient for pain because maintenance dosage doesn't provide pain relief; patients with tolerance to opiate agonists, including those with chronic cancer pain, may require a higher dosage.

• Monitor patients who are pregnant or who have liver or renal impairment for increased adverse effects from methadone because drug may have a prolonged duration and cumulative effect in these patients. Methadone may prolong labor by reducing strength, duration, and frequency of uterine contractions, so expect dosage to be tapered before third trimester of pregnancy. Breast-feeding mothers on maintenance therapy put their infants at risk of withdrawal symptoms if they abruptly stop breastfeeding or discontinue methadone therapy. Methadone also accumulates in CNS tissue, increasing the risk of seizures in infants.

• Check plasma amylase and lipase levels in patients who develop biliary tract spasms because levels may increase up to 15 times normal. Notify prescriber immediately of any significant or sustained increase.

• Monitor patients who have head injuries or other conditions that may increase intracranial pressure (ICP) because methadone may further increase ICP.

• Assess patient for withdrawal symptoms and tolerance to therapy because physiologic dependence can occur with long-term methadone use. Avoid abrupt discontinuation because withdrawal symptoms will occur within 3 to 4 days after last dose.

• Monitor patients, especially the elderly, for cardiac arrhythmias, hypotension, hypovolemia, orthostatic hypotension, and vasovagal syncope because methadone may produce cholinergic effects in patients with cardiac disease, resulting in bradycardia and peripheral vasodilation; dosage decrease may be indicated.

• Monitor patients with prostatic hypertrophy, urethral stricture, or renal disease for urine retention and oliguria because methadone can increase tension of detrusor muscle.

• Be prepared to treat patient's symptoms of anxiety; be aware that anxiety may be confused with symptoms of opioid abstinence and that methadone doesn't have antianxiety effects.

• Monitor patients with seizure disorders because methadone may induce or aggravate seizure activity.

PATIENT TEACHING

• Instruct patient taking oral concentrate form of methadone to dilute it with water or another liquid to a volume of at least 30 ml, and preferably to 90 ml or more, before administration.

• Instruct patient to dissolve dispersible tablets in 120 ml of water or other liquid immediately before administration. Alert patient that if water is used and residue is left in the cup after ingesting, he should add a little more liquid to the cup and drink to ensure all the drug was consumed.

• Advise patient to notify prescriber of all other drugs he's currently taking and to avoid alcohol and other depressants, such as sleeping pills and tranquilizers, because they may increase drug's CNS depressant effects.

• Instruct patient to take drug only as prescribed and not to change dosage without prescriber approval. Inform patient that abrupt cessation of methadone therapy can precipitate withdrawal symptoms. Urge him to notify prescriber if he develops any concerns over therapy.

• Urge patient to notify prescriber if he experiences palpitations, dizziness, light-headedness, or syncope, which may be caused by methadone-induced arrhythmias.

• Instruct patient to avoid potentially hazardous activities or those that require mental alertness because methadone therapy may cause drowsiness or sleepiness.

• Teach patient to change positions slowly to minimize the effects of orthostatic hypotension.

• Instruct patient to notify prescriber of worsening or breakthrough pain because dosage may need to be adjusted.
• Inform parents that a child on methadone maintenance therapy may become unusually excited or restless; advise them to notify prescriber of changes in child's behavior.
• Instruct female patient to notify prescriber immediately if she becomes pregnant during methadone therapy because drug may cause physical dependence in fetus and withdrawal symptoms in neonate.
• Caution patient who is breastfeeding not to stop doing so abruptly and not to stop taking methadone without prescriber's approval because infant may experience withdrawal symptoms.
• Instruct patient or parents to keep methadone out of the reach of children because accidental ingestion can be fatal.

methamphetamine hydrochloride

Desoxyn, Desoxyn Gradumet

Class, Category, and Schedule
Chemical class: Amphetamine
Therapeutic class: CNS stimulant
Pregnancy category: C
Controlled substance schedule: II

Indications and Dosages
➤ *To treat attention-deficit hyperactivity disorder (ADHD)*
EXTENDED-RELEASE TABLETS
Children age 6 and over. 20 to 25 mg daily.
TABLETS
Children age 6 and over. *Initial:* 5 mg once or twice daily. Increased by 5 mg every wk. *Maintenance:* 20 to 25 mg daily in divided doses twice daily.

Route	Onset	Peak	Duration
P.O.	Unknown	Unknown	6–24 hr

Mechanism of Action
May produce CNS stimulation by facilitating release and blocking reuptake of norepinephrine at adrenergic nerve terminals and by stimulating alpha and beta receptors in the peripheral nervous system. Metham-phetamine also promotes dopamine release and blocks its reuptake in the brain's limbic regions. It appears to act mainly in cerebral cortex and, possibly, reticular activating system. Its actions decrease motor restlessness, increase alertness, and reduce drowsiness and fatigue. Peripheral actions include increased blood pressure and mild bronchodilation and respiratory stimulation.

Contraindications
Advanced arteriosclerosis; glaucoma; hypersensitivity to methamphetamine, sympathomimetic amines, or their components; hyperthyroidism; history of drug abuse; moderate to severe hyper-tension; severe agitation; symptomatic cardiovascular disease; use within 14 days of MAO inhibitor

Interaction
DRUGS
ascorbic acid: Decreased methamphetamine absorption and therapeutic effect
beta blockers: Increased risk of heart block, hypotension, and severe bradycardia
CNS stimulants: Increased CNS stimulation and risk of adverse reactions
digoxin, levodopa: Increased risk of arrhythmias
diuretics, other antihypertensives: Possibly decreased antihypertensive effect
ethosuximide, phenobarbital, phenytoin: Possibly delayed absorption of these drugs
haloperidol, phenothiazines: Possibly interference with effects of these drugs and with methamphetamine's CNS stimulant effects
inhalation anesthetics: Increased risk of ventricular arrhythmias
insulin: Altered insulin requirements
lithium: Possibly antagonized CNS stimulant effects of methamphetamine
MAO inhibitors: Possibly severe hyper-tension, risk of hypertensive crisis, increased vaso-pressor effect of methamphetamine
meperidine: Increased risk of hypotension and life-threatening interactions, such as severe respiratory depression and coma
metrizamide (intrathecal): Increased risk of seizures

thyroid hormones: Enhanced effects of both drugs
tricyclic antidepressants: Increased risk of arrhythmias and severe hypertension
urinary acidifiers: Increased metabolism and shortened pharmacologic effects of methamphetamine
urinary alkalinizers: Decreased metabolism and prolonged pharmacologic effects of methamphetamine

FOODS

caffeine: Increased methamphetamine effects

Adverse Reactions

CNS: Dizziness, euphoria, headache, hyperactivity, insomnia, irritability, mania, nervousness, psychotic episodes, restlessness, talkativeness, tremor
CV: Arrhythmias, chest pain, hypertension, hypotension, MI, palpitations, peripheral vasculopathy including Raynaud's phenomenon, tachycardia
EENT: Accommodation abnormality, blurred vision, dry mouth, taste perversion
ENDO: Stunted growth
GI: Abdominal cramps, anorexia, constipation, diarrhea, nausea, vomiting
GU: Impotence, libido changes, priapism
SKIN: Diaphoresis, urticaria
Other: Physical and psychological dependence

Nursing Considerations

• Know that methamphetamine should not be used in a patient (especially a child or an adolescent) with a serious heart condition, such as a structural heart defect, cardiomyopathy, or a serious heart rhythm abnormality.
• Use methamphetamine cautiously in patients with a history of psychiatric problems or suicidal or homicidal tendencies.
• Assess for seizures in patients with a history of seizure disorders because drug may lower seizure threshold.
• Observe patient for evidence of drug tolerance and, possibly, extreme dependence, which may develop after a few weeks. Be aware that methamphetamine abuse may occur.
• Expect treatment for ADHD to include psychological, educational, and social measures in addition to drug therapy.

• Monitor child's growth pattern. If growth appears to be delayed, notify prescriber because methamphetamine therapy may need to be interrupted temporarily.
• Watch for signs of chronic methamphetamine intoxication, including hyperactivity, insomnia, irritability, and personality changes. Notify prescriber if they occur.
• Monitor patient for exertional chest pain, unexplained syncope, and other evidence that could suggest heart disease. If present, notify prescriber. A cardiac evaluation will be needed, and therapy may need to stop.
• Expect drug to be periodically discontinued to assess child's need for drug.
• Notify prescriber if patient exhibits paradoxical aggravation of symptoms or other adverse effects, and expect dosage to be reduced or drug discontinued.

PATIENT TEACHING

• Instruct parent of patient to give methamphetamine at least 6 hours before bedtime to prevent insomnia.
• Explain high risk of abuse with this drug. Instruct parent of patient not to increase dosage unless advised by prescriber and not to give drug to prevent fatigue.
WARNING Advise patient to take methamphetamine exactly as prescribed because misuse may cause serious heart effects or even death.
• Caution parent that patient should not crush or chew E.R. tablets.
• Advise parent that patient should avoid caffeine, which increases drug's effects.
• Instruct parent of patient to report signs of overstimulation, such as diarrhea, hyperactivity, insomnia, and irritability.

methazolamide
MZM, Neptazane

Class and Category

Chemical class: Sulfonamide derivative
Therapeutic class: Antiglaucoma
Pregnancy category: C

Indications and Dosages

➤ *To treat open-angle glaucoma*

TABLETS

Adults. 50 to 100 mg twice daily or three times daily.

Route	Onset	Peak	Duration
P.O.	2–4 hr	6–8 hr	10–18 hr

Mechanism of Action

Inhibits the enzyme carbonic anhydrase, which normally appears in renal proximal tubule cells, choroid plexus of the brain, and ciliary processes of the eye. By inhibiting this enzyme in the eyes, methazolamide decreases aqueous humor secretion, which reduces intraocular pressure.

Contraindications

Cirrhosis; hyperchloremic acidosis; hypersensitivity to methazolamide, other carbonic anhydrase inhibitors, or their components; hypokalemia; hyponatremia; severe adrenocortical, hepatic, or renal impairment

Interaction

DRUGS

amphetamines, anticholinergics, mecamylamine, procainamide, quinidine: Decreased renal clearance of these drugs, increased risk of toxicity
amphotericin B, corticosteroids: Increased risk of severe hypokalemia
barbiturates, carbamazepine, phenytoin, primidone: Increased risk of osteopenia
digoxin: Increased risk of hypokalemia and digitalis toxicity
ephedrine: Possibly prolonged duration of action of ephedrine
insulin, oral antidiabetic drugs: Increased risk of glycosuria and hyperglycemia
lithium: Increased lithium excretion
mannitol: Increased diuresis and further reduction of intraocular pressure
methenamine compounds: Decreased methenamine effectiveness
mexiletine: Possibly impaired renal excretion of mexiletine
neuromuscular blockers: Possibly prolonged duration of action of blockers from methazolamide-induced hypokalemia, increased risk of prolonged respiratory paralysis and depression

salicylates: Possibly CNS depression and metabolic acidosis, increased risk of methazolamide toxicity

Adverse Reactions

CNS: Confusion, depression, drowsiness, fatigue, fever, malaise, paresthesia, seizures, weakness
EENT: Hearing loss, myopia (transient), taste perversion, tinnitus
GI: Anorexia, diarrhea, nausea, vomiting
GU: Crystalluria, nephrotoxicity, renal calculi
SKIN: Photosensitivity, pruritus, rash, Stevens-Johnson syndrome, urticaria
Other: Metabolic acidosis

Nursing Considerations

• Use methazolamide cautiously in patients with obstructive pulmonary disease.
• Monitor fluid intake and output, weight, and serum electrolyte levels during methazolamide therapy.

PATIENT TEACHING

• Direct patient to take methazolamide exactly as prescribed because increasing dosage may lead to metabolic acidosis.
• Advise patient to take drug with food if GI distress occurs.
• Instruct patient to report if rash develops.
• Caution patient to avoid hazardous activities until drug's CNS effects are known.
• Emphasize need to have regular eye examinations during methazolamide therapy.

methenamine hippurate

Hiprex, Urex

methenamine mandelate

Mandelamine

Class and Category

Chemical class: Formaldehyde precursor, hexamethylenetetramine
Therapeutic class: Antibiotic
Pregnancy category: C

Indications and Dosages

➤ *To prevent or suppress frequently recurring UTI caused by a wide variety of gram-negative and gram-positive bacteria (including enterococci,* Escherichia coli, Micrococcus pyogenes, *and staphylococci) in intermittently catheterized patients with neurogenic bladder*

ENTERIC-COATED TABLETS, ORAL SUSPENSION (METHENAMINE MANDELATE)

Adults and adolescents. 1 g four times daily before meals and at bedtime.

Children ages 6 to 12. 500 mg four times daily, or 50 mg/kg daily in divided doses.

Children under age 6. 18.4 mg/kg four timesdaily.

TABLETS (METHENAMINE HIPPURATE)

Adults and adolescents. 1 g twice daily.

Children ages 6 to 12. 0.5 to 1 g every 12 hr.

Mechanism of Action

Hydrolyzes to formaldehyde and ammonia in an acidic environment, such as urine, producing greater amounts of formaldehyde as pH decreases. Formaldehyde has bactericidal action, possibly by denaturing proteins. To facilitate hydrolysis, methenamine is formulated with weak organic acid, such as hippuric acid or mandelic acid.

Contraindications

Concurrent therapy with sulfonamides, hypersensitivity to methenamine, renal insufficiency, severe dehydration, severe hepatic disease

Interaction

DRUGS

bicarbonate-containing antacids, urinary alkalinizers: Decreased methenamine effect

sulfonamides, such as sulfamethizole: Possibly formation of insoluble precipitate in urine

FOODS

milk, milk products, most fruits: Possibly decreased effectiveness of methenamine

Adverse Reactions

CNS: Headache
CV: Edema
EENT: Stomatitis
GI: Abdominal cramps, anorexia, diarrhea, nausea, vomiting

GU: Bladder irritation, crystalluria, dysuria, hematuria, proteinuria, urinary frequency
RESP: Pulmonary hypersensitivity (dyspnea, pneumonitis)
SKIN: Pruritus, rash, urticaria

Nursing Considerations

• Be aware that methenamine is used for prophylaxis; it isn't recommended as primary treatment for UTI.
• Drug shouldn't be given to patients with creatinine clearance less than 50 ml/min/1.73 m^2.
• Before giving first dose, expect to obtain urine specimen for culture and sensitivity tests and to review test results if available.
• Plan to give methenamine mandelate around the clock to maintain a therapeutic blood level.
• Make sure patient receives adequate fluids.
• Expect to repeat culture and sensitivity tests if patient fails to improve.

PATIENT TEACHING

• Instruct patient to take methenamine with food to avoid GI distress.
• Direct patient to drink extra fluids; avoid alkaline foods, such as milk, milk products, and most fruits; and avoid antacids that contain sodium bicarbonate or carbonate during methenamine therapy.
• Instruct patient to report painful urination, rash, or severe GI distress.
• Urge patient to comply with urine testing before and during long-term therapy.

methicillin sodium

Staphcillin

Class and Category

Chemical: Penicillinase-resistant penicillin*Therapeutic:* Antibiotic
Pregnancy category: B

Indications and Dosages

➤ *To treat general infections, such as sepsis, sinusitis, and skin and soft-tissue infections, caused by susceptible organisms (including penicillinase-producing and non–penicillinase-producing strains of* Staphylococcus epidermidis, Staphylococcus saprophyticus, *and* Streptococcus pneumoniae)

M

I.V. INFUSION, I.M. INJECTION

Adults and children weighing 40 kg (88 lb) or more. 1 g every 4 to 6 hr (I.M.) or 1 g every 6 hr (I.V.). *Maximum:* 24 g daily.

Children weighing less than 40 kg. 25 mg/kg every 6 hr.

DOSAGE ADJUSTMENT For adults and children with cystic fibrosis, dosage adjusted to 50 mg/kg every 6 hr.

➤ *To treat bacterial meningitis*

I.V. INFUSION, I.M. INJECTION

Neonates weighing 2 kg (4.4 lb) or more. 50 mg/kg every 8 hr for first wk after birth and then 50 mg/kg every 6 hr.

Neonates weighing less than 2 kg. 25 to 50 mg/kg every 12 hr for first wk after birth and then 50 mg/kg every 8 hr.

Mechanism of Action

Kills bacteria by inhibiting cell wall synthesis. In susceptible bacteria, the rigid, cross-linked cell wall is assembled in several steps. In final stage of cross-linking, methicillin binds with and inactivates penicillin-binding proteins (enzymes responsible for linking cell wall strands), resulting in bacterial cell lysis and death. *Staphylococcus aureus* has developed resistance to methicillin by altering its penicillin-binding proteins.

Incompatibilities

Don't mix methicillin in same syringe or I.V. solution with other drugs. Don't mix methicillin with dextrose solutions because their low acidity may damage drug. Give methicillin at least 1 hour before or after aminoglycosides and at different sites; otherwise, mutual inactivation can occur.

Contraindications

Hypersensitivity to methicillin sodium, other penicillins, or their components

Interaction

DRUGS

aminoglycosides: Substantial aminoglycoside inactivation

chloramphenicol, erythromycins, sulfonamides, tetracyclines: Possibly decreased therapeutic effects of methicillin

methotrexate: Increased risk of methotrexate toxicity

probenecid: Possibly decreased renal clearance, increased blood level, and increased risk of toxicity of methicillin

Adverse Reactions

CNS: Aggressiveness, agitation, anxiety, confusion, depression, headache, seizures

EENT: Oral candidiasis

GI: Abdominal pain, diarrhea, hepatotoxicity, nausea, pseudomembranous colitis, vomiting

GU: Interstitial nephritis, vaginitis

HEME: Leukopenia, neutropenia, thrombocytopenia

SKIN: Exfoliative dermatitis, pruritus, rash, urticaria

Other: Anaphylaxis; infusion-site redness, swelling, and tenderness; injection-site pain, redness, and swelling; serum sicknesslike reaction

Nursing Considerations

WARNING Be aware that methicillin isn't a first-line treatment for the indications above because of the prevalence of methicillin-resistant *Staphylococcus aureus.*

• Before giving first dose, obtain appropriate body fluid or tissue specimens for culture and sensitivity tests, as ordered, and review test results if available.

• Inject I.M. form deep into gluteal muscle.

• In I.V. use, observe infusion site closely for redness, swelling, and tenderness.

• Monitor fluid intake and output and renal function test results during therapy.

• Observe for signs of superinfection, such as diarrhea, vaginal itching, and white patches or sores in mouth or on tongue. Notify prescriber if they occur.

• Closely monitor renal function test results, including serum creatinine level; about one-third of patients have interstitial nephritis after 10 days of methicillin therapy.

• Monitor liver function test results, and report evidence of hepatotoxicity, such as fever and nausea.

PATIENT TEACHING

• Explain that I.M. injection may be painful.

• Unless contraindicated, instruct patient to drink extra fluids during therapy.

• Advise patient to report diarrhea, injection-site pain, mouth sores, or rash.

methimazole
Tapazole

Class and Category

Chemical class: Thioimidazole derivative
Therapeutic class: Antithyroid
Pregnancy category: D

Indications and Dosages

➤ *To treat mild hyperthyroidism*

TABLETS

Adults and adolescents. *Initial:* 15 mg daily as a single dose or in divided doses twice daily for 6 to 8 wk or until euthyroid level is reached. *Maintenance:* 5 to 30 mg daily as a single dose or in divided doses twice daily.
Children. *Initial:* 0.4 mg/kg daily as a single dose or in divided doses twice daily. *Maintenance:* 0.2 mg/kg daily as a single dose or in divided doses twice daily.

➤ *To treat moderate hyperthyroidism*

TABLETS

Adults and adolescents. *Initial:* 30 to 40 mg/day as a single dose or in divided doses twicedaily. for 6 to 8 wk or until euthyroid level is reached. *Maintenance:* 5 to 30 mg daily as a single dose or in divided doses twice daily.
Children. *Initial:* 0.4 mg/kg daily as a single dose or in divided doses twice daily. *Maintenance:* 0.2 mg/kg daily as a single dose or in divided doses twice daily.

➤ *To treat severe hyperthyroidism*

TABLETS

Adults and adolescents. *Initial:* 60 mg daily as a single dose or in divided doses twice daily. for 6 to 8 wk or until euthyroid level is reached. *Maintenance:* 5 to 30 mg daily as a single dose or in divided doses twice daily.
Children. *Initial:* 0.4 mg/kg daily as a single dose or in divided doses twice daily. *Maintenance:* 0.2 mg/kg daily as a single dose or in divided doses twice daily.

➤ *As adjunct to treat thyrotoxicosis*

SUPPOSITORIES

Adults and adolescents. 15 to 20 mg every 4 hr on first day and then adjusted based on patient response.
Children. 0.4 mg/kg daily as a single dose or in divided doses twice daily.

Route	Onset	Peak	Duration
P.O.	5 days	7 wk	Unknown

Mechanism of Action

Directly interferes with thyroid hormone synthesis in the thyroid gland by inhibiting iodide incorporation into thyroglobulin. Iodination of thyroglobulin is an important step in synthesizing the thyroid hormones thyroxine and triiodothyronine. Eventually, thyroglobulin is depleted and the circulating thyroid hormone level drops.

Contraindications

Breastfeeding; hypersensitivity to methimazole, other antithyroid drugs, or their components

Interaction

DRUGS

amiodarone, iodine, potassium iodide: Decreased response to methimazole
digoxin: Possibly increased blood digoxin level
oral anticoagulants: Possibly a need for altered anticoagulant dosage

Adverse Reactions

CNS: Drowsiness, headache, paresthesia, vertigo
CV: Edema
EENT: Loss of taste
ENDO: Hypothyroidism
GI: Diarrhea, indigestion, nausea, vomiting
HEME: Agranulocytosis, aplastic anemia, leukopenia, thrombocytopenia
MS: Arthralgia, myalgia
SKIN: Alopecia, jaundice, pruritus, rash, skin discoloration, urticaria
Other: Lupus-like symptoms, lymphadenopathy

Nursing Considerations

• Closely monitor thyroid function test results during methimazole therapy.
• Check CBC results to detect abnormalities caused by inhibition of myelopoiesis.
• Watch for signs and symptoms of hypothyroidism, such as cold intolerance, depression, and edema.
• Be aware that hyperthyroidism may increase metabolic clearance of beta blockers and theophylline and that dosages of these drugs may need to be reduced as the patient's thyroid condition becomes corrected.

PATIENT TEACHING

• Instruct patient to take drug with meals to avoid adverse GI reactions.

M

• Explain about possible hair loss or thinning during and for months after therapy.
• Instruct patient to notify prescriber immediately about cold intolerance, fever, sore throat, tiredness, and unusual bleeding or bruising.

methocarbamol

Carbacot, Robaxin, Robaxin 750, Skelex

Class and Category

Chemical class: Carbamate derivative of guaifenesin
Therapeutic class: Skeletal muscle relaxant
Pregnancy category: C

Indications and Dosages

➤ *To relieve discomfort caused by acute, painful musculoskeletal conditions*
TABLETS
Adults and adolescents. *Initial:* 1,500 mg four times daily for 2 to 3 days; for severe discomfort, 8,000 mg daily. *Maintenance:* 750 mg every 4 hr, 1,000 mg four times daily, or 1,500 mg three times daily.
I.V. INJECTION (100 MG/ML)
Adults and adolescents. Up to 3,000 mg daily administered at 8-hr intervals for 3 consecutive days. Regimen repeated as prescribed after patient is drug-free for 48 hr.
I.M. INJECTION (100 MG/ML)
Adults and adolescents. 1,000 to 3,000 mg/day administered at 8-hr intervals for 3 consecutive days. Regimen repeated as prescribed after patient is drug-free for 48 hr.
➤ *To provide supportive therapy for tetanus*
TABLETS
Adults and adolescents. 24,000 mg daily given by NG tube.
I.V. INFUSION OR INJECTION (100 MG/ML)
Adults and adolescents. 1,000 to 3,000 mg by infusion or 1,000 to 2,000 mg by direct injection every 6 hr. *Maximum:* 300 mg (3 ml)/min.
Children. 15 mg/kg every 6 hr.

Route	Onset	Peak	Duration
P.O.	30 min	Unknown	Unknown
I.V.	Immediate	Unknown	Unknown

Mechanism of Action

May depress CNS, which leads to sedation and reduced skeletal muscle spasms. Methocarbamol also alters perception of pain.

Contraindications

Hypersensitivity to methocarbamol or its components, renal disease (injectable form)

Interaction

DRUGS
CNS depressants: Increased CNS depression
ACTIVITIES
alcohol use: Increased CNS depression

Adverse Reactions

CNS: Dizziness, drowsiness, fever, headache, light-headedness, seizures (I.V.), syncope, vertigo, weakness
CV: Bradycardia, hypotension, and thrombophlebitis (parenteral)
EENT: Blurred vision, conjunctivitis, diplopia, metallic taste, nasal congestion, nystagmus
GI: Nausea
GU: Black, brown, or green urine
SKIN: Flushing, pruritus, rash, urticaria
Other: Anaphylaxis (parenteral), angioedema, injection-site irritation or pain (I.M.), injection-site sloughing (I.V.)

Nursing Considerations

• If needed, crush methocarbamol tablets and mix with water for administration by NG tube.
• Give I.V. form directly through infusion line at 3 ml/min. To prepare solution, add 10 ml to no more than 250 ml D_5W or normal saline solution. Infuse at no more than 300 mg (3 ml)/min to avoid hypotension and seizures.
• Keep patient recumbent during I.V. administration and for at least 15 minutes afterward. Then have him rise slowly.
• Monitor I.V. site regularly for signs of phlebitis.
• Inject I.M. form deep into large muscle, such as the gluteus. Give no more than 5 ml/dose every 8 hours. One dose is usually adequate.
• Don't give methocarbamol by subcutaneous route.
• Keep epinephrine, antihistamines, and corticosteroids available in case patient experiences anaphylactic reaction.

• Be aware that the parenteral dosage form shouldn't be used in patients with renal dysfunction because the polyethylene glycol 300 vehicle is nephrotoxic.

PATIENT TEACHING
• Tell patient to take drug exactly as prescribed.
• Advise patient to take drug with food or milk to avoid nausea.
• Inform patient that urine may turn green, black, or brown until methocarbamol is discontinued.
• Advise patient to avoid hazardous activities until drug's CNS effects are known.
• Instruct patient to avoid alcohol and other CNS depressants during therapy.

---

methotrexate
(amethopterin)
Rasuvo, Rheumatrex

methotrexate sodium
Folex, Folex PFS, Mexate, Mexate-AQ, Otrexup

Class and Category
Chemical class: Folic acid analogue
Therapeutic class: Antipsoriatic, anti-rheumatic
Pregnancy category: X

Indications and Dosages
➤ *To treat severe psoriasis unresponsive to other therapy*
TABLETS (METHOTREXATE)
Adults. 2.5 to 5 mg every 12 hr for 3 doses/wk, increased as ordered by 2.5 mg/wk. *Maximum:* 20 mg/wk.
I.V. OR I.M. INJECTION (METHOTREXATE SODIUM)
Adults. 10 mg/wk. *Maximum:* 25 mg/wk.
SUBCUTANEOUS INJECTION (OTREXUP, RASUVO)
Adults. 10 to 25 mg weekly. *Maximum:* 30 mg weekly.
➤ *To treat severe rheumatoid arthritis unresponsive to other therapy*
TABLETS (METHOTREXATE)
Adults. 2.5 to 5 mg every 12 hr for 3 doses/wk, increased as ordered by 2.5 mg/wk.

Maximum: 20 mg/wk. Alternatively, 7.5 mg as a single dose weekly.
SUBCUTANEOUS INJECTION (RASUVO)
Adults. 7.5 mg once weekly, then gradually increased to achieve an optimal response. *Maximum:* 20 mg/wk.
➤ *To treat active polyarticular juvenile idiopathic arthritis unresponsive to other therapy*
SUBCUTANEOUS INJECTION (OTREXUP, RASUVO)
Children. 10 mg/m2 once weekly.

Route	Onset	Peak	Duration
P.O., I.V., I.M.	3–6 wk	Unknown	Unknown

Mechanism of Action
May exert immunosuppressive effects by inhibiting replication and function of T and possibly B lymphocytes. Methotrexate also slows rapidly growing cells, such as epithelial skin cells in psoriasis. This action may result from the drug's inhibition of dihydrofolate reductase, the enzyme that reduces folic acid to tetrahydrofolic acid. Inhibition of tetrahydrofolic acid interferes with DNA synthesis and cell reproduction in rapidly proliferating cells.

Contraindications
Breastfeeding, hypersensitivity to metho-trexate or its components, pregnancy

Interaction
DRUGS
bone marrow depressants: Possibly increased bone marrow depression
co-trimoxazole: Possibly increased bone marrow suppression
folic acid: Possibly decreased effectiveness of methotrexate
hepatotoxic drugs: Increased risk of hepatotoxicity
chloramphenicol, neomycin, tetracycline: Possibly decreased methotrexate absorption
NSAIDs, penicillins, phenylbutazone, phenytoin, probenecid, salicylates, sulfonamides: Increased risk of methotrexate toxicity
oral anticoagulants: Increased bleeding risk
proton pump inhibitors such as esomeprazole, omeprazole, pantoprazole: Increased risk of methotrexate toxicities

sulfonamides: Increased risk of hepato-toxicity

theophylline: Possibly increased risk of theophylline toxicity

vaccines: Risk of disseminated infection with live-virus vaccines, risk of suppressed response to killed-virus vaccines

ACTIVITIES

alcohol use: Increased risk of hepatotoxicity

Adverse Reactions

CNS: Aphasia, cerebral thrombosis, chills, dizziness, drowsiness, fatigue, fever, head-ache, hemiparesis, leukoencephalopathy, malaise, paresis, seizures

CV: Chest pain, deep vein thrombosis, hypotension, pericardial effusion, pericarditis, thromboembolism

ENDO: Gynecomastia

EENT: Blurred vision, conjunctivitis, gingivitis, glossitis, pharyngitis, stomatitis, transient blindness, tinnitus

GI: Abdominal pain, anorexia, cirrhosis, diarrhea, elevated liver function test results, enteritis, GI bleeding and ulceration, hepatitis, hepatotoxicity, nausea, pancreatitis, vomiting

GU: Cystitis, hematuria, infertility, menstrual dysfunction, nephropathy, renal failure, tubular necrosis, vaginal discharge

HEME: Anemia, aplastic anemia, leukopenia, neutropenia, pancytopenia, thrombocytopenia

MS: Arthralgia, dysarthria, myalgia, stress fracture

RESP: Dry nonproductive cough, dyspnea, interstitial pneumonitis, pneumonia, pulmonary fibrosis or failure, pulmonary infiltrates

SKIN: Acne, alopecia, altered skin pigmentation, ecchymosis, erythema multiforme, exfoliative dermatitis, furunculosis, necrosis, photosensitivity, pruritus, psoriatic lesions, rash, Stevens-Johnson syndrome, telangiectasia, toxic epidermal necrolysis, ulceration, urticaria

Other: Anaphylaxis, increased risk of infection, lymphadenopathy, lympho-proliferative disease

Nursing Considerations

• Follow facility policy for preparing and handling drug; parenteral form poses a risk of carcinogenicity, mutagenicity, and teratogenicity. Avoid skin contact.

• Monitor results of CBC, chest Xray, liver and renal function tests, and urinalysis before and during treatment.

• Administer subcutaneous injection into patient's abdomen or thigh.

• Increase patient's fluid intake to 2 to 3 L daily, unless contraindicated, to reduce the risk of adverse GU reactions.

• Assess patient for bleeding and infection.

WARNING Expect renal impairment to severely alter drug elimination.

• Be aware that high doses of methotrexate can impair renal elimination by forming crystals that obstruct urine flow. To prevent drug precipitation, alkalinize patient's urine with sodium bicarbonate tablets, as ordered.

• Follow standard precautions because drug can cause immunosuppression.

• If patient becomes dehydrated from vomiting, notify prescriber and expect to withhold drug until patient recovers.

• If patient receives high doses of drug, keep leucovorin readily available as antidote.

• Be aware that methotrexate resistance may develop with prolonged use.

PATIENT TEACHING

• Prepare a calendar of treatment days for patient, and emphasize importance of following instructions exactly.

• Teach patient prescribed weekly subcu-taneous injections, how to administer the injection using the single-dose auto-injector. Tell him to give the injection into his abdomen or thigh and to rotate injection sites.

• Instruct patient to avoid alcohol during methotrexate therapy.

• Encourage frequent mouth care to reduce the risk of mouth sores.

• Instruct patient to use sunblock when exposed to sunlight.

• Advise patient to notify prescriber about bruising, chills, cough, fever, dark or bloody urine, mouth sores, shortness of breath, sore throat, and yellow skin or eyes.

• Urge women of childbearing age to use reliable contraception during methotrexate therapy.

methoxypolyethylene glycol-epoetin beta

Mircera

Class and Category
Chemical class: Continuous erythropoietin receptor activator
Therapeutic class: Antianemic
Pregnancy category: C

Indications and Dosages
➤ *To treat anemia associated with chronic renal failure in dialysis-dependent and dialysis-independent patients*

I.V. INJECTION, SUBCUTANEOUS INJECTION
Adults not currently being treated with an erythropoiesis-stimulating agent. *Initial:* 0.6 mcg/kg every 2 wk, increased or decreased by 25% monthly as needed. *Maintenance:* 1.2 mcg/kg every 4 wk.
Adults stabilized on less than 8,000 units/ wk of epoetin alfa or 40 mcg/wk of darbepoetin alfa. 60 mcg every 2 wk or 120 mcg every 4 wk.
Adults stabilized on 8,000 to 16,000 units/ wk of epoetin alfa or 40 to 80 mcg/wk of darbepoetin alfa. 100 mcg every 2 wk or 200 mcg every 4 wk.
Adults stabilized on more than 16,000 units/wk of epoetin alfa or more than 80 mcg/wk of darbepoetin alfa. 180 mcg every 2 wk or 360 mcg every 4 wk.

DOSAGE ADJUSTMENT If hemoglobin increase is greater than 1 g/dl during any 2-wk period or hemoglobin is increasing and approaching 12 g/dl, dosage reduced by 25%. If hemoglobin continues to increase despite this reduction, drug discontinued until hemoglobin begins to decrease; then drug restarted at a dose 25% less than previously given. If hemoglobin doesn't increase by 1 g/dl after 4 wk of therapy, dosage increased by 25%.

Route	Onset	Peak	Duration
I.V., SubQ	7–15 days	72 hr	72 hr

Mechanism of Action
Stimulates release of reticulocytes from bone marrow into the bloodstream, where they develop into mature RBCs.

Incompatibilities
Don't mix methoxypolyethylene glycol-epoetin beta with any other drug.

Contraindications
Hemoglobin greater than 12 g/dl, hypersensitivity to methoxypolyethylene glycolepoetin beta or its components, red cell aplasia, uncontrolled hypertension

Adverse Reactions
CNS: Headache, seizures, stroke
CV: Chest pain, congestive heart failure, deep vein thrombosis, hypertension, hypotension, MI, tachycardia, vascular access thrombosis
EENT: Nasopharyngitis
GI: Constipation, diarrhea, GI bleeding, vomiting
GU: UTI
HEME: Pure red cell aplasia, severe anemia
MS: Back or limb pain, muscle spasms
RESP: Cough, upper respiratory tract infection
SKIN: Erythema, pruritus, rash
Other: Anaphylaxis, antibody formation to drug

Nursing Considerations
• Use drug cautiously in patients who have conditions that could decrease or delay response to drug, such as aluminum intoxication, folic acid deficiency, hemolysis, infection, inflammation, iron deficiency, malignant neoplasm, osteitis (birrosa cystica), or vitamin B_{12} deficiency.
• Also use drug cautiously in patients with a cardiovascular disorder caused by hypertension, a history of seizures, vascular disease, or a hematologic disorder, such as hypercoagulation, myelodysplastic syndrome or sickle cell disease.
• Be aware that if patient's blood pressure is difficult to control even with drug therapy or dietary measures, dose of methoxypolyethylene glycol-epoetin beta should be reduced or drug withheld until blood pressure is controlled.
• Don't shake vial during preparation to avoid denaturing glycoprotein, inactivating drug. Protect vials and prefilled syringes from light by storing in original cartons.
• Discard unused portion of single-dose vial because it contains no preservatives.

M

WARNING Target hemoglobin shouldn't exceed 12 g/dl because it increases risk of life-threatening adverse cardiovascular effects.

• Monitor drug effectiveness by checking hemoglobin every 2 weeks until stabilized at 10 to 12 g/dl and maintenance dose has been established. Then expect hemoglobin to be monitored at least monthly unless dosage adjustment is needed.

• Expect to give an iron supplement because iron requirements rise when erythropoiesis consumes existing iron stores.

• Notify prescriber if patient has sudden loss of response to drug, evidenced by severe anemia and a low reticulocyte count. Anti-erythropoietin antibody-related anemia may be present, which requires stopping drug and any other erythropoietic proteins.

• Take seizure precautions, especially during the first couple months of therapy.

• Risk of hypertensive or thrombotic complications increases if hemoglobin rises more than 1 g/dl over 2 weeks.

PATIENT TEACHING

• Teach patient how to administer drug and how to dispose of needles properly. Caution against reusing needles.

• Stress importance of complying with dosage regimen and keeping follow-up medical and laboratory appointments.

• Review possible adverse reactions, and urge patient to notify prescriber about chest pain, headache, hives, rapid heartbeat, rash, seizures, shortness of breath, or swelling.

• Advise patient that the risk of seizures is highest during the first couple of months of methoxypolyethylene glycol-epoetin beta therapy. Urge him to avoid hazardous activities during this time.

• Encourage patient to eat iron-rich foods.

methscopolamine bromide

Pamine, Pamine Forte

Class and Category

Chemical class: Quaternary ammonium derivative of scopolamine

Therapeutic class: anticholinergic
Pregnancy category: C

Indications and Dosages

➤ *As adjunct to treat peptic ulcer*

TABLETS

Adults. For mild to moderate symptoms, 2.5 mg 30 min before meals and 2.5 to 5 mg at bedtime; for severe symptoms, 5 mg 30 min. before meals and at bedtime.

Route	Onset	Peak	Duration
P.O.	1 hr	Unknown	4–6 hr

Mechanism of Action

Reduces volume and total acid content of gastric secretions, which may have a beneficial effect in treating peptic ulcer. Drug also reduces GI motility and inhibits salivation, which may have additional benefits.

Contraindications

Glaucoma, hypersensitivity to methscopolamine bromide or its components, intestinal atony (elderly or debilitated patients), myasthenia gravis, obstructive disease of GI or GU tract, paralytic ileus, severe ulcerative colitis, toxic megacolon complicating ulcerative colitis, unstable cardiovascular status in acute hemorrhage

Interaction

DRUGS

antacids: Possibly decreased methscopolamine absorption
anticholinergics, antipsychotics, tricyclic antidepressants: Possibly increased anticholinergic effects

Adverse Reactions

CNS: Confusion, dizziness, drowsiness, headache, insomnia, nervousness, weakness
CV: Palpitations, tachycardia
EENT: Blurred vision, cycloplegia, dry mouth, increased intraocular pressure, loss of taste, pupil dilation
ENDO: Suppression of lactation
GI: Bloating, constipation, nausea, vomiting
GU: Impotence, urinary hesitancy, urine retention
SKIN: Decreased sweating, urticaria
Other: Anaphylaxis

Nursing Considerations
• Use with caution in elderly patients and in patients with autonomic neuropathy, congestive heart failure, coronary artery disease, hepatic or renal disease, hypertension, hyperthyroidism, prostatic hypertrophy, tachycardia, or ulcerative colitis.
• Notify prescriber if diarrhea occurs because it may be an early sign of incomplete intestinal obstruction.

PATIENT TEACHING
• Advise patient to avoid excessive exposure to heat to reduce the risk of heat prostration and heatstroke because methscopolamine decreases sweating.
• Caution patient to avoid antacids because they may interfere with drug's absorption.
• Advise patient to avoid hazardous activities until drug's CNS effects are known.

methsuximide
Celontin

Class and Category
Chemical class: Succinimide derivative
Therapeutic class: Anticonvulsant
Pregnancy category: Not rated

Indications and Dosages
➤ *To treat absence seizures unresponsive to other drugs*

CAPSULES
Adults and children. *Initial:* 300 mg daily. Increased by 150 to 300 mg daily every 1 to 2 wk until control is achieved with minimal adverse reactions. *Maximum:* 1.2 g daily in divided doses.

Mechanism of Action
Elevates seizure threshold and reduces frequency of seizures by depressing motor cortex and elevating threshold of CNS response to convulsive stimuli. Methsuximide is metabolized to active metabolite N-demethylmethsuximide, which may add to the anticonvulsant effects of the drug.

Contraindications
Hypersensitivity to methsuximide, succinimides, or their components

Interaction
DRUGS
carbamazepine, phenobarbital, phenytoin, primidone: Possibly decreased blood methsuximide level
CNS depressants: Possibly increased CNS depression
haloperidol: Altered seizure pattern; possibly decreased blood haloperidol level
loxapine, MAO inhibitors, maprotiline, molindone, phenothiazines, pimozide, thioxanthenes, tricyclic antidepressants: Possibly lowered seizure threshold and reduced therapeutic effect of methsuximide
ACTIVITIES
alcohol use: Possibly increased CNS depression

Adverse Reactions
CNS: Aggressiveness, ataxia, decreased concentration, dizziness, drowsiness, fatigue, fever, headache, insomnia, irritability, mental depression, nightmares, seizures, suicidal ideation
EENT: Periorbital edema, pharyngitis
GI: Abdominal and epigastric pain, abdominal cramps, abnormal liver function test results, anorexia, diarrhea, hiccups, nausea, vomiting
GU: Microscopic hematuria, proteinuria
HEME: Agranulocytosis, aplastic anemia, eosinophilia, leukopenia, pancytopenia
MS: Muscle pain
SKIN: Erythematous and pruritic rash, Stevens-Johnson syndrome, systemic lupus erythematosus, urticaria
Other: Lymphadenopathy

Nursing Considerations
• Monitor CBC and platelet count and assess patient for signs of infection, such as cough, fever, and pharyngitis, because methsuximide may cause blood dyscrasias.
• Monitor liver function test results and urinalysis results in patients with a history of hepatic or renal disease; methsuximide may cause functional changes in liver and kidneys.
• When giving drug to patient with a history of mixed-type epilepsy, institute seizure precautions because drug may increase risk of generalized tonic-clonic seizures.
• Expect the dosage to be carefully and slowly adjusted according to patient's

M

response and needs and withdrawn slowly to avoid precipitating seizures.
- Plan to use 150-mg capsule when making dosage adjustments for small children.
- Notify prescriber if patient develops depression or aggressiveness.
- Monitor patient closely for evidence of suicidal thinking or behavior, especially when therapy starts or dosage changes.

PATIENT TEACHING
- Advise patient to take a missed dose as soon as he remembers unless it's nearly time for the next dose. Warn him not to double the dose.
- Instruct patient to take drug with milk or food to reduce gastric irritation.
- Advise patient to notify prescriber if he develops cough, fever, or pharyngitis.
- Urge patient to avoid alcohol because of increased risk of CNS depression.
- Instruct patient to avoid hazardous activities until drug's adverse effects are known.
- Caution patient not to stop taking drug abruptly to avoid risk of absence seizures.
- Urge caregivers to watch patient closely for evidence of suicidal tendencies, especially when therapy starts or dosage changes, and to report concerns immediately.
- Urge woman who becomes pregnant while taking methsuximide to enroll in the North American antiepileptic drug pregnancy registry by calling 1-888-233-2334. Explain that this registry is collecting information about the safety of antiepileptic drugs during pregnancy.

methyldopa
Aldomet, Apo-Methyldopa (CAN), Dopamet (CAN), Nu-Medopa (CAN)

methyldopate hydrochloride
Aldomet

Class and Category
Chemical class: 3,4-dihydroxyphenylalanine (DOPA) analogue

Therapeutic class: Antihypertensive
Pregnancy category: B (oral form), C (parenteral form)

Indications and Dosages
➤ *To manage hypertension, to treat hypertensive crisis*
ORAL SUSPENSION, TABLETS (METHYLDOPA)
Adults. *Initial:* 250 mg twice daily or three times daily for first 48 hr, increased as ordered after 2 days. *Maintenance:* 500 to 2,000 mg daily in divided doses twice daily to four times daily. *Maximum:* 3,000 mg daily.
Children. *Initial:* 10 mg/kg daily in divided doses twice daily to four times daily for first 48 hr, increased as ordered after 2 days. *Maximum:* 65 mg/kg or 3,000 mg daily.
I.V. INFUSION (METHYLDOPATE HYDROCHLORIDE)
Adults. 250 to 500 mg diluted in D_5W and infused over 30 to 60 min every 6 hr. *Maximum:* 1,000 mg every 6 hr.

Children. 20 to 40 mg/kg infused over 30 to 60 min every 6 hr. *Maximum:* 65 mg/kg or 3,000 mg daily.

Route	Onset	Peak	Duration
P.O.	Unknown	4–6 hr*	12–24 hr†
I.V.	Unknown	4–6 hr	10–16 hr

Mechanism of Action
Is decarboxylated in the body to produce alpha-methylnorepinephrine, a metabolite that stimulates central inhibitory alpha-adrenergic receptors. This action may reduce blood pressure by decreasing sympathetic stimulation of heart and peripheral vascular system.

Incompatibilities
Don't administer methyldopa through same I.V. line as barbiturates or sulfonamides.

Contraindications
Active hepatic disease, hypersensitivity to methyldopa or its components, impaired

---

* For single dose; 2 to 3 days for multiple-doses.
† For single dose; 24 to 48 hr for multiple doses.

hepatic function from previous methyldopa therapy, use within 14 days of MAO inhibitor

Interaction

DRUGS

antihypertensives: Increased hypotension
appetite suppressants, NSAIDs, tricyclic antidepressants: Possibly decreased therapeutic effects of methyldopa
central anesthetics: Possibly need for reduced anesthetic dosage
CNS depressants: Possibly increased CNS depression
haloperidol: Increased risk of adverse CNS effects
levodopa: Possibly decreased therapeutic effects of levodopa and increased risk of adverse CNS effects
lithium: Increased risk of lithium toxicity
MAO inhibitors: Possibly hallucinations, headaches, hyperexcitability, and severe hypertension
oral anticoagulants: Possibly increased therapeutic effects of anticoagulants
sympathomimetics: Possibly decreased therapeutic effects of methyldopa and increased vasopressor effects of sympathomimetics

ACTIVITIES

alcohol use: Possibly increased CNS depression

Adverse Reactions

CNS: Decreased concentration, depression, dizziness, drowsiness, fever, headache, involuntary motor activity, memory loss (transient), nightmares, paresthesia, parkinsonism, sedation, vertigo, weakness
CV: Angina, bradycardia, edema, heart failure, myocarditis, orthostatic hypotension
EENT: Black or sore tongue, dry mouth, nasal congestion
ENDO: Gynecomastia
GI: Constipation, diarrhea, flatulence, hepatic necrosis, hepatitis, nausea, pancreatitis, vomiting
GU: Decreased libido, impotence
HEME: Agranulocytosis, hemolytic anemia, leukopenia, positive Coombs' test, positive tests for ANA and rheumatoid factor, thrombocytopenia
SKIN: Eczema, rash, urticaria
Other: Weight gain

Nursing Considerations
• For I.V. infusion, add methyldopate to 100ml of D_5W and administer over 30 to 60 minutes.
• Expect to monitor CBC and differential results before and periodically during methyldopa therapy.
• Monitor blood pressure regularly during therapy.
• Monitor results of Coombs' test; a positive result after several months of treatment indicates that patient has hemolytic anemia. Expect to discontinue drug.
• Assess for weight gain and edema. If they develop, give a diuretic, as prescribed.
• Notify prescriber if patient has signs of heart failure (dyspnea, edema, hypertension) or involuntary, rapid, jerky movements.
• Be aware that hypertension may return within 48 hours after stopping drug.

PATIENT TEACHING
• Instruct patient to take methyldopa exactly as prescribed and not to skip a dose. Explain that hypertension can return within 48 hours after stopping drug.
• Suggest that patient take drug at bedtime to minimize daytime drowsiness.
• Instruct patient to weigh himself daily and to report a gain of more than 5 lb (2.3 kg) in 2 days.
• Advise patient to change position slowly to minimize orthostatic hypotension.
• Direct patient to notify prescriber about bruising, chest pain, fever, involuntary jerky movements, prolonged dizziness, rash, and yellow eyes or skin.
• Caution patient not to stop drug abruptly; doing so may cause withdrawal symptoms, such as headache, hypertension, increased sweating, nausea, and tremor.

methylnaltrexone bromide
Relistor

Class and Category
Chemical class: Noroxymorphone methobromide

Therapeutic class: Peripheral mu-opioid receptor antagonist
Pregnancy category: B

Indications and Dosages

➤ *To treat opioid-induced constipation in patients receiving palliative care and not responsive to laxative therapy.*

SUBCUTANEOUS INJECTION

Adults weighing more than 114 kg (251 lb). 0.15 mg/kg every other day, as needed. *Maximum:* 0.15 mg/kg daily.
Adults weighing 62 to 114 kg (136 to 251 lb). 12 mg every other day, as needed. *Maximum:* 12 mg daily.
Adults weighing 38 to less than 62 kg (84 to less than 136 lb). 8 mg every other day, as needed. *Maximum:* 8 mg daily.
Adults weighing less than 38 kg. 0.15 mg/ kg every other day, as needed. *Maximum:* 0.15 mg/kg daily.

➤ *To treat opioid-induced constipation in patients with chronic noncancer pain*

SUBCUTANEOUS INJECTION

Adults. 12 mg once daily.

DOSAGE ADJUSTMENT For patients with severe renal failure (creatinine clearance less than 30 ml/min/1.73 m²), dosage reduced by half.

Route	Onset	Peak	Duration
SubQ	Unknown	0.5 hr	Unknown

Mechanism of Action

Binds to peripherally acting mu-opioid receptors in the GI tract, preventing opioid-induced slowing of GI transit time and motility. When transit time and motility is restored to normal, constipation is relieved.

Contraindications

Hypersensitivity to methylnaltrexone bromide or its components, GI obstruction, I.V. administration

Adverse Reactions

CNS: Dizziness
GI: Abdominal pain, diarrhea, flatulence, gastrointestinal perforation, nausea
SKIN: Diaphoresis

Nursing Considerations

• Use methylnaltrexone cautiously in patients with known or suspected lesions of the gastrointestinal (GI) tract as well as conditions that may affect the structural integrity of the GI tract wall, such as diverticular disease, infiltrative GI tract malignancies, Ogilvie's syndrome, peptic ulcer disease, and peritoneal metastases, because of increased risk of GI perforation.

• To determine volume of drug to give patients who weigh more than 114 kg (251lb) or less than 38 kg (84 lb), multiply patient's weight in pounds by 0.0034 and round up to the nearest 0.1 ml. Or. multiply patient's weight in kilograms by 0.0075 and round up to the nearest 0.1 ml. For patients who weigh 62 to 114 kg (136 to 251 lb), injection volume administered should be 0.6 ml. For patients who weigh 38 to less than 62 kg (84 to less than 136 lb), injection volume administered should be 0.4 ml.

• Inspect vial before giving drug to make sure solution is clear and colorless to pale yellow.

• Give drug only as subcutaneous injection into patient's upper arm, abdomen, or thigh and no more than once in 24 hours. Make sure to rotate injection sites.

• Once drug is drawn into syringe, it should be given immediately. However, if needed, it may be stored at room temperature for up to 24 hours.

• Notify prescriber about severe or persistent diarrhea, and expect drug to be discontinued.

• Monitor patient for development of severe, persistent, or worsening abdominal pain because gastrointestinal perforation may occur with severe constipation that has not responded to methylnaltrexone therapy. Notify prescriber immediately and expect drug to be discontinued.

• Monitor patient for symptoms of opioid withdrawal such as abdominal pain, anxiety, chills, diaphoresis, diarrhea, or yawning that has occurred with methylnaltrexone therapy. Patients at greatest risk for opioid withdrawal are those who have disruptions to the blood–brain barrier with opioid administration.

PATIENT TEACHING
• Teach patient or caregiver how to prepare and give methylnaltrexone subcutaneously. Stress need to rotate injection sites.
• Inform patient that a bowel movement may occur within 30 minutes after drug has been administered.
• Advise patient that if severe or persistent diarrhea, abdominal pain, nausea, or vomiting that is new or worsens occurs, prescriber should be notified and drug discontinued.
• Reassure patient that drug is not a controlled substance.
• Tell patient to stop taking methylnaltrexone if she stops taking opioid pain medication.

methylphenidate hydrochloride

Concerta, Daytrana, Metadate, Metadate CD, Metadate ER, Methylin, Methylin ER, PMS-Methylphenidate (CAN), Quillivant XR, Riphenidate (CAN), Ritalin, Ritalin-LA, Ritalin SR (CAN), Ritalin-SR

Class, Category, and Schedule
Chemical class: Piperidine derivative
Therapeutic class: CNS stimulant
Pregnancy category: C
Controlled substance schedule: II

Indications and Dosages
➤ *To treat attention-deficit hyperactivity disorder (ADHD)*
CAPSULES, E.R. TABLETS, ORAL SOLUTION, S.R. TABLETS, TABLETS
Adults and adolescents. 5 to 20 mg twice daily or three times daily *Maximum:* 90 mg daily.

Children ages 6 to 12. 5 mg twice daily before breakfast and lunch; increased by 5 to 10 mg daily at 1-wk intervals. *Maximum:* 60 mg daily.
E.R. ORAL SUSPENSION (QUILLIVANT XR)
Adults and children ages 6 and older. *Initially,* 20 mg once daily in morning; increased weekly in increments of 10 to 20 mg, as needed. *Maximum:* 60 mg daily.
E.R. ONCE-DAILY TABLETS (CONCERTA)
Adults and adolescents. 18 mg daily; increased in 18-mg increments at 1-wk intervals. *Maximum:* 72 mg daily, not to exceed 2 mg/kg daily.
Children ages 6 to 12. 18 mg daily. *Maximum:* 54 mg daily.
E.R. ONCE-DAILY CAPSULES (METADATE CD)
Children age 6 and over. 20 mg daily. Dosage titrated to 40 or 60 mg daily based on individual response. *Maximum:* 60 mg daily.
DOSAGE ADJUSTMENT Dosage reduced or drug stopped if no improvement in 1 mo. When maintenance dosage is achieved with tablets, may be switched to E.R. or S.R. tablets.
TRANSDERMAL PATCH (DAYTRANA)
Adolescents ages 13 to 17, children ages 6 to 12. *Initial:* 10-mg (12.5-cm^2) patch worn 9 hr daily; after 1 wk, increased to 15-mg (18.75-cm^2) patch worn 9 hr daily; after 1 more wk, increased to 20-mg (25-cm^2) patch worn 9 hr daily; after 1 more wk, increased to 30-mg (37.5-cm^2) patch worn 9 hr daily. *Maximum:* 30-mg (37.5-cm^2) patch worn 9 hr daily.
➤ *To treat narcolepsy*
ORAL SOLUTION, TABLETS
Adults and adolescents. 5 to 20 mg twice daily or three times daily. *Maximum:* 90 mg daily.

Route	Onset	Peak	Duration
P.O. (tablets)	Unknown	Unknown	3–6 hr
P.O. (E.R., S.R.)	Unknown	Unknown	About 8 hr
P.O. (E.R. once daily)	Unknown	Unknown	About 12 hr

Mechanism of Action

Blocks the reuptake mechanism of dopaminergic neurons in the cerebral cortex and subcortical structures of the brain, including the thalamus, decreasing motor restlessness and improving concentration.

Methylphenidate also may trigger sympathomimetic activity. This action produces increased motor activity, alertness, mild euphoria, and decreased fatigue in patients with narcolepsy.

Contraindications

Angina pectoris, anxiety, cardiac arrhythmias, depression, fructose intolerance, glaucoma, glucose-galactose malabsorption, heart failure, hypersensitivity to methylphenidate or its components, hyperthyroidism, motor tics, recent MI, severe agitation, severe hypertension, sucrase-isomaltase insufficiency, tension, thyrotoxicosis, Tourette's syndrome or family history of it, use of halogenated anesthetics, use within 14 days of an MAO inhibitor

Interaction

DRUGS

anticholinergics: Possibly increased anticholinergic effects of both drugs
anticonvulsants, oral anticoagulants, phenylbutazone, tricyclic antidepressants: Inhibited metabolism and increased blood levels of these drugs
dopamine agonists and antagonists: Possibly altered effectiveness of these drugs
diuretics, antihypertensives: Decreased therapeutic effects of these drugs
halogenated anesthetics: Possibly sudden decrease in blood pressure during surgery
MAO inhibitors: Possibly increased adverse effects of methylphenidate, possibly severe hypertension

ACTIVITIES

alcohol use: Possibly increased CNS effects; with long-acting forms, possible increased adverse effects

FOODS

caffeine: Increased methylphenidate effects

Adverse Reactions

CNS: Agitation, aggressiveness, anxiety, confusion, depression, dizziness, dyskinesia, emotional lability, fever, hallucinations, headache, hyperactivity, insomnia, irritability, ischemic neurologic defects (reversible), mania, migraine, motor tics, nervousness,

obsessive-compulsive disorder, paresthesia, psychosis, sedation, seizures, stroke, suicidal ideation, transient mood depression, tension, tremor, Tourette's syndrome, vertigo
CV: Angina, arrhythmias, bradycardia, cardiac arrest, chest pain, extrasystoles, hypertension, hypotension, MI, palpitations, peripheral vasculopathy including Raynaud's phenomenon, sudden death, tachycardia
EENT: Accommodation abnormality, blurred vision, diplopia, dry mouth or throat, mydriasis, pharyngitis, rhinitis, sinusitis, vision changes
ENDO: Dysmenorrhea, growth suppression in children with long-term use
GI: Abdominal pain, anorexia, constipation, diarrhea, dyspepsia, hepatotoxicity, nausea, vomiting
GU: Decreased libido, priapism
HEME: Anemia, decreased platelet count, leukopenia, pancytopenia, thrombocytopenia, thrombocytopenic purpura
MS: Arthralgia, myalgia, muscle tightness or twitching
RESP: Increased cough, upper respiratory tract infection
SKIN: Allergic contact dermatitis, alopecia, application-site reactions (transdermal patch), diaphoresis, erythema multiforme, exfoliative dermatitis, pruritus, rash, urticaria
Other: Anaphylaxis, angioedema, physical and psychological dependence, weight loss

Nursing Considerations

WARNING Be aware that methylphenidate may induce CNS stimulation and psychosis and may worsen behavior disturbances and thought disorders in patients who already have psychosis. Use drug cautiously in patients with psychosis.

• Keep in mind that, when signs and symptoms of ADHD occur with acute stress reactions or with preexisting structural cardiac abnormalities or other serious heart problems, methylphenidate usually isn't indicated because of possible worsened reaction or sudden death.

• Reconstitute oral suspension form by first tapping bottle until powder flows freely. Remove bottle cap and add specified amount of water to the drug bottle (53 ml of water to 300-mg drug bottle, 105 ml of water to 600-mg drug bottle, 131 ml of water to 750-mg drug bottle, or 158 ml of water to

900-mg drug bottle). Insert bottle adapter into neck of bottle and replace cap. Shake vigorously using a back and forth motion for at least 10 seconds. Know that reconstituted oral suspension is stable up to 4 months.
- Monitor children and adolescents for first-time psychotic or manic symptoms. If present, notify prescriber and expect drug to be discontinued.

WARNING Know that the E.R. tablet form (Concerta) shouldn't be given to patients with esophageal motility disorders; drug may cause GI obstruction because tablet doesn't change shape in GI tract.
- Monitor blood pressure and pulse rate to detect hypertension and excessive stimulation. Notify prescriber if present. For patient with hypertension, expect to increase antihypertensive dosage or add another antihypertensive to regimen.

WARNING Watch for signs of physical or psychological dependence. Methylphenidate's abuse potential is similar to that of amphetamines; use cautiously in patients with a history of drug abuse.
- Stopping drug abruptly after long-term use may unmask dysphoria, paranoia, severe depression, or suicidal thoughts.
- Monitor growth in children. Report failure to grow or gain weight, and expect to stop drug.
- Watch closely (especially children, adolescents, and young adults), for suicidal tendencies, particularly when therapy starts and dosage changes, because depression may worsen temporarily during these times, possibly leading to suicidal ideation.
- Monitor transdermal patch application site for erythema. If more intense reactions occur with erythema, such as local edema or papule or vesicle formation that doesn't improve within 48 hours after patch is removed from irritated site or that spreads beyond the patch site, further diagnostic testing is required to determine presence of allergic contact dermatitis.
- Patients with allergic contact dermatitis from transdermal patch may develop systemic allergy reaction if methylphenidate is taken by another route, such as by mouth. Monitor patient closely if route of administration changes, and report any evidence of flare-up of previous

dermatitis or positive patch-test sites, generalized skin eruptions in previously unaffected skin, headache, fever, malaise, arthralgia, diarrhea, or vomiting because drug may need to be discontinued.
- Observe patient for paradoxical aggravation of symptoms or other serious adverse reactions. If present, notify prescriber and expect dosage to be reduced or drug discontinued.
- Inspect patient's fingers and toes for signs of peripheral vasculopathy, such as digital ulceration and/or soft tissue breakdown. Although usually mild and intermittent, more severe manifestation may occur. Notify prescriber if present, and expect dose to be reduced or drug discontinued.

PATIENT TEACHING
- Emphasize need to take drug exactly as prescribed because misuse may cause serious adverse cardiovascular reactions, including sudden death.
- For transdermal form, teach patient to apply patch to a clean, dry location in his hip area 2 hours before effect is needed and to remove it 9 hours after application.
- Caution patient to avoid applying patch to skin that's oily, damaged, or irritated and to avoid the waistline, where clothing may dislodge the patch. Tell patient to rotate application sites between hips.
- Instruct patient to apply patch immediately after opening pouch and removing protective liner. Tell him to press patch firmly in place with palm of his hand for about 30 seconds. Reassure patient that exposing site to water shouldn't cause patch to fall off. If a patch does fall off, explain that a new patch may be applied but that the total exposure time for the day shouldn't exceed 9 hours.
- Urge patient not to chew or crush E.R. tablets.
- Tell patient to take tablets at least 6 hours before bedtime to avoid insomnia and to take E.R. once-daily tablets in the morning.
- Advise patient taking E.R. once-daily tablets (Concerta) that he may see intact tablet in stool. Explain that drug is slowly released from nonabsorbable tablet shell.
- Tell patient taking capsule form to swallow it whole or sprinkle contents onto a tablespoon of applesauce and take immediately, followed by a liquid such as water.

• Instruct patient taking E.R. oral suspension form to vigorously shake the bottle for at least 10 seconds before measuring dose to ensure that the proper dose is being taken. Also alert patient taking drug long term, that prescriber may take patient off of drug periodically to determine continued need.

• Direct patient to notify prescriber about excessive nervousness, fever, insomnia, palpitations, rash, or vomiting.

• Warn patient with seizure disorder that drug may cause seizures.

• Inform parents of children on long-term therapy that drug may delay growth.

• Warn male patients and parents of male children that painful or prolonged penile erections may occur while taking the drug, especially after a dosage increase or during period of drug withdrawal. In the event that this happens, immediate medical attention should be sought.

• Instruct patient or parents to monitor fingers and toes for ulceration and/or soft tissue breakdown. If noticed, prescriber should be called. Reassure patient that signs and symptoms generally improve after the dose is reduced or drug is discontinued.

• Urge family or caregiver to watch patient closely for suicidal tendencies, especially when therapy starts or dosage changes and particularly if patient is a child, teenager, or young adult.

methylprednisolone

Medrol, Meprolone

methylprednisolone acetate

depMedalone, Depoject, Depo-Medrol, Depopred, Depo-Predate, Methylcotolone

methylprednisolone sodium succinate

A-methaPred, Solu-Medrol

Class and Category

Chemical class: Synthetic glucocorticoid

Therapeutic class: Anti-inflammatory, immunosuppressant
Pregnancy category: C

Indications and Dosages

➤ *To treat ulcerative colitis*
I.V. INFUSION (METHYLPREDNISOLONE SODIUM SUCCINATE)
Adults. 40 to 120 mg 3 to 7 times/wk for 2 or more wk. Later doses given I.V. or I.M., based on patient's condition and response.
Children. 0.14 to 0.84 mg/kg daily in divided doses every 12 to 24 hr.
➤ *To treat a wide range of immune and inflammatory disorders, including allergic rhinitis, asthma, Crohn's disease, and systemic lupus erythematosus*
TABLETS (METHYLPREDNISOLONE)
Adults. 4 to 48 mg daily as a single dose or in divided doses.
Children. 0.42 to 1.67 mg/kg daily in divided doses three times daily or four times daily.
I.V. INFUSION, I.M. INJECTION (METHYLPREDNISOLONE SODIUM SUCCINATE)
Adults. *Initial:* 10 to 40 mg infused over several min. Later doses given I.V. or I.M., based on patient's condition and response.
Children. 0.14 to 0.84 mg/kg every 12 to 24 hr.
I.M. INJECTION (METHYLPREDNISOLONE ACETATE)
Adults. 40 to 120 mg daily to every 2 wk, according to clinical response.
Children. 0.14 to 0.84 mg/kg every 12 to 24 hr.
INTRA-ARTICULAR, INTRALESIONAL, OR SOFT-TISSUE INJECTION (METHYLPREDNISOLONE ACETATE)
Adults. 4 to 80 mg every 1 to 5 wk, according to clinical response.
➤ *To treat adrenal hyperplasia*
I.M. INJECTION (METHYLPREDNISOLONE ACETATE)
Adults. 40 mg every 2 wk.
Children. 0.14 to 0.84 mg/kg every 12 to 24 hr.
➤ *To treat acute exacerbations of multiple sclerosis*
TABLETS (METHYLPREDNISOLONE)
Adults. 160 mg daily for 7 days followed by 64 mg every other day for 1 mo.
I.V. OR I.M. INJECTION (METHYLPREDNISOLONE ACETATE, METHYLPREDNISOLONE SODIUM SUCCINATE)
Adults. 160 mg daily for 1 wk followed by 64 mg every other day for 1 mo.

➤ *To treat adrenocortical insufficiency*
TABLETS (METHYLPREDNISOLONE), I.M. INJECTION (METHYLPREDNISOLONE SODIUM SUCCINATE)
Children. 0.18 mg/kg daily in divided doses three times daily.
I.M. INJECTION (METHYLPREDNISOLONE ACETATE)
Children. 0.12 mg/kg every 3 days or 0.039 to 0.059 mg/kg daily.

Mechanism of Action

Binds to intracellular glucocorticoid receptors and suppresses inflammatory and immune responses by inhibiting accumulation of neutrophils and monocytes at inflammation sites, stabilizing lysosomal membranes, suppressing the antigen response of macrophages and helper T cells, and inhibiting the synthesis of inflammatory response mediators, such as cytokines, interleukins, and prostaglandins.

Route	Onset	Peak	Duration
P.O.	In 60 min	1–2 hr	1.25–1.5 days
I.V.	Rapid	30 min	Unknown
I.M.	6–48 hr	4–8 days	1–4 wk

Incompatibilities

Don't mix methylprednisolone with any drug without first consulting pharmacist. Don't dilute methylprednisolone acetate with any other drug.

Contraindications

Fungal infection, hypersensitivity to methylprednisolone or its components, idiopathic thrombocytopenic purpura (I.M.), intrathecal administration, premature infants (preparations containing benzyl alcohol)

Interaction
DRUGS
acetaminophen: Increased risk of hepatotoxicity
aminoglutethimide: Possibly loss of methylprednisolone-induced adrenal suppression
amphotericin B, carbonic anhydrase inhibitors: Possibly severe hypokalemia
anabolic steroids, androgens: Increased risk of edema and worsening of acne
anticholinergics: Possibly increased intraocular pressure

asparaginase: Increased risk of hyperglycemia and toxicity
aspirin, NSAIDs: Increased risk of adverse GI effects and bleeding
barbiturates, carbamazepine, phenytoin, rifampin: Decreased blood methylprednisolone level
cholestyramine: Possibly increased methylprednisolone clearance
cyclosporine: Increased risk of seizures
digoxin: Possibly hypokalemia-induced arrhythmias and digitalis toxicity
estrogens, oral contraceptives: Possibly increased therapeutic and toxic effects of methylprednisolone
insulin, oral antidiabetic drugs: Possibly increased blood glucose level
isoniazid: Possibly decreased therapeutic effects of isoniazid
ketoconazole, macrolide antibiotics such as erythromycin and troleandomycin: Decreased methylprednisolone clearance and increased risk of adverse effects
mexiletine: Possibly decreased blood mexiletine level
neuromuscular blockers: Possibly increased neuromuscular blockade, causing respiratory depression or apnea
oral anticoagulants, thrombolytics: Increased risk of GI ulceration and hemorrhage, possibly decreased therapeutic effects of these drugs
potassium supplements: Possibly decreased effects of these supplements
somatrem, somatropin: Possibly decreased therapeutic effects of these drugs
streptozocin: Increased risk of hyperglycemia
troleandomycin: Increased blood methylprednisolone level
vaccines: Decreased antibody response and increased risk of neurologic complications
ACTIVITIES
alcohol use: Increased risk of adverse GI effects and bleeding

Adverse Reactions

CNS: Ataxia, behavioral changes, depression, dizziness, euphoria, fatigue, headache, increased intracranial pressure with papilledema, insomnia, malaise, mood changes, neuropathy, paresthesia, restlessness, seizures, steroid psychosis, syncope, vertigo

CV: Arrhythmias (from hypokalemia), cardiac arrest, edema, fat embolism, heart failure, hypertension, hypertrophic cardiomyopathy (premature infants), hypotension, myocardial rupture following recent MI, tachycardia, thromboembolism, thrombophlebitis
EENT: Exophthalmos, glaucoma, increased intraocular pressure, nystagmus, posterior subcapsular cataracts
ENDO: Adrenal insufficiency, cushingoid symptoms (moon face, buffalo hump, central obesity, supraclavicular fat pad enlargement), diabetes mellitus, growth suppression in children, hyperglycemia, negative nitrogen balance from protein catabolism
GI: Abdominal distention, elevated liver enzymes, hepatomegaly, hiccups, increased appetite, melena, nausea, pancreatitis, peptic ulcer, ulcerative esophagitis, vomiting
GU: Amenorrhea, glycosuria, menstrual irregularities, perineal burning or tingling
HEME: Easy bruising, leukocytosis
MS: Arthralgia; aseptic necrosis of femoral and humeral heads; Charcot-like arthropathy; compression fractures; muscle atrophy, twitching, or weakness; myalgia; osteoporosis; spontaneous fractures; steroid myopathy; tendon rupture
RESP: Pulmonary edema
SKIN: Acne; allergic dermatitis; altered skin pigmentation; diaphoresis; dry, scaly skin; erythema; hirsutism; necrotizing vasculitis; petechiae; purpura; rash; scarring; sterile abscess; striae; subcutaneous fat atrophy; thin, fragile skin; urticaria
Other: Activation of latent infections, anaphylaxis, angioedema, exacerbation of systemic fungal infections, hypernatremia, hypocalcemia, hypokalemia, hypokalemic alkalosis, impaired wound healing, masking of signs of infection, metabolic alkalosis, suppressed skin test reaction, weight gain

Nursing Considerations

• Know that high doses of systemic corticosteroids, including methylprednisolone, should not be used for the treatment of traumatic brain injury because of increased risk of death or in patients with active ocular herpes simplex because of risk of corneal perforation. Preparations containing benzyl alcohol

should not be used to treat pediatric patients because of risk of "gasping syndrome."
• Administer methylprednisolone with extreme caution in patients with a recent myocardial infarction because corticosteroid use may increase risk of left ventricular free wall rupture.
• Use cautiously in patients with congestive heart failure or renal insufficiency because sodium retention and edema can occur in patients taking a corticosteroid. Also use cautiously in patients with peptic ulcer, diverticulitis, fresh intestinal anastomoses, or nonspecific ulcerative colitis; these conditions increase risk of perforation during corticosteroid therapy.
• Give methylprednisolone tablets with food to minimize indigestion and GI irritation. For once-daily dosing, give in the morning to coincide with normal cortisol secretion. Expect prescriber to add an antacid or H_2-receptor antagonist to regimen.
• Discard parenteral products that are discolored or contain particles. Discard any remaining Depo-Medrol suspension after prescribed dose is drawn from vial.
• Inject I.M. form deep into gluteal muscle. Avoid injecting into deltoid muscle because of risk of subcutaneous atrophy.
• Arrange for low-sodium diet with added potassium, as prescribed.
• Protect patient from falling, especially elderly patient at risk for fractures from osteoporosis.
• Closely monitor patient for signs of infection because drug may mask them or may worsen systemic fungal infections or active latent disease. Be aware that chickenpox and measles can become life-threatening in patients taking a corticosteroid.
• Assess for possible depression or psychotic episodes during therapy.
• Monitor blood glucose level; dosage of insulin or oral antidiabetic drug may need to be adjusted in diabetic patient.
WARNING To avoid possibly fatal acute adrenocortical insufficiency, expect to taper long-term therapy when discontinuing it, but expect dosage to be increased during times of stress.
• Be aware that changes in thyroid function, such as development of hypothyroidism or hyperthyroidism, may require dosage

adjustment in chronic therapy because metabolic clearance of methylprednisolone is affected by thyroid activity.
- Avoid skin testing during methylprednisolone therapy because drug may suppress reaction.

PATIENT TEACHING
- Caution patient not to stop taking methylprednisolone abruptly or to change dosage without consulting prescriber.
- Tell patient to take a missed dose as soon as he remembers unless it's nearly time for the next dose. Caution against double-dosing.
- Urge patient to notify prescriber immediately about dark or tarry stools; signs of impending adrenocortical insufficiency, such as anorexia, dizziness, fainting, fatigue, fever, joint pain, muscle weakness, or nausea; and sudden weight gain or swelling.
- Instruct patient not to obtain vaccinations unless approved by prescriber.
- Urge patient to take vitamin D, calcium supplements, or both if recommended by prescriber.
- Inform patient that insomnia and restlessness usually resolve after 1 to 3 weeks.
- Caution patient to avoid people with contagious diseases.
- Explain the need for regular exercise or physical therapy to maintain muscle mass.
- Advise patient to carry medical identification that documents his need for long-term corticosteroid therapy.

---

metoclopramide hydrochloride

Apo-Metoclop (CAN), Maxeran (CAN), Metoclopramide Intensol, Octamide, PMS-Metoclopramide (CAN), Reglan

Class and Category
Chemical class: Benzamide
Therapeutic class: Antiemetic, upper GI stimulant
Pregnancy category: B

Indications and Dosages
➤ *To treat diabetic gastroparesis*

ORAL SOLUTION, ORAL SOLUTION CONCENTRATE, TABLETS
Adults and adolescents. 10 mg 30 min before meals and at bedtime up to four times daily.
I.V. OR I.M. INJECTION
Adults and adolescents. 10 mg three times daily or four times daily for severe symptoms; dosage adjusted as needed.
➤ *To treat gastroesophageal reflux disease*
ORAL SOLUTION, ORAL SOLUTION CONCENTRATE, TABLETS
Adults and adolescents. 10 to 15 mg 30 min before meals and at bedtime.
➤ *To prevent chemotherapy-induced vomiting*
I.V. INFUSION
Adults and adolescents. 3 mg/kg before chemotherapy and then 0.5 mg/kg/hr for 8 hr.
I.V. INJECTION
Adults and adolescents. 1 to 2 mg/kg 30 min before chemotherapy and then repeated every 2 to 3 hr, as needed.
Children. 1 mg/kg as a single dose, repeated in 1 hr. *Maximum:* 2 mg/kg.
➤ *To prevent postoperative nausea and vomiting*
I.M. INJECTION
Adults and adolescents. 10 to 20 mg near end of procedure.
DOSAGE ADJUSTMENT Reduced by half if creatinine clearance is less than 40 ml/min/1.73 m^2.

Mechanism of Action
Antagonizes the inhibitory effect of dopamine on GI smooth muscle. This causes gastric contraction, which promotes gastric emptying and peristalsis, thus reducing gastroesophageal reflux. Metoclopramide also blocks dopaminergic receptors in the chemoreceptor trigger zone, preventing nausea and vomiting.

Route	Onset	Peak	Duration
P.O.	30–60 min	Unknown	1–2 hr
I.V.	1–3 min	Unknown	1–2 hr
I.M.	10–15 min	Unknown	1–2 hr

Incompatibilities
Don't administer metoclopramide through same I.V. line as calcium gluconate,

cephalothin sodium, chloramphenicol sodium, cisplatin, erythromycin lactobionate, furosemide, methotrexate, penicillin G potassium, or sodium bicarbonate.

Contraindications

Concurrent use of butyrophenones, phenothiazines, or other drugs that may cause extrapyramidal reactions; GI hemorrhage, mechanical obstruction, or perforation; hypersensitivity to metoclopramide or its components; pheochromocytoma; seizure disorders

Interaction

DRUGS

anticholinergics, opioid analgesics: Possibly decreased metoclopramide effects
apomorphine: Possibly decreased antiemetic effect of apomorphine, possibly increased CNS depression
bromocriptine, pergolide: Possibly decreased therapeutic effects of these drugs
cimetidine: Possibly decreased absorption and therapeutic effects of cimetidine
CNS depressants: Possibly increased CNS depression
cyclosporine: Increased cyclosporine level
digoxin: Decreased gastric digoxin absorption
levodopa: Possibly decreased levodopa effects
MAO inhibitors: Increased risk of severe hypertension if patient has essential hypertension
mexiletine: Possibly faster mexiletene absorption
succinylcholine: Possibly prolonged therapeutic action of succinylcholine

ACTIVITIES

alcohol use: Risk of excessive sedation

Adverse Reactions

CNS: Agitation, anxiety, depression, dizziness, drowsiness, extrapyramidal reactions (motor restlessness, parkinsonism, tardive dyskinesia), fatigue, headache, insomnia, irritability, lassitude, neuroleptic malignant syndrome, panic reaction, restlessness
CV: AV block, fluid retention, heart failure, hypertension, hypotension, supraventricular tachycardia
EENT: Dry mouth
ENDO: Galactorrhea, gynecomastia
GI: Constipation, diarrhea, nausea
GU: Menstrual irregularities

HEME: Agranulocytosis
SKIN: Rash
Other: Restless leg syndrome

Nursing Considerations

• Use metoclopramide cautiously in patients with hypertension because it may increase catecholamine levels.
WARNING Watch closely for tardive dyskinesia, especially in the elderly, women, and patients with diabetes, because this serious adverse effect is often irreversible even after therapy stops. Therapy lasting longer than 12 weeks isn't recommended because risk of tardive dyskinesia increases the longer the patient takes metoclopramide. Risk also has been linked to total cumulative dose so prescriber must take this into account when setting dosage. At first sign of involuntary movements of face, tongue, or limbs, notify prescriber and expect to discontinue drug.
• Monitor patient with NADH-cytochrome b5 reductase deficiency because metoclopramide increases risk of methemoglobinemia and sulfhemoglobinemia, and patient can't receive methylene blue.
• Assess patient for signs of intestinal obstruction, such as abnormal bowel sounds, diarrhea, nausea, and vomiting, before administering metoclopramide. Notify prescriber if you detect them.
• For I.V. use, you need not dilute doses of 10 mg or less. Give drug over 1 to 2 minutes. For doses larger than 10 mg, dilute in 50 ml normal saline solution, half-normal (0.45) saline solution, D_5W, or lactated Ringer's solution and infuse over at least 15 minutes.
• Avoid rapid I.V. delivery because it may cause anxiety, restlessness, and drowsiness.
WARNING Notify prescriber if patient shows signs of toxicity, such as disorientation, drowsiness, and extrapyramidal reactions.
• Monitor patient, especially one with heart failure or cirrhosis, for possible fluid retention or volume overload due to transient increase in plasma aldosterone level.
• Monitor patient closely for neuroleptic malignant syndrome, a rare but potentially fatal disorder characterized by

hyperthermia, muscle rigidity, altered level of consciousness, irregular pulse or blood pressure, tachycardia, diaphoresis, and arrhythmias.

• Store drug in a light-resistant container; discard if discolored or contains particulate.

PATIENT TEACHING

• Advise against activities that require alertness for about 2 hours after each dose.

• Urge patient to avoid alcohol and CNS depressants while taking metoclopramide. They may increase CNS depression.

• Tell patient to immediately report involuntary movements of face, eyes, tongue, or hands, including lip smacking, chewing, puckering of mouth, frowning, scowling, sticking out tongue, blinking, moving eyes, or shaking arms and legs.

• Explain that stopping metoclopramide may cause withdrawal symptoms that include dizziness, nervousness, and headache.

metolazone
Diulo, Mykrox, Zaroxolyn

Class and Category
Chemical class: Quinazoline derivative
Therapeutic class: Antihypertensive, diuretic
Pregnancy category: B

Indications and Dosages
➤ *To manage mild to moderate hypertension*
EXTENDED TABLETS
Adults. 2.5 to 5 mg daily.
PROMPT TABLETS (MYKROX)
Adults. 0.5 mg daily. *Maintenance:* 0.5 to 1 mg daily. *Maximum:* 1 mg daily.
➤ *To manage edema from heart failure or renal disease*
EXTENDED TABLETS
Adults. 5 to 20 mg daily.

Mechanism of Action
Promotes renal excretion of water and sodium by inhibiting their reabsorption in distal convoluted tubules. The resulting reduction in plasma and extracellular fluid volume reduces blood pressure. Metolazone also helps reduce blood pressure by decreasing peripheral vascular resistance.

Route	Onset	Peak	Duration
P.O.	1 hr	2 hr	12–24 hr

Contraindications
Anuria; hepatic coma; hypersensitivity to metolazone, other sulfonamide derivatives, quinethazones, thiazides, or their components; renal failure

Interaction
DRUGS
allopurinol: Increased risk of hypersensitivity to allopurinol
amiodarone: Increased risk of arrhythmias from hypokalemia
amphotericin B: Increased risk of electrolyte imbalances
anesthetics: Increased effects of anesthetics
antigout drugs: Increased blood uric acid level and risk of gout attack
antihypertensives: Increased hypotension
antineoplastics: Prolonged antineoplastic-induced leukopenia
calcium salts: Increased risk of hypercalcemia
cholestyramine, colestipol: Decreased metolazone absorption
diazoxide: Increased risk of hyperglycemia
digoxin: Increased risk of electrolyte imbalances and digoxin-induced arrhythmias
diuretics: Additive effects of both drugs, possibly leading to severe hypovolemia and electrolyte imbalances
dopamine: Increased diuretic effect
insulin, oral antidiabetic drugs: Decreased effectiveness of these drugs, increased risk of hyperglycemia
lithium: Increased risk of lithium toxicity
methenamine: Decreased metolazone effectiveness from urinary alkalinization
methyldopa: Possibly hemolytic anemia
neuromuscular blockers: Increased risk of hypokalemia and neuromuscular blockade, increased risk of respiratory depression
NSAIDs, sympathomimetics: Possibly decreased metolazone effectiveness
oral anticoagulants: Decreased anticoagulation
vitamin D: Increased vitamin D action, increased risk of hypercalcemia

Adverse Reactions
CNS: Anxiety, chills, depression, dizziness, drowsiness, headache, insomnia, neuropathy, paresthesia, restlessness, syncope, weakness

M

CV: Chest pain, cold extremities, orthostatic hypotension, palpitations, peripheral edema, vasculitis, venous thrombosis
EENT: Bitter taste, blurred vision, dry mouth, epistaxis, pharyngitis, sinus congestion, tinnitus
ENDO: Hyperglycemia
GI: Abdominal pain, anorexia, cholecystitis, constipation, diarrhea, hepatic dysfunction, hepatitis, indigestion, nausea, pancreatitis, vomiting
GU: Decreased libido, glycosuria, impotence
HEME: Agranulocytosis, aplastic anemia, leukopenia, thrombocytopenia
MS: Arthralgia, gout, myalgia
RESP: Cough
SKIN: Dry skin, necrosis, petechiae, photosensitivity, pruritus, rash, urticaria
Other: Hypochloremia, hypokalemia, hyponatremia, hypovolemia, metabolic alkalosis

Nursing Considerations

WARNING Be aware that Mykrox prompt tablets shouldn't be substituted for Diulo or Zaroxolyn extended tablets because they aren't equivalent.
• Anticipate giving metolazone with a loop diuretic if patient responds poorly to loop diuretic alone.
• To monitor drug's diuretic effect, measure fluid intake and output and daily weight.
• If response to 1 mg of Mykrox is inadequate, expect to add another drug rather than increase dosage.
• Monitor blood chemistry test results and assess for evidence of hypochloremia, hypokalemia, and, possibly, mild metabolic alkalosis.
• Monitor serum calcium and uric acid levels, especially if patient has a history of gout or renal calculi. Metolazone may slightly increase calcium reabsorption and decrease uric acid excretion.

PATIENT TEACHING
• Inform patient that metolazone controls but doesn't cure hypertension. Discuss possible need for lifelong therapy and consequences of uncontrolled hypertension.
• Instruct patient to take drug at the same time each day.
• Direct patient to take drug with food or milk to minimize adverse GI reactions.

• Advise patient to change position slowly to minimize orthostatic hypotension.
• Urge patient to notify prescriber about persistent, severe diarrhea, nausea, or vomiting, which can cause dehydration and orthostatic hypotension.
• Emphasize the importance of weight and diet control, especially limiting sodium intake.
• Inform diabetic patient that metolazone may increase blood glucose level and that he should check his level often.

metoprolol succinate
Toprol-XL

metoprolol tartrate
Apo-Metoprolol (CAN), Betaloc (CAN), Betaloc Durules (CAN), Lopresor (CAN), Lopresor SR (CAN), Lopressor, Novometoprol (CAN)

Class and Category
Chemical class: Beta$_1$-adrenergic antagonist
Therapeutic class: Antianginal, antihypertensive, MI prophylaxis and treatment
Pregnancy category: C

Indications and Dosages
➤ *To manage hypertension, alone or with other antihypertensives*
E.R. TABLETS (METOPROLOL SUCCINATE)
Adults. *Initial:* 25 to 100 mg daily, adjusted weekly as prescribed. *Maximum:* 400 mg daily.
E.R. TABLETS (METOPROLOL TARTRATE)
Adults. *Maintenance:* 100 to 400 mg daily to maintain blood pressure control after therapeutic level has been achieved with immediate-release tablets.
TABLETS (METOPROLOL TARTRATE)
Adults. *Initial:* 100 mg daily, adjusted weekly as prescribed. *Maximum:* 450 mg daily as a single dose or in divided doses.
➤ *To treat acute MI or evolving acute MI*
TABLETS (METOPROLOL TARTRATE), I.V. INJECTION (METOPROLOL TARTRATE)
Adults. *Initial:* 5 mg by I.V. bolus every 2 minfor 3 doses followed by 50 mg P.O. for patients who tolerate total I.V. dose (25 to

50 mg P.O. for patients who can't tolerate total I.V. dose) every 6 hr for 48 hr, starting 15 min after final I.V. dose; after 48 hr, 100 mg twice daily followed by maintenance dosage. *Maintenance:* 100 mg P.O. twice daily for at least 3 mo.
➤ *To treat angina pectoris and chronic stable angina*
E.R. TABLETS (METOPROLOL SUCCINATE)
Adults. 100 mg daily, increased weekly as prescribed. *Maximum:* 400 mg daily as a single dose or in divided doses.
E.R. TABLETS (METOPROLOL TARTRATE)
Adults. *Initial:* 100 mg daily, adjusted weekly as prescribed. *Maximum:* 450 mg daily.
TABLETS (METOPROLOL TARTRATE)
Adults. *Initial:* 50 mg twice daily, adjusted weekly as prescribed. *Maximum:* 450 mg daily.
➤ *To treat stable, symptomatic (New York Heart Association [NYHA] class II or III), ischemic, hypertensive, or cardiomyopathic heart failure*
E.R. TABLETS (METOPROLOL SUCCINATE)
Adults. *Initial:* 25 mg daily (NYHA Class II) or 12.5 mg daily (NYHA Class III or more severe heart failure) for 2 wk. Then dosage doubled every 2 wk as tolerated. *Maximum:* 200 mg daily.
DOSAGE ADJUSTMENT For patients with hepatic impairment or the elderly, initial dosage reduced with gradual dose titration.

Route	Onset	Peak	Duration
P.O.	60 min	1–2 hr	Unknown
P.O. (E.R.)	Unknown	6–12 hr	Unknown
I.V.	Unknown	20 min	Unknown

Mechanism of Action
Inhibits stimulation of beta$_1$-receptor sites, located mainly in the heart, resulting in decreased cardiac excitability, cardiac output, and myocardial oxygen demand. These effects help relieve angina. Metoprolol also helps reduce blood pressure by decreasing renal release of renin.

Contraindications
Acute heart failure; pulse less than 45 beats/ minute; cardiogenic shock; hypersensitivity to metoprolol, its components, or other beta blockers; pheochromocytoma; second- or third-degree AV block; severe peripheral arterial disorders; sick sinus syndrome

Interaction
DRUGS
alpha-adrenergic agents such as alpha-methyldopa, betanidine, guanethidine: Possibly increased antihypertensive effects
aluminum salts, barbiturates, calcium salts, cholestyramine, colestipol, NSAIDs, rifampin, salicylates, sulfinpyrazone: Decreased therapeutic effects of metoprolol
amiodarone, digoxin, diltiazem, verapamil: Increased risk of complete AV block
calcium channel blockers: Increased risk of heart failure and increased effects of both drugs
catecholamine-depleting drugs such reserpine, monoamine oxidase (MAO) inhibitors: Possibly additive effect resulting in hypotension or marked bradycardia
cimetidine; CYP2D6 inhibitors such as antiarrhythmics, antidepressants, anti-fungals, antihistamines, antimalarials, antipsychotics, antiretrovirals; hydralazine: Increased plasma metoprolol level causing decrease in the cardioselectivity of metoprolol
clonidine: Increased risk of bradycardia and hypotension; increased risk of rebound hypertension when clonidine is discontinued
digoxin, diltiazem, other beta-blockers, verapamil: Decreased heart rate and slowed atrioventricular conduction
dipyridamole: Possibly altered heart rate
estrogens: Possibly decreased anti-hypertensive effect of metoprolol
ergot alkaloids: Possibly enhanced vasoconstrictive action of ergot alkaolids
general anesthetics: Increased risk of hypotension and heart failure
insulin, oral antidiabetic drugs: Decreased blood glucose control, possibly masking of signs and symptoms of hypoglycemia (by metoprolol)
lidocaine: Increased risk of lidocaine toxicity
neuromuscular blockers: Possibly enhanced and prolonged neuromuscular blockade
other antihypertensives: Additive hypo-tensive effect
phenothiazines: Possibly increased blood levels of both drugs
prazosin: Possibly increased postural hypotensive effect of first dose of prazosin
propafenone: Increased blood level and half-life of metoprolol

M

sympathomimetics, xanthines: Possibly decreased therapeutic effects of both drugs

FOODS

all foods: Increased bioavailability of metoprolol

Adverse Reactions

CNS: Anxiety, confusion, CVA, depression, dizziness, drowsiness, fatigue, hallucinations, headache, insomnia, nightmares, paresthesia, short-term memory loss, somnolence, syncope, tiredness, vertigo, weakness

CV: Angina, arrhythmias (including AV block and bradycardia), arterial insufficiency, cardiac arrest, cardiogenic shock, chest pain, decreased HDL level, increased triglyceride levels, gangrene of extremity, heart failure, hypertension, orthostatic hypotension, palpitations, peripheral edema

EENT: Blurred vision, dry eyes or mouth, nasal congestion, rhinitis, taste disturbance, tinnitus

GI: Constipation, diarrhea, flatulence, heartburn, hepatitis, nausea, vomiting

GU: Decreased libido, impotence

HEME: Agranulocytosis, leukopenia, thrombocytopenia

MS: Arthralgia, back pain, myalgia

RESP: Bronchospasm, dyspnea, shortness of breath

SKIN: Alopecia, diaphoresis, photosensitivity, pruritus, rash, urticaria, worsening of psoriasis

Nursing Considerations

• Know that patients undergoing noncardiac major surgery should not begin a high-dose regimen using extended-release metoprolol because such use in patients with cardiovascular risk factors has been associated with bradycardia, hypotension, stroke, and death. However, also be aware that beta-blocker therapy such as metoprolol that is already in place should not be routinely discontinued prior to major surgery.

• Use metoprolol with extreme caution in patients with bronchospastic disease who don't respond to or can't tolerate other antihypertensives. Expect to give smaller doses more often to avoid the higher plasma levels in longer dosage intervals.

• Use cautiously in patients with hypertension or angina who have congestive

heart failure because beta blockers such as metoprolol can further depress myocardial contractility, worsening heart failure.

• For patient with acute MI who can't tolerate initial dosage or who delays treatment, start with maintenance dosage, as prescribed and tolerated.

• Before starting therapy for heart failure, expect to give a diuretic, an ACE inhibitor, and digoxin to stabilize patient.

• If patient has pheochromocytoma, alpha blocker therapy should start first, followed by metoprolol to prevent paradoxical increase in blood pressure from attenuation of beta-mediated vasodilation in skeletal muscle.

• Be aware that metoprolol dosage for heart failure is highly individualized. Monitor patient for evidence of worsening heart failure during dosage increases. If heart failure worsens, expect to increase diuretic dosage and possibly decrease metoprolol dosage or temporarily discontinue drug, as prescribed. Metoprolol dosage shouldn't be increased until worsening heart failure has been stabilized.

• If patient with heart failure develops symptomatic bradycardia, expect to decrease the metoprolol dosage.

WARNING If dosage exceeds 400 mg daily, monitor patient for bronchospasm and dyspnea because metoprolol competitively blocks $beta_2$-adrenergic receptors in bronchial and vascular smooth muscles.

WARNING When substituting metoprolol for clonidine, expect to gradually reduce clonidine and increase metoprolol dosage over several days. Given together, these drugs have additive hypotensive effects.

• Patients who take metoprolol may be at risk for AV block. If AV block results from depressed AV node conduction, prepare to give appropriate drug, as ordered, or assist with insertion of temporary pacemaker.

• Check for signs of poor glucose control in patient with diabetes mellitus. Metoprolol may interfere with therapeutic effects of insulin and oral antidiabetic drugs. It also may mask evidence of hypoglycemia, such as palpitations, tachycardia, and tremor.

• Monitor patient with hyperthyroidism closely because beta-adrenergic blockers such as metoprolol may mask signs of hyperthyroidism, such as tachycardia. Also know that abrupt discontinuation of metoprolol should be avoided because thyroid storm could be precipitated.

• Monitor patient with peripheral vascular disease for evidence of arterial insufficiency (pain, pallor, and coldness in affected extremity). Metoprolol can precipitate or aggravate peripheral vascular disease.

• Be aware that patients with a history of severe anaphylactic reactions may be more reactive to repeated challenges of the allergen while taking beta-blocker therapy, such as metoprolol, and may be unresponsive to the usual doses of epinephrine used to treat an allergic reaction.

WARNING Expect to taper dosage over 1 to 2 weeks when drug is discontinued; stopping abruptly can cause myocardial ischemia, MI, ventricular arrhythmias, or severe hypertension, especially in patients with cardiac disease. Abrupt withdrawal may also cause thyroid storm in a patient with hyperthyroidism or thyrotoxicosis.

PATIENT TEACHING

• Instruct patient to take metoprolol with food at the same time each day—once daily for E.R. tablets. Explain that he may halve tablets but not chew or crush them.

• Advise patient to notify prescriber if pulse rate falls below 60 beats/minute or is significantly lower than usual.

• Urge diabetic patient to check blood glucose level often during therapy.

• Caution patient not to stop drug abruptly.

---

metronidazole

Apo-Metronidazole (CAN), Flagyl, Flagyl I.V. RTU, Metric 21, MetroGel, MetroGel-Vaginal, Metronidazole 1.3%, Nidagel (CAN), Novonidazol (CAN), Protostat, Trikacide (CAN)

metronidazole hydrochloride

Flagyl I.V.

Class and Category

Chemical class: Nitroimidazole derivative

Therapeutic class: Antibiotic, antiprotozoal
Pregnancy category: B

Indications and Dosages

➤ *To treat systemic anaerobic infections caused by* Bacteroides fragilis, Clostridium difficile, Clostridium perfringens, Eubacterium, Fusobacterium, Peptococcus, Peptostreptococcus,*and* Veillonella *species*

CAPSULES, TABLETS

Adults and adolescents. 7.5 mg/kg up to 1,000 mg every 6 hr for 7 days or longer. *Maximum:* 4,000 mg daily.

Children. 7.5 mg/kg every 6 hr or 10 mg/kg every 8 hr.

I.V. INFUSION

Adults and adolescents. *Initial:* 15 mg/kg and then 7.5 mg/kg up to 1,000 mg every 6 hr for 7 days or longer. *Maximum:* 4,000 mg daily.

Children. 7.5 mg/kg every 6 hr or 10 mg/kg every 8 hr.

➤ *To treat amebiasis (*Entamoeba histolytica*)*

CAPSULES, TABLETS

Adults. 500 to 750 mg three times daily for 5 to 10 days.

Children. 11.6 to 16.7 mg/kg three times daily for 10 days.

➤ *To treat trichomoniasis (*Trichomonas vaginalis*)*

CAPSULES, TABLETS

Adults. 2,000 mg as a single dose, 1,000 mg twice daily for 24 hr, or 250 mg three times daily for 7 days.

Children. 5 mg/kg three times daily for 7 days.

➤ *To prevent perioperative bowel infection*

I.V. INFUSION

Adults and adolescents. 15 mg/kg 1 hr before surgery and then 7.5 mg/kg 6 and 12 hr after initial dose.

➤ *To treat acne in patients with rosacea*

TOPICAL GEL

Adults. Thin film applied to affected area twice daily for 9 wk.

➤ *To treat bacterial vaginosis*

VAGINAL CREAM

Adults. 500 mg (1 applicatorful) once or twice daily for 10 to 20 days.

VAGINAL GEL

Adults. 37.5 mg (1 applicatorful) once or twice daily for 5 days.

M

➤ *To treat bacterial vaginosis in nonpregnant women*
VAGINAL GEL (METRONIDAZOLE 1.3%)
Adults. 65 mg (1 applicatorful) once daily at bedtime.
VAGINAL TABLETS
Adults. 500 mg at bedtime for 10 to 20 days.

Mechanism of Action

Undergoes intracellular chemical reduction during anaerobic metabolism. After metronidazole is reduced, it damages DNA's helical structure and breaks its strands, which inhibits bacterial nucleic acid synthesis and causes cell death.

Incompatibilities

Don't administer I.V. metronidazole with aluminum needles or hubs or through same I.V. line as other drugs.

Contraindications

Breastfeeding, hypersensitivity to metronidazole or its components, trichomoniasis during first trimester of pregnancy

Interaction

DRUGS
cimetidine: Possibly delayed elimination and increased blood level of metronidazole
disulfiram: Possibly combined toxicity, with confusion and psychotic reactions
neurotoxic drugs: Increased risk of neurotoxicity
oral anticoagulants: Possibly increased anticoagulant effect
phenobarbital: Increased metabolism and decreased blood level and half-life of metronidazole
phenytoin: Decreased phenytoin clearance
ACTIVITIES
alcohol use: Possibly disulfiram-like effects

Adverse Reactions

CNS: Aseptic meningitis (parenteral form), ataxia, confusion, depression, dizziness, encephalopathy, fever, headache, incoordination, insomnia, irritability, light-headedness, peripheral neuropathy, seizures (high doses), syncope, weakness, vertigo
EENT: Dry mouth, lacrimation (topical form), metallic taste, nasal congestion, optic neuropathy, pharyngitis

GI: Abdominal cramps or pain, anorexia, diarrhea, nausea, pancreatitis, vomiting
GU: Dark urine, vaginal candidiasis (oral, parenteral, and topical forms); burning or irritation of sexual partner's penis, candidal cervicitis or vaginitis, dysuria, dryness of vagina or vulva, urinary frequency, vulvitis (vaginal form)
HEME: Leukopenia
MS: Back pain, dysarthria
SKIN: Burning or stinging sensation, dry skin (topical form); erythema, flushing, pruritus, rash, Stevens-Johnson syndrome, toxic epidermal necrolysis, urticaria (oral and parenteral forms)
Other: Injection-site edema, pain, or tenderness

Nursing Considerations

• Use cautiously in patients with central nervous system diseases.
• Give I.V. drug by slow infusion over 1 hour; don't give by direct I.V. injection.
• Discontinue primary I.V. infusion during metronidazole infusion.
WARNING If patient has adverse CNS reactions, such as seizures or peripheral neuropathy, tell prescriber and stop drug immediately.
• Monitor patient with severe liver disease because slowed metronidazole metabolism may cause drug to accumulate in body and increase the risk of adverse effects.
• If skin irritation occurs, apply topical metronidazole gel less frequently or discontinue it, as ordered.
• Monitor CBC and culture and sensitivity tests if therapy lasts longer than 10 days or if second course of treatment is needed.
• Monitor patient's neurologic status throughout metronidazole therapy. If abnormal neurologic signs and symptoms occur, notify prescriber and expect to discontinue drug.
PATIENT TEACHING
• Instruct female patient to notify prescriber if she is pregnant, intends to get pregnant, or is breastfeeding.
• Urge patient to take metronidazole at evenly spaced intervals during the day and with food to minimize adverse GI reactions.
• Urge patient to complete the entire course of therapy.

• Caution patient to avoid alcohol during therapy and for at least 3 days afterward.
• Advise patient to avoid hazardous activities until drug's CNS effects are known and to report any abnormal neurologic signs or symptoms, such as weakness, numbness, seizures, or vision changes.
• If patient reports dry mouth, suggest ice chips or sugarless hard candy or gum; suggest a dental visit if dryness lasts longer than 2 weeks.
• Instruct patient to notify prescriber if no improvement occurs within a few days of taking tablets or capsules.
• Direct patient using topical gel to wash hands and affected area with a mild, nonirritating cleaner; to rinse well and pat dry; and then to apply a thin film of drug and wash hands again.
• Advise patient with rosacea to keep topical gel away from his eyes. If drug gets into his eyes, urge him to wash them immediately with large amounts of cool tap water and to call prescriber if eyes continue to hurt or burn.
• Instruct patient with rosacea to notify prescriber if no improvement occurs after 3 weeks of topical use; full therapeutic effect may take 9 weeks.
• Teach patient how to fill, insert, and clean vaginal cream or gel applicator after use. Instruct her to wash her hands before and after administration.
• To help vaginal tablets dissolve, instruct patient to run tap water over unwrapped tablet for a few seconds before insertion.
• Inform patient with trichomoniasis that her male sexual partners should wear condoms during her treatment and that they may need treatment themselves to prevent reinfection.
• Caution patient that vaginal cream and tablets (not gel) may contain oils that damage latex condoms.
• Urge patient to follow up with prescriber to make sure infection is gone.

metyrosine

Demser

Class and Category
Chemical class: Alpha-methyl tyrosine

Therapeutic class: Antipheochromocytoma agent
Pregnancy category: C

Indications and Dosages
➤ *To control hypertension and related symptoms until pheochromocytomectomy is performed, to treat chronic malignant pheochromocytoma*
CAPSULES
Adults and adolescents. *Initial:* 250 mg four times daily, increased as ordered by 250 to 500 mg daily. *Maintenance:* 2,000 to 3,000 mg daily in divided doses four times daily. Preoperative dosage given for at least 7 days. *Maximum:* 4,000 mg daily in divided doses.

Mechanism of Action
Blocks activity of tyrosine hydroxylase, the enzyme that controls rate of catecholamine synthesis. This action decreases production of the catecholamines epinephrine and norepinephrine, which, in patients with pheochromocytoma, are produced in excessive amounts.

Contraindications
Hypersensitivity to metyrosine or its components

Interaction
DRUGS
CNS depressants: Increased sedation
haloperidol, phenothiazines: Increased extrapyramidal effects
ACTIVITIES
alcohol use: Increased sedation

Adverse Reactions
CNS: Anxiety, confusion, depression, disorientation, extrapyramidal reactions (difficulty speaking, drooling, parkinsonism, tremor, trismus), hallucinations, headache, sedation
CV: Peripheral edema
EENT: Dry mouth, nasal congestion, pharyngeal edema
ENDO: Galactorrhea, gynecomastia
GI: Abdominal pain, diarrhea, elevated serum AST level, nausea, vomiting
GU: Crystalluria, dysuria (transient), ejaculation failure, hematuria, impotence, urolithiasis

HEME: Anemia, eosinophilia, thrombocytopenia, thrombocytosis
SKIN: Urticaria

Nursing Considerations

• Expect patient taking metyrosine to experience moderate to severe sedation at low and high dosages. Sedation begins during first 24 hours, peaks after 2 to 3 days, and tends to wane during next few days. It usually subsides after 1 week unless dosage is increased or exceeds 2 g daily.
• Obtain urine specimens as ordered to check for crystalluria and urolithiasis. If crystalluria develops, increase fluid intake to achieve daily urine output of 2,000 ml or more with doses above 2 g daily. If crystalluria persists, reduce dosage or stop drug, as ordered.
• Expect to adjust dosage, as prescribed, based on clinical response and urine catecholamine level.
• If signs and symptoms aren't adequately controlled by metyrosine, expect to add an alpha-adrenergic blocker, such as phenoxybenzamine, as prescribed.

PATIENT TEACHING

• Inform patient about metyrosine's sedative effects. Advise him to avoid alcohol and CNS depressants, which may increase sedation.
• Instruct patient to increase fluid intake, as appropriate.
• Urge patient to report drooling, severe diarrhea, trembling and shaking of hands and fingers, or trouble speaking.
• Inform patient that he may experience changes in sleep pattern for 2 to 3 days after stopping drug.
• Advise patient to keep regular visits with prescriber to monitor progress.

mexiletine hydrochloride

Mexitil

Class and Category

Chemical class: Lidocaine analogue
Therapeutic class: Class IB antiarrhythmic
Pregnancy category: C

Indications and Dosages

➤ *To treat life-threatening ventricular arrhythmias*

CAPSULES

Adults. *Initial:* 200 mg every 8 hr, adjusted, as ordered, by 50 to 100 mg/dose every 2 to 3 days, as tolerated. If patient tolerates 300 mg or less every 8 hr, total dosage may be divided and given every 12 hr. If patient continues to experience arrhythmias, dosage frequency may be changed to four times daily. *Maximum:* 1,200 mg daily when given every 8 hr (400 mg/dose); 900 mg daily when given every 12 hr (450 mg/dose).

➤ *To rapidly control life-threatening ventricular arrhythmias*

CAPSULES

Adults. *Initial:* 400 mg followed by 200 mg after 8 hr. *Maintenance:* 200 mg every 8 hr, adjusted, as ordered, by 50 to 100 mg/dose every 2 to 3 days, as tolerated. If patient tolerates 300 mg or less every 8 hr, total dosage may be divided and given every 12 hr. If patient continues to experience arrhythmias, dosage frequency may be changed to four times daily.

DOSAGE ADJUSTMENT For patients with severe hepatic disease or heart failure, dosage reduced and adjusted every 2 or 3 days.

Route	Onset	Peak	Duration
P.O.	0.5–2 hr	2–3 hr	8–12 hr

Mechanism of Action

Produces antiarrhythmic effect by inhibiting fast sodium channels in myocardial cell membranes, especially in the His-Purkinje system. This action decreases duration of action potential and effective refractory period of His-Purkinje system. The myocardium, which becomes refractory again after resting membrane potential is restored, is less likely to generate and respond to ectopic ventricular impulses.

Contraindications

Cardiogenic shock, second- or third-degree AV block without a pacemaker

Interaction

DRUGS

aluminum- or magnesium-containing antacids: Delayed mexiletine absorption
antiarrhythmics: Increased cardiac effects
cimetidine: Possibly increased or decreased blood mexiletine level

hepatic enzyme inducers: Accelerated metabolism and decreased level of mexiletine
metoclopramide: Accelerated mexiletine absorption
rifampin: Decreased blood mexiletine level
theophylline: Increased theophylline level
urine acidifiers: Accelerated renal excretion of mexiletine
urine alkalinizers: Delayed mexiletine excretion

FOODS
caffeine: Possibly decreased clearance and increased effects of caffeine
foods that may acidify urine (such as cheese, cranberries, eggs, fish, grains, meats, plums, poultry, and prunes): Accelerated renal excretion of mexiletine
foods that may alkalinize urine (such as milk and all vegetables and fruits except cranberries, plums, and prunes): Delayed renal excretion of mexiletine

ACTIVITIES
smoking: Reduced mexiletine half-life

Adverse Reactions

CNS: Confusion, dizziness, fatigue, headache, lack of coordination, light-headedness, nervousness, paresthesia, seizures, sleep disturbance, syncope, tremor, weakness
CV: Atrial arrhythmias, AV conduction disorders, bradycardia, cardiogenic shock, chest pain, heart failure, hypotension, palpitations, PVCs, ventricular arrhythmias (increased)
EENT: Blurred vision, dry mouth, tinnitus
GI: Constipation, diarrhea, heartburn, nausea, vomiting
HEME: Agranulocytosis, leukopenia, thrombocytopenia
RESP: Dyspnea
SKIN: Rash

Nursing Considerations

• If mexiletine is replacing another antiarrhythmic, expect to give first dose 6 to 12 hours after last dose of quinidine sulfate or disopyramide, 3 to 6 hours after last dose of procainamide, or 8 to 12 hours after last dose of tocainide, as prescribed.
• If mexiletine is replacing parenteral lidocaine, expect to reduce or withdraw lidocaine 1 to 2 hours after starting mexiletine, as prescribed.

• Monitor continuous ECG and serum mexiletine level.
• Assess patient for thrombocytopenia, which may occur within a few days after mexiletine therapy starts. Expect platelet count to return to normal within 1 month after mexiletine therapy stops.

PATIENT TEACHING
• Instruct patient to take mexiletine at evenly spaced intervals, to avoid missing doses, and to take drug as prescribed, even if he's feeling well.
• Advise patient to take drug with food to reduce adverse GI reactions.
• Inform patient that nausea and vomiting may occur within 2 hours after dose but tend to lessen as treatment continues.
• Advise patient to avoid hazardous activities until drug's CNS effects are known.
• Teach patient to take his pulse, and advise him to contact prescriber if rate is below 50 beats/minute or rhythm is irregular.
• Urge patient to notify prescriber immediately about chest pain, chills, fast or irregular heartbeat, fever, shortness of breath, and unusual bleeding or bruising.
• Advise patient to avoid greatly increasing intake of foods that may acidify urine (cheese, cranberries, eggs, fish, grains, meats, plums, poultry, prunes) or alkalinize urine (milk, all vegetables, all fruits except cranberries, plums, and prunes).
• Encourage patient to keep regular visits with prescriber to monitor progress.

mezlocillin sodium

Mezlin

Class and Category

Chemical class: Acyclaminopenicillin
Therapeutic class: Antibiotic
Pregnancy category: B

Indications and Dosages

➤ *To treat moderate to severe infections, including bacteremia, bone and joint infections, gynecologic infections (such as endometritis, pelvic cellulitis, and pelvic inflammatory disease), intra-abdominal infections (such as cholangitis, cholecystitis, hepatic abscess, intra-abdominal abscess, and peritonitis), lower respiratory tract infections (such as pneumonia and lung abscess), meningitis, septicemia caused by susceptible bacteria, or skin and soft-tissue infections (such as cellulitis and diabetic foot ulcer); to manage febrile neutropenia*

I.V. INFUSION, I.M. INJECTION
Adults and adolescents. 3 g every 4 hr or 4 g every 6 hr.

➤ *To treat life-threatening infections of the types listed above*

I.V. INFUSION, I.M. INJECTION
Adults and adolescents. Up to 350 mg/kg daily. *Maximum:* 24,000 mg daily.
Children and infants. 50 mg/kg every 4 hr (or infused over 30 min every 4 hr).
Neonates over age 7 days weighing 2,000 g (4.4 lb) or less. 75 mg/kg I.V. every 8 hr.
Neonates age 7 days or less weighing 2,000 g or less. 75 mg/kg I.V. every 12 hr.
Neonates age 7 days or less weighing more than 2,000 g. 75 mg/kg I.V. every 6 hr.

➤ *To treat uncomplicated UTI*

I.V. INFUSION, I.M. INJECTION
Adults. 1.5 to 2 g every 6 hr.

➤ *To treat complicated UTI*

I.V. INFUSION
Adults. 3 g every 6 hr.
DOSAGE ADJUSTMENT Dosing interval extended to 6 to 8 hr if needed for patients with creatinine clearance of 10 to 30 ml/min/1.73 m². Dosing interval extended and dosage reduced to 1.5 to 2 g for patients with creatinine clearance below 10 ml/min/1.73 m².

➤ *To treat uncomplicated gonorrhea caused by susceptible strains of* Neisseria gonorrhoeae

I.V. INFUSION, I.M. INJECTION
Adults. 1 to 2 g as a single dose given with 1 g of probenecid P.O. (or probenecid given up to 30 min before mezlocillin).

➤ *To prevent infection from potentially contaminated surgical procedures*

I.V. INFUSION
Adults. 4 g 30 min before surgery and then 4 g every 6 hr for 2 more doses.

➤ *To prevent infection in cesarean section*

I.V. INFUSION
Adults. 4 g as soon as umbilical cord is clamped; then 4 g every 4 hr for 2 more doses, starting 4 hr after initial dose.

Mechanism of Action
Inhibits bacterial cell wall synthesis. In susceptible bacteria, the rigid, cross-linked cell wall is assembled in several stages. Mezlocillin affects final stage of cross-linking process by binding with and inactivating penicillin-binding proteins (enzymes responsible for linking cell wall strands). This causes bacterial cell lysis and death.

Incompatibilities
Administer mezlocillin at separate sites and at least 1 hour before or after administering aminoglycosides. Don't mix mezlocillin in the same I.V. bag, bottle, or tubing with other drugs.

Contraindications
Hypersensitivity to mezlocillin, other penicillins, or their components

Interaction
DRUGS
aminoglycosides: Substantial aminoglycoside inactivation
chloramphenicol, erythromycins, sulfonamides, tetracyclines: Possibly decreased therapeutic effects of mezlocillin
methotrexate: Increased risk of methotrexate toxicity
probenecid: Increased blood level and prolonged half-life of mezlocillin

Adverse Reactions
CNS: Depression, headache, seizures
EENT: Oral candidiasis
GI: Abdominal pain, diarrhea, pseudomembranous colitis, nausea, vomiting
GU: Vaginitis
HEME: Leukopenia, neutropenia
SKIN: Exfoliative dermatitis, pruritus, rash, urticaria
Other: Anaphylaxis; hypokalemia; injection-site pain, redness, and swelling; serum sicknesslike reaction

Nursing Considerations
WARNING Before starting mezlocillin, make sure patient has had no previous hypersensitivity reactions to penicillins.

• Anticipate that mezlocillin therapy will last for at least 2 days after signs and symptoms have resolved—typically 7 to 10 days, depending on severity of infection. Complicated infections may need longer treatment. Group A beta-hemolytic streptococcal infections usually are treated for at least 10 days to reduce risk of rheumatic fever or glomerulonephritis.
• For I.M. injection, reconstitute each gram of mezlocillin with 3 to 4 ml sterile water for injection and shake vigorously. Inject no more than 2 g into a large muscle, such as the gluteus maximus, over 12 to 15 seconds to minimize discomfort.
• Although drug may be given I.M., expect to use intermittent I.V. infusion, as directed, for serious infections.
• For I.V. use, reconstitute each gram of mezlocillin with 9 to 10 ml sterile water for injection, D₅W, or sodium chloride for injection and shake vigorously. Inject directly into I.V. tubing over 3 to 5 minutes.
• For intermittent infusion, further dilute to desired volume (50 to 100 ml) with an appropriate I.V. solution and administer over 30 minutes. Discontinue other infusions during mezlocillin administration.
• Be aware that mezlocillin powder and reconstituted solution may darken slightly but that potency isn't affected.
• Periodically monitor serum potassium level during long-term therapy, as ordered.
• During long-term therapy, watch for signs and symptoms of superinfection, such as oral candidiasis and vaginitis.

PATIENT TEACHING
• Instruct patient taking mezlocillin to notify prescriber immediately about increased bruising or other bleeding tendencies.
• Advise patient to report diarrhea and to check with prescriber before taking an antidiarrheal medicine because of the risk of masking pseudomembranous colitis.

---

micafungin sodium
Mycamine

Class and Category
Chemical class: Semisynthetic lipopeptide echinocandin
Therapeutic class: Antifungal
Pregnancy category: C

Indications and Dosages
➤ *To treat esophageal candidiasis*
I.V. INFUSION
Adults. 150 mg infused over 1 hr once daily.
Children age 4 months and older weighing more than 30 kg. 2.5 mg/kg infused over 1 hr once daily. *Maximum*: 150 mg once daily.
Children age 4 months and older weighing 30 kg or less. 3 mg/kg infused over 1 hr once daily.
➤ *To prevent* Candida *infection in patients undergoing hematopoietic stem cell transplantation*
I.V. INFUSION
Adults. 50 mg infused over 1 hr once daily.
Children age 4 months and older. 1 mg/kg infused over 1 hr once daily. *Maximum:* 50 mg once daily.
➤ *To treat candidemia, acute disseminated candidiasis, and* Candida *peritonitis and abscesses*
I.V. INFUSION
Adults. 100 mg infused over 1 hr once daily.
Children age 4 months and older. 2 mg/kg infused over 1 hr once daily. *Maximum:* 100 mg once daily.

Mechanism of Action
Inhibits synthesis of 1,3-beta-D-glucan, which is an essential component of the *Candida* fungal cell wall. Without 1,3-beta-D-glucan, the fungal cell dies.

Contraindications
Hypersensitivity to micafungin, its components, or other echinocandins

Incompatibilities
Mixing or infusing with other drugs may cause micafungin to precipitate.

Interaction
DRUGS
immunosuppressants: Possibly additive adverse hematologic effects
itraconazole, nifedipine, sirolimus: Increased plasma levels of these drugs

Adverse Reactions
CNS: Anxiety, delirium, dizziness, dysgeusia, fatigue, fever, headache, insomnia, intracranial hemorrhage, rigors, seizures, somnolence

CV: Arrhythmia, atrial fibrillation, bradycardia, cardiac arrest, deep venous thrombosis, hypertension, hypotension, MI, peripheral edema, phlebitis, tachycardia, shock, vasodilation
EENT: Epistaxis, mucosal inflammation
ENDO: Hypoglycemia, hyperglycemia
GI: Abdominal pain, anorexia, constipation, diarrhea, dyspepsia, elevated liver enzyme levels, hepatic dysfunction, hiccups, hyperbilirubinemia, jaundice, nausea, vomiting
GU: Acute renal failure, anuria, elevated serum creatinine and blood urea levels, oliguria, renal tubular necrosis
HEME: Anemia, coagulopathy, disseminated intravascular coagulation, eosino-philia, hemolytic anemia, leukopenia, lymphopenia, neutropenia, pancytopenia, thrombocytopenia
MS: Arthralgia, back pain
RESP: Apnea, cough, cyanosis, dyspnea, hypoxia, pneumonia, pulmonary embolism
SKIN: Erythema, erythema multiforme, flushing, necrosis, pruritus, rash, Stevens-Johnson syndrome, toxic epidermal necrolysis, urticaria
Other: Acidosis, anaphylaxis, angioedema, bacteremia, hyperkalemia, hypernatremia, hypocalcemia, hypokalemia, hypomagnesemia, hyponatremia, hypophosphatemia, injection-site reactions including phlebitis and thrombophlebitis, sepsis

Nursing Considerations
• Use cautiously in patients with hepatic insufficiency.
• Reconstitute micafungin by adding 5 ml 0.9% sodium chloride injection, USP or 5% dextrose injection, USP solution to each 50-mg vial being used (to yield 10 mg micafungin/ml) and to each 100-mg vial being used (to yield 20 mg micafungin/ml). Swirl vial gently to minimize excessive foaming. For adult patients, add reconstituted solution to 100 ml 0.9% sodium chloride injection, USP or 5% dextrose injection, USP, For pediatric patients, follow manufacturer guidelines for calculating volume to use for dilution. Give solution for both adults and children over 1 hour after flushing an existing intravenous line with 0.9% sodium chloride injection, USP. Protect diluted solution from light,

although the infusion drip chamber or tubing does not need to be covered.
• Administer concentrations greater than 1.5 mg/ml through a central catheter to minimize risk of infusion reactions.
• Monitor infusion rate carefully because infusions that took less than 1 hour to infuse have been associated with more frequent hypersensitivity reactions.
WARNING Monitor patient closely for hypersensitivity reactions, including anaphylaxis and angioedema. Stop infusion immediately if present, notify prescriber, and provide supportive care, as prescribed.
• Monitor patient's liver and renal function closely throughout therapy because liver and renal abnormalities may occur in patients receiving micafungin.
• Monitor hematologic status closely because hematologic abnormalities may occur. If they do, monitor patient closely. If patient's condition worsens, expect micafungin to be discontinued.
PATIENT TEACHING
• Instruct patient to report any infusion-site discomfort immediately.
• Tell patient to report any unusual or persistent signs and symptoms to prescriber.

midazolam hydrochloride
Versed

Class, Category, and Schedule
Chemical class: Benzodiazepine
Therapeutic class: Sedative-hypnotic
Pregnancy category: D
Controlled substance schedule: IV

Indications and Dosages
➤ *To induce preoperative sedation or amnesia, to control preoperative anxiety*
ORAL SOLUTION
Children ages 6 months to 16 years. 0.25 to 0.5 mg/kg as a single dose 30 to 45 min before surgery. *Usual:* 0.5 mg/kg. *Maximum:* 20 mg.
I.V. INJECTION
Adults age 60 and over. 1.5 mg over 2 min immediately before procedure. After 2-min

waiting period, dosage adjusted to desired level in 25% increments, as ordered. *Maximum:* 1 mg in 2 min.
Adults under age 60 and adolescents. Up to 2.5 mg over 2 min immediately before procedure. After 2-min waiting period, dosage adjusted to desired level in 25% increments, as ordered. *Maximum:* 5 mg.
Children ages 6 to 12. Initial: 0.025 to 0.05 mg/kg, up to 0.4 mg/kg, if needed. *Maximum:* 10 mg.
Children ages 6 months to 5 years. *Initial:* 0.05 to 0.1 mg/kg, up to 0.6 mg/kg, if needed. *Maximum:* 6 mg.

I.M. INJECTION
Adults age 60 and over. 0.02 to 0.05 mg/kg as a single dose 30 to 60 min before surgery.
Adults under age 60 and adolescents. 0.07 to 0.08 mg/kg as a single dose 30 to 60 min before surgery.
Children ages 6 months to 12 years. 0.1 to 0.15 mg/kg, up to 0.5 mg/kg for more anxious patients. *Maximum:* 10 mg.
➤ *To relieve agitation and anxiety in mechanically ventilated patients*

I.V. INFUSION
Adults. *Initial:* 0.01 to 0.05 mg/kg infused over several min, repeated at 10- to 15-min intervals until adequate sedation occurs. *Maintenance:* 0.02 to 0.1 mg/kg/hr initially, adjusted to desired level in 25% to 50% increments, as ordered. After achieving desired level of sedation, infusion rate decreased by 10% to 25% every few hr, as ordered, until minimum effective infusion rate is determined.
Children. *Initial:* 50 to 200 mcg/kg over 2 to 3 min followed by 1 to 2 mcg/kg/min by continuous infusion. *Maintenance:* 0.4 to 6 mcg/kg/min.
Infants over age 32 weeks. 1 mcg/kg/min by continuous infusion.
Infants under age 32 weeks. 0.5 mcg/kg/min by continuous infusion.

Route	Onset	Peak	Duration
I.V.*	1.5–5 min	Rapid	2–6 hr
I.M.*	5–15 min	15–60 min	2–6 hr
I.M.†	30–60 min	Unknown	Unknown

---
* For sedation.
† For amnesia.

Mechanism of Action
May exert sedating effect by increasing activity of gamma-aminobutyric acid, a major inhibitory neurotransmitter in the brain. As a result, midazolam produces a calming effect, relaxes skeletal muscles, and—at high doses—induces sleep.

Contraindications
Acute angle-closure glaucoma; alcohol intoxication; coma; hypersensitivity to midazolam, other benzodiazepines, or their components; shock

Interaction
DRUGS
antihypertensives: Increased risk of hypotension
cimetidine, diltiazem, erythromycin, fluconazole, indinavir, itraconazole, ketoconazole, ranitidine, ritonavir, saquinavir, verapamil: Intense and prolonged sedation caused by reduced midazolam metabolism
CNS depressants: Possibly increased CNS and respiratory depression and hypotension
rifampin: Decreased blood midazolam level
FOODS
grapefruit, grapefruit juice: Possibly increased blood midazolam level and risk of toxicity
ACTIVITIES
alcohol use: Possibly intense, prolonged sedative effect and increased respiratory depression and hypotension

Adverse Reactions
CNS: Agitation, delirium, or dreaming during emergence from anesthesia; anxiety; ataxia; chills; combativeness; confusion; dizziness; drowsiness; euphoria; excessive sedation; headache; insomnia; lethargy; nervousness; nightmares; paresthesia; prolonged emergence from anesthesia; restlessness; retrograde amnesia; sleep disturbance; slurred speech; weakness; yawning
CV: Cardiac arrest, hypotension, nodal rhythm, PVCs, tachycardia, vasovagal episodes
EENT: Blurred vision, diplopia, or other vision changes; increased salivation; laryngospasm; miosis; nystagmus; toothache
GI: Hiccups, nausea, retching, vomiting

M

RESP: Airway obstruction, bradypnea, bronchospasm, coughing, decreased tidal volume, dyspnea, hyperventilation, respiratory arrest, shallow breathing, tachypnea, wheezing
SKIN: Pruritus, rash, urticaria
Other: Injection-site burning, edema, induration, pain, redness, and tenderness

Nursing Considerations

• Before giving midazolam, determine whether patient consumes alcohol or takes antihypertensives, antibiotics, or protease inhibitors because these substances can produce an intense and prolonged sedative effect when taken with midazolam.

WARNING I.V. midazolam is given only in hospital or ambulatory care settings that allow continuous monitoring of respiratory and cardiac function. Keep resuscitative drugs and equipment at hand.

• As needed, combine midazolam injection with D_5W, normal saline solution, or lactated Ringer's solution. With D_5W and normal saline, solution is stable 24 hours. With lactated Ringer's, solution is stable 4 hours.

• As needed, mix injection in same syringe with atropine sulfate, meperidine hydrochloride, morphine sulfate, or scopolamine hydrobromide. The resulting solution is stable for 30 minutes.

• Assess level of consciousness frequently because the range between sedation and unconsciousness or disorientation is narrow with midazolam.

• Be aware that recovery time is usually 2 hours but may be up to 6 hours.

PATIENT TEACHING

• Inform patient that he may not remember procedure because midazolam produces amnesia.

• Advise patient to avoid hazardous activities until drug's adverse CNS effects, such as dizziness and drowsiness, have worn off.

• Instruct patient to avoid alcohol and other CNS depressants for 24 hours after receiving drug, as directed by prescriber.

midodrine hydrochloride

ProAmatine

Class and Category

Chemical class: Desglymidodrine prodrug
Therapeutic class: Antihypotensive, vasopressor
Pregnancy category: C

Indications and Dosages

➤ *To treat symptomatic orthostatic hypotension*

TABLETS

Adults. 10 mg three times daily in 3- to 4-hr intervals.

DOSAGE ADJUSTMENT Initial dose possibly reduced to 2.5 mg for patients with renal impairment.

Route	Onset	Peak	Duration
P.O.	Unknown	30 min	2–3 hr

Mechanism of Action

Is broken down into the active metabolite desglymidodrine. Desglymidodrine directly stimulates alpha-adrenergic receptors in arteries and veins. This action increases total peripheral vascular resistance, which in turn increases systolic and diastolic blood pressure.

Contraindications

Acute renal disease, hypersensitivity to midodrine or its components, initial supine systolic pressure above 180 mm Hg, persistent and excessive supine hypertension, pheochromocytoma, severe heart disease, thyrotoxicosis, urine retention

Interaction

DRUGS

beta blockers, digoxin: Enhanced or precipitated bradycardia, AV block, arrhythmias
cimetidine, flecainide, metformin, procainamide, quinidine, ranitidine, triamterene: Possibly decreased renal clearance of these drugs
dihydroergotamine, ephedrine, phenylephrine, phenylpropanolamine, pseudoephedrine: Increased vasopressor effects
doxazosin, prazosin, terazosin: Antagonized midodrine effects
fludrocortisone acetate: Increased risk of supine hypertension

Adverse Reactions

CNS: Anxiety, asthenia, chills, confusion, delusions, dizziness, feeling of pressure or fullness in head, headache, hyperesthesia,

insomnia, nervousness, paresthesia, somnolence
CV: Hypertension (sitting and supine), vasodilation
EENT: Canker sore, dry mouth, vision changes
GI: Flatulence, indigestion, nausea
GU: Dysuria, urinary frequency and urgency, urine retention
MS: Back pain, leg cramps
SKIN: Dry skin, erythema multiforme, facial flushing, piloerection, rash, scalp pruritus

Nursing Considerations
• Monitor hepatic and renal function, as ordered, before and during midodrine therapy.
• Give drug at 3- to 4-hour intervals, if ordered and needed to control symptoms. Don't give after evening meal, less than 4 hours before bed, or more often than every 3 hours.
WARNING Monitor for severe, persistent systolic supine hypertension, which may develop with single doses up to 20 mg.
• Avoid placing patient flat in bed for any length of time. Elevate head of bed when patient is supine.
• Monitor supine and sitting blood pressure often during midodrine therapy.
PATIENT TEACHING
• Instruct patient to take midodrine every 3 to 4 hours during daytime but not to take final dose after evening meal or within 4 hours of going to bed.
• Advise patient to elevate head of bed when he lies supine. Caution him not to remain flat for any length of time.
• Direct patient to notify prescriber immediately about headache, increased dizziness, urine retention, or vision changes.
• Encourage patient to keep follow-up appointments to monitor blood pressure and hepatic and renal function.

miglitol
Glyset

Class and Category
Chemical class: Desoxynojirimycin derivative

Therapeutic class: Alpha-glucosidase inhibitor, antidiabetic drug
Pregnancy category: B

Indications and Dosages
➤ *To manage type 2 diabetes mellitus*
TABLETS
Adults. *Initial:* 25 mg three times daily with first bite of each meal. Or, 25 mg daily, increased gradually to 25 mg three times daily. *Maximum:* 100 mg three times daily.
DOSAGE ADJUSTMENT After 4 to 8 wk, dosage increased, if ordered, to 50 mg three times daily. for about 3 mo; then dosage adjusted based on glycosylated hemoglobin (HbA$_{1C}$) level.

Route	Onset	Peak	Duration
P.O.	Rapid	2–3 hr	Unknown

Mechanism of Action
Inhibits intestinal glucoside hydrolase enzymes, which normally hydrolyze oligosaccharides and disaccharides to glucose and other monosaccharides. This action delays carbohydrate digestion and absorption and reduces postprandial blood glucose level.

Contraindications
Acute or chronic bowel disorder, diabetic ketoacidosis, hypersensitivity to miglitol or its components

Interaction
DRUGS
digestive enzyme preparations, intestinal adsorbents (activated charcoal): Decreased miglitol effects
digoxin: Decreased blood digoxin level
insulin, sulfonylureas: Increased risk and severity of hypoglycemia
propranolol, ranitidine: Decreased bioavailability of these drugs

Adverse Reactions
GI: Abdominal pain or distention, diarrhea, flatulence, hepatotoxicity, ileus including paralytic ileus, nausea, pneumatosis cystoides intestinalis (rare), subileus
HEME: Low serum iron level
SKIN: Rash (transient)

Nursing Considerations
• Use miglitol cautiously in patient with serum creatinine level above 2 mg/dl.

M

• Be aware that some patients with type 2 diabetes also may receive a sulfonylurea or insulin as an adjunct to miglitol therapy. Monitor these patients closely for hypoglycemia because sulfonylureas and insulin may cause hypoglycemia, and miglitol therapy may make it more severe. If hypoglycemia occurs, use an oral glucose product such as dextrose to treat mild-to-moderate hypoglycemia rather than sucrose, whose hydrolysis to glucose and fructose is inhibited by miglitol.
• Give miglitol with first bite of each meal. Drug must have arrived at site of enzymatic action when carbohydrates reach small intestine.
• Review patient's HbA$_{1C}$ level, as appropriate, to monitor long-term glucose control.
• Monitor patient for evidence of overdose, such as transient increases in abdominal discomfort, diarrhea, and flatulence (but not hypoglycemia).
• Monitor patient for constipation, diarrhea, mucus discharge, or rectal bleeding suggestive of pneumatosis cystoides intestinalis. If suspected, notify prescriber and prepare patient for diagnostic imaging, as ordered. If confirmed, expect drug to be discontinued.

PATIENT TEACHING
• Explain that miglitol is an adjunct to diet, which is the primary treatment for type 2 diabetes mellitus.
• Instruct patient to take drug with first bite of each meal.
• Describe signs and symptoms of hypo-glycemia and pathophysiology of diabetes to patient and family members.
• If miglitol is the only drug patient takes to control blood glucose level, explain that it won't cause hypoglycemia.
• If patient takes a sulfonylurea or insulin with miglitol, recommend that he keep a source of glucose readily available to reverse hypoglycemia.
• Explain importance of monitoring blood and urine glucose levels.
• Explain that adverse GI reactions usually decrease in frequency and intensity over time.
• Teach obese patient about weight loss, calorie restriction, diet, and regular exercise, as indicated.

• Instruct patient to report to prescriber persistent or severe constipation, diarrhea, mucus discharge, or rectal bleeding.

milnacipran hydrochloride
Savella

Class and Category
Chemical class: Selective norepinephrine and serotonin reuptake inhibitor
Therapeutic class: Antifibromyalgia
Pregnancy category: C

Indications and Dosages
➤ *To manage fibromyalgia*
TABLETS
Adults and adolescents age 17 and over. *Initial:* 12.5 mg on day one; 12.5 mg twice daily on days 2 and 3; 25 mg twice daily on days 4 through 7; and then 50 mg twice daily, increased, if needed to 100 mg twice daily. *Maximum:* 100 mg twice daily.
DOSAGE ADJUSTMENT For patients with severe renal impairment (creatinine clearance of 5 to 29 ml/min/1.73 m^2), maintenance dosage reduced by half.

Route	Onset	Peak	Duration
P.O.	Unknown	2–4 hr	Unknown

Mechanism of Action
Inhibits reuptake of norepinephrine and serotonin by CNS neurons without affecting uptake of dopamine or other neuro-transmitters, thereby increasing amount of norepinephrine and serotonin available in nerve synapses. Elevated norepinephrine and serotonin levels may improve symptoms of fibromyalgia, including central analgesic effect.

Contraindications
Hypersensitivity to milnacipran or its components, uncontrolled narrow-angle glaucoma, use within 14 days of MAO inhibitor, including intravenous methylene blue and linezolid

Interaction
DRUGS
antipsychotics or other dopamine antagonists, MAO inhibitors, selective serotonin reuptake

inhibitors, serotonin-norepinephrine reuptake inhibitors: Possibly development of serotonin syndrome or neuroleptic malignant syndromelike reactions
aspirin, NSAIDs, warfarin: Increased risk of bleeding
clomipramine: Increased risk of euphoria and postural hypotension
clonidine: Possibly inhibited antihypertensive effect
CNS-active drugs: Possibly increased CNS effects
digoxin (I.V.): Possibly increased risk of postural hypotension and tachycardia
epinephrine, norepinephrine: Increased risk of arrhythmias and paroxysmal hypertension
lithium: Increased risk of serotonin syndrome
MAO inhibitors: Possibly hyperpyretic episodes, hypertensive crisis, serotonin syndrome, and severe seizures
serotonergic drugs such as SSRIs, triptans, and tramadol: Increased risk of hypertension and coronary artery vasoconstriction
ACTIVITIES
alcohol use: Increased risk of liver impairment

Adverse Reactions

CNS: Aggression, anger, anxiety, chills, delirium, depression, dizziness, fatigue, fever, hallucinations, headache, homicidal ideation, hypoesthesia, insomnia, irritability, loss of consciousness, migraine, neuroleptic malignant syndrome, parkinsonism, paresthesia, seizures, serotonin syndrome, suicidal ideation, tremor
CV: Chest pain, hypercholesterolemia, hypertension, hypertensive crisis, increased heart rate, palpitations, peripheral edema, supraventricular tachycardia, tachycardia
EENT: Accommodation abnormality, blurred vision, dry mouth, mydriasis
ENDO: Galactorrhea, hot flashes, hyperprolactinemia
GI: Abdominal distention or pain, anorexia, constipation, diarrhea, dyspepsia, elevated liver enzymes, gastroesophageal reflux, flatulence, hepatitis, jaundice, liver dysfunction, nausea, vomiting
GU: Acute renal failure, cystitis, decreased libido, dysuria, ejaculation disorder, erectile dysfunction, prostatitis, scrotal or testicular pain, testicular swelling, urinary hesitation, urine retention, urethral pain, UTI
HEME: Leukopenia, neutropenia, thrombocytopenia
MS: Rhabdomyolysis
RESP: Dyspnea, upper respiratory infection
SKIN: Erythema multiforme, flushing, hyperhidrosis, night sweats, pruritus, rash, Stevens-Johnson syndrome
Other: Hyponatremia, weight gain or loss

Nursing Considerations

- Because milnacipran may aggravate liver disease, it shouldn't be given to patients with alcohol addiction or chronic liver disease.
- Use cautiously in patients with mild to moderate renal impairment and patients with significant hypertension or cardiac disease. Also use cautiously in patients with a history of dysuria, especially men with prostatic hypertrophy, prostatitis, and other lower urinary tract obstructive disorders.
- At least 14 days should elapse between stopping an MAO inhibitor and starting milnacipran. At least 5 days should elapse between stopping milnacipran and starting an MAO inhibitor.
- Measure patient's blood pressure and heart rate before starting and periodically during milnacipran therapy because drug can raise blood pressure and heart rate. If hypertension or tachycardia occurs and persists, notify prescriber and expect to reduce dosage or discontinue drug.
- Watch closely for suicidal tendencies, especially when therapy starts and dosage changes.

WARNING Monitor patient closely for serotonin syndrome, a rare but serious adverse effect of selective serotonin reuptake inhibitors such as milnacipran. Signs and symptoms include agitation, confusion, diaphoresis, diarrhea, fever, hyperactive reflexes, poor coordination, restlessness, shaking, talking or acting with uncontrolled excitement, tremor, and twitching. In its most severe form, it can resemble neuroleptic malignant syndrome with muscle rigidity, autonomic instability with possible rapid fluctuation of vital signs, and mental status changes. If

M

symptoms occur, notify prescriber immediately, expect to discontinue drug, and provide supportive care.
• Monitor patient's liver function. If jaundice or signs and symptoms of liver dysfunction occur, notify prescriber and expect drug to be discontinued.
• Watch for hypersensitivity reactions, especially in patients with aspirin sensitivity, because drug contains the yellow dye tartrazine.
• Check patient's serum sodium level, as ordered, because drug may cause hyponatremia, especially in elderly patients, patients taking diuretics, and patients who are volume-depleted.
• Expect to taper drug when no longer needed, as ordered, to minimize adverse reactions.

PATIENT TEACHING
• Urge family or caregiver to watch patient closely for suicidal tendencies, especially when therapy starts or dosage changes.
• Caution patient against stopping drug abruptly because serious adverse effects may result.
• Instruct patient to alert all prescribers that he takes milnacipran.
• Tell patient to have his blood pressure monitored regularly throughout milnacipran therapy.
• Advise patient to avoid activities, such as driving, that require alertness until the CNS effects of milnacipran are known.
• Caution patient to avoid aspirin and NSAIDs, if possible, while taking milnacipran.

milrinone lactate

Primacor

Class and Category
Chemical class: Bipyridine derivative
Therapeutic class: Inotropic, vasodilator
Pregnancy category: C

Indications and Dosages
➤ *To provide short-term treatment of acute heart failure*
I.V. INFUSION
Adults. *Loading:* 50 mcg/kg over 10 min (at least 0.375 mcg/kg/min). *Usual:* 0.375 to

0.75 mcg/kg/min. *Maximum:* 1.13 mg/kg daily.

DOSAGE ADJUSTMENT Dosage adjusted according to cardiac output, pulmonary artery wedge pressure (PAWP), and clinical response. If creatinine clearance is 30 to 39 ml/min/1.73 m^2, infusion rate reduced to 0.33 mcg/kg/min; if 20 to 29 ml/min/ 1.73 m^2, to 0.28 mcg/kg/min; if 10 to 19 ml/min/1.73 m^2, to 0.23 mcg/kg/min; and if less than 9 ml/min/1.73 m^2, to 0.2 mcg/kg/min.

Route	Onset	Peak	Duration
I.V.	5–15 min	Unknown	3–6 hr

Incompatibilities
Don't administer milrinone through same I.V. line as furosemide because precipitate will form. Don't add other drugs to premixed milrinone flexible containers.

Contraindications
Hypersensitivity to milrinone or its components

Interaction
DRUGS
antihypertensives: Possibly hypotension

Adverse Reactions
CNS: Headache, tremor
CV: Angina, hypotension, supraventricular arrhythmias, ventricular ectopic activity, ventricular fibrillation, ventricular tachycardia, torsades de pointes
GI: Liver function test abnormalities
HEME: Thrombocytopenia
RESP: Bronchospasm
SKIN: Rash
Other: Anaphylactic shock, hypokalemia, infusion-site reactions (pain, swelling, redness)

Nursing Considerations
• Make sure ECG equipment is available for continuous monitoring during milrinone therapy.
• Discard drug if it's discolored or contains particles.
• For loading dose, infuse undiluted drug directly into I.V. line with compatible infusing solution. For continuous infusion, dilute drug with half-normal (0.45) saline solution, normal saline solution, or D_5W. Dilution isn't needed when using premixed milrinone flexible containers.

Mechanism of Action

An inotropic drug, milrinone increases the force of myocardial contraction—and cardiac output—by blocking the enzyme phosphodiesterase. Normally, this enzymeis activated by hormones binding to cell membrane receptors. As shown below left, phosphodiesterase normally degrades intracellular cAMP, which restricts calciummovement into myocardial cells. By inhibiting phosphodiesterase, as shown below right, milrinone slows the rate of cAMP degradation, increasing the intracellularc AMP level and the amount of calcium that enters myocardial cells. In blood vessels, increased cAMP causes smooth-muscle relaxation, which improves cardiac output by reducing preload and afterload.

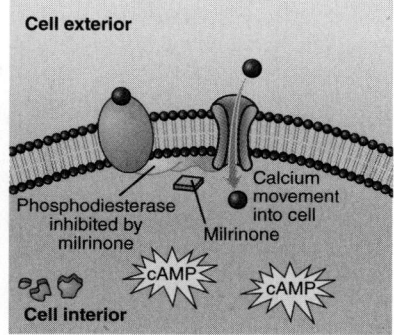

M

- Check platelet count before and periodically during infusion, as ordered. Expect to discontinue drug if platelet count falls below 150,000/mm^3.
- Give loading dose using a controlled-rate infusion device. For continuous infusion, use a calibrated electronic infusion device.
- Monitor cardiac output, pulmonary artery wedge pressure, blood pressure, heart rate, weight, and fluid status during therapy to determine drug effectiveness.
- Monitor renal and liver function test results and serum electrolyte levels. Notify prescriber of abnormalities.
- If severe hypotension develops, notify prescriber at once and expect to stop drug.
- Expect patient to receive digoxin before starting milrinone, which can increase ventricular response rate.

PATIENT TEACHING
- Reassure patient that you will be present and that he will be monitored constantly during therapy.

minocycline
Minocin

minocycline hydrochloride

Alti-Minocycline (CAN), Apo-Minocycline (CAN), Dynacin, Gen-Minocycline (CAN), Minocin, Novo-Minocycline (CAN), Solodyn, Vectrin

Class and Category
Chemical class: Tetracycline
Therapeutic class: Antibiotic, antiprotozoal
Pregnancy category: D

Indications and Dosages
➤ *To treat bartonellosis, brucellosis, chancroid, granuloma inguinale, inclusion conjunctivitis, lymphogranuloma venereum, nongonococcal urethritis, plague, psittacosis, Q fever, relapsing fever, respiratory tract infections*

(including pneumonia), rickettsial pox, Rocky Mountain spotted fever, tularemia, typhus, and UTI caused by gram-negative organisms (including Bartonella bacilliformis, Brucella *species,* Haemophilus ducreyi, Haemophilus influenzae, Vibriocholerae, *and* Yersinia pestis), *susceptible gram-positive organisms (including certain strains of* Streptococcus pneumoniae), *and other organisms (including* Actinomyces *species,* Bacillus anthracis, Borrelia recurrentis, Chlamydia *species,* Mycoplasma pneumoniae, *and* Rickettsiae); *as adjunct to treat intestinal amebiasis and as alternative to treat listeriosis caused by* Listeria monocytogenes, *syphilis caused by* Treponema pallidum, *and yaws caused by* Treponema pertenue *for nonpregnant patients allergic to penicillin*

CAPSULES, ORAL SUSPENSION
Adults and adolescents. *Initial:* 200 mg. *Maintenance:* 100 mg every 12 hr. Or 100 to 200 mg initially followed by 50 mg every 6 hr.
Children over age 8. *Initial:* 4 mg/kg. *Maintenance:* 2 mg/kg every 12 hr.

I.V. INJECTION
Adults and adolescents. *Initial:* 200 mg. *Maintenance:* 100 mg every 12 hr. *Maximum:* 400 mg daily.
Children over age 8. *Initial:* 4 mg/kg. *Maintenance:* 2 mg/kg every 12 hr.
DOSAGE ADJUSTMENT If patient has renal impairment, don't exceed 200 mg daily.
➤ *As adjunct to treat inflammatory acne vulgaris that's unresponsive to oral tetracycline or erythromycin*

CAPSULES, ORAL SUSPENSION
Adults and adolescents. 50 mg once daily to three times daily.
➤ *To treat inflammatory lesions of non-nodular moderate to severe acne vulgaris*

E.R. TABLETS
Adults and adolescents age 12 and over. 1 mg/kg once daily for 12 weeks.
DOSAGE ADJUSTMENT For patient with renal impairment, dosage reduced or time interval between doses extended.
➤ *To treat uncomplicated gonorrhea from* Neisseria gonorrhoeae *in nonpregnant patients allergic to penicillin*

CAPSULES, ORAL SUSPENSION
Adults and adolescents. *Initial:* 200 mg. *Maintenance:* 100 mg every 12 hr for at least 4 days.
➤ *To treat uncomplicated gonococcal urethritis in men*

CAPSULES, ORAL SUSPENSION
Adults and adolescents. 100 mg twice daily for 5 days.
➤ *To treat asymptomatic meningococcal carriers with* Neisseria meningitidis *in nasopharynx*

CAPSULES, ORAL SUSPENSION
Adults and adolescents. 100 mg every 12 hr for 5 days.
Children over age 8.
Initial: 4 mg/kg. *Maintenance:* 2 mg/kg every 12 hr for 5 days.
➤ *To treat infections caused by* Mycobacterium marinum

CAPSULES, ORAL SUSPENSION
Adults. 100 mg every 12 hr for 6 to 8 wk.

Route	Onset	Peak	Duration
P.O.	Unknown	2–4 hr	6–12 hr
I.V.	Unknown	Unknown	6–12 hr

Mechanism of Action
Inhibits bacterial protein synthesis by competitively binding to the 30S ribosomal subunit of the mRNA-ribosome complex of certain organisms.

Incompatibilities
Don't mix minocycline in same syringe with solution that contains calcium because precipitate will form.

Contraindications
Hypersensitivity to minocycline, other tetracyclines, or their components

Interaction
DRUGS
aluminum-, calcium-, or magnesium-containing antacids; calcium supplements; choline and magnesium salicylates; iron-containing preparations; magnesium-containing laxatives; sodium bicarbonate: Possibly formation of nonabsorbable complex, impaired minocycline absorption
cholestyramine, colestipol: Possibly impaired cholestyramine or colestipol absorption

cimetidine: Possibly decreased GI absorption and effectiveness of minocycline
digoxin: Possibly increased blood digoxin level and risk of digitalis toxicity
insulin: Possibly decreased need for insulin
iron salts: Possibly decreased GI absorption and antimicrobial effect of minocycline
lithium: Possibly increased or decreased blood lithium level
methoxyflurane: Increased risk of nephrotoxicity
oral anticoagulants: Possibly potentiated anticoagulant effects
oral contraceptives containing estrogen: Decreased contraceptive effectiveness, increased risk of breakthrough bleeding
penicillin: Interference with bactericidal action of penicillin
vitamin A: Possibly benign intracranial hypertension

Adverse Reactions

CNS: Dizziness, fever, headache, light-headedness, unsteadiness, vertigo
CV: Pericarditis
EENT: Blurred vision, darkened or discolored tongue, glossitis, papilledema, tooth discoloration, vision changes
ENDO: Thyroid function abnormality or cancer
GI: Abdominal cramps or pain, anorexia, diarrhea, dysphagia, enterocolitis, esophageal irritation and ulceration, hepatitis, hepatotoxicity, indigestion, nausea, pancreatitis, pseudomembranous colitis, vomiting
GU: Genital candidiasis, nephrotoxicity
HEME: Eosinophilia, hemolytic anemia, neutropenia, thrombocytopenia, thrombocytopenic purpura
MS: Arthralgia, myopathy (transient)
RESP: Pulmonary infiltrates (with eosinophilia)
SKIN: Erythema multiforme, exfoliative dermatitis, brown pigmentation of skin and mucous membranes, erythematous and maculopapular rash, jaundice, onycholysis, photosensitivity, pruritus, purpura (anaphylactoid), Stevens-Johnson syndrome, urticaria
Other: Anaphylaxis, angioedema, serum sicknesslike reaction, systemic lupus erythematosus exacerbation

Nursing Considerations

• Use minocycline cautiously in patients with renal or hepatic dysfunction and in those taking other hepatotoxic drugs because drug may cause nephrotoxicity or hepatotoxicity.
WARNING Notify prescriber if patient is breastfeeding because drug appears in breastmilk and may have toxic effects.
• Monitor blood, renal, and hepatic tests before and during long-term therapy.
• Shake oral suspension well before use.
• To prepare drug for I.V. use, reconstitute each 100-mg vial with 5 to 10 ml sterile water for injection. Further dilute in 500 to 1,000 ml normal saline solution, D_5W, dextrose 5% in normal saline solution, or Ringer's or lactated Ringer's solution. Administer final dilution immediately, but avoid rapid administration.
• Store reconstituted drug at room temperature and use within 24 hours.
• Assess patient for signs of superinfection; if signs appear, notify prescriber, discontinue minocycline, and start appropriate therapy, as ordered.
• Monitor patient for development of foul-smelling diarrhea, which suggests *Clostridium difficile.* If present, notify prescriber, obtain stool culture, and expect to withhold minocycline and provide supportive care, as indicated and ordered.
• Monitor PT in patient who also takes an anticoagulant during minocycline therapy.
• Monitor patient for signs and symptoms of thyroid cancer such as presence of nodule or alteration in thyroid function in patients receiving minocycline therapy over prolonged periods.
• Monitor patient for headache and blurred vision because benign intracranial hypertension has occurred with the use of tetracyclines. If present, notify prescriber and expect drug to be discontinued.

PATIENT TEACHING
• Instruct patient to shake oral suspension well and to use calibrated measuring device.
• Advise patient to take minocycline with a full glass of water, with food or milk, and in an upright position to minimize esophageal and GI irritation.

M

• Direct patient to take a missed dose as soon as he remembers unless it's nearly time for the next dose. Caution against double-dosing.
• Instruct patient not to take minocycline within 2 hours of an antacid or 3 hours of an iron preparation.
• Urge patient to complete full course of treatment even if he feels better before finishing.
• Instruct patient to notify prescriber if no improvement occurs in a few days.
• Advise patient to avoid prolonged exposure to sun or sunlamps during therapy.
• Counsel female patient to avoid becoming pregnant because minocycline should be avoided, if possible, during tooth development (last half of gestation up to age 8). Drug may permanently turn teeth yellow, gray, or brown and cause enamel hypoplasia. It also may slow skeletal growth and cause congenital anomalies, including limb reduction.
• Encourage patient who uses an oral contraceptive to use additional contraceptive method during minocycline therapy.
• Instruct patient to notify prescriber immediately about blurred vision, dizziness, headache, known or suspected pregnancy, and unsteadiness.
• Explain that diarrhea may occur up to 2 months after completing therapy; urge patient to notify prescriber if it occurs.

minoxidil (oral)
Loniten
minoxidil (topical)
Apo-Gain (CAN), Gen-Minoxidil (CAN), Minox (CAN), Minoxigaine (CAN), Rogaine (CAN), Rogaine ES for Men, Rogaine for Men, Rogaine for Women

Class and Category
Chemical class: Piperidinopyrimidine derivative
Therapeutic class: Antihypertensive (oral), hair-growth stimulant (topical)
Pregnancy category: C

Indications and Dosages
➤ *To manage severe symptomatic hypertension or hypertension with target organ damage that's unresponsive to other treatment*
TABLETS
Adults and adolescents. *Initial:* 5 mg as a single dose or divided doses twice daily. Increased, as directed, after at least 3 days. *Maintenance:* 10 to 40 mg daily. *Maximum:* 100 mg daily.
Children. *Initial:* 0.2 mg/kg daily. Increased, as directed, after at least 3 days. *Maintenance:* 0.25 to 1 mg/kg daily as a single dose or in divided doses twice daily. *Maximum:* 50-mg starting dose, 50 mg daily.
DOSAGE ADJUSTMENT Dosage possibly reduced for elderly patients and those who have renal failure or are having dialysis.
➤ *To treat alopecia*
TOPICAL 2%
Adults up to age 65. 1 ml applied twice daily to area of desired hair growth.
TOPICAL 5%
Adult men up to age 65. 1 ml applied twice daily to area of desired hair growth.

Route	Onset	Peak	Duration
P.O.	30 min	2–3 hr	24–48 hr
Topical 2%	4 mo	1 yr	Unknown
Topical 5%	2 mo	1 yr	Unknown

Mechanism of Action
Reduces blood pressure by inhibiting intracellular phosphodiesterase, an enzyme that facilitates hydrolysis of cAMP and cGMP. This action decreases the intracellular cAMP level, relaxes arterial smooth muscles, and lowers blood pressure. Oral minoxidil produces greater dilation in arteries than in veins. It also reduces peripheral resistance and increases heart rate, cardiac output, and stroke volume.
  Topical minoxidil may cause hair regrowth by increasing cutaneous blood flow and stimulating resting hair follicles.

Contraindications
Acute MI; dissecting aortic aneurysm; hypersensitivity to minoxidil or its components, including propylene glycol; pheochromocytoma; skin irritation or abrasions (topical)

Interaction

DRUGS

guanethidine: Possibly severe hypotension, increased risk of orthostatic hypotension (oral)

nitrates, other hypotension-producing drugs, potent parenteral antihypertensives: Possibly severe hypotension

NSAIDs, sympathomimetics: Decreased antihypertensive effects

topical petrolatum, topical steroids: Increased absorption of topical minoxidil if used on same area

topical retinoids: Increased absorption of topical minoxidil and, possibly, formation of granulation tissue

Adverse Reactions

CNS: Fatigue, paresthesia (oral); light-headedness, neuritis (topical); headache (both)

CV: ECG changes, heart failure, pericardial tamponade, pericarditis, rebound hypertension (oral); cardiac tamponade, hypotension, palpitations, reflex hypertension (topical); angina, edema, fast or irregular heartbeat, pericardial effusion (both)

EENT: Vision changes (topical)

ENDO: Breast tenderness (oral)

GI: Abdominal distention, ascites, nausea, vomiting (oral)

GU: Elevated BUN and serum creatinine levels (oral); sexual dysfunction (topical)

HEME: Leukopenia; thrombocytopenia; transient decrease in hematocrit, hemoglobin, and erythrocyte counts (oral)

RESP: Dyspnea, pulmonary hypertension (oral)

SKIN: Flushing, hyperpigmentation, Stevens-Johnson syndrome (oral); allergic contact dermatitis, alopecia, dry or flaky skin, eczema, erythema, folliculitis, scalp burning (topical); hypertrichosis, rash (both)

Other: Facial edema (topical); sodium and water retention, weight gain (both)

Nursing Considerations

- **WARNING** Be aware that patient who receives guanethidine should be hospitalized before starting oral minoxidil therapy so that his blood pressure can be monitored.
- Be aware that drug isn't usually prescribed for mild hypertension.
- For rapid management of hypertension, expect to adjust dosage up to every 6 hours and to monitor patient as prescribed. Also expect to give a beta blocker and diuretic.
- Monitor progress by measuring blood pressure often and weight daily. Evaluate for signs of fluid and sodium retention and for other systemic adverse reactions.
- Watch for signs of pericardial effusion. Be prepared to stop oral minoxidil, if ordered.
- Expect to discontinue oral minoxidil gradually because abrupt discontinuation may lead to rebound hypertension.
- Apply topical drug only on healthy scalp. Avoid sunburned or abraded scalp.
- Use gloves when applying solution.
- Avoid inhaling mist from spray applicator.
- Expect minoxidil to be least effective in men with mainly frontal hair loss.
- Expect topical form to have little effect on blood pressure in patients who don't have hypertension.

PATIENT TEACHING

- Inform patient that oral minoxidil controls but doesn't cure hypertension.
- Advise him to take tablets at the same time every day.
- Teach patient to take his radial pulse, and advise him to take it daily. Instruct him to notify prescriber if it exceeds normal rate by 20 beats/minute or more.
- Emphasize the importance of daily blood pressure and weight measurements.
- Instruct patient to notify prescriber immediately about bloating, breathing problems, a fast or irregular heartbeat, flushed or red skin, swelling of feet or lower legs, or weight gain of more than 5 lb (2.3 kg) in 1 day.
- Advise patient to have regular checkups with prescriber to monitor progress.
- Urge patient to consult prescriber before taking other prescription or OTC drugs.
- Reassure patient that body hair thickening and darkening reverses after oral minoxidil is discontinued.
- For patient using topical minoxidil, teach proper application technique and provide manufacturer's written instructions. Advise him to wear gloves when applying drug and to make sure hair and scalp are dry first.
- Instruct patient to start applying drug at center of balding area, to let dry for 2 to 4

M

hours, and not to use hairdryer to help it dry faster.

• Warn patient to avoid applying drug to abraded, irritated, or sunburned areas of scalp; to avoid inhaling mist when using a spray applicator; and to avoid getting drug in his eyes, nose, or mouth. If accidental contact does occur, advise him to flush the area with large amounts of cool tap water.

• Instruct patient not to shampoo his hair for at least 4 hours after application and to avoid using other skin products on treated skin. Direct him to avoid using minoxidil for 24 hours before and after chemical hair products, such as dyes and relaxers.

• Caution patient not to use more drug or apply it more often than prescribed and not to apply it to other body areas. Explain the risk of adverse systemic reactions with excessive topical use.

• Tell patient to keep topical minoxidil away from heat or flame because it's flammable.

• Inform patient that minoxidil may stain clothing, hats, or bed linens before it's dry.

• Instruct patient to notify prescriber if burning, itching, or redness develops after application. For severe reactions, advise patient to wash drug off and consult prescriber before applying it again.

• Urge patient to consult prescriber if hair loss continues after 2 weeks or if growth fails to increase in 4 months.

• Inform patient that new hair growth may be lost 3 to 4 months after stopping topical minoxidil and that progressive hair loss will resume.

mipomersen sodium

Kynamro

Class and Category
Chemical class: Synthetic phosphorothioate oligonucleotide sodium salt
Therapeutic class: Antihyperlipidemic
Pregnancy category: B

Indications and Dosages
➤ *To control lipid levels as adjunct to diet and other lipid-lowering treatments in homozygous familial hypercholesterolemia*

SUBCUTANEOUS INJECTION
Adults. 200 milligrams once weekly.

Mechanism of Action
Targets human messenger ribonucleic acid (mRNA) for apo B-100, the principal apolipoprotein of low density lipoproteins (LDL) and its metabolic precursor, very low density lipoprotein (VLDL). Once targeted, translation of the apo B-100 protein is inhibited, resulting in lower lipid levels.

Contraindications
Active liver disease, hypersensitivity to mipomersen or its components, moderate or severe hepatic impairment, unexplained persistent elevations of serum transaminases

Interaction
DRUGS
other hepatotoxic drugs such as acetaminophen, amiodarone, isotretinoin, methotrexate, tamoxifen, tetracyclines: Increased risk of hepatotoxicity and hepatic steatosis
ACTIVITIES
alcohol use: Possibly increased risk of hepatic steatosis

Adverse Reactions
CNS: Chills, fatigue, fever, headache, insomnia
CV: Angina pectoris, hypertension, palpitations, peripheral edema
GI: Abdominal pain, elevated liver enzymes, hepatic steatosis, hepatotoxicity, nausea, transaminase elevations, vomiting
MS: Extremity or musculoskeletal pain
Other: Flulike symptoms; injection-site reactions such as discoloration, erythema, hematoma, local swelling, pain, pruritus, tenderness;

Nursing Considerations
• Know that because mipomersen increases risk of hepatotoxicty, the drug can only be administered through the Kynamro REMS program.

• Determine that patient has had transaminase levels, alkaline phosphatase, and total bilirubin measured prior to initiating mipomersen therapy to rule out liver impairment.

• Administer mipomersen only by subcutaneous route. Never administer drug intramuscularly or intravenously.
• Know that each vial or prefilled syringe contains 200 mg of mipomersen in one milliliter of solution and is intended for single dose only.
• Remove vial or prefilled syringe from refrigerated storage and allow to reach room temperature for at least 30 minutes prior to administration.
• Give injection on the same day every week. If a dose is missed, give injection at least 3 days from the next weekly dose. Administer injection into the patient's abdomen, thigh region, or outer area of the upper arm. Never inject drug in areas of active skin disease or injury such as sunburns, skin rashes, inflammation, skin infections, or active areas of psoriasis. Also, do not inject drug into tattooed skin or scar areas.
• Be aware that transaminase levels should be measured monthly for first year of therapy and then every three months thereafter. If transaminase values are equal to or greater than three times upper limit normal but less than five times upper limit normal, expect to confirm elevation with a repeat measurement within one week. If confirmed, expect dosage to be withheld and additional liver-related tests done, such as measurement of alkaline phosphatase, total bilirubin, and INR. If transaminase elevations are five times or greater, expect drug to be withheld immediately and additional liver-related tests performed. Once transaminases level are less than three times upper limit normal, know that drug may be resumed and liver function assessed more frequently. If transaminase elevations are accompanied by signs of abnormal liver function such as abdominal pain, doubling or greater bilirubin values of upper limit normal, fever, flulike symptoms, jaundice, lethargy, nausea, or vomiting, expect drug to be discontinued.

PATIENT TEACHING
• Remind patient of importance of adhering to the low-fat diet prescribed, as mipomersen therapy is not a replacement for dietary control of fat in her diet.

• Teach patient how to administer a subcutaneous injection and where on body to administer drug. Remind patient to rotate sites and to discard syringe and needle appropriately.
• Warn patient that flulike symptoms may occur within 2 days of injection but does not occur with all injections. If significant, tell patient to notify prescriber.
• Tell patient to inform all prescribers about mipomersen therapy because of potential drug interactions.
• Review signs and symptoms of liver impairment and emphasize importance of reporting such to prescriber. Inform patient of need for blood tests to monitor her liver function and importance of compliance with test schedule.

WARNING Instruct patient not to consume more than one alcoholic beverage daily.

mirabegron

Myrbetriq

M

Class and Category
Chemical class: Beta-3 adrenergic agonist
Therapeutic class: Bladder relaxant
Pregnancy category: C

Indications and Dosages
➤ *To treat overactive bladder with symptoms of urge urinary incontinence, urgency, and urinary frequency*

E.R. TABLETS
Adults. *Initially:* 25 mg once daily, increased as needed to 50 mg once daily.

DOSAGE ADJUSTMENT For patients with severe hepatic or renal impairment, dosage should not exceed 25 mg once daily.

Mechanism of Action
Relaxes the detrusor smooth muscle during the storage phase of the urinary bladder fill-void cycle by activating the beta-3 adrenergic receptor, which increases bladder capacity. With increased bladder capacity, urge sensation is decreased, which in turn decreases urinary frequency.

Contraindications
Hypersensitivity to mirabegron or its components

Interaction
DRUGS
CYP2D6 substrates such as desipramine, flecainide, metoprolol, propafenone, thioridazine: Increased blood levels of these drugs
digoxin: Increased risk of digoxin toxicity

Adverse Reactions
CNS: Dizziness, fatigue, headache
CV: Atrial fibrillation, hypertension, elevated LDH levels, palpitations, tachycardia
EENT: Dry mouth, glaucoma, nasopharyngitis, rhinitis, sinusitis
GI: Abdominal distention or pain, constipation, diarrhea, dyspepsia, elevated liver enzymes, gastritis, nausea
GU: Bladder pain, cystitis, nephrolithiasis, prostate cancer, urinary retention, UTI, vaginal infections, vulvovaginal pruritis
MS: Arthralgia, back pain
SKIN: Pruritis, rash, Stevens-Johnson syndrome
Other: Influenza-like infection

Nursing Considerations
• Know that mirabegron should not be given to patients with severe uncontrolled hypertension (defined as systolic blood pressure 180 mm Hg or higher and/or diastolic blood pressure 110 mm Hg or higher) because drug can increase blood pressure. Monitor patient's blood pressure regularly and report persistent or significant increases to prescriber.
• Be aware that mirabegron should not be given to patients with end stage renal disease or in patients with severe hepatic impairment because drug has not been studied in these conditions, and adverse effects are unknown.
• Use mirabegron cautiously in patients with bladder outlet obstruction and in patients taking antimuscarinic drugs for the treatment of this condition because the drug may cause urinary retention.
• May take up to 8 weeks to observe efficacy with 25 mg strength
PATIENT TEACHING
• Instruct patient to take mirabegron with water and to swallow tablet whole.

Caution patient not to chew, divide, or crush tablets prior to ingesting.
• Warn patient that drug may increase blood pressure. Encourage patient to have his blood pressure checked regularly, especially if he has hypertension.
• Tell patient to notify prescriber if he experiences a decrease in urinary output despite a normal intake.

mirtazapine
Remeron, Remeron SolTab

Class and Category
Chemical class: Piperazinoazepine
Therapeutic class: Antidepressant
Pregnancy category: C

Indications and Dosages
➤ *To treat major depression*
DISINTEGRATING TABLETS, TABLETS
Adults. *Initial:* 15 mg daily, preferably at bedtime. Increased as needed and tolerated at 1- to 2-wk intervals. *Maximum:* 45 mg daily.

Route	Onset	Peak	Duration
P.O.	1–2 wk	6 wk or longer	Unknown

Mechanism of Action
May inhibit neuronal reuptake of norepinephrine and serotonin. By doing so, this tetracyclic antidepressant increases the action of these neurotransmitters in nerve cells. Increased neuronal serotonin and norepinephrine levels may elevate mood.

Contraindications
Hypersensitivity to mirtazapine or its components; use within 14 days of an MAO inhibitor, including intravenous methylene blue and linezolid

Interaction
DRUGS
antihypertensives: Increased hypotensive effects of these drugs or enhanced mirtazapine effects
anxiolytics, hypnotics, other CNS depressants (including sedatives): Increased CNS depression
MAO inhibitors, including linezolid and intravenous methylene blue, other serotonergic

drugs: Possibly hyperpyrexia, hypertension, seizures, and serotonin syndrome
ACTIVITIES
alcohol use: Increased CNS depression

Adverse Reactions

CNS: Agitation, akathisia, amnesia, anxiety, apathy, asthenia, ataxia, cerebral ischemia, chills, confusion, delirium, delusions, depersonalization, depression, dizziness, dream disturbances, drowsiness, dyskinesia, dystonia, emotional lability, euphoria, extrapyramidal reactions, fever, hallucinations, hostility, hyperkinesia, hyperreflexia, hypoesthesia, hypokinesia, lack of coordination, malaise, mania, migraine headache, neuroleptic malignant syndrome-like reactions, neurosis, paranoia, paresthesia, psychomotor restlessness, seizures, serotonin syndrome, somnolence, syncope, tremor, vertigo
CV: Angina, bradycardia, edema, hypercholesterolemia, hypertension, hypertriglyceridemia, hypotension, MI, orthostatic hypotension, peripheral edema, PVCs, torsades de pointes, vasodilation, ventricular arrhythmia
EENT: Accommodation disturbances, conjunctivitis, dry mouth, earache, epistaxis, eye pain, glaucoma, gingival bleeding, glossitis, hearing loss, hyperacusis, keratoconjunctivitis, lacrimation, pharyngitis, sinusitis, stomatitis
ENDO: Breast pain
GI: Abdominal distention and pain, anorexia, cholecystitis, colitis, constipation, elevated ALT level, eructation, increased appetite, nausea, thirst, vomiting
GU: Amenorrhea, cystitis, dysmenorrhea, dysuria, hematuria, impotence, increased libido, leukorrhea, renal calculi, urinary frequency and incontinence, urine retention, UTI, vaginitis
HEME: Agranulocytosis, neutropenia
MS: Arthralgia, back pain, dysarthria, muscle twitching, myalgia, myasthenia, neck pain and rigidity
RESP: Asthma, bronchitis, cough, dyspnea, pneumonia
SKIN: Acne, alopecia, bullous dermatitis, dry skin, erythema multiforme, exfoliative dermatitis, photosensitivity, pruritus, rash, Stevens-Johnson syndrome, toxic epidermal necrolysis

Other: Dehydration, facial edema, flulike symptoms, herpes simplex, hyponatremia, weight change

Nursing Considerations

• Use mirtazapine cautiously in elderly patients and in those receiving concurrent medication known to cause hyponatremia because drug may lower the serum sodium level in these patients.
• Administer mirtazapine before bedtime.
• Expect disintegrating tablet to dissolve on patient's tongue within 30 seconds.
WARNING Don't give drug within 14 days of an MAO inhibitor or concurrent therapy with serotonin-precusors such as L-tryptophan and oxitriptan to avoid serious, possibly fatal, serotonin syndrome reaction. Use drug cautiously in patients receiving other serotonergic drugs such as triptans, lithium, tramadol, St. John's wort, and most tricyclic antidepressants because of increased risk for serotonin syndrome. Know that both disorders can occur as an adverse drug reaction to mirtazapine therapy without the concomitant use of other drugs. Monitor patient closely for signs and symptoms of serotonin syndrome such as change in mental status, alteration in vital signs, neuromuscular abnormalities or gastrointestinal symptoms. Its most severe form resembles neuroleptic malignant syndrome and presents with hyperthermia, muscle rigidity, autonomic instability with possible rapid changes in vital signs and mental status changes. If any of these symptoms occur, notify prescriber immediately, provide supportive care, as ordered, and expect mirtazapine to be discontinued.
• Monitor patient closely, especially during the first few weeks of therapy, for the development of akathisia, an unpleasant or distressing restlessness and need to move, often accompanied by an inability to sit or stand still. Notify prescriber, if present, and know that increasing the dose may worsen patient's condition.
• If patient takes drug for depression, watch closely for suicidal tendencies, especially when therapy starts or dosage changes, because depression may briefly worsen.

• Monitor patient closely for infection (fever, pharyngitis, stomatitis), which may be linked to a low WBC count. If these signs occur, notify prescriber and expect to stop drug.

• Expect mirtazapine therapy to last 6 months or longer for acute depression.

• Be aware that mirtazapine therapy should not be discontinued abruptly because adverse reactions may occur.

PATIENT TEACHING

• Instruct patient not to swallow disintegrating tablet. Tell him to hold tablet on tongue and let it dissolve. Inform him that tablet will dissolve within 30 seconds.

• Inform phenylketonuric patient that mirtazapine disintegrating tablets contain phenlyalanine 2.6 mg per 15-mg tablet, 5.2 mg per 30-mg tablet, and 7.8 mg per 45-mg tablet.

• Advise patient that drug may cause mild pupillary dilation, which may lead to an episode of acute closure glaucoma. Encourage patient to have an eye exam before starting therapy to see if he is at risk.

• Instruct patient to avoid alcohol and other CNS depressants during therapy and for up to 7 days after drug is discontinued.

• Advise patient to avoid hazardous activities until drug's CNS effects are known.

• Direct patient to change position slowly to minimize the effects of orthostatic hypotension.

• Instruct patient to notify prescriber at once about chills, fever, mouth irritation, sore throat, and other signs of infection.

• Encourage patient to visit prescriber regularly during therapy to monitor progress.

• Caution patient not to discontinue mirtazapine therapy abruptly.

misoprostol

Cytotec

Class and Category

Chemical class: Prostaglandin E_1 analogue
Therapeutic class: Antiulcer, gastric antisecretory
Pregnancy category: X

Indications and Dosages

➤ *To prevent NSAID-induced gastric ulcers*

TABLETS

Adults. 200 mcg four times daily or 400 mcg twice daily with food, with last dose at bedtime every day.

DOSAGE ADJUSTMENT Dosage reduced to 100 mcg four times daily if patient can't tolerate 200-mcg dose.

Route	Onset	Peak	Duration
P.O.	30 min	60–90 min	3–6 hr

Mechanism of Action

May protect the stomach from NSAID-induced mucosal damage by increasing gastric mucus production and mucosal bicarbonate secretion. Misoprostol also inhibits gastric acid secretion caused by such stimuli as food, coffee, and histamine.

Contraindications

Hypersensitivity to prostaglandins or their analogues, pregnancy

Interaction

DRUGS

magnesium-containing antacids: Increased misoprostol-induced diarrhea

Adverse Reactions

CNS: Anxiety, asthenia, chills, confusion, depression, drowsiness, dizziness, fatigue, fever, headache, neuropathy, neurosis, rigors, stroke, syncope, thirst
CV: Arrhythmias, chest pain, edema, hypertension, hypotension, increased cardiac enzyme levels, MI, phlebitis, thromboembolism
EENT: Abnormal taste or vision, conjunctivitis, deafness, earache, epistaxis, gingivitis, tinnitus
ENDO: Hyperglycemia
GI: Abdominal pain, constipation, diarrhea, dysphagia, flatulence, GI bleeding or inflammation, hepatobiliary dysfunction, indigestion, nausea, reflux, vomiting
GU: Dysmenorrhea, dysuria, hematuria, hypermenorrhea, impotence, loss of libido, menstrual irregularities, polyuria, urinary tract infection, vaginal bleeding
HEME: Anemia, abnormal differential thrombocytopenia purpura, increased erythrocyte sedimentation rate
MS: Arthralgia, back pain, myalgia, muscle cramps or stiffness

RESP: Bronchitis, bronchospasm, dyspnea, pneumonia, pulmonary embolism, upper respiratory tract infection
SKIN: Alopecia, diaphoresis, dermatitis, pallor, rash
Other: Anaphylaxis, gout, weight changes

Nursing Considerations

WARNING Ask female patient if she is or may be pregnant. If so, notify prescriber because misoprostol may cause uterine bleeding, contractions, spontaneous abortion, and teratogenic effects in the fetus.
• Use drug cautiously in patients with cerebrovascular disease, coronary artery disease, or uncontrolled epilepsy because of the risk of severe complications.
• Also use misoprostol cautiously in patients with inflammatory bowel disease because drug may worsen intestinal inflammation and cause diarrhea. If diarrhea causes severe dehydration, misoprostol may be discontinued.

PATIENT TEACHING

• Caution female patient about risk of taking misoprostol during pregnancy, and urge her to use reliable contraception during therapy. Urge her to notify prescriber at once if she is or might be pregnant.
• Instruct patient to take misoprostol with meals and at bedtime.
• Advise patient that he may take NSAIDs, if prescribed, during misoprostol therapy.
• Explain that diarrhea is dose related and usually resolves after 8 days. Tell patient to avoid magnesium-containing antacids because they may worsen diarrhea and to call prescriber if diarrhea lasts more than 8 days.
• Urge female patient to notify prescriber immediately about postmenopausal bleeding; she may need diagnostic tests.

---

mitoxantrone hydrochloride

Novantrone

Class and Category

Chemical class: Anthracenedione
Therapeutic class: Antineoplastic
Pregnancy category: D

Indications and Dosages

➤ *To reduce neurologic disability and frequency of relapses in patients with secondary (chronic) progressive, progressive relapsing, or worsening relapsing-remitting multiple sclerosis (patients whose neurologic status is significantly abnormal between relapses)*

I.V. INFUSION

Adults. 12 mg/m^2 over 5 to 15 min every 3 mo. *Maximum:* Cumulative dose of 140 mg/m^2.

➤ *As adjunct to treat pain related to advanced hormone-refractory prostate cancer*

I.V. INFUSION

Adults. 12 to 14 mg/m^2 over 5 to 15 min every 21 days.

➤ *As adjunct to treat acute nonlymphocytic leukemia (ANLL)*

I.V. INFUSION

Adults. *Initial:* 12 mg/m^2 over at least 3 min on days 1 to 3 with 100 mg/m^2 of cytarabine as a continuous 24-hr infusion on days 1 to 7. If patient's antileukemic response is inadequate or incomplete, second induction course is given at same dosage. *Maintenance:* 6 wk after induction, 12 mg/m^2 over at least 3 min on days 1 and 2 with 100 mg/m^2 of cytarabine as a continuous 24-hr infusion on days 1 to 5. A second maintenance course is given 4 wk after the first if needed and tolerated.

Mechanism of Action

Binds to DNA, causing cross-linkage and strand breakage, interfering with RNA synthesis, and inhibiting topoisomerase II, an enzyme that uncoils and repairs damaged DNA. Mitoxantrone produces a cytocidal effect on proliferating and nonproliferating cells and doesn't appear to be cell-cycle specific. It's known to inhibit B-cell, T-cell, and macrophage proliferation and impair antigen function.

Incompatibilities

Don't mix mitoxantrone in the same infusion as heparin (because a precipitate may form); don't mix with any other drugs.

Contraindications

Hypersensitivity to mitoxantrone or its components

M

Interaction

DRUGS

allopurinol, colchicine, probenecid, sulfinpyrazone: Possibly interference with antihyperuricemic action of these drugs
blood-dyscrasia–causing drugs (such as cephalosporins and sulfasalazine): Increased risk of leukopenia and thrombocytopenia
bone marrow depressants, such as carboplatin and lomustine: Possibly additive bone marrow depression
daunorubicin, doxorubicin: Increased risk of cardiotoxicity
methotrexate and other antineoplastics: Risk of developing leukemia
vaccines, killed virus: Decreased antibody response to vaccine
vaccines, live virus: Increased risk of replication of and adverse effects of vaccine virus, decreased antibody response to vaccine

Adverse Reactions

CNS: Headache, seizures
CV: Arrhythmias, cardiotoxicity, chest pain, congestive heart failure, decreased left ventricular ejection fraction, ECG changes
EENT: Blue-colored cornea, conjunctivitis, mucositis, stomatitis
GI: Abdominal pain, diarrhea, GI bleeding, nausea, vomiting
GU: Blue-green urine, renal failure
HEME: Acute myelogenous leukemia, leukopenia, other leukemias, thrombocytopenia
MS: Myelodysplasia
RESP: Cough, dyspnea
SKIN: Alopecia, extravasation, jaundice
Other: Allergic reaction, anaphylaxis, hyperuricemia, infection, infusion-site pain or redness

Nursing Considerations

• Before mitoxantrone therapy and before each dose, expect patient to have an ECG and evaluation of left ventricular ejection fraction. Expect to obtain hematocrit, hemoglobin level, and CBC with platelet count. If patient's left ventricular ejection fraction drops below normal, expect drug to be discontinued.
• Be aware that drug shouldn't be given to patient with multiple sclerosis whose neutrophil count is less than 1,500/mm³

or who has a below-normal left ventricular ejection fraction.
• Check liver function test results, as ordered, before each course of therapy. Expect that drug won't be given to multiple sclerosis patient with abnormal liver function.
• Assess patient for cardiac dysfunction throughout therapy. Watch for evidence of cardiotoxicity, such as arrhythmias and chest pain, in patient with heart disease. Risk increases when cumulative dose reaches 140 mg/m² in cancer or 100 mg/m² in multiple sclerosis. Notify prescriber of any significant changes, and expect drug to be discontinued. Be aware that congestive heart failure may occur months or years after drug has been discontinued.
• Anticipate obtaining pregnancy test before each course of therapy for women of childbearing age with multiple sclerosis.
• Follow facility policy for handling antineoplastics. Be aware that manufacturer recommends goggles, gloves, and a gown during drug preparation and delivery.
• Before infusing drug, dilute it in at least 50 ml of normal saline solution or D₅W.
WARNING Drug shouldn't be given intrathecally because paralysis may occur.
• If mitoxantrone solution contacts your skin or mucosa, wash thoroughly with warm water. If it contacts your eyes, irrigate them thoroughly with water or normal saline solution.
• Discard unused diluted solution because it contains no preservatives. After penetration of stopper, store undiluted drug for up to 7 days at room temperature or 14 days refrigerated. Avoid freezing drug.
• If extravasation occurs, stop infusion immediately and notify prescriber. Reinsert I.V. line in another vein and resume infusion. Although mitoxantrone is a nonvesicant, observe the extravasation site for signs of necrosis or phlebitis.
• Monitor patients with chickenpox or recent exposure and patients with herpes zoster for severe, generalized disease.
• Monitor blood uric acid level for hyperuricemia in patients with a history of gout or renal calculi. Expect to give allopurinol, as prescribed, to patients with

leukemia or lymphoma and elevated blood uric acid level to prevent uric acid nephropathy.

WARNING If severe or life-threatening nonhematologic or hematologic toxicity occurs during first induction course, expect to withhold the second course until it resolves.

• If patient develops thrombocytopenia, take precautions per facility policy.

• Assess patient for evidence of infection, such as fever, if leukopenia occurs. Expect to obtain appropriate specimens for culture and sensitivity testing.

• Be aware that patients receiving mitoxantrone in combination with other antineoplastics or radiation therapy or who have multiple sclerosis are at risk for developing secondary leukemia, including acute myelogenous leukemia.

PATIENT TEACHING

• Advise patient to complete dental work, if possible, before treatment begins or defer it until blood counts return to normal; drug may delay healing and cause gingival bleeding. Teach patient proper oral hygiene, and advise use of a toothbrush with soft bristles.

• Urge patient to drink plenty of fluid to increase urine output and uric acid excretion.

• Advise patient to contact prescriber immediately if GI upset occurs, but to continue taking drug unless otherwise directed.

• Emphasize the importance of complying with the dosage regimen and keeping follow-up medical and laboratory appointments.

• Explain that urine may appear blue-green for 24 hours after treatment and that the whites of the eyes may appear blue. Emphasize that these effects are temporary and harmless. Explain that hair loss is possible, but that hair should return after therapy ends.

• Caution patient not to receive immunizations unless approved by prescriber. Also, advise persons who live in same household as patient to avoid receiving immunization with oral polio vaccine. Tell patient to avoid persons who recently received the oral polio vaccine or to wear a mask over his nose and mouth.

• Instruct patient to avoid persons with infections if bone marrow depression occurs. Advise patient to contact prescriber if fever, chills, cough, hoarseness, lower back or side pain, or painful or difficult urination occurs; these changes may signal an infection.

• Tell patient to contact prescriber immediately if he has unusual bleeding or bruising, black or tarry stools, blood in urine or stool, or pinpoint red spots on his skin.

• Urge patient not to touch his eyes or the inside of his nose unless he has just washed his hands.

• Emphasize the need to avoid accidental cuts, as from a razor or fingernail clippers, because of possible excessive bleeding or infection.

• Caution patient to avoid contact sports or activities that may cause bruising or injury.

• Urge patient to comply with yearly examinations after therapy ends to check for late-occurring drug-induced heart problems. Tell patient to report trouble breathing, swelling in legs or ankles, or an uneven or fast heartbeat even after drug has been discontinued.

modafinil
Provigil

Class, Category, and Schedule
Chemical class: Benzhydryl sulfinylacetamide derivative
Therapeutic class: CNS stimulant
Pregnancy category: C
Controlled substance schedule: IV

Indications and Dosages
➤ *To improve daytime wakefulness in patients with narcolepsy, obstructive sleep apnea hypopnea syndrome, and shift work sleep disorder*

TABLETS
Adults and adolescents age 16 and over. 200 mg daily in the morning or 1 hr before starting work shift. *Maximum:* 400 mg daily.

DOSAGE ADJUSTMENT For patients with severe hepatic impairment, dosage should be reduced by 50%.

Mechanism of Action

May inhibit the release of gamma-aminobutyric acid (GABA), the most common inhibitory neurotransmitter, or CNS depressant, in the brain. Modafinil also increases the release of glutamate, an excitatory neurotransmitter, or CNS stimulant, in the thalamus and hippocampus. These two actions may improve wakefulness.

Contraindications

Hypersensitivity to modafinil or its components

Interaction

DRUGS

amitriptyline, citalopram, clomipramine, diazepam, imipramine, propranolol, tolbutamide, topiramate: Possibly prolonged elimination time and increased blood levels of these drugs
carbamazepine: Possibly decreased modafinil effectiveness and decreased blood carbamazepine level
cimetidine, clarithromycin, erythromycin, fluconazole, fluoxetine, fluvoxamine, itraconazole, ketoconazole, nefazodone, sertraline: Possibly inhibited metabolism, decreased clearance, and increased blood level of modafinil
contraceptive-containing implants or devices, oral contraceptives: Possibly contraceptive failure
cyclosporine: Possibly decreased blood cyclosporine level and increased risk of organ transplant rejection
dexamethasone, phenobarbital and other barbiturates, primidone, rifabutin, rifampin: Possibly decreased blood level and effectiveness of modafinil
dextroamphetamine, methylphenidate: Possibly 1-hour delay in modafinil absorption when these drugs are given together
fosphenytoin, mephenytoin, phenytoin: Possibly decreased effectiveness of modafinil, increased blood phenytoin level, and increased risk of phenytoin toxicity
theophylline: Possibly decreased blood level and effectiveness of theophylline
triazolam: Possibly decreased effectiveness of triazolam
warfarin: Possibly decreased warfarin metabolism and increased risk of bleeding

FOODS

all foods: 1-hour delay in modafinil absorption and possibly delayed onset of action
caffeine: Increased CNS stimulation
grapefruit juice: Possibly decreased modafinil metabolism

Adverse Reactions

CNS: Aggressiveness, agitation, anxiety, confusion, delusions, depression, hallucinations, headache, insomnia, mania, nervousness, psychosis, suicidal ideation
GI: Nausea
HEME: Agranulocytosis
SKIN: Drug rash with eosinophilia and systemic symptoms (DRESS), rash, Stevens-Johnson syndrome, toxic epidermal necrolysis
Other: Anaphylaxis, angioedema, infection, multi-organ hypersensitivity

Nursing Considerations

• Modafinil shouldn't be given to patients with mitral valve prolapse syndrome or a history of left ventricular hypertrophy because drug may cause ischemic changes.
• Use cautiously in patients with recent MI or unstable angina because effect of drug is unknown in these disorders.
• Use cautiously in patients with a history of psychosis, depression, or mania because these conditions may worsen during therapy and may require modafinil to be stopped.
WARNING Monitor patient with a history of alcoholism, stimulant abuse, or other substance abuse for compliance with modafinil therapy. Observe for signs of misuse or abuse, including frequent prescription refill requests, increased frequency of dosing, or drug-seeking behavior. Also watch for evidence of excessive modafinil dosage, including aggressiveness, anxiety, confusion, decreased prothrombin time, diarrhea, irritability, nausea, nervousness, palpitations, sleep disturbances, and tremor.
• Be aware that modafinil, like other CNS stimulants, may alter mood, perception, thinking, judgment, feelings, motor skills, and signs that patient needs sleep.
• If giving drug to patient with a history of psychosis, emotional instability, or

psychological illness with psychotic features, be prepared to perform baseline behavioral assessments or frequent clinical observation.

• Stop drug at first sign of rash, and notify prescriber. Although rare, rash may indicate a potentially life-threatening event.

• Monitor patient for signs and symptoms of multisystem organ hypersensitivity, such as fever, rash, myocarditis, hepatitis, hematologic abnormalities, pruritus, asthenia, or any other serious abnormality, because multi-organ hypersensitivity may vary in its presentation. Notify prescriber if suspected, and expect to discontinue drug and provide supportive care, as ordered.

• Watch closely for suicidal tendencies, especially in patients with a psychiatric history.

PATIENT TEACHING

• Inform patient that modafinil can help, but not cure, narcolepsy and that drug's full effects may not be seen right away.

• Advise patient to avoid taking modafinil within 1 hour of eating because food may delay drug's absorption and onset of action. If he drinks grapefruit juice, encourage him to drink a consistent amount daily.

• Instruct patient to stop taking modafinil and to notify prescriber if he develops a rash, fever, or other serious effect.

• Urge patient to report chest pain, depression, anxiety, or evidence of psychosis or mania to prescriber.

• Inform patient that drug can affect concentration and function and can hide signs of fatigue. Urge him not to drive or perform activities that require mental alertness until full CNS effects are known.

• Because alcohol may decrease alertness, advise patient to avoid it while taking modafinil.

• Encourage a regular sleeping pattern.

• Caution patient to avoid excessive intake of foods, beverages, and OTC drugs that contain caffeine because caffeine may lead to increased CNS stimulation.

• Inform female patient that modafinil can decrease the effectiveness of certain contraceptives, including birth control pills and implantable hormonal contraceptives. If she uses such contraceptives, urge her to use an alternate birth control method during modafinil therapy and for up to 1 month after she stops taking the drug.

• Advise patient to keep follow-up appointments with prescriber so that her progress can be monitored.

• Urge family or caregiver to watch patient closely for abnormal behaviors, including suicidal tendencies, especially if patient has a psychiatric history.

moexipril hydrochloride

Univasc

Class and Category

Chemical class: Prodrug of moexiprilat
Therapeutic class: Antihypertensive
Pregnancy category: D

Indications and Dosages

➤ *To manage hypertension without diuretic therapy*

TABLETS

Adults. *Initial:* 7.5 mg daily 1 hr before a meal. *Maintenance:* 7.5 to 30 mg as a single dose or in divided doses twice daily. 1 hr before meals. *Maximum:* 30 mg/day.

DOSAGE ADJUSTMENT For patients with creatinine clearance of less than 40 ml/min/1.73 m², initial dosage reduced to 3.75 mg daily and increased, as ordered, to maximum of 15 mg daily.

➤ *To manage hypertension with diuretic therapy*

TABLETS

Adults. *Initial:* 3.75 mg daily 1 hr before a meal. Increased gradually, as ordered, until blood pressure is controlled.

Route	Onset	Peak	Duration
P.O.	1 hr	3–6 hr	24 hr

Mechanism of Action

Is converted to the active metabolite moexiprilat, which reduces blood pressure by inhibiting ACE activity. ACE normally catalyzes conversion of angiotensin I to angiotensin II—a vasoconstrictor that stimulates aldosterone secretion by adrenal cortex and directly suppresses renin release. Inhibited ACE activity results in decreased peripheral arterial resistance, increased plasma renin activity, and decreased aldosterone secretion. Decreased aldosterone secretion causes water and sodium excretion.

Contraindications
Concurrent aliskiren (in patients with diabetes), history of angioedema with previous ACE inhibitor use, hypersensitivity to moexipril or its components

Interaction
DRUGS
aliskiren (in patients with diabetes), angiotensin receptor blockers, other ACE inhibitors: Increased risk of hyperkalemia, hypotension, and renal dysfunction
allopurinol, bone marrow depressants, corticosteroids (systemic), cytostatic drugs, procainamide: Increased risk of possibly fatal neutropenia or agranulocytosis
antacids: Possibly decreased moexipril bioavailability
cyclosporine, heparin, potassium-containing drugs, potassium-sparing diuretics, potassium supplements: Increased risk of hyperkalemia
digoxin: Possibly increased digoxin level
diuretics, other hypotension-producing drugs: Hypotension, risk of renal failure (from sodium or volume depletion), possibly decreased secondary aldosteronism and hypokalemia caused by diuretics
lithium: Increased blood lithium level and risk of lithium toxicity
NSAIDs: Decreased antihypertensive effect of moexipril; possible decreased renal function in patients who are elderly or have volume-depletion or preexisting renal dysfunction
phenothiazines: Increased pharmacologic effects of moexipril
sympathomimetics: Decreased anti-hypertensive effect of moexipril
sodium aurothiomalate: Possibly nitritoid reaction with facial flushing, nausea, vomiting, and hypotension
FOODS
all foods: Decreased moexipril absorption
low-salt milk, salt substitutes: Possibly hyperkalemia
ACTIVITIES
alcohol use: Possibly hypotension

Adverse Reactions
CNS: Anxiety, chills, confusion, dizziness, drowsiness, fatigue, fever, headache, malaise, mood changes, nervousness, sleep disturbance, stroke, syncope
CV: Angina, arrhythmias, chest pain, hypotension, MI, orthostatic hypotension, palpitations, peripheral edema
EENT: Dry mouth, hoarseness, laryngeal edema, mouth or tongue swelling, pharyngitis, rhinitis, sinusitis, taste perversion, tinnitus
GI: Abdominal distention or pain, anorexia, constipation, diarrhea, dysphagia, elevated liver function test results, hepatitis, increased appetite, nausea, pancreatitis, vomiting
GU: Azotemia, elevated BUN and serum creatinine and uric acid levels, interstitial nephritis, oliguria, proteinuria, renal insufficiency, urinary frequency
HEME: Agranulocytosis, bone marrow depression, elevated erythrocyte sedimentation rate, hemolytic anemia, leukocytosis, leukopenia, neutropenia, thrombocytopenia
MS: Arthralgia, leg heaviness or weakness, myalgia, myositis
RESP: Bronchospasm, cough, dyspnea, upper respiratory tract infection
SKIN: Alopecia, diaphoresis, flushing, onycholysis, pallor, pemphigus, photo-sensitivity, pruritus, rash, Stevens-Johnson syndrome, urticaria
Other: Anaphylaxis, angioedema (of arms, face, larynx, legs, lips, mucous membranes, tongue), flulike symptoms, hyperkalemia, hyponatremia, positive ANA titer

Nursing Considerations
WARNING Contact prescriber if patient is or may be pregnant. Moexipril may cause fetal or neonatal harm or death if used during second or third trimester.
• Be aware that patient who already takes a diuretic should be medically supervised for several hours after first moexipril dose.
• Administer drug 1 hour before meals.
• Monitor blood pressure, leukocyte count, and liver and renal function test results during moexipril therapy.
• Be aware that black patients may be less responsive to antihypertensive effect if moexipril is used alone to control blood pressure.

• Urge female patient to notify prescriber immediately if she is or may be pregnant.
• Instruct patient to take moexipril at the same time each day, 1 hour before meals.
• Direct patient to take a missed dose as soon as he remembers unless it's nearly time for the next dose. Caution against doubling the dose.

WARNING Instruct patient to stop drug and seek immediate medical attention for hoarseness; swelling of tongue, glottis, larynx, face, hands, or feet; or sudden difficulty swallowing or breathing.
• Caution patient not to stop drug without consulting prescriber, even if he feels better.
• Inform patient about possible dizziness, especially after first dose and if he takes a diuretic.
• Advise patient to change position slowly to minimize orthostatic hypotension.
• Caution patient to avoid hazardous activities until drug's CNS effects are known.
• Instruct patient to notify prescriber if he faints or experiences persistent dizziness.
• Instruct patient to report evidence of infection (such as chills, fever, and sore throat), diarrhea, nausea, or vomiting, which may lead to dehydration-induced hypotension.
• Advise patient to avoid alcohol during moexipril therapy because it may cause hypotension.
• Instruct patient to check with prescriber before taking OTC drugs.
• Urge patient to avoid potassium supplements and potassium-containing salt substitutes unless prescriber allows them.
• Advise patient to visit prescriber regularly to monitor progress.
• Discuss importance of weight control and low-salt diet in managing hypertension.

molindone hydrochloride

Moban Concentrate

Class and Category
Chemical class: Dihydroindolone derivative
Therapeutic class: Antipsychotic drug
Pregnancy category: Not rated

Indications and Dosages
➤ *To manage symptoms of psychotic disorders*

ORAL SOLUTION
Adults and children age 12 and over.
Initial: 50 to 75 mg daily in divided doses three times daily or four times daily. Dosage increased to 100 mg daily in 3 to 4 days, as needed. *Maintenance:* For mild psychosis, 5 to 15 mg three times daily or four times daily; for moderate psychosis, 10 to 25 mg three times daily or four times daily; for severe psychosis, 225 mg daily in divided doses. *Maximum:* 225 mg daily.
DOSAGE ADJUSTMENT Initial dosage reduced for elderly or debilitated patients.

Route	Onset	Peak	Duration
P.O.	Unknown	Unknown	24–36 hr

Mechanism of Action
Occupies dopamine receptor sites in the reticular activating and limbic systems in the CNS. By blocking dopamine activity in these areas, molindone reduces the symptoms of psychosis, helping the patient to think and behave more coherently.

Contraindications
Hypersensitivity to molindone, its components, or other antipsychotic drugs, including haloperidol, loxapine, phenothiazines, and thioxanthenes

Interaction
DRUGS
amphetamines: Decreased amphetamine effectiveness, decreased antipsychotic effectiveness of molindone
anesthetics, barbiturates, benzodiazepines, CNS depressants, opioid analgesics: Possibly prolonged and intensified CNS depressant effects
antacids, antidiarrheals: Decreased molindone absorption
anticholinergics, antidyskinetics, antihistamines: Possibly increased anticholinergic effects
beta blockers: Possibly increased effect of beta blocker
bromocriptine: Possibly decreased therapeutic effects of bromocriptine and increased serum prolactin level
extrapyramidal reaction–causing drugs, such as amoxapine, haloperidol, loxapine,

M

metoclopramide, olanzapine, phenothiazines, pimozide, rauwolfia alkaloids, risperidone, tacrine, and thioxanthenes: Increased severity of extrapyramidal effects
insulin, oral antidiabetic drugs: Possibly increased serum glucose level
levodopa: Inhibited antidyskinetic effects of levodopa, possibly decreased antipsychotic effects of molindone
lithium: Increased risk of neurotoxicity, increased extrapyramidal effects
MAO inhibitors, maprotiline, trazodone, tricyclic antidepressants: Possibly prolonged and intensified sedative or anticholinergic effects of all drugs
phenytoin, tetracycline: Interference with absorption of phenytoin and tetracycline

ACTIVITIES
alcohol use: Prolonged and intensified CNS depression

Adverse Reactions

CNS: Depression, drowsiness, euphoria, extrapyramidal reactions (such as akathisia, dystonia, motor restlessness, pseudo-parkinsonism, and tardive dyskinesia), headache, hyperactivity, lack of coordination, neuroleptic malignant syndrome, tiredness
CV: Orthostatic hypotension, tachycardia, unstable blood pressure
EENT: Blinking or eyelid spasm, blurred vision, dry mouth, inability to move eyes, nasal congestion
ENDO: Breast engorgement, lactation
GI: Constipation, nausea
GU: Decreased libido, menstrual irregularities, urine retention
HEME: Agranulocytosis, leukopenia, neutropenia
MS: Muscle spasms of back, face, and neck; muscle twitching; twisting movements of the body; weakness or stiffness of limbs
RESP: Dyspnea
SKIN: Diaphoresis, pallor, rash
Other: Heatstroke

Nursing Considerations

• Molindone shouldn't be used to treat dementia-related psychosis in the elderly because of an increased mortality risk.
• **WARNING** Assess patient for signs and symptoms of neuroleptic malignant syndrome, such as diaphoresis, dyspnea, fatigue, fever, incontinence, pallor, severe

muscle stiffness, tachycardia, and unstable blood pressure; notify prescriber immediately if they occur. Expect to discontinue drug and begin intensive medical treatment. Monitor patient carefully for recurrence if antipsychotic therapy resumes.
• Molindone shouldn't be given to patients who have severe CNS depression or who are comatose because of drug's CNS depressant effects.
• Monitor elderly patients for orthostatic hypotension and symptoms of tardive dyskinesia, including blinking or eyelid spasms, involuntary movements of the limbs, and unusual facial expressions, because these patients may be sensitive to drug's anticholinergic and extrapyramidal effects. Expect to reduce dosage or discontinue drug.
• Give oral solution undiluted or mixed with water, carbonated beverage, fruit juice, or milk.
• Monitor CBC often during first few months of therapy, especially if patient has low WBC count or history of drug-induced leukopenia or neutropenia. If WBC count drops, and especially if neutrophil count drops below 1000/mm³, expect molindone to be discontinued. If neutropenia is significant, also monitor patient for fever or other evidence of infection and provide appropriate treatment, as prescribed.

PATIENT TEACHING
• Instruct patient to follow treatment regimen and to notify prescriber before discontinuing drug because gradual dosage reduction may be needed.
• Instruct patient not to take drug within 2 hours of taking an antacid. Advise him to take drug with food or a full glass of milk or water to reduce gastric irritation.
• Instruct patient to take oral solution undiluted or mixed with water, carbonated beverage, fruit juice, or milk.
• Urge patient to avoid alcohol consumption because of possible additive effects and hypotension.
• Advise patient, especially an elderly patient, to rise slowly from a supine or seated position to avoid feeling dizzy, light-headed, or faint.
• Explain that drug may reduce body's response to heat. Tell patient to avoid

temperature extremes, such as hot showers, tubs, or saunas. Urge caution during exercise.

• Caution patient not to take OTC drugs for colds or allergies during therapy because they can increase the risk of heatstroke and increase anticholinergic effects, such as blurred vision, constipation, dry mouth, and urine retention.

• Inform patient and family members that maximum clinical improvement in symptoms may take several weeks or months.

• Advise female patient of childbearing age to notify prescriber if she intends to become or suspects that she is pregnant during therapy.

mometasone furoate monohydrate

Asmanex, Nasonex

Class and Category
Chemical class: Glucocorticoid
Therapeutic class: Antiasthmatic, anti-inflammatory
Pregnancy category: C

Indications and Dosages
➤ *To manage symptoms of seasonal or perennial allergic rhinitis*
NASAL SPRAY
Adults and children 12 years and over. 100 mcg (2 sprays) in each nostril daily.
Children ages 2 to 12. 50 mcg (1 spray) in each nostril daily.
➤ *To maintain asthma control*
ORAL INHALATION
Adults and children age 12 and over who have been taking bronchodilators alone or inhaled corticosteroids. *Initial:* 220 mcg (1 inhalation) once daily in evening. *Maximum:* 440 mcg (2 inhalations) daily given as 220 mcg (1 inhalation) twice daily or 440 mcg (1 inhalation) once daily.
Adults and children age 12 and over who have taken oral corticosteroids. 440 mcg (2 inhalations) twice daily.
Children ages 4 to 11. 110 mcg (1 inhalation) once daily in evening.

Mechanism of Action
Inhibits the activity of cells and mediators active in the inflammatory response, possibly by decreasing influx of inflammatory cells into nasal passages and thereby decreasing nasal inflammation.

Contraindications
Hypersensitivity to mometasone or its components or to milk proteins; recent septal ulcers, nasal surgery, or nasal trauma; status asthmaticus or other asthma episodes that require emergency care

Adverse Reactions
CNS: Headache
CV: Chest pain
EENT: Cataracts, conjunctivitis, dry mouth, earache, epistaxis, glaucoma, nasal irritation, oral and pharyngeal candidiasis, otitis media, pharyngitis, rhinitis, sinusitis, throat tightness, unpleasant taste
ENDO: Adrenal insufficiency, growth suppression
GI: Diarrhea, dyspepsia, nausea, vomiting
GU: Dysmenorrhea
MS: Arthralgia, decreased bone mineral density, myalgia, pain
RESP: Asthma, bronchitis, bronchospasm, increased cough, upper respiratory tract infection, wheezing
SKIN: Pruritus, rash, urticaria
Other: Anaphylaxis, angioedema, flulike symptoms, viral infection

Nursing Considerations
WARNING Be aware that Asmanex brand of mometasone contains small amounts of lactose, which contains trace levels of milk proteins. Do not administer to patients with a milk protein allergy because anaphylactic reactions have occurred.

• Use mometasone cautiously if patient has tubercular infection; untreated fungal, bacterial, or systemic viral infection; or ocular herpes simplex.

• If patient takes an oral corticosteroid, expect to taper it slowly 1 week after changing to mometasone. If patient takes prednisone, expect to reduce it by no more than 2.5 mg daily at weekly intervals, beginning at least 1 week after mometasone therapy starts. Monitor patient for symptoms of systemically active corticosteroid withdrawal such as joint and muscle pain, lassitude, and depression despite maintenance or even improvement of respiratory symptoms. **WARNING** Assess patient switched from systemic corticosteroid to mometasone for adrenal insufficiency (fatigue, hypotension, lassitude, nausea, vomiting, weakness) during initial treatment and during stress, trauma, surgery, infection or an electrolyte-depleting condition. Notify prescriber immediately if signs or symptoms arise because adrenal insufficiency may be life-threatening. Hypothalamic-pituitary-adrenal axis function may take several months to recover after systemic corticosteroids are discontinued. Abrupt withdrawal of mometasone also may precipitate adrenal insufficiency.

• Notify prescriber immediately if patient has bronchospasm after mometasone oral inhalation, and expect to give a fast-acting inhaled bronchodilator, discontinue mometasone, and use an alternate drug.

• Closely monitor a child's growth pattern; drug may stunt growth.

• Report oropharyngeal candidiasis, and expect patient to receive appropriate antifungal therapy while remaining on mometasone therapy. If candidiasis is severe, however, mometasone therapy may need to be temporarily halted.

PATIENT TEACHING

• For nasal spray, instruct patient to shake container before each use. Instruct her to blow her nose, tilt her head slightly forward, and insert tube into a nostril, pointing toward inner corner of eye, away from nasal septum. Tell her to hold the other nostril closed and spray while inhaling gently. Then have her repeat the procedure in the other nostril.

• For oral inhalation, give patient these instructions for using inhaler: Remove cap only after placing inhaler in an upright position. Twist cap in counterclockwise while holding colored base, making sure indented arrow (on white portion of the inhaler directly above the colored base) is pointing to the dose counter. Removing the cap loads inhaler with drug, and the dose counter on the base will count down by one. Take a full breath in and out, and then place mouthpiece in your mouth. Firmly close your lips around mouthpiece, taking care not to cover ventilation holes on the inhaler. Then take a fast, deep breath. You may not taste, smell, or feel anything with the inhalation. After taking the breath, remove inhaler from your mouth and hold your breath for about 10 seconds. Don't exhale into the inhaler. Wipe the mouthpiece dry, if needed, and replace the cap right away, turning it clockwise as you press down. You should hear a click when the cap is fully closed. Write down the date inhaler is opened, and discard it 45 days from that date or when dose counter reads 00, whichever comes first.

• Instruct patient to gargle or rinse after each use of oral inhaler to help prevent mouth and throat dryness, relieve throat irritation, and prevent oropharyngeal infection.

WARNING Caution patient not to use mometasone oral inhalation to relieve acute bronchospasm and to notify prescriber if rescue inhaler is required more often or doesn't seem to be as effective.

• If patient switches from an oral corticosteroid to mometasone, advise her to carry or wear medical identification indicating the need for supplemental systemic corticosteroids during stress or severe asthma attack. Tell her to seek emergency care if either occurs.

• Instruct patient to contact prescriber if symptoms persist or worsen after 3 weeks.

• Caution patient to avoid exposure to chickenpox and measles and, if exposed, to contact prescriber immediately.

montelukast sodium

Singulair

Class and Category

Chemical class: Leukotriene receptor antagonist
Therapeutic class: Antiasthmatic
Pregnancy category: B

Indications and Dosages
➤ *To prevent or treat asthma*
ORAL GRANULES
Children ages 12 to 23 mo. 4 mg daily in the evening. *Maximum:* 4 mg daily.
CHEWABLE TABLETS
Children ages 6 to 14. 5 mg daily in the evening. *Maximum:* 5 mg daily.
Children ages 2 to 5. 4 mg daily in the evening. *Maximum:* 4 mg daily.
TABLETS
Adults and adolescents age 15 and over. 10 mg daily in the evening. *Maximum:* 10 mg daily.
➤ *To treat seasonal allergic rhinitis*
ORAL GRANULES
Children ages 2 to 5. 4 mg daily.
CHEWABLE TABLETS
Children ages 6 to 14. 5 mg daily.
Children ages 2 to 5. 4 mg daily.
TABLETS
Adults and adolescents age 15 and over. 10 mg daily.
➤ *To treat perennial allergic rhinitis*
ORAL GRANULES
Children ages 6 months to 5 years. 4 mg daily.
CHEWABLE TABLETS
Children ages 6 to 14. 5 mg daily.
Children ages 2 to 5. 4 mg daily.
TABLETS
Adults and adolescents age 15 and over. 10 mg daily.
➤ *To prevent exercise-induced broncho-constriction*
TABLETS
Adults and adolescents age 15 and over. 10 mg at least 2 hr before exercise. *Maximum:* 10 mg in 24 hr.

Route	Onset	Peak	Duration
P.O.	Unknown	Unknown	24 hr

Mechanism of Action
Antagonizes receptors for cysteinyl leukotrienes, produced by arachidonic acid metabolism and released from mast cells, eosinophils, and other cells. When cysteinyl leukotrienes bind to receptors in bronchial airways, they increase endothelial membrane permeability, which leads to airway edema, smooth-muscle contraction, and altered activity of cells in asthma's inflammatory process. Montelukast blocks these effects.

Interaction
DRUGS
phenobarbital: Decreased amount of circulating montelukast

Adverse Reactions
CNS: Aggression, agitation, anxiousness, asthenia, attention disturbance, depression, disorientation, dizziness, dream abnor-malities, drowsiness, fatigue, fever, hallucinations, headache, hostility, hypoesthesia, insomnia, irritability, memory impairment, paresthesia, restlessness, seizures, sleep walking, somnolence, suicidal ideation, tremor
CV: Palpitations, edema
EENT: Dental pain, epistaxis, laryngitis, nasal congestion, otitis media, pharyngitis, sinusitis
GI: Abdominal pain, cholestatic hepatitis, diarrhea, dyspepsia, elevated liver function test results, hepatic eosinophilic infiltration, hepatotoxicity, indigestion, infectious gastroenteritis; diarrhea, nausea, pancreatitis, vomiting
GU: Enuresis (children), pyuria
HEME: Increased bleeding tendency, systemic eosinophilia, thrombocytopenia
MS: Arthralgia, muscle cramps, myalgia
RESP: Cough, upper respiratory tract infection, pulmonary eosinophilia
SKIN: Erythema multiforme, erythema nodosum, pruritus, rash, Stevens-Johnson syndrome, toxic epidermal necrolysis, urticaria
Other: Anaphylaxis, angioedema (in all patients); flulike syndrome, viral infection (in children)

Nursing Considerations
WARNING Montelukast isn't for acute asthma attack or status asthmaticus.
•Montelukast shouldn't be abruptly substituted for inhaled or oral corticosteroids; expect to taper corticosteroid dosage gradually, as directed.
•Monitor patient for adverse reactions, such as cardiac and pulmonary symptoms, eosinophilia, and vasculitis, in patient undergoing corticosteroid withdrawal. Notify prescriber if such reactions occur.
•Watch patient closely for suicidal tendencies during montelukast therapy,

M

especially when therapy starts or dosage changes.

• Monitor patient for adverse neuro-psychiatric effects and notify prescriber if present. Drug may need to be discontinued.

PATIENT TEACHING

• Advise patient to take montelukast daily as prescribed, even when he feels well. Urge him not to decrease dosage or stop taking other prescribed asthma drugs unless instructed by prescriber.

• Caution patient not to use drug for acute asthma attack or status asthmaticus; make sure he has appropriate short-acting rescue drug available.

• Tell parents administering oral granules to pour contents directly into the child's mouth or mix with ice cream or cold or room temperature applesauce, carrots, or rice—but not liquids or other foods—just before administration. Liquids may be given after drug has been administered. Once packet is opened, the full dose must be administered within 15 minutes. Drug must not be stored for future use if mixed with food.

• Instruct patient to notify prescriber if he needs a short-acting inhaled broncho-dilator more often than usual, or more often than prescribed, to control symptoms.

• Teach patient to use a peak flowmeter to determine his personal best expiratory volume.

• Caution patient with aspirin sensitivity to avoid aspirin and NSAIDs during montelukast therapy. Montelukast may not effectively reduce bronchospasm in such a patient.

• Inform patient (or parents of child) with phenylketonuria that chewable tablet contains phenylalanine.

• Instruct patient to notify prescriber if she is or could be pregnant.

• Urge family or caregiver to watch patient closely for abnormal behaviors, including suicidal tendencies, during therapy, and urge them to notify prescriber if present.

• Instruct patient to report increased bleeding tendency or severe skin reaction that occurs without warning immediately to prescriber.

morphine sulfate

Astramorph PF, Avinza, DepoDur, Duramorph, Epimorph (can), Kadian, M-Eslon (can), Morphine Extra-Forte (can), Morphine Forte (can), Morphine H.P. (can), Morphitec (can), MS Contin, MSIR, MS/L, MS/L Concentrate, MS/S, OMS Concentrate, Oramorph SR, Rescudose, RMS Uniserts, Roxanol, Roxanol 100, Roxanol UD, Statex (can)

Class, Category, and Schedule

Chemical class: Phenanthrene derivative
Therapeutic class: Analgesic
Pregnancy category: C
Controlled substance schedule: II

Indications and Dosages

➤ *To relieve acute or chronic moderate to severe pain; as adjunct to treat pulmonary edema caused by left-sided heart failure; to supplement general, local, or regional anesthesia*

CAPSULES, ORAL SOLUTION, SYRUP, TABLETS

Adults. *Initial:* 10 to 30 mg every 4 hr, as needed.

Children. Individualized dosage based on patient's age, size, and need.

I.V. INFUSION

Adults. *Initial:* 15 mg (or more) followed by 0.8 to 10 mg/hr, increased, as needed, for effectiveness. *Maintenance:* 0.8 to 80 mg/hr.

Children. 0.01 to 0.04 mg/kg/hr postoperatively, 0.025 to 2.6 mg/kg/hr for severe chronic cancer pain, or 0.03 to 0.15 mg/kg/hr for sickle cell crisis.

Neonates. *Initial:* 0.010 mg/kg/hr (10 mcg/kg/hr) postoperatively. *Maintenance:* 0.015 to 0.02 mg/kg/hr (15 to 20 mcg/kg/hr).

I.V. INJECTION

Adults. 2.5 to 15 mg injected slowly.

Children. 0.5 to 0.1 mg/kg given slowly.

I.M. OR SUBCUTANEOUS INJECTION

Adults. *Initial:* 10 mg (based on 70-kg [154-lb] adult) every 4 hr. *Maintenance:* 5 to 20 mg.

Children. *Initial:* 0.1 to 0.2 mg/kg every 4 hr. *Maximum:* 15 mg/dose.

EPIDURAL INFUSION (PRESERVATIVE-FREE)

Adults. *Initial:* 2 to 4 mg/24 hr, increased by 1 to 2 mg/24 hr, as directed.

EPIDURAL INJECTION (PRESERVATIVE-FREE)
Adults. *Initial:* 5 mg into lumbar region. If pain isn't relieved after 1 hr, 1- to 2-mg doses given at appropriate intervals to relieve pain. *Maximum:* 10 mg/24 hr.
INTRATHECAL INJECTION (PRESERVATIVE-FREE)
Adults. 0.2 to 1 mg as a single dose.
SUPPOSITORIES
Adults. 10 to 30 mg every 4 hr, as needed.
Children. Individualized dosage based on patient's age, size, and need.
➤ *To manage moderate to severe pain when a continuous, around-the-clock opioid analgesic is needed for an extended period of time*
E.R. CAPSULES (AVINZA)
Adults using morphine as the first opioid analgesic. *Initial:* 30 mg once daily at 24-hour intervals, increased by 30 mg every 4 days, as needed.
Adults converting from other oral morphine formulations: Total previous daily dose every 24 hrs.
Adults converting from parenteral morphine. Highly individualized. *Usual:* 3 times the previous daily parenteral morphine dosage.
Adults converting from other nonmorphine opioids (oral or parenteral). Highly individualized. *Usual:* Half of the estimated daily morphine requirements every 24 hr, and then increased as needed.
E.R. TABLETS (MS CONTIN)
Adults converting from other oral morphine formulations. One-half of patient's previous 24-hr requirements every 12 hr. Alternatively, one-third of patient's previous 24-hr. requirements every 8 hr.
Adults converting from parenteral morphine. Highly individualized. *Usual:* 3 times the previous daily parenteral morphine dosage.
Adults converting from other parenteral or oral nonmorphine opioids. Highly individualized. *Usual:* Half of the estimated daily morphine requirements, and then increased as needed.
➤ *To relieve MI pain*
I.V. INJECTION
Adults. 1 to 4 mg by slow I.V. injection. Repeated up to every 5 min, if needed. *Maximum:* 2 to 15 mg.
➤ *To provide preoperative analgesia*

I.M. OR SUBCUTANEOUS INJECTION
Adults. 5 to 20 mg given 45 to 60 min before surgery.
Children. 0.05 to 0.1 mg/kg given 45 to 60 min before surgery. *Maximum:* 10 mg.
➤ *To provide analgesia during labor*
I.M. OR SUBCUTANEOUS INJECTION
Adults. 10 mg, with subsequent doses based on patient's response.

Route	Onset	Peak	Duration
P.O.	Unknown	1–2 hr	4–5 hr
P.O. (E.R.)	Unknown	Unknown	8–12 hr
I.V.	Unknown	20 min	4–5 hr
I.M.	10–30 min	30–60 min	4–5 hr
SubQ	10–30 min	50–90 min	4–5 hr
Epidural	15–60 min	Unknown	Up to 24 hr
Intrathecal	15–60 min	Unknown	Up to 24 hr
P.R.	20–60 min	Unknown	Unknown

Mechanism of Action
Binds with and activates opioid receptors (mainly mu receptors) in brain and spinal cord to produce analgesia and euphoria.

Contraindications
For all drug forms: Acute or severe bronchial asthma in an unmonitored setting or in the absence of resuscitative equipment, hypersensitivity to morphine or its components, labor (premature delivery), prematurity (in infants), respiratory depression, upper airway obstruction
For E.R. formulations: Paralytic ileus
For oral solution: Acute abdominal disorders, acute alcoholism, alcohol withdrawal syndrome, arrhythmias, brain tumor, head injuries, heart failure caused by chronic lung disease, increased intracranial or cerebrospinal pressure, recent biliary tract surgery, respiratory insufficiency, seizure disorders, severe CNS depression, surgical anastomosis, use within 14 days of an MAO inhibitor
For I.V., I.M., or subcutaneous injection: Acute alcoholism, alcohol withdrawal syndrome, arrhythmias, brain tumor, heart failure caused by chronic lung disease, seizure disorders

M

For epidural or intrathecal injection:
Anticoagulant therapy, bleeding tendency, injection-site infection, parenteral corticosteroid treatment (or other treatment or condition that prohibits drug delivery by intrathecal or epidural route) within 2 weeks

Interaction
DRUGS
amitriptyline, clomipramine, nortriptyline: Increased CNS and respiratory depression
anticholinergics: Possibly severe constipation leading to ileus, urine retention
antidiarrheals (such as loperamide and paregoric): CNS depression, possibly severe constipation
antihistamines, chloral hydrate, glutethimide, MAO inhibitors, methocarbamol: Increased CNS and respiratory depressant effects
antihypertensives, hypotension-producing drugs: Increased hypotension, risk of orthostatic hypotension
bupivacaine: Increased serum morphine level and possibly significant adverse effects
buprenorphine: Decreased therapeutic effects of morphine, increased respiratory depression, possibly withdrawal symptoms
cimetidine: Increased analgesic and CNS and respiratory depressant effects
CNS depressants (antiemetics, general anesthetics, hypnotics, opioids, phenothiazines, sedatives, tranquilizers): Possibly coma, hypotension, respiratory depression, severe sedation
diuretics: Decreased diuretic efficacy
hydroxyzine: Increased analgesic, CNS depressant, and hypotensive effects of morphine
metoclopramide: Possibly antagonized metoclopramide effect on GI motility
mixed agonist-antagonist analgesics: Possibly withdrawal symptoms
naloxone: Antagonized analgesic and CNS and respiratory depressant effects of morphine, possibly withdrawal symptoms
naltrexone: Possibly induction or worsening of withdrawal symptoms if morphine given within 7 to 10 days before naltrexone
neuromuscular blockers: Increased or prolonged respiratory depression
opioid analgesics (such as alfentanil and sufentanil): Increased CNS and respiratory depression, increased hypotension

zidovudine: Decreased zidovudine clearance
ACTIVITIES
alcohol use: Increased CNS and respiratory depression, increased hypotension

Adverse Reactions
CNS: Agitation, amnesia, anxiety, ataxia, chills, coma, confusion, decreased concentration, delirium, delusions, depression, dizziness, dream abnormalities, drowsiness, edema, euphoria, fever, gait disturbance, hallucinations, headache, increased intracranial pressure, insomnia, lethargy, light-headedness, malaise, mood alterations, psychosis, restlessness, rigidity, sedation, seizures, syncope, thinking disturbances, thirst, tremor, unarousable, uncoordinated muscle movements, unresponsiveness, vertigo, weakness
CV: Bradycardia, cardiac arrest, edema, hypertension, hypotension, orthostatic hypotension, palpitations, shock, tachycardia, vasodilation
EENT: Amblyopia, blurred vision, diplopia, dry mouth, eye pain, hiccup, laryngeal edema or laryngospasm (allergic), miosis, nystagmus, rhinitis, taste or voice alteration
ENDO: Hypogonadism
GI: Abdominal cramps or pain, anorexia, biliary tract spasm, constipation, diarrhea, dysphagia, elevated liver function test results, gastroenteritis, gastroesophageal reflux, hiccups, ileus and toxic megacolon (in patients with inflammatory bowel disease), intestinal obstruction, indigestion, nausea, vomiting
GU: Decreased ejaculate potency, decreased libido, difficult ejaculation, dysuria, impotence, menstrual irregularities, oliguria, prolonged labor, urinary hesitancy, urine retention
HEME: Anemia, leukopenia, thrombocytopenia
MS: Arthralgia, decreased bone mineral density, skeletal muscle rigidity
RESP: Apnea, asthma exacerbation, atelectasis, bronchospasm, depressed cough reflex, hypoventilation, pulmonary edema, respiratory arrest and depression, wheezing
SKIN: Diaphoresis, dryness, flushing, pallor, pruritus, rash, urticaria
Other: Allergic reaction; anaphylaxis; facial edema; injection-site edema, pain, rash, or

redness; physical and psychological dependence; weight loss; withdrawal symptoms

Nursing Considerations
• Use extreme caution when administering morphine to patients with conditions accompanied by hypoxia, hypercapnia, or decreased respiratory reserve such as asthma, chronic obstructive pulmonary disease (COPD), or cor pulmonale. This is because, even with usual therapeutic doses, morphine may decrease respiratory drive while simultaneously increasing airway resistance to the point of apnea. Monitor patient's respiratory status closely, especially during the initiation of therapy or following a dose increase.
• Use morphine with extreme caution in patients who may be at risk for carbon dioxide retention (e.g., those with increased intracranial pressure or brain tumors). Monitor for signs of sedation and respiratory depression, especially when initiating therapy. Morphine may reduce respiratory drive, and the resultant carbon dioxide retention can further increase intracranial pressure. Also know that opioids like morphine may obscure signs and symptoms in a patient with a head injury.
• Use cautiously in patients about to undergo surgery of the biliary tract and patients with acute pancreatitis secondary to biliary tract disease because morphine may cause spasm of the sphincter of Oddi.
• Store morphine at room temperature.
• Before giving morphine, make sure opioid antagonist and equipment for oxygen delivery and respiration are available.
• Before therapy, assess patient's drug use, including all prescription and OTC drugs.
• Expect prescriber to usually start patient who has never received opioids on immediate-release form and then switch to E.R. form if therapy must last longer than a few days. Know that Avinza E.R. capsules is an exception to this rule because it may be prescribed to patients as the first opioid analgesic they receive. Expect to give the first dose of Avinza with the last dose of any immediate-release opioid medication because of its extended-release characteristics.

• Keep in mind that when morphine is given by epidural route, dosage must be individualized according to patient's age, body mass, physical status, previous experience with opioids, risk factors for respiratory depression, and drugs to be coadministered before or during surgery.
• Give oral form with food or milk to minimize adverse GI reactions, if needed. Solution can be mixed with fruit juice to improve taste.
• If needed, open E.R. capsules and sprinkle contents on applesauce (at room temperature or cooler) just before giving to patient. Make sure patient doesn't chew or crush capsules or dissolve capsule's pellets in his mouth.
• Be aware that E.R. forms of morphine aren't interchangeable.
• Discard injection solution that is discolored or darker than pale yellow or that contains precipitates that don't dissolve with shaking.
WARNING Don't use highly concentrated solutions (such as 10 to 25 mg/ml) for single-dose I.V., I.M., or subcutaneous administration. These solutions are intended for use in continuous, controlled microinfusion devices.
• For direct I.V. injection, dilute appropriate dose with 4 to 5 ml of sterile water for injection. Inject 2.5 to 15 mg directly into tubing of free-flowing I.V. solution over 4 to 5 minutes. Rapid I.V. injection may increase adverse reactions.
• For continuous I.V. infusion, dilute drug in D_5W and administer with infusion-control device. Adjust dose and rate based on patient response, as prescribed.
• Avoid I.M. route for long-term therapy because of injection-site irritation.
• During subcutaneous injection, take care to avoid injecting drug intradermally.
• For intrathecal injection, expect prescriber to give no more than 2 ml of 0.5-mg/ml solution or 1 ml of 1-mg/ml solution. Expect intrathecal dosage to be about one-tenth of epidural dosage.
• If rectal suppository is too soft to insert, refrigerate for 30 minutes or run wrapped suppository under cold tap water.
WARNING Monitor respiratory and circulatory status carefully and frequently during morphine therapy, especially when

drug therapy is initiated and when patient is being converted to morphine because respiratory depression and severe hypotension can develop. Be especially vigilant with elderly, cachectic, and debilitated patients who are at higher risk. Know that life-threatening depression can occur even when morphine is taken as prescribed and is not misused or abused.

• Monitor patient with seizure disorder for increased seizure activity because morphine may worsen the disorder.

• Monitor patient for excessive or persistent sedation; dosage may need to be adjusted.

• If patient is receiving a continuous morphine infusion, watch for and notify prescriber about new neurologic signs or symptoms. Inflammatory masses (such as granulomas) have caused serious neurologic reactions, including paralysis.

• Expect morphine to cause physical and psychological dependence; watch for drug tolerance and withdrawal, such as body aches, diaphoresis, diarrhea, fever, piloerection, rhinorrhea, sneezing, and yawning.

• If tolerance to morphine develops, expect prescriber to increase dosage.

• Morphine may have a prolonged duration and cumulative effect in patients with impaired hepatic or renal function. It also may prolong labor by reducing strength, duration, and frequency of uterine contractions.

• When discontinuing morphine in patients receiving more than 30 mg daily, expect prescriber to reduce daily dose by about one-half for 2 days and then by 25% every 2 days thereafter until total dose reaches initial amount recommended for patients who haven't received opioids (15 to 30 mg daily). This regimen minimizes the risk of withdrawal symptoms.

PATIENT TEACHING

• Instruct patient to take morphine exactly as prescribed and not to change dosage without consulting prescriber.

• Explain that patient may take tablets or capsules with food or milk to relieve GI distress and may mix oral solution with juice to improve taste.

• Urge patient not to break, chew, or crush E.R. capsules and tablets to avoid rapid release and, possibly, toxicity.

• For patient who has difficulty swallowing, suggest that he open E.R. capsules and sprinkle contents on food or liquids. Urge him to take drug immediately and not let capsule contents dissolve in his mouth.

• Instruct patient to moisten rectal suppository before inserting it.

• Urge patient to avoid alcohol and other CNS depressants during therapy.

• Advise patient to avoid potentially hazardous activities during morphine therapy.

• Tell patient to change positions slowly to minimize the orthostatic hypotension.

• Instruct patient to notify prescriber about worsening or breakthrough pain.

• Explain that morphine may be habit-forming. Urge him to notify prescriber if he experiences anxiety, decreased appetite, excessive tearing, irritability, muscle aches or twitching, rapid heart rate, or yawning.

• Advise female patient to notify prescriber if she becomes pregnant. Regular morphine use during pregnancy may cause physical dependence in fetus and withdrawal in neonate.

• Tell patient to alert all prescribers of morphine use.

• Warn patient not to discontinue morphine use abruptly if more than a few weeks of use has occurred, as withdrawal symptoms may develop.

• Caution patient to keep drug out of reach of children because accidental consumption by a child may be fatal.

moxifloxacin hydrochloride

Avelox, Avelox IV

Class and Category

Chemical class: Fluoroquinolone
Therapeutic class: Antibiotic
Pregnancy category: C

Indications and Dosages

➤ *To treat acute sinusitis caused by* Haemophilus influenzae, Moraxella catarrhalis, *or* Streptococcus pneumoniae; *to treat mild to moderate community-acquired pneumonia caused*

by Chlamydia pneumoniae,
H. influenzae, M. catarrhalis, Mycoplasma pneumoniae, *or* S. pneumoniae *(including penicillin- or multi-drug–resistant strains)*

TABLETS, I.V. INFUSION
Adults. 400 mg every 24 hr for 10 days.
➤ *To treat acute exacerbation of chronic bronchitis caused by* H. influenzae, H. parainfluenzae, Klebsiella pneumoniae, M. catarrhalis, S. pneumoniae, *or* Staphylococcus aureus

TABLETS, I.V. INFUSION
Adults. 400 mg every 24 hr for 5 days.
➤ *To treat uncomplicated skin and soft-tissue infections caused by* S. aureus *or* Streptococcus pyogenes

TABLETS, I.V. INFUSION
Adults. 400 mg every 24 hr for 7 days.
➤ *To treat complicated skin and skin structure infections caused by* S. aureus, E. coli, K. pneumoniae,*or* Enterobacter cloacae

TABLETS, I.V. INFUSION
Adults. 400 mg every 24 hr for 7 to 21 days.
➤ *To treat complicated intra-abdominal infections, including polymicrobial infections such as abscesses caused by* E. coli, Bacteroides fragilis, Streptococcus anginosus, Streptococcus constellatus, Enterococcus faecalis, Proteus mirabilis, Clostridium perfringens, Bacteroides thetaiotaomicron, *or* Peptostreptococcus *species*

TABLETS, I.V. INFUSION
Adults. 400 mg every 24 hr for 5 to 14 days with initial dosage given as I.V. infusion.

Mechanism of Action

Inhibits synthesis of bacterial enzyme DNA gyrase by counteracting excessive super-coiling of DNA during replication or transcription. Inhibiting DNA gyrase causes rapid- and slow-growing bacterial cells to die.

Incompatibilities

Don't infuse I.V. moxifloxacin simultaneously through the same I.V. line with other I.V. substances, additives, or drugs.

Contraindications

Hypersensitivity to moxifloxacin, other fluoroquinolones, or their components; myasthenia gravis

Interaction

DRUGS
aluminum- or magnesium-containing antacids; drug formulations with divalent or trivalent cations, such as didanosine chewable buffered tablets or powder for oral solution;metal cations, such as iron; multivitamins containing iron or zinc; sucralfate: Possibly substantial interference with moxifloxacin absorption, causing low blood moxifloxacin level
class IA antiarrhythmics, such as quinidine; class III antiarrhythmics, such as sotalol; other drugs known to prolong QTc interval, such as disopyramide and pentamidine: Possibly prolonged QTc interval
corticosteroids: Increased risk of Achilles and other tendon ruptures
NSAIDs: Increased risk of CNS stimulation and seizures
warfarin: Possibly increased anticoagulation

Adverse Reactions

CNS: Abnormal gait, altered coordination, confusion, depression, dizziness, fever, hallucinations, headache, increased intracranial pressure (including pseudotumor cerebri), peripheral neuropathy, psychosis, psychotic reaction, seizures, suicidal ideation, syncope, tremors
CV: Hypertension, hypotension, palpitations, peripheral edema, prolonged QTc interval, tachycardia, vasculitis, vasodilation, ventricular tachyarrhythmias
EENT: Altered taste, deafness or other hearing impairments, laryngeal edema, vision loss
ENDO: Hyperglycemia, hypoglycemia
GI: Abdominal pain, abnormal liver function test results, acute hepatic necrosis or failure, cholestatic hepatitis, diarrhea, dyspepsia, hepatic failure, hepatitis, jaundice, nausea, pseudomembranous colitis, vomiting
GU: Acute renal insufficiency or failure, interstitial nephritis
HEME: Agranulocytosis, aplastic anemia, eosinophilia, hemolytic anemia, leukopenia, pancytopenia, prolonged PT, thrombocytopenia
MS: Arthralgia, muscle weakness, myalgia, tendon inflammation, pain, or rupture
RESP: Allergic pneumonitis
SKIN: Photosensitivity, rash, Stevens-Johnson syndrome, toxic epidermal necrolysis

M

Other: Anaphylaxis, anaphylactic shock, angioedema, serum sickness, worsening of myasthenia gravis

Nursing Considerations

- Use cautiously in patients with liver dysfunction, including cirrhosis, because drug may adversely affect liver function.
- Obtain a fluid or tissue specimen for culture and sensitivity, as ordered. Expect to begin therapy before results are available.

WARNING Before starting moxifloxacin therapy, determine if patient takes a class IA antiarrhythmic, such as quinidine; a class III antiarrhythmic, such as sotalol; or other drugs that prolong the QTc interval, such as antipsychotics, cisapride, erythromycin, or tricyclic antidepressants. These drugs should be avoided in patients taking moxifloxacin because they may prolong the QTc interval and lead to life-threatening ventricular tachycardia or torsades de pointes. Monitor patient closely throughout therapy, especially if he has significant bradycardia or acute myocardial ischemia because these conditions increase risk of prolonging the QTc interval.

- Infuse drug over 60 minutes with ready-to-use flexible bags with 400 mg of moxifloxacin in 250 ml of 0.8% saline. Don't dilute further.
- If giving through Y-type tubing or piggyback, stop other solutions during moxifloxacin infusion, and flush the line before and after infusion with a compatible solution, such as normal saline solution, 1M sodium chloride, 5% dextrose, sterile water for injection, 10% dextrose, or lactated Ringer's. Also flush line before and after giving other drugs in same I.V. line.
- Don't refrigerate I.V. moxifloxacin ready-to-use bags because precipitation will occur. Discard any unused portion; premixed bags are for single-use only.
- Expect to obtain a 12-lead ECG to assess patient for prolonged QTc interval. Ask patient if he or a blood relative has a history of prolonged QTc interval. Monitor elderly patients closely; they may have increased risk of prolonged QT interval.

- If patient has hypokalemia, expect to correct it before beginning moxifloxacin therapy to prevent arrhythmias.
- Determine if patient has a history of CNS disorder, such as cerebral arteriosclerosis or epilepsy, because drug may lower seizure threshold. Notify prescriber before starting drug, and take seizure precautions.
- Monitor patient for central nervous adverse reactions such as confusion, depression, dizziness, hallucinations, peripheral neuropathy, suicidal ideation, and tremors. If any occurs, notify prescriber and expect moxifloxacin to be discontinued.
- If profuse, watery diarrhea develops, contact prescriber and expect to obtain a stool specimen to rule out pseudomembranous colitis caused by *Clostridium difficile*. If diarrhea occurs, notify prescriber and expect to withhold moxifloxacin and treat with fluids, electrolytes, protein, and an antibiotic effective against *C. difficile*.
- Monitor serum potassium level, as ordered, during therapy to assess for hypokalemia.
- Keep emergency resuscitation equipment readily available, and observe for evidence of hypersensitivity, such as angioedema, dyspnea, and urticaria. If you suspect anaphylaxis, prepare to give epinephrine, corticosteroids, and diphenhydramine, as prescribed.
- Monitor patients who are prone to tendinitis, such as the elderly, athletes, and those taking corticosteroids, for complaints of tendon pain, inflammation, or rupture. If present, notify prescriber and expect to discontinue moxifloxacin, place patient on bedrest with no exercise of affected limb, and obtain diagnostic tests to confirm rupture.
- Monitor patient's blood glucose, especially in diabetic patients receiving concomitant treatment with an oral hypoglycemic agent or insulin, for changes in blood glucose levels that could become increased or decreased. If dysglycemia occurs, treat according to standard of care and expect that drug may need to be discontinued.

PATIENT TEACHING

- Urge patient to notify prescriber at once about palpitations or fainting because they may indicate a serious arrhythmia.

- Teach patient to take drug at least 4 hours before and 8 hours after aluminum- or magnesium-containing antacids, didanosine chewable buffered tablets or oral solution prepared from powder, multivitamins containing iron or zinc, or sucralfate.
- Urge patient to drink plenty of fluids while taking moxifloxacin.
- Caution patient to stop drug and notify prescriber if he has trouble breathing, a rash, or other signs of an allergic reaction.
- Urge patient to stop any exercise and contact prescriber immediately if he develops tendon inflammation, pain, or rupture.
- Tell patient to notify prescriber if sensory or motor changes occur.
- Caution patient to avoid hazardous activities until adverse CNS effects are known.
- Urge patient to tell prescriber if diarrhea develops, even more than 2 months after moxifloxacin therapy ends.
- Caution patient to complete the prescribed course of therapy even if he feels better before it's completed.
- Tell patient to avoid excessive exposure to sunlight or artificial ultraviolet light because severe sunburn may result. Instruct patient to notify prescriber if sunburn develops because moxifloxacin may need to be discontinued.

mycophenolate mofetil

CellCept, CellCept Oral Suspension

mycophenolate mofetil hydrochloride

CellCept Intravenous

mycophenolic acid

Myfortic

Class and Category

Chemical class: 2-morpholinoethyl ester of mycophenolic acid
Therapeutic class: Immunosuppressant
Pregnancy category: D

Indications and Dosages

➤ *To prevent organ rejection in patients receiving allogenic kidney transplants*

CAPSULES, ORAL SUSPENSION, TABLETS, I.V. INFUSION

Adults. 1 g (over 2 hr for I.V. infusion) twice daily

E.R. TABLETS

Adults. 720 mg twice daily.

SUSPENSION

Children with body surface area less than 1.25 m^2. 600 mg/m^2 twice daily. *Maximum:* 2 g (10 ml) daily.

CAPSULES

Children with body surface area of 1.25 m^2 to 1.5 m^2. 750 mg twice daily.

CAPSULES, TABLETS

Children with body surface area greater than 1.5 m^2. 1 g twice daily.

➤ *To prevent organ rejection in patients receiving allogenic heart transplants*

CAPSULES, ORAL SUSPENSION, TABLETS, I.V. INFUSION

Adults. 1.5 g (over 2 hr for I.V. infusion) twice daily.

➤ *To prevent organ rejection in patients receiving allogenic liver transplants*

I.V. INFUSION

Adults. 1 g infused over 2 hr twice daily.

CAPSULES, ORAL SUSPENSION, TABLETS

Adults. 1.5 g twice daily.

Mechanism of Action

Hydrolyzes to form mycophenolic acid (MPA), which inhibits guanosine nucleotide synthesis and proliferation of T and B lymphocytes. MPA also suppresses antibody formation by B lymphocytes and prevents glycosylation of lymphocyte and monocyte glycoproteins involved in adhesion to endothelial cells. MPA also may inhibit leukocytes from sites of inflammation and graft rejection, which may explain how mycophenolate mofetil prolongs allogeneic transplant survival.

Incompatibilities

Don't mix or give mycophenolate mofetil hydrochloride in same infusion catheter with other I.V. drugs or admixtures.

Contraindications

Hypersensitivity to mycophenolate mofetil, mycophenolic acid, or any of its components; hypersensitivity to polysorbate 80 (I.V. form)

M

Interaction
DRUGS
acyclovir, ganciclovir, probenecid: Increased plasma levels of both drugs
amoxicillin plus clavulanic acid, cholestyramine, cyclosporine, metronidazole, norfloxacin, rifampin: Decreased plasma level of mycophenolate mofetil
antacids with magnesium and aluminum hydroxides, sevelamer: Decreased absorption of oral mycophenolate mofetil
azathioprine: Increased bone marrow suppression
live vaccines: Decreased effectiveness of live vaccines
oral contraceptives: Possibly decreased effectiveness of oral contraceptives
proton pump inhibitors: Possibly decreased effectiveness of mycophenolate mofetil

Adverse Reactions
CNS: Agitation, anxiety, chills, confusion, delirium, depression, dizziness, emotional lability, fever, hallucinations, headache, hypertonia, hypesthesia, insomnia, malaise, meningitis, nervousness, neuropathy, paresthesia, progressive multifocal leukoencephalopathy, psychosis, seizure, somnolence, syncope, thinking abnormality, tremor, vertigo
CV: Angina pectoris, arrhythmias, arterial thrombosis, atrial fibrillation or flutter, bradycardia, cardiac arrest, CV disorder, congestive heart failure, extrasystole, generalized edema, hemorrhage, hypercholesterolemia, hyperlipemia, hypertension, hypotension, increased lactic dehydrogenase, increased SGOT and SGPT, increased venous pressure, infectious endocarditis, orthostatic hypotension, palpitations, pericardial effusion, peripheral edema, peripheral vascular disorder, pulmonary edema or hypertension, supraventricular tachycardia, thrombosis, vasodilation, vasospasm, ventricular extrasystole, ventricular tachycardia
EENT: Amblyopia, cataract, conjunctivitis, deafness, dry mouth, ear disorder or pain, epistaxis, eye hemorrhage, gingivitis, gum hyperplasia, lacrimation disorder, mouth ulceration, oral candidiasis, pharyngitis, rhinitis, sinusitis, stomatitis, tinnitus, vision abnormality, voice alteration

ENDO: Cushing's syndrome, diabetes mellitus, hypercalcemia, hypocalcemia, hypoglycemia, hypothyroidism, parathyroid disorder
GI: Abdomen enlargement or pain, anorexia, ascites, cholangitis, cholestatic jaundice, colitis, constipation, diarrhea, dyspepsia, dysphagia, esophagitis, flatulence, gastritis, gastroenteritis, GI hemorrhage, GI infection, GI candidiasis, hepatitis, hernia, ileus, jaundice, liver damage, liver function test abnormalities, melena, nausea, pancreatitis, peritonitis, rectal disorder, stomach ulcer, vomiting
GU: Albuminuria; bilirubinemia; BK virus-related nephropathy; dysuria; hematuria; hydronephrosis; impotence; increased BUN or creatinine levels; kidney tubular necrosis; nocturia; oliguria; pain; polyomavirus-associated nephropathy; prostatic disorder; pyelonephritis; renal failure; scrotal edema, urinary tract disorder or infection; urine abnormality, frequency, incontinence, or retention
HEME: Anemia, coagulation disorder, hypochromic anemia, increased prothrombin time or thromboplastin time, leukocytosis, leukopenia, polyhemia, pure red cell aplasia, thrombocytopenia
MS: Arthralgia; back, neck or pelvic pain; joint disorder; leg cramps; myalgia; myasthenia; osteoporosis
RESP: Apnea; asthma; atelectasis; bronchitis; cough; dyspnea; hemoptysis; hyperventilation; hypoxia; lung edema; pleural effusion; pneumonia; pneumothorax; pulmonary fibrosis; respiratory acidosis, candidiasis, neoplasm, or pain; sputum increase
SKIN: Abscess; acne; alopecia, cellulite; ecchymosis; fungal dermatitis; hirsutism; pallor; petechia; pruritus; rash; benign neoplasm, carcinoma, hypertrophy, or ulcer; sweating; vesiculobullous rash
Other: Abnormal healing; acidosis; activation of latent infections (such as tuberculosis) or reactivation of hepatitis B or hepatitis C; alkalosis; bacterial, fungal, protozoal, and viral infections, including opportunistic infections; cyst;congenital malformations in unborn child; dehydration; facial edema; flulike syndrome; gout; hiccup; hyperkalemia; hyperuricemia; hypervolemia; hypochloremia;hypokalemia; hypomagnesemia; hyponatremia;

hypoproteinemia; hypophosphatemia; increased alkaline phosphatase; increased gamma glutamyl transpeptidase; loss of pregnancy during first trimester; lymphoma; malignancies; sepsis; thirst; weight gain or loss

Nursing Considerations

• Before starting mycophentolate therapy in a woman of childbearing potential, make sure she has a negative pregnancy test within 1 week of starting therapy, using a test with a sensitivity of at least 25 mIU/ml. Therapy shouldn't start until results are confirmed.

• Expect to give I.V. form within 24 hours of transplantation and for no longer than 14 days. Expect to switch patient to oral form as soon as possible, as ordered.

• Expect to administer oral form of drug as soon as possible following transplantation.

• When preparing oral suspension or I.V. form, avoid inhalation or direct contact with skin or mucous membranes. If contact occurs, wash area thoroughly with soap and water and rinse eyes with water.

• To prepare oral suspension, tap closed bottle several times to loosen powder and then measure 94 ml of water in a graduated cylinder. Add half of the water to the bottle and shake for about 1 minute. Then add remainder of water and shake again for 1 minute. Remove child-resistant cap and push bottle adapter into neck of bottle. Close bottle tightly with child-resistant cap. Be aware that the suspension bottle may become cold immediately after reconstitution.

• Know that oral suspension can be administered by 8F or larger nasogastric tube.

• When giving oral suspension, don't mix with any other drugs. Ask patient about history of phenylketonuria before initial administration because oral suspension contains aspartame.

• Don't open or crush capsules. If necessary, use the oral suspension.

• Handle I.V. form similarly to a chemotherapeutic drug because mycophenolate mofetil is genotoxic and embryotoxic and may have mutagenic properties.

• Know that I.V. form must be reconstituted and diluted to 6 mg/ml

using 5% dextrose injection USP. Inject 14 ml 5% dextrose injection USP into each vial (2 vials will be needed for each 1-g dose; 3 vials for each 1.5-g dose), then shake gently. Further dilute a 1-g dose by adding 2 reconstituted vials to 140 ml of 5% dextrose injection USP; dilute a 1.5-g dose by adding 3 reconstituted vials to 210 ml of 5% dextrose injection USP.

• Be aware that I.V. form should be administered within 4 hours of constitution as an infusion and over no less than 2 hours. Never administer by rapid or bolus I.V. injection.

• Know that cyclosporine and corticosteroids should be used with mycophenolate mofetil therapy.

• Obtain CBC weekly during first month of therapy, twice monthly for the second and third months of therapy, and then monthly through the first year, as ordered. Notify prescriber of any abnormalities. If significant, anticipate dosage reduction if absolutely necessary because reduced immunosuppression increases the risk of organ rejection. Also provide supportive care.

• Monitor patient's serum creatinine levels, as ordered, to detect changes in kidney functionbecause drug may cause polyomavirus-associated nephropathy. Notify prescriber if changes occur and expect dosage to be reduced, if needed.

• Monitor patient closely for adverse reactions because drug has many adverse effects, some of which can be serious or severe.

• Expect to stop drug or reduce the dose and provide supportive care, as ordered, if neutropenia develops.

WARNING Mycophenolate mofetil therapy has been associated with progressive multifocal leukoencephalopathy that can be life-threatening. Monitor patient for hemiparesis, apathy, confusion, cognitive deficiencies, and ataxia. Report suspicions of disorder immediately to prescriber.

PATIENT TEACHING

• Advise women of childbearing age that two forms of contraceptives should be used simultaneously before beginning mycophenolate mofetil therapy and for 6 weeks following discontinuation of therapy because of potential for fetal harm. Inform women who use oral contraceptives that drug may decrease effectiveness of oral contraceptives. Urge patient to notify prescriber immediately if pregnancy occurs.

• Before therapy starts, tell patient about increased risk of lymphomas or other malignancies. Tell patient to report any unusual signs or symptoms to prescriber.

• Tell patient to take oral form of drug on an empty stomach.

• Inform patient prescribed oral suspension that it contains aspartame, which is a source of phenylalanine.

• Instruct patient not to crush tablets or capsules or open capsules.

• Inform patient not to receive live vaccines during therapy. Urge him to avoid people who have received such vaccines or to wear a protective mask when he's around them.

• Tell patient to report any serious or ongoing adverse reactions, especially neurologic abnormalities, to prescriber immediately.

• Caution patient to avoid contact with people who have infections because drug causes immunosuppression.

• Urge patient to report any signs of infection, unexpected bruising or bleeding, or any other sign of bone marrow depression immediately.

• Tell patient that frequent laboratory tests may be needed during therapy. Emphasize that having these tests done is essential to continuing therapy.

• Advise patient to avoid exposure to direct sunlight and UV light and to wear sunscreen when outdoors because of increased risk for skin cancer.

• Advise patient not to take antacids at the same time as oral mycophenolate mofetil because some antacids can decrease drug's absorption.

• Tell patient to report unusual tiredness, lack of energy, paleness, dizziness, or fainting because dosage may need to be reduced or drug discontinued.

• Emphasize importance of follow-up care to monitor the drug's effectiveness and possible adverse effects because of the increased risk for cancer and infections as a result of immunosuppression. Inform patient of the need for periodic laboratory tests.

N O

nabumetone

Relafen

Class and Category

Chemical class: Naphthylalkanone derivative
Therapeutic class: Anti-inflammatory, antirheumatic
Pregnancy category: C (first trimester), Not rated (later trimesters)

Indications and Dosages

➤ *To relieve symptoms of acute and chronic osteoarthritis and rheumatoid arthritis*

TABLETS

Adults. *Initial:* 1 g daily as a single dose or in divided doses twice daily, increased to 1.5 to 2 g daily in divided doses twice daily. *Maintenance:* Adjusted according to clinical response. *Maximum:* 2 g daily.

Mechanism of Action

Blocks activity of cyclooxygenase, the enzyme needed to synthesize prostaglandins, which mediate the inflammatory response and cause local vasodilation, swelling, and pain. Prostaglandins also promote pain transmission from periphery to spinal cord. By blocking cyclooxygenase and inhibiting prostaglandins, the NSAID nabumetone reduces inflammatory symptoms and relieves pain.

Contraindications

Angioedema, asthma, bronchospasm, nasal polyps, rhinitis, or urticaria induced by aspirin, iodides, or other NSAIDs

Interaction

DRUGS

acetaminophen (long-term use): Increased risk of adverse renal effects
anticoagulants, thrombolytics: Increased risk of GI bleeding
antihypertensives: Decreased anti-hypertensive effectiveness
beta blockers: Decreased antihypertensive effects of beta blockers

bone marrow depressants, such as aldesleukin and cisplatin: Increased risk of leukopenia and thrombocytopenia
cefamandole, cefoperazone, cefotetan, plicamycin, valproic acid: Increased risk of hypoprothrombinemia and bleeding
colchicine, other NSAIDs, salicylates: Increased GI irritability and bleeding
cyclosporine, gold compounds, nephrotoxic drugs: Increased risk of nephrotoxicity
digoxin: Increased blood digoxin level and risk of digitalis toxicity
diuretics: Decreased diuretic effectiveness
glucocorticoids, potassium supplements: Increased GI irritability and bleeding
insulin, oral antidiabetic drugs: Increased effects of these drugs; risk of hypoglycemia
lithium: Increased risk of lithium toxicity
methotrexate: Increased risk of methotrexate toxicity
probenecid: Increased risk of nabumetone toxicity

ACTIVITIES

alcohol use: Increased GI irritability and bleeding

Adverse Reactions

CNS: Drowsiness, fatigue, fever, headache, nervousness, seizures, stroke, vertigo
CV: Edema, hypertension, MI, tachycardia
EENT: Dry mouth, pharyngitis, stomatitis, tinnitus
GI: Abdominal pain, anorexia, constipation, diarrhea, diverticulitis, dyspepsia, dysphagia, esophagitis, flatulence, gastritis, gastroenteritis, gastroesophageal reflux disease, GI bleeding and ulceration, hepatic dysfunction, indigestion, jaundice, melena, nausea, perforation of stomach or intestines, stomatitis, vomiting
GU: Albuminuria, azotemia, interstitial nephritis, nephrotic syndrome
HEME: Agranulocytosis, anemia, eosinophilia, granulocytopenia, hemolytic anemia, leukopenia, neutropenia, pancytopenia, thrombocytopenia
MS: Muscle spasms, myalgia
RESP: Asthma, pneumonitis, respiratory depression
SKIN: Alopecia, erythema multiforme, photosensitivity, pruritus, rash, Stevens-Johnson syndrome, toxic epidermal necrolysis
Other: Anaphylaxis, angioedema

N O

Nursing Considerations

- Use nabumetone with extreme caution in patients with a history of ulcer disease or GI bleeding because NSAIDs such as nabumetone increase risk of GI bleeding and ulceration. Expect to use nabumetone for shortest time possible in these patients.
- Be aware that serious GI tract ulceration, bleeding, and perforation may occur without warning symptoms. Elderly patients are at greater risk. To minimize risk, give drug with food. If GI distress occurs, withhold drug and notify prescriber immediately.
- Use nabumetone cautiously in patients with hypertension, and monitor blood pressure closely throughout therapy. Drug may cause hypertension or worsen it.

WARNING Monitor patient closely for thrombotic events, including MI and stroke, because NSAIDs increase the risk.

- Monitor patient—especially if elderly or receiving long-term nabumetone therapy—for less common but serious adverse GI reactions, including anorexia, constipation, diverticulitis, dysphagia, esophagitis, gastritis, gastroenteritis, gastroesophageal reflux disease, hemorrhoids, hiatal hernia, melena, stomatitis, and vomiting.
- Monitor liver function test results because, rarely, elevations may progress to severe hepatic reactions, including fatal hepatitis, liver necrosis, and hepatic failure.
- Monitor BUN and serum creatinine levels in elderly patients, patients taking diuretics or ACE inhibitors, and patients with heart failure, impaired renal function, or hepatic dysfunction; nabumetone may cause renal failure.
- Monitor CBC for decreased hemoglobin and hematocrit; drug may worsen anemia.

WARNING If patient has bone marrow suppression or is receiving treatment with an antineoplastic, monitor laboratory results (including WBC count), and watch for evidence of infection because anti-inflammatory and antipyretic actions of nabumetone may mask signs and symptoms, such as fever and pain.

- Assess patient's skin regularly for signs of rash or other hypersensitivity reaction because nabumetone is an NSAID and may cause serious skin reactions without warning, even in patients with no history of NSAID sensitivity. At first sign of reaction, stop drug and notify prescriber.
- Assess patient for severe hepatic reactions, including jaundice. Stop drug, as prescribed, if symptoms persist.

PATIENT TEACHING

- Instruct patient to take nabumetone with food to reduce GI distress.
- Advise patient to take drug with a full glass of water and to remain upright for 15 to 30 minutes afterward to prevent drug from lodging in esophagus and causing irritation.
- Tell patient not to increase dose or frequency without consulting prescriber.
- Urge patient to avoid alcohol to reduce risk of GI bleeding.
- Inform patient that regular laboratory tests are needed to check for drug toxicity during long-term therapy.
- Caution pregnant patient not to take NSAIDs such as nabumetone during the last trimester because they may cause premature closure of the ductus arteriosus.
- Explain that nabumetone may increase the risk of serious adverse cardiovascular reactions; urge patient to seek immediate medical attention if signs or symptoms arise, such as chest pain, shortness of breath, weakness, and slurring of speech.
- Explain that nabumetone may increase the risk of serious adverse GI reactions; emphasize the importance of seeking immediate medical attention for such signs and symptoms as epigastric or abdominal pain, indigestion, black or tarry stools, or vomiting blood or material that looks like coffee grounds.
- Alert patient to rare, but serious, skin reactions. Urge her to seek immediate medical attention for rash, blisters, itching, fever, or other indications of hypersensitivity.

nadolol

Corgard, Syn-Nadolol (CAN)

Class and Category

Chemical class: Nonselective beta blocker
Therapeutic class: Antianginal, antihypertensive
Pregnancy category: C

Indications and Dosages

➤ *To manage hypertension, alone or with other antihypertensives*

TABLETS

Adults. *Initial:* 40 mg daily, increased by 40 to 80 mg daily every 7 days, as needed. *Maintenance:* 40 to 80 mg daily. *Maximum:* 320 mg daily.

➤ *To manage angina pectoris as long-term therapy*

TABLETS

Adults. *Initial:* 40 mg daily, increased by 40 to 80 mg daily every 3 to 7 days, as needed. *Maintenance:* 40 to 80 mg daily. *Maximum:* 240 mg daily.

DOSAGE ADJUSTMENT Interval possibly increased to every 24 to 36 hr if creatinine clearance is 31 to 50 ml/min/1.73 m^2; to every 24 to 48 hr if it's 10 to 30 ml/min/1.73 m^2; or to every 40 to 60 hr if it's less than 10 ml/min/1.73 m^2.

Route	Onset	Peak	Duration
P.O.	Up to 5 days	4 hr	24 hr

Mechanism of Action

Selectively blocks $alpha_1$ and $beta_2$ receptors in vascular smooth muscle and $beta_1$ receptors in the heart, thereby reducing peripheral vascular resistance and blood pressure. Potent beta blockade decreases cardiac excitability, cardiac output, and myocardial oxygen demand, thus reducing angina. It also prevents reflex tachycardia, which typically occurs with most alpha blockers.

Contraindications

Asthma; bronchospasm; cardiogenic shock; heart failure; hypersensitivity to nadolol, other beta blockers, or their components; second- or third-degree AV block; severe COPD; sinus bradycardia

Interaction

DRUGS

allergen immunotherapy, allergenic extracts for skin testing: Increased risk of serious systemic reactions or anaphylaxis
amiodarone: Increased risk of conduction abnormalities and negative inotropic effects
beta blockers, digoxin: Increased risk of bradycardia
calcium channel blockers: Increased risk of bradycardia

cimetidine: Possibly increased effects of nadolol
clonidine, guanabenz: Impaired blood pressure control
diazoxide, nitroglycerin: Increased risk of hypotension
estrogens, NSAIDs: Possibly reduced antihypertensive effect of nadolol
general anesthetics: Increased risk of hypotension and myocardial depression
insulin, oral antidiabetic drugs: Possibly increased risk of hyperglycemia and impaired recovery from hypoglycemia, masking of signs of hypoglycemia
lidocaine: Increased risk of lidocaine toxicity
neuromuscular blockers: Possibly prolonged action of these drugs
phenothiazines: Possibly increased blood levels of both drugs
reserpine: Increased risk of bradycardia and hypotension
sympathomimetics with alpha- and beta-adrenergic effects, such as pseudoephedrine: Possibly hypertension, excessive bradycardia, and heart block
xanthines, such as theophyllines: Possibly decreased therapeutic effects of both drugs

Adverse Reactions

CNS: Anxiety, depression, dizziness, drowsiness, fatigue, headache, paresthesia, syncope, vertigo, weakness, yawning
CV: Bradycardia, chest pain, edema, heart block, heart failure, hypotension, orthostatic hypotension, ventricular arrhythmias
EENT: Nasal congestion, taste perversion
GI: Dyspepsia, elevated liver function test results, hepatic necrosis, hepatitis, nausea, vomiting
GU: Ejaculation failure, impotence
RESP: Cough, dyspnea, wheezing
SKIN: Jaundice, pruritus, scalp tingling

Nursing Considerations

• Use nadolol cautiously in patients with diabetes mellitus because it may prolong or worsen hypoglycemia by interfering with glycogenolysis.
• Anticipate that drug may worsen psoriasis; in patients with myasthenia gravis, it may worsen muscle weakness and diplopia.
• Be aware that chronic beta blocker therapy such as nadolol is not routinely withheld

prior to major surgery because the benefits outweigh the risks associated with its use with general anesthesia and surgical procedures. **WARNING** Withdraw drug gradually over 2 weeks, or as ordered, to avoid MI caused by unopposed beta stimulation or thyroid storm caused by underlying hyperthyroidism. Expect drug to mask tachycardia caused by hyperthyroidism.

PATIENT TEACHING
• Teach patient how to take her radial pulse, and direct her to do so before each dose of nadolol.
• Instruct patient to notify prescriber if pulse rate falls below 60 beats/minute.
• Caution patient not to stop taking nadolol abruptly or change dosage. Tell her to take a missed dose as soon as possible unless it's within 8 hours of the next scheduled dose.
• Advise patient with diabetes to check blood glucose level often because nadolol may mask signs of hypoglycemia, such as tachycardia.
• Review signs of impending heart failure, and urge patient to notify prescriber immediately if they occur.

nafarelin acetate

Synarel

Class and Category
Chemical class: Decapeptide, gonadotropin-releasing hormone analogue
Therapeutic class: Antiendometriotic, gonadal hormone inhibitor
Pregnancy category: X

Indications and Dosages
➤ *To treat endometriosis*
NASAL INHALATION
Adults. 1 spray (200 mcg) into a nostril every morning and 1 spray into other nostril every evening for up to 6 mo. If amenorrhea doesn't occur in 2 mo, dosage increased, as prescribed, to 800 mcg daily in divided doses.
➤ *To treat gonadotropin-dependent precocious puberty*
NASAL INHALATION
Children at puberty. 2 sprays (400 mcg) into each nostril every morning and

evening. *Maximum:* 1,800 mcg daily in divided doses three times daily.

Mechanism of Action
Stimulates release of the gonadotropins luteinizing hormone (LH) and follicle-stimulating hormone (FSH), which temporarily increase ovarian steroidogenesis. Within 1 month, however, repeated administration of nafarelin halts pituitary gland stimulation and decreases LH and FSH secretion. This action decreases estrogen level, which improves symptoms of endometriosis. In children, repeated nafarelin administration returns LH and FSH to prepubescent levels, stopping development of secondary sex characteristics and slowing bone growth.

Route	Onset	Peak	Duration
Nasal	60–120	20 days[†]	3–6[†] days*

Contraindications
Breastfeeding; hypersensitivity to gonadotropin-releasing hormones, gonadotropin-releasing hormone analogues, nafarelin, or their components; pregnancy; undiagnosed vaginal bleeding

Interaction
DRUGS
nasal decongestants: Possibly impaired nafarelin absorption

Adverse Reactions
CNS: Asthenia, depression, fever, headache, mood changes, paresthesia, seizures, stroke, transient ischemic attack
CV: Chest pain, deep vein thrombosis, edema, hot flashes, myocardial infarction, palpitations
EENT: Eye pain, rhinitis
ENDO: Galactorrhea, gynecomastia, transient increase in pubic hair growth
GI: Hepatic dysfunction
GU: Hypermenorrhea, hypertrophy of female genitalia, impotence, libido changes, menstrual irregularities, ovarian cysts, uterine bleeding, vaginal dryness, vaginal spotting between menses
MS: Arthralgia, decreased bone density, myalgia
RESP: Dyspnea, pulmonary embolism

---

* For gonadal hormone inhibitor effects, 4 wk.
† For antiendometriotic effects.

SKIN: Acne, hirsutism, rash, seborrhea, skin discoloration (brown)
Other: Body odor

Nursing Considerations
• Be aware that pregnancy must be ruled out before nafarelin therapy starts and that drug isn't recommended for use by breastfeeding women.
• Expect to start treatment for endometriosis between days 2 and 4 of menstrual cycle. Menses should cease after 6 weeks of treatment. Continued menses may indicate lack of compliance.
• Be aware that bone loss may increase if endometriosis treatment lasts longer than 6 months. Safety of retreatment after 6 months is unknown.
• Avoid giving nasal decongestant within 2 hours after nafarelin because it may impair nafarelin absorption.
• Be aware that prescriber will regularly monitor serum hormone levels in patient with gonadotropin-dependent precocious puberty, especially during first 6 to 8 weeks of therapy, to ensure rapid suppression of pituitary function.

PATIENT TEACHING
• Instruct patient to comply with prescriber's instructions for administering nafarelin to obtain desired drug effects.
• Instruct patient to tilt her head back while administering nafarelin to enhance absorption; urge her to try not to sneeze afterward.
• Caution patient not to change dosage without consulting prescriber.
• Counsel patient to use nonhormonal contraception and to notify prescriber if she is or could be pregnant.
• Direct patient not to use nasal decongestant within 2 hours after using nafarelin. If rhinitis occurs, urge her to contact prescriber for instructions.
• Teach patient how to cope with adverse reactions to help maximize compliance.
• Inform patient with endometriosis that drug should cause menses to stop. Urge her to notify prescriber if periods fail to stop, even though she's taking drug exactly as prescribed.
• Advise patient with endometriosis to avoid alcohol and tobacco during therapy because they increase bone loss.

• Inform patient with gonadotropin-dependent precocious puberty that signs of puberty will persist during first month of treatment. If they don't resolve within 2 months, advise patient or parents to notify prescriber.
• Tell patient with gonadotropin-dependent precocious puberty that prescriber will assess bone growth velocity and bone age during first 3 to 6 months of therapy.
• Reassure parents of child with precocious puberty that child will resume growing when treatment stops.

nafcillin sodium
Nafcil, Nallpen, Unipen

Class and Category
Chemical class: Penicillin
Therapeutic class: Antibiotic
Pregnancy category: B

Indications and Dosages
➤ *To treat infections caused by penicillinase-producing* Staphylococcus aureus
CAPSULES, TABLETS
Adults and adolescents. 250 to 1,000 mg every 4 to 6 hr. *Maximum:* 6,000 mg daily.
Children over age 1 month. 6.25 to 12.5 mg/kg every 6 hr.
Neonates. 10 mg/kg every 6 to 8 hr.
I.V. INFUSION
Adults and adolescents. 500 to 1,500 mg every 4 hr. *Maximum:* 20,000 mg daily.
Children from birth to age 12. 10 to 20 mg/kg every 4 hr, or 20 to 40 mg/kg every 8 hr.
I.M. INJECTION
Adults and adolescents. 500 mg every 4 to 6 hr. *Maximum:* 12,000 mg daily.
Children over age 1 month. 25 mg/kg every 12 hr.
Neonates. 10 mg/kg every 12 hr.
➤ *To treat streptococcal pharyngitis*
CAPSULES, TABLETS
Children. 250 mg every 8 hr.
➤ *To treat bone and joint infections, endocarditis, meningitis, and pericarditis caused by susceptible organisms*
I.V. INFUSION
Adults and adolescents. 1,500 to 2,000 mg every 4 to 6 hr. *Maximum:* 20,000 mg daily.

N O

I.V. INFUSION, I.M. INJECTION
Children from birth to age 12. 10 to
20 mg/kg every 4 hr or 20 to 40 mg/kg
every 8 hr. *For meningitis in neonates
weighing up to 2 kg (4.4 lb),* 25 to 50 mg/kg
every 12 hr for first week after birth and
then 50 mg/kg every 8 hr. *For neonates
weighing 2 kg or more,* 50 mg/kg every 8 hr
during first week after birth and then
50 mg/kg every 6 hr.

Mechanism of Action
Binds to certain penicillin-binding proteins
in bacterial cell walls, thereby inhibiting the
final stage of bacterial cell wall synthesis.
The result is cell lysis. Nafcillin's action is
bolstered by its chemical composition; its
unique side chain resists destruction by
beta-lactamases.

Incompatibilities
Don't mix nafcillin in same I.V. bag as
aminoglycosides; they're chemically
incompatible.

Contraindications
Hypersensitivity to nafcillin, other
penicillins, or their components

Interaction
DRUGS
aminoglycosides: Substantial mutual
inactivation
*chloramphenicol, erythromycins,
sulfonamides, tetracyclines:* Possibly
decreased therapeutic effects of nafcillin
hepatotoxic drugs: Increased risk of
hepatotoxicity
methotrexate: Increased risk of methotrexate toxicity
probenecid: Increased blood nafcillin level
FOODS
all foods: Decreased nafcillin absorption

Adverse Reactions
CNS: Depression, headache, seizures
EENT: Oral candidiasis
GI: Abdominal pain, diarrhea, nausea,
pseudomembranous colitis, vomiting
GU: Vaginitis
HEME: Leukopenia, neutropenia
SKIN: Exfoliative dermatitis, pruritus, rash,
urticaria
Other: Anaphylaxis; hypokalemia;
injection-site pain, redness, and swelling;
serum sicknesslike reaction

Nursing Considerations
• Obtain body fluid or tissue samples for
culture and sensitivity testing, as
prescribed, and obtain test results, if
possible, before giving nafcillin, as ordered.
• Give capsules or tablets at least 1 hour
before meals or 2 hours afterward.
• For I.M. injection, use only reconstituted
solutions from vials. Inject deep into large
muscle, preferably upper outer quadrant
of gluteus maximus or lateral thigh.
• For intermittent I.V. infusion, infuse over
30 to 60 minutes.
• Give nafcillin at least 1 hour before or
after aminoglycosides, especially if patient
has renal disease.
• When giving nafcillin to patient at risk for
hypertension or fluid overload, be aware
that each gram contains 2.5 mEq sodium.
WARNING Avoid giving nafcillin to
premature neonate if drug was reconstituted with bacteriostatic water that
contains benzyl alcohol. Doing so can
cause potentially fatal metabolic acidosis
and circulatory, CNS, renal, and
respiratory dysfunction.
• Monitor serum nafcillin level closely in
children, as ordered, because liver and
biliary tract, the main routes of nafcillin
elimination, function immaturely in
children.
• Watch for evidence of superinfection, such
as oral candidiasis and pseudomembranous
colitis, especially in elderly, immunocompromised, or debilitated patients who
receive large doses of nafcillin. If profuse,
watery diarrhea develops, contact prescriber
and expect to obtain a stool specimen to
rule out pseudomembranous colitis caused
by *Clostridium difficile.* If diarrhea occurs,
notify prescriber and expect to withhold
nafcillin and treat with fluids, electrolytes,
protein, and an antibiotic effective against
C. difficile.
PATIENT TEACHING
• Instruct patient to take nafcillin capsules
or tablets on an empty stomach.
• Urge patient to complete entire
prescription, even if she feels better.
• Advise patient to notify prescriber if she
experiences chills, fever, GI distress, or rash.
• Urge patient to tell prescriber if diarrhea
develops, even 2 or more months after
nafcillin therapy ends.

nalbuphine hydrochloride

Nubain

Class and Category
Chemical class: Phenanthrene derivative
Therapeutic class: Analgesic, anesthesia adjunct
Pregnancy category: B

Indications and Dosages
➤ *To relieve moderate to severe pain*
I.V., I.M., OR SUBCUTANEOUS INJECTION
Adults weighing 70 kg (154 lb). 10 mg every 3 to 6 hr, as needed. Dosage adjusted for patients weighing more or less.
➤ *As adjunct to anesthesia*
I.V. INJECTION
Adults. 0.3 to 3 mg/kg over 10 to 15 min followed by 0.25 to 0.5 mg/kg, as needed.
DOSAGE ADJUSTMENT For patients who have repeatedly received an opioid agonist, initial dose possibly reduced to 25% of usual. For patients in whom tolerance to drug's effects hasn't developed, maximum usually is 20 mg/dose or 160 mg daily.

Route	Onset	Peak	Duration
I.V.	2–3 min	30 min	3–4 hr
I.M.	In 15 min	1 hr	3–6 hr
SubQ	In 15 min	Unknown	3–6 hr

Mechanism of Action
Binds with and stimulates mu and kappa opiate receptors in the spinal cord and higher levels in the CNS. In this way, nalbuphine alters the perception of and emotional response to pain.

Incompatibilities
Don't give nalbuphine with diazepam or pentobarbital. Use separate I.V. line or flush line well before and after administration.

Contraindications
Hypersensitivity to nalbuphine or its components

Interaction
DRUGS
alfentanil, CNS depressants, fentanyl, sufentanil: Increased risk of hypotension and CNS and respiratory depression

anticholinergics: Increased risk of severe constipation and urine retention
antidiarrheals, such as difenoxin and atropine, loperamide, and paregoric: Increased risk of severe constipation and increased CNS depression
antihypertensives: Increased risk of hypotension
buprenorphine: Possibly decreased therapeutic effects of nalbuphine and increased risk of respiratory depression
hydroxyzine: Increased risk of CNS depression and hypotension
MAO inhibitors: Risk of possibly fatal increased CNS excitation or depression
metoclopramide: Possibly antagonized effects of metoclopramide
naloxone, naltrexone: Decreased pharmacologic effects of nalbuphine
neuromuscular blockers: Increased risk of prolonged CNS and respiratory depression
ACTIVITIES
alcohol use: Increased risk of coma, hypotension, profound sedation, and respiratory depression

Adverse Reactions
CNS: Confusion, depression, dizziness, euphoria, fatigue, hallucinations, headache, nervousness, restlessness, seizures, syncope, tiredness, weakness
CV: Hypertension, hypotension, tachycardia
EENT: Blurred vision, diplopia, dry mouth
GI: Abdominal cramps, anorexia, constipation, nausea, vomiting
GU: Decreased urine output, ureteral spasm
RESP: Dyspnea, pulmonary edema, respiratory depression, wheezing
SKIN: Diaphoresis, flushing, pruritus, rash, sensation of warmth, urticaria
Other: Injection-site burning, pain, redness, swelling, and warmth

Nursing Considerations
• Use nalbuphine cautiously in patients taking other drugs that can cause respiratory depression.
• Keep resuscitation equipment and naloxone readily available to reverse nalbuphine's effects, if needed.
• For direct I.V. injection through an I.V. line with a compatible infusing solution, give drug slowly—no more than 10 mg over 3 to 5 minutes. Inject into

free-flowing normal saline solution, D$_5$W, or lactated Ringer's solution.

• During prolonged use, expect to give a stool softener to minimize constipation.

• If patient is opioid-dependent, expect drug to cause withdrawal symptoms, such as abdominal cramps, anorexia, anxiety, backache, bone or joint pain, confusion, depression, diaphoresis, dysphoria, erythema, fear, fever, irritability, labile blood pressure and pulse, lacrimation, muscle spasms, myalgia, mydriasis, nasal congestion, nausea, opioid craving, piloerection, restlessness, rhinorrhea, sensation of crawling skin, sleep disturbances, tremor, uneasiness, vomiting, and yawning.

WARNING Be aware that drug may obscure neurologic assessment findings if patient has a cerebral aneurysm, head injury, or increased intracranial pressure.

PATIENT TEACHING

• Advise patient to avoid hazardous activities until nalbuphine's CNS effects are known.

• Counsel patient against making important decisions while receiving drug because it may cloud her judgment.

nalidixic acid

NegGram

Class and Category

Chemical class: Naphthyridine derivative quinolone
Therapeutic class: Antibiotic
Pregnancy category: Not rated (first trimester), B (later trimesters)

Indications and Dosages

➤ *To treat UTI caused by gram-negative bacteria, such as most* Enterobacter *species,* Escherichia coli, Klebsiella *species,* Morganella morganii, Proteus mirabilis, Proteus vulgaris, *and* Providencia rettgeri

ORAL SUSPENSION, TABLETS
Adults and children age 12 and over.
Initial: 1,000 mg every 6 hr for 1 to 2 wk.
Maintenance: 500 mg every 6 hr. *Maximum:* 4,000 mg daily.
Children ages 3 months to 12 years.

Initial: 55 mg/kg daily in divided doses four times daily for 1 to 2 wk. *Maintenance:* 33 mg/kg daily in divided doses four times daily.

Mechanism of Action

Inhibits the enzyme DNA gyrase, which is responsible for unwinding and supercoiling of bacterial DNA before it replicates. By inhibiting this enzyme, nalidixic acid causes bacterial cells to die.

Contraindications

Hypersensitivity to nalidixic acid or its components, porphyria, seizure disorder, use with melphalan or other related chemotherapeutic alkylating drugs

Interaction
DRUGS
aluminum-, calcium-, and magnesium-containing antacids; didanosine; multivitamins containing iron or zinc; sucralfate: Possibly interference with nalidixic acid absorption
chloramphenicol, nitrofurantoin, tetracycline: Decreased effects of nalidixic acid
cyclosporine: Possibly increased blood cyclosporine level
melphalan: Possibly increased risk of serious GI toxicity
oral anticoagulants: Increased anticoagulant effects
probenecid: Decreased effects of nalidixic acid and increased risk of adverse reactions
theophylline: Possibly increased blood theophylline level
FOODS
caffeine: Decreased clearance and prolonged half-life of caffeine

Adverse Reactions

CNS: Confusion, drowsiness, hallucinations, headache, increased intracranial pressure with bulging fontanels (infants and children), light-headedness, malaise, paresthesia, peripheral neuropathy, psychosis, restlessness, seizures, tremor, weakness
EENT: Altered color perception, blurred vision, diplopia, halo vision, photophobia
GI: Abdominal pain, diarrhea, nausea, pseudomembranous colitis, vomiting
HEME: Eosinophilia, hemolytic anemia, leukopenia, thrombocytopenia
MS: Tendon rupture

SKIN: Jaundice, photosensitivity, pruritus, rash, Stevens-Johnson syndrome, urticaria
Other: Anaphylaxis, metabolic acidosis

Nursing Considerations

- Be aware that nalidixic acid shouldn't be given to patient with creatinine clearance below 10 ml/min/1.73 m^2 because of the increased risk of drug toxicity, and should be used cautiously in patients with liver disease, epilepsy, glucose-6-phosphate dehydrogenase deficiency, or severe cerebral arteriosclerosis or renal failure.
- Avoid giving drug within 2 hours of didanosine; multivitamins that contain iron or zinc; sucralfate; or antacid that contains aluminum, calcium, or magnesium.
- If nalidixic acid therapy exceeds 2 weeks, monitor patient's blood counts and renal and liver function test results periodically, as ordered.

WARNING Stop nalidixic acid at first sign of hypersensitivity, including rash, because it may indicate anaphylaxis. Reaction may occur with first dose. Expect to give epinephrine and supportive care.

- If patient also takes cyclosporine or theophylline, monitor blood level of these drugs and adjust dosage, as prescribed.
- If patient has a history of seizures or cerebral arteriosclerosis, monitor for seizures during nalidixic acid therapy.
- Notify prescriber if patient has symptoms of peripheral neuropathy (pain, burning, tingling, numbness, weakness, or altered sensations of light touch, pain, temperature, position sense, or vibration sense), which could be permanent; or tendon rupture, which requires immediate rest. In each case, expect to stop nalidixic acid.

PATIENT TEACHING

- Encourage patient to drink plenty of fluids during therapy, unless directed otherwise by prescriber.
- Urge patient to complete entire course of therapy, even if she feels better before it's finished.
- Advise patient to protect skin from sunlight.
- Urge patient to notify prescriber immediately about vision changes or such adverse CNS reactions as confusion, drowsiness, hallucinations, psychosis, and seizures.

- Urge patient to stop drug and notify prescriber if rash or other evidence of hypersensitivity develops.
- Tell patient to take drug at least 2 hours before or after aluminum-, calcium-, or magnesium-containing antacids; didanosine chewable buffered tablets or oral solution prepared from powder; multivitamins that contain iron or zinc; or sucralfate.
- Caution patient to avoid hazardous tasks until CNS effects of drug are known.
- Instruct patient to limit caffeine intake while taking nalidixic acid.
- Tell patient to stop drug and notify prescriber if she develops tendon pain or inflammation or abnormal changes in motor or sensory function.
- Urge patient to notify prescriber if diarrhea develops, even up to 2 months after nalidixic acid therapy stops.

naloxegol

Movantik

Class and Category

Chemical class: PEGylated derivative of naloxone
Therapeutic class: Opioid antagonist on gastrointestinal tract
Pregnancy category: C

Indications and Dosages

➤ *To treat opioid-induced constipation in patients with chronic noncancer pain*
TABLETS
Adults. 25 mg once daily in the morning.
DOSAGE ADJUSTMENT For patients unable to tolerate naloxegol at the normal dose, patients with renal impairment (creatinine clearance less than 60 ml/min), and patients taking moderate CYP3A4 inhibitor drugs such as diltiazem, erythromycin, or verapamil, dosage reduced to 12.5 mg once daily in the morning. If dose is well tolerated in patients with renal impairment, dosage increased to 25 mg once daily in the morning.

Mechanism of Action

Functions as a peripherally acting mu-opioid receptor antagonist in tissues such as the

N
O

gastrointestinal tract, thereby decreasing the constipating effects of opioids.

Contraindications

Concomitant therapy with strong CYP3A4 inhibitors such as clarithromycin and ketoconazole, gastrointestinal obstruction or risk of recurrent obstruction, hypersensitivity to naloxegol or its components

Interaction

DRUGS

CYP3A4 inducers such as carbamazepine, rifampin, St. John's wort: Decreased plasma naloxegol levels and effectiveness
CYP3A4 inhibitors such as clarithromycin, diltiazem, erythromycin, itraconazole, ketoconazole, verapamil: Increased plasma naloxegol levels, possibly increasing risk of adverse reactions including opioid withdrawal
other opioid antagonists: Potential for additive effects and increased risk of opioid withdrawal

FOOD

grapefruit, grapefruit juice: Increased plasma naloxegol levels

Adverse Reactions

CNS: Headache
GI: Abdominal pain, diarrhea, flatulence, nausea, vomiting
SKIN: Diaphoresis
Other: Opioid withdrawal

Nursing Considerations

- Expect all maintenance laxative therapy to be discontinued prior to patient starting naloxegol therapy but know that laxatives may be given, as ordered and if needed, after 3 days of naloxegol therapy.
- Monitor patient for the development of severe, persistent, or worsening abdominal pain because gastrointestinal perforation has occurred with use of another peripherally acting opioid antagonist. If this type of abdominal pain occurs, withhold drug and notify prescriber.
- Monitor patient's reaction to naloxegol therapy, especially in patients who have taken opioids for at least 4 weeks prior to starting naloxegol, because sustained exposure to opioids may cause an increased response to naloxegol.
- Monitor patient for opioid withdrawal symptoms such as abdominal pain, anxiety, chills, diaphoresis, diarrhea, irritability,

and yawning. Clusters of these symptoms may occur with naloxegol therapy, especially if patient is receiving methadone or has a disruption in opioid therapy.
- Know that if opioid therapy is discontinued, naloxegol therapy should be discontinued.

PATIENT TEACHING

- Tell patient to stop all maintenance laxative therapy prior to starting naloxegol therapy. Reassure him laxatives may be used, if needed, after the first 3 days of therapy.
- Instruct patient to take naloxegol at least 1 hour prior to the first meal of the day or 2 hours after the meal.
- Tell patient tablets must be swallowed whole and he should not crush or chew tablets.
- Remind patient not to consume grapefruit or grapefruit juice while taking naloxegol.
- Tell patient to notify prescriber if opioid therapy is discontinued.
- Advise patient to inform prescriber of all medications being taken, including over-the-counter drugs and any new drug therapy begun once naloxegol therapy begins.
- Instruct patient to stop drug and seek medical attention promptly if he develops severe, persistent, or worsening abdominal pain.
- Warn patient that opioid withdrawal symptoms may occur while taking naloxegol and to notify prescriber.
- Caution female patients of childbearing age to notify prescriber immediately if pregnancy is suspected or has occurred, as the drug may precipitate opioid withdrawal in a fetus due to the undeveloped blood–brain barrier.
- Advise females who might wish to nurse their infants not to do so, as the infant may experience opioid withdrawal symptoms because of the drug's presence in breastmilk.

naloxone hydrochloride

Evzio, Narcan

Class and Category

Chemical class: Thebaine derivative

Therapeutic class: Opioid antagonist
Pregnancy category: B

Indications and Dosages

➤ *To treat known or suspected opioid overdose*

I.V., I.M., OR SUBCUTANEOUS INJECTION (NARCAN)
Adults and children age 5 and over weighing more than 20 kg (44 lb). 0.4 to 2 mg repeated every 2 to 3 min, as needed (in divided doses for children). If no response after 10 mg, patient may not have opioid-induced respiratory depression.
Infants and children under age 5. 0.01 mg/ kg as a single dose; if no improvement, 0.1 mg/kg given in divided doses.

I.V., I.M., OR SUBCUTANEOUS INJECTION (NARCAN)
Neonates. 0.01 mg/kg repeated every 2 to 3 min, as needed, until desired response occurs.

I.M. OR SUBCUTANEOUS INJECTION (EVZIO)
Adults and children. 0.4 mg, repeated every 2 to 3 minutes, as needed, until desired response occurs.

➤ *To treat postoperative opioid-induced respiratory depression*

I.V. INJECTION
Adults and adolescents. *Initial:* 0.1 to 0.2 mg every 2 to 3 min until desired response occurs. Additional doses given every 1 to 2 hr, if needed, based on patient response.
Children. *Initial:* 0.005 to 0.01 mg every 2 to 3 min until desired response occurs. Additional doses given every 1 to 2 hr, as needed, based on patient response.

➤ *To reverse opioid-induced asphyxia*

I.V., I.M., OR SUBCUTANEOUS INJECTION
Neonates. *Initial:* 0.01 mg/kg every 2 to 3 min until desired response occurs. Additional doses given every 1 to 2 hr, if needed, based on patient response.

➤ *As adjunct to treat hypotension caused by septic shock*

I.V. INFUSION OR INJECTION
Adults. 0.03 to 0.2 mg/kg over 5 min followed by continuous infusion of 0.03 to 0.3 mg/kg/hr for 1 to 24 hr, as needed, based on patient response.

Route	Onset	Peak	Duration
I.V.	1–2 min	5–15 min	45 min or longer
I.M., SubQ	2–5 min	5–15 min	45 min or longer

Mechanism of Action

Briefly and competitively antagonizes mu, kappa, and sigma receptors in the CNS, thus reversing analgesia, hypotension, respiratory depression, and sedation caused by most opioids. Mu receptors are responsible for analgesia, euphoria, miosis, and respiratory depression. Kappa receptors are responsible for analgesia and sedation. Sigma receptors control dysphoria and other delusional states.

Incompatibilities

Don't mix naloxone with any other solution unless you verify that the drugs are compatible; drug is incompatible with alkaline, bisulfite, and metabisulfite solutions.

Contraindications

Hypersensitivity to naloxone or its components

Interaction

DRUGS
butorphanol, nalbuphine, pentazocine: Reversal of these drugs' analgesic and adverse effects
opioid analgesics: Reversal of these drugs' analgesic and adverse effects, possibly withdrawal symptoms in opioid-dependent patients

Adverse Reactions

CNS: Excitement, irritability, nervousness, restlessness, seizures, tremor, violent behavior
CV: Hypertension (severe), hypotension, ventricular fibrillation, ventricular tachycardia
GI: Nausea, vomiting
RESP: Pulmonary edema
SKIN: Diaphoresis
Other: Withdrawal symptoms

Nursing Considerations

• Keep resuscitation equipment readily available during naloxone administration.
• Administer Narcan brand by I.V. route whenever possible.
• Administer Evzio brand only by I.M. or subcutaneous route following printed instructions on the device label. Be aware that an electronic voice will guide user through each step but if it does not operate properly, the device will still deliver the intended dose. Once the red safety guard is removed, drug must be used immediately or disposed of properly. Do not attempt to replace the red safety guard once it is removed.

N
O

• Upon actuation, Evzio brand will automatically insert the needle I.M. or subcutaneously, deliver 0.4 mg naloxone, and retract needle fully into its housing. Post injection, the black base locks in place, a red indicator appears in the viewing window, and the electronic visual and audible instructions signal that Evzio has delivered the intended dose.

• Give repeat doses as prescribed, depending on patient's response.

• Anticipate that rapid reversal of opioid effects can cause diaphoresis, nausea, and vomiting.

WARNING Watch for withdrawal symptoms, especially when giving naloxone to opioid-dependent patient. Symptoms may include abdominal cramps, anorexia, anxiety, backache, bone or joint pain, confusion, depression, diaphoresis, dysphoria, erythema, fear, fever, irritability, labile blood pressure and pulse, lacrimation, muscle spasms, myalgia, mydriasis, nasal congestion, nausea, opioid craving, piloerection, restlessness, rhinorrhea, sensation of crawling skin, sleep disturbances, tremor, uneasiness, vomiting, and yawning.

• Expect patient with hepatic or renal dysfunction to have increased circulating blood naloxone level.

PATIENT TEACHING

• Inform patient or family that naloxone will reverse opioid-induced adverse reactions.

• Urge opioid-dependent patient to seek drug rehabilitation.

naltrexone hydrochloride

ReVia, Vivitrol

Class and Category

Chemical class: Thebaine derivative
Therapeutic class: Opioid antagonist
Pregnancy category: C

Indications and Dosages

➤ *To treat opioid dependence*
TABLETS
Adults. *Initial:* 25 mg, repeated within 1 hr, if needed and if no withdrawal symptoms occur. *Maintenance:* 50 to 150 mg daily or 350 mg/wk by intermittent dosing regimen.

➤ *To prevent relapse to opioid dependence following opioid detoxification*
I.M. INJECTION
Adults. 380 mg every 4 wk or once monthly.
➤ *As adjunct to treat alcoholism*
TABLETS
Adults. 50 mg daily (up to 100 mg daily for some patients) for 12 wk.
I.M. INJECTION
Adults. 380 mg every 4 wk or once monthly.

Mechanism of Action

Displaces opioid agonists from—or blocks them from binding with—mu, kappa, and delta receptors. Opioid receptor blockade reverses the euphoric effect of opioids. Naltrexone also inhibits the effects of endogenous opioids, thus reducing alcohol craving.

Route	Onset	Peak	Duration
P.O.	15–30 min	In 12 hr	24 hr*
I.M.	Unknown	2 hr	Unknown

Contraindications

Acute hepatitis, acute opioid withdrawal, concurrent use of opioid analgesics (including opioid agonists, such as methadone or levo-alpha-acetyl-methadol [LAAM] or partial agonists such as buprenorphine), failure of naloxone challenge test, hepatic failure, hypersensitivity to naltrexone or its components, opioid dependence, positive urine screen for opioids

Interaction

DRUGS
opioid analgesics: Reversal of analgesic and adverse effects of these drugs, possibly withdrawal symptoms in opioid-dependent patients
thioridazine: Increased somnolence and lethargy

Adverse Reactions

CNS: Abnormal thinking, agitation, anxiety, asthenia, chills, confusion, depression, dizziness, euphoria, fatigue, fever, hallucinations, headache, hyperkinesia, insomnia, irritability, malaise,

---

* For 50 mg; 48 hr for 100 mg; 72 hr for 150 mg.

nervousness, restlessness, somnolence, suicidal ideation, syncope, tremor
CV: Chest pain, edema, hypertension, palpitations, tachycardia
EENT: Blurred vision, burning eyes, conjunctivitis, dry mouth, eyelid swelling, hoarseness, pharyngitis, rhinitis, sneezing, tinnitus, vision abnormalities
ENDO: Hot flashes
GI: Abdominal cramps, anorexia, constipation, diarrhea, elevated liver enzymes, GI ulceration, hepatotoxicity with excessive doses, nausea, vomiting
GU: Difficult ejaculation, urinary frequency
HEME: Idiopathic thrombocytopenic purpura
MS: Arthralgia, back pain or stiffness, joint stiffness, muscle cramps, myalgia
RESP: Cough, dyspnea, eosinophilic pneumonia, upper respiratory tract infection
SKIN: Increased sweating, pruritus, rash
Other: Injection-site reactions, such as pain, tenderness, induration, swelling, erythema, pruritus, bruising; thirst

Nursing Considerations

• Use naltrexone cautiously in patients with severe renal impairment, thrombo-cytopenia, hemophilia, or severe hepatic failure.
• To avoid withdrawal symptoms, wait 7 to 10 days after last opioid dose, as prescribed, before starting naltrexone. Because urine testing isn't always conclusive, prepare patient for naloxone challenge test if there are any doubts about patient's abstinence.
• Give oral drug with food or antacids to decrease adverse GI reactions.
• Dilute parenteral form using only diluent supplied in carton. Inject intramuscularly in gluteal muscle using only needle supplied in carton. Don't substitute any components for components in carton. Store entire dose pack in refrigerator; unrefrigerated drug can be stored at room temperature for no more than 7 days. Avoid administering as a subcutaneous injection because of increased risk of severe injection-site reactions.
• Inspect injection site for reactions, such as tenderness, induration, swelling, or redness. Ask if patient feels pain or itching at the

site. Report any such findings to prescriber because abscesses and site necrosis may occur and require surgical intervention.
WARNING Never give parenteral form intravenously.
• Patients who receive naltrexone and need pain management are more likely to have longer, deeper respiratory depression and histamine-release reactions (such as facial swelling, itching, generalized erythema, and bronchoconstriction) if given an opioid analgesic. Expect alternative analgesics to be used, such as regional analgesia, conscious sedation with a benzodiazepine, nonopioid analgesics, or general anesthesia. If an opioid analgesic must be used, monitor patient closely.
• Watch patient closely for suicidal tendencies throughout naltrexone therapy.
• Anticipate that some patients may need treatment for up to 1 year.
• Be aware that after opioid detoxification, patients may have lowered tolerance to opioids that could result in life-threatening respiratory compromise or circulatory collapse if patient uses previously tolerated doses of opioids.

PATIENT TEACHING
WARNING Caution patient against taking opioids during naltrexone therapy or in the future because she'll be more sensitive to them. In fact, strongly warn patient that taking large doses of heroin or any other opioid (including methadone or LAAM) while taking naltrexone could lead to coma, serious injury, or death.
• Explain that patient may have nausea after first injection but that it is usually mild and subsides within a few days. Most patients don't have nausea with repeat doses.
• Tell patient to report adverse reactions promptly, especially dyspnea, coughing, wheezing, abdominal pain, and jaundice. Also, tell patient to report any injection-site reactions to prescriber, especially if reaction does not improve in 1 month following the injection or worsens as further treatment may be necessary.
• Caution patient to avoid performing hazardous activities, such as driving, until CNS effects of drug are known.
• Urge family or caregiver to watch patient closely for abnormal behaviors, including

N
O

suicidal tendencies, even after patient stops taking naltrexone.
- Inform patient that naltrexone doesn't eliminate or diminish alcohol withdrawal symptoms.
- Urge patient to have comprehensive rehabilitation in addition to receiving naltrexone.
- Inform patient about nonopioid treatments for cough, diarrhea, and pain.
- Warn patient that drug may cause liver damage. Tell her to report any signs of liver dysfunction, such as yellowing of skin or whites of her eyes, anorexia, or digestive problems to prescriber.
- Instruct patient to carry medical identification that lists naltrexone therapy.
- Instruct women of childbearing age to notify prescriber if pregnancy is suspected.

naproxen

Apo-Naproxen (CAN), EC-Naprosyn, Naprosyn, Naprosyn-E (CAN), Naxen (CAN), Novo-Naprox (CAN), Nu-Naprox (CAN)

naproxen sodium

Aleve, Anaprox, Anaprox DS, Apo-Napro-Na (CAN), Naprelan, Naprosyn-SR (CAN), Novo-Naprox Sodium (CAN)

Class and Category

Chemical class: Propionic acid derivative
Therapeutic class: Analgesic, anti-inflammatory, antipyretic
Pregnancy category: C

Indications and Dosages

➤ *To relieve mild to moderate musculoskeletal inflammation, including ankylosing spondylitis, osteoarthritis, and rheumatoid arthritis*

DELAYED-RELEASE TABLETS, ORAL SUSPENSION, TABLETS (NAPROXEN)
Adults. 250 to 500 mg twice daily.
Maximum: 1,500 mg daily for limited periods, as prescribed.

E.R. TABLETS (NAPROXEN SODIUM)
Adults. 750 to 1,000 mg daily.
Maximum: 1,500 mg daily.

TABLETS (NAPROXEN SODIUM)
Adults. 275 to 550 mg twice daily
Maximum: 1,650 mg daily for limited periods, as prescribed.

SUPPOSITORIES (NAPROXEN SODIUM)
Adults. 500 mg at bedtime in addition to daytime P.O. administration. *Maximum:* 1,500 mg daily (P.O. and suppository combined).

➤ *To relieve symptoms of juvenile rheumatoid arthritis and other inflammatory conditions in children*

ORAL SUSPENSION, TABLETS (NAPROXEN)
Children. 10 mg/kg daily in divided doses twice daily.

➤ *To relieve symptoms of acute gouty arthritis*

DELAYED-RELEASE TABLETS, ORAL SUSPENSION, TABLETS (NAPROXEN)
Adults. *Initial:* 750 mg, then 250 mg every 8 hr until symptoms subside.

E.R. TABLETS (NAPROXEN SODIUM)
Adults. *Initial:* 1,000 to 1,500 mg on day 1; then 1,000 mg daily until symptoms subside. *Maximum:* 1,500 mg daily.

TABLETS (NAPROXEN SODIUM)
Adults. *Initial:* 825 mg, then 275 mg every 8 hr until symptoms subside.

➤ *To relieve mild to moderate pain, including acute tendinitis and bursitis, arthralgia, dysmenorrhea, and myalgia*

DELAYED-RELEASE TABLETS (NAPROXEN)
Adults. *Initial:* 1,000 mg daily.
Maximum: 1,500 mg daily.

E.R. TABLETS (NAPROXEN SODIUM)
Adults. *Initial:* 1,100 mg daily, increased as prescribed. *Maximum:* 1,500 mg daily.

ORAL SUSPENSION, TABLETS (NAPROXEN)
Adults. *Initial:* 500 mg, then 250 mg every 6 to 8 hr, as needed. *Maximum:* 1,250 mg daily.

TABLETS (NAPROXEN SODIUM)
Adults. *Initial:* 550 mg, then 275 mg every 6 to 8 hr, as needed. *Maximum:* 1,375 mg daily.

➤ *To relieve fever and mild to moderate musculoskeletal inflammation or pain*

TABLETS (OTC NAPROXEN SODIUM)
Adults. 220 mg every 8 to 12 hr; or 440 mg and 220 mg 12 hr later. *Maximum:* 660 mg daily for 10 days unless directed otherwise.
DOSAGE ADJUSTMENT For patients over age 65, 220 mg every 12 hr. *Maximum:* 440 mg for 10 days unless directed otherwise.

Route	Onset	Peak	Duration
P.O. (naproxen)*	1 hr†	2–4 hr†‡	7–12 hr†
P.O. (naproxen sodium)*	30 min†	1 hr†‡	7–12 hr†

Mechanism of Action

Blocks cyclooxygenase, the enzyme needed to synthesize prostaglandins, which mediate the inflammatory response and cause local vasodilation, swelling, and pain. Thus, naproxen, an NSAID, reduces symptoms of inflammation and relieves pain. Antipyretic action probably stems from effects on the hypothalamus, which increases peripheral blood flow, causing vasodilation and heat dissipation.

Contraindications

Angioedema, asthma, bronchospasm, nasal polyps, rhinitis, or urticaria induced by aspirin, iodides, or other NSAIDs; hypersensitivity to naproxen or its components

Interaction

DRUGS

angiotensin converting enzyme (ACE) inhibitors, angiotensin receptor blockers (ARBs) : Decreased antihypertensive effects; increased risk of renal dysfunction, especially in the elderly and those with volume depletion or impaired renal function
acetaminophen: Increased risk of adverse renal effects with combined long-term use
aluminum hydroxide or magnesium oxide antacids, cholestyramine, sucralfate: Possibly delayed absorption of naproxen
anticoagulants, thrombolytics: Prolonged PT, increased risk of bleeding
antihypertensives: Decreased effectiveness of antihypertensive
aspirin: Decreased aspirin effectiveness from lowered plasma and peak aspirin levels
beta blockers: Decreased antihypertensive effects of these drugs

---

* For antirheumatism, onset is in 14 days, peak is unknown, and duration is 2 to 4 wk.
† For analgesia.
‡ For gout, 1 to 2 days.

bone marrow depressants, such as aldesleukin and cisplatin: Increased risk of leukopenia and thrombocytopenia
cefamandole, cefoperazone, cefotetan, plicamycin, valproic acid: Increased risk of hypoprothrombinemia and bleeding
cimetidine: Altered blood naproxen level
colchicine, glucocorticoids, other NSAIDs, potassium supplements, salicylates: Increased GI irritability and bleeding
cyclosporine, gold compounds, nephrotoxic drugs: Increased risk of nephrotoxicity
digoxin: Increased blood digoxin level and risk of digitalis toxicity
diuretics: Decreased diuretic effectiveness
furosemide: Decreased natriuretic effect
insulin, oral antidiabetic drugs: Increased effectiveness of these drugs; risk of hypoglycemia
lithium: Increased risk of lithium toxicity
methotrexate: Increased risk of methotrexate toxicity
naproxen-containing products: Increased risk of toxicity
phenytoin: Increased blood phenytoin level
probenecid: Increased risk of naproxen toxicity

ACTIVITIES

alcohol use, smoking: Increased risk of naproxen-induced GI ulceration

Adverse Reactions

CNS: Aseptic meningitis, chills, cognitive impairment, decreased concentration, depression, dizziness, dream disturbances, drowsiness, fever, headache, insomnia, light-headedness, malaise, seizures, stroke, vertigo
CV: Edema, heart failure, hypertension, MI, palpitations, tachycardia, vasculitis
EENT: Papilledema, papillitis, retrobulbar optic neuritis, stomatitis, tinnitus, vision or hearing changes
ENDO: Hyperglycemia, hypoglycemia
GI: Abdominal pain, anorexia, colitis, constipation, diarrhea, diverticulitis, dyspepsia, dysphagia, elevated liver function test results, esophagitis, flatulence, gastritis, gastroenteritis, gastroesophageal reflux disease, GI bleeding and ulceration, heartburn, hematemesis, hepatitis, indigestion, melena, nausea, pancreatitis, peptic ulceration, perforation of stomach or intestines, stomatitis, vomiting

GU: Elevated serum creatinine level, glomerulonephritis, hematuria, infertility (in women), interstitial nephritis, menstrual irregularities, nephrotic syndrome, renal failure, renal papillary necrosis
HEME: Agranulocytosis, anemia, aplastic anemia, eosinophilia, granulocytopenia, hemolytic anemia, leukopenia, neutropenia, pancytopenia, thrombocytopenia
MS: Muscle weakness, myalgia
RESP: Asthma, dyspnea, eosinophilic pneumonitis, respiratory depression
SKIN: Alopecia, diaphoresis, ecchymosis, erythema multiforme, photosensitivity, pruritus, pseudoporphyria, purpura, rash, Stevens-Johnson syndrome, systemic lupus erythematosus, toxic epidermal necrolysis, urticaria
Other: Anaphylaxis, angioedema, hyperkalemia

Nursing Considerations

• Use naproxen with extreme caution in patients with a history of ulcer disease or GI bleeding because NSAIDs such as naproxen increase risk of GI bleeding and ulceration. Expect to use naproxen for the shortest time possible in these patients.
• Use naproxen cautiously in patients with hypertension, and monitor blood pressure closely. Drug may cause hypertension or worsen it. Because of naproxen's sodium content, watch for fluid retention.
• Use naproxen cautiously in patients with heart failure, hypovolemia, liver dysfunction, renal dysfunction, salt depletion, or patients taking diuretics and ACE inhibitors or ARBs, and the elderly because of increased risk of renal decompensation.
• Monitor patient for serious GI tract ulceration, bleeding, and perforation, which may occur without warning symptoms. Elderly patients are at greater risk. To minimize risk, give drug with food. If GI distress occurs, withhold drug and notify prescriber immediately.
• Rehydrate a dehydrated patient before giving drug. If patient has renal disease, monitor renal function closely during therapy.
• Naproxen isn't recommended for patients with advanced renal disease.
WARNING Monitor patient closely for thrombotic events, including MI and stroke,

because NSAIDs increase the risk, especially if used in higher doses than recommended or for extended periods of time.
• Monitor patient—especially if elderly or receiving long-term naproxen therapy—for less common but serious adverse GI reactions, including anorexia, constipation, diverticulitis, dysphagia, esophagitis, gastritis, gastroenteritis, gastroesophageal reflux disease, hemorrhoids, hiatal hernia, melena, stomatitis, and vomiting.
• Monitor liver function test results because, in rare cases, elevations may progress to severe hepatic reactions, including fatal hepatitis, liver necrosis, and hepatic failure.
• Monitor BUN and serum creatinine levels in elderly patients, patients taking diuretics or ACE inhibitors, and patients with heart failure, impaired renal function, or hepatic dysfunction; naproxen may cause renal failure.
• Monitor CBC for decreased hemoglobin and hematocrit because drug may worsen anemia.
WARNING If patient has bone marrow suppression or is receiving treatment with an antineoplastic drug, monitor laboratory results (including WBC count), and watch for evidence of infection because anti-inflammatory and antipyretic actions of naproxen may mask signs and symptoms, such as fever and pain.
• Assess patient's skin regularly for signs of rash or other hypersensitivity reaction because naproxen is an NSAID and may cause serious skin reactions without warning, even in patients with no history of NSAID sensitivity. At first sign of reaction, stop drug and notify prescriber.
• Assess drug effectiveness in ankylosing spondylitis, as evidenced by decreased night pain, morning stiffness, and pain at rest; in osteoarthritis: decreased joint pain or tenderness and increased mobility, range of motion, and ability to perform daily activities; in rheumatoid arthritis: increased mobility and decreased joint swelling and morning stiffness; in acute gouty arthritis: decreased heat, pain, swelling, and tenderness in affected joints.
• Tell prescriber if patient complains of vision changes; patient may need ophthalmic exam.

PATIENT TEACHING

• Caution patient not to exceed recommended dosage, take for longer than directed, or take for more than 10 days without consulting prescriber because serious adverse reactions may occur.
• Tell patient to swallow delayed-release tablets whole and not to break, crush, or chew them.
• Advise patient to take drug with food to reduce GI distress.
• Tell patient to take drug with a full glass of water and to remain upright for 15 to 30 minutes after taking it to prevent drug from lodging in esophagus and causing irritation.
• Caution patient to avoid hazardous activities until drug's CNS effects are known.
• Urge patient to keep scheduled appointments with prescriber to monitor progress.
• Tell pregnant patient to avoid taking naproxen-containing products late in pregnancy.
• Explain that naproxen may increase risk of serious adverse cardiovascular reactions; urge patient to seek immediate medical attention if signs or symptoms arise, such as chest pain, shortness of breath, weakness, and slurring of speech.
• Inform patient that naproxen may increase risk of serious adverse GI reactions; stress the importance of seeking immediate medical attention for such signs and symptoms as epigastric or abdominal pain, indigestion, black or tarry stools, or vomiting blood or material that looks like coffee grounds.
• Alert patient to rare but serious skin reactions. Urge her to seek immediate medical attention for rash, blisters, itching, fever, or other indications of hypersensitivity.
• Advise patient to consult prescriber before taking naproxen-containing OTC products if he has asthma, ulcers, bleeding problems, high blood pressure, heart or kidney disease, a need for diuretic therapy, serious adverse effects from previous use of fever reducers or pain relievers, or persistent stomach problems, such as heartburn, upset stomach, or stomach pain.

naratriptan hydrochloride
Amerge

Class and Category
Chemical class: Selective serotonin 5-HT receptor agonist
Therapeutic class: Antimigraine
Pregnancy category: C

Indications and Dosages
➤ *To relieve acute migraine with or without aura*
TABLETS
Adults. 1 to 2.5 mg as a single dose, repeated in 4 hr as needed if only partial relief obtained. *Maximum:* 5 mg daily.
DOSAGE ADJUSTMENT For patients with mild to moderate renal or hepatic impairment, maximum dosage reduced to 2.5 mg daily.

Mechanism of Action
Binds to receptors on intracranial blood vessels and sensory nerves in trigeminal-vascular system to stimulate negative feedback, which halts serotonin release. Thus, naratriptan selectively constricts inflamed and dilated cranial vessels in the carotid circulation and inhibits production of proinflammatory neuropeptides.

Contraindications
Basilar or hemiplegic migraine; cerebrovascular, peripheral vascular, or coronary artery disease (ischemic or vasospastic); hypersensitivity to naratriptan or its components; hypertension (uncontrolled); severe hepatic or renal dysfunction; use within 24 hours of another 5-HT agonist or an ergotamine-containing or ergot-type drug, such as dihydroergotamine or methysergide

Interaction
DRUGS
ergot-containing drugs: Possibly prolonged or additive vasospastic reactions
fluoxetine, fluvoxamine, paroxetine, sertraline: Possibly weakness, hyperreflexia, and incoordination
oral contraceptives: Possibly reduced clearance and increased blood level of naratriptan

other selective serotonin 5-HT receptor agonists (including rizatriptan, sumatriptan, and zolmitriptan): Possibly additive effects
selective serotonin reuptake inhibitors, serotonin norepinephrine reuptake inhibitors, other triptans: Increased risk of serotonin syndrome

Adverse Reactions

CNS: Dizziness, drowsiness, fatigue, malaise, paresthesia
CV: Chest pain, pressure, or heaviness; hypertension, hypertensive crisis
EENT: Decreased salivation, otitis media, pharyngitis, photophobia, rhinitis, throat tightness
GI: Nausea, vomiting
OTHER: Anaphylaxis, angioedema

Nursing Considerations

WARNING Because naratriptan therapy can cause coronary artery vasospasm, monitor patient with coronary artery disease for signs or symptoms of angina while taking drug. Because naratriptan may also cause peripheral vasospastic reactions, such as ischemic bowel disease, monitor patient for abdominal pain and bloody diarrhea.

• Monitor patient for hypertension during naratriptan therapy even in patients with no history of hypertension because drug can cause significant elevation in blood pressure.

• Be prepared to perform complete neurovascular assessment in any patient who reports an unusual headache or who fails to respond to first dose of naratriptan.

WARNING Monitor patient closely for serotonin syndrome if she is taking naratriptan along with a selective serotonin reuptake inhibitor or serotonin norepinephrine reuptake inhibitor. Notify prescriber immediately if the patient exhibits agitation, hallucinations, coma, tachycardia, labile blood pressure, hyperthermia, hyperreflexia, incoordination, nausea, vomiting, or diarrhea because serotonin syndrome can be life-threatening. Provide supportive care.

PATIENT TEACHING

• Inform patient that naratriptan is used to treat acute migraine attacks and that it won't prevent or reduce the number of migraines.

• If patient has no relief from initial dose of naratriptan, instruct her to notify prescriber rather than taking another dose in 4 hours; she may need a different drug.

• Advise patient not to take more than maximum prescribed amount of naratriptan during any 24-hour period or to exceed 10 times or more instances of drug use each month. Overuse can cause headaches to become worse or increase frequency of migraine attacks. Tell patient that if she is using naratriptan 10 times or more in a 30-day period she should notify prescriber, as drug may need to be discontinued. Also tell patient that she may need to be treated for withdrawal symptoms upon discontinuation.

• Advise patient to seek reevaluation by prescriber if she has more than four headaches during any 30-day period while taking naratriptan.

• Urge patient to inform all prescribers that she is receiving naratriptan therapy because serious drug interactions may occur.

natalizumab

Tysabri

Class and Category

Chemical class: Recombinant humanized IgG4K monoclonal antibody
Therapeutic class: Anti-multiple sclerotic
Pregnancy category: C

Indications and Dosages

➤ *To delay physical disability and reduce frequency of clinical exacerbations in relapsing forms of multiple sclerosis; to induce and maintain remission in moderately to severely active Crohn's disease with evidence of inflammation in patients who had inadequate response to or are unable to tolerate conventional therapy and inhibitors of tumor necrosis factor alpha*

I.V. INFUSION

Adults. 300 mg infused over 1 hr every 4 wk.

Route	Onset	Peak	Duration
I.V.	Unknown	24 wk	Unknown

Mechanism of Action

Inhibits migration of leukocytes from vascular space, increasing the number of circulating leukocytes. It does this by binding to integrins on the surface of leukocytes (except neutrophils) and inhibiting adhesion of leukocytes to their counter receptors. In multiple sclerosis, lesions probably occur when activated inflammatory cells, including T-lymphocytes, cross the blood–brain barrier.

Contraindications

History of or presence of progressive multifocal leukoencephalopathy, hypersensitivity to natalizumab or its components

Interaction

DRUGS

antineoplastics, immunosuppressants, immunomodulating agents: Increased risk of life-threatening infection

Adverse Reactions

CNS: Depression, dizziness, encephalitis, fatigue, headache, meningitis, progressive multifocal leukoencephalopathy (PML), rigors, somnolence, suicidal ideation, vertigo
CV: Chest discomfort, peripheral edema
EENT: Sinusitis, tonsillitis, tooth infection
GI: Abdominal discomfort, cholelithiasis, diarrhea, elevated liver enzymes, gastroenteritis, hepatotoxicity, jaundice, nausea
GU: Amenorrhea; dysmenorrhea; irregular menstruation; ovarian cysts; UTI; urinary incontinence, frequency, or urgency; vaginitis
MS: Arthralgia, back or limb pain, joint swelling, muscle cramp
RESP: Cough, pneumonia or other respiratory tract infection
SKIN: Dermatitis, night sweats, pruritus, rash, urticaria
Other: Acute hypersensitivity reaction, anaphylaxis, antibody formation, flulike illness, herpes, immune reconstitution inflammatory syndrome, serious infection, weight gain or loss

Nursing Considerations

• Make sure patient has enrolled in the TOUCH prescribing program before giving natalizumab. Once patient has signed and initialed the TOUCH program enrollment form, place original signed form in the patient's medical record, send a copy to Biogen Idec, and give a copy to patient.
• Be aware that all serious opportunistic and atypical infections must be reported to Biogen Idec at 1-800-456-2255 and the FDA's MedWatch Program at 1-800-FDA-1088.
• Make sure patient with multiple sclerosis has had an MRI of the brain before starting natalizumab therapy. It will help distinguish evidence of multiple sclerosis from PML symptoms if they occur after therapy starts.
• Dilute natalizumab concentrate 300 mg/15 ml in 100 ml of normal saline injection. Gently invert solution to mix completely. Do not shake.
• Following dilution, infuse drug immediately over 1 hour. After infusion, flush line with normal saline injection.
• Do not give natalizumab by I.V. push or bolus injection.
• If not infused right away, refrigerate drug and use within 8 hours.
• Observe patient during and for 1 hour after infusion for hypersensitivity reaction, evidenced by urticaria, dizziness, fever, rash, rigors, pruritus, nausea, flushing, hypotension, dyspnea, and chest pain. Reaction is more likely to occur if natalizumab therapy was interrupted. If hypersensitivity reaction occurs, notify prescriber; expect to withhold drug and provide supportive care.
WARNING Monitor patient closely for evidence of PML, a viral brain infection that may be disabling or fatal, because natalizumab increases the risk. Patients at increased risk include those who have received natalizumab for longer than 2 years, have had prior treatment with an immunosuppressant, and who have anti-JCV antibodies. If patient has unexplained neurologic changes, notify prescriber, withhold natalizumab, and prepare patient for a gadolinium-enhanced brain MRI and possible cerebrospinal fluid analysis, as ordered. Be aware that immune reconstitution inflammatory syndrome may occur in patients who develop PML, even when drug has been discontinued. Monitor such patients for evidence of an overwhelming

inflammatory response either to an opportunistic infection or the paradoxical symptomatic relapse of a prior infection despite it having been treated successfully in the past.
• Expect that patient will be reevaluated 3 months after first infusion, 6 months after first infusion, and every 6 months thereafter.
• Assess patient for evidence of infection because natalizumab may adversely affect immune system, increasing risk of infection. For example, the drug increases the risk for encephalitis and meningitis caused by herpes simplex and varicella zoster viruses that could become life-threatening. If infection occurs, expect to obtain appropriate specimens for culture and sensitivity and to treat accordingly. If infection is serious, expect drug to be discontinued.
• Be aware that if patient with Crohn's disease has no therapeutic response after 12 weeks, natalizumab should be discontinued. If patient is on chronic oral corticosteroid therapy, expect tapering of oral cortico-steroid dose to begin. If patient can't be tapered off oral cortico-steroids within 6 months of starting natalizumab therapy, expect natalizumab to be discontinued. Likewise, if patient needs additional steroid use that extends beyond 3 months in a calendar year to control signs and symptoms of Crohn's disease, expect natalizumab to be discontinued.
• Assess patient's liver function regularly, as ordered, because natalizumab may cause significant liver damage. Expect drug to be discontinued if patient becomes jaundiced or liver enzymes become elevated.
• Ensure that when natalizumab is discontinued, patient completes the "Initial Discontinuation Questionnaire" and then has an appointment in six months to complete the "6-Month Discontinuation Questionnaire."

PATIENT TEACHING
• Instruct patient on benefits and risks of natalizumab therapy, and provide medication guide for patient to read.
• Encourage patient to ask questions before signing the enrollment form.

• Emphasize need to report any worsening symptoms that persist over several days.
• Tell patient to inform all healthcare providers that he is receiving natalizumab therapy.
• Stress the need to have follow-up visits 3 months after first infusion, 6 months after first infusion, and at least every 6 months thereafter.
• Instruct patient to report evidence of allergic reaction such as urticaria, dizziness, fever, rash, rigors, pruritus, nausea, flushing, hypotension, dyspnea, and chest pain.
• Instruct patient to avoid people who have infections. Advise him to report fever, cough, lower-back or side pain, or other unexplained signs and symptoms because they may indicate infection.
• Alert patient that signs and symptoms suggestive of PML can occur up to six months after drug is discontinued and should be reported immediately.

nateglinide
Starlix

Class and Category
Chemical class: Amino acid derivative
Therapeutic class: Antidiabetic
Pregnancy category: C

Indications and Dosages
➤ *To control blood glucose level in type 2 diabetes mellitus, either as monotherapy or with metformin or a thiazolidinedione*
TABLETS
Adults. 120 mg three times daily 1 to 30 min before meals.
DOSAGE ADJUSTMENT Dosage reduced to 60 mg three times daily in patients with near-goal glycosylated hemoglobin (HbA_{1c}) level.

Contraindications
Diabetic ketoacidosis, hypersensitivity to nateglinide or its components, type 1 diabetes mellitus

Route	Onset	Peak	Duration
P.O.	20 min	1 hr	4 hr

DRUGS
corticosteroids, phenytoin, rifampin, somatropin, St. John's wort, sympathomimetics, thiazide diuretics, thyroid products: Possibly reduced hypoglycemic effects of nateglinide
MAO inhibitors, nonselective beta-adrenergic blockers, NSAIDs, salicylates, somatostatin analogues: Possibly additive hypoglycemic effects of nateglinide

Adverse Reactions
CNS: Dizziness
ENDO: Hypoglycemia
GI: Cholestatic hepatitis, diarrhea, elevated liver enzyme levels, jaundice
MS: Accidental trauma, arthropathy, back pain
RESP: Bronchitis, cough, upper respiratory tract infection
SKIN: Pruritus, rash, urticaria
Other: Flulike symptoms

Nursing Considerations
• Give nateglinide 1 to 30 minutes before meals to reduce the risk of hypoglycemia.

• Monitor fasting glucose and HbA$_{1c}$ levels periodically, as ordered, to evaluate treatment effectiveness.
• Monitor patient often in event of fever, infection, trauma, or surgery because transient loss of glucose control may occur, requiring an alteration in therapy.

PATIENT TEACHING
• Instruct patient to take nateglinide 1 to 30 minutes before meals. Advise her to skip scheduled dose if she skips a meal to reduce the risk of hypoglycemia.
• Teach patient to measure blood glucose level and recognize hyperglycemia and hypoglycemia. Advise her to notify prescriber if blood glucose level is abnormal.
• Inform patient that strenuous exercise, insufficient calorie intake, and consumption of alcohol increase risk of hypoglycemia.
• Advise patient to monitor blood glucose level as prescribed and to keep follow-up appointments to monitor HbA$_{1c}$ level because drug may become less effective over time.

Mechanism of Action
Nateglinide stimulates the release of insulin from functioning beta cells of the pancreas. In patients with type 2 diabetes mellitus, a lack of functioning beta cells diminishes blood levels of insulin and causes glucose intolerance. By interacting with the adenosine triphosphatase (ATP)–potassium channel on the beta cell membrane, nateglinide prevents potassium (K^+) from leaving the cell.

This causes the beta cell to depolarize and the cell membrane's calcium channel to open. Consequently, calcium (Ca^{++}) moves into the cell and insulin moves out of it. The extent of insulin release is glucose dependent; the lower the glucose level, the less insulin is secreted from the cell.

By promoting insulin secretion in patients with type 2 diabetes mellitus, nateglinide improves glucose tolerance.

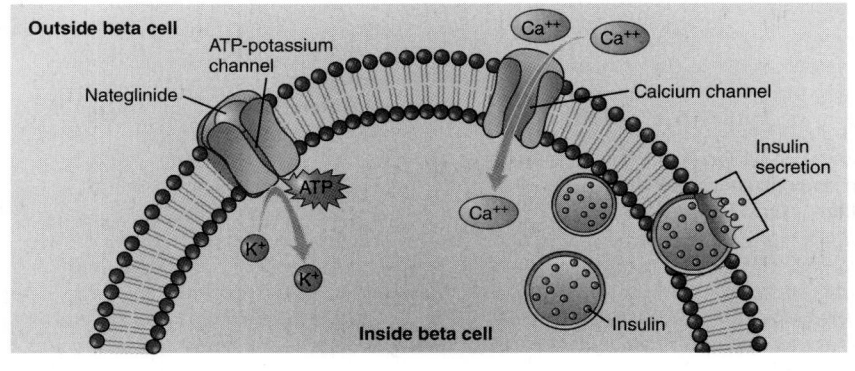

nebivolol hydrochloride

Bystolic

Class and Category

Chemical class: Beta-adrenergic blocker
Therapeutic class: Antihypertensive
Pregnancy category: C

Indications and Dosages

➤ *To treat hypertension*

TABLETS

Adults. *Initial:* 5 mg once daily, increased at 2-wk intervals, as needed. *Maximum:* 40 mg once daily.

DOSAGE ADJUSTMENT For patients with moderate renal impairment (creatinine clearance less than 30 ml/min/1.73 m^2) or moderate hepatic impairment (Child-Pugh Class B), initial dose reduced to 2.5 mg.

Mechanism of Action

May prevent arterial dilation and inhibit renin secretion, although precise mechanism of action isn't known. Negative chronotropic effects may slow resting heart rate, and negative inotropic effects may reduce cardiac output, myocardial contractility, and myocardial oxygen consumption during stress or exercise. All of these actions may work together to lower systolic and diastolic blood pressure.

Route	Onset	Peak	Duration
P.O.	Unknown	1.5–4 hr	Unknown

Contraindications

Advanced AV block, cardiogenic shock, decompensated cardiac failure, hypersensitivity to nebivolol or its components, sick sinus syndrome (unless permanent pacemaker is in place), severe bradycardia, severe hepatic impairment

Interaction

DRUGS

antiarrhythmias such as disopyramide, beta blockers, digoxin, selected calcium antagonists such as diltiazem and verapamil: Increased effect on AV conduction and myocardial depression; increased risk of bradycardia

fluoxetine, paroxetine, propafenone, quinidine: Increased hypertensive effect of nebivolol
guanethidine, reserpine: Possibly excessive reduction of sympathetic activity

Adverse Reactions

CNS: Asthenia, dizziness, fatigue, headache, insomnia, paresthesia, somnolence, syncope, vertigo
CV: Allergic vasculitis, AV block, bradycardia, chest pain, hypercholesterolemia, hyperuricemia, MI, peripheral edema, peripheral ischemia, Raynaud's phenomenon
ENDO: Hyperglycemia, mask symptoms of hypoglycemia
GI: Abdominal pain, diarrhea, elevated liver enzymes, nausea, vomiting
GU: Acute renal failure, elevated BUN level, erectile dysfunction
HEME: Decreased platelet count, thrombocytopenia
RESP: Acute pulmonary edema, bronchospasm, dyspnea
SKIN: Pruritus, psoriasis, rash, urticaria
Other: Angioedema

Nursing Considerations

• Know that patients with bronchospastic disease usually shouldn't be treated with beta blocker therapy such as nebivolol.
• Use nebivolol cautiously in patients with impaired hepatic or renal function.
• Expect to administer an alpha blocker, as ordered, before starting nebivolol therapy in patients with pheochromocytoma.
• Monitor blood pressure and pulse rate often, especially at start of nebivolol therapy and during dosage adjustments. Also monitor fluid intake and output and daily weight, and watch for evidence of heart failure, such as dyspnea, edema, fatigue, and jugular vein distention. If heart failure occurs or worsens, expect drug to be discontinued.
• Be aware that nebivolol shouldn't be stopped abruptly because MI, myocardial ischemia, severe hypertension, or ventricular arrhythmias may result.
• Because of this, expect nebivolol therapy to continue throughout the perioperative period of major surgery. However, monitor patient closely for protracted severe

hypotension and difficulty restarting and keeping a heartbeat. Be prepared to administer a beta agonist such as dobutamine or isoproterenol, as ordered, to reverse the effects of nebivolol, if needed.
• Assess distal circulation and peripheral pulses in patient with peripheral vascular disease because drug can worsen it.
• Be aware that nebivolol may mask tachycardia from hyperthyroidism and that abrupt withdrawal can cause thyroid storm. Drug also can decrease blood glucose level, prolong or mask symptoms of hypoglycemia, promote hyperglycemia in patient with diabetes mellitus, or worsen psoriasis.
• Monitor patient closely for hypersensitivity reactions that may occur with beta blockers, especially patients with a history of severe anaphylactic reactions who may not be responsive to usual doses of epinephrine used to treat allergic reactions.
• Know that an alpha blocker should be initiated, as ordered, prior to the use of nebivolol therapy in a patient with pheochromocytoma.

PATIENT TEACHING
• Instruct patient to take nebivolol exactly as prescribed and not to stop using it abruptly.
• Tell patient to weigh herself daily during nebivolol therapy and to notify prescriber if she gains more than 2 lb (0.9 kg) in 1 day or 5 lb (2.3 kg) in 1 week.
• Advise patient to rise slowly from a seated or lying position to minimize effects of orthostatic hypotension.
• Advise patient to avoid hazardous activities until drug's CNS effects are known.
• Instruct patient to contact prescriber about bleeding or bruising, cough at night, dizziness, edema, rash, shortness of breath, or slow pulse rate.
• Advise diabetic patient to monitor her blood glucose level more often during nebivolol therapy because drug may mask symptoms of hypoglycemia.
• Inform patient with psoriasis that drug may aggravate this condition.

nefazodone hydrochloride

Serzone

Class and Category
Chemical class: Phenylpiperazine derivative
Therapeutic class: Antidepressant
Pregnancy category: C

Indications and Dosages
➤ *To treat major depression*
TABLETS
Adults. *Initial:* 100 mg twice daily, increased by 100 to 200 mg daily every wk, as prescribed. *Maintenance:* 150 to 300 mg twice daily. *Maximum:* 600 mg daily.
DOSAGE ADJUSTMENT Initial dosage possibly reduced to 50 mg twice daily for elderly or debilitated patients; then dosage adjusted as ordered, based on patient response.

Route	Onset	Peak	Duration
P.O.	Several wk	Unknown	Unknown

Mechanism of Action
May inhibit serotonin reuptake at presynaptic neurons, which may increase neuronal level of serotonin, an inhibitory neurotransmitter thought to regulate mood. Nefazodone also may act as a postsynaptic serotonin receptor antagonist, further increasing the amount of synaptic serotonin that's available.

Contraindications
Concurrent use of astemizole, cisapride, or terfenadine; hypersensitivity to nefazodone, other phenylpiperazine antidepressants, or their components; restarting nefazodone therapy that was discontinued because of liver injury; use within 14 days of MAO inhibitor therapy

Interaction
DRUGS
alprazolam, buspirone, carbamazepine, cyclosporine, modafinil, triazolam: Increased blood levels of these drugs
antihypertensives: Increased risk of hypotension
astemizole, cisapride, terfenadine: Increased blood levels of these drugs, prolonged QT interval, and, possibly, serious cardio-

N O

vascular effects, including death from ventricular tachycardia

cilostazol: Decreased cilostazol clearance, increased adverse effects of cilostazol, such as headache

dextromethorphan, sibutramine, tramadol, trazodone: Increased risk of serotonin syndrome

digoxin: Increased blood digoxin level, increased risk of digitalis toxicity

haloperidol: Decreased haloperidol clearance

indinavir: Inhibited indinavir metabolism

levobupivacaine: Increased blood levobupivacaine level, possibly toxicity

lovastatin, simvastatin: Increased risk of rhabdomyolysis and myositis

MAO inhibitors: Possibly fatal reactions, including autonomic instability (with rapidly fluctuating vital signs), hyperthermia, mental status changes (such as severe agitation progressing to delirium and coma), muscle rigidity, and myoclonus

methadone: Increased blood level and adverse effects of methadone, additive CNS effects

nevirapine: Increased nefazodone metabolism, inhibited nevirapine metabolism

ritonavir: Inhibited nefazodone and ritonavir metabolism

sildenafil: Decreased sildenafil clearance

tacrolimus: Decreased tacrolimus clearance and increased adverse effects, including delirium and renal failure

ACTIVITIES

alcohol use: Increased risk of CNS depression

Adverse Reactions

CNS: Abnormal gait, apathy, asthenia, ataxia, chills, confusion, decreased concentration, delusions, depersonalization, dizziness, dream disturbances, euphoria, fever, hallucinations, headache, hostility, hypotonia, insomnia, light-headedness, malaise, memory loss, myoclonic jerks, neuralgia, paranoia, paresthesia, somnolence, suicidal ideation, syncope, tremor, vertigo

CV: Angina, hypertension, hypotension, peripheral edema, orthostatic hypotension, tachycardia, vasodilation, ventricular arrhythmias

EENT: Abnormal vision, blurred vision, conjunctivitis, diplopia, dry eyes and mouth, earache, epistaxis, eye pain, gingivitis, halitosis, hyperacusis, laryngitis, mydriasis, neck rigidity, periodontal abscess, pharyngitis, photophobia, stomatitis, taste perversion, tinnitus, visual field defects

ENDO: Breast pain, gynecomastia, lymphadenopathy

GI: Abdominal distention, colitis, constipation, diarrhea, elevated liver function test results, eructation, esophagitis, gastritis, gastroenteritis, hernia, hepatotoxicity, hiccups, increased appetite, indigestion, life-threatening hepatic failure, nausea, peptic ulcer, rectal bleeding, thirst, vomiting

GU: Abnormal ejaculation; amenorrhea; cystitis; hematuria; hypermenorrhea; impotence; libido changes; nocturia; pelvic pain; polyuria; renal calculi; urinary frequency, incontinence, or urgency; urine retention; UTI; vaginal bleeding; vaginitis

HEME: Anemia, leukopenia

MS: Arthralgia, arthritis, bursitis, dysarthria, gout, muscle stiffness, tenosynovitis

RESP: Asthma, bronchitis, cough, dyspnea, pneumonia

SKIN: Acne, alopecia, dry skin, ecchymosis, eczema, maculopapular rash, photosensitivity, pruritus, rash, urticaria

Other: Allergic reaction, dehydration, infection, serotonin syndrome, weight loss

Nursing Considerations

WARNING Be aware that nefazodone should not be given with astemizole, cisapride, MAO inhibitors, or terfenadine; serious, even fatal, reactions may occur.

WARNING Be aware that life-threatening hepatic failure has occurred during nefazodone therapy, resulting in need for transplant or causing death. Check patient's liver enzymes, as ordered, prior to nefazodone therapy. Know that patients with active liver disease or who have elevated liver enzymes should not begin nefazodone therapy. Monitor patient for signs of hepatic failure, such as the development of anorexia, dark urine, fatigue, jaundice, and malaise during therapy. Expect patient's liver enzymes to be checked regularly and drug to be discontinued if patient exhibits signs and symptoms of liver dysfunction or liver enzymes become elevated.

- Assess for evidence of serotonin syndrome, such as abdominal cramps, aggression, agitation, chills, diarrhea, headache, insomnia, lack of coordination, nausea, palpitations, paresthesia, poor concentration, and worsening of obsessive thoughts.
- Monitor patient closely for suicidal tendencies, especially when therapy starts or dosage changes, because depression may worsen temporarily. Follow facility policy.

PATIENT TEACHING
- Instruct patient to take nefazodone exactly as prescribed and not to alter dosage.
- Urge patient to immediately report evidence of hepatic failure, such as jaundice, dark urine, lack of appetite, nausea, or abdominal pain.
- Inform patient that antidepressant effects may not occur for several weeks and that treatment may last 6 months or longer.
- Caution patient to avoid alcohol during nefazodone therapy.
- Advise patient to avoid hazardous activities until drug's CNS effects are known.
- Suggest that patient try sugarless gum or hard candy for dry mouth. Urge her to notify prescriber if dry mouth persists.
- Urge family or caregiver to watch patient closely for suicidal tendencies, especially when therapy starts or dosage changes.

neomycin sulfate
Mycifradin, Neo-Fradin

Class and Category
Chemical class: Aminoglycoside
Therapeutic class: Antibiotic
Pregnancy category: D

Indications and Dosages
➤ *To suppress intestinal bacterial growth in preoperative bowel preparation*
TABLETS (24-HR REGIMEN)
Adults. 1 g every hr for 4 doses and then 1 g every 4 hr for remainder of 24 hr before

surgery. Or, for 8 a.m. surgery, 1 g of neomycin with erythromycin at 1 p.m., 2 p.m., and 11 p.m. the day before surgery. **Children.** 25 mg/kg at 1 p.m., 2 p.m., and 11 p.m. the day before surgery.
TABLETS (2- TO 3-DAY REGIMEN)
Adults and children. 88 mg/kg every 4 hr in 6 equally divided doses for 2 to 3 days before surgery.
➤ *As adjunct in hepatic encephalopathy*
TABLETS
Adults. 4 to 12 g daily in divided doses every 6 hr for 5 to 6 days.
Children. 50 to 100 mg/kg daily in divided doses every 6 hr for 5 to 6 days.
➤ *To treat infectious diarrhea caused by enteropathic* Escherichia coli
TABLETS
Adults and children. 50 mg/kg daily in divided doses four times daily for 2 to 3 days.

Mechanism of Action
Is transported into bacterial cells, where it competes with messenger RNA to bind with a specific receptor protein on the 30S ribosomal subunit of DNA. This action causes abnormal, nonfunctioning proteins to form. A lack of functional proteins causes bacterial cell death.

Contraindications
Hypersensitivity or serious reaction to neomycin, other aminoglycosides, or their components; inflammatory or ulcerative GI disease; intestinal obstruction

Interaction
DRUGS
digoxin, spironolactone: Possibly reduced absorption rate of these drugs
dimenhydrinate: Possibly masked symptoms of neomycin-induced ototoxicity
methotrexate: Possibly decreased absorption and bioavailability of methotrexate
neuromuscular blockers: Potentiated neuromuscular blockade, increased risk of prolonged respiratory depression
oral anticoagulants: Possibly potentiated anticoagulant effects

Adverse Reactions
EENT: Ototoxicity
GI: Diarrhea, malabsorption syndrome (decreased serum carotene level and xylose absorption, increased fecal fat and

N
O

flatulence), nausea, pseudomembranous colitis, vomiting

GU: Nephrotoxicity

Nursing Considerations

• Monitor patient's BUN and serum creatinine levels to assess renal function before and during neomycin therapy. Expect to decrease dosage or stop drug if nephrotoxicity develops.

• Monitor blood neomycin level, as directed, to assess for therapeutic range of 5 to 10 mcg/ml.

WARNING Neomycin is highly ototoxic and may cause hearing loss and tinnitus.

• Watch for evidence of pseudomembranous colitis, such as severe abdominal cramps and severe, watery diarrhea.

• Anticipate that neomycin's curare-like effect may worsen muscle weakness in patients with neuromuscular disorders, such as myasthenia gravis and parkinsonism.

PATIENT TEACHING

• Urge patient to complete full course of neomycin therapy.

• Unless contraindicated, urge patient to drink plenty of fluids to prevent nephrotoxicity.

• Urge patient undergoing bowel preparation to comply with recommended regimen, including low-residue diet, bisacodyl enema administration, and neomycin use.

• Advise patient to notify prescriber about hearing loss or ringing in ears.

neostigmine bromide

Prostigmin

neostigmine methylsulfate

Bloxiverz, Neostigmine Methylsulfate

Class and Category

Chemical class: Quaternary ammonium compound

Therapeutic class: Anticholinesterase, curare antidote

Pregnancy category: C

Indications and Dosages

➤ *To treat symptoms of myasthenia gravis*

TABLETS (NEOSTIGMINE BROMIDE)

Adults. *Initial:* 15 mg every 3 to 4 hr. Dosage adjusted based on clinical response. *Maintenance:* 150 mg daily in divided doses based on clinical response.

Children. 2 mg/kg daily in 6 to 8 divided doses.

I.M. OR SUBCUTANEOUS INJECTION (NEOSTIGMINE METHYLSULFATE)

Adults. *Initial:* 0.5 mg. Dosage adjusted based on clinical response.

Children. 0.01 to 0.04 mg/kg every 2 to 3 hr.

➤ *To reverse nondepolarizing neuromuscular blockade*

I.V. INJECTION (NEOSTIGMINE METHYLSULFATE)

Adults. 0.5 to 2 mg by slow push, repeated as needed up to 5 mg; 0.6 to 1.2 mg of atropine or 0.2 to 0.6 mg of glycopyrrolate given with or a few minutes before neostigmine, as ordered.

Children. 0.04 mg/kg by slow push; 0.02 mg of atropine/kg is given I.M. or subcutaneously with each dose or alternate doses.

I.V. INJECTION (BLOXIVERZ)

Adults and children. 0.03 mg/kg (drugs with shorter half-lives) or 0.07 mg/kg (drugs with longer half-lives or need for more rapid recovery) infused over at least one minute. *Maximum:* 0.07 mg/kg or 5 mg, whichever is less.

➤ *To prevent postoperative, nonobstructive urine retention and abdominal distention (adynamic ileus)*

I.M. OR SUBCUTANEOUS INJECTION (NEOSTIGMINE METHYLSULFATE)

Adults. 0.25 mg immediately after surgery and repeated every 4 to 6 hr for 2 to 3 days.

➤ *To treat postoperative, nonobstructive urine retention and abdominal distention (adynamic ileus)*

I.M. OR SUBCUTANEOUS INJECTION (NEOSTIGMINE METHYLSULFATE)

Adults. 0.5 mg; injections repeated every 3 hr for at least 5 doses if patient has voided or bladder has emptied within 1 hr.

Route	Onset	Peak	Duration
P.O.	45–75 min*	Unknown	3–6 hr
I.V.	4–8 min†	30 min	2–4 hr

Route	Onset	Peak	Duration
I.M.	20–30 min[†]	30 min	2–4 hr

Mechanism of Action

Inhibits action of cholinesterase, an enzyme that destroys acetylcholine at myoneuronal junctions, thereby increasing acetylcholine accumulation at myoneuronal junctions and facilitating nerve impulse transmission across the junctions. This action:
- helps prevent or relieve urine retention by increasing detrusor muscle tone in the bladder and causing bladder contractions strong enough to induce urination.
- prevents or treats postoperative abdominal distention by increasing gastric motility and tone.
- improves muscle strength and increases muscle response to repetitive nerve stimulation in myasthenia gravis.

Contraindications

Hypersensitivity to neostigmine, other anticholinesterases, bromides, or their components; mechanical obstruction of intestinal or urinary tract; peritonitis

Interaction

DRUGS

aminoglycosides, anesthetics, capreomycin, colistimethate, colistin, lidocaine, lincomycins, polymyxin B, quinine: Increased risk of neuromuscular blockade
anticholinergics: Possibly masked signs of cholinergic crisis
guanadrel, guanethidine, mecamylamine, trimethaphan: Possibly antagonized effects of neostigmine, possibly decreased anti-hypertensive effects
neuromuscular blockers: Possibly prolonged action of depolarizing—and antagonized action of nondepolarizing—neuromuscular blockers
procainamide, quinidine: Possibly antagonized effects of neostigmine
quinine: Decreased neostigmine effectiveness

Adverse Reactions

CNS: Dizziness, drowsiness, headache, seizures, syncope, weakness

---
[*] For adynamic ileus, 2 to 4 hr.
[†] For adynamic ileus, 10 to 30 min.

CV: Arrhythmias (AV block, bradycardia, nodal rhythm, tachycardia), cardiac arrest, ECG changes, hypotension
EENT: Increased salivation, lacrimation, miosis, vision changes
GI: Abdominal cramps, diarrhea, flatulence, increased peristalsis, nausea, vomiting
GU: Urinary frequency
MS: Arthralgia, dysarthria, muscle spasms
RESP: Bronchospasm, dyspnea, increased bronchial secretions, respiratory arrest or depression
SKIN: Flushing, diaphoresis, rash, urticaria

Nursing Considerations

- Be aware that 15-mg oral neostigmine bromide is equivalent to 0.5 mg parenteral neostigmine methylsulfate.
- If also giving atropine, be sure to administer it before neostigmine, as prescribed.
- When giving neostigmine I.V., make sure patient is well ventilated and airway remains patent until normal respiration is assured.
- When administering Bloxiverz, know that a peripheral nerve stimulation device should be used to time the initial dose and any further doses of neostigmine, if needed.
- If patient has myasthenia gravis, give drug night and day, as ordered, with larger portions of daily dose during periods of increased fatigue. If patient's condition becomes refractory to neostigmine, expect to reduce dosage or discontinue drug, as prescribed, for a few days.
- *WARNING* Monitor patient for evidence of neostigmine overdose, which can cause possibly fatal cholinergic crisis (increased muscle weakness, including respiratory muscles). Expect to stop neostigmine and atropine, as ordered.

PATIENT TEACHING

- Instruct patient to take neostigmine exactly as prescribed.
- Advise patient to take drug with food or milk to reduce adverse GI reactions.
- Suggest that patient with myasthenia gravis keep a daily record of doses and adverse reactions during therapy.
- Instruct patient to schedule activities to minimize fatigue.

N
O

nesiritide

Natrecor

Class and Category

Chemical class: Human B-type natriuretic peptide
Therapeutic class: Arterial and venous smooth muscle cell relaxant
Pregnancy category: C

Indications and Dosages

➤ *To reduce dyspnea at rest or with minimal activity in patients with acute decompensated congestive heart failure*

I.V. INFUSION, I.V. INJECTION

Adults. 2-mcg/kg bolus and then continuous infusion of 0.01 mcg/kg/min for up to 48 hr.

Route	Onset	Peak	Duration
I.V.	In 15 min	1 hr	3 hr

Mechanism of Action

Binds to guanylate cyclase receptor of vascular smooth muscle and endothelial cells. This action increases intracellular levels of cyclic guanosine monophosphate, which leads to arterial and venous smooth muscle cell relaxation. Ultimately, nesiritide reduces pulmonary capillary wedge pressure and systemic arterial pressure in patients with congestive heart failure, which decreases the heart's workload and subsequently relieves dyspnea.

Incompatibilities

Don't infuse nesiritide through same I.V. line as bumetanide, enalaprilat, ethacrynate sodium, furosemide, heparin, hydralazine, or insulin because these drugs are chemically and physically incompatible with nesiritide. Don't infuse drugs that contain the preservative sodium metabisulfite through same I.V. line as nesiritide.

Contraindications

Cardiogenic shock, hypersensitivity to nesiritide or its components, persistent systolic blood pressure less than 100 mm Hg

Interaction

DRUGS

ACE inhibitors: Increased risk of symptomatic hypotension

Adverse Reactions

CNS: Anxiety, dizziness, headache, insomnia
CV: Angina, bradycardia, hypotension, PVCs, ventricular tachycardia
GI: Abdominal pain, nausea, vomiting
GU: Elevated serum creatinine level, worsening of renal function
MS: Back pain
Other: Anaphylaxis and other hypersensitivity reactions

Nursing Considerations

WARNING Be aware that nesiritide isn't recommended for patients suspected to have low cardiac filling pressures or patients for whom vasodilating drugs aren't appropriate, such as those with constrictive pericarditis, pericardial tamponade, restrictive or obstructive cardiomyopathy, significant valvular stenosis, or other conditions in which cardiac output depends on venous return.

• Reconstitute 1.5-mg vial by adding 5 ml diluent removed from a 250-ml plastic I.V. bag containing preservative-free D_5W, normal saline solution, dextrose 5% in half-normal (0.45) saline solution, or dextrose 5% in quarter-normal (0.2) saline solution.

• Don't shake vial. Rock it gently so all surfaces, including the stopper, are in contact with diluent to ensure complete reconstitution. Inspect drug for particulate matter and discoloration; if present, discard drug.

• Withdraw entire contents of reconstituted solution and add it to 250-ml plastic I.V. bag used to withdraw diluent to yield a solution of about 6 mcg/ml. Invert I.V. bag several times to ensure complete mixing.

• After preparing infusion bag, withdraw bolus volume from infusion bag and give it over about 60 seconds. Immediately after bolus, infuse drug at 0.1 ml/kg/hr, which will deliver 0.01 mcg/kg/min.

• Prime I.V. tubing with 25 ml of solution before connecting to the I.V. line and before administering the bolus dose or starting the infusion.

• Flush the I.V. line between doses of nesiritide and incompatible drugs.

• Because nesiritide binds to heparin and therefore could bind to the heparin lining

of a heparin-coated catheter, don't give it through a central heparin-coated catheter.
• Store reconstituted vials at room temperature (20° to 25° C [68° to 77° F]) or refrigerate (2° to 8° C [36° to 46° F]) for up to 24 hours.
• Because nesiritide contains no antimicrobial preservatives, discard the reconstituted solution after 24 hours.
• Monitor blood pressure and heart rate and rhythm frequently during therapy.
• If hypotension occurs, notify prescriber and expect to reduce dosage or discontinue the drug. Implement measures to support blood pressure as prescribed.
• Assess patient's breath sounds and respiratory rate, rhythm, depth, and quality frequently during drug therapy.
• Monitor serum creatinine level during and after therapy has been completed. Notify prescriber of abnormal results because nesiritide may decrease renal function.
WARNING Monitor patient for serious hypersensitivity reactions following nesiritide administration. Reactions can become serious, requiring supportive care such as treatment with epinephrine, oxygen, IV fluids, antihistamines, corticosteroids, pressor amines, and airway management.
• Store unopened drug at controlled room temperature or refrigerate. Keep in carton until time of use.

PATIENT TEACHING
• Instruct patient to notify you or another nurse if she becomes dizzy because this may indicate hypotension.
• Reassure patient that her blood pressure, heart rate, and breathing will be monitored frequently.
• Emphasize importance of reporting an allergic reaction immediately.

---

netilmicin sulfate

Netromycin

Class and Category
Chemical class: Aminoglycoside
Therapeutic class: Antibiotic
Pregnancy category: D

Indications and Dosages
➤ *To treat serious systemic infections, such as intra-abdominal infections, lower respiratory tract infections, septicemia, and skin and soft-tissue infections, caused by* Enterobacter aerogenes, Escherichia coli, Klebsiella pneumoniae, Proteus mirabilis, Pseudomonas aeruginosa, Serratia *species, and* Staphylococcus aureus

I.V. INFUSION, I.M. INJECTION
Adults and children age 12 and over. 1.3 to 2.2 mg/kg every 8 hr or 2 to 3.25 mg/kg every 12 hr for 7 to 14 days. *Maximum:* 7.5 mg/kg daily.
Children ages 6 weeks to 12 years. 1.8 to 2.7 mg/kg every 8 hr or 2.7 to 4 mg/kg every 12 hr for 7 to 14 days.
Infants up to age 6 weeks. 2 to 3.25 mg/kg every 12 hr for 7 to 14 days.
➤ *To treat complicated UTI caused by* Citrobacter *species,* Enterobacter *species,* E. coli, K. pneumoniae, P. mirabilis, P. aeruginosa, Serratia *species, and* Staphylococcus *species*

I.V. INFUSION, I.M. INJECTION
Adults and adolescents. 1.5 to 2 mg/kg every 12 hr for 7 to 14 days. *Maximum:* 7.5 mg/kg daily.

Mechanism of Action
Is transported into bacterial cells, where it competes with messenger RNA to bind with a specific receptor protein on the 30S ribosomal subunit of DNA. This action causes abnormal, nonfunctioning proteins to form. A lack of functional proteins causes bacterial cell death.

Incompatibilities
Don't mix netilmicin with beta-lactam antibiotics (penicillins and cephalosporins) because substantial mutual inactivation may result. If prescribed concurrently, administer these drugs at separate sites.

Contraindications
Hypersensitivity to netilmicin, other aminoglycosides, or their components

Interaction
DRUGS
capreomycin, other aminoglycosides: Increased risk of nephrotoxicity, neuromuscular blockade, and ototoxicity

cephalosporins, nephrotoxic drugs: Increased risk of nephrotoxicity
loop diuretics, ototoxic drugs: Increased risk of ototoxicity
methoxyflurane, polymyxins (parenteral): Increased risk of nephrotoxicity and neuromuscular blockade
neuromuscular blockers: Increased neuromuscular blockade

Adverse Reactions
CNS: Disorientation, dizziness, encephalopathy, headache, myasthenia gravis–like syndrome, neuromuscular blockade (acute muscle paralysis and apnea), paresthesia, peripheral neuropathy, seizures, vertigo, weakness
CV: Hypotension, palpitations
EENT: Blurred vision, hearing loss, nystagmus, tinnitus
GI: Diarrhea, elevated liver function tests results, nausea, vomiting
GU: Elevated BUN and serum creatinine levels, nephrotoxicity, oliguria, proteinuria
HEME: Anemia, eosinophilia, leukopenia, prolonged PT, thrombocytopenia, thrombocytosis
MS: Muscle twitching
RESP: Apnea
SKIN: Allergic dermatitis, erythema, pruritus, rash
Other: Angioedema; hyperkalemia; injection-site hematoma, induration, and pain

Nursing Considerations
• To prepare netilmicin for I.V. use, dilute each dose in 50 to 200 ml of suitable diluent, such as normal saline solution, D_5W, or lactated Ringer's solution, and give slowly over 30 to 60 minutes.
• Ensure adequate hydration during therapy to maintain adequate renal function.
• Monitor blood netilmicin level; optimum peak level is 6 to 10 mcg/ml and trough level is 0.5 to 2 mcg/ml.
• Check patient's BUN and serum creatinine levels, urine specific gravity, and creatinine clearance during netilmicin therapy, as ordered.
• Anticipate higher risk of nephrotoxicity in elderly patients, those with impaired renal function, and those who receive high doses or prolonged netilmicin therapy.
• Reduce dosage or discontinue drug, as ordered, if signs of drug-induced auditory

or vestibular toxicity develop; the damage may be permanent.

PATIENT TEACHING
• Encourage patient to drink plenty of fluids during netilmicin therapy.
• Instruct patient to notify prescriber immediately about dizziness, hearing loss, muscle twitching, nausea, numbness and tingling, ringing or buzzing in ears, seizures, significant changes in amount of urine or frequency of urination, and vomiting.
• Urge patient to keep follow-up appointments to monitor progress.

nicardipine hydrochloride
Cardene, Cardene IV, Cardene SR

Class and Category
Chemical class: Dihydropyridine derivative
Therapeutic class: Antianginal, antihypertensive
Pregnancy category: C

Indications and Dosages
➤ *To manage angina pectoris and Prinzmetal's angina, to manage hypertension*
CAPSULES
Adults and adolescents. 20 to 40 mg three times daily, increased every 3 days, as prescribed.
E.R. CAPSULES
Adults. 30 mg twice daily.
I.V. INFUSION
Adults. 0.5 to 2.2 mg/hr by continuous infusion.
➤ *To control acute hypertension*
I.V. INFUSION
Adults. *Initial:* 5 mg/hr by continuous infusion; increased by 2.5 mg/hr every 5 to 15 min, as prescribed. *Maximum:* 15 mg/hr.
DOSAGE ADJUSTMENT For patients with impaired liver function or reduced hepatic blood flow, dosage may be decreased.

Route	Onset	Peak	Duration
P.O.	20 min	1–2 hr	Unknown
P.O. (E.R.)	20 min	1–2 hr	12 hr
I.V.	Immediate	Unknown	Unknown

Mechanism of Action

May slow extracellular calcium movement into myocardial and vascular smooth-muscle cells by deforming calcium channels in cell membranes, inhibiting ion-controlled gating mechanisms, and interfering with calcium release from the sarcoplasmic reticulum. By decreasing the intracellular calcium level, nicardipine inhibits smooth-muscle cell contraction and dilates coronary and systemic arteries. As with other calcium channel blockers, these actions lead to decreased myocardial oxygen requirements and reduced peripheral resistance, blood pressure, and afterload.

Incompatibilities

Don't mix nicardipine with sodium bicarbonate or LR solution, and don't administer through same I.V. line.

Contraindications

Advanced aortic stenosis, hypersensitivity to any calcium channel blocker, second- or third-degree AV block in patient without artificial pacemaker

Interaction

DRUGS

anesthetics (hydrocarbon inhalation): Possibly hypotension
beta blockers, other antihypertensives, prazocin: Increased risk of hypotension
calcium supplements: Possibly impaired action of nicardipine
cimetidine: Increased nicardipine bioavailability
digoxin: Transiently increased blood digoxin level, increased risk of digitalis toxicity
disopyramide, flecainide: Increased risk of bradycardia, conduction defects, and heart failure
estrogens: Possibly increased fluid retention and decreased therapeutic effects of nicardipine
lithium: Increased risk of neurotoxicity
NSAIDs, sympathomimetics: Possibly decreased therapeutic effects of nicardipine
procainamide, quinidine: Possibly prolonged QT interval

FOODS

grapefruit, grapefruit juice: Possibly increased bioavailability of nicardipine

high-fat meals: Decreased blood nicardipine level

ACTIVITIES

alcohol use: Increased hypotensive effect

Adverse Reactions

CNS: Anxiety, asthenia, ataxia, confusion, dizziness, drowsiness, headache, nervousness, paresthesia, psychiatric disturbance, syncope, tremor, weakness
CV: Arrhythmias (bradycardia, tachycardia), chest pain, exacerbation of angina (chronic therapy), heart failure, hypotension, orthostatic hypotension, palpitations, peripheral edema
EENT: Altered taste, blurred vision, dry mouth, epistaxis, gingival hyperplasia, pharyngitis, rhinitis, tinnitus
ENDO: Gynecomastia, hyperglycemia
GI: Anorexia, constipation, diarrhea, elevated liver function test results, indigestion, nausea, thirst, vomiting
GU: Dysuria, nocturia, polyuria, sexual dysfunction, urinary frequency
HEME: Anemia, leukopenia, thrombocytopenia
MS: Joint stiffness, muscle spasms
RESP: Bronchitis, cough, decreased oxygen saturation, upper respiratory tract infection
SKIN: Dermatitis, diaphoresis, erythema multiforme, flushing, photosensitivity, pruritus, rash, Stevens-Johnson syndrome, urticaria
Other: Hypokalemia, injection-site irritation, weight gain

Nursing Considerations

• Check blood pressure and pulse rate before nicardipine therapy begins, during dosage changes, and periodically throughout therapy. During prolonged therapy, periodically assess ECG tracings for arrhythmias and other changes.
• Dilute each 25-mg ampule of nicardipine with 240 ml of solution to yield 0.1 mg/ml. Mixture is stable at room temperature for 24 hours.
• If using premixed nicardipine for intravenous infusion, check strength carefully because drug comes as single strength (20 mg nicardipine in 200 ml of solution, providing 0.1 mg/ml) or double strength (40 mg nicardipine in 200 ml of solution, providing 0.2 mg/ml).

N
O

• Administer continuous infusion by I.V. pump or controller, and adjust according to patient's blood pressure, as prescribed. Be aware that the I.V. dosage should be titrated slowly in patients receiving a beta blocker and in patients with heart failure or significant left ventricular dysfunction because of possible negative inotropic effects.

• Change peripheral I.V. site every 12 hours, if feasible, to minimize peripheral venous irritation.

• Give first dose of oral nicardipine 1 hour before stopping I.V. infusion, as ordered.

• Monitor fluid intake and output and daily weight for signs of fluid retention, which may precipitate heart failure. Also assess for signs of heart failure, such as crackles, dyspnea, jugular vein distention, peripheral edema, and weight gain.

• During prolonged therapy, periodically monitor liver and renal function test results. Anticipate drug dosage to be titrated slowly in these patients. Expect elevated liver function test results to return to normal after drug is discontinued.

• Monitor patient with angina for increases in frequency, duration, or severity of symptoms because with chronic use of oral nicardipine (rarely with I.V. administration), exacerbation of angina may occur.

• Monitor serum potassium level during prolonged therapy. Hypokalemia increases the risk of arrhythmias.

• Because of drug's negative inotropic effect on some patients, closely monitor patients who take a beta blocker or have heart failure or significant left ventricular dysfunction.

WARNING Expect to taper dosage gradually before discontinuing drug. Otherwise, angina or dangerously high blood pressure could result.

PATIENT TEACHING

• Urge patient to take nicardipine as prescribed, even if she feels well.

• Instruct patient to swallow E.R. capsules whole, not to chew, crush, cut, or open them.

• Advise patient not to take drug within 1 hour of eating a high-fat meal or grapefruit product. Urge her not to alter the amount of grapefruit products in her diet without consulting prescriber.

WARNING Caution patient against stopping nicardipine abruptly because angina or dangerously high blood pressure could result.

• Teach patient how to take her pulse, and urge her to notify prescriber immediately if it falls below 50 beats/minute.

• Teach patient how to measure blood pressure, and urge her to do so weekly if drug was prescribed for hypertension. Suggest that she keep a log of blood pressure readings and take it to follow-up visits.

• Advise patient to change position slowly to minimize orthostatic hypotension.

• Urge patient to avoid potentially hazardous activities until drug's CNS effects are known.

• Advise patient to notify prescriber immediately about chest pain that's not relieved by rest or nitroglycerin, constipation, irregular heartbeats, nausea, pronounced dizziness, severe or persistent headache, and swelling of hands or feet.

• Encourage patient to comply with suggested lifestyle changes, such as alcohol moderation, low-sodium or low-fat diet, regular exercise, smoking cessation, stress management, and weight reduction.

• Inform patient that saunas, hot tubs, and prolonged hot showers may cause dizziness or fainting.

• Instruct patient to avoid prolonged sun exposure and to use sunscreen when going outdoors.

niclosamide
Niclocide

Class and Category
Chemical class: Salicylanilide derivative
Therapeutic class: Anthelmintic
Pregnancy category: B

Indications and Dosages
➤ *To treat beef* (Taenia saginata), *fish* (Diphyllobothrium latum), *or pork* (Taenia solium) *tapeworm infestations*
CHEWABLE TABLETS
Adults. 2 g as a single dose; repeated in 7 days, if needed. *Maximum:* 2 g daily.

Children weighing more than 34 kg (75 lb). 1.5 g as a single dose; repeated in 7 days, if needed. *Maximum:* 2 g daily.
Children weighing 11 (24 lb) to 34 kg. 1 g as a single dose; repeated in 7 days, if needed. *Maximum:* 2 g daily.
➤ *To treat dwarf tapeworm* (Hymenolepsis nana) *infestations*
CHEWABLE TABLETS
Adults. 2 g daily for 7 days; repeated in 7 to 14 days, if needed.
Children weighing more than 34 kg. 1.5 g on day 1 and then 1 g daily for next 6 days; repeated in 7 to 14 days, if needed. *Maximum:* 2 g daily.
Children weighing 11 to 34 kg. 1 g on day 1 and then 500 mg daily for the next 6 days; repeated in 7 to 14 days, if needed. *Maximum:* 2 g daily.

Mechanism of Action

May alter anaerobic energy production in tapeworms by inhibiting oxidative phosphorylation in their mitochondria, which decreases synthesis of ATP. Niclosamide causes the scolex (headlike segment) and proximal segment of tapeworm to detach from intestinal wall, which leads to parasite evacuation from intestine through normal peristalsis.

Contraindications

Age under 2 years; hypersensitivity to niclosamide, other anthelmintics, or their components

Interaction

ACTIVITIES
alcohol use: Decreased niclosamide effects

Adverse Reactions

CNS: Dizziness, drowsiness, headache, light-headedness
EENT: Taste perversion
GI: Abdominal distress, anorexia, constipation, diarrhea, nausea, vomiting
SKIN: Anal pruritus, rash

Nursing Considerations

• To identify infestation, collect several stool specimens before starting niclosamide therapy, as ordered, because eggs and parasite segments are released irregularly.
• If patient can't chew tablets thoroughly, crush and give them with small amount of water.

• For young child, crush tablets to fine powder and mix with small amount of water to make paste.
• Be aware that treatment isn't considered successful until stools have shown no eggs or parasites for at least 3 months.

PATIENT TEACHING
• Instruct patient to take niclosamide after a light meal.
• For young child, instruct parent to crush tablets to fine powder and mix with small amount of water to make paste.
• Urge patient to complete entire course of niclosamide therapy.
• Advise patient to avoid hazardous activities until drug's CNS effects are known.
• Advise patient to store niclosamide in a cool, dry, dark place. Caution against storing in bathroom, near kitchen sink, or in other damp places because heat and moisture break down drug.
• Inform patient that stool may need to be examined on day 7 of treatment and again 1 and 3 months after treatment.
• Instruct patient to wash hands thoroughly, to wash all bedding, and to use meticulous personal and environmental hygiene to decrease the risk of autoinfection.
• Caution patient against eating undercooked fish, pork, or beef.

nicotine for inhalation

Nicotrol Inhaler

nicotine nasal solution

Nicotrol NS

nicotine polacrilex

Nicorette, Nicorette Plus (CAN), Thrive

nicotine transdermal system

Habitrol, Nicoderm, NicoDerm CQ, Nicotrol, ProStep

Class and Category

Chemical class: Pyridine alkaloid
Therapeutic class: Smoking cessation adjunct
Pregnancy category: C (nicotine polacrilex),
D (other forms of nicotine)

Indications and Dosages

➤ *To relieve nicotine withdrawal
symptoms, including craving*
CHEWING GUM
Adults. *Initial:* 2 or 4 mg, as needed, or every
1 to 2 hr, adjusted to complete withdrawal by
4 to 6 mo. *Maximum:* 30 pieces of 2-mg gum
daily or 20 pieces of 4-mg gum daily.
NASAL SOLUTION
Adults. 1 to 2 sprays (1 to 2 mg) in each
nostril/hr. *Maximum:* 5 mg/hr or 40 mg
daily for up to 3 mo.
ORAL INHALATION
Adults and adolescents. 6 to 16 cartridges
(24 to 64 mg) daily for up to 12 wk; then
dosage gradually reduced over 12 wk or
less. *Maximum:* 16 cartridges (64 mg) daily
for 6 mo.
TRANSDERMAL SYSTEM
Adults. *Initial:* 14 to 22 mg daily, adjusted
to lower-dose systems over 2 to 5 mo.
DOSAGE ADJUSTMENT For adolescents and
for adults weighing less than 45 kg (100 lb)
and who smoke less than 10 cigarettes daily
or have heart disease, initial dosage reduced
to 11 to 14 mg daily and adjusted to lower-
dose systems over 2 to 5 mo.

Mechanism of Action

Binds selectively to nicotinic-cholinergic
receptors at autonomic ganglia, in the
adrenal medulla, at neuromuscular
junctions, and in the brain. By providing a
lower dose of nicotine than cigarettes, this
drug reduces nicotine craving and
withdrawal symptoms.

Contraindications

Hypersensitivity to nicotine, its
components, or components of transdermal
system; life-threatening arrhythmias;
nonsmokers; recovery from acute MI;
severe angina pectoris; skin disorders
(transdermal); temporomandibular joint
disease (chewing gum)

Interaction

DRUGS
*acetaminophen, beta blockers, imipramine,
insulin, oxazepam, pentazocine,*

theophylline: Possibly increased therapeutic
effects of these drugs (chewing gum, nasal
spray, transdermal system)
alpha blockers, bronchodilators: Possibly
increased therapeutic effects of these drugs
(chewing gum, transdermal system)
bupropion: Potentiated therapeutic effects of
nicotine, possibly increased risk of hypertension
sympathomimetics: Possibly decreased
therapeutic effects of these drugs (chewing
gum, transdermal system)
theophylline, tricyclic antidepressants:
Possibly altered pharmacologic actions of
these drugs (oral inhalation)
FOODS
*acidic beverages (citrus juices, coffee, soft
drinks, tea, wine):* Decreased nicotine
absorption from gum if beverages
consumed within 15 minutes before or
while chewing gum
caffeine: Increased effects of caffeine
(chewing gum, nasal spray, transdermal
system)

Adverse Reactions

CNS: Dizziness, dream disturbances,
drowsiness, headache, irritability, light-
headedness, nervousness (chewing gum,
transdermal system); amnesia, confusion,
difficulty speaking, headache, migraine
headache, paresthesia (nasal spray); chills,
fever, headache, paresthesia (oral
inhalation)
CV: Arrhythmias (all forms); hypertension
(chewing gum, transdermal system);
peripheral edema (nasal spray)
EENT: Increased salivation, injury to teeth
or dental work, mouth injury, oral blistering,
pharyngitis, stomatitis (chewing gum);
altered taste, dry mouth (chewing gum,
transdermal system); altered smell and taste,
burning eyes, dry mouth, earache, epistaxis,
gum disorders, hoarseness, lacrimation,
mouth and tongue swelling, nasal blisters,
nasal irritation or ulceration, pharyngitis,
rhinitis, sinus problems, sneezing, vision
changes (nasal spray); altered taste,
lacrimation, pharyngitis, rhinitis, sinusitis,
stomatitis (oral inhalation)
GI: Eructation (chewing gum); abdominal
pain, constipation, diarrhea, flatulence,
increased appetite, indigestion, nausea,
vomiting (chewing gum, transdermal

system); abdominal pain, constipation, diarrhea, flatulence, hiccups, indigestion, nausea (nasal spray); diarrhea, flatulence, hiccups, indigestion, nausea, vomiting (oral inhalation)
GU: Dysmenorrhea (chewing gum, transdermal system); menstrual irregularities (nasal spray)
MS: Jaw and neck pain (chewing gum); arthralgia, myalgia (chewing gum, transdermal system); arthralgia, back pain, myalgia (nasal spray); back pain (oral inhalation)
RESP: Cough (chewing gum, transdermal system); bronchitis, bronchospasm, chest tightness, cough, dyspnea, increased sputum production (nasal spray); chest tightness, cough, dyspnea, wheezing (oral inhalation)
SKIN: Diaphoresis, erythema, pruritus, rash, urticaria (chewing gum, transdermal system); acne, flushing of face, pruritus, purpura, rash (nasal spray); pruritus, rash, urticaria (oral inhalation)
Other: Allergic reaction (chewing gum, transdermal system); physical dependence (nasal spray); flulike symptoms, generalized pain, withdrawal symptoms (oral inhalation)

Nursing Considerations
• When administering nicotine by oral inhalation, expect optimal effect to result from continuous puffing for 20 minutes.
• To avoid possible burns, remove patch before patient has an MRI.

PATIENT TEACHING
• Instruct patient to read and follow package instructions to obtain best results with nicotine product.
• Advise patient to notify prescriber about other drugs she takes.
• Emphasize that patient must stop smoking as soon as nicotine treatment starts to avoid toxicity.
• Tell patient to stop taking drug and notify prescriber or seek emergency medical care if she develops an allergic reaction such as difficulty breathing or a rash.
• For chewing gum therapy, instruct patient to wait at least 15 minutes after drinking coffee, juice, soft drink, tea, or wine. Advise her to chew gum until she detects a tingling sensation or peppery taste and

then to place gum between her cheek and gum until tingling or peppery taste subsides. Then direct her to move gum to a different site until tingling or taste subsides, repeating until she no longer feels the sensation—usually about 30 minutes. Caution against swallowing the gum. Advise her to stop use and contact prescriber if she experiences oral blistering.
• For nasal spray, tell patient to tilt her head back and spray into a nostril. Caution against sniffing, swallowing, or inhaling spray because nicotine is absorbed through nasal mucosa.
• Warn patient that prolonged use of nasal form may cause dependence.
• For oral inhalation, tell patient to use 6 to 16 cartridges daily to prevent or relieve withdrawal symptoms and craving. Starting with 1 or 2 cartridges daily yields poor success. Direct patient to inhale through device like a cigarette, puffing often for 20 minutes.
• For transdermal system, tell patient not to open package until just before use because nicotine is lost in the air. Advise her to apply system to clean, hairless, dry site on upper outer arm or upper body. Instruct her to change systems and rotate sites every 24 hours and not to use the same site for 7 days. To avoid possible burns, advise patient to remove patch before undergoing any MRI procedure.
WARNING Urge patient to keep all unused nicotine forms safely away from children and pets and to discard used forms carefully. (Enough nicotine may remain in used systems to poison children and pets.) Instruct her to contact a poison control center immediately if she suspects that a child has ingested nicotine.
• Explain to patient with asthma or COPD that nicotine may cause bronchospasm.
• Inform patient that it may take several attempts to stop smoking. Urge her to join a smoking cessation program.

nifedipine
Adalat, Adalat CC, Adalat PA (CAN), Adalat XL (CAN), Apo-Nifed (CAN), Novo-Nifedin (CAN), Nu-Nifed (CAN), Procardia, Procardia XL

Class and Category

Chemical class: Dihydropyridine derivative
Therapeutic class: Antianginal, antihypertensive
Pregnancy category: C

Indications and Dosages

➤ *To manage angina*

CAPSULES (ADALAT, APO-NIFED, NOVO-NIFEDIN, NU-NIFED, PROCARDIA)

Adults. *Initial:* 10 mg three times daily, increased over 1 to 2 wk as needed. *Maintenance:* 10 to 20 mg three times daily *Maximum:* 180 mg daily, 30 mg/dose.

E.R. TABLETS (ADALAT XL, PROCARDIA XL)

Adults. *Initial:* 30 to 60 mg daily, increased or decreased over 7 to 14 days based on patient response. *Maximum:* 90 mg daily.

➤ *To manage hypertension*

E.R. TABLETS (ADALAT CC)

Adults. *Initial:* 30 mg daily. *Maintenance:* 30 to 60 mg daily, increased or decreased over 7 to 14 days based on patient response. *Maximum:* 90 mg daily.

E.R. TABLETS (ADALAT PA)

Adults. *Initial:* 10 to 20 mg twice daily, increased every 3 wk based on patient response. *Maintenance:* 20 mg twice daily. *Maximum:* 80 mg daily.

E.R. TABLETS (ADALAT XL)

Adults. *Initial:* 30 to 60 mg daily, increased or decreased over 7 to 14 days based on patient response. *Maintenance:* 60 to 90 mg daily. *Maximum:* 120 mg daily.

E.R. TABLETS (PROCARDIA XL)

Adults. 30 to 60 mg daily, increased or decreased over 7 to 14 days based on patient response. *Maximum:* 120 mg daily.

DOSAGE ADJUSTMENT Dosage may be reduced for elderly patients and those with heart failure or impaired hepatic or renal function.

Route	Onset	Peak	Duration
P.O. (caps)	20 min	Unknown	Unknown

Mechanism of Action

May slow movement of calcium into myocardial and vascular smooth-muscle cells by deforming calcium channels in cell membranes, inhibiting ion-controlled gating mechanisms, and disrupting calcium release from sarcoplasmic reticulum. Decreasing intracellular calcium level inhibits smooth-muscle cell contraction and dilates arteries, which decreases myocardial oxygen demand, peripheral resistance, blood pressure, and afterload.

Contraindications

Hypersensitivity to a calcium channel blocker, second- or third-degree AV block without artificial pacemaker, sick sinus syndrome

Interaction

DRUGS

anesthetics (hydrocarbon inhalation): Possibly hypotension

antiviral drugs, cimetidine, cisapride, clarithromycin, dalfopristin, diltiazem, erythromycin, fluconazole, fluoxetine, itraconazole, ketoconazole, nefazodone, other antihypertensives, prazocin, quinupristin, timolol, valproic acid, verapamil: Increased risk of hypotension

benazepril: Possibly increased heart rate and hypotensive effect

beta blockers: Increased risk of profound hypotension, heart failure, and worsening of angina

calcium supplements: Possibly interference with action of nifedipine

carbamazepine, NSAIDs, phenobarbital, phenytoin, rifabutin, rifampin, rifapentin, St. John's wort, sympathomimetics: Possibly decreased therapeutic effects of nifedipine

digoxin: Transiently increased blood digoxin level, increased risk of digitalis toxicity

disopyramide, flecainide: Increased risk of bradycardia, conduction defects, and heart failure

doxazocin: Decreased doxazocin effectiveness; increased nifedipine effectiveness

estrogens: Possibly increased fluid retention and decreased nifedipine effects

lithium: Increased risk of neurotoxicity

metformin: Increased metformin absorption and plasma level

tacrolimus: Decreased tacrolimus metabolism

FOODS

grapefruit, grapefruit juice: Possibly increased bioavailability of nifedipine

high-fat meals: Possibly delayed nifedipine absorption

ACTIVITIES

alcohol use: Additive hypotensive effect

Adverse Reactions

CNS: Anxiety, ataxia, confusion, dizziness, drowsiness, headache, nervousness (possibly extreme), nightmares, paresthesia, psychiatric disturbance, syncope, tremor, weakness
CV: Arrhythmias (bradycardia, tachycardia), chest pain, heart failure, hypotension, palpitations, peripheral edema
EENT: Altered taste, blurred vision, dry mouth, epistaxis, gingival hyperplasia, nasal congestion, pharyngitis, sinusitis, tinnitus
ENDO: Gynecomastia, hyperglycemia
GI: Anorexia; constipation; diarrhea; dyspepsia; elevated liver function test results; gastrointestinal bleeding, irritation, or obstruction; hepatitis; nausea; vomiting
GU: Dysuria, nocturia, polyuria, sexual dysfunction, urinary frequency
HEME: Anemia, leukopenia, positive Coombs' test, thrombocytopenia
MS: Joint stiffness, muscle cramps
RESP: Chest congestion, cough, dyspnea, respiratory tract infection, wheezing
SKIN: Acute generalized exanthematous pustulosis, diaphoresis, erythema multiforme, exfoliative dermatitis, flushing, photosensitivity, pruritus, rash, Stevens-Johnson syndrome, toxic epidermal necrolysis, urticaria

Nursing Considerations

• Be aware that patients with galactose intolerance should not take nifedipine because the drug contains lactose. The capsule form of nifedipine should not be used to treat hypertension because its effects on blood pressure are not known.
• Use cautiously in patients with cirrhosis because it is unknown how nifedipine exposure may be altered in these patients.
• When starting and stopping nifedipine therapy, taper it, as prescribed, over 7 to 14 days.
• For closely monitored hospitalized patient with angina, dosage may be increased 10 mg every 4 to 6 hours to control chest pain.
• Because of drug's negative inotropic effect on some patients, frequently monitor heart rate and rhythm, as well as blood pressure, especially in patients who take a beta blocker or have heart failure, significant left ventricular dysfunction, or tight aortic stenosis.
• Monitor fluid intake/output and daily weight; fluid retention may lead to heart failure. Also assess for signs of heart failure, such as crackles, dyspnea, jugular vein distention, peripheral edema, and weight gain.

PATIENT TEACHING
• Instruct patient to swallow E.R. tablets whole, not to crush, chew, or break them. Inform her that their empty shells may appear in stool.
• Urge patient to take nifedipine exactly as prescribed, even when she's feeling well. Advise her to notify prescriber if she misses two or more doses.
• Urge patient not to take drug within 1 hour of a high-fat meal or grapefruit. Urge her not to alter the amount of grapefruit in her diet without consulting prescriber.
WARNING Caution patient against stopping nifedipine abruptly because angina or dangerously high blood pressure could result.
• Teach patient to measure pulse rate and blood pressure, and advise her to call prescriber if they drop below accepted levels. Suggest keeping a log of weekly measurements and taking it to follow-up visits.
• Instruct patient to notify prescriber immediately about chest pain, difficulty breathing, ringing in ears, and swollen gums.
• Advise patient to avoid hazardous activities until drug's CNS effects are known.
• Urge patient to avoid alcoholic beverages because they may worsen dizziness, drowsiness, and hypotension.
• Teach patient to minimize constipation by increasing her intake of fluids, if allowed, and dietary fiber.
• Emphasize the need to comply with prescribed lifestyle changes, such as alcohol moderation, low-fat or low-sodium diet, regular exercise, smoking cessation, stress reduction, and weight reduction.
• Emphasize the need for good oral hygiene and regular dental visits.
• Caution patient that hot tubs, saunas, and prolonged hot showers may cause dizziness and fainting.
• Advise patient to avoid prolonged sun exposure and to wear sunscreen outdoors.

N
O

nisoldipine

Sular

Class and Category

Chemical class: Dihydropyridine derivative
Therapeutic class: Antihypertensive
Pregnancy category: C

Indications and Dosages

➤ To manage hypertension

E.R. TABLETS

Adults. 20 mg daily, increased by 10 mg every 7 days, as prescribed. *Maintenance:* 20 to 40 mg daily. *Maximum:* 60 mg daily.

DOSAGE ADJUSTMENT For patients over age 65 and patients with hepatic impairment, initial dosage reduced to 10 mg daily.

Mechanism of Action

May slow extracellular calcium movement into myocardial and vascular smooth-muscle cells by deforming calcium channels in cell membranes, inhibiting ion-controlled gating mechanisms, and interfering with calcium release from the sarcoplasmic reticulum. By decreasing the intracellular calcium level, nisoldipine inhibits smooth-muscle cell contraction and dilates coronary and systemic arteries. As with other calcium channel blockers, these actions lead to decreased myocardial oxygen requirements and reduced peripheral resistance, blood pressure, and afterload.

Contraindications

Hypersensitivity to calcium channel blocker, second- or third-degree AV block with no artificial pacemaker, sick sinus syndrome

Interaction

DRUGS

beta blockers: Possibly increased risk of hypotension
CYP3A4 inducers such as carbamazepine, phenytoin: Decreased nisoldipine levels and effectiveness
CYP3A4 inhibitors such as azole antifungals, cimetidine, quinidine: Increased blood nisoldipine level; increased risk of adverse reactions
NSAIDs: Decreased antihypertensive effect of nisoldipine

FOODS

grapefruit, grapefruit juice: Possibly increased bioavailability of nisoldipine
high-fat meals: Possibly delayed nisoldipine absorption

ACTIVITIES

alcohol use: Additive hypotensive effect

Adverse Reactions

CNS: Dizziness, headache
CV: Angina, hypotension, palpitations, peripheral edema, vasodilation
EENT: Pharyngitis, sinusitis
GI: Constipation, nausea
RESP: Bronchospasm, dyspnea
SKIN: Rash
Other: Allergic-type reaction

Nursing Considerations

• Monitor pulse rate and rhythm and blood pressure before starting nisoldipine therapy, during dosage adjustments, and periodically throughout therapy.
• Don't break or crush E.R. tablets.
• For optimal absorption, give drug 1 hour before or 2 hours after meals.
• Monitor fluid intake and output and daily weight to assess for signs of fluid retention, which may lead to heart failure. Also assess for signs of heart failure, such as crackles, dyspnea, jugular vein distention, peripheral edema, and weight gain.
• Monitor patient for allergic-type reaction that may include bronchospasm, especially if patient has aspirin sensitivity, because drug contains FD&C yellow no. 5 dye.

PATIENT TEACHING

• Instruct patient to swallow E.R. nisoldipine tablets whole, not to break, crush, or chew them.
• Advise patient to take drug 1 hour before or 2 hours after meals. Urge her not to alter amount of grapefruit products in her diet without consulting prescriber.
• Urge patient to continue taking drug as prescribed, even if she feels well.
WARNING Caution patient against stopping drug abruptly because blood pressure could rise dangerously high.
• Instruct patient to notify prescriber about constipation, difficulty breathing, dizziness, irregular heartbeat, nausea, severe headache, and swelling of hands or feet.
• Teach patient and family how to measure blood pressure, and instruct them to

notify prescriber if systolic blood pressure falls below 90 mm Hg. Suggest that patient keep a log of weekly measurements and take it to follow-up visits.
• Advise patient to change positions slowly to minimize the effects of orthostatic hypotension. Inform her that hot tubs, saunas, and prolonged hot showers may worsen this adverse reaction.
• Caution patient to avoid hazardous activities until drug's CNS effects are known.
• Urge patient to avoid alcohol and OTC alcohol-containing drugs without consulting prescriber. Many OTC preparations can raise blood pressure.
• Emphasize the need to adhere to prescribed lifestyle changes, such as alcohol moderation, low-fat and low-sodium diet, regular exercise, smoking cessation, stress reduction, and weight reduction.

nitrofurantoin

Apo-Nitrofurantoin (CAN), Furadantin, Macrobid, Macrodantin, Novo-Furantoin (CAN)

Class and Category
Chemical class: Nitrofuran derivative
Therapeutic class: Antibiotic
Pregnancy category: B (except near term)

Indications and Dosages
➤ *To treat acute cystitis*
CAPSULES, ORAL SUSPENSION, TABLETS
Adults. 50 to 100 mg every 6 hr. *Maximum:* 600 mg daily or 10 mg/kg daily.
Children over age 1 month. 0.75 to 1.75 mg/kg every 6 hr.
E.R. CAPSULES
Adults and children age 12 and over. 100 mg every 12 hr for 7 days.
➤ *To suppress chronic cystitis*
CAPSULES, ORAL SUSPENSION, TABLETS
Adults. 50 to 100 mg at bedtime.
Maximum: 600 mg daily or 10 mg/kg daily.
Children over age 1 month. 1 mg/kg daily at bedtime.

Mechanism of Action
Inactivates or alters bacterial ribosomal proteins and other macromolecules. This action of nitrofurantoin inhibits bacterial

protein synthesis, aerobic energy metabolism, DNA synthesis, RNA synthesis, and cell wall synthesis. Nitrofurantoin is bacteriostatic at low doses and bactericidal at higher doses.

Contraindications
Age under 1 month, anuria, creatinine clearance less than 60 ml/min/1.73 m^2, history of cholestatic jaundice or hepatic dysfunction with previous nitrofurantoin therapy, hypersensitivity to nitrofurantoin or parabens, oliguria, pregnancy near term

Interaction
DRUGS
hepatotoxic drugs: Increased risk of hepatotoxicity
magnesium trisilicate: Decreased nitrofurantoin absorption
methyldopa, procainamide, hemolytics: Increased risk of toxic effects from nitrofurantoin
nalidixic acid: Possibly impaired therapeutic effects of this drug
neurotoxic drugs: Increased risk of neurotoxicity
probenecid, sulfinpyrazone: Increased blood nitrofurantoin level and increased risk of toxicity

Adverse Reactions
CNS: Chills, confusion, depression, headache, neurotoxicity, peripheral neuropathy
CV: Vasculitis
EENT: Optic neuritis, parotitis, tooth discoloration
GI: Abdominal pain, anorexia, cholestatic jaundice, diarrhea, hepatic necrosis, hepatitis, jaundice, nausea, pancreatitis, pseudomembranous colitis, vomiting
GU: Rust-colored to brown urine
HEME: Aplastic anemia, granulocytopenia, hemolytic anemia, leukopenia, megaloblastic anemia, methemoglobinemia, thrombocytopenia
MS: Arthralgia, myalgia
RESP: Asthma (in asthmatic patients), cyanosis, interstitial pneumonitis (acute), pulmonary fibrosis
SKIN: Alopecia; eczematous, erythematous, or maculopapular eruptions; erythema multiforme; exfoliative dermatitis; pruritus; rash; Stevens-Johnson syndrome

Other: Anaphylaxis, angioedema, drug-induced fever, lupus-like syndrome

Nursing Considerations

• Obtain a specimen of patient's urine for culture and sensitivity tests, as ordered; review test results if possible before giving nitrofurantoin.
• Give drug with food or milk to avoid staining teeth.
• Don't crush or break capsules.
• Shake oral nitrofurantoin suspension before pouring dose, and mix with food or milk, as needed.
• Monitor patient for evidence of super-infection, such as abdominal pain, diarrhea, and fever. If patient develops diarrhea, it may indicate pseudo-membranous colitis caused by *Clostridium difficile.* Notify prescriber and expect to withhold nitrofurantoin and treat with fluids, electrolytes, protein, and an antibiotic effective against *C. difficile.*
• Monitor patient for pulmonary and hepatic abnormalities because rare but severe reactions have occurred with nitrofurantoin use, especially in the elderly.
• Observe patient for changes in nervous function because peripheral neuropathy, although uncommon, may become severe or irreversible. Patients with renal impairment, anemia, diabetes mellitus, electrolyte imbalance, vitamin B deficiency, or debilitating disease are at higher risk for peripheral neuropathy.

PATIENT TEACHING

• Instruct patient to shake nitrofurantoin oral suspension before measuring dose and to take drug with food or milk.
• Caution patient against taking any preparations that contain magnesium trisilicate during therapy.
• Explain that urine may turn brown, orange, or rust-colored during therapy.
• Instruct patient to complete prescribed course of therapy even if symptoms subside before course is completed.
• Urge patient to tell prescriber about diarrhea that's severe or lasts longer than 3 days. Explain that watery or bloody stools can occur 2 or more months after nitrofurantoin therapy and can be serious, requiring prompt treatment.

nitroglycerin
(glyceryl trinitrate)

Deponit, Minitran, Nitro-Bid, Nitrocot, Nitro-Dur, Nitrogard, Nitroglyn E-R, Nitroject, Nitrol, Nitrolingual, NitroMist, Nitrong SR, Nitro-par, Nitrostat, Nitro-time, Transderm-Nitro, Tridil

Class and Category

Chemical class: Nitrate
Therapeutic class: Antianginal, antihypertensive, vasodilator
Pregnancy category: B (Nitrostat), C

Indications and Dosages

➤ *To prevent or treat angina*

E.R. BUCCAL TABLETS

Adults. 1 mg every 5 hr while awake.

E.R. CAPSULES

Adults. 2.5, 6.5, or 9 mg every 12 hr. Frequency of doses increased to every 8 hr based on patient's response.

E.R. TABLETS

Adults. 2.6 or 6.5 mg every 12 hr. Frequency of doses increased to every 8 hr based on patient's response.

S.L. TABLETS

Adults. 0.3 to 0.6 mg, repeated every 5 min. *Maximum:* 3 tabs in 15 min or 10 mg daily.

TRANSDERMAL OINTMENT

Adults. 10 to 20 (15 to 30 mg) every 8 hr. Frequency of doses increased to every 6 hr if angina occurs between doses. *Maximum:* 50 (75 mg)/application.

TRANSDERMAL PATCH

Adults. 0.1 to 0.8 mg/hr, worn 12 to 14 hr.

TRANSLINGUAL SPRAY

Adults. For treatment, 1 or 2 metered doses (0.4 or 0.8 mg) onto or under tongue, repeated every 5 min as needed. For prevention, 1 or 2 metered doses (0.4 or 0.8 mg) onto or under tongue 5 to 10 minutes before activities that could lead to acute attack.

➤ *To prevent or treat angina, to manage hypertension or heart failure*

I.V. INFUSION

Adults. 5 mcg/min, increased by 5 mcg/min every 3 to 5 min to 20 mcg/min, as prescribed, and then by 10 to 20 mcg/min every 3 to 5 min until desired effect occurs.

Mechanism of Action

May interact with nitrate receptors in vascular smooth-muscle cell membranes. This interaction reduces nitroglycerin to nitric oxide, which activates the enzyme guanylate cyclase, increasing intracellular formation of cGMP. Increased cGMP level may relax vascular smooth muscle by forcing calcium out of muscle cells, causing vasodilation. Venous dilation decreases venous return to the heart, reducing left ventricular end-diastolic pressure and pulmonary artery wedge pressure. Arterial dilation decreases systemic vascular resistance, systolic arterial pressure, and mean arterial pressure. Thus, nitroglycerin reduces preload and afterload, decreasing myocardial workload and oxygen demand. It also dilates coronary arteries, increasing blood flow to ischemic myocardial tissue.

Route	Onset	Peak	Duration
P.O.*	3 min	Unknown	5 hr
P.O.†	20–45 min	Unknown	8–12 hr
I.V.	1–2 min	Unknown	3–5 min
S.L.	1–3 min	Unknown	30–60 min
Trans-dermal‡	In 30 min	Unknown	4–8 hr
Trans-dermal§	In 30 min	Unknown	8–24 hr
Trans-lingual	2 to 4 min	Unknown	30–60 min

Incompatibilities

Don't administer I.V. nitroglycerin through I.V. bags or tubing made of polyvinyl chloride. Don't mix drug with other solutions.

Contraindications

Acute MI (S.L.), angle-closure glaucoma, cerebral hemorrhage, concurrent use of phosphodiesterase inhibitors or riociguat, constrictive pericarditis (I.V.), head trauma, hypersensitivity to adhesive in transdermal form, hypersensitivity to nitrates, hypotension

---

* Buccal.
† E.R.
‡ Ointment.
§ Patch.

(I.V.), hypovolemia (I.V.), inadequate cerebral circulation (I.V.), increased intracranial pressure, orthostatic hypotension, pericardial tamponade, severe anemia

Interaction

DRUGS

acetylcholine, norepinephrine: Possibly decreased therapeutic effects of these drugs
heparin: Possibly decreased anticoagulant effect of heparin (I.V. nitroglycerin)
opioid analgesics, other antihypertensives, vasodilators: Possibly increased orthostatic hypotension
phosphodiesterase inhibitors (such as sildenafil, tadalafil, vardenafil), riociguat: Possibly severe hypotensive effect of nitroglycerin
sympathomimetics: Possibly decreased antianginal effect of nitroglycerin and increased risk of hypotension

ACTIVITIES

alcohol use: Possibly increased orthostatic hypotension

Adverse Reactions

CNS: Agitation, anxiety, dizziness, headache, insomnia, restlessness, syncope, weakness
CV: Arrhythmias (including tachycardia), edema, hypotension, orthostatic hypotension, palpitations
EENT: Blurred vision, burning or tingling in mouth (buccal, S.L. forms), dry mouth
GI: Abdominal pain, diarrhea, indigestion, nausea, vomiting
GU: Dysuria, impotence, urinary frequency
HEME: Methemoglobinemia
MS: Arthralgia
RESP: Bronchitis, pneumonia
SKIN: Contact dermatitis (transdermal forms), flushing of face and neck, rash

Nursing Considerations

• Use nitroglycerin cautiously in elderly patients, especially those who are volume-depleted or taking several medications, because of the increased risk of hypotension and falls. Hypotension may be accompanied by angina and paradoxical slowing of the heart rate. Notify prescriber if these occur, and provide appropriate treatment, as ordered.
• Plan a nitroglycerin-free period of about 10 hours each day, as prescribed, to maintain therapeutic effects and avoid tolerance.

N
O

• Place E.R. buccal tablets in buccal pouch with patient in sitting or lying position.
• Don't break or crush E.R. tablets or capsules. Have patient swallow them whole with a full glass of water.
• Place S.L. tablet under patient's tongue and make sure it dissolves completely.
• Be sure to remove cotton from S.L. tablet container to allow quick access to drug.
• When applying transdermal ointment, apply correct amount on dose-measuring paper. Then place paper on hairless area of body and spread in a thin, even layer over an area at least 2ĭ by 3ĭ. Don't place on cuts or irritated areas. Wash your hands after application. Rotate sites. Store at room temperature.
• Open transdermal patch package immediately before use. Apply patch to hairless area, and press edges to seal. Rotate sites. Store at room temperature. If patient needs cardioversion or defibrillation, remove transdermal patch.
• Don't shake translingual spray container before administering. Have patient inhale and hold her breath, and then spray drug under or on her tongue.
• Be aware that I.V. nitroglycerin should be diluted only in D_5W or normal saline solution and shouldn't be mixed with other infusions. The pharmacist should add drug to a glass bottle, not a container made of polyvinyl chloride. Don't use a filter because plastic absorbs drug. Administer with infusion pump.
• Check vital signs before every dosage adjustment and often during therapy.
• Frequently monitor heart and breath sounds, level of consciousness, fluid intake and output, and pulmonary artery wedge pressure, if possible.
• Store premixed containers in the dark; don't freeze them.
WARNING Assess patient for evidence of overdose, such as confusion, diaphoresis, dyspnea, flushing, headache, hypotension, nausea, palpitations, tachycardia, vertigo, vision changes, and vomiting. Treat as prescribed by removing nitroglycerin source, if possible; elevating legs above heart level; and administering an alpha-adrenergic agonist, such as phenylephrine, as prescribed, to treat severe hypotension.

PATIENT TEACHING
• Teach patient to recognize signs and symptoms of angina pectoris, including chest fullness, pain, and pressure, possibly with sweating and nausea. Pain may radiate down left arm or into neck or jaw. Inform women and those with diabetes mellitus or hypertension that they may feel only fatigue and shortness of breath.
• Instruct patient to read and follow package instructions to obtain full benefits of drug.
• To prevent drug tolerance, inform patient that prescriber may order a 10- to 12-hour drug-free period at night (or at another time if she has chest pain at night or in the morning).
• Instruct patient to swallow E.R. tablets or capsules whole—not to break, crush, or chew them—with a full glass of water.
• For sublingual or buccal use, advise patient to place tablet under her tongue or in buccal pouch when angina starts and then to sit or lie down. Instruct her not to swallow drug, but to let it dissolve. Explain that moisture in her mouth helps drug absorption. If angina doesn't subside, instruct patient to place another tablet under her tongue or in buccal pouch after 5 minutes and to repeat, if needed, for three doses total. If pain doesn't subside after 20 minutes, urge patient to call 911 or another emergency service.
• Advise patient to carry S.L. tablets in their original brown bottle in a purse or jacket pocket, but not one that will be affected by body heat. Instruct her to store drug in a dry place at room temperature and to discard cotton from container. Advise her to discard and replace S.L. tablets after 6 months.
• Advise patient using transdermal ointment or patch to rotate sites to avoid skin sensitization.
• Inform patient that swimming or bathing doesn't affect transdermal forms but that hot tubs, saunas, prolonged hot showers, electric blankets, and magnetic therapy over the site may increase drug absorption and cause dizziness and hypotension.
• Caution against inhaling translingual spray. Before first use, tell patient to press actuator button 10 times to prime container and then hold container upright with forefinger on top of actuator button.

Tell her to open her mouth, bring container as close as possible, press actuator button firmly to release spray onto or under tongue, and release button and immediately close her mouth. Remind her to replace plastic cover on container and to not spit out the drug or rinse her mouth for 5 to 10 minutes. Tell her to reprime container by pressing actuator button twice if container hasn't been used for more than 6 weeks. Remind patient to periodically check level of fluid in container. If it reaches the top or middle hole on side of container, more should be obtained. Caution patient not to let level of liquid get to bottom of hole.

• Inform patient that nitroglycerin commonly causes headache, which typically resolves after a few days of continuous therapy. Suggest taking acetaminophen, as needed.

• Advise patient to notify prescriber immediately about blurred vision, dizziness, and severe headache.

• Suggest that patient change positions slowly to minimize orthostatic hypotension.

• Advise patient to avoid hazardous activities until drug's CNS effects are known.

• Urge patient to avoid alcohol and erectile dysfunction drugs during therapy.

nitroprusside sodium

Nipride, Nitropress

Class and Category
Chemical class: Cyanonitrosylferrate
Therapeutic class: Antihypertensive, vasodilator
Pregnancy category: C

Indications and Dosages
➤ *To treat hypertensive crisis and manage severe heart failure*
I.V. INFUSION
Adults and children. *Initial:* 0.25 to 0.3 mcg/kg/min, increased gradually every few minutes until blood pressure reaches desired level. *Maintenance:* 3 mcg/kg/min (range, 0.25 to 10 mcg/kg/min). *Maximum:* 10 mcg/kg/min for 10 min.

Route	Onset	Peak	Duration
I.V.	1–2 min	Immediate	1–10 min

Mechanism of Action
May interact with nitrate receptors in vascular smooth-muscle cell membranes. This action reduces nitroprusside to nitric oxide and then activates intracellular guanylate cyclase, which increases the cGMP level. Increased cGMP level may relax vascular smooth muscle by forcing calcium out of muscle cells. Smooth-muscle relaxation causes arteries and veins to dilate, which reduces peripheral vascular resistance and blood pressure.

Incompatibilities
Don't mix nitroprusside with any other drug.

Contraindications
Acute heart failure with decreased peripheral vascular resistance, congenital optic atrophy, decreased cerebral perfusion, hypersensitivity to nitroprusside or its components, hypertension from aortic coarctation or AV shunting, tobacco-induced amblyopia

Interaction
DRUGS
dobutamine: Increased cardiac output, decreased pulmonary artery wedge pressure
ganglionic blockers, general anesthetics, hypotension-producing drugs: Increased hypotensive effect
sympathomimetics: Decreased antihypertensive effect of nitroprusside

Adverse Reactions
CNS: Anxiety, dizziness, headache, increased intracranial pressure, nervousness, restlessness
CV: Hypotension, tachycardia
ENDO: Hypothyroidism
GI: Abdominal pain, ileus, nausea, vomiting
HEME: Methemoglobinemia
MS: Muscle twitching
SKIN: Diaphoresis, flushing, rash
Other: Infusion-site phlebitis

Nursing Considerations
• Obtain baseline vital signs before administering nitroprusside.
WARNING Don't give drug undiluted. Reconstitute with 2 ml D_5W, and add solution to 250 to 500 ml D_5W to produce 200 mcg/ml or 100 mcg/ml, respectively.

N
O

• Be aware that solution is stable at room temperature for 24 hours when protected from light. Don't use reconstituted solution if it contains particles or is blue, green, red, or darker than faint brown.
• Use an infusion pump. Place opaque cover over infusion container because drug is metabolized by light. I.V. tubing doesn't need to be covered.
• Keep patient supine when starting drug or titrating dose up or down.
• Monitor blood pressure continuously with intra-arterial pressure monitor. Record blood pressure every 5 minutes at start of infusion and every 15 minutes thereafter.
• If patient has severe heart failure, expect to administer an inotropic drug, such as dopamine or dobutamine, as prescribed.
WARNING For patient who receives prolonged nitroprusside therapy or short-term high-dose therapy, watch for evidence of thiocyanate toxicity (ataxia, blurred vision, delirium, dizziness, dyspnea, headache, hyperreflexia, loss of consciousness, nausea, tinnitus, vomiting). Toxicity can cause arrhythmias, metabolic acidosis, severe hypotension, and death.
• Monitor serum thiocyanate level at least every 72 hours; levels above 100 mcg/ml are associated with toxicity.
WARNING Assess patient for evidence of cyanide toxicity (absence of reflexes, coma, distant heart sounds, hypotension, metabolic acidosis, mydriasis, pink skin, shallow respirations, and weak pulse). If you detect such evidence, discontinue nitroprusside, as ordered, and give 4 to 6 mg/kg sodium nitrite over 2 to 4 minutes to convert hemoglobin to methemoglobin. Follow with 150 to 200 mg/kg sodium thiosulfate. Repeat this regimen at half the original doses after 2 hours, as ordered.
PATIENT TEACHING
• Advise patient to change position slowly to minimize dizziness from sudden, severe hypotension.

nizatidine

Apo-Nizatidine (CAN), Axid, Axid AR

Class and Category
Chemical class: Ethenediamine derivative

Therapeutic class: Antiulcer
Pregnancy category: B

Indications and Dosages
➤ *To manage active duodenal ulcer*
CAPSULES
Adults and adolescents. 300 mg at bedtime or 150 mg twice daily for 8 wk.
DOSAGE ADJUSTMENT Dosage reduced to 150 mg daily if creatinine clearance is 20 to 50 ml/min/1.73 m^2; to 150 mg every other day if creatinine clearance is less than 20 ml/min/1.73 m^2.
➤ *To prevent recurrence of duodenal ulcer*
CAPSULES
Adults and adolescents. 150 mg at bedtime.
DOSAGE ADJUSTMENT Dosage reduced to 150 mg every other day for patients with creatinine clearance of 20 to 50 ml/min/ 1.73 m^2; to 150 mg every 3 days for those with creatinine clearance less than 20 ml/ min/1.73 m^2.
➤ *To manage acute benign gastric ulcer*
CAPSULES
Adults and adolescents. 300 mg at bedtime or 150 mg twice daily.
➤ *To manage gastroesophageal reflux disease*
CAPSULES
Adults and adolescents. 150 mg twice daily.
➤ *To prevent or relieve acid indigestion or heartburn*
TABLETS
Adults and adolescents. 75 mg 30 min to 1 hr before meals.

Route	Onset	Peak	Duration
P.O.	Unknown	Unknown	10–12 hr*

Mechanism of Action
Inhibits basal and nocturnal secretion of gastric acid by reversibly and competitively blocking H$_2$ receptors, especially those in gastric parietal cells. Nizatidine also inhibits gastric acid secretion in response to stimuli, including food and caffeine.

Contraindications
Hypersensitivity to nizatidine or other H$_2$-receptor antagonists

---

* For nocturnal acid secretion; up to 4 hr for food-stimulated acid secretion.

Interaction

DRUGS

antacids: Decreased nizatidine bioavailability

itraconazole, ketoconazole: Decreased absorption of these drugs

salicylates: Increased blood level of these drugs

sucralfate: Possibly decreased nizatidine absorption

Adverse Reactions

CNS: Agitation, anxiety, confusion, depression, dizziness, fatigue, fever, hallucinations, headache, insomnia, somnolence

CV: Arrhythmias, chest pain, vasculitis

EENT: Amblyopia, dry mouth, laryngeal edema, pharyngitis, rhinitis, sinusitis

ENDO: Gynecomastia

GI: Abdominal pain, constipation, diarrhea, hepatitis, nausea, vomiting

GU: Decreased libido, hyperuricemia not associated with gout or nephrolithiasis, impotence

HEME: Anemia, aplastic anemia, eosinophilia, hemolytic anemia, leukopenia, neutropenia, pancytopenia, thrombocytopenia

MS: Back pain, myalgia

RESP: Bronchospasm, cough

SKIN: Alopecia, diaphoresis, erythema multiforme, exfoliative dermatitis, jaundice, pruritus, rash, Stevens-Johnson syndrome, toxic epidermal necrolysis, urticaria

Other: Anaphylaxis, angioedema, serum sicknesslike reaction

Nursing Considerations

• Monitor CBC, BUN and serum creatinine levels, and liver function test results before and periodically during nizatidine therapy.

• Don't give within 1 hour of an antacid.

PATIENT TEACHING

• Instruct patient not to take nizatidine within 1 hour of an antacid.

• Urge patient to take nizatidine exactly as prescribed, even if she feels better before prescription is finished. Inform her that ulcer may take up to 8 weeks to heal.

• If patient smokes, urge her to stop because smoking increases gastric acid production.

• Teach patient to minimize constipation by drinking plenty of fluids (if allowed), eating high-fiber foods, and exercising regularly.

• Instruct patient to notify prescriber immediately about abdominal pain, easy bruising, extreme fatigue, yellow skin or sclera, trouble swallowing food, bloody vomitus, or bloody or tarry stools.

• Urge patient not to take nizatidine with other acid reducers.

norepinephrine bitartrate
(levarterenol bitartrate)

Levophed

Class and Category

Chemical class: Catecholamine

Therapeutic class: Cardiac stimulant, vasopressor

Pregnancy category: C

Indications and Dosages

➤ *To treat acute hypotension, cardiogenic shock, and septic shock*

I.V. INFUSION

Adults. *Initial:* 0.5 to 1 mcg/min. Increased, as ordered, until systolic blood pressure reaches desired level. *Maintenance:* 2 to 12 mcg/min.

Children. 0.1 mcg/kg/min. *Maximum:* 1 mcg/kg/min.

➤ *To treat refractory shock*

I.V. INFUSION

Adults. Up to 30 mcg/min.

Route	Onset	Peak	Duration
I.V.	Rapid	Unknown	1–2 min

Mechanism of Action

At more than 4 mcg/min, directly stimulates alpha-adrenergic receptors and inhibits adenyl cyclase, which inhibits cAMP production. Inhibition of cAMP constricts arteries and veins and increases peripheral vascular resistance and systolic blood pressure. At less than 2 mcg/min, norepinephrine directly stimulates beta-adrenergic receptors in the myocardium and increases adenyl cyclase activity, producing positive inotropic and chronotropic effects.

Contraindications

Concurrent use of hydrocarbon inhalation anesthetics, hypersensitivity to norepinephrine or its components, hypovolemia, mesenteric or peripheral vascular thrombosis

Interaction

DRUGS

alpha blockers: Decreased vasopressor effects of norepinephrine
beta blockers: Decreased cardiac-stimulating effect of norepinephrine, possibly decreased therapeutic effects of both drugs
digoxin: Increased risk of arrhythmias, possibly potentiated inotropic effect
doxapram: Possibly increased vasopressor effects of both drugs
ergonovine, ergotamine, methylergonovine, methysergide, oxytocin: Possibly increased vasoconstriction
general anesthetics: Risk of arrhythmias
guanadrel, guanethidine: Increased vasopressor response to norepinephrine, possibly severe hypertension
MAO inhibitors: Possibly life-threatening arrhythmias, hyperpyrexia, severe headache, severe hypertension, and vomiting
maprotiline, tricyclic antidepressants: Possibly potentiated cardiovascular and pressor effects of norepinephrine, including arrhythmias, severe hypertension, and hyperpyrexia
methylphenidate: Possibly potentiated vasopressor effect of norepinephrine
nitrates: Possibly decreased therapeutic effects of both drugs
phenoxybenzamine: Possibly arrhythmias or hypotension
sympathomimetics: Increased risk of adverse cardiovascular effects
thyroid hormones: Increased risk of coronary insufficiency

Adverse Reactions

CNS: Anxiety, dizziness, headache, insomnia, nervousness, tremor, weakness
CV: Angina, bradycardia, ECG changes, edema, hypertension, hypotension, palpitations, peripheral vascular insufficiency (including gangrene), PVCs, sinus tachycardia
GI: Nausea, vomiting
GU: Decreased renal perfusion
RESP: Apnea, dyspnea

SKIN: Pallor
Other: Infusion-site sloughing and tissue necrosis, metabolic acidosis

Nursing Considerations

• Dilute norepinephrine concentrate for infusion in D_5W, dextrose 5% in normal saline solution, or normal saline solution. Dilutions typically range from 16 to 32 mcg/ml.
• Make sure solution contains no particles and isn't discolored before administering.
• Give drug with a flow-control device.
• Check blood pressure every 2 to 3 minutes, preferably by direct intra-arterial monitoring, until stabilized and then every 5 minutes.
WARNING Because extravasation can cause severe tissue damage and necrosis, expect prescriber to give multiple subcutaneous injections of phentolamine (5 to 10 mg diluted in 10 to 15 ml normal saline solution) around extravasated infusion site.
• If blanching occurs along vein, change infusion site and notify prescriber at once.
• Monitor continuous ECG during therapy.
PATIENT TEACHING
• Urge patient to immediately report burning, leaking, or tingling around I.V. site.

norfloxacin

Noroxin

Class and Category

Chemical class: Fluoroquinolone
Therapeutic class: Antibiotic
Pregnancy category: C

Indications and Dosages

➤ *To treat uncomplicated UTI caused by* Escherichia coli, Klebsiella pneumoniae, *or* Proteus mirabilis
TABLETS
Adults. 400 mg every 12 hr for 3 days.
➤ *To treat uncomplicated UTI caused by* Citrobacter freundii, Enterobacter aerogenes, Enterobacter cloacae, Enterococcus faecalis, Proteus *species,* Pseudomonas aeruginosa, Staphylococcus aureus, Staphylococcus

epidermidis, Staphylococcus saprophyticus, *or* Streptococcus agalactiae

TABLETS

Adults. 400 mg every 12 hr for 7 to 10 days.

➤ *To treat complicated UTI caused by* E. coli, E. faecalis, K. pneumoniae, P. aeruginosa, P. mirabilis, *or* Serratia marcescens

TABLETS

Adults. 400 mg every 12 hr for 10 to 21 days. *Maximum:* 800 mg daily.

➤ *To treat uncomplicated gonorrhea*

TABLETS

Adults. 800 mg as a single dose.

➤ *To treat prostatitis caused by* E. coli

TABLETS

Adults. 400 mg every 12 hr for 28 days.

DOSAGE ADJUSTMENT Dosage reduced to 400 mg daily for patients with creatinine clearance of 30 ml/min/1.73 m² or less.

Mechanism of Action

Inhibits the enzyme DNA gyrase, which unwinds and supercoils bacterial DNA before it replicates. By inhibiting this enzyme, norfloxacin interferes with bacterial cell replication and causes cell death.

Contraindications

History of tendinitis or tendon rupture associated with use of fluoroquinolones; hypersensitivity to norfloxacin, other fluoroquinolones, or their components; myasthenia gravis

Interaction

DRUGS

aluminum-, calcium-, or magnesium-containing antacids; ferrous sulfate; magnesium-containing laxatives; sucralfate; zinc: Possibly decreased absorption and blood level of norfloxacin

caffeine, clozapine, ropinirole, tacrine, theophylline, tizanidine: Possibly increased blood level of these drugs

class IA antiarrhythmics, such as quinidine; class III antiarrhythmics, such as sotalol; other drugs known to prolong QTc interval, such as disopyramide and pentamidine: Possibly prolonged QTc interval

cyclosporine: Possibly increased serum creatinine and blood cyclosporine levels

didanosine: Possibly decreased norfloxacin absorption

glyburide: Risk of severe hypoglycemia

nitrofurantoin: Possibly decreased norfloxacin effectiveness

NSAIDs: Possibly increased risk of CNS stimulation and seizures

probenecid: Decreased norfloxacin excretion and risk of toxicity

warfarin: Possibly increased anticoagulant effect and risk of bleeding

FOODS

caffeine: Reduced clearance of caffeine leading to accumulation of caffeine in blood

Adverse Reactions

CNS: Ataxia, confusion, dizziness, drowsiness, fever, Guillain-Barré syndrome, hallucinations, headache, hypoesthesia, insomnia, light-headedness, paresthesia, peripheral neuropathy, psychosis, restlessness, seizures, tremors

CV: Prolonged QT interval, torsades de pointes, vasculitis

EENT: Decreased taste sensation, diplopia, hearing loss, stomatitis, taste perversion, tinnitus, visual changes

GI: Abdominal cramps or pain, acute hepatic necrosis or failure, diarrhea, elevated liver function test results, hepatitis, jaundice, nausea, pancreatitis, pseudo-membranous colitis, vomiting

GU: Interstitial nephritis, renal failure, vaginal candidiasis

HEME: Agranulocytosis, aplastic anemia, hemolytic anemia, leukopenia, neutropenia, pancytopenia, thrombocytopenia

MS: Arthralgia; muscle spasms; myasthenia gravis exacerbation; myalgia; tendinitis; tendon inflammation, pain, or rupture

RESP: Allergic pneumonitis, dyspnea

SKIN: Blisters, diaphoresis, drug rash with eosinophilia and systemic symptoms (DRESS syndrome), erythema, erythema multiforme, exfoliative dermatitis, leukocytoclastic vasculitis, photosensitivity, pruritus, rash, Stevens-Johnson syndrome, toxic epidermal necrolysis, urticaria

Other: Anaphylaxis, angioedema, serum sickness

Nursing Considerations

- Obtain urine specimen for culture and sensitivity tests before starting drug, if possible.
- Determine if patient has a history of CNS disorder because drug may lower seizure

N
O

threshold. Notify prescriber before starting drug, and institute seizure precautions. Also monitor patient during therapy for central nervous system stimulation such as confusion, hallucinations, light-headedness, restlessness, or tremors. If present, notify prescriber, expect drug to be discontinued, provide safety measures and supportive care, as indicated.

WARNING Before starting therapy, determine if patient takes a class IA antiarrhythmic, such as quinidine; a class III antiarrhythmic, such as sotalol; or other drugs that prolong the QTc interval. Also find out if patient has hypokalemia or an underlying QT-interval prolonging condition. These drugs and conditions, especially in the elderly, may prolong the QTc interval and lead to life-threatening ventricular tachycardia or torsades de pointes in a patient taking norfloxacin.

• Give drug on an empty stomach 2 hours before or after antacids, didanosine, sucralfate, or vitamins that contain iron or zinc.

• Keep emergency resuscitation equipment readily available, and watch for signs of hypersensitivity, such as angioedema, dyspnea, jaundice, rash, and urticaria. If you suspect anaphylaxis, prepare to give epinephrine, corticosteroids, and diphenhydramine, as prescribed.

• Notify prescriber if patient has symptoms of peripheral neuropathy (pain, burning, tingling, numbness, weakness, or altered sensations of light touch, pain, tempera-ture, position sense, or vibration sense), which could be permanent. Expect to stop norfloxacin.

• Monitor patients prone to tendinitis, such as the elderly, athletes, and those taking corticosteroids, for complaints of tendon pain, inflammation, or rupture. If present, notify prescriber and expect to discontinue norfloxacin, place patient on bedrest with no exercise of affected limb, and obtain diagnostic tests to confirm rupture.

• Monitor patient for diarrhea, which may indicate pseudomembranous colitis caused by *Clostridium difficile*. If diarrhea occurs, notify prescriber and expect to withhold norfloxacin and treat with fluids, electrolytes, protein, and an antibiotic effective against *C. difficile*.

• Instruct patient to take drug on an empty stomach with a large glass of water to prevent crystalluria. Urge her to drink several glasses of water daily during therapy.

• Instruct patient to take norfloxacin at least 2 hours before or after eating, drinking milk, or taking antacids, didanosine, sucralfate, or vitamins that contain iron or zinc.

• Advise patient to avoid hazardous activities until drug's CNS effects are known.

• Tell patient to stop drug and report tendon pain, inflammation, or abnormal changes in motor or sensory function.

• Urge patient to protect skin from sunlight and to report photosensitivity at once.

• Tell patient to take drug exactly as prescribed, even if symptoms subside.

• Urge patient to tell prescriber about diarrhea that's severe or lasts longer than 3 days. Remind patient that watery or bloody stools can occur 2 or more months after antibiotic therapy and can be serious, requiring prompt treatment.

nortriptyline hydrochloride

Aventyl, Pamelor

Class and Category

Chemical class: Dibenzocycloheptene derivative
Therapeutic class: Antidepressant
Pregnancy category: D

Indications and Dosages

➤ *To treat depression*
CAPSULES, ORAL SOLUTION
Adults. *Initial:* 25 mg three times a day or four times a day. *Maximum:* 150 mg daily.
Adolescents. 25 to 50 mg daily or 1 to 3 mg/kg daily in divided doses.
Children ages 6 to 12. 10 to 20 mg daily or 1 to 3 mg/kg daily in divided doses.
DOSAGE ADJUSTMENT Dosage possibly reduced to 30 to 50 mg daily (in divided doses or at bedtime) for elderly patients.

Route	Onset	Peak	Duration
P.O.	2–3 wk	Unknown	Unknown

Mechanism of Action

May interfere with reuptake of serotonin (and possibly other neurotransmitters) at presynaptic neurons, thus enhancing serotonin's effects at postsynaptic receptors. By restoring normal neurotransmitter levels at nerve synapses, this tricyclic antidepressant may elevate mood.

Contraindications

Acute recovery phase of stroke or MI; hypersensitivity to nortriptyline, other tricyclic antidepressants, or their components; use within 14 days of MAO inhibitor therapy including intravenous methylene blue or linezolid

Interaction

DRUGS

amantadine, anticholinergics, antidyskinetics, antihistamines: Possibly increased anticholinergic effects, confusion, hallucinations, nightmares; increased CNS depression
anticonvulsants: Possibly increased CNS depression and risk of seizures, possibly decreased anticonvulsant effectiveness
antithyroid drugs: Possibly agranulocytosis
barbiturates, carbamazepine: Possibly decreased level and effects of nortriptyline
bupropion, clozapine, cyclobenzaprine, haloperidol, loxapine, maprotiline, molindone, phenothiazines, thioxanthenes: Possibly increased sedative and anticholinergic effects, possibly increased risk of seizures
cimetidine, fluoxetine: Possibly increased blood nortriptyline level and risk of toxicity
clonidine: Possibly decreased antihypertensive effect and increased CNS depression
disulfiram: Possibly delirium
ethchlorvynol: Possibly delirium, increased CNS depression
guanadrel, guanethidine: Possibly decreased antihypertensive effect of these drugs
MAO inhibitors: Increased risk of hypertensive crisis, severe seizures, and death
oral anticoagulants: Possibly increased anticoagulant activity
pimozide, probucol: Possibly arrhythmias
sympathomimetics, including ophthalmic epinephrine and vasoconstrictive local anesthetics: Increased risk of arrhythmias, hyperpyrexia, hypertension, tachycardia
thyroid hormones: Possibly increased therapeutic and toxic effects of both drugs
ACTIVITIES
alcohol use: Increased CNS and respiratory depression, hypertension, alcohol effects

Adverse Reactions

CNS: Ataxia, confusion, delirium, dizziness, drowsiness, excitation, hallucinations, headache, insomnia, nervousness, nightmares, parkinsonism, serotonin syndrome, stroke, suicidal ideation, tremor
CV: Arrhythmias, orthostatic hypotension
EENT: Angle closure glaucoma, blurred vision, dry mouth, increased intraocular pressure, taste perversion
GI: Constipation, diarrhea, heartburn, ileus, increased appetite, nausea, vomiting
GU: Sexual dysfunction, urine retention
HEME: Bone marrow depression
RESP: Wheezing
SKIN: Diaphoresis, urticaria
Other: Weight gain

Nursing Considerations

- Expect to stop MAO inhibitor therapy, including intravenous methylene blue and linezolid, 10 to 14 days before starting nortriptyline.
- Watch patient closely (especially children, adolescents, and young adults), for suicidal tendencies, particularly when therapy starts and dosage changes because depression may worsen temporarily during these times, possibly leading to suicidal ideation.
- Oral solution (10 mg/5 ml) is 4% alcohol.
- **WARNING** Monitor patient for possible serotonin syndrome, characterized by agitation, chills, confusion, diaphoresis, diarrhea, fever, hyperactive reflexes, poor coordination, restlessness, shaking, talking or acting with uncontrolled excitement, tremor, and twitching. Notify prescriber immediately if serotonin syndrome is suspected because it can become life-threatening and expect to discontinue nortriptyline therapy.
- Give nortriptyline with food to reduce GI reactions.
- Monitor blood nortriptyline level; therapeutic range is 50 to 150 ng/ml.
- Monitor ECG tracing to detect arrhythmias.

• Explain that oral solution contains alcohol.
• Discourage alcohol consumption during therapy.
• Explain that improvement may take weeks.
• Advise patient that drug may cause mild pupillary dilation, which may lead to an episode of acute closure glaucoma. Encourage patient to have an eye exam before starting therapy to see if he is at risk.
• Advise patient to avoid hazardous activities until drug's CNS effects are known.
• Urge family or caregiver to watch patient closely for suicidal tendencies, especially when therapy starts or dosage changes and particularly if patient is a child, teenager, or young adult.
• Instruct patient to change position slowly to minimize orthostatic hypotension.
• Suggest that patient minimize constipation by drinking plenty of fluids (if allowed), eating high-fiber foods, and exercising regularly.

nystatin

Mycostatin, Nadostine (CAN), Nilstat, Nystex, Nystop, Pedi-Dri

Class and Category
Chemical class: Amphoteric polyene macrolide
Therapeutic class: Antifungal
Pregnancy category: Not rated (lozenges, oral suspension, tablets, topical), A (vaginal)

Indications and Dosages
➤ To treat oropharyngeal candidiasis (thrush)
LOZENGES (PASTILLES)
Adults and children over age 5. 200,000 to 400,000 units dissolved in mouth 4 or 5 times daily for up to 14 days.
ORAL SUSPENSION
Adults and children. 400,000 to 600,000 units swished and swallowed four times a day until at least 48 hr after symptoms subside.
Infants. 200,000 units to each side of mouth four times a day until at least 48 hr after symptoms subside.

Neonates. 100,000 units applied to each side of mouth four times a day until at least 48 hr after symptoms subside.
TABLETS
Adults and adolescents. 500,000 to 1,000,000 units three times a day until at least 48 hr after symptoms subside.
Children age 5 and over. 500,000 units four times a day until at least 48 hr after symptoms subside.
➤ To treat cutaneous and mucocutaneous candidiasis
CREAM, OINTMENT, POWDER
Adults and children. 100,000 units (1 g) on affected area twice daily or three times a day for at least 2 wk.
➤ To treat vulvovaginal candidiasis
VAGINAL TABLETS
Adults and adolescents. 100,000 units (1 tab) once or twice daily for 14 days.

Mechanism of Action
Binds to sterols in fungal cell membranes, impairing membrane integrity. Cells lose intracellular potassium and other cellular contents and, eventually, die.

Contraindications
Hypersensitivity to nystatin or its components

Adverse Reactions
ENDO: Hyperglycemia (lozenge, oral suspension)
GI: Abdominal pain, diarrhea, nausea, vomiting (oral forms)
GU: Vaginal burning or itching (vaginal form)
SKIN: Irritation (topical forms)

Nursing Considerations
• Prepare nystatin powder for oral suspension for each dose; it has no preservatives.
• Gently rub nystatin cream or ointment into skin at affected area. Keep area dry and avoid occlusive dressings.
• Don't get topical form in patient's eyes.
• When treating candidal infection of feet, dust patient's shoes, socks, and feet.
• For vaginal form, use applicator supplied by manufacturer.
PATIENT TEACHING
• Instruct patient to let nystatin lozenges dissolve slowly in her mouth, not to chew or swallow them.

• Tell patient to swish oral suspension in her mouth as long as possible before swallowing.
• Advise patient to gently rub ointment or cream into skin at affected area, to keep area dry, and to avoid occlusive dressings.
• Caution patient to keep topical from away from her eyes.
• Advise patient with candidal infection of feet to dust her shoes, socks, and feet with nystatin.
• For vaginal form, tell patient to insert with applicator supplied by manufacturer.

octreotide acetate

Sandostatin, Sandostatin LAR Depot

Class and Category
Chemical class: Cyclic octapeptide, somatostatin analogue
Therapeutic class: Antidiarrheal, hormone suppressant
Pregnancy category: B

Indications and Dosages
➤ *To control symptoms associated with vasoactive intestinal peptide tumors (watery diarrhea) and metastatic carcinoid tumors (diarrhea and flushing)*
I.M. INJECTION
Adults currently receiving subcutaneous injections. 20 mg every 4 wk for 2 mo, with subcutaneous doses continued for 2 to 4 wk after I.M. injections start. If patient has positive response to initial 2-mo regimen, dosage reduced to 10 mg every 4 wk. If symptoms persist or increase after initial 2-mo regimen, dosage increased to 30 mg every 4 wk, as prescribed.
SUBCUTANEOUS INJECTION
Adults. *Initial:* 200 to 300 mcg daily in divided doses twice daily to four times a day, for first 2 wk. *Maintenance:* Individualized. *Maximum:* 450 mcg daily.
➤ *To treat symptoms of acromegaly, to suppress the release of growth hormone from pituitary tumors*
I.V. OR SUBCUTANEOUS INJECTION
Adults. *Initial:* 50 mcg three times a day
Usual: 100 mcg three times a day
Maximum: 1,500 mcg daily.

I.M. INJECTION
Adults currently receiving subcutaneous injections. 20 mg every 4 wk for 3 mo; then adjusted as prescribed in response to serum growth hormone level. *Maximum:* 40 mg every 4 wk.

Route	Onset	Peak	Duration
SubQ	Unknown	Unknown	Up to 12 hr

Mechanism of Action
Controls many types of secretory diarrhea by inhibiting secretion of serotonin and pituitary and GI hormones (including insulin, glucagon, growth hormone, thyrotropin, and, possibly, thyroid-stimulating hormone) as well as vasoactive intestinal peptides and pancreatic poly-peptides (including gastrin, secretin, and motilin). Inhibiting serotonin and peptides increases intestinal absorption of water and electrolytes, decreases pancreatic and gastric acid secretions, and increases intestinal transit time by slowing gastric motility.
    By inhibiting hormones involved in vasodilation, octreotide increases splanchnic arterial resistance and decreases GI blood flow, hepatic vein wedge pressure, hepatic blood flow, portal vein pressure, and intravariceal pressure, thus raising seated and standing blood pressures. By inhibiting serotonin secretion, octreotide eases symptoms of acromegaly, including diarrhea, flushing, wheezing, and urinary excretion of 5-hydroxyindoleacetic acid.

Incompatibilities
Don't mix octreotide in same syringe with fat emulsions or total parenteral nutrition solutions.

Contraindications
Hypersensitivity to octreotide or its components

Interaction
DRUGS
beta blockers, calcium channel blockers: Additive cardiovascular effects of these drugs
bromocriptine: Increased blood bromo-criptine level
cisapride: Decreased effectiveness of both drugs
cyclosporine: Decreased cyclosporine level

N
O

diuretics: Increased risk of fluid and electrolyte imbalances
insulin, oral antidiabetic drugs: Increased risk of hypoglycemia
quinidine, terfenadine: Decreased clearance and increased blood levels of these drugs
vitamin B_{12}: Decreased vitamin B_{12} level

Adverse Reactions

CNS: Dizziness, drowsiness, fatigue, headache, intracranial hemorrhage, migraine, paranoia, seizures, suicidal ideation
CV: Arrhythmias (including conduction abnormalities), edema, hypertension, hypotension, MI, orthostatic hypotension, Raynaud's syndrome
EENT: Deafness, epistaxis, glaucoma, retinal vein thrombosis, sinusitis, vision changes
ENDO: Hyperglycemia, hypoglycemia, hypothyroidism, pituitary apoplexy
GI: Abdominal pain, acute cholecystitis, ascending cholangitis, biliary obstruction, cholelithiasis, cholestatic hepatitis, constipation, diarrhea, elevated liver enzymes, flatulence, gastric or peptic ulcer, GI hemorrhage, intestinal obstruction, nausea, pancreatitis, vomiting
GU: Decreased libido, hematuria, increased urine output, renal failure
HEME: Anemia, pancytopenia, thrombocytopenia
MS: Arthropathy, back pain, myalgia
RESP: Status asthmaticus, pulmonary hypertension, upper respiratory tract infection
SKIN: Alopecia, petechiae, pruritus, rash, urticaria
Other: Anaphylaxis, angioedema, dehydration, electrolyte imbalances, flulike symptoms, injection-site irritation or pain

Nursing Considerations

• Give octreotide by I.V. injection only in an emergency, as prescribed.
• To prepare depot injection (long-acting suspension form), let powder and diluent warm to room temperature and then reconstitute according to manufacturer's instructions. Gently inject 2 ml of supplied diluent down side of vial without disturbing depot powder. Let diluent saturate powder. After 2 to 5 minutes, check sides and bottom of vial without inverting it.

Once powder is completely saturated, swirl—don't shake—vial for 30 to 60 seconds to form suspension. Use immediately after reconstituting.
• Don't give depot injection by subcutaneous route; give only by I.M. route and only to patients who respond to and tolerate subcutaneous drug, as prescribed.
• To minimize pain, use smallest injection volume to deliver dose, and rotate injection sites.
• Avoid deltoid site for I.M. use because injection-site reaction and pain may result. Intragluteal injection is recommended.
WARNING To avoid worsening symptoms, expect to continue subcutaneous injections when switching to I.M. injections, as prescribed.
• Be aware that octreotide increases risk of acute cholecystitis, ascending cholangitis, biliary obstruction, cholestatic hepatitis, and pancreatitis.
• Monitor vital signs, bowel sounds, and stool consistency. Assess for abdominal pain and signs of gallbladder disease.
• Monitor serum liver enzyme levels, as appropriate.
• Monitor patient for signs of electrolyte imbalances and dehydration.
• Carefully monitor diabetic patient for altered glucose control.
• Monitor patient's thyroid function, as ordered, because octreotide suppresses secretion of thyroid-stimulating hormone, which may cause hypothyroidism.
• If patient has periodic symptom flare-ups, expect to give additional subcutaneous octreotide temporarily, as prescribed.

PATIENT TEACHING

• Advise patient to change position slowly to minimize orthostatic hypotension.
• Instruct patient to notify prescriber about adverse reactions, especially abdominal pain, which may indicate pancreatitis.
• Urge diabetic patient to check blood glucose level often.
• Caution female patient of childbearing age that drug may restore fertility and, if pregnancy isn't desired, that contraception should be used during octreotide therapy.

ofloxacin

Floxin

Class and Category

Chemical class: Fluoroquinolone
Therapeutic class: Antibiotic
Pregnancy category: C

Indications and Dosages

➤ *To treat acute, uncomplicated cystitis caused by* Escherichia coli *or* Klebsiella pneumoniae

TABLETS, I.V. INFUSION
Adults. 200 mg every 12 hr for 3 days.

➤ *To treat uncomplicated cystitis caused by* Citrobacter diversus, Enterobacter aerogenes, Proteus mirabilis, *or* Pseudomonas aeruginosa

TABLETS, I.V. INFUSION
Adults. 200 mg every 12 hr for 7 days.

➤ *To treat complicated UTI caused by* C. diversus, E. coli, K. pneumoniae, P. mirabilis, *or* P. aeruginosa
Adults. 200 mg every 12 hr for 10 days.

➤ *To treat uncomplicated gonorrhea*

TABLETS, I.V. INFUSION
Adults and adolescents. 400 mg as single dose.

➤ *To treat urethritis or cervicitis caused by* Chlamydia trachomatis *or* Neisseria gonorrhoeae

TABLETS, I.V. INFUSION
Adults and adolescents. 300 mg twice daily for 7 days as an alternative to doxycycline or azithromycin.

➤ *To treat pelvic inflammatory disease caused by susceptible organisms*

TABLETS
Adults and adolescents. 400 mg twice daily with metronidazole P.O. for 10 to 14 days.

I.V. INFUSION
Adults and adolescents. 400 mg every 12 hr with metronidazole I.V.; then switched to oral therapy, as prescribed, after 24 hr. Full course of therapy lasts 14 days.

➤ *To treat prostatitis caused by* E. coli

TABLETS, I.V. INFUSION
Adults. 300 mg every 12 hr for 6 wk.

➤ *To treat lower respiratory tract infections caused by* Haemophilus influenzae *or* Streptococcus

pneumoniae *and skin and soft-tissue infections caused by* Staphylococcus aureus *or* Streptococcus pyogenes

TABLETS, I.V. INFUSION
Adults. 400 mg every 12 hr for 10 days.
DOSAGE ADJUSTMENT If creatinine clearance is 20 to 50 ml/min/1.73 m^2, dosing interval possibly reduced to every 24 hr; if clearance is less than 10 ml/min/1.73 m^2, dosage possibly reduced by 50% and given every 24 hr.

Mechanism of Action

Inhibits synthesis of the bacterial enzyme DNA gyrase by counteracting excessive supercoiling of DNA during replication or transcription. Inhibition of DNA gyrase causes rapid- and slow-growing bacterial cells to die.

Incompatibilities

Don't mix ofloxacin with other I.V. drugs or additives.

Contraindications

Hypersensitivity to ofloxacin, other fluoroquinolones, or their components; myasthenia gravis

Interaction

DRUGS
aluminum-, calcium-, or magnesium-containing antacids; didanosine; ferrous sulfate; magnesium-containing laxatives; multivitamins; sevelamer; sucralfate; zinc: Decreased absorption of oral ofloxacin
probenecid: Decreased ofloxacin excretion, increased risk of toxicity
procainamide: Decreased renal clearance of procainamide
warfarin: Possibly increased anticoagulant activity and risk of bleeding

Adverse Reactions

CNS: Aggressiveness, agitation, ataxia, dizziness, drowsiness, emotional lability, exacerbation of extrapyramidal disorders and myasthenia gravis, fever, headache, incoordination, insomnia, light-headedness, mania, peripheral neuropathy, psychotic reactions, restlessness, stroke, suicidal ideation, syncope
CV: Arrhythmias, prolonged QT interval, severe hypotension, torsades de pointes, vasculitis

N
O

EENT: Blurred vision; diplopia; disturbances in taste, smell, hearing, and equilibrium
ENDO: Hyperglycemia, hypoglycemia
GI: Abdominal cramps or pain, acute hepatic necrosis or failure, diarrhea, hepatitis, jaundice, nausea, pseudomembranous colitis, vomiting
GU: Acute renal insufficiency or failure, interstitial nephritis, renal calculi, vaginal candidiasis
HEME: Agranulocytosis, aplastic or hemolytic anemia, leukopenia, pancytopenia, thrombocytopenia
MS: Arthralgia; myalgia; rhabdomyolysis; tendinitis; tendon inflammation, pain, or rupture
RESP: Allergic pneumonitis, pulmonary edema
SKIN: Blisters, diaphoresis, erythema, erythema multiforme, exfoliative dermatitis, photosensitivity, pruritus, rash, Stevens-Johnson syndrome, toxic epidermal necrolysis, urticaria
Other: Acidosis, anaphylaxis, infusion-site phlebitis, serum sickness

Nursing Considerations
• Because of increased risk of prolonged QT interval, ofloxacin shouldn't be used if patient has had a prolonged QT interval, has an uncorrected electrolyte disorder, or takes a Class IA or III antiarrhythmic. Monitor elderly patients closely because risk of prolonged QT interval may be increased in this group.
• For I.V. infusion, dilute drug in normal saline solution or D_5W to at least 4 mg/ml, and infuse over 60 minutes to minimize the risk of hypotension. Discard unused portion.
• Monitor patient closely for hypersensitivity, which may occur as early as first dose. Reaction may include angioedema, bronchospasm, dyspnea, itching, rash, jaundice, shortness of breath, and urticaria. If these signs or symptoms appear, notify prescriber immediately and expect to discontinue drug.
• Notify prescriber if patient has symptoms of peripheral neuropathy (pain, burning, tingling, numbness, weakness, or altered sensations of light touch, pain, temperature, position sense, or vibration

sense), which could be permanent; tendon rupture (pain and inflammation), which may occur more often in patients (especially elderly ones) taking corticosteroids and requires immediate rest; or a severe photosensitivity reaction. In each case, expect to stop ofloxacin.
• Maintain adequate hydration to prevent development of highly concentrated urine and crystalluria.
• Expect an increased risk of toxicity in severe hepatic disease, including cirrhosis.
• Be aware that ofloxacin may stimulate the CNS and aggravate seizure disorders.
• If diarrhea develops, notify prescriber because it may indicate pseudomembranous colitis. Ofloxacin may need to be discontinued and additional therapy started.
• Be alert for secondary fungal infection.

PATIENT TEACHING
• Encourage patient to take each oral dose with a full glass of water.
• Tell patient to complete full course of ofloxacin therapy exactly as prescribed, even if he feels better before it's complete.
• Urge patient not to take antacids, iron or zinc preparations, or other drugs (such as sucralfate and didanosine), within 2 hours of ofloxacin to prevent decreased or delayed drug absorption.
• Advise patient to avoid hazardous activities until CNS effects of drug are known.
• Tell patient to limit exposure to sun and ultraviolet light to prevent phototoxicity.
• Advise patient to notify prescriber immediately about burning skin, hives, itching, rash, rapid heart rate, abnormal motor or sensory function, and tendon pain.
• Urge patient to seek medical care immediately for trouble breathing or swallowing, which may signal an allergic reaction.
• Instruct diabetic patient who takes insulin or an antidiabetic to notify prescriber immediately if he develops a hypoglycemic reaction; ofloxacin will have to be stopped.
• Advise patient to notify prescriber if diarrhea develops, even up to 2 months after ofloxacin therapy ends. Additional therapy may be needed.

olanzapine

Zydis, Zyprexa

Route	Onset	Peak	Duration
P.O.	1 wk	Unknown	Unknown
I.M.	Unknown	Unknown	Unknown

Class and Category

Chemical class: Thienobenzodiazepine derivative
Therapeutic class: Antipsychotic
Pregnancy category: C

Indications and Dosages

➤ *To treat schizophrenia*

ORALLY DISINTEGRATING TABLETS, TABLETS
Adults. *Initial:* 5 to 10 mg daily.
Maintenance: 10 mg daily. *Maximum:*
20 mg daily.
Adolescents ages 13 to 17. *Initial:* 2.5 to
5 mg daily. *Maintenance:* 10 mg daily.
Maximum: 20 mg daily.

➤ *To treat manic phase of bipolar I*
disorder (manic or mixed episodes)

ORALLY DISINTEGRATING TABLETS, TABLETS
Adults. *Initial:* 10 to 15 mg daily; may be
increased or decreased by 5 mg every 24 hr
as needed and prescribed. *Maintenance:*
5 to 20 mg daily for 3 to 4 wk. *Maximum:*
20 mg daily.
Adolescents ages 13 to 17. *Initial:* 2.5 to
5 mg daily. *Maintenance:* 10 mg daily.
Maximum: 20 mg daily.

➤ *As adjunct to treat bipolar I disorder*

ORALLY DISINTEGRATING TABLETS, TABLETS
Adults. *Initial:* 10 mg daily with lithium or
valproate sodium; may be increased or
decreased by 5 mg every 24 hr, as needed
and prescribed. *Maintenance:* 5 to 20 mg/
day for 6 wk. *Maximum:* 20 mg daily.
DOSAGE ADJUSTMENT Initial dosage possibly
reduced to 5 mg for debilitated patients,
those prone to hypotension, and female
nonsmokers over age 65. Dosage
adjustment for adolescents increased or
decreased, as needed, in increments or
decrements of 2.5 or 5 mg.

➤ *To treat agitation associated with*
schizophrenia and bipolar I mania

I.M. INJECTION
Adults. 5 to10 mg, as needed. Repeat as
needed every 2 to 4 hr.
DOSAGE ADJUSTMENT Dosage decreased to
5 mg for elderly patients and 2.5 mg for
debilitated patients, those prone to hypotension, and female nonsmokers over age 65.

Mechanism of Action

May achieve antipsychotic effects by
antagonizing dopamine and serotonin
receptors. Anticholinergic effects may result
from competitive binding to and antagonism
of the muscarinic receptors M_1 through M_5.

Contraindications

Blood dyscrasias, bone marrow depression,
cerebral arteriosclerosis, coma, coronary
artery disease, hepatic dysfunction, high-
dose CNS depressants, hypersensitivity to
olanzapine or its components, hypertension,
hypotension, myeloproliferative disorders,
severe CNS depression, subcortical brain
damage

Interaction

DRUGS
anticholinergics: Increased anticholinergic
effects, altered thermoregulation
antihypertensives: Increased effects of both
drugs, increased risk of hypotension
benzodiazepines (parenteral): Increased risk
of excessive sedation and cardiorespiratory
depression
carbamazepine, omeprazole, rifampin:
Increased olanzapine clearance
CNS depressants: Additive CNS depression,
potentiated orthostatic hypotension
diazepam: Increased CNS depressant effects
fluvoxamine: Decreased olanzapine
clearance
levodopa: Decreased levodopa efficacy
lorazepam (parenteral): Possibly increased
somnolence with I.M. olanzapine injection
ACTIVITIES
alcohol use: Additive CNS depression,
potentiated orthostatic hypotension
smoking: Decreased blood olanzapine level

Adverse Reactions

CNS: Abnormal gait, agitation, akathisia,
altered thermoregulation, amnesia, anxiety,
asthenia, dizziness, euphoria, fatigue, fever,
headache, hypertonia, insomnia, nervousness, neuroleptic malignant syndrome,
restlessness, somnolence, stuttering, suicidal
ideation, syncope, tardive dyskinesia,
tremor

N
O

CV: Bradycardia, chest pain, hyperlipidemia, hypertension, hypotension, orthostatic hypotension, peripheral edema, tachycardia
EENT: Amblyopia, dry mouth, increased salivation, pharyngitis, rhinitis
ENDO: Hyperglycemia, hyperprolactinemia
GI: Abdominal pain, constipation, dysphagia, elevated liver enzymes, hepatitis, increased appetite, nausea, thirst, vomiting
GU: Urinary incontinence, UTI
HEME: Agranulocytosis, leukopenia, neutropenia
MS: Arthralgia; back, joint, or limb pain; muscle spasms and twitching
RESP: Cough
SKIN: Ecchymosis, photosensitivity, pruritus, urticaria
Other: Anaphylaxis, angioedema, flulike symptoms, weight gain

Nursing Considerations

WARNING Olanzapine shouldn't be used for elderly patients with dementia-related psychosis because drug increases risk of death in these patients.
• Use cautiously in patients with hepatic impairment or conditions associated with limited hepatic functional reserve and in patients who are being treated with potentially hepatotoxic drugs. Also use cautiously in patients with known cardiovascular or cerebrovascular disease and conditions that would predispose patient to hypotension, such as presence of dehydration, hypovole-mia, or treatment with antihypertensive medications because of the increased risk for bradycardia, syncope, and hypotension.
• Reconstitute parenteral olanzapine by dissolving contents of vial in 2.1 ml sterile water to yield 5 mg/ml. Solution should be clear yellow. Use within 1 hour.
• Inject I.M. olanzapine slowly, deep into muscle mass.
• Keep patient recumbent after I.M. injection of olanzapine if drowsiness, dizziness, bradycardia, or hypoventilation occurs. Don't let patient sit or stand up until blood pressure and heart rate have returned to baseline.

• Monitor patient's blood pressure routinely during therapy because olanzapine may cause orthostatic hypotension.
• Olanzapine may worsen such conditions as angle-closure glaucoma, benign prostatic hyperplasia, and seizures.
• Assess daily weight to detect fluid retention or metabolic changes.
• Notify prescriber if patient develops tardive dyskinesia or urinary incontinence.
• Be alert for and immediately report signs of neuroleptic malignant syndrome.
• Watch patient closely (especially children, adolescents, and young adults), for suicidal tendencies, particularly when therapy starts and dosage changes, because depression may worsen temporarily during these times, possibly leading to suicidal ideation.
• Monitor patient's lipid levels throughout therapy, as ordered, because olanzapine may cause significant elevations.
• Monitor patient's blood glucose level routinely because olanzapine may increase risk of hyperglycemia.
• Monitor CBC often during first few months of therapy, especially if patient has low WBC count or history of drug-induced leukopenia or neutropenia. If WBC count declines, and especially if neutrophil count drops below 1,000/mm^3, expect olanzapine to be discontinued. If neutropenia is significant, also monitor patient for fever or other evidence of infection and provide appropriate treatment, as prescribed.
• Be aware that drug may cause hyperprolactinemia, which, in turn, may reduce pituitary gonadotropin secretion. This then inhibits reproductive function by impairing gonadal steroidogenesis in both female and male patients. In addition, longstanding hyperprolactinemia may decrease bone density in patient when it is associated with hypogonadism.

PATIENT TEACHING
• Advise patient to avoid alcohol and smoking during olanzapine therapy.
• Teach patient to open orally disintegrating tablet sachet by peeling back foil on the blister, not by pushing tablet through the foil. Immediately after opening blister, tell him to use dry hands

to remove tablet and place it in his mouth. Explain that tablet will disintegrate rapidly in saliva so he can easily swallow it without liquid.

• Caution patient with phenylketonuria that disintegrating olanzapine tablets contain phenylalanine.

• Urge patient to avoid hazardous activities until drug's CNS effects are known.

• Instruct patient to change position slowly to minimize effects of orthostatic hypotension.

• Encourage patient to weigh self frequently to detect weight gain. If diabetes is present, also instruct patient to monitor blood glucose level closely.

• Urge family or caregiver to watch patient closely for suicidal tendencies, especially when therapy starts or dosage changes and particularly if patient is a child, teenager, or young adult.

• Warn patient that chronic olanzapine therapy may alter reproductive function through olanzapine-induced hyperprolactinemia causing amenorrhea and impotence. If reproductive adverse effects occur, patient should notify prescriber.

• Advise female patient of childbearing age to notify prescriber if she intends to become or suspects that she is pregnant during therapy.

olmesartan medoxomil

Benicar

Class and Category

Chemical class: Angiotensin II receptor antagonist
Therapeutic class: Antihypertensive
Pregnancy category: D

Indications and Dosages

➤ *To manage or as adjunct to manage hypertension*

SUSPENSION, TABLETS

Adults, adolescents, and children age 6 and over who weigh 35 kg (77 lb) or more.*Initial:* 20 mg daily, increased in 2 wk to 40 mg daily, as needed. *Maximum:* 40 mg daily.

Adolescents and children age 6 and over who weigh 20 kg to less than 35 kg (44 to 77 lb). *Initial:* 10 mg daily, increased in 2 wk to 20 mg daily, as needed. *Maximum:* 20 mg daily.

DOSAGE ADJUSTMENT Lower starting dosage is recommended for patients with possible depletion of intravascular volume, such as those treated with diuretics, especially if impaired renal function is present.

Contraindications

Aliskiren therapy in patients with diabetes or renal impairment (GFR less than 60 ml/min), children under age 1, hypersensitivity to olmesartan medoxomil or its components

Interaction

DRUGS

ACE inhibitors, aliskiren (in patients with diabetes or renal impairment), other angiotensin receptor blockers: Increased risk of hyperkalemia, hypotension, and renal dysfunction
colesevelam: Reduced effectiveness of olmesartan
lithium: Increased serum lithium level with possible toxicity
NSAIDs: Increased risk of renal dysfunction in elderly patients and patients who are volume-depleted or have preexisting renal dysfunction; increased antihypertensive effect of olmesartan

Adverse Reactions

CNS: Asthenia, dizziness, fatigue, headache, insomnia, vertigo
CV: Chest pain, hypercholesterolemia, hyperlipidemia, hypertriglyceridemia, peripheral edema, tachycardia
EENT: Pharyngitis, rhinitis, sinusitis
ENDO: Hyperglycemia, hyperuricemia
GI: Abdominal pain, diarrhea, gastroenteritis, indigestion, nausea, sprue-like enteropathy, vomiting
GU: Acute renal failure, elevated BUN and serum creatinine levels, hematuria, UTI
MS: Arthralgia, arthritis, back pain, myalgia, rhabdomyolysis, skeletal pain
RESP: Bronchitis, cough, upper respiratory tract infection
SKIN: Alopecia, pruritus, rash, urticaria

Mechanism of Action
Olmesartan medoxomil blocks angiotensin II from binding to receptor sites in many tissues, including vascular smooth muscle and adrenal glands.

Angiotensin II, a potent vasoconstrictor, is then free to stimulate the adrenal cortex to secrete aldosterone, and the inhibiting effects of angiotensin II reduce blood pressure.

Other: Anaphylaxis, angioedema, hyperkalemia, increased CK level, flulike symptoms, pain

Nursing Considerations
• Expect to provide treatment such as normal saline solution I.V., as prescribed, to correct known or suspected hypovolemia before beginning olmesartan therapy.
• Make 200 ml of a 2-mg/ml suspension for children or adults who cannot swallow tablets by adding 50 ml of purified water to an amber polyethylene terephthalate (PET) bottle containing twenty 20-mg tablets and allow to stand for a minimum of 5 minutes. Shake the container for at least 1 minute and allow the suspension to stand for at least 1 minute. Repeat 1-minute shaking and 1-minute standing for four additional times. Add 100 ml of Ora-Sweet and 50 ml of Ora-Plus to the suspension and shake well for at least 1 minute. Refrigerate the suspension for up to 4 weeks. Shake the suspension well before each use and return promptly to the refrigerator.
• Monitor patient for increased BUN and serum creatinine levels, especially in a patient with impaired renal function,

because drug may cause acute renal failure. If increased levels are significant or persist, notify prescriber immediately.
• Monitor blood pressure frequently to assess effectiveness of therapy. If blood pressure isn't controlled with olmesartan alone, expect to administer a diuretic, such as hydrochlorothiazide, as prescribed.
WARNING Monitor patient's blood pressure frequently if he receives a diuretic or other antihypertensive during olmesartan therapy because of an increased risk of hypotension.
• Expect to discontinue drug temporarily if patient experiences hypotension. Place patient in supine position immediately and prepare to administer normal saline solution I.V., as prescribed. Expect to resume drug therapy after blood pressure stabilizes.
• If patient also receives a diuretic, provide adequate hydration, as appropriate, to help prevent hypovolemia. Watch for evidence of hypovolemia, such as hypotension with dizziness and fainting.
PATIENT TEACHING
• Teach patient, parent, or caregiver how to mix olmesartan suspension if patient is unable to swallow tablets.

• Advise patient to avoid exercise in hot weather and excessive alcohol use to reduce the risk of dehydration and hypotension. Also instruct him to notify prescriber if he has prolonged diarrhea, nausea, or vomiting.

• Caution patient to avoid hazardous activities until drug's CNS effects are known.

• Explain the importance of regular exercise, proper diet, and other lifestyle changes in controlling hypertension.

• Advise female patient to notify prescriber immediately about known or suspected pregnancy. Explain that if she becomes pregnant, prescriber may replace olmesartan with another antihypertensive that's safe to use during pregnancy.

olodaterol
Striverdi Respimat

Class and Category
Chemical class: Long-acting beta$_2$-adrenergic agonist
Therapeutic class: Bronchodilator
Pregnancy category: C

Indications and Dosages
➤ *To treat long-term airflow obstruction in patients with chronic obstructive pulmonary disease*
ORAL INHALATION
Adults. 5 mcg (2 inhalations) once daily at same time each day.

Mechanism of Action
By binding and activating beta$_2$-adrenoceptors in the airways, intracellular adenyl cyclase (an enzyme that mediates the synthesis of cyclic-3', 5' adenosine monophosphate [cAMP]) is stimulated. Elevated levels of cAMP cause bronchodilation by relaxing airway smooth muscle cells.

Contraindications
Asthma without use of a long-term asthma control drug, hypersensitivity to olodaterol or its components

Interaction
DRUGS
adrenergic agents: Potentiated effects

beta blockers: Decreased effectiveness of olodaterol; possibly severe bronchospasm
diuretics, steroids, xanthine derivatives: Increased risk of hypokalemia
drugs known to prolong QT interval, MAO inhibitors, tricyclic antidepressants: Possibly adverse cardiovascular effects
ketoconazole: Possibly increased serum olodaterol level
non-potassium-sparing diuretics: Possibly increased risk of ECG changes and hypokalemia

Adverse Reactions
CNS: Dizziness, fever
CV: Atrial fibrillation, chest pain, ECG changes, palpitations, tachycardia
EENT: Nasopharyngitis
ENDO: Hyperglycemia
GI: Constipation, diarrhea
GU: UTI
MS: Arthralgia, back pain
RESP: Bronchitis, COPD exacerbation, cough, paradoxical bronchospasms, pneumonia, upper respiratory infection
SKIN: Rash
Other: Anaphylaxis, angioedema, hypokalemia

Nursing Considerations
• Know that olodaterol therapy should not be used in patients with acutely deteriorating COPD, which may be a life-threatening condition. It should also not be used for relief of acute episodes of bronchospasm.

• Use caution when administering olodaterol to patients with cardiovascular disorders, such as coronary insufficiency, arrhythmias, hypertension, or hypertrophic obstructive cardiomyopathy; to patients with seizure disorders or thyrotoxicosis; and to patients who are unusually responsive to sympathomimetic amines or are at risk for developing prolonged QT interval.

• Administer olodaterol only by oral inhalation. Remember to prime inhaler before using for the first time.

• Watch patient closely for paradoxical bronchospasm. If present, discontinue olodaterol therapy immediately, notify prescriber, and implement treatment according to standard of care.

N
O

WARNING Monitor patient for worsening or deteriorating asthma because asthma-related deaths have increased in patients receiving salmeterol, a drug in the same class as olodaterol. Be aware that use of long-acting beta$_2$-adrenergic agonists such as olodaterol is contraindicated in patients with asthma without the use of a long-term asthma control medication, such as an inhaled corticosteroid. Monitor patient closely and notify prescriber immediately of any changes in patient's respiratory status.
• Monitor patients with a history of cardiovascular disorders. Notify prescriber of any significant increases in pulse rate or blood pressure or worsening of chronic conditions. Olodaterol may also cause ECG changes such as flattening of the T wave, prolonged QT interval, and ST-segment depression. Drug may need to be discontinued if such reactions occur.
WARNING Watch patient closely for hypersensitivity reactions. If present, stop olodaterol therapy immediately, notify prescriber, and provide emergency treatment according to standard of care.
• Monitor patient's serum potassium level and assess for signs and symptoms of hypokalemia, especially if patient has severe COPD, because hypokalemia may be made worse by hypoxia and concomitant treatment.

PATIENT TEACHING
• Advise patient, especially if she has a significant cardiac history, to inform prescriber of any other drugs she is taking before beginning olodaterol therapy and to keep prescriber informed of any new drug therapies while taking olodaterol.
• Caution patient not to increase olodaterol dosage or frequency without consulting prescriber because serious adverse reactions may occur.
• Instruct patient on how to load the cartridge into the inhaler. Remind patient that after insertion, the unit must be primed before first use by actuating the inhaler toward the ground until an aerosol cloud is visible and then repeating the process three more times. If not used for more than 3 days, remind patient to actuate the inhaler once before use; if not used for more than 21 days, tell patient to prime inhaler as if using for the first time.

• Teach patient how to use inhaler.
• Urge patient to notify prescriber if her symptoms worsen, if olodaterol becomes less effective, or if she needs more inhalations of her prescribed short-acting beta$_2$-agonist than usual. This may indicate that her condition is worsening.
• Instruct patient to notify prescriber immediately if she experiences palpitations, chest pain, rapid heart rate, or other troublesome effects while taking olodaterol because dosage may need to be adjusted.

olsalazine sodium
Dipentum

Class and Category
Chemical class: Salicylate derivative
Therapeutic class: Bowel disease suppressant
Pregnancy category: C

Indications and Dosages
➤ *To maintain remission of ulcerative colitis*
CAPSULES, TABLETS
Adults and adolescents. 500 mg twice daily.

Mechanism of Action
Exerts anti-inflammatory action in GI tract after being converted by colonic bacteria to mesalamine (5-aminosalicylic acid), which inhibits cyclooxygenase. Inhibition of cyclooxygenase reduces prostaglandin production in intestinal mucosa. This in turn reduces production of arachidonic acid metabolites, which may be increased in patients with inflammatory bowel disease. Olsalazine also exerts an anti-inflammatory effect by indirectly inhibiting leukotriene synthesis, which normally catalyzes production of arachidonic acid.

Contraindications
Hypersensitivity to olsalazine, salicylates, or their components

Interaction
DRUGS
6-mercaptopurine, thioguanine: Increased risk of myelosuppression

low-molecular-weight heparins or heparinoids: Increased risk of bleeding after neuraxial anesthesia
oral anticoagulants: Possibly prolonged PT
varicella vaccine: Increased risk of Reye's syndrome

Adverse Reactions

CNS: Anxiety, depression, dizziness, drowsiness, fatigue, fever, headache, insomnia, lethargy, paresthesia, peripheral neuropathy, vertigo
CV: Cardiac arrest, hypotension, myocarditis, pericarditis, prolonged QT interval, second-degree AV block
ENDO: Hot flashes
EENT: Dry eyes and mouth, lacrimation, laryngeal edema, stridor, stomatitis, tinnitus
GI: Abdominal pain, anorexia, cholestatic jaundice, cirrhosis, diarrhea, dyspepsia, elevated liver enzymes, hepatic failure or necrosis, hepatitis, hepatotoxicity, nausea, vomiting
GU: Dysuria, hematuria, interstitial nephritis, nephrotic syndrome, urinary frequency
HEME: Aplastic or hemolytic anemia, lymphopenia, neutropenia, pancytopenia
MS: Arthralgia, joint pain, muscle spasms, myalgia
RESP: Bronchospasm, dyspnea, interstitial lung disease, shortness of breath
SKIN: Acne, alopecia, erythema nodosum, flushing, photosensitivity, pruritus, rash
Other: Anaphylaxis, angioedema, dehydration

Nursing Considerations

• Assess patient for aspirin allergy before giving olsalazine.
• If patient has severe allergies or asthma, watch closely for worsening symptoms during olsalazine therapy, and notify prescriber immediately if they occur.
• Assess quantity and consistency of stools and frequency of bowel movements before, during, and after therapy.
• Give drug with food to decrease adverse GI reactions.
• Monitor skin for adequate hydration.
• Assess patient for abdominal pain and hyperactive bowel sounds.
• Monitor renal and hepatic status in patient with underlying renal or hepatic dysfunc-

tion because drug may further impair these functions.
PATIENT TEACHING
• Instruct patient to take olsalazine with food.
• Urge patient to continue taking drug as prescribed, even if symptoms improve.
• Advise patient to watch for signs of dehydration.
• Tell patient to report unusual, persistent, or severe adverse effects to prescriber.

omalizumab

Xolair

Class and Category

Chemical class: Recombinant IgG1K anti-IgE monoclonal antibody
Therapeutic class: Antiallergenic
Pregnancy category: B

Indications and Dosages

➤ *To treat moderate to severe persistent asthma in patients with positive skin test or in vitro reactivity to a perennial aeroallergen whose symptoms have been inadequately controlled with inhaled corticosteroids*
SUBCUTANEOUS INJECTION
Adults and adolescents age 12 and over. 150 to 375 mg every 2 or 4 wk. Dose and frequency determined by body weight and blood IgE levels.
DOSAGE ADJUSTMENT Dosage adjusted for significant changes in body weight.
➤ *To treat chronic idiopathic urticaria in patients who remain symptomatic despite H_1 antihistamine treatment*
SUBCUTANEOUS INJECTION
Adults and adolescents age 12 and over. 150 mg or 300 mg every 4 wk.

Mechanism of Action

Helps reduce inflammation by binding to circulating IgE and keeping it from binding to mast cells. This action inhibits degranulation and blocks release of histamine and other chemical mediators. In asthma, inflammation results when antigen reexposure causes mast cells to degranulate and release histamine and chemical mediators.

Contraindications

Hypersensitivity to omalizumab or its components

Adverse Reactions

CNS: Dizziness, fatigue, headache, vertigo
EENT: Earache, pharyngitis, sinusitis
MS: Arm or leg pain, arthralgia, fractures
RESP: Upper respiratory tract infection
SKIN: Dermatitis, pruritus, urticaria
Other: Anaphylaxis; generalized pain; injection-site bruising, burning, hive or mass formation, induration, inflammation, itching, pain, redness, stinging, and warmth; malignancies; viral infection

Nursing Considerations

• Record patient's weight, and obtain blood IgE levels, as ordered, before starting omalizumab prescribed to treat asthma; dosage and dosing frequency are based on these factors.
• Reconstitute using sterile water for injection, and allow 15 to 20 minutes (on average) for lyophilized product to dissolve. Draw 1.4 ml sterile water for injection into a 3-ml syringe with a 1-in 18G needle. Place omalizumab vial upright, and inject sterile water into vial using aseptic technique. Gently swirl upright vial for about 1 minute to evenly wet powder. Don't shake. Every 5 minutes, gently swirl for 5 to 10 seconds until solution contains no gel-like particles. Discard if powder takes longer than 40 minutes to dissolve, and start with a new vial. Once reconstituted, solution should be clear or slightly opalescent and may have a few small bubbles or foam around edge of vial. Use omalizumab within 8 hours if refrigerated or 4 hours if stored at room temperature.
• To remove reconstituted omalizumab from vial, invert vial for 15 seconds to let solution drain toward stopper. Using a new 3-ml syringe with a 1-in 18G needle, insert needle into inverted vial and position needle tip at the very bottom of solution in the vial stopper. Then pull plunger all the way back to end of syringe barrel to remove all solution from inverted vial. To obtain full 150-mg dose (1 vial containing 1.2 ml of reconstituted omalizumab), you must withdraw all product from vial before expelling any air or excess solution from syringe.

• Don't give more than 150 mg of omalizumab per injection site.
• Be prepared to inject omalizumab over 5 to 10 seconds because solution is slightly viscous.

WARNING Monitor patient closely for hypersensitivity reactions, particularly for first 2 hours after delivery. Although rare, anaphylaxis has occurred as early as first dose and more than 1 year after starting regular treatment. Keep emergency medication and equipment readily available.

WARNING Monitor patient closely for signs of cancer. Report any abnormal findings to prescriber.

PATIENT TEACHING

• Instruct patient to notify prescriber immediately about possible hyper-sensitivity, such as rash, hives, or difficulty breathing.
• Caution patient that any improvement in his asthma may take time.
• Encourage patient to comply with regularly scheduled prescriber visits.
• Inform patient of risk of malignancy and suggest routine cancer screening.
• Explain that omalizumab isn't used to treat acute bronchospasm or status asthmaticus.
• Tell patient not to abruptly stop any prescribed systemic or inhaled cortico-steroid when starting omalizumab therapy for asthma treatment because steroid dosage must be tapered gradually under prescriber's supervision.
• If female patient becomes pregnant within 8 weeks before or during omalizumab therapy, urge her to enroll in the Xolair Pregnancy Exposure Registry at 1-866-496-5247. Also, tell her to notify prescriber because drug may need to be changed.

omega-3-acid ethyl esters

Lovaza

Class and Category

Chemical class: Ethyl esters of omega-3 fatty acids
Therapeutic class: Lipid regulator

Pregnancy category: C

Indications and Dosages
➤ *As adjunct to diet to reduce triglyceride level that exceeds 500 mg/dl*
CAPSULES
Adults. 4 g once daily or 2 g twice daily.

Mechanism of Action
Omega-3-acid ethyl esters are essential fatty acids that may inhibit very-low-density lipoprotein and triglyceride synthesis in the liver. With less triglyceride synthesis, plasma triglyceride levels decrease.

Contraindications
Hypersensitivity to omega-3-acid ethyl esters or their components

Interaction
DRUGS
anticogulants: Possibly increased bleeding time

Adverse Reactions
CV: Angina pectoris
EENT: Halitosis, nosebleeds, taste perversion
GI: Diarrhea, dyspepsia, eructation, nausea, vomiting
HEME: Prolonged bleeding time
MS: Back pain
SKIN: Bruising, rash
Other: Anaphylaxis, flulike symptoms

Nursing Considerations
• Be aware that drugs known to increase triglyceride levels—such as beta blockers, thiazide diuretics, and estrogens—should be discontinued or changed, if possible, before omega-3 ethyl ester therapy starts.
• Expect to check patient's triglyceride level before starting and periodically throughout omega-3-acid ethyl ester therapy to determine effectiveness.
• Administer drug with meals.
• Expect to stop omega-3-acid ethyl ester therapy after 2 months if patient's trigylceride level doesn't decrease as expected.
• Monitor patient with history of paroxysmal or persistent atrial fibrillation for recurrences of symptomatic atrial fibrillation or flutter, especially within the first 2 to 3 months of initiating omega-3 ethyl ester therapy.

PATIENT TEACHING
• Explain to patient the importance of dietary measures, an exercise program, and controlling other factors—such as blood glucose level—that may contribute to elevated triglyceride levels.
• Advise patient to take drug with meals.
• Explain that patient will need periodic laboratory tests to evaluate therapy.
• Instruct patient to seek immediate medical attention if chest pain occurs.

omega 3-carboxylic acids
Epanova

Class and Category
Chemical class: Fish oil–derived free fatty acids
Therapeutic class: Antihypertriglyceride
Pregnancy category: C

Indications and Dosages
➤ *To reduce triglyceride levels in patients with severe (equal to or greater than 500 mg/dl) hypertriglyceridemia*
CAPSULES
Adults. 2 g or 4 g once daily.

Mechanism of Action
Possibly reduces synthesis of triglycerides in the liver by inhibiting acyl-CoA-1,2 diacylglycerol acyltransferase, increasing mitochondrial and peroxisomal beta oxidation in the liver, decreasing lipogenesis in the liver, and increasing plasma lipoprotein lipase activity.

Contraindications
Hypersensitivity to omega 3-carboxylic acids or its components

Interaction
DRUGS
anticoagulants, antiplatelet agents: Possibly increased risk of bleeding

Adverse Reactions
CNS: Fatigue
CV: Elevated LDL-C levels
EENT: Difficulty swallowing, nasopharyngitis

N
O

GI: Abdominal discomfort, distention, or pain; constipation; diarrhea; eructation; nausea; vomiting
MS: Arthralgia

Nursing Considerations
• Use cautiously in patients with fish and/or shellfish allergy because omega 3-carboxylic acids contain polyunsaturated free fatty acids derived from fish oils and it is not known if cross-sensitivity exists.
• Monitor LDL-C levels, as ordered, periodically during therapy with omega 3-carboxylic acids because drug may increase these levels in some patients.

PATIENT TEACHING
• Instruct patient to swallow capsules whole and not to crush, break open, chew, or dissolve the capsules.
• Inform patient that drug therapy is not a substitution for dietary measures. Adherence to dietary restrictions must be continued.

omeprazole
Losec (CAN), Prilosec, Zegerid

Class and Category
Chemical class: Substituted benzimidazole
Therapeutic class: Antiulcer
Pregnancy category: C

Indications and Dosages
➤ *To treat gastroesophageal reflux disease (GERD) without esophageal lesions, to prevent erosive esophagitis*
DELAYED-RELEASE CAPSULES, DELAYED-RELEASE TABLETS, ORAL SUSPENSION
Adults. 20 mg daily for 4 wk.
➤ *To treat GERD with erosive esophagitis*
DELAYED-RELEASE CAPSULES, DELAYED-RELEASE TABLETS, ORAL SUSPENSION
Adults. 20 mg daily for 4 to 8 wk.
➤ *To treat pediatric GERD and maintenance of healing of erosive esophagitis*
DELAYED-RELEASE CAPSULES (PRILOSEC), ORAL SUSPENSION (PRILOSEC)
Children age 1 to 16 years of age weighing 20 kg (44 lb) or more. *20 mg daily.*
Children age 1 to 16 weighing 10 kg (22 lb) to less than 20 kg (44 lb). *10 mg daily.*

Children age 1 to 16 weighing 5 kg (11 lb) to less than 10 kg (22 lb). *5 mg daily.*
➤ *To provide short-term treatment of active benign gastric ulcer*
DELAYED-RELEASE CAPSULES
Adults. 40 mg daily for 4 to 8 wk.
DELAYED-RELEASE TABLETS
Adults. 20 mg daily for 4 to 8 wk, increased to 40 mg daily, as needed.
➤ *To treat duodenal or gastric ulcer associated with* Helicobacter pylori
DELAYED-RELEASE CAPSULES, ORAL SUSPENSION
Adults. 40 mg daily with clarithromycin for 14 days, followed by 20 mg daily alone for another 14 days. Or, 20 mg twice daily with amoxicillin for 14 days. Or, 20 mg twice daily with amoxicillin and clarithromycin for 10 days.
DELAYED-RELEASE TABLETS
Adults. 20 mg twice daily. with clarithromycin and amoxicillin or metronidazole for 7 days, followed by 20 mg daily for up to 3 wk (for duodenal ulcer) or 20 to 40 mg daily for up to 12 wk (for gastric ulcer).
➤ *To provide long-term treatment of gastric hypersecretory conditions, such as multiple endocrine adenoma syndrome, systemic mastocytosis, and Zollinger-Ellison syndrome*
DELAYED-RELEASE CAPSULES, DELAYED-RELEASE TABLETS
Adults. 60 mg daily or in divided doses, as prescribed. *Maximum:* 120 mg three times daily.

Route	Onset	Peak	Duration
P.O.	1 hr	In 2 hr	72–96 hr

Contraindications
Hypersensitivity to omeprazole, other proton pump inhibitors, substituted benzimidazoles, or their components

Interaction
DRUGS
alprazolam, astemizole, carbamazepine, cisapride, cyclosporine, diazepam, diltiazem, disulfiram, erythromycin, felodipine, lidocaine, lovastatin, midazolam, quinidine, simvastatin, terfenadine, triazolam, verapamil, voriconazole:
Decreased clearance and increased blood levels of these drugs

Mechanism of Action

Omeprazole interferes with gastric acid secretion by inhibiting the hydrogen potassium -adenosine triphosphatase (H + K + -ATPase) enzyme system, or proton pump, in gastric parietal cells. Normally, the proton pump uses energy from hydrolysis of adenosine triphosphate to drive hydrogen (H^+) and chloride (Cl^-) out of parietal cells and into the stomach lumen in exchange for potassium (K^+), which leaves the stomach lumen and enters parietal cells. After this exchange, H^+ and Cl^- combine in the stomach to form hydrochloric acid (HCl), as shown below left. Omeprazole irreversibly blocks the exchange of intracellular H^+ and extracellular K^+, as shown below right. By preventing H^+ from entering the stomach lumen, omeprazole keeps additional HCl from forming.

 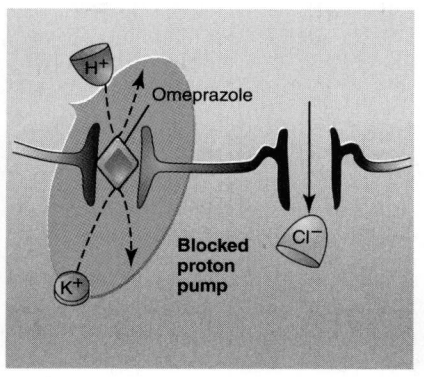

ampicillin, etlontinib, iron salts, itraconazole, ketoconazole, vitamin B_{12}: Impaired absorption of these drugs
atazanavir, nelfinavir: Decreased plasma levels of these agents
cilostazol: Increased blood cilostazol
clopidogrel: Reduced effectiveness of clopidogrel
clarithromycin: Increased blood levels of omeprazole and clarithromycin
digoxin: Increased digoxin bioavailability, possibly digitalis toxicity
levobupivacaine: Increased risk of levobupivacaine toxicity
methotrexate: Possibly delayed methotrexate elimination and increased risk of toxicity
nifedipine: Decreased nifedipine clearance, increased risk of hypotension
phenytoin: Decreased phenytoin clearance, increased risk of phenytoin toxicity
saquinavir: Increased plasma saquinavir level
St John's wort, rifampin: Decreased plasma omeprazole level
sucralfate: Decreased omeprazole absorption
tacrolimus: Possibly increased tacrolimus level
warfarin: Possibly increased risk of abnormal bleeding

Adverse Reactions

CNS: Agitation, asthenia, dizziness, drowsiness, fatigue, headache, psychic disturbance, somnolence
CV: Chest pain, hypertension, peripheral edema
EENT: Anterior ischemic optic neuropathy, optic atrophy or neuritis, stomatitis
ENDO: Hypoglycemia
GI: Abdominal pain, constipation, diarrhea, Clostridium difficile-associated diarrhea, dyspepsia, elevated liver function tests, flatulence, hepatic dysfunction or failure, indigestion, nausea, pancreatitis, vomiting
GU: Interstitial nephritis
HEME: Agranulocytosis, anemia, hemolytic anemia, leukopenia, leukocytosis, neutropenia, pancytopenia, thrombocytopenia
MS: Back pain, bone fracture
RESP: Cough

SKIN: Erythema multiforme, photo-sensitivity, pruritus, rash, Stevens-Johnson syndrome, toxic epidermal necrolysis, urticaria
Other: Anaphylaxis, angioedema, hypomagnesemia, hyponatremia, vitamin B_{12} deficiency (long-term use)

Nursing Considerations
• Give omeprazole before meals, preferably in the morning for once-daily dosing. If needed, also give an antacid, as prescribed.
• If needed, open capsule and sprinkle enteric-coated granules on applesauce or yogurt or mix with water or acidic fruit juice, such as apple or cranberry juice. Give immediately.
• To give drug via NG tube, mix granules in acidic juice because enteric coating dissolves in alkaline pH.
• Because drug can interfere with absorption of vitamin B_{12}, monitor patient for macrocytic anemia.
• Monitor patient for bone fracture, especially in patients receiving multiple daily doses for more than a year because proton pump inhibitors, such as omeprazole, increase risk for osteoporosis-related fractures of the hip, wrist, or spine.
• Be aware that long-term use of omeprazole may increase the risk of gastric carcinoma.
• Know that omeprazole therapy may produce false elevations of serum chromogranin levels, used to help diagnosis presence of neuroendocrine tumors. If test results are high, withhold omeprazole therapy temporarily and repeat test, as ordered.
• If omeprazole is given with antibiotics, watch for diarrhea from *Clostridium difficile.* If diarrhea occurs, notify prescriber and expect to withhold drug and treat with fluids, electrolytes, protein, and an antibiotic effective against *C. difficile.*
• Monitor the patient, especially the patient on long-term therapy, for hypomagnesemia. If patient is to remain on omeprazole long-term, expect to monitor the patient's serum magnesium level, as ordered, and if level becomes low, anticipate magnesium replacement therapy and omeprazole to be discontinued.

PATIENT TEACHING
• Tell patient to take drug before eating—usually before breakfast—and to swallow delayed-release capsules or tablets whole. If needed, patient may sprinkle contents of capsule onto 1 tablespoon of applesauce and swallow immediately without chewing pellets. Tell him to follow with a glass of cool water and not to keep any leftover mixture.
• If patient takes the oral suspension, tell him to empty package into a small cup containing 2 tablespoons of water (no other beverage should be used), stir the mixture well, drink it immediately, refill the cup with water, and drink again.
• Encourage patient to avoid alcohol, aspirin products, ibuprofen, and foods that may increase gastric secretions during therapy. Tell him to notify all prescribers about prescription drug use.
• Advise patient to notify prescriber immediately about abdominal pain or diarrhea.
• Urge female patient of childbearing age to use effective contraception during therapy and to inform prescriber immediately if she is or suspects she may be pregnant.
• Instruct patient to inform all prescribers of omeprazole therapy.

ondansetron hydrochloride
Zofran, Zofran ODT, Zuplenz

Class and Category
Chemical class: Carbazole
Therapeutic class: Antiemetic
Pregnancy category: B

Indications and Dosages
➤ *To prevent chemotherapy-induced nausea and vomiting*
DISINTEGRATING TABLETS, ORAL SOLUTION, TABLETS
Adults and children age 12 and over.
Initial: 8 mg given 30 min before chemotherapy. *After chemotherapy:* 8 mg given 8 hr after initial dose; then 8 mg every 12 hr for 1 to 2 days.
Children ages 4 to 12. *Initial:* 4 mg given 30 min before chemotherapy. *After chemotherapy:*

4 mg given 4 and 8 hr after initial dose; then 4 mg every 8 hr for 1 to 2 days.

ORAL SOLUBLE FILM

Adults receiving highly emetogenic cancer chemotherapy. 24 mg given as three 8-mg films (allowing each 8-mg film to dissolve completely before another given) 30 min before chemotherapy.

Adults and adolescents age 12 and over receiving moderately emetogenic cancer chemotherapy. *Initial:* One 8-mg film given 30 min before chemotherapy and one 8-mg film given 8 hr after the first dose. Then, one 8-mg film given every 12 hr for 1 to 2 days after completion of chemotherapy.

Children ages 4 to 11 receiving moderately emetogenic cancer chemotherapy. *Initial:* One 4-mg film given 30 min before chemotherapy with one 4-mg film given 4 and 8 hr after the first dose. Then, one 4-mg film given every 8 hr for 1 to 2 days after completion of chemotherapy.

I.V. INFUSION

Adults and children ages 6 months to 18 years. Three 0.15-mg/kg doses, each infused over 15 min, starting with first dose given 30 min before chemotherapy and second and third doses given 4 and 8 hours after first dose.

➤ *To prevent nausea and vomiting associated with radiotherapy*

ORAL SOLUBLE FILM

Adults. One 8-mg film given three times a day.

DOSAGE ADJUSTMENT For patient receiving total body irradiation, one 8-mg film given 1 to 2 hr before each fraction of radiotherapy administered each day; for patient receiving single high-dose fraction radiotherapy to the abdomen, one 8-mg film given 1 to 2 hr before radiotherapy, with subsequent doses given every 8 hr after the first dose for 1 to 2 days after completion of radiotherapy; for patient receiving daily fractionated radiotherapy to the abdomen, one 8-mg film given 1 to 2 hr before radiotherapy with subsequent doses given every 8 hr after the first dose for each day radiotherapy is given.

DISINTEGRATING TABLETS, ORAL SOLUTION, TABLETS

Adults and children age 12 and over. *Initial:* 8 mg as a single dose given 1 to 2 hr

before radiation therapy. *Posttherapy:* 8 mg every 8 hr, as needed and tolerated.

➤ *To prevent postoperative nausea and vomiting*

DISINTEGRATING TABLETS, ORAL SOLUTION, TABLETS

Adults. 16 mg as a single dose 1 hr before anesthesia induction.

ORAL SOLUBLE FILM

Adults. 16 mg given as two 8-mg films (first 8-mg film allowed to dissolve completely before second 8-mg film given) 1 hr before induction of anesthesia.

I.V. INJECTION

Adults and children age 12 and over. 4 mg as a single dose over 2 to 5 min just before anesthesia induction or if nausea or vomiting develops shortly after surgery.

Children ages 2 to 12 weighing more than 40 kg (88 lb). 4 mg as a single dose over 2 to 5 min just before anesthesia induction or if nausea or vomiting develops shortly after surgery.

Children ages 1 month to 12 years weighing less than 40 kg. 0.1 mg/kg as a single dose over 2 to 5 min just before or immediately after anesthesia induction or if nausea or vomiting develops shortly after surgery.

I.M. INJECTION

Adults and children age 12 and over. 4 mg as a single dose just before anesthesia induction or if nausea or vomiting develops shortly after surgery.

DOSAGE ADJUSTMENT For patients with hepatic impairment, maximum dosage limited to 8 mg daily I.V. or P.O.

Mechanism of Action

Blocks serotonin receptors centrally in the chemoreceptor trigger zone and peripherally at vagal nerve terminals in the intestine. This action reduces nausea and vomiting by preventing serotonin release in the small intestine (probable cause of chemotherapy- and radiation-induced nausea and vomiting) and by blocking signals to the CNS. Ondansetron may also bind to other serotonin receptors and to mu-opioid receptors.

Incompatibilities

Don't give ondansetron in same I.V. line as acyclovir, allopurinol, aminophylline, amphotericin B, ampicillin, ampicillin and sulbactam, amsacrine, cefepime, cefoperazone, furosemide, ganciclovir, lorazepam, methylprednisolone, mezlocillin, piperacillin, or sargramostim. Alkaline solutions and highly concentrated fluorouracil solutions are physically incompatible.

Contraindications

Concomitant use of apomorphine, congenital long QT syndrome, hypersensitivity to ondansetron or its components

Interaction

DRUGS

cisplatin, cyclophosphamide: Possibly altered blood levels of these drugs
drugs that increase QT interval: Augmented effect on QT interval increasing risk of torsades de pointes

ACTIVITIES

alcohol use: Increased stimulant and sedative effects, including mood and physical sensations

Adverse Reactions

CNS: Agitation, akathisia, anxiety, ataxia, dizziness, drowsiness, dystonia, fever, headache, hypotension, restlessness, seizures, serotonin syndrome, syncope, somnolence, weakness
CV: Arrhythmias, cardiopulmonary arrest (parenteral form), chest pain, hypotension, palpitations, prolonged QT interval, shock, tachycardia, torsades de pointes
EENT: Accommodation disturbances, altered taste, blurred vision, dry mouth, laryngeal edema, laryngospasm, stridor, transient blindness
GI: Abdominal pain, anorexia, constipation, diarrhea, elevated liver enzymes, flatulence, indigestion, intestinal obstruction, thirst
RESP: Bronchospasm, pulmonary embolism, shortness of breath
SKIN: Flushing, hyperpigmentation, maculopapular rash, pruritus, Stevens-Johnson syndrome, toxic epidermal necrolysis, urticaria
Other: Anaphylaxis; angioedema; hiccups; injection-site burning, pain, and redness

Nursing Considerations

WARNING Be aware that oral disintegrating tablets may contain aspartame, which is

metabolized to phenylalanine and must be used cautiously in patients with phenylketonuria.

• Know that if hypokalemia or hypo-magnesemia is present, these electrolyte imbalances should be corrected before ondansetron is administered because of increased risk for QT interval prolon-gation, which could predispose the patient to develop torsades de pointes.

• Place disintegrating tablet or oral soluble film on patient's tongue immediately after opening package. It dissolves in seconds.

• Use calibrated container or oral syringe to measure dose of oral solution.

• Give up to 4 mg I.V. diluted in 50 ml of D_5W or normal saline solution.

• Monitor patient closely for signs and symptoms of hypersensitivity to ondansetron because hypersensitivity reactions, including anaphylaxis and bronchospasm, may occur. If present, discontinue drug, notify prescriber, and provide supportive care.

WARNING Monitor patient closely for serotonin syndrome, which may include agitation, chills, confusion, diaphoresis, diarrhea, fever, hyperactive reflexes, poor coordination, restlessness, shaking, talking or acting with uncontrolled excitement, tremor, and twitching.

• Monitor patient's electrocardiogram, as ordered, and especially in patients with bradyarrhythmias, congestive heart failure, hypokalemia, or hypomagnesemia or in patients taking other medications known to prolong the QT interval because ondansetron therapy can prolong the QT interval resulting in life-threatening arrhythmias such as torsades de pointes. Be aware that no dosage greater than 16 mg should be given intravenously at any one time due to increased risk of prolonged QT interval.

WARNING Be aware that ondansetron may mask symptoms of adynamic ileus or gastric distention after abdominal surgery.

PATIENT TEACHING

• Advise patient to use calibrated container or oral syringe to measure oral solution.

• Instruct patient to place ondansetron disintegrating tablet or oral soluble film on his tongue immediately after opening

package and to let it dissolve on his tongue before swallowing.
• Advise patient to immediately report signs of hypersensitivity, such as rash.
WARNING Advise patients to seek immediate medical attention if the following symptoms occur: changes in mental status, autonomic instability, or neuromuscular symptoms, with or without gastrointestinal symptoms.
• Reassure patient with transient blindness that it will resolve within a few minutes to 48 hours.

oritavancin
Orbactiv

Class and Category
Chemical class: Semisynthetic lipoglycopeptide
Therapeutic class: Antibacterial
Pregnancy category: C

Indications and Dosages
➤ *To treat acute bacterial skin and skin structure infections caused by gram-positive microorganisms such as* Enterococcus faecalis *(vancomycin-susceptible isolates only),* Staphylococcus aureus *(including methicillin-susceptible and methicillin-resistant isolates),* Streptococcus agalactiae, S. anginosus *group* (S. anginosus, S. intermedius, S. constellatus), *and* S. pyogenes
I.V. INFUSION
Adults. 1,200 mg given over 3 hours as a one-time dose.

Mechanism of Action
Kills bacteria by inhibiting cell wall synthesis.

Incompatibilities
Do not mix or administer oritavancin in normal saline solution, as a precipitation of the drug may occur. Also, do not administer with other drugs, including those formulated at a basic or neutral pH, as they may be incompatible with oritavancin.

Contraindications
Hypersensitivity to oritavancin and its components, intravenous unfractionated heparin sodium administration for 48 hours following oritavancin administration

Interaction
DRUGS
CYP2C6 substrates: Possibly decreased or increased CYP2C drug concentration
warfarin: Increased risk of bleeding

Adverse Reactions
CNS: Dizziness, headache
CV: Peripheral edema, tachycardia
ENDO: Hypoglycemia
GI: Diarrhea including *Clostridium difficile*–associated diarrhea, elevated liver enzymes, nausea, vomiting
HEME: Anemia, eosinophilia
MS: Myalgia, osteomyelitis, tenosynovitis
RESP: Bronchospasm, wheezing
SKIN: Erythema multiforme, leucocytoclastic vasculitis, pruritus, rash, urticaria
Other: Angioedema; hyperuricemia; infusion reactions such as erythema, flushing, pruritus, or urticaria; infusion-site extravasation, induration, or phlebitis

Nursing Considerations
• Use oritavancin cautiously in patients with a history of hypersensitivity to glycopeptides because of the possibility of cross-sensitivity.
• Reconstitute drug by adding 40 ml of sterile water for injection to each vial (three vials are needed to provide a dose of 1,200 mg), to provide a 10 mg/ml solution per vial. Gently swirl to avoid foaming and to completely dissolve the powder. Solution should appear clear, colorless to pale yellow.
• Withdraw and discard 120 ml from a 1,000-ml intravenous bag of D_5W (never use normal saline). Then, withdraw 40 ml from each of the three reconstituted vials and add to D_5W intravenous bag to bring bag volume back to 1,000 ml. This will yield a concentration of 1.2 mg/ml. Once mixed in infusion bag, use within 3 hours when stored at room temperature or within 9 hours when refrigerated to allow

N
O

the additional 3 hours needed for administration.

- Flush intravenous line with D₅W solution before and after administering drug.
- Monitor patient closely for signs of bleeding, especially if patient is taking warfarin therapy, because drug may artificially prolong prothrombin time (PT) and INR for up to 24 hours, making monitoring of the effectiveness of warfarin unreliable for at least 24 hours after the administration of oritavancin. Drug may also artificially prolong activated partial thromboplastin time (aPTT) for 48 hours.
- Infuse oritavancin over 3 hours. If patient develops an infusion-related reaction such as flushing, pruritus, or urticaria, slow or stop the infusion and notify prescriber.

WARNING Monitor patient closely for signs of hypersensitivity reactions because some reactions may be serious. If present, discontinue infusion immediately, notify prescriber, and implement appropriate standard of care.

- Assess patient for signs of secondary infection, such as profuse, watery diarrhea. If such diarrhea develops, contact prescriber and expect to obtain a stool specimen to rule out pseudomembranous colitis caused by *Clostridium difficile.* If diarrhea occurs, notify prescriber and expect to withhold drug and treat with fluids, electrolytes, protein, and an antibiotic effective against C. *difficile.*
- Monitor patient for osteomyelitis, as drug has been shown to produce more cases of osteomyelitis than vancomycin used to treat similar infections. If present, be prepared to institute appropriate alternative antibacterial therapy.

PATIENT TEACHING

- Alert patient that an allergic reaction can occur up to a day after oritavancin has been administered. Instruct him to notify prescriber of any signs of an allergic reaction and seek immediate medical attention if signs are severe or prolonged.
- Urge patient to tell prescriber if diarrhea develops, even 2 months or more after oritavancin ends.

orlistat
Alli, Xenical

Class and Category
Chemical class: Lipase inhibitor
Therapeutic class: Antiobesity
Pregnancy category: X

Indications and Dosages
➤ *To promote weight loss in patients with body mass index above 30 kg (66 lb)/m² (27 kg [59.4 lb]/m² in those with diabetes mellitus, hyperlipidemia, or hypertension) and to reduce the risk of weight regain*

GELCAPS
Adults. 120 mg three times a day with fat-containing meals.

Contraindications
Cholestasis, chronic malabsorption syndrome, hypersensitivity to orlistat or its components, pregnancy

Interaction
DRUGS
anticoagulants: Altered therapeutic coagulation
antiepileptics: Possibly increased risk of seizures
cyclosporine: Altered cyclosporine absorption
fat-soluble vitamins: Decreased vitamin absorption, especially vitamin E and beta-carotene
levothyroxine: Possibly decreased levothyroxine effectiveness, resulting in hypothyroidism
pravastatin: Potentiated lipid-lowering effect

Adverse Reactions
CNS: Anxiety, depression, dizziness, fatigue, headache, seizures, sleep disturbance
CV: Pedal edema
EENT: Gingival or tooth disorder, otitis
GI: Abdominal discomfort or pain, acute hepatic failure, cholelithiasis, diarrhea (infectious), elevated liver enzyme levels, fatty or oily stool, fecal incontinence or urgency, flatulence with discharge, hepatitis, heptocellular necrosis, increased frequency of bowel movements, lower gastrointestinal

Mechanism of Action

In the GI tract, orlistat binds with and inactivates gastric and pancreatic enzymes known as lipases, as shown. Normally, lipase enzymes convert ingested triglycerides into absorbable free fatty acids and monoglycerides. By inactivating lipase, orlistat allows undigested triglycerides to pass through the GI tract and exit the body in feces. Blocking the absorption of some of these fats lowers the number of calories received from food, which promotes weight loss.

bleeding, nausea, pancreatitis, rectal pain, vomiting
GU: Elevated urinary oxalate levels, menstrual irregularities, nephrolithiasis, renal failure, UTI, vaginitis
MS: Arthralgia, arthritis, back pain, leg pain, myalgia, tendinitis
RESP: Bronchospasm, respiratory tract infection
SKIN: Dry skin, pruritus, rash, urticaria
Other: Anaphylaxis, angioedema, flulike symptoms

Nursing Considerations

• Use cautiously in patients with a history of hyperoxaluria or calcium oxalate nephrolithiasis, as orlistat may increase levels of urinary oxalate and cause nephrolithiasis and oxalate nephropathy, which may lead to renal failure. Monitor serum creatinine levels closely, as ordered.
• Give orlistat with or up to 1 hour after meals that contain fat.
• Give levothyroxine and orlistat at least 4 hours apart because orlistat may decrease levothyroxine effectiveness, resulting in hypothyroidism.
• Also, give cyclosporine 3 hours after administering orlistat because orlistat can decrease plasma cyclosporine levels.

• Consult prescriber if you think patient has an eating disorder, such as anorexia nervosa or bulimia.
WARNING Monitor patient's liver enzymes, as ordered. Notify prescriber if abnormalities occur and expect to discontinue orlistat immediately. Be aware that severe liver injury has occurred in some patients, resulting in the need for a liver transplant or death.

PATIENT TEACHING
• Instruct patient to take orlistat with or shortly after meals that contain fat.
• Advise patient to take a multivitamin that contains fat-soluble vitamins and beta-carotene at least 2 hours before or after orlistat, if indicated.
• If patient takes levothyroxine, tell him to separate it from orlistat by at least 4 hours.
• Explain orlistat's adverse GI effects and that reducing dietary fat may decrease them. Instruct him to notify prescriber if they become too unpleasant.
• Help patient plan a reduced-fat diet (less than 30% of daily calories) and an exercise program to promote weight loss.
• Advise patient to weigh himself daily, at the same time and wearing similar clothes, to check his progress in losing weight.

• Urge patient to report anorexia, pruritus, jaundice, dark urine, light-colored stools, or right upper quadrant pain immediately to prescriber and to stop taking orlistat.
• Tell patient to notify prescriber if he is receiving drug treatment for seizures. Also, notify prescriber if seizures happen more often or get worse.

orphenadrine citrate
Aniflex, Banflex, Flexoject, Miolin, Mio-Rel, Myotrol, Norflex, Orfro, Orphenate

orphenadrine hydrochloride
Disipal (CAN)

Class and Category
Chemical class: Tertiary amine
Therapeutic class: Skeletal muscle relaxant
Pregnancy category: C

Indications and Dosages
➤ *To relieve muscle spasms in painful musculoskeletal conditions*
E.R. TABLETS (ORPHENADRINE CITRATE)
Adults and adolescents. 100 mg twice daily in the morning and evening.
TABLETS (ORPHENADRINE HYDROCHLORIDE)
Adults and adolescents. 50 mg three times a day. *Maximum:* 250 mg daily.
I.V. OR I.M. INJECTION (ORPHENADRINE CITRATE)
Adults and adolescents. 60 mg every 12 hr, as needed.
DOSAGE ADJUSTMENT Dosage reduced to 25 to 50 mg three times a day or four times a day if patient also receives aspirin and caffeine.

Route	Onset	Peak	Duration
P.O.	In 1 hr	Unknown	4–6 hr*
I.V.	Immediate	Unknown	4–6 hr
I.M.	30 min	Unknown	4–6 hr

Mechanism of Action
May reduce muscle spasms by acting on cerebral motor centers or medulla. Post-ganglionic anticholinergic effects and some antihistaminic and local anesthetic

_____
* 12 hr for extended-release.

action contribute to skeletal muscle relaxation.

Contraindications
Angle-closure glaucoma; hypersensitivity to orphenadrine or its components; myasthenia gravis; obstruction of bladder neck, duodenum, or pylorus; prostatic hypertrophy; stenosing peptic ulcers

Interaction
DRUGS
amantadine, amitriptyline, amoxapine, antimuscarinics, atropine, bupropion, carbinoxamine, chlorpromazine, clemastine, clomipramine, clozapine, cyclobenzaprine, diphenhydramine, disopyramide, doxepin, imipramine, maprotiline, mesoridazine, methdilazine, nortriptyline, phenothiazines, procainamide, promazine, promethazine, protriptyline, thioridazine, triflupromazine, trimeprazine, trimipramine: Possibly additive anticholinergic effects
CNS depressants: Increased CNS depression
haloperidol: Increased schizophrenic symptoms, possibly tardive dyskinesia
propoxyphene: Increased risk of anxiety, confusion, and tremor
ACTIVITIES
alcohol use: Increased CNS depression

Adverse Reactions
CNS: Agitation, confusion, dizziness, drowsiness, light-headedness, syncope, tremor
CV: Palpitations, tachycardia
EENT: Blurred vision, dry eyes and mouth, increased contact lens awareness
GI: Abdominal distention, constipation, nausea, vomiting
GU: Urine retention

Nursing Considerations
• Be aware that orphenadrine shouldn't be given to patients with tachycardia or cardiac insufficiency.
• Give I.V. form over 5 minutes with patient in supine position. Have patient stay in this position for 5 to 10 minutes to minimize adverse reactions. Then help him to sitting position.
• Be aware that drug can aggravate myasthenia gravis and cause tachycardia.
• Anticipate that drug's anticholinergic effects may cause blurred vision, dry eyes, and increased contact lens awareness.

PATIENT TEACHING
• Advise patient to avoid hazardous activities until drug's CNS effects are known.
• Explain that dry mouth may occur, and suggest increased fluid intake, ice chips, and sugarless candy or gum.
• Suggest that patient (especially one who wears contact lenses) use artificial tears to avoid discomfort from dry eyes.

oxacillin sodium
Bactocill, Prostaphlin

Class and Category
Chemical class: Penicillin
Therapeutic class: Antibiotic
Pregnancy category: B

Indications and Dosages
➤ *To treat bacteremia, bone and joint infections (such as osteomyelitis and infectious arthritis), CNS infections (such as ventriculitis and meningitis), endocarditis, septicemia, skin and soft-tissue infections, upper and lower respiratory tract infections, and UTI caused by penicillinase-producing strains of* Staphylococcus *or other susceptible organisms*

CAPSULES, ORAL SOLUTION
Adults and children weighing 40 kg (88 lb) or more. 500 to 1,000 mg every 4 to 6 hr. *Maximum:* 6 g daily.
Children weighing less than 40 kg. 50 to 100 mg/kg daily in divided doses every 4 to 6 hr.

➤ *To treat mild to moderate infections caused by penicillinase-producing strains of* Staphylococcus *or other susceptible organisms*

I.V. INFUSION, I.M. INJECTION
Adults and children weighing 40 kg or more. 250 to 500 mg every 4 to 6 hr.
Infants and children weighing less than 40 kg. 50 mg/kg daily in divided doses every 4 to 6 hr.
Neonates over age 7 days weighing more than 2,000 g. 25 to 50 mg/kg every 6 hr.
Neonates over age 7 days weighing less than 2,000 g. 25 to 50 mg/kg every 8 hr.

Neonates age 7 days and under weighing more than 2,000 g. 25 to 50 mg/kg every 8 hr.
Neonates age 7 days and under weighing 2,000 g or less. 25 to 50 mg/kg every 12 hr.

➤ *To treat severe infections caused by penicillinase-producing strains of* Staphylococcus *or other susceptible organisms*
I.V. INFUSION, I.M. INJECTION
Adults and children weighing 40 kg or more. 1,000 mg every 4 to 6 hr.
Infants and children weighing less than 40 kg. 100 to 200 mg/kg daily in divided doses every 4 to 6 hr.
Neonates over age 7 days weighing more than 2,000 g. 25 to 50 mg/kg every 6 hr.
Neonates over age 7 days weighing less than 2,000 g. 25 to 50 mg/kg every 8 hr.
Neonates age 7 days and under weighing more than 2,000 g. 25 to 50 mg/kg every 8 hr.
Neonates age 7 days and under weighing 2,000 g or less. 25 to 50 mg/kg every 12 hr.

➤ *To treat endocarditis caused by methicillin-susceptible* Staphylococcus aureus *in patients without a prosthetic valve*
I.V. INFUSION
Adults. 2 g every 4 hr for 4 to 6 wk.
➤ *To treat endocarditis caused by methicillin-susceptible* S. aureus *in patients with a prosthetic valve*
I.V. INFUSION
Adults. 2 g every 4 hr for at least 6 wk.

Mechanism of Action
Inhibits bacterial cell wall synthesis. In susceptible bacteria, the rigid, cross-linked cell wall is assembled in several steps. Oxacillin affects final stage of cross-linking process by binding with and inactivating penicillin-binding proteins (enzymes responsible for linking the cell wall strands). This action causes bacterial cell lysis and death.

Incompatibilities
Don't give oxacillin at same time or in same admixture as aminoglycosides because they are chemically and physically incompatible and will inactivate each other.

Contraindications
Hypersensitivity to oxacillin, penicillins, or their components

Interaction

DRUGS

aminoglycosides: Inactivation of both drugs
chloramphenicol, erythromycins,
sulfonamides, tetracyclines: Decreased
therapeutic effects of oxacillin
oral contraceptives: Decreased contraceptive
efficacy
probenecid: Increased blood oxacillin level

FOODS

all foods: Altered absorption of oxacillin

Adverse Reactions

CNS: Anxiety, depression, fatigue,
hallucinations, headache, seizures
EENT: Oral candidiasis
GI: Diarrhea, nausea, pseudomembranous
colitis, vomiting
GU: Interstitial nephritis, vaginal candidiasis
HEME: Agranulocytosis, anemia,
granulocytopenia, neutropenia
SKIN: Exfoliative dermatitis, pruritus, rash,
urticaria
Other: Anaphylaxis

Nursing Considerations

• Administer oxacillin at least 1 hour before
other antibiotics.
• Give oral forms on an empty stomach,
preferably 1 hour before or 2 hours
after ameal, to prevent impaired absorption.
• Before reconstitution, tap bottle several
times to loosen powder. For I.M. injection,
reconstitute with sterile water for
injection, half-normal (0.45) saline
solution, or normal saline solution. Shake
until solution is clear.
• For I.V. infusion, reconstitute only with
normal saline solution or D_5W.
• When giving drug to patient at risk for
hypertension or fluid overload, be aware
that each gram of oxacillin contains
4.02 mEq of sodium.
• Monitor patient closely for diarrhea, which
may indicate pseudomembranous colitis
caused by *Clostridium difficile.* If diarrhea
occurs, notify prescriber and expect to
withhold oxacillin and treat with fluids,
electrolytes, protein, and an antibiotic
effective against *C. difficile.*

PATIENT TEACHING

• Advise patient to take oxacillin on an
empty stomach.
• Instruct patient to notify prescriber
immediately should a rash develop.

• Advise female patient who uses an oral
contraceptive to use an additional
contraceptive method during oxacillin
therapy.
• Urge patient to tell prescriber about
diarrhea that's severe or lasts longer than
3 days. Remind patient that watery or
bloody stools can occur 2 or more months
after antibiotic therapy and can be serious,
requiring prompt treatment.

oxandrolone
Oxandrin

Class, Category, and Schedule

Chemical class: Testosterone derivative
Therapeutic class: Appetite stimulant
Pregnancy category: X
Controlled substance schedule: III

Indications and Dosages

➤ *To promote weight gain after chronic
infection, extensive surgery, failure to
maintain weight despite no evidence of
pathology, or severe trauma; to offset
protein catabolism from prolonged use
of corticosteroids*

TABLETS

Adults. 2.5 to 20 mg in divided doses given
twice daily to four times a day for 2 to 4 wk;
intermittent therapy repeated as prescribed.
Maximum: 20 mg daily.
Children. 0.1 mg/kg daily; intermittent
therapy repeated as prescribed.
DOSAGE ADJUSTMENT Dosage shouldn't
exceed 5 mg twice daily for elderly patients.

Mechanism of Action

Promotes tissue-building processes and
reverses catabolic or tissue-depleting
processes by promoting protein
anabolism.

Contraindications

Breast cancer (males); breast cancer with
hypercalcemia (females); hypersensitivity to
oxandrolone, anabolic steroids, or their
components; nephrosis; pregnancy; prostate
cancer

Interaction

DRUGS

corticosteroids: Increased risk of edema and
severe acne

hepatotoxic drugs: Increased risk of hepato-toxicity
insulin, oral antidiabetic drugs: Possibly hypoglycemia
NSAIDs, oral anticoagulants, salicylates: Increased anticoagulant effects
sodium-containing drugs: Increased risk of edema
somatrem, somatropin: Possibly accelerated epiphyseal closure
warfarin: Increased warfarin half-life and risk of bleeding
FOODS
high-sodium foods: Increased risk of edema

Adverse Reactions

CNS: Depression, excitement, insomnia
CV: Decreased serum HDL level, edema, hyperlipidemia, hypertension
ENDO: Feminization in postpubertal males (epididymitis, gynecomastia, impotence, oligospermia, priapism, testicular atrophy); glucose intolerance; virilism in females (acne, clitoral enlargement, decreased breast size, deepened voice, diaphoresis, emotional lability, flushing, hirsutism, hoarseness, libido changes, male-pattern baldness, menstrual irregularities, nervousness, oily skin or hair, vaginal bleeding, vaginitis, weight gain), virilism in prepubertal males (acne, decreased ejaculatory volume, penis enlargement, prepubertal closure of epiphyseal plates, unnatural growth of body and facial hair)
GI: Diarrhea, elevated liver function test results, hepatocellular carcinoma, nausea, vomiting
GU: Benign prostatic hyperplasia, prostate cancer, urinary frequency, urine retention (elderly men)
HEME: Iron deficiency anemia, leukemia, prolonged bleeding time
SKIN: Jaundice
Other: Fluid retention, hypercalcemia (females), physical and psychological dependence, sodium retention

Nursing Considerations

• Use oxandrolone cautiously in patients with heart disease because drug has hypercholesterolemic effects.
• Provide adequate calories and protein, as ordered, to maintain a positive nitrogen balance during oxandrolone therapy.

• Anticipate an increased risk of fluid and sodium retention in patients with cardiac, hepatic, or renal dysfunction.
• Weigh patient daily to detect fluid retention. If patient has fluid retention, expect a sodium-restricted diet or diuretics.
WARNING Be aware that oxandrolone may suppress spermatogenesis in males and cause permanent virilization in females.
• Monitor blood glucose level frequently in patient with diabetes mellitus.
• If patient takes an oral anticoagulant, check INR or PT as ordered.
PATIENT TEACHING
• Advise patient to consume a diet high in protein and calories to achieve maximum therapeutic effect of oxandrolone.
• Urge patient to weigh himself daily during therapy and to report swelling or unexplained weight gain at once.
• Explain that drug may alter libido.
• Inform woman that drug may cause permanent physical changes, such as clitoral enlargement, deepened voice, and hair growth.
• Advise female patient of childbearing age that she must use contraception during oxandrolone therapy and should notify prescriber immediately about suspected or known pregnancy.
• Instruct diabetic patient to monitor blood glucose level frequently.
• If patient takes warfarin, advise bleeding precautions (such as an electric shaver and soft toothbrush). Tell patient to notify prescriber immediately if bleeding occurs.

oxaprozin
Daypro

Class and Category

Chemical class: Proprionic acid derivative
Therapeutic class: Anti-inflammatory, antirheumatic
Pregnancy category: C (first trimester), Not rated (later trimesters)

Indications and Dosages

➤ *To treat rheumatoid arthritis*
TABLETS
Adults. 1,200 mg daily. Dosage adjusted based on response. *Maximum:* 1,800 mg

daily or 26 mg/kg daily (whichever is less) in divided doses twice daily or three times a day.

➤ *To treat osteoarthritis*

TABLETS

Adults. 600 to 1,200 mg daily. *Maximum:* 1,800 mg daily or 26 mg/kg (whichever is less) in divided doses twice daily or three times a day.

DOSAGE ADJUSTMENT Initial loading dose of 1,200 to 1,800 mg possibly given to speed onset of action. Initial dose limited to 600 mg daily for patients with renal impairment.

Route	Onset	Peak	Duration
P.O.	In 7 days	Unknown	Unknown

Mechanism of Action

Blocks cyclooxygenase, the enzyme needed to synthesize prostaglandins, which mediate the inflammatory response and cause local vasodilation, swelling, and pain. By blocking cyclooxygenase and prosta-glandins, the NSAID oxaprozin relieves pain.

Contraindications

Angioedema, asthma, bronchospasm, nasal polyps, rhinitis, or urticaria induced by aspirin, iodides, or other NSAIDs

Interaction

DRUGS

ACE inhibitors, antihypertensives: Decreased antihypertensive response, possibly impaired renal function

acetaminophen: Increased risk of adverse renal effects with long-term use of both drugs

anticoagulants, thrombolytics: Prolonged PT, increased risk of bleeding

beta blockers: Decreased antihypertensive effect

bone marrow depressants: Increased risk of leukopenia and thrombocytopenia

cefamandole, cefoperazone, cefotetan, plicamycin, valproic acid: Increased risk of hypoprothrombinemia and bleeding

cimetidine: Decreased oxaprozin clearance

corticosteroids, potassium supplements: Increased risk of adverse GI effects

digoxin: Increased blood digoxin level and risk of digitalis toxicity

diuretics: Possibly decreased diuretic effect

insulin, oral antidiabetic drugs: Increased effects of these drugs; risk of hypoglycemia

lithium: Increased blood lithium level

methotrexate: Increased blood methotrexate level and risk of methotrexate toxicity

other NSAIDs, salicylates: Increased GI irritability and bleeding

probenecid: Increased risk of oxaprozin toxicity

ACTIVITIES

alcohol use, smoking: Increased risk of adverse GI effects

Adverse Reactions

CNS: Aseptic meningitis, cerebral hemorrhage, confusion, dizziness, drowsiness, fatigue, headache, insomnia, ischemic stroke, nervousness, sedation, transient ischemic attacks, vertigo, weakness

CV: Deep vein thrombosis, hypertension, hypotension, MI, peripheral edema

EENT: Tinnitus

ENDO: Hypoglycemia

GI: Abdominal pain, constipation, diarrhea, dyspepsia, elevated liver function test results, GI bleeding or ulceration, hepatitis, jaundice, liver failure, nausea, perforation of stomach or intestine, vomiting

GU: Acute renal failure, dysuria, interstitial nephritis, urinary frequency

HEME: Agranulocytosis, anemia, aplastic anemia, leukopenia, pancytopenia, thrombocytopenia

SKIN: Alopecia, erythema multiforme, exfoliative dermatitis, maculopapular rash, photosensitivity, Stevens-Johnson syndrome, toxic epidermal necrolysis

Other: Anaphylaxis, angioedema

Nursing Considerations

• Use oxaprozin with extreme caution in patients with a history of ulcer disease or GI bleeding because NSAIDs, such as oxaprozin, increase risk of GI bleeding and ulceration. Expect to use oxaprozin for the shortest time possible in these patients.

• Be aware that serious GI tract ulceration, bleeding, and perforation may occur without warning symptoms. Elderly patients are at greater risk. To minimize risk, give drug with food. If GI distress occurs, withhold drug and notify prescriber at once.

• Use oxaprozin cautiously in patients with hypertension, and monitor blood pressure closely throughout therapy. Drug may cause hypertension or worsen it.

WARNING Monitor patient closely for thrombotic events, including MI and stroke, because NSAIDs increase the risk.

WARNING If patient has bone marrow suppression or is receiving antineoplastic drug therapy, monitor laboratory results (including WBC count), and watch for evidence of infection because anti-inflammatory and antipyretic actions of oxaprozin may mask signs and symptoms, such as fever and pain.

• Especially if patient is elderly or taking oxaprozin long-term, watch for less common but serious adverse GI reactions, including anorexia, constipation, diverticulitis, dysphagia, esophagitis, gastritis, gastroenteritis, gastroesophageal reflux disease, hemorrhoids, hiatal hernia, melena, stomatitis, and vomiting.

• Monitor liver function test results because, in rare cases, elevated levels may progress to severe hepatic reactions, including fatal hepatitis, liver necrosis, and hepatic failure.

• Monitor BUN and serum creatinine levels in patients with heart failure, impaired renal function, or hepatic dysfunction; those taking diuretics or ACE inhibitors; and elderly patients because drug may cause renal failure.

• Monitor CBC for decreased hemoglobin level and hematocrit because drug may worsen anemia.

• Assess patient's skin routinely for rash or other signs of hypersensitivity reaction because oxaprozin and other NSAIDs may cause serious skin reactions without warning, even in patients with no history of NSAID hypersensitivity. Stop drug at first sign of reaction, and notify prescriber.

PATIENT TEACHING

• Instruct patient to take oxaprozin exactly as prescribed.

• Advise patient to take drug with a full glass of water and to stay upright for 15 to 30 minutes afterward to keep drug from lodging in esophagus and causing irritation.

• Urge patient to avoid alcohol as well as aspirin and other NSAIDs during oxaprozin therapy to avoid bleeding complications.

• Advise patient to avoid excessive sun exposure to reduce the risk of photosensitivity.

• Caution patient to avoid hazardous activities until drug's CNS effects are known.

• Inform patient that risk of bleeding may continue up to 2 weeks after stopping drug.

• Explain that oxaprozin may increase the risk of serious adverse cardiovascular reactions; urge patient to seek immediate medical attention if signs or symptoms arise, such as chest pain, shortness of breath, weakness, and slurring of speech.

• Inform patient that oxaprozin also may increase the risk of serious adverse GI reactions; stress need to seek immediate medical attention for such signs and symptoms as epigastric or abdominal pain, indigestion, black or tarry stools, or vomiting blood or material that looks like coffee grounds.

• Alert patient to rare but serious skin reactions. Urge him to seek immediate medical attention for rash, blisters, itching, fever, or other indications of hypersensitivity.

oxazepam

Apo-Oxazepam (CAN), Novoxapam (CAN), Serax

Class, Category, and Schedule

Chemical class: Benzodiazepine
Therapeutic class: Antianxiety, sedative hypnotic
Pregnancy category: Not rated
Controlled substance schedule: IV

Indications and Dosages

➤ *To treat anxiety*

CAPSULES, TABLETS

Adults. 10 to 15 mg three times a day or four times a day for mild to moderate anxiety; up to 30 mg three times a day or four times a day for severe anxiety.

➤ *To help manage acute alcohol withdrawal symptoms*

CAPSULES, TABLETS
Adults. 15 to 30 mg three times a day or four times a day.
DOSAGE ADJUSTMENT For elderly or debilitated patients, initial dose of 10 mg three times a day increased cautiously to 15 mg three times a day or four times a day.

Mechanism of Action
May potentiate the effects of gamma-aminobutyric acid (GABA) and other inhibitory neurotransmitters by binding to specific benzodiazepine receptors in limbic and cortical areas of the CNS. GABA inhibits excitatory stimulation, which helps control emotional behavior. The limbic system contains highly dense areas of benzodiazepine receptors, which may explain oxazepam's antianxiety effects.

Contraindications
Acute angle-closure glaucoma; concurrent use of itraconazole or ketoconazole; hypersensitivity to oxazepam, benzo-diazepines, or their components; psychoses

Interaction
DRUGS
cimetidine, oral contraceptives: Impaired metabolism and elimination of oxazepam
clozapine: Increased risk of respiratory depression and arrest
CNS depressants: Increased risk of apnea and CNS depression
levodopa: Decreased therapeutic effects of levodopa
probenecid: Increased therapeutic effects of oxazepam and risk of oversedation
ACTIVITIES
alcohol use: Increased risk of apnea and CNS depression

Adverse Reactions
CNS: Anxiety (in daytime), ataxia, confusion, depression, dizziness, drowsiness, fatigue, headache, insomnia, nightmares, sleep disturbance, slurred speech, syncope, talkativeness, tremor, vertigo
GI: Nausea
Other: Drug tolerance, physical and psychological dependence, withdrawal symptoms

Nursing Considerations
WARNING Oxazepam may cause physical and psychological dependence.
• Be aware that drug shouldn't be stopped abruptly after prolonged use; doing so may cause seizures or withdrawal symptoms, such as insomnia, irritability, and nervousness.
• Be aware that withdrawal symptoms can occur when therapy lasts only 1 or 2 weeks.
WARNING Monitor respiratory status in patients with pulmonary disease (such as severe COPD), respiratory depression, or sleep apnea; drug may worsen ventilatory failure.
• Expect an increased risk of falls among elderly patients from impaired cognition and motor function. Take safety precautions.
• Be aware that drug may worsen acute intermittent porphyria, myasthenia gravis, and severe renal impairment.
• Expect patient with late-stage Parkinson's disease to experience decreased cognition or coordination and, possibly, increased psychosis.
PATIENT TEACHING
• Instruct patient to take oxazepam exactly as prescribed and not to stop taking it without consulting prescriber.
• Caution patient about possible drowsiness and reduced coordination.
• Urge patient to avoid alcohol, which increases oxazepam's sedative effects.

oxcarbazepine
Trileptal

Class and Category
Chemical class: Tricyclic iminostilbene derivative
Therapeutic class: Anticonvulsant
Pregnancy category: C

Indications and Dosages
➤ *As adjunct to treat partial seizures*
ORAL SUSPENSION, TABLETS
Adults and adolescents over age 16. *Initial:* 300 mg twice daily. Dosage increased by 600 mg/ day every wk. *Usual:* 1,200 mg daily. *Maximum:* 2,400 mg daily.

Children ages 4 to 16. *Initial:* 4 to 5 mg/kg twice daily to maximum initial dose of 600 mg daily. *Usual:* 900 mg daily for children weighing 20 to 29 kg (44 to 64 lb); 1,200 mg daily for those weighing 29.1 to 39 kg (65 to 86 lb); 1,800 mg daily for those weighing more than 39 kg. *Maximum:* 1,800 mg daily.
DOSAGE ADJUSTMENT For patients with creatinine clearance less than 30 ml/min/1.73 m², usual initial dosage reduced by 50%.
➤ *As monotherapy to treat partial seizures*
ORAL SUSPENSION, TABLETS
Adults and adolescents over age 16.
Initial: 300 mg twice daily Dosage increased by 300 mg/ day every 3 days, as needed. *Usual:* 1,200 mg daily. *Maximum:* 2,400 mg daily.
Children ages 4 to 16. *Initial:* 4 to 5 mg/kg twice daily, increased by 5 mg/kg daily every third day to maximum maintenance dosage, as needed. *Maximum:* 900 mg daily for children weighing 20 to 24.9 kg (44 to 55 lb); 1,200 mg daily for those weighing 25 to 34.9 kg (55 to 77 lb); 1,500 mg daily for those weighing 35 to 49.9 kg (77 to 110 lb); 1,800 mg daily for those weighing 50 to 59.9 kg (110 to 132 lb); 2,100 mg daily for those weighing 60 to 70 kg (132 to 154 lb).
➤ *To convert to monotherapy in treating partial seizures*
ORAL SUSPENSION, TABLETS
Adults and adolescents over age 16.
Initial: 300 mg twice daily. Dosage increased by 600 mg daily every wk over 2 to 4 wk, as needed, while dosage of other anticonvulsant is reduced. *Usual:* 1,200 mg daily. *Maximum:* 2,400 mg daily.
Children ages 4 to 16. *Initial:* 4 to 5 mg/kg twice daily, increased by 10 mg/kg daily weekly as needed to maximum maintenance dosage while dosage of other anticonvulsant is reduced over 3 to 6 wk. *Maximum:* 900 mg daily for children weighing 20 to 24.9 kg (44 to 55 lb); 1,200 mg daily for those weighing 25 to 34.9 kg (55 to 77 lb); 1,500 mg daily for those weighing 35 to 49.9 kg (77 to 110 lb); 1,800 mg daily for those weighing 50 to 59.9 kg (110 to 132 lb); 2,100 mg daily for those weighing 60 to 70 kg (132 to 154 lb).

Mechanism of Action
May prevent or halt seizures by closing or blocking sodium channels in neuronal cell membrane. By preventing sodium from entering the cell, oxcarbazepine may slow nerve impulse transmission, thus decreasing the rate at which neurons fire.

Contraindications
Hypersensitivity to carbamazepine, oxcarbazepine, or their components

Interaction
DRUGS
carbamazepine, phenobarbital, phenytoin, valproic acid: Decreased blood oxcarbazepine level, possibly increased blood levels of phenobarbital and phenytoin
cyclosporine, dihydropyridine calcium antagonists, oral contraceptives: Decreased effectiveness of these drugs
felodipine, verapamil: Decreased blood levels of these drugs
ACTIVITIES
alcohol use: Possibly additive CNS depressant effects

Adverse Reactions
CNS: Abnormal gait, ataxia, dizziness, fatigue, fever, headache, somnolence, suicidal ideation, tremor
EENT: Abnormal vision, diplopia, nystagmus, rhinitis
ENDO: Hypothyroidism
GI: Abdominal pain, elevated liver enzymes, indigestion, nausea, pancreatitis, vomiting
HEME: Agranulocytosis, aplastic anemia, leukopenia, pancytopenia
SKIN: Erythema multiforme, rash, Stevens-Johnson syndrome, toxic epidermal necrolysis
Other: Anaphylaxis, drug reaction with eosinophilia and systemic symptoms (DRESS), hyponatremia, multi-organ hypersensitivity

Nursing Considerations
• Know that patient with allergic reaction to carbamazepine may have hypersensitivity to oxcarbazepine.
• Monitor serum sodium level for signs of hyponatremia, especially during first 3 months.
• Monitor therapeutic oxcarbazepine levels during initiation and titration, and expect to adjust dosage accordingly.
• Implement seizure precautions as needed, especially in patients who are pregnant,

because physiological changes during pregnancy may cause oxcarbazepine levels to decrease gradually throughout pregnancy, increasing the risk of seizures. Patient should also be monitored closely throughout the postpartum period for adverse reactions, as the level of oxcarbazepine may return to normal after delivery.

• Monitor patient's skin closely. If a reaction develops, notify prescriber at once because skin reactions caused by oxcarbazepine may be serious or life-threatening. Be aware that patients carrying the HLA-B*1502 allele may be at increased risk for Stevens-Johnson syndrome or toxic epidermal necrolysis.

WARNING Watch closely for evidence of multi-organ hypersensitivity, such as fever, rash, organ dysfunction, lymphadeno-pathy, hepatitis, liver function abnormalities, hematologic abnormalities, pruritus, nephritis, oliguria, hepatorenal syndrome, arthralgia, and asthenia. If suspected, notify prescriber and expect to stop drug. Provide supportive care, as prescribed.

• Monitor patient closely for evidence of suicidal thinking or behavior, especially when therapy starts or dosage changes.

PATIENT TEACHING

• Teach patient to shake suspension well and prepare dose immediately afterward. Tell him to then withdraw prescribed amount using supplied oral dosing syringe. Instruct him to mix dose in a small glass of water just before taking it, or tell him that he can swallow drug directly from syringe. Instruct him to close bottle and rinse syringe with warm water and let it dry thoroughly.

• Inform patient that he may experience dizziness, double vision, and unsteady gait.

• Instruct patient not to drink alcohol during oxcarbazepine therapy.

• Alert patient to possibility of hyper-sensitivity or serious skin reactions and importance of reporting them to prescriber.

• Warn patient to notify prescriber immediately if he develops a fever; rash; swelling of face, eyes, lips, tongue; difficulty swallowing or breathing; or other evidence of hypersensitivity because

drug may need to be stopped and emergency medical care given.

• Alert woman of childbearing age that oxcarbazepine may render hormonal contraceptives ineffective. Urge patient to use an additional or a different contraceptive during oxcarbazepine therapy.

• Urge caregivers to watch patient closely for evidence of suicidal tendencies, especially when therapy starts or dosage changes, and to report concerns to prescriber at once.

• Urge female patient who becomes pregnant while taking oxcarbazepine to enroll in the North American antiepileptic drug pregnancy registry by calling 1-888-233-2334. Explain that the registry is collecting information about the safety of antiepileptic drugs during pregnancy.

oxtriphylline

Apo-Oxtriphylline (CAN), Choledyl, Choledyl SA

Class and Category

Chemical class: Xanthine derivative
Therapeutic class: Bronchodilator
Pregnancy category: C

Indications and Dosages

➤ *To treat acute asthma, bronchospasm due to chronic bronchitis or COPD*

DELAYED-RELEASE TABLETS

Adults and children age 6 and over. 300 mg daily for 3 days; then increased to 400 mg daily for 3 days. *Maintenance:* 600 mg daily in divided doses every 6 to 8 hr.

E.R. TABLETS

Adults and children age 6 and over. 300 mg daily for 3 days; then increased to 400 mg daily for 3 days. *Maintenance:* 600 mg daily in divided doses every 12 hr.

Mechanism of Action

Inhibits phosphodiesterase enzymes, causing bronchodilation. Normally, these enzymes inactivate cAMP and cGMP, which are responsible for bronchial smooth-muscle relaxation. Other mechanisms of action may include calcium translocation, prostaglandin antagonism, catecholamine stimulation, inhibition of cGMP metabolism, and adenosine receptor antagonism.

Contraindications

Hypersensitivity to oxtriphylline, xanthines, or their components; peptic ulcer; seizure disorder unless controlled by an anti-convulsant

Interaction

DRUGS

activated charcoal, aminoglutethimide, barbiturates, ketoconazole, rifampin, sulfinpyrazone, sympathomimetics: Decreased blood theophylline level
allopurinol, beta blockers (nonselective), calcium channel blockers, cimetidine, corticosteroids, disulfiram, ephedrine, influenza virus vaccine, interferon, macrolides, mexiletine, oral contraceptives, quinolones, thiabendazole: Increased blood theophylline level
benzodiazepines, propofol: Possibly antagonized sedative effects of these drugs
carbamazepine, isoniazid, loop diuretics: Possibly altered blood theophylline level
halothane anesthetics: Increased risk of cardiotoxicity
hydantoins: Possibly decreased blood hydantoin level
ketamine: Increased risk of seizures
lithium: Decreased blood lithium level
neuromuscular blockers: Possibly reversal of neuromuscular blockade
tetracyclines: Possibly increased adverse effects of theophylline

FOODS

all foods: Altered bioavailability and absorption of E.R. oxtriphylline
charcoal broiled beef; low-carbohydrate, high-protein diet: Increased theophylline elimination
high-carbohydrate, low-protein diet: Decreased elimination and prolonged half-life of theophylline

ACTIVITIES

alcohol use: Increased CNS effects, especially with elixir
smoking (1 or more packs daily): Decreased effects of oxtriphylline

Adverse Reactions

CNS: Anxiety, dizziness, headache, insomnia, restlessness, seizures
CV: Hypotension, palpitations, sinus tachycardia

EENT: Unpleasant taste
GI: Anorexia, diarrhea, nausea, vomiting
RESP: Tachypnea
SKIN: Alopecia, flushing, rash

Nursing Considerations

• Be aware that oxtriphylline contains 64% anhydrous theophylline, so dosage is based on equivalent of 5 to 6 mg of anhydrous theophylline/kg.
• Be aware that food delays absorption of delayed-release and E.R. forms and that large volumes of fluid may increase absorption.
• Know that delayed-release and E.R. preparations vary in their absorption rate.
• Monitor blood theophylline level because toxicity may develop at a level only slightly above therapeutic.

PATIENT TEACHING

• If patient complains of GI discomfort, suggest taking drug with or just after meals.
• Urge patient to stop smoking and to notify prescriber about changes in smoking habits. Also instruct him to avoid alcohol during oxtriphylline therapy.
• Encourage patient to keep follow-up appointments for laboratory studies.

oxybutynin chloride

Ditropan, Ditropan XL, Gelnique 10%, Oxytrol

Class and Category

Chemical class: Tertiary amine
Therapeutic class: Antispasmodic
Pregnancy category: B

Indications and Dosages

➤ *To treat overactive bladder, including neurogenic bladder, with urinary frequency, urgency, or incontinence from involuntary contraction of detrusor muscle*

E.R. TABLETS (DITROPAN XL)

Adults. *Initial:* 5 mg daily, adjusted by 5 mg/ wk, as prescribed. *Maximum:* 30 mg daily.

SYRUP, TABLETS (DITROPAN)

Adults. 5 mg twice daily or three times a day. *Maximum:* 5 mg four times a day or 20 mg daily.

Children age 5 and over. 5 mg twice daily. *Maximum*: 15 mg three times a day.

TRANSDERMAL SYSTEM (OXYTROL)

Adults. System supplying 3.9 mg daily, applied twice weekly.

TOPICAL GEL (GELNIQUE)

Adults. 1 sachet (containing 100 mg/g oxybutynin chloride gel) applied once daily to dry, intact skin on the abdomen, upper arms, shoulders, or thighs.

DOSAGE ADJUSTMENT For elderly patients, possibly 2.5 mg twice daily initially, increased to maximum of 5 mg three timesa day, as prescribed.

Route	Onset	Peak	Duration
P.O.	30–60 min	3–6 hr	6–10 hr
Transdermal	Unknown	24–48 hr	96 hr

Mechanism of Action

Exerts antimuscarinic (atropine-like) and potent direct antispasmodic (papaverine-like) actions on smooth muscle in the bladder and decreases detrusor muscle contractions. The result is increased bladder capacity and a decreased urge to void.

Contraindications

Acute hemorrhage, angle-closure glaucoma, gastric retention (gel form), GI obstruction, hypersensitivity to oxybutynin or its components, ileus, intestinal atony in elderly or debilitated patients, myasthenia gravis, obstructive uropathy, toxic megacolon with ulcerative colitis, urine retention (gel form)

Interaction

DRUGS

amantadine, amitriptyline, amoxapine, antimuscarinics, brompheniramine, bupropion, carbinoxamine, chlorpheniramine, chlorpromazine, clemastine, clomipramine, clozapine, cyclobenzaprine, dimenhydrinate, diphenhydramine, disopyramide, doxepin, doxylamine, imipramine, maprotiline, mesoridazine, methdilazine, nortriptyline, procainamide, promazine, promethazine, protriptyline, thioridazine, triflupromazine, trimeprazine, trimipramine: Increased anticholinergic effects
CNS depressants: Increased sedation
ketoconazole: Possibly altered total absorption rate and blood level of ketoconazole

opioid agonists: Increased depressive effects on GI motility and bladder function
parasympathomimetics: Decreased antimuscarinic action of oxybutynin

ACTIVITIES

alcohol use: Increased sedation

Adverse Reactions

CNS: Agitation, asthenia, confusion, depression, dizziness, drowsiness, fatigue, hallucinations, headache, insomnia, memory impairment, nervousness, psychosis, restlessness, seizures, somnolence, thirst
CV: Arrhythmias, chest discomfort, edema, hypertension, hypotension, palpitations, peripheral edema, QT-interval prolongation, tachycardia, vasodilation
EENT: Blurred vision; cycloplegia; dry eyes, mouth, nose, and throat; glaucoma; keratoconjunctivitis sicca; eye irritation; mydriasis; nasopharyngitis; rhinitis; sinusitis
ENDO: Hot flashes, hyperglycemia, suppression of lactation
GI: Abdominal pain, anorexia, constipation, decreased GI motility, diarrhea, dysphagia, esophagitis, flatulence, gastroesophageal reflux, indigestion, nausea, vomiting
GU: Cystitis, dysuria, impotence, urinary hesitancy, urine retention, UTI
MS: Arthralgia, arthritis, back pain
RESP: Asthma, bronchitis, cough, dysphonia, upper respiratory tract infection
SKIN: Decreased sweating, dry skin, flushing, pruritus, rash, urticaria
Other: Anaphylaxis, angioedema, application-site reactions (anesthesia, dermatitis, erythema, irritation, papules, pruritus), flulike symptoms, fungal infections, heatstroke

Nursing Considerations

• Use oxybutynin cautiously in patients with diarrhea because it may signal incomplete GI obstruction, especially in patients with colostomy or ileostomy. Also use cautiously in patients with dementia because drug may aggravate symptoms.
• Use cautiously in patients with myasthenia gravis or GI disorders because drug may adversely affect these conditions.
• Assess urinary symptoms before and after treatment.

• Make sure patient swallows E.R. tablets whole and doesn't crush, chew, or divide them. Expect to see portions of drug in stool.

• Apply transdermal system to dry, intact skin of abdomen, hip, or buttock; avoid using same site for at least 7 days by rotating sites.

• Apply gel form to dry, intact skin on patient's abdomen, upper arms, shoulders, or thighs. Rotate application sites.

WARNING Monitor patient for angioedema of the face, lips, tongue and/or larynx, even after just the first dose. If present, notify prescriber, stop oxybutynin therapy, as ordered, and provide emergency supportive care.

WARNING Watch for adverse cardiovascular reactions in patients with arrhythmias, coronary artery disease, heart failure, or hypertension because drug's anti-muscarinic effects may increase their risk.

• Decreased GI motility can cause adynamic ileus; assess for abdominal pain and ileus.

• Be aware that drug may aggravate benign prostatic hyperplasia, gastroesophageal reflux disease, and hyperthyroidism.

• Monitor patient for anticholinergic CNS effects, such as hallucinations, agitation, confusion and somnolence, especially in the first few months of therapy or when dosage is increased. If such effects occur, notify prescriber and expect dosage to be reduced or drug discontinued.

PATIENT TEACHING

• Instruct patient to take oxybutynin on an empty stomach. If adverse GI reactions develop, suggest taking drug with food or milk.

• Advise patient to swallow tablets whole and not to chew, crush, or break them.

• Instruct patient how to apply transdermal system or gel. Tell her to apply to clean, dry skin, avoiding areas that have been recently shaved or have open sores or rashes. Remind patient to wash hands after handling product.

• Warn patient that gel is flammable and that she should avoid open fire or smoking until gel has dried. Also tell patient to avoid bathing, swimming, showering, exercising, or immersing application site in water for 1 hour after application and to cover site with clothing once gel has dried.

• Warn of possible decreased alertness, and advise patient against performing hazardous activities until drug's CNS effects are known.

• Caution patient to avoid strenuous exercise and excessive sun exposure because of increased risk of heatstroke.

• Urge patient to avoid alcohol during therapy.

• Instruct patient to seek immediate emergency care if he experiences swelling of his face, lips, tongue, or throat, or if he has difficulty breathing.

oxycodone hydrochloride

Oxecta, OxyContin, Roxicodone

Class, Category, and Schedule

Chemical class: Phenanthrene derivative
Therapeutic class: Analgesic
Pregnancy category: Not rated
Controlled substance schedule: II

Indications and Dosages

➤ *To relieve moderate to severe pain*
ORAL SOLUTION (ROXICODONE)
Adults. 5 mg every 3 to 6 hr, as needed, and increased as needed.
TABLETS (ROXICODONE)
Adults. 5 mg every 3 to 6 hr or 10 mg every 6 to 8 hr, as needed.
TABLETS (OXECTA)
Adults. 5 to 15 mg every 4 to 6 hr, as needed.
➤ *To manage moderate to severe pain when a continuous around-the-clock opioid analgesic is needed for an extended period of time*
CONTROLLED-RELEASE TABLETS, E.R. TABLETS (OXYCONTIN)
Adults who haven't received opioids before. *Initial:* 10 mg every 12 hr, increased every 1 to 2 days, as needed.
Adults converting from other oral oxycodone formulations or other opioids. Highly individualized. *Usual:* Half the 24-hr oxycodone dose every 12 hr.
Adults converting from fentanyl transdermal patch. Highly individualized.

Usual: 10 mg oxycodone for each 25 mcg/hr of fentanyl patch dosage every 12 hr, beginning 18 hr after removing patch.
DOSAGE ADJUSTMENT For patients with hepatic impairment, one-third to one-half the usual starting dose and then adjusted, as needed.

Route	Onset	Peak	Duration
P.O.	10–15 min	1 hr	3–4 hr

Mechanism of Action

Alters perception of and emotional response to pain at spinal cord and higher levels of CNS by blocking release of inhibitory neurotransmitters, such as gamma-aminobutyric acid and acetylcholine.

Contraindications

Acute or severe bronchial asthma or hypercarbia in an unmonitored setting or in the absence of resuscitative equipment, gastrointestinal obstruction, hypersensitivity to oxycodone or its components, paralytic ileus, significant respiratory depression

Interaction

DRUGS
anticholinergics: Possibly severe constipation and ileus
antidiarrheals: Possibly severe constipation and additive CNS depression
antihypertensives: Possibly exaggerated antihypertensive effects and risk of orthostatic hypotension
butorphanol, pentazocine: Possibly acute withdrawal symptoms in opioid-dependent patients, decreased analgesic effects
carbamazepine, phenytoin, primidone, rifampin: Possibly need for increased oxycodone dosage to achieve analgesia and prevent withdrawal symptoms in opioid-dependent patients
cimetidine: Possibly apnea, confusion, disorientation, and seizures from respiratory depression and impaired CNS function
CNS depressants: Possibly increased CNS and respiratory depression and orthostatic hypotension that could result in life-threatening reactions
CYP3A4 inhibitors such as azole-antifungal drugs, macrolide antibiotics, and protease inhibitors: Possibly increased plasma oxycodone levels and prolonged opioid effects

MAO inhibitors: Possibly fatal reactions, including cardiac arrest, coma, respiratory depression, seizures, and severe hypertension
nalbuphine, nalmefene, naloxone, naltrexone: Blocked oxycodone effects, withdrawal symptoms in opioid-dependent patients
ACTIVITIES
alcohol use: Additive CNS and respiratory depressive effects

Adverse Reactions

CNS: Abnormal dreams, anxiety, asthenia, chills, dizziness, drowsiness, euphoria, excitation, headache, insomnia, nervousness, sedation, seizures, somnolence, syncope, twitching
CV: Bradycardia, chest pain, hypotension, orthostatic hypotension, palpitations
EENT: Blurred vision, choking or difficulty swallowing tablets (OxyContin), dry eyes or mouth, lens opacities, miosis
ENDO: Syndrome of inappropriate antidiuretic hormone secretion
GI: Abdominal pain, anorexia, constipation, diarrhea, dyspepsia, dysphagia, elevated liver function test results, gastritis, hiccups, ileus, nausea, vomiting
GU: Amenorrhea, decreased libido, erectile dysfunction, oliguria, urinary hesitancy, urine retention
RESP: Dyspnea, respiratory depression
SKIN: Diaphoresis, pruritus, rash
Other: Anaphylaxis, drug tolerance, hyponatremia, physical and psychological dependence, withdrawal symptoms

Nursing Considerations

• Use extreme caution when administering oxycodone to patients with conditions accompanied by hypoxia or decreased respiratory reserve such as asthma, chronic obstructive pulmonary disease (COPD), or cor pulmonale. This is because even with usual therapeutic dosages, oxycodone may decrease respiratory drive while simultaneously increasing airway resistance to the point of apnea. Monitor patient's respiratory status closely, especially in elderly, cachectic, and debilitated patients and in patients with chronic pulmonary disease. Respiratory depression may occur at any time, but it is most likely to occur during the initiation of therapy or following a dose increase. Have resuscitative equipment nearby.

• Use oxycodone with extreme caution in patients who may be at risk for carbon dioxide retention (e.g., those with increased intracranial pressure or brain tumors). Monitor for signs of sedation and respiratory depression, especially when initiating therapy. Oxycodone may reduce respiratory drive, and the resultant carbon dioxide retention can further increase intracranial pressure. Also know that opioids like oxycodone may obscure signs and symptoms in a patient with a head injury.

• Assess patient's pain level regularly, and give drug as prescribed before pain becomes severe.

• Be careful to have patient swallow one controlled-release tablet (OxyContin) at a time, with enough water to ensure complete swallowing immediately after the patient places the tablet in his mouth; otherwise, choking on tablets or difficulty swallowing the tablets may occur due to the swelling and hydrogelling property of the tablet if left in the mouth too long.

• Be prepared to adjust dosage for patient who hasn't previously received opioids, as prescribed, until he can tolerate drug effects.

• Expect to give controlled-release tablets only to opioid-tolerant patients who need at least 160 mg daily.

WARNING Monitor patient closely for respiratory depression, especially in elderly, cachectic, or debilitated patients; when initiating and titrating dosages; or when other drugs that depress respiration are given together. Report respiratory depression immediately, because respiratory arrest can occur. Be prepared to provide supportive care.

• Monitor patient's blood pressure closely, especially when initiating oxycodone therapy and when titrating the dose, because oxycodone may cause severe hypotension and syncope in ambulatory patients due to its vasodilatory effects. Risk of hypotension is greater in patients who already have been compromised by a reduced blood volume or concurrent administration of certain CNS depressant drugs, such as general anesthetics and phenothiazines.

• Assess patient for possible paradoxical excitation during dosage titration.

• Assess patient for abdominal pain because oxycodone may mask underlying GI disorders.

• Monitor patients with seizure disorders closely because oxycodone may induce or aggravate seizures.

WARNING Be aware that oxycodone has a high potential for abuse.

WARNING Be aware that abuse of crushed controlled-release tablets poses a hazard of overdose and death. If you suspect abuse and determine that patient also is abusing alcohol or illicit substances, notify prescriber immediately because risk of overdose and death is increased. If you suspect parenteral abuse, be aware that tablet excipients, especially talc, may result in local tissue necrosis, infection, pulmonary granulomas, endocarditis, and valvular heart injury.

PATIENT TEACHING

WARNING Strongly warn patient to swallow oxycodone tablets whole and not to break, chew, or crush them because taking broken, chewed, or crushed tablets leads to rapid release and absorption of a potentially fatal dose.

• Instruct patient not to take oxycodone more often than prescribed and not to stop abruptly after long-term use.

• Caution patient prescribed controlled-release tablets to take one tablet at a time; not to presoak, lick, or otherwise wet the tablet prior to placing in his mouth; and to take each tablet with enough water to ensure complete swallowing of tablet.

• Instruct patient to avoid alcohol and hazardous activities during therapy.

• Tell patient to notify prescriber about signs of possible toxicity or hypersensitivity, such as excessive light-headedness, extreme dizziness, itching, swelling, and trouble breathing.

• Warn patient to keep drug out of reach of children because ingestion of the drug by a child can be fatal.

oxymetholone

Anadrol-50, Anapolon-50 (can)

Class, Category, and Schedule

Chemical class: Testosterone derivative

Therapeutic class: Antianemic, antiangioedema (hereditary)
Pregnancy category: X
Controlled substance schedule: III

Indications and Dosages

➤ *To treat acquired and congenital aplastic anemias, anemias caused by deficient RBC production, bone marrow failure anemias, hypoplastic anemias caused by myelotoxic drugs, and myelofibrosis; to prevent or treat hereditary angioedema*

TABLETS
Adults and children. 1 to 2 mg/kg daily for 3 to 6 mo. *Maximum:* 5 mg/kg daily.

Mechanism of Action

Combats anemia by increasing production of erythropoietin, a precursor of RBCs. Oxymetholone also increases hemoglobin level and RBC volume.

Contraindications

Breast or prostate cancer in men, hypercalcemia in women with breast cancer, hypersensitivity to oxymetholone or anabolic steroids, nephrosis, nephrotic phase of nephritis, pregnancy, severe hepatic dysfunction

Interaction

DRUGS
corticosteroids: Increased risk of edema and severe acne
hepatotoxic drugs: Increased risk of hepatotoxicity
insulin, oral antidiabetic drugs: Possibly hypoglycemia
NSAIDs, oral anticoagulants, salicylates: Increased anticoagulant effects
sodium-containing drugs: Increased risk of edema
somatrem, somatropin: Possibly accelerated epiphyseal maturation
FOODS
high-sodium foods: Increased risk of edema

Adverse Reactions

CNS: Depression, excitement, insomnia
CV: Decreased serum HDL level, edema, hyperlipidemia, hypertension
ENDO: Feminization in postpubertal males (epididymitis, gynecomastia, impotence, oligospermia, priapism, testicular atrophy), glucose intolerance, virilism in females (acne, clitoral enlargement, decreased breast size, deepened voice, diaphoresis, emotional lability, flushing, hirsutism, hoarseness, libido changes, male-pattern baldness, menstrual irregularities, nervousness, oily hair or skin, vaginal bleeding, vaginitis, weight gain), virilism in prepubertal males (acne, decreased ejaculatory volume, penis enlargement, prepubertal closure of epiphyseal plates, unnatural growth of body and facial hair)
GI: Diarrhea, elevated liver function test results, hepatocellular carcinoma, nausea, vomiting
GU: Benign prostatic hyperplasia, prostate cancer, urinary frequency, urine retention (elderly men)
HEME: Iron deficiency anemia, leukemia, prolonged bleeding time
SKIN: Jaundice
Other: Fluid retention, hypercalcemia (females), physical and psychological dependence, sodium retention

Nursing Considerations

• Be aware that oxymetholone shouldn't be used in patients with a history of hyper-calcemia because drug may exacerbate this condition or in patients with prostate problems because drug may promote benign or cancerous tumor growth.
• Anticipate increased risk of fluid and sodium retention in patients with cardiac, hepatic, or renal dysfunction. Monitor for signs and symptoms of fluid retention.
• Monitor daily weight. Expect to place patient with fluid retention on sodium-restricted diet or diuretics, as prescribed.
WARNING Be aware that oxymetholone may suppress spermatogenesis in males and cause permanent virilization in females.
PATIENT TEACHING
• Advise patient to consume a diet high in protein and calories to achieve maximum therapeutic effect of oxymetholone.
• Instruct patient to check his weight daily during oxymetholone therapy and to notify prescriber immediately about swelling or unexplained weight gain.
• Inform patient that drug may alter libido.
• Advise diabetic patient to monitor blood glucose levels frequently because drug may increase hypoglycemic effect of antidiabetic drugs.

• Inform female patient that drug may cause permanent physical changes, such as clitoral enlargement, deepened voice, and unnatural hair growth.
• Advise female patient of childbearing age to use contraception during therapy and to notify prescriber immediately about suspected or known pregnancy.

oxymorphone hydrochloride

Numorphan, Opana, Opana ER

Class, Category, and Schedule

Chemical class: Phenanthrene derivative
Therapeutic class: Analgesic
Pregnancy category: Not rated
Controlled substance schedule: II

Indications and Dosages

➤ *To relieve moderate to severe pain*
TABLETS
Adults. *Initial:* 5 to 20 mg every 4 to 6 hr, as needed.
➤ *To relieve moderate to severe pain in patients requiring continuous, around-the-clock opioid treatment for an extended time*
E.R. TABLETS (OPANA ER)
Adults receiving an opioid for first time. *Initial:* 5 mg every 12 hr, increased as needed in 5- to 10-mg increments for each 12-hr dose every 3 to 7 days.
Adults converting from an oral immediate release oxymorphone formulation: *Initial:* Half the patient's total daily oral dose of immediate-release formulation every 12 hours.
Adults converting from parenteral oxymorphone. *Initial:* 10 times the patient's total daily parenteral oxymorphone dose divided by 2 to provide 2 equally divided doses given 12 hr apart daily.
Adults converting from other oral opioids. Highly individualized.
DOSAGE ADJUSTMENT For opioid-naive patients with mild hepatic impairment or who have a creatinine clearance less than 50 ml/min/1.73 m^2 or for opioid-naive patients over the age of 65, initial dosage started at 5 mg. For patients on prior opioid

therapy with creatinine clearance less than 50 ml/min/1.73 m^2 or who are over the age of 65, initial dosage decreased by 50%. For patients receiving other CNS depressants, dosage started at one-third to one-half the usual starting dose.
➤ *To relieve moderate to severe pain, to relieve anxiety in patients with dyspnea from pulmonary edema caused by acute left ventricular dysfunction*
I.V. INJECTION
Adults. *Initial:* 0.5 mg, repeated every 3 to 6 hr, as needed.
I.M. OR SUBCUTANEOUS INJECTION
Adults. *Initial:* 1 to 1.5 mg, repeated every 3 to 6 hr, as needed.
SUPPOSITORIES
Adults. 5 mg every 4 to 6 hr, as needed.
➤ *To relieve obstetric pain during labor*
I.M. INJECTION
Adults. 0.5 to 1 mg as a single dose.

Mechanism of Action

Alters perception of and emotional response to pain at spinal cord and higher levels of CNS by blocking release of inhibitory neurotransmitters, such as gamma-aminobutyric acid and acetylcholine.

Contraindications

Acute or severe asthma; hypercarbia; hypersensitivity to oxymorphone, other morphine analogues, or their components; moderate to severe hepatic impairment; paralytic ileus; pulmonary edema from a chemical respiratory irritant; severe respiratory depression; upper airway obstruction

Route	Onset	Peak	Duration
I.V.	5–10 min	15–30 min	3–4 hr
I.M.	10–15 min	30–90 min	3–6 hr
SubQ	10–20 min	30–90 min	3–6 hr
P.R.	15–30 min	2 hr	3–6 hr

Interaction

DRUGS
anticholingerics: Increased risk of urine retention, severe constipation
antidiarrheals, antiperistaltics: Increased risk of severe constipation, CNS depression
antihypertensives, diuretics, hypotension-producing drugs: Increased hypotensive effects

N
O

buprenorphine: Reduced oxymorphone effectiveness if buprenorphine is given first, possibly withdrawal symptoms in oxymorphone-dependent patients
CNS depressants: Additive CNS and respiratory depressant effects, increased risk of habituation
hydroxyzine, other opioid analgesics: Increased analgesia, CNS depression, and hypotensive effects
MAO inhibitors: Increased risk of unpredictable, severe, sometimes fatal adverse reactions
metoclopramide: Antagonized effects of metoclopramide on GI motility
naloxone: Antagonized analgesic, CNS, and respiratory depressant effects of oxymorphone
naltrexone: Withdrawal symptoms in oxymorphone-dependent patients
neuromuscular blockers: Additive respiratory depression
ACTIVITIES
alcohol use: Additive CNS and respiratory depressant effects, increased risk of habituation

Adverse Reactions

CNS: Agitation, asthenia, CNS depression, confusion, delusions, depersonalization, dizziness, drowsiness, euphoria, fatigue, hallucinations, headache, insomnia, light-headedness, nervousness, nightmares, restlessness, seizures, somnolence, tiredness, tremor, weakness
CV: Bradycardia, hypertension, hypotension, palpitations, tachycardia
EENT: Blurred vision, diplopia, dry mouth, laryngeal edema, laryngospasm, miosis, tinnitus
GI: Abdominal cramps or pain, anorexia, bilary colic, constipation, elevated serum amylase level, hepatotoxicity, ileus, nausea, spasm of the sphincter of Oddi (E.R. tablets), vomiting
GU: Decreased urine output, dysuria, urinary frequency and hesitancy, urine retention
MS: Muscle rigidity (with large doses), uncontrolled muscle movements
RESP: Apnea, atelectasis, bradypnea, bronchospasm, dyspnea, irregular breathing, respiratory depression, wheezing
SKIN: Dermatitis, diaphoresis, erythema, flushing of face, pruritus, urticaria

Other: Angioedema; injection-site burning, pain, redness, and swelling; psychological and physical dependence

Nursing Considerations

• Use extreme caution when administering oxymorphone to patients with conditions accompanied by hypoxia or decreased respiratory reserve, such as asthma, chronic obstructive pulmonary disease (COPD), or cor pulmonale. This is because oxymorphone, even with usual therapeutic dosages, may decrease respiratory drive while simultaneously increasing airway resistance to the point of apnea. Monitor patient's respiratory status closely, especially in elderly, cachectic, and debilitated patients and in patients with chronic pulmonary disease. Respiratory depression may occur at any time, but it is most likely to occur during the initiation of therapy or following a dose increase. Have resuscitative equipment nearby.
• Use oxymorphone with extreme caution in patients who may be at risk for carbon dioxide retention (e.g., those with increased intracranial pressure or brain tumors). Monitor for signs of sedation and respiratory depression, especially when initiating therapy. Oxymorphone may reduce respiratory drive, and the resultant carbon dioxide retention can further increase intracranial pressure. Also know that opioids like oxymorphone may obscure signs and symptoms in a patient with a head injury.
• Use cautiously in patients with mild hepatic impairment because drug is metabolized in liver; impaired renal function because drug is excreted by kidneys; and biliary tract disease because drug may cause spasm of sphincter of Oddi.
• Use cautiously in patients receiving mixed agonist-antagonist opioid analgesics because these drugs may reduce analgesic effect of oxymorphone or may cause withdrawal symptoms.
• Use cautiously in elderly patients because plasma oxymorphone levels in the elderly are higher than in younger patients.
• Oral hydromorphone shouldn't be used "as needed" or for first 24 hours after surgery in patients not already taking opioids

because of the risk of over-sedation and respiratory depression.

• If patient is being converted from one form of drug to another, watch closely for analgesic effectiveness and adverse reactions.

• Taper dosage, as ordered, before stopping therapy to prevent withdrawal in physically dependent patients.

WARNING Monitor patient closely for respiratory depression, especially in elderly, cachectic, or debilitated patients; when initiating or titrating dosages; or when other drugs that depress respiration are given together. Report respiratory depression immediately, because respiratory depression may occur. Be prepared to provide supportive care.

• Monitor patient's blood pressure closely, especially when initiating oxymorphone therapy and when titrating the dose because oxymorphone may cause severe hypotension and syncope in ambulatory patients due to its vasodilatory effects. Risk of hypotension is greatest in patients who already have been compromised by a reduced blood volume or concurrent administration of certain CNS depressant drugs, such as general anesthetics and phenothiazines.

• Monitor patient for signs of excessive opioid-related adverse reactions. If present, notify prescriber and expect next dose to be reduced.

• Monitor urinary and bowel status; constipation may be so severe it causes ileus.

• Offer fluids to relieve dry mouth.

• Be aware that a new formulation of Opana ER has been developed to be crush-resistant to prevent the patient from obtaining a rapid drug release.

PATIENT TEACHING

• Instruct patient to take oxymorphone exactly as prescribed and not to stop abruptly; warn that drug can cause physical dependence.

• Emphasize importance of taking drug before pain becomes severe.

• Instruct patient prescribed oxymorphone in tablet form to take it on an empty stomach.

• Tell patient prescribed extended-release tablet form not to break, chew, dissolve, or crush tablets before taking them because doing so will lead to a rapid drug release and increased risk of a potentially fatal dose. Also, alert patient that sometimes

the inactive ingredients may be eliminated as a soft mass in the stool, which may resemble the original tablet and is harmless. Reassure patient that the active ingredient has already been absorbed.

• Instruct patient to store suppositories in refrigerator.

• Encourage patient to increase fluid and fiber intake during therapy to prevent constipation.

• Emphasize need to avoid alcohol and CNS depressants during therapy because of risk of severe life-threatening adverse reactions.

• Caution patient to avoid potentially hazardous activities until drug's CNS effects are known.

• Advise female patient to stop drug and notify prescriber about known or suspected pregnancy.

• Warn patient to keep drug out of the reach of children, as accidental ingestion may be fatal.

oxytetracycline

Terramycin I.M.

oxytetracycline hydrochloride

Terramycin

Class and Category

Chemical class: Tetracycline derived from *Streptomyces rimosus*
Therapeutic class: Antibiotic, antiprotozoal
Pregnancy category: D

Indications and Dosages

➤ *To treat systemic bacterial and protozoal infections, such as bronchitis, chlamydial infection, Lyme disease, nongonococcal urethritis, rickettsial infection, traveler's diarrhea, and UTI*

CAPSULES (OXYTETRACYCLINE HYDROCHLORIDE)

Adults and adolescents. 250 to 500 mg every 6 hr. *Maximum:* 4,000 mg daily.

Children ages 8 to 12. 6.25 to 12.5 mg/kg every 6 hr.

I.M. INJECTION (OXYTETRACYCLINE)

Adults and adolescents. 100 mg every 8 hr, 150 mg every 12 hr, or 250 mg daily. *Maximum:* 500 mg daily.

Children ages 8 to 12. 5 to 8.3 mg/kg every 8 hr or 7.5 to 12.5 mg/kg every 12 hr. *Maximum:* 250 mg daily.

DOSAGE ADJUSTMENT Dosage possibly reduced for patients with renal impairment.

➤ *To treat brucellosis*

CAPSULES (OXYTETRACYCLINE HYDROCHLORIDE)
Adults and adolescents. 500 mg every 6 hr for 3 wk with 1,000 mg of streptomycin I.M. every 12 hr in wk 1 and daily in wk 2. *Maximum:* 4,000 mg daily.

➤ *To treat uncomplicated gonorrhea*

CAPSULES (OXYTETRACYCLINE HYDROCHLORIDE)
Adults and adolescents. *Initial:* 1,500 mg, then 500 mg every 6 hr to total of 9,000 mg for full course of treatment.

➤ *To treat syphilis*

CAPSULES (OXYTETRACYCLINE HYDROCHLORIDE)
Adults and adolescents. 500 to 1,000 mg every 6 hr for 10 to 15 days to total of 30 to 40 g for full course of treatment.

Mechanism of Action

Binds with ribosomal subunits of susceptible bacteria and alters cytoplasmic membrane, inhibiting bacterial protein synthesis and rendering the organism ineffective.

Contraindications

Hypersensitivity to tetracyclines or their components

Interaction

DRUGS
antacids, calcium supplements, cholestyramine, choline salicylates, colestipol, iron supplements, magnesium salicylates: Possibly decreased absorption of oxytetracycline
digoxin: Increased blood digoxin level
lithium: Altered blood lithium level
methoxyflurane: Increased risk of nephrotoxicity
oral anticoagulants: Increased anticoagulant effects
oral contraceptives: Decreased contraceptive effectiveness, increased risk of break-through bleeding and pregnancy
penicillins: Decreased bactericidal effects of penicillins
sodium bicarbonate: Possibly decreased absorption of oral oxytetracycline
vitamin A: Increased risk of benign intracranial hypertension

FOODS
all foods, especially dairy products: Possibly interference with oxytetracycline absorption

Adverse Reactions

CNS: Dizziness, light-headedness, tiredness, unsteadiness, weakness
EENT: Darkened, discolored, or sore tongue; stomatitis, tooth discoloration (in infants and children under age 8)
GI: Abdominal cramps, diarrhea, indigestion, nausea, thirst, vomiting
GU: Urinary frequency
SKIN: Photosensitivity
Other: Superinfection

Nursing Considerations

WARNING Be aware that oxytetracycline shouldn't be given to premature infants because it may impair skeletal growth or to children under age 8 because it may permanently discolor teeth and cause enamel hypoplasia.

• For an adult, give I.M. injection in upper outer quadrant of buttocks or mid-lateral thigh; deltoid muscle may be used but only if well developed. In children, give injection only in mid-lateral thigh.

• Be aware that patient should be switched from parenteral to oral form as soon as possible.

PATIENT TEACHING

• Instruct patient to take oxytetracycline capsules 1 hour before meals and 3 hours before or after other drugs and dairy products.

• Advise patient to take drug with a full glass of water and in an upright position to minimize adverse GI reactions.

• Urge patient to complete entire course of oxytetracycline therapy, even if he feels better beforehand.

• Caution patient to avoid hazardous activities until drug's CNS effects are known.

• Advise patient to avoid excessive sun exposure and to protect skin when outdoors.

• Urge female patient who uses oral contraceptives to use an additional form of birth control during oxytetracycline therapy.

• Advise patient to discard outdated capsules because drug may become toxic.

P

paliperidone
Invega, Invega Sustenna

Class and Category
Chemical class: Benzisoxazole derivative
Therapeutic class: Antipsychotic (Atypical)
Pregnancy category: C

Indications and Dosages
➤ *To treat schizophrenia; to treat schizoaffective disorder as monotherapy or as an adjunct to mood stabilizers or antidepressants*
E.R. TABLETS (INVEGA)
Adults. *Initial:* 6 mg once daily in the morning; then increased or decreased in increments of 3 mg daily every 6 or more days, as needed. *Maximum:* 12 mg daily.
Adolescents 12 to 17. *Initial:* 3 mg once daily; then increased in increments of 3 mg daily every 6 or more days, as needed.
DOSAGE ADJUSTMENT For patients with mild renal impairment (creatinine clearance 50 to 79 ml/min/1.73 m^2), maximum dosage is 6 mg daily. For patients with moderate to severe renal impairment (creatinine clearance less than 50 ml/min/1.73 m^2), maximum dosage is 3 mg daily.
I.M. INJECTION (INVEGA SUSTENNA)
Adults. *Initial:* 234 mg on day 1 and 156 mg 1 wk later. *Maintenance:* 117 mg monthly. Maintenance dosage decreased or increased monthly according to patient's response and tolerance. Maintenance dosage may be decreased to as low as 39 mg monthly for treatment of schizophrenia or 78 mg for treatment of schizoaffective disorder or increased to a maximum dose of 234 mg monthly.
DOSAGE ADJUSTMENT For patient with mild renal impairment (creatinine clearance equal to or greater than 50 ml/min but less than 80 ml/min, initial dosage decreased to 156 mg on day 1 and second dose given 1 wk later decreased to 117 mg, followed by 78 mg monthly. For patient receiving a strong CYP3A4 inducer such as carbamazepine, rifampin, or St. John's wort, dosage may need to be increased, and when the strong CYP3A4 inducer is discontinued, dosage of paliperidone may need to be decreased.

➤ *To treat schizoaffective disorder*
E.R. TABLETS
Adults. *Initial:* 6 mg once daily; then increased in increments of 3 mg daily every 5 or more days, as needed. *Maximum:* 12 mg daily.
DOSAGE ADJUSTMENT For patients with mild renal impairment (creatinine clearance 50 to 79 ml/min/1.73 m^2), maximum dosage is 6 mg daily. For patients with moderate to severe renal impairment (creatinine clearance less than 50 ml/min/1.73 m^2), maximum dosage is 3 mg daily.

Route	Onset	Peak	Duration
P.O.	Unknown	24 hr	Unknown
I.M.	1 day	13 days	126 days

Mechanism of Action
The main active metabolite of risperidone, paliperidone selectively blocks serotonin and dopamine receptors in mesocortical tract of CNS to suppress psychotic symptoms.

Contraindications
AV block, cardiac arrhythmias, congenital heart disease, history of congenital long-QT syndrome; hypersensitivity to paliperidone, risperidone, or its components

Interaction
DRUGS
antiarrhythmics of class IA (such as quinidine, procainamide) and class III (such as amiodarone, sotalol), antibiotics (such as gatifloxacin, moxifloxacin), antipsychotics (such as chlorpromazine, thioridazine): Increased risk of QT interval prolongation
antihypertensives: Increased antihypertensive effects
bromocriptine, levodopa, pergolide: Possibly antagonized effects of these drugs
CNS depressants: Additive CNS depression
CYP3A4 and P-gp strong inducers (carbamazepine, rifampin, St. John's wort): Decreased plasma paliperidone level and effectiveness
paroxetine: Possible increased blood paliperidone level

P

ACTIVITIES

alcohol use: CNS depression

Adverse Reactions

CNS: Agitation, akathisia, anxiety, asthenia, bradykinesia, cogwheel rigidity, CVA, dizziness, drooling, dyskinesia, dystonia, extrapyramidal disorder, fatigue, fever, headache, hyperkinesia, hypertonia, insomnia, lethargy, neuroleptic malignant syndrome, nuchal rigidity, parkinsonism, psychomotor hyperactivity, restlessness, seizures, somnolence, suicidal ideation, syncope, tardive dyskinesia, transient ischemic attack, tremor, vertigo

CV: Bradycardia, bundle branch block, elevated cholesterol and triglyceride level, first-degree heart block, hypertension, orthostatic hypotension, palpitations, peripheral edema, prolonged QT interval, tachycardia, venous thrombosis

EENT: Blurred vision, dry mouth, eye movement disorder, nasal congestion, nasopharyngitis, oromandibular dystonia, pharyngolaryngeal pain, salivary hypersecretion, swollen tongue

ENDO: Breast pain or tenderness, gynecomastia, hyperglycemia, hyperprolactinemia

GI: Abdominal discomfort, constipation, diarrhea, dyspepsia, flatulence, ileus, nausea, small intestinal obstruction, upper abdominal pain, vomiting

GU: Erectile dysfunction, menstrual abnormalities, priapism, urinary incontinence or retention, UTI

HEME: Agranulocytosis, leukopenia, neutropenia, thrombocytopenia, thrombotic thrombocytopenic purpura

MS: Arthralgia; back or limb pain; dysarthria; joint stiffness; muscle rigidity, spasms, tightness, or twitching; myalgia; torticollis, trismus

RESP: Cough, dyspnea, upper respiratory tract infection

SKIN: Drug eruption, pruritus, rash, urticaria

Other: Anaphylaxis, angioedema, injection-site reactions, weight gain

Nursing Considerations

• Paliperidone shouldn't be used to treat dementia-related psychosis in the elderly because of an increased mortality risk. Parenteral paliperidone is not recommended for patients with moderate to severe renal impairment.

• Drug shouldn't be given if patient has a condition that severely narrows GI tract because tablet doesn't change shape as it passes and could cause blockage.

• Be aware that the long-acting preparation (Invega Sustenna) should be initiated only after patient has been established with oral paliperidone or oral risperidone therapy.

• Administer parenteral paliperidone slowly as a deep intramuscular injection. The first two injections should be administered in the deltoid muscle; thereafter, the injection may be administered in the deltoid or gluteal muscle. Use a 1.5-inch 22G needle for gluteal administration or, if the patient weighs more than 200 pounds, for injecting drug into the deltoid muscle. If patient weighs less than 200 pounds, use a 1-inch 23G needle when administering drug in the deltoid muscle.

• Know that if the due date for the second parenteral dose is missed, the recommended re-initiation depends on the length of time that has elapsed since the patient's first injection. To avoid missing the second dose, the prescriber may order the parenteral dose to be given up to 7 days before or after the due date.

• Be aware that a dosage adjustment may be necessary for the patient receiving the parenteral form of the drug if more than 6 weeks has elapsed since the last injection.

• Be aware that when a patient who has been taking a long-acting injectable antipsychotic consistently is now switching to parenteral paliperidone therapy, the first dose of paliperidone is given in place of the next scheduled injection of the other medication. Parenteral paliperidone therapy is then continued at monthly intervals. The one-week initiation dosing is not required.

WARNING Immediately notify prescriber and expect to stop drug if patient shows signs of neuroleptic malignant syndrome (altered mental status, autonomic instability, hyperpyrexia, muscle rigidity). Patients at risk for developing neuroleptic malignant syndrome are patients with

Parkinson's disease or dementia with Lewy bodies because these patients can experience increased sensitivity to paliperidone.

• Monitor patient for involuntary, dyskinetic movements. Notify prescriber if present, and expect to stop therapy. In some cases, therapy may need to continue despite tardive dyskinesia.

• Monitor blood glucose level because drug increases risk of hyperglycemia and possible ketoacidosis or hyperosmolar coma.

• Dosage adjustments of paliperidone may be needed when carbamazepine therapy is started or discontinued because of carbamazepine's interaction with paliperidone.

• Check CBC often during first few months of therapy, especially if patient has low WBC count or history of drug-induced leukopenia or neutropenia. If WBC count declines, and especially if neutrophil count goes 1,000/mm^3, expect to stop drug. If neutropenia is significant, also watch for evidence of infection and provide appropriate treatment, as prescribed.

• Watch patient closely for suicidal tendencies, especially when therapy starts or dosage changes.

PATIENT TEACHING

• Instruct patient to take tablet whole with liquid. Caution against chewing, splitting, or crushing it because it's designed to release drug at a controlled rate.

• Explain that shell of tablet will be eliminated in stool and that patient need not worry if he sees tablet in stool.

• Urge patient to rise slowly from sitting or lying to minimize orthostatic hypotension.

• Caution patient to avoid hazardous activities until CNS effects of drug are known.

• Advise patient to avoid activities that may cause overheating, such as exercising strenuously, being exposed to extreme heat, or becoming dehydrated.

• Urge family or caregiver to watch patient closely for suicidal tendencies, especially when therapy starts or dosage changes.

• Advise female patient of childbearing age to notify prescriber if she intends to become or suspects that she is pregnant during therapy because neonates exposed to paliperidone during the third trimester of pregnancy are at risk for extrapyramidal and/or withdrawal symptoms following delivery.

• Alert the patient who experiences hyperprolactinemia as a result of paliperidone therapy that reproductive function may become impaired. If this is a concern for the patient, she should consult prescriber.

palonosetron hydrochloride

Aloxi

Class and Category

Chemical class: Selective serotonin subtype 3 (5-HT$_3$) receptor antagonist
Therapeutic class: Antiemetic
Pregnancy category: B

Indications and Dosages

➤ *To prevent acute and delayed nausea and vomiting from chemotherapy*

CAPSULES

Adults. 0.5 mg 1 hr before chemotherapy.

I.V. INJECTION

Adults. 0.25 mg over 30 sec about 30 min before start of chemotherapy.

Infants 1 month of age and older, children, and adolescents ages 12 to 17. 20 mcg/kg over 15 min about 30 min before start of chemotherapy. *Maximum:* 1.5 mg.

➤ *To prevent postoperative nausea and vomiting for up to 24 hr after surgery*

I.V. INJECTION

Adults. 0.75 mg over 10 sec immediately before induction of anesthesia.

Incompatibilities

Palonosetron shouldn't be mixed with any other drug.

Contraindications

Hypersensitivity to palonosetron or its components

Adverse Reactions

CNS: Anxiety, dizziness, drowsiness, fatigue, headache, insomnia, serotonin syndrome, weakness

P

CV: Bradycardia, hypotension, prolonged QT interval, tachycardia
GI: Abdominal pain, constipation, diarrhea
SKIN: Dermatitis, pruritus, rash
Other: Hyperkalemia, hypersensitivity reaction, injection-site reaction (burning, induration, discomfort, pain)

Nursing Considerations

• Use palonosetron cautiously in patients who have or may develop prolonged cardiac conduction intervals—especially QT interval—such as those with congenital QT syndrome, hypokalemia, or hypomagnesemia; those taking a diuretic known to induce electrolyte abnormalities, an antiarrhythmic, or another drug that may prolong QT interval; and those who have received cumulative high-dose anthracycline therapy. With these patients, obtain a baseline ECG before giving palonosetron; repeat the ECG 15 minutes or 24 hours after giving drug, as ordered. Notify prescriber of any delayed conduction.

• Flush I.V. line with normal saline solution before and after giving I.V. palonosetron.

• Closely monitor any patient hypersensitive to other selective serotonin receptor antagonists for a similar reaction. If a reaction occurs, notify prescriber immediately.

WARNING Monitor patient closely for serotonin syndrome, which is characterized by agitation, coma, hallucinations, labile blood pressure, tachycardia, hyperthermia, hyperreflexia, incoordination, nausea, vomiting, or diarrhea. Notify prescriber immediately because serotonin syndrome may be life threatening, and provide supportive care.

PATIENT TEACHING
• Advise patient to avoid hazardous activities until drug's CNS effects are known.
• Instruct patient to notify prescriber of any hypersensitivity reaction, such as rash or allergic dermatitis.

pamidronate disodium
Aredia

Class and Category
Chemical class: Bisphosphonate
Therapeutic class: Antihypercalcemic, bone resorption inhibitor
Pregnancy category: D

Indications and Dosages
➤ *To treat cancer-induced hypercalcemia that's inadequately managed by oral hydration alone*
I.V. INFUSION
Adults. 60 to 90 mg over 2 to 24 hr as a single dose when corrected serum calcium level is 12 to 13.5 mg/dl; 90 mg over 2 to 24 hr when corrected serum calcium level is greater than 13.5 mg/dl. May be repeated as prescribed after 7 days if hypercalcemia recurs.
DOSAGE ADJUSTMENT For patients with renal failure, dosage is limited to 30 mg over 4 to 24 hr, as prescribed. For patients with cardiac or renal failure, drug is given in a smaller volume of fluid or at a slower rate, as prescribed.
➤ *To treat moderate to severe Paget's disease of bone*
I.V. INFUSION
Adults. 30 mg daily over 4 hr on 3 consecutive days for a total dose of 90 mg. Repeated as needed and tolerated.
➤ *To treat osteolytic bone metastases of breast cancer*
I.V. INFUSION
Adults. 90 mg over 2 hr every 3 to 4 wk.
➤ *To treat osteolytic bone metastases of multiple myeloma*
I.V. INFUSION
Adults. 90 mg over 4 hr every mo.

Mechanism of Action
Inhibits bone resorption, possibly by impairing attachment of osteoclast precursors to mineralized bone matrix, thus reducing the rate of bone turnover in Paget's disease and osteolytic metastases. Pamidronate also reduces the flow of calcium from resorbing bone into bloodstream.

Incompatibilities
Don't mix pamidronate with calcium-containing infusion solutions, such as Ringer's solution.

Contraindications
Hypersensitivity to pamidronate, other bisphosphonates, or their components

Interaction
DRUGS
calcium-containing preparations; vitamin D preparations, such as calcifediol and calcitriol: Antagonized pamidronate effects when used to treat hypercalcemia
thalidomide: Increased risk of renal dysfunction in patients with multiple myeloma

Adverse Reactions
CNS: Confusion, fever, psychosis, visual hallucinations
CV: Hypotension
EENT: Conjunctivitis, ocular inflammation
GI: Abdominal cramps, anorexia, GI bleeding, indigestion, nausea, vomiting
GU: Azotemia, focal segmental glomerulosclerosis, glomerulonephropathies, nephrotic syndrome, hematuria, nephritis, renal toxicity leading to failure, renal tubular disorders

HEME: Leukopenia, lymphopenia
MS: Atypical fractures of femur; muscle spasms or stiffness; osteonecrosis (mainly of jaw); severe bone, joint or muscle pain
RESP: Adult respiratory distress syndrome, dyspnea, interstitial lung disease
SKIN: Pruritus, rash
Other: Anaphylaxis, angioedema, flulike symptoms, hyperkalemia, hypernatremia, hypocalcemia, hypokalemia, hypomagnesemia, hypophosphatemia, injection-site pain and swelling, reactivation of herpes simplex and zoster infections

Nursing Considerations
• Make sure patient has had a dental checkup before invasive dental procedures during pamidronate therapy, especially if he has cancer; is receiving chemotherapy, head or neck radiation, or a corticosteroid;

Mechanism of Action
Chemotherapy may induce nausea and vomiting by irritating the small intestine's mucosa, causing mucosal enterochromaffin cells to release serotonin (5-HT$_3$). The 5-HT$_3$ stimulates sympathetic receptors on afferent vagal nerve endings, and the vagus nerve causes the vomiting reflex.

Palonosetron selectively blocks these 5-HT$_3$ receptors. By keeping the vagus nerve from inducing the vomiting reflex, drug reduces or prevents nausea and vomiting. It also may block 5-HT$_3$ receptors centrally, in the brain's chemoreceptor trigger zone.

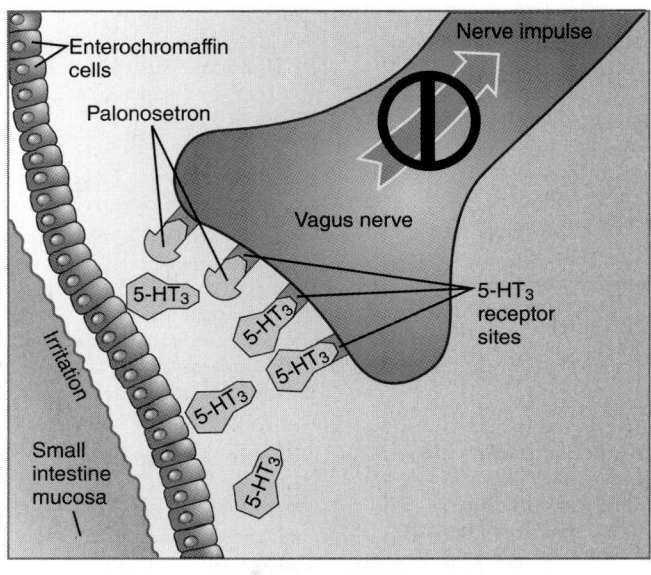

P

or has poor oral hygiene. Risk of osteo-necrosis is increased in these patients.

• Obtain serum creatinine level before each treatment. Notify prescriber of abnormal results because drug may need to be withheld or dosage adjusted until creatinine level returns to normal.

WARNING Don't give more than 90 mg at any one time because of increased risk of serious adverse effect on kidneys.

• Monitor patient's serum electrolytes including calcium, phosphate, and magnesium; CBC differential; and hematocrit and hemoglobin levels, as ordered throughout therapy because abnormalities may occur.

• Monitor patient for hypocalcemia, especially if patient has had thyroid surgery.

• Stay alert for fever during first 3 days of therapy, especially in patients receiving high doses. If fever develops, obtain patient's CBC with differential, as ordered.

• Assess patient with anemia, leukopenia, or thrombocytopenia for worsening of the condition during first 2 weeks of therapy.

PATIENT TEACHING

• Emphasize need to comply with prescribed administration schedule for pamidronate.

• Advise patient to avoid calcium and vitamin D supplements during therapy.

• Instruct patient on proper oral hygiene and on need to notify prescriber about invasive dental procedures.

• Advise women of childbearing age to alert prescriber if she suspects or knows she is pregnant.

• Instruct patient to report to prescriber any new or unusual pain in hip or thigh in the absence of trauma.

---

pancreatin

Donnazyme: *500 mg pancreatin, 1,000 units lipase, 12,500 units protease, 12,500 units amylase*
Hi-Vegi-Lip: *2,400 mg pancreatin, 4,800 units lipase, 60,000 units protease, 60,000 units amylase*
4X Pancreatin: *2,400 mg pancreatin, 12,000 units lipase, 60,000 units protease, 60,000 units amylase*

8X Pancreatin: *7,200 mg pancreatin, 22,500 units lipase, 180,000 units protease, 180,000 units amylase*
Pancrezyme 4X: *2,400 mg pancreatin, 12,000 units lipase, 60,000 units protease, 60,000 units amylase*

Class and Category

Chemical class: Pancreatic enzyme
Therapeutic class: Digestant, pancreatic enzyme replacement
Pregnancy category: C

Indications and Dosages

➤ *To treat pancreatic insufficiency, including steatorrhea*

CAPSULES, TABLETS

Adults. 8,000 to 24,000 units of lipase with meals or snacks, adjusted as prescribed, according to need for steatorrhea control. For severe insufficiency, up to 36,000 units of lipase with meals or snacks.

Mechanism of Action

Releases the enzymes pancreatin, lipase, amylase, and protease, mainly in the duodenum and upper jejunum. These enzymes facilitate the hydrolysis of fats into glycerol and fatty acids, starches into dextrins and sugars, and proteins into peptides. Pancreatin acts locally in the GI tract but is quickly inactivated by gastric acid.

Contraindications

Acute exacerbation of chronic pancreatic disease; acute pancreatitis; hypersensitivity to pancreatin, pancrelipase, or pork

Interaction

DRUGS

acarbose, miglitol: Decreased effectiveness of these drugs
aluminum hydroxide, H$_2$-receptor antagonists, omeprazole, sodium bicarbonate: Increased gastric pH, prolonged enzymatic action of pancreatin
calcium carbonate– and magnesium hydroxide–containing antacids: Decreased pancreatin effectiveness
iron supplements: Decreased iron absorption

Adverse Reactions

EENT: Stomatitis
GI: Abdominal cramps or pain, diarrhea, intestinal obstruction, nausea
SKIN: Rash, urticaria
Other: Hyperuricemia

Nursing Considerations

WARNING Don't administer pancreatin to patient who is allergic to pork.

• Assess patient for GI disturbances and hyperuricemia when giving high doses of pancreatin.

• If patient opens capsules and sprinkles contents on food, watch for signs or symptoms of sensitization (chest tightness, dyspnea, nasal congestion, wheezing), which may result from repeated inadvertent inhalation of powder.

• Be aware that brands of pancreatin aren't interchangeable because the same doses don't contain equivalent amounts of drug.

PATIENT TEACHING

• Instruct patient to take pancreatin before or with meals or snacks to maximize effectiveness.

• To prevent capsule or tablet from lodging in esophagus, advise patient to take drug with a beverage while sitting upright, to swallow it quickly, and to follow with 1 or 2 mouthfuls of solid food.

• Caution patient not to chew tablets; doing so may irritate mouth, lips, and tongue.

• If patient has trouble swallowing capsules, advise her to open capsule and sprinkle its contents on food without inhaling them.

• Caution patient not to take antacids that contain calcium carbonate or magnesium hydroxide during therapy.

pancrelipase

Cotazym: *8,000 units lipase, 30,000 units protease, 30,000 units amylase*
Cotazym-S: *5,000 units lipase, 20,000 units protease, 20,000 units amylase*
Creon: *6,000 units lipase, 19,000 units protease, 30,000 units amylase*
Creon: *12,000 units lipase, 38,000 units protease, 60,000 units amylase*
Creon: *24,000 units lipase, 76,000 units protease, 120,000 units amylase*
Ilozyme: *11,000 units lipase, 30,000 units protease, 30,000 units amylase*
Ku-Zyme HP: *8,000 units lipase, 30,000 units protease, 30,000 units amylase*
Pancrease: *4,500 units lipase, 25,000 units protease, 20,000 units amylase*
Pancrease MT 4: *4,000 units lipase, 12,000 units protease, 12,000 units amylase*
Pancrease MT 10: *10,000 units lipase, 30,000 units protease, 30,000 units amylase*
Pancrease MT 16: *16,000 units lipase, 48,000 units protease, 48,000 units amylase*
Pancrease MT 20: *20,000 units lipase, 44,000 units protease, 56,000 units amylase*
Pancreaze MT 4: *4,200 units lipase, 10,000 units protease, 17,500 units amylase*
Pancreaze MT 10: *10,500 units lipase, 25,000 units protease, 43,750 units amylase*
Pancreaze MT 16: *16,800 units lipase, 40,000 units protease, 70,000 units amylase*
Pancreaze MT 20: *21,000 units lipase, 37,000 units protease, 61,000 units amylase*
Pertzye: *8,000 units lipase, 28,750 units protease, 30,250 units amylase*
Pertzye: *16,000 units lipase, 57,500 units protease, 60,500 units amylase*
Protilase: *4,000 units lipase, 25,000 units protease, 20,000 units amylase*
Ultrase MT 12: *12,000 units lipase, 39,000 units protease, 39,000 units amylase*
Ultrase MT 20: *20,000 units lipase, 65,000 units protease, 65,000 units amylase*
Ultresa: *13,800 units lipase, 27,600 units protease, 27,600 units amylase*
Ultresa: *20,700 units lipase, 41,400 units protease, 41,400 units amylase*
Utresa: *23,000 units lipase, 46,000 units protease, 46,000 units amylase*
Viokace: *10,440 units lipase, 39,150 units protease, 39,150 units amylase*
Viokace: *20,880 units lipase, 78,300 units protease, 78,300 units amylase*
Viokase Tablets: *8,000 units lipase, 30,000 units protease, 30,000 units amylase*
Viokase Powder: *16,800 units lipase, 70,000 units protease, 70,000 units amylase*
Zenpep: *5,000 units lipase, 17,000 units protease, 27,000 units amylase*
Zenpep: *10,000 units lipase, 34,000 units protease, 55,000 units amylase*

Zenpep: 15,000 units lipase, 51,000 units protease, 82,000 units amylase
Zenpep: 20,000 units lipase, 68,000 units protease, 109,000 units amylase
Zymase: 12,000 units lipase, 24,000 units protease, 24,000 units amylase

Class and Category
Chemical class: Porcine pancreatic enzyme
Therapeutic class: Pancreatic enzyme replacement
Pregnancy category: C

Indications and Dosages
➤ *To treat exocrine pancreatic insufficiency, including steatorrhea*
CAPSULES, POWDER, TABLETS
Adults and children age 4 and over. *Initial:* 500 lipase units/kg per meal, adjusted as needed and tolerated. *Maximum:* 2,500 lipase units/kg per meal (or less than or equal to 10,000 lipase units/kg per day), or less than 4,000 lipase units/g fat ingested per day.
Children ages 1 to 4. *Initial:* 1,000 lipase units/kg per meal, adjusted as needed and tolerated. *Maximum:* 2,500 lipase units/kg per meal (or less than or equal to 10,000 lipase units/kg per day), or less than 4,000 lipase units/g fat ingested per day.
Infants up to 12 months. 2,000 to 4,000 lipase units per 120 ml of formula or per breastfeeding.
DELAYED-RELEASE CAPSULES
Adults and children age 4 and over. *Initial:* 500 lipase units/kg per meal, adjusted as needed and tolerated. *Maximum:* 2,500 lipase units/kg per meal (or less than or equal to 10,000 lipase units/kg/per day), or less than 4,000 lipase units/g fat ingested per day.
Children ages 1 to 4. *Initial:* 1,000 lipase units/kg per meal, adjusted as needed and tolerated. *Maximum:* 2,500 lipase units/kg per meal (or less than or equal to 10,000 lipase units/kg per day), or less than 4,000 lipase units/g fat ingested per day.
Infants up to 12 months. 3,000 lipase units per 120 ml of formula or per breastfeeding.
➤ *To treat exocrine pancreatic insufficiency due to chronic pancreatitis or pancreatectomy*
DELAYED-RELEASE CAPSULES (CREON)
Adults. Highly individualized.

Mechanism of Action
Releases high levels of the enzymes lipase, amylase, and protease, mainly in duodenum and upper jejunum. These enzymes facilitate hydrolysis of fats into glycerol and fatty acids, starches into dextrins and sugars, and proteins into peptides.

Contraindications
Acute exacerbation of chronic pancreatic disease; acute pancreatitis; hypersensitivity to pancreatin, pancrelipase, or pork

Interaction
DRUGS
acarbose, miglitol: Decreased effectiveness of these drugs
aluminum hydroxide, H_2-receptor antagonists, omeprazole, sodium bicarbonate: Increased gastric pH, prolonged enzymatic action of pancrelipase
calcium carbonate– and magnesium hydroxide–containing antacids: Decreased pancrelipase effectiveness
iron supplements: Decreased iron absorption

Adverse Reactions
CNS: Dizziness, headache
EENT: Blurred vision, nasopharyngitis, stomatitis
ENDO: Hyperglycemia, hypoglycemia
GI: Abdominal cramps, distention, or pain; abnormal feces; constipation; diarrhea; distal intestinal obstruction syndrome; elevated liver enzymes; fibrosing colonopathy; flatulence; intestinal obstruction; nausea; vomiting
HEME: Anemia
MS: Muscle spasm, myalgia
RESP: Asthma, cough
SKIN: Pruritus, rash, urticaria
Other: Anaphylaxis, hyperuricemia

Nursing Considerations
WARNING Don't administer pancrelipase to patient who is allergic to pork.
• Know that children older than 12 months and younger than 4 years who weigh less than 8 kg, and children 4 years and older weighing less than 16 kg, should not receive Pertzye brand of pancrelipase; nor should children older than 12 months and younger than 4 years who weigh under 14 kg, or children 4 years and older weighing less than 28 kg, receive Ultresa brand of

pancrelipase because capsule dosage strength in these products cannot adequately provide correct dosing for these children.

• Use with caution in patients with gout, renal impairment, or hyperuricemia because porcine-derived pancreatic enzyme products contain purines that may increase blood uric acid levels.

• Be aware that brands of pancrelipase aren't interchangeable because the same doses don't contain equivalent amounts of drug.

• Mix powder with fluid or soft, nondairy food.

• If needed, open capsules or delayed-release capsules and mix contents (enteric-coated spheres, microspheres, or microtablets) with liquid or soft food that requires no chewing. Give immediately because enteric coating will dissolve after prolonged contact with foods at a pH greater than 6. Do not mix contents directly into formula or breastmilk because effectiveness may be diminished. Instead, mix in a small amount of applesauce or other acidic food such as baby food, bananas, or pears, or place contents of capsule directly into infant's mouth, followed by breastmilk or formula.

• If patient opens capsules and sprinkles contents on food, assess for signs of sensitization (chest tightness, dyspnea, nasal congestion, wheezing), which may result from repeated inadvertent inhalation of powder.

• Give drug before or with meals and snacks, and follow with a glass of water or juice.

• Expect drug to cause stomatitis if held in mouth.

• Monitor patient for allergic reactions when beginning therapy. Although rare, severe allergic reactions including anaphylaxis, asthma, hives, and pruritus may occur. Notify prescriber immediately and provide supportive care.

• Check stool for fecal fat content, as ordered.

• Monitor patient for iron deficiency anemia because serum iron level may decline during pancrelipase therapy.

• Monitor blood glucose levels more frequently in patients at risk for abnormal blood glucose levels because glycemic control may be affected by administration of pancreatic enzyme replacement therapy.

WARNING Monitor patient, especially children with cystic fibrosis, for abdominal pain because fibrosing colonopathy, although rare, may occur over a prolonged period of time, especially when doses of pancreatic enzyme products exceed 6,000 lipase units/kg per meal.

PATIENT TEACHING

• Instruct patient to take pancrelipase before or with meals and snacks and to follow with a glass of water or juice.

• Instruct patient not to chew capsules or capsule contents or to crush tablets; patient should swallow immediately because drug may cause irritation if held in mouth.

• Urge patient not to inhale powder from delayed-release capsules; doing so may cause chest tightness, shortness of breath, stuffy nose, trouble breathing, and wheezing.

• Inform patient that sneezing and tearing also may result from contact with powder.

• Caution patient not to use antacids; they may decrease drug effectiveness.

• Inform patient that her stool may have foul smell.

pantoprazole sodium

Pantoloc (CAN), Protonix, Protonix I.V.

Class and Category

Chemical class: Substituted benzimidazole
Therapeutic class: Antiulcer, gastric acid proton pump inhibitor
Pregnancy category: B

Indications and Dosages

➤ *To treat gastroesophageal reflux disease (GERD)*

DELAYED-RELEASE TABLETS
Adults. 40 mg daily for up to 8 wk. Repeated for another 4 to 8 wk if healing doesn't occur.

DELAYED-RELEASE ORAL SUSPENSION
Adults. 40 mg daily given 30 minutes before a meal for up to 8 wk. Repeated for another 4 to 8 wk if healing doesn't occur.
I.V. INFUSION
Adults. 40 mg daily infused over 2 min or 15 min for 7 to 10 days, followed by oral doses.
➤ *To maintain healing of erosive esophagitis and reduce relapse of daytime and nighttime symptoms in patients with GERD*
DELAYED-RELEASE TABLETS
Adults. 40 mg daily for up to 12 mo.
DELAYED-RELEASE ORAL SUSPENSION
Adults. 40 mg daily given 30 minutes before a meal for up to 12 mo.
➤ *To treat pathological hypersecretion associated with Zollinger-Ellison syndrome or other neoplastic conditions*
I.V. INFUSION
Adults. 80 mg every 12 hr infused over 2 min or 15 min; adjusted based on patient's acid output measurements up to 80 mg every 8 hr.

Route	Onset	Peak	Duration
P.O.	1 day	1 wk	1 wk
I.V.	1 day	Unknown	1 wk

Mechanism of Action

Interferes with gastric acid secretion by inhibiting the hydrogen-potassium-adenosine triphosphatase (H^+-K^+-ATPase) enzyme system, or proton pump, in gastric parietal cells. Normally, the proton pump uses energy from hydrolysis of ATPase to drive H^+ and chloride (Cl^-) out of parietal cells and into the stomach lumen in exchange for potassium (K^+), which leaves the stomach lumen and enters parietal cells. After this exchange, H^+ and Cl^- combine in the stomach to form hydrochloric acid (HCl). Pantoprazole irreversibly inhibits the final step in gastric acid production by blocking the exchange of intracellular H^+ and extracellular K^+, thus preventing H^+ from entering the stomach and additional HCl from forming.

Incompatibilities

Midazolam and products containing zinc may cause precipitation or discoloration.

Contraindications

Hypersensitivity to pantoprazole, substituted benzimidazoles (omeprazole, lansoprazole, rabeprazole sodium), or their components

Interaction
DRUGS
ampicillin, cyanocobalamin, digoxin, iron salts, ketoconazole: Possibly impaired absorption of these drugs
atazanavir: Significantly decreased atazanavir level
digoxin, diuretics : Increased risk of hypomagnesemia
methotrexate: Increased risk of methotrexate toxicities
mycophenolate mofetil: Decreased plasma level and effectiveness of pantoprazole
warfarin: Increased INR, PT, and bleeding risk

Adverse Reactions

CNS: Anxiety, asthenia, confusion, dizziness, fatigue, hallucinations, headache, hypertonia, hypokinesia, insomnia, malaise, migraine, somnolence, speech disorder, vertigo
CV: Chest pain, hypercholesterolemia, hyperlipidemia
EENT: Anterior ischemic optic neuropathy, blurred vision, increased salivation, pharyngitis, rhinitis, sinusitis, taste disorder, tinnitus
ENDO: Hyperglycemia
GI: Abdominal pain, atrophic gastritis, *Clostridum difficile*–associated diarrhea, constipation, diarrhea, elevated liver enzymes, flatulence, gastroenteritis, hepatic failure, hepatotoxicity, indigestion, jaundice, nausea, pancreatitis, vomiting
GU: Elevated serum creatinine level, interstitial nephritis
HEME: Agranulocytosis, pancytopenia
MS: Arthralgia, back or neck pain, bone fracture, rhabdomyolysis
RESP: Bronchitis, dyspnea, increased cough, upper respiratory tract infection
SKIN: Erythema multiforme, rash, Stevens-Johnson syndrome, toxic epidermal necrolysis
Other: Anaphylaxis, angioedema, elevated creatine kinase and phosphokinase levels, flulike symptoms, generalized pain,

hyperuricemia, hypomagnesemia, hyponatremia, infection, injection-site reaction, weight changes

Nursing Considerations

• Ensure the continuity of gastric acid suppression during transition from oral to I.V. pantoprazole (or vice versa) because even a brief interruption of effective suppression can lead to serious complications.

• Don't give pantoprazole within 4 weeks of testing for *Helicobacter pylori* because antibiotics, proton pump inhibitors, and bismuth preparations suppress *H. pylori* and may lead to false-negative results. Drug also may cause false-positive results in urine screening tests for tetrahydrocannabinol. Consult guidelines for pantoprazole use before testing.

• Administer delayed-release oral suspension 30 minutes before a meal mixed in apple juice or applesauce or, if given through a nasogastric tube, mixed in apple juice only. Do not mix the oral suspension in liquids other than apple juice, or foods other than applesauce because proper pH is necessary for stability. When mixing with applesauce, administer within 10 minutes and encourage patient to take repeated sips of water to make sure granules are washed down into the stomach. When mixing with apple juice, use only one teaspoon of apple juice to mix granules in, stir for 5 seconds (granules will not dissolve) and give immediately to patient to drink. After administration, rinse the container once or twice with more apple juice and give to patient to drink to ensure full dose has been given.

• Flush I.V. line with D_5W, normal saline solution, or lactated Ringer's injection before and after giving drug.

• When giving I.V. over 2 minutes, reconstitute with 10 ml of normal saline injection. Solution may be stored up to 2 hours at room temperature.

• When giving I.V. over 15 minutes, reconstitute with 10 ml normal saline injection. Then, further reconstitute with 100 ml (for GERD) or 80 ml (for pathological hypersecretion in Zollinger-Ellison syndrome) of D_5W, normal saline

injection, or lactated Ringer's injection. Solution may be stored up to 2 hours before further dilution and up to 22 hours before use.

• Expect to monitor PT or INR during therapy if patient takes an oral anticoagulant.

• Be aware if therapy lasts more than 3 years, patient may not be able to absorb vitamin B_{12} because of hypochlorhydria or achlorhydria. Treatment for cyanocobalamin deficiency may be needed.

• Monitor patient for bone fracture, especially in patients receiving multiple daily doses for more than a year because proton pump inhibitors, such as pantoprazole, increase risk of osteoporosis-related fractures of the hip, wrist, or spine.

• Monitor patient for diarrhea from *Clostridium difficile* which can occur with or without antibiotics in patients taking pantoprazole. If severe diarrhea occurs, notify prescriber and expect to withhold drug and treat with fluids, electrolytes, protein, and an antibiotic effective against *C. difficile*.

• Monitor the patient, especially the patient on long-term therapy for hypomagnesemia. If patient is to remain on pantoprazole long-term, expect to monitor the patient's serum magnesium level, as ordered, and if level becomes low, anticipate magnesium replacement therapy to be given and pantoprazole to be discontinued.

PATIENT TEACHING

• Instruct patient to swallow pantoprazole tablets whole and not to chew or crush them.

• Tell patient to take delayed-release oral suspension 30 minutes before a meal mixed in apple juice or applesauce; no other liquid or food should be used. When mixing with applesauce, tell patient to take mixture within 10 minutes and then to take repeated sips of water to make sure granules are washed down into the stomach. When mixing with apple juice, tell patient to use only one teaspoon of apple juice to mix granules in, stir for 5 seconds (granules will not dissolve) and drink immediately. After drinking, tell

P

patient to rinse the container once or twice with more apple juice and then drink to ensure full dose has been given.
• Advise patient to expect relief of symptoms within 2 weeks of starting therapy.
• Advise patient who takes warfarin to follow bleeding precautions and to notify prescriber immediately if bleeding occurs.
• Instruct patient to notify prescriber if diarrhea occurs and becomes prolonged or severe.

paricalcitol

Zemplar

Class and Category

Chemical class: Sterol derivative, vitamin D analogue
Therapeutic class: Antihyperparathyroid
Pregnancy category: Not rated

Indications and Dosages

➤ *To prevent and treat secondary hyperparathyroidism in patients with chronic renal failure stage 3 or 4*

I.V. INJECTION

Adults. *Initial:* 0.04 to 0.1 mcg/kg (2.8 to 7 mcg) no more than every other day at any time during dialysis. *Maintenance:* If initial dosage doesn't produce a satisfactory response, 2 to 4 mcg given every 2 to 4 wk. *Maximum:* 0.24 mcg/kg/dose or up to 16.8 mcg/dose.

Children age 5 and over. *Initial:* 0.04 mcg/kg three times weekly if baseline intact parathyroid hormone (iPTH) level is less than 500 pg/ml, or 0.08 mcg/kg three times weekly if baseline iPTH level equals or exceeds 500 pg/ml. *Maintenance:* If initial dosage isn't adequate, adjust in 0.04-mcg/kg increments as needed.

DOSAGE ADJUSTMENT If serum PTH level remains the same or increases, dosage is increased. If PTH level decreases by less than 30%, dosage is increased. If PTH level decreases by 30% to 60%, dosage is maintained. If PTH level decreases by more than 60%, dosage is decreased. If PTH level is 1.5 to 3 times the upper limit of normal, dosage is maintained.

DOSAGE ADJUSTMENT Dosage is immediately reduced or drug stopped if serum calcium level is elevated or serum calcium-phosphorus product exceeds 75. Dosage restarted at a lower dose when these levels return to normal.

CAPSULES

Adults. *Initial:* If baseline iPTH level is less than 500 pg/ml, 1 mcg daily or 2 mcg three times weekly, doses separated by at least 1 day. If iPTH level exceeds 500 pg/ml, 2 mcg daily or 4 mcg three times weekly, doses separated by at least 1 day. *Maintenance:* Dosage adjusted in 1-mcg increments based on iPTH level relative to baseline.

Route	Onset	Peak	Duration
I.V.	Unknown	Unknown	15 hr

Mechanism of Action

Reduces serum PTH level by an unknown mechanism. In chronic renal failure, decreased renal synthesis of vitamin D leads to chronic hypocalcemia. In response, parathyroid glands secrete PTH to stimulate vitamin D synthesis, but serum calcium levels can't normalize because of renal failure.

Contraindications

Evidence of vitamin D toxicity, hypercalcemia, hypersensitivity to paricalcitol or components

Interaction

DRUGS

aluminum-containing preparations such as antacids or phosphate binders: Possibly increased blood levels of aluminum and aluminum bone toxicity
atazanavir, clarithromycin, indinavir, itraconazole, ketoconazole, nefazodone, nelfinavir, ritonavir, saquinavir, telithromycin, voriconazole: Increased effects of oral paricalcitol
digoxin: Possibly increased risk of digitalis toxicity
drugs, such as cholestyramine, that impair absorption of fat-soluble vitamins: Possibly impaired absorption of oral paricalcitol
vitamin D or its derivatives (prescription-based doses): Increased risk of hypercalcemia

Adverse Reactions

CNS: Agitation, anxiety, asthenia, chills, confusion, CVA, delirium, depression, dizziness, fatigue, fever, gait disturbance, headache, insomnia, light-headedness, malaise, myoclonus, neuropathy, nervousness, paresthesia, restlessness, syncope, thirst, unresponsive to stimuli, vertigo
CV: Arrhythmia, atrial flutter, cardiac arrest, cardiomyopathy, chest pain, congestive heart failure, hypertension, hypotension, MI, orthostatic hypotension, palpitations, peripheral edema
EENT: Amblyopia, conjunctivitis, dry mouth, glaucoma, ear discomfort, epistaxis, laryngeal edema, ocular hyperemia, pharyngitis, retinal abnormality, rhinitis, sinusitis, taste perversion
ENDO: Breast tenderness, hypercalcemia, hyperparathyroidism, hypocalcemia, hypoparathyroidism, hypoglycemia
GI: Abdominal discomfort or pain, anorexia, constipation, diarrhea, dyspepsia, dysphagia, elevated liver enzymes, gastritis, gastroenteritis, gastroesophageal reflux disease, GI bleeding, intestinal ischemia, nausea, rectal hemorrhage, vomiting
GU: Abnormal kidney function, elevated blood creatinine level, erectile dysfunction, renal failure, uremia, UTI
HEME: Anemia, lymphadenopathy, prolonged bleeding time
MS: Back pain, joint stiffness, leg cramps, muscle twitching, myalgia
RESP: Increased cough, dyspnea, orthopnea, pneumonia, pulmonary edema, wheezing
SKIN: Acne, alopecia, burning sensation, ecchymosis, hirsutism, hypertrophy, night sweats, pruritus, rash (including vesiculobullous), ulceration, urticaria
Other: Acidosis, allergic reaction, angioedema, dehydration, generalized edema, gout, injection-site pain or swelling, hyperkalemia, hyperphosphatemia, hypervolemia, hypokalemia, infections, influenza, sepsis, weight loss

Nursing Considerations

- Before giving drug, look for particles and discoloration; if present, discard drug.
- Give as I.V. bolus; discard unused portion.
- **WARNING** Paricalcitol may lead to vitamin D toxicity and hypercalcemia requiring emergency intervention. Early evidence includes arthralgia, constipation, dry mouth, headache, metallic taste, myalgia, nausea, somnolence, vomiting, and weakness. Late evidence includes albuminuria, anorexia, arrhythmias, azotemia, conjunctivitis (calcific), decreased libido, elevated BUN and serum ALT and AST levels, vascular calcification, hypercholesterolemia, hypertension, hyperthermia, irritability, mild acidosis, nephrocalcinosis, nocturia, pancreatitis, photophobia, polydipsia, polyuria, pruritus, rhinorrhea, and weight loss.
- If toxicity occurs, notify prescriber immediately and expect to decrease or stop drug. Place patient on bed rest and give fluids, low-calcium diet, and a laxative, as prescribed. If patient has a hypercalcemic crisis and dehydration, expect to infuse normal saline solution and a loop diuretic to prompt renal calcium excretion.
- Expect to check patient's serum PTH level, serum calcium, and serum phosphorus levels at least every 2 weeks for 3 months during the initial dosing of paricalcitol or following any dose adjustment, then monthly for 3 months, and then every 3 months thereafter.
- Know that increased serum creatinine levels may occur with paricalcitol therapy and will decrease the patient's estimated glomerular filtration rate, which is especially significant for pre-dialysis patients.
- If patient also takes digoxin, monitor her for evidence of digitalis glycoside toxicity, which is potentiated by hypercalcemia.
- Store drug at 25° C (77° F).

PATIENT TEACHING
- Advise patient to follow a diet high in calcium and low in phosphorus.
- Explain that phosphate binders may be needed to control serum phosphorus level.
- Review early evidence of hypercalcemia and vitamin D toxicity, such as feeling tired or unusually thirsty or experiencing difficulty thinking clearly, loss of appetite, nausea, vomiting, constipation, increased urination, and weight loss. Tell patient to contact prescriber immediately if it develops.

P

• Urge patient to avoid hazardous activities until drug's CNS effects are known.
• If patient takes digoxin, explain evidence of toxicity and the need to contact prescriber immediately if it develops.

paroxetine hydrochloride
Paxil, Paxil CR

paroxetine mesylate
Brisdelle, Pexeva

Class and Category
Chemical class: Phenylpiperidine derivative
Therapeutic class: Antidepressant, anti-obsessional, antipanic
Pregnancy category: D

Indications and Dosages
➤ *To treat major depression*
C.R. TABLETS
Adults. *Initial:* 25 mg daily, increased as prescribed and tolerated by 12.5 mg daily every wk. *Maximum:* 62.5 mg daily.
ORAL SUSPENSION, TABLETS
Adults. *Initial:* 20 mg daily, increased as prescribed and tolerated by 10 mg daily every wk. *Maximum:* 50 mg daily.
➤ *To treat obsessive-compulsive disorder*
ORAL SUSPENSION, TABLETS
Adults. *Initial:* 20 mg daily, increased as prescribed and tolerated by 10 mg daily every wk. *Usual:* 20 to 60 mg daily. *Maximum:* 60 mg daily.
➤ *To treat panic disorder*
C.R. TABLETS
Adults. *Initial:* 12.5 mg daily, increased by 12.5 mg daily every wk as needed. *Maximum:* 75 mg daily.
ORAL SUSPENSION, TABLETS
Adults. *Initial:* 10 mg daily, increased as prescribed and tolerated by 10 mg daily every wk. *Usual:* 10 to 60 mg daily. *Maximum:* 60 mg daily.
➤ *To treat social anxiety disorder*
C.R. TABLETS
Adults. *Initial:* 12.5 mg daily, increased by 12.5 mg daily every wk as needed. *Maximum:* 37.5 mg daily.

ORAL SUSPENSION, TABLETS (PAXIL)
Adults. *Initial:* 20 mg daily, increased as prescribed and tolerated by 10 mg daily every wk. *Usual:* 20 to 60 mg daily. *Maximum:* 60 mg daily.
➤ *To treat generalized anxiety disorder*
ORAL SUSPENSION, TABLETS (PAXIL)
Adults. *Initial:* 20 mg daily, increased as prescribed and tolerated by 10 mg daily every wk. *Usual:* 20 to 50 mg daily. *Maximum:* 60 mg daily.
➤ *To treat posttraumatic stress disorder*
ORAL SUSPENSION, TABLETS (PAXIL)
Adults. *Initial:* 20 mg daily, increased as prescribed and tolerated by 10 mg daily every wk. *Usual:* 20 to 50 mg daily. *Maximum:* 50 mg daily.
➤ *To treat premenstrual dysphoric disorder*
C.R. TABLETS
Adults. *Initial:* 12.5 mg daily in the morning, increased as needed after 1 wk to 25 mg daily. Or, 12.5 mg daily in the morning only during luteal phase of menstrual cycle (2-wk period before onset of monthly cycle), increased as needed after 1 wk to 25 mg daily in the morning during luteal phase of menstrual cycle.
DOSAGE ADJUSTMENT For patients who are elderly, debilitated, or have creatinine clearance less than 30 ml/min/1.73 m², initially 10 mg daily; maximum, 40 mg daily. Avoid C.R. form. For patients taking C.R. tablets with creatinine clearance less than 30 ml/min/1.73 m², initially 12.5 mg daily; maximum, 50 mg daily.
➤ *To treat moderate to severe vasomotor symptoms associated with menopause*
CAPSULES (BRISDELLE)
Adults. 7.5 mg once daily at bedtime.

Route	Onset	Peak	Duration
P.O.	1–4 wk	Unknown	Unknown

Mechanism of Action
Exerts antidepressant, antiobsessional, and antipanic effects by potentiating serotonin activity in CNS and inhibiting serotonin reuptake at presynaptic neuronal membrane. Blocked serotonin reuptake increases levels and prolongs activity of serotonin at synaptic receptor sites.

Contraindications

Hypersensitivity to paroxetine or its components, pimozide or thioridazine therapy, use within 14 days of an MAO inhibitor including linezolid or I.V. methylene blue

Interaction

DRUGS

antacids: Hastened release of C.R. paroxetine

aspirin, NSAIDs, warfarin: Increased anticoagulant activity and risk of bleeding

astemizole: Increased risk of arrhythmias

atomoxetine; risperidone; other drugs metabolized by CYP2D6, such as amitriptyline, desipramine, fluoxetine, imipramine, phenothiazines, tamoxifen, type IC antiarrhythmics: Increased plasma levels of these drugs

barbiturates, fosamprenavir, primidone, ritonavir: Decreased plasma paroxetine level

cimetidine: Possibly increased blood paroxetine level

cisapride, fentanyl, isoniazid, linezolid, methylene blue (I.V.), MAO inhibitors, procarbazine, St John's wort, triptans, tryptophan: Possibly increased risk of serotonin syndrome

codeine, haloperidol, metoprolol, perphenazine, propranolol, risperidone, thioridazine: Decreased metabolism and increased effects of these drugs

cyproheptadine: Decreased paroxetine effects

dextromethorphan: Decreased dextromethorphan metabolism and increased risk of toxicity

digoxin: Possibly decreased digoxin effects

encainide, flecainide, propafenone, quinidine: Potentiated toxicity of these drugs

lithium: Possibly increased blood paroxetine level, increased risk of serotonin syndrome

methadone: Decreased methadone metabolism, increased risk of adverse effects

phenytoin: Possibly phenytoin toxicity

pimozide: Increased risk of prolonged QT interval

procyclidine: Increased blood procyclidine level and anticholinergic effects

tamoxifen: Decreased tamoxifen effectiveness

theophylline: Possibly increased blood theophylline level and risk of toxicity

thioridazine: Increased thioridazine level, possibly leading to prolonged QT interval and life-threatening ventricular arrhythmias

tramadol: Increased risk of serotonin syndrome and seizures

tricyclic antidepressants: Increased metabolism and blood antidepressant levels; increased risk of toxicity, including seizures

Adverse Reactions

CNS: Agitation, akathisia, asthenia, confusion, decreased concentration, dizziness, drowsiness, emotional lability, hallucinations, headache, insomnia, mania, neuroleptic malignant syndrome, psychomotor agitation, restlessness, serotonin syndrome, somnolence, suicidal ideation, tremor

CV: Palpitations, tachycardia torsades de pointes, ventricular fibrillation, ventricular tachycardia

EENT: Angle closure glaucoma, blurred vision, dry mouth, rhinitis, taste perversion

GI: Abdominal cramps or pain, anorexia, constipation, diarrhea, flatulence, nausea, vomiting

GU: Decreased libido, difficult ejaculation, impotence, sexual dysfunction, urine retention

MS: Back pain, bone fracture, myalgia, myasthenia, myopathy

SKIN: Diaphoresis, rash, Stevens-Johnson syndrome

Other: Weight gain or loss

Nursing Considerations

- Be aware that Brisdelle is not used to treat any psychiatric condition because it contains a lower dose of paroxetine.
- Shake oral suspension well. Measure with an oral syringe or calibrated device.
- Don't give enteric-coated form with antacids.
- Watch for akathisia (inner sense of restlessness) and psychomotor agitation, especially during the first few weeks of therapy.
- Watch patient closely (especially children, adolescents, and young adults), for suicidal tendencies, particularly when therapy starts and dosage changes, because depression may worsen temporarily

during these times, possibly leading to suicidal ideation.
• Watch for mania, which may result from any antidepressant in a susceptible patient.
• Monitor patient closely for evidence of GI bleeding, especially if patient also takes a drug known to cause GI bleeding, such as aspirin, an NSAID, or warfarin.

WARNING Monitor patient closely for serotonin syndrome exhibited by agitation, hallucinations, coma, tachycardia, labile blood pressure, hyperthermia, hyper-reflexia, incoordination, nausea, vomiting, or diarrhea. Notify prescriber immediately because serotonin syndrome may be life-threatening, and provide supportive care.

WARNING Be aware that serotonin syndrome in its most severe form may resemble neuroleptic malignant syndrome, which includes hyperthermia, muscle rigidity, and autonomic instability with possibly rapid changes in vital signs and mental status. Stop drug immediately, and provide supportive care.
• To minimize adverse reactions, expect to taper drug rather than stop it abruptly.
• Be aware that pathological fractures have been associated with antidepressant therapy. Monitor patient for unexplained bone pain, joint tenderness, swelling, or bruising.

PATIENT TEACHING
• Advise patient to take paroxetine in the morning to minimize insomnia and to take it with food if adverse GI reactions develop.
• Instruct patient to avoid taking C.R. paroxetine within 2 hours of an antacid.
• Tell patient to swallow C.R. tablets whole and not to cut, crush, or chew them.
• Advise patient that drug may cause mild pupillary dilation, which may lead to an episode of acute closure glaucoma. Encourage patient to have eye exam before starting therapy to see if he is at risk.
• Suggest that patient avoid hazardous activities until drug's CNS effects are known.
• Tell family or caregiver to observe patient closely for suicidal tendencies, especially when therapy starts or dosage changes and especially if patient is a child, teenager, or young adult.

• Explain that full effect may take 4 weeks.
• Urge patient to avoid alcohol during therapy; effects with paroxetine are unknown.
• Tell patient not to take aspirin or NSAIDs during therapy because they increase the risk of bleeding. If patient takes warfarin, tell her to use bleeding precautions and to notify prescriber at once if bleeding occurs.
• Inform patient that episodes of acute depression may persist for months or longer and that they require continued follow-up.
• Instruct patient not to stop drug abruptly but to taper dosage as instructed.
• Alert female patients of childbearing age that paroxetine may cause birth defects and persistent pulmonary hypertension in the newborn if taken during the first trimester of pregnancy. Emphasize the need to use effective contraception and to notify prescriber if pregnancy occurs or is suspected.
• Caution patient to alert all prescribers about paroxetine therapy because of potentially serious drug interactions.
• Tell patient to notify prescriber if she develops unexplained bone pain, joint tenderness, swelling, or bruising.

pegfilgrastim
Neulasta

Class and Category
Chemical class: Recombinant granulocyte colony-stimulating factor conjugate
Therapeutic class: Antineutropenic, hematopoietic stimulator
Pregnancy category: C

Indications and Dosages
➤ *To reduce the risk of infection, as manifested by febrile neutropenia, after myelosuppressive chemotherapy*
SUBCUTANEOUS INJECTION
Adults. 6 mg with each chemotherapy cycle.

Mechanism of Action
Induces formation of neutrophil progenitor cells by binding to receptors on granulocytes, which then divide. Pegfilgrastim also

potentiates the effects of mature neutrophils, thus reducing fever and the risk of infection from severe neutropenia. It is pharmacologically identical to human granulocyte colony-stimulating factor.

Contraindications
Hypersensitivity to filgrastim, pegfilgrastim, or their components or to proteins derived from *Escherichia coli*

Interaction
DRUGS
lithium: Increased neutrophil production

Adverse Reactions
CNS: Fever
GI: Elevated liver function test results, splenic rupture, splenomegaly
GU: Elevated uric acid level
HEME: Leukocytosis, sickle cell crisis
MS: Bone pain
RESP: Acute respiratory distress syndrome, dyspnea, hypoxia, pulmonary infiltrates
SKIN: Acute febrile neutrophilic dermatosis (Sweet's syndrome), cutaneous vasculitis, erythema, flushing, rash, urticaria
Other: Anaphylaxis, angioedema, antibody formation to pegfilgrastim, injection-site reactions (pain, induration, erythema)

Nursing Considerations
• Avoid giving pegfilgrastim for 14 days before and 24 hours after cytotoxic chemotherapy.
• Check CBC, hematocrit, and platelet count before and periodically during therapy.
• Let drug warm to room temperature before injection. Use prefilled syringe and needles.
• Don't shake the solution.
• Discard drug that contains particles, is discolored, or was stored more than 48 hours at room temperature.
WARNING If signs of allergy occur, stop pegfilgrastim infusion and notify prescriber at once. If anaphylaxis occurs, give antihistamine, epinephrine, corticosteroid, and bronchodilator, as ordered.
WARNING Patients receiving filgrastim (parent drug) have had splenic rupture and acute respiratory distress syndrome. Assess patient for fever, respiratory distress, and upper abdominal or shoulder tip pain.

• Assess patients with sickle cell disease for signs of sickle cell crisis; urge hydration.
• Give nonopioid and opioid analgesics, as ordered, if patient experiences bone pain.
• Store drug at 2° to 8° C (36° to 46° F), and protect from freezing and light.
• Be aware that needle cover contains dry natural rubber and should not be handled by persons with a latex allergy.
PATIENT TEACHING
• Urge patient to report promptly any potentially serious reactions (trouble breathing, rash, chest tightness, left upper abdominal pain, shoulder tip pain) and evidence of infection (fever, chills).
• If patient will self-administer, teach her how to prepare, give, and store drug.
• Alert her that needle cover contains dry natural rubber and should not be handled if she has a latex allergy.
• Tell patient to rotate injection sites among thigh, abdomen (except for 2 inches around navel), buttocks, and outer, upper arms. Caution her to avoid tender, hard, red, or bruised areas.
• Urge patient to discard used needles and syringes in a puncture-resistant container and not to reuse them.
• Emphasize the importance of follow-up tests.
• Advise patient to store pegfilgrastim in refrigerator and not to freeze it. Tell her to discard drug if left unrefrigerated for more than 48 hours.

peginesatide
Omontys

P

Class and Category
Chemical class: Synthetic pegylated dimeric peptide
Therapeutic class: Antianemic
Pregnancy category: C

Indications and Dosages
➤ *To treat anemia due to chronic kidney disease in patients on dialysis*
I.V. OR SUBCUTANEOUS INJECTION
Adults not currently treated with another erythropoiesis-stimulating agent (ESA).
0.04 mg/kg once monthly.
Adults converting from epoetin alfa.
Based on the weekly dose of epoetin alfa at

the time of substitution, first dose given 1 wk after the last epoetin alfa dose was administered and then continued monthly. **Adults converting from darbepoetin alfa.** Based on the weekly dose of darbepoetin alfa at the time of substitution, first dose given at the next scheduled dose of darbepoetin alfa in place of it.

DOSAGE ADJUSTMENT For patient experiencing a rapid rise in hemoglobin (more than 1 g/dl in the 2 wk prior to the next dose or more than 2 g/dl in 4 wk), dosage reduced by 25% or more. For the patient whose hemoglobin level is approaching or exceeding 11 g/dl, dosage reduced or drug withheld until hemoglobin levels begin to decrease. If drug was withheld, dosage restarted at a dosage that is 25% less than the previously administered dose. For patient who does not exhibit at least an increase in hemoglobin of more than 1 g/dl after 4 wk of therapy, dosage increased by 25%.

Mechanism of Action

Binds to and activates the human erythropoietin receptor and stimulates erythropoiesis in human red cell precursors to raise the reticulocyte count, which in turn increases hemoglobin.

Incompatibilities

Do not mix peginesatide with other drug solutions.

Contraindications

Hypersensitivity to peginesatide or any of its components, uncontrolled hypertension

Adverse Reactions

CNS: Fever, headache, seizures, stroke
CV: Arteriovenous fistula-site complication, hypertension, hypotension, MI, thromboembolism
GI: Diarrhea, nausea, vomiting
MS: Arthralgia, back or extremity pain, muscle spasms
RESP: Bronchospasms, cough, dyspnea, upper respiratory tract infection
SKIN: Generalized pruritus
Other: Anaphylaxis, angioedema, hyperkalemia, infusion reactions, peginesatide-specific binding antibodies

Nursing Considerations

• Be aware that peginesatide therapy should not be used in patients with cancer whose

anemia is not due to chronic renal failure, because peginesatide may increase risk of tumor progression or recurrence.

• Know that the iron status of the patient must be assessed before and during treatment with peginesatide. If patient has a vitamin deficiency, a metabolic or chronic inflammatory condition, or a bleeding condition, expect these conditions to be treated and corrected before peginesatide treatment is begun.

• Obtain baseline blood pressure measurements prior to peginesatide therapy being started and regularly thereafter because drug may increase blood pressure. If blood pressure becomes difficult to control during drug therapy, notify prescriber and expect drug to be withheld or dosage reduced.

• Know that peginesatide is initiated only in patients receiving dialysis and when the patient's hemoglobin level is less than 10 g/dl. Know that dosage increase should not be done more frequently than once every four weeks.

• Expect patient being converted from epoetin alfa or darbepoetin to maintain the same route of administration.

• Use peginesatide cautiously in patients with a history of cardiovascular disease or stroke, in patients with an insufficient hemoglobin response to other erythropoiesis-stimulating agents, and in patients who have a rate of hemoglobin rise of greater than 1 g/dl over 2 weeks with peginesatide therapy, because risk of developing life-threatening cardiovascular adverse effects or stroke is increased in these situations and death may occur.

• Use cautiously in patients receiving peginesatide who undergo coronary artery bypass graft surgery, because the risk of death is increased, and in patients who are undergoing orthopedic procedures because of increased risk for deep venous thrombosis.

• Do not dilute peginesatide or administer concurrently with other drugs.

• Monitor patient closely for allergic reactions to drug because serious and life-threatening hypersensitivity reactions may occur including anaphylaxis, angioedema, bronchospasm, generalized pruritis, and/ or hypotension. At the first sign of

hypersensitivity, notify prescriber and expect to provide supportive care.
• Expect patients to have adjustments made in their dialysis medications after peginesatide therapy is begun. Patients on hemodialysis may need increased anti-coagulation with heparin to prevent clotting of the extracorporeal circuit during hemodialysis.
• Monitor patient's hemoglobin response at least every 2 weeks, as ordered, until stable and then at least monthly thereafter because death, serious adverse cardio-vascular effects and stroke have occurred when the hemoglobin level became higher than 11 g/dl. Be aware that a patient who does not respond adequately over a 12-week escalation period should not have dosage increased further because effectiveness will not improve and risk of adverse reactions increases. Expect dose in this case to be the lowest possible to maintain a hemoglobin level low enough to reduce the need for red blood cell transfusions. If responsiveness does not improve, expect peginesatide therapy to be discontinued.
• Monitor patient's transferrin saturation and serum ferritin during therapy. Expect to give supplemental iron therapy when serum ferritin is less than 100 mcg/L or when serum transferrin saturation is less than 20%.
• Store unused drug contained in a multiple dose vial at 36° F to 46° F (2° C to 8° C) and discard after 28 days from date of opening vial or expiration date, whichever comes first. Remember to protect drug from light and store in original carton.

PATIENT TEACHING
• Instruct patient how to administer peginesatide subcutaneously, if prescribed, including how to withdraw drug solution into the syringe, how to administer a subcutaneous injection, sites to use and need for site rotation, storage of drug (in original carton), and proper disposal of equipment.
• Advise patient that if a dose is missed he should take it as soon as possible, and then restart peginesatide at the prescribed once-a-month schedule.
• Alert patient with a history of high blood pressure to comply with his antihypertensive therapy and dietary restrictions and to monitor his blood pressure regularly.
• Tell patient with a seizure disorder to alert prescriber of any new-onset neurologic symptoms or change in seizure frequency.
• Inform patient that he will need regular laboratory tests, and emphasize the importance of complying with testing schedule.

penbutolol sulfate
Levatol

Class and Category
Chemical class: Nonselective beta-adrenergic blocker
Therapeutic class: Antihypertensive
Pregnancy category: Not rated

Indications and Dosages
➤ *To manage hypertension*
TABLETS
Adults. 20 mg daily.
DOSAGE ADJUSTMENT For elderly patients, dosage individualized according to sensitivity to drug.

Route	Onset	Peak	Duration
P.O.	Unknown	1.5–3 hr	Unknown

Mechanism of Action
May reduce blood pressure by competing with beta-adrenergic receptor agonists, which helps reduce cardiac output, decrease sympathetic outflow to peripheral blood vessels, and inhibit renin release by kidneys.

Contraindications
Asthma, bradycardia (fewer than 45 beats/min), cardiogenic shock, heart failure, hypersensitivity to penbutolol or its components, second- or third-degree AV block

Interaction
DRUGS
allergen immunotherapy, allergenic extracts for skin testing: Increased risk of serious systemic reaction or anaphylaxis
amiodarone: Additive depressant effect on cardiac conduction, negative inotropic effects

P

anesthetics (hydrocarbon inhalation): Increased risk of myocardial depression and hypotension
calcium channel blockers, clonidine, diazoxide, guanabenz, other hypotension-producing drugs, reserpine: Additive hypotension and possibly other beta blocker effects
cimetidine: Possibly increased blood penbutolol level
digoxin: Increased risk of bradycardia
estrogens: Decreased antihypertensive effect of penbutolol
fentanyl and its derivatives: Possibly increased risk of initial bradycardia after induction doses of fentanyl derivative (with long-term penbutolol use)
insulin, oral antidiabetic drugs: Possibly impaired glucose control and masking of hypoglycemia symptoms such as tachycardia
lidocaine: Decreased lidocaine clearance, increased risk of lidocaine toxicity
MAO inhibitors: Increased risk of significant hypertension
neuromuscular blockers: Possibly potentiated and prolonged action of these drugs
NSAIDs: Possibly decreased hypotensive effect of penbutolol
other beta blockers: Additive beta blocker effects
phenothiazines: Increased blood levels of both drugs
phenytoin (parenteral): Additive cardiac depressant effects
sympathomimetics, xanthines: Possibly inhibited effects of penbutolol and these drugs

Adverse Reactions

CNS: Anxiety, depression, dizziness, drowsiness, fatigue, insomnia, lightheadedness, nervousness, syncope, weakness
CV: Bradycardia, chest pain, edema, peripheral vascular insufficiency
EENT: Nasal congestion
GI: Constipation, diarrhea, epigastric pain, nausea, vomiting
GU: Impotence
RESP: Bronchospasm, dyspnea

Nursing Considerations

• Expect varied drug effectiveness in elderly patients, who may be more sensitive to antihypertensive effects because of reduced drug clearance by kidneys.

WARNING Avoid stopping penbutolol abruptly; doing so may precipitate MI, myocardial ischemia, severe hypertension, or ventricular arrhythmias, particularly in patients with cardiovascular disease. However, be aware that use of a beta blocker such as penbutolol may impair the ability of the heart to respond to reflex adrenergic stimuli, increasing the risks of general anesthesia and surgical procedures. Watch for tachycardia because drug may also mask some signs of hyperthyroidism. Abrupt withdrawal of drug in patients with hyperthyroidism or thyrotoxicosis can precipitate thyroid storm.

• Monitor blood pressure and cardiac output, as appropriate, in patients who have a history of systolic heart failure or left ventricular dysfunction. Drug's negative inotropic effect can depress cardiac output.

• Monitor patients with diabetes mellitus who take antidiabetics because penbutolol can prolong hypoglycemia or promote hyperglycemia. It also can mask evidence of hypoglycemia, especially tachycardia, palpitations, and tremor.

• Watch for impaired circulation in elderly patients with age-related peripheral vasculardisease or patients with Raynaud's phenomenon. Elderly patients are also at increased risk for beta blocker–induced hypothermia.

• Monitor drug refill frequency to help determine patient compliance.

PATIENT TEACHING

• Instruct patient to take penbutolol at the same time every day and not to change dosage without consulting prescriber.

• Advise patient not to stop taking drug abruptly, but to taper dosage gradually under prescriber's supervision.

• Instruct patient with diabetes mellitus to regularly monitor blood glucose level and test urine for ketones.

• Advise patient to consult prescriber before taking OTC drugs, especially cold products.

• Urge patient to avoid hazardous activities until CNS effects of drug are known.

• Instruct patient to inform prescriber of chest pain, fainting, light-headedness, or shortness of breath, any of which may indicate the need for a dosage change.

• Inform patient that penbutolol doesn't cure hypertension. Encourage her to follow recommended diet and lifestyle changes.

penicillamine
Cuprimine, Depen

Class and Category
Chemical class: Degradation product of penicillin
Therapeutic class: Antirheumatic, anti-urolithic, chelating agent
Pregnancy category: D

Indications and Dosages
➤ *To treat cystinuria*
CAPSULES, TABLETS
Adults and adolescents. 500 mg four times a day
Children. 7.5 mg/kg four times a day
➤ *To treat rheumatoid arthritis*
CAPSULES, TABLETS
Adults and adolescents. *Initial:* 125 or 250 mg daily. Dosage increased by 125 or 250 mg daily every 2 to 3 mo. *Maximum:* 1,500 mg daily.
➤ *To treat Wilson's disease*
CAPSULES, TABLETS
Adults and adolescents. Dosage individualized up to 2 g daily in divided doses four times a day by measuring urinary copper excretion.
DOSAGE ADJUSTMENT For elderly patients, 125 mg daily initially, then increased by 125 mg daily every 2 to 3 mo, up to maximum of 750 mg daily. For pregnant women, maximum dose of 1 g daily. For women having planned cesarean section, dosage limited to 250 mg daily during last 6 wk of pregnancy and until wound healing completed.

Mechanism of Action
Combines with copper to form a ring-shaped complex that's excreted in urine, thereby reducing copper levels in the body. Penicillamine also lowers urine cystine levels by binding with cystine to form penicillamine-cysteine disulfide,

---

* For rheumatoid arthritis; 1 to 3 mo for Wilson's disease.

which is more soluble than cystine and more easily excreted in urine. The decrease in urine cystine level also helps prevent formation of cystine calculi and may help existing cystine calculi dissolve over time. In addition, penicillamine improves lymphocyte function by reducing IgM rheumatoid factor and immune complexes in serum and synovial fluid, which may play a role in treatment of rheumatoid arthritis.

Route	Onset	Peak	Duration
P.O.	2–3 mo	Unknown	Unknown

Contraindications
Hypersensitivity to penicillin, penicillamine, or their components; penicillamine-related aplastic anemia or agranulocytosis; renal insufficiency (for patients with rheumatoid arthritis)

Interaction
DRUGS
4-aminoquinolines, bone marrow depressants, gold compounds, immunosuppressants (excluding glucocorticoids), phenylbutazone: Possibly increased risk of serious hematologic or renal adverse reactions
iron supplements: Possibly decreased effectiveness of penicillamine
pyridoxine: Decreased effectiveness of pyridoxine, possibly increased risk of anemia or peripheral neuritis reaction

Adverse Reactions
CNS: Agitation, anxiety, fever, mental changes, myasthenic syndrome, neuropathy
EENT: Altered or loss of taste, optic neuritis, stomatitis, tinnitus
GI: Anorexia, diarrhea, hepatic dysfunction, intrahepatic cholestasis, mild epigastric pain, pancreatitis, nausea, toxic hepatitis, vomiting
GU: Glomerulonephropathy, hematuria, proteinuria, renal failure
HEME: Agranulocytosis, aplastic anemia, hemolytic anemia, leukopenia, thrombocytopenia
MS: Arthralgia, dystonia, muscle weakness

P

SKIN: Pemphigus, pruritus, rash, urticaria
Other: Lupus-like symptoms, lymphadenopathy

Nursing Considerations

- Use penicillamine cautiously in elderly patients because they're at greater risk for rash, altered taste, and renal impairment.
- Give penicillamine 1 hour before or 2 hours after meals and at least 1 hour before or after any other drug, food, or milk. Give last dose of day at least 3 hours after evening meal to maximize absorption.
- For patient who has difficulty swallowing capsules or tablets, open capsule and mix contents in 15 to 30 ml of pureed fruit or fruit juice to mask drug's sulfur odor. Alternatively, ask pharmacist to prepare elixir for oral administration.
- Expect to give 25 mg pyridoxine, as prescribed, to patients receiving penicillamine because penicillamine increases intake requirements for this vitamin.
- Watch for febrile reactions in patients who developed a fever during previous penicillamine therapy. Expect to stop drug if patient develops drug-induced fever.
- Assess skin and mucous membranes for possible sensitivity reactions, such as skin lesions and mouth ulcers. Be prepared to discontinue drug as prescribed.
- Expect to monitor urine laboratory test results twice weekly during first month of therapy, then every 2 weeks for next 5 months, and monthly thereafter. Watch for proteinuria or hematuria, which may precipitate nephrotic syndrome, especially in patients with renal disease or history of renal insufficiency. Also, weigh patient daily, watch for edema, and monitor intake and output because penicillamine may worsen underlying renal disease.
- **WARNING** Monitor patient's WBC and differential cell count, hemoglobin, and platelet count, as ordered, and assess skin, lymph nodes, and body temperature for abnormalities twice weekly during first month of therapy, then every 2 weeks for next 5 months, and monthly thereafter because drug may cause potentially serious hematologic reactions.
- Because of the potential for cross-sensitivity between penicillamine and penicillin, monitor for allergic reaction in patients with a history of penicillin allergy.
- Notify prescriber if patient reports decreased sense of taste, especially for salty and sweet foods. Expect normal taste sensation to be restored (except in patients with Wilson's disease) by giving of 5 to 10 mg of copper a day, as prescribed.
- Monitor patients with diabetes mellitus for reduced insulin requirements to prevent risk of nighttime hypoglycemia because penicillamine may promote formation of anti-insulin antibodies.
- Check liver function tests, as ordered, every 6 months (every 3 months for first year if patient has Wilson's disease) during penicillamine therapy because drug may cause serious hepatic dysfunction.

PATIENT TEACHING

- Advise patient to take penicillamine on an empty stomach.
- Instruct men and nonpregnant women with cystinuria to increase fluid intake and follow prescribed low-methionine diet to minimize cystine production and enhance drug's effectiveness. Urge patient to drink about 1 pint of fluid at bedtime and again during the night because this is when urine is more concentrated.
- Tell patient to notify prescriber immediately if he develops a fever, sore throat, chills, bruising, or bleeding because drug may need to be stopped.
- Instruct patient being treated for Wilson's disease to follow a diet low in copper, avoiding such foods as broccoli, chocolate, copper-enriched cereals, liver, molasses, mushrooms, nuts, and shellfish. Inform her that it may take 1 to 3 months of therapy for her condition to improve.
- Advise patient to consult prescriber before having dental work done during penicillamine therapy because drug can promote mouth ulcers.
- Instruct patient to avoid consuming iron during penicillamine therapy because iron can decrease drug's effectiveness.
- Explain that sense of taste may decrease during penicillamine therapy. Advise patient to notify prescriber if it becomes intolerable.

• Inform patient with rheumatoid arthritis that improvement may take 2 to 3 months of therapy.
• Caution female patient to notify prescriber immediately if she becomes or may be pregnant because dosage may need to be reduced to prevent serious birth defects.

penicillin G benzathine

Bicillin C-R, Bicillin C-R 900/300, Bicillin L-A, Megacillin (CAN), Permapen

penicillin G potassium

Megacillin (CAN), Pentids, Pfizerpen

penicillin G procaine

Ayercillin (CAN), Crysticillin 300 AS, Pfizerpen-AS, Wycillin

penicillin G sodium

penicillin V potassium

Apo-Pen-VK (CAN), Beepen-VK, Betapen-VK, Ledercillin VK, Nadopen-V 200 (CAN), Nadopen-V 400 (CAN), Novo-Pen-VK (CAN), Nu-Pen VK (CAN), Pen Vee (CAN), Pen Vee K, V-Cillin K (CAN), Veetids

Class and Category
Chemical class: Penicillin
Therapeutic class: Antibiotic
Pregnancy category: B

Indications and Dosages
➤ To treat systemic infections caused by gram-positive organisms (including Bacillus anthracis, uorynebacterium diphtheriae, enterococci, Listeria monocytogenes, Staphylococcus aureus,and S. epidermidis), gram-negative organisms (including Neisseria gonorrhoeae, N. meningitidis, Pasteurella multocida, and Streptobacillus moniliformis [rat-bite fever]), and gram-positive anaerobes (including Actinomyces israelii [actinomycosis], Clostridium perfringens, C. tetani, Peptococcus species, Peptostreptococcusspecies, and spirochetes, especially Treponema carateum [pinta], T. pallidum, and u. pertenue [yaws])

ORAL SOLUTION, TABLETS (PENICILLIN G POTASSIUM)
Adults and adolescents. 200,000 to 500,000 units (125 to 312 mg) every 4 to 6 hr. Maximum: 2 million units daily.
Children. 4,167 to 15,000 units/kg every 4 hr, 6,250 to 22,500 units/kg every 6 hr, or 8,333 to 30,000 units/kg every 8 hr.

TABLETS (PENICILLIN V POTASSIUM)
Adults and adolescents. 200,000 to 800,000 units (125 to 500 mg) every 6 to 8 hr. Maximum: 11,520,000 units (7,200 mg) daily
Children. 4,167 to 13,280 units (2.5 to 8.3 mg)/kg every 4 hr, 6,250 to 20,000 units (3.75 to 12.5 mg)/kg every 6 hr, or 8,333 to 26,720 units (5 to 16.7 mg)/kg every 8 hr.

I.V. INFUSION, I.M. INJECTION (PENICILLIN G POTASSIUM, PENICILLIN G SODIUM)
Adults and adolescents. 1 to 5 million units every 4 to 6 hr. Maximum: 80 million units daily.
Children. 8,333 to 16,667 units/kg every 4 hr or 12,500 to 25,000 units/kg every 6 hr.
Premature and full-term neonates. 30,000 units/kg every 12 hr.

I.M. INJECTION (PENICILLIN G PROCAINE)
Adults and adolescents. 600,000 to 1,200,000 units daily in divided doses every 12 to 24 hr.

➤ To treat moderately severe to severe streptococcal infections

I.M. INJECTION (PENICILLIN G BENZATHINE)
Adults and children weighing more than 45 kg (100 lb). 1.2 million units as a single injection.
Children weighing 27 to 45 kg (59 to 100 lb). 900,000 units as a single injection.
Children weighing less than 27 kg. 300,000 to 600,000 units as single injection.

➤ To treat congenital syphilis

I.M. INJECTION (PENICILLIN G BENZATHINE: BICILLIN L-A ONLY)
Children under age 2. 50,000 units/kg as a single injection.

P

➤ *To treat syphilis of less than 1 year's duration*

I.M. INJECTION (PENICILLIN G BENZATHINE: BICILLIN L-A ONLY)

Adults and adolescents. 2.4 million units as a single injection.
Children. 50,000 units/kg up to adult dosage as a single injection. *Maximum:* 2.4 million units/dose.

➤ *To treat syphilis of more than 1 year's duration*

I.M. INJECTION (PENICILLIN G BENZATHINE: BICILLIN L-A ONLY)

Adults and adolescents. 2.4 million units every wk for 3 wk.
Children. 50,000 units/kg every wk for 3 wk.

➤ *To treat bacterial meningitis*

I.V. INFUSION, I.M. INJECTION (PENICILLIN G POTASSIUM)

Adults. 50,000 units/kg every 4 hr or 24 million units daily in divided doses every 2 to 4 hr.

Mechanism of Action

Inhibits final stage of bacterial cell wall synthesis by competitively binding to penicillin-binding proteins inside the cell wall. Penicillin-binding proteins are responsible for various steps in bacterial cell wall synthesis. By binding to these proteins, penicillin leads to cell wall lysis.

Incompatibilities

Don't mix any penicillin in the same syringe or container with aminoglycosides because aminoglycosides will be inactivated. Don't mix penicillin G with drugs that may result in a pH below 5.5 or above 8.

Contraindications

Hypersensitivity to penicillin or its components

Interaction

DRUGS

ACE inhibitors, potassium-containing drugs, potassium-sparing diuretics: Increased risk of hyperkalemia (penicillin G potassium)
chloramphenicol, erythromycin, sulfonamides, tetracycline, thrombolytics: Possibly interference with penicillin's bactericidal effect
cholestyramine, colestipol: Possibly impaired absorption of oral penicillin G

methotrexate: Decreased methotrexate clearance, increased risk of toxicity
oral contraceptives: Decreased contraceptive effectiveness (with penicillin V)
probenecid: Increased blood penicillin level

FOODS

acidic beverages, such as fruit juices: Possibly altered effects of oral penicillin G

Adverse Reactions

CNS: Confusion, dizziness, dysphasia, hallucinations, headache, lethargy, sciatic nerve irritation, seizures
CV: Labile blood pressure, palpitations
EENT: Black "hairy" tongue, oral candidiasis, stomatitis, taste perversion
GI: Abdominal pain, diarrhea, elevated liver function test results (transient), indigestion, nausea, pseudomembranous colitis
GU: Interstitial nephritis (acute), vaginal candidiasis
MS: Muscle twitching
SKIN: Rash
Other: Electrolyte imbalances; injection-site necrosis, pain, or redness

Nursing Considerations

• Obtain body tissue and fluid samples for culture and sensitivity tests as ordered before giving first dose. Expect to begin drug therapy before test results are known.
• Reconstitute vials of penicillin for injection with sterile water for injection, D_5W, or sodium chloride for injection.
• Administer penicillin at least 1 hour before other antibiotics.
• Inject I.M. form deep into large muscle mass. Apply ice to relieve pain.
WARNING Give penicillin G benzathine and penicillin G procaine only by deep I.M. injection; I.V. injection may be fatal, and intra-arterial injection may cause extensive tissue and organ necrosis.
• Be aware that I.M. drug is absorbed slowly, which may make allergic reactions difficult to treat.
• Assess patient for signs of secondary infection, such as profuse, watery diarrhea.If such diarrhea develops, contact prescriber and expect to obtain a stool specimen to rule out pseudomembranous colitis caused by *Clostridium difficile*. If diarrhea occurs, notify prescriber and expect to withhold pencillin and treat with

fluids, electrolytes, protein, and an antibiotic effective against *C. difficile.*

• Monitor serum sodium level and assess for early signs of heart failure in patients receiving high doses of penicillin G sodium.

• When giving penicillin G potassium to patient at risk for hypertension or fluid overload, be aware that each gram of pencillin G potassium also contains 1.02 mEq of sodium.

PATIENT TEACHING

• Instruct patient to report previous allergies to penicillins and to notify prescriber immediately about adverse reactions, including fever.

• Advise patient who uses oral contraceptives to use an additional form of contraception during penicillin V therapy.

• Urge patient to tell prescriber if diarrhea develops, even 2 months or more after penicillin therapy ends.

pentazocine lactate

Talwin

Class, Category, and Schedule

Chemical class: Synthetic opioid
Therapeutic class: Analgesic
Pregnancy category: C
Controlled substance schedule: IV

Indications and Dosages

➤ *To relieve moderate to severe pain*
I.V., I.M., OR SUBCUTANEOUS INJECTION
Adults. *Initial:* 30 mg every 3 to 4 hr, as needed. *Maximum:* 30 mg/single dose I.V., 60 mg/single dose I.M. or subcutaneously, or 360 mg/24 hr for all parenteral forms.
➤ *To relieve obstetric pain*
I.V. INJECTION
Adults. 20 mg when contractions become regular; repeated 2 or 3 times every 2 to 3 hr, as needed.
I.M. INJECTION
Adults. 30 mg as a single dose.

Route	Onset	Peak	Duration
I.V.	2–3 min	15–30 min	2–3 hr
I.M., SubQ	15–20 min	30–60 min	2–3 hr

Mechanism of Action

Binds with opioid receptors, mainly kappa and sigma receptors, at many CNS sites to alter perception of and emotional response to pain.

Incompatibilities

Don't mix pentazocine in same syringe with a soluble barbiturate because precipitation will occur.

Contraindications

Hypersensitivity to pentazocine or its components

Interaction

DRUGS

anticholinergics: Increased risk of urine retention and severe constipation
antidiarrheals, antiperistaltics: Increased risk of severe constipation and CNS depression
antihypertensives, diuretics, other hypotension-producing drugs: Additive hypotensive effects
buprenorphine: Decreased pentazocine effectiveness, increased respiratory depression
CNS depressants: Increased CNS depression, increased risk of habituation
hydroxyzine, other opioid analgesics: Increased analgesia, CNS depression, and hypotensive effects
MAO inhibitors: Increased risk of unpredictable, severe, even fatal adverse reactions
metoclopramide: Antagonized metoclopramide effects on GI motility
naloxone: Antagonized analgesic, CNS, and respiratory depressant effects of pentazocine
naltrexone: Withdrawal symptoms in patients physically dependent on pentazocine
neuromuscular blockers: Increased respiratory depression

ACTIVITIES

alcohol use: Additive CNS depression and increased risk of habituation
smoking: Decreased effectiveness

Adverse Reactions

CNS: Chills, confusion, depression, dizziness, drowsiness, euphoria, fatigue, headache, increased intracranial pressure, hallucinations, insomnia, light-headedness, nervousness, nightmares, paresthesia, restlessness, seizures, syncope, weakness

P

CV: Hypertension, hypotension, tachycardia
EENT: Blurred vision, diplopia, dry mouth, laryngeal edema, laryngospasm, miosis
GI: Anorexia, biliary tract spasm, constipation, diarrhea, hepatotoxicity, nausea, vomiting
GU: Decreased urine output, dysuria, urinary frequency, urine retention
HEME: Agranulocytosis, transient eosinophilia
MS: Muscle rigidity (with large doses)
RESP: Atelectasis, bronchospasm, depressed respirations, dyspnea, hypoventilation, wheezing
SKIN: Diaphoresis, erythema multiforme, facial flushing, pruritus, rash, Stevens-Johnson syndrome, toxic epidermal necrolysis, urticaria
Other: Anaphylaxis, facial edema; injection-site burning, pain, redness, or swelling; physical and psychological dependence

Nursing Considerations

• Use pentazocine with extreme caution in patients with head injury, intracranial lesion, or increased intracranial pressure. Drug may mask neurologic evidence.
• Use pentazocine cautiously: in patients physically dependent on opioid agonists because drug may prompt withdrawal symptoms; in patients with acute MI because drug's cardiovascular effects can increase cardiac workload; in patients with renal or hepatic dysfunction because drug is metabolized in liver and excreted in urine; and in patients with respiratory conditions or who are debilitated or elderly because drug depresses respiratory system.
• When giving repeated parenteral doses, use I.M. or I.V. route when possible and as prescribed because subcutaneous route may cause severe tissue damage at injection site. Rotate I.M. sites to avoid tissue damage.
• After giving parenteral form, expect to taper dosage gradually, as prescribed, to reduce the risk of withdrawal symptoms.

PATIENT TEACHING
• Caution patient that prolonged use of pentazocine may result in dependence.

• Advise patient to avoid hazardous activities until drug's CNS effects are known.
• Caution patient not to use alcohol or OTC drugs without consulting prescriber.
• Advise patient to report possible allergic reaction, such as a rash or itching.

pentobarbital sodium

Nembutal, Nova Rectal (CAN), Novopentobarb (CAN)

Class, Category, and Schedule
Chemical class: Barbiturate
Therapeutic class: Anticonvulsant, sedative-hypnotic
Pregnancy category: D
Controlled substance schedule: II (oral, parenteral), III (rectal)

Indications and Dosages
➤ *To provide daytime sedation*
ELIXIR
Adults. 20 mg three times a day or four times a day.
Children. 2 to 6 mg/kg daily.
SUPPOSITORIES
Adults. 30 mg twice daily to four times a day.
Children. 2 mg/kg three times a day.
➤ *To provide short-term treatment of insomnia*
CAPSULES, ELIXIR
Adults. 100 mg at bedtime.
I.V. INJECTION
Adults. *Initial:* 100 mg, with additional small doses at 1-min intervals, as prescribed. *Maximum:* 500 mg.
I.M. INJECTION
Adults. 150 to 200 mg at bedtime.
SUPPOSITORIES
Adults and adolescents over age 14. 120 to 200 mg at bedtime.
Children ages 12 to 14. 60 to 120 mg at bedtime.
Children ages 5 to 12. 60 mg at bedtime.
Children ages 1 to 4. 30 to 60 mg at bedtime.
Infants ages 2 months to 1 year. 30 mg at bedtime.

➤ *To provide preoperative sedation*
CAPSULES, ELIXIR
Adults. 100 mg before surgery.
Children. 2 to 6 mg/kg before surgery.
Maximum: 100 mg/dose.
I.M. INJECTION
Adults. 150 to 200 mg before surgery.
Children. 2 to 6 mg/kg before surgery.
Maximum: 100 mg/dose.
SUPPOSITORIES
Children ages 12 to 14. 60 to 120 mg before surgery.
Children ages 5 to 12. 60 mg before surgery.
Children ages 1 to 4. 30 to 60 mg before surgery.
Infants ages 2 months to 1 year. 30 mg before surgery.

➤ *To provide emergency treatment of seizures associated with eclampsia, meningitis, status epilepticus, tetanus, or toxic reactions to local anesthetics or strychnine*
I.V. INJECTION
Adults. 100 mg, with additional small doses at 1-min intervals, as prescribed. *Maximum:* 500 mg.
Children. 50 mg, with additional small doses at 1-min intervals, as prescribed, until desired effect occurs.
I.M. INJECTION
Children. 50 mg, with additional small doses at 1-min intervals, as prescribed, until desired effect occurs.
DOSAGE ADJUSTMENT Dosage possibly reduced for elderly or debilitated patients and those with hepatic dysfunction.

Route	Onset	Peak	Duration
P.O., P.R.	15–60 min	1–4 hr	3–4 hr
I.V.	In 1 min	Unknown	15 min
I.M.	10–25 min	Unknown	3–4 hr

Mechanism of Action
Inhibits ascending conduction in reticular formation, which controls CNS arousal to produce drowsiness, hypnosis, and sedation. Pentobarbital also decreases spread of seizure activity in cortex, thalamus, and limbic system. It promotes an increased threshold for electrical stimulation in the motor cortex, which may contribute to anticonvulsant effects.

Contraindications
Hepatic disease; history of addiction to hypnotics or sedatives; hypersensitivity to pentobarbital, barbiturates, or their components; nephritis; porphyria; severe respiratory disease with airway obstruction or dyspnea

Interaction
DRUGS
acetaminophen: Possibly decreased effects of acetaminophen (long-term pentobarbital use)
carbamazepine, chloramphenicol, corticosteroids, cyclosporine, dacarbazine, digoxin, disopyramide, doxycycline, griseofulvin, metronidazole, oral contraceptives, phenylbutazone, quinidine, theophyllines, vitamin D: Decreased effectiveness of these drugs
CNS depressants: Increased CNS depression and risk of habituation
divalproex sodium, valproic acid: Increased risk of CNS toxicity and neurotoxicity
guanadrel, guanethidine: Possibly increased risk of orthostatic hypotension
halogenated hydrocarbon anesthetic: Increased risk of hepatotoxicity (with long-term pentobarbital use)
haloperidol: Possibly decreased blood haloperidol level, possibly altered seizure pattern or frequency
hydantoins: Possibly interference with hydantoin metabolism
leucovorin: Possibly decreased anticonvulsant effect of pentobarbital
maprotiline: Possibly enhanced CNS depression and decreased therapeutic effects of pentobarbital
mexiletine: Possibly decreased blood mexiletine level
oral anticoagulants: Possibly decreased effects of these drugs, possibly increased risk of bleeding when pentobarbital stops
tricyclic antidepressants: Possibly decreased therapeutic effects of these drugs
ACTIVITIES
alcohol use: Increased CNS depression

Adverse Reactions
CNS: Agitation, anxiety, ataxia, confusion, delusions, depression, dizziness, drowsiness, fever, hallucinations, headache, insomnia, irritability, nervousness, nightmares, paradoxical stimulation, seizures, syncope, tremor

P

CV: Orthostatic hypotension
EENT: Vision changes
GI: Anorexia, constipation, hepatic dysfunction, nausea, vomiting
HEME: Agranulocytosis
MS: Arthralgia, bone pain, muscle twitching or weakness
RESP: Respiratory depression
SKIN: Exfoliative dermatitis, rash, Stevens-Johnson syndrome
Other: Physical and psychological dependence, weight loss

Nursing Considerations
• Use pentobarbital with extreme caution in patients with depression, a history of drug abuse, or suicidal tendencies.
• Use drug cautiously in elderly or debilitated patients and those with acute or chronic pain because it may induce paradoxical stimulation.
• When using I.V. route, inject drug at 50 mg/min or less to avoid adverse respiratory and circulatory reactions.
• If patient shows premonitory signs of hepatic coma, withhold drug and notify prescriber immediately.
• Monitor I.V. site closely and avoid extravasation. Drug is highly alkaline and may cause local tissue damage and necrosis.

PATIENT TEACHING
• Inform patient that pentobarbital is habit-forming, and stress the importance of taking it exactly as prescribed.
• Instruct patient who takes elixir form to use a calibrated measuring device and to close container tightly after use.
• Instruct patient who uses suppositories to refrigerate them.
• Advise patient to avoid hazardous activities until drug's CNS effects are known.
• Urge patient to avoid alcohol and other CNS depressants because they may increase drug's adverse CNS effects.

pentosan polysulfate sodium
Elmiron

Class and Category
Chemical class: Low-molecular-weight heparin-like compound
Therapeutic class: Local anti-inflammatory (bladder-specific)
Pregnancy category: B

Indications and Dosages
➤ *To relieve bladder discomfort or pain caused by interstitial cystitis*
CAPSULES
Adults. 100 mg three times a day for up to 3 mo, possibly followed by another 3 mo if no improvement and no adverse reactions.

Mechanism of Action
Adheres to mucosal membrane of bladder wall and may block irritating solutes from reaching cells, thereby decreasing local pain and discomfort.

Contraindications
Hypersensitivity to pentosan, other structurally related compounds, or their components

Interaction
DRUGS
alteplase (recombinant), aspirin (high doses), heparin, oral anticoagulants, streptokinase: Increased risk of hemorrhage

Adverse Reactions
CNS: Depression, dizziness, emotional lability, headache
GI: Abdominal pain, diarrhea, elevated liver enzyme levels, hepatic dysfunction, indigestion, nausea, rectal hemorrhage
HEME: Unusual bleeding or bruising
SKIN: Alopecia, rash

Nursing Considerations
• Use pentosan with extreme caution in patients with conditions that increase bleeding risk, such as aneurysm, diverticula, GI ulceration, hemophilia, polyps, and thrombocytopenia (especially heparin-induced).
• Use drug cautiously in patients with hepatic dysfunction because drug is desulfated in liver and spleen.
• Monitor patient for abnormal bleeding, such as unexplained bruises and epistaxis, because drug is a weak anticoagulant.

• Instruct patient to take pentosan with a full glass of water at least 1 hour before or 2 hours after meals.
• Explain the pattern of exacerbations and remissions with interstitial cystitis. Reassure patient that symptoms should improve within 3 months after starting pentosan therapy.
• Advise patient to take bleeding precautions during therapy, such as using an electric shaver and a soft-bristled toothbrush.
• If alopecia develops, explain that it's usually confined to a single area.

pentoxifylline

Trental

Class and Category

Chemical class: Xanthine derivative
Therapeutic class: Blood viscosity reducer
Pregnancy category: C

Indications and Dosages

➤ *To treat peripheral vascular disease*

E.R. TABLETS

Adults. 400 mg three times a day with meals.

DOSAGE ADJUSTMENT For patients who have severe renal impairment (creatinine clearance below 30 ml/min), dosage reduced to 400 mg once a day. For patients who experience adverse GI or CNS reactions, dosage may be reduced to 400 mg twice daily.

Route	Onset	Peak	Duration
P.O.	2–4 wk	Unknown	Unknown

Mechanism of Action

Relieves symptoms of peripheral vascular disease by:
• reducing blood viscosity by decreasing plasma fibrinogen level and inhibiting RBC and platelet aggregation
• improving erythrocyte flexibility by inhibiting phosphodiesterase and increasing the amount of cAMP in RBCs
• decreasing peripheral vascular resistance and improving microcirculatory blood flow and tissue oxygenation.

Contraindications

Hypersensitivity to pentoxifylline, methylxanthines (such as caffeine, theophylline, and theobromine), or their components; recent cerebral or retinal hemorrhage

Interaction

DRUGS

antihypertensives: Potentiated antihypertensive effects
heparin, oral anticoagulants, other platelet aggregation inhibitors, plicamycin, thrombolytics, valproic acid: Increased risk of bleeding
cimetidine: Increased blood pentoxifylline level, increased risk of adverse effects
sympathomimetics, xanthines: Enhanced CNS stimulation
vitamin K antagonists: Increased anticoagulant activity

ACTIVITIES

smoking: Possibly decreased therapeutic effects of pentoxifylline

Adverse Reactions

CNS: Agitation, anxiety, aseptic meningitis, confusion, depression, dizziness, drowsiness, headache, insomnia, malaise, nervousness, seizures, tremor
CV: Angina, arrhythmia, chest pain, edema, hypotension, palpitation, tachycardia
EENT: Bad taste, blurred vision, conjunctivitis, dry mouth, earache, epistaxis, excessive salivation, laryngitis, nasal congestion, scotoma, sore throat, swollen neck glands
GI: Abdominal discomfort, anorexia, belching, bloating, cholecystitis, constipation, diarrhea, dyspepsia, elevated liver enzymes, flatus, hepatitis, indigestion, jaundice, nausea, vomiting
HEME: Aplastic anemia, decreased serum fibrinogen, leukemia, leukopenia, pancytopenia, purpura, thrombocytopenia
RESP: Dyspnea
SKIN: Brittle nails, flushing, pruritus, rash, urticaria
Other: Anaphylaxis, angioedema, flulike symptoms, thirst, weight changes

Nursing Considerations

• Use pentoxifylline cautiously in elderly patients and those with hepatic or renal dysfunction.

P

• Give drug with meals and an antacid, if needed, to reduce adverse GI reactions. **WARNING** Monitor patient closely for hypersensitivity reactions that could be life-threatening. At the first sign of anaphylactic or anaphylactoid reaction, stop pentoxifylline therapy, notify prescriber, and provide supportive care.

PATIENT TEACHING
• Instruct patient to swallow pentoxifylline E.R. tablets whole and not to crush, break, or chew them.
• Advise patient to take drug with meals to reduce GI irritation. If adverse GI reactions occur anyway, advise her to also take an antacid with meals.
• Although symptoms may not improve for several weeks, urge patient to continue taking drug as prescribed to achieve maximum therapeutic effect.
• Instruct patient not to smoke during therapy because smoking constricts blood vessels and may reduce drug effectiveness.
• Urge patient to report adverse reactions; dosage may need reduction.

perampanel

Fycompa

Class and Category
Chemical class: Benzonitrile hydrate
Therapeutic class: Anticonvulsant
Pregnancy category: C

Indications and Dosages
➤ *Adjunct therapy for treatment of partial-onset seizures in patients with epilepsy*

TABLETS
Adults and children 12 years and older (not receiving enzyme-inducing AED).
Initial: 2 mg once daily at bedtime, then increased every week in increments of 2 mg per day to a daily dose of 4 mg to 8 mg daily at bedtime. As needed, dosage may then be increased every week in increments of 2 mg per day to a daily dose of 10 mg to 12 mg once daily at at bedtime. *Usual:* 8 mg to 12 mg once daily at at bedtime.
Maximum: 12 mg daily at bedtime.
DOSAGE ADJUSTMENT For elderly patients, dosage titration done every 2 wk. For

patients already receiving enzyme-inducing AEDs such as carbamazepine, oxcarbazepine, or phenytoin, initial dosage begun at 4 mg once daily at hs. When enzyme-inducing therapy is discontinued or introduced anew, dosage adjustment may be required. For patients with mild to moderate hepatic impairment, dosage titration done every 2 wk in 2 mg increments until target dose is achieved. For patients with mild hepatic impairment, maximum daily dosage is 6 mg daily at hs; for patients with moderate hepatic impairment, maximum daily dosage is 4 mg daily at hs. For patients with moderate renal impairment, a slower titration may be considered.

Mechanism of Action
Acts as a noncompetitive antagonist on the AMPA glutamate receptor on postsynaptic neurons. Glutamate is the primary excitatory neurotransmitter in the central nervous system. By preventing glutamate action, the central nervous system experiences less stimulation, resulting in less seizure activity in the brain.

Contraindications
Hypersensitivity to perampanel or its components

Interaction
DRUGS
CNS depressants: Possibly increased CNS depression
cytochrome P450 (CYP) inducers such as carbamazepine, phenytoin, oxcarbazepine, rifampin, St. John's wort: Significant decreased plasma perampanel levels
implant or oral contraceptives containing levonorgestrel: Possibly less effectiveness of contraceptive
ACTIVITIES
alcohol: Possibly increased CNS depression

Adverse Reactions
CNS: Abnormal coordination, affect lability, aggression, agitation, anger, anxiety, asthenia, ataxia, belligerence possibly leading to physical assault and homicidal ideation, confusion, depression, dizziness, euphoria, fatigue, gait disturbance, headache, hostility, hypersomnia, hypoaesthesia, increased fall risk, irritability, memory impairment, mood alteration, paresthesia, somnolence, suicidal

ideation, worsening of preexisting
psychiatric conditions, vertigo
CV: Peripheral edema
EENT: Blurred vision, diplopia,
oropharyngeal pain
GI: Constipation, nausea, vomiting
MS: Arthralgia; back, extremity or
musculoskeletal pain; dysarthria; myalgia
RESP: Cough, upper respiratory infections
Other: Hyponatremia, weight gain

Nursing Considerations

• Monitor patient closely for adverse
reactions, especially the patient receiving
12 mg/day because of increased risk of
adverse reactions at that dosage.
• Monitor patient for psychiatric and
behavioral reactions, as perampanel may
induce serious reactions leading to
hostility and even become life-threatening,
with possibility of physical assault or
homicidal ideation occurring. These
adverse reactions have occurred in
patients without prior psychiatric history,
prior aggressive behavior, or concomitant
use of medications associated with
hostility and aggression. Patients with
preexisting psychiatric conditions
sometimes become worse, and use of
alcohol significantly worsens mood and
increases anger. Most often these reactions
appear within the first 6 weeks of therapy,
although new events may occur at any
time during therapy. Notify prescriber
immediately if adverse psychiatric or
behavioral reactions occur. Perampanel
dosage may need to be reduced or drug
therapy temporarily withheld or
discontinued.
• Monitor patient closely for depression that
may lead to suicidal ideation, especially
when perampanel therapy is begun and
when dosage is increased.
• Monitor patient, especially the elderly, for
dizziness and gait disturbance. Encourage
patient to ask for help when getting out of
bed or chair or when ambulating,
especiallyduring the titration phase. Notify
prescriber if such reactions occur, as
dosage may need to be altered or drug
discontinued.
• Be aware that perampanel therapy
increases risk of falls, especially in the
elderly. Monitor patient's movements

closely and put safety measures in place to
help prevent falls.
• Monitor patient's weight because drug can
cause weight gain.
• Expect to withdraw perampanel therapy
gradually when discontinued, if possible,
because abrupt withdrawal can increase
risk of seizures.

PATIENT TEACHING

• Advise patient to take drug exactly as
prescribed.
• Caution patient to avoid performing
activities that require alertness, such as
driving, until effects of drug are known.
• Instruct patient to avoid ingesting alcohol
products while taking perampanel because
the combination can significantly worsen
mood and increase anger, which may lead
to physical assault and homicidal ideation.
• Instruct patient and family members or
caregivers to be on the alert for new onset
or worsening of depression, any unusual
changes in mood or behavior, or
expressions of thoughts about self-harm,
especially when dosage of drug is being
increased or higher doses are prescribed.
Report changes to prescriber immediately.
• Warn patient and family that perampanel
may increase risk of falls. Safety measures
should be implemented to reduce risk.

perindopril erbumine

Aceon

Class and Category

Chemical class: Perindoprilat prodrug
Therapeutic class: Antihypertensive
Pregnancy category: D

Indications and Dosages

➤ *To manage hypertension*
TABLETS
Adults. *Initial:* 4 mg daily as a single dose or
in divided doses twice daily, increased as
prescribed until blood pressure is controlled
or maximum dosage is reached. *Maintenance:*
4 to 8 mg daily. *Maximum:* 8 mg daily.
DOSAGE ADJUSTMENT If patient takes a
diuretic, initial dosage possibly reduced to
2 to 4 mg daily; if patient has renal failure,
initial dosage possibly reduced to 2 mg daily.

P

➤ *To reduce risk of cardiovascular death or nonfatal MI in patients with stable coronary artery disease*

TABLETS

Adults. *Initial:* 4 mg daily for 2 wk; then increased to 8 mg daily. *Maintenance:* 8 mg daily.

DOSAGE ADJUSTMENT If patient is elderly, 2 mg daily for 1 wk, increased to 4 mg daily for 1 wk and then to 8 mg daily if tolerated.

Mechanism of Action

Is converted to the active metabolite perindoprilat, which competes with angiotensin I binding sites, blocking conversion of angiotensin I to angiotensin II, a potent vaso-constrictor. As a result, this ACE inhibitor reduces vasoconstriction and blood pressure. Decreased angiotensin II also reduces aldo-sterone secretion, increasing renal excretion of water and sodium.

Contraindications

Concurrent aliskiren therapy in patients with diabetes or renal impairment (GRF less than 60 ml/min); history of angioedema with ACE inhibitor treatment; hypersensitivity to perindopril, other ACE inhibitors, or their components

Interaction

DRUGS

aliskiren (patients with diabetes or renal impairment), angiotensin-converting-enzyme (ACE) inhibitors, angiotensin receptor blockers (ARDs): Increased risks of hyperkalemia, hypotension, or changes in renal function such as acute renal failure
diuretics: Increased risk of hypotension
lithium: Increased blood lithium level and risk of toxicity
potassium-sparing diuretics, potassium supplements: Increased risk of hyperkalemia
NSAIDs: Increased risk of renal impairment in patients who are elderly, volume-depleted, or already have renal dysfunction
sodium aurothiomalate: Increased risk of nitritoid reaction with facial flushing, nausea, vomiting, and hypotension

Adverse Reactions

CNS: Amnesia, anxiety, dizziness, fatigue, fever, headache, hypertonia, migraine, syncope, vertigo

CV: Chest pain, ECG changes, heart murmur, hypotension, orthostatic hypotension, palpitations, PVCs
EENT: Conjunctivitis, earache, epistaxis, hoarseness, pharyngitis, rhinitis, sinusitis, sneezing, tinnitus
GI: Abdominal pain, diarrhea, elevated liver function test results, flatulence, increased appetite, indigestion
GU: Flank pain, renal calculi, urinary frequency and urgency, vaginitis
HEME: Hematoma, leukopenia, neutropenia
MS: Arthritis, back pain, gout, limb pain, myalgia, neck pain
RESP: Cough
SKIN: Canker sores, diaphoresis, dry skin, ecchymosis, erythema, pruritus, rash
Other: Angioedema, facial edema

Nursing Considerations

• Use cautiously with heart failure, renal artery stenosis, or renal dysfunction.
• Also use cautiously in elderly patients, and watch closely for adverse effects such as dizziness or vertigo, because these patients have an increased risk of falling.
• Monitor patients with hepatic dysfunction for enhanced therapeutic drug effects because drug's bioavailability is increased.
• Monitor serum potassium level to detect hyperkalemia, especially in patients with renal insufficiency or diabetes mellitus, and those who use a potassium-containing salt substitute or take a potassium-sparing diuretic or potassium supplement.

PATIENT TEACHING

• Instruct patient to take perindopril exactly as prescribed, even if she feels well.
WARNING Urge patient to stop taking drug and notify prescriber immediately if she experiences signs of angioedema.
• Advise patient to notify prescriber at once about fever, sore throat, or other signs that may indicate neutropenia.
• Urge patient to avoid potassium supplements and potassium-containing salt substitutes unless prescriber approves.
• Instruct patient to avoid hazardous activities until drug's CNS effects are known.
• Advise woman to report promptly suspected, known, or intended pregnancy. Drug will need to be discontinued.

perphenazine

Apo-Perphenazine (CAN), PMS Perphenazine (CAN), Trilafon, Trilafon Concentrate

Class and Category

Chemical class: Piperazine phenothiazine
Therapeutic class: Antiemetic, antipsychotic *Pregnancy category:* Not rated

Indications and Dosages

➤ *To treat psychotic disorders*

ORAL SOLUTION

Hospitalized adults and adolescents. 8 to 16 mg twice daily to four times a day, adjusted as needed and tolerated. *Maximum:* 64 mg daily.

TABLETS

Adults and adolescents. 4 to 16 mg twice daily to four times daily, adjusted as needed and tolerated. *Maximum:* 64 mg daily.

I.M. INJECTION

Adults and adolescents. 5 to 10 mg every 6 hr, adjusted as needed and tolerated. *Maximum:* 15 mg daily for outpatients, 30 mg daily for hospitalized patients.

➤ *To treat severe nausea and vomiting*

TABLETS

Adults and adolescents. 8 to 16 mg daily in divided doses, decreased as appropriate. *Maximum:* 24 mg daily.

I.V. INFUSION OR INJECTION

Adults and adolescents. 1 mg every 1 to 2 min, up to 5 mg total.

I.M. INJECTION

Adults and adolescents. 5 mg, increased to 10 mg as ordered for rapid control of severe vomiting. *Maximum:* 15 mg daily for outpatients, 30 mg daily for hospitalized patients.

DOSAGE ADJUSTMENT Initial dose possibly reduced and gradually increased for elderly, emaciated, or debilitated patients. Adolescents may need low adult dosage.

Route	Onset	Peak	Duration
P.O.	Several wk	4–7 days	Unknown
I.M.	Unknown	1–2 hr	6 hr

Mechanism of Action

Depresses areas of the brain that control activity and aggression, including cerebral cortex, hypothalamus, and limbic system, by an unknown mechanism. Perphenazine also prevents nausea and vomiting by inhibiting or blocking dopamine receptors in medullary chemoreceptor trigger zone and peripherally by blocking vagus nerve in the GI tract.

Incompatibilities

Don't mix perphenazine oral solution with beverages that contain caffeine or tannins (such as coffee, colas, and teas) or pectinates (such as apple juice) because they're physically incompatible.

Contraindications

Blood dyscrasias; bone marrow depression; cerebral arteriosclerosis; coma; concurrent use of CNS depressants (large doses); coronary artery disease; hepatic impairment; hypersensitivity to perphenazine, other phenothiazines, or their components; myeloproliferative disorders; severe CNS depression; severe hypertension or hypotension; subcortical brain damage

Interaction

DRUGS

aluminum- and magnesium-containing antacids, antidiarrheals (adsorbent): Decreased absorption of oral perphenazine
amantadine, anticholinergics, antidyskinetics, antihistamines: Increased adverse anticholinergic effects
amphetamines: Decreased therapeutic effects of both drugsanticonvulsants: Decreased seizure threshold, inhibited metabolism and toxicity of anticonvulsant
antithyroid drugs: Increased risk of agranulocytosis
apomorphine: Additive CNS depression, decreased emetic response to apomorphine if perphenazine is given first
appetite suppressants (except phenmetrazine): Antagonized anorectic effect of appetite suppressants
beta blockers: Increased blood levels of both drugs and risk of arrhythmias, hypotension, irreversible retinopathy, and tardive dyskinesia
bromocriptine: Possibly interference with bromocriptine's effects

P

CNS depressants: Increased CNS and respiratory depression and hypotensive effects
dopamine: Antagonized peripheral vasoconstriction with high doses of dopamine
ephedrine: Decreased vasopressor response to ephedrine
epinephrine: Blocked alpha-adrenergic effects of epinephrine, possibly causing severe hypotension and tachycardia
hepatotoxic drugs: Increased risk of hepatotoxicity
hypotension-causing drugs: Increased risk of severe orthostatic hypotension
levodopa: Inhibited antidyskinetic effects of levodopa
lithium: Possibly neurotoxicity (disorientation, extrapyramidal symptoms, unconsciousness)
maprotiline, selective serotonin reuptake inhibitors, tricyclic antidepressants: Prolonged and intensified sedative and anticholinergic effects of these drugs or perphenazine
metrizamide: Decreased seizure threshold
opioid analgesics: Increased CNS and respiratory depression, increased risk of orthostatic hypotension and severe constipation
ototoxic drugs, especially antibiotics: Possibly masking of some symptoms of ototoxicity, such as dizziness, tinnitus, and vertigo
probucol, other drugs that prolong QT interval: Prolonged QT interval, which may increase risk of ventricular tachycardia
thiazide diuretics: Possibly hyponatremia and water intoxication
ACTIVITIES
alcohol use: Increased CNS and respiratory depression, hypotensive effects, and risk of heatstroke

Adverse Reactions

CNS: Behavioral changes, cerebral edema, dizziness, drowsiness, extrapyramidal reactions (such as akathisia, dystonia, pseudoparkinsonism), fever, headache, neuroleptic malignant syndrome, seizures, suicidal ideation, syncope, tardive dyskinesia (persistent)
CV: Bradycardia, cardiac arrest, hypertension, hypotension, orthostatic hypotension, tachycardia

EENT: Blurred vision, dry mouth, glaucoma, laryngeal edema, miosis, mydriasis, nasal congestion, ocular changes (corneal opacification, retinopathy)
ENDO: Decreased libido, galactorrhea, gynecomastia, syndrome of inappropriate ADH secretion
GI: Anorexia, constipation, diarrhea, fecal impaction, nausea, vomiting
GU: Bladder paralysis, ejaculation failure, menstrual irregularities, polyuria, urinary frequency, urinary incontinence, urine retention
HEME: Agranulocytosis, eosinophilia, hemolytic anemia, leukopenia, pancytopenia, thrombocytopenic purpura
RESP: Asthma
SKIN: Diaphoresis, eczema, erythema, exfoliative dermatitis, hyperpigmentation, jaundice, pallor, photosensitivity, pruritus, urticaria
Other: Anaphylaxis, angioedema

Nursing Considerations

• Perphenazine shouldn't be used to treat dementia-related psychosis in the elderly because of an increased mortality risk.
• Use perphenazine cautiously in patients with depression or hepatic, pulmonary, or renal dysfunction and in elderly patients, who are at increased risk for increased plasma concentrations and tardive dyskinesia.
• For I.V. use, dilute drug to 0.5 mg/ml with sodium chloride for injection. Protect solution from light. Slight yellowing is acceptable, but discard solution if it's markedly discolored or contains precipitate.
• Obtain blood samples for CBC and liver and renal function tests, as ordered, to detect adverse reactions.
• Monitor temperature frequently, and notify prescriber if it rises; a significant increase suggests drug intolerance.
• Monitor blood pressure of patient who takes large doses of perphenazine, especially if surgery is indicated, because of the increased risk of hypotension.
• Watch patient closely (especially children, adolescents, and young adults), for suicidal tendencies, particularly when perphenazine therapy starts and dosage changes, because depression may worsen temporarily during these times, possibly leading to suicidal ideation.

PATIENT TEACHING

- Instruct patient to take drug exactly as prescribed to ensure optimal effectiveness and minimize adverse reactions.
- Remind patient who takes oral solution to use a calibrated measuring device.
- Instruct patient taking oral solution to dilute every 5 ml (teaspoon) of drug in 2 fluid oz of water, milk, tomato juice, fruit juice (except apple), soup, or carbonated beverage. Caution against using beverages that contain caffeine or tannins (cola, coffee, tea).
- Caution patient not to spill oral solution on skin or clothing because it can cause contact dermatitis and damage clothing.
- Urge patient to avoid alcohol and other CNS depressants during perphenazine therapy and to avoid hazardous activities until drug's CNS effects are known.
- Advise patient to avoid excessive sun exposure and to protect skin when outdoors.
- Instruct patient to notify prescriber about persistent or severe adverse reactions.
- Urge patient to comply with long-term follow-up to detect adverse reactions and determine possible need for perphenazine dosage adjustments.
- Urge family or caregiver to watch patient closely for suicidal tendencies, especially when therapy starts or dosage changes and particularly if patient is a child, teenager, or young adult.

phenazopyridine hydrochloride

Azo-Standard, Baridium, Eridium, Geridium, Phenazo (CAN), Phenazodine, Pyridiate, Pyridium, Urodine, Urogesic, Viridium

Class and Category

Chemical class: Azo dye
Therapeutic class: Urinary analgesic
Pregnancy category: B

Indications and Dosages

➤ *To relieve burning and pain on urination, and urinary frequency and urgency*

TABLETS

Adults and adolescents. 200 mg three times daily with or without food for no longer than 2 days.
Children. 4 mg/kg three times daily with food for no longer than 2 days.

Mechanism of Action

Exerts a topical or local anesthetic effect on urinary tract mucosa as drug is excreted in urine. Phenazopyridine's exact mechanism is unknown.

Contraindications

Hypersensitivity to phenazopyridine or its components, renal insufficiency

Adverse Reactions

CNS: Headache
GI: Indigestion, nausea, vomiting
GU: Reddish orange urine
SKIN: Pruritus, rash
Other: Discoloration of body fluids

Nursing Considerations

- Notify prescriber if yellowish skin or sclerae develop in patient taking phenazopyridine because this may indicate drug accumulation from impaired renal excretion. Expect prescriber to discontinue drug.
- Be aware that phenazopyridine treatment should be limited to 2 days in patients with UTI.

PATIENT TEACHING

- Instruct patient not to take drug for longer than 2 days and to notify prescriber if symptoms persist beyond that time.
- If GI distress develops, advise patient to take drug with meals.
- Inform patient that drug turns urine orange to red and may discolor other body fluids, such as tears.
- Advise patient not to wear contact lenses during therapy because they may become stained.

phenelzine sulfate

Nardil

Class and Category

Chemical class: Hydrazine derivative
Therapeutic class: Antidepressant
Pregnancy category: C

Indications and Dosages

➤ *To treat depression*

Mechanism of Action

Phenelzine relieves symptoms of unipolar depressive disorders by inhibiting the enzyme monoamine oxidase (MAO). Normally, MAO breaks down monoamineneurotransmitters, such as serotonin, as shown below left. By inhibiting this enzyme, phenelzine increases the concentration of serotonin in the vesicles of monoamine nerve endings, allowing more serotonin to be released and engage with receptors on postsynaptic cells, as shown below right. A serotonin deficiency may be responsible in part for endogenous depression.

TABLETS

Adults. *Initial:* 1 mg/kg daily, increased gradually as prescribed and tolerated. *Maintenance:* 45 mg daily. *Maximum:* 90 mg daily.

DOSAGE ADJUSTMENT For elderly patients, initially may be reduced to 0.8 to 1 mg/kg daily in divided doses, increased as ordered and tolerated to maximum of 60 mg daily.

Route	Onset	Peak	Duration
P.O.	7–10 days	4–8 wk	10 days

Contraindications

Cardiovascular disease; cerebrovascular disease; heart failure; hepatic disease; history of headaches; hypersensitivity to phenelzine or its components; hypertension; pheochromocytoma; severe renal impairment; use of anesthetics, antihypertensives, bupropion, buspirone, carbamazepine, CNS depressants, cyclobenzaprine, dextromethorphan, meperidine, selective serotonin-reuptake inhibitors, sympathomimetics, or tricyclic antidepressants; use within 14 days of other MAO inhibitor

Interaction

DRUGS

anticholinergics, antidyskinetics, anti-histamines: Increased anticholinergic effect, prolonged CNS depression (antihistamines)

anticonvulsants: Increased CNS depression, possibly altered pattern of seizures

beta blockers: Increased risk of bradycardia

bromocriptine: Possibly interference with bromocriptine effects

bupropion: Increased risk of bupropion toxicity

buspirone: Increased risk of hypertension

caffeine-containing drugs: Increased risk of dangerous arrhythmias and severe hypertension

carbamazepine, cyclobenzaprine, maprotiline, other MAO inhibitors: Increased risk of hyperpyretic crisis, hypertensive crisis, severe seizures, and death; altered pattern of seizures (with carbamazepine)

CNS depressants: Increased CNS depression

dextromethorphan: Increased risk of excitation, hypertension, and hyper-pyrexia

diuretics: Increased hypotensive effect

doxapram: Increased vasopressor effects of either drug

fluoxetine: Increased risk of agitation, confusion, GI symptoms, hyperpyretic episodes, hypertensive crisis, potentially fatal serotonin syndrome, restlessness, and severe seizures.
guanadrel, guanethidine: Increased risk of hypertension
haloperidol, loxapine, molindone, phenothiazines, pimozide, thioxanthenes: Prolonged and intensified anticholinergic, hypotensive, and sedative effects of these drugs or phenelzine
insulin, oral antidiabetic drugs: Increased hypoglycemic effects
levodopa: Increased risk of sudden, moderate to severe hypertension
local anesthetics (with epinephrine or levonordefrin): Possibly severe hypertension
meperidine, other opioid analgesics: Increased risk of coma, hyperpyrexia, hypotension, immediate excitation, rigidity, seizures, severe hypertension, severe respiratory depression, sweating, vascular collapse, and death
methyldopa: Increased risk of hallucinations, headache, hyperexcitability, and severe hypertension
methylphenidate: Increased CNS stimulant effect of methylphenidate
metrizamide: Decreased seizure threshold, increased risk of seizures
oral anticoagulants: Increased anticoagulant activity
paroxetine, sertraline, trazodone, tricyclic antidepressants: Increased risk of potentially fatal serotonin syndrome
phenylephrine (nasal or ophthalmic): Potentiated vasopressor effect of phenylephrine
rauwolfia alkaloids: Increased risk of moderate to severe hypertension, CNS depression (when phenelzine is added to rauwolfia alkaloid therapy), CNS excitation and hypertension (when rauwolfia alkaloid is added to phenelzine therapy)
spinal anesthetics: Increased risk of hypotension
succinylcholine: Possibly increased neuromuscular blockade of succinylcholine
sympathomimetics: Prolonged and intensified cardiac stimulant and vasopressor effects

tryptophan: Increased risk of confusion, disorientation, hyperreflexia, hyperthermia, hyperventilation, mania or hypomania, and shivering

FOODS
foods and beverages high in tyramine or other pressor amines, such as aged cheese; beer; fava beans or other broad beans; cured meat or sausage; liqueurs; overripe fruit; red and white wine; reduced-alcohol and alcohol-free beer and wine; sauerkraut; sherry; smoked or pickled fish, meats, and poultry; yeast or protein extracts: Increased risk of sudden, severe hypertension

ACTIVITIES
alcohol use: Increased CNS depressant effects and hypertensive crisis

Adverse Reactions

CNS: Agitation, dizziness, drowsiness, headache, overstimulation, restlessness, sedation, sleep disturbance, suicidal ideation, weakness
CV: Bradycardia, edema, hypertensive crisis, orthostatic hypotension, palpitations, tachycardia
EENT: Blurred vision, dry mouth, photophobia
ENDO: Hypoglycemia in diabetic patients
GI: Abdominal pain, constipation, diarrhea, elevated liver function test results, increased appetite, nausea
GU: Impotence, priapism, sexual dysfunction, urinary frequency, urine retention
MS: Muscle twitching
SKIN: Diaphoresis, rash
Other: Hypernatremia, weight gain

Nursing Considerations

- Use phenelzine cautiously in patients with epilepsy because drug may alter seizure threshold.
- Use phenelzine cautiously in patients with diabetes mellitus because insulin sensitivity may increase, predisposing patient to hypoglycemia.
- Expect to observe some therapeutic effect within 7 to 10 days, but keep in mind that full effect may not occur for 4 to 8 weeks.
- Monitor cardiovascular status closely for changes in heart rate (especially if patient receives more than 30 mg daily) and signs

P

of life-threatening hypertensive crisis. Question patient often about headaches and palpitations. If either occurs, notify prescriber and expect to discontinue drug.
• Keep phentolamine readily available to treat hypertensive crisis. Give 5 mg by slow I.V., as prescribed, to reduce blood pressure without causing excessive hypotension. Use external cooling measures, as prescribed, to manage fever.
• To avoid hypertensive crisis, expect to wait 10 to 14 days, as prescribed, when switching patient from one MAO inhibitor to another or when switching from a dibenzazepine-related drug, such as amitriptyline or perphenazine.
• Watch closely for suicidal tendencies, especially in children, adolescents, and young adults and especially when therapy starts or dosage changes.

PATIENT TEACHING
• Inform patient and family members that therapeutic effects of phenelzine may take several weeks to appear and that she should continue taking drug as prescribed.
• Caution patient to rise slowly from a lying or sitting position to minimize effects of orthostatic hypotension.

WARNING Instruct patient to avoid the following foods, beverages, and drugs during phenelzine therapy and for 2 weeks afterward: alcohol-free and reduced-alcohol beer and wine; appetite suppressants; beer; broad beans; cheese (except cottage and cream cheese); chocolate and caffeine in large quantities; dry sausage (including Genoa salami, hard salami, pepperoni, and Lebanon bologna); hay fever drugs; inhaled asthma drugs; liver; meat extract; OTC cold and cough preparations (including those containing dextromethorphan), nasal decongestants (tablets, drops, or spray); pickled herring; products that contain tryptophan; protein-rich foods that may have undergone protein changes by aging, pickling, fermenting, or smoking; sauerkraut; sinus drugs; weight-loss preparations; yeast extracts (including brewer's yeast in large quantities); yogurt; and wine.
• Advise patient to inform all healthcare providers (including dentists) that she takes an MAO inhibitor because certain drugs are contraindicated within 2 weeks.

• Urge patient to avoid hazardous activities until drug's CNS effects are known.
• Emphasize the importance of reporting headaches and other unusual, persistent, or severe symptoms.
• Tell family or caregiver to watch closely for suicidal tendencies, especially in children, adolescents, and young adults and especially when therapy starts or dosage changes.
• Urge patient with diabetes who's taking insulin or an oral antidiabetic to check blood glucose level often during therapy because phenelzine may affect glucose control.

phenobarbital
Ancalixir (CAN), Barbita, Solfoton

phenobarbital sodium
Luminal

Class, Category, and Schedule
Chemical class: Barbiturate
Therapeutic class: Anticonvulsant, sedative-hypnotic
Pregnancy category: D
Controlled substance schedule: IV

Indications and Dosages
➤ *To treat seizures*
CAPSULES, ELIXIR, TABLETS
Adults. 60 to 250 mg daily as a single dose or in divided doses.
Children. 1 to 6 mg/kg daily as a single dose or in divided doses.
I.V. INJECTION
Adults. 100 to 320 mg, repeated as needed. *Maximum:* 600 mg daily.
Children. *Initial:* 10 to 20 mg/kg as a single dose. *Maintenance:* 1 to 6 mg/kg daily.
➤ *To treat status epilepticus*
I.V. INFUSION OR INJECTION
Adults. 10 to 20 mg/kg given slowly and repeated as needed.
Children. 15 to 20 mg/kg over 10 to 15 min.
➤ *To provide short-term treatment of insomnia*
CAPSULES, ELIXIR, TABLETS
Adults. 100 to 320 mg at bedtime.
I.V., I.M., OR SUBCUTANEOUS INJECTION
Adults. 100 to 325 mg at bedtime.

➤ *To provide daytime sedation*
CAPSULES, ELIXIR, TABLETS
Adults. 30 to 120 mg daily in divided doses .twice daily or three times a day.
Children. 2 mg/kg three times a day.
I.V., I.M., OR SUBCUTANEOUS INJECTION
Adults. 30 to 120 mg daily in divided doses twice daily or three times a day.
➤ *To provide preoperative sedation*
CAPSULES, ELIXIR, TABLETS
Children. 1 to 3 mg/kg before surgery.
I.M. INJECTION
Adults. 130 to 200 mg 60 to 90 min before surgery.
I.V. OR I.M. INJECTION
Children. 1 to 3 mg/kg 60 to 90 min before surgery.
DOSAGE ADJUSTMENT Dosage possibly reduced for elderly or debilitated patients to minimize confusion, depression, and excitement.

Route	Onset	Peak	Duration
P.O.	20–60 min	Unknown	Unknown
I.V.	5 min	30 min	4–6 hr
I.M., SubQ	5–20 min	Unknown	4–6 hr

Mechanism of Action
Inhibits ascending conduction of impulses in the reticular formation, which controls CNS arousal to produce drowsiness, hypnosis, and sedation. Phenobarbital also decreases the spread of seizure activity in cortex, thalamus, and limbic system. It promotes an increased threshold for electrical stimulation in the motor cortex, which may contribute to its anticonvulsant properties.

Contraindications
Hepatic disease; history of addiction to hypnotics or sedatives; hypersensitivity to phenobarbital, other barbiturates, or their components; nephritis; porphyria; severe respiratory disease with airway obstruction or dyspnea

Interaction
DRUGS
acetaminophen: Decreased acetaminophen effectiveness with long-term phenobarbital therapy
amphetamines: Delayed intestinal absorption of phenobarbital

anesthetics (halogenated hydrocarbon): Possibly hepatotoxicity
anticonvulsants (hydantoin): Unpredictable effects on metabolism of anticonvulsant
anticonvulsants (succinimide), including carbamazepine: Decreased blood levels and elimination half-lives of these drugs
calcium channel blockers: Possibly excessive hypotension
carbonic anhydrase inhibitors: Enhanced osteopenia induced by phenobarbital
chloramphenicol, corticosteroids, cyclosporine, dacarbazine, digoxin, metronidazole, quinidine: Decreased effectiveness of these drugs from enhanced metabolism
CNS depressants: Additive CNS depression
cyclophosphamide: Possibly reduced half-life and increased leukopenic activity of cyclophosphamide
disopyramide: Possibly ineffectiveness of disopyramide
doxycycline, fenoprofen: Shortened half-life of these drugs
griseofulvin: Possibly decreased absorption and effectiveness of griseofulvin
guanadrel, guanethidine: Possibly increased orthostatic hypotension
haloperidol: Decreased seizure threshold, decreased blood haloperidol level
ketamine (high doses): Increased risk of hypotension and respiratory depression
leucovorin: Interference with phenobarbital's anticonvulsant effect
levothyroxine, oral contraceptives, phenylbutazone, tricyclic antidepressants: Decreased effectiveness of these drugs
loxapine, phenothiazines, thioxanthenes: Decreased seizure threshold
MAO inhibitors: Prolonged phenobarbital effects, possibly altered pattern of seizure activity
maprotiline: Increased CNS depression, decreased seizure threshold at high doses, decreased phenobarbital effectiveness
methoxyflurane: Possibly hepatotoxicity and nephrotoxicity
methylphenidate: Increased risk of phenobarbital toxicity
mexiletine: Decreased blood mexiletine level
oral anticoagulants: Decreased anticoagulant activity, increased risk of bleeding when phenobarbital is discontinued
pituitary hormones (posterior): Increased risk of arrhythmias and coronary insufficiency

P

primidone: Altered pattern of seizures, increased CNS effects of both drugs
valproate, valproic acid: Decreased phenobarbital metabolism, increased risk of barbiturate toxicity
vitamin D: Decreased phenobarbital effectiveness
xanthines: Increased xanthine metabolism, antagonized hypnotic effect of phenobarbital
ACTIVITIES
alcohol use: Additive CNS depression

Adverse Reactions
CNS: Anxiety, depression, dizziness, drowsiness, headache, irritability, lethargy, mood changes, paradoxical stimulation, sedation, vertigo
CV: Hypotension, sinus bradycardia
EENT: Miosis, ptosis
GI: Constipation, diarrhea, nausea, vomiting
GU: Decreased libido, impotence, sexual dysfunction
MS: Arthralgia, bone tenderness
RESP: Bronchospasm, respiratory depression
SKIN: Dermatitis, photosensitivity, rash, urticaria
Other: Injection-site phlebitis (I.V.), physical and psychological dependence

Nursing Considerations
• Be aware that phenobarbital shouldn't be given during third trimester of pregnancy because repeated use can cause dependence in neonate. It also shouldn't be given to breastfeeding women because it may cause CNS depression in infants.
• Use I.V. route cautiously in patients with CV disease, hypotension, pulmonary disease, or shock because drug may cause adverse hemodynamic or respiratory effects.
• Because drug can cause respiratory depression, assess respiratory rate and depth beforeuse, especially in patient with bronchopneumonia, pulmonary disease, respiratory tract infection, or status asthmaticus.
• Give elixir undiluted or mix with water, milk, or fruit juice. Use a calibrated device to measure doses.
• If necessary, crush tablets and mix with food or fluids.

• Reconstitute sterile powder with at least 10 ml sterile water for injection. Don't use reconstituted solution if it fails to clear within 5 minutes. Further dilute prescribed dose with normal saline solution or D_5W and infuse over 30 to 60 minutes.
• Don't give more rapidly than 60 mg/min by I.V. injection.
• During I.V. use, monitor blood pressure, respiratory rate, and heart rate and rhythm. Anticipate increased risk of hypotension, even at recommended rate. Keep resuscitation equipment readily available.
• During I.M. use, don't inject more than 5 ml into any one I.M. site to prevent sterile abscess formation.
• Be aware that drug may cause physical and psychological dependence.
• Expect that phenobarbital's CNS effects may exacerbate major depression, suicidal tendencies, or other mental disorders.
• Take safety precautions for elderly patients, as appropriate, because they're more likely to experience confusion, depression, and excitement as adverse CNS reactions.
• Anticipate that phenobarbital may cause paradoxical stimulation in children.
• Be aware that drug may trigger signs and symptoms in patients with acute intermittent porphyria.
PATIENT TEACHING
• Instruct patient to take phenobarbital elixir undiluted or to mix it with water, milk, or fruit juice. Advise her to use a calibrated device to measure doses.
• If patient has trouble swallowing tablets, suggest crushing and adding to food or fluid.
• Caution patient about possible drowsiness and reduced alertness. Advise her to avoid potentially hazardous activities until drug's CNS effects are known.
• Urge patient to avoid alcohol during therapy.
• Inform parents that a child may react with paradoxical excitement. Tell them to notify prescriber if this occurs.
• Instruct woman to report suspected, known, or intended pregnancy. Advise against breastfeeding during therapy.

phentolamine mesylate

Regitine

Class and Category

Chemical class: Imidazoline
Therapeutic class: Antihypertensive,
diagnostic aid, vasodilator
Pregnancy category: Not rated

Indications and Dosages

➤ *To diagnose pheochromocytoma*
I.V. INJECTION
Adults. 2.5 mg as a single dose. After
negative result, test repeated with 5-mg
dose, if indicated.
Children. 1 mg as a single dose. After
negative result, test repeated with 0.1-mg/
kg dose, if indicated.
➤ *To manage hypertension before or*
during pheochromocytomectomy
I.V. OR I.M. INJECTION
Adults. 5 mg 1 to 2 hr before surgery,
repeated as needed. During surgery, 5 mg
I.V., as needed.
Children. 1 mg 1 to 2 hr before surgery,
repeated as needed. During surgery, 1 mg
I.V., as needed.
➤ *To prevent dermal necrosis or sloughing*
after extravasation of I.V.
norepinephrine
I.V. INJECTION
Adults, children, and infants. 10 mg/L of
I.V. fluid that contains norepinephrine at
rate determined by patient response.
➤ *To treat dermal necrosis or sloughing*
after extravasation of I.V. norepinephrine
INTRADERMAL INJECTION
Adults. 5 to 10 mg in 10 ml of normal
saline solution infiltrated in affected area
within 12 hr of extravasation.
Children. 0.1 to 0.2 mg/kg. *Maximum:*
10 mg.

Mechanism of Action

Blocks the actions of circulating
epinephrine and norepinephrine by
antagonizing alpha$_1$ and alpha$_2$ receptors.
Phentolamine causes peripheral
vasodilation through direct relaxation of
vascular smooth muscle and alpha
blockade. Positive inotropic and
chronotropic effects increase cardiac output.
A positive inotropic effect primarily raises
blood pressure, but in larger doses,
phentolamine causes peripheral
vasodilation and can reduce blood pressure.
   In patients with pheochromocytoma,
phentolamine causes systolic and diastolic
blood pressures to fall dramatically. In those
without pheochromocytoma, it causes blood
pressure to fall or rise slightly or remain the
same.

Contraindications

Angina, hypersensitivity to phentolamine or
its components, MI

Interaction

DRUGS
antihypertensives: Additive hypotensive
effect
dopamine: Antagonized vasopressor activity
of dopamine
epinephrine, methoxamine, norepinephrine,
phenylephrine: Inhibited alpha adrenergic
effects of these drugs
metaraminol: Possibly decreased vasopressor
effect of metaraminol
ACTIVITIES
alcohol use: Additive vasodilation, increased
risk of hypotension and tachycardia

Adverse Reactions

CNS: Dizziness
CV: Angina; arrhythmias, including
tachycardia; hypotension
EENT: Nasal congestion
GI: Diarrhea, nausea, vomiting
GU: Ejaculation disorders, priapism
MS: Muscle weakness
SKIN: Flushing

Nursing Considerations

• Reconstitute each 5-mg vial phentolamine
  with 1 ml sterile water for injection.
• Use reconstituted solution immediately;
  don't store unused portion.
• Dilute 5 to 10 mg of reconstituted solution
  in 500 ml D$_5$W. Inspect drug for particles
  and discoloration before administering.
• When diagnosing pheochromocytoma,
  hold nonessential drugs, as ordered, for at
  least 24 hours (preferably 48 to 72) before
  test.
• Before giving I.V. test dose for pheochromocytoma, place patient in supine position
  and assess baseline blood pressure with

P

readings every 10 minutes for at least 30 minutes.
- In pheochromocytoma, expect excessive hypotension after patient receives drug.
- Take safety precautions according to facility policy if patient experiences dizziness.

PATIENT TEACHING
- Instruct patient to move slowly after phentolamine administration to minimize dizziness and avoid falls.

phenylephrine hydrochloride

Alconefrin Nasal Drops 12, Alconefrin Nasal Drops 25, Alconefrin Nasal Drops 50, Alconefrin Nasal Spray 25, Doktors, Duration, Neo-Synephrine, Neo-Synephrine Nasal Drops, Neo-Synephrine Nasal Jelly, Neo-Synephrine Nasal Spray, Neo-Synephrine Pediatric Nasal Drops, Nostril Spray Pump, Nostril Spray Pump Mild, Rhinall, Rhinall-10 Children's Flavored Nose Drops, Vicks Sinex

Class and Category

Chemical class: Sympathomimetic amine
Therapeutic class: Antiarrhythmic, decongestant, vasoconstrictor, vasopressor
Pregnancy category: C (parenteral), Not rated (nasal)

Indications and Dosages

➤ *To manage mild to moderate hypotension*
I.V. INJECTION
Adults. *Initial:* 0.1 to 0.5 mg. *Usual:* 0.2 mg, repeated no more than every 10 to 15 min.
I.M. OR SUBCUTANEOUS INJECTION
Adults. *Initial:* 1 to 5 mg. *Usual:* 2 to 5 mg (range, 1 to 10 mg), repeated no more than every 10 to 15 min, as prescribed.
➤ *To treat severe hypotension or shock*
I.V. INFUSION
Adults. *Initial:* 100 to 180 mcg/min (0.1 to 0.18 mg/min) until blood pressure is stable. *Maintenance:* 40 to 60 mcg/min (0.04 to 0.06 mg/min). Infusion concentration and flow rate adjusted as needed, based on patient response.
➤ *To prevent hypotension during spinal anesthesia*

I.M. OR SUBCUTANEOUS INJECTION
Adults. 2 to 3 mg 3 or 4 min before injection of spinal anesthetic.
Children. 0.5 to 1 mg for each 11.3 kg (25 lb).
➤ *To treat hypotension during spinal anesthesia*
I.V. INJECTION
Adults. *Initial:* 0.2 mg, increased by no more than 0.2 mg, as needed. *Maximum:* 0.5 mg/dose.
Children. 0.5 to 1 mg for each 11.3 kg (25 lb).
➤ *To treat paroxysmal supraventricular tachycardia*
I.V. INJECTION
Adults. *Initial:* Up to 0.5 mg by rapid injection; later doses increased 0.1 to 0.2 mg higher than preceding dose, as needed.
Maximum: 1 mg/dose.
➤ *To treat sinus, nasal, and eustachian tube congestion*
NASAL JELLY OR SOLUTION
Adults and children age 12 and over. 2 or 3 drops or sprays of 0.25% or 0.5% solution every 4 hr, as needed, or small quantity of 0.5% nasal jelly in each nostril every 3 to 4 hr, as needed A 1% solution may be used for severe congestion.
Children ages 6 to 12. 2 or 3 drops or sprays of 0.25% solution in each nostril every 4 hr, as needed.
Children ages 2 to 6. 2 or 3 drops or sprays of 0.125% or 0.16% solution in each nostril every 4 hr, as needed.

Mechanism of Action

Directly stimulates alpha-adrenergic receptors and inhibits the intracellular enzyme adenyl cyclase, which then inhibits production of cAMP. Inhibition of cAMP causes arterial and venous constriction and increases peripheral vascular resistance and systolic blood pressure. With greater-than-therapeutic doses, phenylephrine directly stimulates beta-adrenergic receptors in the myocardium, which increases activity of adenyl cyclase and produces positive inotropic and chrono-tropic effect. Intranasal use directly stimulates alpha-adrenergic receptors on the nasal mucosa, constricting local vessels and decreasing blood flow and mucosal edema.

Route	Onset	Peak	Duration
I.V.	Immediate	Unknown	15–20 min
I.M.	10–15 min	Unknown	30 min–2 hr
SubQ	10–15 min	Unknown	50 min–1 hr
Nasal	Unknown	Unknown	30 min–4 hr

Incompatibilities

Don't combine nasal form with alkalis, butacaine, ferrous salts, metals, or oxidizing agents.

Contraindications

Hypersensitivity to bisulfites, phenylephrine, or their components; severe coronary artery disease or hypertension; use within 14 days of MAO inhibitor; ventricular tachycardia

Interaction

DRUGS

alpha blockers, haloperidol, loxapine, phenothiazines, thioxanthenes: Possibly decreased vasoconstrictor effect of phenylephrine; decreased decongestant effect of nasal phenylephrine (with phenothiazines)
antihypertensives, diuretics: Possibly decreased antihypertensive effects
atropine: Possibly enhanced vasopressor effect of phenylephrine
beta blockers: Decreased therapeutic effects of both drugs
bretylium: Possibly potentiated vasopressor effect and arrhythmias
doxapram: Increased vasopressor effect of both drugs
ergot alkaloids: Possibly cerebral blood vessel rupture, increased vasopressor effect, peripheral vascular ischemia, and gangrene (with ergotamine)
guanadrel, guanethidine: Increased vasopressor effect of phenylephrine, increased risk of severe hypertension and arrhythmias
hydrocarbon inhalation anesthetics: Increased risk of serious arrhythmias
MAO inhibitors: Increased and prolonged cardiac stimulation, increased vasopressor effect, increased risk of severe cardiovascular and cerebrovascular effects, hyperpyrexia, vomiting
maprotiline, tricyclic antidepressants: Increased risk of severe cardiovascular

effects (including arrhythmias, hyperpyrexia, severe hypertension); possibly increased or decreased sensitivity to I.V. phenylephrine
mecamylamine, methyldopa: Decreased hypotensive effects of these drugs, increased vasopressor effect of phenylephrine
nitrates: Possibly decreased vasopressor effect of phenylephrine and decreased antianginal effect of nitrates
oxytocin: Possibly severe, persistent hypertension
phenoxybenzamine: Decreased vasoconstrictor effect of phenylephrine, possibly hypotension and tachycardia
theophylline: Possibly enhanced toxicity (including cardiotoxicity); decreased theophylline level (with nasal phenylephrine)
thyroid hormones: Increased cardiovascular effects of both drugs
urinary acidifiers: Possibly increased elimination and decreased therapeutic effects (with nasal phenylephrine)
urinary alkalizers: Possibly decreased elimination and toxic effects (with nasal phenylephrine)

Adverse Reactions

CNS: Dizziness, headache, insomnia, nervousness, paresthesia, restlessness, sleep disturbance (nasal), tremor, weakness
CV: Angina, bradycardia, hypertension, hypotension, palpitations, peripheral vasoconstriction that may lead to necrosis or gangrene, tachycardia, ventricular arrhythmias
EENT: Burning, dry, or stinging nasal mucosa; rebound congestion; and rhinitis (nasal forms)
GI: Nausea, vomiting
RESP: Dyspnea
SKIN: Extravasation with tissue necrosis and sloughing, pallor
Other: Allergic reaction

Nursing Considerations

• Don't dilute phenylephrine for I.M. or subcutaneous use.
• To reduce the risk of tissue extravasation, don't inject subcutaneous drug intradermally.
• For I.V. use, dilute with D_5W or sodium chloride for injection and prepare as prescribed—usually 10 mg/500 ml.

P

• After nasal application, rinse spray bottle tip or nasal dropper with hot water and dry with clean tissue. Wipe tip of nasal jelly tube with clean tissue.

• To prevent transmission of infection, don't use nasal form on more than one patient.

• Assess for signs and symptoms of angina, arrhythmias, and hypertension because phenylephrine may increase myocardial oxygen demand and the risk of proarrhythmias and blood pressure changes.

WARNING If patient has thyroid disease, watch for increased sensitivity to catecholamines and possible thyrotoxicity or cardiotoxicity.

WARNING Be aware that extravasation may cause tissue necrosis, gangrene, and other reactions around injection site. Expect to use phentolamine if extravasation occurs.

PATIENT TEACHING

• If patient uses nasal form, explain that excessive use may cause rebound congestion. Urge her not to exceed recommended dosage and to use for only 3 to 5 days.

• Teach patient who uses nasal form how to care for spray bottle, dropper, or tube.

• Advise patient to avoid hazardous activities until drug's CNS effects are known.

phenytoin

Dilantin-30 (CAN), Dilantin-125, Dilantin Infatabs

phenytoin sodium

Dilantin, Dilantin Kapseals, Phenytex

Class and Category

Chemical class: Hydantoin derivative
Therapeutic class: Anticonvulsant
Pregnancy category: C

Indications and Dosages

➤ *To treat tonic-clonic, simple, or complex partial seizures in patients who have had no prior treatment*

CHEWABLE TABLETS, ORAL SUSPENSION (PHENYTOIN)

Adults and adolescents. *Initial:* 125 mg suspension or 100 to 125 mg tablet three

times a day, adjusted every 7 to 10 days as needed and tolerated.

Children. *Initial:* 5 mg/kg daily in divided doses twice daily or three times a day, adjusted as needed and tolerated. *Maintenance:* 4 to 8 mg/kg daily in divided doses twice daily or three times daily. *Maximum:* 300 mg daily.

EXTENDED CAPSULES (PHENYTOIN SODIUM)

Adults and adolescents. *Initial:* 100 mg three times daily, adjusted every 7 to 10 days as needed and tolerated. *Maintenance:* Once seizures are controlled, adjusted dosage given daily if needed and tolerated.

DOSAGE ADJUSTMENT For hospitalized patients without hepatic or renal disease, oral loading dose of 400 mg followed in 2 hr by 300 mg, and then followed in 2 more hr by another 300 mg, for a total of 1 g.

Children. *Initial:* 5 mg/kg daily in divided doses twice daily or three times a day, adjusted as needed and tolerated. *Maintenance:* 4 to 8 mg/kg daily in divided doses twice daily or three times a day. *Maximum:* 300 mg daily.

PROMPT CAPSULES (PHENYTOIN SODIUM)

Adults and adolescents. 100 mg three times a day, adjusted every 7 to 10 days as needed and tolerated.

Children. *Initial:* 5 mg/kg daily in divided doses twice daily or three times a day, adjusted as needed and tolerated. *Maintenance:* 4 to 8 mg/kg daily in divided doses twice daily or three times a day. *Maximum:* 300 mg daily.

➤ *To treat status epilepticus*

I.V. INJECTION (PHENYTOIN SODIUM)

Adults and adolescents. *Initial:* 15 to 20 mg/ kg by slow push in 50 ml sodium chloride injection at no more than 50 mg/ min. *Maintenance:* Beginning within 12 to 24 hr of initial dose, 5 mg/kg daily P.O. in divided doses twice daily to four times a day or 100 mg I.V. every 6 to 8 hr.

Children. 15 to 20 mg/kg at no more than 1 mg/kg/min. *Maximum:* 50 mg/min.

DOSAGE ADJUSTMENT For elderly or very ill patients and those with CV or hepatic disease, dosage reduced to 25 mg/min, as prescribed, or possibly as low as 5 to 10 mg/ min to reduce the risk of adverse reactions.

➤ *To prevent or treat seizures during neurosurgery*

I.V. INJECTION (PHENYTOIN SODIUM)
Adults. 100 to 200 mg every 4 hr at no more than 50 mg/min during or immediately after neurosurgery.

Mechanism of Action
Limits the spread of seizure activity and the start of new seizures by regulating voltage-dependent sodium and calcium channels in neurons, inhibiting calcium movement across neuronal membranes, and enhancing sodium-potassium ATP activity in neurons and glial cells. These actions all help stabilize the neurons.

Incompatibilities
Don't mix phenytoin in same syringe with any other drugs or with any I.V. solutions other than sodium chloride for injection because precipitate will form.

Contraindications
Adams-Stokes syndrome, delavirdine therapy, hypersensitivity to phenytoin or its components, SA block, second- or third-degree heart block, sinus bradycardia

Interaction
DRUGS
acetaminophen: Possibly hepatotoxicity, decreased acetaminophen effects
activated charcoal, antacids, calcium salts, enteral feedings, sucralfate: Decreased absorption of oral phenytoin
albendazole: Decreased plasma albendazole levels
allopurinol, benzodiazepines, chloramphenicol, cimetidine, disulfiram, fluconazole, isoniazid, itraconazole, methylphenidate, metronidazole, miconazole, omeprazole, phenacemide, ranitidine, sulfonamides, trazodone, trimethoprim: Decreased metabolism and increased effects of phenytoin
amiodarone, antiepileptic agents such as ethosuximide, felbamate, methsuximide, oxcarbazepine, or topiramate; capecitabine; chloramphenicol; chlordiazepoxide; disulfiram; estrogens; fluorouracil; fluoxetine; fluvastatin; fluvoxamine; H₂-antagonists such as cimetidine; halothane; isoniazid; methsuximide, methylphenidate; omeprazole; phenothiazines; salicylates; sertraline; succinimides; sulfonamides; ticlopidine; tolbutamide; trazodone; warfarin: Possibly increased blood phenytoin level

antiepileptics such as felbamate, topiramate, oxcarbazepine, quetiapine; certain HIV antivirals such as amprenavir, efavirenz, indinavir, lopinavir/ritonavir, nelfinavir, ritonavir, saquinavir: Decreased plasma concentrations of these drugs
antifungals (azole): Increased blood phenytoin level, decreased blood antifungal level
antineoplastics, carbamazepine, diazepam, diazoxide, folic acid, fosamprenavir, nelfinavir, nitrofurantoin, pyridoxine, reserpine, rifampin, ritonavir, St. John's wort, sucralfate, theophylline, vigabatrin: Decreased phenytoin effects
barbiturates: Variable effects on blood phenytoin level
bupropion, clozapine, loxapine, MAO inhibitors, maprotiline, molindone, pheno-thiazines, pimozide, thioxanthenes, tricyclic antidepressants: Decreased seizure threshold, decreased anticonvulsant effects
calcium channel blockers: Increased metabolism and decreased effects of these drugs, possibly increased blood phenytoin level
carbamazepine: Decreased blood level and effects of carbamazepine, possibly phenytoin toxicity
carbonic anhydrase inhibitors: Increased risk of osteopenia from phenytoin
chlordiazepoxide, diazepam: Possibly increased blood phenytoin level, decreased effects of these drugs
clonazepam: Possibly decreased blood level and effects of clonazepam, possibly phenytoin toxicity
corticosteroids, cyclosporine, dicumarol, digoxin, disopyramide, doxycycline, estrogens, furosemide, irinotecan, lamotrigine, levodopa, methadone, metyrapone, mexiletine, oral contraceptives, paclitaxel, quinidine, rifampin, sertraline, sirolimus, tacrolimus, teniposide, theophylline: Increased metabolism and decreased effects of these drugs
dopamine: Increased risk of severe hypotension and bradycardia (with I.V. phenytoin)
fluoxetine: Increased blood phenytoin level and risk of phenytoin toxicity
folic acid, leucovorin: Decreased blood phenytoin level, increased risk of seizures

P

fosamprenavir: Possibly decreased concentration of active metabolite, amprenavir
fosamprenavir/ritonavir: Possibly increased concentration of active metabolite, amprenavir
haloperidol: Decreased effects of haloperidol, decreased anticonvulsant effect of phenytoin
halothane anesthetics: Increased risk of hepatotoxicity and phenytoin toxicity
ifosfamide: Decreased phenytoin effects, possibly increased toxicity
influenza virus vaccine: Possibly decreased phenytoin effects
insulin, oral antidiabetic drugs: Possibly hyperglycemia, increased blood phenytoin level (with tolbutamide)
levonorgestrel, mebendazole, streptozocin, sulfonylureas: Decreased effects of these drugs
lidocaine, propranolol (possibly other beta blockers): Increased cardiac depressant effects (with I.V. phenytoin), possibly decreased blood level and increased adverse effects of phenytoin
lithium: Increased risk of lithium toxicity, increased risk of neurologic symptoms with normal blood lithium level
meperidine: Increased metabolism and decreased effects of meperidine, possibly meperidine toxicity
methadone: Possibly increased metabolism of methadone and withdrawal symptoms
neuromuscular blockers: Shorter duration of action and decreased effects of neuromuscular blockers
oral anticoagulants: Decreased metabolism and increased effects of phenytoin; early increase and then decrease in anticoagulation
paroxetine: Decreased bioavailability of both drugs
phenobarbital, sodium valproate, valproic acid: Increased or decreased serum phenytoin levels; unpredictable phenytoin effects on these drugs
phenylbutazone, salicylates: Increased phenytoin effects, possibly phenytoin toxicity
primidone: Increased primidone effects, possibly primidone toxicity
rifampin: Increased hepatic metabolism of phenytoin
vitamin D: Possibly decreased vitamin D effects, resulting in rickets or osteomalacia (with long-term use of phenytoin)

warfarin : Increased or decreased therapeutic response of warfarin
ACTIVITIES
alcohol use: Additive CNS depression, increased blood phenytoin levels with acute alcohol use; decreased blood phenytoin levels with chronic alcohol use

Adverse Reactions
CNS: Ataxia, confusion, depression, dizziness, drowsiness, excitement, fever, headache, involuntary motor activity, lethargy, nervousness, peripheral neuropathy, restlessness, slurred speech, suicidal ideation, tremor, vertigo, weakness
CV: Cardiac arrest, hypotension, periarteritis nodosa, vasculitis
EENT: Amblyopia, conjunctivitis, diplopia, earache, epistaxis, eye pain, gingival hyperplasia, hearing loss, loss of taste, nystagmus, pharyngitis, photophobia, rhinitis, sinusitis, taste perversion, tinnitus
ENDO: Gynecomastia, hyperglycemia
GI: Abdominal pain, acute hepatic failure, anorexia, constipation, diarrhea, epigastric pain, jaundice, hepatic dysfunction, hepatic necrosis, hepatitis, nausea, vomiting
GU: Glycosuria, Peyronie's disease, priapism, renal failure
HEME: Acute intermittent porphyria (exacerbation), agranulocytosis, anemia, eosinophilia, leukopenia, pancytopenia, thrombocytopenia
MS: Arthralgia, arthropathy, bone fractures, decreased bone mineral density, muscle twitching, osteomalacia, polymyositis
RESP: Apnea, asthma, bronchitis, cough, dyspnea, hypoxia, increased sputum production, pneumonia, pneumothorax, pulmonary fibrosis
SKIN: Exfoliative dermatitis, maculopapular or morbilliform rash, purpuric dermatitis, Stevens-Johnson syndrome, toxic epidermal necrolysis, unusual hair growth, urticaria
Other: Drug reaction with eosinophilia and systemic symptoms (DRESS), facial feature coarsening or enlargement, immunoglobulin abnormalities, injection-site pain, lupuslike symptoms, lymphadenopathy, polyarteritis, weight gain or loss

Nursing Considerations

WARNING Patients of Asian ancestry who have the genetic allelic variant HLA-B 1502 develop serious and sometimes fatal dermatologic reactions ten times more often than people without this variant when given carbamazepine, another antiepileptic drug. Because early data suggest a similar effect with phenytoin, this drug shouldn't be used as a substitute for carbamazepine in these patients.

• Be aware that preferred administration routes for phenytoin are oral and I.V. injection. With I.M. administration, phenytoin has a variable absorption rate.

• If patient has difficulty swallowing, open prompt (rapid-release) capsules and mix contents with food or fluid.

• Shake oral suspension before measuring dose, and use a calibrated measuring device.

• To minimize GI distress, give phenytoin with or just after meals.

• Inspect I.V. form for particles and discoloration before administering.

WARNING Avoid rapid I.V. injection because it may cause cardiac arrest, CNS depression, or severe hypotension.

• To decrease vein irritation, follow I.V. injection with flush of sodium chloride for injection through same I.V. catheter.

• Continuously monitor ECG tracings and blood pressure when administering I.V. phenytoin.

• Frequently assess I.V. site for signs of extravasation because drug can cause tissue necrosis.

• If patient has an NG tube in place, minimize drug absorption by polyvinyl chloride tubing by diluting suspension threefold with sodium chloride for injection, D_5W, or sterile water. After administration, flush tube with at least 20 ml diluent.

• Separate oral phenytoin administration by at least 2 hours from antacids and calcium salts.

• Expect continuous enteral feedings to disrupt phenytoin absorption and, possibly, reduce blood phenytoin level. Discontinue tube feedings 1 to 2 hours before and after phenytoin administration, as prescribed. Anticipate giving increased phenytoin doses to compensate for reduced bioavailability during continuous tube feedings.

• Monitor phenytoin level. Therapeutic level ranges from 10 to 20 mcg/L.

WARNING Monitor patient's hematologic status during therapy because phenytoin can cause blood dyscrasias. A patient with a history of agranulocytosis, leukopenia, or pancytopenia may have an increased risk of infection because phenytoin can cause myelosuppression.

• Anticipate that drug may worsen intermittent porphyria.

• Frequently monitor blood glucose level of patient with diabetes mellitus because drug can stimulate glucagon secretion and impair insulin secretion, either of which can raise blood glucose level.

• Monitor thyroid hormone levels in patient receiving thyroid replacement therapy because phenytoin may decrease circulating thyroid hormone levels and increase thyroid-stimulating hormone level.

• Be aware that long-term phenytoin therapy may increase patient's requirements for folic acid or vitamin D supplements. However, keep in mind that a diet high in folic acid may decrease seizure control.

• Monitor patient closely for evidence of suicidal thinking or behavior, especially when therapy starts or dosage changes.

PATIENT TEACHING

• Instruct patient to crush or thoroughly chew phenytoin chewable tablets before swallowing or to shake oral solution well.

• Advise patient to take drug exactly as prescribed; she should not change brands, dosage, or stop taking drug unless instructed by prescriber.

• Instruct patient to avoid taking antacids or calcium products within 2 hours of phenytoin.

• Urge patient to avoid alcohol during therapy.

• Caution patient to avoid hazardous activities until drug's CNS effects are known.

• Inform patient with diabetes mellitus about the increased risk of hyperglycemia and the possible need for increased antidiabetic drug dosage during therapy. Advise her to check blood glucose level often.

P

- Emphasize the importance of good oral hygiene, and encourage patient to inform her dentist that she's taking phenytoin.
- Encourage patient to obtain medical identification that indicates her diagnosis and drug therapy.
- Urge caregivers to watch patient closely for evidence of suicidal tendencies, especially when therapy starts or dosage changes, and to report concerns at once to prescriber.
- Encourage woman who becomes pregnant while taking phenytoin to enroll in the North American antiepileptic drug pregnancy registry by calling 1-888-233-2334. Explain that the registry is collecting information about the safety of antiepileptic drugs during pregnancy.

physostigmine salicylate
Antilirium

Class and Category
Chemical class: Salicylic acid derivative
Therapeutic class: Anticholinergic antidote, cholinesterase inhibitor
Pregnancy category: Not rated

Indications and Dosages
➤ *To counteract toxic anticholinergic effects (anticholinergic syndrome)*
I.V. OR I.M. INJECTION
Adults and adolescents. 0.5 to 2 mg at no more than 1 mg/min; then 1 to 4 mg, repeated every 20 to 30 min as needed.
Children. 0.02 mg/kg I.V., at no more than 0.5 mg/min, repeated every 5 to 10 min as needed. *Maximum:* 2 mg/dose.

Mechanism of Action
Inhibits destruction of acetylcholine by acetylcholinesterase. This action increases acetylcholine concentration at cholinergic transmission sites and prolongs and exaggerates effects of acetylcholine that are blocked by toxic doses of anticholinergics.

Route	Onset	Peak	Duration
I.V.	3–8 min	5 min	30–60 min
I.M.	3–8 min	20–30 min	30–60 min

Contraindications
Asthma; cardiovascular disease; diabetes mellitus; gangrene; GI or GU obstruction; hypersensitivity to physostigmine, sulfites, or their components

Interaction
DRUGS
choline esters: Enhanced effects of carbachol and bethanechol with concurrent use of physostigmine, enhanced effects of acetylcholine and methacholine with prior use of physostigmine
succinylcholine: Prolonged neuromuscular paralysis

Adverse Reactions
CNS: CNS stimulation, fatigue, hallucinations, restlessness, seizures (with too-rapid I.V. delivery), weakness
CV: Bradycardia (with too-rapid I.V. delivery), irregular heartbeat, palpitations
EENT: Increased salivation, lacrimation, miosis
GI: Abdominal pain, diarrhea, nausea, vomiting
GU: Urinary urgency
MS: Muscle twitching
RESP: Bronchospasm, chest tightness, dyspnea (with too-rapid I.V. administration), increased bronchial secretions, wheezing
SKIN: Diaphoresis

Nursing Considerations
- Use physostigmine cautiously in patients with bradycardia, epilepsy, or Parkinson's disease.
- Avoid rapid I.V. delivery, which may lead to bradycardia, respiratory distress, or seizures.
- Check pulse and respiratory rates, blood pressure, and neurologic status often.
- Monitor ECG tracing during I.V. use.
- Closely monitor patient with asthma for asthma attack because physostigmine may precipitate attack by causing bronchoconstriction.
- Watch for seizures in patient with a history of seizures because physostigmine can induce seizures by stimulating CNS.
WARNING Be alert for life-threatening cholinergic crisis, which may indicate

physostigmine overdose and may include confusion, diaphoresis, hypotension, miosis, muscle weakness, nausea, paralysis(including respiratory paralysis), salivation, seizures, sinus bradycardia, and vomiting. If you detect such signs, prepare to give atropine (the antidote) and use resuscitation equipment. Keep in mind that atropine counteracts only muscarinic cholinergic effects; paralytic effects may continue.

PATIENT TEACHING
• Reassure patient that vital signs will be monitored often to help prevent or detect adverse reactions.
• Instruct patient to notify prescriber at once about evidence of cholinergic crisis.

pindolol

Novopindol (CAN), SynPindol (CAN), Visken

Class and Category
Chemical class: Nonselective beta blocker
Therapeutic class: Antihypertensive
Pregnancy category: B

Indications and Dosages
➤ *To manage hypertension*
TABLETS
Adults. *Initial:* 5 mg twice daily, increased by 10 mg daily every 3 to 4 wk, as prescribed. *Maintenance:* 10 to 30 mg daily. *Maximum:* 60 mg daily (U.S.), 45 mg daily (Canada).

Route	Onset	Peak	Duration
P.O.	Unknown	1–2 hr	Up to 24 hr

Mechanism of Action
Blocks sympathetic stimulation of $beta_1$ receptors in the heart and $beta_2$ receptors in vascular and bronchial smooth muscle by competing with adrenergic neurotransmitters, such as catecholamines. Pindolol's negative chronotropic effects slow the resting heart rate and reduce exercise-induced tachycardia. Its negative inotropic effects reduce cardiac output, myocardial contractility, systolic and diastolic blood pressure, and myocardial oxygen consumption during stress or exercise.

Among beta blockers, pindolol has the most intrinsic sympathomimetic activity and nonselective antagonism.

Contraindications
Advanced AV block; asthma; bronchospasm; cardiogenic shock; heart failure; hepatic disease; hypersensitivity to pindolol, other beta blockers, or their components; hypotension (with systolic pressure less than 100 mm Hg); sinus bradycardia

Interaction
DRUGS
allergy extracts or immunotherapy, iodinated contrast media: Increased risk of systemic reaction or anaphylaxis
aluminum salts, barbiturates, calcium salts, certain penicillins, cholestyramine, colestipol, NSAIDs, rifampin, salicylates, sulfinpyrazone: Decreased blood level and effects of pindolol
antihypertensives: Additive hypotensive effect
beta blockers, digoxin: Increased risk of bradycardia
calcium channel blockers, quinidine: Possibly increased effects of both drugs, symptomatic bradycardia (with diltiazem or verapamil), excessive hypertension or heart failure (with nifedipine)
cimetidine: Increased blood pindolol level
epinephrine: Possibly hypertension followed by bradycardia
ergotamine: Possibly severe peripheral vasoconstriction with pain and cyanosis
estrogens: Decreased antihypertensive effect
fentanyl, fentanyl derivatives: Risk of bradycardia after anesthesia induction
insulin, oral antidiabetic drugs: Masked symptoms of hypoglycemia, increased risk of hyperglycemia
lidocaine: Increased risk of lidocaine toxicity
MAO inhibitors: Possibly hypertension
neuromuscular blockers: Possibly increased or prolonged neuromuscular blockade
phenothiazines: Increased blood levels of both drugs
phenytoin: Possibly increased cardiac depressant effects
prazosin, reserpine: Increased risk of orthostatic hypotension, bradycardia (with reserpine)

P

quinolones: Possibly increased bioavailability of pindolol
xanthines: Possibly decreased effects of both drugs, decreased xanthine clearance

Adverse Reactions
CNS: Anxiety, confusion, depression, dizziness, fatigue, fever, hallucinations, hypothermia, insomnia, memory loss, paresthesia, peripheral neuropathy, stroke, syncope, weakness
CV: Arrhythmias (including AV block and bradycardia), chest pain, decreased peripheral circulation, heart failure, hyperlipidemia, hypotension, MI, orthostatic hypotension, peripheral edema and ischemia, thrombosis of renal or mesenteric artery
EENT: Pharyngitis
ENDO: Hyperglycemia, hypoglycemia
GI: Colitis (ischemic), constipation, diarrhea, elevated liver function test results, gastritis, nausea, pancreatitis, vomiting
GU: Cystitis, decreased libido, renal colic, renal failure, urinary frequency, urine retention, UTI
HEME: Agranulocytosis, bleeding, eosinophilia, leukopenia, nonthrombo-cytopenic purpura, thrombocytopenia, thrombocytopenic purpura, unusual bleeding or bruising
MS: Arthralgia, back pain
RESP: Bronchospasm, pulmonary edema, pulmonary emboli
SKIN: Acne; alopecia; crusted, red, or scaly skin; diaphoresis; eczema; exfoliative dermatitis; hyperpigmentation; pruritus; purpura; rash
Other: Angioedema, positive ANA titer

Nursing Considerations
• Check blood pressure and pulse rate often, especially at start of pindolol therapy. Also monitor fluid intake and output and daily weight, and assess for evidence of heart failure, such as dyspnea, edema, fatigue, and jugular vein distention.
• Be aware that drug shouldn't be stopped abruptly because MI, myocardial ischemia, severe hypertension, or ventricular arrhythmias may result.
• Expect to discontinue drug up to 2 days before surgery, as prescribed, to reduce the risk of heart failure.

• Assess distal circulation and peripheral pulses in patient with Raynaud's phenomenon or other peripheral vascular disorder because drug can worsen these conditions.
• Be aware that pindolol can mask tachycardia from hyperthyroidism; abrupt withdrawal can cause thyroid storm. Drug also may potentiate diplopia and muscle weakness in patient with myasthenia gravis; decrease blood glucose level, prolong or mask symptoms of hypoglycemia, and promote hyper-glycemia in patient with diabetes mellitus; and worsen psoriasis.
PATIENT TEACHING
• Instruct patient to weigh herself daily during pindolol therapy and to notify prescriber if she gains more than 2 lb (0.9 kg) in 1 day or 5 lb (2.3 kg) in 1 week.
• Caution patient not to stop drug abruptly.
• Advise patient to rise slowly from a seated or lying position to minimize effects of orthostatic hypotension.
• Advise patient to avoid hazardous activities until drug's CNS effects are known.
• Instruct patient to contact prescriber about bleeding or bruising, cough at night, depression, dizziness, edema, rash, short-ness of breath, slow pulse rate, or sore throat.
• Advise diabetic patient to monitor her blood glucose level more often during pindolol therapy because drug may mask symptoms of hypoglycemia.
• Inform patient with psoriasis that drug may aggravate this condition.

pioglitazone hydrochloride

Actos

Class and Category
Chemical class: Thiazolidinedione
Therapeutic class: Antidiabetic
Pregnancy category: C

Indications and Dosages
➤ *To achieve glucose control in type 2 diabetes mellitus as monotherapy or in*

combination with insulin, metformin, or a sulfonylurea
TABLETS
Adults. *Initial:* 15 or 30 mg daily. *Maximum:* 45 mg daily.
DOSAGE ADJUSTMENT For patients with congestive heart failure, starting dose is 15 mg once daily. For patients receiving concomitant gemfibrozil or other strong CYP2C8 inhibitors, maximum dose should not exceed 15 mg once daily. For patients taking insulin, insulin dosage decreased by 10% to 25%, as prescribed, once glucose level reaches 100 mg/dl or less. If hypoglycemia occurs, dosage of any concurrent antidiabetic is reduced, as prescribed.

Mechanism of Action
Decreases insulin resistance by enhancing the sensitivity of insulin-dependent tissues, such as adipose tissue, skeletal muscle, and the liver, and reduces glucose output from the liver. Drug activates peroxisome proliferator-activated receptor-gamma (PPARg) receptors, which modu-late transcription of insulin-responsive genes involved in glucose control and lipid metabolism. In this way, pioglitazone reduces hyperglycemia, hyperinsulinemia, and hypertriglyceridemia in patients with type 2 diabetes mellitus and insulin resistance. However, to work effectively, pioglitazone needs endogenous insulin. Unlike sulfonylureas, it doesn't increase pancreatic insulin secretion.

Contraindications
Diabetic ketoacidosis, hypersensitivity to pioglitazone or its components, New York Heart Association (NYHA) Class III or IV heart failure, severe hepatic dysfunction, type 1 diabetes mellitus

Interaction
DRUGS
gemfibrozil and other strong CYP2C8 inhibitors: Increased pioglitazone effect
insulin, oral antidiabetic agents: Possible increased risk of hypoglycemia
ketoconazole: Possibly decreased metabolism of pioglitazone
oral contraceptives: Possibly decreased effectiveness of oral contraceptives
rifampin: Possibly altered glucose control

Adverse Reactions
CNS: Headache
CV: Congestive heart failure, edema
EENT: Blurred vision, decreased visual acuity, macular edema, pharyngitis, sinusitis, tooth disorders
HEME: Decreased hemoglobin level and hematocrit
MS: Fractures, myalgia
RESP: Upper respiratory tract infection
Other: Weight gain

Nursing Considerations
• Be aware that pioglitazone isn't recommended for patients with symptomatic heart failure. It is also not recommended in patients with active bladder cancer because there is insufficient information regarding the drug's role in promoting bladder tumors and should only be used with extreme caution in patients with a history of bladder cancer.
• Be prepared to monitor liver function test results before therapy begins, every 2 months during first year, and annually thereafter, as ordered, because drug is extensively metabolized in the liver. Expect to stop drug if jaundice develops or ALT values exceed 2.5 times normal.
WARNING Monitor patient for signs and symptoms of congestive heart failure—such as shortness of breath, rapid weight gain, or edema—because pioglitazone can cause fluid retention that may lead to or worsen heart failure. Notify prescriber immediately of any deterioration in the patient's cardiac status, and expect to discontinue the drug, as ordered.
• Assess for signs and symptoms of hypoglycemia, especially if patient is also taking another antidiabetic drug.
• Monitor fasting glucose level, as ordered, to evaluate effectiveness of therapy.
• Monitor glycosylated hemoglobin level to assess drug's long-term effectiveness.
PATIENT TEACHING
• Emphasize the need for patient to continue exercise program, diet control, and weight management during pioglitazone therapy.
• Advise patient to notify prescriber immediately if she experiences shortness of breath, fluid retention, or sudden weight gain because drug may need to be discontinued.

- Urge patient to report vision changes promptly and expect to have an eye examination by an ophthalmologist, regardless of when the last examination occurred.
- Instruct patient to keep appointments for liver function tests, as ordered, typically every 2 months during first year of therapy and annually thereafter.
- Inform female patient who uses oral contraceptives that drug decreases their effectiveness; suggest that she use another method of contraception while taking pioglitazone.
- Also inform female patient that she may be at risk for fractures during pioglitazone therapy, and urge her to take safety precautions to prevent falls and other injuries.

piperacillin sodium

Pipracil

Class and Category

Chemical class: Piperazine derivative of ampicillin, acylureidopenicillin
Therapeutic class: Antibiotic
Pregnancy category: B

Indications and Dosages

➤ *To treat moderate to severe bacterial infections, including bone and joint infections, gynecologic infections, intra-abdominal infections, lower respiratory tract infections, septicemia, and skin and soft-tissue infections, caused by susceptible strains of* Acinetobacter *species,* anaerobic cocci, Bacteroides *species,* Enterobacter *species,* Escherichia coli, Haemophilus influenzae, Klebsiella *species,* Proteus *species,* Pseudomonas aeruginosa, *and* Serratia *species*

I.V. INFUSION

Adults and adolescents. 12 to 18 g daily or 200 to 300 mg/kg daily in divided doses every 4 to 6 hr. *Maximum:* 24 g daily.

➤ *To treat bacterial meningitis*

I.V. INFUSION

Adults and adolescents. 4 g every 4 hr or 75 mg/kg every 6 hr. *Maximum:* 24 g daily.

➤ *To treat uncomplicated UTI and community-acquired pneumonia caused*

by susceptible organisms, including E. coli, Klebsiella *species, and* Serratia *species*

I.V. INFUSION, I.M. INJECTION

Adults. 6 to 8 g daily or 100 to 125 mg/kg daily in divided doses every 6 to 12 hr.

➤ *To treat complicated UTI caused by susceptible organisms, including* Acinetobacter *species,* Klebsiella *species, and* Serratia *species*

I.V. INFUSION

Adults. 8 to 16 g daily or 125 to 200 mg/kg daily in divided doses every 6 to 8 hr.

➤ *To treat uncomplicated gonorrhea caused by susceptible strains of* Neisseria gonorrhoeae

I.M. INJECTION

Adults. 2 g as a single dose 30 min after 1-g dose of probenecid P.O.

➤ *To provide surgical prophylaxis in intra-abdominal procedures, including GI and biliary surgery*

I.V. INFUSION

Adults. 2 g 20 to 30 min before anesthesia, 2 g during surgery, and 2 g every 6 hr for 24 hr after surgery.

➤ *To provide surgical prophylaxis in abdominal hysterectomy*

I.V. INFUSION

Adults. 2 g 20 to 30 min before anesthesia, 2 g just after surgery, and 2 g 6 hr later.

➤ *To provide surgical prophylaxis in vaginal hysterectomy*

I.V. INFUSION

Adults. 2 g 20 to 30 min before anesthesia, then 2 g 6 and 12 hr after initial dose.

➤ *To provide surgical prophylaxis in cesarean section*

I.V. INFUSION

Adults. 2 g after cord is clamped, then 2 g 4 and 8 hr after initial dose.

Mechanism of Action

Binds to specific penicillin-binding proteins and inhibits the third and final stage of bacterial cell wall synthesis by interfering with an autolysin inhibitor. Uninhibited autolytic enzymes destroy the cell wall and result in cell lysis.

Incompatibilities

Don't mix piperacillin sodium in same container with aminoglycosides because of chemical incompatibility (depending on concentrations, diluents, pH, and temperature). Don't mix with solutions that contain only sodium bicarbonate because of chemical instability.

Contraindications

Hypersensitivity to cephalosporins, penicillins, or their components

Interaction

DRUGS

aminoglycosides: Additive or synergistic effects against some bacteria, possibly mutual inactivation

anti-inflammatory drugs (including aspirin and NSAIDs), heparin, oral anticoagulants, platelet aggregation inhibitors, sulfinpyrazone, thrombolytics: Increased risk of bleeding

hepatotoxic drugs (including labetalol and rifampin): Increased risk of hepatotoxicity

methotrexate: Increased blood methotrexate level and risk of toxicity

probenecid: Increased blood piperacillin level and risk of toxicity

vecuronium: Possibly prolonged perioperative neuromuscular blockade of vecuronium

Adverse Reactions

CNS: Dizziness, fever, hallucinations, headache, lethargy, seizures, stroke
CV: Cardiac arrest, hypotension, palpitations, tachycardia, vasodilation, vasovagal reactions
EENT: Oral candidiasis, pharyngitis
GI: Diarrhea, epigastric distress, intestinal necrosis, nausea, pseudomembranous colitis, vomiting
GU: Hematuria, impotence, nephritis, neurogenic bladder, priapism, proteinuria, renal failure, vaginal candidiasis
HEME: Agranulocytosis, eosinophilia, hemolytic anemia, leukopenia, neutropenia, pancytopenia, prolonged bleeding time, thrombocytopenia
MS: Arthralgia
RESP: Dyspnea, pulmonary embolism, pulmonary hypertension
SKIN: Exfoliative dermatitis, mottling, rash, toxic epidermal necrolysis, urticaria
Other: Anaphylaxis; facial edema; hypokalemia; hyponatremia; injection-site pain, phlebitis, and skin ulcer; superinfection

Nursing Considerations

• Expect to obtain blood, sputum, or other samples for culture and sensitivity testing before giving piperacillin and to start therapy before results are available.
• Be aware that sunlight may darken piperacillin powder for dilution but won't alter drug potency.
• For initial dilution for I.V. infusion, reconstitute each gram of drug with at least 5 ml sterile water for injection, sodium chloride for injection, D_5W, dextrose 5% in normal saline solution, or bacteriostatic water that contains parabens or benzyl alcohol. Shake solution vigorously after adding diluent, and inspect for particles and discoloration before giving.
• For further dilution, use sodium chloride for injection, D_5W, dextrose 5% in normal saline solution, lactated Ringer's solution, or dextran 6% in normal saline solution. Solutions diluted with lactated Ringer's solution should be given within 2 hours.
• For intermittent infusion, infuse appropriate dose over 20 to 30 minutes.
• Give aminoglycosides 1 hour before or after piperacillin; use a separate site, I.V. bag, and tubing.
• For I.M. injection, reconstitute each gram of piperacillin with at least 2 ml of an appropriate diluent listed above.
• Don't give more than 2 g I.M. in one site. Use deltoid area cautiously and only if well developed to avoid injuring radial nerve.
• Watch for bleeding or excessive bruising because drug can decrease platelet aggregation, especially in patients with renal failure. If bleeding occurs, notify prescriber and expect to stop piperacillin.
• Monitor CBC regularly, as ordered, to detect hematologic abnormalities, such as leukopenia and neutropenia.
• Monitor serum potassium level to detect hypokalemia from urinary potassium loss.
• Check for diarrhea during and after therapy because it may indicate pseudomembranous colitis caused by *Clostridium difficile.* If diarrhea occurs, notify prescriber and expect to withhold piperacillin and treat with fluids, electrolytes, protein, and an antibiotic effective against *C. difficile.*

P

• Watch for hypersensitivity reactions, especially if patient has cystic fibrosis. Notify prescriber, and expect to stop drug.

PATIENT TEACHING

• Advise patient to consult prescriber before using OTC drugs during piperacillin therapy because of the risk of interactions.

• Inform patient that increased bruising may occur if she takes anti-inflammatory drugs during piperacillin therapy.

• Advise patient to notify prescriber about signs of superinfection, such as white patches on tongue or in mouth.

• Urge patient to tell prescriber about diarrhea that's severe or lasts longer than 3 days. Remind patient that watery or bloody stools can occur 2 or more months after antibiotic therapy and can be serious, requiring prompt treatment.

• Instruct patient to complete full course of therapy, even if symptoms subside.

---

pirbuterol acetate

Maxair, Maxair Autohaler

Class and Category

Chemical class: Sympathomimetic amine
Therapeutic class: Bronchodilator
Pregnancy category: C

Indications and Dosages

➤ *To prevent or treat bronchospasm caused by COPD, to treat bronchospasm caused by asthma*

ORAL INHALATION

Adults and adolescents. 1 or 2 inhalations (200 to 400 mcg) every 4 to 6 hr. *Maximum:* 12 inhalations (2.4 mg) daily.

Route	Onset	Peak	Duration
Oral inhalation	In 5 min	In 30–90 min	3–6 hr

Mechanism of Action

Attaches to $beta_2$ receptors on bronchial cell membranes, which stimulates the intracellular enzyme adenyl cyclase to convert adenosine triphosphate (ATP) to cAMP. The increased intracellular level of cAMP relaxes bronchial smooth-muscle cells and inhibits histamine release. Pirbuterol also stabilizes mast cells and inhibits the release of histamine.

Contraindications

Hypersensitivity to pirbuterol or its components, tachycardia

Interaction

DRUGS

beta-adrenergic bronchodilators: Additive effects
beta blockers (ophthalmic): Possibly decreased pirbuterol effects, increased risk of bronchospasm
beta blockers (systemic): Decreased effects of both drugs, increased risk of bronchospasm
MAO inhibitors, tricyclic antidepressants: Potentiated cardiovascular effects

Adverse Reactions

CNS: Anxiety, confusion, depression, dizziness, headache, nervousness, tiredness, tremor
CV: Arrhythmias (including PVCs and tachycardia), chest pain, ECG changes (including flattening of T waves, prolonged QT interval, and ST-segment depression), hypotension, palpitations
EENT: Dry mouth
GI: Abdominal cramps, diarrhea, nausea, vomiting
RESP: Bronchospasm, cough
SKIN: Alopecia, rash, urticaria
Other: Facial edema, hypokalemia

Nursing Considerations

• For patient with a cardiovascular disorder, such as arrhythmia, hypertension, or ischemic cardiac disease, monitor blood pressure and heart rate and rhythm to detect significant changes after pirbuterol use.

• Be aware that elderly patients have greater risk of adverse reactions than younger adults.

WARNING Stop giving drug and notify prescriber immediately if patient has paradoxical bronchospasm, a life-threatening adverse reaction.

PATIENT TEACHING

• Teach patient how to use an inhaler and spacer correctly, and urge her to keep the inhaler readily available at all times.

• Recommend the use of an autohaler if patient has trouble coordinating inhalations with a regular inhaler.

• Advise patient to clean the inhaler's mouthpiece at least once daily.

- Caution patient against overusing drug because doing so may increase adverse reactions.
- Teach patient how to use peak flow meter and determine her personal best reading.

WARNING Advise patient to notify prescriber if symptoms worsen, if bronchospasm occurs more frequently, if she needs to use the inhaler more often, or if the inhaler becomes less effective.

piroxicam

Apo-Piroxicam (CAN), Feldene, Novo-Pirocam (CAN), Nu-Pirox (CAN), PMS-Piroxicam (CAN)

Class and Category
Chemical class: Oxicam derivative
Therapeutic class: Anti-inflammatory, antirheumatic
Pregnancy category: Not rated

Indications and Dosages
➤ *To treat acute and chronic osteoarthritis and rheumatoid arthritis*

CAPSULES
Adults. *Initial:* 20 mg once daily or 10 mg twice daily.

Mechanism of Action
Blocks the activity of cyclooxygenase, the enzyme needed for prostaglandin synthesis. Prostaglandins, important mediators of the inflammatory response, cause local vasodilation with swelling and pain. By blocking cyclooxygenase activity and inhibiting prostaglandins, this NSAID reduces inflammatory symptoms and pain.

Route	Onset	Peak	Duration
P.O.	Unknown	Several	Unknown days to 1 wk*

Contraindications
Angioedema, asthma, bronchospasm, nasal polyps, rhinitis, or urticaria induced by aspirin, iodides, or other NSAIDs; hypersensitivity to piroxicam or its components

Interaction
DRUGS
acetaminophen: Possibly increased adverse renal effects with long-term use of both drugs

---
* With severe inflammation, 2 wk or more.

antihypertensives: Possibly decreased or reversed effects of antihypertensives
aspirin, other NSAIDs: Increased risk of bleeding and adverse GI effects, possibly increased blood piroxicam level
cefamandole, cefoperazone, cefotetan: Increased risk of hypoprothrombinemia and bleeding
colchicine: Increased risk of GI bleeding, hemorrhage, and ulcers
corticosteroids, potassium supplements: Increased risk of adverse GI effects
cyclosporine: Increased risk of nephrotoxicity from both drugs, increased blood cyclosporine level
diuretics: Decreased antihypertensive, diuretic, and natriuretic effects of diuretics
gold compounds, nephrotoxic drugs: Increased risk of adverse renal effects
heparin, oral anticoagulants, thrombolytics: Increased anticoagulant effects, increased risk of hemorrhage
insulin, oral antidiabetic drugs: Possibly increased hypoglycemic effect of these drugs
lithium: Possibly increased blood lithium level and toxicity
methotrexate: Decreased methotrexate clearance and increased risk of methotrexate toxicity
platelet aggregation inhibitors: Increased risk of bleeding and GI ulceration or hemorrhage
plicamycin, valproic acid: Increased risk of hypoprothrombinemia and GI bleeding, hemorrhage, and ulceration
probenecid: Possibly increased blood level, effectiveness, and risk of toxicity of piroxicam
ACTIVITIES
alcohol use: Increased risk of adverse GI effects

Adverse Reactions
CNS: Anxiety, aseptic meningitis, asthenia, cerebral hemorrhage, confusion, depression, dizziness, dream disturbances, drowsiness, fever, headache, insomnia, ischemic stroke, malaise, nervousness, paresthesia, somnolence, syncope, transient ischemic attack, tremor, vertigo
CV: Deep vein thrombosis, edema, heart failure, hypertension, MI, peripheral edema, tachycardia

EENT: Blurred vision, dry mouth, epistaxis, glossitis, stomatitis, tinnitus
ENDO: Hypoglycemia
GI: Abdominal pain; anorexia; constipation; diarrhea; elevated liver function test results; esophagitis; flatulence; gastritis; GI bleeding, perforation, or ulceration; heartburn; hematemesis; hepatitis; indigestion; jaundice; liver failure; melena; nausea; vomiting
GU: Acute renal failure, cystitis, dysuria, elevated serum creatinine level, hematuria, interstitial nephritis, nephrotic syndrome, oliguria, polyuria, proteinuria, renal failure or insufficiency
HEME: Agranulocytosis, anemia, aplastic anemia, coagulation abnormalities, eosinophilia, leukopenia, pancytopenia, thrombocytopenia
RESP: Asthma, dyspnea
SKIN: Alopecia, diaphoresis, ecchymosis, erythema, erythema multiforme, exfoliative dermatitis, photosensitivity, pruritus, purpura, rash, Stevens-Johnson syndrome, toxic epidermal necrolysis, urticaria
Other: Anaphylaxis, angioedema, flulike symptoms, hyperkalemia, infection, sepsis, weight loss or gain

Nursing Considerations
• Administer piroxicam with food to decrease GI upset.
• Use piroxicam with extreme caution in patients with a history of ulcer disease or GI bleeding because NSAIDs such as piroxicam increase risk of GI bleeding and ulceration. Expect to use piroxicam for the shortest time possible in these patients.
• Be aware that serious GI tract ulceration, bleeding, and perforation may occur without warning symptoms. Elderly patients are at greater risk. To minimize risk, give drug with food. If GI distress occurs, withhold drug and notify prescriber at once.
• Use piroxicam cautiously in patients with hypertension, and monitor blood pressure closely throughout therapy. Drug may cause hypertension or worsen it.
WARNING Monitor patient closely for thrombotic events, including MI and stroke, because NSAIDs increase the risk.
WARNING If patient has bone marrow suppression or is receiving antineoplastic

drug therapy, monitor laboratory results (including WBC count), and watch for evidence of infection because anti-inflammatory and antipyretic actions of piroxicam may mask signs and symptoms, such as fever and pain.
• Especially if patient is elderly or taking drug long term, watch for less common but serious adverse GI reactions, including anorexia, constipation, diverticulitis, dysphagia, esophagitis, gastritis, gastro-enteritis, gastroesophageal reflux disease, hemorrhoids, hiatal hernia, melena, stomatitis, and vomiting.
• Monitor liver function test results because, rarely, elevated levels may progress to severe hepatic reactions, including fatal hepatitis, liver necrosis, and hepatic failure.
• Monitor BUN and serum creatinine levels in patients with heart failure, impaired renal function, or hepatic dysfunction; those taking diuretics or ACE inhibitors; and elderly patients because drug may cause renal failure.
• Monitor CBC for decreased hemoglobin level and hematocrit because drug may worsen anemia.
• Assess patient's skin routinely for rash or other signs of hypersensitivity reaction because piroxicam and other NSAIDs may cause serious skin reactions without warning, even in patients with no history of NSAID hypersensitivity. Stop drug at first sign of reaction, and notify prescriber.
WARNING Be aware that drug may cause premature closure of ductus arteriosus in growing fetus during third trimester of pregnancy. Be prepared to suggest referral for high-risk pregnancy.

PATIENT TEACHING
• Advise patient to take piroxicam with meals to minimize GI distress. Also direct her to take drug with a full glass of water and to remain upright for 30 minutes afterward to decrease risk of drug lodging in esophagus and causing irritation.
• Instruct patient to swallow capsules whole and not to crush, break, chew, or open them.
• Advise patient to avoid alcohol, aspirin, and other NSAIDs, unless prescribed, while taking piroxicam.

- Caution patient to avoid hazardous activities until drug's CNS effects are known.
- If patient also takes an anticoagulant, advise her to watch for and immediately report bleeding problems, such as bloody or tarry stools and bloody vomitus.
- If patient also takes insulin or an oral antidiabetic, advise her to closely monitor blood glucose level to prevent hypoglycemia. Urge her to carry candy or other simple sugars to treat mild hypoglycemia. Advise her to notify prescriber if hypoglycemic episodes are frequent or severe.
- Explain that piroxicam may increase risk of serious adverse cardiovascular reactions; urge patient to seek immediate medical attention if signs or symptoms arise, such as chest pain, shortness of breath, weakness, and slurring of speech.
- Tell patient that piroxicam may increase risk of serious adverse GI reactions; stress the need to seek immediate medical attention for such signs and symptoms as epigastric or abdominal pain, indigestion, black or tarry stools, or vomiting blood or material that looks like coffee grounds.
- Alert patient to possibility of rare but serious skin reactions. Urge her to seek immediate medical care for rash, blisters, itching, fever, or other signs of hypersensitivity.
- Instruct female patient to consult prescriber if she becomes pregnant because drug may cause premature closure of ductus arteriosus in growing fetus.

pitavastatin
Livalo

Class and Category
Chemical class: HMG-CoA reductase inhibitor
Therapeutic class: Antihyperlipidemic, statin
Pregnancy category: X

Indications and Dosages
➤ *To decrease elevated total cholesterol, LDL, apolipoprotein u, and triglyceride levels; to increase HDL level as adjunct to diet in patients with primary hyperlipidemia or mixed dyslipidemia*

TABLETS
Adults. *Initial:* 2 mg once daily, increased as needed. *Maximum:* 4 mg once daily
DOSAGE ADJUSTMENT For patients with moderate renal impairment (glomerular filtration rate 30 to 60 ml/min/1.73 m^2) or patients receiving dialysis, initial dosage reduced to 1 mg once daily, with maximum of 2 mg once daily. For patients taking erythromycin, dosage shouldn't exceed 1 mg daily; for patients taking rifampin, dosage shouldn't exceed 2 mg daily.

Route	Onset	Peak	Duration
P.O.	Unknown	1 hr	Unknown

Mechanism of Action
Reduces plasma cholesterol and lipoprotein levels by inhibiting HMG-CoA reductase and cholesterol synthesis in the liver. Consequently, number of LDL receptors on liver cells increases, and LDL uptake and breakdown are enhanced. With sustained inhibition of cholesterol synthesis in the liver, levels of very low-density lipoproteins are decreased.

Contraindications
Active liver disease (including unexplained persistent LFT elevation), breastfeeding, concurrent cyclosporine therapy, hypersensitivity to pitavastatin or its components, women who are pregnant or may become pregnant

Interaction
DRUGS
colchicine, fibrates such as gemfibrozil: Increased risk of myopathy, including rhabdomyolysis
cyclosporine, erythromycin, lopinavir and ritonavir, rifampin: Increased pitavastatin exposure
niacin: Increased risk of adverse skeletal muscle effects

Adverse Reactions
CNS: Asthenia, confusion, cognitive impairment, depression, dizziness, fatigue, headache, hypoesthenia, insomnia, malaise, memory loss
EENT: Nasopharyngitis
ENDO: Elevated glycosylated hemoglobin level, hyperglycemia

P

GI: Abdominal discomfort or pain, constipation, diarrhea, dyspepsia, elevated liver enzyme levels, hepatic failure, hepatitis, jaundice, nausea
GU: Acute renal failure, erectile dysfunction, myoglobinuria
MS: Arthralgia, back or extremity pain, muscle spasms, myopathy, myositis, rhabdomyolysis
RESP: Interstitial lung disease
SKIN: Pruritus, rash, urticaria
Other: Elevated creatine phosphokinase level, influenza

Nursing Considerations
• Be aware that pitavastatin isn't recommended for patients with severe renal impairment who aren't on dialysis and for patients currently receiving lopinavir and ritonavir therapy because of increased risk of serious adverse effects.
• Note that pravastatin, another HMG-CoA reductase inhibitor, sounds similar to pitavastatin and could be confusing. Make sure of correct drug before giving.
• Monitor liver function test results before pravastatin therapy starts and as indicated during therapy.
• Use pitavastatin cautiously in patients with risk factors for myopathy, such as those over age 65, presence of renal impairment, being inadequately treated for hypothyroidism, or concurrent use of niacin-containing products or fibrates. Monitor patient throughout therapy for muscular complaints and an elevated blood creatine kinase level, as ordered. Drug should be discontinued if patient's creatine kinase level becomes markedly elevated, or if myopathy is suspected or confirmed.
• Expect to monitor patient's lipid levels after 4 weeks of therapy to determine drug effectiveness and periodically thereafter, as ordered. Expect dosage to be adjusted if lipid levels remain elevated.
PATIENT TEACHING
• Emphasize that pitavastatin is an adjunct to, not a substitute for, a low-cholesterol diet.
• Tell patient to take drug at the same day to maintain its effects.
• Instruct patient to report unexplained muscle pain, tenderness, or weakness, especially if accompanied by malaise or fever.

• Advise patient to limit alcohol ingestion while taking pitavastatin because alcohol-induced liver dysfunction may be difficult to differentiate from pitavastatin-induced liver dysfunction.
• Instruct patient to consult prescriber before taking OTC niacin products because of increased risk of adverse muscle effects.
• Caution women of childbearing age that drug is contraindicated in pregnancy because drug could be harmful to the baby. If pregnancy is suspected, patient should notify prescriber immediately.

polymyxin B sulfate
Aerosporin

Class and Category
Chemical class: Bacillus polymyxa derivative
Therapeutic class: Antibiotic
Pregnancy category: Not rated

Indications and Dosages
➤ *To treat infections resistant to less toxic drugs, such as bacteremia, septicemia, and UTI caused by susceptible organisms, including* Enterobacter aerogenes, Escherichia coli, Haemophilus influenzae, *and* Klebsiella pneumoniae
I.V. INFUSION
Adults and children age 2 and over. 15,000 to 25,000 units/kg daily in divided doses every 12 hr or as a continuous infusion.
Maximum: 2 million units daily.
Infants and children under age 2. Up to 40,000 units/kg daily in divided doses every 12 hr or as a continuous infusion.
I.M. INJECTION
Adults and children age 2 and over. 25,000 to 30,000 units/kg daily in divided doses every 4 to 6 hr. *Maximum:* 2 million units daily.
Infants and children under age 2. Up to 40,000 units/kg daily in divided doses every 4 to 6 hr.
DOSAGE ADJUSTMENT Dosage reduced by 50% for patients with creatinine clearance of 5 to 20 ml/min/1.73 m^2; by 85% for patients with creatinine clearance of less than 5 ml/min/1.73 m^2.

➤ *To prevent bacteriuria and bacteremia in patients with an in-dwelling catheter*
BLADDER IRRIGATION
Adults and children age 2 and over.
Combination of 200,000 units (20 mg) polymyxin B sulfate and 57 mg neomycin sulfate added to 1,000 ml normal saline solution daily as a continuous bladder irrigation for up to 10 days; rate adjusted as prescribed, based on patient's urine output.
➤ *To treat meningitis caused by susceptible strains of* Pseudomonas aeruginosa *or* H. influenzae
INTRATHECAL INJECTION
Adults and children age 2 and over. 50,000 units daily for 3 to 4 days, then 50,000 units every other day for at least 2 wk after CSF cultures are negative and glucose content is normal.
Infants and children under age 2. 20,000 units daily for 3 to 4 days, then 25,000 units every other day for at least 2 wk after CSF cultures are negative and glucose content is normal.

Mechanism of Action

Binds to cell membrane phospholipids in gram-negative bacteria, increasing permeability of cell membrane. Polymyxin B also acts as a cationic detergent, altering osmotic barrier of membrane and causing essential intracellular metabolites to leak out. Both actions lead to cell death.

Incompatibilities

Don't mix polymyxin B sulfate with amphotericin B, calcium salts, chloramphenicol, chlorothiazide, heparin sodium, magnesium salts, nitrofurantoin, penicillins, prednisolone, and tetracyclines. They're incompatible.

Contraindications

Hypersensitivity to polymyxin B or its components

Interaction

DRUGS
general anesthetics, neuromuscular blockers, skeletal muscle relaxants: Increased or prolonged skeletal muscle relaxation, possibly respiratory paralysis
nephrotoxic and neurotoxic drugs (such as aminoglycosides, amphotericin B, colistin, sodium citrate, streptomycin, tobramycin,

and vancomycin): Increased risk of nephrotoxicity and neurotoxicity

Adverse Reactions

CNS: Ataxia, confusion, dizziness, drowsiness, fever, giddiness, headache, increased leukocyte and protein levels in CSF, neurotoxicity, paresthesia (circumoral or peripheral), slurred speech
CV: Thrombophlebitis
EENT: Blurred vision, nystagmus
GU: Albuminuria, azotemia, cylindruria, decreased urine output, hematuria, nephrotoxicity
HEME: Eosinophilia
RESP: Respiratory muscle paralysis
SKIN: Rash, urticaria
Other: Anaphylaxis, drug-induced fever, facial flushing, injection-site pain, stiff neck (with intrathecal injection), superinfection

Nursing Considerations

• Be aware that patients receiving polymyxin B sulfate are hospitalized to allow appropriate supervision.
• Obtain blood, urine, or other samples for culture and sensitivity tests, as ordered, before giving drug. Expect to start drug before results are known. Keep in mind that baseline renal function tests should have been performed before administration. Check test results, if available, and notify prescriber of abnormalities.
• For I.M. injection, reconstitute sterile powder with 2 ml of sterile water for injection or sodium chloride for injection.
• Be aware that I.M. route isn't usually recommended (especially for infants and children) because it can cause severe pain at injection site.
• For I.V. infusion, dissolve polymyxin B in 300 to 500 ml of D_5W and infuse over 60 to 90 minutes.
• For intrathecal route, add 10 ml sodium chloride for injection to polymyxin B vial.
• Inspect for particles and discoloration before giving drug.
• During therapy, monitor renal function, including BUN and serum creatinine levels, especially in patients with a history of renal insufficiency.
WARNING Be aware that declining urine output and rising BUN level suggest nephrotoxicity, which also is characterized

P

by albuminuria, azotemia, cylindruria, excessive excretion of electrolytes, hematuria, leukocyturia, and rising blood drug level. Notify prescriber immediately if you detect any of these signs.

WARNING Notify prescriber immediately if patient experiences blurred vision, circumoral or peripheral paresthesia, confusion, dizziness, drowsiness, facial flushing, giddiness, myasthenia, nystagmus, or slurred speech. These may be signs of neurotoxicity, a serious adverse reaction that may lead to respiratory arrest or paralysis if untreated.

• Assess for signs of superinfection, such as mouth sores, severe diarrhea, and white patches on tongue or in mouth, especially in debilitated or elderly patients.

• Monitor fluid intake and output and provide adequate fluids to reduce the risk of nephrotoxicity.

PATIENT TEACHING

• Encourage patient to maintain adequate fluid intake during polymyxin B therapy.

• Instruct patient to notify prescriber at once about diarrhea, mouth sores, or vaginitis, possible early signs of super-infection.

posaconazole
Noxafil

Class and Category
Chemical class: Triazole
Therapeutic class: Antifungal
Pregnancy category: C

Indications and Dosages

➤ *To prevent invasive aspergillus and candida infections in patients at high risk because of severe immuno-compromise from such conditions as graft-versus-host disease with hematopoietic stem-cell transplant or hematologic malignancies with prolonged neutropenia from chemotherapy*

ORAL SUSPENSION

Adults and adolescents. 200 mg (5 ml) three times a day until recovery from neutropenia or immunosuppression.

Delayed Release Tablets

Adults and adolescents. *Initial:* 300 mg twice daily on first day, followed by 300 mg once daily starting on second day until recovery from neutropenia or immunosuppression.

I.V. INFUSION

Adults. *Initial:* 300 mg infused over 90 min via a central venous line or over 30 min for a peripheral venous line twice daily on first day, followed by 300 mg infused over 90 min via a central venous line or over 30 min for a peripheral venous line once daily starting on second day until recovery from neutropenia or immunosuppression.

➤ *To treat oropharyngeal candidiasis*

ORAL SUSPENSION

Adults. *Initial:* 100 mg (2.5 ml) twice daily on first day, followed by 100 mg (2.5 ml) once daily for 13 days.

➤ *To treat oropharyngeal candidiasis refractory to itraconazole and or fluconazole*

ORAL SUSPENSION

Adults. 400 mg (10 ml) twice daily until underlying condition improves.

Route	Onset	Peak	Duration
P.O.	Unknown	3–5 hr	Unknown

Mechanism of Action
Blocks synthesis of ergosterol, an essential component of fungal cell membrane, by inhibiting 14 alpha-demethylase, an enzyme needed for conversion of lanosterol to ergosterol. Lack of ergosterol increases cellular permeability, and cell contents leak.

Incompatibilities
Do not dilute posaconazole in any solution other than 5% dextrose in water or 0.9% sodium chloride. Also do not administer any drug not on the approved manufacturer list (see Nursing Considerations for approved listing). Doing so may cause particulate formation.

Contraindications
Concurrent therapy with atorvastatin, lovastatin, simvastatin, sirolimus; hypersensitivity to posaconazole, its components, or other azole antifungals; use with ergot alkaloids or CYP3A4 substrates such as astemizole, cisapride, halofantrine, pimozide, quinidine, and terfenadine

Interaction

DRUGS

astemizole, cisapride, halofantrine, pimozide, quinidine, terfenadine: Increased risk of prolonged QT interval and torsades de pointes
atazanavir, atorvastatin, calcium channel blockers, cyclosporine, midazolam, phenytoin, rifabutin, ritonavir, simvastatin, sirolimus, tacrolimus: Increased plasma levels of these drugs, with increased risk of adverse reactions
cimetidine, efavirenz, fosamprenavir, phenytoin, rifabutin: Possibly decreased plasma level of posaconazole
digoxin: Increased risk of digitalis toxicity
ergot alkaloids: Increased plasma ergot alkaloid level and increased risk of ergotism
esomeprazole, metoclopramide: Possible breakthrough fungal infections
HMG-CoA reductase inhibitors: Increased plasma statin level and increased risk of rhabdomyolysis
vinca alkaloids: Increased plasma vinca alkaloid level and increased risk of neurotoxicity

Adverse Reactions

CNS: Anxiety, asthenia, dizziness, fatigue, fever, headache, insomnia, rigors, tremor, weakness
CV: Edema, hypertension, hypotension, QT-interval prolongation, tachycardia
EENT: Blurred vision, epistaxis, herpes simplex, mucositis, pharyngitis, taste perversion
ENDO: Hyperglycemia, hypocalcemia
GI: Abdominal pain, anorexia, bilirubinemia, constipation, diarrhea, dyspepsia, elevated liver enzyme levels, hepatomegaly, jaundice, nausea, vomiting
GU: Acute renal failure, elevated blood creatinine level, vaginal hemorrhage
HEME: Anemia, neutropenia, thrombocytopenia
MS: Arthralgia, back or musculoskeletal pain
RESP: Coughing, dyspnea, pneumonia, upper respiratory tract infection
SKIN: Diaphoresis, petechiae, pruritus, rash
Other: Bacteremia, cytomegalovirus infection, dehydration, hypokalemia, hypomagnesemia, weight loss

Nursing Considerations

• Use cautiously in patients who have had a hypersensitivity reaction to other azoles because of risk for cross-sensitivity.
• Use cautiously in patients with hepatic or renal dysfunction. Know that posaconazole injection should be avoided, if possible, in patients with moderate or severe renal impairment (GFR less than 50 ml/min). If not possible, expect to monitor serum creatinine levels, as ordered, and if increases occur, anticipate patient being switched to oral posaconazole therapy.
• Use cautiously in patients with potentially proarrhythmic conditions because posaconazole may prolong QT interval.
• Obtain baseline assessment of liver function and check periodically during therapy. If elevations occur or patient has evidence of abnormal liver function, notify prescriber.
• Shake oral suspension well before administering. Use only the spoon provided in the package to measure dosage. Each dose should be administered during or immediately following (within 20 minutes) a full meal to enhance absorption. If patient cannot eat a full meal, administer drug with a liquid nutritional supplement or an acidic carbonated beverage.
• Administer delayed-release tablets with food.
• Do not interchange delayed-release tablet and oral suspension because of differences in the dosing of each formulation.
• Prepare parenteral form of posaconazole by first removing vial from refrigerator and allowing it to warm to room temperature. Transfer 16.7 ml of the drug solution to an intravenous bag or bottle containing about 150 ml of 5% dextrose in water or 0.9% sodium chloride. Once mixed, use immediately, or refrigerate for up to 24 hours. Discard any unused solution.
• Know that the following drugs and solutions may be infused at the same time through the same intravenous line or cannula with posaconazole: amikacin, caspofungin, ciprofloxacin, daptomycin, dextrose in water 5%, dobutamine,

P

famotidine, filgrastim, gentamicin, hydromorphone, levofloxacin, lorazepam, meropenem, micafungin, morphine sulfate, norepinephrine bitartrate, potassium chloride, sodium chloride 0.9%, and vancomycin. All other solutions and drugs may result in particulate formation and should not be co-administered through the same intravenous line or cannula.

• Administer drug through a 0.22-micron polyethersulfone (PES) or polyvinylidene difluoride (PVD) filter using a central venous line by slow infusion over 90 minutes. Never administer drug by bolus injection. If a central venous line is not available, drug may be administered through a peripheral venous catheter only as a single dose in advance of a central venous line being placed or to bridge the period during which a central venous line is replaced or is in use for other treatment. When administering the drug through a peripheral venous catheter, infuse the drug over 30 minutes.

• Monitor patient experiencing severe diarrhea or vomiting for breakthrough fungal infections.

PATIENT TEACHING

• Advise patient prescribed oral suspension form to use the measuring spoon supplied by manufacturer and to rinse it with water after each use.

• Instruct patient to take posaconazole oral suspension with or within 20 minutes after a full meal or liquid nutritional supplement to increase drug absorption. Tell patient that he also may take posaconazole with an acidic carbonated beverage such as ginger ale.

• Advise patient prescribed delayed-release tablets to take with food; to swallow tablets whole; and to not divide, crush, or chew tablets.

• Tell patient to report severe diarrhea or vomiting because these conditions may interfere with drug effectiveness.

potassium acetate

(contains 2 or 4 mEq of elemental potassium per 1 ml of injection)

potassium bicarbonate

(contains 6.5 mEq of elemental potassium per tablet, 20 or 25 mEq of elemental potassium per effervescent tablet for oral solution)
K+Care ET, K-Electrolyte, K-Ide, Klor-Con/EF, K-Lyte, K-Vescent

potassium bicarbonate and potassium chloride

(contains 20 mEq of elemental potassium per 2.8-g granule packet; 20, 25, or 50 mEq of elemental potassium per effervescent tablet for oral solution)
Klorvess Effervescent Granules, K-Lyte/Cl, K-Lyte/Cl 50, Neo-K (CAN), Potassium Sandoz (CAN)

potassium bicarbonate and potassium citrate

(contains 25 or 50 mEq of elemental potassium per effervescent tablet for oral solution)
Effer-K, K-Lyte DS

potassium chloride

(contains 8 or 10 mEq of elemental potassium per E.R. capsule; 6.7, 8, 10, 12, or 20 mEq of elemental potassium per E.R. tablet; 10, 20, 30, or 40 mEq of elemental potassium per 15 ml of oral solution; 10, 15, 20, or 25 mEq of elemental potassium per packet for oral solution; 20 mEq of elemental potassium per packet for oral suspension; 0.1, 0.2, 0.3, 0.4, 1.5, 2, 3, or 10 mEq of elemental potassium per 1 ml of injection)
Apo-K (CAN), Cena-K, Gen-K, K-8, K-10 (CAN), K+ 10, Kalium Durules (CAN), Kaochlor 10%, Kaochlor S-F 10%, Kaon-Cl, Kato, Kay Ciel, K+ Care, KCL 5% (CAN), K-Dur, K-Ide, K-Lease, K-Long (CAN), K-Lor, Klor-Con 10, Klor-Con Powder, Klor-

Con/25 Powder, Klorvess 10% Liquid, Klotrix, K-Lyte/Cl Powder, K-Med 900 (CAN), K-Norm, K-Sol, K-Tab, Micro-K, Micro-K 10, Potasalan, Roychlor 10% (CAN), Rum-K, Slow-K, Ten-K

potassium citrate

(contains 5 mEq or 10 mEq of elemental potassium per tablet)
Urocit-K

potassium gluconate

(contains 20 mEq of elemental potassium per 15 ml of elixir; 2, 2.3, or 2.5 mEq of elemental potassium per tablet)
Glu-K, Kaon, Kaylixir, K-G Elixir, Potassium-Rougier (can)

potassium gluconate and potassium chloride

(contains 20 mEq of elemental potassium per 15 ml of oral solution; 20 mEq of elemental potassium per 5-g packet for oral solution)
Kolyum

potassium gluconate and potassium citrate

(contains 20 mEq of elemental potassium per 15 ml of oral solution)
Twin-K

trikates

(contains 15 mEq of elemental potassium per 5 ml of oral solution)
Tri-K

Class and Category

Chemical class: Electrolyte cation
Therapeutic class: Electrolyte replacement
Pregnancy category: C

Indications and Dosages

➤ *To prevent or treat hypokalemia in patients who can't ingest sufficient*

dietary potassium or who are losing potassium because of a condition (such as hepatic cirrhosis or prolonged vomiting) or drug (such as potassium-wasting diuretics or certain antibiotics)

EFFERVESCENT TABLETS (POTASSIUM BICARBONATE)
Adults and adolescents. 25 to 50 mEq/g once or twice daily, as needed and tolerated.
Maximum: 100 mEq daily.

EFFERVESCENT TABLETS (POTASSIUM BICARBONATE AND POTASSIUM CHLORIDE)
Adults and adolescents. 20, 25, or 50 mEq once or twice daily, as needed and tolerated.
Maximum: 100 mEq daily.

EFFERVESCENT TABLETS (POTASSIUM BICARBONATE AND POTASSIUM CITRATE)
Adults and adolescents. 25 or 50 mEq once or twice daily, as needed and tolerated.
Maximum: 100 mEq daily.

ELIXIR (POTASSIUM GLUCONATE)
Adults and adolescents. 20 mEq twice daily to four times daily, as needed and tolerated. *Maximum:* 100 mEq daily.
Children. 2 to 3 mEq/kg daily in divided doses.

E.R. CAPSULES (POTASSIUM CHLORIDE)
Adults and adolescents. 40 to 100 mEq daily in divided doses twice daily or three times a day for treatment; 16 to 24 mEq daily in divided doses twice daily or three times a day for prevention.
Maximum: 100 mEq daily.

E.R. TABLETS (POTASSIUM CHLORIDE)
Adults and adolescents. 6.7 to 20 mEq three times a day*Maximum:* 100 mEq daily.

GRANULE PACKETS (POTASSIUM BICARBONATE AND POTASSIUM CHLORIDE)
Adults and adolescents. 20 mEq once or twice daily, as needed and tolerated.
Maximum: 100 mEq daily.

GRANULES FOR ORAL SUSPENSION (POTASSIUM CHLORIDE)
Adults and adolescents. 20 mEq 1 to 5 times/day, as needed. *Maximum:* 100 mEq daily.

ORAL SOLUTION (POTASSIUM CHLORIDE)
Adults and adolescents. 20 mEq once daily to four times a day, as needed and tolerated.
Maximum: 100 mEq daily.

P

Children. 1 to 3 mEq/kg daily in divided doses.

ORAL SOLUTION (POTASSIUM GLUCONATE AND POTASSIUM CHLORIDE, POTASSIUM GLUCONATE AND POTASSIUM CITRATE)
Adults and adolescents. 20 mEq twice daily to four times a day, as needed and tolerated. *Maximum:* 100 mEq daily.
Children. 2 to 3 mEq/kg daily in divided doses.

POWDER PACKET FOR ORAL SOLUTION (POTASSIUM CHLORIDE)
Adults. 15 to 25 mEq twice daily to four times a day, as needed and tolerated. *Maximum:* 100 mEq daily.
Children. 1 to 3 mEq/kg daily in divided doses, as needed and tolerated.

POWDER PACKET FOR ORAL SOLUTION (POTASSIUM GLUCONATE AND POTASSIUM CHLORIDE)
Adults and adolescents. 20 mEq dailyTo four times a day, as needed and tolerated. *Maximum:* 100 mEq daily.
Children. 2 to 3 mEq/kg daily in divided doses.

ORAL TRIKATES SOLUTION (POTASSIUM ACETATE, POTASSIUM BICARBONATE, AND POTASSIUM CITRATE)
Adults and adolescents. 15 mEq three times a day to four times a day, as needed and tolerated. *Maximum:* 100 mEq daily.
Children. 2 to 3 mEq/kg daily in divided doses.

TABLETS (POTASSIUM GLUCONATE)
Adults and adolescents. 5 to 10 mEq twice daily to four times a day, as needed and tolerated. *Maximum:* 100 mEq daily.

I.V. INFUSION (POTASSIUM ACETATE AND POTASSIUM CHLORIDE)
Adults and adolescents with serum potassium level above 2.5 mEq/L. Up to 10 mEq/ hr. *Maximum:* 200 mEq daily.
Adults and adolescents with serum potassium level below 2 mEq/L, ECG changes, or paralysis. Up to 20 mEq/hr. *Maximum:* 400 mEq daily.
Children. 3 mEq/kg daily.
DOSAGE ADJUSTMENT Dosage adjusted as prescribed based on patient's ECG patterns and serum potassium level.
➤ *To treat renal tubular acidosis with calcium stones, hypocitraturic calcium oxalate nephrolithiasis of any etiology, and uric acid lithiasis with or without calcium stones*

TABLETS (POTASSIUM CITRATE)
Adults. For patients with severe hypocitraturia, 15 mEq four times a day with meals or 20 mEq three times a day with meals. For patients with mild to moderate hypocitraturia, 10 mEq three times a day with meals.

Mechanism of Action
Acts as the major cation in intracellular fluid, activating many enzymatic reactions essential for physiologic processes, including nerve impulse transmission and cardiac and skeletal muscle contraction. Potassium also helps maintain electroneutrality in cells by controlling exchange of intracellular and extracellular ions. It also helps maintain normal renal function and acid-base balance.

Incompatibilities
Don't mix potassium chloride for injection in same syringe with amino acid solutions, lipid solutions, or mannitol because these drugs may precipitate from solution. Administration with blood or blood products can cause lysis of infused RBCs.

Contraindications
Acute dehydration, Addison's disease (untreated), concurrent use of potassium-sparing diuretics, crush syndrome, disorders that may delay drug passing through GI tract (potassium citrate), heat cramps, hyperkalemia, hypersensitivity to potassium salts or their components, peptic ulcer disease (potassium citrate), renal impairment with azotemia or oliguria, severe hemolytic anemia, UTI (potassium citrate)

Interaction
DRUGS
ACE inhibitors, beta blockers, blood products, cyclosporine, heparin, NSAIDs, potassium-containing drugs, potassium-sparing diuretics: Increased risk of hyperkalemia
amphotericin B, corticosteroids (glucocorticoids, mineralocorticoids), gentamicin, penicillins, polymyxin B: Possibly hypokalemia
anticholinergics, drugs with anticholinergic activity: Increased risk of GI ulceration, stricture, and perforation

calcium salts (parenteral): Possibly arrhythmias
digoxin: Increased risk of digitalis toxicity
insulin, laxatives, sodium bicarbonate: Decreased serum potassium level
sodium polystyrene sulfonate: Possibly decreased serum potassium level and fluid retention
thiazide diuretics: Possibly hyperkalemia when diuretic is discontinued
FOODS
low-salt milk, salt substitutes: Increased risk of hyperkalemia

Adverse Reactions
CNS: Confusion, paralysis, paresthesia, weakness
CV: Arrhythmias, ECG changes
EENT: Throat pain when swallowing
GI: Abdominal pain; bloody stools; diarrhea; flatulence; GI bleeding, perforation, or ulceration; intestinal obstruction; nausea; vomiting
RESP: Dyspnea
SKIN: Rash
Other: Hyperkalemia

Nursing Considerations
• Administer oral potassium with or immediately after meals.
• Mix potassium chloride for oral solution or potassium gluconate elixir in cold water, orange juice, tomato juice (if patient isn't sodium restricted), or apple juice, and stir for 1 full minute before administering.
• Mix potassium bicarbonate, potassium bicarbonate and potassium chloride, and potassium bicarbonate and potassium citrate effervescent tablets with cold water and allow to dissolve completely.
• Be aware that liquid form of oral potassium is prescribed for patients with delayed gastric emptying, esophageal compression, or intestinal obstruction or stricture to decrease the risk of tissue damage.
WARNING Be aware that direct injection of a potassium concentrate may be immediately fatal. Dilute potassium concentrate for injection with adequate volume of solution before I.V. use. Maximum suggested concentration is 40 mEq/L, although stronger concentrations (up to 80 mEq/L) may be used for severe hypokalemia.

Inappropriate solutions or improper technique may cause extravasation, fever, hyperkalemia, hypervolemia, I.V. site infection, phlebitis, venospasm, and venous thrombosis.
• Infuse potassium slowly to avoid phlebitis and decrease risk of adverse cardiac reactions. Keep in mind that different forms of potassium salts contain different amounts of elemental potassium per gram and that not all forms are dosage equivalent.
• Monitor serum potassium level before and during administration of I.V. potassium.
WARNING Be aware that some forms of potassium contain tartrazine, which may cause an allergic reaction, such as asthma. Some forms may also contain aluminum, which may become toxic in a patient with impaired renal function.
• Regularly assess patient for signs of hypokalemia, such as arrhythmias, fatigue, and weakness, and for signs of hyperkalemia, such as arrhythmias, confusion, dyspnea, and paresthesia.
• Because adequate renal function is needed for potassium supplementation, monitor serum creatinine level and urine output during administration. Notify prescriber about signs of decreased renal function.
PATIENT TEACHING
• Inform patient that potassium is part of a normal diet and that most meats, seafoods, fruits, and vegetables contain sufficient potassium to meet recommended daily intake. Also advise her not to exceed recommended daily amount of potassium.
• Teach patient the correct way to take prescribed potassium. This can vary from swallowing a tablet with a full glass of water to mixing certain preparations with half to full glass of cold water or juice.
• Caution patient not to crush or chew E.R. forms unless instructed otherwise.
• Instruct patient to take drug with or right after food.
• Teach patient how to take her radial pulse, and advise her to notify prescriber about significant changes in heart rate or rhythm.
• Advise patient to watch stools for changes in color and consistency and to notify prescriber if they become black, tarry, or red.

P

• Inform patient that although she may see waxy form of E.R. tablet in stools, she has received all of the potassium.

• Urge patient to keep follow-up laboratory appointments as directed by prescriber to determine serum potassium level.

potassium iodide
(KI, SSKI)
Pima, Thyro-Block

Class and Category
Chemical class: Iodine
Therapeutic class: Antithyroid, radiation protectant
Pregnancy category: D

Indications and Dosages
➤ *To prepare for thyroidectomy*
ORAL SOLUTION
Adults and children. 50 to 250 mg three times a day for 10 to 14 days before surgery.
➤ *To manage thyrotoxic crisis*
ORAL SOLUTION
Adults. 50 to 250 mg three times a day or 500 mg every 4 hr.
➤ *To protect thyroid gland during radiation exposure*
ORAL SOLUTION, SYRUP, TABLETS
Adults and adolescents. 100 to 150 mg 24 hr before administration of or exposure to radioactive isotopes of iodine and daily for 3 to 10 days afterward. *Maximum:* 12 g daily.
Children age 1 and over. 130 mg daily for 10 days after administration of or exposure to radioactive isotopes of iodine.
Children under age 1. 65 mg daily for 10 days after administration of or exposure to radioactive isotopes of iodine.

Route	Onset	Peak	Duration
P.O.*	24 hr	10–15 days	Up to 6 wk

Mechanism of Action
Inhibits release of thyroid hormone into circulation, thus alleviating symptoms caused by excessive thyroid hormone stimulation. Potassium iodide also blocks

---
* For antithyroid effects.

thyroid uptake of radioactive iodine isotopes released as a result of radiation exposure.

Contraindications
Acute bronchitis, Addison's disease, dehydration, heat cramps, hyperkalemia, hypersensitivity to iodides or their components, hyperthyroidism, iodism, renal impairment, tuberculosis

Interaction
DRUGS
antithyroid drugs, lithium: Increased risk of hypothyroidism and goiter
captopril, enalapril, lisinopril, potassium-sparing diuretics: Increased risk of hyperkalemia

Adverse Reactions
CNS: Confusion, fatigue, headache, heaviness or weakness in legs, paresthesia
CV: Irregular heartbeat
EENT: Burning in mouth or throat, increased salivation, metallic taste, sore teeth or gums
GI: Diarrhea, epigastric pain, indigestion, nausea, vomiting
HEME: Eosinophilia
MS: Arthralgia
SKIN: Acneiform lesions, urticaria
Other: Angioedema, lymphadenopathy

Nursing Considerations
• Be aware that potassium iodide shouldn't be given to patients with tuberculosis because drug may cause pulmonary irritation and increased secretions.
WARNING Monitor serum potassium level regularly in patients with renal impairment because of the risk of hyperkalemia.
• Monitor thyroid function test results periodically to assess drug's effectiveness.
PATIENT TEACHING
• Advise patient taking potassium iodide oral solution or syrup to use a calibrated measuring device to ensure accurate doses.
• Urge patient to mix solution or syrup in a full glass (8 oz) of water, fruit juice, milk, or broth to improve taste and lessen GI reactions. Advise patient taking tablet form to dissolve each tablet in half a glass (4 oz) of water or milk before ingestion.

• If crystals form in solution, advise patient to place the closed container in warm water and gently shake to dissolve.
• Instruct patient to discard bottle and obtain a new one if solution turns brownish yellow.

potassium phosphates

K-Phos Original, Neutra-Phos-K

potassium and sodium phosphates

K-Phos M.F., K-Phos-Neutral, K-Phos No. 2, Neutra-Phos

sodium phosphates

Class and Category
Chemical class: Anion, soluble salts
Therapeutic class: Antiurolithic, electrolyte replenisher, urinary acidifier
Pregnancy category: C

Indications and Dosages
➤ *As adjunct to treat UTI, to prevent renal calculus formation*
MONOBASIC TABLETS (POTASSIUM PHOSPHATES)
Adults and adolescents. 1 g in 180 to 240 ml water four times a day, after meals and at bedtime.
MONOBASIC TABLETS (POTASSIUM AND SODIUM PHOSPHATES)
Adults and adolescents. 250 mg in 240 ml water four times a day, after bedtime. Dosage interval may be increased to every 2 hr if urine is difficult to acidify. *Maximum:* 2 g/24 hr.
➤ *To prevent or treat hypophosphatemia*
CAPSULES (POTASSIUM PHOSPHATES)
Adults and children age 4 and over. 1.45 g in 75 ml water or juice four times a day, after meals and at bedtime.
Children up to age 4. 200 mg in 60 ml water or juice four times a day, after meals and at bedtime.
CAPSULES (POTASSIUM AND SODIUM PHOSPHATES)
Adults and children age 4 and over. 1.25 g in 75 ml water or juice four times a day, after meals and at bedtime.

Children up to age 4. 200 mg in 60 ml water or fruit juice four times a day, after meals and at bedtime.
MONOBASIC TABLETS (POTASSIUM PHOSPHATES)
Adults and children age 4 and over. 1 g in 180 to 240 ml water four times a day, after meals and at bedtime.
Children up to age 4. 200 mg in 60 ml water four times a day, after meals and at bedtime.
MONOBASIC TABLETS (POTASSIUM AND SODIUM PHOSPHATES)
Adults and children age 4 and over. 250 mg in 240 ml water four times a day, after meals and at bedtime.
Children up to age 4. 200 mg in 60 ml water four times a day, after meals and at bedtime.
ORAL SOLUTION (POTASSIUM PHOSPHATES, POTASSIUM AND SODIUM PHOSPHATES)
Adults and children age 4 and over. 250 mg four times a day, after meals and at bedtime.
Children up to age 4. 200 mg four times a day, after meals and at bedtime.
TABLETS (POTASSIUM AND SODIUM PHOSPHATES)
Adults and children age 4 and over. 250 mg in a full glass of water four times a day, after meals and at bedtime.
Children up to age 4. 200 mg in 60 ml water four times a day, after meals and at bedtime.
I.V. INFUSION (SODIUM PHOSPHATES)
Adults and adolescents. 10 to 15 mmol (310 to 465 mg) daily.
Children. 1.5 to 2 mmol (46.5 to 62 mg)/kg daily.

Mechanism of Action
Reverses symptoms of hypophosphatemia by replenishing the body's supply of phosphate; acidifies urine by causing hydrogen to be exchanged for sodium in renal distal tubule; and inhibits formation of calcium renal calculi by preventing solidification of calcium oxalate.

Incompatibilities
Don't add phosphates to calcium- or magnesium-containing solutions because precipitate may form.

Contraindications
Hyperkalemia (potassium formulations), hypernatremia (sodium formulations), hyperphosphatemia, magnesium ammonium

P

phosphate urolithiasis accompanied by infection, severe renal insufficiency, UTI caused by urea-splitting organisms

Interaction
DRUGS
ACE inhibitors, cyclosporine, heparin (long-term use), NSAIDs, potassium-containing drugs, potassium-sparing diuretics: Increased risk of hyperkalemia (potassium forms only)
aluminum- or magnesium-containing antacids: Possibly impaired phosphate absorption
anabolic steroids, androgens, corticosteroids, estrogens: Increased risk of edema (sodium formulations only)
calcium-containing drugs: Increased risk of calcium deposition in soft tissues
iron supplements: Decreased absorption of oral iron
phosphate-containing drugs, vitamin D: Increased risk of hyperphosphatemia
salicylates: Increased blood salicylate level
zinc supplements: Reduced zinc absorption
FOODS
low-salt milk, salt substitutes: Increased risk of hyperkalemia
oxalates (in spinach and rhubarb), phyates (in bran and whole grains): Decreased absorption of phosphate

Adverse Reactions
CNS: Anxiety, confusion, dizziness, fatigue, headache, paresthesia, seizures, tremor, weakness
CV: Arrhythmias, edema of legs, tachycardia
GI: Diarrhea, epigastric pain, nausea, thirst, vomiting
GU: Decreased urine output
MS: Muscle cramps or weakness
RESP: Dyspnea
Other: Hyperkalemia, hypernatremia, hyperphosphatemia, hypocalcemia, weight gain

Nursing Considerations
• Monitor serum phosphorus level, as appropriate, in patient who receives phosphates and has a condition that may be associated with elevated phosphorus level, such as chronic renal disease, hypoparathyroidism, and rhabdomyolysis; phosphates may further increase serum phosphorus level.

• Monitor serum calcium level, as appropriate, in patient who receives phosphates and has a condition that may be associated with a low calcium level, such as acute pancreatitis, chronic renal disease, hypoparathyroidism, osteomalacia, rhabdomyolysis, and rickets; phosphates may further decrease serum calcium level.
• Monitor serum potassium level, as appropriate, if patient who receives potassium phosphate has a condition linked to elevated potassium level, such as acute dehydration, adrenal insufficiency, extensive tissue breakdown (as in severe burns), myotonia congenita, pancreatitis, rhabdomyolysis, and severe renal insufficiency; she may have increased risk of hyperkalemia.
• Monitor serum sodium level in patient who receives sodium phosphates and has a condition that may be worsened by sodium excess, such as heart failure, hypernatremia, hypertension, peripheral or pulmonary edema, preeclampsia, renal impairment, and severe hepatic disease.
• Monitor urine pH, as ordered, to assess effectiveness of drug used to acidify urine.
• When administering sodium phosphates, monitor ECG tracing frequently during I.V. infusion to detect arrhythmias.
PATIENT TEACHING
• Instruct patient to take phosphates after meals to avoid GI upset and decrease laxative effect.
• Emphasize importance of not swallowing capsules or tablets whole; instead, advise patient to soak tablets in water or fruit juice for 2 to 3 minutes to dissolve them.
• Suggest chilling diluted drug to improve flavor, but caution against freezing.
• Encourage increased intake of fluids (8 oz/ hour, if not contraindicated) to prevent renal calculi.
• Urge patient to notify prescriber immediately about muscle weakness or cramps, unexplained weight gain, or shortness of breath.
• Instruct patient who needs an iron supplement to take it 1 to 2 hours after taking phosphates.

pralidoxime chloride

(2-PAM chloride, 2-pyridine aldoxime methochloride)
Protopam Chloride

Class and Category

Chemical class: Quaternary ammonium oxime
Therapeutic class: Anticholinesterase antidote
Pregnancy category: C

Indications and Dosages

➤ *As adjunct to reverse organophosphate pesticide toxicity*

I.V. INFUSION

Adults. *Initial:* 1 to 2 g in 100-ml normal saline solution infused over 15 to 30 min until muscarinic signs and symptoms disappear; may be repeated in 1 hr and then every 10 to 12 hr if muscle weakness persists

Children. *Initial:* 20 to 50 mg/kg (not to exceed 2,000 mg/dose) in 100-ml normal saline solution infused over 15 to 30 min followed by a continuous infusion of 10 to 20 mg/kg/hr. Alternatively, an initial intermittent infusion of 20 to 50 mg/kg (not to exceed 2,000 mg/dose) given over 15 to 30 min. Dosage may be repeated in 1 hr and then every 10 to 12 hr if muscle weakness persists.

DOSAGE ADJUSTMENT For patient with pulmonary edema, dosage given slowly (over not less than 5 min) as a 50 mg/ml solution in water.

I.M. INJECTION

Adults and children weighing 40 kg or more. For mild symptoms, 600 mg (2 ml). May repeat dose after 15 min and again after an additional 15 min, as needed. If at any time after the first dose patient develops severe symptoms, two additional 600-mg doses may be given in rapid succession for a total cumulative dose of 1,800 mg. For severe symptoms, 600 mg (2 ml) administered 3 times in rapid succession for a total dose of 1,800 mg. For persistent symptoms after 3 injections of 600 mg each have been given, series may be repeated beginning about 1 hr after administration of the last injection.

Children weighing less than 40 kg. For mild symptoms, 15 mg/kg. May repeat dose after 15 min and again after an additional 15 min, as needed. If at any time after the first dose patient develops severe symptoms, two additional 15-mg/kg doses may be given in rapid succession for a total cumulative dose of 45 mg/kg. For severe symptoms, 15 mg/kg administered 3 times in rapid succession for a total dose of 45mg/ kg. For persistent symptoms after 3 injections of 15 mg/kg each have been given, series may be repeated beginning about 1 hr after administration of the last injection.

➤ *To treat anticholinesterase overdose secondary to myasthenic drugs (including ambenonium, neostigmine, and pyridostigmine)*

I.V. INJECTION

Adults. *Initial:* 1 to 2 g, followed by 250 mg every 5 min.

➤ *To treat exposure to nerve agents*

I.V. INJECTION

Adults. *Initial:* 1 atropine-containing autoinjector followed by 1 pralidoxime-containing autoinjector as soon as atropine's effects are evident; both injections repeated every 15 min for 2 additional doses if nerve agent symptoms persist.

DOSAGE ADJUSTMENT Dosage reduced for patients with renal insufficiency.

Mechanism of Action

Reverses muscle paralysis by removing phosphoryl group from inhibited cholinesterase molecules at neuromuscular junction of skeletal and respiratory muscles. Reactivation of cholinesterase restores body's ability to metabolize acetylcholine, which is inhibited by organophosphate pesticides, anticholinesterase overdose, or nerve agent poisoning.

Contraindications

Hypersensitivity to pralidoxime chloride or its components

Interaction

DRUGS

aminophylline, morphine, phenothiazines, reserpine, succinylcholine, theophylline: Increased symptoms of organophosphate poisoning

P

barbiturates: Potentiated barbiturate effects

Adverse Reactions

CNS: Dizziness, drowsiness, headache
CV: Increased systolic and diastolic blood pressure, tachycardia
EENT: Accommodation disturbances, blurred vision, diplopia
GI: Nausea, vomiting
MS: Muscle weakness
RESP: Hyperventilation
Other: Injection-site pain

Nursing Considerations

• Be aware that pralidoxime must be given within 36 hours of toxicity to be effective and atropine must be given as soon as possible after hypoxemia is improved.
• Use drug with extreme caution in patients with myasthenia gravis being treated for organophosphate poisoning because pralidoxime may precipitate myasthenic crisis.
• Reconstitute drug according to manufacturer's guidelines and administration route.
• For intermittent intravenous infusion, further dilute with normal saline solution to 100 ml and infuse over 15 to 30 minutes. Rate should not exceed 200 mg/minute.
• Avoid too-rapid intravenous delivery, which may cause hypertension, laryngospasm, muscle spasms, neuromuscular blockade, and tachycardia. Also be sure to avoid intradermal injection.
• If intravenous route is not feasible, expect to administer the drug intramuscularly or subcutaneously.
• Closely monitor neuromuscular status during therapy.
• Monitor BUN and serum creatinine levels, as appropriate, in patients with renal insufficiency because drug is excreted in urine.
• When pralidoxime is administered with atropine, expect signs of atropination, such as dry mouth and nose, flushing, mydriasis, and tachycardia, to occur earlier than might be expected when atropine is given alone.

PATIENT TEACHING
• Inform patient receiving I.M. pralidoxime that she'll experience pain at the injection site for 40 to 60 minutes afterward.

• Reassure patient that she'll be closely monitored throughout therapy.

pramipexole dihydrochloride

Mirapex, Mirapex ER

Class and Category

Chemical class: Benzothiazolamine derivative
Therapeutic class: Antidyskinetic
Pregnancy category: C

Indications and Dosages

➤ *To treat Parkinson's disease, with or without concurrent levodopa therapy*

TABLETS
Adults. *Initial:* 0.125 mg three times a day for 1 wk, increased weekly thereafter as follows: for week 2, 0.25 mg three times a day; for week 3, 0.5 mg three times a day; for week 4, 0.75 mg three times a day; for week 5, 1 mg three times a day.; for week 6, 1.25 mg three times a day; and for week 7, 1.5 mg three times a day. *Maintenance:* 1.5 to 4.5 mg daily in divided doses three times a day.
Maximum: 4.5 mg daily.

DOSAGE ADJUSTMENT For patients with renal impairment, dosage reduced as follows: for creatinine clearance of 35 to 59 ml/min/ 1.73 m², initial dose of 0.125 mg twice daily, maximum of 3 mg daily; for creatinine clearance of 15 to 34 ml/min/1.73 m², initial dose of 0.125 mg daily, maximum of 1.5 mg daily. Drug shouldn't be given to patients with creatinine clearance of less than 15 ml/min/1.73 m².

E.R. TABLETS
Adults. *Initial:* 0.375 mg once daily, increased every 5 to 7 days, first to 0.75 mg and then by 0.75-mg increments, as needed. *Maximum:* 4.5 mg daily.

DOSAGE ADJUSTMENT For patients with moderate renal impairment (creatinine clearance between 30 and 50 ml/min/ 1.73 m²), initial dosage taken every other day with dosage adjustment done after 1 wk in increments of 0.375 mg only, as needed, to maximum dosage of 2.25 mg daily.
➤ *To treat restless legs syndrome*

TABLETS
Adults. *Initial:* 0.125 mg once daily, 2 to 3 hr before bedtime. Increased in 4 to 7 days to 0.25 mg once daily 2 to 3 hr before bedtime, as needed. Further increased in 4 to 7 days to 0.5 mg once daily 2 to 3 hr before bedtime, as needed.
DOSAGE ADJUSTMENT For patients with moderate to severe renal impairment (creatinine clearance 20 to 60 ml/min/1.73 m²) dosage interval for titration, if needed, increased to 14 days.

Mechanism of Action
May stimulate dopamine receptors in the brain, thereby easing symptoms of Parkinson's disease, which is thought to be caused by a dopamine deficiency.

Contraindications
Hypersensitivity to pramipexole or its components

Interaction
DRUGS
carbidopa, levodopa: Possibly increased peak blood levodopa level and potentiation of levodopa's dopaminergic adverse effects
diltiazem, quinidine, quinine, ranitidine, triamterene, verapamil: Decreased pramipexole clearance
haloperidol, metoclopramide, phenothiazines, thioxanthenes: Decreased pramipexole effectiveness

Adverse Reactions
CNS: Abnormal behavior, amnesia, anxiety, asthenia, compulsive behaviors such as pathological gambling or uncontrollable shopping, confusion, dream disturbances, drowsiness, dyskinesia, dystonia, fatigue, fever, hallucinations, headache, insomnia, malaise, paranoia, restlessness, syncope
CV: Edema, orthostatic hypotension
EENT: Diplopia, dry mouth, rhinitis, vision changes
ENDO: Inappropriate antidiuretic hormone secretion (SIADH)
GI: Anorexia, constipation, dysphagia, nausea, vomiting
GU: Altered libido, hypersexuality, impotence, urinary frequency, urinary incontinence
MS: Arthralgia, myalgia, myasthenia
RESP: Pneumonia

SKIN: Diaphoresis, pruritis, rash
Other: Eating disorders (binge or compulsive eating, hyperphagia), intense urges for certain activities (such as gambling and sex), weight gain or loss

Nursing Considerations
• Use pramipexole cautiously in patients with hallucinations, hypotension, or retinal problems (such as macular degeneration). Drug may worsen these conditions.
• Also use cautiously in patients with renal impairment because pramipexole elimination may be decreased.
• Take safety precautions per facility policy until drug's CNS effects are known.
• Avoid stopping pramipexole abruptly because doing so may cause a symptom complex resembling neuroleptic malignant syndrome and consisting of hyperpyrexia, muscle rigidity, altered level of consciousness, and autonomic instability.
• Be aware that patient may be switched overnight from immediate-release pramipexole tablets to the extended-release tablets at the same daily dose. However, monitor effectiveness to determine if dosage adjustment may be necessary.
• Assess patient for skin changes regularly because melanomas may occur at a higher rate in patients with Parkinson's disease. It isn't clear if this is a result of the disease or drugs used to treat it.
PATIENT TEACHING
• Advise patient to take pramipexole with meals if nausea occurs.
• Caution patient about possible dizziness, drowsiness, or light-headedness, which may result from orthostatic hypotension. Advise her not to rise quickly from a lying or sitting position to minimize these effects.
• Instruct patient to notify prescriber immediately about vision problems or urinary frequency or incontinence.
• Inform patient that improvement in motor performance and activities of daily living may take 2 to 3 weeks.
• Urge patient to have regular skin examinations by a dermatologist or other qualified health professional.
• Advise patient and his family to notify prescriber about onset of intense and compulsive urges, such as eating binges,

pathological gambling, compulsive shopping, or hypersexuality. Dosage may need to be reduced or drug discontinued.
• Caution patient not to stop taking pramipexole abruptly.

pramlintide acetate
Symlin

Class and Category
Chemical class: Synthetic analogue of human amylin, a pancreatic beta cell hormone
Therapeutic class: Antidiabetic
Pregnancy category: C

Indications and Dosages
➤ *To achieve euglycemia in patients with type 1 diabetes who use mealtime insulin therapy but have not achieved desired glucose control*

SUBCUTANEOUS INJECTION
Adults. *Initial:* 15 mcg just before major meal swith 50% reduced dosage of preprandial rapid-acting or short-acting insulin, including fixed-mix insulins such as 70/30. When nausea has abated at least 3 days, dosage increased in increments of 15 mcg. *Maintenance:* 30 to 60 mcg before major meals.

DOSAGE ADJUSTMENT Dosage decreased to 30 mcg if nausea occurs and persists at higher dosages.

➤ *To achieve euglycemia in patients with type 2 diabetes who use mealtime insulin, with or without a sulfonylurea and/or metformin, and have not achieved desire glucose control*

SUBCUTANEOUS INJECTION
Adults. *Initial:* 60 mcg immediately before major meals combined with dosage reduction of preprandial rapid-acting or short-acting insulin, including fixed-mix insulins such as 70/30, by 50%. When nausea has been absent for 3 to 7 days, dosage increased to 120 mcg before major meals.

DOSAGE ADJUSTMENT Dosage decreased to 60 mcg before major meals if nausea occurs and persists with 120-mcg dosage.

Route	Onset	Peak	Duration
SubQ	Unknown	19–21 min	3 hr

Mechanism of Action
Slows the rate at which food is released from stomach to small intestine, thus reducing initial postprandial rise in serum glucose level. Pramlintide also suppresses glucagon secretion and promotes satiety, thus furthering weight loss, which also lowers serum glucose level.

Pramlintide is a synthetic analogue of amylin, a naturally occurring neuro-endocrine hormone secreted with insulin by pancreatic beta cells. In diabetes, secretion of insulin and amylin is reduced or absent.

Contraindications
Gastroparesis, hypersensitivity to pramlintide, cresol or its components; hypoglycemia unawareness

Incompatibilities
Don't mix in same syringe as insulin because pharmacokinetic parameters of pramlintide become altered.

Interaction
DRUGS
drugs that alter GI motility (such as anti-cholinergics) or slow intestinal absorption of nutrients (such as alpha-glucosidase inhibitors): Altered effects of these drugs
oral drugs: Delayed absorption

Adverse Reactions
CNS: Dizziness, fatigue, headache
EENT: Blurred vision, pharyngitis
ENDO: Insulin-induced hypoglycemia
GI: Abdominal pain, anorexia, nausea, pancreatitis, vomiting
MS: Arthralgia
RESP: Coughing
SKIN: Diaphoresis
Other: Hypersensitivity reactions; local injection-site reaction, such as redness, swelling, or pruritus

Nursing Considerations
• Because of the risks involved with pramlintide therapy, insulin-using patients with type 1 or 2 diabetes must have failed to achieve adequate glycemic control despite individualized insulin manage-ment and must be receiving ongoing care with guidance of insulin prescriber and a diabetes educator before pramlintide is prescribed.

• Expect that certain patients won't be prescribed pramlintide because its risks may outweigh its benefits. These include patients with poor compliance with current insulin regimen, poor compliance with monitoring blood glucose level, a glycosylated hemoglobin greater than 9%, recurrent severe hypoglycemia that required assistance during past 6 months, hypoglycemia unawareness, gastroparesis, concurrent therapy with drugs that stimulate GI motility, and pediatric patients.

• Before pramlintide therapy starts, make sure patient's pre-meal insulin dosage has been reduced by 50%.

• Give drug immediately before main meals.

• Monitor patient's pre- and post-meal blood glucose levels regularly to determine effectiveness of pramlintide and insulin therapy and to detect hypoglycemia.

• For 3 hours after each dose of pramlintide, monitor patient closely for hypoglycemia, which may be severe, especially in patients with type 1 diabetes. Effects may include hunger, headache, sweating, tremor, irritability, and trouble concentrating. They may occur with a rapid decrease in blood glucose level regardless of glucose values.

• Although pramlintide doesn't cause hypoglycemia, its use with insulin increases the risk of insulin-induced severe hypoglycemia, which can result in loss of consciousness, coma, or seizures. If hypoglycemia occurs, provide supportive care, including glucagon if prescribed, and notify prescriber. Expect insulin dosage accompanying pramlintide to be reduced.

• Keep in mind that early warning symptoms of hypoglycemia may be different or less severe if patient has had diabetes for a long time; has diabetic nerve disease; takes a beta blocker, clonidine, guanethidine, or reserpine; or is under intensified diabetes control.

• Closely monitor patients taking oral antidiabetics, ACE inhibitors, disopyramide, fibrates, fluoxetine, MAO inhibitors, pentoxifylline, propoxyphene, salicylates, or sulfonamide antibiotics because of an increased risk of hypoglycemia.

• Expect pramlintide to be stopped if patient develops recurrent hypoglycemia that requires medical assistance, develops persistent nausea, or becomes noncompliant with therapy or follow-up visits.

PATIENT TEACHING

• Alert patient that insulin-induced hypoglycemia may occur within 3 hours of injecting pramlintide. Review signs and symptoms and appropriate treatment. Tell patient to notify prescriber if hypoglycemia occurs because insulin dosage will need to be reduced.

• Emphasize need to monitor blood glucose level often, especially before and after eating.

• Tell patient to inject drug subcutaneously immediately before major meals using an insulin syringe to draw up dose and using the same technique as with insulin administration, including rotating sites. Or, if patient has been prescribed the Symlin Pen injector, show her how to use it. Advise patient to inject drug into her abdomen or thigh and not to use her arm as an injection site because absorption may be too variable.

• Warn patient not to mix pramlintide and insulin together in the same syringe.

• Warn patient that nausea is common with pramlintide; urge her to notify prescriber because dosage may need to be decreased.

• Caution patient that if she misses a dose, she should skip the missed dose and continue with the next scheduled dose.

• Instruct patient to keep unopened pramlintide vials in the refrigerator; vials that have been opened may be kept in the refrigerator or at room temperature. Vials should be discarded 28 days after opening.

• Caution patient to avoid hazardous activities that require mental alertness until effects of pramlintide are known.

• Reassure patient that pramlintide won't alter her awareness of or her body's response to insulin-induced hypoglycemia.

• Alert patient that she'll need close follow-up care, at least weekly until a target dose of pramlintide has been reached, she's tolerating the drug well, and her blood glucose level is stable.

• Instruct women of childbearing age to notify prescriber about planned,

P

suspected, or known pregnancy because drug therapy will need to be adjusted.
• Explain that local injection-site reactions, such as redness, swelling or itching, may occur but usually resolve in a few weeks.
• Instruct patient using the SymlinPen to never share it with anyone else, even if the needle has been changed, because of a risk for transmission of blood-borne pathogens.

prasugrel
Effient

Class and Category
Chemical class: Thienopyridine
Therapeutic class: Platelet activation and aggregation inhibitor, antiplatelet
Pregnancy category: B

Indications and Dosages
➤ *To reduce rate of thrombotic cardio-vascular events in patients with acute coronary syndrome who will be managed with percutaneous coronary intervention because of unstable angina, non-ST-elevation MI, or ST-elevation MI*

TABLETS
Adults. *Initial:* 60 mg as a loading dose and then 10 mg once daily. *Maintenance:* 10 mg once daily.
DOSAGE ADJUSTMENT For patients weighing less than 60 kg (132 lb), daily maintenance dosage may be reduced to 5 mg once daily.

Route	Onset	Peak	Duration
P.O.	2 hr	30 min	7–10 days

Mechanism of Action
After forming active metabolite, irreversibly binds to ADP receptors on platelets to inhibit platelet activation and aggregation for the lifetime of the platelet, which is 7 to 10 days. Without platelet activation and aggregation, thrombus cannot form.

Contraindications
Active bleeding, history of transient ischemic attack or stroke, hypersensitivity to prasugrel or its components

Interaction
DRUGS
fibrinolytic agents, heparin, NSAIDs (chronic use), warfarin: Increased risk of bleeding

Adverse Reactions
CNS: Dizziness, fatigue, fever, headache, intracranial hemorrhage
CV: Atrial fibrillation, bradycardia, hypercholesterolemia, hyperlipidemia, hypertension, hypotension, peripheral edema
EENT: Epistaxis, retinal hemorrhage
GI: Diarrhea, GI or retroperitoneal hemorrhage, hepatic dysfunction, nausea
HEME: Anemia, leukopenia, mild to life-threatening bleeding, severe thrombo-cytopenia, thrombotic thrombocytopenic purpura
MS: Back or limb pain
RESP: Cough, dyspnea, hemoptysis
SKIN: Subcutaneous hematoma, rash
Other: Allergic reaction, anaphylaxis, angioedema, malignancies, noncardiac chest pain

Nursing Considerations
• Be aware that patient should be receiving daily aspirin therapy (75 mg or 325 mg) throughout prasugrel therapy.
• Drug isn't recommended for patients age 75 or older (except in high-risk situations such as the presence of diabetes or history of previous MI) or in patients who have active bleeding or a history of a transient ischemic attack or stroke. Monitor patients closely who have other risk factors for bleeding, which include a body weight less than 60 kg, a history of bleeding, or concurrent use of drugs that increase risk of bleeding, such as warfarin, heparin, fibrinolytic therapy, or chronic use of NSAIDs.
• Prasugrel shouldn't be given to patients likely to undergo emergency coronary artery bypass graft (CABG) surgery because of increased bleeding risk. Drug should be discontinued at least 7 days before any surgery.
WARNING Monitor patient closely for bleeding because prasugrel can cause life-threatening hemorrhage. Report hypo-tension in patients who have recently undergone coronary angiography, percutaneous coronary intervention, CABG surgery, or other surgical procedures while taking drug. In this setting, expect therapy to continue because stopping prasugrel,

especially in first few weeks after acute coronary syndrome, increases the risk of adverse cardiovascular effects.

- Because prasugrel inhibits platelet aggregation for the lifetime of the platelet, which is 7 to 10 days, withholding a dose is unlikely help in managing a bleeding event or the risk of bleeding associated with an invasive procedure. Expect to administer exogenous platelets but only 6 hours after prasugrel loading dose or 4 hours after maintenance dose was given.
- Monitor patient's CBC regularly, as ordered, watching for evidence of thrombotic thrombocytopenic purpura, such as fever, neurologic abnormalities, renal dysfunction, and abnormal blood counts. Notify prescriber immediately because condition can be fatal. Expect to implement emergency treatment, such as plasmapheresis.

PATIENT TEACHING

- Emphasize importance of taking prasugrel exactly as prescribed, without lapses in therapy, for drug to be effective and adverse reactions to be reduced.
- Instruct patient to take daily dose of aspirin as prescribed.
- Discourage use of NSAIDs, including OTC products, during prasugrel therapy because of risk of bleeding.
- Caution patient that bleeding may last longer than usual. Instruct him to report unusual bleeding or bruising.
- Instruct patient to inform healthcare providers that he takes prasugrel.
- Urge patient to take precautions against bleeding, such as using an electric shaver and a soft-bristled toothbrush.
- Advise patient to avoid activities that could cause traumatic injury and bleeding.
- Advise patient to seek immediate medical care if swelling of his face or throat occurs or if any signs of an allergic reaction develops that is persistent or becomes worse.

pravastatin sodium

Pravachol

Class and Category

Chemical class: Mevinic acid derivative
Therapeutic class: Antihyperlipidemic
Pregnancy category: X

Indications and Dosages

➤ *To prevent coronary and cardiovascular events in patients at risk, to treat hyperlipidemia*

TABLETS

Adults. *Initial:* 10 to 40 mg daily at bedtime, increased every 4 wk, as needed. *Maintenance:* 10 to 80 mg at bedtime.

DOSAGE ADJUSTMENT For patients with significant renal or hepatic impairment, those taking immunosuppressants, and elderly patients, initial dosage reduced to 10 mg daily at bedtime. For elderly patients and those taking immunosuppressants, maintenance dosage usually limited to 20 mg daily. For patients taking clarithromycin, dosage limited to 40 mg once daily.

➤ *To treat pediatric heterozygous familial hypercholesterolemia*

TABLETS

Adolescents ages 14 to 18. 40 mg daily at bedtime.

Children ages 8 to 14. 20 mg daily at bedtime.

Mechanism of Action

Inhibits cholesterol synthesis in liver by blocking the enzyme needed to convert hydroxymethylglutaryl-CoA (HMG-CoA) to mevalonate, a cholesterol precursor. When cholesterol synthesis is blocked, the liver also increases breakdown of LDL cholesterol.

Contraindications

Active hepatic disease or unexplained, persistent elevated liver function test results; breastfeeding; hypersensitivity to pravastatin or its components; pregnancy

Interaction

DRUGS

cholestyramine, colestipol: Decreased pravastatin bioavailability
clarithromycin, colchicine, cyclosporine, erythromycin, gemfibrozil, immuno-suppressants, niacin, other fibrates: Increased risk of rhabdomyolysis and acute renal failure

oral anticoagulants: Increased bleeding or prolonged PT

Adverse Reactions

CNS: Anxiety, asthenia, chills, confusion, cognitive impairment, cranial nerve dysfunction, depression, dizziness, fatigue, headache, malaise, memory loss, nervousness, peripheral nerve palsy, sleep disturbance
CV: Angina pectoris, chest pain, vasculitis
EENT: Blurred vision, diplopia, rhinitis
ENDO: Abnormal thyroid function, elevated glycosylated hemoglobin levels, gynecomastia, hyperglycemia
GI: Abdominal pain, cholestatic jaundice, cirrhosis, constipation, diarrhea, elevated liver function test results, flatulence, fulminant hepatic necrosis, heartburn, hepatoma, hepatic failure, hepatitis, indigestion, nausea, pancreatitis, vomiting
GU: Dysuria, nocturia, urinary frequency
HEME: Hemolytic anemia, positive ANA, ESR elevation, purpura
MS: Arthralgia, musculoskeletal cramps or pain, myalgia, myopathy, polymyalgia rheumatica, rhabdomyolysis
RESP: Cough, dyspnea, upper respiratory tract infection
SKIN: Dermatomyositis, erythema multiforme, photosensitivity, rash, Stevens-Johnson syndrome, toxic epidermal necrolysis
Other: Anaphylaxis, angioedema, lupuslike syndrome

Nursing Considerations

• Use pravastatin cautiously in patients with renal or hepatic impairment and in elderly patients.
• Monitor liver function test results before pravastatin therapy starts and as indicated during therapy.
• Give drug 1 hour before or 4 hours after giving cholestyramine or colestipol.
• Report unexplained muscle aches or weakness and significant increases in creatine kinase level to prescriber because in rare instances drug causes rhabdomyolysis with acute renal failure caused by myoglobinuria. Expect to stop drug and provide supportive care.
• Monitor patient's BUN and serum creatinine levels periodically for abnormal elevations.

• Monitor blood lipoprotein level, as indicated, to evaluate response to therapy.

PATIENT TEACHING
• Instruct patient to take drug at bedtime, without regard to meals.
• Caution patient not to perform hazardous activities such as driving until effects of drug is known.
• Advise patient to notify prescriber at once about muscle pain, tenderness, weakness, and other evidence of myopathy.
• Urge woman of childbearing age to use a reliable method of contraception during pravastatin therapy and to notify prescriber at once if she becomes pregnant or thinks she may be pregnant.
• Instruct patient not to stop taking pravastatin without consulting prescriber, even when cholesterol level returns to normal.

prazosin hydrochloride

Minipress

Class and Category

Chemical class: Quinazoline derivative
Therapeutic class: Antihypertensive
Pregnancy category: C

Indications and Dosages

➤ *To manage hypertension*

CAPSULES
Adults. *Initial:* 1 mg twice daily or three times a day. *Maintenance:* 6 to 15 mg daily in divided doses twice daily or three times a day. *Maximum:* 40 mg daily.
Children.
Initial: 50 to 400 mcg/kg daily in divided doses twice daily or three times a day. *Maximum:* 7 mg/dose, 15 mg daily.

TABLETS
Adults. *Initial:* 0.5 mg twice daily or three times a day for at least 3 days; then increased to 1 mg twice daily or three times a day, if tolerated, for an additional 3 days. Subsequent dosages adjusted gradually, as needed and tolerated. *Maintenance:* 6 to 15 mg daily in divided doses twice daily or three times a day.
Maximum: 40 mg daily.

Children. *Initial:* 50 to 400 mcg/kg daily in divided doses twice daily or three times a day. *Maximum:* 7 mg/dose, 15 mg daily.

DOSAGE ADJUSTMENT For elderly patients and those with renal impairment, initial dosage possibly reduced to 1 mg once to twice daily.

Route	Onset	Peak	Duration
P.O.	0.5–1.5 hr	2–4 hr*	7–10 hr

Mechanism of Action

Selectively and competitively inhibits alpha$_1$-adrenergic receptors. This action promotes peripheral arterial and venous dilation and reduces peripheral vascular resistance, thereby lowering blood pressure.

Contraindications

Hypersensitivity to prazosin, other quinazolines, or their components

Interaction

DRUGS

antihypertensives, beta blockers, diuretics, phosphodiesterase-5 inhibitors: Increased risk of hypotension and syncope
dopamine: Antagonized peripheral vasoconstrictive effect of dopamine (high doses)
ephedrine: Decreased vasopressor response to ephedrine
epinephrine: Possibly severe hypotension and tachycardia
metaraminol: Decreased vasopressor effect of metaraminol
methoxamine, phenylephrine: Possibly decreased vasopressor effect and shortened duration of action of these drugs
NSAIDs, sympathomimetics: Decreased effectiveness of prazosin

ACTIVITIES

alcohol use: Increased hypotensive effects

Adverse Reactions

CNS: Asthenia, dizziness, drowsiness, fatigue, headache, insomnia, malaise, nervousness, syncope
CV: Angina, bradycardia, edema, orthostatic hypotension, palpitations, vasculitis

* For a single dose; 3 to 4 wk for multiple doses.

EENT: Dry mouth, eye pain
ENDO: Gynecomastia
GI: Nausea
GU: Urinary frequency, urinary incontinence
SKIN: Urticaria
Other: Hypersensitivity reaction

Nursing Considerations

• Use prazosin cautiously in patients with renal impairment because of increased sensitivity to prazosin's effects; in those with angina pectoris because drug may induce or aggravate angina; in those with narcolepsy because prazosin may worsen cataplexy; and in elderly patients because they're at increased risk for drug-induced hypotension.
• Monitor blood pressure regularly to evaluate effectiveness of therapy.

PATIENT TEACHING

• Instruct patient who is starting prazosin to take drug at bedtime to minimize effects of first-dose hypotension.
• Emphasize need to take drug even if feeling well.
• Advise patient to avoid drinking alcohol, standing for long periods, and exercising in hot weather because these activities increase risk of orthostatic hypotension.
• Suggest rising slowly from lying or sitting position to minimize orthostatic hypotension.
• Urge patient to avoid hazardous activities until drug's CNS effects are known.
• Advise patient to notify prescriber immediately about adverse reactions, especially dizziness and fainting.
• Instruct patient not to take any drugs, including OTC forms, without consulting prescriber, to avoid serious interactions.

P

prednisolone

Cotolone, Delta-Cortef, Prelone

prednisolone acetate

Articulose-50, Flo-Pred, Key-Pred, Predacort 50, Predalone 50, Predate 50, Predcor-25, Predcor-50, Pred-Ject 50

prednisolone sodium phosphate

Orapred ODT, Pediapred

prednisolone tebutate

Nor-Pred T.B.A., Predalone T.B.A., Predate TBA, Predcor-TBA

Class and Category
Chemical class: Glucocorticoid
Therapeutic class: Anti-inflammatory, immunosuppressant
Pregnancy category: C

Indications and Dosages
➤ *To treat adrenal insufficiency and acute and chronic inflammatory and immunosuppressive disorders*
SYRUP, TABLETS (PREDNISOLONE); DISINTEGRATING TABLETS, ORAL SOLUTION (PREDNISOLONE SODIUM PHOSPHATE); ORAL SUSPENSION (PREDNISOLONE ACETATE)
Adults and adolescents. 5 to 60 mg daily or in divided doses. *Maximum:* 250 mg daily.
I.M. INJECTION (PREDNISOLONE ACETATE)
Adults and adolescents. 4 to 60 mg daily.
INTRA-ARTICULAR, INTRALESIONAL, OR SOFT-TISSUE INJECTION (PREDNISOLONE ACETATE, PREDNISOLONE TEBUTATE)
Adults and adolescents. 4 to 100 mg of prednisolone acetate, repeated as needed, or 4 to 40 mg of prednisolone tebutate, repeated every 1 to 3 wk, as needed.
➤ *To treat adrenocortical insufficiency in children*
SYRUP, TABLETS (PREDNISOLONE); DISINTEGRATING TABLETS, ORAL SOLUTION (PREDNISOLONE SODIUM PHOSPHATE); ORAL SUSPENSION (PREDNISOLONE ACETATE)
Children. 0.14 mg/kg daily in divided doses three times a day.
I.M. INJECTION (PREDNISOLONE ACETATE)
Children. 0.14 mg/kg over a 24-hr period in divided doses three times a day every third day.
➤ *To treat acute exacerbations of multiple sclerosis*
SYRUP, TABLETS (PREDNISOLONE);DISINTEGRATING TABLETS, ORAL SOLUTION (PREDNISOLONE SODIUM

PHOSPHATE); ORAL SUSPENSION (PREDNISOLONE ACETATE)
Adults. 200 mg daily for 1 wk, followed by 80 mg every other day for 1 mo.

Route	Onset	Peak	Duration
P.O.*	Unknown	1–2 hr	1.25–1.5 days
I.M.†	Slow	Unknown	Unknown
Intra-articular, intra-lesional, soft-tissue injection‡	1–2 days	Unknown	1–3 wk

Mechanism of Action
Binds to intracellular glucocorticoid receptors and suppresses inflammatory and immune responses by:
• inhibiting neutrophil and monocyte accumulation at inflammation site and suppressing their phagocytic and bactericidal activity
• stabilizing lysosomal membranes
• suppressing antigen response of macrophages and helper T cells
• inhibiting synthesis of inflammatory response mediators, such as cytokines, interleukins, and prostaglandins.

Contraindications
Hypersensitivity to prednisolone or its components, idiopathic thrombocytopenic purpura (I.M. form), systemic fungal infection

Interaction
DRUGS
acetaminophen: Possibly hepatotoxicity (long-term use or high acetaminophen doses)
acetazolamide: Possibly hypernatremia or edema
amphotericin B (parenteral): Possibly severe hypokalemia
anabolic steroids, androgens: Possibly edema and severe acne
anticholinergics: Increased intraocular pressure

---

* Prednisolone
† Prednisolone acetate
‡ Prednisolone tebutate

asparaginase: Increased hyperglycemic effect of asparaginase, possibly neuropathy and disturbances in erythropoiesis
carbonic anhydrase inhibitors: Possibly hypocalcemia, hypokalemia, and osteoporosis
digoxin: Possibly arrhythmias and digitalis toxicity from hypokalemia
diuretics: Possibly decreased natriuretic and diuretic effects of diuretics, severe hypokalemia (with potassium-depleting diuretics)
ephedrine: Increased metabolic clearance of prednisolone
estrogens, oral contraceptives: Decreased clearance, increased elimination half-life, and increased therapeutic and toxic effects of prednisolone
folic acid: Increased folic acid requirements (with long-term prednisolone use)
heparin, oral anticoagulants, streptokinase, urokinase: Possibly decreased anticoagulant effect and increased risk of GI ulceration and bleeding
immunosuppressants: Increased risk of infection, lymphomas, and other lymphoproliferative disorders
isoniazid: Decreased blood isoniazid level
mexiletine: Possibly accelerated metabolism and decreased blood level of mexiletine
neuromuscular blockers: Increased neuromuscular blockade
NSAIDs: Increased risk of GI ulceration and bleeding, possibly added therapeutic effect when NSAIDs are used to treat arthritis
potassium supplements: Decreased effectiveness of both drugs
rifampin, other hepatic enzyme inducers: Decreased prednisolone effect
ritodrine: Increased risk of pulmonary edema in pregnant women
salicylates: Possibly decreased blood salicylate level, increased risk of GI ulceration and bleeding
sodium-containing drugs: Possibly edema and hypertension
somatrem, somatropin: Inhibited growth response to somatrem or somatropin
streptozocin: Increased risk of hyperglycemia
toxoids, vaccines: Possibly loss of antibody response, increased risk of neurologic complications

tricyclic antidepressants: Possibly worsened adverse psychiatric effects of prednisolone
troleandomycin: Increased therapeutic and toxic effects of prednisolone
FOODS
sodium-containing foods: Increased risk of edema and hypertension
ACTIVITIES
alcohol use: Increased risk of GI ulceration and bleeding

Adverse Reactions

CNS: Euphoria, headache, insomnia, nervousness, psychosis, restlessness, seizures, vertigo
CV: Edema, heart failure, hypertension
EENT: Cataracts, exophthalmos, glaucoma, increased ocular pressure
ENDO: Adrenal insufficiency, Cushing's syndrome, growth suppression in children, hyperglycemia
GI: Anorexia, GI bleeding and ulceration, increased appetite, indigestion, intestinal perforation, nausea, pancreatitis, vomiting
GU: Menstrual irregularities
MS: Avascular necrosis of joints, bone fractures, muscle atrophy or weakness, myalgia, osteoporosis, tendon rupture (local injection only)
SKIN: Acne; cutaneous or subcutaneous atrophy (with frequent repository injections); diaphoresis; ecchymosis; flushing; petechiae; striae; thin, fragile skin
Other: Delayed wound healing, hypernatremia, hypokalemia, injection-site scarring, negative nitrogen balance

Nursing Considerations

WARNING Avoid using prednisolone in patients with a history of active tuberculosis because drug can reactivate the disease.
• Give once-daily doses in the morning to mirror body's normal cortisol secretion.
• Inspect injectable form for particulates and discoloration before administering.
• For I.M. injection, shake suspension well before withdrawing. Keep in mind that I.M. injections are contraindicated in patients with idiopathic thrombocytopenic purpura.
• For intra-articular injection, attach a 20G to 24G needle to empty syringe, using aseptic technique, so prescriber can remove a few drops of synovial fluid to

P

confirm that needle is in the joint. The aspirating syringe is then exchanged with a prenisolone-filled syringe to inject drug into joint.
• Because prednisolone can produce many adverse reactions, assess patient regularly for evidence of such reactions, including heart failure and hypertension. Also monitor patient's intake, output, and daily weight.
• Monitor growth pattern in children; prednisolone may retard bone growth.
• Prolonged use may cause hypothalamic-pituitary-adrenal suppression.
WARNING Withdraw drug gradually, as ordered, if therapy lasts longer than 2 weeks. Stopping abruptly may cause acute adrenal insufficiency or, possibly, death.
• Be aware that patient may be at risk for emotional instability or psychic disturbance while taking prednisolone, especially if predisposed to them or taking high doses.

PATIENT TEACHING
• Instruct patient to take oral prednisolone with food to decrease stomach upset and to take once-daily dose in the morning.
• Emphasize need to take drug exactly as prescribed; taking too much increases risk of serious adverse reactions.
• Instruct patient taking orally disintegrating tablets to remove tablet from blister pack only when ready to take drug and to place tablet on tongue. Warn her not to split, cut, or break tablets.
• Caution patient not to discontinue drug abruptly.
• Urge patient to avoid alcohol during therapy because of increased risk of GI ulcers and bleeding.
• Urge patient to avoid hazardous activities until drug's CNS effects are known.
• Advise patient to avoid people with contagious infections because drug has an immunosuppressant effect. Urge her to notify prescriber immediately about exposure to measles or chickenpox.
• Caution against receiving vaccinations or other immunizations and coming in contact with people who have recently received oral poliovirus vaccine.
• Teach patient about potential side effects of prednisolone therapy, including

restlessness, mood swings, nervousness, and delayed wound healing.
• Instruct patient to notify prescriber immediately about joint pain, swelling, tarry stools, and visual disturbances. Also instruct her to report signs of infection or injury for up to 12 months after therapy.
• Advise patient to restrict joint use after intra-articular injection and to obtain activity guidelines from prescriber.
• Instruct diabetic patient to check her blood glucose level often because prednisolone may cause hyperglycemia.
• Advise patient to comply with follow-up visits to assess drug's effectiveness and detect adverse reactions.
• Urge patient to carry medical identification revealing prednisolone therapy.

prednisone

Apo-Prednisone (CAN), Deltasone Liquid Pred, Meticorten, Orasone 1, Orasone 5, Orasone 10, Prednicen-M, Prednicot, Prednisone Intensol, Rayos, Sterapred, Sterapred DS, Winpred (CAN)

Class and Category

Chemical class: Glucocorticoid
Therapeutic class: Anti-inflammatory, immunosuppressant
Pregnancy category: Not rated for oral solution, syrup, tablets; D for delayed-release tablets

Indications and Dosages

➤ *To treat adrenal insufficiency and acute and chronic inflammatory and immunosuppressive disorders*
DELAYED-RELEASE TABLETS, ORAL SOLUTION, SYRUP, TABLETS
Adults and adolescents. 5 to 60 mg daily as a single dose or in divided doses. *Maximum:* 250 mg daily.
➤ *To treat adrenogenital syndrome*
DELAYED-RELEASE TABLETS, ORAL SOLUTION, SYRUP, TABLETS
Adults and adolescents. 5 to 10 mg daily.
Children. 5 mg/m^2 daily in divided doses twice daily.
➤ *To treat acute exacerbations of multiple sclerosis*

DELAYED-RELEASE TABLETS, ORAL SOLUTION, SYRUP, TABLETS
Adults. 200 mg daily for 1 wk, then 80 mg every other day for 1 mo. *Maximum:* 250 mg daily.
➤ *To treat nephrosis in children*
DELAYED-RELEASE TABLETS, ORAL SOLUTION, SYRUP, TABLETS
Children age 10 and over. 20 mg four times a day.
Children ages 4 to 10. 15 mg four times a day.
Children ages 18 months to 4 years. 7.5 to 10 mg four times a day.
➤ *To treat rheumatic carditis, leukemia, and tumors in children*
DELAYED-RELEASE TABLETS, ORAL SOLUTION, SYRUP, TABLETS
Children. 0.5 mg/kg four times a day for 2 to 3 wk; then 0.375 mg/kg four times a day for 4 to 6 wk.
➤ *As adjunct to treat tuberculosis in children (with concurrent antitubercular therapy)*
DELAYED-RELEASE TABLETS, ORAL SOLUTION, SYRUP, TABLETS
Children. 0.5 mg/kg four times a day for 2 mo.

Route	Onset	Peak	Duration
P.O.	Rapid	1–2 hr	1.25–1.5 days

Mechanism of Action
Binds to intracellular glucocorticoid receptors and suppresses inflammatory and immune responses by:
- inhibiting neutrophil and monocyte accumulation at inflammation site and suppressing their phagocytic and bactericidal activity
- stabilizing lysosomal membranes
- suppressing antigen response of macrophages and helper T cells
- inhibiting synthesis of inflammatory response mediators, such as cytokines, interleukins, and prostaglandins.

Contraindications
Hypersensitivity to prednisone or its components, systemic fungal infection

Interaction
DRUGS
acetaminophen: Possibly hepatotoxicity (long-term use or high acetaminophen doses)
acetazolamide sodium: Possibly hypernatremia or edema
amphotericin B (parenteral): Possibly severe hypokalemia
anabolic steroids, androgens: Possibly edema and severe acne
antacids: Decreased absorption of prednisone (with long-term use)
anticholinergics: Increased intraocular pressure
asparaginase: Increased hyperglycemic effect of asparaginase, possibly neuropathy and disturbances in erythropoiesis
carbonic anhydrase inhibitors: Possibly hypocalcemia, hypokalemia, and osteoporosis
digoxin: Possibly arrhythmias and digitalis toxicity from hypokalemia
diuretics: Possibly decreased natriuretic and diuretic effects of diuretics, severe hypokalemia (with potassium-depleting diuretics)
ephedrine: Increased metabolic clearance of prednisone
estrogens, oral contraceptives: Decreased clearance, increased elimination half-life, and increased therapeutic and toxic effects of prednisone
folic acid: Increased folic acid requirements (with long-term prednisone use)
heparin, oral anticoagulants, streptokinase, urokinase: Possibly decreased anticoagulant effect and increased risk of GI ulceration and bleeding
immunosuppressants: Increased risk of infection, lymphomas, and other lymphoproliferative disorders
isoniazid: Decreased blood isoniazid level
mexiletine: Possibly accelerated metabolism and decreased blood level of mexiletine
neuromuscular blockers: Increased neuromuscular blockade
NSAIDs: Increased risk of GI ulceration and bleeding, possibly added therapeutic effect when NSAIDs are used to treat arthritis
potassium supplements: Decreased effectiveness of both drugs
ritodrine: Increased risk of pulmonary edema in pregnant women
salicylates: Possibly decreased blood salicylate level, increased risk of GI ulceration and bleeding
sodium-containing drugs: Possibly edema and hypertension

P

somatrem, somatropin: Inhibited growth response to somatrem or somatropin
streptozocin: Increased risk of hyperglycemia
toxoids, vaccines: Possibly loss of antibody response, increased risk of neurologic complications
tricyclic antidepressants: Possibly exacerbated adverse psychiatric effects of prednisone
troleandomycin: Increased therapeutic and toxic effects of prednisone

FOODS
sodium-containing foods: Increased risk of edema and hypertension

ACTIVITIES
alcohol use: Increased risk of GI ulceration and bleeding

Adverse Reactions

CNS: Euphoria, headache, insomnia, nervousness, psychosis, restlessness, seizures, vertigo
CV: Edema, heart failure, hypertension
EENT: Cataracts, exophthalmos, glaucoma, increased ocular pressure
ENDO: Adrenal insufficiency, Cushing's syndrome, growth suppression in children, hyperglycemia
GI: Anorexia, GI bleeding and ulceration, increased appetite, indigestion, intestinal perforation, nausea, pancreatitis, vomiting
GU: Menstrual irregularities
MS: Avascular necrosis of joints, bone fractures, muscle atrophy or weakness, myalgia, osteoporosis
SKIN: Acne; diaphoresis; ecchymosis; flushing; petechiae; striae; thin, fragile skin
Other: Delayed wound healing, hypernatremia, hypokalemia, negative nitrogen balance

Nursing Considerations

• Administer once-daily doses of prednisone in the morning to match body's normal cortisol secretion schedule.
• Because prednisone can produce many adverse reactions, assess regularly for signs and symptoms of such reactions as heart failure and hypertension. Also monitor fluid intake and output and daily weight.
• Monitor growth pattern in children. Prednisone may retard bone growth.
• Be aware that prolonged use of prednisone may cause hypothalamic-pituitary-adrenal suppression.

WARNING Withdraw prednisone gradually, as ordered, if therapy lasts longer than 2 weeks. Stopping abruptly may cause acute adrenal insufficiency and, possibly, death.

PATIENT TEACHING
• Instruct patient to take prednisone with food to decrease GI distress and to take once-daily dose in the morning.
• Emphasize importance of taking drug exactly as prescribed; taking more than prescribed increases risk of serious adverse reactions.
• Tell patient prescribed delayed-release tablet form not to break, divide, or chew tablet because the delayed-release action is dependent on an intact coating.
• Caution patient not to stop drug abruptly.
• Urge patient to avoid alcohol during therapy because of increased risk of GI ulcers and bleeding.
• Urge patient to avoid hazardous activities until drug's CNS effects are known.
• Advise patient to avoid people with contagious infections because drug has an immunosuppressant effect. Urge her to notify prescriber immediately about possible exposure to measles or chickenpox.
• Caution against receiving vaccinations or other immunizations and coming in contact with people who have recently received oral poliovirus vaccine.
• Instruct patient to notify prescriber immediately about joint pain, swelling, tarry stools, and visual disturbances. Also instruct her to report signs of infection or injury for up to 12 months after therapy.
• Instruct diabetic patient to check blood glucose level often because prednisone may cause hyperglycemia.
• Advise patient to comply with follow-up visits to assess drug effectiveness and detect adverse reactions.
• Urge patient to carry medical identification revealing prednisone therapy.

pregabalin
Lyrica

Class and Category
Chemical class: Structural derivative of gamma-aminobutyric acid (GABA)
Therapeutic class: Analgesic, anticonvulsant
Pregnancy category: C

Indications and Dosages

➤ *To relieve neuropathic pain associated with diabetic peripheral neuropathy*

CAPSULES, ORAL SOLUTION

Adults. *Initial:* 50 mg three times a day, increased to 100 mg three times a day, within 1 wk as needed.

➤ *To relieve postherpetic neuralgia; as adjunct therapy to manage partial-onset seizures*

CAPSULES, ORAL SOLUTION

Adults. *Initial:* 75 mg twice daily or 50 mg three times a day, increased to 150 mg twice daily or 100 mg three times a day within 1 week as needed. Then increased to 300 mg twice daily or 200 mg three times a day in 2 to 4 weeks as needed.

➤ *To manage fibromyalgia*

CAPSULES, ORAL SOLUTION

Adults. *Initial:* 75 mg twice daily, increased to 150 mg twice daily in 1 wk, as needed, and then to 225 mg twice daily in 1 wk as needed. *Maximum:* 450 mg daily.

➤ *To manage neuropathic pain associated with spinal cord injury*

CAPSULES, ORAL SOLUTION

Adults. *Initial:* 75 mg twice daily, increased to 150 mg twice daily in 1 wk, as needed, and then to 300 mg twice daily after 2 to 3 wks, as needed.

DOSAGE ADJUSTMENT If creatinine clearance is 30 to 60 ml/min/1.73 m^2, daily dosage reduced by 50%. If clearance is 15 to 30 ml/min/1.73 m^2, daily dosage reduced by 75% and frequency reduced to once or twice daily. If clearance is less than 15 ml/min/1.73 m^2, daily dosage reduced to as low as 25 mg daily. If patient is having hemodialysis, daily dosage is reduced and supplemental dose given immediately after every 4-hour hemodialysis session as follows: If reduced daily dosage is 25 mg daily, give supplemental dose of 25 to 50 mg. If reduced daily dosage is 25 to 50 mg daily, give supplemental dose of 50 to 75 mg. If reduced daily dosage is 75 mg, give supplemental dose of 100 to 150 mg.

Route	Onset	Peak	Duration
P.O.	Unknown	1.5 hr	Unknown

Mechanism of Action

Binds to alpha$_2$-delta site, an auxiliary subunit of voltage calcium channels, in CNS tissue where it may reduce calcium-dependentrelease of several neurotransmitters, possibly by modulating calcium channel function. With fewer neurotransmitters, pain sensation and seizure activity decline.

Contraindications

Hypersensitivity to pregabalin or its components

Interaction

DRUGS

ACE inhibitors: Increased risk of pregabalin-induced angioedema

CNS depressants: Additive CNS effects such as somnolence

lorazepam, oxycodone: Additive effects on cognitive and gross motor function

thiazolidinedione antidiabetics: Possibly increased risk of peripheral edema and weight gain

ACTIVITIES

alcohol use: Additive effects on cognitive and gross motor function

Adverse Reactions

CNS: Abnormal gait, amnesia, anxiety, asthenia, ataxia, balance disorder, confusion, depression, difficulty concentrating, dizziness, euphoria, extrapyramidal syndrome, fatigue, fever, headache, hypertonia, hypesthesia, incoordination, intracranial hypertension, myoclonus, nervousness, neuropathy, paresthesia, psychotic depression, schizophrenic reaction, somnolence, stupor, suicidal ideation, tremor, twitching, vertigo

CV: Chest pain, heart failure, peripheral edema, ventricular fibrillation

EENT: Amblyopia, blurred vision, conjunctivitis, decreased visual acuity, diplopia, dry mouth, nystagmus, otitis media, sinusitis, tinnitus, visual field defect

ENDO: Gynecomastia, hypoglycemia

GI: Abdominal distention or pain, constipation, diarrhea, flatulence, gastroenteritis, GI hemorrhage, increased appetite, nausea, vomiting

GU: Acute renal failure, anorgasmia, decreased libido, glomerulitis, impotence, nephritis, urinary frequency, urinary incontinence, urine retention

P

HEME: Decreased platelet count, leukopenia, thrombocytopenia
MS: Arthralgia, back pain, elevated creatine kinase level, leg or muscle cramps, myalgia, myasthenia
RESP: Apnea, dyspnea
SKIN: Ecchymosis, exfoliative dermatitis, pruritus
Other: Anaphylaxis, angioedema, facial edema, hypersensitivity reaction, Stevens-Johnson syndrome, weight gain

Nursing Considerations
• Pregabalin therapy should be stopped gradually over at least 1 week to decrease risk of seizure activity and avoid unpleasant symptoms such as diarrhea, headache, insomnia, and nausea.
• If patient has evidence of hypersensitivity (red skin, urticaria, rash, dyspnea, facial swelling, wheezing), stop drug at once, notify prescriber, and give supportive care.
• Monitor patient closely for adverse reactions. Notify prescriber if significant adverse reactions persist.
• Monitor patient closely for evidence of suicidal thinking or behavior, especially when therapy starts or dosage changes.

PATIENT TEACHING
• Warn against stopping pregabalin abruptly.
• Urge patient to avoid hazardous activities until she knows how drug affects her.
• Instruct patient to notify prescriber if she has changes in vision or unexplained muscle pain, tenderness, or weakness, especially if these muscle symptoms are accompanied by malaise or fever.
• Alert patient that drug may cause edema and weight gain.
• If patient also takes a thiazolidinedione antidiabetic, tell her these effects may be intensified. If significant, tell patient to notify prescriber.
• Inform male patient who plans to father a child that drug could impair his fertility.
• Instruct diabetic patients to inspect their skin while taking pregabalin.
• Urge caregivers to watch patient closely for evidence of suicidal tendencies, especially when therapy starts or dosage changes and to report concerns at once to prescriber.
• Urge woman who becomes pregnant while taking pregabalin for seizures to enroll in the North American antiepileptic drug pregnancy registry by calling 1-888-233-2334. Explain that the registry is collecting information about the safety of antiepileptic drugs during pregnancy

primidone

Apo-Primidone (CAN), Myidone, Mysoline, PMS Primidone (CAN), Sertan (CAN)

Class and Category
Chemical class: Prodrug of phenobarbital
Therapeutic class: Anticonvulsant
Pregnancy category: Not rated

Indications and Dosages
➤ *To manage generalized tonic-clonic seizures, nocturnal myoclonic seizures, complex partial seizures, and simple partial seizures caused by epilepsy*
CHEWABLE TABLETS, ORAL SUSPENSION, TABLETS
Adults and children age 8 and over.
Initial: 100 or 125 mg at bedtime for first 3 days; then increased to 100 or 125 mg twice daily for next 3 days, followed by 100 or 125 mg three times a day for next 3 days. On 10th day, begin maintenance dosage as prescribed. *Maintenance:* 250 mg three times a day or four times a day, adjusted as needed. *Maximum:* 2 g daily.
Children up to age 8. *Initial:* 50 mg at bedtime for first 3 days; then increased to 50 mg twice daily for next 3 days, followed by increase to 100 mg twice daily for next 3 days. On 10th day, begin maintenance dosage. *Maintenance:* 125 to 250 mg three times a day, adjusted as needed.

Mechanism of Action
Prevents seizures by decreasing excitability of neurons and increasing motor cortex's threshold of electrical stimulation.

Contraindications
Hypersensitivity to primidone, phenobarbital, or their components; porphyria

Interaction
DRUGS
acetaminophen: Decreased acetaminophen effectiveness, increased risk of hepatotoxicity
adrenocorticoids, chloramphenicol, cyclosporine, dacarbazine, disopyramide,

doxycycline, levothyroxine, metronidazole, mexiletine, oral anticoagulants, oral contraceptives (estrogen-containing), quinidine, tricyclic antidepressants: Decreased effectiveness of these drugs
amphetamines: Possibly delayed absorption of primidone
anticonvulsants: Possibly altered pattern of seizures
carbamazepine: Decreased effectiveness of primidone
carbonic anhydrase inhibitors: Increased risk of osteopenia
CNS depressants: Possibly enhanced CNS and respiratory depressant effects of both drugs
cyclophosphamide: Reduced half-life and increased leukopenic activity of cyclophosphamide
enflurane, halothane, methoxyflurane: Increased risk of hepatotoxicity; increased risk of nephrotoxicity (with methoxyflurane)
fenoprofen: Decreased elimination half-life of fenoprofen
folic acid: Increased folic acid requirements
griseofulvin: Decreased antifungal effects of griseofulvin
guanadrel, guanethidine: Possibly aggravated orthostatic hypotension
haloperidol, loxapine, maprotiline, molindone, phenothiazines, thioxanthenes: Possibly lowered seizure threshold and increased CNS depression
leucovorin: Possibly decreased anticonvulsant effects of primidone (with large doses)
MAO inhibitors: Possibly prolonged primidone effects and altered seizure pattern
methylphenidate: Possibly increased blood primidone level, resulting in toxicity
phenobarbital: Increased sedative effects of either drug, possibly altered seizure pattern
phenylbutazone: Decreased primidone effectiveness, increased metabolism and decreased half-life of phenylbutazone
rifampin: Decreased blood primidone level
valproic acid: Increased blood primidone level, leading to increased CNS depression and neurotoxicity; decreased valproic acid half-life and increased hepatotoxicity risk

vitamin D: Decreased effects of vitamin D
xanthines: Increased metabolism and clearance of xanthines (except dyphylline)
ACTIVITIES
alcohol use: Possibly increased CNS and respiratory depressant effects of primidone

Adverse Reactions
CNS: Ataxia, confusion, dizziness, drowsiness, excitement, mental changes, mood changes, restlessness
EENT: Diplopia, nystagmus
GI: Anorexia, nausea, vomiting
GU: Impotence
RESP: Dyspnea
Other: Folic acid deficiency

Nursing Considerations
• Monitor blood levels of primidone and phenobarbital (its active metabolite), as ordered, to determine therapeutic level or detect toxic levels.
• Anticipate that drug may cause confusion, excitement, or mood changes in elderly patients and children.
• Assess for signs of folic acid deficiency: mental dysfunction, neuropathy, tiredness, and weakness.
PATIENT TEACHING
• Instruct patient to crush primidone tablets and mix with food or fluids, as needed.
• Advise patient taking oral suspension to shake bottle well and measure doses with a calibrated device.
• Suggest that patient take drug with meals to minimize adverse GI reactions.
• Urge patient not to stop taking primidone abruptly because doing so can precipitate seizures.
• Caution patient about possible decreased alertness.
• Advise her to avoid hazardous activities until drug's CNS effects are known.
• Urge patient to avoid consuming alcohol and other CNS depressants during primidone therapy.

probenecid
Benemid, Benuryl (CAN), Probalan

Class and Category
Chemical class: Sulfonamide derivative
Therapeutic class: Antibiotic adjunct, antigout, uricosuric
Pregnancy category: Not rated

Indications and Dosages
➤ *To treat chronic gouty arthritis and hyperuricemia due to chronic gout*
TABLETS
Adults and adolescents. *Initial:* 250 mg twice daily for 1 wk; then increased to maintenance dosage. *Maintenance:* 500 mg twice daily; if not effective or 24-hr uric acid excretion isn't greater than 700 mg, dosage increased by 500 mg/day every 4 wk, as needed, up to a maximum of 3 g daily. If no acute attacks of gout occur over next 6 mo and serum uric acid level is within normal limits, dosage decreasedby 500 mg every 6 mo until lowest effective maintenance dose is reached.
Maximum: 3 g daily.
DOSAGE ADJUSTMENT Dosage possibly increased for patients with mild renal dysfunction, except for elderly patients, who require a dosage reduction.
➤ *As adjunct to antibiotic therapy with penicillins and some cephalosporins*
TABLETS
Adults, adolescents age 14 and over, and children weighing more than 50 kg (110 lb). 500 mg four times a day; if given with I.V. or I.M. antibiotic, administer at least 30 min before antibiotic.
Children ages 2 to 14 weighing up to 50 kg. 25 mg/kg as single dose, then 10 mg/kg four times a day; if given with I.V. or I.M. antibiotic, give at least 30 min before antibiotic.
➤ *As adjunct to treat sexually transmitted diseases*
TABLETS
Adults and adolescents. 1 g as single dose, given with appropriate antibiotic.
➤ *As adjunct to treat pediatric gonorrhea*
TABLETS
Postpubertal children and children weighing more than 45 kg (99 lb). 1 g as single dose, given with appropriate antibiotic.
➤ *As adjunct to treat neurosyphilis*

TABLETS
Adults and adolescents. 500 mg four times a day with 1 daily dose (2.4 million units) of penicillin G procaine for 10 to 14 days.

Route	Onset	Peak	Duration
P.O.	Unknown	30 min*	8 hr†

Mechanism of Action
Increases urinary excretion of uric acid and lowers serum uric acid level, which may prevent or resolve urate deposits, tophus formation, and joint changes. Eventually, incidence of acute gout attacks decreases. Probenecid also inhibits renal excretion of penicillins and some cephalosporins, thereby increasing their serum concentration and prolonging their duration of action.

Contraindications
Age less than 2 years, blood dyscrasias, hypersensitivity to probenecid or its components, renal calculi (urate)

Interaction
DRUGS
acyclovir: Decreased renal tubular secretion of acyclovir
allopurinol: Additive antihyperuricemic effects
aminosalicylate sodium, cephalosporins, ciprofloxacin, clofibrate, dapsone, ganciclovir, imipenem, methotrexate, nitrofurantoin, norfloxacin, penicillins: Increased and possibly prolonged blood levels of these drugs, increased risk of toxicity
antineoplastics (rapidly cytolytic): Possibly uric acid nephropathy
diazoxide, mecamylamine, pyrazinamide: Increased risk of hyperuricemia, decreased probenecid effectiveness
dyphylline: Increased half-life of dyphylline
furosemide: Increased blood furosemide level
heparin: Increased and prolonged anti-coagulant effect
indomethacin, ketoprofen, other NSAIDs: Possibly increased adverse effects

---
* For renal clearance of uric acid; 2 hr for effect on blood antibiotic level.
† For effect on blood antibiotic level; unknown for renal clearance of uric acid.

lorazepam, oxazepam, temazepam: Increased effects of these drugs, possibly excessive sedation
riboflavin: Decreased GI absorption of riboflavin
rifampin, sulfonamides: Increased blood levels of these drugs and, possibly, toxicity
salicylates: Decreased uricosuric effects of probenecid
sodium benzoate and sodium phenylacetate: Decreased renal elimination of these drugs
sulfonylureas: Increased sulfonylurea half-life
thiopental: Prolonged thiopental effect
zidovudine: Increased risk of zidovudine toxicity

ACTIVITIES
alcohol use: Increased risk of hyperuricemia, decreased probenecid effectiveness

Adverse Reactions
CNS: Dizziness, headache
EENT: Sore gums
GI: Anorexia, nausea, vomiting
GU: Hematuria, renal calculi (urate), renal colic, urinary frequency
MS: Costovertebral pain; joint pain, redness, and swelling
SKIN: Facial flushing, pruritus, rash, urticaria

Nursing Considerations
• Be aware that probenecid therapy shouldn't start until acute gout attack has subsided. If acute attack starts during therapy, continue therapy as prescribed.
• Use drug cautiously in patients with peptic ulcer disease.
• Expect to give sodium bicarbonate (3 to 7.5 g daily) or potassium citrate (7.5 g daily), as prescribed, to keep urine alkaline and prevent renal calculus formation.
• Monitor CBC, serum uric acid level, and liver and renal function test results during therapy.
• Closely monitor patients receiving intermittent therapy because they're more likely to develop allergic reactions.
• Check blood glucose level often in diabetic patient who takes a sulfonylurea because of the risk of drug interactions.

PATIENT TEACHING
• Advise patient to take probenecid with meals to minimize GI distress.
• Encourage patient to increase fluid intake (up to 3 L daily, if not contraindicated) to help prevent renal calculus formation.
• Instruct patient to notify prescriber immediately if she has signs of an acute gout attack (joint pain, swelling, and redness) or of renal calculi (flank pain and blood in urine).
• Caution patient against taking salicylates while taking probenecid. Instead, advise acetaminophen to treat mild pain or fever.

procainamide hydrochloride

Procan SR, Promine, Pronestyl, Pronestyl-SR

Class and Category
Chemical class: Ethyl benzamide monohydrochloride
Therapeutic class: Antiarrhythmic
Pregnancy category: C

Indications and Dosages
➤ *To treat life-threatening ventricular arrhythmias*
CAPSULES, TABLETS
Adults. 50 mg/kg daily in 8 divided doses (every 3 hr), adjusted as needed and tolerated. *Maximum:* 6 g daily (maintenance).
Children. 12.5 mg/kg four times a day.
E.R. TABLETS
Adults. *Maintenance:* 50 mg/kg daily in divided doses four times a day (every 6 hr), adjusted as needed and tolerated. *Maximum:* 6 g daily (maintenance).
I.V. INFUSION OR INJECTION
Adults. *Initial:* 100 mg diluted in D_5W and given at no more than 50 mg/min. Repeated every 5 min until arrhythmia is controlled or maximum total dose of 1 g is reached. Or, 10 to 15 mg/kg I.V. bolus given at 25 to 50 mg/min. *Maintenance:* 1 to 4 mg/min by continuous infusion.
I.M. INJECTION
Adults. 50 mg/kg daily in divided doses every 3 to 6 hr.

P

➤ *To treat ventricular extrasystoles and arrhythmias associated with anesthesia and surgery*

I.V. INFUSION OR INJECTION

Adults. *Initial:* 100 mg diluted in D_5W and given at no more than 50 mg/min. Dosage repeated every 5 min until arrhythmia is controlled or maximum total dose of 1 g is reached. Or, 10 to 15 mg/kg I.V. bolus given at 25 to 50 mg/min. *Maintenance:* 1 to 4 mg/min by continuous infusion.

I.M. INJECTION

Adults. 100 to 500 mg every 3 to 6 hr.

DOSAGE ADJUSTMENT For elderly patients or those with cardiac or hepatic insufficiency, dosage possibly reduced or dosing intervals increased. For patients with creatinine clearance less than 50 ml/min/1.73 m^2, initial dosage reduced to 1 to 2 mg/min.

Route	Onset	Peak	Duration
P.O.	Unknown	Unknown	60–90 min
P.O. (E.R.)	Unknown	60–90 min	Unknown
I.V.	Unknown	Immediate	Unknown
I.M.	10–30 min	15–60 min	Unknown

Mechanism of Action

Prolongs recovery period after myocardial repolarization by inhibiting sodium influx through myocardial cell membranes. This action prolongs refractory period, causing myocardial automaticity, excitability, and conduction velocity to decline.

Contraindications

Complete heart block, concurrent therapy with a CYP2D6 inhibitor and hypersensitivity to procainamide or its components, systemic lupus erythematosus, torsades de pointes

Interaction

DRUGS

antiarrhythmics: Additive cardiac effects
anticholinergics, antidyskinetics, antihistamines: Possibly intensified atropine-like adverse effects, increased risk of ileus
antihypertensives: Additive hypotensive effects
antimyasthenics: Possibly antagonized effect of antimyasthenic on skeletal muscle

bethanechol: Possibly antagonized cholinergic effect of bethanechol
bone marrow depressants: Possibly increased leukopenic or thrombocytopenic effects
bretylium: Possibly decreased inotropic effect of bretylium and enhanced hypotension
neuromuscular blockers: Possibly increased or prolonged neuromuscular blockade
pimozide: Possibly prolonged QT interval, leading to life-threatening arrhythmias

Adverse Reactions

CNS: Chills, disorientation, dizziness, light-headedness
CV: Heart block (second-degree), hypotension, pericarditis, prolonged QT interval, tachycardia
EENT: Bitter taste
GI: Abdominal distress, anorexia, diarrhea, nausea, vomiting
HEME: Agranulocytosis, neutropenia, thrombocytopenia
MS: Arthralgia, myalgia
RESP: Pleural effusion
SKIN: Pruritus, rash
Other: Drug-induced fever

Nursing Considerations

• Place patient in a supine position before giving procainamide I.M. or I.V. to minimize hypotensive effects. Monitor blood pressure often and ECG tracings continuously during administration and for 30 minutes afterward.
• Inspect parenteral solution for particles and discoloration before giving drug; discard if particles are present or solution is darker than light amber.
• When possible, give drug by I.V. infusion or injection, as prescribed, rather than by I.M. injection.
• If drug is to be given I.M. and patient's platelet count is below 50,000/mm^3, notify prescriber at once because patient may develop bleeding, bruising, or hematomas from procainamide-induced bone marrow suppression and thrombocytopenia. Expect to give procainamide I.V.
• For I.V. injection, dilute procainamide with D_5W according to manufacturer's instructions before administration.

• For I.V. infusion, dilute 200 to 1,000 mg of procainamide to a concentration of 2 or 4 mg/ml using 50 to 500 ml of D_5W.
• Administer I.V. infusion with an infusion pump or other controlled-delivery device.
• Don't exceed 500 mg in 30 minutes by I.V. infusion or 50 mg/min by I.V. injection because heart block or cardiac arrest may occur.
• Anticipate that patient has reached maximum clinical response when ventricular tachycardia resolves, hypotension develops, or QRS complex is 50% wider than original width.
• Expect to give first oral dose 3 to 4 hours after last I.V. dose.

PATIENT TEACHING
• Instruct patient to swallow E.R. procainamide tablets whole, without breaking, crushing, or chewing them.
• If patient has trouble swallowing, tell her to crush regular-release tablets or open capsules and mix contents with food or fluid.
• Instruct patient to take drug 1 hour before or 2 hours after meals with a full glass of water. Inform her that she may take drug with food if GI irritation develops.
• Urge patient to obtain needed dental work before therapy starts or after blood count returns to normal because drug can cause myelosuppression and increased risk of bleeding and infection. Encourage good oral hygiene during therapy, and urge patient to consult prescriber before having dental procedures.
• Advise patient to notify prescriber immediately about bruising, chills, diarrhea, fever, or rash.

prochlorperazine
Compazine, Stemetil (CAN)
prochlorperazine edisylate
Compazine
prochlorperazine maleate
Compazine Spansule, Nu-Prochlor (CAN), Stemetil (CAN)

Class and Category
Chemical class: Phenothiazine, piperazine
Therapeutic class: Antianxiety, antiemetic, antipsychotic
Pregnancy category: Not rated

Indications and Dosages
➤ *To control nausea and vomiting related to surgery*
I.V. INFUSION OR INJECTION (PROCHLORPERAZINE EDISYLATE)
Adults and adolescents. 5 to 10 mg at a rate not to exceed 5 mg/ml 15 to 30 min before anesthesia or during or after surgery, as needed. Dosage repeated once, if necessary. *Maximum:* 10 mg/dose, 40 mg daily.
I.M. INJECTION (PROCHLORPERAZINE EDISYLATE)
Adults and adolescents. 5 to 10 mg 1 to 2 hr before anesthesia or during or after surgery, as needed. Repeated once in 30 min, if needed. *Maximum:* 10 mg/dose, 40 mg daily.
➤ *To control severe nausea and vomiting*
E.R. CAPSULES (PROCHLORPERAZINE MALEATE)
Adults and adolescents. 15 to 30 mg daily in the morning, or 10 mg every 12 hr. *Maximum:* 40 mg daily.
ORAL SOLUTION (PROCHLORPERAZINE EDISYLATE)
Adults and adolescents. 5 to 10 mg three times a day or four times a day. *Maximum:* 40 mg daily.
Children weighing 18 to 39 kg (40 to 86 lb). 2.5 mg three times a day or 5 mg twice daily. *Maximum:* 15 mg daily.
Children weighing 14 to 18 kg (31 to 40 lb). 2.5 mg twice daily or three times a day. *Maximum:* 10 mg daily.
Children weighing 9 to 14 kg (20 to 31 lb). 2.5 mg once or twice daily. *Maximum:* 7.5 mg daily.
TABLETS (PROCHLORPERAZINE MALEATE)
Adults and adolescents. 5 to 10 mg three times a day or four times a day. *Maximum:* 40 mg daily.
I.V. INFUSION OR INJECTION (PROCHLORPERAZINE EDISYLATE)
Adults and adolescents. 2.5 to 10 mg at a rate not to exceed 5 mg/min. *Maximum:* 40 mg daily.
I.M. INJECTION (PROCHLORPERAZINE EDISYLATE)
Adults and adolescents. 5 to 10 mg every 3 to 4 hr, as needed. *Maximum:* 40 mg daily.
Children ages 2 to 12. 132 mcg/kg/dose to maximum of 10 mg on day 1; then

P

increased as needed. *Maximum:* On day 1, 10 mg; thereafter, 25 mg daily for children ages 6 to 12, 20 mg daily for children ages 2 to 6.

SUPPOSITORIES (PROCHLORPERAZINE)
Adults and adolescents. 25 mg twice daily.
Children weighing 18 to 39 kg. 2.5 mg three times a day or 5 mg twice daily. *Maximum:* 15 mg daily.
Children weighing 14 to 18 kg. 2.5 mg twice daily or three times a day. *Maximum:* 10 mg daily.
Children weighing 9 to 14 kg. 2.5 mg once or twice daily. *Maximum:* 7.5 mg daily.
➤ *To manage psychotic disorders, such as schizophrenia*

ORAL SOLUTION (PROCHLORPERAZINE EDISYLATE)
Adults and adolescents. 5 to 10 mg three times a day or four times a day, increased gradually every 2 to 3 days, as needed and tolerated. *Maximum:* 150 mg daily.
Children ages 2 to 12. 2.5 mg twice daily or three times a day.
Maximum: On day 1, 10 mg for all children; thereafter, 25 mg daily for children ages 6 to 12, 20 mg daily for children ages 2 to 6.

TABLETS (PROCHLORPERAZINE MALEATE)
Adults and adolescents. 5 to 10 mg three times a day or four times a day, increased gradually every 2 to 3 days, as needed and tolerated. *Maximum:* 150 mg daily.

I.M. INJECTION (PROCHLORPERAZINE EDISYLATE)
Adults and adolescents.
Initial: 10 to 20 mg, repeated every 2 to 4 hr, as needed, to bring symptoms under control (usually 3 to 4 doses). *Maintenance:* 10 to 20 mg every 4 to 6 hr. *Maximum:* 200 mg daily.
Children ages 2 to 12. 132 mcg/kg/dose on day 1; then increased as needed. *Maximum:* On day 1, 10 mg for all children; thereafter, 25 mg daily for children ages 6 to 12, 20 mg/day for children ages 2 to 6.
➤ *To treat anxiety short-term*

E.R. CAPSULES (PROCHLORPERAZINE MALEATE)
Adults and adolescents. 15 mg daily in the morning, or 10 mg every 12 hr. *Maximum:* 20 mg/day for no longer than 12 wk.

ORAL SOLUTION, TABLETS (PROCHLORPERAZINE EDISYLATE)
Adults and adolescents. 5 mg three times a day or four times a day.
Maximum: 20 mg daily for no longer than 12 wk.

I.V. INFUSION OR INJECTION (PROCHLORPERAZINE EDISYLATE)
Adults and adolescents. 2.5 to 10 mg at no more than 5 mg/min. *Maximum:* 40 mg daily.

I.M. INJECTION (PROCHLORPERAZINE EDISYLATE)
Adults and adolescents. 5 to 10 mg every 3 to 4 hr, as needed.
DOSAGE ADJUSTMENT Initial dose usually reduced and subsequent dosage increased more gradually for elderly, emaciated, and debilitated patients.

Mechanism of Action

Alleviates psychotic symptoms by blocking dopamine receptors, depressing release of selected hormones, and producing alpha-adrenergic blocking effect in the brain.

Prochlorperazine also alleviates nausea and vomiting by centrally blocking dopamine receptors in the medullary chemoreceptor trigger zone and by peripherally blocking the vagus nerve in the GI tract.

Anticholinergic effects and alpha-adrenergic blockade reduce anxiety by decreasing arousal and filtering internal stimuli to the brain stem reticular activating system.

Route	Onset	Peak	Duration
P.O., I.V., I.M., P.R.	Up to several wk*	Up to 6 mo	Unknown

Incompatibilities

Don't mix prochlorperazine in same syringe with other drugs. Precipitate may form when prochlorperazine edisylate is mixed in same syringe with morphine sulfate.

Contraindications

Age less than 2 years, blood dyscrasias, bone marrow depression, cerebral arteriosclerosis, coma, coronary artery disease, hepatic dysfunction, hypersensitivity to pheno-thiazines, myeloproliferative disorders, pediatric surgery, severe CNS depression, severe hypertension or hypotension, subcortical brain damage, use of large quantities of CNS depressants, weight less than 9 kg (20 lb)

---

* For antipsychotic effects; unknown for other indications.

Interaction

DRUGS

aluminum- or magnesium-containing antacids, antidiarrheals (adsorbent): Possibly inhibited absorption of oral prochlorperazine

amantadine, anticholinergics, antidyskinetics, antihistamines: Possibly intensified anticholinergic adverse effects, increased risk of prochlorperazine-induced hyperpyretic effect

amphetamines: Decreased stimulant effect of amphetamines, decreased antipsychotic effect of prochlorperazine

anticonvulsants: Lowered seizure threshold

antithyroid drugs: Increased risk of agranulocytosis

apomorphine: Possibly decreased emetic response to apomorphine, additive CNS depression

appetite suppressants: Possibly antagonized anorectic effect of appetite suppressants (except for phenmetrazine)

astemizole, cisapride, disopyramide, erythromycin, pimozide, probucol, procainamide: Additive QT interval prolongation, increased risk of ventricular tachycardia

beta blockers: Increased risk of additive hypotensive effects, irreversible retinopathy, arrhythmias, and tardive dyskinesia

bromocriptine: Decreased effectiveness of bromocriptine

CNS depressants: Additive CNS depression

dopamine: Possibly antagonized peripheral vasoconstriction (high doses of dopamine)

ephedrine, epinephrine: Decreased vasopressor effects of these drugs

hepatotoxic drugs: Increased risk of hepatotoxicity

hypotension-producing drugs: Possibly severe hypotension with syncope

levodopa: Inhibited antidyskinetic effect of levodopa

lithium: Reduced absorption of oral prochlorperazine, increased lithium excretion, increased extrapyramidal effects, possibly masking of early symptoms of lithium toxicity

MAO inhibitors, maprotiline, tricyclic antidepressants: Possibly prolonged and intensified anticholinergic and sedative effects, increased antidepressant level, inhibited prochlorperazine metabolism,

increased risk of neuroleptic malignant syndrome

mephentermine: Possibly antagonized antipsychotic effect of prochlorperazine and vasopressor effect of mephentermine

metrizamide: Increased risk of seizures

opioid analgesics: Increased risk of CNS and respiratory depression, orthostatic hypotension, severe constipation, urine retention

ototoxic drugs: Possibly masking of some symptoms of ototoxicity, such as dizziness, tinnitus, and vertigo

phenytoin: Possibly inhibited phenytoin metabolism, increased risk of phenytoin toxicity

thiazide diuretics: Possibly potentiated hyponatremia and water intoxication

ACTIVITIES

alcohol use: Additive CNS depression

Adverse Reactions

CNS: Akathisia, altered temperature regulation, dizziness, drowsiness, extrapyramidal reactions (such as dystonia, pseudoparkinsonism, tardive dyskinesia)

CV: Hypotension, orthostatic hypotension, tachycardia

EENT: Blurred vision, dry mouth, nasal congestion, ocular changes, pigmentary retinopathy

ENDO: Galactorrhea, gynecomastia

GI: Constipation, epigastric pain, nausea, vomiting

GU: Dysuria, ejaculation disorders, menstrual irregularities, urine retention

SKIN: Decreased sweating, photosensitivity, pruritus, rash

Other: Weight gain

Nursing Considerations

• Prochlorperazine shouldn't be used to treat dementia-related psychosis in the elderly because of increased mortality risk.

• Avoid contact between skin and solution forms of prochlorperazine because contact dermatitis could result.

• Inject I.M. form slowly, deep into upper outer quadrant of buttocks. Keep patient supine for 30 minutes after injection to minimize hypotensive effects.

• Rotate I.M. injection sites to prevent irritation and sterile abscesses.

P

• Be aware that I.V. form may be given undiluted as injection or diluted in isotonic solution as infusion (mesylate form requires dilution in at least 1 L). Both forms should be given at no more than 5 mg/minute.

• Protect prochlorperazine from light.

• Parenteral solution may develop slight yellowing that won't affect potency. Don't use if discoloration is pronounced or precipitate is present.

• Expect antipsychotic effects to occur in 2 to 3 weeks, although range is days to months.

WARNING Monitor closely for numerous adverse reactions that may be serious.

• Adverse effects may occur up to 12 weeks after discontinuation of E.R. capsules.

PATIENT TEACHING

• Instruct patient to take prochlorperazine with food or a full glass of milk or water to minimize GI distress.

• Advise patient to swallow E.R. capsules whole, not to crush or chew them.

• Instruct patient using suppository to refrigerate it for 30 minutes or hold it under running cold water before removing the wrapper if it softens during storage.

• Teach patient correct administration technique for suppository.

• Caution patient on long-term therapy not to stop prochlorperazine abruptly; doing so may lead to such adverse reactions as nausea, vomiting, and trembling.

• Urge patient to avoid alcohol and OTC drugs that may contain CNS depressants.

• Advise patient to rise slowly from lying and sitting positions to minimize effects of orthostatic hypotension.

• Urge patient to avoid hazardous activities because of the risk of drowsiness and impaired judgment and coordination.

• Instruct patient to avoid excessive sun exposure and to wear sunscreen outdoors.

• Urge patient to notify prescriber about involuntary movements and restlessness.

• Explain that adverse effects may occur up to 12 weeks after stopping E.R. capsules.

progestins

hydroxyprogesterone caproate

Gesterol LA 250, Hy/Gestrone, Hylutin, Prodrox, Pro-Span

levonorgestrel

Norplant System

medrogestone

Colprone (CAN)

medroxy progesterone acetate

Alti-MPA (CAN), Amen, Curretab, Cycrin, Depo-Provera, Gen-Medroxy (CAN), Novo-Medrone (CAN), Provera

megestrol acetate

Apo-Megestrol (CAN), Megace, Megace OS (CAN)

norethindrone

Aygestin, Norlutate (CAN)

norgestrel

Ovrette

progesterone

Crinone, Gesterol 50, PMS-Progesterone (CAN), Prometrium

Class and Category

Chemical class: Progesterone derivative, steroid hormone

Therapeutic class: Antianorectic, anti-cachectic, antineoplastic, ovarian hormone replacement

Pregnancy category: D (hydroxyprogesterone, megestrol [tablets], progesterone); X (levonorgestrel, medroxyprogesterone [parenteral], megestrol [parenteral and suspension], norethindrone, norgestrel); NR (medrogestone, medroxyprogesterone [tablets])

Indications and Dosages

➤ *To treat renal cancer*
I.M. INJECTION (MEDROXYPROGESTERONE)
Adults and adolescents. *Initial:* 400 mg to 1 g every wk until improvement and stabilization. *Maintenance:* 400 mg or more every mo.

➤ *To treat breast cancer*
TABLETS (MEGESTROL)
Adults and adolescents. 160 mg daily as single dose or in divided doses.

➤ *To treat endometrial cancer*
TABLETS (MEGESTROL)
Adult and adolescent women. 40 to 320 mg daily in divided doses.
I.M. INJECTION (MEDROXYPROGESTERONE)
Adults and adolescents.
Initial: 400 mg to 1 g every wk until improvement and stabilization.
Maintenance: 400 mg or more every mo.

➤ *To treat anorexia, cachexia, or significant weight loss in patients who have AIDS*
SUSPENSION (MEGESTROL)
Adults and adolescents. 800 mg daily for the first mo, and then 400 or 800 mg daily for the next 3 mo.

➤ *To treat endometriosis*
TABLETS (NORETHINDRONE ACETATE)
Adult and adolescent women. *Initial:* 5 mg daily for 2 wk, increased by 2.5 mg daily at 2-wk intervals to total dose of 15 mg daily. *Maintenance:* 15 mg daily for 6 to 9 mo unless temporarily discontinued because of breakthrough menstrual bleeding.

➤ *As adjunct to treat endometrial shedding in menopausal women*
TABLETS (MEDROGESTONE)
Adult and adolescent women. 5 to 10 mg daily on days 15 through 25 of menstrual cycle.

➤ *To treat secondary amenorrhea*
TABLETS (MEDROGESTONE)
Adult and adolescent women. 5 to 10 mg daily on days 15 through 25 of menstrual cycle.
TABLETS (MEDROXYPROGESTERONE)
Adult and adolescent women. 5 to 10 mg daily for 5 to 10 days, starting anytime during menstrual cycle.
TABLETS (NORETHINDRONE ACETATE)
Adult and adolescent women. 2.5 to 10 mg daily on days 5 through 25 of menstrual cycle. Or, 2.5 to 10 mg daily for 5 to 10 days during last half of menstrual cycle.

CAPSULES (PROGESTERONE)
Adult and adolescent women. 400 mg daily in evening for 10 days.
I.M. INJECTION (HYDROXYPROGESTERONE)
Adult and adolescent women. 375 mg as one-time dose.
I.M. INJECTION (PROGESTERONE)
Adult and adolescent women. 5 to 10 mg daily for 6 to 10 days. Or, 100 to 150 mg injected as single dose.
VAGINAL GEL (PROGESTERONE)
Adult and adolescent women. 45 mg (1 applicatorful of 4% vaginal gel) every other day for up to 6 doses. Dosage increased, as needed, to 90 mg (1 applicatorful of 8% vaginal gel) every other day for up to 6 doses.

➤ *To treat dysfunctional uterine bleeding*
TABLETS (MEDROGESTONE)
Adult and adolescent women. 5 to 10 mg daily on days 15 through 25 of menstrual cycle.
TABLETS (MEDROXYPROGESTERONE)
Adult and adolescent women. 5 to 10 mg daily for 5 to 10 days, starting on day 16 or 21 of menstrual cycle.
TABLETS (NORETHINDRONE ACETATE)
Adult and adolescent women. 2.5 to 10 mg daily on days 5 through 25 of menstrual cycle. Or, 2.5 to 10 mg daily for 5 to 10 days during last half of menstrual cycle.
I.M. INJECTION (HYDROXYPROGESTERONE)
Adult and adolescent women. 375 mg as one-time dose.
I.M. INJECTION (PROGESTERONE)
Adult and adolescent women. 5 to 10 mg daily for 6 consecutive days.

➤ *To induce menses*
TABLETS (MEDROGESTONE)
Adult and adolescent women. 5 to 10 mg daily on days 15 through 25 of the menstrual cycle.
TABLETS (MEDROXYPROGESTERONE)
Adult and adolescent women. 10 mg daily for 10 days, starting on day 16 of menstrual cycle. Repeated for 2 or more cycles if bleeding is satisfactorily controlled.
I.M. INJECTION (HYDROXYPROGESTERONE)
Adult and adolescent women. 125 to 250 mg on day 10 of menstrual cycle, repeated every 7 days until suppression is no longer desired.

➤ *To prevent pregnancy (postcoital)*

P

Adult and adolescent women. 0.75 mg as soon as possible within 72 hr of intercourse. Second dose given 12 hr later.
➤ *To prevent pregnancy*
TABLETS (NORETHINDRONE)
Adult and adolescent women. 0.35 mg daily, starting on day 1 of menstrual cycle and continuing uninterrupted through the year, whether or not menstrual bleeding occurs.
TABLETS (NORGESTREL)
Adult and adolescent women. 0.075 mg daily starting on day 1 of menstrual cycle and continuing uninterrupted throughout the year, whether or not menstrual bleeding occurs.
I.M. INJECTION (MEDROXYPROGESTERONE)
Adult and adolescent women. 150 mg every 3 mo.
SUBDERMAL IMPLANT (LEVONORGESTREL)
Adult and adolescent women. One set of implants surgically inserted every 2 yr.

Mechanism of Action

Progestins may diminish response to endogenous hormones in tumor cells by decreasing the number of steroid hormone receptors, causing a direct cytotoxic or antiproliferative effect on cell cycle growth and increased terminal cell differentiation. At higher doses, some progestins decrease adrenal production of estradiol and androstenedione, which may decrease estrogen- or testosterone-sensitive tumors. Megestrol stimulates appetite and metabolic effects, which promotes weight gain. Progestins also bind to cytosolic receptors that are loosely bound in cell nucleus, increasing protein synthesis and improving cachexia.

Progestins affect other hormones, especially estrogen, by reducing availability or stability of hormone receptor complex, shutting off estrogen-responsive genes, or causing negative feedback mechanism that decreases number of functioning estrogen receptors. These actions allow menstrual cycle to function normally, alleviating amenorrhea and dysfunctional uterine bleeding and inducing menses. Progestins also act to transform proliferative uterine endometrium into a more differentiated, secretory one, which is the basis for using

medroxyprogesterone to treat some types of amenorrhea. In a normal ovulatory cycle not resulting in pregnancy, decline in progesterone secretion caused by degeneration of corpus luteum in late luteal phase results in endometrial sloughing. A similar sloughing occurs after 5 to 10 days of medroxy-progesterone, provided that adequate estrogen-stimulated proliferation has occurred during follicular phase.

Selected progestins also inhibit secretion of gonadotropins from pituitary gland, which prevents ovulation, follicular maturation, thickening of cervical mucus to prevent sperm penetration, and creation of an atrophic endometrium, resulting in contraceptive effect.

Contraindications

Active thromboembolic disorder; thrombophlebitis; significant hepatic disease; hypersensitivity to peanuts (progesterone), progestins, or their components; known or suspected breast cancer; pregnancy; undiagnosed genital, uterine, or urinary tract bleeding

Interaction
DRUGS
aminoglutethimide: Possibly decreased blood level of medroxyprogesterone
carbamazepine, phenobarbital, phenytoin, rifabutin, rifampin: Possibly decreased effectiveness of progestin
thyroid hormone: Decreased thyroid hormone effectiveness

Adverse Reactions

CNS: Altered or reduced coordination or speech, depression, dizziness, drowsiness, fatigue, headache, irritability, migraine, mood changes, nervousness, postmeno-pausal dementia, syncope, unusual tiredness or weakness
CV: Fluid retention; hypotension; numbness or pain in chest, arm, or leg; thromboembolism
ENDO: Adrenal insufficiency or suppression, breast pain or tenderness, Cushing's syndrome, decreased T_3 resin uptake, delayed return of fertility in women, elevated thyroid-binding globulin, galactorrhea, hyperglycemia, vaginal spotting

EENT: Gingival bleeding, swelling, or tenderness; vision changes or loss
GI: Abdominal cramps or pain, diarrhea, nausea, vomiting
GU: Amenorrhea, breakthrough bleeding or metromenorrhagia, decreased libido, hypermenorrhea, ovarian enlargement or cysts
HEME: Clotting and bleeding abnormalities
MS: Back pain, decreased bone density, osteoporosis, osteoporotic fractures
RESP: Dyspnea
SKIN: Acne, alopecia, melasma, rash
Other: Anaphylaxis; facial fullness; hot flashes; injection- or implantation-site irritation, pain, or redness; weight gain

Nursing Considerations

• Be aware that progestin/estrogen therapy shouldn't be used to prevent cardio-vascular disease or dementia.
• Know that women who currently have or have had breast cancer should not be given hormone contraceptives, including medroxyprogesterone, as a contraceptive injection because breast cancer may be hormonally sensitive.
• Use progestins cautiously in patients with risk factors for arterial vascular disease, such as hypertension, diabetes mellitus, tobacco use, hypercholesterolemia, obesity, systemic lupus erythematosus, or a family or personal history of venous thromboembolism. Drug worsen these conditions.
• Use progestins cautiously in patients who have CNS disorders, such as seizures or depression, because progestins may worsen these conditions.
• Be aware that drug causes significant loss of bone mineral density in adolescence and early adulthood and isn't recommended for long-term contraception. If other contraceptive methods are inadequate, evaluate bone mineral density routinely, as ordered.
• Confirm that patient isn't pregnant before giving progestin as a contraceptive.
• Shake container vigorously for at least 1 minute before giving medroxy-progesterone acetate injection suspension or megestrol acetate oral suspension.

• Inject parenteral medroxyprogesterone slowly, over 5 to 7 seconds, into deltoid muscle. Don't inject into gluteal muscle to lessen absorption problems that may occur when patient sits on injection site. Pat site lightly after injection; don't rub it.
• Be aware that cyclical use of progestins is based on a menstrual cycle of 28 days.
WARNING Notify prescriber immediately if patient develops sudden vision loss, abnormal protrusion of eyeball, diplopia, papilledema, migraine, or other signs of thrombotic events. Expect to discontinue progestin if such signs occur.
• Monitor patient for adrenal suppression, especially with megestrol therapy. If suspected, notify prescriber.
• Expect to stop progestin/estrogen therapy in any woman who develops evidence of cancer; cardiovascular disease such as CVA, MI, pulmonary embolism, or venous thrombosis; or dementia.
PATIENT TEACHING
• Explain risks of progestin/estrogen therapy, including breast, endometrial, or ovarian cancer; cardiovascular disease; dementia; and gallbladder disease, especially in postmenopausal women.
• Instruct woman to notify prescriber if uterine bleeding continues longer than 3 months or if menstruation is delayed by 45 days.
• Warn patient taking progestin for noncontraceptive purposes to use a contraceptive method to prevent pregnancy because drug may harm fetus.
• Advise female patient to contact prescriber immediately if she suspects pregnancy or misses a menstrual period.
• Emphasize importance of using a second method of birth control when taking other drugs that could reduce contraceptive effectiveness of progestins.
• Advise patient that some products may contain peanut oil. If she is allergic to peanuts, tell her to contact pharmacist to find out if prescribed progestin product contains peanut oil.
• Advise female patient who vomits shortly after taking progestin-only oral contra-ceptive pill not to take another

P

dose immediately thereafter but to wait until next scheduled dose before resuming therapy and to use an additional contraceptive method for 48 hours afterward.

• Caution female patient who vomits within 1 hour of taking progestin for emergency contraception to contact prescriber about whether to repeat dose.

• Teach woman how to use vaginal gel, if prescribed. Tell her to avoid using other vaginal products for 6 hours before and after to ensure gel's complete absorption.

• Direct patient to alert all prescribers about progestin therapy because certain blood tests may be affected.

• Emphasize importance of good dental hygiene and regular dental checkups because elevated progestin level increases growth of normal oral flora, which may lead to gum tenderness, bleeding, or swelling.

• Caution postmenopausal women about increased risk of dementia associated with progestin therapy.

promethazine hydrochloride

Anergan 25, Anergan 50, Antinaus 50, Histantil (CAN), Pentazine, Phenazine 25, Phenazine 50, Phencen-50, Phenerzine, Phenoject-50, Pro-50, Promacot, Pro-Med 50, Promet, Prorex-25, Prorex-50, Prothazine, Shogan, V-Gan-25, V-Gan-50

Class and Category

Chemical class: Phenothiazine derivative
Therapeutic class: Antiemetic, antihistamine, antivertigo, sedative-hypnotic
Pregnancy category: C

Indications and Dosages

➤ *To prevent or treat motion sickness*
SYRUP, TABLETS
Adults and adolescents. 25 mg 30 to 60 min before travel and repeated 8 to 12 hr later, if needed. *Maximum:* 150 mg daily.

➤ *To treat vertigo*
SYRUP, TABLETS
Adults and adolescents. 25 mg twice daily, as needed.
Maximum: 150 mg daily.
Children age 2 and over. 0.5 mg/kg or 10 to 25 mg every 12 hr, as needed.
SUPPOSITORIES
Adults and adolescents. 25 mg twice daily, as needed.
Maximum: 150 mg daily.
Children age 2 and over. 0.5 mg/kg or 12.5 to 25 mg every 12 hr.

➤ *To prevent or treat nausea and vomiting in certain types of anesthesia and surgery*
SYRUP, TABLETS
Adults and adolescents. *Initial:* 25 mg; then 10 to 25 mg every 4 to 6 hr, as needed.
Maximum: 150 mg daily.
Children age 2 and over. 0.25 to 0.5 mg/kg or 10 to 25 mg every 4 to 6 hr, as needed.
I.V. OR I.M. INJECTION
Adults and adolescents. 12.5 to 25 mg every 4 hr, as needed. *Maximum:* 150 mg daily.
I.M. INJECTION
Children age 2 and over. 0.25 to 0.5 mg/kg or 12.5 to 25 mg every 4 to 6 hr, as needed.
SUPPOSITORIES
Adults and adolescents. *Initial:* 25 mg; then 12.5 to 25 mg every 4 to 6 hr, as needed.
Maximum: 150 mg daily.
Children age 2 and over. 0.25 to 0.5 mg/kg or 12.5 to 25 mg every 4 to 6 hr.

➤ *To treat signs and symptoms of allergic response*
SYRUP, TABLETS
Adults and adolescents. 10 to 12.5 mg four times a daybefore meals and at bedtime, as needed. Or, 25 mg at bedtime, as needed.
Maximum: 150 mg daily.
Children age 2 and over. 0.125 mg/kg every 4 to 6 hr or 5 to 12.5 mg three times a day, as needed. Or, 0.5 mg/kg or 25 mg at bedtime, as needed.
I.V. INJECTION
Adults and adolescents. 25 mg, repeated within 2 hr, as needed.
I.M. INJECTION, SUPPOSITORIES
Adults and adolescents. 25 mg, repeated in 2 hr, as needed. *Maximum:* 150 mg daily.
Children age 2 and over. 0.125 mg/kg every 4 to 6 hr or 6.25 to 12.5 mg three times a day,as needed. Or, 0.5 mg/kg or 25 mg at bedtime, as needed.

➤ *To provide nighttime, preoperative, or postoperative sedation*
SYRUP, TABLETS
Adults and adolescents. 25 to 50 mg as a single dose. *Maximum:* 150 mg daily.
Children age 2 and over. 0.5 to 1 mg/kg or 10 to 25 mg as a single dose. Or, for preoperative sedation, 1.1 mg/kg along with 1.1 mg/kg of meperidine and appropriate dose of an atropine-like drug.
I.V. INJECTION
Adults and adolescents. 25 to 50 mg as a single dose. Or, for preoperative and postoperative sedation, 25 to 50 mg combined with appropriately reduced dosages of analgesics and anticholinergics.
I.M. INJECTION, SUPPOSITORIES
Adults and adolescents. 25 to 50 mg as a single dose. Or, for preoperative and postoperative sedation, 25 to 50 mg combined with appropriately reduced dosages of analgesics and anticholinergics.
Children age 2 and over. 0.5 to 1 mg/kg or 12.5 to 25 mg as a single dose. Or, for preoperative sedation, 1.1 mg/kg along with 1.1 mg/kg of meperidine and an appropriate dose of an atropine-like drug.
➤ *To relieve apprehension and promote sleep the night before surgery*
SYRUP, TABLETS, SUPPOSITORIES
Adults and adolescents. 50 mg along with 50 mg of meperidine and an appropriate dose of an atropine-like drug at bedtime on the night before surgery.
DOSAGE ADJUSTMENT Dosage usually decreased for elderly patients.
➤ *To provide obstetric sedation*
I.V. OR I.M. INJECTION
Adults and adolescents. 50 mg for early stages of labor, followed by 1 or 2 doses of 25 to 75 mg after labor is established, repeated every 4 hr during normal labor.

Route	Onset	Peak	Duration
P.O.	15–60 min	Unknown	4–6 hr
I.V.	3–5 min	Unknown	4–6 hr
I.M., P.R.	20 min	Unknown	4–6 hr

Mechanism of Action

Competes with histamine for H_1-receptor sites, thereby antagonizing many histamine effects and reducing allergy signs and symptoms. Promethazine also prevents motion sickness, nausea, and vertigo by acting centrally on medullary chemoreceptive trigger zone and by decreasing vestibular stimulation and labyrinthine function in the inner ear. It also promotes sedation and relieves anxiety by blocking receptor sites in CNS, directly reducing stimuli to the brain.

Contraindications

Angle-closure glaucoma; benign prostatic hyperplasia; bladder neck obstruction; bone marrow depression; breastfeeding; children under age 2; coma; hypersensitivity or history of idiosyncratic reaction to promethazine, other phenothiazines, or their components; hypertensive crisis; lower respiratory tract disorders (including asthma) when used as an antihistamine; pyloroduodenal obstruction; stenosing peptic ulcer; use of large quantities of CNS depressants

Interaction

DRUGS
amphetamines: Decreased stimulant effect of amphetamines
anticholinergics: Possibly intensified anticholinergic adverse effects
anticonvulsants: Lowered seizure threshold
appetite suppressants: Possibly antagonized anorectic effect of appetite suppressants
beta blockers: Increased risk of additive hypotensive effects, irreversible retinopathy, arrhythmias, and tardive dyskinesia
bromocriptine: Decreased effectiveness of bromocriptine
CNS depressants: Additive CNS depression
dopamine: Possibly antagonized peripheral vasoconstriction (high doses of dopamine)
ephedrine, metaraminol, methoxamine: Decreased vasopressor response to these drugs
epinephrine: Blocked alpha-adrenergic effects of epinephrine, increased risk of hypotension
guanadrel, guanethidine: Decreased antihypertensive effects of these drugs
hepatotoxic drugs: Increased risk of hepatotoxicity
hypotension-producing drugs: Possibly severe hypotension with syncope
levodopa: Inhibited antidyskinetic effects of levodopa

P

MAO inhibitors: Possibly prolonged and intensified anticholinergic and CNS depressant effects of promethazine
metrizamide: Increased risk of seizures
ototoxic drugs: Possibly masking of some symptoms of ototoxicity, such as dizziness, tinnitus, and vertigo
quinidine: Additive cardiac effects
riboflavin: Increased riboflavin requirement

ACTIVITIES
alcohol use: Additive CNS depression

Adverse Reactions
CNS: Akathisia, CNS stimulation, confusion, dizziness, drowsiness, dystonia, euphoria, excitation, fatigue, hallucinations, hysteria, incoordination, insomnia, irritability, nervousness, neuroleptic malignant syndrome, paradoxical stimulation, pseudoparkinsonism, restlessness, sedation, seizures, syncope, tardive dyskinesia, tremor
CV: Bradycardia, hypertension, hypotension, tachycardia
EENT: Blurred vision; diplopia; dry mouth, nose, and throat; nasal congestion; tinnitus; vision changes
ENDO: Hyperglycemia
GI: Anorexia, cholestatic jaundice, ileus, nausea, rectal burning or stinging (suppository form), vomiting
GU: Dysuria
HEME: Agranulocytosis, leukopenia, thrombocytopenia, thrombocytopenic purpura
RESP: Apnea, respiratory depression, tenacious bronchial secretions
SKIN: Dermatitis, diaphoresis, jaundice, photosensitivity, rash, urticaria
Other: Angioedema, paradoxical reactions

Nursing Considerations
• Use promethazine cautiously in children and elderly patients because they may be more sensitive to its effects, patients with cardiovascular disease or hepatic dysfunction because of potential adverse effects, patients with asthma because of anticholinergic effects, and patients with seizure disorders or those who take drugs that may affect seizure threshold because drug may lower seizure threshold.
• Inject I.M. form deep into large muscle mass, and rotate sites.

WARNING Avoid inadvertent intra-arterial injection of promethazine because it can cause arteriospasm. Also avoid injecting drug under skin; severe tissue damage and gangrene may develop from impaired circulation.
• Give I.V. injection at no more than 25 mg/min; rapid I.V. administration may produce a transient drop in blood pressure.
WARNING Monitor respiratory function because drug may suppress cough reflex and cause thickening of bronchial secretions, aggravating such conditions as asthma and COPD. Rarely, it may depress respirations and induce apnea.
• Monitor patient's hematologic status as ordered because promethazine may cause bone marrow depression, especially when used with other known marrow-toxic agents. Assess patient for signs and symptoms of infection or bleeding.
WARNING Monitor patient for evidence of neuroleptic malignant syndrome, such as fever, hypertension or hypotension, involuntary motor activity, mental changes, muscle rigidity, tachycardia, and tachypnea. Be prepared to provide supportive treatment and drug therapy, as prescribed.
• Be aware that patient shouldn't have intradermal allergen tests within 72 hours of receiving promethazine because drug may significantly alter flare response.

PATIENT TEACHING
• Tell patient to use a calibrated device to ensure accurate doses of promethazine syrup.
• Teach patient correct administration technique for suppository, if needed.
• Advise patient to avoid OTC drugs unless approved by prescriber.
• Instruct patient to notify prescriber immediately if she has involuntary movements and restlessness.
• Urge patient to avoid alcohol and other CNS depressants during therapy.
• Instruct patient to avoid hazardous activities until drug's CNS effects are known.
• Suggest rinsing and use of sugarless gum or hard candy to relieve dry mouth.
• Urge patient to avoid excessive sun exposure and to use sunscreen when outdoors.

propafenone hydrochloride

Rythmol, Rythmol SR

Class and Category
Chemical class: 3-Phenylpropriophenone
Therapeutic class: Class IC antiarrhythmic
Pregnancy category: C

Indications and Dosages
➤ To treat life-threatening ventricular arrhythmias
TABLETS
Adults. *Initial:* 150 mg every 8 hr; after 3 or 4 days, increased to 225 mg every 8 hr (U.S.) or 300 mg every 12 hr (Canada), as needed; after an additional 3 or 4 days, further increased to 300 mg every 8 hr, as needed. *Maximum:* 900 mg daily.
➤ To prolong time of recurrence of symptomatic atrial fibrillation in patients with episodic atrial fibrillation who do not have structural heart disease
E.R. CAPSULES
Adults. *Initial:* 225 mg every 12 hr, increased after 5 or more days to 325 mg every 12 hr, as needed, and further increased to 425 mg every 12 hr, as needed.
DOSAGE ADJUSTMENT For patient with hepatic impairment, dosage may need to be reduced.

Mechanism of Action
Prolongs recovery period after myocardial repolarization by inhibiting sodium influx through myocardial cell membranes. This action prolongs the refractory period, causing myocardial automaticity, excitability, and conduction velocity to decline.

Contraindications
Bronchospastic disorders, such as asthma; Brugada syndrome; cardiogenic shock; concurrent use of both a CYP2D6 inhibitor and a CYP3A4 inhibitor (Rythmol SR); electrolyte imbalances; heart failure (uncontrolled); hypersensitivity to propafenone or its components; severe hypotension or obstructive pulmonary disease; sinus bradycardia or AV conduction disturbances (without artificial pacemaker)

Interaction
DRUGS
amiodarone: Possibly altered cardiac conduction and repolarization; possibly increased blood propafenone level
anesthetics (local): Increased risk of adverse CNS effects
antiarrhythmics, fluoxetine: Increased propafenone level and adverse CV effects
cimetidine, erythromycin, ketoconazole, paroxetine, ritonavir, saquinavir, sertraline: Possibly increased blood propafenone level
class IA and class III antiarrhythmics, oral macrolides, phenothiazines, tricyclic antidepressants: Possibly increased risk of prolonged QT interval
CYP2D6 inhibitors and CYP3A4 inhibitors combined: Significantly increased concentration of propafenone, increasing risk of proarrhythmias and other adverse reactions
desipramine: Possibly increased blood level of desipramine or propafenone
digoxin: Increased risk of digitalis toxicity
haloperidol, imipramine, venlafaxine: Possibly increased levels of these drugs
metoprolol, propranolol: Increased blood level and half-life of these drugs
orlistat: Possibly decreased absorption of propafenone
quinidine: Decreased propafenone metabolism
rifampin: Possibly decreased propafenone level
warfarin: Increased blood warfarin level and risk of bleeding
FOODS
grapefruit juice: Possibly increased blood propafenone level

Adverse Reactions
CNS: Anxiety, depression, dizziness, fatigue, headache, somnolence, tremor, weakness
CV: Angina, atrial flutter, AV block, bradycardia, chest pain, edema, heart failure, hypotension, irregular heartbeat, palpitations, prolonged QT interval, tachycardia, ventricular arrhythmias, worsened supraventricular arrhythmias
EENT: Altered taste, blurred vision, dry mouth
GI: Constipation, diarrhea, flatulence, nausea, vomiting

P

GU: Decreased sperm count, hematuria
HEME: Agranulocytosis
MS: Muscle weakness
RESP: Dyspnea, rales, upper respiratory tract infection, wheezes
SKIN: Ecchymosis, rash
Other: elevated blood alkaline phosphatase, exacerbation of myasthenia gravis, influenza, positive ANA titers

Nursing Considerations
• Assess patient for electrolyte imbalances, such as hyperkalemia, before starting propafenone or any antiarrhythmic to reduce risk of adverse cardiac reactions.
• Use propafenone cautiously in patients with heart failure or myocardial dysfunction because beta-blocking activity may further depress myocardial contractility.
• Use cautiously in patients with renal impairment because about 50% of the drug's metabolites are excreted in the urine, increasing risk of propafenone overdose.
• Monitor ECG tracings, blood pressure, and pulse rate, particularly at start of therapy and with dosage increases. Expect propafenone to be discontinued if Brugada syndrome is confirmed with ECG changes.
• Monitor patient for signs of infection such as fever, sore throat, or chills because propafenone may cause agranulocytosis, particularly during the initial 3 months of therapy. If present, notify prescriber.

PATIENT TEACHING
• Instruct patient to take a missed dose if she remembers within 4 hours; otherwise, tell her to skip missed dose and to resume the regular dosing schedule.
• Advise patient not to stop propafenone or change dosage without asking prescriber.
• Urge patient to carry medical identification showing she that takes propafenone.
• Advise patient to avoid hazardous activities until drug's CNS effects are known.
• Urge patient to increase fluid intake and dietary fiber if she becomes constipated.
• Explain that drug may cause an unusual taste. Advise patient to notify prescriber if taste interferes with compliance.
• Tell patient to notify prescriber promptly of any signs of infection such as fever, sore throat, or chills.

propantheline bromide
Pro-Banthine, Propanthel (CAN)

Class and Category
Chemical class: Quaternary amine
Therapeutic class: Anticholinergic
Pregnancy category: C

Indications and Dosages
➤ *As adjunct to treat peptic ulcer disease*
TABLETS
Adults. 15 mg three times a day before meals and 30 mg at bedtime, adjusted as needed and tolerated. *Maximum:* 120 mg daily.
Children. 0.375 mg/kg four times a day, adjusted as needed and tolerated.
DOSAGE ADJUSTMENT For elderly patients with mild symptoms or patients of below-average weight, dosage possibly reduced to 7.5 mg three times a day or four times a day.

Mechanism of Action
Prevents the neurotransmitter acetylcholine from combining with receptors on postganglionic parasympathetic nerve terminal, thereby reducing smooth-muscle spasms in the GI system, slowing GI motility, and inhibiting gastric acid secretion. All these effects help to heal peptic ulcers.

Route	Onset	Peak	Duration
P.O.	Unknown	Unknown	6 hr

Contraindications
Adhesions between iris and lens, angle-closure glaucoma, hemorrhage accompanied by hemodynamic instability, hepatic dysfunction, hypersensitivity to propantheline or its components, ileus, myasthenia gravis, myocardial ischemia, obstructive GI or urinary disease, renal dysfunction, severe ulcerative colitis, tachycardia

Interaction
DRUGS
amantadine, other anticholinergics, tricyclic antidepressants: Additive anticholinergic effects
antacids, antidiarrheals (adsorbent): Possibly reduced absorption of propantheline

antimyasthenics: Possibly further reduction in intestinal motility
atenolol: Increased effects of atenolol
cyclopropane: Possibly ventricular arrhythmias
digoxin: Possibly digitalis toxicity
haloperidol: Decreased antipsychotic effect of haloperidol in schizophrenic patients
ketoconazole: Decreased ketoconazole absorption
metoclopramide: Possibly decreased metoclopramide effect on GI motility
opioid analgesics: Increased risk of severe constipation and urine retention
phenothiazines: Possibly decreased antipsychotic effects
potassium chloride: Possibly increased severity of potassium chloride–induced GI ulceration, stricture, or perforation
urinary alkalizers: Delayed urinary excretion of propantheline

Adverse Reactions
CNS: Dizziness, excitement, insomnia, nervousness, paradoxical CNS stimulation
CV: Palpitations, tachycardia
EENT: Blurred vision; dry mouth, nose, and throat
GI: Constipation, dysphagia, heartburn, ileus, nausea, vomiting
GU: Impotence, urinary hesitancy, urine retention
SKIN: Decreased sweating, dry skin, flushing

Nursing Considerations
• Don't administer propantheline within 1 hour of antacids or antidiarrheals.
• Monitor elderly patients closely; they may respond to usual dose with agitation, confusion, drowsiness, or excitement.
WARNING Drug can interfere with sweating reflex, increasing the risk of heatstroke.
PATIENT TEACHING
• Instruct patient to take propantheline 30 to 60 minutes before meals and at bedtime, as prescribed.
• Inform patient that drug may cause dizziness. Urge her to avoid hazardous activities until drug's CNS effects are known.
• Encourage patient to increase fluid and fiber intake to decrease constipation. Instruct her to report persistent constipation and urine retention.

• Advise patient to avoid excessive exposure to heat to reduce risk of heat prostration and heatstroke.
• Suggest that patient relieve dry mouth with frequent rinsing and sugar-free hard candy or gum.

propofol
(disoprofol)
Diprivan

Class and Category
Chemical class: 2,6-diisopropylphenol derivative *Therapeutic class:* Sedative-hypnotic
Pregnancy category: B

Indications and Dosages
➤ *To provide sedation for critically ill patients in intensive care*
I.V. INFUSION
Adults. 2.8 to 130 mcg/kg/min. *Usual:* 27 mcg/kg/min.
DOSAGE ADJUSTMENT For elderly, debilitated, or American Society of Anesthesiologists Physical Status (ASA-PS) III or IV patients, induction dose decreased and maintenance rate slower.

Mechanism of Action
Decreases cerebral blood flow, cerebral metabolic oxygen consumption, and intracranial pressure and increases cerebrovascular resistance, which may play a role in propofol's hypnotic effects.

Route	Onset	Peak	Duration
I.V.	Within 40 sec	Unknown	3–5 min

Incompatibilities
Don't mix propofol with other drugs before giving. Don't give propofol through same I.V. line as blood or plasma products because globular component of emulsion will aggregate.

Contraindications
Hypersensitivity to propofol or its components, to eggs or egg products, or to soybeans or soy products

Interaction

DRUGS

CNS depressants: Additive CNS depressant, respiratory depressant, and hypotensive effects; possibly decreased emetic effects of opioids

droperidol: Possibly decreased control of nausea and vomiting

ACTIVITIES

alcohol use: Additive CNS depressant, respiratory depressant, and hypotensive effects

Adverse Reactions

CV: Bradycardia, hypotension
GI: Nausea, vomiting
MS: Involuntary muscle movement (transient)
RESP: Apnea
Other: Anaphylaxis, injection-site burning, pain, or stinging

Nursing Considerations

• Use propofol cautiously in patients with cardiac disease, peripheral vascular disease, impaired cerebral circulation, or increased intracranial pressure because drug may aggravate these disorders.
• To dilute before administration, use only D₅W for final solution of 2 mg/ml or more.
• Consult prescriber about pretreating injection site with 1 ml of 1% lidocaine to minimize pain, burning, or stinging that may occur. If ordered, lidocaine shouldn't be added to propofol solution in quantities greater than 20 mg/200 mg propofol because emulsion may become unstable. Giving drug through a larger vein in forearm or antecubital fossa also may minimize injection-site discomfort.
• Shake container well before using, administer drug promptly after opening, and use vial for a single patient. Use prefilled syringes within 6 hours of opening.
• Use a drop counter, syringe pump, or volumetric pump to safely control infusion rate. Don't infuse drug through filter with a pore size of less than 5 microns; doing so could cause emulsion to break down.
• Discard unused portion of propofol solution plus reservoirs, I.V. tubing, and solutions immediately after or within 12 hours of administration (6 hours if propofol was transferred from original

container) to prevent bacterial growth in stagnant solution. Also, protect solution from light.
• Dosage must be tapered before stopping therapy. Stopping abruptly will cause rapid awakening, anxiety, agitation and resistance to mechanical ventilation.
• Expect patient to recover from sedation within 8 minutes.

WARNING Monitor patient for propofol infusion syndrome, especially with prolonged high-dose infusions. It may cause severe metabolic acidosis, hyperkalemia, lipemia, rhabdomyolysis, hepatomegaly and cardiac and renal failure. Alert prescriber at once and be prepared to provide emergency supportive care as ordered.

PATIENT TEACHING

• Urge patient and family to voice concerns and ask questions before administration.
• Reassure patient that she'll be monitored closely during administration and that vital functions will be supported as needed.

propranolol hydrochloride

Apo-Propranolol (CAN), Detensol (CAN), Inderal, Inderal LA, InnoPran XL, Novopranol (CAN), pms Propranolol (CAN)

Class and Category

Chemical class: Beta-adrenergic blocker
Therapeutic class: Antianginal, antiarrhythmic, antihypertensive, anti-MI, antimigraine, antitremor, hypertrophic cardiomyopathy, and pheochromocytoma therapy adjunct
Pregnancy category: C

Indications and Dosages

➤ *To manage hypertension*

E.R. TABLETS

Adults. *Initial:* 80 mg daily, increased gradually up to 160 mg daily. *Maximum:* 640 mg daily.

XL TABLETS (INNOPRAN XL)

Adults. *Initial:* 80 mg once daily at bedtime, increased, as needed, to 120 mg once daily at bedtime.

ORAL SOLUTION, TABLETS
Adults. *Initial:* 40 mg twice daily, increased gradually to 120 to 240 mg daily, as needed. *Maximum:* 640 mg daily.
Children. *Initial:* 0.5 to 1 mg/kg daily in divided doses twice daily to four times a day, adjusted as needed. *Maintenance:* 2 to 4 mg/kg daily in divided doses twice daily.
➤ *To treat chronic angina*
E.R. TABLETS
Adults. *Initial:* 80 mg daily, increased every 3 to 7 days, as prescribed. *Maximum:* 320 mg/day.
ORAL SOLUTION, TABLETS
Adults. 80 to 320 mg daily in divided doses twice daily, three times a day, or four times a day.
➤ *To treat supraventricular arrhythmias and ventricular tachycardia*
ORAL SOLUTION, TABLETS
Adults. 10 to 30 mg three times a day. or four times a day, adjusted as needed.
I.V. INJECTION
Adults. 1 to 3 mg at a rate not to exceed 1 mg/min; repeated after 2 min and again after 4 hr, as needed.
Children. 0.01 to 0.1 mg/kg at a rate not to exceed 1 mg/min; repeated every 6 to 8 hr, as needed. *Maximum:* 1 mg/dose.
➤ *To control tremor*
ORAL SOLUTION, TABLETS
Adults. *Initial:* 40 mg twice daily, adjusted as needed and prescribed. *Maximum:* 320 mg daily.
➤ *To prevent vascular migraine headaches*
E.R. TABLETS
Adults. *Initial:* 80 mg daily, increased gradually, as needed. *Maximum:* 240 mg daily.
ORAL SOLUTION, TABLETS
Adults. *Initial:* 20 mg four times a day, increased gradually, as needed. *Maximum:* 240 mg daily.
➤ *As adjunct to treat hypertrophic cardiomyopathy*
ORAL SOLUTION, TABLETS
Adults. 20 to 40 mg three times a day or four times a day adjusted, as needed.
➤ *As adjunct to manage pheochromocytoma*
ORAL SOLUTION, TABLETS
Adults. For operable tumors, 20 mg three times a day to 40 mg three times a day or four times a day for 3 days before surgery, concurrently with an alpha blocker. For

inoperable tumors, 30 to 160 mg daily in divided doses.
➤ *To prevent MI*
ORAL SOLUTION, TABLETS
Adults. 180 to 240 mg daily in divided doses.
DOSAGE ADJUSTMENT Dosage increased or decreased for elderly patients, depending on sensitivity to propranolol.

Route	Onset	Peak	Duration
P.O.	Unknown	1–1.5 hr*	Unknown

Mechanism of Action

Through beta-blocking action, propranolol:
• prevents arterial dilation and inhibits renin secretion, resulting in decreased blood pressure (in hypertension and pheochromocytoma) and relief of migraine headaches
• decreases heart rate, which helps resolve tachyarrhythmias
• improves myocardial contractility, which helps ease symptoms of hypertrophic cardiomyopathy
• decreases myocardial oxygen demand, which helps prevent anginal pain and death of myocardial tissue.
In addition, peripheral beta-adrenergic blockade may play a role in propranolol's ability to alleviate tremor.

Contraindications

Asthma, cardiogenic shock, greater than first-degree AV block, sick sinus syndrome, or sinus bradycardia (unless pacemaker in place); heart failure (unless secondary to tachyarrhythmia responsive to propranolol), hypersensitivity to propranolol or its components

Interaction
DRUGS
ACE inhibitors: Increased risk of hypotension, especially in presence of acute MI
allergen immunotherapy, allergenic extracts for skin testing: Increased risk of serious systemic adverse reactions or anaphylaxis
amiodarone: Additive depressant effects on conduction, negative inotropic effects

---

* For regular-release form; unknown for E.R. form.

P

anesthetics (hydrocarbon inhalation): Increased risk of myocardial depression and hypotension

beta blockers: Additive beta blockade effects

bupivacaine, lidocaine, mepivacaine: Decreased clearance of these drugs, possibly increased risk of toxicity

calcium channel blockers, clonidine, diazoxide, guanabenz, reserpine, other hypotension-producing drugs: Additive hypotensive effect and, possibly, other beta blockade effects

catecholamine-depleting drugs, such as reserpine: Increased risk of hypotension, bradycardia, vertigo, syncope, and orthostatic hypotension

cimetidine: Possibly interference with propranolol clearance

digitalis glycosides: Increased risk of bradycardia

diltiazem: Increased risk of bradycardia, hypotension, high-degree heart block, and heart failure

dobutamine, isoproterenol: Reversed effects of propranolol

doxazosin, terazosin: Increased risk of orthostatic hypotension

epinephrine: Increased risk of uncontrolled hypertension

estrogens: Decreased antihypertensive effect of propranolol

fentanyl, fentanyl derivatives: Possibly increased risk of initial bradycardia after induction doses of fentanyl or a derivative (with long-term propranolol use)

glucagon: Possibly blunted hyperglycemic response

insulin, oral antidiabetic drugs: Possibly impaired glucose control, masking of tachycardia in response to hypoglycemia

MAO inhibitors, tricyclic antidepressants: Increased risk of significant hypertension

neuroleptic drugs: Increased risk of hypotension and cardiac arrest

neuromuscular blockers: Possibly potentiated and prolonged action of these drugs

NSAIDs: Possibly decreased hypotensive effects

phenothiazines: Increased blood levels of both drugs

phenytoin: Additive cardiac depressant effects (with parenteral phenytoin)

prazosin: Increased risk of first-dose hypotension

propafenone: Increased blood level and half-life of propranolol

quinidine: Increased propranolol level, resulting in higher degrees of beta blockade and orthostatic hypotension

sympathomimetics, xanthines: Possibly mutual inhibition of therapeutic effects

thyroxine: Possibly decreased T_3 level

verapamil: Increased risk of bradycardia, heart failure, and cardiovascular collapse

warfarin: Increased risk of bleeding

ACTIVITIES

alcohol: Possibly increased plasma propranolol level

nicotine chewing gum, smoking cessation, smoking deterrents: Increased therapeutic effects of propranolol

Adverse Reactions

CNS: Anxiety, depression, dizziness, drowsiness, fatigue, fever, insomnia, lethargy, nervousness, weakness

CV: AV conduction disorders, cold limbs, heart failure, hypotension, sinus bradycardia

EENT: Dry eyes, laryngospasm, nasal congestion, pharyngitis

GI: Abdominal pain, constipation, diarrhea, nausea, vomiting

GU: Impotence, Peyronie's disease, sexual dysfunction

HEME: Agranulocytosis, nonthrombocytopenic purpura, thrombocytopenic purpura

MS: Muscle weakness, myopathy, myotonia

RESP: Bronchospasm, dyspnea, respiratory distress, wheezing

SKIN: Alopecia, erythema multiforme, erythematous rash, exfoliative dermatitis, psoriasiform rash, Stevens-Johnson syndrome, toxic epidermal necrolysis, urticaria

Other: Anaphylaxis, flulike symptoms, systemic lupuslike reaction

Nursing Considerations

• Use propranolol cautiously in patients with bronchospastic lung disease because it may induce asthmatic attack, and in patients with underlying skeletal muscle disease; isolated reports of myopathy and myotonia have occurred with propranolol use.

• Monitor blood pressure, apical and radial pulses, fluid intake and output, daily weight, respiration, and circulation in extremities before and during therapy.
• Give I.V. injection at no more than 1 mg/minute.
WARNING Monitor ECG continuously, as ordered, when giving I.V. injection. Have emergency drugs and equipment available in case of hypotension or cardiac arrest.
• Protect injection solution from light.
• Because drug's negative inotropic effect can depress cardiac output, monitor cardiac output in patients with heart failure, particularly those with severely compromised left ventricular dysfunction.
• Be aware that propranolol can mask tachycardia in hyperthyroidism and that abrupt withdrawal in patients with hyperthyroidism or thyrotoxicosis can cause thyroid storm.
• Monitor diabetic patient taking an antidiabetic because propranolol can prolong hypoglycemia or promote hyperglycemia. It also can mask signs of hypoglycemia, especially tachycardia, palpitations, and tremor, but it doesn't suppress diaphoresis or hypertensive response to hypoglycemia.
WARNING Be aware that stopping drug abruptly, even for surgery, may cause myocardial ischemia, MI, ventricular arrhythmias, or severe hypertension, especially in patients with cardiac disease. However, be aware that the heart may not be able to respond to reflex adrenergic stimuli normally during surgery, which increases the risks of general anesthesia and surgical procedures. It also may cause increased intraocular pressure to return. Dosage should be reduced gradually.

PATIENT TEACHING
• Instruct patient to take propranolol at the same time every day.
• Caution patient not to change dosage without consulting prescriber and not to stop taking drug abruptly.
• Advise patient to notify prescriber immediately if she has shortness of breath.
• Instruct diabetic patient to check blood glucose level and urine for ketones regularly.

• Advise patient to consult prescriber before taking OTC drugs, especially cold products.
• Urge patient to avoid hazardous activities until CNS effects of drug are known.
• Advise smoker to notify prescriber immediately if she stops smoking because cessation may decrease drug metabolism, calling for dosage adjustments.
• Tell patient to notify prescriber if she is or could be pregnant because drug may need to be discontinued.

propylthiouracil (PTU)
Propyl-Thyracil (CAN)

Class and Category
Chemical class: Thiourea derivative
Therapeutic class: Antithyroid
Pregnancy category: D

Indications and Dosages
➤ *To treat hyperthyroidism*
TABLETS
Adults and adolescents. *Initial:* For mild to moderate hyperthyroidism, 300 to 900 mg daily in 1 to 4 divided doses until patient becomes euthyroid; for severe hyperthyroidism, 300 to 1,200 mg daily in 1 to4 divided doses until patient becomes euthyroid. *Maintenance:* 50 to 600 mg daily in 1 to 4 divided doses.
Children age 10 and over. *Initial:* 50 to 300 mg daily in 1 to 4 divided doses. *Maintenance:* Adjusted based on response to initial dosage.
Children ages 6 to 10. *Initial:* 50 to 150 mg/day in 1 to 4 divided doses. *Maintenance:* Adjusted based on response to initial dosage.
Neonates. 10 mg/kg daily in divided doses.
➤ *As adjunct to treat thyrotoxic crisis*
TABLETS
Adults and adolescents. 200 to 400 mg every 4 hr on day 1 plus other measures. Dosage gradually decreased as crisis subsides.
DOSAGE ADJUSTMENT If creatinine clearance is 10 to 50 ml/min/1.73 m^2, recommended dosage reduced by 25%; if creatinine clearance is less than 10 ml/min/1.73 m^2, recommended dosage reduced by 50%.

P

Route	Onset	Peak	Duration
P.O.	Unknown	17 wk	Unknown

Mechanism of Action

Inhibits conversion of peripheral thyroxine to triiodothyronine by interfering with incorporation of iodide into thyroglobulin; drug remains iodinated and degraded in thyroid gland. Diversion of oxidized iodine away from thyroglobulin diminishes thyroid hormone synthesis and levels of circulating thyroid hormone.

Contraindications

Breastfeeding, hypersensitivity to propylthiouracil or its components

Interaction

DRUGS

amiodarone, iodinated glycerol, iodine, potassium iodide: Decreased efficacy of propylthiouracil
digoxin: Risk of digitalis toxicity
oral anticoagulants: Possibly enhanced anticoagulant effect
sodium iodide 131 (radioactive iodine, ^{131}I): Decreased thyroid uptake of ^{131}I

Adverse Reactions

CNS: Dizziness, drowsiness, headache, neuritis, paresthesia, peripheral neuropathy, vertigo
CV: Edema, periarteritis, vasculitis
EENT: Taste perversion or loss
ENDO: Hypothyroidism
GI: Abdominal pain, acute liver failure, epigastric distress, hepatitis, hepatotoxicity, nausea, vomiting
GU: Glomerulonephritis, nephritis
HEME: Agranulocytosis, aplastic anemia, bleeding, granulopenia, hypoprothrombinemia, leukopenia, thrombocytopenia
MS: Arthralgia, joint redness or swelling, myalgia
RESP: Interstitial pneumonitis
SKIN: Alopecia, erythema nodosum, exfoliative dermatitis, pruritus, rash, urticaria
Other: Drug fever, lupuslike symptoms

Nursing Considerations

• Ensure that patient, parents, or caregivers have been informed about the risk of liver failure, especially in children, before administering propylthiouracil.

• Monitor CBC, PT, and liver and thyroid function test results in patients taking propylthiouracil. Elevated serum triiodothyronine (T_3) level may be the sole indicator of inadequate treatment.

• Expect to stop drug 3 to 4 days before ^{131}I treatment to prevent decreased thyroid uptake of ^{131}I; therapy may be resumed 3 to 5 days after radiation, if needed.

• Serum T_3 and thyroxine levels should decrease after about 3 weeks of therapy.

• Expect to decrease beta blocker or theophylline dosage once patient is euthyroid.

• Monitor liver function, especially during first 6 months of therapy, because drug may cause liver failure, need for liver transplant, or death. Expect to stop drug at first sign of liver dysfunction (fatigue, weakness, vague abdominal pain, loss of appetite, itching, easy bruising, jaundice) and obtain liver functions tests and ALT and AST levels, as ordered.

PATIENT TEACHING

• Instruct patient to take drug with meals to decrease risk of adverse GI reactions.

• Urge patient to avoid dietary sources of iodine, such as iodized salt and shellfish.

• Tell patient to check pulse rate and weight daily and to report increased heart rate and excessive weight loss to prescriber.

• Urge patient to report signs and symptoms of infection, such as fever and sore throat, or signs and symptoms that could reflect hepatic dysfunction, such as anorexia and right-upper-quadrant pain.

• Instruct patient to notify prescriber immediately if she becomes pregnant.

• Advise patient to report signs and symptoms of hypothyroidism, such as cold intolerance, depression, and increased fatigue.

• Tell patient to ask prescriber before using OTC cold drugs (some contain iodides).

• Advise patient to notify prescriber immediately if he has fatigue, weakness, vague abdominal pain, loss of appetite, itching, easy bruising, or yellowing of eyes or skin.

protamine sulfate

Class and Category
Chemical class: Simple low-molecular-weight protein
Therapeutic class: Heparin antagonist
Pregnancy category: C

Indications and Dosages
➤ *To treat heparin toxicity or hemorrhage associated with heparin therapy*
I.V. INJECTION
Adults and children. 1 mg for each 100 units of heparin to be neutralized, or as indicated by coagulation test results. *Maximum:* 100 mg (within 2-hr period).

Route	Onset	Peak	Duration
I.V.	5 min	Unknown	2 hr

Mechanism of Action
Neutralizes anticoagulant activity. A strong basic polypeptide, protamine combines with strongly acidic heparin complex to form an inactive stable salt, thereby neutralizing anticoagulant activity of both drugs.

Incompatibilities
Don't mix protamine sulfate in same syringe with other drugs unless they're known to be compatible. Several cephalosporins, penicillins, and other antibiotics are incompatible.

Contraindications
Allergy to fish, hypersensitivity to protamine or its components

Interaction
DRUGS
heparin: Neutralized anticoagulant effect of both drugs

Adverse Reactions
CNS: Weakness
CV: Bradycardia, hypertension, hypotension, shock
GI: Nausea, vomiting
HEME: Unusual bleeding or bruising
RESP: Dyspnea, pulmonary edema (noncardiogenic), pulmonary hypertension
SKIN: Flushing, sensation of warmth
Other: Anaphylaxis

Nursing Considerations
• Expect to administer I.V. protamine undiluted. However, dilute drug if needed (for patients other than neonates) with 5 ml of bacteriostatic water for injection containing 0.9% benzyl alcohol. For neonates, reconstitute with preservative-free sterile water for injection.
• Inject drug slowly at 5 mg/minute; administer no more than 50 mg in 10 minutes or 100 mg in 2 hours.
WARNING Be aware that rapid delivery may cause severe hypotension and anaphylaxis.
• Be prepared to obtain coagulation studies (APTT, activated clotting time) 5 to 15 minutes after giving drug and to repeat them in 2 to 8 hours to detect heparin-rebound hypotension, shock, and bleeding.
• Monitor vital signs, hemodynamic parameters, and fluid intake and output, and assess for flushing sensation.
• Have fluids—epinephrine 1:1,000, dobutamine, or dopamine—available for allergic or hypotensive reactions.
• Be aware that men with vasectomy have an increased risk of hypersensitivity reaction because of possible accumulation of antiprotamine antibodies.
PATIENT TEACHING
• Instruct patient to report adverse reactions immediately.

protriptyline hydrochloride
Triptil (CAN), Vivactil

P

Class and Category
Chemical class: Dibenzocycloheptene derivative
Therapeutic class: Antidepressant
Pregnancy category: Not rated

Indications and Dosages
➤ *To treat depression*
TABLETS
Adults. *Initial:* 5 to 10 mg three times a day or four times a day, increased every wk by 10 mg daily, as needed. *Maximum:* 60 mg daily.
Children age 12 and over. *Initial:* 5 mg three times a day, increased as needed.

DOSAGE ADJUSTMENT For elderly patients, initial dosage limited to 5 mg three times a day, then adjusted, as needed.

Route	Onset	Peak	Duration
P.O.	2–3 wk	Unknown	Unknown

Mechanism of Action

May block reuptake of norepinephrine and serotonin (and possibly other neurotransmitters) at neuronal membranes, thus enhancing their effects at postsynaptic receptors. These neurotransmitters may play a role in relieving depression symptoms.

Contraindications

Acute recovery phase after MI, hypersensitivity to protriptyline or its components, use within 14 days of MAO inhibitor therapy

Interaction

DRUGS

amantadine, anticholinergics, antidyskinetics, antihistamines: Additive anticholinergic effects, potentiated effects of antihistamines or protriptyline, possibly impaired detoxification of atropine and related drugs
anticonvulsants: Possibly lowered seizure threshold and decreased anticonvulsant effectiveness; enhanced CNS depression
antithyroid drugs: Possibly agranulocytosis
barbiturates, carbamazepine: Decreased therapeutic effects of protriptyline
bupropion, clozapine, cyclobenzaprine, haloperidol, loxapine, maprotiline, molindone, phenothiazines, thioxanthenes: Prolonged and intensified anticholinergic and sedative effects, lowered seizure threshold, increased risk of neuroleptic malignant syndrome; increased blood protriptyline level and inhibited phenothiazine metabolism (with phenothiazine use)
cimetidine: Increased risk of protriptyline toxicity
clonidine, guanadrel, guanethidine: Decreased hypotensive effects; increased CNS depression (with clonidine use)
CNS depressants: Possibly serious potentiation of CNS and respiratory depression and hypotensive effect
disulfiram, ethchlorvynol: Possibly transient delirium; increased CNS depression (with ethchlorvynol use)

fluoxetine: Increased protriptyline level
MAO inhibitors: Increased risk of hyperpyretic crisis, severe seizures, and death
methylphenidate: Possibly antagonized effects of methylphenidate and increased blood protriptyline level
metrizamide: Increased risk of seizures
naphazoline, oxymetazoline, phenylephrine, xylometazoline: Possibly increased vasopressor effects of these drugs
oral anticoagulants: Possibly increased anticoagulant activity
pimozide, probucol: Possibly prolonged QT interval and ventricular tachycardia
sympathomimetics: Possibly potentiated cardiovascular effects, decreased vasopressor effects of ephedrine and mephentermine
thyroid hormones: Increased therapeutic and toxic effects of both drugs

ACTIVITIES

alcohol use: Possibly increased response to alcohol

Adverse Reactions

CNS: Agitation, ataxia, confusion, dizziness, drowsiness, exacerbation of psychosis, extrapyramidal reactions, fatigue, lack of coordination, paresthesia, peripheral neuropathy, suicidal ideation, tremor, weakness
CV: Arrhythmias, including heart block and tachycardia; hypertension; hypotension; MI; orthostatic hypotension; palpitations; stroke
EENT: Angle closure glaucoma, black tongue, blurred vision, dry mouth, increased intraocular pressure, lacrimation, stomatitis, tongue swelling
ENDO: Hyperglycemia, hypoglycemia
GI: Abdominal cramps, anorexia, constipation, diarrhea, epigastric discomfort, hepatic dysfunction, nausea, vomiting
GU: Impotence, libido changes, nocturia, urinary frequency and hesitancy, urine retention
SKIN: Diaphoresis, petechiae, photosensitivity, rash, urticaria
Other: Facial edema, weight gain or loss

Nursing Considerations

• Use protriptyline cautiously in patients with a history of seizures because drug can lower seizure threshold.

- Use cautiously in patients with a history of urine retention or increased intraocular pressure because of drug's autonomic activity.

WARNING Avoid giving protriptyline with an MAO inhibitor. If patient is being switched from an MAO inhibitor to protriptyline, make sure MAO inhibitor has been discontinued for 14 days before starting protriptyline.

- Watch patients closely (especially children, adolescents, and young adults) for suicidal tendencies, particularly when therapy starts or dosage changes, because depression may worsen temporarily during these times, possibly leading to suicidal ideation.

PATIENT TEACHING

- Inform patient that protriptyline therapy may take several weeks to reach full effect.
- Advise patient that drug may cause mild pupillary dilation, which may lead to an episode of acute closure glaucoma. Encourage patient to have an eye exam before starting therapy to see if he is at risk.
- Instruct patient to avoid hazardous activities until drug's CNS effects are known.
- Advise patient to change position slowly to minimize orthostatic hypotension.
- Urge patient to avoid alcohol while taking drug.
- Suggest drinking water and using sugarless gum or hard candy to relieve dry mouth.
- Advise patient to avoid sunlight and tanning booths and to wear protective clothing, a hat, and sunscreen when outdoors.
- Instruct diabetic patient to check blood glucose level frequently during first few weeks of protriptyline therapy.
- Urge family or caregiver to watch patient for suicidal tendencies, especially when therapy starts or dosage changes and particularly if patient is a child, teenager, or young adult.

pyrazinamide

pms-Pyrazinamide (CAN), Tebrazid (CAN)

Class and Category

Chemical class: Pyrazine analogue of nicotinamide
Therapeutic class: Antitubercular
Pregnancy category: C

Indications and Dosages

➤ *As adjunct to treat tuberculosis, along with other antitubercular drugs*

TABLETS

Adults and children. 15 to 30 mg/kg daily; or, 50 to 70 mg/kg 2 or 3 times/wk. *Maximum:* For daily regimen, 2 g daily; for twice/wk regimen, 4 g daily; for 3-times/wk regimen, 3 g daily.

DOSAGE ADJUSTMENT For patients with HIV infection, 20 to 30 mg/kg daily for first 2 mo of therapy.

Mechanism of Action

Inhibits growth of *Mycobacterium tuberculosis* by decreasing pH level; exhibits bactericidal or bacteriostatic action, depending on blood pyrazinamide level.

Contraindications

Acute gout, hypersensitivity to pyrazinamide or its components, severe hepatic damage

Interaction

DRUGS

allopurinol, colchicine, probenecid, sulfinpyrazone: Possibly increased blood uric acid level and decreased antigout efficacy
cyclosporine: Possibly decreased blood level and therapeutic effects of cyclosporine

Adverse Reactions

CNS: Fever
GI: Anorexia, hepatotoxicity, nausea, vomiting
GU: Dysuria
HEME: Porphyria
MS: Arthralgia, gout, myalgia
SKIN: Acne, photosensitivity, pruritus, rash, urticaria

Nursing Considerations

- Review liver function test results before and every 2 to 4 weeks during therapy.
- Be aware that drug can affect the accuracy of certain urine ketone strip test results.
- Because drug is metabolized by liver, monitor patient for evidence of hepatotoxicity, such as darkened urine, fever,

jaundice, malaise, nausea, severe pain in feet or toes, and vomiting.

PATIENT TEACHING
• Explain importance of complying with long-term pyrazinamide therapy.
• Tell diabetic patient about possible changes in ketone measurement during therapy.
• Instruct patient to report dark urine, fever, malaise, nausea, severe pain in feet or toes, vomiting, and yellowing of skin or eyes.
• Inform patient of need for regular blood tests and follow-up visits with prescriber.
• Urge patient to minimize exposure to sun and to wear protective clothing, hat, sunglasses, and sunscreen when outdoors.

pyridostigmine bromide

Mestinon, Mestinon-SR (CAN), Mestinon Timespans, Regonol (CAN)

Class and Category
Chemical class: Bromide dimethylcarbamate
Therapeutic class: Antimyasthenic
Pregnancy category: Not rated

Indications and Dosages
➤ *To treat symptoms of myasthenia gravis*
E.R. TABLETS
Adults and adolescents. 180 to 540 mg once or twice daily (at least 6 hr between doses).
SYRUP, TABLETS
Adults and adolescents. *Initial:* 30 to 60 mg every 3 to 4 hr, adjusted as needed. *Maintenance:* 60 mg to 1.5 g daily.
Children. 7 mg/kg daily in 5 or 6 divided doses.
I.V. OR I.M. INJECTION
Adults and adolescents. 2 mg every 2 to 3 hr.
I.M. INJECTION
Neonates of myasthenic mothers. 0.05 to 0.15 mg/kg every 4 to 6 hr.
➤ *To reverse the effects of neuromuscular blockers*
I.V. INJECTION
Adults and adolescents. 10 to 20 mg after 0.6 to 1.2 mg of I.V. atropine has been given.

dosage adjustment Dosage possibly reduced for patients with renal impairment.

Mechanism of Action
Improves muscle strength compromised by myasthenia gravis or neuromuscular blockade by competing with acetylcholine for its binding site on acetylcholinesterase. This action potentiates the effects of acetylcholine on skeletal muscle and the GI tract. Inhibited destruction of acetylcholine allows freer transmission of nerve impulses across the neuromuscular junction.

Route	Onset	Peak	Duration
P.O.	30–45 min	1–2 hr	3–6 hr
P.O. (E.R.)	30–60 min	1–2 hr	6–12 hr
I.V.	2–5 min	Unknown	2–4 hr
I.M.	15 min	Unknown	2–4 hr

Contraindications
Hypersensitivity to pyridostigmine or its components, mechanical obstruction of GI or urinary tract

Interaction
DRUGS
aminoglycosides (systemic), anesthetics (hydrocarbon inhalation), capreomycin, lidocaine (I.V.), lincomycins, polymyxins, quinine: Possibly antagonized effect of pyridostigmine on skeletal muscle; possibly decreased neuromuscular blocking activity of these drugs (with large doses of pyridostigmine)
anesthetics (local): Inhibited neuronal transmission, increased anesthesia effects
anticholinergics: Possibly masked pyridostigmine overdose; reduced intestinal motility
cholinesterase inhibitors: Increased risk of additive toxicity
edrophonium: Possibly worsening of status
guanadrel, guanethidine, mecamylamine, neuromuscular blockers, procainamide: Possibly prolonged phase I blocking effect or reversal of nondepolarization blockade
quinidine, trimethaphan: Possibly antagonized effects of pyridostigmine

Adverse Reactions
EENT: Increased salivation, lacrimation, miosis

GI: Abdominal cramps, diarrhea, increased peristalsis, nausea, vomiting
GU: Urinary frequency, incontinence, or urgency
MS: Fasciculations, muscle spasms or weakness
RESP: Increased tracheobronchial secretions
SKIN: Diaphoresis

Nursing Considerations

• Use pyridostigmine cautiously in patients with renal disease because drug is mainly excreted unchanged by kidneys. Monitor BUN and serum creatinine levels.

WARNING Maintain a rigid dosing schedule because a missed or late dose can precipitate myasthenic crisis.

• Observe for cholinergic reactions when administering drug I.V. or I.M.

WARNING Pyridostigmine overdose may obscure diagnosis of myasthenic crisis because main symptom in both is muscle weakness. Treat cholinergic crisis by stopping anticholinesterase, giving atropine as prescribed, and helping with endotracheal intubation and mechanical ventilation, if needed.

• Be aware that reversal of neuromuscular blockade usually occurs in 15 to 30 minutes. Be prepared to maintain patent airway and ventilation until normal voluntary respiration returns completely. Assess respiratory measurements and muscle tone with peripheral nerve stimulator device, as indicated.

PATIENT TEACHING

• Instruct patient to take pyridostigmine as directed and on schedule. Explain that a late or missed dose can precipitate a crisis. Suggest the use of a battery-operated alarm clock as a reminder.

• Tell patient to take drug with a full glass of water or with food or milk if GI distress occurs.

• Warn patient not to crush or chew E.R. tablets.

• Ask patient to record pyridostigmine dosage, times taken, and drug effects to help determine optimal dosage and schedule.

• Urge patient to carry medical identification describing her condition and drug regimen.

➤━━━━━━━━━━━━━━━◄

P

QRS

quazepam
Doral

Class, Category, and Schedule
Chemical class: Benzodiazepine
Therapeutic class: Sedative-hypnotic
Pregnancy category: X
Controlled substance schedule: IV

Indications and Dosages
➤ *To treat insomnia*
TABLETS
Adults. 15 mg at bedtime.
DOSAGE ADJUSTMENT In elderly and
debilitated patients, dosage may be reduced
to 7.5 mg at bedtime after 1 or 2 nights of
therapy.

Mechanism of Action
May antagonize mu receptors at limbic,
thalamic, and hypothalamic regions of the
brain, blocking release of such inhibitory
neurotransmitters as gamma-aminobutyric
acid (GABA) and acetylcholine. Central
receptors interact with GABA receptors,
allowing for greater influx of chloride into
the neuron, thereby suppressing neuronal
excitability. GABA effects may inhibit spinal
afferent pathways and block the cortical and
limbic arousal that normally occurs when
reticular pathways are stimulated. These
effects result in various levels of CNS
depression, including sleep.

Contraindications
Hypersensitivity to quazepam or its
components, pregnancy, sleep apnea
(known or suspected)

Interactions
DRUGS
addictive drugs: Possibly habituation
carbamazepine: Decreased blood quazepam
level, possibly increased blood
carbamazepine level
*cimetidine, diltiazem, disulfiram,
erythromycin, fluoxetine, fluvoxamine,
isoniazid, itraconazole, ketoconazole,
nefazodone, oral contraceptives,*

propoxyphene, ranitidine, verapamil:
Possibly potentiated effects of quazepam
clozapine: Possibly syncope, with respiratory
depression or arrest
CNS depressants, tricyclic antidepressants:
Increased CNS depression
*CYP2B6 substrates such as bupropion and
efavirenz:* Possibly increased plasma levels
of these agents leading to increased risk of
adverse effects
digoxin: Possibly increased blood digoxin
level and risk of digitalis toxicity
levodopa: Possibly decreased therapeutic
effects of levodopa
phenytoin: Increased risk of phenytoin
toxicity
theophyllines: Possibly antagonized effects
of quazepam
zidovudine: Increased risk of zidovudine
toxicity
FOODS
grapefruit juice: Increased quazepam level
ACTIVITIES
alcohol use: Additive CNS depression
smoking: Possibly decreased effectiveness of
quazepam

Adverse Reactions
CNS: Abnormal complex behaviors, such as
sleep driving; amnesia (anterograde);
anxiety; ataxia; confusion; depression;
dizziness; drowsiness; euphoria; fatigue;
headache; light-headedness; paresthesia;
slurred speech; suicidal ideation; tremor;
weakness
CV: Chest pain, palpitations, tachycardia
EENT: Blurred vision, dry mouth, hyperacusis, photophobia, throat tightness,
worsening of glaucoma
GI: Abdominal cramps, constipation,
diarrhea, heartburn, nausea, thirst,
vomiting
GU: Renal dysfunction, urinary incontinence, urine retention
MS: Muscle spasms
RESP: Dyspnea, increased tracheobronchial
secretions
Other: Anaphylaxis, angioedema

Nursing Considerations
• Use quazepam cautiously in patients with
angle-closure glaucoma because of drug's
anticholinergic effects; in patients with
hepatic dysfunction because this
condition may prolong quazepam's

half-life; in patients with myasthenia gravis because drug may worsen condition; in patients with severe COPD because adverse effects of quazepam may compromise respiratory function; in patients with renal dysfunction because accumulation of metabolites may result in toxicity; and in elderly patients because of age-related decreases in hepatic, renal, and cardiac function.

WARNING Monitor patient closely for signs and symptoms of hypersensitivity reactions, such as dyspnea, throat tightness, nausea, vomiting, and swelling. If present, discontinue quazepam immediately, notify prescriber, and provide supportive care.

WARNING Notify prescriber if eye pain develops in patient with angle-closure glaucoma.

WARNING Be aware that quazepam may intensify signs and symptoms of depression. Monitor patient closely for evidence of suicidal ideation, and institute suicide precautions, as needed.

PATIENT TEACHING
• Instruct patient to stop taking quazepam and seek emergency care if she has trouble breathing, throat tightness, nausea, vomiting, or abnormal swelling.
• Advise patient that drug may cause abnormal behaviors during sleep, such as driving a car, eating, talking on the phone, or having sex without recall of the event. If family members notice such behavior, or if patient sees evidence of it upon awakening, prescriber should be notified.
• Urge patient to avoid consuming alcohol during quazepam therapy because sedation and risk of abnormal behaviors, such as sleep driving, may increase.
• Instruct patient not to stop drug abruptly after prolonged use (6 weeks or more).
• Instruct female patient of childbearing age to use effective contraception during therapy and to notify prescriber immediately of known or suspected pregnancy.
• Urge family or caregiver to watch patient closely for suicidal tendencies, especially when therapy starts or dosage changes.

quetiapine fumarate
Seroquel, Seroquel XR

Class and Category
Chemical class: Dibenzothiazepine derivative
Therapeutic class: Antipsychotic
Pregnancy category: C

Indications and Dosages
➤ *To treat schizophrenia*
TABLETS
Adults. *Initial:* 25 mg twice daily on day 1. Increased by 25 to 50 twice daily or three times a day on days 2 and 3. *Usual:* 300 to 400 mg daily by day 4, in divided doses twice daily or three times a day. Increased every 2 days in increments of 25 to 50 mg twice daily, as needed. *Maximum:* 800 mg daily.
E.R. TABLETS
Adults. *Initial:* 300 mg once daily in evening. Dosage increased daily in increments up to 300 mg, as needed. *Maximum:* 800 mg daily.
➤ *To manage psychotic disorders other than schizophrenia*
TABLETS
Adults. *Initial:* 25 mg twice daily on day 1. Dosage increased by 25 to 50 mg twice daily or three times a day on days 2 and 3. *Usual:* 300 to 400 mg daily by day 4, in divided doses twice daily or three times a day. Dosage increased every 2 days in increments of 25 to 50 mg twice daily, as needed. *Maximum:* 800 mg daily.
➤ *To treat depressive episodes in bipolar disorder*
TABLETS
Adults. *Initial:* On day 1, 50 mg once at bedtime; day 2, 100 mg once at bedtime; day 3, 200 mg once at bedtime; day 4, 300 mg once at bedtime. *Maintenance:* 300 mg once daily at bedtime.
E.R. TABLETS
Adults. *Initial:* 50 mg once daily in evening on day 1, followed by 100 mg once daily in evening on day 2, 200 mg once daily in evening on day 3, and 300 mg once daily in evening on day 4 and thereafter.
➤ *As adjunct therapy with antidepressants to treat major depressive disorder*

E.R. TABLETS

Adults. *Initial:* 50 mg once daily in evening, increased to 150 mg once daily in evening on day 3. *Maximum:* 300 mg daily in evening.

➤ *To treat acute manic episodes in bipolar I disorder*

TABLETS

Adults. 50 mg twice daily, increased to 200 mg twice daily. on day 4 (in increments no greater than 100 mg daily) and then further increased to 400 mg twice daily on day 6 (in increments no greater than 200 mg daily), as needed.

➤ *To treat acute manic episodes in bipolar I disorder as monotherapy; as adjunct with lithium or divalproex to treat acute manic episodes in bipolar I disorder*

E.R. TABLETS

Adults. *Initial:* 300 mg once daily in evening on day 1, followed by 600 mg once daily in evening on day 2 and 200 to 400 mg twice daily on day 3 and thereafter. *Maintenance:* 200 to 400 mg twice daily.

DOSAGE ADJUSTMENT For elderly patients and patients with hepatic impairment, initial dosage no higher than 50 mg once daily and increased in increments of 50 mg/day depending on response and tolerance.

Mechanism of Action

May produce antipsychotic effects by interfering with dopamine binding to dopamine type 2 (D_2)-receptor sites in the brain and by antagonizing serotonin 5-HT_2, dopamine type 1 (D_1), histamine H_1, and adrenergic alpha$_1$ and alpha$_2$ receptors.

Contraindications

Hypersensitivity to quetiapine or its components

Interactions

DRUGS

antibiotics such as gatifloxacin or moxifloxacin; antipsychotic drugs such as chlorpromazine, thioridazine, ziprasidone; class 1A antiarrythmics such as quinidine or procainamide; class III antiarrythmics such as amiodarone or sotatol; levomethadyl acetate, methadone, pentamidine: Possibly increased risk of prolonged QT interval *antihypertensives:* Possibly enhanced antihypertensive effects of these drugs

cimetidine, erythromycin, fluconazole, itraconazole, ketoconazole: Decreased clearance and possibly increased effects of quetiapine
CNS depressants: Possibly increased CNS depression
lorazepam: Possibly increased effects of lorazepam
phenytoin, thioridazine: Increased clearance and possibly decreased effectiveness of quetiapine

ACTIVITIES

alcohol use: Possibly enhanced CNS depression

Adverse Reactions

CNS: Depression, dizziness, drowsiness, dystonia, extrapyramidal reactions, hypertonia, hypothermia, lethargy, restless leg syndrome, retrograde amnesia, somnolence, suicidal ideation, tardive dyskinesia
CV: Cardiomyopathy, hypercholesterolemia, myocarditis, orthostatic hypotension, palpitations
EENT: Dry mouth, nasal congestion, pharyngitis, rhinitis
ENDO: Galactorrhea, hyperglycemia, syndrome of inappropriate ADH secretion
GI: Anorexia, constipation, indigestion, pancreatitis
GU: Nocturnal enuresis
HEME: Agranulocytosis, decreased platelet count, leukopenia, neutropenia
MS: Dysarthria, muscle weakness, rhabdomyolysis
RESP: Cough, dyspnea
SKIN: Diaphoresis, Stevens-Johnson syndrome, toxic epidermal necrolysis
Other: Anaphylaxis, flulike symptoms, hyponatremia, weight gain

Nursing Considerations

WARNING Quetiapine shouldn't be used for elderly patients with dementia-related psychosis because drug increases the risk of death in these patients.

• Know that quetiapine should not be given to patients who have a history of cardiac arrhythmias, such as bradycardia, or who experience hypokalemia or hypomagnesemia. The drug also should not be used with other drugs that prolong the QT interval or in a patient who has a congenital prolongation of the QT interval

Q
R
S

because quetiapine may increase the QT interval, which may increase the risk of torsades de pointes and/or sudden death.
- Use quetiapine cautiously in patients who have a history of cardiovascular disease, a family history of QT prolongation, or in patients who are elderly or take medications that may cause an electrolyte imbalance, such as diuretics, or who have congestive heart failure or heart hypertrophy, because these factors may increase the risk of a prolonged QT interval. Also use cautiously in cardiac patients because quetiapine may cause orthostatic hypotension.
- Monitor patients (particularly young adults) closely for suicidal tendencies, especially when therapy starts or dosage changes, because depression may worsen temporarily during these times.

WARNING Monitor patient taking quetiapine for predisposing factors for neuroleptic malignant syndrome, such as heat stress, physical exhaustion, dehydration, and organic brain disease. Neuroleptic malignant syndrome includes hyperpyrexia, muscle rigidity, altered mental status, and autonomic instability (which may include irregular pulse or blood pressure, tachycardia, diaphoresis, and arrhythmias).
- Monitor patient for signs of tardive dyskinesia, a potentially irreversible complication characterized by involuntary, dyskinetic movements of tongue, mouth, jaw, eyelids, or face. Notify prescriber if such signs develop, because quetiapine therapy may need to be stopped.
- Monitor patient for orthostatic hypotension, especially during initial dosage titration period. Be prepared to correct underlying conditions, such as hypovolemia and dehydration, before starting quetiapine therapy, as prescribed.
- Monitor patient for prolonged abnormal muscle contractions, especially during the first few days of quetiapine therapy, in male patients and in younger patients.
- Assess patient for hypothyroidism because drug can cause dose-dependent decreases in total and free thyroxine (T_4) levels.
- Monitor laboratory results during first 3 weeks of therapy for transient elevations in hepatic enzyme levels. Notify prescriber if they persist or worsen.

- Monitor patient's blood glucose and lipid levels routinely, as ordered, because drug increases the risk of hyperglycemia and hypercholesterolemia.
- Check CBC often during the first few months of therapy, as ordered, in patients with a low white blood cell count or a history of drug-induced hematologic problems. If counts drop or patient develops a fever or other signs of infection, notify prescriber and expect to discontinue drug and provide supportive care.
- Expect to gradually taper off quetiapine therapy when discontinued, as ordered, to avoid acute withdrawal symptoms such as insomnia, nausea, and vomiting.

PATIENT TEACHING
- Instruct patient to take quetiapine with food to reduce stomach upset.
- Advise patient not to stop taking quetiapine suddenly because doing so may exacerbate his symptoms or produce withdrawal symptoms.
- Inform patient that quetiapine therapy may cause dizziness or drowsiness. Advise him not to drive or perform other activities that require alertness until drug's full CNS effects are known.
- Instruct patient to rise slowly from a seated or lying position to reduce the risk of dizziness or fainting.
- Caution patient to avoid consuming alcoholic beverages because they can increase dizziness and drowsiness.
- Urge family or caregiver to watch patient closely for suicidal tendencies, especially when therapy starts or dosage changes and particularly if patient is a young adult.
- Encourage patient on long-term therapy to have regular eye examinations so that cataracts can be detected.
- Advise patient to contact prescriber if his pulse rate becomes abnormally slow or irregular.
- Alert patient that a false positive drug test for methadone or tricyclic antidepressants may occur with quetiapine use.

quinapril hydrochloride

Accupril

Class and Category

Chemical class: Ethylester of quinaprilat
Therapeutic class: Antihypertensive
Pregnancy category: D

Indications and Dosages

➤ *To treat hypertension*

TABLETS

Adults. *Initial:* 10 or 20 mg daily, adjusted every 2 wk based on clinical response. *Maintenance:* 20 to 80 mg daily or in divided doses twice daily.

DOSAGE ADJUSTMENT Initial dosage reduced to 5 mg daily for patients who are dehydrated from previous diuretic therapy, those who are still receiving diuretic therapy, and those with creatinine clearance of 30 to 60 ml/min/1.73 m². Dosage reduced to 2.5 mg daily for patients with creatinine clearance of 10 to 30 ml/min/1.73 m².

Route	Onset	Peak	Duration
P.O.	In 1 hr	2–4 hr	Up to 24 hr

Mechanism of Action

Blocks conversion of angiotensin I to angiotensin II, leading to vasodilation, and reduces aldosterone secretion, which prevents water retention. Quinapril also reduces peripheral arterial resistance. These combined actions lead to a reduction in blood pressure.

Contraindications

Aliskiren therapy in patients with diabetes or patients with renal impairment (GRF less than 60 ml/min), history of angioedema related to previous treatment with ACE inhibitor, hypersensitivity to quinapril or its components

Interactions

DRUGS

aliskiren (patients with diabetes and/or renal impairment), angiotensin receptor blockers, other ACE inhibitors: Increased risk of hyperkalemia, hypotension, and renal dysfunction
allopurinol, bone marrow depressants, corticosteroids (systemic), procainamide: Increased risk of fatal neutropenia or agranulocytosis
CNS depressants, other hypotension-producing drugs: Additive hypotensive effects

cyclosporine, potassium preparations, potassium-sparing diuretics: Possibly hyperkalemia
lithium: Possibly increased blood lithium level and risk of toxicity
mTOR inhibitors such as temsiroimus: Increased risk of angioedema
NSAIDs: Decreased antihypertensive effect of quinapril; increased risk of renal dysfunction in the elderly or patients who are volume-depleted or have preexisting renal dysfunction
sodium aurothiomalate: Possibly nitritoid reactions such as facial flushing, nausea, vomiting, and hypotension
sympathomimetics: Decreased antihypertensive effect of quinapril
tetracyclines: Reduced tetracycline absorption

FOODS

low-salt milk, salt substitutes: Increased risk of hyperkalemia

ACTIVITIES

alcohol use: Additive hypotensive effects

Adverse Reactions

CNS: Depression, dizziness, drowsiness, fatigue, fever, headache, insomnia, light-headedness, malaise, paresthesia, sleep disturbance, syncope, vertigo
CV: Chest pain, hypotension, orthostatic hypotension, palpitations, tachycardia
EENT: Amblyopia, dry mouth, loss of taste, pharyngitis
GI: Abdominal pain, constipation, diarrhea, indigestion, nausea, vomiting
GU: Impotence
MS: Arthralgia, back pain, myalgia
RESP: Cough, dyspnea
SKIN: Alopecia, diaphoresis, flushing, photosensitivity, pruritus, rash, urticaria
Other: Anaphylaxis, angioedema

Nursing Considerations

• Use quinapril cautiously in patients with renal impairment.
WARNING Patients with heart failure, hyponatremia, or severe volume or salt depletion; those who've recently received intensive diuresis or an increase in diuretic dosage; and those undergoing dialysis may be at risk for excessive hypotension. Monitor blood pressure often for first 2 weeks of therapy and whenever quinapril or diuretic dosage increases. If excessive

**Q
R
S**

hypotension occurs, notify prescriber immediately, place patient in a supine position, and, if prescribed, infuse normal saline solution.

WARNING Because of the risk of angio-edema, be prepared to discontinue drug and administer emergency measures, including subcutaneous epinephrine 1:1,000 (0.3 to 0.5 ml), if swelling of tongue, glottis, or larynx causes airway obstruction. Know that patients with a history of angioedema unrelated to ACE inhibitor therapy may be at increased risk of angioedema while receiving quinapril.

• Monitor blood pressure often to assess drug's effectiveness.

PATIENT TEACHING

• Instruct patient to notify prescriber immediately and stop taking quinapril if he has swelling of the face, eyes, lips, or tongue or difficulty breathing.

• Explain that drug may cause dizziness and light-headedness, especially for first few days of therapy. Advise patient to avoid hazardous activities until drug's CNS effects are known and to notify prescriber if he faints.

• Inform women of childbearing age of risks of taking quinapril during pregnancy. Caution her to use effective contraception and to notify prescriber immediately of known or suspected pregnancy.

• Advise patient having surgery or anesthesia to tell specialist that he takes quinapril.

• Instruct patient to consult prescriber before using potassium supplements or salt substitutes that contain potassium.

---

quinidine gluconate

Quinaglute Dura-tabs, Quinate (CAN), Quin-Release

quinidine polygalacturonate

Cardioquin

quinidine sulfate

Apo-Quinidine (CAN), Novoquinidin (CAN), Quinidex Extentabs

Class and Category

Chemical class: Dextrorotatory isomer of quinine
Therapeutic class: Class IA antiarrhythmic
Pregnancy category: C

Indications and Dosages

➤ *To prevent or treat cardiac arrhythmias, including established atrial fibrillation, atrial flutter, paroxysmal atrial fibrillation, paroxysmal atrial tachycardia, paroxysmal atrioventricular junctional rhythm, paroxysmal ventricular tachycardia not associated with complete heart block, and premature atrial and ventricular contractions*

E.R. TABLETS (QUINIDINE GLUCONATE)
Adults. 324 to 660 mg every 8 to 12 hr.
Maximum: 1,944 mg daily.

E.R. TABLETS (QUINIDINE SULFATE)
Adults. 300 to 600 mg every 8 to 12 hr.

TABLETS (QUINIDINE GLUCONATE)
Adults. *Initial:* 325 mg every 2 to 3 hr for 5 to 8 doses, gradually increasing dosage as needed and prescribed. *Maintenance:* 325 to 488 mg tthree times a day or four times a day.

TABLETS (QUINIDINE POLYGALACTURONATE)
Adults. *Initial:* 275 to 825 mg every 3 to 4 hr for 3 or 4 doses, then increased by 137.5 to 275 mg every 3rd or 4th dose until rhythm is restored or toxic effects occur. *Maintenance:* 275 mg twice daily or three times a day.

TABLETS (QUINIDINE SULFATE)
Adults. *Initial:* For premature atrial and ventricular contractions, 200 to 300 mg three times a day or four times a day; for paroxysmal supraventricular tachycardia, 400 to 600 mg every 2 to 3 hr until terminated; for atrial flutter, individual titration after digitalization; for conversion of atrial fibrillation, 200 mg every 2 to 3 hr for 5 to 8 doses, followed by subsequent daily increases, as needed. *Maintenance:* 200 to 400 mg three times a day or four times a day.
Children. 6 mg/kg 5 times daily.

I.V. INFUSION (QUINIDINE GLUCONATE)
Adults. 800 mg in 40 ml of D_5W at up to 0.25 mg/kg/min.

I.M. INJECTION (QUINIDINE SULFATE)
Adults. 190 to 380 mg every 2 to 4 hr.
Maximum: 3 g daily.

Route	Onset	Peak	Duration
P.O.	Unknown	Unknown	6–8 hr
P.O. (E.R.)	Unknown	Unknown	12 hr

Mechanism of Action

Depresses excitability, conduction velocity, and contractility of the myocardium and increases the effective refractory period, thus suppressing arrhythmic activity in the atria, ventricles, and His-Purkinje system.

Contraindications

Digitalis toxicity; history of quinidine-induced thrombocytopenic purpura or torsades de pointes; hypersensitivity to quinidine, other cinchona derivatives, or their components; long-QT syndrome; myasthenia gravis; pacemaker-dependent conduction disturbances

Interactions

DRUGS

antiarrhythmics, phenothiazines, rauwolfia alkaloids: Additive cardiac effects
anticholinergics: Possibly intensified atropine-like adverse effects
antimyasthenics: Antagonized antimyasthenic effects on skeletal muscle
barbiturates, rifampin: Possibly accelerated elimination and decreased effectiveness of quinidine
cimetidine: Increased elimination half-life, possibly leading to quinidine toxicity
digoxin: Possibly digitalis toxicity
hepatic enzyme inducers: Possibly decreased blood quinidine level
neuromuscular blockers: Possibly potentiated neuromuscular blockade
oral anticoagulants: Additive hypoprothrombinemia, increased risk of bleeding
pimozide: Risk of arrhythmias
quinine: Increased risk of quinidine toxicity
urinary alkalizers (such as antacids, carbonic anhydrase inhibitors, citrates, sodium bicarbonate, thiazide diuretics): Increased renal tubular reabsorption of quinidine, possibly leading to quinidine toxicity
verapamil: Possibly AV block, bradycardia, pulmonary edema, significant hypotension, and ventricular tachycardia

Adverse Reactions

CNS: Anxiety, asthenia, ataxia, confusion, delirium, difficulty speaking, dizziness, drowsiness, extrapyramidal reactions, fever, headache, hypertonia, syncope, vertigo
CV: Complete heart block, orthostatic hypotension, palpitations, peripheral edema, prolonged QT interval, torsades de pointes, vasculitis, ventricular arrhythmias, widening QRS complex
EENT: Blurred vision, change in color perception, diplopia, dry mouth, hearing loss (high-frequency), pharyngitis, photophobia, rhinitis, tinnitus
GI: Abdominal pain, anorexia, constipation, diarrhea, indigestion, nausea, vomiting
HEME: Agranulocytosis, hemolytic anemia, leukopenia, neutropenia, thrombocytopenia, thrombocytopenic purpura
MS: Arthralgia, myalgia
RESP: Dyspnea
SKIN: Diaphoresis, eczema, exfoliative dermatitis, flushing, hyperpigmentation, photosensitivity, pruritus, psoriasis, purpura, rash, urticaria
Other: Angioedema, flulike symptoms, weight gain

Nursing Considerations

• Give I.M. form of quinidine undiluted.
• For intermittent I.V. infusion, dilute drug in 40 ml of D_5W and administer using an infusion pump at a rate of 0.25 mg/kg/min or less. Rapid administration may cause hypotension. Monitor ECG tracings and blood pressure throughout administration.
• Monitor therapeutic blood level of quinidine, as ordered.
• Monitor heart rate and rhythm closely because quinidine may cause serious adverse reactions and can be cardiotoxic, especially at dosages exceeding 2.4 g daily. Implement continuous cardiac monitoring, as ordered.
• Assess for early signs and symptoms of cinchonism, including blurred vision, change in color perception, confusion, diplopia, headache, and tinnitus, which may indicate quinidine toxicity.

PATIENT TEACHING

• Advise patient to take quinidine at the same times every day and at evenly spaced intervals.

• Instruct patient to swallow E.R. tablets whole, with a full glass of water, preferably while sitting upright.
• Advise patient to take drug with food if GI upset occurs.
• Urge patient to inform prescriber immediately of blurred or double vision, change in color perception, confusion, diarrhea, fever, headache, loss of hearing, or tinnitus.

rabeprazole sodium
AcipHex

Class and Category
Chemical class: Substituted benzimidazole
Therapeutic class: Antiulcer
Pregnancy category: C

Indications and Dosages
➤ *To provide short-term treatment of erosive esophagitis or ulcerative gastroesophageal reflux disease (GERD)*
DELAYED-RELEASE TABLETS
Adults. For mild to moderate disease, 20 mg daily for 4 to 8 wk; course may be repeated if healing has not occurred at the end of 8 wk. For severe reflux with ulceration or stricture formation, 40 mg daily for 4 to 8 wk.
➤ *To treat symptomatic GERD*
DELAYED-RELEASE TABLETS
Adults and adolescents age 12 and over. 20 mg daily for 4 wk. Course may be repeated if symptoms aren't completely resolved.
DELAYED-RELEASE CAPSULES
Children ages 1 to 11 weighing 15 kg (33 lbs) or more. 10 mg once daily 30 min before a meal for up to 12 wks.
Children ages 1 to 11 weighing less than 15 kg (33 lbs). 5 mg once daily 30 min before a meal up to 12 wks. Increased to 10 mg once daily, as needed.
➤ *To provide maintenance treatment of erosive esophagitis or GERD*
DELAYED-RELEASE TABLETS
Adults. 20 mg daily.
➤ *To promote healing of duodenal ulcer, as adjunct to treat* Helicobacter pylori–*positive duodenal ulcer*

DELAYED-RELEASE TABLETS
Adults. 20 mg daily after breakfast for up to 4 wk for ulcer healing and 2 wk when used with antibiotic therapy for H. pylori.
➤ *As adjunct to reduce the risk of duodenal ulcer recurrence by eradicating* H. pylori
DELAYED-RELEASE TABLETS
Adults. 20 mg twice daily with morning and evening meals in conjunction with amoxicillin 1000 mg twice daily for 7 days and clarithromycin 500 mg twice daily for 7 days.
➤ *To treat hypersecretory conditions, such as Zollinger-Ellison syndrome*
DELAYED-RELEASE TABLETS
Adults. *Initial:* 60 mg daily; may be increased, if needed, to 100 mg daily or 60 mg twice daily.
DOSAGE ADJUSTMENT Dosage reduction may be needed in severe hepatic dysfunction.

Mechanism of Action
Decreases gastric acid secretion by suppressing its release at the secretory surface of gastric parietal cells. Rabeprazole also increases gastric pH and decreases basal acid output, which helps to heal ulcerated areas. In gastric parietal cells, it's transformed to an active sulfonamide, which increases the clearance rate of *Helicobacter pylori.*

Contraindications
Hypersensitivity to rabeprazole, other substituted benzimidazoles (omeprazole, lansoprazole), or their components

Interactions
DRUGS
cyclosporine: Possibly inhibited cyclosporine metabolism
digoxin: Increased risk of digitalis toxicity
methotrexate: Increased risk of methotrexate toxicities
warfarin: Possibly increased PT, INR

Adverse Reactions
CNS: Coma, delirium, disorientation, dizziness, headache, malaise
GI: Abdominal pain, *Clostridium difficile*-associated diarrhea, diarrhea, jaundice, nausea, vomiting
GU: Interstitial nephritis
HEME: Agranulocytosis, hemolytic anemia, leukopenia, pancytopenia, thrombocytopenia

MS: Bone fracture, rhabdomyolysis
RESP: Bronchospasm, interstitial pneumonia
SKIN: Erythema multiforme, rash, Stevens-Johnson syndrome, toxic epidermal necrolysis, urticaria
Other: Anaphylaxis, angioedema, hyperammonemia, hypomagnesemia, vitamin B_{12} deficiency (long-term use)

Nursing Considerations

• Use rabeprazole cautiously in patients with hepatic dysfunction.
• Expect to monitor serum gastrin level in long-term therapy to detect elevation.
• Closely monitor Japanese men receiving rabeprazole for adverse reactions because they're more likely than other patients to have increased blood drug levels.
• Monitor patient for bone fracture, especially in patient receiving multiple daily doses for more than a year because proton pump inhibitors like rabeprazole increase risk of osteoporosis-related fractures of the hip, wrist, and spine.
• Monitor patient for diarrhea because *diarrhea including Clostridium difficile-*associated diarrhea may occur with rabeprazole therapy. Notify prescriber if persistent or severe diarrhea develops.
• Monitor patient's magnesium level, as ordered, because hypomagnesemia may occur with rabeprazole therapy that has lasted longer than 3 months, although most cases have occurred after therapy had been given for more than a year. Notify prescriber if magnesium level drops below normal, as hypomagnesemia may cause tetany, arrhythmias, and seizures. Expect patient to receive magnesium replacement and drug to be discontinued.

PATIENT TEACHING
• Instruct patient to swallow delayed-release rabeprazole tablets whole and not to chew, crush, or split tablets.
• Instruct parents whose child is prescribed delayed-release capsules to make sure that child swallows capsule whole and does not chew or crush granules. If patient is unable to swallow capsule, tell parents that delayed-release capsules may be opened and contents may be sprinkled on a small amount of soft food such, as applesauce or yogurt. Contents may also be emptied into a small amount of liquid, such as infant formula, apple juice, or pediatric electrolyte solution. The dose should be taken within 15 minutes of preparation. Remind parents that food or liquid used to mix granules in should be at or below room temperature. Unused mixture should be discarded.
• Inform patients with hypersecretory conditions, such as Zollinger-Ellison syndrome, that treatment can last for a year or longer.
• Advise patient to contact prescriber if he develops diarrhea, abdominal pain, and fever that does not improve.

raloxifene hydrochloride
(keoxifene hydrochloride)

Evista

Class and Category

Chemical class: Benzothiophene derivative
Therapeutic class: Osteoporosis prophylactic
Pregnancy category: X

Indications and Dosages

➤ *To prevent osteoporosis in postmenopausal women; to reduce risk of invasive breast cancer in postmenopausal women with osteoporosis; to reduce risk of invasive breast cancer in postmenopausal women at high risk*

TABLETS
Adults. 60 mg daily.

Mechanism of Action

Prevents osteoporosis by binding to estrogen receptors, which decreases bone resorption and increases bone mineral density in postmenopausal women.

Contraindications

History of thromboembolic disease, hypersensitivity to raloxifene or its components, pregnancy

Interactions

DRUGS
ampicillin, cholestyramine: Decreased raloxifene absorption
warfarin: Possibly decreased PT

Q
R
S

Adverse Reactions

CNS: Depression, fever, insomnia, migraine, stroke
CV: Chest pain, hot flashes, peripheral edema, thromboembolism, thrombophlebitis
EENT: Laryngitis, pharyngitis, sinusitis
ENDO: Hot flashes
GI: Abdominal pain, cholelithiasis, flatulence, indigestion, nausea, vomiting
GU: Cystitis, infertility, leukorrhea, UTI, vaginitis
MS: Arthralgia, arthritis, leg cramps or spasms, myalgia
RESP: Cough, pneumonia, pulmonary embolism
SKIN: Diaphoresis, rash
Other: Flulike symptoms, weight gain

Nursing Considerations

• Use cautiously in patients who smoke or have a history of stroke, TIA, atrial fibrillation, or hypertension because raloxifene may increase the risk of stroke.
• Use cautiously in patients with renal impairment because effects of raloxifene on renal system are unknown.
WARNING Monitor patient's limbs for impaired circulation and pain (possible thromboembolism).
• Expect prescriber to stop drug at least 72 hours before and during periods of prolonged immobilization. Resume raloxifene therapy as prescribed after patient is fully ambulatory.
PATIENT TEACHING
• Advise patient to avoid lengthy immobility during travel while taking raloxifene because of the increased risk of thrombo-embolism.
• Instruct patient to report adverse reactions to prescriber immediately, especially leg pain or swelling, sudden chest pain, shortness of breath, coughing up blood, or a sudden change in vision.
• Emphasize the importance of compliance with long-term raloxifene therapy.
• Advise patient that postmenopausal women require an average of 1,500 mg of elemental calcium and 400 to 800 international units of vitamin D daily. Vitamin D requirement is increased in women over age 70, women with GI malabsorption syndromes, and women who are chronically ill or nursing-home bound. Review dietary sources of calcium and vitamin D, and have patient discuss supplements with prescriber, as needed.

ramelteon
Rozerem

Class and Category

Chemical class: Melatonin receptor agonist
Therapeutic class: Hypnotic
Pregnancy category: C

Indications and Dosages

➤ *To treat insomnia in patients having difficulty falling asleep*
TABLETS
Adults. 8 mg 30 min before at bedtime.

Route	Onset	Peak	Duration
P.O.	Unknown	0.5–1.5 hr	Unknown

Mechanism of Action

Binds to melatonin receptors MT1 and MT2 in the suprachiasmatic nucleus (SCN) of the hypothalamus. The SCN regulates the sleep–wake cycle, and endogenous melatonin probably is involved in maintaining the circadian rhythm underlying that cycle.

Contraindications

Concurrent therapy with fluvoxamine, history of angioedema with previous ramelteon treatment, hypersensitivity to ramelteon or its components, severe hepatic dysfunction

Interactions

DRUGS
benzodiazepines, melatonin, other sedative-hypnotics: Possible additive sedative effects
donepezil, doxepin, fluconazole, fluvoxamine, ketoconazole: Increased plasma ramelteon levels
rifampin: Decreased ramelteon effectiveness
ACTIVITIES
alcohol use: Possibly additive CNS effect

Adverse Reactions

CNS: Agitation, amnesia, anxiety, bizarre behavior, complex behaviors such as sleep driving, depression, dizziness, fatigue,

hallucinations, headache, insomnia exacerbation, mania, somnolence, suicidal ideation
EENT: Throat tightness
ENDO: Decreased testosterone level, increased prolactin level
GI: Diarrhea, dysgeusia, nausea, vomiting
MS: Arthralgia, myalgia
RESP: Dyspnea, upper respiratory tract infection
Other: Anaphylaxis, angioedema

Nursing Considerations
• Be aware that ramelteon therapy is not recommended for patients with severe sleep apnea or COPD because its effects have not been studied in these patient populations.
• Use cautiously in patients with mild to moderate hepatic dysfunction. Drug is contraindicated in severe hepatic dysfunction.
• Ramelteon is the first approved hypnotic not classified as a controlled substance.
WARNING Monitor patient closely for hypersensitivity reactions such as dyspnea, throat tightness, nausea, vomiting, and swelling. If present, discontinue ramelteon immediately, notify prescriber, and provide supportive care.
• Watch patient closely for suicidal tendencies, particularly when therapy starts and dosage changes, because depression may worsen temporarily during these times, possibly leading to suicidal ideation.
PATIENT TEACHING
• Instruct patient not to take ramelteon with or immediately after eating a high-fat meal.
• Caution patient to avoid potentially hazardous activities after taking ramelteon; drug's intended effect is to decrease alertness.
• Advise patient that drug may cause abnormal behaviors during sleep, such as driving a car, eating, talking on the phone, or having sex without any recall of the event. If family members notice any such behavior or patient sees evidence of such behavior upon awakening, prescriber should be notified.
• Advise limiting alcohol during therapy.

• Tell patient to notify prescriber if insomnia worsens or new signs or symptoms occur.
• Inform patient that drug may affect reproductive hormones; urge patient to report cessation of menses or galactorrhea (females) or decreased libido or problems with infertility.
• Urge family or caregiver to watch patient closely for suicidal tendencies, especially when therapy starts or dosage changes.

ramipril
Altace

Class and Category
Chemical class: Ethylester of ramiprilat
Therapeutic class: Antihypertensive
Pregnancy category: D

Indications and Dosages
➤ *To treat heart failure after MI*
CAPSULES
Adults. *Initial:* 1.25 to 2.5 mg twice daily. *Maintenance:* 5 mg twice daily.
➤ *To treat hypertension*
CAPSULES
Adults. *Initial:* 2.5 mg daily. *Maintenance:* 2.5 to 20 mg once daily or in divided doses twice daily.
DOSAGE ADJUSTMENT Initial dosage reduced to 1.25 mg daily for patients dehydrated from diuretics, those receiving diuretics, and those with creatinine clearance less than 40 ml/min/1.73 m^2; dosage then slowly increased until blood pressure is under control or maximum daily dose of 5 mg is reached. Dosage also reduced to 1.25 mg daily for patients with heart failure post myocardial infarction who cannot tolerate the initial dosage of 2.5 mg once daily.

Route	Onset	Peak	Duration
P.O.	1–2 hr	4–6.5 hr	24 hr

Mechanism of Action
Blocks conversion of angiotensin I to angiotensin II, causing vasodilation, and reduces aldosterone secretion, which prevents water retention. Ramipril also reduces peripheral arterial resistance. Combined, these actions reduce blood pressure.

Q
R
S

Contraindications

Aliskiren therapy in patients with diabetes or patients with renal impairment (GRF less than 60 ml/min), history of angioedema, hypersensitivity to ramipril, its components, or any other ACE inhibitors

Interactions

DRUGS

aliskiren (patients with diabetes and/or renal impairment), angiotensin receptor blockers, other ACE inhibitors: Increased risk of hyperkalemia, hypotension, and renal dysfunction
allopurinol, bone marrow depressants, corticosteroids (systemic), procainamide: Increased risk of fatal neutropenia or agranulocytosis
CNS depressants, other hypotension-producing drugs: Additive hypotensive effect
cyclosporine, potassium preparations, potassium-sparing diuretics: Possibly hyperkalemia
insulin, oral antidiabetics: Increased risk of hypoglycemia
lithium: Increased risk of lithium toxicity
mTOR inhibitors such as temsiroimus: Increased risk of angioedema
NSAIDs: Decreased antihypertensive effect of ramipril; increased risk of renal dysfunction in the elderly and patients with volume depletion or preexisting renal dysfunction
sodium aurothiomalate: Increased risk of nitritoid reaction (facial flushing, nausea, vomiting, hypotension)
sympathomimetics: Decreased antihypertensive effect of ramipril
telmisartan: Possibly increased risk of adverse effects, especially renal dysfunction
tetracyclines: Reduced tetracycline absorption

FOODS

low-salt milk, salt substitutes: Increased risk of hyperkalemia

ACTIVITIES

alcohol use: Additive hypotensive effects

Adverse Reactions

CNS: Depression, dizziness, drowsiness, fatigue, fever, headache, insomnia, light-headedness, malaise, paresthesia, sleep disturbance, syncope, vertigo
CV: Chest pain, hypotension, orthostatic hypotension, palpitations, tachycardia

EENT: Amblyopia, dry mouth, loss of taste, pharyngitis
GI: Abdominal pain, constipation, diarrhea, elevated liver function test results, hepatic failure, hepatitis, nausea, vomiting
GU: Acute renal failure, elevated BUN and serum creatinine levels, impotence, oliguria, progressive azotemia
HEME: Agranulocytosis, anemia, bone marrow depression, pancytopenia
MS: Arthralgia, back pain, myalgia
RESP: Cough, dyspnea
SKIN: Alopecia, diaphoresis, flushing, jaundice, onycholysis, pemphigoid, photosensitivity, pruritus, rash, Stevens-Johnson syndrome, toxic epidermal necrolysis, urticaria
Other: Angioedema

Nursing Considerations

• Use ramipril cautiously in patients with renal or hepatic impairment.
WARNING Patients with dehydration, heart failure, or hyponatremia; those who've recently received intensive diuresis or an increase in diuretic dosage; and those having dialysis may risk excessive hypotension. Monitor such patients closely the first 2 weeks of therapy and whenever ramipril or diuretic dosage increases. If excessive hypotension occurs, notify prescriber immediately, place patient in a supine position, and, if prescribed, infuse normal saline solution.
WARNING Because of the risk of angioedema, be prepared to stop drug and provide emergency measures, including subcutaneous epinephrine 1:1,000 (0.3 to 0.5 ml), if swelling of tongue, glottis, or larynx causes airway obstruction.
• Monitor blood pressure frequently during therapy to assess drug's effectiveness.
• Monitor patient's renal and hepatic function closely during therapy. If patient develops jaundice or marked elevations of hepatic enzymes, notify prescriber and expect ramipril to be discontinued.

PATIENT TEACHING

• Advise patient to stop taking ramipril and inform prescriber immediately if she experiences swelling of the face, eyes, lips, or tongue or has difficulty breathing.
• Explain that drug may cause dizziness and light-headedness, especially during first

few days of therapy. Instruct patient to notify prescriber immediately if she faints.
• Inform female patient of childbearing age of the risks of taking ramipril during pregnancy. Caution patient to use effective contraception and to report known or suspected pregnancy immediately.
• Urge patient to tell providers that she takes ramipril before having surgery or anesthesia.
• Tell patient to ask prescriber before using supplements or salt substitutes that contain potassium.

ranitidine hydrochloride

Apo-Ranitidine (CAN), Gen-Ranitidine (CAN), Novo-Ranitidine (CAN), Nu-Ranit (CAN), Zantac, Zantac EFFERdose Tablets, Zantac 150 GELdose, Zantac 300 GELdose

Class and Category

Chemical class: Aminoalkyl-substituted furan derivative
Therapeutic class: Antiulcer agent, gastric acid secretion inhibitor
Pregnancy category: B

Indications and Dosages

➤ *To prevent duodenal and gastric ulcers*
CAPSULES, EFFERVESCENT GRANULES, EFFERVESCENT TABLETS, SYRUP, TABLETS
Adults and adolescents. 150 mg at bedtime.
➤ *To provide short-term treatment of active duodenal and benign gastric ulcers*
CAPSULES, EFFERVESCENT GRANULES, EFFERVESCENT TABLETS, SYRUP, TABLETS
Adults and adolescents. 150 mg twice daily for gastric ulcers; 150 mg twice daily or 300 mg at bedtime for duodenal ulcers.
Children ages 1 month to 16 years. 2 to 4 mg/kg twice daily up to 300 mg daily. *Maintenance:* 2 to 4 mg/kg daily up to 150 mg daily.
CONTINUOUS I.V. INFUSION
Adults and adolescents. 6.25 mg/hr. *Maximum:* 400 mg daily.
INTERMITTENT I.V. INFUSION
Adults and adolescents. 50 mg diluted to total volume of 100 ml and infused over 15 to 20 min every 6 to 8 hr. *Maximum:* 400 mg daily.

Children. 2 to 4 mg/kg daily diluted to a suitable volume and infused over 15 to 20 min.
I.V. INJECTION
Adults and adolescents. 50 mg diluted to total volume of 20 ml and injected slowly over no less than 5 min every 6 to 8 hr. *Maximum:* 400 mg daily.
I.M. INJECTION
Adults and adolescents. 50 mg every 6 to 8 hr. *Maximum:* 400 mg daily.
➤ *To treat acute gastroesophageal reflux disease*
CAPSULES, EFFERVESCENT GRANULES, EFFERVESCENT TABLETS, SYRUP, TABLETS
Adults and adolescents. 150 mg twice daily.
EFFERVESCENT TABLETS
Children ages 1 month to 16 years. 2.5 to 5 mg/kg twice daily.
INTERMITTENT I.V. INFUSION
Children. 2 to 8 mg/kg diluted to suitable volume and infused over 15 to 20 min three times daily.
➤ *To treat erosive esophagitis*
CAPSULES, EFFERVESCENT GRANULES, EFFERVESCENT TABLETS, SYRUP, TABLETS
Adults and adolescents. 150 mg four times a day.
EFFERVESCENT TABLETS
Children ages 1 month to 16 years. 2.5 to 5 mg/kg twice daily.
➤ *To treat hypersecretory gi conditions, such as Zollinger-Ellison syndrome, systemic mastocytosis, and multiple endocrine adenoma syndrome*
CAPSULES, EFFERVESCENT GRANULES, EFFERVESCENT TABLETS, SYRUP, TABLETS
Adults and adolescents. *Initial:* 150 mg twice daily, adjusted as needed. *Maximum:* 6 g daily in divided doses.
CONTINUOUS I.V. INFUSION
Adults and adolescents. *Initial:* 1 mg/kg/hr, increased by 0.5 mg/kg/hr up to 2.5 mg/kg/hr.
Maximum: 400 mg daily.
INTERMITTENT I.V. INFUSION
Adults. 50 mg diluted to total volume of 100 ml and infused over 15 to 20 min every 6 to 8 hr. *Maximum:* 400 mg daily.
I.V. INJECTION
Adults and adolescents. 50 mg diluted to total of 20 ml and injected slowly over at least 5 min every 6 to 8 hr. *Maximum:* 400 mg daily.

Q
R
S

I.M. INJECTION
Adults. 50 mg every 6 to 8 hr.
➤ *To prevent acid indigestion, heartburn, and sour stomach caused by eating certain foods or drinking certain beverages*
TABLETS
Adults and adolescents. 75 mg 30 to 60 min before food or beverages expected to cause symptoms. *Maximum:* 150 mg daily over no more than 2 continuous wk.
➤ *To treat acid indigestion, heartburn, and sour stomach*
TABLETS
Adults and adolescents. 75 mg when symptoms start; repeated once within 24 hr, if needed.
DOSAGE ADJUSTMENT For patients whose creatinine clearance is less than 50 ml/min/1.73 m², 150 mg P.O. every 24 hr with dosage interval increased thereafter to every 12 hr, as needed. Or 50 mg I.V. every 18 to 24 hr with dosage interval increased to every 12 hr, as needed. Dosage reduction may also be necessary for patients with hepatic dysfunction.

Route	Onset	Peak	Duration
P.O., I.V., I.M.	Unknown	1–3 hr	13 hr

Mechanism of Action
Inhibits basal and nocturnal secretion of gastric acid and pepsin by competitively inhibiting the action of histamine at H_2 receptors on gastric parietal cells. This action reduces total volume of gastric juices and, thus, irritation of GI mucosa.

Contraindications
Acute porphyria, hypersensitivity to ranitidine or its components

Interactions
DRUGS
antacids: Decreased ranitidine absorption
atazanavir, delavirdine, diazepam, gefitinib, itraconazole, ketoconazole, sucralfate: Decreased absorption of these drugs
bone marrow depressants: Increased risk of neutropenia or other blood dyscrasias
glipizide, glyburide, metoprolol, midazolam, nifedipine, phenytoin, theophylline, triazolam: Increased effects of these drugs, possibly leading to toxic reactions

procainamide: Possibly increased risk of procainamide toxicity
warfarin: Possibly altered PT
ACTIVITIES
alcohol use: Increased blood alcohol level (with oral ranitidine)

Adverse Reactions
CNS: Dizziness, drowsiness, fever, headache, insomnia
CV: Vasculitis
GI: Abdominal distress, constipation, diarrhea, nausea, vomiting
GU: Acute interstitial nephritis, impotence
MS: Arthralgia, myalgia
RESP: Bronchospasm
SKIN: Alopecia, erythema multiforme, rash
Other: Anaphylaxis, angioedema

Nursing Considerations
• Be aware that ranitidine must be diluted for I.V. use if not using premixed solution. For I.V. injection, dilute to total of 20 ml with normal saline solution, D_5W, $D_{10}W$, lactated Ringer's solution, or 5% sodium bicarbonate. For I.V. infusion, dilute to total volume of 100 ml of same solutions.
• Give I.V. injection at no more than 4 ml/min, intermittent I.V. infusion at 5 to 7 ml/min, and continuous I.V. infusion at 6.25 mg/hr (except with hypersecretory conditions, when initial infusion rate is 1 mg/kg/hr, gradually increased after 4 hours, as needed, in increments of 0.5 mg/kg/hr).
• Don't add additives to premixed solution.
• Stop primary I.V. solution infusion during piggyback administration.
PATIENT TEACHING
• Tell patient to dissolve 150-mg effervescent tablets or granules in 6 to 8 oz water or 25-mg effervescent tablets in at least 5 ml water.
• Advise patient (or parent) to wait until effervescent tablet is completely dissolved before taking (or giving to child or infant).
• Caution patient not to chew effervescent tablets, swallow them whole, or let them dissolve on the tongue.
• Alert patients with phenylketonuria that effervescent tablets and granules contain phenylalanine.
• Tell patient that she may take drug with food.
• Tell patient to stop taking ranitidine and contact prescriber if she has trouble

swallowing, vomits blood, or passes black or bloody stools.

• If needed, advise patient to take antacids, 2 hours before or after ranitidine; advise against taking other acid reducers with drug.

• If patient takes drug to prevent heartburn, tell her to contact prescriber about frequent chest pain or wheezing with heartburn; stomach pain; unexplained weight loss; nausea; vomiting; heartburn lasting more than 3 months; heartburn with light-headedness, dizziness, or sweating; chest or shoulder pain with shortness of breath, sweating, light-headedness, or pain spreading to arms, neck, or shoulders. These problems may be serious.

• Inform patient that healing of an ulcer may require 4 to 8 weeks of therapy.

ranolazine
Ranexa

Class and Category
Chemical class: Piperazineacetamide
Therapeutic class: Antianginal
Pregnancy category: C

Indications and Dosages
➤ *To treat chronic angina*
E.R. TABLETS
Adults. *Initial:* 500 mg twice daily, increased to 1,000 mg twice daily, as needed. *Maximum:* 1,000 mg twice daily.
DOSAGE ADJUSTMENT For patients taking a moderate CYP3A inhibitor, such as diltiazem, erythromycin, fluconazole or verapamil, maximum dosage reduced to 500 mg twice daily.

Route	Onset	Peak	Duration
P.O.	Unknown	2–5 hr	Unknown

Mechanism of Action
Exerts anti-ischemic and antianginal effects by an unknown mechanism not dependent on reductions in heart rate or blood pressure. Ranolazine inhibits cardiac late sodium current, but how this action inhibits angina symptoms is also unknown.

Contraindications
Hypersensitivity to ranolazine or its components, liver cirrhosis, use of CYP3A inducers or strong inhibitors

Interactions
DRUGS
CYP2D6 such as antipsychotics, metoprolol, tricyclic antidepressants: Increased plasma levels of these drugs
CYP3A inducers, such as carbamazepine, phenobarbital, phenytoin, rifabutin, rifampin, rifapentin, St. John's wort: Decreased blood ranolazine level and decreased effectiveness
CYP3A substrates, such as cyclosporine, lovastatin, simvastatin, sirolimus, tacrolimus: Possibly increased blood levels of these drugs
CYP3A inhibitors, such as clarithromycin, diltiazem, erythromycin, fluconazole, indinavir, itraconazole, ketoconazole, nefazodone, nelfinavir, ritonavir, saquinavir, verapamil: Increased blood ranolazine level and increased risk of adverse reactions
digoxin: Increased blood digoxin level
ACTIVITIES
grapefruit juice, grapefruit containing products: Increased blood ranolazine level and increased risk of adverse reactions

Adverse Reactions
CNS: Abnormal coordination, asthenia, confusion, dizziness, hallucination, headache, hypoesthesia, paresthesia, syncope, tremor, vertigo
CV: Bradycardia, hypotension, orthostatic hypotension, palpitations, peripheral edema, QT-interval prolongation
EENT: Blurred vision, dry mouth, tinnitus
GI: Abdominal pain, anorexia, constipation, dyspepsia, nausea, vomiting
GU: Dysuria, elevated blood urea and creatinine levels, hematuria, renal failure, urinary retention
HEME: Eosinophilia, leukopenia, pancytopenia, thrombocytopenia
RESP: Dyspnea, pulmonary fibrosis
SKIN: Diaphoresis, pruritus, rash
Other: Angioedema

Nursing Considerations
• Monitor patient's QT interval, as ordered, because ranolazine prolongs it in a dose-related manner.

Q
R
S

- Assess effectiveness of ranolazine at preventing anginal pain.
- Know that acute renal failure may occur in some patients with severe renal impairment (creatinine clearance less than 30 ml/min) while taking drug. Monitor patient's serum creatinine levels and blood urea nitrogen after drug therapy begins and then periodically, as ordered. If elevations occur, notify prescriber and expect drug to be discontinued.
- Monitor patient's serum, magnesium, potassium, and liver enzyme levels.

PATIENT TEACHING
- Instruct patient to take ranolazine exactly as prescribed.
- Inform patient that drug may be taken with or without food.
- Caution patient to swallow tablets whole and not to crush, break, or chew them.
- Advise patient to limit the amount of grapefruit and grapefruit juice consumed while taking this drug.
- Advise patient to notify prescriber if serious or persistent adverse reactions occur.
- Instruct patient to notify all prescribers of ranolazine use.

rasagiline
Azilect

Class and Category
Chemical class: Propargylamine
Therapeutic class: Irreversible MAO inhibitor
Pregnancy category: C

Indications and Dosages
➤ *To treat idiopathic Parkinson's disease as initial monotherapy in early-stage disease; adjunct in patients not taking levodopa*

TABLETS
Adults. 1 mg once daily.

➤ *As adjunct with levodopa or levodopa and carbidopa in treatment of later-stage idiopathic Parkinson's disease*

TABLETS
Adults. 0.5 mg once daily increased to 1 mg once daily, as needed.

DOSAGE ADJUSTMENT For patients with mild hepatic failure, dosage shouldn't exceed 0.5 mg daily.

Mechanism of Action
Inhibits metabolic degradation of catecholamines and serotonin in the CNS and peripheral tissues, increasing extracellular dopamine level in the striatum. The increased dopamine level helps control alterations in voluntary muscle movement (such as tremors and rigidity) in Parkinson's disease because dopamine, a neurotransmitter, is essential for normal motor function. By stimulating peripheral and central dopaminergic 2 (D_2) receptors on postsynaptic cells, dopamine inhibits firing of striatal neurons (such as cholinergic neurons), improving motor function.

Route	Onset	Peak	Duration
P.O.	Unknown	1 hr	Unknown

Contraindications
Acute MI; angina; cardiac arrhythmias; coronary artery disease; cerebrovascular disease; elective surgery that requires general anesthesia; hypersensitivity to rasagiline or its components; pheochromocytoma; moderate to severe hepatic impairment; stroke; use within 14 days of cyclobenzaprine, dextromethorphan, MAO inhibitors, meperidine, mirtazapine, tramadol, methadone, propoxyphene, St. John's wort, or sympathomimetic amines

Interactions
DRUGS
ciprofloxacin and other CYP1A2 inhibitors: Increased rasagiline plasma level
dextromethorphan: Increased risk of psychosis or bizarre behavior
levodopa, levodopa and carbidopa: Increased risk of dyskinesias
MAO inhibitors, sympathomimetics: Increased risk of hypertensive crisis
meperidine, methadone, propoxyphene, tramadol: Increased risk of life-threatening adverse reactions characterized by coma, severe hypertension or hypotension, severe respiratory depression, seizures, malignant hyperpyrexia, excitation, and peripheral vascular collapse
selective serotonin reuptake inhibitors, tetracyclic antidepressants, tricyclic antidepressants: Increased risk of severe

CNS toxicity with hyperpyrexia, behavioral and mental status changes, diaphoresis, muscle rigidity, hypertension, syncope, and possible death

Adverse Reactions

CNS: Abnormal dreams, amnesia, anxiety, asthenia, ataxia, cerebral ischemia, coma, compulsive behaviors (binge eating, increased sexual urges, intense urges to spend money), confusion, daytime sleepiness, depression, difficulty thinking, dizziness, dyskinesia, dystonia, fever, hallucinations, headache, malaise, manic depressive reaction, nightmares, paresthesia, psychotic-like behavior, seizures, serotonin syndrome, somnolence, stroke, stupor, syncope, vertigo
CV: Angina, bundle branch heart block, chest pain, heart failure, MI, hypertensive crisis, postural hypotension, thrombophlebitis, ventricular tachycardia or fibrillation
EENT: Blurred vision, conjunctivitis, dry mouth, gingivitis, hemorrhage, laryngeal edema, retinal detachment or hemorrhage, rhinitis
GI: Abdominal pain, anorexia, constipation, diarrhea, dyspepsia, dysphagia, epistaxia, gastroenteritis, gastrointestinal hemorrhage, intestinal obstruction or perforation, liver function test abnormalities, nausea, vomiting
GU: Acute renal failure, albuminuria, decreased libido, hematuria, impotence, incontinence, priapism
HEME: Anemia, leukopenia, thrombocytopenia
MS: Arthralgia, arthritis, bone necrosis, bursitis, leg cramps, myasthenia, neck pain or stiffness, tenosynovitis
RESP: Apnea, asthma, cough, dyspnea, pleural effusion, pneumothorax, interstitial pneumonia
SKIN: Alopecia, carcinoma, diaphoresis, ecchymosis, exfoliative dermatitis, pruritus, ulcer, vesiculobullous rash
Other: Angioedema, flu syndrome, hypersensitivity reaction, hypocalcemia, weight loss

Nursing Considerations

WARNING Monitor patient's blood pressure closely throughout therapy. Notify prescriber immediately if patient has evidence of hypertensive crisis, such as blurred vision, chest pain, difficulty thinking, stupor or coma, seizures, severe headache, neck stiffness, nausea, vomiting, palpitations or signs and symptoms suggesting a stroke. Expect to stop drug immediately if these occur.

• Keep phentolamine readily available to treat hypertensive crisis. Give 5 mg by slow I.V. infusion, as prescribed, to reduce blood pressure without causing excessive hypotension. Use external cooling measures, as prescribed, to manage fever.

• Monitor patient receiving rasagline with levodopa for worsening of preexisting dyskinesia. If it occurs, notify prescriber and expect levodopa dosage to be decreased.

• Be aware that patient may experience orthostatic hypotension, especially in the first 2 months of rasagiline therapy and that it may also occur while patient is supine.

PATIENT TEACHING

WARNING Inform patient taking recommended dosage of rasagiline that dietary tyramine restriction is no longer needed except for avoidance of very tyramine-rich foods such as aged cheese (e.g., Stilton), which may increase blood pressure greatly. If patient doesn't feel well soon after eating a suspected high-tyramine meal, he should contact prescriber immediately.

• Remind patient not to exceed the recommended dose because of risk of hypertension.

• Advise patient to stop taking rasagline and to notify prescriber immediately if he develops blurred vision, chest pain, trouble thinking, stupor or coma, seizures, severe headache, stiff neck, nausea, vomiting, palpitations, or evidence of stroke.

WARNING Monitor patient closely for serotonin syndrome, a rare but serious adverse effect of rasagiline. Signs and symptoms include agitation, confusion, diaphoresis, diarrhea, fever, hyperactive reflexes, poor coordination, restlessness, shaking, talking or acting with uncontrolled excitement, tremor, and twitching. If symptoms occur, notify prescriber immediately, expect to discontinue drug, and provide supportive care.

Q
R
S

- Suggest that patient change position slowly to minimize orthostatic hypotension.
- Alert patient that drug may cause hallucinations or changes in behavior that may be severe, especially at the initiation of drug therapy or when an increase in dosage occurs. If they occur, tell patient to notify prescriber promptly.
- Alert patient and caregivers that drug may cause impulsive or compulsive behaviors such as binge eating, increased sexual activities, gambling, or spending money inappropriately. If any questionable behavior occurs, instruct patient or caregiver to notify prescriber, as dosage may need to be adjusted or drug discontinued.
- Instruct patient to notify all prescribers of rasagline therapy, especially if antidepressants or antibiotics such as ciprofloxacin or a similar drug are being considered, and to avoid taking any over the counter cold medications.
- Caution patient not to perform hazardous activities until CNS effects of drug are known. Some patients have fallen asleep without warning while engaged in activities of daily living, including driving.

remifentanil hydrochloride

Ultiva

Class, Category, and Schedule

Chemical class: Fentanyl analogue
Therapeutic class: Anesthesia adjunct
Pregnancy category: C
Controlled substance schedule: II

Indications and Dosages

➤ *As adjunct to induce general anesthesia*

INTERMITTENT I.V. INFUSION

Adults and children age 2 and over. 0.5 to 1 mcg/kg plus inhalation or I.V. anesthetic.

➤ *To maintain general anesthesia*

INTERMITTENT I.V. INFUSION

Adults and children age 2 and over. 0.05 to 0.2 mcg/kg, followed by 0.5 to 1 mcg/kg every 2 to 5 min, as needed.

➤ *To continue analgesic effect in immediate postoperative period*

CONTINUOUS I.V. INFUSION

Adults and children age 2 and over. *Initial:* 0.1 mcg/kg/min, adjusted by 0.025 mcg/kg/min every 5 min, as prescribed, to balance level of analgesia and respiratory rate. *Maximum:* 0.2 mcg/kg/min.

➤ *To supplement local or regional anesthesia in a monitored anesthetic setting*

I.V. INFUSION

Adults and children age 2 and over. *With a benzodiazepine:* 0.05 mcg/kg/min, starting 5 min before placement of local or regional block; after placement of block, decreased to 0.025 mcg/kg/min and then further adjusted every 5 min in increments of 0.025 mcg/kg/min, as needed. *Without a benzodiazepine:* 0.1 mcg/kg/min, starting 5 min before placement of local or regional block; after placement of block, decreased to 0.05 mcg/kg/min and then further adjusted every 5 min in increments of 0.025 mcg/kg/min, as needed.

I.V. INJECTION

Adults and children age 2 and over. *With a benzodiazepine:* 0.5 mcg/kg over 30 to 60 sec as a single dose 60 to 90 sec before local anesthetic is administered. *Without a benzodiazepine:* 1 mcg/kg administered over 30 to 60 sec as a single dose 60 to 90 sec before local anesthetic is administered.

DOSAGE ADJUSTMENT For elderly patients, starting dose possibly reduced by half. If patient is more than 30% over ideal body weight, starting dose based on ideal body weight.

Route	Onset	Peak	Duration
I.V.	1 min	1–2 min	5–10 min

Incompatibilities

Don't give remifentanil through same I.V. line as blood because nonspecific esterases in blood products may inactivate drug.

Contraindications

Epidural or intrathecal administration, hypersensitivity to fentanyl analogues

Interactions

DRUGS

anesthetics (barbiturate, inhalation), benzodiazepines, propofol: Possibly synergistic effects, increasing risk of hypotension and respiratory depression

Mechanism of Action

Remifentanil decreases transmission and perception of pain by stimulating m_u-opioid receptors in neurons. This action decreases the activity of adenyl cyclase in neurons, which in turn decreases cAMP production. With less cAMP available, potassium (K^+) is forced out of neurons, and calcium (Ca^{++}) is prevented from entering neurons. As a result, neuron excitability declines, and fewer neurotransmitters (such as substance P) leave the neurons, thereby decreasing pain transmission.

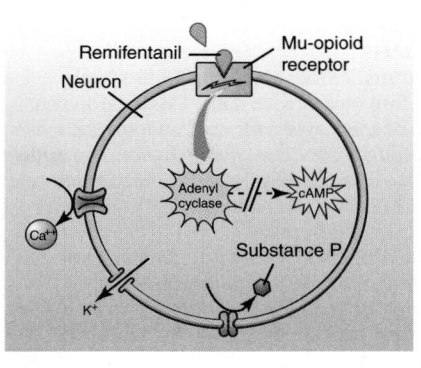

atropine, glycopyrrolate: Possibly reversal of remifentanil-induced bradycardia
ephedrine, epinephrine, norepinephrine: Possibly reversal of remifentanil-induced hypotension
neuromuscular blockers: Prolonged skeletal muscle rigidity caused by remifentanil
opioid antagonists: Possibly reversal of remifentanil's effects

Adverse Reactions

CNS: Headache, shivering
CV: Asystole, bradycardia, hypotension
GI: Nausea, vomiting
MS: Skeletal muscle rigidity
RESP: Apnea, cough, dyspnea, respiratory depression, stridor, wheezing
Other: Anaphylaxis

Nursing Considerations

• Inject remifentanil into I.V. tubing at or as close as possible to venous cannula.
• Use infusion device to deliver continuous infusion.
• Monitor vital signs and oxygenation continuously during administration.
• Expect analgesic effects to dissipate rapidly when drug is discontinued. Expect to start adequate postoperative analgesia, as prescribed, before stopping drug.
WARNING After stopping drug, clear I.V. tubing to prevent inadvertent later delivery.
• Monitor respiratory status continuously because of risk of respiratory depression from residual effects of other anesthetics for up to 30 minutes after infusion stops.
PATIENT TEACHING
• Explain expected drug effects to patient, and reassure her that she'll be monitored continuously during drug administration.

repaglinide

Prandin

Class and Category

Chemical class: Meglitinide
Therapeutic class: Antidiabetic
Pregnancy category: C

Indications and Dosages

➤ *To achieve glucose control in type 2 diabetes mellitus as monotherapy in patients whose glycosylated hemoglobin (Hba_{1c}) level is less than 8%*
TABLETS
Adults. *Initial:* 0.5 mg 15 to 30 min before meals twice daily. Dosage doubled, as needed, every wk until adequate glucose response obtained. *Maintenance:* 0.5 to 4 mg/dose up to four times a day. *Maximum:* 16 mg daily in divided doses of not more than 4 mg/dose.
➤ *To achieve glucose control in type 2 diabetes mellitus as monotherapy in patients whose Hba_{1c} is 8% or greater and in combination with metformin or thiazolidinedione (pioglitazone*

Q
R
S

hydrochloride, rosiglitazone maleate) therapy

TABLETS

Adults. *Initial:* 1 or 2 mg 15 to 30 min before meals twice daily. Dosage doubled, as needed, every wk until adequate glucose response obtained. *Maintenance:* 1 to 4 mg/ dose up to four times a day. *Maximum:* 16 mg daily in divided doses of not more than 4 mg/dose.

DOSAGE ADJUSTMENT For patients with moderate to severe hepatic or renal impairment, increased time between dosage adjustments.

Stimulates release of insulin from functioning pancreatic beta cells. In patients with type 2 diabetes mellitus, a shortage of these cells decreases blood insulin levels and causes glucose intolerance. By interacting with the adenosine triphosphatase (ATP)– potassium channel on the beta cell membrane, repaglinide prevents potassium from leaving the cell. This causes the beta cell to depolarize and the cell membrane's calcium channel to open. As a result, calcium moves into the cell and insulin moves out. The extent of insulin release is glucose dependent; the lower the glucose level, the less insulin is secreted from the cell.

Contraindications

Concurrent therapy with gemfibrozil, diabetic ketoacidosis, hypersensitivity to repaglinide or its components, severe hepatic or renal impairment, type 1 diabetes mellitus

Interactions

DRUGS

barbiturates, carbamazepine, rifampin, troglitazone: Possibly increased repaglinide metabolism

beta blockers, chloramphenicol, clarithromycin, cyclosporine, deferasirox, MAO inhibitors, NSAIDs, oral anticoagulants, probenecid, salicylates, sulfonamides, trimethoprim: Enhanced hypoglycemic effects

calcium channel blockers, corticosteroids, diuretics, estrogens, isoniazid, niacin, oral contraceptives, phenothiazines, phenytoin, sympathomimetics, thyroid hormones: Possibly loss of glucose control

erythromycin, ketoconazole, miconazole: Possibly inhibited repaglinide metabolism

gemfibrozil, montelukast, trimethoprim: Increased blood repaglinide level, resulting in enhanced and prolonged blood glucose– lowering effects

NPH insulin: Possibly increased risk of angina

OATP1B1 inhibitors such as cyclosporine, trimethoprim: Increased plasma repaglinide level

Adverse Reactions

CNS: Headache
CV: Angina
EENT: Rhinitis, sinusitis
ENDO: Hypoglycemia
GI: Diarrhea, elevated liver enzymes, hepatitis, nausea, pancreatitis
HEME: Hemolytic anemia, leukopenia, thrombocytopenia
MS: Arthralgia, back pain
RESP: Bronchitis, upper respiratory tract infection
SKIN: Alopecia, Stevens-Johnson syndrome
Other: Anaphylaxis

Nursing Considerations

• Be aware that repaglinide shouldn't be used with NPH insulin because the combination may increase the risk of angina.

• Expect to check HbA_{1c} level every 3 months, as ordered, to assess patient's long-term control of blood glucose level.

• During times of increased stress, such as from infection, surgery, or trauma, monitor blood glucose level often and assess need for additional insulin.

PATIENT TEACHING

• Instruct patient to take repaglinide 15 to 30 minutes before meals and to skip dose whenever she skips a meal.

• Explain that repaglinide is an adjunct to diet in managing type 2 diabetes mellitus.

• Inform patient that changes in blood glucose level may cause blurred vision or visual disturbances, especially when repaglinide therapy starts. Reassure him that these changes are usually transient.

• Teach patient how to monitor her blood glucose level and when to notify prescriber about changes.

• Review signs and symptoms of hyperglycemia and hypoglycemia with patient and family. Instruct patient to notify prescriber immediately if she

experiences anxiety, confusion, dizziness, excessive sweating, headache, increased thirst, increased urination, or nausea.
• Advise patient to wear or carry identification indicating that she has diabetes. Encourage her to carry candy or other simple carbohydrates with her to treat mild episodes of hypoglycemia.
• Inform patient that her HbA$_{1c}$ level will be tested every 3 to 6 months until her blood glucose level is controlled.

reserpine

Novoreserpine (CAN), Reserfia (CAN), Serpalan, Serpasil (CAN)

Class and Category
Chemical class: Rauwolfia alkaloid
Therapeutic class: Antihypertensive
Pregnancy category: C

Indications and Dosages
➤ *To treat hypertension*
TABLETS
Adults. 0.1 to 0.25 mg daily.
Children. 0.005 to 0.02 mg/kg daily once daily or in divided doses twice daily.
DOSAGE ADJUSTMENT Lower dosage possibly required for elderly or severely debilitated patients.

Route	Onset	Peak	Duration
P.O.	Days–3 wk	3–6 wk	1–6 wk

Contraindications
Active peptic ulcer, electroconvulsive therapy, hypersensitivity to reserpine or its components, mental depression (current or history of), ulcerative colitis

Interactions
DRUGS
anticholinergics: Decreased effectiveness of anticholinergics
barbiturates: Increased CNS depression
beta blockers: Additive and, possibly, excessive beta-adrenergic blockade
bromocriptine: Possibly interference with bromocriptine's effects
digoxin, procainamide, quinidine: Increased risk of arrhythmias

hypotension-producing drugs: Increased antihypertensive effect; increased risk of orthostatic hypotension or bradycardia (with guanadrel or guanethidine)
levodopa: Decreased levodopa effectiveness
MAO inhibitors: Increased risk of severe hypertension and hyperpyrexia, additive CNS depression
NSAIDs: Decreased antihypertensive effect
sympathomimetics: Increased vasopressor effects, decreased antihypertensive effect
ACTIVITIES
alcohol use: Increased CNS depression

Adverse Reactions
CNS: Anxiety, depression, dizziness, drowsiness, headache, nervousness, nightmares, sleep disturbance, syncope, weakness
CV: Arrhythmias, such as bradycardia; chest pain; peripheral edema
EENT: Conjunctival injection, dry mouth, epistaxis, glaucoma, hearing loss, nasal congestion, optic atrophy, uveitis
ENDO: Breast engorgement
GI: Abdominal cramps or pain, anorexia, diarrhea, increased gastric secretions, melena, nausea, vomiting
GU: Decreased libido, galactorrhea, gynecomastia, impotence
MS: Myalgia
RESP: Dyspnea
SKIN: Purpura
Other: Weight gain

Nursing Considerations
• If patient has a history of depression, use reserpine cautiously because it may cause depression masked as somatic complaints.
• Monitor blood pressure frequently during drug therapy.
• Alert anesthesiologist if patient is scheduled for surgery. Drug may cause circulatory instability even if withheld before procedure.
PATIENT TEACHING
• Instruct patient to take reserpine with food or milk to minimize stomach upset.
• Caution patient about possible drowsiness, and advise her to avoid potentially hazardous activities until drug's CNS effects are known.
• Explain the need for frequent appointments to monitor blood pressure and adjust dosage at start of therapy.

Mechanism of Action
Reserpine reduces blood pressure by decreasing norepinephrine stores in presynaptic sympathetic neurons.

Normally, when a nerve impulse activates a sympathetic neuron, the nerve ending releases norepinephrine, which stimulates alpha or beta receptors on target cell membranes, as shown below left. Stimulation of alpha receptors may produce vasoconstriction; stimulation of beta receptors may increase heart rate and force of myocardial contraction, which raises cardiac output. Through a reuptake mechanism, some norepinephrine returns to the neuron and is stored in vesicles for reuse.

Reserpine displaces norepinephrine from vesicles in the nerve fiber, and MAO degrades the displaced norepinephrine, as shown below right. These actions reduce the amount of norepinephrine available to stimulate postsynaptic alpha and beta receptors, reducing tesamorelin egrifta vasoconstriction, cardiac output, and blood pressure.

reteplase
Retavase

Class and Category
Chemical class: Recombinant plasminogen activator (r-PA)
Therapeutic class: Thrombolytic
Pregnancy category: C

Indications and Dosages
➤ *To improve ventricular function, prevent heart failure, and reduce mortality after acute MI*
I.V. INJECTION
Adults. 10 units over 2 min; repeated after 30 min.

Mechanism of Action
Converts plasminogen to plasmin, which works to break up fibrin clots that have formed in the coronary arteries. Elimination of the clots improves cardiac blood and oxygen flow to the area, thus improving ventricular function.

Incompatibilities
Don't add other drugs to reteplase injection solution or administer them through same I.V. line as reteplase.

Contraindications
Active internal bleeding, aneurysm, arteriovenous malformation, bleeding diathesis, brain tumor, history of stroke or other cerebrovascular disease, hypersensitivity to reteplase or its components, intracranial or intraspinal surgery or trauma during previous 2 months, severe uncontrolled hypertension (systolic 200 mm Hg or higher, diastolic 110 mm Hg or higher)

Interactions
DRUGS
antifibrinolytics (including aminocaproic acid, aprotinin, and tranexamic acid): Decreased effectiveness of reteplase

antineoplastics, antithymocyte globulin, certain cephalosporins (such as cefamandole, cefoperazone, and cefotetan), heparin, oral anticoagulants, platelet aggregation inhibitors (such as abciximab, aspirin, and dipyridamole), strontium-89 chloride, sulfinpyrazone, valproic acid: Increased risk of bleeding

Adverse Reactions

CNS: Intracranial hemorrhage
GI: GI bleeding, nausea, vomiting
HEME: Thrombocytopenia
RESP: Hemoptysis
SKIN: Bleeding from wounds, ecchymosis, hematoma, purpura
Other: Allergic reaction, injection-site bleeding

Nursing Considerations

• Expect to start reteplase, as prescribed, as soon as possible after MI symptoms begin.
• Closely monitor patient with atrial fibrillation, severe hypertension, or other cardiac disease for signs and symptoms of cerebral embolism.
• To reconstitute, use diluent, syringe, needle, and dispensing pin provided. Withdraw 10 ml of preservative-free sterile water for injection. Remove and discard needle from syringe, and connect dispensing pin to syringe. Remove protective cap from spike end of dispensing pin, and insert spike into reteplase vial. Inject 10 ml of sterile water into the vial. With the spike still in the vial, swirl gently to dissolve the powder. Don't shake. Expect to see slight foaming. Let the vial stand for several minutes. When the bubbles dissipate, withdraw 10 ml of reconstituted solution into the syringe (about 0.7 ml may remain in the vial). Now detach the syringe from the dispensing pin and attach the 20G needle.
• Use the solution within 4 hours. Discard if it's discolored or contains particulates.
• Don't give heparin and reteplase in the same solution. Instead, flush the heparin line with normal saline solution or D_5W before and after reteplase injection.
• Because fibrin is lysed during therapy, closely monitor all possible bleeding sites (catheter insertions, arterial and venous punctures, cutdowns, and needle punctures).

• Avoid I.M. injections, venipunctures, and nonessential handling of patient during therapy.
• If arterial puncture is needed, use an arm vessel that can be compressed, if possible. After sample is obtained, apply pressure for at least 30 minutes; then apply a pressure dressing. Check site often for bleeding.
• If bleeding occurs and can't be controlled by local pressure, notify prescriber immediately. Be prepared to stop anticoagulant therapy immediately and to discontinue second reteplase bolus, as prescribed.
• Anticipate that reperfusion arrhythmias, such as premature ventricular contractions or ventricular tachycardia, may follow coronary thrombolysis.

PATIENT TEACHING
• Advise patient to report adverse reactions immediately.

rifampin
(rifampicin)
Rifadin, Rifadin IV, Rimactane, Rofact (CAN)m

Class and Category

Chemical class: Semisynthetic antibiotic derivative of rifamycin
Therapeutic class: Antimycobacterial antitubercular
Pregnancy category: C

Indications and Dosages

➤ *As adjunct to treat tuberculosis caused by all strains of* Mycobacterium tuberculosis

CAPSULES, ORAL SUSPENSION, I.V. INFUSION
Adults. 10 mg/kg daily with other antitubercular drugs for 2 mo. *Maximum:* 600 mg daily.
Infants and children. 10 to 20 mg/kg daily in combination with other antitubercular drugs for 2 mo. *Maximum:* 600 mg daily.
➤ *To eliminate meningococci from nasopharynx of asymptomatic carriers of* Neisseria meningitidis

CAPSULES, ORAL SUSPENSION, I.V. INFUSION
Adults. 600 mg every 12 hr for 2 days (total of 4 doses).

Q
R
S

Infants age 1 month and over and children. 10 mg/kg every 12 hr for 2 days (total of 4 doses). *Maximum:* 600 mg daily. **Infants under age 1 month.** 5 mg/kg every 12 hr for 2 days (total of 4 doses). *Maximum:* 600 mg daily.

DOSAGE ADJUSTMENT For patients with hepatic impairment, maximum of 8 mg/kg daily. For patients with creatinine clearance of 10 ml/min/1.73 m² or less, recommended dosage usually decreased by 50%.

Mechanism of Action

Inhibits bacterial and mycobacterial RNA synthesis by binding to DNA-dependent RNA polymerase, thereby blocking RNA transcription. Exhibits dose-dependent bactericidal or bacteriostatic action. Rifampin is highly effective against rapidly dividing bacilli in extracellular cavitary lesions, such as those found in the nasopharynx.

Incompatibilities

Don't administer rifampin in the same I.V. line as diltiazem.

Contraindications

Concurrent use of nonnucleoside reverse transcriptase inhibitors or protease inhibitors by patients with HIV, hypersensitivity to rifamycins

Interactions

DRUGS

aminophylline, oxtriphylline, theophylline: Increased metabolism and clearance of these theophylline preparations

anesthetics (hydrocarbon inhalation, except isoflurane), hepatotoxic drugs, isoniazid: Increased risk of hepatotoxicity

antiviral drugs such as atazanavir, darunavir, fosamprenavir, saquinavir, tipranavir: Decreased plasma concentration of antiviral drugs

atovaquone: Decreased plasma atovaquone levels and increased plasma rifampin levels

beta blockers, chloramphenicol, clofibrate, corticosteroids, cyclosporine, dapsone, digitalis glycosides, disopyramide, hexobarbital, itraconazole, ketoconazole, mexiletine, oral anticoagulants, oral antidiabetic drugs, phenytoin, propafenone, quinidine, tocainide, verapamil (oral): Increased metabolism, resulting in lower blood levels of these drugs

bone marrow depressants: Increased leukopenic or thrombocytopenic effects

clofazimine: Reduced absorption of rifampin, delaying its peak concentration and increasing its half-life

diazepam: Enhanced diazepam elimination, resulting in decreased drug effectiveness

estramustine, estrogens, oral contraceptives: Decreased estrogenic effects

methadone: Possibly impaired absorption of methadone, leading to withdrawal symptoms

probenecid: Increased blood level or prolonged duration of rifampin, increasing risk of toxicity

nonnucleoside reverse transcriptase inhibitors, protease inhibitors (indinavir, nelfinavir, ritonavir, saquinavir): Accelerated metabolism of these drugs (by patients with HIV), resulting in subtherapeutic levels; delayed metabolism of rifampin, increasing risk of toxicity

trimethoprim: Increased elimination and shortened elimination half-life of trimethoprim

vitamin D: Increased metabolism and decreased efficacy of vitamin D, leading to decreased serum calcium and phosphate levels and increased parathyroid hormone levels

ACTIVITIES

alcohol use: Increased risk of hepatotoxicity

Adverse Reactions

CNS: Ataxia, behavioral changes, chills, confusion, difficulty concentrating, dizziness, drowsiness, fatigue, fever, generalized numbness, headache, paresthesia, psychoses

CV: Hypotension, myopathy, vasculitis

EENT: Conjunctivitis, discolored saliva, tears, and sputum; mouth or tongue soreness; periorbital edema

ENDO: Adrenal insufficiency, blood glucose alterations (patients with diabetes), visual disturbances

GI: Abdominal cramps, anorexia, diarrhea, discolored feces, elevated liver function test results, epigastric discomfort, flatulence, heartburn, hepatitis, nausea, pseudomembranous colitis, vomiting

GU: Acute renal failure or tubular necrosis, discolored urine, elevated BUN and serum uric acid, hematuria, interstitial nephritis, menstrual disturbances, renal insufficiency

HEME: Agranulocytosis, decreased hemoglobin, disseminated intravascular coagulation, eosinophilia, hemolytic anemia, leukopenia
MS: Arthralgia, extremity pain, muscle weakness, myalgia
RESP: Shortness of breath, wheezing
SKIN: Discolored skin and sweat, erythema multiforme, flushing, pemphigoid reaction, pruritus, rash, Stevens-Johnson syndrome, toxic epidermal necrolysis, urticaria
Other: Anaphylaxis, facial edema, flulike symptoms

Nursing Considerations
• Obtain blood samples or other specimens for culture and sensitivity testing, as ordered, before giving rifampin and throughout therapy to monitor response to drug.
• Expect to monitor liver function test results before and every 2 to 4 weeks during therapy. Immediately report abnormalities.
• Use rifampin cautiously in patients with diabetes mellitus because rifampin therapy may make diabetes management more difficult because of its effect on blood glucose levels.
• For I.V. infusion, reconstitute by adding 10 ml sterile water for injection to 600-mg vial of rifampin. Swirl gently to dissolve. Withdraw appropriate dose and add to 500 ml D$_5$W (preferred solution) or normal saline solution and infuse over 3 hours. Or, withdraw appropriate dose and add to 100 ml D$_5$W (preferred solution) or normal saline solution and infuse over 30 minutes. Use reconstituted drug promptly because rifampin may precipitate out of D$_5$W solution after 4 hours. In normal saline solution, drug is stable up to 24 hours at room temperature.
• Be aware that patient receiving intermittent therapy (once or twice weekly) is at increased risk for adverse reactions.
• Expect drug to discolor skin and body fluids reddish orange to reddish brown.
• Be aware that rifampin can cause myelosuppression and increase risk of infection. Notify prescriber immediately if signs of infection, such as fever, develop.

• Instruct patient to take rifampin 1 hour before or 2 hours after a meal with a full glass of water.
• Emphasize the need to take drug exactly as prescribed. Explain that interruptions can lead to increased adverse reactions.
• Explain that drug may turn urine, feces, saliva, sputum, sweat, tears, and skin reddish orange to reddish brown.
• Caution patient against wearing soft contact lenses during therapy because drug may permanently stain them.
• Advise patient who takes an oral contraceptive to use an additional form of birth control during rifampin therapy.
• Urge patient to notify prescriber about flulike symptoms, anorexia, darkened urine, fever, joint pain or swelling, malaise, nausea, vomiting, and yellowish skin or eyes, which may indicate hepatitis.
• Advise patient to avoid alcohol during rifampin therapy.
• Instruct patient to notify prescriber if no improvement occurs within 2 to 3 weeks.
• Inform patient with diabetes mellitus that rifampin therapy may affect his blood glucose levels and to monitor his blood glucose levels closely.

riluzole
Rilutek

Class and Category
Chemical class: Benzothiazole
Therapeutic class: Amyotrophic lateral sclerosis treatment agent
Pregnancy category: C

Indications and Dosages
➤ *To treat amyotrophic lateral sclerosis*
TABLETS
Adults. 50 mg every 12 hr.

Mechanism of Action
Inhibits release of glutamic acid, an excitatory amino acid neurotransmitter, in the CNS, thus reducing its effects on target cells. Glutamic acid affects degeneration of neurons; reducing its level may help slow amyotrophic lateral sclerosis.

Q
R
S

Contraindications

Hypersensitivity to riluzole or its components

Interactions

DRUGS

allopurinol, hepatotoxic drugs, methyldopa, sulfasalazine: Increased risk of hepatotoxicity
amitriptyline, phenacetin, quinolones, tacrine, theophylline: Delayed elimination of riluzole
omeprazole, rifampin: Increased riluzole clearance

FOODS

charbroiled foods: Increased riluzole elimination

ACTIVITIES

alcohol use: Increased risk of hepatotoxicity
smoking: Increased riluzole elimination

Adverse Reactions

CNS: Asthenia, dizziness, headache, insomnia, paresthesia (circumoral), somnolence, spasticity, vertigo
CV: Peripheral edema
EENT: Dry mouth, rhinitis, stomatitis
GI: Abdominal pain, anorexia, constipation, diarrhea, elevated liver function test results, flatulence, hepatitis, indigestion, nausea, vomiting
HEME: Neutropenia
MS: Back or muscle pain or stiffness
RESP: Dyspnea, hypersensitivity pneumonitis, increased cough, interstitial lung disorder, pneumonia
SKIN: Alopecia, eczema, pruritus
Other: Anaphylaxis

Nursing Considerations

• Use riluzole cautiously in patients with impaired hepatic or renal function.
• Also use cautiously in elderly patients, women, and Japanese patients because of increased risk of toxicity from decreased drug clearance.
• Monitor liver function test results before and during riluzole therapy.
• Monitor patient for respiratory symptoms, such as dry cough or dyspnea. Notify prescriber if present, and expect patient to have a chest X-ray, as ordered. If evidence of interstitial lung disease or hypersensitivity pneumonitis is present, expect riluzole to be discontinued immediately.

PATIENT TEACHING

• Instruct patient to take riluzole regularly, every 12 hours, either 1 hour before or 2 hours after a meal, and at the same time each day.
• Instruct patient to store riluzole at room temperature, protected from bright light.
• Urge patient to minimize alcohol, smoking, and charred foods because they speed drug excretion.
• Tell patient to report fever, cough, or difficulty breathing.

risedronate sodium
Actonel, Atelvia

Class and Category

Chemical class: Pyridinyl bisphosphonate
Therapeutic class: Bone resorption inhibitor
Pregnancy category: C

Indications and Dosages

➤ *To treat Paget's disease of bone when serum alkaline phosphatase level is at least twice normal and patient is symptomatic or at risk for complications*
TABLETS (ACTONEL)
Adults. 30 mg daily for 2 mo. Repeated after 2 mo if relapse occurs or if serum alkaline phosphatase level fails to normalize.
➤ *To prevent or treat glucocorticoid-induced osteoporosis*
TABLETS (ACTONEL)
Adults. 5 mg daily. Or, for postmenopausal osteoporosis, 35 mg once/wk or 75 mg taken on 2 consecutive days once/mo.
➤ *To prevent or treat postmenopausal osteoporosis*
TABLETS (ACTONEL)
Adults. 5 mg daily. Or, 35 mg once weekly, 75 mg taken on 2 consecutive days once a month, or 150 mg once a month
➤ *To treat osteoporosis in women*
E.R. TABLETS (ATELVIA)
Adults. 35 mg (1 tablet) once weekly.
➤ *To treat osteoporosis in men*
TABLETS (ACTONEL)
Adults. 35 mg once weekly.

Route	Onset	Peak	Duration
P.O.	Unknown	3 mo	16 mo

Mechanism of Action

Hinders excessive bone remodeling characteristic of Paget's disease by binding to bone and reducing the rate at which osteoclasts are resorbed by bone.

Contraindications

Esophageal abnormalities that delay esophageal emptying, such as stricture or achalasia; hypersensitivity to risedronate or its components; inability to stand or sit upright for at least 30 minutes; hypocalcemia

Interactions

DRUGS

aspirin, NSAIDs: Increased risk of GI irritation
calcium-containing preparations, including antacids: Impaired absorption of risedronate
FOODS
all foods: Decreased risedronate bioavailability

Adverse Reactions

CNS: Anxiety, asthenia, depression, dizziness, fatigue, headache, insomnia, sciatica, syncope, vertigo, weakness
CV: Chest pain, hypercholesterolemia, hypertension, peripheral edema, vaso-dilation
EENT: Amblyopia, cataract, dry eyes, nasopharyngitis, painful swallowing, pharyngitis, rhinitis, sinusitis, tinnitus
GI: Abdominal pain, colitis, constipation, diarrhea, dyspepsia, dysphagia, eructation, esophagitis, esophageal or gastric ulcers, flatulence, gastritis, nausea, vomiting
GU: UTI
MS: Arthralgia; atypical femur fractures; back, limb, neck, or shoulder pain; jaw osteonecrosis; leg cramps or spasms; myasthenia; myalgia; osteoarthritis; retrosternal pain
RESP: Asthma exacerbation; bronchitis; cough; pneumonia; severe incapacitating bone, joint, or muscle pain; upper respiratory tract infection
SKIN: Bullous reaction, pruritus, rash
Other: Anaphylaxis, angioedema, flulike symptoms, hypersensitivity reaction, hypocalcemia

Nursing Considerations

- Risedroante isn't recommended for patients with severe renal impairment.
- Make sure patient has had a dental checkup before having invasive dental procedures during risedronate therapy, especially if patient has cancer; is receiving chemotherapy, head or neck radiation, or a corticosteroid; or has poor oral hygiene because risk of osteonecrosis is increased in these patients.
- Give supplemental calcium and vitamin D, as prescribed, during risedronate therapy if patient's dietary intake is inadequate.
- Give calcium supplements and antacids at different time of day than risedronate administration to avoid impaired drug absorption and altered effectiveness.
- Watch for rare, but possibly severe hypersensitivity reactions such as rash, bullous skin reactions, and angioedema.

PATIENT TEACHING

- Instruct patient to take risedronate at least 1 hour before first food or drink of day (except water) while in an upright position and with 6 to 8 oz of water. Caution against lying down for at least 30 minutes after taking drug to keep it from lodging in esophagus and causing irritation. Also instruct patient not to chew or suck on tablet because doing so may irritate mouth or throat.
- Advise patient to stop taking risedronate and to notify prescriber if she develops dysphagia, pain while swallowing, retrosternal pain, or new or worsening heartburn.
- Alert patient that drugs in the same class as risedronate have caused severe bone, joint, or muscle pain. If such symptoms appear while taking risedronate, advise patient to contact prescriber.
- If patient takes 35 mg once weekly and misses a dose, tell her to take it the morning after she remembers and then to take the next dose on its usual day. If patient takes 75 mg on 2 consecutive days once monthly and she misses both doses with more than 7 days until the next scheduled dose, tell her to take the first missed dose on the morning after she remembers and the second dose the following day. If she misses only one of the two doses, tell her to take it the morning after she remembers and then resume her normal schedule. If patient takes 150 mg once monthly and misses a dose, urge her to contact prescriber for instructions. Caution

Q
R
S

patient not to take more than 150 mg within a 7-day period and not to take two tablets of any strength on the same day.
• Tell patient to take calcium supplements or antacids at different times than risedronate.
• Urge women of childbearing age to tell prescriber about planned, suspected, or known pregnancy because of risk to fetal skeleton.
• Tell patient to stop risedronate and contact prescriber about swelling or skin abnormalities.
• Instruct patient about proper oral hygiene and about the need to notify prescriber about invasive dental procedures.
• Instruct patient to notify prescriber immediately of any new thigh or groin pain that might be reflective of an atypical femur fracture.

risperidone
Risperdal, Risperdal Consta

Class and Category
Chemical class: Benzisoxazole derivative
Therapeutic class: Antipsychotic
Pregnancy category: C

Indications and Dosages
➤ *To manage psychotic disorders*
ORAL SOLUTION, ORALLY DISINTEGRATING TABLETS, TABLETS
Adults. 1 mg twice daily on day 1; 2 mg twice daily on day 2; 3 mg twice daily on day 3. Or, 2 mg daily on day 1; 4 mg daily on day 2; 6 mg daily on day 3. Then increased by 1 to 2 mg daily at 1- to 2-wk intervals, as needed. *Maximum:* 16 mg daily.
Adolescents ages 13 to 17. *Initial:* 0.5 mg once daily, increased as needed every 24 hr in 0.5- to 1-mg increments. *Maximum:* 3 mg once daily.
I.M. INJECTION (RISPERDAL CONSTA)
Adults. *Initial:* 25 mg every 2 wk, increased as needed every 4 wk to 37.5 or 50 mg. *Maximum:* 50 mg every 2 wk.
➤ *To treat bipolar mania*
ORAL SOLUTION, ORALLY DISINTEGRATING TABLETS, TABLETS
Adults. *Initial:* 2 or 3 mg daily, increased as needed by 1 mg daily up to 6 mg. *Maximum:* 6 mg daily for no more than 3 wk.

Children and adolescents ages 10 to 17. *Initial:* 0.5 mg once daily, increased as needed every 24 hr in 0.5- to 1-mg increments. *Maximum:* 2.5 mg once daily.
➤ *To treat bipolar mania as monotherapy or as adjunct to lithium or valproate therapy*
I.M. INJECTION (RISPERDAL CONSTA)
Adults. 25 mg every 2 wk., increased, as needed to 37.5 mg or 50 mg. *Maximum:* 50 mg every 2 wk.
DOSAGE ADJUSTMENT Initially 0.5 mg twice daily for elderly or debilitated patients, those with renal or hepatic impairment, and those at risk for hypotension. Increased by 0.5 mg twice daily every wk, as needed. Given daily after target dosage maintained for 2 or 3 days. Maximum for patients with severe hepatic dysfunction, 4 mg daily; for elderly patients, 3 mg daily. Initially 12.5 mg for patients receiving drug I.M. who have renal or hepatic impairment, take other drugs that increase risperidone blood level, or have a history of tolerating psychotropic drugs poorly. For adolescents and children with persistent somnolence, dose may be split and given twice daily.
➤ *To treat irritability associated with autistic disorder*
ORAL SOLUTION, ORALLY DISINTEGRATING TABLETS, TABLETS
Children age 5 and over and adolescents weighing less than 20 kg (44 lb). *Initial:* 0.25 mg daily, increased after 4 days to 0.5 mg daily. Dosage further increased, as needed in 2 wk intervals in 0.25 mg increments.
Children age 5 and over and adolescents weighing 20 kg or more. *Initial:* 0.5 mg daily, increased after 4 days to 1 mg daily. Dosage further increased, as needed in 2 wk intervals in 0.5 mg increments.

Mechanism of Action
Selectively blocks serotonin and dopamine receptors in the mesocortical tract of the CNS to suppress psychotic symptoms.

Incompatibilities
Don't mix oral solution with cola or tea.

Contraindications
Hypersensitivity to risperidone or its components

Interactions
DRUGS
antihypertensives: Increased antihypertensive effects
bromocriptine, levodopa, pergolide: Possibly antagonized effects of these drugs
carbamazepine: Increased risperidone clearance with long-term concurrent use
clozapine: Decreased risperidone clearance with long-term concurrent use
CNS depressants: Additive CNS depression
fluoxetine, paroxetine: Increased plasma risperidone level
ACTIVITIES
alcohol use: Additive CNS depression

Adverse Reactions
CNS: Abnormal coordination, aggressiveness, agitation, akathisia, anxiety, asthenia, confusion, decreased concentration, depression, dizziness, dream disturbances, drooling, drowsiness, dyskinesia, dystonia, fatigue, fever, headache, hypothermia, insomnia, lassitude, malaise, mania, memory loss, nervousness, neuroleptic malignant syndrome, paresthesia, parkinsonism, restlessness, seizures, shaking of head repeatedly, somnolence, tardive dyskinesia, tremor, vertigo
CV: Atrial fibrillation, bradycardia, bundle branch block, cardiopulmonary arrest, chest pain, elevated triglyceride levels, first-degree AV block, hypercholesterolemia, orthostatic hypotension, palpitations, QT-interval prolongation, tachycardia
EENT: Conjunctivitis, decreased or increased salivation, dry mouth, ear pain, epistaxis, nasal congestion, pharyngitis, retinal artery occlusion, rhinitis, sinusitis, taste alteration, vision changes
ENDO: Diabetic ketoacidosis (patients with diabetes), elevated prolactin level, galactorrhea, hyperglycemia, hyperprolactinemia, hypoglycemia, inappropriate antidiuretic hormone secretion (SIADH), pituitary adenoma, precocious puberty
GI: Abdominal pain, anorexia, constipation, diarrhea, gastritis, ileus, indigestion, intestinal obstruction, jaundice, nausea, pancreatitis, vomiting
GU: Amenorrhea, decreased libido, delayed ejaculation, dysmenorrhea, dysuria, glucosuria, hypermenorrhea, incontinence, increased appetite, polyuria, priapism, sexual dysfunction, urinary incontinence or retention, UTI
HEME: Agranulocytosis, anemia, leukopenia, neutropenia, thrombocytopenia
MS: Arthralgia; back, buttock, or neck pain; dysarthria; muscle weakness; myalgia
RESP: Cough, dyspnea, pulmonary embolism, sleep apnea, upper respiratory tract infection
SKIN: Alopecia, diaphoresis, dry skin, eczema, hyperpigmentation, photosensitivity, pruritus, rash, seborrhea
Other: Anaphylaxis; angioedema; infections; influenza; injection-site induration, pain, redness, or swelling; weight gain or loss

Nursing Considerations
• Use risperidone cautiously in debilitated patients, elderly patients, and patients with hepatic or renal dysfunction or hypotension because of their increased sensitivity to the drug. Also use risperidone cautiously in patients with a history of seizures; although rare, seizures may occur in those with schizophrenia.
WARNING Be aware that risperidone should not be used to treat elderly patients with dementia-related psychosis because it increases risk of death in these patients.
• Be aware that oral risperidone or another antipsychotic should be continued for 3 weeks after long-acting I.M. form of risperidone is first administered to provide an adequate therapeutic plasma level until risperidone release from injection site has begun. If the patient has never received oral risperidone, an oral trial should be prescribed before use of I.M. form to determine patient's tolerance of the drug.
• Remove I.M. form from refrigerator and allow it to come to room temperature before reconstitution. Follow manufacturer's guidelines for reconstitution, using only the diluent supplied in the dose pack.
• Give I.M. form using only the needle supplied in the dose pack. Inject entire contents of syringe into the upper outer quadrant of gluteal area within 2 minutes of reconstitution. If drug can't be given

Q
R
S

right after reconstitution, shake the upright vial vigorously back and forth until particles are resuspended. Discard reconstituted drug if not used within 6 hours. Never administer I.M. form intravenously.

• Monitor for orthostatic hypotension, especially in patients with cardiac or cerebrovascular disease.

WARNING Immediately notify prescriber and expect to stop giving risperidone if patient shows evidence of neuroleptic malignant syndrome (altered mental status, autonomic instability, hyperpyrexia, muscle rigidity), which can be fatal.

• Monitor patient's blood glucose and lipid levels as ordered because drug increases the risk of hyperglycemia and hyper-cholesterolemia.

• Monitor patient's CBC, as ordered, because serious adverse hematologic reactions may occur, such as agranulo-cytosis, leukopenia, or neutropenia. More frequent monitoring during the first few months of risperidone therapy is recommended for patients with a history of drug-induced leukopenia or neutropenia, or those who have had a significantly low WBC count in the past. If abnormalities occur during therapy, monitor patient for fever or other signs of infection, notify prescriber, and expect drug to be discontinued if severe.

PATIENT TEACHING

• Instruct patient to dilute risperidone oral solution with water, coffee, orange juice, or low-fat milk, but not with cola or tea.

• Tell patient prescribed orally disintegrating tablets to break open the blister unit with dry hands by peeling the foil back to expose the tablet. Emphasize the importance of not pushing tablet through the foil because this could damage the tablet. Once patient has removed tablet, she should place immediately on her tongue, where it will dissolve within seconds. Tell patient not to chew orally disintegrating tablet or attempt to spit it out of her mouth.

• Urge patient to avoid alcohol because of its additive CNS effects.

• Caution diabetic patient to monitor blood glucose level closely because risperidone may increase it.

rivaroxaban
Xarelto

Class and Category
Chemical class: Factor Xa inhibitor
Therapeutic class: Antithrombolytic
Pregnancy category: C

Indications and Dosages
➤ *To reduce the risk of stroke and systemic embolism in patients with nonvalvular atrial fibrillation*
TABLETS
Adults with creatinine clearance greater than 50 ml/min. 20 mg once daily with evening meal.
Adults with creatinine clearance between 15 ml/min and 50 ml/min. 15 mg once daily with evening meal.
➤ *To prevent deep vein thrombosis, which may lead to pulmonary embolism in patients undergoing knee or hip replacement surgery*
TABLETS
Adults. 10 mg once daily begun 6 to 10 hours after surgery once hemostasis has been established and given for 12 days after knee replacement surgery and given 35 days after hip replacement surgery.
➤ *To treat deep vein thrombosis or pulmonary embolism*
TABLETS
Adults. 15 mg twice daily with food for 21 days, followed by 20 mg once daily with food.
➤ *To reduce risk of recurrence of deep vein thrombosis or pulmonary embolism*
TABLETS
Adults. 20 mg once daily with food.

Mechanism of Action
Selectively blocks the active site of factor Xa, which plays a central role in the cascade of blood coagulation. Without the action of factor Xa, blood clotting is impaired.

Contraindications
Active pathological bleeding, hyper-sensitivity to rivaroxaban or its components

Interaction
DRUGS
anticoagulants, aspirin, clopidogrel, NSAIDs, other platelet aggregation inhibitors: Possibly increased bleeding risk

cabamazepine, phenytoin, rifampin, St. John's wort: Decreased effectiveness of rivaroxaban
clarithromycin, conivaptan, diltiazem, dronedarone, erythromycin, fluconazole, ketoconazole, indinavir/ritonavir, itraconazole, lopinavir/ritonavir, ritonavir, verapamil: Increased rivaroxaban exposure resulting in increased bleeding risk

Adverse Reactions
CNS: Cerebral hemorrhage, epidural hematoma, hemiparesis, subdural hematoma, syncope
GI: Cholestasis, cytolytic hepatitis, gastrointestinal bleeding, jaundice, retroperitoneal hemorrhage
HEME: Agranulocytosis, excessive bleeding, including hemorrhage, thrombocytopenia
MS: Extremity pain, muscle spasm
RESP: Pulmonary hemorrhage with or without bronchiectasis
SKIN: Pruritus, Stevens-Johnson syndrome
Other: Anaphylaxis, angioedema

Nursing Considerations
• Know that rivaroxaban used to reduce the risk of stroke and systemic embolism in nonvalvular atrial fibrillation should not be given to patients with moderate or severe hepatic impairment, to patients with any hepatic disease associated with coagulopathy, and to patients with a creatinine clearance that is less than 15 ml/min. Monitor patient's hepatic and renal function, as ordered, throughout rivaroxaban therapy.
• Know that rivaroxaban used to prevent or treat deep vein thrombosis, to treat pulmonary embolism, and to reduce risk of recurrence of deep vein thrombosis or pulmonary embolism should not be given to patients with a creatinine clearance less than 30 ml/min.
• Be aware that rivaroxaban should not be given to patients with prosthetic heart valves or as an alternative to unfractionated heparin in patients with pulmonary embolism who are hemodynamically unstable or who may receive thrombolysis or pulmonary embolectomy.

• Be aware that rivaroxaban should be used cautiously during pregnancy because the effects in pregnancy have not been studied.
• Monitor patient closely for signs and symptoms of a hypersensitivity reaction because severe hypersensitivity reactions have occurred following rivaroxaban therapy.
• Be aware that manufacturer guidelines should be followed when patient is switching from or to other anticoagulants. For example, when patient is switching from warfarin to rivaroxaban therapy, expect warfarin to be discontinued and rivaroxaban started when the International Normalized Ratio (INR) is below 3. For patients currently receiving an anticoagulant other than warfarin, such as low-molecular-weight heparin or non-warfarin oral anticoagulant, expect to start rivaroxaban therapy within 2 hours of the next scheduled evening administration of the drug, and plan to omit administration of the other anticoagulant, as ordered. For unfractionated heparin being administered by continuous infusion, expect to stop the infusion and start rivaroxaban therapy at the same time. For patients currently taking rivaroxaban and transitioning to an anticoagulant with rapid onset, expect rivaroxaban to be discontinued and the first dose of the other anticoagulant to be given at the time the next rivaroxaban would have been given.
• Administering rivaroxaban via a nasogastric tube or gastric feeding tube requires tablets to be crushed and suspended in 50 ml of water. Following administration, enteral feeding should be given immediately.
• Monitor patient's renal function, as ordered. Expect rivaroxaban to be discontinued if acute renal failure occurs.
WARNING Monitor patient closely for bleeding as rivaroxaban therapy may cause life-threatening bleeding. Expect drug to be discontinued with active pathological hemorrhage because there is no antidote for rivaroxaban.
• Expect rivaroxaban to be discontinued 24 hours before an invasive procedure or surgery, if possible and restarted after adequate hemostasis has been established after the invasive surgery or procedure.

• Know that if patient has an epidural catheter inserted, it should not be removed any earlier than 18 hours after the last rivaroxaban dose was administered, and the next rivaroxaban dose should not be administered any earlier than 6 hours after the removal of the catheter because an epidural or spinal hematoma can occur and can result in long-term or permanent paralysis. If traumatic puncture occurs, know that rivaroxaban should be withheld for 24 hours.

• Be aware that if rivaroxaban is discontinued and adequate alternative anticoagulation is not present, the risk for thrombosis increases. Monitor patient closely.

PATIENT TEACHING

• Emphasize the importance of taking rivaroxaban exactly as prescribed.

• Instruct patient taking 15-mg or 20-mg tablets to take with food; 10-mg tablets do not need to be taken with food. For patient unable to swallow tablets, tell patient to crush tablets and mix with applesauce immediately prior to taking and then follow with food.

• Tell patient not to stop taking rivaroxaban without first consulting prescriber.

• Instruct patient with atrial fibrillation to take the drug with the evening meal.

• Advise patient to report any unusual bleeding or bruising to the prescriber. Inform patient that it may take longer for him to stop bleeding and to take bleeding precautions, such as avoiding the use of a razor and using a soft-bristle toothbrush.

• Tell patient to alert all prescribers to use of rivaroxaban therapy before any invasive procedure, including dental work, is scheduled.

• Caution patient not to take any medication, including over the counter and herbal medicines, without first consulting with prescriber.

• Advise female patient to notify prescriber immediately if pregnancy is suspected or known.

rivastigmine tartrate

Exelon, Exelon Patch

Class and Category

Chemical class: Carbamate derivative
Therapeutic class: Antidementia
Pregnancy category: B

Indications and Dosages

➤ *To treat Alzheimer's-type dementia*

CAPSULES, ORAL SOLUTION

Adults. *Initial:* 1.5 mg twice daily Dosage increased by 3 mg daily every 2 wk, as needed. *Maximum:* 12 mg daily.

TRANSDERMAL

Adults. *Initial:* 4.6 mg/24 hr. After 4 wk, increased to 9.5 mg/24 hr for patients with mild to moderate Alzheimer's disease and 13.5 mg/24 hr for patients with severe Alzheimer's disease. When therapeutic effect begins to decrease in patients with mild to moderate Alzheimer's disease, dosage increased to 13.5 mg/24 hr. *Maximum:* 13.5 mg/24 hr.

➤ *To treat mild to moderate dementia in Parkinson's disease*

CAPSULES, ORAL SOLUTION

Adults. *Initial:* 1.5 mg twice daily. Dosage increased by 3 mg daily every 4 wk, as needed. *Maximum:* 12 mg daily.

TRANSDERMAL

Adults. *Initial:* 4.6 mg/24 hr. After 4 wk, increased to 9.5 mg/24 hr. When therapeutic effect begins to decrease, dosage increased to 13.5 mg/24 hr. *Maximum:* 13.5 mg/24 hr.

➤ *To convert patient from oral to transdermal rivastigmine therapy*

TRANSDERMAL

Adults. If total oral dosage was less than 6 mg daily, use 4.6 mg/24 hr, with first transdermal patch applied the day after the last oral dose. If total oral dosage was 6 to 12 mg daily, use 9.5 mg/24 hr, with first transdermal patch applied the day after the last oral dose.

DOSAGE ADJUSTMENT If patient develops adverse effects (such as nausea or vomiting) during oral therapy, treatment should be stopped for several doses, as prescribed, restarted at lowest dose, and increased by 3 mg daily every 2 wk, as needed. If patient develops adverse effects during transdermal therapy, treatment should be discontinued for several days and restarted at same or next lower dose level. For patient with moderate to severe renal impairment, or mild to moderate hepatic impairment, 4.6 mg/24 hr patch used for both initial and maximum dose. For patients with low body weight of less than 50 kg (110 lbs) and experiencing excessive nausea and vomiting, maintenance dose kept at 4.6 mg/24 hr

Mechanism of Action

May slow the decline of cognitive function in patients with Alzheimer's disease by increasing acetylcholine concentration at cholinergic transmission sites. This action prolongs and exaggerates the effects of acetylcholine that are otherwise blocked by toxic levels of anticholinergics. The cognitive decline in these patients is partially related to cholinergic deficits along neuronal pathways projecting from the basal forebrain to the cerebral cortex and hippocampus that are involved in memory, attention, learning, and cognition.

Contraindications

History of application-site reactions suggestive of allergic contact dermatitis (for patch form); hypersensitivity to carbamate derivatives, rivastigmine, or their components

Interactions

DRUGS

anticholinergics: Possibly decreased effectiveness of anticholinergics
bethanechol, succinylcholine: Possibly synergistic effects

Adverse Reactions

CNS: Aggression, anxiety, asthenia, confusion, depression, dizziness, extrapyramidal movements, fatigue, fever, hallucinations, headache, insomnia, malaise, parkinsonism, seizures, somnolence, tremor
CV: Hypertension
EENT: Rhinitis
GI: Abdominal pain, abnormal liver function tests, anorexia, constipation, diarrhea, duodenal ulcers, flatulence, hepatitis, indigestion, nausea, vomiting
GU: UTI
SKIN: Disseminated cutaneous hypersensitivity reactions, increased sweating, reaction at patch application site (pruritus, redness, swelling), Stevens-Johnson syndrome
Other: Dehydration, flulike symptoms, weight loss

Nursing Considerations

WARNING Be aware that rivastigmine should be started at lowest recommended dosage and adjusted to effective maintenance dosage because initial therapy at high dosage can cause serious adverse GI reactions, including anorexia, nausea, and weight loss. Also, a higher than recommended starting dosage may cause severe vomiting and possibly esophageal rupture. If treatment is interrupted for longer than several days, expect to restart at lowest recommended dosage.

• Be aware that drug shouldn't be stopped abruptly because doing so may increase behavioral disturbances and precipitate a further decline in cognitive function.
• Monitor respiratory status of patients with pulmonary disease, including asthma, chronic bronchitis, and emphysema, because rivastigmine has a weak affinity for peripheral cholinesterase, which may increase bronchoconstriction and bronchial secretions.
• Monitor patient for adequate urine output because cholinomimetics, such as rivastigmine, may induce or exacerbate urinary tract or bladder obstruction.
• Monitor patients with Parkinson's disease for exaggerated parkinsonian symptoms, which may result from drug's increased cholinergic effects on CNS.

WARNING Monitor patient closely for hypersensitivity skin reactions regardless of route of administration. If suspected, notify prescriber, and expect drug to be discontinued.

PATIENT TEACHING
• Explain to patient and family that rivastigmine can't cure Alzheimer's or Parkinson's disease but may slow the progressive deterioration of memory and improve patient's ability to perform activities of daily living.
• Teach patient and family how to administer oral solution, if prescribed, emphasizing need to use the oral dosing syringe provided. Explain that dose may be swallowed directly from the syringe or mixed into a small glass of water, cold fruit juice, or soda; stirred; and then drunk.
• Explain that oral drug should be taken with food to reduce adverse GI effects.

• Instruct patient or caregiver to apply transdermal patch to clean, dry, hairless, intact skin in a location, such as the back, that won't be rubbed by tight clothing and won't be affected by lotion, cream, or powder. Tell patient to remove the old patch before applying a new one and to use a new application site daily. Caution against using the same site within 14 days.
• Tell patient applying transdermal patch to press patch firmly against skin until the edges stick well. Reassure patient that patch may be worn while swimming or bathing.
• Instruct a family member to supervise patient's use of rivastigmine.
• Urge caregiver to contact prescriber and to withhold drug if patient stops taking it for more than several days.
• •Emphasize importance of inspecting skin for signs of an allergic reaction, such as presence of rash, reddness, or itching. If present, instruct patient or family to notify prescriber, as drug will need to be discontinued.

rizatriptan benzoate
Maxalt, Maxalt-MLT

Class and Category
Chemical class: Selective 5-hydroxytryptamine
Therapeutic class: Antimigraine
Pregnancy category: C

Indications and Dosages
➤ *To relieve acute migraine headache*
DISINTEGRATING TABLETS, TABLETS
Adults. 5 to 10 mg when migraine headache starts; repeated every 2 hr, as needed. *Maximum:* 30 mg daily.
Children age 6 to 17 years weighing 40 kg (88 lb) or more. 10 mg when migraine headache starts.
Children age 6 to 17 years weighing less than 40 kg (88 lb). 5 mg when migraine headache starts.
DOSAGE ADJUSTMENT For patients taking propranolol, initial dosage reduced to 5 mg, then repeated every 2 hr, as needed, up to maximum of 15 mg daily.

Mechanism of Action
Binds to selective 5-hydroxytryptamine receptor sites on cerebral blood vessels, causing vessels to constrict. This may decrease the characteristic pulsing sensation and thus relieve the pain of migraine headaches. Rizatriptan may also relieve pain by inhibiting the release of proinflammatory neuropeptides and reducing transmission of trigeminal nerve impulses from sensory nerve endings during a migraine attack.

Contraindications
Basilar or hemiplegic migraine, hypersensitivity to rizatriptan or its components, ischemic coronary artery disease, uncontrolled hypertension, use within 14 days of MAO inhibitor therapy, use within 24 hours of other serotonin-receptor agonists or ergotamine-containing or ergot-type drugs

Interactions
DRUGS
ergot-containing drugs: Prolonged vasospastic reactions
MAO inhibitors, propranolol: Increased blood rizatriptan level
selective serotonin reuptake inhibitors, serotonin norepinephrine reuptake inhibitors, other triptans: Increased risk of serotonin syndrome
serotonin-receptor agonists: Additive vasospastic effects

Adverse Reactions
CNS: Altered temperature sensation, anxiety, asthenia, ataxia, chills, confusion, depression, disorientation, dizziness, dream disturbances, drowsiness, euphoria, fatigue, hangover, headache, hypoesthesia, insomnia, mental impairment, nervousness, paresthesia, somnolence, tremor, vertigo
CV: Arrhythmias, such as bradycardia and tachycardia; chest pain; hot flashes; hypertension; palpitations
EENT: Blurred vision; burning eyes; dry eyes, mouth, and throat; earache; eye pain or irritation; lacrimation; nasal congestion and irritation; pharyngeal edema; pharyngitis; tinnitus; tongue swelling
GI: Abdominal distention, constipation, diarrhea, dysphagia, flatulence, heartburn, indigestion, nausea, thirst, vomiting

GU: Menstrual irregularities, polyuria, urinary frequency
MS: Arthralgia; dysarthria; muscle spasms, stiffness, or weakness; myalgia
RESP: Dyspnea, upper respiratory tract infection, wheezing
SKIN: Diaphoresis, flushing, pruritus, rash, urticaria
Other: Angioedema, dehydration, facial edema

Nursing Considerations

• Use rizatriptan cautiously in patients with renal or hepatic dysfunction because of impaired drug metabolism or excretion. Monitor patient's BUN and serum creatinine levels and liver function test results, as appropriate.

• Also use cautiously in patients with peripheral vascular disease because drug may cause vasospastic reactions, leading to vascular and colonic ischemia with abdominal pain and bloody diarrhea. Assess peripheral circulation and bowel sounds frequently during therapy.

• Assess patient's cardiovascular status and institute continuous ECG monitoring, as ordered, immediately after giving rizatriptan in patients with cardiovascular risk factors, because of possible asymptomatic cardiac ischemia.

• Monitor blood pressure regularly in patients with hypertension because rizatriptan may increase blood pressure.

WARNING Monitor patient closely for serotonin syndrome if she is taking rizatriptan along with a selective serotonin reuptake inhibitor or serotonin norepinephrine reuptake inhibitor. Notify prescriber immediately if the patient exhibits agitation, hallucinations, coma, tachycardia, labile blood pressure, hyperthermia, hyperreflexia, incoordination, nausea, vomiting, or diarrhea, as serotonin syndrome can be life-threatening. Provide supportive care.

PATIENT TEACHING

• Instruct patient taking rizatriptan-disintegrating tablets to remove tablet from blister pack with dry hands just before taking, to place tablet on tongue, and to allow it to dissolve and be swallowed with saliva.

• Advise phenylketonuric patient not to use disintegrating tablet form because it contains phenylalanine.

• Instruct patient to seek emergency care immediately if cardiac symptoms, such as chest pain, occur after administration.

• Caution patient about possible adverse CNS reactions, and advise her to avoid potentially hazardous activities until drug's CNS effects are known.

• Urge patient to inform all prescribers of rizatriptan therapy because serious drug interactions may occur.

roflumilast
Daliresp

Class and Category
Chemical class: Selective phosphodiesterase 4 inhibitor
Therapeutic class: Antipulmonic obstructive agent
Pregnancy category: C

Indications and Dosages
➤ *To reduce the risk of COPD exacerbations in patients with severe COPD associated with chronic bronchitis and a history of exacerbations*

TABLETS
Adults. 500 mcg daily.

Mechanism of Action
Increases intracellular cyclic AMP in lung cells by inhibiting a major cyclic AMP-metabolizing enzyme in lung tissue to improve pulmonary function

Contraindications
Hypersensitivity to roflumilast or its components, moderate to severe liver impairment

Interaction
DRUGS
CYP450 inhibitors or dual inhibitors (both CYP34A and CYP1A2), such as cimetidine, erythromycin, enoxacin, fluvoxamine, ketoconazole; oral contraceptives containing gestodene and ethinyl estradiol: Increased roflumilast exposure with increased risk of adverse effects
cytochrome P450 enzyme inducers, such as carbamazepine, phenobarbital, phenytoin,

Q
R
S

rifampicin: Decreased effectiveness of roflumilast

Adverse Reactions
CNS: Anxiety, depression, dizziness, headache, insomnia, suicidal ideation, tremor
CV: Atrial fibrillation
EENT: Rhinitis, sinusitis
GI: Abdominal pain, acute pancreatitis, anorexia, diarrhea, dyspepsia, gastritis, nausea, vomiting
GU: Acute renal failure, UTI
MS: Back pain, muscle spasms
Other: Influenza, weight loss

Nursing Considerations
• Monitor effectiveness of roflumilast to reduce COPD exacerbations.
• Watch patient closely for suicidal tendencies because roflumilast has been associated with an increase in psychiatric adverse reactions, such as insomnia and depression, as well as suicidal ideation.
• Monitor patient's weight and notify prescriber if significant weight loss occurs.
PATIENT TEACHING
• Tell family or caregiver to monitor patient for suicidal tendencies because drug may worsen depression during roflumilast and increase suicidal thinking.
• Warn patient that roflumilast is not a bronchodilator and should not be used to relieve acute bronchospasm.

ropinirole hydrochloride
Requip

Class and Category
Chemical class: Nonergot alkaloid dopamine agonist
Therapeutic class: Antidyskinetic
Pregnancy category: C

Indications and Dosages
➤ *To treat signs and symptoms of Parkinson's disease*
TABLETS
Adults. *Initial:* 0.25 mg three times a day. Dosage titrated upward every wk according to the following schedule: 0.25 mg three

times a day in wk 1; 0.5 mg three times a day in wk 2; 0.75 mg three times a day in wk 3; 1 mg three times a day in wk 4. After wk 4, dosage increased by 1.5 mg daily every wk up to 9 mg daily, then by 3 mg/day up to 24 mg daily. *Maximum:* 24 mg/day.
E.R. TABLETS
Adults. *Initial:* 2 mg once daily for 1 to 2 wk, increased, as needed, in increments of 2 mg/day at 1 wk or longer intervals. *Maximum:* 24 mg/day.
DOSAGE ADJUSTMENT For patient with end-stage renal disease on hemodialysis, dosage titration is based on tolerability and need for efficacy; maximum total daily dose reduced to 18 mg daily.
➤ *To treat moderate to severe primary restless legs syndrome*
TABLETS
Adults. *Initial:* 0.25 mg 1 to 3 hr before bedtime. Dosage increased on day 3 to 0.5 mg and then to 1 mg at beginning of week 2 (day 8). If needed, dosage further increased in 0.5-mg increments every wk for 5 wk. *Maximum:* 4 mg daily.
DOSAGE ADJUSTMENT For patients with end-stage renal disease on hemodialysis, dosage titration is based on tolerability and need for efficacy, with recommended maximum total daily dose reduced to 3 mg daily.

Mechanism of Action
Directly stimulates postsynaptic dopamine type 2 (D_2) receptors within the brain and acts as an agonist at peripheral D_2 receptors. These actions inhibit the firing of striatal cholinergic neurons, thus helping to control alterations in voluntary muscle movement (such as tremors and rigidity) associated with Parkinson's disease.

Contraindications
Hypersensitivity to ropinirole or its components

Interactions
DRUGS
carbamazepine, cimetidine, ciprofloxacin, clarithromycin, diltiazem, enoxacin, erythromycin, fluvoxamine, mexiletine, norfloxacin, omeprazole, phenobarbital, phenytoin, rifampin, ritonavir, troleandomycin: Altered drug clearance and increased blood level of ropinirole

chlorprothixene, domperidone, droperidol, haloperidol, metoclopramide, phenothiazines, thiothixene: Possibly decreased effectiveness of ropinirole
CNS depressants: Additive effects
ethinyl estradiol: Possibly reduced clearance of ropinirole
ACTIVITIES
alcohol use: Additive effects

Adverse Reactions

CNS: Asthenia, compulsive behaviors, confusion, dizziness, dyskinesia, falling asleep during activities of daily living, fatigue, hallucinations, headache, hypoesthesia, malaise, neuralgia, paresthesia, psychotic-like behaviors, rigors, somnolence, syncope, transient ischemic attack, vertigo
CV: Acute coronary syndrome, angina, bradycardia, cardiac failure, chest pain, hypertension, MI, orthostatic hypotension, palpitations, peripheral edema, sick sinus syndrome, tachycardia
EENT: Abnormal vision, dry mouth, nasal congestion, nasopharyngitis, rhinitis, tooth-ache
GI: Abdominal pain, constipation, diarrhea, dyspepsia, gastric hemorrhage, gastroenteritis, indigestion, intestinal obstruction, ischemic hepatitis, nausea, pancreatitis, vomiting
GU: Elevated BUN level, erectile dysfunction, UTI
HEME: Anemia
MS: Arthralgia; arthritis; exacerbation of restless leg syndrome in the early-morning hours or earlier onset of symptoms in the evening with increase in symptoms or spread of symptoms to other extremities; limb pain; muscle cramps, spasms, or stiffness; myalgia; neck pain; osteoarthritis; tendinitis
RESP: Asthma, bronchitis, cough, upper respiratory tract infection
SKIN: Diaphoresis, flushing, hot flashes, melanoma, night sweats, rash
Other: Influenza, intense urges to perform certain activities (such as gambling or sex), viral infection, weight loss

Nursing Considerations

WARNING Expect to reassess patient for excessive sedation periodically during therapy. Excessive, acute drowsiness may arise as late as 1 year after starting therapy.

• When ropinirole is given as adjunct to levodopa, expect concurrent dosage of levodopa to be gradually decreased as tolerated.
• Expect to stop ropinirole gradually over 7 days, as follows: over first 4 days, reduce from three times a day to twice daily; during last 3 days, reduce to once daily, followed by complete withdrawal of drug.
WARNING Watch for altered mental status during drug withdrawal. Rapid dose reduction may lead to a symptom complex resembling neuroleptic malignant syndrome that includes fever, muscle rigidity, altered level of consciousness, and autonomic instability.
• Watch for orthostatic hypotension, especially in patient with early Parkinson's disease. Orthostatic hypotension can occur more than 4 weeks after start of therapy or after a dosage reduction because ropinirole may impair systemic regulation of blood pressure.
• Monitor patient for hallucinations, especially if patient has Parkinson's disease, is elderly, or takes levodopa.
• Monitor patient for worsening of preexisting dyskinesia; ropinirole may potentiate dopaminergic adverse effects of levodopa.
• Avoid giving CNS depressants, sleep aids, and other CNS-interacting drugs during ropinirole therapy because they increase the risk of somnolence.
• Assess patient for skin changes regularly because risk of melanoma is higher in patients with Parkinson's disease. It isn't clear whether this results from disease or from the drugs used to treat it.
PATIENT TEACHING
• Inform patient with Parkinson's disease that ropinirole helps to improve muscle control and movement but doesn't cure Parkinson's disease.
• Encourage patient to take ropinirole with food to decrease risk of adverse GI effects.
• Caution patient to avoid hazardous activities until CNS effects of drug—including sedation—are known.
• If patient falls asleep during normal activities, advise her to notify prescriber.
• Urge patient to avoid consuming alcohol and other sedating drugs (such as sleep aids) during therapy because they may increase drug's CNS depressant effects.

Q
R
S

• If patient has restless legs syndrome, explain that symptoms might appear in early morning or have an earlier onset in the evening or even the afternoon during ropinirole therapy and could be worse or spread to other limbs. Urge patient to notify prescriber if this occurs.
• Instruct patient to change positions slowly to minimize effect on blood pressure.
• Urge patient to have regular skin examinations by a dermatologist or other qualified health professional.
• Advise patient to notify prescriber about intense urges (as for gambling or sex) because dosage may need to be reduced or drug discontinued.

rosiglitazone maleate

Avandia

Class and Category
Chemical class: Thiazolidinedione
Therapeutic class: Antidiabetic drug
Pregnancy category: C

Indications and Dosages
➤ *To achieve glucose control in type 2 diabetes mellitus as monotherapy or in combination with metformin*
TABLETS
Adults. *Initial:* 4 mg once daily or 2 mg twice daily, increased to 8 mg once daily or 4 mg twice daily. if glucose control is inadequate after 12 wk. *Maximum:* 8 mg daily.
➤ *To achieve glucose control in type 2 diabetes mellitus in combination with insulin therapy*
TABLETS
Adults. 4 mg daily with no change in insulin dosage. Insulin dosage decreased by 10% to 25% if hypoglycemia occurs, or fasting plasma concentrations decrease to less than 100 mg/dl with combination therapy.

Mechanism of Action
Increases tissue sensitivity to insulin. This peroxisome proliferator-activated receptor agonist regulates the transcription of insulin-responsive genes found in key target tissues, such as adipose tissue, skeletal muscle, and

the liver. Enhanced tissue sensitivity to insulin lowers the blood glucose level.

Contraindications
Hypersensitivity to rosiglitazone or its components, New York Heart Association (NYHA) class III or IV heart failure

Interactions
DRUGS
CYP2C8 inducers, such as rifampin: Possibly decreased effects of rosiglitazone
CYP2C8 inhibitors, such as gemfibrozil: Possibly increased effects of rosiglitazone

Adverse Reactions
CNS: CVA, fatigue, headache
CV: Angina, congestive heart failure, edema, hypertension, myocardial ischemia or infarction
EENT: Blurred vision, decreased visual acuity, macular edema, nasopharyngitis, sinusitis
ENDO: Hyperglycemia, hypoglycemia
GI: Diarrhea, elevated liver enzymes, hepatotoxicity
HEME: Anemia
MS: Arthralgia, back pain, fracture (especially upper arm, hand, foot)
RESP: Dyspnea, upper respiratory tract infection
MS: Bone fracture (especially upper arm, hand, foot)
SKIN: Pruritus, rash, Stevens-Johnson syndrome, urticaria
Other: Anaphylaxis, angioedema, weight gain

Nursing Considerations
• Give rosiglitazone cautiously in patients with edema, heart failure, or hepatic impairment because of potential adverse reactions.
• Be aware that drug isn't recommended for patients with symptomatic heart failure.
• Evaluate patient's liver function before starting drug and periodically throughout therapy, as ordered. Notify prescriber about abnormalities, such as nausea, vomiting, abdominal pain, fatigue, anorexia, and dark urine. Drug may need to be stopped.
WARNING Monitor patient for evidence of congestive heart failure—such as shortness of breath, rapid weight gain, or edema—because rosiglitazone can cause fluid

retention that may lead to or worsen heart failure. Notify prescriber immediately if the patient's cardiac status deteriorates, and expect to stop the drug, as ordered.

• Know that patients taking rosiglitazone and insulin together have an increased risk of experiencing a myocardial infarction or stroke. Monitor these patients closely for any signs and symptoms of these disorders. If present, notify prescriber, expect to stop rosiglitazone and provide appropriate medical care as indicated and ordered.

• Monitor fasting glucose and glycosylated hemoglobin A_{1c} levels periodically, as ordered, to evaluate rosiglitazone effectiveness.

• Be aware that drug is effective only in the presence of endogenous insulin.

PATIENT TEACHING

• Emphasize the need to follow an exercise program and a diet control program during rosiglitazone therapy.

• Advise patient to notify prescriber immediately if she has shortness of breath, fluid retention, or sudden weight gain, because drug may need to be discontinued.

• Instruct patient to have liver function tests, as prescribed, about every 2 months for first year and then annually.

• Inform premenopausal, anovulatory patient that drug may induce ovulation, increasing risk of pregnancy.

• Urge patient, especially women, to take precautions against falling or experiencing trauma; drug increases risk of fractures, particularly of the upper arm, hand, and foot.

rosuvastatin calcium

Crestor

Class and Category

Chemical class: HMG-CoA reductase inhibitor
Therapeutic class: Antihyperlipidemic
Pregnancy category: X

Indications and Dosages

➤ *To treat hyperlipidemia, mixed dyslipidemia, hypertriglyceridemia, and*

primary dysbetalipoproteinemia (type III hyperlipoproteinemia); to slow the progression of atherosclerosis; to prevent primary cardiovascular disease (reduce the risk of stroke, myocardial infarction, or need for arterial revascularization procedures) in patients without clinically evident CAD but with increased risk factors of cardiovascular disease such as age (men 50 years and older; women 60 years and older), hsCRP of 2 mg/l or greater, and the presence of at least one additional cardiovascular disease risk factor such as hypertension, low HDL-C, smoking, or a family history of premature CAD

TABLETS

Adults with LDL-C level of 190 mg/dl or below. *Initial:* 10 mg daily, increased every 2 to 4 wk, as needed. *Maximum:* 40 mg daily.

Adults with LDL-C level greater than 190 mg/dl. *Initial:* 20 mg daily, increased every 2 to 4 wk, as needed. *Maximum:* 40 mg daily.

➤ *To treat homozygous familial hypercholesterolemia*

TABLETS

Adults. *Initial:* 20 mg daily, increased every 2 to 4 wk, as needed. *Maximum:* 40 mg daily.

➤ *To treat heterozygous familial hypercholesterolemia*

TABLETS

Children age 10 and over and adolescents at least 1 year post-menarche. 5 to 20 mg daily, increased q 4 wk, as needed. Maximum: 20 mg daily.

DOSAGE ADJUSTMENT For patients taking cyclosporine, dosage shouldn't exceed 5 mg daily. For Asian patients, initial dosage should be limited to 5 mg daily. For patients taking gemfibrozil or combined atazanavir and ritonavir or lopinavir and ritonavir, 10 mg daily. For patients with severe renal impairment (creatinine clearance greater than 30 ml/min/1.73 m^2) who aren't having hemodialysis, dosage should start at 5 mg daily but not exceed 10 mg daily. For patients taking niacin or fenofibrate, dosage reduction should be considered.

Route	Onset	Peak	Duration
P.O.	Unknown	3–5 hr	Unknown

Mechanism of Action

Cholesterol and triglycerides circulate in the blood as part of lipoprotein complexes. Rosuvastatin inhibits the enzyme 3-hydroxy-3-methylglutaryl-coenzyme A (HMG-CoA) reductase. This inhibition reduces lipid levels by increasing the number of hepatic low-density-lipoprotein (LDL) receptors on the cell surface to increase uptake and catabolism of LDL. It also inhibits hepatic synthesis of very-low-density lipoprotein (VLDL), which decreases the total number of VLDL and LDL particles.

Contraindications

Active liver disease, breast-feeding, hypersensitivity to rosuvastatin or its components, pregnancy, unexplained persistent elevations of serum transaminase levels

Interactions

DRUGS

antacids: Decreased blood rosuvastatin level if given within 2 hours of rosuvastatin
atazanavir/ritonavir, cyclosporine, gemfibrozil, lopinavir/ritonavir, niacin (equal to or greater than 1g/day), other lipid-lowering drugs: Increased rosuvastatin level and risk of myopathy
azole antifungals, clarithromycin, daruavir/ ritonavir, erythromycin, fenofibrates, fosamprenavir, fosamprenavir/ritonavir, saquinavir/ritonavir, telaprevir, tipranavir/ ritonavir: Possibly increased risk of myopathy
oral contraceptives: Increased blood ethinyl estradiol and norgestrel levels
warfarin: Increased INR

Adverse Reactions

CNS: Asthenia, cognitive impairment, confusion, depression, dizziness, headache, hypertonia, insomnia, memory loss, nightmares, paresthesia, peripheral neuropathy
CV: Chest pain, hypertension, peripheral edema
EENT: Pharyngitis, rhinitis, sinusitis
ENDO: Elevated glycosylated hemoglobin levels, gynecomastia, hyperglycemia, thyroid function abnormalities
GI: Abdominal pain, constipation, diarrhea, elevated liver function test results, gastroenteritis, hepatic failure, hepatitis, jaundice, nausea, pancreatitis
GU: Acute renal failure, proteinuria, UTI
HEME: Thrombocytopenia
MS: Arthralgia, arthritis, back pain, immune-mediated necrotizing myopathy, myalgia, myopathy, rhabdomyolysis
RESP: Bronchitis, increased cough
SKIN: Rash, urticaria
Other: Angioedema, flulike symptoms, generalized pain, infection

Nursing Considerations

• Use rosuvastatin cautiously in patients who consume large quantities of alcohol or who have a history of liver disease, because drug is contraindicated in patients with active liver disease or unexplained persistent elevations of transaminaselevels.
• Also use cautiously in patients with risk factors for myopathy, such as renal impairment, advanced age, and hypothyroidism.
• If ALT or AST levels increase to more than three times the normal range, expect dosage to be reduced or drug discontinued.
• Monitor serum lipoprotein level, as ordered, to evaluate response to therapy.
• Expect rosuvastatin to be discontinued if patient develops markedly elevated creatinine kinase levels, or if myopathy is diagnosed or suspected. Drug may be temporarily withheld if patient develops any condition that may be related to myopathy or that predisposes her to renal failure, such as sepsis, hypotension, major surgery, trauma, uncontrolled seizures, or severe metabolic, endocrine, or electrolyte disorders.
• Obtain baseline liver function test results and expect to monitor them thereafter, as indicated. Notify prescriber if proteinuria or hematuria appears on patient's routine urinalysis, because rosuvastatin dosage may need to be reduced.

PATIENT TEACHING

• Encourage patient to follow a low-fat, low-cholesterol diet.
• Tell patient who takes rosuvastatin to wait at least 2 hours before taking antacids.
• Instruct patient to notify prescriber immediately about muscle pain, tenderness, or weakness, especially if

accompanied by malaise or fever. He should also tell the prescriber if these symptoms occur even after drug is discontinued.

• Encourage patient or family to notify prescriber if patient begins to notice new onset or worsening of memory loss, forgetfulness, or confusion.

• Tell woman of childbearing age about the need to use reliable contraceptive method while taking drug. Instruct her to notify prescriber at once if she suspects she may be pregnant.

• Instruct patient with diabetes to test his blood glucose regularly and have a HbA1c level checked routinely.

rotigotine

Neupro

Class and Category
Chemical class: Nonergoline dopamine agonist
Therapeutic class: Antidyskinetic
Pregnancy category: C

Indications and Dosages
➤ *To treat signs and symptoms of idiopathic Parkinson's disease*
TRANSDERMAL
Adults in early-stage. *Initial:* Apply 2 mg every 24 hr once daily, increased weekly in increments of 2 mg every 24 hr, as needed. *Maximum:* 6 mg every 24 hr.
Adults in advanced stage. *Initial:* Apply 4 mg every 24 hr once daily, increased weekly in increments of 2 mg every 24 hr, as needed. *Maximum:* 8 mg every 24 hr.
➤ *To treat moderate-to-severe primary restless leg syndrome*
TRANSDERMAL
Adults. *Initial:* Apply 1 mg every 24 hr once daily, increased weekly in increments of 1 mg every 24 hr, as needed. *Maximum:* 3 mg every 24 hr.

Mechanism of Action
Thought to stimulate dopamine receptors within the caudate-putamen in the brain. Increased dopamine levels helps relieve the signs and symptoms associated with Parkinson's disease and restless leg syndrome.

Contraindications
Hypersensitivity to rotigotine or the components of the transdermal system.

Interaction
DRUGS
dopamine antagonists (antipsychotics or metoclopramide): Possibly diminish effectiveness of rotigotine

Adverse Reactions
CNS: Abnormal dreams, aggressive behavior, agitation, asthenia, balance disorder, compulsive behaviors, confusion, delusions, depression, disorientation, dizziness, dysesthesias, dyskinesia, excessive sleepiness, fatigue, hallucinations, headache, insomnia, lethargy, paranoid ideation, paraesthesia, psychotic-like behavior, sleep disorders, somnolence, syncope, tremor, vertigo
CV: Cardiac valvulopathy, ECG T-wave abnormality, hiccups, hypertension, orthostatic hypotension, pericarditis, peripheral edema, tachycardia
EENT: Dry mouth, nasal or sinus congestion, nasopharyngitis, pharyngolaryngeal pain, sinusitis, tinnitus
ENDO: Hot flashes
GI: Anorexia, constipation, diarrhea, dyspepsia, nausea, retroperitoneal fibrosis, vomiting
GU: Erectile dysfunction
HEME: Decreased serum ferritin level
MS: Arthralgia, exacerbation or worsening of restless leg syndrome, musculoskeletal pain, muscle spasms
RESP: Cough, pleural effusion or thickening, pulmonary infiltrates, upper respiratory infection
SKIN: Erythema, hyperhidrosis, melanoma, pruritis
Other: Application-site reactions (erythemia, edema, pruritis, rash), weight gain or loss

Nursing Considerations
• Be aware that patients should be screened for a history of sleep disorders and usage of concomitant sedating medications because the risk of falling asleep with or without warning signs of sleepiness increases when these risk factors are present.
• Use caution when administering rotigotine to a patient with severe cardiovascular disease because syncope can occur. Also

Q
R
S

monitor patient for fluid retention, especially in a patient with a history of congestive heart failure.
• Monitor patient closely after rotigotine treatment is started for signs and symptoms of an allergic reaction to rotigotine or sulfite because the drug does contain a sulfite. Know that sulfite sensitivity is more frequent in asthmatic patients than in nonasthmatic patients.
• Take blood pressure and pulse frequently because drug can cause a significant increase in blood pressure, and pulse may become higher than 100 beats/minute. Also watch for orthostatic hypotension, especially in patients with early Parkinson's disease and in all patients during dosage titration.
• Monitor patient for dyskinesia, which may occur with rotigotine use. Notify prescriber if present because dosage adjustment may be needed or drug discontinued.
• Monitor patient for hallucinations, especially if patient has Parkinson's disease, is elderly, or takes levodopa.
• Expect to gradually stop rotigotine therapy, as ordered. For patient with Parkinson's disease, daily dose reduced by a maximum of 2mg in 24 hours every other day until complete withdrawal of rotigotine is achieved. For patient with restless leg syndrome, daily dose reduced by 1 mg every 24 hours every other day, until complete withdrawal of rotigotine is achieved.

PATIENT TEACHING
• Alert patient to the possibility of application-site reactions such as redness, itchiness, puffiness, or a rash. Using a different site when applying the patch can reduce these adverse effects. If application-site reactions become severe, tell patient to notify the prescriber.
• Caution patient to avoid performing hazardous activities, such as driving
• until effects of drug are known.
• Inform him that some patients taking rotigotine have fallen asleep during activities of daily living, sometimes without warning.
• Warn patient and family that drug may cause compulsive behaviors such as intense urges to gamble, shop, have sex, or binge eating. Prescriber should be notified if compulsive behaviors are exhibited.

rufinamide
Banzel

Class and Category
Chemical class: Triazole derivative
Therapeutic class: Anticonvulsant
Pregnancy category: C

Indications and Dosages
➤ *As adjunct treatment of seizures associated with Lennox-Gastaut syndrome*
TABLETS
Adults. *Initial:* 200 to 400 mg twice daily, increased in daily increments of 200 to 400 mg twice daily, every 2 days until reaching 1,600 mg twice daily. *Maximum:* 1,600 mg twice daily.
Children age 4 and over. *Initial:* 5 mg/kg twice daily, increased in daily increments of 5 mg/kg twice daily. every 2 days until reaching 22.5 mg/kg twice daily or 1600 mg twice daily, whichever is less.
DOSAGE ADJUSTMENT For patients undergoing dialysis, dosage may need to be increased. For patients also receiving valproate, initial dosage reduced to less than 400 mg daily.

Route	Onset	Peak	Duration
P.O.	Unknown	4–6 hr	Unknown

Mechanism of Action
Unknown, although rufinamide is known to slow sodium channel recovery from inactivation after a prolonged prepulse and to limit repetitive firing of sodium-dependent action potentials in neurons in the brain. These actions may help limit seizure activity.

Contraindications
Familial short-QT syndrome, hypersensitivity to rufinamide or its components

Interactions
DRUGS
contraceptives containing ethinyl estradiol and norethindrone: Decreased effectiveness of the oral contraceptive
phenytoin: Increased plasma phenytoin level and risk of adverse reactions

valproate: Increased plasma rufinamide level and risk of adverse reactions
ACTIVITIES
alcohol use: Increased CNS effects

Adverse Reactions

CNS: Aggression, anxiety, ataxia, attention disturbance, dizziness, fatigue, headache, hyperactivity, seizures, somnolence, status epilepticus, suicidal ideation, tremor, vertigo
CV: First-degree AV block, right bundle branch block
EENT: Sinusitis
ENDO: Blurred vision, diplopia, naso-pharyngitis, nystagmus
GI: Abdominal pain, anorexia, constipation, dyspepsia, nausea, vomiting
GU: Dysuria, enuresis, hematuria, incontinence, nephrolithiasis, pollakiuria, polyuria
HEME: Anemia, leukopenia, lymph-adenopathy, neutropenia, thrombocytopenia
MS: Back pain
RESP: Bronchitis
SKIN: Pruritus, rash
Other: Multiorgan hypersensitivity

Nursing Considerations

• Administer rufinamide with food because absorption is increased.
• Monitor patient's QT interval regularly, as ordered, because rufinamide may shorten the QT interval and possibly predispose patient to ventricular fibrillation if the interval falls below 300 msec.
WARNING Watch closely for multi-organ hypersensitivity, especially if patient develops a rash. Although uncommon, it may cause serious adverse effects, such as urticaria, facial edema, fever, elevated eosinophils or liver enzymes, hematuria, stupor, lymphadenopathy and severe hepatitis, in addition to rash. Notify prescriber at once if such changes appear, and expect to stop drug and provide supportive care.
• Watch closely for suicidal tendencies, especially when therapy starts and dosage changes and particularly in children and adolescents.
• To stop therapy, expect to taper dosage to minimize adverse effects rather than stopping abruptly.

PATIENT TEACHING
• Make sure patient receives medication guide describing drug use and possible suicidal tendencies.
• Instruct patient to take drug exactly as prescribed and to take each dose with food. If patient has trouble swallowing tablets, tell him they may be crushed.
• Inform woman that rufinamide decreases effectiveness of contraceptives containing ethinyl estradiol and norethindrone. Tell her to use a different contraceptive during therapy and to contact prescriber immediately if she thinks she's pregnant.
• Tell patient to report a rash accompanied by fever or other symptoms immediately.
• Warn family or caregiver to watch patient for suicidal tendencies, especially when therapy starts or dosage changes, and particularly if patient is a child or adolescent.
• Advise patient to avoid hazardous activities until drug's CNS effects are known.
• Caution patient not to stop taking drug abruptly. Explain that gradual tapering helps to avoid withdrawal symptoms.
• Explain that alcohol consumption may intensify drug effects.

salmeterol xinafoate
Serevent Diskus

Class and Category
Chemical class: Sympathomimetic amine
Therapeutic class: Bronchodilator
Pregnancy category: C

Indications and Dosages
➤ *To prevent asthma-induced bronchospasm*
ORAL INHALATION POWDER
Adults and children age 4 and over. 1 inhalation (50 mcg) every 12 hr.
➤ *To prevent COPD-induced bronchospasm*
ORAL INHALATION POWDER
Adults. 1 inhalation (50 mcg) every 12 hr.
➤ *To prevent exercise-induced bronchospasm*

ORAL INHALATION POWDER
Adults and children age 4 and over.
1 inhalation (50 mcg) at least 30 min before exercise.

Route	Onset	Peak	Duration
Inhalation	10–20 min	3–4 hr	12 hr

Mechanism of Action
Attaches to beta$_2$ receptors on bronchial cell membranes, stimulating the intracellular enzyme adenylate cyclase to convert adenosine triphosphate to cAMP. The resulting increase in intracellular cAMP level relaxes bronchial smooth-muscle cells, stabilizes mast cells, and inhibits histamine release.

Contraindications
Hypersensitivity to salmeterol or its components, to treat asthma without use of a long-term asthma control medication

Interactions
DRUGS
atazanavir, clarithromycin, indinavir, itraconazole, ketoconazole, nefazodone, nelfinavir, ritonavir, saquinavir, telithromycin: Possibly increased risk of adverse cardiovascular effects
beta blockers: Mutual inhibition of therapeutic effects
loop or thiazide diuretics: Increased risk of hypokalemia and potentially life-threatening arrhythmias
MAO inhibitors, tricyclic antidepressants: Potentiated adverse vascular effects, such as hypertensive crisis

Adverse Reactions
CNS: Dizziness, fever, headache, nervousness, paresthesia, tremor
CV: Palpitations, tachycardia
EENT: Dry mouth, nose, and throat; sinus problems
GI: Nausea
MS: Arthralgia
RESP: Cough, paradoxical bronchospasm
SKIN: Contact dermatitis, eczema, rash, urticaria
Other: Angioedema, generalized aches and pains

Nursing Considerations
• Be aware that salmeterol shouldn't be used to relieve bronchospasm quickly because

of its prolonged onset of action and that patients already taking drug twice daily shouldn't take additional doses for exercise-induced bronchospasm.

WARNING Be aware that a recent study suggests that asthma-related deaths may increase in asthmatics receiving salmeterol. Know that salmeterol should not be used in patients whose asthma is adequately controlled on low- or medium-dose inhaled corticosteroids and it should only be used as additional therapy for patients with asthma who are currently taking but are not adequately controlled on long-term asthma control medication, such as an inhaled corticosteroid. Monitor this patient population closely throughout salmeterol therapy, and notify prescriber immediately of any changes in patient's respiratory status. Expect to discontinue use as soon as possible.

• Watch for arrhythmias and changes in blood pressure after use in patients with cardiovascular disorders, including ischemic cardiac disease, hypertension, and arrhythmias, because of drug's beta-adrenergic effects.

• Monitor patient's compliance. Expect adults with poor compliance and children and adolescents who require the addition of a long-acting beta agonist such as salmeterol to be prescribed a combination product containing both an inhaled corticosteroid and a long-acting beta agonist to increase compliance.

• Be aware that Serevent Diskus delivers full dose of salmeterol in only one inhalation.

WARNING Stop salmeterol immediately and notify prescriber if patient develops paradoxical bronchospasm. Risk is greatest with first use of a new canister or vial used as an inhalant.

PATIENT TEACHING
• Advise patient who is using salmeterol to prevent asthma-induced bronchospasm to take doses 12 hours apart for optimum effect. Caution against using drug more than every 12 hours.

• Teach patient how to use the diskus by instructing him to slide the lever only once when preparing dose to avoid wasting doses. Advise him to exhale immediately before using the diskus and then to place mouthpiece to his lips and inhale through his mouth, not his nose. Then he should remove mouthpiece from his mouth, hold his breath for at least 10 seconds, and exhale slowly.

• Advise patient to rinse mouth with water after each dose to minimize dry mouth.

• Advise patient to discard diskus 6 weeks after removing it from overwrap or when dose indicator reads zero.

• Instruct patient to notify prescriber if he needs four or more oral inhalations of rapid-acting inhaled bronchodilator a day for 2 or more consecutive days, or if he uses more than one canister of rapid-acting bronchodilator in an 8-week period.

• Caution patient not to use other drugs to treat his underlying respiratory condition without consulting prescriber and to let all prescribers know that he takes salmeterol.

---

salsalate
(salicylic acid)

Amigesic, Anaflex 750, Argesic-SA, Disalcid, Marthritic, Mono-Gesic, Salflex, Salsitab

Class and Category

Chemical class: Salicylic acid ester
Therapeutic class: Analgesic, anti-inflammatory
Pregnancy category: C

Indications and Dosages

➤ *To relieve symptoms of rheumatoid arthritis and related rheumatic disorders*

CAPSULES

Adults and adolescents. *Initial:* 1 g three times a day; dosage then titrated, as needed.

TABLETS

Adults and adolescents. *Initial:* 0.5 to 1 g twice daily or three times a day; dosage then titrated, as needed.

Route	Onset	Peak	Duration
P.O.	Unknown	2–3 wk	Unknown

Mechanism of Action

Exerts peripherally induced analgesic and anti-inflammatory effects by blocking pain impulses and inhibiting prostaglandin synthesis.

Contraindications

Bleeding disorders; hypersensitivity to NSAIDs, salicylates, or their components

Interactions

DRUGS

acetaminophen: Increased risk of renal dysfunction with prolonged use of both drugs
anticoagulants, thrombolytics: Increased risk and severity of GI bleeding
antiemetics: Masked symptoms of salicylate-induced ototoxicity
bismuth subsalicylate: Increased risk of salicylate toxicity with large doses of salsalate
cefamandole, cefoperazone, cefotetan, platelet aggregation inhibitors, plicamycin, valproic acid: Possibly hypoprothrombinemia
corticosteroids: Possibly decreased blood salsalate level; additive therapeutic effects when both drugs are used to treat arthritis
furosemide: Increased risk of ototoxicity and salicylate toxicity
hydantoins: Possibly decreased hydantoin metabolism, leading to toxicity
insulin, oral antidiabetic drugs: Potentiated hypoglycemic effect
laxatives (cellulose-containing): Possibly reduced salsalate effectiveness due to impaired absorption
methotrexate: Increased risk of methotrexate toxicity
NSAIDs: Increased risk of adverse GI effects
ototoxic drugs, vancomycin: Increased risk of ototoxicity
probenecid, sulfinpyrazone: Decreased uricosuric effects
topical salicylic acid, other salicylates: Increased risk of salicylate toxicity if significant quantities are absorbed
urinary acidifiers (ammonium chloride, ascorbic acid, potassium or sodium phosphates): Decreased salicylate excretion, possibly leading to salicylate toxicity
urinary alkalizers (antacids [long-term high-dose use], carbonic anhydrase inhibitors, citrates, sodium bicarbonate): Increased salicylate excretion, leading to reduced effectiveness and shortened half-life; increased risk of salicylate toxicity with

Q
R
S

carbonic anhydrase inhibitor–induced metabolic acidosis
vitamin K: Increased vitamin K requirements
ACTIVITIES
alcohol use: Increased risk of GI bleeding

Adverse Reactions

CNS: CNS depression, confusion, dizziness, drowsiness, fever, headache, lassitude
EENT: Hearing loss, tinnitus, vision changes
GI: Anorexia, diarrhea, epigastric discomfort, GI bleeding, heartburn, hepatotoxicity, indigestion, nausea, thirst, vomiting
HEME: Hemolytic anemia, leukopenia, prolonged bleeding time, thrombocytopenia
SKIN: Diaphoresis, purpura, rash, urticaria
Other: Angioedema, Reye's syndrome

Nursing Considerations

• Avoid using salsalate in patients with hypoprothrombinemia or vitamin K deficiency because drug's hypoprothrombinemic effect may precipitate bleeding.
• Monitor hepatic and renal function, as appropriate, during long-term therapy.
• Assess for signs and symptoms of GI bleeding, such as abdominal pain or black, tarry stools, especially in patient with peptic ulcer disease.
• Assess for symptoms of ototoxicity, such as ringing or roaring in ears.
PATIENT TEACHING
• Instruct patient to take salsalate with food or a full glass of water and to remain upright for 1 hour after administration to prevent drug from lodging in esophagus and causing irritation.
• Inform patient that therapeutic response may not occur for 2 to 3 weeks.
• Urge patient to notify prescriber immediately of abdominal pain or black, tarry stools; these symptoms may indicate GI bleeding or drug toxicity.

sapropterin
dihydrochloride

Kuvan

Class and Category

Chemical class: Synthetic tetrahydrobiopterin salt
Therapeutic class: Phenylalanine reducer
Pregnancy category: C

Indications and Dosages

➤ *To reduce blood phenylalanine level in patients with hyperphenylalaninemia from tetrahydrobiopterin-responsive phenylketonuria, with phenylalanine-restricted diet*
TABLETS
Adults and children age 4 and over.
Initial: 10 mg/kg daily with dosage increased or decreased after 1 wk based on response and then periodically adjusted, as needed. Expect to discontinue drug if levels fail to increase after 1 mo of therapy at 20 mg/kg/day. *Maintenance:* 5 to 20 mg/kg daily. *Maximum:* 20 mg/kg daily.

Mechanism of Action

As a synthetic form of tetrahydrobiopterin, the cofactor of the enzyme phenylalanine hydroxylase (PAH), sapropterin hydroxylates phenylalanine to form tyrosine. This improves the oxidative metabolism of phenylalanine, which decreases blood phenylalanine.

Contraindications

Hypersensitivity to sapropterin or its components

Interactions

DRUGS
folate metabolism inhibitors, such as methotrexate: Possibly decreased effectiveness of sapropterin
levodopa: Possibly increased risk of irritability, overstimulation, or seizures
sildenafil, tadalafil, vardenafil: Possibly additive vasorelaxation effect leading to hypotension

Adverse Reactions

CNS: Agitation, dizziness, fever, headache, irritability, over stimulation, seizures
CV: MI, peripheral edema
EENT: Nasal congestion, pharyngolaryngeal pain, rhinorrhea

GI: Abdominal pain, diarrhea, elevated liver enzymes, gastrointestinal bleeding, nausea, vomiting
GU: Polyurina
HEME: Bleeding, neutropenia
MS: Arthralgia
RESP: Cough, respiratory failure, upper respiratory infection
SKIN: Rash

Nursing Considerations

• Use cautiously in patients with hepatic impairment because impaired phenylalanine metabolism may be linked to hepatic damage.
• Administer drug at same time each day.
• Dissolve tablets in 4 to 8 ounces of water or apple juice, which may take a few minutes. Stirring or crushing tablets will hasten process. Know that tablets may not dissolve completely. Give solution within 15 minutes with food. If there are particles left in glass after administration, add more water or apple juice and have patient drink again to ensure a complete dose.
• Monitor patient's blood phenylalanine level regularly, as ordered.
• Expect drug to be discontinued if patient's blood phenylalanine level doesn't decrease after 1 month at maximum dosage.
• Continue to restrict dietary phenylalanine intake.

PATIENT TEACHING

• Tell patient to dissolve tablets in 4 to 8 ounces water or apple juice, which may take a few minutes. Advise him to stir or crush tablets to hasten process and to drink solution within 15 minutes of dissolving. Explain that tablets may not completely dissolve and that he can drink solution with particles floating in it. After drinking solution, tell him to add more water or apple juice if any particles are clinging to glass and drink again.
• Emphasize to patient or caregiver the importance of continuing dietary restriction of phenylalanine intake.
• Emphasize continued need for periodic blood tests to determine drug effectiveness.
• Tell patient to take a missed dose as soon as he remembers, unless it's almost time for the next dose. Warn patient not to take more than 1 dose per day.

saxagliptin monohydrate

Onglyza

Class and Category

Chemical class: Dipeptidyl peptidase-4 inhibitor
Therapeutic class: Antidiabetic
Pregnancy category: B

Indications and Dosages

➤ *To improve blood glucose control in type 2 diabetes mellitus as adjunct to diet and exercise*

TABLETS

Adults. 2.5 mg or 5 mg once daily
DOSAGE ADJUSTMENT For patients with moderate or severe renal impairment (creatinine clearance 50 ml/min/1.73 m^2 or less), patients with end-stage renal disease, patients having hemodialysis, and patients receiving strong CYP3A4/5 inhibitors, dosage shouldn't exceed 2.5 mg once daily.

Route	Onset	Peak	Duration
P.O.	Unknown	2 hr	24 hr

Mechanism of Action

Incretin hormones, such as glucose-dependent insulintropic polypeptide (GIP) and glucagons-like peptide-1 (GLP-1), are released into bloodstream from small intestine in response to meals. Upon arrival at the pancreas, they stimulate pancreatic beta cells to release insulin. GLP-1 also reduces glucagon secretion from pancreatic alpha cells, which reduces hepatic glucose production. Incretin hormones become inactivated within minutes of release by the enzyme, dipeptidyl peptidase-4. Saxagliptin inhibits this enzyme, thereby slowing inactivation of incretin hormones, which provides more time for them to increase insulin levels and blunt glucagon secretion. More insulin and less hepatic glucose production work together to lower blood glucose levels.

Contraindications

Hypersensitivity to saxagliptin or its components

Q
R
S

Interactions
DRUGS
aprepitant, diltiazem, erythromycin, fluconazole, fosamprenavir, verapamil: Possibly increased plasma saxagliptin level
atazanavir, clarithromycin, indinavir, itraconazole, ketoconazole, nefazodone, nelfinavir, ritonavir, saquinavir, telithromycin: Increased plasma saxagliptin level
insulin, sulfonylureas: Increased risk of hypoglycemia
FOODS
grapefruit juice: Possibly increased plasma saxagliptin levels

Adverse Reactions
CNS: Headache
CV: Peripheral edema
EENT: Sinusitis, nasopharyngitis
ENDO: Hypoglycemia
GI: Acute pancreatitis, abdominal pain, gastroenteritis, vomiting
GU: Elevated plasma creatinine level, UTI
HEME: Lymphopenia
RESP: Upper respiratory tract infection
SKIN: Exfoliative skin conditions, rash, urticaria
Other: Anaphylaxis, angioedema, facial edema

Nursing Considerations
• Know that saxagliptin shouldn't be used to treat type 1 diabetes mellitus or diabetic ketoacidosis.
• Use cautiously in patients who have experienced angioedema with another dipeptidyl peptidase-4 inhibitor because it is not known if a cross-sensitivity reaction may occur with saxagliptin.
• Obtain a serum creatinine level, as ordered, before starting saxagliptin therapy and then periodically thereafter to monitor patient's renal function.
• Monitor patient closely for hypersensitivity to saxagliptin, especially within the first 3 months of therapy beginning with first dose. These reactions can be serious and life-threatening and may include anaphylaxis, angioedema, and exfoliative skin conditions. Discontinue saxagliptin immediately if hypersensitivity occurs, and notify prescriber.

• Monitor patient's blood glucose level and hemoglobin A_{1C} to assess effectiveness of saxagliptin therapy.
• Watch for hypoglycemia in patients taking insulin or other antidiabetics, such as sulfonylureas. Expect dosage of insulin or other antidiabetics, such as sulfonylureas, to be decreased to reduce risk of hypoglycemia.
• Monitor patient for signs and symptoms of acute pancreatitis such as severe, sharp pain in the upper abdominal accompanied by nausea, vomiting, and fever. If present, notify prescriber, expect to stop saxagliptin, as ordered, and provide supportive care, as indicated and ordered.

PATIENT TEACHING
• Emphasize that saxagliptin isn't a replacement for diet and exercise therapy.
• Explain importance of self-monitoring glucose levels during saxagliptin therapy.
• Teach patient to recognize hypoglycemia and how to treat it if it should occur. Urge him to carry glucose with him at all times in case hypoglycemia occurs.
• Instruct patient to notify prescriber if fever, trauma, infection, illness, surgery, or other stress occurs because blood glucose control may be altered, requiring temporary insulin therapy.
• Instruct patient to seek immediate medical attention if he experiences persistent, acute abdominal pain, nausea, vomiting, and fever, as well as any sign of hypersensitivity, such as rash, skin flaking or peeling, hives, swelling of any area on skin or face, or difficulty breathing or swallowing.

scopolamine hydrobromide
scopolamine transdermal system
Transderm-Scop, Transderm-V (CAN)

Class and Category
Chemical class: Belladonna alkaloid, tertiary amine

Therapeutic class: Anesthesia adjunct, anticholinergic, antiemetic, antispasmodic, antivertigo
Pregnancy category: C

Indications and Dosages

➤ *To treat biliary tract disorders, enuresis, nausea and vomiting, and nocturia*

I.V., I.M., OR SUBCUTANEOUS INJECTION (HYDROBROMIDE)

Adults and adolescents. 300 to 600 mcg (0.3 to 0.6 mg) as a single dose.
Children. 6 mcg (0.006 mg)/kg as a single dose.

➤ *To prevent excessive salivation and respiratory tract secretions during anesthesia*

I.M. INJECTION (HYDROBROMIDE)

Adults and adolescents. 0.2 to 0.6 mg 30 to 60 min before induction of anesthesia.
Children ages 8 to 12. 0.3 mg 45 to 60 min before induction of anesthesia.
Children ages 3 to 8. 0.2 mg 45 to 60 min before induction of anesthesia.
Children ages 7 months to 3 years. 0.15 mg 45 to 60 min before induction of anesthesia.
Infants ages 4 to 7 months. 0.1 mg 45 to 60 min before induction of anesthesia.

➤ *As adjunct to anesthesia to induce sleep and calmness*

I.V., I.M., OR SUBCUTANEOUS INJECTION (HYDROBROMIDE)

Adults and adolescents. 0.6 mg three times a day or four times a day.

➤ *As adjunct to anesthesia to induce amnesia*

I.V., I.M., OR SUBCUTANEOUS INJECTION (HYDROBROMIDE)

Adults and adolescents. 0.32 to 0.65 mg.

➤ *To prevent nausea, vomiting, and vertigo associated with motion sickness*

TRANSDERMAL SYSTEM

Adults and adolescents. 1 U.S. transdermal system (0.5 mg) applied behind ear for 3-day period, beginning at least 4 hr before antiemetic effect is required. Or, 1 Canadian transdermal system (1 mg) applied behind ear for 3-day period, beginning at least 12 hr before antiemetic effect is required.

DOSAGE ADJUSTMENT Dosage reduction possible for elderly patients because of their increased sensitivity to scopolamine.

Contraindications

Angle-closure glaucoma; hemorrhage with hemodynamic instability; hepatic dysfunction; hypersensitivity to barbiturates, scopolamine, other belladonna alkaloids, or their components; ileus; intestinal atony; myasthenia gravis; myocardial ischemia; obstructive GI disease, such as pyloric stenosis; obstructive uropathy, as in prostatic hyperplasia; renal impairment; tachycardia; toxic megacolon; ulcerative colitis

Route	Onset	Peak	Duration
I.V., I.M., SubQ*	30 min	1–2 hr	4–6 hr
I.V.†	10 min	50–80 min	2 hr
I.M.‡	15–30 min	Unknown	4 hr
Trans-dermal	4 hr	Unknown	72 hr

Mechanism of Action

Competitively inhibits acetylcholine at autonomic postganglionic cholinergic receptors. Because the most sensitive receptors are in the salivary, bronchial, and sweat glands, this action reduces secretions from these glands. Scopolamine reduces GI smooth-muscle tone; decreases gastric secretions and GI motility; reduces bladder detrusor muscle tone; reduces nasal, oropharyngeal, and bronchial secretions; and decreases airway resistance by relaxing smooth muscles in the bronchi and bronchioles.

Scopolamine also blocks neural pathways in the inner ear to relieve motion sickness and depresses the cerebral cortex to produce sedation and hypnotic effects.

Interactions

DRUGS

adsorbent antidiarrheals, antacids: Decreased absorption and therapeutic effects of scopolamine
anticholinergics (other): Possibly intensified anticholinergic effects

---

* For inhibition of saliva.
† For amnesia.
‡ For antiemesis.

**Q
R
S**

antimyasthenics: Possibly reduced intestinal motility
CNS depressants: Possibly potentiated effects of either drug, resulting in additive sedation
cyclopropane: Increased risk of ventricular arrhythmias (with I.V. scopolamine)
haloperidol: Decreased antipsychotic effect of haloperidol
ketoconazole: Decreased ketoconazole absorption
lorazepam (parenteral): Possibly hallucinations, irrational behavior, and sedation
metoclopramide: Possibly antagonized effect of metoclopramide on GI motility
opioid analgesics: Increased risk of severe constipation and ileus
potassium chloride: Possibly increased severity of potassium chloride–induced GI lesions
urinary alkalizers (antacids, carbonic anhydrase inhibitors, citrates, sodium bicarbonate): Delayed excretion of scopolamine, possibly leading to increased therapeutic and adverse effects
ACTIVITIES
alcohol use: Additive CNS effects

Adverse Reactions
CNS: Dizziness, drowsiness, euphoria, insomnia, memory loss, paradoxical stimulation
CV: Palpitations, tachycardia
EENT: Blurred vision; dry eyes, mouth, nose, and throat; mydriasis
GI: Constipation, dysphagia
GU: Urinary hesitancy, urine retention
SKIN: Decreased sweating, dry skin, flushing
Other: Injection-site irritation or redness

Nursing Considerations
• For I.V. injection, dilute scopolamine with sterile water for injection.
• Assess for bladder distention and monitor urine output because drug's antimuscarinic effects can cause urine retention.
• Monitor for pain. In presence of pain, drug may act as a stimulant and produce delirium if used without morphine or meperidine.
• Monitor heart rate for transient tachycardia, which may occur with high doses of drug. Rate should return to normal within 30 minutes.

PATIENT TEACHING
• Instruct patient to apply scopolamine transdermal patch on hairless area behind ear and to wash hands thoroughly with soap and water before and after applying.
• Advise patient to avoid hazardous activities until drug's CNS effects are known.
• Instruct patient to avoid alcohol while taking oral forms of scopolamine.
• If patient complains of dry eyes, suggest lubricating drops.

secobarbital sodium
Novosecobarb (CAN), Seconal

Class, Category, and Schedule
Chemical class: Barbiturate
Therapeutic class: Sedative-hypnotic
Pregnancy category: D
Controlled substance schedule: II

Indications and Dosages
➤ *To induce sedation before surgery*
CAPSULES
Adults. 200 to 300 mg 1 to 2 hr before surgery.
Children. 2 to 6 mg/kg 1 to 2 hr before surgery. *Maximum:* 100 mg.
➤ *To provide short-term treatment of insomnia*
CAPSULES
Adults. 100 mg at bedtime.
➤ *To relieve apprehension, daytime anxiety, and tension*
CAPSULES
Adults. 30 to 50 mg three times a day or four times a day.
Children. 2 mg/kg three times a day.
DOSAGE ADJUSTMENT Reduced dosage required for elderly or debilitated patients and those with renal or hepatic dysfunction.

Route	Onset	Peak	Duration
P.O.	10–15 min	15–30 min	1–4 hr

Mechanism of Action
Inhibits upward conduction of nerve impulses to the reticular formation of the brain, thereby disrupting impulse transmission to the cortex. This action depresses the CNS, producing drowsiness, hypnosis, and sedation.

Contraindications

History of barbiturate addiction; hypersensitivity to secobarbital, other barbiturates, or their components; nephritis; porphyria; severe hepatic or respiratory impairment

Interactions

DRUGS

acetaminophen, adrenocorticoids, beta blockers, chloramphenicol, cyclosporine, dacarbazine, digoxin, disopyramide, estrogens, metronidazole, oral anticoagulants, oral contraceptives, quinidine, thyroid hormones, tricyclic antidepressants: Decreased effectiveness of these drugs

addictive drugs: Increased risk of addiction

calcium channel blockers: Possibly excessive hypotension

carbamazepine, succinimide anticonvulsants: Decreased blood levels and increased elimination of these drugs

carbonic anhydrase inhibitors: Increased risk of osteopenia

CNS depressants: Increased CNS depressant effects

cyclophosphamide: Increased risk of leuko-penic activity and reduced half-life of cyclophosphamide

divalproex sodium, valproic acid: Increased CNS depression and neurologic toxicity

doxycycline, fenoprofen: Increased elimi-nation of these drugs

general anesthetics (enflurane, halothane, methoxyflurane): Increased risk of hepatotoxicity; increased risk of nephro-toxicity (with methoxyflurane)

griseofulvin: Decreased griseofulvin absorption

guanadrel, guanethidine: Possibly increased orthostatic hypotension

haloperidol: Possibly altered pattern or frequency of seizures, decreased blood haloperidol level

ketamine: Increased risk of hypotension or respiratory depression (when secobarbital is used as preanesthetic)

leucovorin (large doses): Decreased anticonvulsant effect of secobarbital

loxapine, phenothiazines, thioxanthenes: Possibly lowered seizure threshold

MAO inhibitors: Possibly prolonged CNS depressant effects of secobarbital

maprotiline: Increased CNS depressant effect; possibly lowered seizure threshold and decreased anticonvulsant effect with high doses of maprotiline

methylphenidate: Increased risk of barbi-turate toxicity

mexiletine: Decreased blood mexiletine level

phenylbutazone: Decreased effectiveness of secobarbital

posterior pituitary hormones: Increased risk of arrhythmias and coronary insufficiency

primidone: Increased sedative effect of either drug, change in seizure pattern

vitamin D: Decreased vitamin D effects

xanthines (aminophylline, oxtriphylline, theophylline): Increased metabolism of xanthines (except dyphylline), decreased hypnotic effect of secobarbital

FOODS

caffeine: Increased caffeine metabolism, decreased hypnotic effect of secobarbital

ACTIVITIES

alcohol use: Increased CNS depression

Adverse Reactions

CNS: Anxiety, clumsiness, confusion, depression, dizziness, drowsiness, hangover, headache, insomnia, irritability, lethargy, nervousness, nightmares, paradoxical stimulation, syncope

CV: Hypotension

EENT: Laryngospasm

GI: Anorexia, constipation, nausea, vomiting

MS: Arthralgia, muscle weakness

RESP: Apnea, bronchospasm, respiratory depression

SKIN: Jaundice

Other: Drug dependence, weight loss

Nursing Considerations

• Be aware that prolonged use of secobarbital may lead to tolerance and physical and psychological dependence.

WARNING To avoid withdrawal symptoms, expect to taper drug after long-term therapy. Withdrawal symptoms usually appear 8 to 12 hours after stopping drug and may include anxiety, insomnia, muscle twitching, nausea, orthostatic hypotension, vomiting, weakness, and

Q
R
S

weight loss. Severe symptoms may include delirium, hallucinations, and seizures. Generalized tonic-clonic seizures may occur within 16 hours or up to 5 days after last dose.

• Assess patient for signs and symptoms of barbiturate toxicity, including dyspnea, severe confusion, and severe drowsiness. Notify prescriber immediately if they appear because barbiturate toxicity may be life-threatening.

• Expect prescriber to provide patient with the least possible quantity of secobarbital to minimize the risk of acute or chronic overdosage. For patients who are depressed, suicidal, or drug-dependent or who have a history of drug abuse, institute precautions to prevent drug hoarding and overdosage.

PATIENT TEACHING
• Instruct patient to take secobarbital exactly as prescribed because of the risk of addiction.

• Inform patient that taking drug with food may reduce adverse GI effects.

• Advise patient to avoid alcohol and caffeine and potentially hazardous activities during therapy.

• Inform patient about possible hangover effect.

• If patient takes an oral contraceptive, recommend using an additional form of birth control during therapy.

• Caution patient not to stop taking drug abruptly.

• Instruct patient to notify prescriber of bone pain, muscle weakness, or unexplained weight loss during therapy.

selegiline hydrochloride

Apo-Selegiline (CAN), Carbex, Eldepryl, Gen-Selegiline (CAN), NOVO-Selegiline (CAN), Nu-Selegiline (CAN), SD Deprenyl (CAN), Selegiline-5 (CAN), Zelapar

selegiline transdermal system

Emsam

Class and Category
Chemical class: Phenethylamine derivative
Therapeutic class: Antidepressant (Emsam), antidyskinetic
Pregnancy category: C

Indications and Dosages
➤ *As adjunct to carbidopa-levodopa therapy to treat Parkinson's disease*
CAPSULES, TABLETS
Adults. 10 mg once daily, or 5 mg twice daily with breakfast and lunch.
DOSAGE ADJUSTMENT For patient with levodopa-induced adverse effects, 2.5 mg four times a day.
➤ *As adjunct to carbidopa-levodopa therapy to treat Parkinson's disease in patients whose response to therapy has deteriorated*
ORALLY DISINTEGRATING TABLETS (ZELAPAR)
Adults. *Initial:* 1.25 mg once daily before breakfast for at least 6 wk; then increased to 2.5 mg once daily, as needed.
➤ *To treat depression*
TRANSDERMAL SYSTEM (EMSAM)
Adults. *Initial:* 6 mg/24 hr with patch applied daily to upper torso, upper thigh, or outer surface of upper arm. Increased every 2 wk in increments of 3 mg/24 hr, as needed.
Maximum: 12 mg/24 hr.

Mechanism of Action
Reduces dopamine metabolism by noncompetitively inhibiting the brain enzyme monoamine oxidase type B. This increases the amount of dopamine available to relieve symptoms of parkinsonism. Selegiline's metabolites may also enhance dopamine transmission by inhibiting its reuptake at synapses.

Contraindications
Hypersensitivity to selegiline or its components; pheochromocytoma; use within 14 days of meperidine; use within 10 days of general anesthesia; use with carbamazepine, oxcarbazepine, selective serotonin reuptake inhibitors (fluoxetine, paroxetine, sertraline), dual serotonin and norepinephrine reuptake inhibitors (duloxetine, venlafaxine), tricyclic antidepressants (amitriptyline, bupropion, imipramine), analgesics (tramadol, pro-poxyphene), dextromethorphan; use with

St. John's wort, mirtazapine, cyclo-benzaprine, oral selegline, other MAO inhibitors, sympathomimetic amines (Emsam only)

Interactions
DRUGS
carbamazepine, oxcarbazepine: Increased blood selegiline level
fluoxetine, fluvoxamine, nefazodone, paroxetine, sertraline, venlafaxine: Increased risk of adverse reactions similar to those of serotonin syndrome (confusion, hypomania, restlessness, myoclonus), autonomic instability, delirium, muscle rigidity, and severe agitation
levodopa: Increased risk of confusion, dyskinesia, hallucinations, nausea, and orthostatic hypotension
meperidine, possibly other opioid agonists: Increased risk of diaphoresis, excitation, muscle rigidity, and severe hypertension
sympathomimetics: Increased risk of severe hypertension
tricyclic antidepressants: Possibly serious CNS reactions, including decreased level of consciousness, hyperpyrexia, hypertension, muscle rigidity, seizures, and syncope
FOODS
caffeine: Increased risk of hypertension
foods that contain tyramine or other high-pressor amines: Increased risk of sudden and severe hypertension
ACTIVITIES
alcohol use: Increased risk of hypertension

Adverse Reactions
CNS: Anxiety, chills, confusion, dizziness, drowsiness, dyskinesia, euphoria, extrapyramidal reactions, falling asleep during activities of daily living, fatigue, hallucinations, headache, insomnia, irritability, lethargy, memory loss, mood changes, nervousness, paresthesia, restlessness, suicidal ideation, syncope, tremor, weakness
CV: Arrhythmias, chest pain, hypertension, orthostatic hypotension, palpitations, peripheral edema
EENT: Altered taste, blepharospasm, blurred vision, burning lips or mouth, diplopia, dry mouth, pharyngitis, sinusitis, tinnitus

GI: Abdominal pain, anorexia, constipation, diarrhea, GI bleeding, heartburn, nausea, vomiting
GU: Dysuria, urinary hesitancy, urinary urgency, urine retention
MS: Arthralgia, back and leg pain, muscle fatigue and spasms, neck stiffness
RESP: Asthma
SKIN: Diaphoresis, photosensitivity, rash
Other: Application site reactions (Emsam), intense urges to perform certain activities (such as gambling or sex)

Nursing Considerations
• Assess patient for mental status and mood changes because selegiline can worsen such conditions as dementia, severe psychosis, tardive dyskinesia, and tremor. Be especially alert for suicidal tendencies, particularly when therapy starts or dosage changes.
• Monitor patient who is also taking levodopa for levodopa-induced adverse reactions, including confusion, dyskinesia, hallucinations, nausea, and orthostatic hypotension.
• Monitor for decreased symptoms of Parkinson's disease to evaluate drug's effectiveness.
• Be aware that drug can reactivate gastric ulcers because it prevents breakdown of gastric histamine. Assess for related signs and symptoms, such as abdominal pain.
• Assess patient for skin changes regularly because risk of melanoma is increased in patients with Parkinson's disease. It isn't clear whether increase results from disease or drugs used to treat it.
PATIENT TEACHING
• Caution patient to take only prescribed amount because increased dosage may cause severe adverse reactions.
• Advise patient to avoid taking selegiline in the late afternoon or evening because it may interfere with sleep.
• For orally disintegrating tablets, tell patient to take it before breakfast without any liquid. Caution him not to push tablet through the foil on the blister pack but instead to peel back the foil with dry hands and gently remove the tablet. He should then immediately place the tablets on top of his tongue and let it disintegrate. Advise him not to drink or ingest any

Q
R
S

food for 5 minutes before and after taking the drug.
- If patient will use transdermal form, explain how and where to apply patch, stressing need to rotate sites. Tell patient to wash hands well after application and to dispose of removed patch immediately.
- Emphasize that only one patch may be worn at a time. If a patch falls off, tell patient to apply a new patch to a new site and to resume previous schedule.
- Urge patient to avoid tyramine-rich foods and beverages during and for 2 weeks after stopping selegiline therapy unless patient is prescribed the lowest dosage of transdermal system (6 mg per 24 hours), which doesn't require diet modification. Review which foods are considered tyramine-rich.
- Instruct patient to immediately report severe headache, neck stiffness, racing heart, palpitations, or other sudden or unusual symptoms.
- Caution patient to avoid exposing transdermal patch to sources of direct heat, such as heating pads, electric blankets, heat lamps, saunas, hot tubs, and prolonged sunlight exposure.
- Tell patient not to cut transdermal patch into smaller pieces.
- Urge caregiver to monitor patient closely for suicidal tendencies, especially when therapy starts or dosage changes.
- Urge patient to avoid hazardous activities until drug's CNS effects are known.
- Advise patient to change positions slowly to minimize the effects of orthostatic hypotension.
- Suggest that patient elevate his legs when sitting to reduce ankle swelling.
- Urge patient to avoid excessive sun exposure.
- Instruct patient to notify prescriber if symptoms develop that could indicate overdose, including muscle twitching and eye spasms.
- Urge patient to notify prescriber if dry mouth lasts longer than 2 weeks. Advise him to have routine dental checkups.
- Urge patient to have regular skin examinations done by a dermatologist or other qualified health professional.

- Advise patient to notify prescriber about intense urges (as for gambling or sex) because dosage may need to be reduced or drug discontinued.

sertraline hydrochloride
Zoloft

Class and Category
Chemical class: Naphthylamine derivative
Therapeutic class: Antidepressant, anti-obsessant, antipanic
Pregnancy category: C

Indications and Dosages
➤ *To treat major depression*
ORAL CONCENTRATE, TABLETS
Adults. *Initial:* 50 mg daily, increased after several wk in increments of 50 mg daily every wk, as needed. *Maximum:* 200 mg daily.
➤ *To treat obsessive-compulsive disorder*
ORAL CONCENTRATE, TABLETS
Adults and adolescents. *Initial:* 50 mg daily, increased after several wk in increments of 50 mg daily every wk, as needed.
Maximum: 200 mg daily.
Children ages 6 to 12. *Initial:* 25 mg daily, increased every wk, as needed. *Maximum:* 200 mg daily.
➤ *To treat panic disorder, with or without agoraphobia; to treat posttraumatic stress disorder*
ORAL CONCENTRATE, TABLETS
Adults. *Initial:* 25 mg daily, increased to 50 mg daily after 1 wk; then increased by 50 mg daily every wk, as needed.
Maximum: 200 mg daily.
DOSAGE ADJUSTMENT Initial dosage reduction recommended for elderly patients and those with hepatic impairment.
➤ *To treat premenstrual dysphoric disorder (pmdd)*
ORAL CONCENTRATE, TABLETS
Adult women. *Initial:* 50 mg daily in morning or evening throughout menstrual cycle; or, 50 mg daily in morning or evening during luteal phase of menstrual cycle only. Dosage increased each

menstrual cycle in 50-mg increments up to 150 mg daily, or each luteal phase up to 100 mg daily, as needed. Once 100-mg daily dosage established for luteal phase, each successive cycle requires a 50-mg titration step for 3 days at the beginning of each luteal phase.
Maximum: 150 mg daily for dosing throughout menstrual cycle, or 100 mg daily for dosing during luteal phase only.

Route	Onset	Peak	Duration
P.O.	2–4 wk*	Unknown	Unknown

Mechanism of Action
Inhibits reuptake of the neurotransmitter serotonin by CNS neurons, thereby increasing the amount of serotonin available in nerve synapses. An elevated serotonin level may result in elevated mood and reduced depression. This action may also relieve symptoms of other psychiatric conditions attributed to serotonin deficiency.

Contraindications
Concurrent use of disulfiram (oral concentrate) or pimozide; hypersensitivity to sertraline or its components; use within 14 days of an MAO inhibitor, including intravenous methylene blue and linezolid for antiobsessant effect, longer than 4 wk.

Interactions
DRUGS
antidopaminergics, antipsychotics, moclobemide, serotonergics such as 5-HT agonists,buspirone, fenfluramine, fentanyl, lithium, St. John's wort, triptans, tryptophan: Increased risk of potentially fatal serotonin syndrome
aspirin, NSAIDs, warfarin: Increased anticoagulant activity and risk of bleeding
astemizole, terfenadine: Possibly increased blood levels of these drugs, leading to increased risk of arrhythmias
cimetidine: Increased sertraline half-life
MAO inhibitors: Possibly hyperpyretic episodes, hypertensive crisis, serotonin syndrome, and severe seizures
serotonin and norepinephrine reuptake inhibitors: Increased risk of bleeding, especially GI bleeding

tolbutamide: Possibly hypoglycemia
tricyclic antidepressants: Possibly impaired metabolism of tricyclic antidepressants, resulting in increased risk of toxicity

Adverse Reactions
CNS: Abnormal dreams, aggressiveness, agitation, amnesia, anxiety, apathy, cerebrovascular spasm, delusions, depression, dizziness, drowsiness, emotional lability, euphoria, extrapyramidal symptoms, fatigue, fever, hallucination, headache, hyperkinesia, insomnia, nervousness, neuroleptic malignant syndrome-like reaction, paranoid reaction, paresthesia, psychosis, serotonin syndrome, suicidal ideation, tremor, weakness, yawning
CV: Atrial arrhythmias, AV block, bradycardia, palpitations, prolonged QT interval, torsades de pointes, vasculitis, ventricular tachycardia
EENT: Abnormal accommodation, acute closure glaucoma, cataract, conjunctivitis, blindness, dry mouth, earache, epistaxis, eye pain, optic neuritis, rhinitis, sinusitis, teeth grinding, tinnitus, vision changes
ENDO: Hyperglycemia, hyper-prolactinemia, hypothyroidism, syndrome of inappropriate ADH secretion
GI: Abdominal cramps or pain, anorexia, constipation, diarrhea, elevated liver enzymes, flatulence, hepatic dysfunction including failure, hepatitis, increased appetite, indigestion, nausea, pancreatitis, vomiting
GU: Acute renal failure, anorgasmia; decreased libido; ejaculation disorders; impotence; leucorrhea; menstrual disorders; polyuria; urinary frequency, incontinence, or retention; vaginal hemorrhage
HEME: Agranulocytosis, aplastic anemia, leucopenia, pancytopenia, thrombo-cytopenia
MS: Arthralgia, dystonia, muscle cramps or weakness, myalgia
RESP: Bronchospasm, coughing, dyspnea, pulmonary hypertension
SKIN: Diaphoresis, flushing, photo-sensitivity, purpura, rash, severe cutaneous disorders, Stevens-Johnson syndrome
Other: Anaphylaxis, angioedema, lupus-like syndrome, serum sickness, weight loss

Q
R
S

---

* For antidepressant and antipanic effects;

1060 selegiline hydrochloride

Nursing Considerations
- Be aware that sertraline should not be given to patients with congenital long QT syndrome, bradycardia, hypokalemia or hypomagnesemia, recent acute myocardial infarction, or uncompensated heart failure because of increased risk of prolonged QT interval and torsades de pointes. It should also not be given to patients who are taking other drugs that prolong the QT interval. Expect hypokalemia and hypomagnesemia to be corrected before sertraline therapy is begun.
- Monitor liver function test results and BUN and serum creatinine levels, as appropriate, in patients with hepatic or renal dysfunction.

WARNING Monitor patient closely for evidence of serotonin syndrome, such as agitation, hallucinations, coma, tachycardia, labile blood pressure, hyperthermia, hyperreflexia, incoordination, nausea, vomiting, and diarrhea. Serotonin syndrome in its most severe form can resemble neuroleptic malignant syndrome, which includes hyperthermia, muscle rigidity, autonomic instability, possibly rapid changes in vital signs, and mental status changes. Notify prescriber immediately because serotonin syndrome reactions that resemble neuroleptic malignant syndrome may be life-threatening. Be prepared to provide supportive care.

- Monitor patient for hypo-osmolarity of serum and urine and for hyponatremia, which may indicate sertraline-induced syndrome of inappropriate ADH secretion.
- Be aware that effective antidepressant therapy can promote development of mania in predisposed people. If mania develops, notify prescriber immediately and expect to withhold sertraline.
- Watch closely for suicidal tendencies, especially when therapy starts and dosage changes and especially in children and adolescents.
- Monitor patient closely for evidence of GI bleeding, especially if patient takes a drug known to cause it, such as aspirin, an NSAID, a serotonin or norepinephrine reuptake inhibitor, or warfarin.

- When therapy stops, expect to taper dosage to minimize adverse effects rather than stopping drug abruptly.

PATIENT TEACHING
- Advise patient that drug may cause mild pupillary dilation, which may lead to an episode of acute closure glaucoma. Encourage patient to have an eye exam before starting therapy to see if he is at risk.
- Teach patient to dilute oral concentrate before taking it. Tell him to use supplied dropper to remove prescribed amount and mix it with 4 oz (one-half cup) of water, ginger ale, lemon or lime soda, lemonade, or orange juice. Warn him not to mix oral concentrate with anything else. Explain that it's normal for mixture to be slightly hazy.
- Tell patient to take dose immediately after mixing it.
- If patient has latex sensitivity, advise him to use an alternate dispenser because the supplied dropper dispenser contains dry natural rubber.
- Advise patient to avoid hazardous activities until drug's CNS effects are known.

WARNING Tell patient that sertraline increases the risk of serotonin syndrome and reactions that resemble neuroleptic malignant syndrome, rare but serious complications, when taken with some other drugs. Teach patient to recognize signs and symptoms of serotonin syndrome and neuroleptic malignant syndrome, and advise him to notify prescriber immediately if they occur.

- Warn family or caregiver to watch patient closely for evidence of suicidal thinking or behavior, especially when therapy starts or dosage changes, and especially if patient is a child or adolescent.
- Caution patient not to stop taking drug abruptly. Explain that gradual tapering helps to avoid withdrawal symptoms.
- Instruct female patients to notify prescriber if they are or could be pregnant and to discuss benefits and risks of continuing sertraline therapy throughout the pregnancy.
- Advise patient to consult prescriber before taking any OTC product, especially aspirin products or NSAIDs.

• Alert patient that false-positive urine testing for benzodiazepines may occur while taking sertraline, requiring a more sensitive test to be performed.

sevelamer hydrochloride

Renagel

sevelamer carbonate

Renvela

Class and Category
Chemical class: Polyallylamine-epichlorhydrin polymer
Therapeutic class: Antihyperphosphatemic
Pregnancy category: C

Indications and Dosages
➤ To lower serum phosphate level during end-stage renal disease

CAPSULES (RENAGEL)
Adults. 2 capsules (806 mg) three times a day if serum phosphorus level is 6 to 7.5 mg/dl; 3 capsules (1,209 mg) three times a day if serum phosphorus level is 7.6 to 8.9 mg/dl; or 4 capsules (1,612 mg) three times a day if serum phosphorus level is 9 mg/dl or more. Dosage increased or decreased gradually by 1 capsule (403 mg)/ meal, as needed.
Maximum: 30 capsules (12.1 g) daily.

TABLETS (RENVELA)
Adults. 1 tablet (800 mg) three times a day with meals if serum phosphorus level is 5.5 mg/dl to 7.5 mg/dl; or 2 tablets (1,600 mg) three times a day with meals if serum phosphorus level is 7.5 mg/dl or greater. Dosage increased or decreased gradually by 1 tablet (800 mg)/meal at 2-wk intervals, as needed.
DOSAGE ADJUSTMENT For patients being switched from calcium acetate to sevelamer carbonate, 1 tablet of sevelamer (800 mg) can be substituted for every 1 tablet of calcium (667 mg) being taken.

POWDER FOR SUSPENSION (RENVELA)
Adults. 0.8 g three times a day with meals if serum phosphorus level is 5.5 mg/dl to 7.5

mg/dl; or 1.6 g three times a day with meals if serum phosphorus level is 7.5 mg/dl or greater. Dosage increased or decreased gradually by 0.8 g/meal at 2-wk intervals, as needed.
DOSAGE ADJUSTMENT For patients being switched from calcium acetate to sevelamer carbonate, 1 packet of 0.8 g strength powder can be substituted for every 1 tablet (667 mg) being taken.

Mechanism of Action
Inhibits phosphate absorption in the intestine by binding dietary phosphate, thereby lowering serum phosphorus level.

Contraindications
Fecal impaction, GI obstruction, hypersensitivity to sevelamer or its components, hypophosphatemia, ileus

Interactions
DRUGS
antiarrhythmics, anticonvulsants, digoxin, levothyroxine, liothyronine, quinolones, tetracyclines, theophylline, warfarin: Possibly altered absorption of these drugs
phosphate salts, phosphorus salts: Neutralized therapeutic effects of sevelamer
ciprofloxacin: Decreased ciprofloxacin effectiveness

Adverse Reactions
CNS: Headache, fever
CV: Hypertension, hypotension, thrombosis
EENT: Nasopharyngitis
GI: Abdominal pain, constipation (severe), diarrhea, dysphagia, fecal impaction, flatulence, ileus, indigestion, intestinal obstruction or perforation, nausea, vomiting
RESP: Bronchitis, dyspnea, increased cough, upper respiratory tract infection
MS: Arthralgia, back or limb pain
SKIN: Pruritus, rash
Other: Infection

Nursing Considerations
• Give other drugs at least 1 hour before or 3 hours after sevelamer to prevent interaction.
• Suggest suspension form be used in patients with swallowing disorders because tablet may get stuck in the esophagus in these individuals, and they

Q
R
S

may require hospitalization and emergency intervention to remove it.
• Be aware that severe hypophosphatemia may occur in patient with dysphagia, major GI tract surgery, or severe GI motility disorder (including severe constipation) because drug prevents phosphate absorption.
• Monitor blood pressure frequently.
• Monitor serum phosphorus level to determine drug's effectiveness; monitor other serum electrolyte levels, especially bicarbonate and chloride, to detect imbalances.

PATIENT TEACHING
• Tell patient to take drug with meals and to swallow capsules or tablets whole with water and not to open, break, or chew them.
• Instruct patient taking suspension form to mix entire contents of each packet of powder thoroughly with the amount of water indicated on packet. More than one packet can be mixed together. He should stir the mixture vigorously, even though it does not dissolve, and drink entire preparation immediately or up to 30 minutes later (but he will need to stir the mixture again vigorously right before drinking if it was not consumed immediately).
• Caution patient to take other drugs 1 hour before or 3 hours after sevelamer.
• Review symptoms of thrombosis, and advise patient to report them immediately.
• Instruct patient to report severe or prolonged constipation to prescriber because additional treatment may be needed to prevent serious complications.

---

sildenafil citrate
Revatio, Viagra

Class and Category
Chemical class: Pyrazolopyrimidinone derivative
Therapeutic class: Antihypertensive (pulmonary arterial), anti-impotence
Pregnancy category: B

Indications and Dosages
➤ *To treat erectile dysfunction*

TABLETS (VIAGRA)
Adults. 50 mg daily, taken 1 hr before sexual activity; increased as prescribed, based on clinical response. *Maximum:* 100 mg daily.
DOSAGE ADJUSTMENT Initially 25 mg for elderly patients, those with hepatic cirrhosis or creatinine clearance less than 30 ml/min/ 1.73 m², and those taking potent cytochrome P-450 3A4 inhibitors or ritonavir. Dosage reduced to 25 mg if taken within 4 hr of an alpha blocker. *Maximum:* 25 mg/48 hr.
➤ *To treat pulmonary arterial hypertension in order to improve exercise ability and delay clinical worsening of condition in patients classified as group 1 by the World Health Organization*
ORAL SUSPENSION, TABLETS (REVATIO)
Adults. 5 mg or 20 mg three times a day.
I.V. INJECTION (REVATIO)
Adults. 2.5 mg or 10 mg administered as bolus three times a day.

Route	Onset	Peak	Duration
P.O.	In 30 min	Unknown	4 hr

Mechanism of Action
Enhances the effect of nitric oxide released in the penis by stimulation. Nitric oxide increases cGMP level, relaxes smooth muscle, and increases blood flow to the corpus cavernosum, thus producing an erection.

Contraindications
Continuous or intermittent nitrate therapy, hypersensitivity to sildenafil or components

Interactions
DRUGS
barbiturates, bosentan, carbamazepine, efavirenz, nevirapine, phenytoin, rifabutin, rifampin: Altered plasma level of either drug
cimetidine, erythromycin, itraconazole, ketoconazole, mibefradil: Prolonged sildenafil effect
doxazosin and other alpha-blockers: Increased risk of symptomatic hypotension
nitrates: Profound hypotension
protease inhibitors: Increased sildenafil effect rifampin: Decreased sildenafil effect

FOODS

high-fat meals: Drug absorption delayed by up to 60 minutes

Adverse Reactions

CNS: Cerebrovascular, intracerebral, or subarachnoid hemorrhage; dizziness; headache; migraine; seizures; syncope; transient global amnesia, transient ischemic attack

CV: Heart failure, hypertension, hypotension, myocardial infarction or ischemia, orthostatic hypotension, palpitations, sudden cardiac death, tachycardia, vaso-occlusive crisis (presence of sickle cell disease), ventricular arrhythmias

EENT: Blurred vision; change in color perception; diplopia; epistaxis; hearing loss; increased intraocular pressure; nasal congestion; nonarteritic anterior ischemic optic neuropathy; ocular burning, pressure, redness or swelling; paramacular edema; photophobia; retinal vascular bleeding or disease; tinnitus, visual decrease or temporary vision loss; vitreous detachment

ENDO: Uncontrolled diabetes mellitus

GI: Diarrhea, indigestion

GU: Cystitis, dysuria, painful erection, priapism, UTI

MS: Arthralgia, back pain

RESP: Pulmonary hemorrhage, upper respiratory tract infection

SKIN: Flushing, photosensitivity

Nursing Considerations

• Use sildenafil cautiously in patients with renal or hepatic dysfunction, elderly patients, and men with penile abnormalities that may predispose them to priapism. In addition, use cautiously in patients who have suffered a myocardial infarction, stroke, or life-threatening arrhythmia within the last 6 months or in patients with resting hypotension (blood pressure less than 90/50), hypertension (blood pressure greater than 170 or 110), cardiac failure, coronary artery disease causing unstable angina, retinitis pigmentosa, or sickle cell or related anemias, as sildenafil therapy has not been studied in these patient groups.

• Also use cautiously in patients with left ventricular outflow obstruction, such as aortic stenosis and idiopathic hypertrophic subaortic stenosis, and those with severely impaired autonomic control of blood pressure because these conditions increase patient's sensitivity to vasodilators such as sildenafil.

• To reconstitute powder for oral suspension, tap the bottle to release the powder, then remove the cap. Accurately measure out 60 ml of water and pour the water into the bottle, replace the cap, and shake the bottle vigorously for a minimum of 30 seconds. Solution should be clear and colorless and contain 10 mg sildenafil per 12.5 ml of solution. Store drug at room temperature. Discard any remaining oral suspension 60 days after constitution.

• Monitor patient's blood pressure and heart rate and rhythm before and often during therapy.

• Monitor vision, especially in patients over age 50; who have diabetes, hypertension, coronary artery disease, or hyperlipidemia; or who smoke, because sildenafil rarely may cause nonarteritic anterior ischemic optic neuropathy that may lead to decreased vision or permanent vision loss.

WARNING Monitor patient being treated for pulmonary hypertension secondary to sickle cell disease for vaso-occlusive crisis (severe pain and change in color and temperature if extremity is involved). Notify prescriber immediately and prepare to provide supportive care.

PATIENT TEACHING

• Explain that sildenafil used to treat erectile dysfunction may be taken up to 4 hours before sexual activity, but that taking it 1 hour beforehand provides the most effective results.

WARNING Warn patient not to take sildenafil if he also takes any form of organic nitrate, either continuously or intermittently, or other PDE5 inhibitors, including REVATIO (a sildenafil product used to treat another condition), because profound hypotension and death could result. Also caution patient taking sildenafil for erectile dysfunction not to take more than 25 mg within 4 hours of an alpha blocker, such as doxazosin, because symptomatic orthostatic hypotension can occur.

Q
R
S

• Instruct patient prescribed oral suspension form how to mix it, store it, and discard any remaining suspension after 60 days. Stress importance of using the oral dosing syringe that accompanies the drug to measure dosage.

• Tell patient to stop taking drug and contact prescriber if vision decreases suddenly in one or both eyes or if he has a loss of hearing, possibly with tinnitus and dizziness.

• Advise patient taking sildenafil for erectile dysfunction to seek sexual counseling to enhance the drug's effects.

• To avoid possible penile damage and permanent loss of erectile function, urge patient to notify prescriber immediately if erection is painful or lasts longer than 4 hours.

• Instruct diabetic patient to monitor his blood glucose level frequently because drug may affect glucose control.

silodosin
Rapaflo

Class and Category
Chemical class: Highly selective alpha$_1$-adrenergic receptor blocker
Therapeutic class: Benign prostatic anti-hyperplasia agent
Pregnancy category: B

Indications and Dosages
➤ *To treat symptomatic benign prostatic hyperplasia*
CAPSULES
Adult men. 8 mg daily. *Maximum:* 8 mg daily.
DOSAGE ADJUSTMENT For patients with moderate renal impairment (creatinine clearance between 30 and 50 ml/min), dosage reduced to 4 mg daily.

Mechanism of Action
Binds to postsynaptic alpha$_1$ adreno-receptors located in the prostate gland, bladder base and neck, and prostatic capsule and urethra. Blocking action at these adrenoreceptor sites causes relaxation of smooth muscle in the local area, which improves urine flow and reduces other benign prostatic hyperplasia symptoms.

Contraindications
Hypersensitivity to silodosin and its components, severe hepatic insufficiency (Child-Pugh score 10 or above), severe renal insufficiency (creatinine clearance less than 30 ml/min/1.73 m^2), use with strong CYP3A4 inhibitors such as clarithromycin, ketoconazole, itraconazole, and ritonavir

Interactions
DRUGS
alpha blockers: Possibly increased effects and risk of adverse reactions
antihypertensives: Increased risk of dizziness and orthostatic hypotension
cyclosporine, CYP3A4 inhibitors such as clarithromycin, diltiazem, erythromycin, itraconazole, ketoconazole, ritonavir: Possibly increased serum silodosin levels and risk of adverse reactions
PDE5 inhibitors: Possibly increased risk of orthostatic hypotension

Adverse Reactions
CNS: Asthenia, dizziness, headache, insomnia, syncope
CV: Orthostatic hypotension
EENT: Nasal congestion, nasopharyngitis, rhinorrhea, sinusitis
GI: Abdominal pain, diarrhea, elevated liver enzymes, impaired hepatic function, jaundice
GU: Elevated prostate specific antigen level, retrograde ejaculation
SKIN: Pruritus, purpura, rash, toxic skin eruption, urticaria
Other: Angioedema

Nursing Considerations
• Use cautiously in patients with mild renal impairment and mild or moderate hepatic impairment. Patients with moderate renal impairment need dosage adjustment.

• Monitor patient's blood pressure for reduction, especially if he takes an antihypertensive with silodosin.

PATIENT TEACHING
• Instruct patient to take drug with a meal.

• Tell patient who has difficulty swallowing capsules that he may carefully open the capsule and sprinkle the powder on a tablespoonful of applesauce and take within 5 minutes without chewing. He should then drink an 8-oz glass of cool water immediately afterwards. Inform him

that the applesauce should not be hot and it should be soft enough to be swallowed without chewing.
• Advise patient to avoid hazardous activities until drug's CNS effects are known.
• Advise patient planning cataract surgery or other ocular procedure to tell ophthalmologist that he takes silodosin or has taken it in the past because of potential adverse reactions.

simvastatin

Zocor

Class and Category
Chemical class: Synthetically derived fermentation product of *Aspergillus terreus*
Therapeutic class: Antihyperlipidemic
Pregnancy category: X

Indications and Dosages
➤ *To treat hyperlipidemia*
TABLETS
Adults. *Initial:* 20 to 40 mg daily in the evening. Dosage adjusted at 4-wk intervals, as needed, to achieve target LDL-cholesterol level. *Maintenance:* 5 to 80 mg daily. *Maximum:* 80 mg daily.
DOSAGE ADJUSTMENT Patients who have severe renal insufficiency should initially receive 5 mg simvastatin daily and be increased as needed to no more than 10 mg daily. Maximum dosage of 10 mg daily should also not be exceeded in patients who are also taking fibrates other than gemfibrozil or niacin. Maximum dosage of 10 mg daily should not be exceeded in patients taking verapamil or diltiazem and 20 mg daily should not be exceeded in patients taking amiodarone, amlodipine, or ranolazine. For patients taking voriconazole, dosage may need to be reduced. For Chinese patients, maximum dosage of 80 mg daily reduced if patient is also taking 1 gram or more daily of niacin.
➤ *To treat homozygous familial hypercholesterolemia*
TABLETS
Adults. 40 mg daily in the evening, or 80 mg/day in 3 divided doses—20 mg, 20 mg, and 40 mg (in the evening). Dosage

adjusted every 4 wk, as needed, to achieve target LDL-cholesterol level. *Maintenance:* 5 to 40 mg/day. *Maximum:* 80 mg daily, although this is not recommended for any patients not currently taking it without problems.
DOSAGE ADJUSTMENT Patients who have severe renal insufficiency should initially receive 5 mg simvastatin daily and be increased as needed to no more than 10 mg daily. Maximum dosage of 10 mg daily should also not be exceeded in patients who are also taking fibrates other than gemfibrozil or niacin. Maximum dosage of 10 mg daily should not be exceeded in patients taking diltiazem or verapamil; 20 mg daily should not be exceeded in patients taking amiodarone, amlodipine, or ranolazine. For patients taking voriconazole, dosage may need to be reduced. For Chinese patients, maximum dosage of 80 mg daily reduced if patient is also taking 1 gram or more daily of niacin.
➤ *To treat adolescent heterozygous familial hypercholesterolemia*
TABLETS
Children ages 10 to 17 at least 1 year postmenarche. *Initial:* 10 mg daily in the evening. Adjusted every 4 wk, as needed, to achieve target LDL-cholesterol level. *Maintenance:* 10 to 40 mg daily. *Maximum:* 40 mg daily.
DOSAGE ADJUSTMENT For patients with renal impairment, initial dosage reduced to 5 mg daily. For patients who take diltiazem, dronedarone, or verapamil, daily dosage should not exceed 10 mg; for patients who take amiodarone, amlodipine, or ranolazine, daily dosage should not exceed 20 mg. For patients who take voriconazole, dosage may need to be reduced. For patient with homozygous familial hypercholesterolemia taking lomitapide, daily dosage should not exceed 20 mg. For patients with homozygous familial hypercholesterolemia who have been taking 80 mg of simvastatin for 12 months or longer and have no evidence of muscle toxicity, daily dosage should not exceed 40 mg when taking lomitapide.

Mechanism of Action
Interferes with the hepatic enzyme hydroxymethylglutaryl-coenzyme A

Q
R
S

reductase. This action reduces the formation of mevalonic acid, a cholesterol precursor, thus interrupting the pathway necessary for cholesterol synthesis. When the cholesterol level declines in hepatic cells, LDLs are consumed, which in turn reduces the levels of circulating total cholesterol and serum triglycerides.

Route	Onset	Peak	Duration
P.O.	2 wk	4–6 wk	Unknown

Contraindications

Active hepatic disease; breastfeeding; concurrent use with strong CYP3A4 inhibitors such as boceprevir, clarithromycin, erythromycin, HIV protease inhibitors, itraconazole, ketoconazole, nefazodone, posaconazole, telaprevir, or telithromycin; concurrent use with cobicistat-containing products, cyclosporine, danazol, or gemfibrozil; hypersensitivity to simvastatin or its components; pregnancy

Interactions

DRUGS
amiodarone, amlodipine, antiretroviral protease inhibitors including combinations (amprenavir,boceprevir, indinavir, nelfinavir, ritonavir, saquinavi, telaprevir), azole antifungals, boceprevir, cobicistat-containing products, clarithromycin, colchicine, cyclosporine, danazol, dronedarone, erythromycin, gemfibrozil and other fibrates, itraconazole, ketoconazole, nefazodone, niacin (1 g daily or more), posaconazole, ranolazine, telithromycin, verapamil, voriconazole: Increased risk of myopathy or rhabdomyolysis
azole antifungals, cyclosporine, gemfibrozil, immunosuppressants, macrolide antibiotics (including erythromycin), niacin, verapamil: Increased risk of acute renal failure
bile acid sequestrants, cholestyramine, colestipol: Decreased simvastatin bioavailability
digoxin: Possibly slight elevation in blood digoxin level
diltiazem, lomitapide, verapamil: Possibly increased blood simvastatin level, increased risk of myopathy
oral anticoagulants: Increased bleeding or prolonged PT

FOODS
grapefruit juice (1 or more quarts daily): Increased risk of myopathy or rhabdomyolysis

Adverse Reactions

CNS: Asthenia, cognitive impairment, dizziness, fatigue, headache, insomnia, vertigo
CV: Atrial fibrillation, chest pain, edema
EENT: Cataracts, rhinitis, sinusitis
ENDO: Elevated hemoglobin A1C levels, hyperglycemia
GI: Abdominal pain, constipation, diarrhea, elevated liver function test results, flatulence, gastritis, heartburn, hepatic failure, indigestion, nausea, pancreatitis, vomiting
GU: Erectile dysfunction, UTI
MS: Immune-mediated necrotizing myopathy, myalgia, myopathy, rhabdomyolysis
RESP: Bronchitis, interstitial lung disease, upper respiratory tract infection
SKIN: Eczema, pruritus, rash

Nursing Considerations

• Use simvastatin cautiously in elderly patients and those with renal or hepatic impairment.
• Know that 80 mg of simvastatin should be used rarely, since it is associated with a high risk of myopathy. If 40 mg of simvastatin is not sufficiently efficacious, then an alternative agent should be used.
• Also, use cautiously in Chinese patients who are receiving more than 20 mg daily of simvastatin and are also receiving lipid-modifying doses of niacin-containing products because of increased risk for myopathy. Know that these patients should not receive 80 mg of simvastatin daily if they are taking concurrently 1 gram or more of a niacin-containing product.
• Give drug 1 hour before or 4 hours after giving bile acid sequestrant, cholestyramine, or colestipol.
• Monitor serum lipoprotein level, as ordered, to evaluate response to therapy.
• Expect to obtain liver function tests prior to initiation of simvastatin therapy and then thereafter, as needed.
• Monitor patient for elevated CPK level (as ordered) or for muscle pain, tenderness, or

weakness and other symptoms of myopathy; if left unchecked, the more serious form—rhabdomyolysis—may occur, which may lead to renal failure. If CPK level is significantly elevated or patient has symptoms of myopathy, notify prescriber and expect to withhold drug, as ordered.

PATIENT TEACHING
• Urge patient to take drug in the evening.
• Urge patient to follow low-fat, cholesterol-lowering diet.
• Urge patient to notify prescriber immediately about muscle pain, tenderness, or weakness and other symptoms of myopathy and symptoms of abnormal liver function such as anorexia, dark urine, fatigue, right upper abdominal discomfort, or yellowing of skin.
• Inform female patient of childbearing age of need to use reliable contraceptive method while taking drug. Instruct her to notify prescriber at once if she suspects pregnancy.
• Advise patient to avoid grapefruit juice to decrease risk of drug toxicity.
• Inform patient with diabetes of need to test his blood sugar regularly and to obtain an HbA1c periodically.
• Encourage patient or family to notify prescriber if patient develops or exhibits worsening memory loss, forgetfulness, and confusion.
• Alert patient of increased risk for myopathy if he takes 80 mg of simvastatin daily.

sirolimus
(rapamycin)
Rapamune

Class and Category
Chemical class: Macrocyclic lactone
Therapeutic class: Immunosuppressant
Pregnancy category: C

Indications and Dosages
➤ *To prevent rejection of kidney transplantation*
ORAL SOLUTION
Adults and adolescents over age 13 weighing 40 kg (88 lb) or more. *Initial:* 6-mg loading dose. *Maintenance:* 2 mg daily.

Adolescents over age 13 weighing less than 40 kg. *Initial:* 3-mg/m^2 loading dose. *Maintenance:* 1 mg/m^2 daily.
dosage adjustment Maintenance dosage reduced by one-third for patients with impaired hepatic function. Maintenance dosage increased by as much as 400% for patients discontinuing concomitant cyclosporine therapy in order to maintain blood sirolimus trough level of 12 to 24 nanograms/ml.

Route	Onset	Peak	Duration
P.O.	Unknown	Unknown	Up to 6 mo after discontinuation

Mechanism of Action
Inhibits activation and proliferation of T lymphocytes and antibody production. Sirolimus also inhibits cell cycle progression from the G1 to the S phase, possibly by inhibiting a key regulatory kinase believed to suppress cytokine-driven T-cell proliferation.

Contraindications
Hypersensitivity to sirolimus or its components, malignancy

Interactions
DRUGS
aminoglycosides, amphotericin B, cyclosporine: Possibly impaired renal function
bromocriptine, cimetidine, cisapride, clarithromycin, clotrimazole, cyclosporine, danazol, diltiazem, erythromycin, fluconazole, indinavir, itraconazole, ketoconazole, metoclopramide, nicardipine, ritonavir, troleandomycin, verapamil: Possibly increased blood sirolimus level and toxicity
calcineurin inhibitors: Increased risk of deteriorating renal function, serum lipid abnormalities, or development of UTI, hemolytic uremic syndrome (HUS), thrombotic thrombocytopenic purpura (TTP), or thrombotic microangiopathy (TMA)
carbamazepine, phenobarbital, phenytoin, rifabutin, rifapentin, St. John's wort: Possibly decreased blood sirolimus level
corticosteroids: Increased risk of deteriorating renal function, serum lipid abnormalities, and UTI

Q
R
S

HMG-CoA reductase inhibitors: Increased risk of rhabdomyolysis when administered concurrently with sirolimus and cyclosporine
rifampin: Significantly increased sirolimus clearance
vaccines (killed virus): Possibly decreased immune response to vaccines
vaccines (live virus): Increased risk of contracting disease from live virus
FOODS
grapefruit juice: Possibly decreased metabolism of sirolimus
high-fat diet: Reduced rate of sirolimus absorption

Adverse Reactions

CNS: Asthenia, fever, headache, insomnia, progressive multifocal leukoencephalopathy (PML), tremor
CV: Atrial fibrillation, chest pain, hyperlipidemia, hypersensitivity vasculitis, hypertension, pericardial effusion, peripheral edema
ENDO: Hyperglycemia
GI: Abdominal pain, ascites, constipation, diarrhea, elevated liver enzymes, hepatotoxicity, nausea, vomiting
GU: Azoospermia, BK viral nephritis, elevated serum creatinine level, focal segmental glomerulosclerosis, menstrual disorders, nephrotic syndrome, ovarian cysts, proteinuria, UTI
HEME: Anemia, neutropenia, pancytopenia, thrombocytopenia
MS: Arthralgia, low back or flank pain, joint abnormality
RESP: Dyspnea on exertion, interstitial lung disease, pleural effusion, pulmonary hemorrhage
SKIN: Acne, cancer, exfoliative dermatitis, rash
Other: Anaphylaxis; angioedema; delayed wound healing; hypercholesterolemia; hypokalemia; hypophosphatemia; increased susceptibility to infection, including opportunistic infections such as tuberculosis and activation of latent viral infections; lymphedema; lymphoma; weight gain or loss

Nursing Considerations

• Be aware that sirolimus isn't recommended in liver or lung transplant patients.

• Use sirolimus cautiously in patients who are receiving other drugs known to adversely affect renal function, such as aminoglycosides and amphotericin B; together, they may further decrease renal function.
• Monitor patients with existing or recent (including recent exposure to) chickenpox and patients with herpes zoster for worsening symptoms because they have an increased risk of developing severe generalized disease while taking sirolimus.
• Mix oral sirolimus with at least 2 oz (60 ml) of water or orange juice in a glass or plastic container. Don't dilute drug in grapefruit juice or any other liquid.
• Stir well and have patient drink solution immediately. Then rinse glass with at least 4 oz (120 ml) of additional liquid, stir well, and have patient drink that liquid to make sure that all of drug is taken.
• Give initial dose as soon after transplantation as possible and daily dose 4 hours after cyclosporine, as prescribed.
• Monitor whole blood sirolimus concentrations, as ordered, in patients receiving concentrated form of drug, patients weighing less than 40 kg (88 lb), patients with hepatic impairment, and those receiving potent CYP3A4 inducers or inhibitors concurrently.
• When using trough level to determine drug's effectiveness, keep in mind that dosage adjustment should be made only after other factors are taken into account, such as signs, symptoms, and tissue biopsy findings. Keep in mind that interpretation methods vary among laboratories and values aren't interchangeable.
• Monitor serum creatinine level, as ordered, because BK virus associated nephropathy has occurred with sirolimus therapy. In addition, patients receiving sirolimus and cyclosporine may develop impaired renal function. Notify prescriber of any increases in serum creatinine level because sirolimus or cyclosporine dosage may need to be adjusted or drug discontinued.
• Monitor patient for urinary protein excretion, as ordered. If protein appears in urine, sirolimus may be discontinued.

- Monitor patient for signs and symptoms of infection and check CBC results, as ordered, to detect sirolimus-induced blood dyscrasias or changes in neutrophil count, which may indicate infection.
- For patients with hyperlipidemia, be prepared to institute dietary changes, an exercise program, or a lipid-lowering drug regimen if blood cholesterol or triglyceride levels increase because drug may aggravate hyperlipidemia.

PATIENT TEACHING
- Advise patient to take sirolimus consistently either with or without food (but not food high in fat) to prevent changes in absorption rate.
- Instruct patient to take daily dose with at least 2 oz (60 ml) of water or orange juice. Caution him not to dilute drug in grapefruit juice or any other liquid. Advise him to stir mixture well and drink immediately, then to add at least another 4 oz (120 ml) of liquid to empty container, stir mixture again, and drink that liquid to ensure that he has swallowed all of drug.
- Urge patient to avoid people with colds, flu, or other infections because immunosuppression makes him more vulnerable.
- Instruct patient not to take live vaccines, such as measles, mumps, rubella, oral polio, bacille Calmette-Guérin, yellow fever, varicella, and TY21a typhoid, during sirolimus therapy.
- Inform patient that sirolimus therapy may increase his risk of skin cancer. Tell him to avoid prolonged sun exposure, tanning booths, and sun lamps. He should use a sunscreen with a high protection factor and wear protective clothing when outdoors.
- Advise patient to keep follow-up appointments for blood tests, as ordered.

sitagliptin

Januvia

Class and Category
Chemical class: Beta amino acid derivative
Therapeutic class: Antidiabetic
Pregnancy category: C

Indications and Dosages
➤ *To achieve control of glucose level in type 2 diabetes mellitus as monotherapy or with metformin or other thiazolidinediones*

TABLETS
Adults. 100 mg once daily.

DOSAGE ADJUSTMENT For patients with moderate renal insufficiency (creatinine clearance 30 to 50 ml/min/1.73 m²), dosage reduced to 50 mg once daily; for patients with severe renal insufficiency (creatinine clearance less than 30 ml/min/1.73 m²) or end-stage renal disease requiring hemodialysis or peritoneal dialysis, dosage reduced to 25 mg once daily.

Route	Onset	Peak	Duration
P.O.	Unknown	1–4 hr	Unknown

Mechanism of Action
Inhibits the dipeptidyl peptidase-4 enzyme to slow inactivation of incretin hormones. These hormones are released by the intestine throughout the day but increase in response to a meal. When blood glucose level is normal or increased, incretin hormones increase insulin synthesis and release from pancreatic beta cells. One type of incretin hormone, glucagon-like peptide (GLP-1) also lowers glucagon secretion from pancreatic alpha cells, which reduces hepatic glucose production. These combined actions decrease blood glucose level in type 2 diabetes.

Contraindications
Diabetic ketoacidosis, hypersensitivity to sitagliptin or its components, type 1 diabetes

Interactions
DRUGS
ACE inhibitors, disopyramide, fibric acid derivatives, fluoxetine, sulfonylureas: Possibly increased hypoglycemic effects
beta blockers: Possibly prolonged hypoglycemia or promotion of hyper-glycemia
digoxin: Slightly increased plasma digoxin level
estrogens, oral contraceptives, phenytoin, progestins, thiazide diuretics, triamterene: Possibly decreased hypoglycemic effects

Adverse Reactions
CNS: Headache
EENT: Nasopharyngitis

Q
R
S

GI: Abdominal pain, acute pancreatitis, constipation, diarrhea, elevated hepatic enzymes, nausea, vomiting
GU: Acute renal failure, worsening renal function
RESP: Upper respiratory tract infection
MS: Arthralgia, back or extremity pain, myalgia
SKIN: Cutaneous vasculitis, rash, Stevens-Johnson syndrome, urticaria
Other: Anaphylaxis, angioedema

Nursing Considerations
• Assess patient's renal function before starting sitagliptin therapy, as ordered, and periodically thereafter. In moderate to severe renal dysfunction, dosage will be reduced.
• Monitor patient for hypersensitivity reactions that, although uncommon, may be severe. If present, notify prescriber and expect sitagliptin to be discontinued.
• Monitor patient's blood glucose level, as ordered, to determine effectiveness of sitagliptin therapy.

PATIENT TEACHING
• Emphasize the need to follow an exercise program and a diet control program during sitagliptin therapy.
• Warn patient not to split, crush, or chew the tablet before swallowing.
• Advise patient to notify prescriber immediately if she has trouble breathing, or has hives, rash, or swelling.
• Inform patient that periodic blood tests will be done to determine effectiveness of drug and to assess kidney function.
• Teach patient how to monitor blood glucose level and when to report changes.
• Caution patient that taking other drugs in addition to sitagliptin to control his diabetes may lead to hypoglycemia. Review signs, symptoms, and appropriate prescribed treatment with him.
• Instruct patient to contact prescriber if he develops other illnesses, such as infection, or experiences trauma or surgery because his diabetes medication may need adjustment.
• Advise patient to carry identification indicating that she has diabetes.
• Instruct patient to stop taking sitagliptin and report persistent severe abdominal pain, possibly radiating to the back and accompanied by vomiting.

sodium bicarbonate
Arm and Hammer Pure Baking Soda, Bell/ans, Citrocarbonate, Soda Mint

Class and Category
Chemical class: Electrolyte
Therapeutic class: Antacid, electrolyte replenisher, systemic and urinary alkalizer
Pregnancy category: C

Indications and Dosages
➤ *To treat hyperacidity*
EFFERVESCENT POWDER
Adults and adolescents. 3.9 to 10 g in a glass of water after meals. *Maximum:* 19.5 g daily.
Children ages 6 to 12. 1 to 1.9 g in a glass of water after meals.
ORAL POWDER
Adults and adolescents. One-half tsp in a glass of water every 2 hr, as needed. *Maximum:* 4 tsp daily in patients up to age 60.
TABLETS
Adults and adolescents. 325 mg to 2 g daily to four times a day, as needed. *Maximum:* 16 g daily.
Children ages 6 to 12. 520 mg, repeated once after 30 min, as needed.
➤ *To provide urinary alkalization*
ORAL POWDER
Adults and adolescents. 1 tsp in a glass of water every 4 hr. *Maximum:* 4 tsp daily in patients up to age 60.
TABLETS
Adults and adolescents. *Initial:* 4 g, then 1 to 2 g every 4 hr. *Maximum:* 16 g daily.
Children. 23 to 230 mg/kg daily, adjusted as needed.
I.V. INFUSION
Adults and children. 2 to 5 mEq/kg over 4 to 8 hr.
➤ *To treat metabolic acidosis during cardiac arrest*
I.V. INJECTION
Adults and children. *Initial:* 1 mEq/kg, followed by 0.5 mEq/kg every 10 min while arrest continues.
➤ *To treat less urgent forms of metabolic acidosis*
I.V. INFUSION
Adults and children. 2 to 5 mEq/kg over 4 to 8 hr.

DOSAGE ADJUSTMENT Dosage reduction possible for elderly patients because of age-related renal impairment.

Mechanism of Action

Increases plasma bicarbonate level, buffers excess hydrogen ions, and raises blood pH, thereby reversing metabolic acidosis. Sodium bicarbonate also increases the excretion of free bicarbonate ions in urine, raising urine pH; increased alkalinity of urine may help to dissolve uric acid calculi. In addition, it relieves symptoms of hyperacidity by neutralizing or buffering existing stomach acid, thereby increasing the pH of stomach contents.

Incompatibilities

Don't admix I.V. form of sodium bicarbonate in same solution or administer through same I.V. line as other drugs because precipitate may form.

Contraindications

Hypocalcemia in which alkalosis may lead to tetany; hypochloremic alkalosis secondary to vomiting, diuretics, or nasogastric suction; preexisting metabolic or respiratory alkalosis

Interactions
DRUGS

amphetamines, quinidine: Decreased urinary excretion of these drugs, possibly resulting in toxicity
anticholinergics: Decreased anticholinergic absorption and effectiveness
calcium-containing products: Increased risk of milk-alkali syndrome
chlorpropamide, lithium, salicylates, tetracyclines: Increased renal excretion and decreased absorption of these drugs
ciprofloxacin, norfloxacin, ofloxacin: Decreased solubility of these drugs, leading to crystalluria and nephrotoxicity
citrates: Increased risk of systemic alkalosis; increased risk of calcium calculus formation and hypernatremia in patients with history of uric acid calculi
digoxin: Possibly elevated digoxin level
enteric-coated drugs: Increased risk of gastric or duodenal irritation from rapid removal of enteric coating
ephedrine: Increased ephedrine half-life and duration of action

H₂-receptor antagonists, iron supplements or preparations, ketoconazole: Decreased absorption of these drugs
mecamylamine: Decreased excretion and prolonged effect of mecamylamine
methenamine: Decreased methenamine effectiveness
mexiletine: Possibly mexiletine toxicity
potassium supplements: Decreased serum potassium level
sucralfate: Interference with binding of sucralfate to gastric mucosa
urinary acidifiers (ammonium chloride, ascorbic acid, potassium and sodium phosphates): Counteracted effects of urinary acidifiers
FOODS
dairy products: Increased risk of milk-alkali syndrome with prolonged use of sodium bicarbonate

Adverse Reactions
CNS: Mental or mood changes
CV: Irregular heartbeat, peripheral edema (with large doses), weak pulse
EENT: Dry mouth
GI: Abdominal cramps, thirst
MS: Muscle spasms, myalgia
SKIN: Extravasation with necrosis, tissue sloughing, or ulceration

Nursing Considerations
• Monitor sodium intake of patient taking sodium bicarbonate because effervescent powder contains 700.6 mg of sodium/3.9 g; oral powder contains 952 mg of sodium/tsp; and tablets contain 325 mg/3.9-mEq tablet, 520 mg/6.2-mEq tablet, and 650 mg/7.7-mEq tablet.
• For I.V. infusion, dilute drug with normal saline solution, D₅W, or other standard electrolyte solution before administration.
• Avoid rapid I.V. infusion, which can cause severe alkalosis. Be aware that during cardiac arrest, risk of death from acidosis may outweigh risks of rapid infusion.
• Monitor urine pH, as ordered, to determine drug's effectiveness as urine alkalizer.
• If patient on long-term sodium bicarbonate therapy is consuming calcium or milk, watch for milk-alkali syndrome, characterized by anorexia, confusion, headache, hypercalcemia, metabolic acidosis, nausea, renal insufficiency, and vomiting.

Q
R
S

• Be aware that parenteral forms are hypertonic and that increased sodium intake can produce edema and weight gain.
• Assess I.V. site often for evidence of extravasation. If it occurs, notify prescriber at once and remove I.V. catheter. Elevate the limb, apply warm compresses, and expect prescriber to administer a local injection of hyaluronidase or lidocaine.

PATIENT TEACHING
• Advise patient not to take sodium bicarbonate with large amounts of dairy products or for longer than 2 weeks, unless directed by prescriber.
• Caution patient not to take more drug than prescribed to avoid adverse reactions.
• Direct patient not to take drug within 2 hours of other oral drugs.
• Advise patient to avoid taking other prescribed or OTC drugs without prescriber's approval because many drugs interact with sodium bicarbonate.

sodium ferric gluconate

(contains 62.5 mg elemental iron per 5 ml)
Ferrlecit

Class and Category
Chemical class: Iron salt, mineral
Therapeutic class: Antianemic
Pregnancy category: B

Indications and Dosages
➤ *To treat iron deficiency anemia in patients receiving long-term hemodialysis and erythropoietin*

I.V. INFUSION OR INJECTION
Adults. 125 mg of elemental iron. *Usual:* Minimum cumulative dose of 1 g elemental iron given over eight sequential dialysis treatments. Dosage repeated at lowest dosage needed to maintain target levels of hemoglobin and hematocrit and acceptable limits of blood iron level.

Mechanism of Action
Acts to replenish iron stores lost during hemodialysis as a result of increased blood loss or increased iron utilization from epoetin therapy. Iron is an essential component of hemoglobin, myoglobin, and several enzymes, including cytochromes, catalase, and peroxidase, and is needed for catecholamine metabolism and normal neutrophil function. Sodium ferric gluconate also normalizes RBC production by binding with hemoglobin or being stored as ferritin in reticuloendothelial cells of the liver, spleen, and bone marrow.

Incompatibilities
Don't mix sodium ferric gluconate with other drugs or parenteral nutrition solutions for I.V. infusion.

Contraindications
Anemia other than iron deficiency, hypersensitivity to iron salts or their components, iron overload

Interactions
DRUGS
oral iron preparations: Possibly reduced absorption of oral iron supplements

Adverse Reactions
CNS: Asthenia, dizziness, fatigue, fever, headache, hypertonia, nervousness, paresthesia, syncope
CV: Chest pain, generalized edema, hypertension, hypotension, tachycardia
EENT: Dry mouth
GI: Abdominal pain, diarrhea, nausea, vomiting
HEME: Hemorrhage
MS: Back pain, leg cramps
RESP: Cough, dyspnea, upper respiratory tract infection, wheezing
SKIN: Diaphoresis, pruritus
Other: Anaphylaxis, generalized pain, hyperkalemia, hypersensitivity, infusion or injection-site reaction

Nursing Considerations
• To reconstitute sodium ferric gluconate for I.V. infusion, dilute prescribed dosage in 100 ml of normal saline solution immediately before infusion. Infuse over 1 hour. Discard any unused diluted solution.
• Inspect drug for particles and discoloration before administration and discard if present.
• Give undiluted drug by slow I.V. injection at up to 12.5 mg/min, not to exceed 125 mg per injection.

• Be aware that most patients need a minimum cumulative dose of 1 gram of elemental iron administered over eight sequential dialysis treatments.

WARNING Assess patient for evidence of allergic reaction, including chills, facial flushing, pruritus, and rash, and of a hypersensitivity reaction, including diaphoresis, dyspnea, nausea, severe lower back pain, vomiting, and wheezing. Discontinue drug and notify prescriber immediately if patient develops an allergic or hypersensitivity reaction, and be prepared to provide emergency interventions.

WARNING Assess blood pressure often after drug administration because hypotension may occur and may be related to infusion rate or total cumulative dose. Avoid rapid infusion, and be prepared to provide I.V. fluids for volume expansion.

• Expect to monitor blood hemoglobin level, hematocrit, serum ferritin level, and transferrin saturation, as ordered, before, during, and after sodium ferric gluconate therapy. Make sure serum iron level is tested 48 hours after last dose. To prevent iron toxicity, notify prescriber and expect to end therapy if blood iron level is normal or elevated.

• Assess patient for possible iron overload, characterized by bleeding in GI tract and lungs, decreased activity, pale conjunctivae, and sedation.

PATIENT TEACHING

• Warn patient not to take any oral iron preparations during sodium ferric gluconate therapy without first consulting prescriber.

• Inform patient that symptoms of iron deficiency may include decreased stamina, learning problems, shortness of breath, and fatigue.

sodium phenylbutyrate

Buphenyl

Class and Category

Chemical class: Phenylacetate prodrug

Therapeutic class: Antihyperammonemic
Pregnancy category: C

Indications and Dosages

➤ *As adjunct to treat urea cycle disorders in combination with low-protein diet*

POWDER, TABLETS

Adults and children weighing more than 20 kg (44 lb). 9.9 to 13 g/m^2 daily in 4 to 6 divided doses with meals.

Children weighing up to 20 kg. 450 to 600 mg/kg daily in 4 to 6 divided doses with meals.

Mechanism of Action

Provides alternate pathway for eliminating waste nitrogen by forming phenylacetate, an active metabolite that conjugates with glutamine to produce phenylacetyl-glutamine, which is excreted by the kidneys.

Contraindications

Acute hyperammonemia, hypersensitivity to sodium phenylbutyrate or its components

Interactions

DRUGS

corticosteroids: Increased serum ammonia level

haloperidol, valproate: Increased risk of hyperammonemia

probenecid: Decreased excretion of conjugated product of sodium phenylbutyrate

Adverse Reactions

CNS: Depression, disorientation, fatigue, headache, light-headedness, memory loss, syncope
CV: Arrhythmias
EENT: Hypoacusis, taste perversion
GI: Abdominal pain, anorexia, constipation, elevated liver function test results, gastritis, nausea, peptic ulcer, rectal bleeding, vomiting
GU: Amenorrhea, menstrual irregularities
HEME: Anemia, aplastic anemia, leukocytosis, leukopenia, thrombocytopenia
SKIN: Rash
Other: Body odor, hyperchloremia, hypoalbuminemia, hypophosphatemia, metabolic acidosis, metabolic alkalosis, weight gain

Q
R
S

Nursing Considerations

• Mix powder form of sodium phenyl-butyrate with food or liquid, but not with acidic beverages such as coffee and tea.

• Be aware that drug shouldn't be used to treat acute hyperammonemia, which is a medical emergency.

• Monitor patient with history of heart failure or severe renal failure for fluid retention because of drug's sodium content.

PATIENT TEACHING

• Instruct patient to take sodium phenyl-butyrate with meals but not to mix it with acidic beverages such as coffee and tea.

• Advise patient to comply with follow-up laboratory tests, as prescribed.

• Urge patient to notify prescriber immediately about changes in body odor because they may signal metabolic imbalance.

sodium polystyrene sulfonate

Kayexalate, K-Exit (CAN), Kionex, PMS-Sodium Polystyrene Sulfonate (CAN), SPS Suspension

Class and Category

Chemical class: Sulfonated cation-exchange resin
Therapeutic class: Antihyperkalemic
Pregnancy category: C

Indications and Dosages

➤ *To treat hyperkalemia*

ORAL POWDER, SUSPENSION

Adults. 15 g (4 level tsp) once daily to four times a day.
Maximum: 40 g four times a day.
Children. 1 g/kg/dose, as needed.

RECTAL POWDER, SUSPENSION

Adults. 25 to 100 g as retention enema, as needed.
Children. 1 g/kg/dose as retention enema, as needed.

Route	Onset	Peak	Duration
P.O.	2–12 hr	Unknown	Unknown

Mechanism of Action

Releases sodium ions in exchange for other cations in intestines. Resin enters large intestine and releases sodium ions in exchange for hydrogen ions. As the resin moves through the intestines, hydrogen ions are then exchanged for potassium ions, which are in greater concentration. Bound resin leaves the body in feces, carrying potassium and other ions with it, thereby reducing serum potassium level.

Contraindications

Hypersensitivity to sodium polystyrene sulfonate or its components, hypokalemia, obstructive bowel disease, reduced intestinal motility in neonates, oral administration in neonates

Interactions

DRUGS

aluminum hydroxide: Increased risk of intestinal obstruction
antacids, laxatives: Increased risk of metabolic alkalosis
potassium-sparing diuretics, potassium supplements: Increased risk of fluid retention

Adverse Reactions

CV: Peripheral edema
GI: Abdominal cramps, anorexia, colonic necrosis, constipation, diarrhea, epigastric pain, fecal impaction, GI bleeding, indigestion, intestinal necrosis, ischemic colitis, nausea, perforation, vomiting
GU: Decreased urine output
Other: Hypernatremia, hypocalcemia, hypokalemia, hypomagnesemia, weight gain

Nursing Considerations

• Know that sodium polystyrene sulfonate should not be given to a patient who has not had a bowel movement post-surgery, or in patients who are at risk for developing constipation or impaction (including patients with a history of impaction, chronic constipation, inflammatory bowel disease, ischemic colitis, vascular intestinal atherosclerosis, previous bowel resection or bowel obstruction) because these factors increase the risk for intestinal necrosis, which may be life-threatening.

- Use sodium polystyrene sulfonate cautiously in patients with heart failure, hypertension, or marked edema.
- Be aware that drug is available as powdered resin or as solution that contains sorbitol to facilitate movement of resin through intestines. As a result, patient may experience abdominal cramps, diarrhea, nausea, and vomiting.
- Because the drug doesn't take effect for several hours, be aware that it's inappropriate for treating acute, life-threatening hyperkalemia.
- If patient has hypokalemia or hypocalcemia, notify prescriber immediately and expect to withhold drug because it reduces potassium and calcium levels. Evidence of hypokalemia includes abdominal cramps, acidic urine, anorexia, drowsiness, ECG changes, hypotension, hypoventilation, muscle weakness, and tachycardia. Evidence of hypocalcemia includes abdominal pain, agitation, anxiety, ECG changes, hypotension, muscle twitching, psychosis, seizures, and tetany.
- To give powdered resin as oral suspension, mix powder in water, syrup, or food and give promptly, being sure to follow full aspiration precautions (such as keeping patient in an upright position while giving drug). If needed, administer through gastric feeding tube.
- Precede rectal administration with a cleansing enema, as ordered.
- When giving rectally, suspend powdered resin in 100 ml of aqueous solution warmed to body temperature, in bag connected to soft, large (French 28) catheter. Have patient lie on his left side with his lower leg straight and upper leg flexed or with his knees to his chest. Gently insert the tube into the rectum and well into the sigmoid colon. The solution should flow into the colon by way of gravity and be retained for 30 to 60 minutes or longer, if possible. After patient is unable to retain the solution any longer, administer a non-sodium-containing cleansing enema, as prescribed.
- Use of sorbitol with sodium polystyrene sulfonate isn't recommended because of increased risk of colonic necrosis and other serious GI effects, such as bleeding, ischemic colitis, and perforation.

- After administration, assess for constipation and fecal impaction. If either occurs, notify prescriber, expect drug to be discontinued, and provide care, as ordered, to relieve constipation or fecal impaction.

PATIENT TEACHING
- Instruct patient not to mix oral form of sodium polystyrene sulfonate with foods and liquids high in potassium content, such as bananas and orange juice.
- If patient will self-administer rectal solution, teach the correct technique and body position. Remind him to let the solution flow into the colon by gravity and to retain it for at least 30 to 60 minutes, longer if possible.
- Advise patient to notify prescriber immediately about abdominal cramps, nausea, and vomiting.

sodium thiosalicylate

Rexolate, Tusal

Class and Category

Chemical class: Salicylic acid derivative
Therapeutic class: Analgesic, anti-inflammatory
Pregnancy category: Not rated

Indications and Dosages

➤ *To relieve symptoms of acute gout*
I.V. OR I.M. INJECTION
Adults. *Initial:* 100 mg every 3 to 4 hr for 2 days; then 100 mg daily.
➤ *To relieve pain from musculoskeletal conditions*
I.V. OR I.M. INJECTION
Adults. 50 to 100 mg daily or every other day.
➤ *To relieve symptoms of osteoarthritis*
I.V. OR I.M. INJECTION
Adults. 100 mg 3 times/wk for several wk, then once/wk, usually up to a total dosage of 2.5 g. After 1 to 2 wk, another course of treatment may be given.
➤ *To treat rheumatic fever*
I.V. OR I.M. INJECTION
Adults. *Initial:* 100 to 150 mg every 4 to 8 hr for 3 days, then 100 mg twice daily.

Q
R
S

Mechanism of Action

Exerts peripherally induced analgesic and anti-inflammatory effects by blocking pain impulses and inhibiting prostaglandin synthesis.

Contraindications

GI bleeding; hemophilia; hemorrhage; hypersensitivity to sodium thiosalicylate, NSAIDs, or their components; Reye's syndrome

Interactions
DRUGS

ACE inhibitors, beta blockers: Decreased antihypertensive effect of these drugs
activated charcoal: Decreased sodium thiosalicylate absorption
antacids, urinary alkalizers: Increased excretion of sodium thiosalicylate, leading to reduced drug effectiveness and shortened half-life
carbonic anhydrase inhibitors (such as acetazolamide): Increased risk of salicylate toxicity; possibly displacement of acetazolamide from protein-binding sites, resulting in toxicity
corticosteroids: Possibly increased sodium thiosalicylate excretion
insulin, oral antidiabetic drugs: Altered glucose control (with large sodium thiosalicylate doses)
loop diuretics: Possibly decreased effectiveness of loop diuretics in patients with renal or hepatic impairment
methotrexate: Increased risk of methotrexate toxicity
nizatidine: Increased blood sodium thiosalicylate level
probenecid, sulfinpyrazone: Decreased uricosuric effects
spironolactone: Possibly inhibited diuretic effect of spironolactone
urinary acidifiers (including ammonium chloride, ascorbic acid, methionine): Decreased sodium thiosalicylate excretion, possibly leading to salicylate toxicity
ACTIVITIES
alcohol use: Increased risk of gastrointestinal ulceration

Adverse Reactions

GI: Anorexia, diarrhea, GI bleeding, heartburn, hepatotoxicity, indigestion, nausea, thirst, vomiting

HEME: Leukopenia, platelet dysfunction, prolonged bleeding time, thrombocytopenia
RESP: Bronchospasm
SKIN: Rash, urticaria
Other: Angioedema

Nursing Considerations

• Use drug cautiously in patients with asthma, chronic urticaria, or nasal polyps because these patients are more prone to hypersensitivity.
• Expect to monitor hepatic and renal function during long-term drug therapy.
• After repeated use or large doses, look for signs of salicylate toxicity: CNS depression, confusion, diaphoresis, diarrhea, difficulty hearing, dizziness, headache, hyperventilation, lassitude, tinnitus, and vomiting. .
• Be aware that tinnitus usually means that the blood sodium thiosalicylate level has reached or exceeded the upper limit for therapeutic effects.
PATIENT TEACHING
• Instruct patient to notify prescriber immediately about bleeding or symptoms of salicylate toxicity.

solifenacin succinate

VESIcare

Class and Category

Chemical class: Muscarinic receptor antagonist
Therapeutic class: Bladder antispasmodic
Pregnancy category: C

Indications and Dosages

➤ *To treat overactive urinary bladder with symptoms of urge incontinence, urgency, and frequency*
TABLETS
Adults. 5 mg daily; if tolerated well, increased to 10 mg daily.
DOSAGE ADJUSTMENT For patients with severe renal impairment or moderate hepatic impairment or patients taking ketoconazole or other potent CYP3A4 inhibitors, dosage limited to 5 mg daily.

Route	Onset	Peak	Duration
P.O.	Unknown	3–8 hr	Unknown

Mechanism of Action
Antagonizes the effect of acetylcholine on muscarinic receptors in detrusor muscle, decreasing the muscle spasms that cause inappropriate bladder emptying. This action increases bladder capacity and volume, which relieves the sensation of urgency and frequency and enhances bladder control.

Contraindications
Gastric retention, hypersensitivity to solifenacin or its components, uncontrolled angle-closure glaucoma, urine retention

Interactions
DRUGS
ketoconazole, other potent CYP3A4 inhibitors: Possibly decreased metabolism of solifenacin and increased risk of adverse effects

Adverse Reactions
CNS: Confusion, delirium, depression, dizziness, fatigue, hallucinations, headache, somnolence
CV: Atrial fibrillation, hypertension, palpitations, prolonged QT interval, peripheral edema, tachycardia, torsades de pointes
EENT: Blurred vision, dry eyes or mouth, glaucoma, pharyngitis
GI: Abdominal pain, anorexia, constipation, elevated liver enzyme levels, gastroesophageal reflux disease, ileus, indigestion, nausea, vomiting
GU: Renal impairment, UTI, urinary retention
MS: Muscle weakness
RESP: Airway obstruction from angio-edema, cough, dysphonia
SKIN: Erythema multiforme, exfoliative dermatitis, pruritus, rash, urticaria
Other: Anaphylaxis, angioedema, flulike symptoms, hyperkalemia

Nursing Considerations
• Use cautiously in patients with ulcerative colitis, intestinal atony, or myasthenia gravis because solifenacin may decrease GI motility; in patients with significant bladder outflow obstruction because

solifenacin may cause urine retention; in patients with hepatic impairment because solifenacin is metabolized in the liver; and in patients with renal impairment because solifenacin excretion may be impaired.
• Monitor patient closely, even after first dose, for hypersensitivity reactions. Although uncommon, anaphylactic reactions and angioedema have occurred with solifenacin therapy. Be prepared to manage these life-threatening reactions and expect drug to be discontinued if they occur.
• Monitor patient for signs of anti-cholinergic CNS adverse reactions, especially after treatment is begun or dosage increased.
• Monitor elderly patients, especially those age 75 and over, for adverse reactions because they're at increased risk for solifenacin-induced adverse reactions.
PATIENT TEACHING
• Instruct patient to take solifenacin with a full glass of water and to swallow the tablet whole.
• Caution patient to avoid exertion in a warm or hot environment because sweating may be delayed, which could increase body temperature and increase risk of heatstroke.
• Advise patient to avoid potentially hazardous activities until drug's CNS effects are known.
• Inform patient that alcohol may cause drowsiness, and urge patient to limit or avoid alcoholic beverages while taking solifenacin.

sotalol hydrochloride

Betapace, Betapace AF, Sotacor (CAN), Sotylize

Class and Category
Chemical class: Methanesulfonanilide
Therapeutic class: Class III antiarrhythmic
Pregnancy category: B

Indications and Dosages
➤ *To treat life-threatening ventricular arrhythmias*

Q
R
S

TABLETS

Adults. *Initial:* 80 mg once or twice daily, increased, as needed, in increments of 80 mg every 3 days provided patient's QT interval is less than 500 ms. *Maintenance:* 160 to 320 mg daily in divided doses twice daily or three times a day. *Maximum:* 640 mg daily.

Children. Highly individualized based on age and body surface area.

DOSAGE ADJUSTMENT If creatinine clearance is 30 to 60 ml/min/1.73 m^2, dosage interval extended to every 24 hr; if creatinine clearance is less than 30 ml/min/1.73 m^2, dosage interval extended to every 36 to 48 hr, according to response; if creatinine clearance less than 10 ml/min/1.73 m^2, dosage adjusted as prescribed.

➤ *To maintain normal sinus rhythm in patients with highly symptomatic atrial fibrillation who are currently in sinus rhythm*

TABLETS

Adults. *Initial:* If creatinine clearance is 40 to 60 ml/min/1.73 m^2, 80 mg daily; if creatinine clearance exceeds 60 ml/min/1.73 m^2, 80 mg twice daily. *Maintenance:* After at least 3 days (five or six doses given daily), if 80-mg dose is tolerated and QT interval less than 500 msec, dosage maintained and patient discharged. Or hospitalized patient monitored closely to determine maintenance dosage while dosage increased to 120 mg twice daily for 3 days (five or six doses if daily dosing). *Maximum:* 160 mg twice daily if creatinine clearance exceeds 60 ml/min/1.73 m^2.

DOSAGE ADJUSTMENT If 80-mg once or twice daily doesn't reduce frequency of atrial fibrillation relapses and is tolerated without excessive QT-interval prolongation (greater than 520 msec), dosage increased to 120 mg once or twice daily, depending on creatinine clearance. If 120-mg dose doesn't reduce frequency of early relapse and is tolerated using same criteria, dosage increased to 160 mg once or twice daily, depending on creatinine clearance.

DOSAGE ADJUSTMENT If QT interval is 520 msec or more, dosage reduced until it returns to less than 520 msec. If QT interval exceeds 520 msec with lowest maintenance dosage of 80 mg, drug discontinued. If

renal function deteriorates, daily dose reduced by half and given daily.

Route	Onset	Peak	Duration
P.O.	Unknown	2–3 hr	Unknown

Mechanism of Action

Combines class II and class III antiarrhythmic activity to increase sinus cycle length. This beta blocker decreases AV nodal conduction and increases AV nodal refractoriness. Suppression of SA node automaticity and AV node conductivity decreases atrial and ventricular ectopy.

Contraindications

Asthma, atrial arrhythmias (if baseline QT interval exceeds 450 msec or creatinine clearance is less than 40 ml/min/1.73 m^2), cardiogenic shock, congenital or acquired QT syndromes, COPD, heart failure (unless it results from tachyarrhythmia that's treatable by sotalol), hypersensitivity to sotalol or its components, second- or third-degree AV block without functioning pacemaker, sinus bradycardia

Interactions

DRUGS

allergen immunotherapy, allergenic extracts for skin testing: Increased risk of serious systemic adverse reaction or anaphylaxis
amiodarone: Additive depressant effect on conduction, negative inotropic effect
anesthetics (hydrocarbon inhalation): Increased risk of myocardial depression and hypotension
antacids: Altered sotalol effectiveness
astemizole, class I antiarrhythmics, phenothiazines, terfenadine, tricyclic antidepressants: Prolonged QT interval, life-threatening torsades de pointes
beta blockers (other): Additive beta blockade
beta$_2$-receptor stimulants: Decreased effectiveness of these drugs
calcium channel blockers, clonidine, diazoxide, guanabenz, reserpine and other antihypertensives: Additive antihypertensive effect and, possibly, other beta-blocking effects
cimetidine: Possibly impaired sotalol clearance
digoxin: Increased risk of bradycardia

glucagon: Possibly blunted hyperglycemic response
insulin, oral antidiabetic drugs: Impaired glucose control, increased risk of hyperglycemia
lidocaine: Decreased lidocaine clearance, increased risk of lidocaine toxicity
MAO inhibitors: Increased risk of significant hypertension
neuromuscular blockers: Possibly potentiated and prolonged neuromuscular blockade
phenothiazines: Increased blood levels of both drugs
propafenone: Increased blood level and half-life of sotalol
sympathomimetics, xanthines: Possibly mutual inhibition of therapeutic effects

Adverse Reactions

CNS: Anxiety, depression, dizziness, drowsiness, fatigue, insomnia, lethargy, nervousness, weakness
CV: AV conduction disorders, bradycardia, heart failure, hypotension, peripheral vascular insufficiency
EENT: Nasal congestion
ENDO: Hyperglycemia, hypoglycemia
GI: Abdominal pain, constipation, diarrhea, nausea, vomiting
GU: Sexual dysfunction
MS: Muscle weakness
RESP: Bronchospasm, dyspnea, wheezing

Nursing Considerations

• Expect to obtain baseline creatinine clearance and QT interval before starting sotalol and periodically throughout therapy, as ordered.
• Monitor blood pressure, apical and radial pulses, fluid intake and output, daily weight, respiratory rate, and circulation in limbs before and during sotalol therapy.
• If prescriber is stopping amiodarone, be aware that sotalol shouldn't be started until QT interval has returned to baseline because of possible adverse cardiac effects.
• Be aware that stopping sotalol abruptly may cause life-threatening reactions. For this reason, chronic beta blocker therapy such as sotalol is not routinely withheld prior to major surgery. However, be aware that the impaired ability of the heart to

respond to reflex adrenergic stimuli may increase the risks of general anesthesia and surgical procedures.
• Monitor serum electrolyte levels because drug can increase risk of torsades de pointes in patients with electrolyte imbalances, especially hypokalemia or hypomagnesemia.
• Assess carefully if patient has diabetes mellitus or thyrotoxicosis because they may mask hypoglycemia and hyperthyroidism.

PATIENT TEACHING
• Advise patient to notify prescriber immediately if he has difficulty breathing.
• Urge patient to consult prescriber before taking OTC drugs, especially cold remedies, which may decrease sotalol's effectiveness.
• Urge patient to avoid hazardous activities until drug's CNS effects are known.

---

sparfloxacin
Zagam

Class and Category
Chemical class: Fluoroquinolone
Therapeutic class: Antibiotic
Pregnancy category: C

Indications and Dosages
➤ *To treat community-acquired pneumonia caused by* Chlamydia pneumoniae, Haemophilus influenzae, H. parainfluenzae, Moraxella catarrhalis, Mycoplasma pneumoniae, *or* streptococcus pneumoniae *and acute bacterial exacerbations of chronic bronchitis caused by* C. pneumoniae, Enterobacter cloacae, H. influenzae, H. parainfluenzae, Klebsiella pneumoniae, M. catarrhalis, Staphylococcus aureus, *or* S. pneumoniae

TABLETS
Adults. 400 mg on day 1, followed by 200 mg/day for 10 days.
DOSAGE ADJUSTMENT For patients with creatinine clearance less than 50 ml/min/1.73 m^2, 400 mg on day 1 and then dosing interval extended to 200 mg every 48 hr for 9 days.

Q
R
S

Mechanism of Action
Causes bacterial cells to die by inhibiting the enzyme DNA gyrase, which is responsible for unwinding and supercoiling bacterial DNA before it replicates.

Contraindications
History of photosensitivity, hypersensitivity to quinolone derivatives, job or lifestyle that precludes compliance with measures to prevent phototoxicity, prolonged QTc interval or use of drugs that can prolong QTc interval

Interactions
DRUGS
aluminum-, calcium-, or magnesium-containing antacids; ferrous sulfate; magnesium-containing laxatives; sucralfate; zinc: Decreased bioavailability of sparfloxacin
amiodarone, astemizole, bepridil, cisapride, class IA antiarrhythmics (disopyramide, quinidine, procainamide), class III antiarrhythmics (ibutilide, sotalol), erythromycin, pentamidine, phenothiazines, terfenadine, tricyclic antidepressants, other drugs that can prolong QTc interval: Possibly prolonged QTc interval and torsades de pointes

Adverse Reactions
CNS: Asthenia, cerebral thrombosis, dizziness, drowsiness, headache, insomnia, light-headedness, nervousness, seizures, somnolence
CV: Cardiopulmonary arrest, embolism, prolonged QTc interval, torsades de pointes, vasodilation
EENT: Laryngeal edema, taste perversion
GI: Abdominal pain, diarrhea, hepatic necrosis or failure, hepatitis, intestinal perforation, nausea, pseudomembranous colitis, vomiting
GU: Acute renal failure, vaginal candidiasis
HEME: Agranulocytosis, hemolytic anemia, pancytopenia, thrombocytopenia
MS: Rhabdomyolysis, tendinitis, tendon rupture
RESP: Interstitial pneumonia, pulmonary edema
SKIN: Photosensitivity, pruritus, rash, Stevens-Johnson syndrome, toxic epidermal necrolysis
Other: Acidosis, anaphylaxis, angioedema, squamous cell carcinoma

Nursing Considerations
- Use sparfloxacin cautiously in patients with known or suspected CNS disorders because of risk of seizures. Institute seizure precautions according to facility policy.
- Monitor renal and liver function test results, as appropriate, during prolonged therapy.
- Measure QTc interval regularly because sparfloxacin has been found to increase QTc interval and risk of torsades de pointes.
- Severe diarrhea may indicate pseudomembranous colitis; give fluid, electrolyte, and protein replacement, as ordered.

PATIENT TEACHING
- Urge patient to avoid potentially hazardous activities until sparfloxacin's CNS effects are known.
- Advise patient to notify prescriber at once about aching or throbbing tendon pain.
- Instruct patient to wait 4 hours after taking sparfloxacin before taking antacids that contain aluminum, calcium, or magnesium; laxatives that contain magnesium; or vitamins that contain iron or zinc.
- Caution patient to avoid exposure to sunlight, bright natural light, and other sources of ultraviolet light during therapy and for 5 days afterward. Urge him to wear sunscreen and protective clothing when outdoors.
- Urge patient to notify prescriber at first sign of photosensitivity reaction (blistering, burning or swelling sensation, itching, rash, redness).

spectinomycin hydrochloride
Trobicin

Class and Category
Chemical class: Aminocyclitol, aminoglycoside derivative
Therapeutic class: Antibiotic
Pregnancy category: Not rated

Indications and Dosages
➤ *To treat acute endocervical, rectal, and urethral gonorrhea caused by susceptible strains of* Neisseria gonorrhoeae

I.M. INJECTION
Adults and children weighing 45 kg (99 lb) or more. 2 g as a single dose, repeated as prescribed for adult if reinfection occurs or is strongly suspected. *Maximum:* 4 g for adults, 2 g for children.
Children weighing less than 45 kg (except infants). 40 mg/kg as a single dose.

Mechanism of Action
Binds to negatively charged sites on bacterial outer cell membrane, disrupting cell integrity, and binds to bacterial ribosomal subunits, inhibiting protein synthesis. Both actions lead to bacterial cell death.

Contraindications
Hypersensitivity to spectinomycin or its components

Adverse Reactions
CNS: Dizziness, insomnia
GI: Abdominal cramps, nausea, vomiting
Other: Injection-site pain

Nursing Considerations
• To reconstitute spectinomycin, add 3.2 ml bacteriostatic water for injection (with benzyl alcohol) to each 2-g vial or 6.2 ml of diluent to each 4-g vial. Shake vial vigorously before withdrawing dose.
• Administer I.M. injection deep into large muscle mass, preferably upper outer quadrant of gluteal muscle.

PATIENT TEACHING
• Tell patient he'll be tested for syphilis at the start of treatment and 3 months later because spectinomycin treatment may mask or delay syphilis symptoms.
• Explain risk factors for sexually transmitted diseases, and teach correct condom use.
• Advise patient to encourage sexual partner to be tested for gonorrhea.
• Instruct patient to notify prescriber if signs and symptoms persist after a few days.

spironolactone
Aldactone, Novospiroton (CAN)

Class and Category
Chemical class: Aldosterone antagonist

Therapeutic class: Aldosterone antagonist, antihypertensive, diagnostic aid for primary hyperaldosteronism, diuretic
Pregnancy category: Not rated

Indications and Dosages
➤ *To treat edema cause by heart failure, hepatic cirrhosis, or nephrotic syndrome*
TABLETS
Adults. *Initial:* 25 to 200 mg daily in divided doses twice daily to four times a day for at least 5 days. *Maintenance:* 75 to 400 mg daily in divided doses twice daily to four times a day. *Maximum:* 400 mg daily.
Children. *Initial:* 1 to 3 mg/kg daily as a single dose or in divided doses twice daily to four times a day for at least 2 wk; adjusted, as needed, after 5 days. *Maximum:* 3 times initial dose.
➤ *To treat hypertension*
TABLETS
Adults. *Initial:* 50 to 100 mg daily as a single dose or in divided doses twice daily to four times a day for at least 2 wk; gradually adjusted every 2 wk, as needed, to control blood pressure, up to 200 mg daily. *Maximum:* 400 mg daily.
Children. *Initial:* 1 to 3 mg/kg daily as a single dose or in divided doses twice daily to four times a day for at least 2 wk; adjusted, as needed, after 5 days. *Maximum:* 3 times initial dose.
➤ *To aid in the diagnosis of primary hyperaldosteronism*
TABLETS
Adults. For long test, 400 mg daily in divided doses twice daily to four times a day for 3 to 4 wk; for short test, 400 mg daily in divided doses twice daily to four times a day for 4 days.
➤ *To treat primary hyperaldosteronism*
TABLETS
Adults. 100 to 400 mg daily in divided doses twice daily to four times a day before surgery. *Maximum:* 400 mg daily.
DOSAGE ADJUSTMENT Long-term maintenance dosage decreased for patients at risk for complications during surgery.
➤ *To substitute as therapy for diuretic-induced hypokalemia*
TABLETS
Adults. 25 to 100 mg daily as a single dose or in divided doses twice daily to four times a day. *Maximum:* 400 mg daily.

Q
R
S

Route	Onset	Peak	Duration
P.O.*	Unknown	2–3 days	2–3 days

Contraindications

Acute renal insufficiency, Addison's disease or other conditions associated with hyperkalemia, anuria, concomitant use of eplerenone, hyperkalemia, hypersensitivity to spironolactone or its components

Interactions

DRUGS

ACE inhibitors, aldosterone blockers, angiotensin II antagonists, cyclosporine, heparin and low molecular weight heparin, NSAIDs, indomethacin, other potassium-sparing diuretics, potassium-containing drugs, potassium supplements: Increased risk of severe hyperkalemia
cholestyramine: Increased risk of hyperkalemic metabolic acidosis
digoxin: Possibly increased half-life of digoxin
exchange resins (sodium cycle), such as sodium polystyrene sulfonate: Increased risk of hypokalemia and fluid retention
heparin, oral anticoagulants: Decreased anticoagulant effect of these drugs
hypotension-producing drugs: Possibly potentiated antihypertensive or diuretic effect of spironolactone
lithium: Possibly lithium toxicity
NSAIDs, sympathomimetics: Decreased antihypertensive effect of spironolactone
FOODS
high potassium diet, low-salt milk, salt substitutes: Increased risk of severe hyperkalemia

Adverse Reactions

CNS: Dizziness, encephalopathy, fatigue, headache, lethargy, somnolence
EENT: Increased intraocular pressure, nasal congestion, tinnitus, vision changes
ENDO: Breast pain, gynecomastia
GI: Abdominal pain, anorexia, constipation, diarrhea, flatulence, nausea, vomiting
GU: Impotence
HEME: Agranulocytosis, aplastic anemia, leucopenia, neutropenia, thrombocytopenia
RESP: Cough, dyspnea

---

* For diuretic effect; others unknown

MS: Arthralgia, back and leg pain, leg cramps, muscle weakness, myalgia
SKIN: Alopecia, drug rash with eosinophilia and systemic symptoms (DRESS), pruritus, Stevens-Johnson syndrome, toxic epidermal necrolysis
Other: Electrolyte disturbances including dilutional hyponatremia, hyperkalemia, and hyperchloremic metabolic acidosis

Nursing Considerations

• Be aware that for children or patients who have trouble swallowing, pharmacist may crush spironolactone tablets, mix with flavored syrup, and dispense as a suspension. It's stable for 1 month when refrigerated.
• In diagnosing primary aldosteronism, test is considered positive if patient's serum potassium level rises when spironolactone is given and falls when it's discontinued.
• Expect to evaluate patient's serum potassium level 1 week after spironolactone therapy begins, after each dosage adjustment, monthly for the first 3 months, quarterly for 1 year, and then every 6 months thereafter or as ordered. Notify prescriber if level exceeds 5 mEq/L or patient's renal function deteriorates (serum creatinine level exceeding 4 mg/dl). If patient has severe heart failure, follow closely because hyperkalemia may be fatal in such patients.
• Evaluate spironolactone's effectiveness by assessing blood pressure and edema.
• Stop drug for several days, as prescribed, before patient undergoes adrenal vein catheterization to measure serum aldosterone level and plasma renin activity.

PATIENT TEACHING

• Instruct patient to take spironolactone with meals or milk.
• If patient can't swallow tablets, mention that pharmacist can crush and mix them with a flavored syrup as a suspension.
• Teach patient who takes spironolactone for hypertension how to measure his blood pressure. Urge him to monitor it regularly and report pressure greater than 140 mm Hg systolic or 90 mm Hg diastolic to prescriber.
• Caution patient that he may experience dizziness during spironolactone therapy if fluid balance is altered.

Mechanism of Action

Normally, aldosterone attaches to receptors on the walls of distal convoluted tubule cells, causing sodium (Na^+) and water (H_2O) reabsorption in the blood, as shown at left. Spironolactone competes with aldosterone for these receptors, thereby preventing sodium and water reabsorption and causing their excretion through the distal convoluted tubules, as shown below right. Increased urinary excretion of sodium and water reduces blood volume and blood pressure.

• Warn patient to avoid performing hazardous activities, such as driving, until adverse effects of drug are known.
• Instruct patient to inform prescriber of any new condition or new drug therapy, including over-the-counter medications, so that prescriber can evaluate if the patient is at increased risk for hyperkalemia.

streptokinase
Kabikinase, Streptase

Class and Category
Chemical class: Purified beta-hemolytic *Streptococcus* filtrate
Therapeutic class: Thrombolytic
Pregnancy category: C

Indications and Dosages
➤ *To lyse coronary artery thrombi*
I.V. INFUSION
Adults. 1,500,000 international units within 60 min of event.
INTRACORONARY INFUSION
Adults. 20,000-international unit bolus, followed by 2,000 international units/min

for 60 min for total dose of 140,000 international units.
➤ *To lyse acute arterial thromboembolism or thrombosis, acute pulmonary embolism, or deep vein thrombosis*
I.V. INFUSION
Adults. 250,000-international unit bolus over 30 min, followed by 100,000 international units/hr for 24 to 72 hr.
➤ *To clear an occluded arteriovenous cannula*
I.V. INJECTION
Adults. 100,000 to 250,000 international units instilled slowly into each occluded lumen.

Mechanism of Action
Binds to fibrin in thrombus and converts trapped plasminogen to plasmin. Plasmin breaks down fibrin, fibrinogen, and other clotting factors, thereby dissolving the thrombus.

Route	Onset	Peak	Duration
I.V.	Immediate	20–120 min	4 hr

Incompatibilities
Don't mix streptokinase in the same syringe or give through the same I.V. line as other drugs.

Q
R
S

Contraindications

Active internal bleeding, AV malformation or aneurysm, bleeding diathesis, history of stroke or intracranial or intraspinal surgery within the previous 2 months, hypersensitivity to streptokinase or its components, intracranial cancer, severe uncontrolled hypertension

Interactions

DRUGS

anticoagulants, enoxaparin, heparin, NSAIDs, platelet aggregation inhibitors: Increased risk of bleeding
antifibrinolytics: Antagonized effects of both drugs
antihypertensives: Increased risk of severe hypotension, especially when streptokinase is administered rapidly to treat coronary artery occlusion
cefamandole, cefoperazone, cefotetan, plicamycin, valproic acid: Possibly hypoprothrombinemia and increased risk of severe hemorrhage
corticosteroids, ethacrynic acid, salicylates: Possibly GI ulceration or bleeding

Adverse Reactions

CNS: Chills, fever
CV: Arrhythmias, hypotension
HEME: Unusual bleeding or bruising

Nursing Considerations

• Obtain hematocrit, platelet count, APTT, PT, and INR, as ordered, before giving streptokinase.
• To prevent foaming, don't shake drug during reconstitution.
• Check frequently for bleeding at I.V. site and for blood in urine and stool. Perform neurologic assessment to detect intracranial bleeding.
• If serious spontaneous bleeding (not controlled by local pressure) occurs, stop streptokinase infusion immediately and notify prescriber.
• Monitor heart rate and rhythm by continuous ECG, as ordered.
• Treat fever with acetaminophen, as prescribed, rather than aspirin to reduce the risk of bleeding.

PATIENT TEACHING

• Explain to patient that he'll be on bed rest during streptokinase therapy.

• Inform patient that minor bleeding may occur at arterial puncture or surgical sites. Reassure him that appropriate care measures will be taken if bleeding occurs.
• Advise patient to wear or carry medical alert identification stating that he takes streptokinase.
• Inform patient that if he experiences chest pain within 12 months of therapy, he should notify healthcare providers that he has received streptokinase because repeated administration within 12 months may be ineffective.

streptomycin sulfate

Class and Category

Chemical class: Aminoglycoside
Therapeutic class: Antibiotic
Pregnancy category: D

Indications and Dosages

➤ *To treat gram-negative bacillary bacteremia, meningeal infections, pneumonia, systemic infections, and UTI caused by susceptible strains of* Aerobacter aerogenes, Brucella, Calymmatobacterium granulomatis, Enterococcus faecalis, Escherichia coli, Haemophilus ducreyi, H. influenzae, Klebsiella pneumoniae, *and* Proteus

I.M. INJECTION

Adults. 1 to 2 g daily in divided doses every 6 to 12 hr. *Maximum:* 2 g daily.
Children. 20 to 40 mg/kg daily in divided doses every 6 to 12 hr.

➤ *As adjunct to treat endocarditis caused by* Streptococcus viridans *or* E. faecalis

I.M. INJECTION

Adults. 1 g twice daily for 1 wk (*S. viridans*) or 2 wk (*E. faecalis*) with penicillin. Then, 500 mg twice daily for 1 wk (*S. viridans*) or 4 wk (*E. faecalis*).

➤ *As adjunct to treat tuberculosis caused by* Mycobacterium tuberculosis

I.M. INJECTION

Adults. 1 g daily with other antibiotics; dosage reduced to 1 g 2 or 3 times/wk, as appropriate and prescribed. *Maximum:* 2 g daily.
Children. 20 mg/kg daily with other antibiotics. *Maximum:* 1 g daily.

DOSAGE ADJUSTMENT For elderly patients, dosage decreased to 500 to 750 mg daily in combination with other antibiotics.

➤ *To treat plague caused by* Yersinia pestis

I.M. INJECTION

Adults. 2 g daily in 2 equally divided doses for at least 10 days.

Children. 30 mg/kg daily in divided doses twice daily or three times a day for 10 days.

➤ *To treat tularemia caused by* Francisella tularensis

I.M. INJECTION

Adults. 1 to 2 g daily in divided doses for 7 to 14 days.

DOSAGE ADJUSTMENT If creatinine clearance is 50 to 80 ml/min/1.73 m^2, dosage reduced to 7.5 mg/kg I.M. every 24 hr; if 10 to 49 ml/min/1.73 m^2, 7.5 mg/kg I.M. every 24 to 72 hr; if less than 10 ml/min/1.73 m^2, 7.5 mg/kg I.M. every 72 to 96 hr.

Mechanism of Action

Binds to negatively charged sites on the bacteria's outer cell membrane, disrupting cell integrity. Streptomycin also binds to bacterial ribosomal subunits and inhibits protein synthesis. Both actions lead to bacterial cell death.

Incompatibilities

Don't mix streptomycin in same solution or administer through same I.V. line as other antibiotics.

Contraindications

Hypersensitivity to streptomycin or other aminoglycosides

Interactions

DRUGS

antimyasthenics: Possibly decreased effect of antimyasthenics on skeletal muscle

beta-lactam antibiotics: Inactivation of streptomycin

capreomycin, other aminoglycosides: Increased potential for ototoxicity, nephro- toxicity, and neuromuscular blockade

indomethacin (I.V.): Decreased renal clearance of streptomycin when given to premature neonates, possibly leading to aminoglycoside toxicity

methoxyflurane, polymyxins (parenteral): Increased risk of nephrotoxicity and neuromuscular blockade

nephrotoxic and ototoxic drugs: Increased risk of nephrotoxicity and ototoxicity

neuromuscular blockers: Increased neuromuscular blockade

Adverse Reactions

CNS: Clumsiness, dizziness, neurotoxicity, paresthesia, peripheral neuropathy, seizures, unsteadiness, vertigo

EENT: Hearing loss, sensation of fullness in ears, tinnitus, vision loss

GI: Anorexia, nausea, thirst, vomiting

GU: Decreased or increased urine output, nephrotoxicity

MS: Muscle twitching

SKIN: Erythema, pruritus, rash, urticaria

Nursing Considerations

• Use streptomycin cautiously in patients with renal impairment. In severely uremic patients, single dose can produce high blood level of drug for several days; cumulative effects may produce ototoxicity.

• Expect prescriber to order baseline renal function studies and to assess cranial nerve VIII function (responsible for hearing) at start of streptomycin therapy to allow for later comparisons.

• Monitor serum peak and trough levels, as ordered, to ensure adequate, but not toxic, drug level.

• Be aware that streptomycin should be given only by I.M. injection.

• To reconstitute streptomycin, add between 4.2 and 4.5 ml of sodium chloride for injection or sterile water for injection to each 1-g vial to provide a concentration of 200 mg/ml, or add between 3.2 and 3.5 ml of diluent to each 5-g vial to provide a concentration of 250 mg/ml. Alternatively, add 6.5 ml of diluent to each 5-g vial to provide a concentration of 500 mg/ml.

• Don't give more than 500 mg/ml.

• Rotate injection sites to prevent sterile abscess formation.

PATIENT TEACHING

• Advise patient to refrigerate streptomycin solution at 36° to 46° F (2° to 8° C).

• Inform patient that treatment for tuber- culosis lasts at least 1 year.

• Urge patient to notify prescriber if he has fullness or ringing in ears, hearing loss, or vertigo.

Q
R
S

sucralfate

Apo-sucralfate (CAN), Carafate, Sulcrate (CAN), Sulcrate Suspension Plus (CAN)

Class and Category

Chemical class: Disulfated disaccharide, aluminum salt
Therapeutic class: Antiulcer
Pregnancy category: B

Indications and Dosages

➤ *To prevent duodenal ulcer*

TABLETS

Adults and adolescents. 1 g twice daily.

➤ *To treat active duodenal ulcer*

ORAL SUSPENSION

Adults and adolescents. 1 g four times a day 1 hr before meals and at bedtime for 4 to 8 wk, possibly less. Or, 2 g twice daily on empty stomach on waking and at bedtime for 4 to 8 wk, possibly less.

TABLETS

Adults and adolescents. 1 g four times a day 1 hr before meals and at bedtime for 4 to 8 wk, possibly less.

Mechanism of Action

May react with hydrochloric acid in the stomach to form a complex that buffers acid. The complex adheres electrostatically to proteins on the ulcer's surface and creates a protective barrier at the ulcer site. Sucralfate also inhibits back-diffusion of hydrogen ions and adsorbs pepsin and bile acids, actions that promote healing of an existing duodenal ulcer and prevent ulcer formation.

Interactions

DRUGS

aluminum-containing drugs (such as antacids, antidiarrheals, buffered aspirin with aluminum, and vaginal douches): Possibly aluminum toxicity in patients with renal failure
antacids: Possibly interference with binding of sucralfate to GI mucosa
cimetidine, ciprofloxacin, digoxin, norfloxacin, ofloxacin, phenytoin, ranitidine, tetracycline, theophylline: Decreased bioavailability of these drugs

Adverse Reactions

CNS: Dizziness, drowsiness, headache, insomnia, light-headedness, vertigo
EENT: Dry mouth
ENDO: Hyperglycemia
GI: Constipation, diarrhea, indigestion, nausea, vomiting
MS: Back pain
RESP: Bronchospasm, dyspnea
SKIN: Pruritus, rash, urticaria
OTHER: Anaphylaxis, angioedema

Nursing Considerations

• Use sucralfate cautiously in patients with chronic renal failure because of increased risk of aluminum toxicity.
• Administer drug to patient when he has an empty stomach.
• Monitor diabetic patient's blood glucose level closely because sucralfate may cause hyperglycemia significant enough to require an adjustment of antidiabetic drug therapy prescribed.

PATIENT TEACHING

• Instruct patient to take sucralfate on an empty stomach at least 1 hour before meals and at bedtime.
• Advise patient not to take antacids within 30 minutes of sucralfate.
• Caution patient to check with prescriber before taking another drug within 2 hours of sucralfate.

sucroferric oxyhydroxide

Velphoro

Class and Category

Chemical class: Polynuclear iron(III) oxyhydroxide
Therapeutic class: Phosphate binder
Pregnancy category: B

Indications and Dosages

➤ *To control serum phosphorus levels in patients with chronic kidney disease on dialysis*

TABLETS

Adults. *Initial:* 500 mg three times daily with meals, increasing or decreasing dosage in 500-mg increments weekly, as needed.

Maintenance: 1,500 to 2,000 mg daily.
Maximum: 3,000 mg daily.

Mechanism of Action

Phosphate binding takes place by ligand exchange between hydroxyl groups and/or water in sucroferric oxyhydroxide and phosphate in the diet. The bound phosphate is eliminated in feces. Both serum phosphorus levels and calcium phosphorus product levels are reduced as a consequence of the reduced dietary phosphate absorption.

Contraindications

Hypersensitivity to sucroferric oxyhydroxide or its components

Interaction

DRUGS

calcitriol, ciprofloxacin, digoxin, doxycycline, enalapril, furosemide, HMG-CoA reductase inhibitors, hydrochlorothiazide, levothyroxine, losartan, metoprolol, nifedipine, omeprazole, quinidine, warfarin: Absorption of these drugs may be affected

Adverse Reactions

EENT: Abnormal drug distaste
GI: Dark-colored feces, diarrhea, nausea

Nursing Considerations

• Give sucroferric oxyhydroxide with meals and administer all other oral drugs prescribed for the patient at a different time because absorption of the other drugs may be affected.
• Monitor patient's serum phosphorus levels regularly, as ordered, to determine drug effectiveness and need for dosage adjustments.
• Monitor patients who develop peritonitis during peritoneal dialysis, patients with significant gastric or hepatic disorders or following major gastrointestinal surgery, and patients who have a history of hemochromatosis or other diseases characterized by iron accumulation because sucroferric oxyhydroxide effects on these conditions are not known.

Patient Teaching

• Instruct patient to take sucroferric oxyhydroxide with meals.
• Tell patient tablets must be chewed and not swallowed whole. Tell him the tablets

may be crushed to aid chewing and swallowing them.
• Inform patient that drug may cause discolored (black) stool but this effect is harmless.
• Instruct patient to take any concomitant drug therapy at least 2 hours before sucroferric oxyhydroxide.

sulfadiazine

Class and Category

Chemical class: Sulfonamide
Therapeutic class: Antibiotic, antiprotozoal
Pregnancy category: C

Indications and Dosages

➤ *To treat asymptomatic carriers of meningitis*

TABLETS

Adults and adolescents. 1 g every 12 hr for 2 days.
Children ages 1 to 12. 500 mg every 12 hr for 2 days.
Children ages 2 to 12 months. 500 mg daily for 2 days.

➤ *To prevent recurrent rheumatic fever*

TABLETS

Adults and adolescents. 500 mg daily (for patients weighing less than 30 kg [66 lb]) to 1 g daily (for patients weighing 30 kg or more).

➤ *To treat inclusive nocardiosis*

TABLETS

Adults and adolescents. 4 to 8 g daily for at least 6 wk.

➤ *As adjunct to treat toxoplasmosis in patients with AIDS*

TABLETS

Adults and adolescents. 1 to 2 g every 6 hr, with 50 to 100 mg daily of pyrimethamine and 10 to 25 mg daily of leucovorin.
Children age 2 months and over. 50 mg/kg twice daily for 12 mo, together with 2 mg/kg daily of pyrimethamine for 2 days, then 1 mg/kg/day of pyrimethamine for 2 to 6 mo, then 1 mg/kg daily of pyrimethamine 3 times/wk for remainder of 12 mo; in addition, 5 mg of leucovorin given 3 times/wk for 12 mo. *Maximum:* 6 g daily.

➤ *To treat toxoplasmosis in pregnant women after week 16 of gestation*

Q
R
S

TABLETS

Adults. 1 g every 6 hr, together with 25 mg daily of pyrimethamine and 5 to 15 mg daily of leucovorin.

Mechanism of Action

Inhibits para-aminobenzoic acid, a bacterial enzyme responsible for synthesizing folic acid, which susceptible bacteria require for growth. By inactivating bacteria, sulfadiazine prevents or alleviates infection.

Contraindications

Breastfeeding; hypersensitivity to sulfadiazine, its components, or other chemically related drugs, such as sulfonamides; pregnancy at term

Interactions

DRUGS

bone marrow depressants: Increased risk of leukopenic or thrombocytopenic effects

cyclosporine: Decreased blood cyclosporine level, increased risk of nephrotoxicity

estrogen-containing oral contraceptives: Increased risk of breakthrough bleeding and pregnancy

hemolytics: Increased risk of adverse effects

hepatotoxic drugs: Increased risk of hepatotoxicity

hydantoins, oral anticoagulants, oral antidiabetic drugs: Increased or prolonged effects of these drugs, possibly toxicity

indomethacin, probenecid, salicylates: Increased blood level of free sulfadiazine caused by displacement from plasma protein–binding sites

methotrexate: Increased risk of leukopenic or thrombocytopenic effects of methotrexate

phenylbutazone, sulfinpyrazone: Increased blood sulfadiazine level

uricosuric drugs: Potentiated uricosuric action

Adverse Reactions

CNS: Dizziness, fatigue, fever, headache, lethargy, weakness

EENT: Pharyngitis

GI: Anorexia, diarrhea, dysphagia, nausea, vomiting

GU: Crystalluria

HEME: Agranulocytosis, aplastic anemia, hemolytic anemia, leukopenia, thrombocytopenia, unusual bleeding or bruising

MS: Arthralgia, myalgia

SKIN: Blisters, erythema, jaundice, pallor, photosensitivity, pruritus, rash

Other: Drug-induced fever

Nursing Considerations

• Use sulfadiazine cautiously in patients with blood dyscrasias or megaloblastic anemia from folate deficiency because drug may cause blood dyscrasias; in those with G6PD deficiency because hemolysis may occur; in those with hepatic or renal impairment because of increased risk of toxicity; and in those with porphyria because drug may precipitate an acute attack.

• Obtain blood sample for CBC and body tissue or fluid specimen for culture and sensitivity tests, as ordered, before giving drug. Expect first dose to be given before results are available.

WARNING Monitor patient for drug-induced fever, which may develop 7 to 10 days after starting sulfadiazine therapy. Signs and symptoms may include abdominal pain, anorexia, ataxia, depression, diarrhea, headache, insomnia, nausea, peripheral neuropathy, tinnitus, and vomiting.

• Monitor fluid intake and output during therapy. Altered fluid balance may increase risk of crystalluria.

• Frequently monitor blood glucose level, and assess for signs and symptoms of hypoglycemia in patients who take an oral antidiabetic drug. Be prepared to respond if hypoglycemia develops.

PATIENT TEACHING

• Instruct patient to take sulfadiazine exactly as prescribed and to complete the full course, even if he feels better.

• Advise patient to take drug with a full glass of water and to drink plenty of fluids during therapy.

• Urge patient to notify prescriber if urine turns reddish brown; this may indicate crystalluria.

• Inform patient about possible dizziness, and urge him to avoid potentially hazardous activities until drug's CNS effects are known.

• Advise patient to avoid prolonged exposure to sunlight and to wear sunscreen and protective clothing when outdoors.

• Urge patient who takes oral contraceptives to use an additional method of birth control during therapy.
• Advise patient who takes an oral antidiabetic drug to check his blood glucose level frequently because of the increased risk of hypoglycemia during therapy.

sulfamethizole
Thiosulfil Forte

Class and Category
Chemical class: Sulfonamide
Therapeutic class: Antibiotic
Pregnancy category: C

Indications and Dosages
➤ *To treat cystitis and other UTIS caused by* Enterobacter *species,* Escherichia coli, Klebsiella *species,* Proteus mirabilis, P. vulgaris, *or* Staphylococcus aureus
TABLETS
Adults. 0.5 to 1 g every 6 to 8 hr.
Children age 2 months and over. 7.5 to 11.25 mg/kg every 6 hr.
DOSAGE ADJUSTMENT Dosage usually reduced for patients with impaired renal function.

Mechanism of Action
Inhibits para-aminobenzoic acid, a bacterial enzyme responsible for synthesizing folic acid, which susceptible bacteria require for growth. By inactivating bacteria, sulfamethizole prevents or alleviates infection.

Contraindications
Breastfeeding; hypersensitivity to sulfamethizole, its components, or other chemically related drugs, such as sulfonamides; pregnancy at term

Interactions
DRUGS
bone marrow depressants: Increased risk of leukopenic or thrombocytopenic effects
cyclosporine: Decreased blood cyclosporine level, increased risk of nephrotoxicity
estrogen-containing oral contraceptives: Increased risk of breakthrough bleeding and pregnancy
hemolytics: Increased risk of adverse effects

hepatotoxic drugs: Increased risk of hepatotoxicity
hydantoins, oral anticoagulants, oral antidiabetic drugs: Increased or prolonged effects of these drugs, possibly toxicity
indomethacin, probenecid, salicylates: Increased blood level of free sulfamethizole caused by displacement from plasma protein–binding sites
methotrexate: Increased risk of leukopenic or thrombocytopenic effects of methotrexate
phenylbutazone, sulfinpyrazone: Increased blood sulfamethizole level
uricosuric drugs: Potentiated uricosuric action

Adverse Reactions
CNS: Dizziness, fatigue, fever, headache, lethargy, weakness
EENT: Pharyngitis
GI: Anorexia, diarrhea, dysphagia, nausea, vomiting
GU: Crystalluria
HEME: Agranulocytosis, aplastic anemia, hemolytic anemia, leukopenia, thrombocytopenia, unusual bleeding or bruising
MS: Arthralgia, myalgia
SKIN: Blisters, erythema, jaundice, pallor, photosensitivity, pruritus, rash
Other: Drug-induced fever

Nursing Considerations
• Use sulfamethizole cautiously in patients with blood dyscrasias or megaloblastic anemia from folate deficiency because drug may cause blood dyscrasias; in those with G6PD deficiency because hemolysis may occur; in those with hepatic or renal impairment because of increased risk of toxicity; and in those with porphyria because drug may precipitate an acute attack.
• Obtain blood sample for CBC and body tissue or fluid specimen for culture and sensitivity tests, as ordered, before giving drug. Expect first dose to be given before results are available.
WARNING Monitor patient for drug-induced fever, which may develop 7 to 10 days after sulfamethizole starts. Signs and symptoms include abdominal pain, anorexia, ataxia, depression, diarrhea, headache, insomnia,

Q
R
S

nausea, peripheral neuropathy, tinnitus, and vomiting.
• Monitor fluid intake and output during therapy. Altered fluid balance may increase risk of crystalluria.
• Frequently monitor blood glucose level and assess for signs and symptoms of hypoglycemia in patients who take an oral antidiabetic drug. Be prepared to respond if hypoglycemia develops.

PATIENT TEACHING
• Instruct patient to take sulfamethizole exactly as prescribed and to complete the full course even if he feels better.
• Advise patient to take drug with a full glass of water and to drink plenty of fluids during therapy.
• Urge patient to notify prescriber if urine turns reddish brown; this may indicate crystalluria.
• Inform patient about possible dizziness, and urge him to avoid hazardous activities until drug's CNS effects are known.
• Advise patient to avoid prolonged exposure to sunlight and to wear sunscreen and protective clothing when outdoors.
• Urge patient who takes oral contraceptives to use an additional method of birth control during therapy.
• Advise patient who takes an oral antidiabetic drug to check his blood glucose level frequently because of the increased risk of hypoglycemia during therapy.

sulfamethoxazole

Apo-Sulfamethoxazole (CAN), Gantanol, Urobak

Class and Category
Chemical class: Sulfonamide
Therapeutic class: Antibiotic, antiprotozoal
Pregnancy category: C

Indications and Dosages
➤ *To treat chlamydial conjunctivitis; malaria (as adjunct to quinine sulfate and pyrimethamine); toxoplasmosis (as adjunct to pyrimethamine); and UTI, including pyelonephritis and cystitis, caused by susceptible organisms*

TABLETS
Adults. *Initial:* 2 g, followed by 1 g every 8 to 12 hr.
Children age 2 months and over. *Initial:* 50 to 60 mg/kg, then 25 to 30 mg/kg every 12 hr. *Maximum:* 2 g for initial dose, 75 mg/kg daily for subsequent doses.
DOSAGE ADJUSTMENT Dosage reduction usually needed for patients with impaired renal function.
➤ *To treat uncomplicated urethritis, cervicitis, and proctitis caused by Chlamydia trachomatis*
TABLETS
Adults. 1 g every 12 hr for 10 days.
DOSAGE ADJUSTMENT For patients with creatinine clearance of 10 to 30 ml/min/1.73 m², recommended dose reduced by 50% or dosing interval extended; for creatinine clearance of less than 10 ml/min/1.73 m², recommended dose reduced by 75% or dosing interval extended, as prescribed.

Mechanism of Action
Inhibits para-aminobenzoic acid, a bacterial enzyme responsible for synthesizing folic acid, which susceptible bacteria require for growth. By inactivating bacteria, sulfamethoxazole prevents or alleviates infection.

Contraindications
Breastfeeding; hypersensitivity to sulfamethoxazole, its components, or other chemically related drugs, such as sulfonamides; pregnancy at term

Interactions
DRUGS
bone marrow depressants: Increased risk of leukopenic or thrombocytopenic effects
cyclosporine: Decreased blood cyclosporine level, increased risk of nephrotoxicity
estrogen-containing oral contraceptives: Increased risk of breakthrough bleeding and pregnancy
hemolytics: Increased risk of adverse effects
hepatotoxic drugs: Increased risk of hepatotoxicity
hydantoins, oral anticoagulants, oral antidiabetic drugs: Increased or prolonged effects of these drugs, possibly toxicity
indomethacin, probenecid, salicylates: Increased blood level of free

sulfamethoxazole caused by displacement from plasma protein-binding sites
methotrexate: Increased risk of leukopenic or thrombocytopenic effects of methotrexate
phenylbutazone, sulfinpyrazone: Increased blood sulfamethoxazole level
uricosuric drugs: Potentiated uricosuric action

Adverse Reactions

CNS: Dizziness, fatigue, fever, headache, lethargy, weakness
EENT: Pharyngitis
GI: Anorexia, diarrhea, dysphagia, nausea, vomiting
GU: Crystalluria
HEME: Agranulocytosis, aplastic anemia, hemolytic anemia, leukopenia, thrombocytopenia, unusual bleeding or bruising
MS: Arthralgia, myalgia
SKIN: Blisters, erythema, jaundice, pallor, photosensitivity, pruritus, rash
Other: Drug-induced fever

Nursing Considerations

• Use sulfamethoxazole cautiously in patients with blood dyscrasias or megaloblastic anemia from folate deficiency because drug may cause blood dyscrasias; in those with G6PD deficiency because hemolysis may occur; in those with hepatic or renal impairment because of increased risk of toxicity; and in those with porphyria because drug may precipitate an acute attack.
• Obtain blood sample for CBC and body tissue or fluid specimen for culture and sensitivity tests, as ordered, before giving drug. Expect first dose to be given before results are available.
WARNING Monitor patient for drug-induced fever, which may develop 7 to 10 days after sulfamethoxazole starts. Signs and symptoms include abdominal pain, anorexia, ataxia, depression, diarrhea, headache, insomnia, nausea, peripheral neuropathy, tinnitus, and vomiting.
• Monitor fluid intake and output during therapy. Altered fluid balance may increase risk of crystalluria.
• Frequently monitor blood glucose level and assess for signs and symptoms of

hypoglycemia in patients who take an oral antidiabetic drug. Be prepared to respond if hypoglycemia develops.

PATIENT TEACHING

• Instruct patient to take sulfamethoxazole exactly as prescribed and to complete the full course even if he feels better.
• Advise patient to take drug with a full glass of water and to drink plenty of fluids during therapy.
• Urge patient to notify prescriber if urine turns reddish brown; this may indicate crystalluria.
• Inform patient about possible dizziness, and urge him to avoid potentially hazardous activities until drug's CNS effects are known.
• Advise patient to avoid prolonged exposure to sunlight and to wear sunscreen and protective clothing when outdoors.
• Urge patient who takes oral contraceptives to use an additional method of birth control during therapy.
• Advise patient who takes an oral antidiabetic drug to check his blood glucose level frequently because of increased risk of hypoglycemia during therapy.

sulfasalazine

Alti-Sulfasalazine (CAN), Azulfidine, Azulfidine EN-Tabs, PMS-Sulfasalazine (CAN), PMS-Sulfasalazine E.C. (CAN), Salazopyrin EN-Tabs (CAN), S.A.S.-500 (CAN), S.A.S. Enteric-500 (CAN)

Class and Category

Chemical class: Salicylate, sulfonamide
Therapeutic class: Anti-inflammatory, antirheumatic, immunomodulator
Pregnancy category: B

Indications and Dosages

➤ *To treat inflammatory bowel diseases, such as ulcerative colitis, and to maintain or prolong remission*
DELAYED-RELEASE TABLETS, TABLETS
Adults and adolescents. *Initial:* 500 to 1,000 mg every 6 to 8 hr. Or 500 mg every 6 to 12 hr to decrease adverse

GI reactions. *Maintenance:* 500 mg every 6 hr.
Children over age 6. *Initial:* 6.7 to 10 mg/kg every 4 hr, 10 to 15 mg/kg every 6 hr, or 13.3 to 20 mg/kg every 8 hr. *Maintenance:* 7.5 mg/kg every 6 hr.
➤ *To treat rheumatoid arthritis*
DELAYED-RELEASE TABLETS, TABLETS
Adults. *Initial:* 500 to 1,000 mg daily during wk 1, increased by 500 mg daily every wk, as needed, up to 2,000 mg daily in divided doses. If no response after 12 wk, increased to 3,000 mg daily. *Maintenance:* 1,000 mg every 12 hr. *Maximum:* 3,000 mg daily.
➤ *To treat juvenile rheumatoid arthritis in patients who have not responded to salicylates or other NSAIDS*
DELAYED-RELEASE TABLETS
Children ages 6 to 16. 30 to 50 mg/kg daily in divided doses twice daily. *Maximum:* 2 g daily.

Mechanism of Action
As a prodrug of sulfapyridine and 5-aminosalicylic acid (mesalamine), delivers more sulfapyridine and mesalamine to the colon than either metabolite could provide alone. Sulfapyridine provides antibacterial action along the intestinal wall; mesalamine inhibits cyclooxygenase, thereby decreasing the production of arachidonic acid metabolites and reducing colonic inflammation.

Contraindications
Hypersensitivity to salicylates, sulfasalazine, sulfonamides, chemically related drugs, or their components; intestinal or urinary obstruction; porphyria

Interactions
DRUGS
bone marrow depressants: Increased leukopenic and thrombocytopenic effects of both drugs
digoxin: Possibly inhibited absorption and decreased blood level of digoxin
folic acid (vitamin B_9): Decreased folic acid absorption
hepatotoxic drugs: Increased risk of hepatotoxicity
hydantoins, oral anticoagulants, oral antidiabetic drugs: Increased, prolonged, or toxic effects of these drugs

methotrexate, phenylbutazone, sulfinpyrazone: Possibly potentiated effects of these drugs

Adverse Reactions
CNS: Ataxia, chills, depression, fatigue, fever, Guillain-Barré syndrome, headache, insomnia, meningitis, peripheral neuropathy, seizures, vertigo, weakness
CV: Myocarditis, pericarditis, vasculitis
EENT: Hearing loss, orange-yellow tears, oropharyngeal pain, pharyngitis, tinnitus
GI: Abdominal pain, anorexia, cirrhosis, diarrhea, elevated liver enzymes, hepatitis, hepatotoxicity, indigestion, jaundice, nausea, pancreatitis, ulcerative colitis exacerbation, vomiting
GU: Crystalluria, decreased ejaculatory volume, male infertility, nephritis, nephrolithiasis, nephrotic syndrome, orange-yellow urine, toxic nephrosis
HEME: Agranulocytosis, aplastic anemia, Heinz body or hemolytic anemia, hematophagic histiocytosis, leukopenia, neutropenia, thrombocytopenia, unusual bleeding or bruising
MS: Arthralgia, rhabdomyolysis
RESP: Cyanosis, eosinophilic infiltration, idiopathic pulmonary fibrosis, lymphocytic interstitial pneumonitis, pleuritis pneumonia
SKIN: Alopecia, drug rash with eosinophilia and systemic symptoms (DRESS), erythema multiforme, exfoliative dermatitis, epidermal necrolysis, photosensitivity, pruritus, purpura, rash, Stevens-Johnson syndrome, toxic epidermal necrolysis, urticaria
Other: Anaphylaxis, angioedema, folate deficiency, infections (serious), lupus erythematosus-like syndrome, mononucleosis-like syndrome, sepsis, serum sickness syndrome

Nursing Considerations
• Use sulfasalazine cautiously in patients with a history of recurring or chronic infections because drug may predispose patient to infections. Monitor patients for new infections throughout therapy. If present, notify prescriber.
• Monitor CBC, liver function test results, and BUN and serum creatinine levels before and periodically during prolonged sulfasalazine therapy.

- Be aware that sulfasalazine doses over 4 g or a blood level over 50 mcg/ml increases the risk of adverse and toxic reactions.
- Monitor fluid intake and output and urine color, pH, and consistency. Acidic urine may require alkalization to prevent crystalluria.
- Be aware that measurements, by liquid chromatography, of urinary normetanephrine may cause a false-positive test result.

WARNING Monitor patient, especially during the first month of sulfasalazine therapy, for hypersensitivity reactions that may become life-threatening. At first sign of rash, mucosal lesions or any other sign of hypersensitivity, stop sulfasalazine therapy and notify prescriber.

PATIENT TEACHING

- Instruct patient to take sulfasalazine with meals, milk, or an antacid to decrease GI distress, and to swallow tablets whole.
- Advise patient to prevent crystalluria by taking drug with a full glass of water and drinking at least 64 oz of fluid per day.
- Instruct patient and family to administer drug around the clock.
- Inform patient that symptom relief may take 2 to 5 days for ulcerative colitis and 4 to 12 weeks for rheumatoid arthritis.
- Alert patient that drug may turn urine and skin orange-yellow.
- Advise contact lens wearer to consider wearing glasses during therapy because drug can permanently stain contact lenses yellow.
- Instruct patient to avoid prolonged sun exposure and to wear protective clothing and sunscreen when outdoors.
- Advise patient to brush with a soft-bristled toothbrush and to use dental floss and toothpicks gently because leukopenic and thrombocytopenic drug effects increase risk of infection and gingival bleeding.
- Urge patient to return for laboratory tests and follow-up visits to monitor drug's effect.
- Instruct patient to report sore throat; fever; paleness; skin abnormalities such as skin blistering, discoloration, rash or hives; or jaundice. These may be signs of serious adverse effects. Explain that prescriber may order tests to determine their cause and that drug may be discontinued until test results are known.

- Instruct mothers who are breastfeeding to stop taking sulfasalzine or stop breastfeeding immediately if their infant develops bloody stools or diarrhea, and to notify prescriber.

sulfinpyrazone

Anturane, Apo-Sulfinpyrazone (CAN), Novopyrazone (CAN)

Class and Category

Chemical class: Pyrazalone derivative
Therapeutic class: Antigout, uricosuric
Pregnancy category: Not rated

Indications and Dosages

➤ *To treat chronic or intermittent gouty arthritis*

CAPSULES, TABLETS

Adults. *Initial:* 100 to 200 mg twice daily, increased by 200 mg daily every 2 to 4 days, as needed. *Maintenance:* 100 to 200 mg twice daily. *Maximum:* 400 mg twice daily during wk 1; then 200 to 400 mg twice daily until serum urate level is controlled.

Route	Onset	Peak	Duration
P.O.	Unknown	Unknown	4–10 hr

Mechanism of Action

Inhibits renal tubular reabsorption of uric acid, thereby increasing uric acid excretion and decreasing serum urate level. Decreased serum urate level prevents urate deposition, tophus formation, and chronic joint changes. It also helps resolve existing urate deposits and eventually reduces the number of gouty arthritis attacks.

Contraindications

Active peptic ulcer disease, blood dyscrasias, hypersensitivity to sulfinpyrazone or its components, symptoms of GI inflammation or ulceration

Interactions

DRUGS

acetaminophen: Increased risk of hepatotoxicity, decreased acetaminophen effects

Q
R
S

aminosalicylate sodium: Increased blood level and prolonged duration of this drug, possibly leading to toxicity
antineoplastics: Increased risk of uric acid nephropathy
bismuth subsalicylate and other salicylates: Decreased sulfinpyrazone effects
cefamandole, cefoperazone, cefotetan, moxalactam, plicamycin, valproic acid: Possibly hypoprothrombinemia, increased risk of severe hemorrhage
diazoxide, mecamylamine, pyrazinamide: Possibly increased serum uric acid level
hydantoins: Increased blood hydantoin level, possibly leading to hydantoin toxicity
niacin: Possibly decreased uricosuric effect of sulfinpyrazone
nitrofurantoin: Decreased nitrofurantoin effectiveness, possibly nitrofurantoin toxicity
NSAIDs, oral anticoagulants, platelet aggregation inhibitors, thrombolytics: Increased risk of bleeding
oral antidiabetic drugs: Increased risk of hypoglycemia
probenecid: Increased sulfinpyrazone effects
theophylline: Possibly decreased blood theophylline level
verapamil: Increased clearance and decreased bioavailability of verapamil
ACTIVITIES
alcohol use: Possibly increased serum uric acid level

Adverse Reactions
CNS: Dizziness
EENT: Tinnitus
GI: Abdominal pain, epigastric discomfort, GI bleeding, indigestion, nausea, vomiting
GU: Dysuria, flank pain, hematuria, renal calculi, renal colic, renal failure
HEME: Agranulocytosis, anemia, aplastic anemia, leukopenia, thrombocytopenia
MS: Arthralgia, gouty arthritis (acute attack)
RESP: Bronchospasm, dyspnea, wheezing
SKIN: Erythema, rash

Nursing Considerations
• Expect to start with full maintenance dose, as ordered, for patient being switched to sulfinpyrazone from another uricosuric.
• Monitor serum uric acid level periodically, as ordered, to evaluate drug effectiveness.

• Assess for signs of acute gouty arthritis, especially during first few months of sulfinpyrazone therapy.
PATIENT TEACHING
• Instruct patient to take sulfinpyrazone with food, milk, or an antacid to prevent GI distress.
• Emphasize the importance of taking drug every day, even when feeling better, to prevent acute gouty arthritis attacks.
• Inform patient that acute gouty arthritis may worsen during initial therapy but should improve as treatment continues. Explain that he may not experience drug's full therapeutic effect for 6 months.
• If an acute gouty arthritis attack occurs, advise patient to seek additional treatment but to continue taking sulfinpyrazone, as prescribed, to help prevent exacerbation.
• Advise patient to drink at least 80 oz of fluids per day to decrease the risk of renal calculus formation.
• Instruct patient to consult prescriber before taking OTC products that contain aspirin or acetaminophen.
• Advise patient to avoid alcohol while taking sulfinpyrazone.
• Encourage patient to return for ordered follow-up laboratory tests to check for blood dyscrasias.

sulfisoxazole
Apo-Sulfisoxazole (CAN), Gantrisin, Novo-Soxazole (CAN), Sulfizole (CAN)

sulfisoxazole acetyl
Gantrisin

Class and Category
Chemical class: Sulfonamide
Therapeutic class: Antibiotic, antiprotozoal
Pregnancy category: C

Indications and Dosages
➤ *To treat nocardiosis; plague; malaria (as adjunct to quinine sulfate and pyrimethamine); and UTI, including pyelonephritis and cystitis, caused by susceptible organisms*
ORAL SUSPENSION, ORAL SYRUP, TABLETS
Adults and adolescents. *Initial:* 2 to 4 g daily in divided doses. *Maintenance:* 4 to

8 g daily in divided doses every 4 to 6 hr. *Maximum:* 8 g daily.
Children over age 2 months. *Initial:* 75 mg/kg, followed by 120 to 150 mg/kg daily in divided doses every 4 to 6 hr. *Maximum:* 6 g daily.

➤ *To treat uncomplicated cystitis in women*
ORAL SUSPENSION, ORAL SYRUP, TABLETS
Adults. 2 g as a single dose.

➤ *To treat acute or recurrent otitis media in combination with erythromycin in penicillin-allergic patients*
ORAL SUSPENSION, ORAL SYRUP, TABLETS
Children. 150 mg of sulfisoxazole/kg daily and 50 mg of erythromycin/kg daily in divided doses four times a day.

➤ *To treat lymphogranuloma venereum*
ORAL SUSPENSION, ORAL SYRUP, TABLETS
Adults. 500 mg every 6 hr for 21 days.

➤ *To treat uncomplicated urethritis, cervicitis, or proctitis caused by* Chlamydia trachomatis
ORAL SUSPENSION, ORAL SYRUP, TABLETS
Adults. 500 mg every 6 hr.

DOSAGE ADJUSTMENT For patients with renal impairment, dosing interval changed to every 8 to 24 hr, as prescribed.

Mechanism of Action

Inhibits para-aminobenzoic acid, a bacterial enzyme responsible for synthesizing folic acid, which susceptible bacteria require for growth. By inactivating bacteria, sulfisoxazole prevents or alleviates infection.

Contraindications

Breastfeeding; hypersensitivity to sulfisoxazole, other chemically related drugs, such as sulfonamides, or their components; pregnancy at term

Interactions
DRUGS

bone marrow depressants, methotrexate: Increased risk of leukopenia or thrombocytopenia
cyclosporine: Increased risk of nephrotoxicity
diuretics: Increased incidence of thrombocytopenic purpura
hemolytics (such as doxapram and methyldopa): Increased risk of toxic reaction
hepatotoxic drugs (such as amiodarone): Increased risk of hepatotoxicity

hydantoins, oral anticoagulants, oral antidiabetic drugs: Increased or prolonged effects of these drugs, possibly toxicity
indomethacin, probenecid, salicylates: Increased blood sulfisoxazole level
oral contraceptives: Increased risk of breakthrough bleeding with long-term sulfisoxazole use
phenylbutazone, sulfinpyrazone: Risk of increased blood sulfisoxazole level
thiopental: Increased anesthetic effect of thiopental
tolbutamide: Prolonged half-life of tolbutamide
uricosurics: Potentiated uricosuric action

Adverse Reactions

CNS: Dizziness, fatigue, fever, headache, lethargy, weakness
EENT: Pharyngitis
GI: Anorexia, diarrhea, dysphagia, nausea, vomiting
GU: Crystalluria
HEME: Agranulocytosis, aplastic anemia, hemolytic anemia, leukopenia, thrombocytopenia, unusual bleeding or bruising
MS: Arthralgia, myalgia
SKIN: Blisters, erythema, jaundice, pallor, photosensitivity, pruritus, rash
Other: Drug-induced fever

Nursing Considerations

• Use sulfisoxazole cautiously in patients with blood dyscrasias or megaloblastic anemia from folate deficiency because drug may cause blood dyscrasias; in those with G6PD deficiency because hemolysis may occur; in those with hepatic or renal impairment because of increased risk of toxicity; and in those with porphyria because drug may precipitate acute attack.
• Obtain blood sample for CBC and tissue or fluid specimen for culture and sensitivity testing, as ordered, before beginning sulfisoxazole therapy. Expect to give first dose before results are available.
• ***WARNING*** Expect prescriber to discontinue sulfisoxazole if patient exhibits signs of blood dyscrasias, including fever, jaundice, maculopapular or other rash, pallor, pharyngitis, or purpura.
• Monitor CBC often, as appropriate, during treatment for signs of adverse reactions.

Q
R
S

• Closely monitor patients with AIDS, who are at increased risk for adverse reactions. **WARNING** Monitor patient for drug-induced fever, which may develop 7 to 10 days after sulfisoxazole starts. Signs and symptoms include abdominal pain, anorexia, ataxia, depression, diarrhea, headache, insomnia, nausea, peripheral neuropathy, tinnitus, and vomiting.

• Monitor fluid intake and output. Unless contraindicated, provide sufficient fluids to maintain a daily urine output of at least 1,200 ml.

• For otitis media caused by *Haemophilus influenzae*, expect to give drug with erythromycin, as prescribed.

• Frequently monitor blood glucose level and assess for signs of hypoglycemia in patients who take oral antidiabetic drugs.

PATIENT TEACHING

• Instruct patient to take sulfisoxazole exactly as prescribed and to complete the full course of therapy even if he feels better.

• Advise patient to take drug with a full glass of water.

• Inform patient that tablet may be chewed or crushed and mixed with liquid to ease swallowing.

• Advise patient to shake oral suspension well before use and to measure oral suspension or syrup dose with calibrated device to ensure accuracy.

• Inform patient that oral suspension or syrup form of drug may be stored at room temperature.

• Advise patient to drink 2 to 3 L of fluid daily to maintain hydration, unless contraindicated.

• Caution patient to avoid hazardous activities until drug's CNS effects are known.

• Instruct patient who takes an oral antidiabetic to check her blood glucose level often because of the risk of hypoglycemia.

• Advise patient to avoid prolonged exposure to sunlight and to use sunscreen and wear protective clothing when outdoors.

sulindac

Apo-Sulin (CAN), Clinoril, Novo-Sundac (CAN)

Class and Category

Chemical class: Pyrroleacetic acid derivative
Therapeutic class: Antigout, anti-inflammatory, antirheumatic
Pregnancy category: Not rated

Indications and Dosages

➤ *To decrease pain and inflammation in ankylosing spondylitis, acute attacks of gout or pseudogout, bursitis, moderately painful arthralgia, osteoarthritis, rheumatoid arthritis, and tendinitis*

TABLETS

Adults and adolescents over age 14. *Initial:* 150 to 200 mg twice daily, adjusted based on patient's response. *Maximum:* 200 mg twice daily.

➤ *To relieve symptoms of acute gouty arthritis, acute subacromial bursitis, and supraspinatus tendinitis*

TABLETS

Adults and adolescents over age 14. 200 mg twice daily for 7 to 14 days; decreased to lowest effective dosage after satisfactory response occurs.

DOSAGE ADJUSTMENT For elderly patients, dosage reduced to 50% of usual adult dosage, if needed.

Mechanism of Action

May block the activity of cyclooxygenase, an enzyme needed to synthesize prostaglandins, which mediate the inflammatory response and cause local vasodilation, swelling, and pain. By blocking cyclooxygenase and inhibiting prostaglandins, this NSAID reduces inflammatory symptoms and pain.

Route	Onset	Peak	Duration
P.O.	In 1 wk*	2–3 wk*	Unknown

Contraindications

Angioedema, asthma, bronchospasm, nasal polyps, rhinitis, or urticaria induced by aspirin, iodides, or other NSAIDs

Interactions

DRUGS

acetaminophen, cyclosporine, gold compounds, nephrotoxic drugs: Increased risk of adverse renal effects

* For antirheumatic effects; unknown for antigout or anti-inflammatory effects.

angiotensin-converting enzyme (ACE)
inhibitors, angiotensin II antagonists:
Decreased antihypertensive effect of these
drugs; increased risk of renal impairment in
patients with already compromised renal
function
antacids: Decreased blood level and effects
of sulindac
antihypertensives: Risk of decreased
antihypertensive effect
aspirin, salicylates: Decreased sulindac
effects, increased risk of GI hemorrhage
bone marrow depressants: Increased risk of
leukopenia and thrombocytopenia
cefamandole, cefoperazone, cefotetan,
colchicine, oral anticoagulants, plicamycin,
thrombolytics, valproic acid: Increased risk
of bleeding
cimetidine, ranitidine: Increased
bioavailability of both drugs
digoxin: Increased blood digoxin level and
risk of digitalis toxicity
dimethyl sulfoxide (DMSO): Decreased
sulindac effectiveness, possibly peripheral
neuropathy with topical application of DMSO
diuretics: Possibly decreased loop diuretic
effects and increased thiazide diuretic effects
glucocorticoids, other NSAIDs, potassium
supplements: Increased risk of adverse GI
effects
hydantoins: Increased blood hydantoin level
and risk of phenytoin toxicity
insulin, oral antidiabetic drugs: Increased
risk of hypoglycemia
lithium: Possibly increased blood level and
toxic effects of lithium
methotrexate: Decreased methotrexate
excretion, possibly leading to toxicity
platelet aggregation inhibitors: Increased risk
of bleeding, additive effects of these drugs
probenecid: Increased blood level and
adverse and toxic effects of sulindac
ACTIVITIES
alcohol use: Increased risk of adverse GI
effects, including GI bleeding

Adverse Reactions

CNS: Aseptic meningitis, cerebral
hemorrhage, chills, drowsiness, fever,
headache, ischemic stroke, malaise,
nervousness, transient ischemic attack
CV: Deep vein thrombosis, edema, heart
failure, hypertension, MI, palpitations,
peripheral edema, vasculitis

EENT: Tinnitus
ENDO: Hypoglycemia
GI: Abdominal cramps or pain, anorexia,
constipation, diarrhea, esophageal
irritation, flatulence, gastritis, gastrointestinal bleeding or ulceration, hepatic
failure, hepatitis, hepatotoxicity,
indigestion, jaundice, liver failure, nausea,
perforation of stomach or intestines,
vomiting
GU: Acute renal failure, decreased urine
output, interstitial nephritis, nephrotic
syndrome, polyuria, proteinuria
HEME: Agranulocytosis, aplastic anemia,
leukopenia, pancytopenia
RESP: Bronchial spasm, dyspnea,
pulmonary edema, wheezing
SKIN: Diaphoresis, erythema multiforme,
exfoliative dermatitis, maculopapular rash,
pruritus, purpura, Stevens-Johnson syndrome,
toxic epidermal necrolysis, urticaria
Other: Anaphylaxis, angioedema, facial
edema, hypersensitivity syndrome

Nursing Considerations

• Use sulindac with extreme caution in
patients with a history of ulcer disease
or GI bleeding because NSAIDs such as
sulindac increase risk of GI bleeding
and ulceration. Expect to use sulindac
for the shortest time possible in these
patients.
• Be aware that serious GI tract ulceration,
bleeding, and perforation may occur
without warning symptoms. Elderly
patients are at greater risk. To minimize
risk, give drug with food. If GI distress
occurs, withhold drug and notify
prescriber at once.
• Use sulindac cautiously in patients with
hypertension, and monitor blood pressure
closely throughout therapy. Drug may
cause hypertension or worsen it.
WARNING Monitor patient closely for
thrombotic events, including MI and
stroke, because NSAIDs increase the
risk.
• If patient has systemic lupus
erythematosus and mixed connective
tissue disease, monitor him closely
because sulindac increases the risk of
aseptic meningitis.
WARNING If patient has bone marrow
suppression or is receiving antineoplastic

Q
R
S

drug therapy, monitor laboratory results (including WBC count), and watch for evidence of infection because anti-inflammatory and antipyretic actions of sulindac may mask signs and symptoms, such as fever and pain.

• Especially if patient is elderly or taking sulindac long term, watch for less common but serious adverse GI reactions, including anorexia, constipation, diverticulitis, dysphagia, esophagitis, gastritis, gastroenteritis, gastroesophageal reflux disease, hemorrhoids, hiatal hernia, melena, stomatitis, and vomiting.

• Monitor liver function test results because, in rare cases, elevated levels may progress to severe hepatic reactions, including fatal hepatitis, liver necrosis, and hepatic failure.

• Watch BUN and serum creatinine levels in elderly patients; those with heart failure, impaired renal function, or hepatic dysfunction; and those taking diuretics or ACE inhibitors; because drug may cause renal failure.

• Monitor CBC for decreased hemoglobin and hematocrit because drug may worsen anemia.

• Assess patient's skin routinely for rash or other signs of hypersensitivity reaction because sulindac and other NSAIDs may cause serious skin reactions without warning, even in patients with no history of NSAID hypersensitivity. Stop drug at first sign of reaction, and notify prescriber.

WARNING Monitor patient for adventitious breath sounds and dyspnea; sulindac may cause fluid retention, which may precipitate heart failure in susceptible patients.

• Expect patient to undergo audiometric examinations before and periodically during prolonged therapy, as ordered.

• Monitor patient for evidence of hypersensitivity syndrome, which could become life-threatening. Report multiple occurring and multi-organ adverse reactions to prescriber and expect drug to be discontinued. Be prepared to provide emergency supportive care, as ordered.

PATIENT TEACHING

• Instruct patient to take sulindac exactly as prescribed. Explain that higher doses don't increase effectiveness and may increase risk of adverse reactions.

• Advise patient to crush tablet and mix with food, if needed, to aid in swallowing.

• Instruct patient to take drug with or immediately after meals to decrease GI distress, to take with a full glass of water, and to remain upright for 20 to 30 minutes after administration to prevent drug from lodging in esophagus and causing esophageal irritation.

• Urge patient to notify prescriber immediately of chills, fever, rash, or sweating, which may indicate hypersensitivity.

• Advise patient to consult prescriber before using acetaminophen, alcohol, aspirin, other NSAIDs, or any OTC drugs during sulindac therapy.

• Caution patient to avoid hazardous activities until drug's CNS effects are known.

• Explain the need for periodic physical examinations and laboratory tests during prolonged therapy to monitor drug effectiveness.

• Inform patient that sulindac may increase the risk of serious adverse cardiovascular reactions; urge patient to seek immediate medical attention if signs or symptoms arise, such as chest pain, shortness of breath, weakness, and slurring of speech.

• Tell patient that sulindac also may increase the risk of serious adverse GI reactions; stress the need to seek immediate medical attention for such signs and symptoms as epigastric or abdominal pain, indigestion, black or tarry stools, or vomiting blood or material that looks like coffee grounds.

• Alert patient to the possibility of rare but serious hypersensitivity reactions. Urge him to seek immediate medical attention for rash, blisters, itching, fever, or other indications of hypersensitivity.

sumatriptan succinate

Alsuma, Imitrex, Sumatriptan, Sumavel Dose Pro

sumatriptan iontophoretic transdermal system

Zecuity

Class and Category

Chemical class: Serotonin 5-HT_1-receptor agonist
Therapeutic class: Antimigraine
Pregnancy category: C

Indications and Dosages

➤ *To relieve acute migraine attacks, with or without aura*

TABLETS

Adults. 25 to 100 mg as a single dose as soon as possible after onset of symptoms, repeated every 2 hr, as needed. *Maximum:* 300 mg daily.

DOSAGE ADJUSTMENT For patients with hepatic dysfunction, 50 mg is maximum single dose.

SUBCUTANEOUS INJECTION

Adults. *Initial:* 6 mg, repeated after 1 or 2 hr, as needed. *Maximum:* 2 (6-mg) injections/24 hr with dosages separated by at least 1 hr. If migraine symptoms return after initial subcutaneous injection, 50 mg P.O. every 2 hr up to 200 mg daily.

DOSAGE ADJUSTMENT For patients also taking MAO inhibitors or experiencing dose-related adverse reactions, dosage reduced.

NASAL SPRAY

Adults. 1 or 2 sprays (5 or 10 mg) into one nostril as a single dose or 1 spray (20 mg) into one nostril as a single dose. One additional dose may be taken if another attack occurs after at least 2 hr. *Maximum:* 40 mg daily.

TRANSDERMAL

Adults. *Initial:* 6.5-mg patch , repeated in 2 hr, as needed. *Maximum:* 2 (6.5 mg)

patches/24 hours with dosages separated by at least 2 hr.

➤ *To relieve cluster headaches*

SUBCUTANEOUS INJECTION

Adults. *Initial:* 6 mg, repeated after 1 or 2 hr, as needed. *Maximum:* 2 (6-mg) injections/24 hr with dosages separated by at least 1 hr.

DOSAGE ADJUSTMENT For patients also taking MAO inhibitors, dosage reduced.

Route	Onset	Peak	Duration
P.O.	In 30 min	2–4 hr	Up to 24 hr
SubQ	In 10 min	1–2 hr	Up to 24 hr
Nasal	In 15 min	Unknown	Up to 24 hr

Mechanism of Action

May stimulate 5-HT_1 receptors, causing selective vasoconstriction of inflamed and dilated cranial blood vessels in carotid circulation, thus decreasing carotid arterial blood flow and relieving acute migraines.

Contraindications

Allergic contact dermatitis (transdermal form only), basilar or hemiplegic migraine, cardiovascular disease, hypersensitivity to sumatriptan or its components, ischemic heart disease, Prinzmetal's angina, use within 24 hours of ergotamine-containing or ergot-type drugs or another serotonin 5-HT_1 receptor agonist such as triptans (with exception of a single dose of another sumatriptan product, provided the doses are separated by at least 1 hour or 2 hours for transdermal route), use within 14 days of MAO inhibitor therapy

Interactions

DRUGS

antidepressants, lithium: Increased risk of serious adverse effects
ergotamine-containing drugs: Possibly additive or prolonged vasoconstrictive effects
fluoxetine, fluvoxamine, paroxetine, sertraline: Possibly incoordination, hyper-reflexia, and weakness
MAO inhibitors: Risk of decreased sumatriptan clearance, increased risk of serious adverse effects
selective serotonin reuptake inhibitors, serotonin norepinephrine reuptake inhibitors,

Q R S

other triptans: Increased risk of serotonin syndrome

Adverse Reactions

CNS: Anxiety, atypical sensations, dizziness, drowsiness, fatigue, fever, headache, malaise, sedation, serotonin syndrome, seizures, vertigo, weakness
CV: Arrhythmias; chest heaviness, pain, pressure, or tightness; coronary artery vasospasm; ECG changes; hypertension; hypotension; palpitations; peripheral vascular ischemia
EENT: Abnormal vision, blindness or partial vision loss, jaw or mouth discomfort, nasal burning (P.O., subcutaneous), nasal irritation (nasal), nose or throat discomfort, photophobia (P.O., subcutaneous), taste perversion (nasal), tongue numbness or soreness
GI: Abdominal discomfort, bloody diarrhea, colonic ischemia, dysphagia
MS: Jaw discomfort, muscle cramps, myalgia, neck pain or stiffness
SKIN: Allergic or site dermatitis, diaphoresis, erythema, flushing, pallor, photosensitivity (P.O., subcutaneous), pruritus, rash, urticaria
Other: Injection-site burning, pain, and redness

Nursing Considerations

• Be aware that sumatriptan shouldn't be given to elderly patients because they're more likely to have decreased hepatic function, coronary artery disease (CAD), and more pronounced blood pressure increases.
• Assess patient for chest pain, and monitor blood pressure in patients with CAD before and for at least 1 hour after sumatriptan administration.
• Don't give sumatriptan within 24 hours of another 5-HT$_1$-receptor agonist, such as naratriptan, rizatriptan, or zolmitriptan with the exception of a single dose of another sumatriptan product, provided the doses are separated by at least 1 hour (2 hours for transdermal patch). Don't give an ergotamine-containing or ergot-type drug within 24 hours of sumatriptan therapy. Doing so increases risk of serious adverse interactions and effects.

• After nasal administration, rinse tip of bottle with hot water (don't suction water into bottle) and dry with a clean tissue. Replace cap after cleaning.
• Inspect injection solution for particles and discoloration before administering. Discard solution if you detect these changes.
• Be aware that drug shouldn't be administered I.V. because this may precipitate coronary artery vasospasm.
• Apply transdermal patch to patient's upper arm or thigh only. Do not cut patch. Apply patch to dry, intact, nonirritated skin on a site that is relatively hair-free and is without scars, tattoos, abrasions, or other skin conditions. Do not apply to a previous application site until the site remains erythema-free for at least 3 days. Once applied, push the activation button, which will cause the red light emitting diode (LED) to turn on. Know that the patch must be activated within 15 minutes of assembly. Once dosing is complete, the activation light will turn off. Patch should remain in place for 4 hours or until the light has turned off. Medical tape can be used to secure the patch. Dispose of patch by folding so the adhesive side sticks to itself, and safely discard.
• Be aware that no more than 4 patches should be used in one month.
• Assess patients with risk factors for CAD for arrhythmias, chest pain, and other signs of heart disease.
• For patients with seizure disorder, institute seizure precautions according to facility policy because sumatriptan may lower seizure threshold.
WARNING Monitor patient closely for serotonin syndrome exhibited by agitation, hallucinations, coma, tachycardia, labile blood pressure, hyperthermia, hyperreflexia, incoordination, nausea, vomiting, or diarrhea. Notify prescriber immediately because serotonin syndrome may be life threatening and provide supportive care.

PATIENT TEACHING
• Advise patient to use sumatriptan as soon as possible after the onset of migraine symptoms.

- Urge patient to contact prescriber and avoid taking sumatriptan if headache symptoms aren't typical.
- Remind patient not to exceed prescribed daily dosage. Inform him that overuse of the drug for 10 or more days per month may lead to exacerbation of headache and may require detoxification. If his use of the drug increases, advise him to notify his prescriber.
- Advise patient to swallow tablets whole and drink fluids to disguise unpleasant taste.
- Show patient suitable sites for subcutaneous injection, and teach him how to load, administer, and discard auto-injector. Or, explain how to administer drug using needle-free drug delivery system, Sumavel DosePro. (Snap off plastic tip, flip back lever into active position, and press end of device to the skin of abdomen or thigh.)
- Instruct patient to administer no more than two subcutaneous doses in 24 hours and not to take a second dose if first dose doesn't provide significant relief.
- Teach patient how to use the transdermal patch as prescribed. Tell patient to apply transdermal patch to upper arm or thigh only. Warn him not cut patch. Instruct him to apply patch to dry, intact, nonirritated skin on a site that is relatively hair-free and is without scars, tattoos, abrasions, or other skin conditions. He should not apply patch to a previous application site until the site remains erythema-free for at least 3 days. Once applied, patient should push the activation button, which will cause the red light emitting diode (LED) to turn on. Inform him that the patch must be activated within 15 minutes of assembly. Once dosing is complete, the activation light will turn off. Tell him that patch should remain in place for 4 hours or until the light has turned off. Medical tape can be used to secure the patch. Teach him how to dispose of the used patch, keeping it away from children and pets. Inform patient that no more than 4 patches should be used in one month.
- Inform patient that he may experience burning, pain, and redness for 10 to 30 minutes after subcutaneous injection.

Suggest that he apply ice to relieve pain and redness.
- Teach patient how to use nasal form correctly.
- To avoid cross-contamination, advise patient not to use the same nasal container for more than one person.
- Encourage patient to lie down in a dark, quiet room after taking drug to help relieve migraine.
- Instruct patient to seek emergency care for chest, jaw, or neck tightness after drug use because drug may cause coronary artery vasospasm; subsequent doses may require ECG monitoring.
- Urge patient to report palpitations or rash to prescriber.
- Advise patient to avoid potentially hazardous activities until drug's CNS effects are known.
- Alert patient with seizure disorder that drug may lower seizure threshold.
- Encourage yearly ophthalmologic examinations for patients who require prolonged drug therapy.
- Inform woman who is breastfeeding that she should avoid breastfeeding for 12 hours after treatment with sumatriptan to minimize infant exposure to the drug.
- Urge patient to inform all prescribers of sumatriptan therapy because of potentially dangerous drug interactions.

suvorexant
Belsomra

Class and Category
Chemical class: Antagonism of orexin receptors
Therapeutic class: Hypnotic
Pregnancy category: C
Controlled substance schedule: IV

Indications and Dosages
➤ *To treat insomnia characterized by difficulties with sleep onset and/or sleep maintenance*

TABLETS
Adults. 10 mg once per night within 30 minutes of bedtime and with at least 7 hours remaining for sleep; increased, as

needed, to 20 mg once daily. *Maximum:* 20 mg once daily at night.
DOSAGE ADJUSTMENT For patients taking moderate CYP3A inhibitors, dosage reduced to 5 mg once per night, with maximum dosage not exceeding 10 mg once per night. For patients taking CNS depressants concurrently, dosage may need to be decreased.

Mechanism of Action
Antagonism of orexin receptors blocks the binding of wake-promoting neuropeptides orexin A and orexin B to produce sleep.

Contraindications
Hypersensitivity to suvorexant and its components, narcolepsy

Interaction
DRUGS
CYP3A inducers: Decreased effectiveness of suvorexant
CYP3A inhibitors: Increased effect of suvorexant and incidence of adverse reactions
digoxin: Increased serum digoxin levels
other CNS depressants (benzodiazepines, opioids, tricyclic antidepressants): Additive CNS depression; increased risk of abnormal thinking and behavioral changes
ACTIVITIES
alcohol use: Additive CNS depression; increased risk of abnormal thinking and behavioral changes

Adverse Reactions
CNS: Abnormal dreams, amnesia, anxiety, cataplexy-like behaviors (mild), dizziness, hallucinations, headache, impaired daytime wakefulness, leg weakness (temporarily) sleep paralysis (temporarily), somnolence, suicidal ideation, worsening of depression
EENT: Dry mouth
GI: Diarrhea
RESP: Cough, upper respiratory tract infection
Other: Physical and psychological dependence

Nursing Considerations
• Use suvorexant with extreme caution in patients with a history of drug or alcohol abuse because of risk of addiction.

• Use suvorexant cautiously in elderly or debilitated patients and those with depression or impaired respiratory function.
• Monitor obese patients and women closely for adverse effects because these patients are at increased risk. Be aware that there is a dosage relationship to development of adverse reactions in general.
• Monitor respiratory status, especially in patients with respiratory compromise, who are at increased risk for respiratory depression.
• Watch patient closely for suicidal tendencies, particularly when therapy starts and dosage changes, because depression may worsen temporarily during these times, possibly leading to suicidal ideation.

Patient Teaching
• Tell patient to take drug 30 minutes before bedtime on an empty stomach with at least 7 hours remaining for sleep time.
• Caution patient to avoid potentially hazardous activities after taking suvorexant; drug's intended effect is to decrease alertness. Tell patient that CNS depressant effects may persist in some patients for up to several days after the drug is discontinued.
• Advise patient that drug may cause abnormal behaviors during sleep that extend into daytime, causing wakefulness impairment. Such behaviors may include driving a car, eating, talking on the phone, or having sex without any recall of the event. If family members notice any such behavior or patient sees evidence of such behavior upon awakening, drug should be withheld and prescriber notified.
• Advise limiting alcohol during therapy.
• Tell patient to notify prescriber if insomnia worsens or new signs or symptoms occur.
• Urge family or caregiver to watch patient closely for suicidal tendencies, especially when therapy starts or dosage changes.

T

tacrine hydrochloride
(tetrahydroamino-acridine, THA)

Cognex

Class and Category
Chemical class: Monoamine acridine
Therapeutic class: Dementia treatment
Pregnancy category: C

Indications and Dosages
➤ *To treat mild to moderate Alzheimer's-type dementia*

CAPSULES
Adults. *Initial:* 10 mg four times a day for 4 wk, increased to 20 mg four times a day and adjusted every 4 wk as prescribed. *Maximum:* 160 mg daily in 4 divided doses.

Contraindications
Hypersensitivity to tacrine, other acridine derivatives, or their components; jaundice from previous tacrine use; serum bilirubin level that exceeds 3 mg/dl

Interaction
DRUGS
anticholinergics: Decreased effects of both drugs
cholinergics, other cholinesterase inhibitors: Increased effects of these drugs and tacrine, possibly leading to toxicity
cimetidine: Increased blood tacrine level, possibly leading to toxicity
neuromuscular blockers: Prolonged or exaggerated muscle relaxation
NSAIDs: Increased gastric acid secretion, possibly GI irritation and bleeding
theophylline: Increased blood theophylline level, possibly leading to toxicity
FOODS
all foods: Reduced tacrine bioavailability

Mechanism of Action
Tacrine may relieve dementia in patients with Alzheimer's disease by increasing theacetylcholine level in the CNS. In Alzheimer's disease, some cholinergic neurons lose their ability to function, which decreases the acetylcholine level. The remaining functioning cholinergic neurons release acetylcholine, but it's enzymatically broken down by cholinesterases into acetic acid and choline, as shown below left. Without acetylcholine to activate muscarinic (M) and nicotinic (N) receptors on postsynaptic cell membranes, nerve transmission and excitability decrease.

Tacrine binds with and inhibits cholinesterases, making more intact acetylcholineavailable in cholinergic synapses, as shown below right. This prolongs and enhances acetylcholine's effects, which increases nerve transmission and reduces symptoms of dementia.

ACTIVITIES

smoking: Possibly decreased tacrine effectiveness

Adverse Reactions

CNS: Agitation, anxiety, asthenia, ataxia, confusion, depression, dizziness, fatigue, hallucinations, headache, hostility, insomnia, seizures, somnolence, syncope, tremor

CV: Arrhythmias, chest pain, conduction disturbances, hypertension, hypotension, palpitations, peripheral edema, sick sinus syndrome

EENT: Rhinitis

GI: Abdominal pain, anorexia, constipation, diarrhea, elevated liver function test results, flatulence, indigestion, nausea, vomiting

GU: Bladder obstruction, urinary frequency and incontinence, UTI

MS: Back pain, muscle stiffness, myalgia

RESP: Asthma, cough, upper respiratory tract infection, wheezing

SKIN: Flushing, jaundice, purpura, rash

Other: Weight loss

Nursing Considerations

• In patients with asthma, monitor for wheezing and increased mucus production because tacrine may increase bronchoconstriction and bronchial secretions.

• Expect to monitor hepatic enzyme levels (specifically ALT), as ordered, every other week from at least week 4 to week 16 of tacrine therapy.

• If patient has elevated serum ALT level, monitor her for signs and symptoms of hepatitis, such as jaundice and right-upper-quadrant pain. ALT level should return to normal 4 to 6 weeks after therapy stops.

• Once ALT level returns to normal, expect to begin tacrine therapy again (starting at 10 mg q.i.d.) as prescribed, and check patient's hepatic enzyme levels weekly for 16 weeks, monthly for 2 months, and then every 3 months thereafter, as ordered.

• Monitor patient for bradyarrhythmias, conduction disturbances, and sick sinus syndrome because tacrine may have a vagotonic effect on the heart rate.

WARNING Be aware that tacrine's cholinergic effects may exacerbate seizures or parkinsonian symptoms.

• Monitor patient's urine output and assess for abdominal distention and abnormal bowel sounds because drug's cholinergic effects may exacerbate conditions involving urinary tract or GI obstruction or ileus.

• Be aware that patients with peptic ulcer disease and those receiving NSAIDs are at increased risk for developing diarrhea, nausea, and vomiting because tacrine increases gastric acid secretion.

• Assess patient for increased signs and symptoms because drug becomes less effective as Alzheimer's disease progresses and the number of intact cholinergic neurons declines.

PATIENT TEACHING

• Instruct patient to take tacrine on an empty stomach, and advise caregiver to make sure that the patient swallows the drug.

• If patient experiences GI distress, suggest taking drug with meals. Mention that drug's effects may be delayed.

• Urge patient to seek assistance when walking and changing position until drug's effects are known. Instruct her to avoid potentially hazardous activities during this period.

• Advise patient not to smoke because it decreases drug's effectiveness.

• Caution patient not to stop taking drug abruptly. Doing so may impair cognitive ability.

• Inform caregiver that tacrine will become less effective as Alzheimer's disease progresses.

• Urge caregiver to make sure patient returns regularly for follow-up visits and laboratory tests to monitor drug effectiveness.

tacrolimus

Astagraf XL, Hecoria, Prograf

Class and Category

Chemical class: Macrolide

Therapeutic class: Immunosuppressant

Pregnancy category: C

Indications and Dosages

➤ *To prevent organ rejection in patients undergoing allogeneic liver, kidney, or heart transplantation*

CAPSULES (HECORIA, PROGRAF)
Adults having kidney transplantation in combination with azathioprine. 0.2 mg/ kg/day given in two equally divided doses every 12 hr beginning only after renal function has recovered (serum creatinine level of 4 mg/dl or less).

Adults having kidney transplantation in combination with MMF/IL-2 receptor antagonist therapy. 0.1 mg/kg/day given in two equally divided doses every 12 hr beginning only after renal function has recovered (serum creatinine level of 4 mg/ dl or less).

DOSAGE ADJUSTMENT FOR PROGRAF Black patients may need higher doses after kidney transplantation to attain comparable trough concentrations compared to Caucasian patients.

Adults having liver transplantation. 0.10 to 0.15 mg/kg/day given in two equally divided doses every 12 hr. Administer 6 hr after transplantation.

Children having liver transplantation. 0.15 to 0.20 mg/kg/day given in two equally divided doses every 12 hr. Administer 6 hr after transplantation.

Adults having heart transplantation. 0.075 mg/kg/day given in two equally divided doses every 12 hr. Administer first dose 6 hr after transplantation.

I.V. INFUSION (PROGRAF)
Adults having kidney or liver transplantation. 0.03 to 0.05 mg/kg/day as a continuous infusion beginning no sooner than 6 hr after transplantation.

Adults having heart transplantation. 0.0187 to 0.025 mg/kg/day as a continuous infusion beginning no sooner than 6 hr after transplantation.

Children having liver transplantation. 0.03 to 0.05 mg/kg/day as a continuous infusion beginning no sooner than 6 hr after transplantation.

DOSAGE ADJUSTMENT FOR HECORIA, PROGRAF Therapy delayed up to 48 hours or longer in patients with postoperative oliguria. For patients with hepatic or renal impairment, dosage kept at lower end of range with possible need for further reduction.

➤ *To prevent organ rejection in patients undergoing allogeneic kidney transplantation*

EXTENDED-RELEASE CAPSULES (ASTAGRAF XL)
Adults with basiliximab induction. 0.15 mg/kg/day 1 hr before a meal or 2 hr after a meal and started prior to or within 48 hr of completion of transplant procedure, but may be delayed until renal function has recovered.

Adults without basliximab induction. Pre-operatively: 0.1 mg/kg/day 1 hr before a meal or 2 hr after a meal. Post-operatively: 0.2 mg/kg/day.

DOSAGE ADJUSTMENT FOR ASTAGRAF XL Black patients may need higher doses to attain comparable trough concentrations compared to Caucasian patients. For patients with post-operative oliguria, initial dose administered no sooner than 6 hr and within 48 hr of transplantation, but may be delayed until renal function shows evidence of recovery. For patients who have developed nephrotoxicity, dosage reduced. For patients with severe hepatic impairment, lower dosage may be required.

Mechanism of Action
Inhibits T-lymphocyte activation, possibly by binding to an intracellular protein, FKBP-12. This binding results in formation of a complex of tacrolimus-FKBP-12, calcium, calmodulin, and calcineurin, which inhibits phosphatase activity of calcineurin. This inhibition may prevent dephosphorylation and translocation of nuclear factor of activated T-cells, a nuclear component thought to initiate gene transcription for the formation of lymphokines. The result is inhibition of T-lymphocyte activation, which produces immunosuppression.

Incompatibilities
Don't store diluted drug in PVC containers because of increased instability of tacrolimus and possible extraction of phthalates. Don't mix or co-infuse tacrolimus with solutions of pH 9 or greater, such as with acyclovir or ganciclovir, because of chemical instability of tacrolimus in alkaline media.

Contraindications
Breastfeeding, hypersensitivity to tacrolimus or its components,

T

hypersensitivity to polyoxyl 60 hydrogenated castor oil (parenteral form), ocular exposure, within 24 hours of cyclosporine therapy

Interaction

DRUGS

aminoglycosides, amphotericin B, cisplatin, cyclosporine, other nephrotoxic drugs: Increased risk of renal impairment
amiodrone, CYP3A4 inducers or inhibitors that has potential to prolong QT interval: Possibly prolonged QT interval
amiodrone, boceprevir, bromocriptine, chloramphenicol, cimetidine, cisapride, clarithromycin, clotrimazole, cyclosporine, danazol, diltiazem, erythromycin, ethinyl estradiol, fluconazole, ganciclovir, itraconazole, ketoconazole, lansoprazole, magnesium-aluminum-hydroxide, metoclopramide, methylprednisolone, nefazodone, nicardipine, nifedipine, nelfinavir, omeprazole, protease inhibitors, ritonavir, telaprevir, troleandomycin, verapamil, voriconazole: Possibly increased blood tacrolimus level
carbamazepine, caspofungin, phenobarbital, phenytoin, rifabutin, rifampin, sirolimus, St. John's wort: Possibly decreased blood tacrolimus level
mycophenolic acid: Possibly increased plasma mycophenolic acid level
phenytoin: Possibly increased blood phenytoin level
sirolimus: Increased risk of wound healing complications, renal dysfunction, and insulin-dependent posttransplant diabetes mellitus
vaccines (live or killed): Possibly suppressed immune response and increased adverse effects of vaccine

ACTIVITIES

alcohol use (Astagraf XL): Increased rate of release of tacrolimus

FOODS

grapefruit juice: Possibly increased blood tacrolimus trough levels in liver transplant patients
high-fat foods: Decreased absorption of oral tacrolimus

Adverse Reactions

CNS: Asthenia, fever, dizziness, headache, hemiparesis, insomnia, jittery feeling, leukoencephalopathy, mental changes, mutism, neurotoxicity, paresthesia, posterior reversible encephalopathy syndrome, progressive multifocal leukoencephalopathy, seizures, speech disorder, stroke, syncope, tremor
CV: Atrial and ventricular arrhythmias, cardiac arrest, chest pain, hyper-cholesterolemia, hyperlipemia, hypertension, hypertriglyceridemia, myocardial hypertrophy or ischemia, MI, pericardial effusion, peripheral edema, QT-interval prolongation, torsades de pointes, venous thrombosis
EENT: Blindness, cortical blindness, deafness, hearing loss, photophobia
ENDO: Cushingoid features, diabetes mellitus, hot flashes, hyperglycemia
GI: Abdominal pain, anorexia, ascites, bile duct stenosis, colitis, constipation, diarrhea, dyspepsia, enterocolitis, gastric ulcer, gastroenteritis, gastroesophageal reflux disease, gastrointestinal perforation, hepatic impairment or toxicity, impaired gastric emptying, nausea, pancreatitis, venoocclusive liver disease, vomiting
GU: Acute renal failure, BK virus nephropathy, elevated creatinine and BUN levels, hemorrhagic cystitis, hemolytic-uremic syndrome, micturition abnormality, nephrotoxicity, oliguria, renal impairment, UTI
HEME: Agranulocytosis, anemia, decreased platelet count, disseminated intravascular coagulation, hemolytic anemia, leuko-cytosis, neutropenia, pancytopenia, pure red cell aplasia, thrombocytopenia
MS: Arthralgia, back pain
RESP: Acute respiratory distress syndrome, atelectasis, bronchitis, cough increase, dyspnea, interstitial lung disease, lung infiltration, pleural effusion, respiratory distress or failure
SKIN: Flushing, malignancy, pruritus, rash, Stevens-Johnson syndrome, toxic epidermal necrolysis
Other: Anaphylaxis, cytomegalovirus infection, hyperkalemia, hypokalemia, hypomagnesemia, hypophosphatemia, impaired wound healing, lymphoproliferative or malignant disorders, multi-organ failure, opportunistic infections (including activation of latent viral infections), primary graft dysfunction, weight loss

Nursing Considerations

• Know that tacrolimus should not be given to patients with congenital long QT syndrome because of increased risk of life-threatening ventricular arrhythmias.
• Don't start tacrolimus therapy within 24 hours of cyclosporine, and vice versa. If tacrolimus or cyclosporine blood levels are elevated beyond 24 hours of either drug being discontinued, the other drug should not be started until elevation is resolved.
• Be aware that I.V. tacrolimus therapy should only be given if patient can't tolerate oral tacrolimus. Patient should be switched to oral therapy as soon as possible.
• Do not interchange oral immediate-release capsules with oral extended-release capsules.
• Know that drug should not be used simultaneously with cyclosporine, but when used to prevent kidney transplant rejection, it is recommended to be used concomitantly with mycophenolate mofetil. When Hecoria or Prograf formula is used to prevent either kidney or heart transplant rejection, azathioprine may be substituted for mycophenolate mofetil.
• Expect to give drug with adrenal corticosteroid therapy.
• Dilute intravenous drug with normal saline solution or 5% dextrose to 0.004 to 0.02 mg/ml following manufacturer guidelines. Once diluted, drug should be stored in glass or polyethylene containers (not PVC, because of decreased stability and possible extraction of phthalates). Discard after 24 hours if not used.
• When converting patient from parenteral to oral therapy after heart transplantation, expect to give oral form 8 to 12 hours after infusion is discontinued.
• Be aware that children having liver transplantation usually need higher doses of tacrolimus than adults.
WARNING Closely monitor patient for anaphylaxis at least during first 30 minutes of I.V. administration. Make sure emergency equipment and drugs, such as aqueous solution of epinephrine and oxygen, are immediately available.
• Monitor patient's blood tacrolimus trough levels regularly, as ordered. Higher trough levels increase risk of toxicity.

• Monitor blood pressure, especially in patients with history of hypertension, because drug can worsen this condition.
• Monitor results of liver and renal function tests, as ordered, to detect signs of decreased function.
• Know that tacrolimus may increase serum cholesterol, lipid, and triglyceride levels.
• Monitor patient's blood glucose level closely because tacrolimus may cause post-transplant diabetes mellitus with the need for insulin therapy, especially in black and Hispanic patients.
• Monitor patient's serum potassium level, as ordered, because drug can alter it.
• Watch for evidence of neurotoxicity, especially in patients receiving high doses of drug. Evidence of encephalopathy includes headache, impaired consciousness, loss of motor function, psychiatric disturbance, seizures, and tremors.
WARNING Monitor patient's ECG and electrolytes, as ordered, periodically throughout tacrolimus therapy because drug may prolong the QT interval, especially in patients with electrolyte disturbances, congestive heart failure, bradyarrhythmias and concomitant use of certain antiarrhythmic drugs.

PATIENT TEACHING

• Advise patient to take oral doses of Prograf, 12 hours apart, at same time each day on an empty stomach. Advise patient to take oral doses of Astagraf XL once daily in the morning either 1 hour before a meal or 2 hours after a meal on an empty stomach. Tell patient to swallow capsule whole and not to chew, divide, or crush capsule.
• Tell patient to avoid consuming grapefruit juice or alcohol while taking tacrolimus.
• Advise patient not to stop taking drug without consulting prescriber.
• Instruct patient not to receive virus vaccines during therapy. Urge him to avoid people who have received such vaccines or to wear a protective mask when he's around them.
• Caution patient to avoid having contact with people who have infections during therapy because tacrolimus causes immunosuppression.

T

• Emphasize the importance of having repeated laboratory tests while taking tacrolimus, and urge compliance.
• Inform patient that tacrolimus therapy may result in insulin-dependent diabetes. Tell him to report frequent urination or an increase in thirst, hunger, or fatigue.
• Instruct patient to limit exposure to direct sunlight and to wear protective clothing and use sunscreen when exposure can't be avoided.

tadalafil
Adcirca, Cialis

Class and Category
Chemical class: Phosphodiesterase inhibitor
Therapeutic class: Anti-impotence
Pregnancy category: B

Indications and Dosages
➤ *To treat erectile dysfunction*
TABLETS
Adults. *Initial:* 10 mg taken 1 hr before sexual activity; dosage decreased to 5 mg or increased to 20 mg, as prescribed, based on clinical response. *Maximum:* 20 mg daily. Or, 2.5 mg once daily, increased to 5 mg once daily, if needed.
DOSAGE ADJUSTMENT For patients who take drug on an as-needed basis and are taking potent CYP3A4 inhibitors such as itraconazole, ketoconazole, or ritonavir, dosage shouldn't exceed 10 mg every 72 hr. For patients taking potent CYP3A4 inhibitors and drug once daily, the maximum recommended dose is 2.5 mg daily. For patients with a creatinine clearance of 30 to 50 ml/min, who take drug on an as-needed basis, initial dosage decreased to 5 mg daily and maximum dosage not to exceed 10 mg every 48 hr. For patients with a creatinine clearance of less than 30 ml/min or who are on hemodialysis, who take drug on an as-needed basis, maximum dose should not exceed 5 mg every 72 hr. Once daily dosing is not recommended for patients with a creatinine clearance less than 30 ml/min. For patients with mild to moderate hepatic dysfunction who take drug on an as-needed basis, dosage should not exceed 10 mg once every day.

➤ *To treat benign prostatic hyperplasia*
TABLETS
Adults. 5 mg once daily at approximately the same time every day.
DOSAGE ADJUSTMENT For patients taking potent CYP3A4 inhibitors such as itraconazole, ketoconazole, or ritonavir, dosage reduced to 2.5 mg daily. For patients with a creatinine clearance of 30 to 50 mg/ml, initial dosage reduced to 2.5 mg once daily with possible increase to 5 mg, based upon individual response. Drug is not recommended for patients with a creatinine clearance less than 30 ml/min for this indication.

➤ *To treat benign prostatic hyperplasia and erectile dysfunction*
TABLETS
Adults. 5 mg once daily, at approximately the same time every day without regard to timing of sexual activity.
DOSAGE ADJUSTMENT For patients taking potent CYP3A4 inhibitors such as itraconazole, ketoconazole, or ritonavir, dosage reduced to 2.5 mg daily. For patients with a creatinine clearance of 30 to 50 mg/ml, initial dosage reduced to 2.5 mg once daily with possible increase to 5 mg, based upon individual response. Drug is not recommended for patients with a creatinine clearance less than 30 ml/min for this indication.

➤ *To treat pulmonary arterial hypertension in order to improve exercise ability in patients classified as group 1 by the world health organization*
TABLETS (ADCIRCA)
Adults. 40 mg once daily.
DOSAGE ADJUSTMENT For patients with mild to moderate hepatic or renal impairment or who have already taken ritonavir for at least 1 week, initial dosage of 20 mg once daily and then increased as tolerated. For patient already taking tadalafil and being prescribed ritonavir, tadalafil temporarily discontinued for at least 24 hours before ritonavir starts. Then, after at least 1 week of ritonavir, tadalafil restarted at 20 mg once daily and then increased to 40 mg once daily, as tolerated.

Route	Onset	Peak	Duration
P.O.	Unknown	30 min–6 hr	Unknown

Mechanism of Action

Enhances the effect of nitric oxide released in the penis during sexual stimulation. Nitric oxide activates the enzyme guanylate cyclase, which causes increased levels of cGMP in the corpus cavernosum. This leads to increased blood flow to the penis, thus producing an erection.

Contraindications

Continuous or intermittent nitrate therapy, hypersensitivity to tadalafil or its components, retinitis pigmentosa

Interaction

DRUGS

carbamazepine, phenytoin, phenobarbitol: Possibly decreased tadalafil effects
doxazosin, tamsulosin and other alpha blockers: Increased risk of symptomatic hypotension
erythromycin, itraconazole, ketoconazole, ritonavir: Prolonged tadalafil effects
nitrates: Profound hypotension
protease inhibitors (other than ritonavir): Possibly prolonged tadalafil effects
rifampin: Decreased tadalafil effects

FOODS

grapefruit juice: Possibly prolonged tadalafil effects

ACTIVITIES

alcohol use: Potentiated blood pressure–lowering effects

Adverse Reactions

CNS: Asthenia, dizziness, fatigue, headache, hypesthesia, insomnia, migraine, paresthesia, seizures, somnolence, stroke, syncope, transient global amnesia, vertigo
CV: Angina pectoris, chest pain, hypotension, hypertension, MI, postural hypotension, palpitations, sudden cardiac death, tachycardia
EENT: Blurred vision, changes in color vision, conjunctivitis, dry mouth, epistaxis, eyelid swelling, eye pain, hearing or visual loss, increased lacrimation, nasal congestion, nasopharyngitis, nonarteritic anterior ischemic optic neuropathy, pharyngitis, retinal artery or vein occlusion, visual field defects
GI: Abnormal liver function studies, diarrhea, dysphagia, dyspepsia, esophagitis, gastroesophageal reflux, gastritis, increased gamma-glutamyl transpeptidase levels, nausea, upper abdominal pain, vomiting
GU: Priapism, spontaneous penile erection, UTI
MS: Arthralgia, back or neck pain, extremity pain, myalgia
RESP: Bronchitis, cough, dyspnea, upper respiratory tract infection
SKIN: Diaphoresis, exfoliative dermatitis, flushing, pruritus, rash, Stevens-Johnson syndrome, urticaria
Other: Facial edema, flulike symptoms, hypersensitivity reactions

Nursing Considerations

• Know that patients with hereditary degenerative retinal disorders, including retinitis pigmentosa, should not receive tadalafil because of the risk of serious ophthalmic adverse reactions.
• Patients with severe hepatic or renal impairment should not receive tadalafil because its effects in these patients are unknown.
• Use tadalafil cautiously in patients with left ventricular outflow obstruction, such as aortic stenosis and idiopathic hypertrophic subaortic stenosis, and those with severely impaired autonomic control of blood pressure because these conditions increase sensitivity to vasodilators, such as tadalafil.
• Use tadalafil cautiously in patients with conditions that may predispose them to priapism, such as sickle cell anemia, multiple myeloma, leukemia, or penile deformities (such as angulation, cavernosal fibrosis, or Peyronie's disease).
• Monitor blood pressure and heart rate and rhythm before and during therapy.

PATIENT TEACHING

• Explain that, when used as needed to treat erectile dysfunction, tadalafil should be taken 1 hour before sexual activity to provide the most effective results. Alternatively, if the patient chooses to take a smaller dose of tadalfil daily, encourage him to take it at about the same time every day, regardless of the timing of sexual activity.
WARNING Tell patient not to take tadalafil if he takes any form of organic nitrate, either continuously or intermittently, because profound hypotension and death could result.

T

• If patient takes tadalafil to treat erectile dysfunction, advise him to obtain sexual counseling to help enhance the drug's effects.
• To avoid possible penile damage and permanent loss of erectile function, urge patient to notify prescriber immediately if erection is painful or lasts longer than 4 hours.
• Advise patient to limit alcohol consumption while taking tadalafil.
WARNING Tell patient to seek immediate medical attention if he experiences a sudden loss of vision in one or both eyes or hearing loss that may be accompanied by tinnitus and dizziness.

tamoxifen citrate

Apo-Tamox (CAN), Gen-Tamoxifen (CAN), Nolvadex, Novo-Tamoxifen (CAN), Tamofen (CAN), Tamone (CAN)

Class and Category
Chemical class: Triphenylethylene derivative
Therapeutic class: Nonsteroidal antiestrogen agent, partial estrogen agonist
Pregnancy category: D

Indications and Dosages
➤ *To treat metastatic breast cancer in men and women; to treat node-negative breast cancer in women, or node-positive breast cancer in postmenopausal women, after total or segmental mastectomy, axillary dissection, and breast irradiation*
TABLETS
Adults. 20 to 40 mg daily. Dosages greater than 20 mg administered twice daily.
➤ *To reduce the risk of invasive breast cancer in women with ductal carcinoma in situ (DCIS) after surgery and radiation, to reduce the risk of breast cancer in women at high risk*
TABLETS
Adults. 20 mg daily for 5 yr.

Mechanism of Action
May block the effects of estrogen on breast tissue by competing with estrogen for estrogen-receptor binding sites. Estrogen may stimulate the growth of cancer cells.

Contraindications
Hypersensitivity to tamoxifen or its components; women at high risk for breast cancer and women with ductal carcinoma in situ and a history of deep vein thrombosis or pulmonary embolus or who need coumarin-type anticoagulant therapy; use with anastrozole therapy

Interaction
DRUGS
bromocriptine: Possibly increased blood tamoxifen level
estrogens: Possibly altered therapeutic effect of tamoxifen
warfarin and other coumarin-type anticoagulants: Increased anticoagulant effect of these drugs

Adverse Reactions
CNS: Confusion, depression, dizziness, fatigue, headache, light-headedness, somnolence, stroke, weakness
CV: Edema, hyperlipidemia, thrombosis
EENT: Keratopathy, ocular toxicity (including cataracts), optic neuritis, retinopathy
GI: Elevated liver function test results, hepatotoxicity, nausea, vomiting
GU: Endometrial cancer, endometrial hyperplasia, endometrial polyps, genital itching, menstrual irregularities, ovarian cysts, uterine malignancies, vaginal discharge (females); impotence, decreased libido (males)
HEME: Anemia, leukopenia, thrombocytopenia
MS: Transient bone or tumor pain
RESP: Pulmonary embolism
SKIN: Bullous pemphigoid, dry skin, erythema multiforme, rash, Stevens-Johnson syndrome, thinning hair
Other: Angioedema, hot flashes, hypercalcemia, weight gain

Nursing Considerations
WARNING Make sure that patient has been informed about serious or potentially life-threatening adverse effects associated with tamoxifen before therapy begins. Be aware that women with ductal carcinoma in situ and those at high risk for breast cancer are more likely to develop uterine cancer, stroke, or pulmonary emboli than others receiving tamoxifen.

• If patient is premenopausal, begin drug therapy in the middle of menstruation; if patient's menstrual cycles are irregular, verify that she has had a negative pregnancy test before therapy starts.
• Expect patient to undergo an ophthalmic examination before and periodically during tamoxifen therapy. Also expect to monitor patient for adverse ocular reactions, such as cataracts.
• Assess patient for signs and symptoms of thromboembolic events, such as shortness of breath, leg pain, and change in mental status.
• Periodically monitor patient's platelet and WBC counts, cholesterol and triglyceride levels, and liver function test results, as ordered.
• Monitor blood calcium level and assess patient for signs and symptoms of hypercalcemia, such as nausea, vomiting, and thirst; tamoxifen may cause hypercalcemia in breast cancer patients with bone metastasis within a few weeks of starting treatment.
• Store tamoxifen in a closed, light-resistant container at room temperature.

PATIENT TEACHING
• Advise patient to swallow tamoxifen tablet whole with water.
• Instruct premenopausal patient to use a nonhormonal form of contraception, such as a condom or diaphragm, during tamoxifen therapy. Emphasize that she shouldn't become pregnant while taking drug and for 2 months afterward. Advise her to notify prescriber at once if she becomes pregnant during therapy.
• Inform patient of the most common side effects—hot flashes, vaginal discharge, and irregular menses.
• Urge patient to immediately notify prescriber if she notices a rash, itching, difficulty breathing, or facial swelling because they may signify a hypersensitivity reaction.
• Advise patient to notify prescriber if she experiences leg pain or calf swelling during tamoxifen therapy because they may indicate a blood clot.
• Instruct patient to report signs of hepatotoxicity, such as tiredness, nausea, yellow skin, and flulike symptoms.

• Advise patient to have regular gynecologic exmainations and to notify prescriber about abnormal symptoms, including abdominal or pelvic pain, new breast lumps, and unusual vaginal discharge or bleeding.
• Urge patients who take tamoxifen for prophylaxis to have regular mammograms because tamoxifen doesn't prevent all cancers.
• Emphasize the importance of taking tamoxifen regularly. Urge patient to consult prescriber if adverse reactions, such as nausea and vomiting, are interfering with dosage schedule. These symptoms may be a sign of hypercalcemia.
• Inform women who wish to breastfeed that tamoxifen may appear in breastmilk and cause serious adverse effects in the infant.

tamsulosin hydrochloride
Flomax

Class and Category
Chemical class: Sulfamoylphenethylamine derivative
Therapeutic class: Benign prostatic hyperplasia (BPH) treatment
Pregnancy category: B

Indications and Dosages
➤ *To treat BPH*
CAPSULES
Adults. *Initial:* 0.4 mg daily 30 min after a meal for 2 to 4 wk, increased to 0.8 mg daily if no response to initial dosage. *Maximum:* 0.8 mg daily.

Mechanism of Action
Blocks alpha$_1$-adrenergic receptors in the prostate. This action inhibits smooth-muscle contraction in the prostate, prostatic capsule, prostatic urethra, and bladder neck, which improves the rate of urine flow and reduces symptoms of BPH.

Contraindications
Hypersensitivity to tamsulosin, quinazolines, or their components

T

Interaction
DRUGS
alpha blockers: Additive effects of both drugs
cimetidine: Risk of decreased tamsulosin
clearance
*CYP2D6 inhibitors (such as fluoxetine,
paroxetine, terbinafine), CYP3A4 inhibitors
(such as erythromycin, ketoconazole):*
Possibly increased plasma tamsulosin level
phosphodiesterase-5 inhibitors: Increased
risk of hypotension

Adverse Reactions
CNS: Asthenia, dizziness, drowsiness,
headache, insomnia, syncope, vertigo
CV: Arrhythmia, atrial fibrillation, chest
pain, orthostatic hypotension, palpitations,
tachycardia
EENT: Amblyopia, diplopia, dry mouth,
epistaxis, intraoperative floppy iris
syndrome (during cataract and glaucoma
surgery), pharyngitis, rhinitis, visual
impairment
GI: Constipation, diarrhea, nausea, vomiting
GU: Decreased libido, ejaculation disorders,
priapism
MS: Back pain
RESP: Dyspnea, respiratory impairment
SKIN: Dermatitis exfoliative,
desquamation, erythema multiforme,
pruritus, rash, Stevens-Johnson syndrome,
urticaria
Other: Angioedema

Nursing Considerations
• Be aware that prostate cancer should be
ruled out before tamsulosin therapy
begins.
• Give drug about 30 minutes after the same
meal each day.
• If patient takes drug on an empty
stomach, monitor his blood pressure
because of the increased risk of orthostatic hypotension.
• If patient doesn't take drug for several
days, resume therapy at 0.4 mg/dose, as
prescribed.
PATIENT TEACHING
• Instruct patient not to open, crush, or chew
tamsulosin capsules and to take drug about
30 minutes after the same meal each day.
• Instruct patient to notify prescriber if he
misses several days of therapy, and caution
him against restarting drug at previous
dosage.

• Advise patient to avoid potentially
hazardous activities until drug's CNS
effects are known. Mention the need for
caution if dosage is increased.
• Advise patient to change position slowly,
especially after initial dose and each
dosage increase, to minimize effects of
orthostatic hypotension.
• Tell patient to inform ophthalmologist of
tamsulosin therapy because drug may
increase risk for complications with
cataract surgery.

tapentadol
Nucynta, Nucynta ER

Class, Category, and Schedule
Chemical class: Mu-opioid agonist
Therapeutic class: Centrally acting synthetic
analgesic
Pregnancy category: C
Controlled substance schedule: II

Indications and Dosages
➤ *To relieve moderate to severe acute pain*
TABLETS
Adults. 50 mg to 100 mg repeated every
4 to 6 hr, as needed. *Maximum:* 700 mg on
first day; 600 mg daily thereafter
DOSAGE ADJUSTMENT On first day of
therapy, second dose may be given as soon
as 1 hour after first dose, if needed. For
patients with moderate hepatic impairment
(Child-Pugh Class B), dosage should not
exceed 50 mg for each episode, and
intervals between doses should be at least
8 hours.
E.R. TABLETS
**Adults currently not taking opioid
analgesics.** *Initial:* 50 mg twice daily,
increased as needed. *Maximum:* 250 mg
twice daily.
Adults currently taking opioid analgesics.
Initial: 50 mg followed by dosage increased,
as needed with subsequent doses split into
two equal doses given twice daily.
Maximum: 250 mg twice daily.
DOSAGE ADJUSTMENT For patients with
moderate hepatic impairment, initial
dosage reduced to 50 mg once daily and
increased as needed to maximum dosage of
100 mg once daily.

➤ *To relieve neuropathic pain associated with diabetic peripheral neuropathy when a continuous, around-the-clock opioid analgesic is needed for an extended period of time*

E.R. TABLETS

Adults currently not taking opioid analgesics. *Initial:* 50 mg twice daily, increased as needed no sooner than every 3 days. *Maximum:* 250 mg twice daily.

Adults currently taking opioid analgesics. *Initial:* 50 mg followed by dosage increased, as needed no sooner than every 3 days with subsequent doses split into two equal doses given twice daily. *Maximum:* 250 mg twice daily.

DOSAGE ADJUSTMENT For patients with moderate hepatic impairment, initial dosage reduced to 50 mg once daily and increased as needed to maximum dosage of 100 mg once daily.

Route	Onset	Peak	Duration
P.O.	Unknown	1 hr	4 hr

Mechanism of Action

Binds with and activates opioid receptors (mainly mu receptors) in brain and spinal cord and inhibits norepinephrine reuptake to produce analgesia.

Contraindications

Acute or severe bronchial asthma, hypercapnia or significant respiratory depression not monitored or without available resuscitation equipment; gastrointestinal obstruction including paralytic ileus; hypersensitivity to tapentadol or its components; within 14 days of MAO inhibitor therapy

Interaction

DRUGS

CNS depressants: Increased risk of life-threatening effects from respiratory or CNS depression

MAO inhibitors: Possibly hyperpyretic episodes, hypertensive crisis, serotonin syndrome, and severe seizures

serotonergics: Increased risk of potentially fatal serotonin syndrome

ACTIVITIES

alcohol use: Increased serum tapentadol level possibly resulting in fatal overdose from CNS and respiratory depression, risk of CNS depression

Adverse Reactions

CNS: Abnormal dreams, anxiety, confusion, dizziness, fatigue, hallucinations, headache, insomnia, lethargy, panic attack, seizure, serotonin syndrome, somnolence, suicidal ideation, syncope, tremor
CV: Hypotension, palpitations
EENT: Dry mouth, nasopharyngitis
ENDO: Hot flash
GI: Constipation, dyspepsia, diarrhea, nausea, vomiting
GU: Anorexia, UTI
MS: Arthralgia
RESP: Respiratory depression, upper respiratory infection
SKIN: Diaphoresis, pruritus, rash, urticaria
Other: Anaphylaxis including anaphylactic shock, anagioedema, physical or psychological dependence, withdrawal

Nursing Considerations

• Be aware that tapentadol isn't recommended for patients with severe renal impairment (creatinine clearance less than 30 ml/min/1.73 m^2) or severe hepatic dysfunction (Child-Pugh Class C).

• Use tapentadol with extreme caution in patients with hypoxia, hypercapnia, or decreased respiratory reserve such as may occur in asthma, COPD, cor pulmonale, severe obesity, sleep apnea syndrome, myxedema, kyphoscoliosis, CNS depression, or coma. Also use cautiously in patients with head injury or conditions in which increased intracranial pressure may occur because drug may obscure the signs and symptoms. Also use cautiously in patients with mild to moderate renal or hepatic dysfunction and in patients with biliary tract disease, including acute pancreatitis, because drug may cause spasm of the sphincter of Oddi.

• Expect to begin tapentadol therapy at lower doses in elderly patients because of age-related decreased renal and hepatic function.

WARNING Monitor patient's respiratory rate, depth, and effort during tapentadol therapy because drug may cause respiratory depression, especially in elderly or debilitated patients and in those who have conditions accompanied by hypoxia,

T

hypercapnia, or upper airway obstruction. If respiratory rate drops below 10 breaths per minute, notify prescriber, expect drug to be discontinued, and provide needed supportive care, which may include an opioid antagonist such as naloxone, as ordered.

• Monitor patient's blood pressure closely, especially when initiating tapentadol therapy and when titrating the dose because the drug may cause severe hypotension and syncope in ambulatory patients due to its vasodilatory effects. Risk of hypotension is greatest in patients who already have been compromised by a reduced blood volume or concurrent administration of certain CNS depressant drugs such as general anesthetics and phenothiazines.

• Monitor patients with seizure disorders closely because tapentadol may induce or aggravate seizures.

• Monitor patient for evidence of physical and psychological dependence.

WARNING Watch patient closely for evidence of serotonin syndrome, which can be life-threatening. Report mental status changes (agitation, hallucinations, coma), autonomic instability (tachycardia, labile blood pressure, hyperthermia), neuromuscular abnormalities (hyperreflexia, incoordination) or GI disturbances (nausea, vomiting or diarrhea).

• Don't stop tapentadol abruptly if used on a regular basis because withdrawal symptoms may occur.

• Be aware that tapentadol shouldn't be used during or just before labor and delivery.

• Watch patient closely for suicidal tendencies, particularly when therapy starts and after dosage changes.

PATIENT TEACHING

• Instruct patient to take tapentadol exactly as prescribed and not to adjust dose or frequency without consulting prescriber.

• Tell patient prescribed E.R. tablet form, to take tablet whole and not to cut, crush, dissolve, or chew the tablet because doing so could be fatal.

• Advise patient to avoid hazardous activities until drug's CNS effects are known.

• Caution patient to avoid alcohol or other CNS depressants while taking tapentadol.

• Advise patient who has been taking tapentadol regularly not to stop taking it abruptly; instead, patient should taper drug use gradually, based on prescriber instructions, to reduce the risk of withdrawal symptoms.

• Urge family or caregiver to watch patient closely for suicidal tendencies, especially when therapy starts or after dosage changes.

• Tell female patient to notify prescriber if pregnancy occurs, as prolonged use of tapentadol during pregnancy can result in neonatal opioid withdrawal syndrome, which may be life threatening.

• Caution patient to keep drug out of the hands of children because accidental ingestion could be fatal.

tedizolid
Sivextro

Class and Category
Chemical class: Oxazolidinone
Therapeutic class: Antibacterial
Pregnancy category: C

Indications and Dosages
➤ *To treat acute bacterial skin and skin structure infections caused by the following gram-positive microorganisms:* Enterococcus faecalis, Staphylococcus aureus *(including methicillin-resistant and methicillin-susceptible isolates),* Streptococcus agalactiae, S. anginosus group *(including* S. anginosus, S. intermedius, *and* S. constellatus), *and* S. pyogenes

TABLETS
Adults. 200 mg once daily for 6 days.
I.V. INFUSION
Adults. 200 mg infused over 1 hour once daily for 6 days.

Mechanism of Action
Causes cell wall lysis and subsequent death of bacteria cell

Incompatibilities
Do not dilute tedizolid with any solution containing divalent cations (i.e., Ca^{2+}, Mg^{2+}), including lactated Ringer's injection and Hartmann's solution because of

incompatibilities. Do not mix tedizolid with other drugs or reconstitute drug with any solution other than sterile water for injection because incompatibilities are unknown.

Contraindications
Hypersensitivity to tedizolid and its components

Adverse Reactions
CNS: Dizziness, headache, hypoesthesia, insomnia, paresthesia, peripheral neuropathy, VII nerve paralysis
CV: Hypertension, palpitations, tachycardia
EENT: Blurred vision, optic neuropathy, oral candidiasis, visual impairment, vitreous floaters
GI: *Clostridium difficile*–associated diarrhea, diarrhea, elevated liver enzymes, nausea, vomiting
GU: Vulvovaginal mycotic infection
HEME: Anemia; decreased absolute neutrophil count, hemoglobin, platelet count, or white blood cell count
SKIN: Dermatitis, flushing, pruritus, urticaria
Other: Hypersensitivity, infusion-related reactions

Nursing Considerations
• Be aware that tedizolid may not be effective in the treatment of bacterial skin and skin structure infections in patients with neutropenia and should not be used.
• Reconstitute each vial with 4 ml of sterile water for injection. Gently swirl the contents (do not shake to minimize foaming) and let the vial stand until the cake has completely dissolved and any foam disperses. May be stored at room temperature or in the refrigerator for up to 24 hours.
• Withdraw 4 ml of reconstituted solution from vial (do not invert the vial during extraction). Slowly inject the 4 ml of reconstituted solution into an intravenous bag containing 250 ml of 0.9% sodium chloride. Invert bag gently to mix (do not shake).
• Administer parenteral form as an intravenous infusion over 1 hour. Never administer as an intravenous push or bolus. If the intravenous line is used for subsequent infusions of any other drugs, flush the line before and after tedizolid infusion with 0.9% sodium chloride injection, USP.
• Assess patient for signs of secondary infection, such as profuse, watery diarrhea. If such diarrhea develops, contact prescriber and expect to obtain a stool specimen to rule out pseudomembranous colitis caused by *Clostridium difficile.* If diarrhea occurs, notify prescriber and expect to withhold drug and treat with fluids, electrolytes, protein, and an antibiotic effective against *C. difficile.*
PATIENT TEACHING
• Tell patient receiving oral tedizolid that it may be taken without regard to food.
• Instruct patient that if he misses a dose, to take it as soon as possible anytime up to 8 hours prior to his next scheduled dose. If less than 8 hours remain before the next dose, he should skip the missed dose and take the next dose on schedule.
• Stress the importance of completing the prescribed 6 days of therapy.
• Urge patient to tell prescriber if diarrhea develops, which may occur even as late as 2 or more months after tedizolid therapy has ended.

telavancin
Vibativ

Class and Category
Chemical class: Lipoglycopeptide
Therapeutic class: Antibacterial
Pregnancy category: C

Indications and Dosages
➤ *To treat complicated skin and skin structure infections caused by gram-positive organisms* (Staphylococcus aureus, Streptococcus pyogenes, Streptococcus agalactiae, Streptococcus anginosus *group [includes* S. anginosus, S. intermedius, *and* S. constellatus*]), or* Enterococcus faecalis *(vancomycin-susceptible isolates only)*
I.V. INFUSION
Adults. 10 mg/kg administered over 60 min every 24 hours for 7 to 14 days

T

➤ *To treat hospital-acquired and ventilator-associated bacterial pneumonia caused by Staphylococcus aureus when alternative treatments are not suitable*

I.V. INFUSION

Adults. 10 mg/kg administered over 60 min every 24 hours for 7 to 21 days.

DOSAGE ADJUSTMENT For patients with creatinine clearance of 30 to 50 ml/min/1.73 m², dosage reduced to 7.5 mg/kg every 24 hours. For patient with creatinine clearance of at least 10 but less than 30 ml/min/1.73 m², 10 mg/kg every 48 hours.

Route	Onset	Peak	Duration
I.V.	Unknown	1–2 hr	24 hr

Mechanism of Action

Inhibits cell wall synthesis and alters the permeability of bacterial membranes, causing cell wall lysis and cell death. Telavancin is a lipoglycopeptide antibacterial that's a synthetic derivative of vancomycin.

Incompatibilities

Don't mix telavancin with other drugs or IV solutions containing additives. If administration must be through the same IV line, flush the line with 5% dextrose injection, 0.9% sodium chloride injection, or lactated Ringer's injection before and after infusing telavancin.

Contraindications

Hypersensitivity to telavancin or its components, intravenous unfractionated heparin sodium

Interaction

DRUGS

ACE inhibitors, loop diuretics, NSAIDs: Increased risk of nephrotoxicity

drugs known to prolong the QT interval, such as clarithromycin, disopyramide, erythromycin, quinidine: Increased risk of prolonged QT interval

Adverse Reactions

CNS: Dizziness, rigors
CV: Prolonged QT interval
EENT: Taste disturbance
GI: Abdominal pain, anorexia, diarrhea, *Clostridium difficile*–associated diarrhea, nausea, vomiting
GU: Elevated creatinine level, foamy urine, nephrotoxicity such as renal failure, impairment, or insufficiency
HEME: Abnormal coagulation test results (aPTT, activated clotting time, coagulation-based factor X activity assay, INR, and PT)
SKIN: Pruritus, rash
Other: Infusion-related reactions such as erythema or pain

Nursing Considerations

• Know that telavancin isn't recommended for patients with congenital long-QT syndrome, uncompensated heart failure, or severe left ventricular hypertrophy or who currently have a prolonged QT interval because it may prolong the QT interval, causing life-threatening complications.

• Know that use of intravenous unfractionated heparin sodium is contraindicated wtih telavancin because the activated partial thromboplastin time (aPTT) test results may be falsely prolonged for up to 18 hours after telavancin administration.

• Use cautiously in patients taking drugs known to prolong the QT interval because of increased the risk of a prolonged QT interval.

• Make sure woman of childbearing age has a negative pregnancy test result before starting telavancin because of risk of fetal harm.

• Obtain baseline serum creatinine level before telavancin therapy starts, and monitor it throughout therapy, as ordered, because drug may cause nephrotoxicity, especially in patients with preexisting renal disease, diabetes mellitus, congestive heart failure, or hypertension and in patients taking such nephrotoxic drugs as NSAIDs, ACE inhibitors, and loop diuretics. If renal function declines, notify prescriber and expect to discontinue telavancin.

• Dilute a 250-mg vial with 15 ml or a 750-mg vial with 45 ml of a diluent such as 5% dextrose injection, sterile water for injection, or 0.9% sodium chloride injection to obtain a solution of 15 mg/ml. When ready to administer drug, further dilute doses of 150 mg to 800 mg in 100 to 250 ml of 5% dextrose injection, 0.9% sodium chloride injection, or lactated Ringer's

injection before infusion. Doses less than 150 mg or greater than 800 mg should be further diluted in a volume that yields a final concentration of 0.6 to 0.8 mg/ml.
- Infuse telavancin over 60 minutes because more rapid infusion may cause a reaction like red-man syndrome, which causes flushing of upper body, urticaria, pruritus, or rash. If present, stop or slow infusion to resolve.
- Use telavancin within 4 hours of the time it is reconstituted in the vial (including its transfer to an infusion bag for further dilution) if kept at room temperature and 72 hours if refrigerated. Discard if time limit exceeds these parameters.
- Monitor patient for diarrhea, which may range from mild to severe and may occur up to 2 months after antibiotic is discontinued. Report diarrhea and, if *C. difficile* is suspected, expect telavancin to be discontinued. Provide supportive care, such as fluid and electrolyte replacement, protein supplementation, antibiotic therapy to treat *C. difficile,* and possibly surgical intervention, as needed.
- Be aware that while telavancin doesn't interfere with coagulation, it does interfere with certain tests used to monitor coagulation, such as PT, INR, APTT, activated clotting time, and coagualtion-based factor Xa tests. Collect blood samples for coagulation tests as close as possible to administration of next dose of telavancin to minimize interference.

PATIENT TEACHING
- Instruct women of childbearing age to use effective contraception during telavancin therapy.
- Caution patient that diarrhea may occur up to 2 months after antibiotic has been discontinued and to report any persistent or severe episodes to prescriber.
- Warn patient that drug may cause urine to be foamy and taste to be altered.
- Advise patient to alert all prescribers that he takes telavancin because some drugs may interact with it, causing serious adverse effects.

telithromycin

Ketek

Class and Category
Chemical class: Semisynthetic ketolide
Therapeutic class: Antibiotic
Pregnancy category: C

Indications and Dosages
➤ *To treat mild to moderate community-acquired pneumonia caused by* Streptococcus pneumoniae, Haemophilus influenzae, Moraxella catarrhalis, Chlamydophila pneumoniae, *or* Mycoplasma pneumoniae

TABLETS
Adults. 800 mg once daily P.O. for 7 to 10 days.
DOSAGE ADJUSTMENT For patients with severe renal impairment, including patients on dialysis, dosage reduced to 600 mg once daily for 7 to 10 days. For patients with severe renal impairment and coexisting hepatic impairment, dosage reduced to 400 mg once daily for 7 to 10 days.

Route	Onset	Peak	Duration
P.O.	Unknown	1 hr	Unknown

Mechanism of Action
Binds to domains II and V of the 50S ribosomal subunit in many aerobic, anaerobic, gram-positive, and gram-negative bacteria of the respiratory tract. Telithromycin may also inhibit the assembly of nascent ribosomal units. These actions inhibit RNA-dependent protein synthesis in bacterial cells, causing them to die.

Contraindications
Cisapride or pimozide therapy; history of hepatitis or jaundice associated with use of telithromycin or any macrolide antibiotic; hypersensitivity to telithromycin, macrolide antibiotics, or their components; myasthenia gravis

Interaction
DRUGS
atorvastatin, lovastatin, midazolam, pimozide, simvastatin: Possibly increased blood levels of these drugs
cisapride, dofetilide, procainamide, quinidine: Increased risk of prolonged QT interval
colchicine: Increased blood colchicine levels with risk of colchicine toxicity

T

itraconazole, ketoconazole: Increased blood level of telithromycin
oral anticoagulants: Possibly potentiated effects of oral anticoagulants
rifampin: Decreased blood level of telithromycin
sotalol: Decreased sotalol absorption
theophylline: Increased risk of adverse GI reactions

Adverse Reactions
CNS: Dizziness, fatigue, headache, insomnia, somnolence, transient loss of consciousness, vertigo
CV: Atrial arrhythmias, prolonged QT interval, torsades de pointes
EENT: Blurred vision, difficulty focusing eyes, diplopia, dry mouth, glossitis, oral candidiasis, stomatitis
GI: Abdominal distention or pain, anorexia, constipation, diarrhea, elevated liver function test results, flatulence, fulminant hepatitis, gastroenteritis, gastritis, hepatic failure or necrosis, hepatitis, nausea, pseudomembranous colitis, taste perversion, vomiting
GU: Vaginal candidiasis, vaginitis, vaginosis (fungal)
HEME: Increased platelet count
MS: Exacerbated myasthenia gravis, muscle cramps
RESP: Acute respiratory failure
SKIN: Diaphoresis, rash
Other: Angioedema, anaphylaxis

Nursing Considerations
• Be aware that telithromycin therapy shouldn't be used in patients who have congenital prolonged QT interval or ongoing proarrhythmic conditions (such as uncorrected hypokalemia or hypomagnesemia, or serious bradycardia) or in those receiving concurrent therapy with class IA or class III antiarrhythmics because telithromycin increases the risk of QT-interval prolongation, which may lead to ventricular arrhythmias, including torsades de pointes.
• Before administering the first telithromycin dose, expect to obtain respiratory specimens for culture and sensitivity testing.
• Monitor patient closely for diarrhea, which may indicate pseudomembranous colitis. If it occurs, notify prescriber and expect to

withhold drug and give fluids, electrolytes, protein, and an antibiotic effective against *Clostridium difficile.*
WARNING Monitor patient's liver studies for abnormalities, and assess patient for evidence of liver dysfunction, such as fatigue, malaise, anorexia, nausea, jaundice, acholic stools, and liver tenderness, because telithromycin may cause potentially life-threatening acute hepatic failure and severe liver damage.

PATIENT TEACHING
• Emphasize need to take drug for prescribed duration, even if patient feels better before prescription is finished.
• Caution patient to avoid hazardous activities until drug's CNS and visual effects are known. Explain that telithromycin can cause trouble focusing eyes, especially for first 30 minutes after a dose.
• Instruct patient to notify prescriber if visual disturbances occur, and tell her to avoid quick changes in viewing near and distant objects.
• Tell patient to alert prescriber if she faints because drug may alter heart rhythm.
• Caution patient to notify prescriber immediately about fatigue, malaise, anorexia, nausea, abdominal tenderness, yellow skin, or changes in stool appearance.

telmisartan
Micardis

Class and Category
Chemical class: Nonpeptide angiotensin II antagonist
Therapeutic class: Antihypertensive
Pregnancy category: D

Indications and Dosages
➤ *To manage hypertension, alone or with other antihypertensives*
TABLETS
Adults. *Initial:* 40 mg daily. *Maintenance:* 20 to 80 mg daily. *Maximum:* 80 mg daily.
➤ *To reduce risk of MI, stroke, or death from cardiovascular causes in patients at high risk who are unable to take ACE inhibitors*

TABLETS
Adults age 55 and over. 80 mg once daily.

Route	Onset	Peak	Duration
P.O.	Unknown	In 4 wk	Unknown

Mechanism of Action

Blocks angiotensin II from binding to receptor sites in many tissues, including vascular smooth muscle and adrenal glands. This action inhibits the vasoconstrictive and aldosterone-secreting effects of angiotensin II, which reduces blood pressure.

Contraindications

Concurrent aliskiren therapy in patients with diabetes or renal impairment (GFR less than 60 ml/min.), hypersensitivity to telmisartan or its components

Interaction

DRUGS
ACE inhibitors, aliskiren, other angiotensin receptor blockers: Increased risk of hypotension, hyperkalemia, and renal dysfunction
digoxin: Increased peak blood digoxin level and risk of digitalis toxicity
diuretics, other antihypertensives: Enhanced hypotensive effect
lithium: Increased serum lithium levels and toxicity
NSAIDs: Increased risk of renal dysfunction in elderly patients and those with volume depletion and existing renal dysfunction
ramipril: Increased serum ramipril level; decreased telmisartan level

Adverse Reactions

CNS: Asthenia, dizziness, fatigue, headache, syncope, weakness
CV: Atrial fibrillation, bradycardia, chest pain, congestive heart failure, hypertension, hypotension, MI, orthostatic hypotension, peripheral edema
EENT: Pharyngitis, sinusitis
ENDO: Hypoglycemia (in diabetics)
GI: Abdominal pain, diarrhea, elevated liver enzyme levels, indigestion, nausea, vomiting
GU: Acute renal failure, erectile dysfunction, renal dysfunction, UTI
HEME: Anemia, eosinophilia, thrombocytopenia

MS: Back pain, leg or muscle cramps, myalgia, tendon pain, tendinitis, tenosynovitis
RESP: ACE cough, upper respiratory tract infection
SKIN: Diaphoresis, erythema, rash, urticaria
Other: Anaphylaxis, angioedema, elevated uric acid level, flulike symptoms, hyperkalemia, hypovolemia

Nursing Considerations

• Give telmisartan cautiously to patients with dehydration or hyponatremia.
• Expect prescriber to add a diuretic to regimen if patient's blood pressure isn't well controlled by telmisartan.
• Check patient's blood pressure regularly. Be prepared to treat symptomatic hypotension by placing patient in supine position and giving normal saline solution, as ordered.
• Monitor BUN and serum creatinine levels and urine output in patients with impaired renal function because they're at increased risk for oliguria, progressive azotemia, and possibly acute renal failure.
• Monitor liver function test results, as appropriate, and assess for evidence of drug toxicity in patients with severe hepatic disease because they're at increased risk for toxicity from increased drug accumulation.
• Avoid using telmisartan in pregnant women during second and third trimesters because drug can increase the risk of fetal harm.

PATIENT TEACHING
• Advise patient to avoid hazardous activities until telmisartan's CNS effects are known.
• Instruct patient to change position slowly to minimize effects of orthostatic hypotension.
• Urge patient to immediately notify prescriber about diarrhea, dizziness, severe nausea, or vomiting.
• Instruct patient to consult prescriber before taking any new drug.
• Advise patient to drink adequate amounts of fluid during hot weather and when exercising.
• Advise female patients of childbearing age to notify presciber immediately about known or suspected pregnancy.

T

temazepam

Apo-Temazepam (CAN),
Novo-Temazepam (CAN), Restoril

Class, Category, and Schedule
Chemical class: Benzodiazepine
Therapeutic class: Sedative-hypnotic
Pregnancy category: X
Controlled substance schedule: IV

Indications and Dosages
➤ *To provide short-term management of insomnia*
CAPSULES
Adults. 7.5 to 30 mg 30 min before bedtime. *Maximum:* 30 mg daily.
DOSAGE ADJUSTMENT For elderly or debilitated patients, 7.5 mg 30 min before bedtime. *Maximum:* 15 mg daily.

Mechanism of Action
May potentiate the effects of gamma-aminobutyric acid (GABA) and other inhibitory neurotransmitters by binding to specific benzodiazepine receptor sites in limbic and cortical areas of the CNS. By binding to these receptor sites, temazepam increases GABA's inhibitory effects and blocks cortical and limbic arousal.

Contraindications
Hypersensitivity to temazepam, other benzodiazepines, or their components; pregnancy

Interaction
DRUGS
antihistamines (such as brompheniramine, carbinoxamine, chlorpheniramine, clemastine, cyproheptadine, diphenhydramine, trimeprazine), anxiolytics, barbiturates, general anesthetics, opioid analgesics, phenothiazines, promethazine, sedative-hypnotics, tramadol, tricyclic antidepressants: Increased sedation or respiratory depression
clozapine: Risk of respiratory depression or arrest
digoxin: Increased risk of elevated blood digoxin level and digitalis toxicity
flumazenil: Increased risk of withdrawal symptoms
levodopa: Possibly decreased levodopa effects
oral contraceptives: Decreased response to temazepam
phenytoin: Possibly phenytoin toxicity
probenecid: Increased response to temazepam
zidovudine: Possibly zidovudine toxicity
ACTIVITIES
alcohol use: Increased CNS depression and risk of apnea
smoking: Increased temazepam clearance

Adverse Reactions
CNS: Aggressiveness, anxiety (in daytime), ataxia, complex behaviors (such as sleep driving), confusion, decreased concentration, depression, dizziness, drowsiness, euphoria, fatigue, headache, insomnia, nightmares, slurred speech, suicidal ideation, syncope, talkativeness, tremor, vertigo, wakefulness during last third of night
CV: Palpitations, tachycardia
EENT: Abnormal or blurred vision, increased salivation, throat tightness
GI: Abdominal pain, constipation, diarrhea, hepatic dysfunction, nausea, thirst, vomiting
GU: Decreased libido
HEME: Agranulocytosis, anemia, leukopenia, neutropenia, thrombocytopenia
MS: Muscle spasm or weakness
RESP: Dyspnea, increased bronchial secretions
SKIN: Diaphoresis, flushing, jaundice, pruritus, rash
Other: Anaphylaxis, angioedema, physical and psychological dependence

Nursing Considerations
• Use temazepam cautiously in patients with a history of depression or suicidal thoughts.
WARNING Monitor patient closely for evidence of hypersensitivity reaction, such as dyspnea, throat tightness, nausea, vomiting, and swelling. If present, discontinue temazepam immediately, notify prescriber, and provide supportive care.
• Watch patient closely for suicidal tendencies, particularly when therapy starts and dosage changes, because depression may worsen temporarily during these times and could lead to suicidal ideation.
WARNING Monitor patient for evidence of physical and psychological dependence during therapy.

- Implement safety precautions, according to facility policy, especially in elderly patients, because they're more sensitive to drug's CNS effects.
- Assess patients with respiratory depression, severe COPD, or sleep apnea for signs of ventilatory failure.
- Be aware that temazepam can aggravate acute intermittent porphyria, myasthenia gravis, and severe renal impairment.
- Be aware that temazepam may cause worsening psychosis or deterioration of cognition or coordination in patients with late-stage Parkinson's disease.
- Be aware that drug shouldn't be discontinued abruptly, even after only 1 to 2 weeks of therapy, because doing so may cause seizures or withdrawal symptoms, such as insomnia, irritability, and nervousness.

PATIENT TEACHING
- Instruct patient to take temazepam exactly as prescribed and not to stop or change dosage without consulting prescriber.
- Explain the risks associated with abrupt cessation, including abdominal cramps, acute sense of hearing, confusion, depression, nausea, numbness, perceptual disturbances, photophobia, sweating, tachycardia, tingling, trembling, and vomiting.
- Advise patient to avoid consuming alcohol because it increases drug's sedative effects and the risk of such abnormal behaviors as sleep driving.
- Caution patient about possible drowsiness. Advise her to avoid potentially hazardous activities until drug's CNS effects are known.
- Urge patient to notify prescriber immediately about excessive drowsiness, nausea, and known or suspected pregnancy.
- Instruct patient to stop taking temazepam and seek emergency care if she experiences difficulty breathing, throat tightness, nausea, vomiting, or abnormal swelling.
- Advise patient that drug may cause abnormal behaviors during sleep, such as driving a car, eating, talking on the phone, or having sex without any recall of the event. If family notices any such behavior or patient sees evidence of such behavior upon awakening, the prescriber should be notified.
- Urge family or caregiver to watch patient closely for suicidal tendencies, especially when therapy starts or dosage changes.

tenecteplase
TNKase

Class and Category
Chemical class: Purified glycoprotein
Therapeutic class: Thrombolytic
Pregnancy category: C

Indications and Dosages
➤ *To reduce mortality associated with acute MI*
I.V. INJECTION
Adults. Single bolus administered over 5 sec in individualized dosage based on patient's weight, as follows: 30 mg (6 ml) for patients weighing less than 60 kg (132 lb); 35 mg (7 ml) for patients weighing 60 to 69 kg (132 to 152 lb); 40 mg (8 ml) for patients weighing 70 to 79 kg (154 to 174 lb); 45 mg (9 ml) for patients weighing 80 to 89 kg (176 to 196 lb); 50 mg (10 ml) for patients weighing 90 kg (198 lb) or more.
Maximum: 50 mg total dose.

Mechanism of Action
Binds to fibrin and converts plasminogen to plasmin. Plasmin breaks down fibrin, fibrinogen, and other clotting factors, resulting in dissolution of a coronary artery thrombus.

Incompatibilities
Don't administer tenecteplase through an I.V. line containing dextrose because precipitation may occur.

Contraindications
Active internal bleeding, aneurysm, arteriovenous malformation, bleeding disorders, brain tumor, history of cerebrovascular accident, hypersensitivity to tenecteplase or its components, intracranial or intraspinal surgery or trauma within past 2 months, severe uncontrolled hypertension

Interaction
DRUGS
abciximab, aspirin, clopidogrel, dipyridamole, heparin, oral anticoagulants, ticlopidine: Possibly increased risk of bleeding

Adverse Reactions

CNS: Intracranial hemorrhage
EENT: Epistaxis, gingival bleeding, pharyngeal bleeding
GI: GI and retroperitoneal bleeding
GU: Genitourinary bleeding, prolonged or heavy menstrual bleeding
HEME: Hematoma
RESP: Hemoptysis
SKIN: Bleeding at puncture sites, surgical incision sites, or venous cutdown sites

Nursing Considerations

WARNING Reconstitute tenecteplase for injection immediately before use because drug contains no antibacterial preservatives. If reconstituted drug isn't used immediately, refrigerate vial at 36° to 46° F (2° to 8° C). Discard solution if not used within 8 hours.

• To reconstitute and administer drug, use supplied 10-ml syringe with dual cannula device. Withdraw 10 ml of supplied (preservative-free) sterile water for injection into syringe, and inject entire contents into vial containing tenecteplase dry powder, directing stream of diluent into powder. Gently swirl—don't shake—vial until contents are completely dissolved. If slight foaming occurs during reconstitution, allow drug to stand undisturbed for a few minutes to allow large bubbles to dissipate. Then withdraw prescribed dose of tenecteplase from reconstituted drug in vial, using supplied syringe. Make sure that reconstituted preparation is a colorless to pale yellow transparent solution. Discard any unused solution.

• Give drug as a single I.V. bolus over 5 seconds. Although supplied syringe is intended for use with needleless I.V. systems, be aware that it is also compatible with a conventional needle. Follow manufacturer's directions for use with each system. Flush any dextrose-containing I.V. lines with saline solution before and after administering tenecteplase.

WARNING Monitor patient for evidence of GI bleeding, including bloody or black, tarry stools; bloody or coffee-ground vomitus; and severe stomach pain. Notify prescriber immediately if any of these signs or symptoms develops.

• Assess tenecteplase injection site for signs and symptoms of hematoma, including deep, dark purple bruises under skin and itching, pain, redness, or swelling. Also monitor patient for superficial bleeding, delayed bleeding at puncture sites, and bleeding from surgical incisions.

• Assess for signs and symptoms of intracranial bleeding (such as decreased level of consciousness), retroperitoneal bleeding (such as abdominal pain or swelling and back pain), genitourinary bleeding (such as hematuria), or respiratory tract bleeding (such as hemoptysis). Notify prescriber immediately if patient develops any of these signs or symptoms.

• If serious bleeding (not controllable by local pressure) occurs, expect to discontinue concomitant heparin or oral antiplatelet therapy immediately.

• If possible, avoid I.M. injections and nonessential handling of patient for first few hours after drug administration.

• If arterial puncture becomes necessary during first few hours after tenecteplase administration, expect to use an upper extremity that's accessible to manual compression. Apply pressure for at least 30 minutes after procedure, use a pressure dressing, and frequently monitor puncture site for signs of bleeding.

PATIENT TEACHING

• Advise patient to immediately report any bleeding, including from nose or gums.

• Instruct patient to limit physical activity during tenecteplase administration to reduce the risk of injury or bleeding.

terazosin hydrochloride

Hytrin

Class and Category

Chemical class: Quinazoline derivative
Therapeutic class: Antihypertensive, benign prostatic hyperplasia (BPH) treatment
Pregnancy category: C

Indications and Dosages

➤ *To manage hypertension*

CAPSULES

Adults. *Initial:* 1 mg at bedtime. *Maintenance:* 1 to 5 mg daily as a single dose or in divided doses every 12 hr. *Maximum:* 20 mg daily.

➤ *To treat symptomatic BPH*

CAPSULES

Adults. *Initial:* 1 mg at bedtime, increased in increments to 2 mg, 5 mg, and then 10 mg, as needed, based on symptom improvement and urine flow rate. *Maintenance:* 5 to 10 mg daily as a single dose or in divided doses every 12 hr. *Maximum:* 20 mg daily.

Route	Onset	Peak	Duration
P.O.	15 min	2–3 hr	24 hr

Mechanism of Action

Blocks postsynaptic alpha$_1$-adrenergic receptors in many tissues, including vascular smooth muscle, the bladder neck, and the prostate. This action promotes vasodilation, which reduces blood pressure and improves urine flow.

Contraindications

Hypersensitivity to terazosin, other quinazolines, or their components

Interaction

DRUGS

clonidine: Possibly decreased clonidine effects
diuretics, other antihypertensives: Additive hypotensive effect
dopamine: Risk of decreased terazosin effects and antagonized vasoconstrictive effect of dopamine (in high doses)
epinephrine: Risk of decreased terazosin effects, possibly severe hypotension and tachycardia
indomethacin, other NSAIDs: Altered terazosin effects related to sodium and fluid retention
methoxamine, phenylephrine: Decreased vasopressor effects, and shortened duration of action of these drugs
phosphodiesterase-5 inhibitors, verapamil: Additive blood pressure–lowering effects and symptomatic hypotension
sympathomimetics: Decreased terazosin effects

Adverse Reactions

CNS: Asthenia, dizziness, headache, lethargy, nervousness, paresthesia, somnolence, syncope, vertigo

CV: Chest pain, hypotension, orthostatic hypotension, palpitations, peripheral edema, sinus tachycardia
EENT: Blurred vision, dry mouth, intraoperative floppy iris syndrome, nasal congestion, sinusitis
GI: Constipation, diarrhea, nausea, vomiting
MS: Arthralgia, back pain
Other: Flulike symptoms, weight gain

Nursing Considerations

• Be aware that prostate cancer should be ruled out before giving terazosin for BPH.
• Expect prescriber to reduce terazosin dosage if a diuretic or another antihypertensive is added to patient's regimen.
• Monitor blood pressure 2 to 3 hours after initial dose because of possible first-dose hypotension and again after 24 hours to evaluate patient's response.
• If patient requires administration by feeding tube, place capsule in 60 ml of warm tap water. Stir until capsule shell dissolves and liquid contents are released into water (5 to 10 minutes).
• Be aware that elderly patients may have exaggerated hypotension and other adverse reactions.

PATIENT TEACHING

• Instruct patient to take terazosin at the same time each night.
• Explain possible first-dose hypotension. Advise patient to change position and rise slowly to prevent syncope early in therapy. Suggest sitting or lying down if dizziness or light-headedness occurs.
• Advise patient to avoid hazardous activities until drug's CNS effects are known.
• Instruct patient to notify prescriber if she misses several doses in a row; caution her against resuming therapy at previous dose.
• Inform patient that drug may take 2 to 6 weeks to improve urinary hesitancy.
• Advise patient to avoid alcohol use, prolonged standing, and excessive exercise or exposure to hot weather because these activities can worsen orthostatic hypotension.
• Emphasize the importance of regular follow-up visits with prescriber to evaluate patient's response to drug.

T

terbinafine hydrochloride

Lamisil

Class and Category

Chemical class: Allylamine derivative
Therapeutic class: Antifungal
Pregnancy category: B

Indications and Dosages

➤ *To treat onychomycosis of fingernails and toenails*

TABLETS
Adults and adolescents. 125 mg twice daily or 250 mg daily for 6 to 12 wk.
DOSAGE ADJUSTMENT For patients with stable chronic hepatic dysfunction or renal dysfunction (creatinine clearance less than 50 ml/min/1.73 m^2 or serum creatinine greater than 3.4 mg/dl), dosage reduced by 50%.

Mechanism of Action

Inhibits the conversion of squalene mono-oxygenase to squalene epoxidase, a key enzyme in fungal biosynthesis. The resulting squalene accumulation weakens cell membranes and creates a deficiency of ergosterol, the fungal membrane component necessary for normal fungal growth.

Contraindications

Hypersensitivity to terbinafine or its components

Interaction

DRUGS
beta blockers, class 1C antiarrhythmics such as flecainide and propafenone, MAO inhibitors (type B), selective serotonin reuptake inhibitors, tricyclic antidepressants: Possibly increased blood levels of these drugs
cimetidine, other hepatic enzyme inhibitors: Significantly decreased terbinafine clearance, possibly increased adverse reactions
cyclosporine: Increased clearance of cyclosporine and decreased effectiveness of cyclosporine
CYP2C and CYP3A4 inhibitors such as amiodarone and ketoconazole: Possibly significant increased systemic exposure of terbinafine

hepatotoxic drugs: Increased risk of hepatotoxicity
rifampin: Increased clearance and decreased effectiveness of terbinafine
warfarin: Altered prothrombin time
FOODS
caffeine: Decreased caffeine clearance
ACTIVITIES
alcohol use: Increased risk of severe hepatitis

Adverse Reactions

CNS: Depression, fatigue, fever, headache, malaise, vertigo
CV: Myocarditis, pericarditis, vasculitis
EENT: Hearing impairment, loss of smell, reduced visual acuity, taste perversion, tinnitus, visual field defect
GI: Abdominal pain, anorexia, diarrhea, elevated liver function test results, flatulence, hepatic failure, hepatitis, indigestion, nausea, pancreatitis, vomiting
GU: Nephritis
HEME: Agranulocytosis, anemia, severe neutropenia, pancytopenia, thrombocytopenia
MS: Arthralgia, elevated creatine phosphokinase, myalgia, rhabdomyolysis
RESP: Pneumonitis
SKIN: Acute genralized exanthematous pustulosis, alopecia, cutaneous lupus erythematosus, drug reaction with eosinophilia and systemic symptoms (DRESS), exacerbation of psoriasis, exfoliative dermatitis, photosensitivity, psoriasiform eruptions, pruritus, rash, Stevens-Johnson syndrome, toxic epidermal necrolysis, urticaria,
Other: Anaphylaxis, angioedema, influenza-like illness, serum sickness-like reaction, systemic lupus erythematosus

Nursing Considerations

• Because terbinafine has been linked to serious adverse hepatic effects, expect to send nail specimens for laboratory testing to confirm onychomycosis before starting therapy.
• Be aware that drug shouldn't be given to patients with chronic or active hepatic disease or renal impairment.
• Monitor patient for hepatic failure (anorexia, dark urine, fatigue, jaundice, nausea, pale stools, right upper abdominal pain, and vomiting). Expect to stop drug and obtain liver function tests if these problems develop.

WARNING Monitor patient for serious skin or hypersensitivity reactions such as Stevens-Johnson syndrome or drug reaction with eosinophilia and systemic symptoms (DRESS) syndrome. Know that in addition to skin abnormalities such as rash and urticaria, DRESS may also involve one or more organs. If hypersensitivity reactions progress or persistent, notify prescriber and expect drug to be discontinued.

PATIENT TEACHING
• Instruct patient to space terbinafine doses evenly if taking drug more than once a day.
• Emphasize the need to complete the full course of terbinafine therapy to prevent relapse of infection.
• Discourage consumption of alcohol during therapy.
• Tell patient to contact prescriber if onychomycosis doesn't improve in a few weeks.
• Instruct patient to avoid direct sunlight or UV light and to wear sunscreen when outdoors.
• Tell patient to watch for skin reactions, such as hives, itching, or rash suggestive of a hypersensitivity reaction. If present, tell patient to notify prescriber.

terbutaline sulfate

Brethaire, Brethine, Bricanyl, Bricanyl Turbuhaler (CAN)

Class and Category
Chemical class: Sympathomimetic amine
Therapeutic class: Bronchodilator
Pregnancy category: B

Indications and Dosages
➤ *To prevent or reverse bronchospasm from asthma, bronchitis, or emphysema*

TABLETS (BRETHINE, BRICANYL)
Adults and adolescents age 15 and over. 2.5 to 5 mg three times a day at 6-hr intervals while awake. *Maximum:* 15 mg daily.
Children ages 12 to 15. 2.5 mg three times a day at 6-hr intervals while awake. *Maximum:* 7.5 mg daily.

Children ages 6 to 11. 50 to 75 mcg/kg three times a day at 6-hr intervals while awake. *Maximum:* 150 mcg/kg/dose or 5 mg daily.

SUBCUTANEOUS INJECTION (BRICANYL)
Adults and children age 12 and over.
Initial: 0.25 mg, repeated in 15 to 30 min as needed. *Maximum:* 0.5 mg/4-hr period.
Children ages 6 to 12. 5 to 10 mcg (0.005 to 0.01 mg)/kg every 15 to 20 min, up to 3 doses. *Maximum:* 400 mcg (0.4 mg)/dose.

INHALATION AEROSOL (BRETHAIRE)
Adults and children. 2 inhalations (400 mcg) every 4 to 6 hr, as needed.

INHALATION AEROSOL (BRICANYL TURBUHALER)
Adults and children. 1 inhalation (500 mcg), repeated after 5 min, as needed. *Maximum:* 6 inhalations daily.

Route	Onset	Peak	Duration
P.O.	30–90 min	2–3 hr	4–8 hr
SubQ	15–30 min	30–60 min	1.5–4 hr
Inhalation	In 5 min	30–90 min	3–6 hr

Mechanism of Action
Stimulates beta$_2$-adrenergic receptors in the lungs, which is believed to increase production of cAMP. The increased cAMP level relaxes bronchial smooth muscles, thereby increasing bronchial airflow and relieving bronchospasm.

Contraindications
Hypersensitivity to terbutaline, other sympathomimetic amines, or their components

Interaction
DRUGS
antihypertensives, diuretics: Decreased antihypertensive effect
beta blockers: Mutual inhibition of therapeutic effects, increased risk of bronchospasm
CNS stimulants: Additive CNS stimulation, possibly resulting in adverse effects
digoxin: Increased risk of arrhythmias, possibly digitalis toxicity
halogenated anesthetics: Possibly ventricular arrhythmias

MAO inhibitors: Possibly potentiated action of terbutaline; headache, hyperpyrexia, hypertension, possible hypertensive crisis
maprotiline, tricyclic antidepressants: Possibly potentiated action of terbutaline
nitrates: Decreased effectiveness of nitrates
ritodrine: Increased effects of either drug and potential for adverse effects
sympathomimetics: Increased CNS stimulation and risk of adverse cardiovascular effects, including prolonged QT interval
thyroid hormones: Increased effects of either drug, risk of coronary insufficiency in patients with coronary artery disease
xanthines (theophylline): Increased CNS stimulation and other additive toxic effects

FOODS
caffeine: Increased CNS stimulation and other additive toxic effects

Adverse Reactions
CNS: Anxiety, dizziness, drowsiness, headache, insomnia, light-headedness, nervousness, restlessness, tremor, weakness
CV: Chest pain, irregular heartbeat, palpitations, tachycardia
EENT: Dry mouth, taste perversion
ENDO: Hyperglycemia
GI: Heartburn, nausea, vomiting
MS: Muscle spasms
RESP: Dyspnea
SKIN: Diaphoresis, flushing, rash

Nursing Considerations
• Use terbutaline cautiously in patients with cardiovascular disease because drug can adversely affect cardiovascular function. Monitor patient's heart rate and rhythm and blood pressure, and assess for chest pain.
• For subcutaneous use, inject into lateral deltoid area.
• Assess patient's respiratory rate, depth, and quality; oxygen saturation; and activity tolerance at regular intervals because continuous use of beta$_2$-agonists for 12 months or longer accelerates the decline in pulmonary function.

PATIENT TEACHING
• Teach patient how to use terbutaline aerosol inhaler or give subcutaneous injection, as needed.
• Instruct patient not to increase dose or frequency without consulting prescriber.

• Urge patient to seek immediate medical attention if symptoms worsen.
• Inform patient that she may experience transient nervousness or tremors during terbutaline therapy.

teriflunomide
Aubagio

Class and Category
Chemical class: 4-trifluoromethylphenyl amide
Therapeutic class: Anti–multiple sclerotic agent
Pregnancy category: X

Indications and Dosages
TABLETS
Adults. 7 mg or 14 mg once daily.

Mechanism of Action
Inhibits dihydroorotate dehydrogenase, a mitochondrial enzyme involved in de novo pyrimidine synthesis to possibly reduce the number of activated lymphocytes in the central nervous system responsible for the signs and symptoms of multiple sclerosis.

Contraindications
Concurrent therapy with leflunomide, hypersensitivity to teriflunomide or its components, pregnancy, severe hepatic impairment, women of childbearing age not using reliable contraception

Interaction
DRUGS
alosetron, caffeine, duloxetine, theophylline, tizanidine: Reduced effectiveness of these drugs
ethinylestradiol, levonorgestrel: Increased risk of adverse reactions related to these drugs
paclitaxel, pioglitazone, repaglinide, rosiglitazone: Possibly increased exposure of these drugs with potential for leading to adverse effects
warfarin: Decreased peak international normalized ratio

Adverse Reactions
CNS: Anxiety, burning sensation, headache, paresthesia, peripheral neuropathy, sciatica
CV: Hypertension, palpitations

EENT: Blurred vision, conjunctivitis, oral herpes, sinusitis, toothache
GI: Abdominal distention, diarrhea, elevated liver enzymes, gastroenteritis, hepatic dysfunction or failure, nausea, upper abdominal pain
GU: Acute uric acid nephropathy, cystitis, elevated serum creatinine levels, transient acute renal failure
HEME: Leukopenia, neutropenia
MS: Manifestation of carpal tunnel syndrome, musculoskeletal pain, myalgia
RESP: Bronchitis, upper respiratory infection
SKIN: Acne, alopecia, pruritus
Other: Hyperkalemia, influenza-like symptoms, onset of seasonal allergies, weight loss

Nursing Considerations

• Know that teriflunomide isn't recommended for patients with severe immunodeficiency, bone marrow dysplasia, or severe, uncontrolled infections because of its immunosuppressant effect. It is also not recommended for patients with liver disease or those with a serum alanine aminotransferase level greater than two times the upper level normal prior to initiation of therapy because drug may worsen liver dysfunction.
• Obtain a pregnancy test on all women of child bearing age, as ordered, prior to starting teriflunomide therapy. Know that drug should not be started if pregnancy is suspected or confirmed and in women who refuse to use a reliable contraceptive.
• Use cautiously in patients who are over 60 years of age, patients with diabetes, or in patients taking concomitant neurotoxic drugs because of an increased risk of developing peripheral neuropathy. If peripheral neuropathy occurs during teriflunomide therapy, notify prescriber and expect drug to be discontinued and possibly cholestyramine washout ordered.
• Test patient for latent tuberculosis before starting leflunomide, as ordered. If positive, expect standard medical treatment to be given before teriflunomide therapy starts.
• Obtain baseline blood pressure before starting teriflunomide, and monitor

periodically thereafter because drug may cause hypertension.
• Assess liver enzyme (ALT and AST) levels at start of therapy, monthly during first 6 months, and if stable, every 6 to 8 weeks thereafter, as ordered. If levels become elevated greater than threefold upper level normal, notify prescriber and expect teriflunomide therapy to be withheld until underlying cause is determined. If the elevation is thought to be teriflunomide induced, expect to start cholestyramine washout, as ordered, and monitor liver test weekly until normalized. If another cause is found for the elevation, expect to resume teriflunomide therapy.
• Ensure that a complete CBC has been done within the past 6 months of starting teriflunomide therapy to use as a baseline. Repeat CBC, as ordered, thereafter if signs and symptoms of bone marrow suppression occur.
• Notify prescriber if patient develops a serious infection or skin condition because drug may need to be interrupted and cholestyramine or charcoal given to eliminate drug rapidly.
WARNING Monitor patient's respiratory function closely because drug may cause interstitial lung disease that could become life-threatening. If patient develops a cough and dyspnea, notify prescriber; drug may need to be stopped, and patient may need cholestyramine or charcoal to eliminate drug rapidly.
• Check patient's serum potassium level, as ordered, if symptoms of hyperkalemia or acute renal failure occur.
PATIENT TEACHING
• Tell patient to report signs of respiratory dysfunction, such as cough and dyspnea.
WARNING Caution woman of childbearing potential not to become pregnant while taking drug because of the high risk of birth defects. Emphasize importance of using reliable forms of birth control and to notify prescriber immediately if pregnancy is suspected.
• Instruct patient to report signs of hepatotoxicity, such as yellow skin or eyes, darkened urine, and fatigue.

T

• Advise patient to avoid live vaccines during teriflunomide therapy.
• Instruct patient to notify prescriber if she develops an infection or skin condition.

teriparatide
Forteo

Class and Category
Chemical class: Recombinant human parathyroid hormone (PTH)
Therapeutic class: Bone growth and density regulator
Pregnancy category: C

Indications and Dosages
➤ *To treat osteoporosis in postmenopausal women and primary or hypogonadal osteoporosis in men at high risk for fracture; to treat men and women with glucocorticoid-induced osteoporosis at high risk for fracture*
SUBCUTANEOUS INJECTION
Adults. 20 mcg daily for up to 2 yr.

Route	Onset	Peak	Duration
SubQ	2 hr	4–6 hr	16–24 hr

Contraindications
Hypersensitivity to teriparatide or its components

Interaction
DRUGS
digitalis glycosides: Possibly increased risk of digitalis toxicity

Adverse Reactions
CNS: Asthenia, depression, dizziness, headache, insomnia, paresthesia, syncope, vertigo
CV: Angina pectoris, chest pain, hypertension, transient orthostatic hypotension
EENT: Pharyngitis, rhinitis, taste perversion, tooth disorder
ENDO: Transient hypoparathyroidism
GI: Constipation, diarrhea, indigestion, vomiting
MS: Arthralgia, muscle cramps or spasms in back or leg, neck pain
RESP: Cough, dyspnea, pneumonia
SKIN: Diaphoresis, pruritus, rash, urticaria

Other: Angioedema, generalized pain, injection-site reactions (erythema, localized bruising, minor bleeding, pain, pruritus, swelling), transient hypercalcemia or hypocalcemia

Nursing Considerations
WARNING Be aware that teriparatide shouldn't be used to treat patients at risk for osteosarcoma (such as those with Paget's disease or a metabolic bone disease other than osteoporosis), unexplained elevations of alkaline phosphatase, open epiphyses, or prior skeletal radiation or malignancy.
WARNING Be aware that patients with hypercalcemia shouldn't receive teriparatide because drug may worsen hypercalcemia.
• Use drug cautiously in patients with active or recent urolithiasis because drug could worsen this condition.
• Monitor patient closely for allergic reactions because teriparatide is a peptide agent.
• Monitor patient's blood calcium level, and notify prescriber of any elevation; in persistent hypercalcemia, the drug may need to be stopped.
• Monitor patient's blood pressure during the first several doses of drug therapy because of a risk of transient orthostatic hypotension. If this occurs, place patient in a reclining position and alert prescriber.

PATIENT TEACHING
• Teach patient how to administer teriparatide by subcutaneous injection and how to properly use the delivery pen device and dispose of needles. Advise her not to share pen device with others.
• Inform patient that each delivery pen can be used for up to 28 days after the first injection but then should be discarded even if it still contains solution.
• Instruct patient to store the delivery pen in the refrigerator and to recap it when not in use to protect it from damage and light.
• Tell patient that delivery pen may be used immediately after removal from refrigerator and should be put back in refrigerator as soon as the injection is given.

Mechanism of Action

Teriparatide, which contains recombinant PTH, stimulates new bone growth andincreases bone density. In a patient with osteoporosis, bone density and mass arediminished by an imbalance between bone destruction and formation. Normally, osteoclasts break down and resorb bone, leaving behind a cavity in a section of bone. Then bone-building cells, called osteoblasts, line the walls of the cavity and stimulate new bone formation. PTH stimulates these actions by attaching to receptors on osteoclasts and osteoblasts, as shown below. Teriparatide binds to cell-surface receptors on osteoblasts and preferentially stimulates osteoblastic over osteoclastic activity. Also, the drug increases the amount of circulating calcium available for bone formation by increasing the intestinal absorption of calcium and phosphate, thus enhancing the rate of calcium resorption from bone, increasing the reabsorption of calcium, and inhibiting the reabsorption of phosphate in the kidneys. These actions stimulate new bone formation and increase bone density to reduce osteoporotic bone changes.

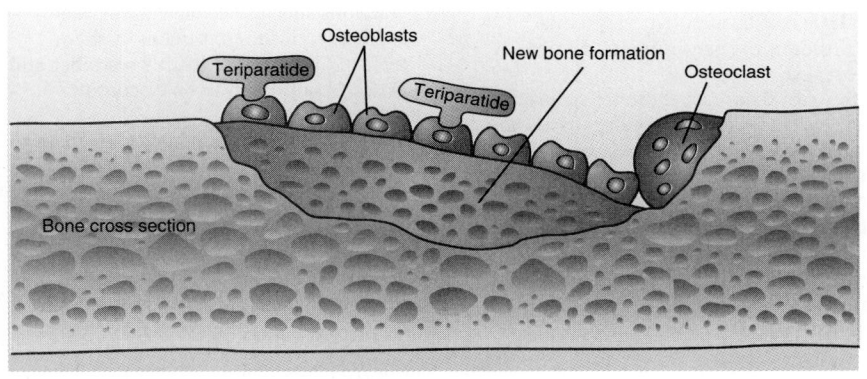

- Instruct patient to inject drug into thigh or abdominal wall and to rotate injection sites.
- Caution patient to administer drug in a room where she can immediately sit or lie down if light-headedness or palpitations occur. Advise her to notify prescriber if these symptoms persist or worsen.
- Instruct patient to notify prescriber of persistent symptoms of hypercalcemia, such as nausea, vomiting, constipation, lethargy, and muscle weakness.
- Caution patient about potential developing osteosarcoma.

tesamorelin
Egrifta

Class and Category

Chemical class: Recombinant DNA product
Therapeutic class: Growth hormone releasing factor analog
Pregnancy category: X

Indications and Dosages

➤ *To reduce excess abdominal fat in HIV-infected patients with lipodystrophy*

SUBCUTANEOUS INJECTION
Adults. 2 mg once daily.

Mechanism of Action

Stimulates growth hormone secretion, which is both anabolic and lipolytic. By interacting with specific receptors on adipocytes, fat breakdown occurs.

Contraindications

Active malignancy; disruption of the hypothalamic-pituitary axis due to hypophysectomy, hypopituitarism, pituitary

T

tumor or surgery, head irradiation or head trauma; hypersensitivity to tesamorelin or its components; pregnancy

Interaction

DRUGS

anticonvulsants, corticosteroids, cyclosporine, sex steroids: Possibly altered metabolization of these drugs

glucocorticoids: Possibly decreased effectiveness requiring larger dosages

Adverse Reactions

CNS: Depression, hypoesthesia, insomnia, paresthesia, peripheral neuropathy
CV: Chest pain, hypertension, palpitations, peripheral edema
ENDO: Hot flashes, hyperglycemia
GI: Abdominal pain (upper), dyspepsia, nausea, vomiting
MS: Arthralgia, carpel tunnel syndrome, elevated blood creatine phosphokinase, extremity pain, joint stiffness or swelling, muscle spasms or strain, musculoskeletal pain or stiffness, myalgia
SKIN: Erythema, flushing, night sweats, pruritus, rash, urticaria
Other: Anti-tesamorelin IgG antibodies, injection-site reactions (erythema, hemorrhage, irritation, pain, pruritis, rash, swelling, urticaria)

Nursing Considerations

• Do not administer tesamorelin to any patient with an active malignancy, and expect drug to be discontinued if patient becomes critically ill for any reason during tesamorelin therapy.
• Use cautiously in patients with a history of nonmalignant neoplasms or patients with a history of treated and stable malignancies because tesamorelin therapy could reactivate the underlying malignancy.
• Evaluate patient's glucose status prior to initating tesamorelin therapy to obtain a baseline because the drug may cause glucose intolerance. Continue to monitor glucose levels throughout therapy and treat accordingly, as prescribed.
• Follow instructions provided with the medication for reconstituting tesamorelin. Once reconsituted, drug must be administered immediately. If a delay occurs, the reconstituted solution must be discarded.

• Administer as a subcutaneous injection into the abdomen. Rotate sites to different areas of the abdomen. Do not inject drug into scar tissue, bruises, or the navel.
• Monitor serum IGF-1 levels, as ordered, because tesamorelin stimulates growth hormone production and increases serum IGF-1 levels. If persistent elevations occur (greater than 3 SDS), notify prescriber because drug may need to be discontinued.
• Ensure patient with diabetes undergoes ophthalmologic examinations regularly because drug may cause retinopathy to develop or worsen because of the increased drug-induced IGF-1 levels.
• Monitor patient closely for hypersensitivity reactions such as the development of erythema, flushing, pruritus, rash, or urticaria. If present, notify prescriber and expect tesamorelin to be discontinued.

PATIENT TEACHING

• Teach patient how to reconstitute drug and administer a subcutaneous injection. Emphasize importance of rotating sites within the abdomen to reduce incidence of injection reactions.
• Instruct patient to notify prescriber immediately and to stop taking tesamorelin if he develops a hypersensitivity reaction such as a rash or hives.
• Inform patient with diabetes that drug may alter his glucose control and that he should test his blood glucose regularly. Medical attention should be sought if glucose control becomes affected.

tetracycline hydrochloride

Achromycin, Achromycin V, Apo-Tetra (CAN), Novo-Tetra (CAN), Nu-Tetra (CAN), Panmycin, Robitet, Sumycin, Tetracap, Tetracyn, Tetracyn 500

Class and Category

Chemical class: Chlortetracycline derivative
Therapeutic class: Antibiotic
Pregnancy category: D

Indications and Dosages

➤ *To treat actinomycosis caused by susceptible organisms*

CAPSULES, ORAL SUSPENSION, TABLETS
Adults and adolescents. 250 to 500 mg every 6 hr or 500 to 1,000 mg every 12 hr. *Maximum:* 4 g daily.
Children age 8 and over. 6.25 to 12.5 mg/kg every 6 hr or 12.5 to 25 mg/kg every 12 hr.
➤ *To treat acne vulgaris*
CAPSULES, ORAL SUSPENSION, TABLETS
Adults and adolescents. *Initial:* 500 to 2,000 mg daily in divided doses until improvement occurs (usually in 3 wk); then dosage reduced gradually. *Maintenance:* 125 to 1,000 mg daily. *Maximum:* 4 g daily.
➤ *To treat brucellosis caused by susceptible organisms*
CAPSULES, ORAL SUSPENSION, TABLETS
Adults and adolescents. 500 mg every 6 hr for 3 wk, given with 1 g of streptomycin I.M. every 12 hr in week 1 and daily in week 2. *Maximum:* 4 g daily.
Children ages 8 to 12. 6.25 to 12.5 mg/kg every 6 hr, or 12.5 to 25 mg/kg every 12 hr.
➤ *To treat gonorrhea caused by* Neisseria gonorrhoeae
CAPSULES, ORAL SUSPENSION, TABLETS
Adults and adolescents. 1,500 mg, then 500 mg every 6 hr for 5 days. *Maximum:* 4 g daily.
➤ *To treat syphilis caused by* Treponema pallidum
CAPSULES, ORAL SUSPENSION, TABLETS
Adults and adolescents. 500 mg every 6 hr for 15 days (for early syphilis) or 30 days (for late syphilis). *Maximum:* 4 g daily.
Children ages 9 to 12. 6.25 to 12.5 mg/kg every 6 hr, or 12.5 to 25 mg/kg every 12 hr.
➤ *To treat uncomplicated endocervical, rectal, or urethral infections caused by* Chlamydia trachomatis
CAPSULES, ORAL SUSPENSION, TABLETS
Adults and adolescents. 500 mg four times a day for at least 7 days. *Maximum:* 4 g daily.
DOSAGE ADJUSTMENT For patients with renal impairment, dosage possibly reduced because of extended half-life.

Mechanism of Action

Exerts a bacteriostatic effect against a wide variety of gram-positive and gram-negative organisms by passing through the bacterial lipid bilayer, where it binds reversibly to 30S ribosomal subunits. Bound tetracycline blocks the binding of aminoacyl transfer RNA to messenger RNA, thus inhibiting bacterial protein synthesis.

Contraindications

Hypersensitivity to tetracycline or its components

Interaction

DRUGS
aluminum-, calcium-, or magnesium-containing antacids; iron supplements (oral); magnesium-containing laxatives; magnesium salicylate; multivitamins (containing manganese or zinc salts); sodium bicarbonate: Possibly impaired absorption of oral tetracycline and formation of nonabsorbable complexes
cholestyramine, colestipol: Possibly impaired absorption of oral tetracycline
digoxin: Possibly increased digoxin level
methoxyflurane: Possibly nephrotoxicity
oral contraceptives (containing estrogen): Possibly reduced contraceptive reliability and increased risk of breakthrough bleeding (with long-term tetracycline use)
penicillins: Possibly decreased bactericidal effect of penicillins
vitamin A: Possibly benign intracranial hypertension
FOODS
dairy products and other foods: Possibly impaired absorption of oral tetracycline

Adverse Reactions

CNS: Dizziness, light-headedness, unsteadiness
EENT: Darkened or discolored tongue, enamel hypoplasia, oral candidiasis, tooth discoloration (in children)
GI: Abdominal pain, diarrhea, hepatotoxicity, nausea, rectal candidiasis, vomiting
GU: Vaginal candidiasis
SKIN: Photosensitivity

Nursing Considerations

• Avoid giving tetracycline to children under age 8 because drug may cause permanent brown or yellow tooth discoloration and enamel hypoplasia.
• Be aware that tooth discoloration and enamel hypoplasia may occur in breastfeeding infants, along with inhibition of linear skeletal growth, oral and vaginal candidiasis, and photosensitivity.

T

• To reduce the risk of esophageal irritation or ulceration, avoid bedtime dosing of tetracycline for patient with esophageal obstruction or compression.

• Assess for photosensitivity, which can develop within a few minutes or up to several hours after exposure to sunlight or other ultraviolet (UV) light. Effects may last for 1 to 2 days after discontinuation of drug.

• Be aware that citric acid in tetracycline preparations may accelerate drug deterioration and that using outdated drug may cause Fanconi's syndrome, characterized by multiple defects in renal tubular function. Symptoms include acidosis, bicarbonate wasting, glycosuria, hypokalemia, osteomalacia, and phosphaturia.

PATIENT TEACHING

• Instruct patient to take oral tetracycline at least 1 hour before meals or 2 hours after meals because dairy products and some foods may interfere with absorption.

• Advise patient to take each dose with a full glass of water while in an upright position to avoid esophageal or GI irritation.

• Instruct patient taking oral suspension to shake container well before measuring dose and to use a calibrated measuring device.

• Advise patient to avoid taking other drugs, including OTC antacids and other preparations, within 3 hours of oral tetracycline.

• Urge patient to complete entire course of tetracycline therapy even if she feels better.

• Caution her to avoid direct sunlight or UV light and to wear sunscreen when outdoors.

• Advise women who use oral contraceptives containing estrogen to use another method of contraception while taking tetracycline because contraceptives may be less effective. Tell patient to notify prescriber immediately if pregnancy is suspected or known.

• Emphasize the need to discard outdated tetracycline because of the risk of toxic effects.

• Encourage patient to take safety precautions if she experiences dizziness or other adverse CNS reactions.

theophylline

Aerolate, Aerolate III, Aerolate Jr., Aerolate Sr., Apo-Theo LA (CAN), Asmalix, Elixophyllin, Lanophyllin, PMS Theophylline (CAN), Pulmophylline (CAN), Quibron-T Dividose, Quibron-T/SR Dividose, Respbid, Slo-Bid Gyrocaps, Slo-Phyllin, Theo-24, Theo-SR (CAN), Theobid Duracaps, Theochron, Theoclear, Theoclear LA, Theo-Dur, Theolair, Theolair-SR, Theovent Long-Acting, T-Phyl, Truxophyllin, Uni-Dur, Uniphyl

Class and Category
Chemical class: Xanthine derivative
Therapeutic class: Bronchodilator
Pregnancy category: C

Indications and Dosages
➤ *As loading dose to treat reversible airway obstruction in patients not currently receiving theophylline*
CAPSULES, ELIXIR, ORAL SOLUTION, SYRUP, TABLETS
Adults and children. 5 mg/kg as a single dose.
I.V. INFUSION
Adults and children. 5 mg/kg infused over 20 to 30 min.
➤ *As partial loading dose to treat reversible airway obstruction in patients currently receiving theophylline*
CAPSULES, ELIXIR, ORAL SOLUTION, SYRUP, TABLETS, I.V. INFUSION
Adults and children. Individualized dosage based on blood theophylline level, as prescribed. Loading dose based on principle that 0.5 mg/kg of theophylline will produce a 1-mcg/ml increase in blood theophylline level.
➤ *To provide maintenance treatment of reversible airway obstruction associated with asthma or COPD*
CAPSULES, TABLETS
Adults and children weighing more than 45 kg (99 lb). *Initial:* 300 mg daily in equally divided doses every 6 to 8 hr; after 3 days, if tolerated, increased to 400 mg daily in divided doses every 6 to 8 hr; after 3 more days, if tolerated, increased to

600 mg daily in divided doses every 6 to 8 hr. Dosages above 600 mg daily are based on blood theophylline level and clinical response.

Children age 1 and over weighing 45 kg or less. *Initial:* 12 to 14 mg/kg daily up to maximum of 300 mg daily in equally divided doses every 4 to 6 hr; after 3 days, if tolerated, increased to 16 mg/kg up to maximum of 400 mg daily in equally divided doses every 4 to 6 hr; after 3 more days, if tolerated, 20 mg/kg daily up to maximum of 600 mg daily in equally divided doses every 4 to 6 hr. Dosages above 600 mg daily are based on blood theophylline level and clinical response.

ELIXIR

Adults. *Initial:* 300 mg daily in equally divided doses every 6 to 8 hr; after 3 days, if tolerated, increased to 400 mg daily in divided doses every 6 to 8 hr; after 3 more days, if tolerated, increased to 600 mg daily in divided doses every 6 to 8 hr. Dosages above 600 mg daily are based on blood theophylline level and clinical response.

E.R. CAPSULES OR TABLETS

Adults and children weighing 45 kg or more. *Initial:* 300 mg daily in equally divided doses every 8 to 12 hr; after 3 days, if tolerated, increased to 400 mg daily in divided doses every 8 to 12 hr; after 3 more days, if tolerated, increased to 600 mg daily in divided doses every 8 to 12 hr. Dosages above 600 mg daily are based on blood theophylline level and clinical response.

Children age 1 and over weighing less than 45 kg. *Initial:* 12 to 14 mg/kg daily up to maximum of 300 mg daily in equally divided doses every 8 to 12 hr; after 3 days, if tolerated, increased to 16 mg/kg up to maximum of 400 mg daily in equally divided doses every 8 to 12 hr; after 3 more days, if tolerated, dosage increased to 20 mg/kg daily up to maximum of 600 mg daily in equally divided doses every 8 to 12 hr. Dosages above 600 mg daily are based on blood theophylline level and clinical response.

ORAL SOLUTION, SYRUP

Adults and children weighing more than 45 kg. *Initial:* 300 mg daily in equally divided doses every 6 to 8 hr; after 3 days, if tolerated, increased to 400 mg daily in divided doses every 6 to 8 hr; after 3 more

days, if tolerated, increased to 600 mg daily in divided doses every 6 to 8 hr. Dosages above 600 mg daily are based on blood theophylline level and clinical response.

Children age 1 and over weighing 45 kg or less. *Initial:* 12 to 14 mg/kg daily up to maximum of 300 mg daily in equally divided doses every 4 to 6 hr; after 3 days, if tolerated, increased to 16 mg/kg up to a maximum of 400 mg daily in equally divided doses every 4 to 6 hr; after 3 more days, if tolerated, dosage increased to 20 mg/kg daily up to maximum of 600 mg daily in equally divided doses every 4 to 6 hr. Dosages above 600 mg daily are based on blood theophylline level and clinical response.

Full-term infants ages 26 to 52 weeks. Dosage individualized in mg/kg daily, as prescribed, and administered in equally divided doses every 6 hr.

Full-term infants up to age 26 weeks. Dosage individualized in mg/kg daily, as prescribed, and administered in equally divided doses every 8 hr.

Premature infants age 24 days and over. 1.5 mg/kg every 12 hr.

Premature infants under age 24 days. 1 mg/kg every 12 hr.

I.V. INFUSION

Adults and adolescents age 16 and over. 0.4 mg/kg/hr for nonsmokers, 0.7 mg/kg/hr for smokers.

DOSAGE ADJUSTMENT For elderly patients and adults with cardiac decompensation, cor pulmonale, or hepatic impairment, I.V. dosage reduced to 0.2 mg/kg/hr.

Children ages 9 to 16. 0.7 mg/kg/hr.

Children ages 1 to 9. 0.8 mg/kg/hr.

Full-term infants up to age 1. Dosage individualized in mg/kg daily as prescribed.

Mechanism of Action

Inhibits phosphodiesterase enzymes, causing bronchodilation. Normally, these enzymes inactivate cAMP and cGMP, which are responsible for bronchial smooth-muscle relaxation. Theophylline also may cause calcium translocation, antagonize prostaglandins and adenosine receptors, stimulate catecholamines, and inhibit cGMP metabolism.

Incompatibilities

Don't mix parenteral theophylline solution with any additives. Don't infuse

T

theophylline through same I.V. line as Hetastarch (Hespan), a colloidal plasma volume expander, which is incompatible with theophylline.

Contraindications

Hypersensitivity to theophylline or its components, peptic ulcer disease, uncontrolled seizure disorder

Interaction

DRUGS

adenosine: Decreased adenosine effectiveness

allopurinol, cimetidine, ciprofloxacin, clarithromycin, disulfiram, enoxacin, erythromycin, fluvoxamine, interferon alpha (human recombinant), methotrexate, mexiletine, pentoxifylline, propafenone, propranolol, tacrine, thiabendazole, ticlopidine, troleandomycin, verapamil: Increased blood theophylline level and risk of toxicity

aminoglutethimide, carbamazepine, isoproterenol (I.V.), moricizine, oral contraceptives (containing estrogen), phenobarbital, phenytoin, rifampin: Decreased blood theophylline level and possibly drug effectiveness

benzodiazepines: Possibly reversal of benzodiazepine sedation

beta blockers: Possibly decreased bronchodilator effect of theophylline

ephedrine: Increased adverse effects, including insomnia, nausea, and nervousness

halothane anesthetics: Increased risk of ventricular arrhythmias

ketamine: Lowered seizure threshold

lithium: Decreased lithium effectiveness

neuromuscular blockers: Possibly antagonized neuromuscular blockade

sucralfate: Decreased absorption of oral theophylline

FOODS

high-carbohydrate, low-protein diet: Possibly decreased theophylline elimination

low-carbohydrate, high-protein diet; daily intake of charbroiled beef: Possibly increased theophylline elimination

ACTIVITIES

alcohol use: Increased blood theophylline level and risk of toxicity

smoking: Increased drug clearance, decreased drug effectiveness

Adverse Reactions

CNS: Agitation, anxiety (I.V. form), behavioral changes, confusion, disorientation, headache, insomnia, nervousness, nonconvulsive status epilepticus, seizures, tremor

CV: Hypotension, tachycardia, ventricular arrhythmias

ENDO: Hyperglycemia

GI: Abdominal pain, diarrhea, heartburn, nausea, vomiting

GU: Increased urine output

Other: Hypercalcemia

Nursing Considerations

• Be aware that ideal body weight is used to calculate theophylline dosages because drug doesn't bind well in body fat.

• Be aware that E.R. capsules and tablets shouldn't be used for oral loading doses.

• Infuse theophylline loading dose, bolus, or intermittent infusion at a rate that doesn't exceed 25 mg/min.

• Administer continuous theophylline infusion with rate-controlled infusion device.

• Monitor blood theophylline level, as ordered, to gauge therapeutic level and detect toxicity.

• Frequently assess heart rate and rhythm because theophylline can exacerbate existing arrhythmias.

• Be especially alert for signs of toxicity in patient with acute pulmonary edema, hypothyroidism, influenza vaccination, prolonged fever, sepsis with multiple organ failure, shock, or viral pulmonary infection because of decreased drug clearance.

• Monitor blood theophylline level in patients with uncorrected acidemia because they have an increased risk of toxicity.

• Expect patient with cystic fibrosis or hyperthyroidism to have increased theophylline clearance and decreased drug effectiveness. Monitor blood theophylline level, as ordered.

• Suspect toxicity if patient experiences vomiting, and be prepared to obtain blood theophylline level.

PATIENT TEACHING

• Instruct patient to swallow theophylline tablets whole and not to chew or crush them, unless scored for breaking.

• Explain that patient may open capsules and mix contents with soft food but that she shouldn't chew or crush granules.
• Instruct patient to take drug with a full glass of water on an empty stomach (30 to 60 minutes before meals or 2 hours after meals). However, suggest that she take drug with food or antacids if GI distress occurs.
• Encourage patient to take drug at the same times every day.
• Advise patient to notify prescriber if she develops a fever, makes a significant dietary change, or starts or stops smoking or taking other drugs because these factors may alter blood theophylline level.
• Tell female patient to notify prescriber if she is or cold be pregnant.

thiethylperazine maleate
Torecan

Class and Category
Chemical class: Piperazine phenothiazine
Therapeutic class: Antiemetic
Pregnancy category: Not rated

Indications and Dosages
➤ *To treat nausea and vomiting*
TABLETS, I.M. INJECTION, SUPPOSITORIES
Adults and adolescents. 10 mg once daily to three times a day. *Maximum:* 30 mg daily.

Route	Onset	Peak	Duration
P.O.	30–60 min	Unknown	4 hr

Mechanism of Action
Relieves nausea and vomiting by centrally blocking dopamine receptors in the medullary chemoreceptor trigger zone.

Contraindications
Breastfeeding; coma; hypersensitivity to thiethylperazine, sulfites, tartrazine dye, or their components; jaundice; severe CNS depression

Interaction
DRUGS
aluminum- or magnesium-containing antacids, antidiarrheals (adsorbent): Decreased absorption of thiethylperazine
anticonvulsants (including barbiturates): Lowered seizure threshold
antihistamines, tricyclic antidepressants: Additive CNS and GI effects, including ileus and severe constipation
antihypertensives: Enhanced hypotensive effect of both drugs
antimuscarinics (including antiparkinsonian drugs, MAO inhibitors, meperidine, and phenothiazines): Additive GI effects, including ileus and severe constipation
appetite suppressants: Decreased anorectic effect
barbiturates, benzodiazepines, CNS depressants, general anesthetics, opioid analgesics: Additive CNS effects
beta blockers: Increased blood levels of both drugs; additive hypotensive effects; possibly arrhythmias, irreversible retinopathy, and tardive dyskinesia
bromocriptine: Possibly decreased effectiveness of bromocriptine
hepatotoxic drugs: Increased risk of hepatotoxicity
levodopa: Decreased effectiveness of levodopa
lithium: Possibly acute encephalopathy
methoxsalen, porfimer: Possibly increased photosensitivity
metrizamide: Increased risk of seizures
ototoxic drugs: Possibly masked symptoms of ototoxicity (dizziness, tinnitus, and vertigo)
phenytoin: Increased risk of phenytoin toxicity
quinidine: Possibly adverse cardiac effects
riboflavin: Increased requirements for riboflavin
sympathomimetics: Reduced vasopressor response and duration of action of sympathomimetics
tramadol: Additive CNS effects, increased risk of seizures
ACTIVITIES
alcohol use: Additive CNS effects

Adverse Reactions
CNS: Confusion, dizziness, EEG abnormalities, extrapyramidal reactions (dystonia, pseudoparkinsonism), sedation
CV: ECG changes, hypotension, orthostatic hypotension, tachycardia
EENT: Blurred vision, dry mouth
ENDO: Gynecomastia
GI: Constipation, increased appetite

GU: Darkened urine, ejaculation disorders, menstrual irregularities, urine retention
HEME: Agranulocytosis, leukopenia (transient)
SKIN: Contact dermatitis, photosensitivity
Other: Weight gain

Nursing Considerations

- Avoid using thiethylperazine in patients with neurologic impairment because drug can disrupt central temperature regulation.
- Avoid inadvertent I.V. administration of thiethylperazine; injection is for I.M. administration only.
- Keep patient in recumbent position for 30 to 60 minutes after I.M. injection to minimize the risk of hypotension.
- Be aware that parenteral preparations contain sulfites and that tablets contain tartrazine dye.
- Moisten suppository with water or water-soluble lubricant before insertion. If suppository has softened excessively, chill for 30 minutes or run under cold water before removing wrapper.
- Avoid skin contact with drug to prevent contact dermatitis.
- Because thiethylperazine may cause reactions from anticholinergic effects and adrenergic blockade, assess for blurred vision, constipation, dry mouth, impotence, urine retention (from cholinergic activity) and priapism (from alpha-adrenergic blockade).
- During prolonged therapy, assess for visual disturbances because drug may cause corneal keratopathy and retinal discoloration (pigmentary retinopathy).
- **WARNING** Be aware that thiethylperazine may cause neuroleptic malignant syndrome, a rare but extremely serious reaction characterized by cardiovascular instability, decreased level of consciousness, extrapyramidal effects, and hyperpyrexia.
- Monitor CBC with differential, as ordered, because drug may worsen existing blood dyscrasias, such as agranulocytosis, neutropenia, and thrombocytopenia, in patients with bone marrow suppression. Be aware that drug may worsen angle-closure glaucoma, encephalopathy, organic or traumatic brain damage, or tardive dyskinesia.

- When possible, avoid combining thiethylperazine with CNS depressants because these drugs may potentiate thiethylperazine's effects.
- Monitor patient with cardiac disease for exaggerated cardiovascular reactions.
- Implement seizure precautions and monitor for seizures in patients with known seizure disorder because drug may lower seizure threshold.
- Implement safety precautions, according to facility policy, for elderly patients. They may be especially sensitive to drug's sedative and extrapyramidal effects.
- Be prepared to discontinue drug 48 hours before myelography and to resume drug 24 to 48 hours afterward to minimize the risk of seizures.
- Be aware that photosensitivity may turn patient's skin yellow-brown, gray, or purple because of hyperpigmentation.
- Be aware that drug shouldn't be given to pregnant patient because it may cause jaundice and extrapyramidal symptoms in her neonate.

PATIENT TEACHING

- Instruct patient to stay recumbent for 1 hour after taking thiethylperazine to minimize effects of orthostatic hypotension.
- Advise patient to notify prescriber immediately about adverse CNS reactions, decreased urine output, or vision changes.
- Urge patient to avoid alcohol use and potentially hazardous activities during therapy.
- Encourage patient to avoid excessive sun exposure and to use sunscreen when she's outdoors.
- Advise patient on long-term therapy to have periodic eye examinations to detect possible eye disorders.

thiopental sodium
Pentothal

Class, Category, and Schedule
Chemical class: Barbiturate
Therapeutic class: Anticonvulsant, sedative-hypnotic
Pregnancy category: C
Controlled substance: Schedule III

Indications and Dosages

➤ *To control seizures from anesthesia or other causes*

I.V. INJECTION

Adults. *Initial:* 75 to 125 mg (3 to 5 ml of 2.5% solution) as soon as possible after onset of seizure. *Maximum:* 250 mg given over 10 min.

➤ *To facilitate narcoanalysis*

I.V. INFUSION OR INJECTION

Adults. Dosage individualized based on patient's age, condition, sex, and weight; injected at 100 mg/min (4 ml/min of 2.5% solution) with patient counting backwards from 100. Expect to discontinue injection once patient becomes confused with her counting but is still awake. Or, use 0.2% concentration in D_5W for injection and infuse at 50 ml/min.

➤ *To treat cerebral hypertension*

I.V. INFUSION OR INJECTION

Adults. 1.5 to 3.5 mg/kg, repeated as needed, to reduce elevated intracranial pressure (ICP).

Route	Onset	Peak	Duration
I.V.	10–40 sec	Unknown	10–30 min

Mechanism of Action

Depresses the CNS and may inhibit ascending transmission of impulses in the reticular formation. Thiopental may enhance or mimic inhibitory action of gamma-aminobutyric acid, thereby causing anti-convulsant effect and producing sedation and hypnosis. Thiopental may reduce ICP by increasing cerebral vascular resistance, which decreases cerebral blood flow and volume.

Incompatibilities

Don't mix thiopental with acidic I.V. drugs or solutions, succinylcholine, or tubocurarine.

Contraindications

History of porphyria; hypersensitivity to thiopental, its components, or other barbiturates

Interaction

DRUGS

clonidine, CNS depressants, guanabenz, magnesium sulfate, methyldopa, metyrosine, pargyline, rauwolfia alkaloids: Additive CNS depressant effects

diazoxide, diuretics, guanadrel, guanethidine, mecamylamine, trimethaphan: Possibly additive hypotensive effect

ketamine: Increased risk of hypotension or respiratory depression; possibly countered hypnotic effect of thiopental

phenothiazines: Possibly increased CNS depression or excitation, increased hypotensive effect

ACTIVITIES

alcohol use: Additive CNS depressant effects

Adverse Reactions

CNS: Agitation, anxiety, seizures

CV: Bradycardia, hypotension, shock, tachycardia, thrombophlebitis

GI: Hiccups

RESP: Apnea, bronchospasm, cough, laryngospasm, respiratory depression, wheezing

SKIN: Hives, itching, rash, redness

Other: Angioedema

Nursing Considerations

• Before administering thiopental, expect to premedicate patient with an anti-cholinergic, such as atropine or glycopyrrolate, to minimize secretions.

• Be prepared to administer a test dose of 25 to 75 mg (1 to 3 ml of 2.5% solution) to determine tolerance or sensitivity. Expect to observe patient for at least 1 minute after administering test dose.

• Dilute drug with a compatible I.V. solution before administering, such as D_5W for injection, normal saline solution for injection, or sterile water for injection. Be aware that sterile water for injection shouldn't be used to prepare 0.2% or 0.4% solution because it would result in a hypotonic solution and cause hemolysis.

• To prepare 0.2% solution, dilute 1 g of thiopental with 500 ml of compatible diluent to produce a final concentration of 2 mg/ml.

• To prepare 0.4% solution, dilute 1 g thiopental with 250 ml compatible diluent or 2 g thiopental with 500 ml compatible diluent to produce a final concentration of 4 mg/ml.

• To prepare 2.5% solution, dilute 1 g of thiopental with 40 ml of compatible diluent or 5 g of thiopental with 200 ml of compatible diluent to produce a final concentration of 25 mg/ml.

T

• Inspect solution for particles before administration. Use solution within 24 hours of reconstitution, and discard unused portion after 24 hours.
• Monitor patient's blood and tissue oxygenation and vital signs during I.V. administration. Keep emergency equipment and drugs nearby in case respiratory depression occurs.
• If patient has a history of CV disease or hypotension, monitor her for CV depressant effects, such as bradycardia, hypotension, or shock.
• In patient with a history of seizures, institute seizure precautions according to facility protocol.
• Monitor respiratory rate, rhythm, and quality for signs of respiratory depression in debilitated patient or one with a history of respiratory disease.
• Monitor patient's neurologic status every hour, or as ordered, in patient with increased ICP.

PATIENT TEACHING
• Explain the need for frequent hemo-dynamic monitoring.
• Advise patient to use caution when driving or performing tasks that require alertness for at least 24 hours after receiving thiopental.
• Instruct patient not to consume alcohol or other CNS depressants for at least 24 hours after thiopental administration (unless prescribed) because they increase the effects of thiopental.
• Instruct patient to report persistent drowsiness, rash, severe dizziness, or skin lesions to prescriber.

thioridazine
Mellaril (CAN), Mellaril-S, Novo-Ridazine (CAN)

thioridazine hydrochloride
Apo-Thioridazine (CAN), Mellaril, Mellaril Concentrate, Novo-Ridazine (CAN), PMS Thioridazine

Class and Category
Chemical class: Piperidine phenothiazine

Therapeutic class: Antipsychotic drug
Pregnancy category: Not rated

Indications and Dosages
➤ *To treat schizophrenia in patients unresponsive to other antipsychotic drugs*
ORAL SOLUTION, ORAL SUSPENSION, TABLETS
Adults and adolescents. *Initial:* 50 to 100 mg three times a day gradually increased, as needed and tolerated. *Maintenance:* 200 to 800 mg daily in two to four divided doses. *Maximum:* 800 mg daily.
Children ages 2 to 12. *Initial:* 0.5 mg/kg daily in divided doses, gradually increased, as needed and tolerated. *Maximum:* 3 mg/kg daily.

Route	Onset	Peak	Duration
P.O.	Up to several wk	6 wk– 6 mo	Unknown

Mechanism of Action
Depresses areas of the brain that control activity and aggression, including the cerebral cortex, hypothalamus, and limbic system by blocking postsynaptic dopamine$_2$ (D_2) receptors. Drug may relieve anxiety by indirectly reducing arousal and increasing filtration of internal stimuli to the brain stem reticular activating system.

Contraindications
Coma; concurrent use of drugs that inhibit the metabolism of thioridazine, such as fluoxetine, fluvoxamine, paroxetine, pindolol, and propranolol; concurrent use of drugs that prolong the QT interval; concurrent use of high doses of a CNS depressant; history of arrhythmias; hypersensitivity to thioridazine, other phenothiazines, or their components; prolonged QT interval; reduced cytochrome P450 2D6 activity; severe CNS depression; severe hypertensive or hypotensive cardiac disease

Interaction
DRUGS
amandadine, antihistamines, anti-muscarinics, clozapine, cyclobenzaprine, diphenoxylate, disopyramide, maprotiline: Additive anticholinergic effects

amiodarone, bepridil, cisapride, disopyramide, erythromycin, flecainide, grepafloxacin, ibutilide, pimozide, probucol, procainamide, quinidine, sotalol, sparfloxacin, tocainide: Possibly prolonged QT interval
amphetamine, chlorpromazine, dextroamphetamine: Possibly decreased effects of these drugs and thioridazine
antacids, antidiarrheals (adsorbent), kaolin, rifabutin, rifampin, rifapentine: Reduced bioavailability of thioridazine
anxiolytics, benzodiazepines, clonidine, dronabinol, guanabenz, guanfacine, opioid analgesics, phenothiazines, sedative-hypnotics: Possibly increased CNS effects or hypotension
barbiturates, fosphenytoin, phenytoin, valproic acid: Increased CNS depression, lowered seizure threshold
bromocriptine: Possibly decreased effectiveness of bromocriptine
carbamazepine: Possibly decreased blood thioridazine level
charcoal: Reduced thioridazine absorption
dopamine, droperidol, haloperidol, metoclopramide, metyrosine: Possibly increased adverse CNS effects
ephedrine, epinephrine, norepinephrine, phenylephrine: Possibly severe hypotension, MI, or tachycardia
fluoxetine, fluvoxamine, other cytochrome P450 2D6 inhibitors, paroxetine, pindolol: Inhibited metabolism of thioridazine, leading to elevated blood thioridazine level
general anesthetics: Possibly potentiated CNS depression
guanadrel, guanethidine, methyldopa: Inhibited hypotensive effect of these drugs
levodopa, pergolide, pramipexole, ropinirole: Possibly inhibited antiparkinsonian response
lithium (high doses): Risk of encephalopathic syndrome (characterized by confusion, elevated liver function test results and fasting blood glucose level, extrapyramidal symptoms, fever, lethargy, leukocytosis, and weakness)
MAO inhibitors: Possibly exaggerated extrapyramidal reactions
methoxsalen, oral contraceptives, porfimer, sulfonamides, sulfonylureas, tetracyclines, thiazide diuretics, vitamin A analogues: Possibly increased photosensitivity

propranolol: Increased blood propranolol and thioridazine levels, increased CNS effects, hypotension
tramadol: Increased blood tramadol level, possibly increased risk of seizures
trazodone: Possibly additive hypotension
ACTIVITIES
alcohol use: Additive CNS effects

Adverse Reactions
CNS: Akathisia, altered temperature regulation, depression, dizziness, drowsiness, extrapyramidal reactions (dystonia, laryngospasm, motor restlessness, pseudoparkinsonism), headache, insomnia
CV: ECG changes, hypertension, hypotension, prolonged QT interval, torsades de pointes, ventricular tachycardia
EENT: Blurred vision, change in color perception, dry mouth, impaired night vision, mydriasis, photophobia
ENDO: Breast engorgement, galactorrhea
GI: Constipation, ileus, nausea
GU: Amenorrhea, decreased libido, ejaculation disorders, impotence, menstrual irregularities, priapism, urine retention
HEME: Agranulocytosis, anemia, aplastic anemia, eosinophilia, leukocytosis, leukopenia, pancytopenia, thrombocytopenia
SKIN: Hyperpigmentation, jaundice, photosensitivity
Other: Weight gain

Nursing Considerations
WARNING Expect to give thioridazine only if patient has failed to respond to therapy with at least two other antipsychotic drugs because thioridazine may prolong the QT interval and has been associated with torsades de pointes and sudden death.
WARNING Thioridazine shouldn't be used to treat elderly patients with dementia-related psychosis because drug increases the risk of death in these patients.
• Obtain baseline and serial ECG tracings and serum potassium levels, as ordered. Notify prescriber if QT interval is greater than 500 msec or if potassium level is abnormal, and expect to discontinue drug immediately.
• Frequently monitor blood pressure and assess for chest pain in patients with heart disease because thioridazine has caused

T

hypotension and has precipitated angina on occasion. Also monitor urine output in patients with benign prostatic hyperplasia because drug can worsen urine retention.

• Be aware that high doses and large dosage changes in patient with a seizure disorder may lower seizure threshold. Institute seizure precautions, as appropriate, according to facility policy.

• Administer drug with food, milk, or a full glass of water to minimize GI distress.

• Measure oral suspension using calibrated measuring device. Dilute with 60 to 120 ml of fruit juice, distilled water, or acidified tap water immediately before administration.

• Don't give thioridazine oral suspension with carbamazepine oral suspension; a rubbery orange precipitate may form in stool.

• To prevent contact dermatitis, don't let oral solution come in contact with skin.

• Administer antacid or adsorbent antidiarrheal at least 1 hour before or 2 hours after thioridazine.

WARNING Be aware that thioridazine can cause neuroleptic malignant syndrome—most commonly in male patients. Signs and symptoms include altered level of consciousness, altered mental status, autonomic instability (diaphoresis, hypotension or hypertension, sinus tachycardia), hyperthermia, and severe extrapyramidal dysfunction. Acute renal failure, increased serum creatine phosphokinase level, and leukocytosis also have occurred. Notify prescriber immediately if such symptoms develop, and be prepared to discontinue therapy.

• Be aware that drug shouldn't be discontinued abruptly. Sudden withdrawal of thioridazine may produce transient dizziness, nausea, tremor, and vomiting.

• Assess for eye pain because drug's anticholinergic effects can worsen angle-closure glaucoma.

• Promptly investigate and report blurred vision, defective color perception, or impaired night vision because of the risk of pigmentary retinopathy.

• Expect prescriber to discontinue thioridazine and order CBC if patient experiences signs of infection. Also expect drug therapy to be stopped 48 hours before myelography and resumed 24 to 48 hours afterward.

• Monitor patient for signs and symptoms of tardive dyskinesia—such as uncontrollable movements of the arms, face, or legs—even after treatment stops. Notify prescriber if they develop.

PATIENT TEACHING

• Instruct patient to take thioridazine exactly as prescribed and not to stop taking drug without consulting prescriber because of the risk of withdrawal symptoms.

• Instruct patient to notify prescriber immediately if she develops unusual symptoms, such as dizziness, palpitations, and syncope, because they may indicate the presence of torsades de pointes.

• Advise patient not to take drug within 2 hours of an antacid.

• Caution patient to avoid alcohol use, which increases thioridazine's sedative effects, and to avoid hazardous activities if drowsiness occurs.

• Urge patient to notify prescriber immediately if she experiences blurred vision, defective color perception, difficulty with nighttime vision, excessive drowsiness, nausea, sore throat, or other signs of infection. Thioridazine treatment may be discontinued.

• Advise female patient to use effective contraception while taking drug because its fetal effects are unknown. Instruct her to inform prescriber immediately of known or suspected pregnancy.

• Because drug may alter temperature regulation, encourage patient to avoid exposure to extreme temperatures during therapy.

• Advise patient to wear protective dark glasses to minimize the effects of adverse vision reactions.

• If patient requires long-term therapy, explain the risk of tardive dyskinesia, and urge her to notify prescriber immediately if she develops uncontrollable movements of her arms, face, or legs.

• Instruct patient to tell other prescribers that she's taking thioridazine before she takes any new drug.

thiothixene

Navane

thiothixene hydrochloride

Navane, Thiothixene HCl Intensol

Class and Category

Chemical class: Thioxanthene derivative
Therapeutic class: Antipsychotic
Pregnancy category: Not rated

Indications and Dosages

➤ *To treat psychotic disorders, such as acute psychosis, psychotic depression, and schizophrenia*

CAPSULES (THIOTHIXENE), ORAL SOLUTION (THIOTHIXENE HYDROCHLORIDE)

Adults and children age 12 and over.
Initial: 2 mg three times a day (for mild conditions) or 5 mg twice daily (for more severe conditions), increased every wk, as needed. *Usual:* 10 to 40 mg daily in divided doses. *Maximum:* 60 mg daily (for severe conditions).

DOSAGE ADJUSTMENT For elderly patients, lowest effective dosage used for maintenance therapy; maximum dosage limited to 30 mg/day. For some patients, one daily dose possibly used for maintenance therapy.

I.M. INJECTION (THIOTHIXENE HYDROCHLORIDE)
Adults. *Initial:* 4 mg twice daily to four times a day. *Optimal:* 4 mg every 6 to 12 hr. *Usual:* 16 to 20 mg daily in divided doses. *Maximum:* 30 mg daily.

Mechanism of Action

Increases dopamine turnover by blocking postsynaptic dopamine receptors in the mesolimbic system. Eventually, dopamine neurotransmission decreases, resulting in antipsychotic effects.

Contraindications

Blood dyscrasias, coma, hypersensitivity to thiothixene or its components, Parkinson's disease, severe CNS depression, shock, use of quinidine

Interaction

DRUGS
amphetamines: Decreased effectiveness of either drug
antacids, antidiarrheals (adsorbent): Possibly reduced bioavailability of thiothixene
antihistamines, tricyclic antidepressants: Additive anticholinergic effects, causing severe constipation, ileus, or increased intraocular pressure
bromocriptine: Possibly increased serum prolactin level and decreased effectiveness of bromocriptine
carbamazepine: Possibly decreased blood thiothixene level
dopamine: Decreased vasoconstrictive effect of dopamine (in high doses)
ephedrine, phenylephrine: Possibly reduced vasopressor response
epinephrine: Possibly epinephrine reversal, leading to severe hypotension, tachycardia, and possibly MI
erythromycin: Increased adverse effects of thiothixene
general anesthetics, opioid analgesics, tramadol: Additive CNS effects, increased risk of seizures
guanadrel, guanethidine: Possibly decreased antihypertensive effect of these drugs
hypotensive drugs: Possibly excessive hypotension
levodopa: Possibly reduced effectiveness of levodopa
lithium: Possibly encephalopathic syndrome (with a blood level that exceeds 12 mEq/L)
MAO inhibitors: Possibly exaggerated extrapyramidal reactions
metaraminol, methoxamine, norepinephrine: Possibly reduced vasopressor response
pergolide: Possibly reduced effectiveness of pergolide
propranolol: Possibly seizures and increased hypotension
quinidine: Additive orthostatic hypotension, possibly prolonged QT interval

ACTIVITIES
alcohol use: Additive CNS effects, increased risk of seizures
smoking: Possibly decreased blood thiothixene level

T

Adverse Reactions

CNS: Agitation, akathisia, drowsiness, dystonia, fatigue, insomnia, light-headedness, neuroleptic malignant syndrome, paradoxical exacerbation of psychotic disorder, restlessness, seizures, syncope, tardive dyskinesia, weakness
CV: ECG changes, edema, hypotension, peripheral edema, tachycardia
EENT: Blurred vision, dry mouth, increased salivation, miosis, mydriasis, nasal congestion, retinopathy
ENDO: Breast engorgement, galactorrhea, hyperglycemia, hypoglycemia
GI: Anorexia, constipation, diarrhea, elevated liver function test results, ileus, increased appetite, nausea, vomiting
GU: Amenorrhea, glycosuria, impotence, priapism
HEME: Agranulocytosis, anemia, eosinophilia, hemolytic anemia, leukocytosis, leukopenia, neutropenia, pancytopenia, thrombocytopenia
SKIN: Contact dermatitis, decreased sweating, photosensitivity, pruritus, rash
Other: Hyperuricemia, weight gain

Nursing Considerations

WARNING Thiothixene shouldn't be used to treat elderly patients with dementia-related psychosis because drug increases the risk of death in these patients.
• Administer thiothixene capsules with food or milk if needed to minimize GI distress.
• Don't give drug within 1 hr of an antacid.
• Dilute oral solution with 60 to 120 ml of fruit or tomato juice, milk, soup, water, or a carbonated beverage. Measure dose and administer using a calibrated measuring device. Avoid spilling solution on skin because drug may cause contact dermatitis.
• Avoid inadvertent I.V. delivery of thiothixene. It's intended for I.M. use.
• Be aware that I.M. administration usually is reserved for acute, severe agitation or for patients who can't take oral preparations.
• Maintain patient in recumbent position for 30 minutes after I.M. injection to minimize orthostatic hypotension.
• Assess patient for early signs of potentially irreversible tardive dyskinesia, a syndrome of involuntary rhythmic movements of the face, jaw, mouth, or tongue.

WARNING Be aware that drug can precipitate neuroleptic malignant syndrome, a serious condition characterized by altered mental status, arrhythmias, diaphoresis, hyperpyrexia, muscle rigidity, and tachycardia, especially in patients with hyperthyroidism or thyrotoxicosis. Symptoms may be severe enough to cause life-threatening respiratory depression.
• Monitor patient's serum calcium level because hypocalcemia may lead to dystonic reactions.
• Keep in mind that hypotension from thiothixene may precipitate angina in patients with known cardiac disease.

WARNING Be aware that drug-induced adverse CNS reactions may mimic or suppress neurologic evidence of CNS disorders, such as brain tumor, encephalitis, encephalopathy, meningitis, Reye's syndrome, and tetanus.
• Monitor for extrapyramidal symptoms—particularly dystonias—in children with acute illnesses, including CNS infections, dehydration, gastroenteritis, measles, or varicella-zoster infections.
• Monitor patient's CBC, as ordered, because serious adverse hematologic reactions may occur, such as agranulocytosis, leukopenia, and neutropenia. More frequent monitoring during first few months of thiothixene therapy is recommended for patients with a history of drug-induced leukopenia or neutropenia or who have had a significantly low WBC count in the past. If abnormalities occur during therapy, monitor patient for fever or other signs of infection, notify prescriber, and expect drug to be discontinued if abnormalities are severe.
• Implement seizure precautions in patients with a history of seizures or EEG abnormalities because thiothixene can lower the seizure threshold.
• Assess patient for eye pain because thiothixene's anticholinergic effects may worsen angle-closure glaucoma. Assess patient with benign prostatic hyperplasia for urine retention.

PATIENT TEACHING
• Fully inform patient facing long-term thiothixene therapy about risk of developing tardive dyskinesia.

• Advise patient to avoid exposure to sunlight or ultraviolet light, and to apply sunscreen when outdoors.
• Urge patient to avoid smoking or to begin a smoking cessation program while taking thiothixene.
• Encourage patient to avoid extreme temperature changes during drug therapy to prevent hyperthermia or hypothermia caused by decreased sweating.
• Instruct patient to immediately report sore throat or other signs of infection.

thyroid USP

Armour Thyroid, Thyrar, Thyroid Strong, Westhroid

Class and Category
Chemical class: Porcine thyroid gland hormone
Therapeutic class: Thyroid hormone replacement
Pregnancy category: A

Indications and Dosages
➤ *To treat hypothyroidism without myxedema*
TABLETS
Adults and children. *Initial:* 60 mg daily, increased by 30 mg daily every mo as needed. *Maintenance:* 60 to 120 mg daily.
➤ *To treat hypothyroidism or myxedema in patients with cardiovascular disease*
TABLETS
Adults. *Initial:* 15 mg daily; daily dosage doubled every 2 wk, as indicated to achieve desired response, up to 180 mg daily. *Maintenance:* 60 to 180 mg daily.
➤ *To treat congenital hypothyroidism (cretinism) or severe hypothyroidism in children and infants*
TABLETS
Children and infants. *Initial:* 15 mg daily; daily dosage doubled every 2 wk, as indicated to achieve desired response, up to 180 mg daily. If desired response isn't achieved, dosage further increased by 30 to 60 mg daily. *Maintenance:* Individualized.

Mechanism of Action
Stimulates growth and maturation of tissues, increases energy expenditure, and affects all enzyme actions through several mechanisms. Thyroid hormone:
• regulates cell differentiation and proliferation
• aids in myelination of nerves and development of axonal and dendritic processes in the nervous system
• enhances protein and carbohydrate metabolism by promoting metabolic processes that increase gluconeogenesis and protein synthesis and facilitate the mobilization of glycogen stores.

Contraindications
Acute MI not associated with hypothyroidism, hypersensitivity to thyroid USP or its components, obesity treatment, untreated thyrotoxicosis

Interaction
DRUGS
barbiturates, carbamazepine, phenytoin, rifampin: Possibly increased catabolism of thyroid hormone
cholestyramine, colestipol: Decreased effectiveness of thyroid hormone
corticosteroids: Decreased metabolism of corticosteroids
estrogens: Possibly increased circulating concentrations of thyroxine-binding globulin, decreased effectiveness of thyroid hormone
insulin, oral antidiabetic drugs: Possibly altered blood glucose control
ketamine: Risk of marked hypertension and tachycardia
oral anticoagulants: Altered anticoagulant effect
sympathomimetics: Increased adverse cardiovascular effects
tricyclic antidepressants: Increased therapeutic and toxic effects of both drugs
FOODS
all foods: Possibly altered absorption of thyroid hormone

Adverse Reactions
CNS: Headache, insomnia, nervousness, tremor
CV: Angina; arrhythmias, including atrial fibrillation and sinus tachycardia; palpitations
ENDO: Hyperthyroidism
GI: Diarrhea, vomiting
GU: Menstrual irregularities

T

SKIN: Alopecia, diaphoresis
Other: Heat intolerance, weight loss

Nursing Considerations

• Avoid giving oral thyroid hormone with food because it may alter drug absorption.
• Don't give thyroid hormone within 5 hours of cholestyramine or colestipol. Giving them together can reduce hormone absorption.
WARNING Be aware that thyroid hormone therapy can unmask or worsen adrenal insufficiency, precipitate adrenal crisis in patients with uncontrolled adrenal insufficiency, and increase the risk of arrhythmias in patients with coronary artery disease.
• Monitor blood glucose level often because thyroid hormone therapy can unmask or exacerbate symptoms of other endocrine disorders and also may alter antidiabetic drug dosage requirements in patients with diabetes mellitus. Be aware that withdrawal of thyroid hormone can precipitate a hypoglycemic response in susceptible patients.

PATIENT TEACHING
• Tell patient to take thyroid hormone on an empty stomach at the same time each day.
• Advise her to inform prescriber immediately and seek medical attention if she experiences chest pain, nervousness, or sweating.
• Instruct patient who uses cholestyramine or colestipol not to take these drugs within 5 hours of thyroid dose.
• Inform patient that full effects may not be evident for 1 to 3 weeks.
• Instruct patient with diabetes mellitus to monitor blood glucose level frequently.

thyrotropin (thyroid-stimulating hormone, TSH)

Thytropar

thyrotropin alfa

Thyrogen

Class and Category

Chemical class: Recombinant glycoprotein of human TSH
Therapeutic class: Diagnostic aid
Pregnancy category: C

Indications and Dosages

➤ *To provide diagnostic follow-up of patients with well-differentiated thyroid carcinoma*

I.M. INJECTION (THYROTROPIN ALFA)
Adults and adolescents age 16 and over.
0.9 mg every 24 hr for 2 doses or every 72 hr for 3 doses. Scanning or serum thyroglobulin testing performed 72 hr after last injection.

➤ *To provide differential diagnosis of subclinical hypothyroidism or low thyroid reserve*

I.M. OR SUBCUTANEOUS INJECTION (THYROTROPIN)
Adults and adolescents age 16 and over.
10 international units daily for 1 to 3 days, followed by radioactive iodine study 24 hr after last injection. No response indicates thyroid failure; substantial response indicates pituitary failure.

➤ *To determine thyroid status in patients receiving thyroid hormone, to differentiate between primary and secondary hypothyroidism*

I.M. OR SUBCUTANEOUS INJECTION (THYROTROPIN)
Adults and adolescents age 16 and over.
10 international units daily for 1 to 3 days.

➤ *To aid in diagnosing thyroid carcinoma remnant after surgery*

I.M. OR SUBCUTANEOUS INJECTION (THYROTROPIN)
Adults and adolescents age 16 and over.
10 international units daily for 3 to 7 days.

➤ *As adjunct for radioiodine ablation of thyroid tissue remnants in patients who have undergone a near-total or total thyroidectomy for well-differentiated thyroid cancer and who have no evidence of metastatic thyroid cancer*

I.M. INJECTION (THYROTROPIN ALFA)
Adults. 0.9 mg, followed by a second 0.9 mg 24 hr later, followed by radioiodine administration 24 hr later.

Mechanism of Action

Stimulates production of thyroglobulin by active thyroid tissue and enhances uptake of iodine, synthesis of thyroid precursor hormones (monoiodotyrosine, diiodotyrosine, and levothyroxine), and release of triiodothyronine (T_3) and thyroxine (T_4) from the thyroid gland into systemic circulation. Thyrotropin also binds with thyroid cancer tissue and stimulates iodine uptake in radioactive iodine imaging to detect cancer cells in euthyroid patients after near-total or total thyroidectomy.

Contraindications

Coronary thrombosis, hypersensitivity to thyrotropin or its components, uncorrected adrenal insufficiency

Adverse Reactions

CNS: Asthenia, dizziness, fatigue, fever, headache, hemiparesis, hemiplegia, insomnia, paresthesia, stroke, unilateral weakness
CV: Atrial arrhythmias, hypercholesterolemia
EENT: Nasopharyngitis
ENDO: Hyperthyroidism
GI: Diarrhea, nausea, vomiting
RESP: Respiratory distress
SKIN: Flushing, pruritus, rash, urticaria
Other: Flulike symptoms; sudden, rapid, painful enlargement of locally recurring papillary carcinoma

Nursing Considerations

WARNING Be aware that thyrotropin can unmask or worsen adrenal insufficiency, precipitate adrenal crisis in patients with uncontrolled adrenal insufficiency, and increase the risk of arrhythmias in patients with coronary artery disease.
• Use cautiously in patients who have been previously treated with bovine TSH and, in particular, those patients who have experienced hypersensitivity reactions to bovine TSH. Also use cautiously in elderly patients and patients with dialysis-dependent end-stage renal disease, heart disease, and patients with significant residual thyroid tissue.
• Reconstitute thyrotropin solution with manufacturer-provided diluent, which contains no preservatives.
• Administer I.M. thyrotropin injections to the buttocks.
WARNING Avoid inadvertent I.V. or intradermal injection of thyrotropin.

I.V. administration may result in severe reactions, including diaphoresis, hypotension, nausea, tachycardia, and vomiting. Intradermal injection may damage tissue at injection site.
• Monitor patient closely, especially during first 24 hours after drug administration, because patients have died (rarely) during this time. Know that patients who have not had their thyroid gland removed prior to thyrotropin therapy; patients with distant metastatic thyroid cancer; or patients with known heart disease, extensive metastatic disease, or other known serious underlying illness may require hospitalization for initiation of thyrotropin therapy.
• Assess patient frequently for signs and symptoms of stroke or other neurologic abnormalities for several days because of increased risk of such events occurring within 20 minutes to 3 days after thyrotropin therapy has been initiated.
• Expect to administer glucocorticoids prior to beginning thyrotropin therapy in patients with distant metastatic thyroid cancer whose local tumor expansion may compromise vital anatomic structures such as the trachea, central nervous system, or lungs because sudden, rapid, and painful enlargement of locally recurring papillary carcinoma may occur within 12 to 48 hours of thyrotropin therapy. Also monitor patient for dyspnea, stridor, or dysphonia. If present, notify prescriber immediately.
• Check for chest pain and increased heart rate, especially in patients with cardiac or coronary artery disease, including angina, hypertension, and recent acute MI, and in patients with residual thyroid tissue. Drug may increase serum thyroid hormone level.

PATIENT TEACHING
• Advise patient to continue taking prescribed thyroid hormone replacement while receiving injections of thyrotropin alfa unless otherwise directed by prescriber.
• If patient is scheduled for radioactive iodine test, tell her to follow a low-iodine diet. Inform patient that testing may take 5 to 12 days to complete.

T

• Instruct patient to seek immediate emergency care if signs and symptoms of a stroke or other adverse nervous system reactions occur.

tiagabine hydrochloride

Gabitril

Class and Category
Chemical class: Nipecotic acid derivative
Therapeutic class: Anticonvulsant
Pregnancy category: C

Indications and Dosages
➤ *As adjunct to treat partial seizures*
TABLETS
Adults. *Initial:* 4 mg daily; increased by 4 mg/wk up to 16 mg daily, then dosage increased by 4 to 8 mg every wk until desired response occurs. *Usual:* 32 to 56 mg daily. *Maximum:* 56 mg daily in 2 to 4 divided doses.
Children ages 12 to 18. *Initial:* 4 mg daily for 1 wk, then increased by 4 to 8 mg/ wk until desired response occurs. *Maximum:* 32 mg daily in 2 to 4 divided doses.
DOSAGE ADJUSTMENT For patients with impaired hepatic function, dosage individualized and reduced, or interval extended if needed, because of reduced drug clearance.

Mechanism of Action
Appears to inhibit neuronal and glial uptake of gamma-aminobutyric acid (GABA), the major inhibitory neuro-transmitter in the CNS. Tiagabine makes more GABA available in the CNS to open chloride channels in postsynaptic membranes, thereby leading to membrane hyperpolarization and preventing transmission of nerve impulses.

Contraindications
Hypersensitivity to tiagabine or its components

Interaction
DRUGS
benzodiazepines, CNS depressants: Possibly additive CNS depression

carbamazepine, phenobarbital, phenytoin: Possibly decreased tiagabine effectiveness
ACTIVITIES
alcohol use: Possibly additive CNS depression

Adverse Reactions
CNS: Amnesia, anxiety, asthenia, ataxia, confusion, depression, dizziness, drowsi-ness, EEG abnormalities, hostility, impaired cognition, insomnia, light-headedness, paresthesia, seizures, status epilepticus, suicidal ideation, tremor, weakness
EENT: Pharyngitis, stomatitis
GI: Abdominal pain, diarrhea, increased appetite, nausea, vomiting
GU: UTI
MS: Dysarthria
SKIN: Ecchymosis, rash

Nursing Considerations
• Give tiagabine with food.
WARNING Expect to taper dosage gradually, as prescribed, because stopping drug abruptly may increase seizure frequency.
• Take seizure precautions because tiagabine has caused seizures and status epilepticus in patients with no history of seizures.
• Watch patient closely for evidence of suicidal tendencies, especially when therapy starts or dosage changes, and report concerns at once.
PATIENT TEACHING
• Instruct patient to take drug with food.
• Advise patient to avoid hazardous activities until drug's CNS effects are known. Also urge her to avoid alcohol use.
• If patient takes a CNS depressant, explain that drug may increase depressant effect.
• Instruct patient not to stop taking tiagabine abruptly. Explain that prescriber usually tapers dosage over 4 weeks to reduce the risk of withdrawal seizures.
• Urge caregivers to watch patient closely for evidence of suicidal tendencies, especially when therapy starts or dosage changes, and to report concerns immediately.
• Encourage woman who becomes pregnant while taking tiagabine to enroll in the North American antiepileptic drug pregnancy registry by calling 1-888-233-

2334. Explain that the registry is collecting information about the safety of anti-epileptic drugs during pregnancy.

ticagrelor
Brilinta

Class and Category
Chemical class:
Cyclopentyltriazolopyrimidine inhibitor
Therapeutic class: Platelet inhibitor
Pregnancy category: C

Indications and Dosages
➤ *To reduce the rate of thrombotic cardiovascular events in patients with acute coronary syndrome (unstable angina, non-ST elevation myocardial infarction, or ST elevation myocardial infarction)*
TABLETS
Adults. *Initial:* 180 mg as a loading dose followed by 90 mg twice daily.

Mechanism of Action
Reversibly interacts with the platelet P2Y12 ADP-receptor to prevent platelet activation.

Contraindications
Active bleeding, history of intracranial hemorrhage, hypersensitivity to ticagrelor or its components, severe hepatic impairment
Interaction
DRUGS
aspirin (daily doses above 100 mg): Reduced effectiveness of ticagrelor
CYP3A inducers such as carbamazepine, dexamethasone, phenobarbital, phenytoin, rifampin: Elevated ticagrelor levels and risk of adverse effects
CYP3A inhibitors such as atazanavir, clarithromycin, indinavir, itraconazole, ketoconazole, nefazodone, nelfinavir, ritonavir, saquinavir, voriconazole: Substantially reduced blood ticagrelor levels and effectiveness
digoxin: Altered blood digoxin levels
lovastatin, sinvastatin: Increased serum levels of these drugs

Adverse Reactions
CNS: Dizziness, fatigue, headache, intracranial bleeding

CV: Atrial fibrillation, bradycardia, chest pain, hypertension, hypotension (may be severe), intracardial bleed with cardiac tamponade
EENT: Epistaxis, intraocular bleeding with permanent vision loss
ENDO: Gynecomastia
GI: Diarrhea, nausea
GU: Elevated serum creatinine level
HEME: Minor or major bleeding
MS: Back or noncardiac chest pain
RESP: Cough, dyspnea
SKIN: Bruising
Other: Angioedema, elevated uric acid, hypovolemic shock

Nursing Considerations
• Be aware that aspirin is used with ticagrelor therapy. Expect to administer 325 mg of aspirin initially followed by a maintenance dose of aspirin of 75 to 100 mg daily. Know that a patient who has already received a loading dose of clopidogrel may be started on ticagrelor therapy immediately.
• Monitor patient closely for bleeding tendencies. Know that risk of bleeding increases with ticagrelor use in older patients as well as patients with a history of bleeding disorders, performance of percutaneous invasive procedures and concomitant use of drugs that increase the risk of bleeding such as anticoagulant and fibrinolytic therapy, higher doses of aspirin, and chronic use of nonsteroidal anti-inflammatory drugs.
• Be prepared to discontinue ticagrelor therapy, as ordered, five days before surgery, if possible.
• Be suspicious of bleeding in a patient who becomes hypotensive and has recently undergone coronary angiography, PCI, CABG, or other surgical procedures, even if the patient does not have any signs of bleeding. Notify prescriber immediately if patient becomes hypotensive and expect to provide supportive care.
• Monitor patient for dyspnea that may occur with ticagrelor therapy. If dyspnea is determined to be caused by the drug, expect to continue therapy as no specific treatment is needed and often resolves on its own.

T

• Avoid abrupt interruption of ticagrelor therapy because doing so increases the risk of myocardial infarction, stent thrombosis, and death.

PATIENT TEACHING
• Warn patient not to discontinue ticagrelor therapy abruptly because of increased risk of life-threatening adverse effects.
• Advise patient to seek immediate emergency care if bleeding occurs and is serious.
• Instruct patient to take bleeding precautions such as avoiding the use of a razor and brushing teeth with a soft-bristled toothbrush.
• Tell patient to alert all prescribers of ticagrelor therapy.

ticarcillin disodium

Ticar

Class and Category
Chemical class: Penicillin
Therapeutic class: Antibiotic
Pregnancy category: B

Indications and Dosages
➤ *To treat moderate to severe infections, such as bacteremia, diabetic foot ulcers, empyema, intra-abdominal infections, lower respiratory tract infections (including pneumonia), lung abscess, peritonitis, pulmonary infections due to complications of cystic fibrosis (including bronchiectasis and pneumonia), septicemia, and skin and soft-tissue infections (including cellulitis) caused by susceptible organisms*

I.V. INFUSION
Adults and children. 200 to 300 mg/kg daily in divided doses every 4 to 6 hr. *Usual:* 3 g every 4 hr or 4 g every 6 hr.
➤ *To treat uncomplicated UTI*
I.V. INFUSION, I.M. INJECTION
Adults and children weighing 40 kg (88 lb) or more. 1 g every 6 hr.
Children over age 1 month and weighing less than 40 kg. 50 to 100 mg/kg daily in divided doses every 6 to 8 hr.
➤ *To treat complicated UTI*
I.V. INFUSION
Adults and children. 150 to 200 mg/kg in equally divided doses every 4 to 6 hr. *Usual:* 3 g every 6 hr.

DOSAGE ADJUSTMENT For patients with creatinine clearance of 30 to 60 ml/min/1.73 m^2, 2 g I.V. every 4 hr; with creatinine clearance of 10 to 30 ml/min/1.73 m^2, 2 g I.V. every 8 hr; with creatinine clearance of less than 10 ml/min/1.73 m^2, 2 g I.V. every 12 hr or 1 g I.M. every 6 hr.

Mechanism of Action
Inhibits bacterial cell wall synthesis by binding to specific penicillin-binding proteins inside the bacterial cell wall. Ultimately, this leads to cell wall lysis and death.

Incompatibilities
Don't administer ticarcillin through the same I.V. line as amikacin, gentamicin, or tobramycin. Don't give within 1 hr of aminoglycosides.

Contraindications
Hypersensitivity to ticarcillin, penicillins, or their components

Interaction
DRUGS
aminoglycosides: Additive or synergistic activity against some bacteria; possibly mutual inactivation when infused simultaneously via Y-site
anticoagulants: Possibly interference with platelet aggregation, prolonged PT
methotrexate: Prolonged blood methotrexate level, increased risk of methotrexate toxicity
probenecid: Prolonged blood ticarcillin level

Adverse Reactions
CV: Thrombophlebitis, vasculitis
GI: Elevated liver function test results, nausea, pseudomembranous colitis, vomiting
GU: Proteinuria
HEME: Anemia, eosinophilia, hemorrhage, leukopenia, neutropenia, prolonged bleeding time, thrombocytopenia
SKIN: Erythema nodosum, exfoliative dermatitis, pruritus, rash, toxic epidermal necrolysis, urticaria
Other: Anaphylaxis, hypernatremia, hypokalemia, injection-site pain, superinfection

Nursing Considerations
• Obtain body fluid or tissue samples for culture and sensitivity testing, as ordered.

Review test results, if possible, before giving first dose of ticarcillin.
• Don't inject more than 2 g of drug at any one I.M. injection site.
• Reconstitute each gram of ticarcillin with 4 ml of compatible diluent. Further dilute reconstituted I.V. solution to 10 to 100 mg/ml with compatible I.V. solution. To minimize vein irritation, don't exceed concentration of 100 mg/ml. Concentrations of 50 mg/ml or greater are preferred. Infuse appropriate I.V. dose over 30 to 120 minutes.
• Check for local injection-site reaction, including thrombophlebitis, during therapy.
• Be aware that ticarcillin may worsen symptoms in patients with a history of GI disease or colitis.
• For patients with renal impairment, take seizure precautions, according to facility policy, because of increased risk of seizures.
• Monitor patient closely for diarrhea, which may indicate pseudomembranous colitis caused by *Clostridium difficile.* If diarrhea occurs, notify prescriber and expect to withhold ticarcillin and treat with fluids, electrolytes, protein, and an antibiotic effective against *C. difficile.*
• Also look for signs of superinfection, such as oral candidiasis and rash in breast-feeding infant.
• Monitor serum electrolyte levels for hypernatremia due to drug's high sodium content and for hypokalemia due to increased urinary potassium loss.
WARNING Monitor patient's platelet count, PT, and APTT because ticarcillin may increase bleeding time and, in rare cases, may induce thrombocytopenia.

PATIENT TEACHING
• Emphasize the need to take full course of ticarcillin exactly as prescribed, even if feeling better.
• Urge patient to report past allergies to penicillins and to notify prescriber at once about adverse reactions, including fever.
• Advise patient to decrease sodium intake to reduce the risk of electrolyte imbalance.
• Instruct patient to report diarrhea that's severe or prolonged. Remind patient that watery or bloody stools can occur 2 or more months after antibiotic therapy and can be serious, requiring prompt treatment.

ticlopidine hydrochloride
Ticlid

Class and Category
Chemical class: Thienopyridine derivative
Therapeutic class: Antithrombotic, platelet aggregation inhibitor
Pregnancy category: B

Indications and Dosages
➤ *To reduce the risk of initial thrombotic stroke in patients who have experienced transient ischemic attack, to reduce the risk of recurrent stroke in patients who have previously experienced thrombotic stroke*
TABLETS
Adults. 250 mg twice daily.
➤ *As adjunct to reduce the risk of subacute stent thrombosis after successful coronary stent implantation*
TABLETS
Adults. 250 mg b.i.d. with antiplatelet doses of aspirin for up to 30 days after successful stent implantation.

Route	Onset	Peak	Duration
P.O.	2–4 days	8–11 days	1–2 wk

Contraindications
Coagulopathy, GI bleeding, hematologic disorders related to hematopoiesis (including history of thrombotic thrombocytopenic purpura, neutropenia, and thrombocytopenia), hemophilia, hypersensitivity to ticlopidine or its components, intracranial bleeding, retinal bleeding, severe hepatic disease

Interaction
DRUGS
aluminum- and magnesium-containing antacids: Possibly decreased peak blood ticlopidine level
antineoplastics, antithymocyte globulin, heparin, NSAIDs, oral anticoagulants, platelet aggregation inhibitors, salicylates, strontium-89 chloride, thrombolytics: Increased risk of bleeding
cimetidine: Reduced clearance of ticlopidine, increased risk of adverse reactions

T

Mechanism of Action

Normally, platelets don't adhere to blood vessel walls. However, when a thrombotic stroke or other disorder damages blood vessel walls, platelets are activated andadhere within seconds. Once activated, platelets release adenosine diphosphate (ADP). This causes fibrinogen to bind to glycoprotein IIb/IIIa (GP IIb/IIIa) receptors on the surface of activated platelets and connect with other activated platelets. Then a thrombus forms.

Ticlopidine inhibits the release of ADP from activated platelets, which prevents fibrinogen from binding to GP IIb/IIIa receptors on the surface of activated platelets, as shown below. This action prevents platelets from aggregating to form a thrombus, which prevents thrombosis of an implanted stent or recurrence of stroke.

cyclosporine, digoxin: Decreased blood level and possibly reduced effects of these drugs
porfimer: Decreased effectiveness of porfimer photodynamic therapy
xanthines (aminophylline, oxytriphylline, theophylline): Decreased theophylline clearance, increased risk of toxicity

Adverse Reactions

CNS: Dizziness
CV: Hypercholesterolemia, vasculitis
EENT: Tinnitus
GI: Abdominal pain, anorexia, diarrhea, elevated liver function test results, flatulence, indigestion, nausea, vomiting
HEME: Agranulocytosis, aplastic anemia, hemolysis, hemolytic anemia, neutropenia, pancytopenia, thrombocytopenia, thrombotic thrombocytopenia, thrombotic thrombocytopenic purpura
SKIN: Pruritus, purpura, rash
Other: Hyponatremia, serum sickness-like reaction

Nursing Considerations

• Give ticlopidine with food to maximize GI absorption and minimize any GI distress.

• Avoid I.M. injections of other drugs because excessive bleeding, bruising, or hematoma may occur.
• During first 3 months of therapy, monitor CBC every 2 weeks, as ordered (more frequently in patients with depressed neutrophil count).
• Be aware that ticlopidine therapy typically is used for patients with stroke or an increased risk of stroke who can't tolerate aspirin because of the risk of neutropenia or agranulocytosis.
WARNING Be aware that ticlopidine therapy irreversibly affects platelet aggregation. Expect prescriber to discontinue drug 10 to 14 days before surgical procedures to prevent uncontrolled bleeding.
• Monitor serum cholesterol level during first month of ticlopidine therapy for expected increase. Hypercholesterolemia may persist for duration of treatment.

PATIENT TEACHING
• Urge patient to take ticlopidine with food.
• Inform patient that she may be at increased risk for infection because drug

may decrease WBC or platelet count, especially in first 3 months of therapy.
• Advise patient to notify prescriber immediately if she has chills, fever, or sore throat.
• Urge patient to keep scheduled appointments for blood tests to detect abnormalities.
• Instruct patient to apply prolonged pressure to injured areas because bleeding may take longer than usual to stop. Urge her to immediately report to prescriber any unusual bleeding or bruising.

tigecycline
Tygacil

Class and Category
Chemical class: Glycylcycline
Therapeutic class: Antibiotic
Pregnancy category: D

Indications and Dosages
➤ *To treat complicated skin and skin structure infections caused by* Escherichia coli, Enterococcus faecalis *(vancomycin-susceptible isolates only),* Staphylococcus aureus *(methicillin-susceptible and resistant isolates),* Streptococcus agalactiae, Streptococcus anginosus *group (includes* S. anginosus, S. intermedius, *and* S. constellatus*),* Streptococcus pyogenes, *and* Bacteroides fragilis; *to treat complicated intra-abdominal infections caused by* Citrobacter freundii, Enterobacter cloacae, E. coli, Klebsiella oxytoca, Klebsiella pneumoniae, Enterococcus faecalis *(vancomycin-susceptible isolates only),* S. aureus *(methicillin-susceptible isolates only),* S. anginosus *group,* B. fragilis, Bacteroides thetaiotaomicron, Bacteroides uniformis, Bacteroides vulgatus, Clostridium perfringens, *and* Peptostreptococcus micros; *to treat community-acquired bacterial pneumonia caused by* Streptococcus pneumoniae *(penicillin-susceptible isolates), including cases with concurrent bacteremia,* Haemophilus influenzae *(beta-lactamase negative isolates), and* Legionella pneumophila

I.V. INFUSION
Adults. *Initial:* 100 mg infused over 30 to 60 min followed by 50 mg infused over 30 to 60 min every 12 hr for 5 to 14 days for complicated skin and skin structure infections and intra-abdominal infections (7 to 14 days for community-acquired bacterial pneumonia).
DOSAGE ADJUSTMENT For patients with severe hepatic impairment, initial dosage of 100 mg should be followed by a reduced maintenance dosage of 25 mg every 12 hr.

Mechanism of Action
Inhibits protein translation in bacteria by binding to the 30S ribosomal subunit, which prevents binding of aminoacyl tRNA molecules to the ribosome complex, thus interfering with protein synthesis. Through this bacteriostatic action, bacteria are weakened.

Incompatibilities
Don't give amphotericin B, chlorpromazine, methylprednisolone, or voriconazole simultaneously through the same Y-site.

Contraindications
Hypersensitivity to tigecycline or its components

Adverse Reactions
CNS: Asthenia, chills, dizziness, fever, headache, insomnia, somnolence
CV: Bradycardia, hypertension, hypotension, peripheral edema, phlebitis, septic shock, tachycardia, thrombophlebitis, vasodilation
EENT: Dry mouth, taste perversion
ENDO: Hyperglycemia, hypoglycemia
GI: Abdominal pain, acute pancreatitis, anorexia, cholestasis (hepatic), constipation, diarrhea, dyspepsia, elevated liver enzyme levels, hepatic dysfunction or failure, jaundice, nausea, pancreatitis, pseudo-membranous colitis, vomiting
GU: Elevated BUN and creatinine levels, vaginal candidiasis
HEME: Anemia, increased PT, leukocytosis, thrombocythemia
MS: Back pain
RESP: Increased cough, dyspnea
SKIN: Diaphoresis, photosensitivity, pruritus, rash, Stevens-Johnson Syndrome
Other: Anaphylaxis, hypersensitivity reaction, hypocalcemia; hypokalemia;

hyponatremia; hypoproteinemia; injection-site reaction, such as edema, phlebitis, inflammation, and pain

Nursing Considerations

• Know that tigecycline should only be prescribed when alternative treatments are not suitable because an increase in all-cause mortality has been observed in clinical trials.

• Obtain body tissue and fluid samples for culture and sensitivity tests as ordered before giving first dose of tigecycline. Expect to begin drug therapy before test results are known.

• Avoid giving tigecycline to children under age 8 because drug may cause permanent brown or yellow tooth discoloration and enamel hypoplasia.

• Use tigecycline cautiously in patients hypersensitive to tetracycline antibiotics because glycylcycline antibiotics are structurally similar to tetracyclines.

• Also use cautiously in patients with complicated intra-abdominal infections secondary to intestinal perforation because of the risk of septic shock.

• Determine whether female patients could be pregnant before starting tigecycline therapy because the drug may cause harm to fetus.

• Reconstitute each vial of tigecycline with 5.3 ml of 0.9% sodium chloride injection or 5% dextrose injection to achieve a concentration of 10 mg/ml. Note that the color will be yellow to orange. If it's not, the solution should be discarded. Immediately withdraw reconstituted solution from the vial and add to a 100-ml I.V. bag for infusion. Drug may be stored in the I.V. bag at room temperature for up to 6 hours or refrigerated up to 24 hours before use.

• If the patient's I.V. line is used to infuse other drugs, flush the line with either 0.9% sodium chloride injection or 5% dextrose injection before and after tigecycline infusion.

• Infuse tigecycline over 30 to 60 minutes.

• Monitor patient closely for diarrhea, which may indicate pseudomembranous colitis, which is known to occur with many antibiotics. If diarrhea occurs during tigecycline therapy, notify prescriber and

expect to withhold drug. Expect to treat psuedomembranous colitis, if confirmed, with fluids, electrolytes, protein, and an antibiotic effective against *Clostridium difficile.*

• Monitor patient for adverse reactions, keeping in mind the similarity between tigecycline and tetracycline.

• Assess patient for superinfection, such as vaginal candidiasis, that may result from overgrowth of nonsusceptible organisms, including fungi. If signs of infection are present, notify prescriber and provide supportive care, as prescribed.

• Monitor patient's liver function closely. If enzyme levels become elevated, notify prescriber because dosage may need to be decreased or drug discontinued.

• Be aware that adverse reactions may continue after therapy stops.

PATIENT TEACHING

• Instruct patient to report adverse reactions, especially hypersensitivity reactions, such as a rash or itching, as well as diarrhea.

• Tell patient to report discomfort at the infusion site because the site may need to be changed.

• Urge patient to report diarrhea that's severe or prolonged. Remind patient that watery or bloody stools can occur 2 or more months after antibiotic therapy and can be serious, requiring prompt treatment.

tiludronate disodium

(contains 200 mg of tiludronic acid per tablet)
Skelid

Class and Category

Chemical class: Aminobiphosphonate
Therapeutic class: Bone resorption inhibitor
Pregnancy category: C

Indications and Dosages

➤ *To treat Paget's disease in patients with serum alkaline phosphatase levels at least twice the upper limit of normal, who are symptomatic or at risk for future complications of the disease*

TABLETS

Adults. *Initial:* 400 mg of tiludronic acid daily 2 hr before or after meals for 3 mo. *Maximum:* 400 mg of tiludronic acid daily.

Mechanism of Action

Reduces the activity of cells that cause bone loss and increases bone mass. Tiludronate may act by inhibiting osteoclast activity on newly formed bone resorption surfaces. This activity reduces the number of sites at which bone is remodeled. When bone formation exceeds bone resorption at these remodeling sites, bone mass increases. Tiludronate may also inhibit bone destruction by binding to hydroxyapatite crystals, which give bone its rigidity.

Contraindications

Creatinine clearance less than 30 ml/min/1.73 m², esophageal abnormalities that delay esophageal emptying, hypersensitivity to tiludronate or its components, inability to stand or sit upright for at least 30 minutes

Interaction

DRUGS

aluminum- or magnesium-containing antacids, mineral supplements (such as calcium, iron), salicylates, salicylate-containing compounds: Decreased absorption of tiludronate

indomethacin: Possibly increased bioavailability of tiludronate

FOODS

all foods and beverages (except plain water): Decreased absorption of tiludronate

Adverse Reactions

CNS: Dizziness, headache
CV: Chest pain, edema
EENT: Cataracts, conjunctivitis, difficulty swallowing, glaucoma, pharyngitis, rhinitis
GI: Diarrhea, esophageal irritation and ulceration, flatulence, indigestion, nausea, vomiting
MS: Arthralgia, atypical femoral fractures, back pain, myalgia, osteonecrosis of jaw, retrosternal pain
RESP: Cough, upper respiratory tract infection
SKIN: Rash
Other: Flulike symptoms

Nursing Considerations

• Be prepared to monitor serum calcium levels before, during, and after tiludronate therapy because drug may exacerbate such conditions as hyperparathyroidism, hypocalcemia, and vitamin D deficiency. Ensure adequate dietary intake of calcium and vitamin D during and after treatment. If hypocalcemia occurs, expect to administer a calcium supplement, as prescribed.

• Use cautiously in patients with active upper gastrointestinal conditions such as Barrett's esophagus, dysphagia, other esophageal disease, gastritis, duodenitis, or ulcers because tiludronate therapy may worsen these conditions because of its irritating effect on upper GI mucosa.

WARNING To help minimize tiludronate's irritation on the patient's upper GI mucosa, have patient take drug with full glass of plain water and remain upright for at least 30 minutes.

PATIENT TEACHING

• Instruct patient to take drug with 6 to 8 oz of plain water on an empty stomach (at least 2 hours before or after beverages, food, other drugs, or mineral supplements, including mineral water) because food and beverages may severely reduce drug's effect. Also, advise her to remain upright for at least 30 minutes after taking drug.

• Advise patient not to chew or suck on tablet to reduce the risk of esophageal irritation.

• Instruct patient to notify prescriber immediately if she develops signs or symptoms of esophageal irritation, such as trouble swallowing or painful swallowing, retrosternal pain, or worsening heartburn; these may indicate a serious esophageal disorder.

• Caution patient not to take salicylate-containing drugs, such as aspirin, during tiludronate therapy.

• Encourage patient to maintain adequate vitamin D and calcium intake during tiludronate therapy. Calcium supplements should not be taken within 2 hours before or 2 hours after taking tiludronate. Aluminum- or magnesium-containing antacids should also be taken at least 2 hours after taking tiludronate.

T

• Instruct patient to notify prescriber of new or worsening groin or thigh pain.

timolol maleate

Apo-Timol (CAN), Blocadren, Novo-Timol (CAN)

Class and Category

Chemical class: Beta blocker
Therapeutic class: Antihypertensive, MI prophylactic, vascular headache prophylactic
Pregnancy category: C

Indications and Dosages

➤ *To manage hypertension*

TABLETS

Adults. *Initial:* 10 mg twice daily, increased every wk as prescribed. *Maintenance:* 20 to 40 mg daily in divided doses. *Maximum:* 60 mg daily.

➤ *To provide long-term prophylaxis after MI*

TABLETS

Adults. 10 mg twice daily, beginning 1 to 4 wk after MI and continuing for at least 2 yr.

➤ *To prevent migraine headache*

TABLETS

Adults. *Initial:* 10 mg twice daily. *Maintenance:* 20 mg daily in divided doses. *Maximum:* 30 mg daily; discontinued after 8 wk, as prescribed, if maximum dose is ineffective.

Route	Onset	Peak	Duration
P.O.	30 min	1–2 hr	4–8 hr

Mechanism of Action

Selectively blocks alpha$_1$ and beta$_2$ receptors in vascular smooth muscle and beta$_1$ receptors in the heart. This reduces peripheral vascular resistance and blood pressure and relieves migraine headaches. Timolol's potent beta blockade prevents the reflex tachycardia that typically occurs with most alpha blockers, and decreases cardiac excitability, cardiac output, and myocardial oxygen demand, thus preventing MI.

Contraindications

Acute bronchospasm; asthma; cardiogenic shock; children; COPD (severe); heart failure; hypersensitivity to timolol, other beta blockers, or their components; second- or third-degree AV block; severe sinus bradycardia

Interaction

DRUGS

allergen immunotherapy, allergenic extracts for skin testing: Increased risk of serious systemic adverse reactions or anaphylaxis
amiodarone: Additive depressant effect on cardiac conduction, negative inotropic effect
anesthetics (hydrocarbon inhalation): Increased risk of myocardial depression and hypotension
beta blockers: Additive beta blockade effects
calcium channel blockers, clonidine, diazoxide, guanabenz, reserpine, other hypotension-producing drugs: Additive hypotensive effect and, possibly, other beta blockade effects
cimetidine: Possibly interference with timolol clearance
estrogens: Decreased antihypertensive effect of timolol
fentanyl, fentanyl derivatives: Possibly increased risk of initial bradycardia after induction doses of fentanyl or derivative (with long-term timolol use)
glucagon: Possibly blunted hyperglycemic response
insulin, oral antidiabetic drugs: Possibly masking of tachycardia in response to hypoglycemia, impaired glucose control
lidocaine: Decreased lidocaine clearance, increased risk of lidocaine toxicity
MAO inhibitors: Increased risk of significant hypertension
neuromuscular blockers: Possibly potentiated and prolonged action of these drugs
NSAIDs: Possibly decreased hypotensive effect
phenothiazines: Increased blood levels of both drugs
phenytoin (parenteral): Additive cardiac depressant effect
sympathomimetics, xanthines: Possibly mutual inhibition of therapeutic effects

Adverse Reactions

CNS: Asthenia, decreased concentration, depression, dizziness, fatigue, fever, hallucinations, headache, insomnia,

nervousness, nightmares, paresthesia, stroke, syncope, vertigo
CV: Angina, arrhythmias, bradycardia, cardiac arrest, chest pain, edema, palpitations, Raynaud's phenomenon, vasodilation
EENT: Diplopia, dry eyes, eye irritation, ptosis, tinnitus, vision changes
ENDO: Hyperglycemia, hypoglycemia
GI: Abdominal pain, diarrhea, hepatomegaly, indigestion, nausea, vomiting
GU: Decreased libido, impotence
MS: Arthralgia, decreased tolerance to exercise, extremity pain, muscle weakness
RESP: Bronchospasm, cough, crackles, dyspnea
SKIN: Alopecia, diaphoresis, hyperpigmentation, pruritus, purpura, rash
Other: Anaphylaxis, weight loss

Nursing Considerations
WARNING Be aware that timolol may mask evidence of acute hypoglycemia in diabetic patient. It also may mask certain signs of hyperthyroidism, such as tachycardia.
• Be aware that timolol may prolong hypoglycemia by interfering with glycogenolysis or may promote hyperglycemia by decreasing tissue sensitivity to insulin.
• Monitor blood pressure and cardiac output, as appropriate, for patient with a history of systolic heart failure or left ventricular dysfunction because timolol's negative inotropic effect can depress cardiac output.
WARNING Timolol shouldn't be discontinued abruptly because this may produce MI, myocardial ischemia, severe hypertension, or ventricular arrhythmias, particularly in patient with known cardiovascular disease.
• Expect varied drug effectiveness in elderly patients; they may be less sensitive to drug's antihypertensive effect or more sensitive because of reduced drug clearance.
• Monitor for impaired circulation in elderly patients with age-related peripheral vascular disease or patients with Raynaud's phenomenon. Such patients may experience exacerbated symptoms

from increased alpha stimulation. Elderly patients also are at increased risk for beta blocker–induced hypothermia.
• If timolol worsens skin condition, such as psoriasis, notify prescriber.
PATIENT TEACHING
• Instruct patient taking timolol to inform prescriber of chest pain, fainting, lightheadedness, or shortness of breath, which may indicate the need for dosage change.
• Caution patient not to stop taking drug abruptly. Timolol dosage must be tapered gradually under prescriber's supervision.
• Instruct patient with diabetes to monitor blood glucose level often during therapy.
• Warn patient with psoriasis about possible flare-ups of skin condition.

tinidazole
Tindamax

Class and Category
Chemical class: Synthetic nitroimidazole
Therapeutic class: Antiprotozoal
Pregnancy category: C

Indications and Dosages
➤ *To treat trichomoniasis caused by* Trichomonas vaginalis
TABLETS
Adults. 2 g one time with food.
➤ *To treat giardiasis caused by Giardia* duodenalis (G. lamblia)
TABLETS
Adults. 2 g one time with food.
Children age 4 and over. 50 mg/kg (up to 2 g) one time with food.
➤ *To treat intestinal amebiasis caused by* Entamoeba histolytica
TABLETS
Adults. 2 g daily for 3 days with food.
Children age 4 and over. 50 mg/kg (up to 2 g) daily for 3 days with food.
➤ *To treat amebic liver abscess caused by* entamoeba histolytica
TABLETS
Adults. 2 g daily for 3 to 5 days with food.
Children age 4 and over. 50 mg/kg (up to 2 g) daily for 3 to 5 days with food.
DOSAGE ADJUSTMENT For patients receiving hemodialysis, an additional dose equivalent to one-half the dose prescribed should be

given after the dialysis treatment on the days dialysis is performed.

Mechanism of Action

Undergoes intracellular chemical reduction during anaerobic metabolism. After tinidazole is reduced, it damages DNA's helical structure and breaks its strands, which inhibits bacterial nucleic acid synthesis and causes cell death.

Contraindications

Breastfeeding, hypersensitivity to tinidazole or its components, treatment of trichomoniasis during first trimester of pregnancy

Interaction

DRUGS

cholestyramine: Possibly decreased bioavailability of tinidazole
cimetidine, ketoconazole: Possibly delayed elimination and increased blood level of tinidazole
cyclosporine, tacrolimus: Possibly increased serum cyclosporine and tacrolimus levels
disulfiram: Possibly combined toxicity, resulting in confusion and psychosis
fluorouracil: Possibly decreased fluorouracil clearance
lithium: Possibly increased serum lithium levels
oral anticoagulants: Possibly increased anticoagulant effect
oxytetracycline: Possibly diminished effect of tinidazole
phenobarbital, phenytoin, rifampin: Possibly increased metabolism and decreased blood level of tinidazole

ACTIVITIES

alcohol use: Possibly disulfiram-like effects

Adverse Reactions

CNS: Ataxia, dizziness, coma, confusion, depression, drowsiness, fatigue, fever, headache, insomnia, malaise, peripheral neuropathy, seizures, vertigo, weakness
CV: Palpitations
EENT: Dry mouth, excessive salivation, furry tongue, metallic or bitter taste, oral candidiasis, pharyngitis, stomatitis, tongue discoloration
GI: Abdominal cramps, anorexia, constipation, diarrhea, epigastric discomfort, flatulence, hepatic abnormalities, indigestion, nausea, thirst, vomiting

GU: Darkened urine, dysuria, increased vaginal discharge, menorrhagia, UTI, vaginal candidiasis or odor, vulvo-vaginal discomfort
HEME: Reversible thrombocytopenia, transient leukopenia or neutropenia
MS: Arthralgia, arthritis, myalgia, pelvic pain
RESP: Bronchospasm, dyspnea, upper respiratory tract infection
SKIN: Diaphoresis, erythema multiforme, flushing, pruritus, rash, Stevens-Johnson syndrome, urticaria
Other: Angioedema

Nursing Considerations

• Use tinidazole cautiously in patients with CNS disease or blood dyscrasias because tinidazole's adverse effects may worsen these disorders. Also use cautiously in patients with hepatic impairment because a chemically related drug has reduced elimination.
• Take seizure precautions. If a seizure or other abnormal neurologic symptoms occur, notify prescriber and expect to stop drug.
• Treat a patient diagnosed with trichomoniasis and her sexual partner with the same dose of tinidazole and at the same time, as ordered, because trichomoniasis is a sexually transmitted disease.
• Monitor patient's total WBC count and differential if retreatment with tinidazole is needed because adverse hematologic reactions may occur with repeated use.

PATIENT TEACHING

• Tell patient to take tinidazole with food to minimize gastric discomfort.
• Instruct patient unable to swallow tablets to crush tinidazole and mix in artificial cherry syrup and then take with food.
• Advise patient to avoid alcohol while taking tinidazole and for 3 days afterward because alcohol can cause intense flushing.
• Tell patient to alert prescriber before taking tinidazole if she thinks or knows she is pregnant because tinidazole crosses the placental barrier during the first trimester and its effects on the fetus are unknown.
• Instruct breastfeeding patient not to breastfeed during therapy and for 3 days after taking last dose.

tinzaparin sodium

Innohep

Class and Category

Chemical class: Low–molecular-weight heparin
Therapeutic class: Anticoagulant, antithrombotic
Pregnancy category: B

Indications and Dosages

➤ *As adjunct to treat pulmonary thromboembolism and acute symptomatic deep vein thrombosis*

SUBCUTANEOUS INJECTION

Adults. 175 anti-Xa international units/kg daily for at least 6 days. *Maximum:* 18,000 to 21,000 anti-Xa international units daily.

Route	Onset	Peak	Duration
SubQ	2–3 hr	4–6 hr	24 hr

Mechanism of Action

Potentiates the action of antithrombin III, a coagulation inhibitor. By binding with antithrombin III, tinzaparin rapidly binds with and inactivates clotting factors (primarily fibrin and factor Xa). Without thrombin, fibrinogen can't convert to fibrin and clots can't form.

Contraindications

Active major bleeding; heparin-induced thrombocytopenia (current or past); hypersensitivity to tinzaparin or its components, other low–molecular-weight heparins, sulfites, benzyl alcohol, or pork products

Interaction

DRUGS

alteplase, anistreplase, aspirin, dextran, dipyridamole, NSAIDs, oral anticoagulants, streptokinase, sulfinpyrazone, urokinase: Possibly increased risk of bleeding and risk of spinal or epidural hematomas

Adverse Reactions

CNS: Confusion, dizziness, epidural or spinal hematoma, headache, insomnia, intracranial hemorrhage, paralysis
CV: Angina, hypertension, hypotension, tachycardia
EENT: Epistaxis, gingival bleeding, pharyngeal bleeding
GI: Constipation, elevated liver function test results, GI and retroperitoneal bleeding, hematemesis, nausea, vomiting
GU: Hematuria, genitourinary bleeding, prolonged or heavy menstrual bleeding, UTI
HEME: Anemia, thrombocytopenia, unusual bruising
MS: Back pain
RESP: Dyspnea, hemoptysis, pulmonary embolism
SKIN: Bleeding at puncture sites, surgical incision sites, or venous cutdown sites; rash
Other: Injection-site hematoma, including itching, pain, redness, and swelling

Nursing Considerations

• Use tinzaparin with extreme caution in patients who are elderly and have renal insufficiency because drug may increase the risk of death.
• Expect warfarin therapy to begin within 1 to 3 days of tinzaparin use.
• Monitor patient's INR. Expect therapy to continue until INR reaches 2.0 for 2 consecutive days.
WARNING Monitor patient for evidence of GI bleeding, including bloody or black, tarry stools; bloody or coffee-ground vomitus; and severe stomach pain. Notify prescriber immediately if patient develops any of these signs or symptoms.
• Assess tinzaparin injection site for signs and symptoms of hematoma, including deep, dark purple bruises under skin and itching, pain, redness, or swelling.
• Assess patient for evidence of intracranial bleeding (such as decreased level of consciousness), retroperitoneal bleeding (such as abdominal pain or swelling and back pain), genitourinary bleeding (such as hematuria), or respiratory tract bleeding (such as hemoptysis). Notify prescriber immediately about any of these signs or symptoms.
• If serious bleeding (not controllable by local pressure) occurs, expect to discontinue any concomitant warfarin or antiplatelet drugs immediately.
• Expect to treat bleeding by administering 1 mg of protamine sulfate 1% solution I.V. per 100 anti-Xa international units of tinzaparin, as prescribed.

T

- If possible, avoid giving I.M. injections to patient receiving tinzaparin. If arterial puncture becomes necessary during tinzaparin therapy, expect to apply pressure after procedure and to monitor puncture site frequently for signs of bleeding.
- Monitor patient's laboratory tests for elevated liver enzyme levels. If significant elevations persist or worsen, notify prescriber immediately.

WARNING Monitor patient receiving tinzaparin and epidural or spinal anesthesia or when a spinal puncture is performed because spinal hematomas can occur, causing long-term or permanent paralysis. Watch for evidence of neurologic impairment, such as changes in sensory or motor function. If present, notify prescriber immediately because urgent care is needed to minimize effects of hematoma. Use of indwelling epidural catheters, concurrent use of other drugs that affect hemostatis, a history of traumatic or repeated epidural or spinal punctures, or a history of spinal deformity or spinal surgery increases the risk of spinal or epidural hematomas in patients receiving tinzaparin.

PATIENT TEACHING
- Advise patient who is receiving tinzaparin to immediately report any bleeding, including from nose or gums.
- Instruct patient to limit physical activity during tinzaparin administration to reduce the risk of injury or bleeding.
- Urge female patient to notify prescriber if she is or could be pregnant.

tiotropium bromide
Spiriva HandiHaler, Spiriva Respimat

Class and Category
Chemical class: Nonane bromide monohydrate
Therapeutic class: Anticholingeric, bronchodilator
Pregnancy category: C

Indications and Dosages
➤ *To prevent bronchospasm associated with COPD, including chronic bronchitis and emphysema; to reduce COPD exacerbations*

ORAL INHALATION (HANDIHALER)
Adults. 18 mcg (2 inhalations) once daily
ORAL INHALATION (RESPIMAT)
Adults. 5 mcg (2 inhalations) once daily. *Maximum:* 5 mcg every 24 hr.

Mechanism of Action
Prevents acetylcholine from attaching to muscarinic receptors on membranes of smooth-muscle cells. By blocking acetylcholine's effects in the bronchi and bronchioles, tiotropium relaxes smooth muscles and causes bronchodilation.

Contraindications
Hypersensitivity to atropine or its derivatives, including ipratropium, tiotropium, or their components

Interaction
DRUGS
anticholinergics: Possibly increased anticholinergic effects

Adverse Reactions
CNS: Depression, difficulty speaking, dizziness, paresthesia, stroke
CV: Angina, atrial fibrillation, chest pain, hypercholesterolemia, palpitations, peripheral edema, supraventricular tachycardia, tachycardia
EENT: Application site irritation (glossitis, mouth ulceration, pharyngolaryngeal pain), blurred vision, cataract, dry mouth, epistaxis, eye pain, glaucoma, hoarseness, laryngitis, oral candidiasis, pharyngitis, rhinitis, sinusitis, stomatitis, throat irritation, visual halos
ENDO: Hyperglycemia
GI: Abdominal pain, constipation, dysphagia, gastroesophageal reflux, indigestion, intestinal obstruction, ileus, vomiting
GU: Urinary difficulty, urine retention, UTI
MS: Arthritis, leg or skeletal pain, myalgia
RESP: Cough, paradoxical bronchospasm, upper respiratory tract infection
SKIN: Pruritus, rash, urticaria
Other: Allergic reaction, angioedema, candidiasis, flulike symptoms, infection

Nursing Considerations
- Use tiotropium cautiously in patients with angle-closure glaucoma, benign prostatic hyperplasia, or bladder neck obstruction.

WARNING Monitor patient closely after giving first dose of tiotropium for immediate hypersensitivity reactions, including angioedema and paradoxical bronchospasm. If reaction occurs, notify prescriber and expect to stop tiotropium and provide supportive care. Because atropine is of a similar structure, monitor patients hypersensitive to atropine closely when giving tiotropium because of potential for similar hypersensitivity reactions. Also use tiotropium cautiously in patients who have severe hypersensitivity to milk proteins.

• Monitor patient's renal function, as ordered, especially in patients with moderate to severe renal impairment, because tiotropium is excreted mainly by the kidneys.

• Monitor patient's pulmonary function, as ordered, to evaluate the effectiveness of tiotropium.

PATIENT TEACHING

• Caution patient not to use tiotropium to treat acute bronchospasm and that drug should not be used more often than every 24 hours.

• Instruct patient on the proper use of the HandiHaler inhalation device, if prescribed. Tell patient to place the capsule into the center chamber of the inhalation device and then to press and release the button on the side of the inhalation device to pierce the capsule. Then have the patient exhale completely, close her lips around the mouthpiece, inhale slowly and deeply, and hold her breath for as long as is comfortable.

• Alert patient that the HandiHaler device should not be used to take any other drug and that the tiotropium capsule must be taken only using the device and never swallowed.

• Tell patient not to expose capsules used in the HandiHaler device to air until ready for use. To remove a capsule from the blister pack, tell patient to open the foil only as far as the stop line to avoid exposing the rest of the capsules in the blister pack to air. Instruct patient used in the HandiHaler device to discard capsules if they are inadvertently exposed to air and won't be used immediately.

• Advise patient to keep powder found in the capsule used with the HandiHaler

device out of her eyes because it may irritate them or blur her vision.

• Tell patient prescribed the Respimat inhaler to insert the cartridge into the inhaler prior to first use and prime the device by actuating the inhaler (pointed toward the ground) until an aerosol cloud is visible and then repeat the process three more times. Remind patient that if the inhaler is not used for more than 3 days, the inhaler should be actuated once prior to use; if not used for more than 21 days, the inhaler should be activated three times prior to use.

• Inform patient that the Respimat inhaler should not be used to take any other drug.

• Instruct patient to rinse her mouth after each treatment to help minimize throat dryness and irritation.

• Advise patient to tell prescriber about decreased response to tiotropium as well as difficulty urinating, eye pain, palpitations, and vision changes.

tirofiban hydrochloride

Aggrastat

Class and Category
Chemical class: Tyrosine derivative
Therapeutic class: Platelet aggregation inhibitor
Pregnancy category: B

Indications and Dosages
➤ *To treat acute coronary syndrome*
I.V. INFUSION
Adults. 0.4 mcg/kg/min for 30 min, followed by 0.1 mcg/kg/min.
DOSAGE ADJUSTMENT For patients with creatinine clearance of less than 30 ml/min/1.73 m^2, infusion rate reduced by one-half.

Route	Onset	Peak	Duration
I.V.	Immediate	30 min	4–8 hr

Mechanism of Action
Binds to glycoprotein IIb/IIIa receptor sites on the surface of activated platelets. Circulating fibrinogen can bind to these receptor sites and link platelets together, forming a clot that

eventually blocks a coronary artery. By binding to receptor sites, tirofiban prevents the normal binding of fibrinogen and other factors and inhibits platelet aggregation.

Incompatibilities
Don't infuse tirofiban in same I.V. line with any drug other than atropine sulfate, dobutamine, dopamine, epinephrine hydrochloride, furosemide, heparin, lidocaine, midazolam hydrochloride, morphine sulfate, nitroglycerin, potassium chloride, propranolol hydrochloride, or famotidine (Pepcid injection).

Contraindications
Acute pericarditis; arteriovenous malformation; coagulopathy; stroke that occurred within previous 30 days or a history of hemorrhagic stroke; GI or GU bleeding; hemophilia; history of thrombocytopenia after tirofiban use; hypersensitivity to tirofiban or its components; intracranial aneurysm or mass, intracranial bleeding, retinal bleeding, aortic dissection, or any evidence of active abnormal bleeding within previous 30 days; major surgery or trauma within previous 6 weeks; severe uncontrolled hypertension (systolic blood pressure above 180 mm Hg, diastolic blood pressure above 110 mm Hg)

Interaction
DRUGS
antineoplastics, antithymocyte globulin, NSAIDs, oral anticoagulants, platelet aggregation inhibitors, strontium-89 chloride, thrombolytics: Increased risk of bleeding
levothyroxine, omeprazole: Increased rate of tirofiban clearance
porfimer: Decreased effectiveness of porfimer photodynamic therapy
salicylates: Increased risk of bleeding, possibly hypoprothrombinemia

Adverse Reactions
CNS: Chills, dizziness, fever, headache, intracranial hemorrhage
CV: Edema, hemopericardium, peripheral edema, sinus bradycardia
GI: Hematemesis, nausea, retroperitoneal bleeding, vomiting
GU: Hematuria, pelvic pain
HEME: Severe thrombocytopenia with chills, fever, and possibly fatal bleeding complications

RESP: Pulmonary hemorrhage
SKIN: Diaphoresis, rash, urticaria
Other: Allergic reaction, anaphylaxis, infusion site bleeding

Nursing Considerations
WARNING Dilute 50-ml vial of tirofiban before use; don't dilute 500-ml container because it holds premixed solution ready for I.V. infusion. Don't use solution unless it's clear and the seal is intact.
• If prescribed, give tirofiban with heparin for 48 to 108 hours. Expect to continue infusion throughout angiography and for 12 to 24 hours after angioplasty or atherectomy.
WARNING If patient is also receiving a heparin infusion, expect to monitor APTT before treatment, 6 hours after heparin infusion starts, and regularly thereafter. Expect to adjust heparin dosage to maintain APTT at about two times the control. Notify prescriber immediately if patient develops an abnormally high APTT. Also, assess patient for signs and symptoms of abnormal bleeding and report them to prescriber immediately because potentially life-threatening bleeding may occur.
• After cardiac catheterization or percutaneous transluminal coronary angioplasty, keep patient on bed rest with head of bed elevated. Ensure hemostasis of percutaneous site for at least 4 hours before discharge. Minimize invasive procedures, including epidural proce-dures, to reduce the risk of bleeding.
• Monitor patient's platelet count, hemoglobin level, and hematocrit, as ordered. Expect to discontinue tirofiban if patient's platelet count is less than 90,000/mm^3. Expect to give a platelet transfusion, as prescribed, if platelet count falls below 50,000/mm^3.
PATIENT TEACHING
• Advise patient to immediately report any bleeding, bruising, headache, pain, or swelling during I.V. infusion of tirofiban.

tizanidine hydrochloride
Zanaflex

Class and Category
Chemical class: Imidazoline
Therapeutic class: Antispasmodic
Pregnancy category: C

Indications and Dosages
➤ *To manage acute and intermittent increases of muscle tone with spasticity*
TABLETS
Adults. 4 mg every 6 to 8 hr, as needed, increased gradually by 2 to 4 mg/dose, as needed and as prescribed. *Maximum:* 36 mg daily or 3 doses daily.

Mechanism of Action
Reduces spasticity by decreasing the release of excitatory amino acids. This alpha$_2$-adrenergic agonist's action increases presynaptic inhibition of spinal motor neurons, with the greatest effects on polysynaptic pathways.

Route	Onset	Peak	Duration
P.O.	Unknown	1–2 hr	3–6 hr

Contraindications
Hypersensitivity to tizanidine or its components, use with ciprofloxacin or fluvoxamine

Interaction
DRUGS
acetaminophen: Delayed peak effects of acetaminophen
alpha$_2$-adrenergic agonists: Possibly significant hypotension
antihypertensives: Additive hypotensive effects
CYP1A2 inhibitors (such as acyclovir, amiodarone, cimetidine, famotidine, mexiletine, propafenone, ticlopidine, verapamil, zileuton), fluoroquinolones (including ciprofloxacin, fluvoxamine): Possibly increased plasma tizanidine level; increased risk of hypotension and sedation
oral contraceptives: Decreased tizanidine clearance
rofecoxib: Possibly increased adverse reactions
ACTIVITIES
alcohol use: Increased adverse effects of tizanidine, additive CNS depression

Adverse Reactions
CNS: Anxiety, delusions, drowsiness, dyskinesia, fatigue, fever, hallucinations, slurred speech

CV: Orthostatic hypotension
EENT: Dry mouth, pharyngitis, rhinitis
GI: Abdominal pain, anorexia, constipation, diarrhea, dyspepsia, elevated liver function test results, hepatic failure, hepatomegaly, nausea, vomiting
GU: Urinary frequency, UTI
MS: Back pain, muscle weakness, myasthenia
SKIN: Diaphoresis, jaundice, rash, ulceration

Nursing Considerations
• Be aware that extreme caution is required if tizanidine is prescribed for a patient with hepatic impairment because the drug is extensively metabolized in the liver.
• Monitor hepatic and renal function for first 6 months and periodically thereafter.
• Expect prolonged drug use to inhibit saliva.
• Be aware that tizanidine should be stopped slowly to prevent withdrawal and rebound hypertension, tachycardia, and hypertonia.
PATIENT TEACHING
• Caution patient not to stop taking tizanidine suddenly to prevent adverse effects.
• Advise patient to change positions slowly to minimize effects of orthostatic hypotension.
• Urge patient to avoid alcohol during drug therapy because of its additive CNS effects.
• Tell patient to notify prescriber or a dentist if dry mouth lasts longer than 2 weeks.
• Instruct patient to inform all prescribers and pharmacists about any drug he starts or stops taking.

tobramycin sulfate
Bethkis, Kitabis Pak, Nebcin, Tobi, Tobi Podhaler, Tobramycin

Class and Category
Chemical class: Aminoglycoside
Therapeutic class: Antibiotic
Pregnancy category: D

Indications and Dosages
➤ *To treat bacteremia; bone and joint, gynecologic, intra-abdominal, lower respiratory tract, skin and soft-tissue, and urinary tract infections; endocar-*

ditis; meningitis; neonatal sepsis; pyelonephritis; and septicemia caused by susceptible strains of Acinetobacter *species,* Aeromonas *species,* Citrobacter *species,* Enterobacter *species,* Escherichia coli, Haemophilus influenzae *(beta lactamase–negative and –positive),* Klebsiella *species,* Morganella morganii, Proteus mirabilis, Proteus vulgaris, Providencia rettgeri, Pseudomonas aeruginosa, Salmonella *species,* Serratia *species,* Shigella *species,* Staphylococcus aureus, *and* Staphylococcus epidermidis; *to treat febrile neutropenia*

I.V. INFUSION, I.M. INJECTION (NEBCIN, TOBRAMYCIN)
Adults. 3 to 6 mg/kg daily in divided doses every 8 to 12 hr.
Children over age 5. 2 to 2.5 mg/kg every 8 hr.
Children under age 5. 2.5 mg/kg every 8 to 16 hr.
Neonates over age 7 days weighing more than 2 kg (4.4 lb). 2.5 mg/kg every 8 hr.
Neonates over age 7 days weighing 1.2 to 2 kg (2.6 to 4.4 lb). 2.5 mg/kg every 8 to 12 hr.
Neonates age 7 days and under weighing 2 kg or more. 2.5 mg/kg every 12 hr.
Neonates age 7 days and under weighing 1.2 to 2 kg. 2.5 mg/kg every 12 to 18 hr.
Preterm neonates weighing 1 to 1.2 kg (2.2 to 2.6 lb). 2.5 mg/kg every 18 to 24 hr.
Preterm neonates weighing less than 1 kg. 3.5 mg/kg every 24 hr.
➤ *To treat pulmonary infection caused by* P. aeruginosa *in patients with cystic fibrosis*

I.V. INFUSION (NEBCIN, TOBRAMYCIN)
Adults and children. 2.5 to 3.3 mg/kg every 8 hr; dosage adjusted to achieve peak blood drug level of 8 to 12 mcg/ml and trough blood drug level below 2 mcg/ml.
INHALATION (BETHKIS, KITABIS PAK, NEBCIN, TOBRAMYCIN)
Adults and children over age 6. 1 ampule (300 mg) twice daily in alternating periods of 28 days on and 28 days off.
INHALATION (TOBI PODHALER)
Adults and children 6 years and older. Four 28 mg capsules inhaled using

Podhaler every 12 hr in alternating periods of 28 days on and 28 days off.
➤ *To treat meningitis caused by susceptible organisms*
INTRATHECAL INJECTION (TOBRAMYCIN)
Adults. 4 to 8 mg daily with parenteral therapy.
Children. 1 to 2 mg daily with parenteral therapy.
➤ *To treat systemic infection*
INTRAPERITONEAL INFUSION (TOBRAMYCIN)
Adults and children. 1.5 to 2 mg/kg.
➤ *To treat dialysis-associated peritonitis in patients with end-stage renal disease*
INTRAPERITONEAL INFUSION (TOBRAMYCIN)
Adults and children. 4 to 8 mg/L in each dialysate exchange bag, increased, as prescribed, 6 to 8 mg/L in documented *Pseudomonas* infection or to 20 mg/L administered in one exchange bag daily.
DOSAGE ADJUSTMENT For patients with renal impairment, dosage possibly reduced.

Mechanism of Action
Inhibits bacterial protein synthesis by binding irreversibly to one of two aminoglycoside-binding sites on the 30S ribosomal subunit, resulting in bacteriostatic effects. Bactericidal effects may stem from tobramycin's ability to accumulate within cells so that the intracellular drug level exceeds the extracellular level.

Incompatibilities
Don't mix tobramycin in same solution with parenteral aminoglycosides or beta-lactam antibiotics because mutual inactivation may result. Don't dilute or mix inhalation solution in nebulizer with dornase alfa.

Contraindications
Concurrent cidofovir, ethacrynic acid, furosemide, intravenous mannitol, or urea therapy; hypersensitivity to tobramycin, aminoglycosides, sodium bisulfite, or their components

Interaction
DRUGS
acyclovir, aminoglycosides, amphotericin B, carboplatin, cisplatin, NSAIDs, vancomycin: Additive nephrotoxicity
carbenicillin, ticarcillin: Possibly inactivation of tobramycin

dimenhydrinate: Possibly masking of symptoms of ototoxicity
ethacrynic acid, furosemide: Additive ototoxicity
general anesthetics, neuromuscular blockers: Possibly increased neuromuscular blockade

Adverse Reactions

CNS: Confusion, dizziness, headache, inability to speak, lethargy, neurotoxicity, vertigo
EENT: Hearing loss, tinnitus
GI: *Clostridium difficile*–associated diarrhea, diarrhea, elevated liver function test results, nausea, vomiting
GU: Elevated BUN and serum creatinine levels, nephrotoxicity, oliguria, proteinuria, renal failure
HEME: Anemia, leukocytosis, leukopenia, neutropenia, thrombocytopenia
RESP: Bronchospasm
SKIN: Exfoliative dermatitis, pruritus, rash, urticaria
Other: Hypocalcemia, hypokalemia, hypomagnesemia, hyponatremia, injection-site pain

Nursing Considerations

• Obtain fluid and tissue samples for culture and sensitivity testing before and during tobramycin therapy, as ordered. Review results, if available, before therapy starts.
• After reconstituting drug for intravenous administration with 30 ml of sterile or bacteriostatic water for injection, dilute further with normal saline solution or D_5W.
• Give each I.V. dose over 20 to 60 minutes.
WARNING Don't infuse tobramycin over less than 20 minutes to avoid neuromuscular blockade and excessive peak drug level.
• Don't expose ampules for inhalation solution to intense light. Refrigerate them at 36° to 46° F (2° to 8° C).
• Capsules for inhalation should be stored in the blister and each capsule removed immediately before use. Always administer tobramycin by Podhaler last, if other inhaled medications are being administered.
• Because drug can cause bilateral and irreversible hearing loss, assess for early signs of cochlear and vestibular ototoxicity, including high-frequency hearing loss and vertigo.

• Monitor serum calcium, magnesium, potassium, and sodium levels to detect electrolyte imbalances.
WARNING Be alert for allergic reactions, including anaphylaxis, because some forms of drug contain sodium bisulfite.
• Stop tobramycin therapy 7 days before starting cidofovir therapy, as prescribed. Know that diuretics can increase risk of aminoglycoside toxicity by altering antibiotic concentrations in serum and tissue and therefore should not be administered with tobramycin.
• Watch for signs of nephrotoxicity, such as elevated BUN and serum creatinine levels.
• Expect dehydration to increase the risk of nephrotoxicity.
WARNING Monitor patient with myasthenia gravis or parkinsonism for increased muscle weakness because of tobramycin's potential curare-like effect.
• Monitor patient closely for diarrhea, which may indicate pseudomembranous colitis caused by *C. difficile.* If diarrhea occurs, notify prescriber, expect to withhold tobramycin, and treat with fluids, electrolytes, protein, and an antibiotic effective against *C. difficile.*

PATIENT TEACHING
• Instruct patient on how to administer drug by inhalation. For inhaled tobramycin using ampules, instruct patient to inhale over 10 to 15 minutes, using a handheld nebulizer with a compressor. For inhaled tobramycin using capsules, instruct patient always to store capsules in the blister, not to remove capsules until immediately before use, and to use only with the Podhaler.
• Teach patient how to use nebulizer while sitting or standing upright and to breathe normally through its mouthpiece. Nose clips may help patient breathe through her mouth.
• Instruct patient to disinfect her nebulizer every other treatment day by boiling the nebulizer parts (except tubing) for a full 10 minutes and then drying the parts on a clean, lint-free cloth.
• Urge patient to immediately report high-frequency hearing loss and vertigo.
• Instruct female patient to notify prescriber immediately about known or suspected pregnancy because drug poses danger to fetus.

T

• Urge patient to tell prescriber about diarrhea that's severe or lasts longer than 3 days. Remind patient that watery or bloody stools may occur 2 or more months after antibiotic therapy and may be serious, requiring prompt treatment.

tocainide hydrochloride

Tonocard

Class and Category
Chemical class: Lidocaine analogue
Therapeutic class: Class IB antiarrhythmic
Pregnancy category: C

Indications and Dosages
➤ *To treat life-threatening, sustained ventricular tachycardia*

TABLETS
Adults. *Initial:* 400 mg every 8 hr.
Maintenance: 1.2 to 1.8 g daily in divided doses every 8 hr.

DOSAGE ADJUSTMENT Dosage possibly reduced by 25% if creatinine clearance is 10 to 30 ml/min/1.73 m² and by 50% if creatinine clearance is less than 10 ml/min/1.73 m².

Route	Onset	Peak	Duration
P.O.	Unknown	0.5–2 hr	8 hr

Mechanism of Action
Combines with fast sodium channels in myocardial cell membranes, which inhibits sodium influx into cells and decreases ventricular depolarization, automaticity, and excitability during diastole.

Contraindications
Hypersensitivity to tocainide or its components, second- or third-degree AV block without ventricular pacemaker

Interaction
DRUGS
antiarrhythmics: Possibly additive cardiac effects, additive toxicity
beta blockers: Increased cardiac index, left ventricular pressures, and pulmonary artery wedge pressures

cimetidine: Possibly decreased blood tocainide level
rifampin: Accelerated hepatic metabolism of tocainide, reduced tocainide effectiveness

Adverse Reactions
CNS: Agitation, anxiety, ataxia, coma, confusion, depression, dizziness, fatigue, hallucinations, headache, mood changes, nervousness, paresthesia, psychosis, seizures, sleep disturbance, syncope, tremor, vertigo
CV: AV conduction disorders, bradycardia, chest pain, heart failure, hypertension, hypotension, palpitations, prolonged QT interval, PVCs, tachycardia, ventricular fibrillation
EENT: Blurred vision, vision changes
GI: Anorexia, diarrhea, nausea, vomiting
HEME: Agranulocytosis, anemia, aplastic anemia, bone marrow depression, hemolysis, leukopenia, neutropenia, thrombocytopenia
RESP: Pulmonary edema, fibrosis, and hypersensitivity (pneumonitis); respiratory arrest
SKIN: Diaphoresis, exfoliative dermatitis, pruritus, rash, skin lesions, urticaria

Nursing Considerations
• Monitor CBC with differential weekly during first 3 months of tocainide treatment and routinely thereafter to detect blood dyscrasias. Although rare, agranulocytosis, anemia, aplastic anemia, bone marrow depression, hemolysis, leukopenia, neutropenia, or thrombocytopenia may be fatal. Expect findings to normalize about 1 month after therapy stops.
• Maintain continuous cardiac monitoring or obtain periodic ECG tracings, as ordered, to assess drug effectiveness.
• Watch for tremor, a possible sign of maximum dosing.
• Assess patient for additive adverse cardiac effects, especially if tocainide is used with another antiarrhythmic.
• Be aware that tocainide is secreted in breastmilk and has the potential to cause serious adverse reactions in breastfeeding infants.

PATIENT TEACHING
• Inform patient that electrophysiologic studies may be performed before tocainide therapy starts.

• Tell patient to notify prescriber about tremor because dosage may need adjustment.
• Explain that chest X-rays may be needed if adverse pulmonary reactions occur.
• Inform patient that ambulatory monitoring may be needed to verify antiarrhythmic response.
• Emphasize the importance of keeping all scheduled appointments for follow-up blood tests.

tocilizumab

Actemra

Class and Category

Chemical class: Recombinant human anti-human interleukin 6 (IL-6) monoclonal antibody
Therapeutic class: Biologic disease-modifying antirheumatic drug (DMARD)
Pregnancy category: C

Indications and Dosages

➤ *To treat moderate to severe active rheumatoid arthritis as monotherapy in patients who have had an inadequate response to one or more Disease-Modifying Anti-Rheumatic Drugs (DMARDs) or as adjunct with methotrexate or other DMARDs*

I.V. INFUSION

Adults. 4 mg/kg over 60 min every 4 wk, increased, as needed, to 8 mg/kg over 60 min every 4 wk. *Maximum:* 800 mg per infusion.

SUBCUTANEOUS INJECTION

Adults weighing 100 kg (220 lbs) or more. 162 mg every wk.
Adults weighing less than 100 kg (220 lbs). 162 mg every other wk, followed by increased dosage frequency to every wk, as needed.

DOSAGE ADJUSTMENT Interruption of dosing may be needed to manage dose-related laboratory abnormalities, including elevated liver enzymes, neutropenia, and thrombocytopenia.
DOSAGE ADJUSTMENT Dosage reduced from 8 mg/kg to 4 mg/kg for management of dose-related laboratory changes, including elevated liver enzymes (AST or ALT 1 to

3 times the upper limit of normal), neutropenia (absolute neutrophil count approaching 1,000/mm^3), or thrombocytopenia (platelet count approaching 100,000/mm^3).

➤ *To treat active systemic juvenile idiopathic arthritis as monotherapy or as adjunct with methotrexate*

I.V. INFUSION

Children age 2 and older weighing 30 kg (66 lbs) or more. 8 mg/kg over 60 min every 2 wks.
Children age 2 and older weighing less than 30 kg (66 lbs). 12 mg/kg over 60 min every 2 wks.

DOSAGE ADJUSTMENT Interruption of dosing may be needed to manage dose-related laboratory abnormalities including elevated liver enzymes, neutropenia, and thrombo-cytopenia.

➤ *To treat polyarticular juvenile idiopathic arthritis*

I.V. INFUSION

Children age 2 and older weighing 30 kg (66 lb) or more. 8 mg/kg over 60 min every 4 wks.
Children age 2 and older weighing less than 30 kg (66 lb). 10 mg/kg over 60 min every 4 wks.

DOSAGE ADJUSTMENT Interruption of dosing may be needed to manage dose-related laboratory abnormalities, including elevated liver enzymes, neutropenia, and thrombo-cytopenia.

Mechanism of Action

Binds to interleukin 6 (IL-6) receptors to interrupt signaling through them. IL-6 is a proinflammatory cytokine produced by various cells, such as T- and B-cells, lymphocytes, monocytes, and fibroblasts. It is also produced by synovial and endothelial cells, leading to local production of IL-6 in joints affected by inflammatory processes such as rheumatoid arthritis. Binding of IL-6 receptors prevents inflammation-related signals from being relayed, which reduces inflammatory response and relieves signs and symptoms of rheumatoid arthritis.

Incompatibilities

Don't mix tocilizumab with other drugs.

T

Contraindications

Hypersensitivity to tocilizumab or its components, absolute neutrophil count below 2,000/mm³, platelet count below 100,000/mm³, ALT or AST above 1.5 times upper limit of normal

Interaction

DRUGS

anti-CD20 monoclonal antibodies, IL-1R antagonists, selective co-stimulation modulators, TNF antagonists: Increased risk of immunosuppression and infection
atorvastatin; cytochrome P-450 substrates with a narrow therapeutic index such as cyclosporine, theophylline, warfarin; CYP3A4 substrates such as lovastatin, oral contraceptives, simvastain; omeprazole: Possibly decreased plasma levels of these drugs with decreased effectiveness
live vaccines: Increased risk of adverse vaccine effects

Adverse Reactions

CNS: Dizziness, headache
CV: Elevated lipid levels, hypertension
EENT: Nasopharyngitis, oral ulceration
GI: Diverticulitis, elevated liver enzymes, gastritis, gastroenteritis, perforation, upper abdominal pain
GU: UTI
HEME: Neutropenia, thrombocytopenia
MS: Bacterial arthritis
RESP: Bronchitis, pneumonia, upper respiratory tract infection
SKIN: Cellulitis, generalized erythema, pruritus, rash, Stevens-Johnson syndrome, urticaria
Other: Anaphylaxis, anti-tocilizumab antibodies, herpes zoster, malignancies, opportunistic infections including activation of latent infections, sepsis, tuberculosis with pulmonary or extrapulmonary disease

Nursing Considerations

• Tocilizumab may be used as monotherapy to treat rheumatoid arthritis, or together with methotrexate or other nonbiological DMARDs.
• Tocilizumab isn't recommended for patients with active liver disease or impairment because drug may adversely affect liver function.

• Make sure patient has a tuberculin skin test before therapy starts. If skin test is positive, tuberculosis treatment will need to be started before tocilizumab therapy can begin. Even patients who have tested negative for tuberculosis may develop tuberculosis during therapy. Monitor patient for persistent cough, wasting or weight loss, and low-grade fever; report such findings to prescriber.

WARNING If patient has evidence of an active infection when drug is prescribed, therapy shouldn't start until infection has been treated. Monitor all patients for infections, including invasive fungal infections such as aspergillosis, candidiasis, or pneumocystis; or bacterial, myobacterial, protozoal, or viral opportunistic infections during and after therapy, especially patients who are taking immunosuppressants. If a serious infection develops, expect prescriber to interrupt drug therapy until infection is controlled.

• Obtain a baseline of patient's absolute neutrophil count, platelet count, and liver enzymes before starting tocilizumab therapy, as ordered. Therapy shouldn't begin if patient's absolute neutrophil count is below 2,000/mm³, platelet count below 100,000/mm³ or ALT or AST level is above 1.5 times the upper limit of normal. Monitor these values, as ordered, every 4 to 8 weeks (2 to 4 weeks for systemic juvenile idiopathic arthritis), and report abnormalities. Dosage adjustment may be required or drug may need to be discontinued if abnormalities occur.

• Use tocilizumab cautiously in patients with recurrent infection or increased risk of infection, patients who live in regions where tuberculosis and histoplasmosis are endemic, and patients with a history of CNS demyelinating disorders because they may occur, although rarely, during tocilizumab therapy.

• When preparing to give tocilizumab intravenously, use either a 100-ml infusion bag or bottle (patients weighing 30 kg or more) or a 50-ml infusion bag or bottle (patients weighing less than 30 kg) containing 0.9% sodium chloride injection. Begin by withdrawing a volume equal to the volume of tocilizumab solution (patient's dose). Slowly add drug

from each vial into infusion bag or bottle and gently invert bag to mix while avoiding foaming. Discard any unused drug left in vials. Once fully diluted, solution may be stored in the refrigerator or at room temperature for up to 24 hours.
• Give tocilizumab with an infusion set, and never as I.V. push or bolus. Don't infuse concurrently with other drugs in same I.V. line.
• Know that when transitioning from intravenous therapy to subcutaneous therapy, the first subcutaneous dose should be given instead of next scheduled intravenous dose.

WARNING Stop tocilizumab immediately and notify prescriber if patient has an allergic reaction. Provide supportive care, as needed.

PATIENT TEACHING
• Instruct patient or caregiver on how to administer drug subcutaneously, if prescribed. Remind patient or caregiver to rotate sites and never give injection into moles, scars, or areas where the skin is tender, bruised, red, hard, or not intact. Tell how to dispose of syringe properly and to keep syringes, including those discarded, out of reach of children and pets.
• Review the signs and symptoms of an allergic reaction (rash, swollen face, difficulty breathing), and tell patient to seek emergency care immediately if these occur.
• Inform patient that infections, including activation of latent infections such as tuberculosis, may occur during tocilizumab therapy. Instruct him to report unusual, persistent, or severe signs and symptoms to prescriber.
• Instruct patient to contact a healthcare provider immediately about severe, persistent abdominal pain because it could reflect GI perforation.
• Advise patient to avoid people with infections and to have all prescribed laboratory tests performed.
• Inform patient that risk of developing a malignancy is higher in patients taking tocilizumab, but it is still rare. Emphasize importance of follow-up visits and reporting any unusual or sudden signs or symptoms.

• Caution against receiving live-virus vaccines while taking tocilizumab.
• Advise patient to inform all healthcare providers about tocilizumab use and to inform prescriber about any OTC medications being taken, including herbal remedies and vitamin and mineral supplements.
• Urge woman who becomes pregnant while receiving tocilizumab to contact prescriber and to join the pregnancy registry by calling 1-877-311-8972 so exposure to tocilizumab can be monitored.

tofacitinib citrate
Xeljanz

Class and Category
Chemical class: Citrate salt
Therapeutic class: Antirheumatic
Pregnancy category: C

Indications and Dosages
➤ *To treat moderate to severe active rheumatoid arthritis as monotherapy in patients who have had an inadequate response or intolerance to methotrexate; adjunct to methotrexate or other nonbiologic disease modifying antirheumatic drugs (DMARDs).*
TABLETS
Adults. 5 mg twice daily.
DOSAGE ADJUSTMENT For patients with moderate or severe renal insufficiency, moderate hepatic impairment, concomitant use of CYP3A4 inhibitors such as ketoconazole, or concomitant use with one or more drugs that result in both moderate inhibition of CYP3A4 and potent inhibition of CYP2C19 such as fluconazole, dosage interval decreased to once daily.

Mechanism of Action
Modulates the signaling pathway by inhibiting the enzyme, Janus kinase (JAK). JAK is an intracellular enzyme which transmits signals arising from cytokine or growth factor–receptor interactions on the cellular membrane to influence cellular processes of hematopoiesis and immune cell function. Inhibiting the phosphorylation and activation of Signal Transducers and Activator

of Transcription (STATs) needed to influence cellular processes lessens some of the signs and symptoms of rheumatoid arthritis.

Contraindications

Hypersensitivity to tofacitinib or its components

Interaction

DRUGS

azathioprine, cyclosporine, tacrolimus: Potentiated immunosuppression
CYP3A4 potent inducers such as rifampin: Possibly loss or reduced effectiveness of tofacitinib
P450(CYP)3A4 potent inhibitors such as ketoconazole, moderate CYP34A inhibitors/ potent CYP2C19 inhibitors such as fluconazole: Increased tofacitinib exposure and adverse drug reactions
live vaccines: Increased risk of infection

Adverse Reactions

CNS: Fatigue, fever, headache, insomnia, paresthesia
CV: Elevated lipid levels, hypertension, peripheral edema
EENT: Esophageal candidiasis, naso-pharyngitis, sinus congestion
GI: Abdominal pain, diarrhea, dyspepsia, elevated liver enzymes, gastritis, hepatic steatosis, liver injury, nausea, vomiting
GU: UTI
MS: Arthralgia, joint swelling, musculo-skeletal pain, tendonitis
HEME: Anemia, lymphocytosis, neutropenia
RESP: Cough, dyspnea, pneumonia, pneumocystosis, upper respiratory infection
SKIN: Cellulitis, erythema, multidermatomal herpes zoster, rash, pruritus
Other: Bacteria, myobacterial, invasive fungal, viral or other opportunistic infections such as tuberculosis and other mycobacterial infections, cryptococcus, cytomegalovirus, or BK viral infection; dehydration; Epstein Barre Virus–associated post-transplant lymphoproliferative disorder; herpes zoster; lymphoproliferative disorder; malignancies such as breast, lung, gastric, colorectal, renal cell, prostate, lymphoma, and malignant melanoma

Nursing Considerations

• Be aware tofacitinib therapy should not be given to a patient who has an active infection, including localized infections.
• Know that tofacitinib should not be given to patients with severe hepatic impairment; tofacitinib should not be initiated in patients with a lymphocyte count less than 500 cells/mm³, an absolute neutrophil count (ANC) less than 1,000 cells/mm³, or hemoglobin levels less than 9g/dl.
• Screen patient for viral hepatitis, as ordered, prior to starting tofacitinib therapy.
• Check to be sure that the patient has been tested for latent or active tuberculosis before tofacitinib therapy begins. Antituberculosis therapy might be prescribed for patients with a past history of latent or active tuberculosis if completion of treatment cannot be verified. Also, patients who have a negative test for latent tuberculosis may also be prescribed antituberculosis therapy if they have risk factors for tuberculosis.
• Use extreme caution when administering drug to patients with a history of chronic or recurrent infections, exposure to tuberculosis, history of a serious or an opportunistic infection, have resided or traveled in areas of endemic tuberculosis or endemic mycoses, or have underlying conditions that may predispose them to infection.
• Use cautiously in patients with a known malignancy, other than successfully treated nonmelanoma skin cancer. The prescriber may choose to discontinue the drug in patients who develop a malignancy during tofacitinib therapy.
• Use cautiously in patients who may be at increased risk for gastrointestinal perforation, such as a patient with a history of diverticulitis. Monitor patient closely throughout tofacitinib therapy. Notify prescriber if patient experiences new onset abdominal symptoms suggestive of perforation.
• Check with patient to be sure past immunizations received are in line with current immunization guidelines before starting tofacitinib therapy. If the patient needs further immunizations, ensure that it is done before drug therapy begins.

• Obtain a CBC to determine patient's baseline, as ordered. Once the baseline is established, expect prescriber to order a lymphocyte level every 3 months; an ANC level after 4 to 8 weeks of therapy and then every 3 months; and a hemoglobin level after 4 to 8 weeks and then every 3 months. These test results will guide the prescriber in making modifications in the patient's treatment plan.

• Monitor the patient's liver enzymes routinely, as ordered, because drug has been associated with liver damage. Alert prescriber of any abnormalities and expect drug to be withheld during the investigation as to the cause of the elevated liver enzymes. If no other cause can be found, expect prescriber to discontinue the drug.

• Know that viral reactivation, including herpes virus reactivation (herpes zoster), has occurred with tofacitinib therapy.

• Expect prescriber to order a lipid profile on the patient 4 to 8 weeks after tofacitinib therapy has begun, because the drug has caused increases in lipid parameters generally within the first 6 weeks of therapy. Expect to manage hyperlipidemia, if present, according to clinical guidelines, as prescribed.

• Monitor patient for signs and symptoms of infection during and after tofacitinib therapy. Notify prescriber if an infection develops and expect to obtain a complete blood count, if ordered. Be aware that drug should be discontinued if the patient has a lymphocyte count or ANC count less than 500. If the patient has an ANC level between 500 and 1,000 or a hemoglobin level greater than a 2 g/dl decrease or less than 8.0 g/dl, expect drug therapy to be interrupted until the ANC and hemoglobin levels have returned to target range.

PATIENT TEACHING

• Instruct patient to take tofacitinib exactly as prescribed.

• Review infection control measures with patient as well as the signs and symptoms of an infection. If an infection occurs, tell patient to notify prescriber immediately.

• Make sure patient understands the serious adverse reactions associated with tofacitinib such as the development of malignancies and serious infections.

• Inform women of childbearing age to notify prescriber if pregnancy is suspected or known because drug effect on the fetus is unknown. Tell her that if she does get pregnant while taking tofacitinib, she should consult the prescriber to learn how she can be added to the pregnancy registry sponsored by Pfizer, the maker of tofacitinib, or if she prefers, tell the patient she may call Pfizer directly at 1-877-311-8972.

• Encourage patient to comply with laboratory blood tests needed to monitor patient's reaction to tofacitinib.

• Advise patient at increased risk for skin cancer to have a periodic skin examination.

tolazamide
Tolinase

Class and Category
Chemical class: First-generation sulfonylurea
Therapeutic class: Antidiabetic
Pregnancy category: C

Indications and Dosages
➤ *As adjunct to treat type 2 diabetes mellitus that's uncontrolled by diet and exercise*

TABLETS
Adults. *Initial:* 100 mg daily with breakfast if fasting blood glucose level is less than 200 mg/dl; 250 mg daily if fasting blood glucose level is more than 200 mg/dl. Dose adjusted every wk by 100 to 250 mg, if needed. Doses greater than 500 mg daily are divided and given every 12 hr. *Maximum:* 1,000 mg daily.
DOSAGE ADJUSTMENT If patient takes more than 40 units daily of insulin, initial dosage increased to 250 mg daily and insulin dosage decreased by 50%.

Route	Onset	Peak	Duration
P.O.	Unknown	3–4 hr	10–20 hr

Mechanism of Action
Stimulates insulin release from beta cells in the pancreas. Tolazamide also increases peripheral tissue sensitivity to insulin either by enhancing insulin binding to cellular receptors or by increasing the number of insulin receptors.

T

Contraindications

Diabetic coma; diabetic ketoacidosis; hypersensitivity to tolazamide, sulfonylureas, or their components; pregnancy; sole therapy for type 1 diabetes mellitus

Interaction

DRUGS

ACE inhibitors, anabolic steroids, androgens, azole antifungals, bromocriptine, chloramphenicol, clofibrate, disopyramide, guanethidine, H$_2$-receptor antagonists, insulin, magnesium salts, MAO inhibitors, methyldopa, octreotide, oxyphenbutazone, phenylbutazone, probenecid, quinidine, salicylates, sulfonamides, tetracycline, theophylline, tricyclic antidepressants, urinary acidifiers: Increased risk of hypoglycemia
asparaginase, calcium channel blockers, cholestyramine, clonidine, corticosteroids, danazol, diazoxide, estrogen, glucagon, hydantoins, isoniazid, lithium, morphine, nicotinic acid, oral contraceptives, phenothiazines, rifabutin, rifampin, sympathomimetics, thiazide diuretics, thyroid drugs, urinary alkalizers: Increased risk of hyperglycemia
beta blockers: Possibly hyperglycemia or masking of signs and symptoms of hypoglycemia
digoxin: Increased risk of digitalis toxicity
pentamidine: Initial hypoglycemia and then hyperglycemia if beta cell damage occurs

ACTIVITIES

alcohol use: Altered blood glucose control (usually hypoglycemia), possibly disulfiram-like reaction

Adverse Reactions

CNS: Dizziness, fatigue, headache, malaise, paresthesia, vertigo
ENDO: Hypoglycemia
GI: Anorexia, cholestasis, heartburn, nausea, vomiting
HEME: Agranulocytosis, aplastic anemia, hemolysis, hemolytic anemia, leukopenia, thrombocytopenia
MS: Muscle weakness
SKIN: Erythema, photosensitivity, pruritus, rash, urticaria

Nursing Considerations

• When switching an insulin-treated patient with type 2 diabetes, expect to start tolazamide at 100 mg daily if patient takes less than 20 units daily of insulin, or 250 mg daily if patient takes 20 to 40 units daily of insulin.
• Anticipate that patient receiving tolazamide may need temporary insulin treatment during periods of physiologic stress, such as fever, surgery, systemic infection, and trauma.
• For patient over age 65, expect to start tolazamide at 100 mg daily.
• Assess elderly patients for signs of hypoglycemia because they're more susceptible to drug's hypoglycemic effect. Anticipate that hypoglycemia may be more difficult to detect.
• Assess patient with thyroid disease for altered blood glucose control because thyroid hormone increases GI absorption of glucose.
• Expect prescriber to stop tolazamide 2 weeks before pregnant patient delivers her neonate to minimize the risk of prolonged hypoglycemia in neonate.

PATIENT TEACHING

• Advise patient to avoid alcohol while taking tolazamide.
• Teach patient and family members how to monitor blood glucose level and how to recognize signs of hypoglycemia and hyperglycemia.
• Instruct patient to treat mild hypoglycemia with fruit juice or other simple sugars.

tolbutamide

Apo-Tolbutamide (CAN),
Novo-Butamide (CAN), Orinase

Class and Category

Chemical class: First-generation sulfonylurea
Therapeutic class: Antidiabetic
Pregnancy category: C

Indications and Dosages

➤ *As adjunct to treat type 2 diabetes mellitus that's uncontrolled by diet and exercise*

TABLETS

Adults. *Initial:* 1 to 2 g daily in divided doses twice daily or three times a day.

Maintenance: 0.25 to 2 g daily. *Maximum:*
3 g daily.

Route	Onset	Peak	Duration
P.O.	Unknown	3–4 hr	6–12 hr

Mechanism of Action

Stimulates insulin release from beta cells in
the pancreas. Tolbutamide also increases
peripheral tissue sensitivity to insulin either
by enhancing insulin binding to cellular
receptors or by increasing the number of
insulin receptors.

Contraindications

Diabetes complicated by pregnancy;
diabetic coma; diabetic ketoacidosis;
hypersensitivity to tolbutamide,
sulfonylureas, or their components; sole
therapy for type 1 diabetes mellitus

Interaction

DRUGS

*ACE inhibitors, anabolic steroids, androgens,
azole antifungals, bromocriptine,
chloramphenicol, clofibrate, disopyramide,
guanethidine, H₂-receptor antagonists,*

*H_2-receptor antagonists,
insulin, magnesium salts, MAO inhibitors,
methyldopa, octreotide, oxyphenbutazone,
phenylbutazone, probenecid, quinidine,
salicylates, sulfonamides, tetracycline,
theophylline, tricyclic antidepressants,
urinary acidifiers:* Increased risk of
hypoglycemia

*asparaginase, calcium channel blockers,
cholestyramine, clonidine, corticosteroids,
danazol, diazoxide, estrogen, glucagon,
hydantoins, isoniazid, lithium, morphine,
nicotinic acid, oral contraceptives,
phenothiazines, rifabutin, rifampin,
sympathomimetics, thiazide diuretics,
thyroid drugs, urinary alkalizers:* Increased
risk of hyperglycemia

beta blockers: Possibly hyperglycemia or
masking of signs and symptoms of
hypoglycemia

digoxin: Increased risk of digitalis toxicity

pentamidine: Initial hypoglycemia and then
hyperglycemia if beta cell damage occurs

ACTIVITIES

alcohol use: Altered blood glucose control
(usually hypoglycemia), possibly
disulfiram-like reaction

Adverse Reactions

CNS: Dizziness, fatigue, headache, malaise,
paresthesia, vertigo

ENDO: Hypoglycemia

GI: Anorexia, cholestasis, heartburn,
nausea, vomiting

HEME: Agranulocytosis, aplastic anemia,
hemolysis, hemolytic anemia, leukopenia,
thrombocytopenia

MS: Muscle weakness

SKIN: Erythema, photosensitivity, pruritus,
rash, urticaria

Nursing Considerations

• If patient takes 20 units or less of insulin
daily, expect a possible transfer from
insulin to tolbutamide. If patient takes
more than 20 units of insulin daily, expect
to reduce insulin dosage as tolbutamide
therapy starts.

• Anticipate that patient receiving
tolbutamide may need temporary insulin
treatment during periods of physiologic
stress, such as fever, surgery, systemic
infection, or trauma.

• Assess elderly patients for signs of
hypoglycemia because they're more
susceptible to drug's hypoglycemic effect.
Anticipate that hypoglycemia may be
more difficult to detect.

• Assess patient with thyroid disease for
altered blood glucose control because
thyroid hormone increases GI absorption
of glucose.

• Expect prescriber to stop tolbutamide
2 weeks before pregnant patient delivers
her neonate to minimize the risk of
prolonged hypoglycemia in neonate.

PATIENT TEACHING

• Advise patient to avoid alcohol while
taking tolbutamide.

• Teach patient and family members how to
monitor blood glucose level and recognize
signs of hypoglycemia and hyperglycemia.

• Instruct patient to treat mild
hypoglycemia with fruit juice or other
simple sugars.

T

tolcapone

Tasmar

Class and Category
Chemical class: Nitrobenzophenone
Therapeutic class: Antidyskinetic
Pregnancy category: C

Indications and Dosages
➤ As adjunct (with levodopa and carbidopa) to treat Parkinson's disease

TABLETS
Adults. *Initial:* 100 mg three times a day. *Maximum:* 200 mg three times a day.

Mechanism of Action
Prolongs plasma half-life of levodopa by inhibiting catechol-O-methyltransferase (COMT), an enzyme responsible for metabolizing catecholamines—including dopa, dopamine, epinephrine, norepinephrine, and their hydroxylated metabolites. COMT inhibition decreases the metabolizing enzyme for levodopa, which yields a more sustained plasma levodopa level, making more available for diffusion into the CNS to be converted to dopamine.

Contraindications
Confusion, hyperpyrexia, or rhabdomyolysis with previous use of tolcapone; hepatic dysfunction; hypersensitivity to tolcapone or its components

Interaction
DRUGS
desipramine: Possibly increased frequency of adverse effects
levodopa: Increased levodopa bioavailability, with increased risk of orthostatic hypotension and syncope
MAO inhibitors: Possibly inhibited catecholamine metabolism

Adverse Reactions
CNS: Aggression, agitation, confusion, delirium, delusions, disorientation, dizziness, drowsiness, dyskinesia, fatigue, fever, hallucinations, headache, lethargy, loss of balance, paranoid ideation, psychotic-like behavior, somnolence
CV: Chest pain, orthostatic hypotension
EENT: Dry mouth
GI: Abdominal pain, acute fulminant liver failure, anorexia, cholestasis, constipation, diarrhea, elevated liver function test results, vomiting
GU: Bright yellow urine, hematuria

MS: Muscle cramps, rhabdomyolysis
RESP: Dyspnea, upper respiratory tract infection
SKIN: Diaphoresis, jaundice
Other: Intense urges to perform certain activities excessively (such as binge eating, gambling, sex, or spending money)

Nursing Considerations
• Ensure that patient has had the risks of tolcapone therapy explained fully to him and has signed the acknowledgment form before starting therapy.
• Know that tolcapone should not be given to patient with a major psychotic disorder because of the increased risk of exacerbating psychosis.
• Use cautiously in patient with severe dyskinesia or dystonia because drug is known to cause rhabdomyolysis.
• Monitor liver function test results, as ordered, during tolcapone therapy to detect hepatic impairment. Expect to discontinue drug if patient's liver enzymes exceed twice the upper limit of normal or if patient has any signs or symptoms of liver dysfunction, such as persistent nausea, fatigue, lethargy, anorexia, jaundice, dark urine, pruritus, or right upper quadrant tenderness.
• Assess patient for hallucinations, new or worsening mental status, or behavioral changes during tolcapone therapy or after starting or increasing the dose, especially in patients over age 75. If present, notify prescriber as dosage may need to be reduced or drug discontinued.
• Anticipate that drug may precipitate or exaggerate preexisting dyskinesia.
• Expect tolcapone to be discontinued if no improvement occurs after 3 weeks of drug therapy.
• Assess patient for skin changes regularly because risk of melanoma in higher in patients with Parkinson's disease. It isn't clear whether risk results from disease or drugs used to treat it.

PATIENT TEACHING
• Inform patient that urine may turn bright yellow during tolcapone therapy.
• Advise patient to avoid hazardous activities until drug's CNS effects are known. Inform patient that tolcapone therapy may cause

him to fall asleep suddenly during activities of daily living without warning and can occur for the first time even a year after therapy has begun. If this happens, tell patient to notify prescriber and continue to avoid hazardous activities until pescriber has deemed such activities safe. Also warn patient and family that hallucinations, new or worsening mental status, and behavioral changes have occurred with use of tolcapone, especially in patients over the age of 75.

• Urge patient to notify prescriber immediately about darkened urine, decreased appetite, fatigue, jaundice, lethargy, and right-sided abdominal pain.

• Caution patient not to stop taking drug abruptly. Explain that prescriber will supervise tapering of drug dosage.

• Urge patient to have regular follow-up appointments and laboratory tests.

• Urge patient to have regular skin examinations by a dermatologist or other qualified health professional.

• Advise patient to notify prescriber about intense urges that result in performing certain behaviors excessively (such as binge eating, uncontrolled gambling, sex, or spending money) because dosage may need to be reduced or drug discontinued.

tolmetin

Novo-Tolmetin (CAN), Tolectin DS, Tolectin 200, Tolectin 400 (CAN), Tolectin 600

Class and Category

Chemical class: Pyrroleacetic acid derivative
Therapeutic class: Anti-inflammatory
Pregnancy category: C (first trimester), Not rated (later trimesters)

Indications and Dosages

➤ *To relieve moderate pain from rheumatoid arthritis and osteoarthritis*

CAPSULES, TABLETS

Adults. *Initial:* 400 mg three times a day. *Maintenance:* 600 to 1,800 mg daily in divided doses three times a day or four times a day. *Maximum:* 2,000 mg daily for rheumatoid arthritis, 1,600 mg daily for osteoarthritis.

➤ *To treat juvenile rheumatoid arthritis*

CAPSULES, TABLETS

Children over age 2. *Initial:* 20 mg/kg daily in divided doses three times a day or four times a day. *Maintenance:* 15 to 30 mg/kg daily in divided doses. *Maximum:* 30 mg/kg daily.

Route	Onset	Peak	Duration
P.O.	Unknown	1–2 wk	Unknown

Mechanism of Action

Blocks cyclooxygenase, the enzyme needed to synthesize prostaglandins, which mediate the inflammatory response and cause local vasodilation, swelling, and pain. Prostaglandins also promote pain transmission from the periphery to the spinal cord. By blocking cyclooxygenase and inhibiting prostaglandins, tolmetin reduces inflammatory symptoms and relieves pain.

Contraindications

Angioedema, asthma, bronchospasm, nasal polyps, rhinitis, or urticaria caused by aspirin, iodides, or other NSAIDs

Interaction

DRUGS

ACE inhibitors, beta blockers: Decreased effectiveness of these drugs, possibly reduced renal function
alendronate, corticosteroids, other NSAIDs, salicylates: Possibly adverse GI effects
anticoagulants, platelet aggregation inhibitors, thrombolytics: Additive inhibition of platelet aggregation; prolonged bleeding time
antineoplastics, antithymocyte globulin, strontium-89 chloride: Increased risk of bleeding
cidofovir: Possibly nephrotoxicity
cyclosporine: Potentiated cyclosporine nephrotoxicity
digoxin: Increased blood digoxin level
lithium: Possibly lithium toxicity
methotrexate: Increased or prolonged blood methotrexate level

ACTIVITIES

alcohol use: Increased risk of adverse GI effects

Adverse Reactions

CNS: Aseptic meningitis, cerebral hemorrhage, ischemic stroke, depression,

T

dizziness, drowsiness, fatigue, headache, transient ischemic attack, weakness
CV: Chest pain, deep vein thrombosis, edema, hypertension, MI, peripheral edema
EENT: Tinnitus
ENDO: Hypoglycemia
GI: Abdominal pain; constipation; diarrhea; elevated liver function test results; flatulence; gastritis; GI bleeding, perforation, or ulceration; hepatitis; indigestion; jaundice; liver failure; nausea; peptic ulcer disease; vomiting
GU: Acute renal failure, dysuria, elevated BUN level, hematuria, interstitial nephritis, nephrotic syndrome, nephrotoxicity, proteinuria, UTI
HEME: Agranulocytosis, aplastic anemia, hemolytic anemia, leukopenia, pancytopenia, prolonged bleeding time
SKIN: Erythema multiforme, exfoliative dermatitis, maculopapular rash, Stevens-Johnson syndrome, toxic epidermal necrolysis, urticaria
Other: Anaphylaxis, angioedema, weight gain or loss

Nursing Considerations

• Give tolmetin with food or milk to reduce adverse GI reactions.
• Assess patient for improvement within 7 days and progressive improvement over several successive weeks.
• Use tolmetin with extreme caution in patients with a history of ulcer disease or GI bleeding because NSAIDs such as tolmetin increase the risk of GI bleeding and ulceration. Expect to use tolmetin for the shortest time possible in these patients.
• Be aware that serious GI tract ulceration, bleeding, and perforation may occur without warning symptoms. Elderly patients are at greater risk. To minimize risk, give drug with food. If GI distress occurs, withhold drug and notify prescriber at once.
• Use tolmetin cautiously in patients with hypertension, and monitor blood pressure closely throughout therapy. Drug may cause hypertension or worsen it.
WARNING Monitor patient closely for thrombotic events, including MI and stroke, because NSAIDs increase the risk.
WARNING If patient has bone marrow suppression or is receiving antineoplastic

drug therapy, monitor laboratory results (including WBC count), and watch for evidence of infection because anti-inflammatory and antipyretic actions of tolmetin may mask signs and symptoms, such as fever and pain.
• Especially if patient is elderly or taking tolmetin long-term, watch for less common but serious adverse GI reactions, including anorexia, constipation, diverticulitis, dysphagia, esophagitis, gastritis, gastroenteritis, gastroesophageal reflux disease, hemorrhoids, hiatal hernia, melena, stomatitis, and vomiting.
• Monitor liver function test results because, rarely, elevated levels may progress to severe hepatic reactions, including fatal hepatitis, liver necrosis, and hepatic failure.
• Monitor BUN and serum creatinine levels in patients with heart failure, impaired renal function, or hepatic dysfunction; those taking diuretics or ACE inhibitors; and elderly patients because drug may cause renal failure.
• Monitor CBC for decreased hemoglobin and hematocrit because drug may worsen anemia.
• Assess patient's skin routinely for rash or other signs of hypersensitivity reaction because tolmetin and other NSAIDs may cause serious skin reactions without warning, even in patients with no history of NSAID hypersensitivity. Stop drug at first sign of reaction, and notify prescriber.
• Assess invasive sites or wounds for bleeding and bruising from drug's effects on platelets.

PATIENT TEACHING
• Tell patient to take drug with food or milk.
• Urge patient to limit sodium intake because drug may cause fluid retention.
• Tell patient to avoid alcohol during therapy.
• Teach patient how to perform proper oral hygiene, and advise her to have needed dental work done before tolmetin therapy starts because of the increased risk of bleeding.
• Explain that tolmetin may increase the risk of serious adverse cardiovascular reactions; urge patient to seek immediate medical attention if signs or symptoms arise, such as chest pain, shortness of breath, weakness, and slurring of speech.

• Tell patient that tolmetin also may increase the risk of serious adverse GI reactions; stress the need to seek immediate medical attention for such signs and symptoms as epigastric or abdominal pain, indigestion, black or tarry stools, or vomiting blood or material that looks like coffee grounds.
• Alert patient to the possibility of rare but serious skin reactions. Urge her to seek immediate medical attention for rash, blisters, itching, fever, or other indications of hypersensitivity.

tolterodine tartrate

Detrol, Detrol LA

Class and Category

Chemical class: Prodrug of 5-hydroxymethyltolterodine
Therapeutic class: Antispasmodic
Pregnancy category: C

Indications and Dosages

➤ *To treat overactive bladder*

TABLETS

Adults. 2 mg twice daily. Reduced to 1 mg twice daily based on patient response and tolerance.

DOSAGE ADJUSTMENT Dosage reduced to 1 mg twice daily for patients with significant hepatic or renal dysfunction and for patients who are also receiving cytochrome P-450 3A4 inhibitors, such as clarithromycin, erythromycin, and the antifungals itraconazole, ketoconazole, and miconazole.

E.R. TABLETS

Adults. 4 mg daily. Reduced to 2 mg daily based on individual response and tolerance.

Mechanism of Action

Exerts antimuscarinic (atropine-like) and potent direct antispasmodic (papaverine-like) actions on smooth muscle in the bladder, which decreases detrusor muscle contractions. This helps reduce urinary frequency and urgency as well as urge-related incontinence.

Contraindications

Gastric retention; hypersensitivity to tolterodine tartrate, its components, or to

fesoterodine fumarate extended-release tablets; uncontrolled angle-closure glaucoma; urine retention

Interaction

DRUGS

clarithromycin, erythromycin, itraconazole, ketoconazole, miconazole: Possibly increased blood tolterodine level
class IA antiarrhythmics (such as quinidine, procainamide) or class III antiarrhythmics (such as amiodarone, sotalol): Possibly increased risk of prolonged QT interval
fluoxetine: Possibly decreased tolterodine metabolism

Adverse Reactions

CNS: Confusion, disorientation, dizziness, drowsiness, fatigue, hallucinations, headache, memory impairment, somnolence, worsening of dementia
CV: Chest pain, edema, hypertension, palpitations, QT interval prolongation, tachycardia
EENT: Abnormal vision, blurred vision, dry eyes, dry mouth
GI: Abdominal pain, constipation, diarrhea, flatulence, indigestion, nausea
GU: Dysuria, urine retention, UTI
Other: Anaphylaxis, angioedema, flulike symptoms

Nursing Considerations

• Use cautiously in patients with decreased GI motility, myasthenia gravis, or narrow-angle glaucoma because tolterodine could make these conditions worse.
WARNING Monitor patients with a history of bladder outflow obstruction for decreased urine output or bladder distention because tolterodine poses a risk of urine retention.
• Monitor patients with a history of GI obstructive disorders, such as pyloric stenosis, for abdominal distention or bloating because of increased risk of gastric retention.
• Be aware that drug's antimuscarinic effects may produce blurred vision, dizziness, and drowsiness. If these occur, institute fall precautions according to facility policy.

PATIENT TEACHING

• Instruct patient taking tolterodine to report immediately to prescriber any difficulty urinating or infrequent urination, as well as difficulty breathing or

T

swelling that involves the face, lips, throat or tongue, and to seek emergency medical care.

• Advise patient not to drive or perform activities that require high alertness until drug's CNS and vision effects are known. Instruct her to notify prescriber if dizziness or blurred vision persists.

• Encourage patient to use sugarless candy, gum, or ice to relieve dry mouth. Advise her to notify prescriber or dentist if dry mouth persists or worsens over 2 weeks.

tolvaptan

Samsca

Class and Category
Chemical class: Nonpeptide vasopressin receptor antagonist
Therapeutic class: Antihyponatremic
Pregnancy category: C

Indications and Dosages
➤ To treat significant hypervolemic and euvolemic hyponatremia (serum sodium level less than 125 mEq/l or symptomatic but less-marked hyponatremia that has resisted correction with fluid restriction), including patients with heart failure or syndrome of inappropriate antidiuretic hormone (SIADH)

TABLETS
Adults. Initial: 15 mg once daily, increased after at least 24 hours to 30 mg once daily. Maximum: 60 mg once daily for 30 days or less.

Mechanism of Action
Raises serum sodium levels by increasing urine output and decreasing urine osmolality. Tolvaptan does this by preventing attachment of vasopressin to vasopressin V2 receptors on cell membranes in the nephron's collecting duct. Without vasopressin activity, urinary water excretion increases.

Contraindications
Acute need to raise serum sodium urgently; anuria; concomitant use of strong CYP3A inhibitors such as clarithromycin,

ketoconazole, indinavir, itraconazole, nefazodone, nelfinavir, ritonavir, saquinavir, telithromycin; hypovolemic hypontremia; hypersensitivity to tolvaptan or its components; inability of patient to sense or respond appropriately to thirst

Interaction
DRUGS
ACE inhibitors, angiotensin receptor blockers, potassium sparing diuretics, potassium supplements: Increased risk of hyperkalemia
CYP3A inducers such as barbiturates, carbamazepine, phenytoin, rifabutin, rifampin, rifapentin, St. John's wort: Decreased serum tolvaptan level and decreased effectiveness
CYP3A inhibitors such as aprepitant, clarithromycin, diltiazem, erythromycin, fluconazole, ketoconazole, indinavir, itraconazole, nefazodone, nelfinavir, ritonavir, saquinavir, telithromycin, verapamil; P-gp inhibitors such as cyclosporine: Increased serum tolvaptan level and risk of adverse reactions
digoxin: Increased digoxin level
desmopressin: Possibly altered desmopressin activity
FOODS
grapefruit juice: Increased serum tolvaptan level

Adverse Reactions
CNS: Asthenia, CVA, fever, osmotic demyelination syndrome, thirst
CV: Deep vein thrombosis, intracardiac thrombus, ventricular fibrillation
EENT: Dry mouth
ENDO: Diabetic ketoacidosis, hyper-glycemia
GI: Anorexia, constipation, gastrointestinal bleeding, hepatic dysfunction, ischemic colitis, nausea
GU: Nocturia, polyuria, urethral or vaginal hemorrhage
HEME: Disseminated intravascular coagulation, prolonged prothrombin time
MS: Rhabdomyolysis
RESP: Pulmonary embolism, respiratory failure
SKIN: Rash
Other: Anaphylaxis, dehydration, hyperkalemia, hypernatremia, hyponatremia, hypovolemia, osmotic demyelination syndrome (with too rapid correction of hyponatremia)

Nursing Considerations

• Be aware that tolvaptan should not be given to patients with a creatine clearance of less than 10ml/min because no benefit can be expected in patients who are anuric.

• Use cautiously in patients with cirrhosis because of increased risk of GI bleeding.

WARNING Give tolvaptan, initially or if reintroduced, in a hospital setting because too-rapid correction of hyponatremia (more than 12 mEq/L in 24 hour) causes osmotic demyelination (affective changes, coma, dysarthria, dysphagia, lethargy, mutism, spastic quadriparesis, seizures, death). If present, notify prescriber immediately and expect to stop tolvaptan and give hypotonic fluids.

• Monitor fluid and electrolyte balance regularly, especially when starting tolvaptan and adjusting dosage, as ordered. If patient develops hypernatremia, notify prescriber and expect to decrease dose or withhold drug and modify the patient's free-water intake or infusion, as ordered.

• Don't restrict fluids during first 24 hours of therapy because doing so may increase the risk of overly-rapid correct of serum sodium, hypovolemia, and dehydration.

• Use of hypertonic saline isn't recommended during tolvaptan therapy because effects are unknown.

• Monitor patient for signs and symptoms of hepatic dysfunction such as anorexia, dark urine, fatigue, jaundice, and right upper abdominal pain; if present, notify prescriber, and obtain liver enzymes immediately, as ordered. Be aware that to minimize risk of liver injury, drug should not be given longer than 30 days. If hepatic dysfunction is confirmed, expect drug to be discontinued. Know that if the cause of hepatic dysfunction is found to be due to something other than tolvaptan therapy, expect drug to be resumed.

PATIENT TEACHING

• Instruct patient to consume fluids according to thirst during first 24 hours of therapy and not to try to limit fluid intake.

• When drug is discontinued, tell patient that he'll need to resume fluid restriction and will need continued monitoring of sodium level and fluid status.

• Tell patient to notify prescriber if he experiences dark urine or yellowing of skin and eyes, fatigue, loss of appetite, or right upper abdominal pain.

topiramate
Qudexy XR, Topamax, Trokendi XR

Class and Category

Chemical class: Sulfamate-substituted monosaccharide
Therapeutic class: Anticonvulsant
Pregnancy category: D

Indications and Dosages

➤ *To treat partial-onset or primary generalized tonic-clonic seizures*

CAPSULES

Adults and children age 10 and over. *Initial:* 25 mg twice daily in morning and evening. Increased by 25 mg daily for wks 2, 3, and 4. Increased by 50 mg daily for wks 5 and 6. *Maintenance:* 200 mg twice daily in morning and evening.

Children age 2 to 10 years of age. *Initial:* 25 mg once daily in evening for wk 1. Increased to 25 mg twice daily in morning and evening for wk 2. Increased thereafter by 25 to 50 mg/day each subsequent wk, as tolerated, over the next 5 wks. *Maintenance for patient weighing up to 11 kg:* 75 mg to 125 mg twice daily. *Maintenance for patient weighing 12 to 22 kg:* 100 mg to 150 mg twice daily. *Maintenance for patient weighing 23 to 31 kg:* 100 mg to 175 mg twice daily. *Maintenance for patient weighing 32 to 38 kg:* 125 mg to 175 mg twice daily. *Maintenance for patient weighing more than 38 kg:* 125 mg to 200 mg twice daily.

EXTENDED-RELEASE CAPSULES

Adults and children age 10 and over. *Initial:* 50 mg once daily for wk 1; 100 mg once daily for wk 2; 150 mg once daily for wk 3; 200 mg once daily for wk 4; 300 mg once daily for wk 5; and 400 mg once daily for wk 6 and beyond. *Maintenance:* 400 mg once daily.

T

➤ *As adjunct to treat partial seizures and primary generalized tonic-clonic seizures*

CAPSULES, TABLETS

Adults and adolescents age 17 and over. *Initial:* 25 to 50 mg daily in divided doses twice daily. for 1 wk. Increased by 25 to 50 mg daily every wk thereafter until maintenance dose is reached. *Maintenance:* 200 to 400 mg daily in divided doses twice daily.

Children ages 2 to 16. *Initial:* 25 mg or less at bedtime for 1 wk. Increased every 1 to 2 wk by 1 to 3 mg/kg daily in divided doses twice daily until maintenance dose is reached. *Maintenance:* 5 to 9 mg/kg daily in divided doses twice daily.

EXTENDED-RELEASE CAPUSLES

Adults and adolescents age 17 and over. *Initial:* 25 mg to 50 mg once daily, increased weekly in increments of 25 mg to 50 mg once daily, as needed. *Maximum:* 400 mg once daily.

Children age 6 to 16 years of age. *Initial:* 1 mg/kg/day to 3 mg/kg/day once daily at night for 1 wk, increased every 1 to 2 wks in increments of 1 mg/kg/day, as needed. *Maximum:* 9 mg/kg/day.

➤ *As adjunct to treat seizures associated with Lennox-Gastaut syndrome*

CAPSULES, TABLETS

Children ages 2 to 16. 25 mg at bedtime for 1 wk. Increased every 1 to 2 wk by 1mg/kg to 3 mg/kg daily in divided doses twice daily until maintenance dose is reached *Maintenance:* 5 mg/kg to 9 mg/kg daily in divided doses twice daily.

EXTENDED-RELEASE CAPUSLES

Adults and adolescents age 17 and over. *Initial:* 25 mg to 50 mg once daily, increased weekly in increments of 25 mg to 50 mg once daily, as needed. *Maximum:* 400 mg once daily.

Children age 6 to 16 years of age. *Initial:* 1 mg/kg/day to 3 mg/kg/day once daily at night for 1 wk, increased every 1 to 2 wks in increments of 1 mg/kg/day, as needed. *Maximum:* 9 mg/kg/day.

➤ *To prevent migraine headache*

CAPSULES, TABLETS (TOPAMAX)

Adults and children age 12 and over. *Initial:* 25 mg daily in evening for 1 wk; then 25 mg twice daily morning and evening for 1 wk; then 25 mg in morning and 50 mg in evening for 1 wk, then 50 mg twice daily in morning and evening. *Maintenance:* 50 mg twice daily.

DOSAGE ADJUSTMENT For patients with moderate to severe renal impairment, dosage possibly reduced by 50%. For patients undergoing hemodialysis, a supplemental dose may be required during a prolonged period of dialysis.

Mechanism of Action

May block the spread of seizures by reducing the length and frequency of excitatory transmission. Topiramate increases the availability of the inhibitory neurotransmitter gamma-aminobutyric acid by blocking voltage-sensitive sodium channels. This action promotes the movement of chloride ions into neurons.

Contraindications

Hypersensitivity to topiramate or its components, metabolic acidosis with concurrent metformin use (Trokendi XR), recent alcohol use defined as within 6 hours prior to and 6 hours after taking topiramate (Trokendi XR)

Interaction

DRUGS

antihistamines, barbiturates, benzodiazepines, CNS depressants, opioid analgesics, skeletal muscle relaxants, tricyclic antidepressants: Additive CNS depression

carbamazepine: Decreased blood topiramate level

carbonic anhydrase inhibitors: Increased risk of renal calculus formation

digoxin: Possibly decreased blood digoxin level

ethinyl estradiol: Increased risk of break-through bleeding

oral contraceptives: Increased risk of breakthrough bleeding, decreased contraceptive efficacy

phenobarbital: Altered blood phenobarbital level

phenytoin: Decreased blood level of topiramate

probenecid: Possibly blocked renal tubular reabsorption of topiramate and decreased blood topiramate level

valproic acid: Decreased blood levels of both drugs, increased risk of hyper-ammonemia or hypothermia

ACTIVITIES
alcohol use: Additive CNS depression

Adverse Reactions

CNS: Agitation, anxiety, asthenia, ataxia, confusion, decreased concentration, depression, dizziness, encephalopathy, fatigue, fever, hallucinations, headache, hyperthermia, hypoesthesia, insomnia, irritability, memory loss, mood changes, nervousness, paresthesia, psychomotor slowing, psychosis, slurred speech, somnolence, suicidal ideation, syncope, tremor
CV: Cardiac arrest, chest pain, hot flashes, hypertension, hypotension, palpitations, vasodilation
EENT: Blurred vision, diplopia, dry mouth, gingivitis, hearing loss, maculopathy, nystagmus, periorbital pain, pharyngitis, rhinitis, secondary angle-closure glaucoma with acute myopia, sinusitis, taste perversion, tinnitus, tongue edema, vision changes including visual field defects
ENDO: Breast pain, hyperglycemia
GI: Abdominal pain, anorexia, constipation, diarrhea, flatulence, gastroenteritis, gastroesophageal reflux, hepatic failure, hepatitis, indigestion, nausea, pancreatitis, vomiting
GU: Cystitis, decreased libido, dysmenorrhea, dysuria, frequent urination, impotence, menstrual irregularities, renal calculi, renal tubular acidosis, UTI, vaginitis
HEME: Anemia, bleeding events (mild to severe), leukopenia
MS: Arthralgia, back pain, leg cramps or pain, muscle weakness
RESP: Bronchitis, cough, dyspnea, pulmonary embolism, upper respiratory tract infection
SKIN: Acne, alopecia, decreased sweating, erythema multiforme, pemphigus, pruritus, rash, Stevens-Johnson syndrome, toxic epidermal necrolysis
Other: Dehydration, hyperammonemia, metabolic acidosis, weight gain or loss

Nursing Considerations

• Obtain baseline serum bicarbonate level before topiramate therapy and monitor periodically throughout therapy, as ordered.

• Use topiramate cautiously in patients with inborn errors of metabolism or impaired hepatic function, or those who are taking valproic acid; these patients may be at higher risk for hyperammonemia, with or without encephalopathy, while taking topiramate. In addition, hypothermia may occur in patients taking valproic acid concomitantly. If present, notify prescriber and expect topiramate or valproic acid therapy to be discontinued.

• Give capsule with water and have patient swallow it whole. If needed, open capsules and empty contents onto a spoonful of soft food. Discard unused portion.

• Never store food sprinkled with drug for use at a later time.

WARNING Anticipate an increase in seizure activity if topiramate therapy for seizures stops abruptly. Take seizure precautions, as appropriate. Expect drug to be withdrawn gradually if time permits.

• If patient reports ocular pain or decreased visual acuity, notify prescriber immediately; topiramate may cause increased intraocular pressure and secondary angle-closure glaucoma as well as visual field defects. Expect to stop drug immediately.

• If patient has a history of renal calculi, assess for signs of recurrence.

• Monitor patient for bleeding events, especially patients who have conditions that increase risk of bleeding, who take drugs that cause thrombocytopenia such as other antiepileptic drugs, or who take drugs that affect platelet function or coagulation such as aspirin, nonsteroidal anti-inflammatory drugs, selective serotonin reuptake inhibitors, or anticoagulants.

PATIENT TEACHING

• Instruct patient to swallow topiramate tablets whole.

• Urge patient to avoid potentially hazardous activities until drug's CNS effects are known.

• Advise patient to watch for decreased sweating and significantly increased body temperature, especially during hot weather, and to notify prescriber immediately if they occur.

T

• Tell patient to maintain adequate fluid intake to minimize the risk of developing kidney stones.
• Instruct patient to avoid alcohol use completely within 6 hours before and after taking topiramate.
• Advise female patient of possible breakthrough bleeding. If she takes an oral contraceptive, encourage her to use another form of contraception during therapy.
• Caution patient not to stop taking topiramate abruptly because seizures may occur. Instead, patient should expect drug to be withdrawn gradually if it needs to be discontinued.
• Instruct patient to seek immediate emergency care for blurred vision, other visual disturbances, or periorbital pain.
• Tell patient to notify prescriber if he develops unexplained lethargy, vomiting, or changes in mental status.
• Urge caregivers to watch patient closely for evidence of suicidal tendencies, especially when topiramate therapy starts or dosage changes, and to report concerns at once to prescriber.
• Counsel female patient of childbearing age to use effective birth control, as topiramate therapy may cause cleft lip or palate if the fetus is exposed to drug in utero.
• Urge woman who becomes pregnant while taking topiramate to enroll in the North American antiepileptic drug pregnancy registry by calling 1-888-233-2334. Explain that the registry is collecting information about the safety of antiepileptic drugs during pregnancy.

torsemide

Demadex

Class and Category

Chemical class: Anilinopyridine sulfonylurea derivative
Therapeutic class: Antihypertensive, diuretic
Pregnancy category: B

Indications and Dosages

➤ *To treat edema in heart failure*

TABLETS, I.V. INJECTION
Adults. *Initial:* 10 to 20 mg daily, adjusted by doubling, as prescribed, to achieve desired effect. *Maximum:* 200 mg daily.
➤ *To treat edema in chronic renal failure*
TABLETS, I.V. INJECTION
Adults. *Initial:* 20 mg daily, adjusted by doubling, as prescribed, to achieve desired effect. *Maximum:* 200 mg daily.
➤ *To treat ascites, alone or with amiloride or spironolactone*
TABLETS, I.V. INJECTION
Adults. *Initial:* 5 to 10 mg daily. *Maximum:* 40 mg daily.
➤ *To manage hypertension*
TABLETS
Adults. *Initial:* 5 mg daily, increased to 10 mg daily after 4 to 6 wk, if response is inadequate. *Maximum:* 10 mg daily.

Route	Onset	Peak	Duration
P.O.	1 hr	1–2 hr	6–8 hr
I.V.	10 min	1 hr	6–8 hr

Mechanism of Action

Blocks active sodium and chloride reabsorption in the ascending loop of Henle by promoting rapid excretion of water, sodium, and chloride. Torsemide also increases the production of renal prostaglandins, increasing the plasma renin level and renal vasodilation. As a result, blood pressure falls, reducing preload and afterload.

Contraindications

Hypersensitivity to torsemide, sulfonamides, or their components

Interaction

DRUGS
ACE inhibitors, antihypertensives: Additive hypotension
amiloride, spironolactone, triamterene: Possibly counteracted torsemide-induced hypokalemia
amphotericin B: Increased risk of nephrotoxicity and severe, prolonged hypokalemia or hypomagnesemia
cisplatin: Increased risk of significant hypokalemia or hypomagnesemia, possibly permanent ototoxicity

cortisone, fluorocortisone, hydrocortisone: Increased risk of sodium retention and hypokalemia
digoxin: Increased risk of arrhythmias and digitalis toxicity due to hypokalemia or hypomagnesemia
indomethacin: Possibly decreased diuretic and antihypertensive effects of torsemide and increased risk of renal failure
lithium: Possibly lithium toxicity
metolazone, thiazide diuretics: Increased risk of severe fluid and electrolyte loss
neuromuscular blockers: Possibly increased neuromuscular blockade due to hypokalemia
probenecid: Possibly decreased diuretic effect of torsemide
quinidine and other ototoxic drugs: Increased risk of ototoxicity
salicylates: Increased risk of salicylate toxicity
ACTIVITIES
alcohol use: Additive diuresis and, possibly, dehydration

Adverse Reactions
CNS: Dizziness, drowsiness, fatigue, headache, insomnia, lethargy, nervousness, restlessness, weakness
CV: Chest pain, ECG abnormalities, edema, hypotension, tachycardia
EENT: Dry mouth, hearing loss, ototoxicity, pharyngitis, rhinitis, tinnitus
GI: Constipation, diarrhea, indigestion, nausea, pancreatitis, thirst, vomiting
GU: Azotemia (prerenal), oliguria, urinary frequency
MS: Muscle spasms, myalgia
RESP: Cough
SKIN: Stevens-Johnson syndrome, toxic epidermal necrolysis
Other: Hypochloremia, hypokalemia, hypomagnesemia, hyponatremia, hypovolemia

Nursing Considerations
• Inject I.V. torsemide slowly over 2 minutes. Flush I.V. line with normal saline solution before and afterward.
• Don't exceed 200 mg in a single I.V. dose of torsemide.
• Monitor patient's serum electrolyte levels and fluid intake and output to detect hypovolemia.
WARNING Expect torsemide-induced electrolyte imbalances, such as hypokalemia

and hypomagnesemia, to increase the risk of toxicity and fatal arrhythmias in a patient who takes a digitalis glycoside. Hypokalemia also potentiates the neuromuscular blockade effects of nondepolarizing neuromuscular blockers.
PATIENT TEACHING
• Advise patient to change position slowly to minimize the effects of orthostatic hypotension.
• Instruct patient to notify prescriber at once about drowsiness, dry mouth, hearing changes, lethargy, muscle pain, nausea, restlessness, thirst, vomiting, or weakness.
• Advise diabetic patient to monitor her blood glucose level often because drug may raise it.

tramadol hydrochloride

ConZip, Rybix ODT, Ryzolt, Ultram, Ultram ER

Class and Category
Chemical class: Cyclohexanol
Therapeutic class: Analgesic
Pregnancy category: C
Controlled substance schedule: IV

Indications and Dosages
➤ *To relieve moderate to moderately severe pain*
TABLETS
Adults and adolescents over age 16. 50 to 100 mg every 4 to 6 hr, as needed. *Maximum:* 400 mg daily.
DOSAGE ADJUSTMENT If patient has hepatic impairment, dosage reduced to 50 mg every 12 hr. If patient is age 75 or over, maximum dosage reduced to 300 mg daily. If creatinine clearance is 30 ml/min/1.73 m^2 or less, interval increased to every 12 hr and maximum dosage limited to 200 mg daily.
E.R. TABLETS
Adults. 100 mg once daily, increased in 100-mg increments once daily every 5 days, as needed. *Maximum:* 300 mg once daily.
ORALLY DISINTEGRATING TABLETS
Adults and adolescents age 17 and over who do not require a rapid onset of analgesic effect. *Initial:* 50 mg once daily,

T

increased, as needed, on day 4 to 50 mg twice daily, then increased, as needed, on day 7 to 50 mg three times daily, then increased, as needed, on day 10 to 50 mg four times daily. After titration, 50 mg to 100 mg as needed every 4 to 6 hr. *Maximum:* 400 mg daily.

Adults and adolescents age 17 and over who require a rapid onset of analgesic effect. 50 mg to 100 mg every 4 to 6 hr, as needed. *Maximum:* 400 mg daily.

DOSAGE ADJUSTMENT For patients with creatinine clearance less than 30 ml/min, dosing interval increased to 12 hr with maximum daily dosage not to exceed 200 mg. For patients with cirrhosis, dosage reduced to 50 mg every 12 hr. For patients over 75 years of age, maximum dosage reduced to 300 mg daily.

Mechanism of Action
Binds with mu receptors and inhibits the reuptake of norepinephrine and serotonin, which may account for tramadol's analgesic effect.

Route	Onset	Peak	Duration
P.O.	1 hr	2–3 hr	7–14 hr

Contraindications
Alcohol intoxication; excessive use of central-acting analgesics, hypnotics, opioids, or other psychotropic drugs; hypersensitivity to tramadol or its components; use within 14 days of MAO inhibitor therapy

Interaction
DRUGS
alpha blockers, CYP2D6 and CYP3A4 inhibitors (amitriptyline, erythromycin, fluoxetine, paroxetine, quinidine), linezolid, lithium, MAO inhibitors, St. John's wort, selective serotonin and norepinephrine reuptake inhibitors, tricyclic antidepressants, triptans: Increased risk of serotonin syndrome
amiodarone, cimetidine, clomipramine, desipramine, fluphenazine, haloperidol, propafenone, quinidine, ritonavir, thioridazine: Decreased analgesia, increased adverse effects of tramadol
amitriptyline, amphetamines, antipsychotics, bupropion, cyclobenzaprine, dextro-amphetamine, erythromycin, fluoxetine, ketoconazole, paroxetine, quinidine,

MAO inhibitors, naloxone, tricyclic antidepressants: Increased risk of seizures
carbamazepine: Increased tramadol metabolism
CNS depressants such as barbiturates, benzodiazepines, opioid analgesics, phenothiazines, sedative-hypnotics, tranquilizers: Additive CNS depression
general anesthetics: Increased CNS and respiratory depression
phenothiazines, rifampin: Additive CNS depression, increased risk of seizures
warfarin: Possibly increased INR
ACTIVITIES
alcohol use: Additive CNS depression

Adverse Reactions
CNS: Agitation, anxiety, asthenia, depression, dizziness, emotional lability, euphoria, fatigue, fever, hallucinations, headache, hypertonia, hypoesthesia, insomnia, lethargy, nervousness, paresthesia, restlessness, rigors, seizures, serotonin syndrome, somnolence, suicidal ideation, tremor, vertigo, weakness
CV: Chest pain, orthostatic hypotension, vasodilation
EENT: Blurred vision, dry mouth, nasal or sinus congestion, sore throat, vision changes
ENDO: Hot flashes
GI: Abdominal pain, anorexia, constipation, diarrhea, indigestion, nausea, vomiting
GU: Urinary frequency, urine retention
MS: Arthralgia; back, limb, or neck pain
RESP: Cough, dyspnea
SKIN: Diaphoresis, dermatitis, flushing, pruritus, rash
Other: Flulike illness, physical and psychological dependence

Nursing Considerations
• Be aware that tramadol shouldn't be given to patients with a history of anaphylactoid reactions to codeine or other opioids.
• Avoid giving tramadol to patients with acute abdominal conditions because it may mask evidence and disrupt assessment of the abdomen.
• Because tramadol may lead to physical and psychological dependence, assess patient for evidence of dependence or abuse before giving first dose of tramadol.

Avoid giving drug to patients with a history of dependence on other opioids.
• Use tramadol cautiously in patients who are taking tranquilizers or antidepressant drugs and in patients who use alcohol in excess or who suffer from emotional disturbance or depression.
• After patient receives first tramadol dose, watch for allergic reactions, including angioedema, bronchospasm, pruritus, Stevens-Johnson syndrome, toxic epidermal necrolysis, and urticaria. Also watch for signs and symptoms of anaphylaxis, such as dyspnea and hypotension.
WARNING Monitor patient closely for evidence of serotonin syndrome, such as agitation, hallucinations, coma, tachycardia, labile blood pressure, hyperthermia, hyperreflexia, incoordination, nausea, vomiting, or diarrhea. Notify prescriber at once because serotonin syndrome may be life threatening. Be prepared to discontinue drug and provide supportive care.
• If patient has respiratory depression, assess respiratory status often, and expect to give a nonopioid analgesic—not tramadol.
• If patient develops respiratory depression, expect to give naloxone. Watch for seizures because naloxone may increase this risk. Take seizure precautions.
• Assess respiratory status often if patient has increased intracranial pressure or head injury because of possible increased carbon dioxide retention and CSF pressure, either of which may cause respiratory depression. Also, be aware that tramadol may constrict pupils, obscuring evidence of intracranial complications.
WARNING Watch for seizures in patients with epilepsy, a history of seizures, or an increased risk of seizures, such as those with head injury, metabolic disorders, alcohol or drug withdrawal, or CNS infection.
• Expect to taper tramadol rather than stopping it abruptly to avoid such acute withdrawal symptoms as anxiety, diarrhea, insomnia, nausea, pain, panic attacks, paresthesias, piloerection, rigors, sweating, tremor, and upper respiratory symptoms.
• Monitor patient closely for evidence of suicidal thinking or behavior, especially when therapy starts or dosage changes.

PATIENT TEACHING
• Urge patient to follow prescribed dose limits and dosing intervals to prevent respiratory depression and seizures.
• Instruct patient prescribed extended-release form to swallow tablet whole and not to chew, crush, or split tablet.
• Instruct patient prescribed orally disintegrating tablets to place the tablet on his tongue until it is completely dissolved, which may take up to a minute, and then swallow it. Tablet may be taken with or without water but tablet must be completely dissolved before water is taken.
• Caution patient not to stop tramadol abruptly.
• Instruct patient to avoid hazardous activities until drug's CNS effects are known.
• Advise patient to avoid alcohol while taking tramadol.
• Urge patient to notify prescriber about known, suspected, or intended pregnancy.
• Urge caregivers to watch patient closely for evidence of suicidal tendencies, especially when therapy starts or dosage changes and to report concerns at once to prescriber.
• Tell patient to notify prescriber immediately if he develops any sudden onset, unusual, persistent, or severe adverse reactions.
• Instruct patient to inform all prescribers of tramadol therapy because of potential drug interactions.

trandolapril
Mavik

Class and Category
Chemical class: ACE inhibitor (nonsulfhydryl-containing)
Therapeutic class: Antihypertensive, vasodilator
Pregnancy category: D

Indications and Dosages
➤ *To manage hypertension*
TABLETS
Adults. *Initial:* 1 mg daily, increased every wk based on clinical response. Dosage may be given in two daily doses if antihypertensive effect diminishes before 24 hr. *Usual:* 2 to 4 mg daily. *Maximum:* 8 mg daily.

DOSAGE ADJUSTMENT Initial dosage increased to 2 mg daily for blacks with hypertension. Initial dosage reduced to 0.5 mg for patients also receiving a diuretic, those with a creatinine clearance of less than or equal to 30 ml/min/1.73 m^2, and those with cirrhosis.

➤ *To treat heart failure after MI*

TABLETS

Adults. *Initial:* 1 mg daily. *Usual:* 4 mg or more daily. *Maximum:* 8 mg daily.

Route	Onset	Peak	Duration
P.O.	2 hr	8 hr	24 hr

Mechanism of Action

Reduces blood pressure by inhibiting the conversion of angiotensin I to angiotensin II. Angiotensin II is a potent vasoconstrictor that stimulates the renal cortex to secrete aldosterone. Decreased release of aldosterone reduces sodium and water retention and increases their excretion, thereby reducing blood pressure. Trandolapril may also inhibit renal and vascular production of angiotensin II.

Contraindications

Aliskiren therapy in patients with diabetes or renal impairment (GFR less than 60 ml/min), hereditary or idiopathic angioedema, history of angioedema related to previous treatment with ACE inhibitor, hypersensitivity to trandolapril or its components

Interaction

DRUGS

aliskiren (in patients with diabetes), angiotensin receptor blockers, other ACE inhibitors: Increased risk of hyperkalemia, hypotension, and renal dysfunction
allopurinol, bone marrow depressants (such as methotrexate), corticosteroids (systemic), cytostatic drugs, procainamide: Increased risk of potentially fatal neutropenia or agranulocytosis
antacids: Decreased blood trandolapril level
cyclosporine, potassium-containing drugs, potassium-sparing diuretics, potassium supplements: Increased risk of hyperkalemia
diuretics, other antihypertensives: Increased hypotensive effects
inhalation anesthetics (selected): Enhanced hypotensive effect of selected inhalation anesthetics

insulin, oral hypoglycemic agents: Possibly increased risk of hypoglycemia
lithium: Increased blood lithium level and risk of lithium toxicity
NSAIDs: Possibly reduced antihypertensive effects; increased risk of renal dysfunction especially in the elderly and patients with volume-depletion or preexisting renal dysfunction
sodium aurothiomalate: Increased risk of nitroid reactions, such as facial flushing, nausea, vomiting, and hypotensionsympathomimetics: Possibly reduced antihypertensive effects

FOODS

high-potassium diet, low-sodium milk, potassium-containing salt substitutes: Increased risk of hyperkalemia

ACTIVITIES

alcohol use: Possibly increased hypotensive effect

Adverse Reactions

CNS: Anxiety, depression, dizziness, drowsiness, fatigue, fever, hallucination, headache, insomnia, malaise, paresthesia, stroke, syncope, transient ischemic attack, vertigo
CV: Angina, arrhythmia, bradycardia, cardiac failure, chest pain, edema, first-degree AV block, hypotension, MI, myocardial ischemia, orthostatic hypotension, palpitations, tachycardia, ventricular tachycardia
EENT: Dry mouth, epistaxis, loss of taste, throat inflammation
GI: Abdominal cramps, distention, or pain; constipation; diarrhea; dyspepsia; elevated liver enzymes; hepatitis; jaundice; nausea; pancreatitis; vomiting
GU: Decreased libido, elevated blood urea nitrogen and creatinine, impotence, renal failure
HEME: Agranulocytosis, decreased leukocytes or neutrophils, pancytopenia, thrombocytopenia
MS: Extremity pain, muscle cramps, myalgia
RESP: Bronchitis, cough, dyspnea, upper respiratory tract infection
SKIN: Alopecia, diaphoresis, flushing, pemphigus, pruritus, rash, Stevens-Johnson syndrome, toxic epidermal necrolysis
Other: Angioedema, elevated SGOT levels, gout, hyperkalemia, hypocalcemia, hyponatremia

Nursing Considerations

WARNING Closely monitor blood pressure during first 2 weeks of therapy and whenever dosage is adjusted, especially in patients with heart failure, hyponatremia, or severe volume or sodium loss. If excessive hypotension occurs, notify prescriber immediately, place patient in supine position, and infuse I.V. normal saline solution, as prescribed.

WARNING Be alert for signs and symptoms of angioedema. If swelling of tongue, glottis, or larynx causes airway obstruction, notify prescriber and be prepared to discontinue drug and administer emergency measures, including subcutaneous epinephrine 1:1,000 (0.3 to 0.5 ml).

• Continue to monitor patient's blood pressure to assess drug's long-term effectiveness.

PATIENT TEACHING

• Instruct patient to notify prescriber immediately and stop taking trandolapril if she experiences swelling of face, eyes, lips, or tongue or has difficulty breathing.

• Explain that drug may cause dizziness and light-headedness, especially during first few days of therapy. Advise patient to avoid driving and other potentially hazardous activities until drug's CNS effects are known and to notify prescriber immediately if she faints.

• Inform female patient of childbearing age about risks of taking trandolapril during pregnancy. Urge her to use effective contraceptive method and to notify prescriber immediately if she becomes or thinks she might be pregnant.

• Advise patient planning to undergo surgery or anesthesia to inform specialist that she's taking trandolapril.

• Instruct patient to consult prescriber before using potassium supplements or salt substitutes containing potassium.

• Inform patient about possible loss of taste, which may result in weight loss. Reassure her that loss of taste is usually reversed after 2 to 3 months.

tranexamic acid

Cyklokapron, Lysteda

Class and Category

Chemical class: Synthetic lysine amino acid derivative
Therapeutic class: Antifibrinolytic
Pregnancy category: B

Indications and Dosages

➤ *To treat cyclic heavy menstrual bleeding*
TABLETS
Adults. 1,300 mg three times daily for a maximum of 5 days during monthly menstruation

DOSAGE ADJUSTMENT For patient with a serum creatinine level above 1.4 mg/dl but equal to or less than 2.8 mg/dl, 1,300 mg two times a day for a maximum of 5 days during menstruation; for patient with a serum creatinine level above 2.8 mg/dl but equal to or less than 5.7 mg/dl, 1,300 mg once daily for a maximum of 5 days during menstruation; for patient with a serum creatinine level above 5.7 mg/dl, 650 mg once daily for a maximum of 5 days during menstruation.

➤ *To treat patients with hemophilia to reduce or prevent hemorrhage and reduce need for replacement therapy during and following tooth extraction*
I.V. INFUSION
Adults. *Initial:* 10 mg/kg immediately before tooth extraction together with replacement therapy, followed by 10 mg/kg three times a day or four times a day, as needed, for up to 8 days.

DOSAGE ADJUSTMENT For patients with moderate to severe renal impairment, dosage frequency decreased according to serum creatinine level.

Mechanism of Action

Displaces plasminogen from surface of fibrin by binding to high-affinity lysine site of plasminogen. This diminishes dissolution of hemostatic fibrin, which decreases bleeding.

Route	Onset	Peak	Duration
P.O.	Unknown	3 hr	Unknown

Contraindications

Active thromboembolic disease; history or intrinsic risk of thrombosis or thrombo-embolism, including retinal vein or artery occlusion; hypersensitivity to tranexamic acid or its components; use of combination hormonal contraception

T

Incompatibilities

Do not administer tranexamic acid intravenously with blood or solutions containing penicillin.

Interaction

DRUGS

anti-inhibitor coagulant concentrates, factor IX complex concentrates, hormonal contraceptives: Increased thrombotic risk
tissue plasminogen activators: Possibly decreased effectiveness of both tranexamic acid and the tissue plasminogen activator
tretinoin (oral): Possibly exacerbation of the procoagulant effect of tretinoin

Adverse Reactions

CNS: Cerebral thrombosis, dizziness, fatigue, headache, migraine, seizures
CV: Deep vein thrombosis, MI
EENT: Central retinal artery and vein obstruction, feeling of tightness in throat, impaired color vision, ligneous conjunctivitis, nasal and sinus congestion, sinusitis, visual abnormalities
GI: Abdominal pain, diarrhea, nausea, vomiting
GU: Acute renal cortical necrosis
HEME: Anemia
MS: Arthralgia, back pain, muscle cramps and spasms, myalgia
RESP: Dyspnea, pulmonary embolism, respiratory congestion
SKIN: Allergic skin reactions, facial flushing
Other: Anaphylaxis, multiple allergies including seasonal

Nursing Considerations

• Tranexamic acid therapy isn't recommended for women who use hormonal contraceptives or who take factor IX complex concentrates or anti-inhibitor coagulant concentrates because of the increased risk of thromboembolism, especially if she is obese, a smoker, or over the age of 35.
• Use tranexamic acid cautiously in patients with acute promyelocytic leukemia who are taking oral tretinoin for remission induction; they could be susceptible to possible exacerbation of the procoagulant effect of tretinoin.
• Cerebral edema and cerebral infarction may occur in women taking tranexamic acid if a subarachnoid hemorrhage occurs.

WARNING Monitor patient closely for allergic reactions to tranexamic acid such as dyspnea, a feeling of tightness in the throat, and facial flushing that may require emergency medical treatment.

PATIENT TEACHING

• Instruct patient to swallow tranexamic acid tablets whole, without chewing or breaking them. Therapy shouldn't exceed 5 days during menstruation.
• Tell patient to seek emergency care immediately if she has any signs of allergic reaction, especially dyspnea, a feeling of tightness in the throat, and facial flushing; she should stop taking drug.
• Advise patient to report any changes in vision or ocular discomfort.

tranylcypromine sulfate

Parnate

Class and Category

Chemical class: Nonhydrazine derivative
Therapeutic class: Antidepressant
Pregnancy category: Not rated

Indications and Dosages

➤ *To treat major depressive episodes without melancholia*

TABLETS

Adults and adolescents over age 16.
30 mg/ day in divided doses. After first 2 wk, increased by 10 mg every 1 to 2 wk, as needed. *Maintenance:* 10 to 40 mg daily. *Maximum:* 60 mg daily.
DOSAGE ADJUSTMENT For elderly patients, initial dosage possibly reduced to 2.5 to 5 mg daily and increased by 2.5 to 5 mg every 3 to 4 days, as needed; maximum dosage 45 mg daily. Alternative therapies should be carefully considered for patients over age 60.

Mechanism of Action

Reversibly binds to MAO, reducing its activity and resulting in increased levels of neurotransmitters, including dopamine, epinephrine, and norepinephrine. This regulation of CNS neurotransmitters helps ease depression.

Route	Onset	Peak	Duration
P.O.	7–10 days	4–8 wk	10 days

Contraindications

Cardiovascular disease; cerebrovascular disease; heart failure; hepatic disease; history of headaches; hypersensitivity to tranylcypromine or its components; hypertension; pheochromocytoma; severe renal impairment; use of anesthetics, antihypertensives, bupropion, buspirone, carbamazepine, CNS depressants, cyclobenzaprine, dextromethorphan, meperidine, other MAO inhibitors, selective serotonin-reuptake inhibitors, selective norepinephrine reuptake inhibitors, sympathomimetics, or tricyclic antidepressants

Interaction

DRUGS

amoxapine, bupropion, maprotiline, selective norepinephrine reuptake inhibitors, selective serotonin reuptake inhibitors, trazodone, tricyclic antidepressants: Increased risk of severe hypertensive crisis, increased anticholinergic effects
anticonvulsants: Additive CNS depression
antihistamines: Possibly prolonged anti-cholinergic and CNS depressant effects
antipsychotics: Additive anticholinergic, hypotensive, and sedative effects
beta blockers: Possibly worsened bradycardia
bromocriptine: Increased blood prolactin level and interference with bromocriptine effects
buspirone: Increased blood pressure
dextroamphetamine, isometheptene, local anesthetics, naphazoline, oxymetazoline, psychostimulants, sympathomimetics including amphetamines, tetrahydrozoline, xylometazoline: Increased risk of severe hypertensive reaction
dextromethorphan, tryptophan: Increased risk of serotonin syndrome
diuretics: Additive hypotensive effects
doxapram: Increased vasopressor effects
furazolidone, procarbazine, selegiline: Increased risk of severe hyperpyretic or hypertensive crisis, seizures, or death
guanadrel, guanethidine: Increased risk of moderate to severe hypertension

insulin, oral antidiabetic drugs: Possibly prolonged hypoglycemic response
levodopa: Increased vasopressor effects, hypertension, adverse cardiovascular effects
meperidine: Increased risk of coma, diaphoresis, excitation, hypertension, rigidity, severe respiratory depression, shock, and, possibly, death
methyldopa: Increased risk of hallucinations
metrizamide, tramadol: Increased risk of seizures
succinylcholine: Possibly prolonged succinylcholine effects
FOODS
aged cheese; avocados; bananas; fava or broad beans; cured sausage (bologna, pepperoni, salami, and summer sausage) or other meat; overripe fruit; pickled fish, meats, or poultry; protein extract; smoked fish, meats, or poultry; soy sauce; yeast extract; and other foods high in pressor amines, such as tyramine: Increased risk of sudden, severe hypertension
caffeine-containing beverages and foods: Increased risk of severe hypertensive crisis and dangerous arrhythmias
ACTIVITIES
alcohol-containing products that also may contain tyramine, such as beer (including reduced-alcohol and alcohol-free beer), wine (red and white), sherry, hard liquor, liqueurs: Increased risk of hypertensive crisis

Adverse Reactions

CNS: Anxiety, chills, dizziness, drowsiness, fever, headache, insomnia, intracranial hemorrhage, paresthesia, restlessness, suicidal ideation, tremor, weakness
CV: Bradycardia, chest pain, edema, hypertensive crisis, orthostatic hypotension, palpitations, tachycardia
EENT: Blurred vision, dry mouth, mydriasis, photophobia, tinnitus
GI: Abdominal pain, anorexia, constipation, diarrhea, nausea, vomiting
GU: Ejaculation disorders, impotence, urine retention
HEME: Agranulocytosis, anemia, leuko-penia, thrombocytopenia
MS: Muscle spasms, myoclonus, neck stiffness
SKIN: Clammy skin, diaphoresis

T

Nursing Considerations

• Monitor patient's blood pressure during tranylcypromine therapy to detect hypertensive crisis and to decrease the risk of orthostatic hypotension.

WARNING Notify prescriber immediately if patient has evidence of hypertensive crisis, such as chest pain, headache, neck stiffness, and palpitations. Expect to stop drug right away.

• Anticipate that therapeutic response may not occur for up to 4 weeks.

• Expect drug to aggravate symptoms of Parkinson's disease, including muscle spasms, myoclonic movement, and tremor.

• Keep dietary restrictions in place for at least 2 weeks after stopping tranylcypromine because of the slow recovery from drug's enzyme-inhibiting effects.

• Expect to stop tranylcypromine 10 days before elective surgery, as prescribed, to avoid hypotension.

• Be aware that abrupt cessation of drug can precipitate original symptoms.

• Check diabetic patient's blood glucose level often to detect loss of control.

• Anticipate that coadministration with a selective serotonin reuptake inhibitor may cause confusion, seizures, severe hypertension, and other, less severe symptoms.

• Monitor severely depressed patients, including children and teens, for suicidal tendencies. Take safety measures, and notify prescriber immediately.

• Assess patient for sudden insomnia. If it develops, notify prescriber and be prepared to administer drug early in the day.

PATIENT TEACHING

• Instruct patient to avoid foods that contain cheese and that are high in tyramine, such as anchovies, avocadoes, bananas, beer, canned figs, caviar, Chianti wine, chocolate, dried fruit, fava beans, liqueurs, meat tenderizers, overripe fruit, pickled herring, raspberries, sauerkraut, sherry, sour cream, soy sauce, yeast extract, and yogurt while taking tranylcypromine.

• Urge patient to continue dietary restrictions for at least 2 weeks after tranylcypromine therapy stops.

• Advise patient to notify prescriber at once about chest pain, dizziness, headache, nausea, neck stiffness, palpitations, rapid heart rate, sweating, and vomiting.

• Urge patient to avoid alcohol and excessive caffeine intake during therapy.

• Urge patient to change position slowly to minimize orthostatic hypotension.

• Advise patient to avoid hazardous activities until drug's CNS effects are known.

• Caution patient not to take any other prescribed or OTC drugs without consulting prescriber.

• Caution patient not to stop drug abruptly to avoid recurrence of original symptoms.

• Instruct female patient to use effective contraception during tranylcypromine therapy to prevent fetal abnormalities. Urge her to notify prescriber immediately about known or suspected pregnancy.

WARNING Urge parents to watch their child or adolescent closely for abnormal thinking or behavior or increased aggression or hostility. Stress importance of notifying prescriber about unusual changes.

trazodone hydrochloride

Oleptro

Class and Category

Chemical class: Triazolopyridine derivative
Therapeutic class: Antidepressant, anxiolytic
Pregnancy category: C

Indications and Dosages

➤ *To treat major depression*

E.R. TABLETS

Adults. *Initial:* 150 mg once daily, increased by 75 mg daily every 3 days, as needed. *Maximum:* 375 mg daily.

Mechanism of Action

Blocks serotonin reuptake along the presynaptic neuronal membrane, causing an antidepressant effect. Trazodone exerts an alpha-adrenergic blocking action and produces modest histamine blockade, causing a sedative effect. It also inhibits the vasopressor response to norepinephrine, which reduces blood pressure.

Route	Onset	Peak	Duration
P.O.	1–2 wk	Unknown	Unknown

Contraindications

Hypersensitivity to trazodone or its components, recovery from acute MI, use within 14 days of an MAO inhibitor including intravenous methylene blue and linezolid

Interaction

DRUGS

aspirin, NSAIDs: Possibly increased risk of bleeding
barbiturates and other CNS depressants: Enhanced effect of CNS depressants
carbamazepine: Decreased trazodone level
CYP3A4 inhibitors such as indinavir, ketoconazole, and ritonavir: Possibly increased plasma trazodone levels with increased risk of adverse reactions
digoxin, phenytoin: Possibly increased blood levels of these drugs and increased risk of toxicity
MAO inhibitors: Increased serotonin effects
serotonergic drugs: Increased risk of serotonin syndrome
warfarin: Altered anticoagulation response
ACTIVITIES
alcohol use: Increased CNS depression, risk of respiratory depression and hypotension

Adverse Reactions

CNS: Abnormal coordination or dreams, agitation, anxiety, aphasia, ataxia, balance disorder, chills, confusion, CVA, dizziness, drowsiness, extrapyramidal symptoms, fatigue, hallucinations, headache, insomnia, light-headedness, memory impairment, migraine, nervousness, paresthesia, paranoid reaction, psychosis, seizures, serotonin syndrome, somnolence, stupor, suicidal ideation, syncope, tardive dyskinesia, tremor, vertigo, weakness
CV: Arrhythmias, congestive heart failure, edema, hypotension, orthostatic hypotension, palpitations, prolonged QT interval, vasodilation
EENT: Angle closure glaucoma, blurred vision, diplopia, dry mouth
ENDO: Inappropriate ADH syndrome
GI: Abdominal pain, cholestasis, constipation, diarrhea, elevated bilirubin or liver enzymes, indigestion, jaundice, nausea, vomiting

GU: Anorgasmia; ejaculation disorders; decreased libido; priapism; urinary incontinence, retention, or urgency
HEME: Hemolytic anemia, leukocytosis
MS: Back pain, myalgia
RESP: Apnea, dyspnea
SKIN: Alopecia, hirsutism, night sweats, pruritus, psoriasis, rash, urticaria
Other: Hyponatremia

Nursing Considerations

• Use trazodone cautiously in patients with cardiac disease because drug can cause arrhythmias.
• Give trazodone shortly after the patient has a meal or light snack to reduce nausea.
• Give larger portion of daily dose at bedtime if drowsiness occurs.
• Because trazadone's mechanism of action is similar to that of selective serotonin reuptake inhibitors, expect high doses (6 to 8 mg/kg) to increase blood serotonin level and low doses (0.05 to 1 mg/kg) to decrease blood serotonin level.
• Expect most patients who respond to trazodone to do so by the end of the second week of therapy.
• Closely monitor depressed patients for suicidal thoughts and tendencies. Notify prescriber if they occur, and take suicide precautions according to facility policy.
WARNING Monitor patient closely for serotonin syndrome exhibited by agitation, hallucinations, coma, tachycardia, labile blood pressure, hyperthermia, hyperreflexia, incoordination, nausea, vomiting, or diarrhea. Notify prescriber immediately because serotonin syndrome may be life threatening and provide supportive care.
WARNING Be aware that serotonin syndrome in its most severe form may resemble neuroleptic malignant syndrome, which includes hyperthermia, muscle rigidity, and autonomic instability with possibly rapid changes in vital signs and mental status. Stop drug immediately and provide supportive care.
• Be aware that adverse CNS reactions usually improve after patient completes a few weeks of therapy.
WARNING Be aware that trazodone therapy may increase the risk of priapism.

T

- Urge patient to avoid taking trazodone on an empty stomach because doing so may increase the risk of dizziness or light-headedness.
- Advise patient that drug may cause mild pupillary dilation, which may lead to an episode of acute closure glaucoma. Encourage patient to have an eye exam before starting therapy to see if he is at risk.
- Caution patient to avoid potentially hazardous activities during therapy.
- Advise patient not to fast during trazodone therapy because of possible adverse CNS reactions.
- Instruct male patient to notify prescriber immediately about priapism.
- Caution patient not to take aspirin or nonsteroidal anti-inflammatory agents without first discussing use with the prescriber.
- Instruct patient not to stop trazodone therapy abruptly.
- Urge family and caregivers to watch patient closely for abnormal thinking or behavior or increased aggression or hostility. Emphasize importance of notifying prescriber about unusual changes.

triamcinolone

Aristocort, Aristopak, Atolone, Kenacort, Nasacort AQ

triamcinolone acetonide

AllerNaze, Kenalog-10, Kenalog-40, Ken-Jec-40, Nasacort, Nasacort Allergy 24 Hour, Nasacort HFA

triamcinolone diacetate

Acetocot, Amcort, Aristocort, Aristocort Forte, Articulose-LA, Cenocort Forte, Cinalone 40, Clinacort, Kenacort Diacetate, Tilone, Tramacort-D, Triam-Forte, Triamolone 40, Tristoject

triamcinolone hexacetonide

Aristospan

Class and Category

Chemical class: Synthetic glucocorticoid
Therapeutic class: Anti-inflammatory, immunosuppressant
Pregnancy category: C (nasal and oral inhalation), Not rated (oral and parenteral)

Indications and Dosages

➤ *To prevent bronchospasm or provide long-term corticosteroid treatment to control asthma*

ORAL INHALATION (TRIAMCINOLONE ACETONIDE)
Adults and children age 12 and over.
Initial: 2 metered sprays (200 mcg) three times a day or four times a day. *Maintenance:* Individualized dosage given twice daily. *Maximum:* 16 metered sprays daily in divided doses.
Children ages 6 to 11. 2 to 4 metered sprays (200 to 400 mcg) twice daily to four times a day. *Maximum:* 12 metered sprays daily.

➤ *To treat acute rheumatic carditis, berylliosis, and Hodgkin's disease; as adjunct to treat fulminating or disseminated pulmonary tuberculosis (with appropriate antituberculosis therapy)*

SYRUP (TRIAMCINOLONE DIACETATE), TABLETS (TRIAMCINOLONE)
Adults and children age 12 and over.
Initial: 4 to 48 mg daily as a single dose or in divided doses. Some patients may require an initial dose of 60 mg.
Children under age 12. 0.42 to 1.7 mg/kg daily as a single dose or in divided doses.

I.M. INJECTION (TRIAMCINOLONE ACETONIDE: KENALOG-40 ONLY)
Adults and children age 12 and over. 40 to 80 mg every 4 wk, as needed.
Children ages 6 to 11. 40 mg every 4 wk, as needed, or 30 to 200 mcg/kg every 1 to 7 days.

I.M. INJECTION (TRIAMCINOLONE DIACETATE)
Adults and children age 12 and over.
40 mg every wk, or 4 to 7 times the daily P.O. dose as a single injection every 4 days to every 4 wk.
Children ages 6 to 11. 40 mg/wk.

➤ *To relieve inflammation caused by acute gouty arthritis, acute nonspecific tenosynovitis, acute or subacute bursitis, epicondylitis, osteoarthritis, post-traumatic osteoarthritis, rheumatoid arthritis, and synovitis*

SYRUP (TRIAMCINOLONE DIACETATE)
Adults and children age 12 and over. 4 to 48 mg daily as a single dose or in divided doses, adjusted, as prescribed, to lowest effective dose based on clinical response.

TABLETS (TRIAMCINOLONE)
Adults and children age 12 and over. 8 to 16 mg daily in divided doses three times a day or four times a day, adjusted, as prescribed, to lowest effective dose based on clinical response.

SYRUP (TRIAMCINOLONE DIACETATE), TABLETS (TRIAMCINOLONE)
Children ages 6 to 11. 0.42 to 1.7 mg/kg daily as a single dose or in divided doses, adjusted based on clinical response.

I.M. INJECTION (TRIAMCINOLONE ACETONIDE: KENALOG-40 ONLY)
Adults and children age 12 and over. 40 to 80 mg every 4 wk.
Children ages 6 to 11. 40 mg every 4 wk.

I.M. INJECTION (TRIAMCINOLONE DIACETATE)
Adults and children age 6 and over. 40 mg every wk as single injection, repeated every 4 wk, as needed.

INTRA-ARTICULAR OR INTRABURSAL INJECTION (TRIAMCINOLONE ACETONIDE)
Adults and children age 6 and over. 2.5 to 15 mg, as needed.

INTRA-ARTICULAR OR INTRASYNOVIAL INJECTION (TRIAMCINOLONE DIACETATE)
Adults. 5 to 40 mg, repeated as prescribed every 1 to 8 wk, as needed.

INTRA-ARTICULAR INJECTION (TRIAMCINOLONE HEXACETONIDE)
Adults. 2 to 20 mg, repeated as prescribed every 3 to 4 wk, as needed.

➤ *To treat primary (Addison's disease) or secondary adrenocortical insufficiency*

SYRUP (TRIAMCINOLONE DIACETATE)
Adults and children age 12 and over. 4 to 12 mg daily as a single dose or in divided doses.

SYRUP (TRIAMCINOLONE DIACETATE), TABLETS (TRIAMCINOLONE)
Children ages 6 to 11. 0.12 mg (base)/kg daily as a single dose or in divided doses.

➤ *To treat inflammatory dermatoses*

TABLETS (TRIAMCINOLONE)
Adults and children age 12 and over. 8 to 16 mg daily. *Usual:* 1 to 2 mg daily.

➤ *To treat disseminated lupus erythematosus*

TABLETS (TRIAMCINOLONE)
Adults and children age 12 and over. 20 to 30 mg daily. *Usual:* 3 to 30 mg daily.

➤ *To treat nephrotic syndrome*

TABLETS (TRIAMCINOLONE)
Adults and children age 12 and over. 16 to 20 mg daily.

➤ *To relieve symptoms of perennial and seasonal allergic rhinitis*

TABLETS (TRIAMCINOLONE)
Adults and children age 12 and over. 8 to 12 mg daily. *Usual:* 2 to 6 mg daily.
Children ages 6 to 11. 0.42 to 1.7 mg/kg daily as a single dose or in divided doses.

NASAL INHALATION (NASACORT)
Adults and children age 12 and over.
Initial: 220 mcg daily in 2 sprays (55 mcg each)/nostril. *Maintenance:* 110 mcg daily in 1 spray (55 mcg)/nostril. *Maximum:* 440 mcg (8 sprays daily).

NASAL INHALATION (NASACORT AQ, NASACORT ALLERGY 24 HOUR)
Adults and children age 12 and over.
Initial: 110 mcg daily in 2 sprays (55 mcg each)/nostril. *Maintenance:* 55 mcg daily in 1 spray/nostril. *Maximum:* 220 mcg or 4 sprays daily.
Children ages 6 to 11. 110 mcg daily in 1 spray (55 mcg each)/nostril. *Maximum:* 220 mcg or 4 sprays daily.
Children ages 2 to 5. 110 mcg daily in 1 spray (55 mcg)/nostril. *Maximum:* 110 mcg or 2 sprays daily.

NASAL INHALATION (NASACORT HFA)
Adults and children age 12 and over.
Initial: 220 mcg daily in 2 sprays (55 mcg each)/nostril. May be increased to 440 mcg daily in 4 sprays/nostril, as needed.
Children ages 6 to 11. 220 mcg daily in 2 sprays (55 mcg each)/nostril.

NASAL INHALATION (ALLERNAZE)
Adults and children age 12 and over.
Initial: 200 mcg daily in 2 sprays (50 mcg each)/nostril. *Maximum:* 400 mcg daily in 4 sprays (50 mcg each)/nostril or divided into 2 daily doses.

➤ *To treat chronic idiopathic thrombocytopenic purpura*

T

TABLETS (TRIAMCINOLONE)
Adults and children age 12 and over.
0.8 mg/kg daily.

Route	Onset	Peak	Duration
P.O. (tablets)	Unknown	1–2 hr	2.25 days
Unknown			
I.M.*	24–48 hr	Unknown	1–6 wk
I.M.†	Slow	Unknown	4 days–4 wk
Inhalation-	12 hr	3–4 hr	Unknown
Intra-articular, intra-bursal*	Unknown	Unknown	Several wk
Intra-articular, intra-synovial†	Unknown	Unknown	1–8 wk

Mechanism of Action
Inhibits the release of prostaglandins and leukotrienes, thus reducing immediate and late-phase allergic responses in chronic asthma. Triamcinolone also:
• decreases peribronchial edema and mucus secretion by inhibiting the binding of allergens to immunoglobulin E antibodies on the surface of mast cells, thereby inactivating the release of chemotactic substances
• decreases inflammation by interfering with leukocyte adhesion to capillary walls
• inhibits the release of leukocytic acid hydrolases, preventing macrophage accumulation at the infection site
• inhibits histamine and kinin release, preventing the formation of scar tissue

Incompatibilities
Don't mix triamcinolone hexacetonide with parenteral local anesthetics because precipitation can occur.

Contraindications
Acute status asthmaticus (inhalation form), administered as an intrathecal injection,

---

* Acetonide.
† Diacetate.

hypersensitivity to triamcinolone or its components, live-virus vaccine therapy, systemic fungal infection (except Aristocort Forte when administered as an intra-articular injection for localized joint conditions), idiopathic thrombocytopenic purpura (given as I.M. injection)

Interaction
DRUGS
amphotericin B, ethacrynic acid, furosemide, thiazide diuretics: Increased potassium-wasting effect, severe hypokalemia
aspirin: Increased blood salicylate level, increased risk of salicylate toxicity
cholinesterase inhibitors: Increased risk of severe muscle weakness in patients with myasthenia gravis
digitalis glycosides: Increased risk of arrhythmias and digitalis toxicity
estrogens: Increased triamcinolone effects
hepatic enzyme inducers such as barbiturates, carbamazepine, phenytoin, rifampin: Increased triamcinolone metabolism with decreased effectiveness
hepatic enzyme inhibitors such as ketoconazole, macrolide antibiotics: Decreased triamcinolone clearance, increased risk of adverse effects
insulin, oral antidiabetic drugs: Increased blood glucose level
isoproterenol: Increased risk of cardio-toxicity
live-virus vaccines: Decreased antibody response, increased risk of neurologic complications
neuromuscular blockers: Increased risk of hypokalemia and enhanced neuromuscular blockade
NSAIDs: Increased risk of adverse GI effects
toxoids: Decreased resistance to toxoids

Adverse Reactions
CNS: Depression, dizziness, emotional lability, exacerbated psychosis, fatigue, headache, increased intracranial pressure with papilledema (pseudotumor cerebri) usually following discontinuation of drug, insomnia, malaise, neuritis, neuropathy, paresthesia, personality changes, psychiatric disorders, restlessness, seizures, vertigo
CV: Edema, heart failure, hypertension

EENT: Altered sense of smell or taste, cataracts, dry mouth, epistaxis (nasal form), glaucoma, hoarseness, nasal congestion, nasal irritation (inhalation form), nasal septal perforation (nasal form), oropharyngeal candidiasis, pharyngitis, posterior subcapsular cataracts, rhinorrhea, secondary ocular infection, sinusitis, sneezing
ENDO: Cushing's syndrome, diabetes mellitus, growth retardation (children)
GI: Abdominal pain, constipation, diarrhea, dyspepsia, esophageal ulceration, gastritis, nausea, vomiting
GU: Altered motility and number of spermatozoa, cystitis, renal disease, UTI, vaginitis
MS: Bone mineral density loss, bursitis, muscle wasting or weakness, myalgia, osteoporosis, tenosynovitis
RESP: Asthma, bronchitis, bronchospasm (inhalation form), chest congestion, dyspnea, increased cough
SKIN: Ecchymosis, petechiae (parenteral form), photosensitivity, pruritus, rash, striae, urticaria
Other: Anaphylaxis; angioedema; decreased resistance to infections; facial edema; flu syndrome; herpes infection; hiccups; impaired wound healing; injection-site atrophy, induration, pain, soreness, and sterile abscess; moon face; weight gain

Nursing Considerations
• Be aware that high doses of corticosteroids such as triamcinolone aren't recommended for patients with cranial trauma who don't require a corticosteroid for another condition because they increase risk of death.
• Triamcinolone should be administered with extreme caution, if at all, in patients who have active or quiescent tuberculosis infection of the respiratory tract, untreated fungal or bacterial infection, systemic viral or parasitic infection, or ocular herpes simplex because this drug can make these infections worse.
• Use cautiously in patients with ocular herpes simplex because of possible corneal perforation. Be aware that drug should not be used in active ocular herpes simplex.
• Use cautiously in patients with active or latent peptic ulcer, diverticulitis, fresh intestinal anastomoses, and nonspecific ulcerative colitis; there is increased risk of a perforation for these patients. Be aware that signs of peritoneal irritation following gastrointestinal perforation in patients receiving steroid therapy may be minimal or absent.
• Monitor patient with cirrhosis carefully for an enhanced drug effect because increased metabolism of steroids may occur in the presence of cirrhosis.
• Give oral form of triamcinolone with meals to minimize GI distress.
• Use calibrated device to measure liquid doses.
• If necessary, crush tablets and mix with food or fluids.
• Know that triamcinolone acetonide parenteral formulation with trade name Kenalog-40 can be administered I.M. Other parenteral triamcinolone acetonide forms should never be injected I.M. Shake I.M. suspension thoroughly before drawing it into syringe.
• Be aware that specialized training may be needed to administer parenteral triamcinolone.
• Don't administer parenteral forms of triamcinolone intravenously.
WARNING Know that drug should not be administered via the intrathecal or epidural route because severe neurologic adverse reactions may occur
• Know that drug should not be administered intra-articularly into an infected site, and injection into a previously infected joint is usually not recommended.
• Be aware that triamcinolone may reactivate tuberculosis in patients who have a history of it.
• Monitor patient for hypersensitivity. Although rare, triamcinolone has caused anaphylaxis that ended in death. Notify prescriber immediately if hypersensitivity occurs; expect to discontinue triamcinolone therapy and provide emergency supportive care.
• Monitor patients, especially infants, closely for gasping syndrome because parenteral triamcinolone contains benzyl alcohol. Exposure to high doses may result in toxicity evidenced by life-threatening hypotension and metabolic acidosis.

T

WARNING Know that patients on cortico-steroid therapy require an increased dosage of rapidly acting corticosteroids when unusual stress is anticipated, during the stressful event, and for a period after the stressful situation. Assess patient for signs and symptoms of adrenal insufficiency (fatigue, hypotension, lassitude, nausea, vomiting, and weakness) during times of stress, such as infection, surgery, or trauma. Notify prescriber immediately if you detect these signs and symptoms because adrenal insufficiency may be life threatening. Drug-induced secondary adrenocortical insufficiency may be minimized by gradual reduction of dosage.

• Be aware that, although rare, bone mineral density loss and osteoporosis may occur, which may increase risk of fractures, especially in patients on prolonged triamcinolone therapy.

• Adjust triamcinolone dosage, as prescribed, in patients with changes in thyroid status because metabolic clearance of corticosteroids is decreased in hypo-thyroid patients and increased in hyperthyroid patients.

• Assess patient for signs and symptoms of infection (fever, malaise, abnormal symptoms in particular body system) because steroid therapy such as triamcinolone increases risk of susceptibility to infections, especially with higher dosages.

PATIENT TEACHING

• Caution patient not to adjust dosage for prescription triamcinolone without consulting prescriber and to follow dosage recommendations when using an over-the-counter preparation.

• Teach patient how to administer nasal aerosols properly, using manufacturer's instructions, to avoid nasal irritation.

• Instruct patient to dispose of aerosol canister after 240 uses (100 uses for Nasacort HFA) because dosage may not be correct after that time.

• Teach patient how to use nasal spray, including how to prime spray pump bottle before use. Caution patient to not to get nasal spray in eyes. If this occurs, patient should rinse his eyes well with water.

• Inform patient that maximum benefit of triamcinolone therapy may not occur for up to 2 weeks.

• Advise patient to notify prescriber immediately if asthma fails to respond to inhaled drug; additional systemic therapy may be needed.

• Caution patient to avoid exposure to people who have chickenpox or measles, as well as other contagious infections, throughout triamcinolone therapy and for 12 months afterward.

• Advise patient to have periodic eye examinations during long-term therapy because triamcinolone can cause glaucoma or ocular nerve damage.

triamterene
Dyrenium

Class and Category
Chemical class: Pterdine derivative
Therapeutic class: Diuretic
Pregnancy category: B

Indications and Dosages
➤ *To treat edema in cirrhosis, heart failure, and nephrotic syndrome*
CAPSULES
Adults. *Initial:* 25 to 100 mg daily. *Maximum:* 300 mg daily.

Mechanism of Action
Inhibits sodium reabsorption in distal convoluted tubules and cortical collecting ducts, causing sodium and water loss and enhancing potassium retention.

Route	Onset	Peak	Duration
P.O.	2–4 hr	1 to several days	7–9 hr

Contraindications
Anuria, diabetic nephropathy or renal disease linked to renal insufficiency, hyperkalemia (potassium level of 5.5 mEq/L or more), hypersensitivity to triamterene or its components, severe hepatic dysfunction

Interaction

DRUGS
ACE inhibitors, amiloride, angiotensin-II receptor antagonists, cyclosporine, heparin, potassium-containing drugs, potassium salts, potassium supplements, spironolactone: Increased risk of hyperkalemia
amantadine: Decreased amantadine clearance, possibly amantadine toxicity
antihypertensives: Increased antihypertensive effect
diuretics: Increased diuretic effect
folic acid: Possibly antagonized action of folic acid
indomethacin: Increased risk of renal impairment
lithium: Increased risk of lithium toxicity
NSAIDs: Decreased diuretic effect of triamterene, increased risk of hyperkalemia
oral antidiabetic drugs: Altered blood glucose control

Adverse Reactions
CNS: Dizziness, fatigue, headache, weakness
EENT: Dry mouth
ENDO: Hyperglycemia, hypoglycemia
GI: Diarrhea, nausea, vomiting
GU: Azotemia, elevated BUN and serum creatinine levels, renal calculi
SKIN: Jaundice, photosensitivity, rash

Nursing Considerations
• Be aware that triamterene shouldn't be given to patient with creatinine clearance below 10 ml/min/1.73 m^2 because this condition increases the risk of drug-induced hyperkalemia.
• Monitor serum potassium level during therapy, especially in patient with renal impairment or diabetes mellitus. Also monitor patient's BUN and serum creatinine levels to assess renal function and prevent hyperkalemia.
• Monitor patient for irregular heartbeat, which is usually the first sign of hyperkalemia.
• If you suspect hyperkalemia, obtain an ECG tracing, as ordered. A widened QRS complex or an arrhythmia requires prompt additional therapy.
• Monitor laboratory test results and watch for signs of metabolic or respiratory acidosis, which may occur suddenly in

patient with cardiac disease or uncontrolled diabetes mellitus.
• Monitor patient's serum uric acid and sodium levels, as ordered, because triamterene may reduce uric acid clearance and increase the risk of gout and hyperuricemia. This drug also may worsen preexisting hyponatremia.
• Monitor CBC with differential because drug may increase the risk of megalo-blastic anemia in patient with folic acid deficiency.

PATIENT TEACHING
• Advise patient to take triamterene with food or milk.
• Instruct patient to avoid exposure to excessive heat or sunlight to prevent dehydration and, possibly, photo-sensitivity.
• Explain to patient with a history of gout that drug may increase the risk of attack.
• Advise patient to notify prescriber about ineffective diuresis and unexplained weight gain during therapy.

triazolam

Alti-Triazolam (CAN), Apo-Triazo (CAN), Gen Triazolam (CAN), Halcion, Novo-Triolam (CAN)

Class, Category, and Schedule
Chemical class: Benzodiazepine
Therapeutic class: Sedative-hypnotic
Pregnancy category: X
Controlled substance schedule: IV

Indications and Dosages
➤ *To provide short-term management of insomnia*

TABLETS
Adults. 0.125 to 0.25 mg at bedtime. *Maximum:* 0.5 mg daily (for patients with inadequate response to usual dose).
DOSAGE ADJUSTMENT For elderly or debilitated patients, initial dosage reduced to 0.125 mg at bedtime and maximum dosage limited to 0.25 mg daily.

Route	Onset	Peak	Duration
P.O.	15–30 min	Unknown	Unknown

T

Mechanism of Action

Potentiates effects of the inhibitory neurotransmitter gamma-aminobutyric acid, which increases inhibition of the ascending reticular activating system and produces varying levels of CNS depression, including sedation, hypnosis, skeletal muscle relaxation, anticonvulsant activity, and coma.

Contraindications

Concurrent therapy with azoles such as fluconazole, itraconazole, ketoconazole, or nefazodone, and selected HIV protease inhibitors such as indinavir, lopinavir, nelfinavir, ritonavir, or saquinavir; hypersensitivity to triazolam, other benzodiazepines, or their components; pregnancy

Interaction

DRUGS

anxiolytics, barbiturates, brompheniramine, carbinoxamine, cetirizine, chlorpheniramine, clemastine, cyproheptadine, dimenhydrinate, diphenhydramine, doxylamine, general anesthetics, methdilazine, opioid analgesics, sedative-hypnotics, phenothiazines, promethazine, tramadol, tricyclic antidepressants, trimeprazine: Increased sedation, respiratory depression

azoles such as itraconazole, ketoconazole, or nefazodone; selected HIV protease inhibitors such as indinavir, lopinavir, nelfinavir, ritonavir, or saquinavir: Possibly increased plasma triazolam levels and increased risk of adverse reactions

cimetidine, diltiazem, disulfiram, erythromycin, probenecid, verapamil: Increased sedation

flumazenil: Increased risk of withdrawal symptoms

oral contraceptives: Increased blood triazolam level

FOODS

grapefruit juice: Increased blood triazolam level and sedation

ACTIVITIES

alcohol use: Increased sedation, respiratory depression

Adverse Reactions

CNS: Anxiety, ataxia, complex behaviors (such as sleep driving), confusion, depression, dizziness, drowsiness, fatigue, headache, insomnia, nightmares, syncope, talkativeness, tremor, vertigo

EENT: Throat tightness

GI: Nausea, vomiting

RESP: Dyspnea

Other: Anaphylaxis, angioedema, physical and psychological dependence

Nursing Considerations

• Be aware that triazolam shouldn't be discontinued abruptly, even after only 1 to 2 weeks of therapy. Doing so can cause withdrawal symptoms, including abdominal cramps, confusion, depression, diaphoresis, hyperacusis, insomnia, irritability, nausea, nervousness, paresthesia, perceptual disturbances, photophobia, tachycardia, tremor, and vomiting.

WARNING Assess patient for signs of physical and psychological dependence, and notify prescriber if they occur.

• Monitor patient's respiratory rate and depth and ABG results, as appropriate, because drug may worsen ventilatory failure in patient with pulmonary disease, such as severe COPD, respiratory depression, or sleep apnea. Use drug cautiously in patients with acute intermittent porphyria, myasthenia gravis, and severe renal impairment because it may aggravate these conditions.

• Take safety precautions for elderly patients because triazolam may impair cognitive and motor function and increase the risk for falls.

• Use drug cautiously in patients with advanced Parkinson's disease because it may worsen cognition, coordination, and psychosis.

WARNING Monitor patient closely for hypersensitivity reactions such as dyspnea, throat tightness, nausea, vomiting, and swelling. If present, stop triazolam immediately, notify prescriber, and provide supportive care.

PATIENT TEACHING

• Instruct patient to take triazolam exactly as prescribed and not to stop taking it abruptly because of the risk of having withdrawal symptoms.

• Instruct patient to stop taking triazolam and seek emergency care if she has trouble breathing, throat tightness, nausea, vomiting, or abnormal swelling.

- Advise patient that drug may cause abnormal behaviors during sleep, such as driving a car, eating, talking on the phone, or having sex without any recall of the event. If family notices any such behavior or patient sees evidence of such behavior upon awakening, the prescriber should be notified.
- Caution patient about possible drowsiness during therapy.
- Urge patient to avoid alcohol consumption because it increases drug's sedative effects and risk of abnormal behaviors, such as sleep driving.
- Advise patient to notify prescriber about excessive drowsiness, known or suspected pregnancy, and nausea.

trifluoperazine hydrochloride

Apo-Trifluoperazine (CAN), PMS-Trifluoperazine (CAN)

Class and Category
Chemical class: Piperazine phenothiazine
Therapeutic class: Antianxiety, antipsychotic
Pregnancy category: Not rated

Indications and Dosages
➤ *To treat psychotic disorders*
SYRUP, TABLETS
Adults and adolescents. *Initial:* 2 to 5 mg twice daily, increased gradually, as needed. *Maintenance:* 15 to 20 mg daily. *Maximum:* 40 mg daily.
Children age 6 and over. *Initial:* 1 mg daily or in divided doses twice daily, increased gradually, as needed.
I.M. INJECTION
Adults and adolescents. 1 to 2 mg every 4 to 6 hr, as needed. *Maximum:* 10 mg daily.
Children age 6 and over. 1 mg daily or in divided doses twice daily, as needed.
➤ *To relieve anxiety*
SYRUP, TABLETS, I.M. INJECTION
Adults and adolescents. *Initial:* 1 to 2 mg daily, increased gradually, as needed. *Maximum:* 6 mg daily for 12 wk.

Mechanism of Action
Blocks postsynaptic dopamine receptors, increasing dopamine turnover and decreasing dopamine neurotransmission. This action may depress the areas of the brain that control activity and aggression, including the cerebral cortex, hypothalamus, and limbic system. Trifluoperazine may relieve anxiety by indirectly reducing arousal and increasing the filtering of internal stimuli to the reticular activating system.

Contraindications
Blood dyscrasias; bone marrow depression; cerebral arteriosclerosis; coma; coronary artery disease; hepatic dysfunction; hypersensitivity to trifluoperazine, other phenothiazines, or their components; myeloproliferative disorders; severe hypertension or hypotension; significant CNS depression; subcortical brain damage; use of high doses of CNS depressants

Interaction
DRUGS
adsorbent antidiarrheals, aluminum- and magnesium-containing antacids: Possibly inhibited absorption of oral trifluoperazine
amantadine, anticholinergics, antidyskinetics, antihistamines: Possibly intensified adverse anticholinergic effects, increased risk of trifluoperazine-induced hyperpyrexia
amphetamines: Decreased stimulant effect of amphetamines, decreased antipsychotic effect of trifluoperazine
anticonvulsants: Lowered seizure threshold
antithyroid drugs: Increased risk of agranulocytosis
apomorphine: Possibly decreased emetic response to apomorphine, additive CNS depression
appetite suppressants: Decreased effects of appetite suppressants
astemizole, cisapride, disopyramide, erythromycin, pimozide, probucol, procainamide, quinidine: Prolonged QT interval, increased risk of ventricular tachycardia
beta blockers: Increased blood levels of both drugs, possibly leading to additive hypotensive effect, arrhythmias, irreversible retinopathy, and tardive dyskinesia
bromocriptine: Impaired therapeutic effects of bromocriptine

T

CNS depressants: Additive CNS depression
ephedrine, metaraminol: Decreased vasopressor response to ephedrine
epinephrine: Blocked alpha-adrenergic
effects of epinephrine
*extrapyramidal reaction–causing drugs
(droperidol, haloperidol, metoclopramide,
metyrosine, risperidone):* Increased severity
and frequency of extrapyramidal reactions
hepatotoxic drugs: Increased risk of hepatotoxicity
hypotension-producing drugs: Possibly
severe hypotension with syncope
levodopa: Decreased antidyskinetic effect of
levodopa
lithium: Reduced absorption of oral
trifluoperazine, possibly encephalopathy
and additive extrapyramidal effects
*MAO inhibitors, maprotiline, tricyclic
antidepressants:* Possibly prolonged and
intensified sedative and anticholinergic
effects, increased blood level of antidepressants, impaired trifluoperazine
metabolism, increased risk of neuroleptic
malignant syndrome
mephentermine: Decreased antipsychotic
effect of trifluoperazine and vasopressor
effect of mephentermine
methoxamine, phenylephrine: Decreased
vasopressor effect and shortened duration
of action of these drugs
metrizamide: Increased risk of seizures
opioid analgesics: Increased risk of CNS and
respiratory depression, orthostatic hypotension, severe constipation, and urine
retention
ototoxic drugs: Possibly masking of some
symptoms of ototoxicity, such as dizziness,
tinnitus, and vertigo
phenytoin: Lowered seizure threshold;
inhibited phenytoin metabolism, possibly
leading to phenytoin toxicity
photosensitizing drugs: Possibly additive
photosensitivity and intraocular photo-
chemical damage to choroid, lens, or retina
thiazide diuretics: Possibly hyponatremia
and water intoxication
ACTIVITIES
alcohol use: Increased CNS and respiratory
depression, increased hypotensive effect

Adverse Reactions

CNS: Akathisia, altered temperature
regulation, dizziness, drowsiness,
extrapyramidal reactions (dystonia,
pseudoparkinsonism, tardive dyskinesia)
CV: Hypotension, orthostatic hypotension,
tachycardia
EENT: Blurred vision, dry mouth, nasal
congestion, ocular changes (deposits of fine
particles in cornea and lens), pigmentary
retinopathy
ENDO: Galactorrhea, gynecomastia
GI: Constipation, epigastric pain, nausea,
vomiting
GU: Ejaculation disorders, menstrual
irregularities, urine retention
SKIN: Contact dermatitis, decreased
sweating, photosensitivity, pruritus, rash
Other: Injection-site irritation and sterile
abscess, weight gain

Nursing Considerations

WARNING Trifluoperazine shouldn't be
used to treat elderly patients with
dementia-related psychosis because drug
increases the risk of death in these
patients
• Use trifluoperazine cautiously in patients
with glaucoma because of drug's anticholinergic effect.
• Before administration, observe parenteral
solution, which may turn slightly yellow
without altering its potency. Don't use
solution if discoloration is pronounced or
precipitate is present.
• For I.M. administration, inject drug slowly
and deep into upper outer quadrant of the
buttocks. Keep patient in a supine position
for 30 minutes after injection to minimize
hypotensive effect.
• Rotate I.M. injection sites to avoid
irritation and sterile abscesses.
WARNING Watch closely for tardive
dyskinesia, which may continue after
treatment stops. Signs include uncontrolled movements of arms, body, cheeks,
jaw, legs, mouth, or tongue. Notify
prescriber if such signs occur.
• Closely monitor elderly patients and
severely ill or dehydrated children. They're
at increased risk for certain adverse CNS
reactions.
• To prevent contact dermatitis, avoid skin
contact with oral or injection solution.
PATIENT TEACHING
• Instruct patient to take trifluoperazine
exactly as prescribed and not to stop

taking drug abruptly or without consulting prescriber.
• Advise patient to take drug with food or a full glass of milk or water to minimize adverse GI reactions.
• Urge patient to consult prescriber before using other drugs because of possible interactions.
• Instruct patient to notify prescriber immediately if she experiences difficulty swallowing or speaking and her tongue protrudes from her mouth.
• Caution patient to avoid alcohol during therapy.
• Advise patient to avoid potentially hazardous activities until drug's CNS effects are known.
• Instruct patient to change position slowly to minimize effects of orthostatic hypotension.
• Urge patient to avoid exposure to the sun and extreme heat because drug may cause photosensitivity and interfere with thermoregulation. Encourage her to wear sunscreen when outdoors.

triflupromazine
Vesprin

Class and Category
Chemical class: Phenothiazine
Therapeutic class: Antiemetic, antipsychotic
Pregnancy category: Not rated

Indications and Dosages
➤ *To treat psychotic disorders*
I.M. INJECTION
Adults and adolescents. 60 mg, as needed. *Maximum:* 150 mg daily.
Children age 30 months and over. 0.2 to 0.25 mg/kg, as needed. *Maximum:* 10 mg daily.
➤ *To treat nausea and vomiting*
I.V. INJECTION
Adults. 1 mg, as needed. *Maximum:* 3 mg daily.
I.M. INJECTION
Adults and adolescents. 5 to 15 mg every 4 hr. *Maximum:* 60 mg daily.
Children age 30 months and over. 0.2 to 0.25 mg/kg, as needed. *Maximum:* 10 mg daily.

Mechanism of Action
Blocks postsynaptic dopamine receptors, increasing dopamine turnover and decreasing dopamine neurotransmission. This action may depress the areas of the brain that control activity and aggression, including the cerebral cortex, hypothalamus, and limbic system. Triflupromazine also prevents nausea and vomiting by inhibiting or blocking dopamine receptors in the medullary chemoreceptor trigger zone and, peripherally, by blocking the vagus nerve in the GI tract.

Contraindications
Blood dyscrasias, bone marrow depression, cerebral arteriosclerosis, coma or severe CNS depression, concurrent use of large amount of CNS depressants, coronary artery disease, hepatic dysfunction, hypersensitivity to phenothiazines, severe hypertension or hypotension, subcortical brain damage

Interaction
DRUGS
amantadine, anticholinergics, antidyskinetics, antihistamines: Possibly intensified adverse anticholinergic effects and increased risk of triflupromazine-induced hyperpyrexia
amphetamines: Decreased stimulant effect of amphetamines, decreased antipsychotic effect of triflupromazine
anticonvulsants: Lowered seizure threshold
antithyroid drugs: Increased risk of agranulocytosis
apomorphine: Possibly decreased emetic response to apomorphine, additive CNS depression
appetite suppressants: Decreased anorectic effect of appetite suppressants
astemizole, cisapride, disopyramide, erythromycin, pimozide, probucol, procainamide, quinidine: Prolonged QT interval, increased risk of ventricular tachycardia
beta blockers: Increased blood levels of both drugs, possibly leading to additive hypotensive effect, arrhythmias, irreversible retinopathy, and tardive dyskinesia
bromocriptine: Impaired therapeutic effects of bromocriptine
CNS depressants: Additive CNS depressant effects

T

ephedrine: Decreased vasopressor response to ephedrine
epinephrine: Blocked alpha-adrenergic effects of epinephrine
extrapyramidal reaction–causing drugs (droperidol, haloperidol, metoclopramide, metyrosine, risperidone): Increased severity and frequency of extrapyramidal reactions
hepatotoxic drugs: Increased risk of hepatotoxicity
hypotension-producing drugs: Possibly severe hypotension with syncope
levodopa: Decreased antidyskinetic effect of levodopa
lithium: Possibly encephalopathy and additive extrapyramidal effects
MAO inhibitors, maprotiline, tricyclic antidepressants: Increased CNS depression, impaired triflupromazine metabolism, increased risk of neuroleptic malignant syndrome
mephentermine: Possibly antagonized antipsychotic effect of triflupromazine and vasopressor effect of mephentermine
metaraminol: Decreased vasopressor effect of metaraminol
methoxamine, phenylephrine: Decreased vasopressor effect and shortened duration of action of these drugs
metrizamide: Increased risk of seizures
opioid analgesics: Increased risk of CNS and respiratory depression, orthostatic hypotension, severe constipation, and urine retention
ototoxic drugs: Possibly masking of some symptoms of ototoxicity, such as dizziness, tinnitus, and vertigo
phenytoin: Lowered seizure threshold; inhibited phenytoin metabolism, possibly leading to phenytoin toxicity
photosensitizing drugs: Possibly additive photosensitivity and intraocular photo-chemical damage to choroid, lens, or retina
thiazide diuretics: Possibly hyponatremia and water intoxication
ACTIVITIES
alcohol use: Increased CNS and respiratory depression, increased hypotensive effect

Adverse Reactions

CNS: Akathisia, altered temperature regulation, dizziness, drowsiness, extrapyramidal reactions (dystonia, pseudoparkinsonism, tardive dyskinesia)
CV: Hypotension, orthostatic hypotension, tachycardia
EENT: Blurred vision, dry mouth, nasal congestion, ocular changes (deposits of fine particles in cornea and lens), pigmentary retinopathy
ENDO: Galactorrhea, gynecomastia
GI: Constipation, epigastric pain, nausea, vomiting
GU: Ejaculation disorders, menstrual irregularities, urine retention
SKIN: Decreased sweating, photosensitivity, pruritus, rash
Other: Injection-site irritation and sterile abscess, weight gain

Nursing Considerations

• Use triflupromazine cautiously in patients with glaucoma because of drug's anti-cholinergic effects.
• Before administration, observe parenteral solution, which may turn slightly yellow without altering potency. Don't use solution if discoloration is pronounced or precipitate is present.
• Don't let solution come in contact with your skin because contact dermatitis may occur.
• For I.M. administration, slowly inject triflupromazine deep into upper outer quadrant of buttocks. Keep patient supine for 30 minutes afterward to minimize hypotensive effect.
• Rotate I.M. injection sites to avoid irritation and sterile abscesses.
WARNING Watch closely for tardive dyskinesia, which may continue after treatment stops. Signs include uncontrolled movements of arms, body, cheeks, jaw, legs, mouth, or tongue. Notify prescriber if such signs occur.
• Closely monitor elderly patients and severely ill or dehydrated children. They're at increased risk for certain adverse CNS reactions.
PATIENT TEACHING
• Instruct patient to change position slowly to minimize effects of orthostatic hypotension.
• Urge patient to avoid potentially hazardous activities until triflupromazine's CNS effects are known.
• Instruct patient to notify prescriber immediately if she experiences difficulty

swallowing or speaking and her tongue protrudes from her mouth.
• Caution patient to avoid alcohol during therapy.
• Urge patient to avoid exposure to the sun and extreme heat because drug may cause photosensitivity and interfere with thermoregulation. Encourage her to wear sunscreen when outdoors.

trihexyphenidyl hydrochloride

Apo-Trihex (CAN), Artane, PMS Trihexyphenidyl (CAN), Trihexane, Trihexy

Class and Category
Chemical class: Tertiary amine
Therapeutic class: Antidyskinetic
Pregnancy category: C

Indications and Dosages
➤ *To treat parkinsonism*
ELIXIR, TABLETS
Adults. *Initial:* 1 to 2 mg on day 1, divided into 3 equal doses and given with meals. Total daily dose increased by 2 mg every 3 to 5 days until desired response or maximum dose is reached. *Maximum:* 15 mg daily.
E.R. CAPSULES
Adults. 5 mg after breakfast; additional 5 mg 12 hr later, as needed. *Maximum:* 15 mg daily.
➤ *To treat drug-induced extrapyramidal symptoms*
TABLETS
Adults. 1 mg daily, increased to 5 to 15 mg/day, as needed, to control symptoms.

Route	Onset	Peak	Duration
P.O.	1 hr	Unknown	6–12 hr

Mechanism of Action
Blocks acetylcholine's action at cholinergic receptor sites, which restores normal dopamine and acetylcholine balance in the brain, relaxing muscle movement and decreasing drooling, rigidity, and tremor. Drug also may inhibit reuptake and storage of dopamine, prolonging its action.

Contraindications
Achalasia, bladder neck or prostatic obstruction, narrow-angle glaucoma, hypersensitivity to trihexyphenidyl or its components, megacolon, myasthenia gravis, pyloric or duodenal obstruction, stenosing peptic ulcer

Interaction
DRUGS
amantadine, anticholinergics, MAO inhibitors, tricyclic antidepressants: Increased anticholinergic effects
antidiarrheals (adsorbent): Possibly decreased therapeutic effects of trihexyphenidyl
chlorpromazine: Decreased blood chlorpromazine level
CNS depressants: Increased sedative effect
levodopa: Increased efficacy of levodopa
ACTIVITIES
alcohol use: Increased sedation

Adverse Reactions
CNS: Confusion, dizziness, drowsiness, nervousness
EENT: Blurred vision; dry eyes, mouth, nose, or throat; mydriasis
GI: Constipation, nausea, vomiting
GU: Dysuria, urine retention
SKIN: Decreased sweating

Nursing Considerations
• Use trihexyphenidyl cautiously in patients with cardiovascular, hepatic, or renal disorders. Patients with cardiovascular disorders, such as atherosclerosis, hypertension, and ischemic heart disease, are at risk for tachycardia and coronary ischemia from drug's positive chronotropic effects. Hepatic and renal dysfunction increase the risk of adverse reactions.
• Before therapy begins, assess patient's muscle rigidity and tremor to establish a baseline. During therapy, reassess patient to detect improvement in these signs and evaluate drug effectiveness.
• Obtain patient's intraocular pressure before and periodically during trihexyphenidyl therapy, as ordered, because drug can precipitate incipient glaucoma.
PATIENT TEACHING
• Instruct patient to take trihexyphenidyl after meals.

• Teach patient not to break or chew E.R. capsules.
• Instruct patient to use calibrated device to measure elixir.
• Advise patient to avoid potentially hazardous activities until drug's CNS effects are known.
• Advise patient with dry eyes or increased contact lens awareness to use lubricating drops or stop wearing contact lenses during drug therapy.
• Caution patient being treated for parkinsonism not to stop taking trihexyphenidyl suddenly because doing so may worsen symptoms.
• Advise patient to maintain adequate hydration and avoid exercising during hot weather because trihexyphenidyl increases the risk of heatstroke.

trimethobenzamide hydrochloride

Benzacot, Tebamide, Tigan, Tribenzagan, Trimazide

Class and Category

Chemical class: Ethanolamine derivative
Therapeutic class: Antiemetic
Pregnancy category: Not rated

Indications and Dosages

➤ *To treat nausea and vomiting*

CAPSULES

Adults and adolescents. 250 mg every 6 to 8 hr, as needed.
Children weighing 15 to 45 kg (33 to 99 lb). 100 to 200 mg every 6 to 8 hr, as needed.

I.M. INJECTION

Adults and adolescents. 200 mg every 6 to 8 hr, as needed.

DOSAGE ADJUSTMENT For patient with renal impairment, dosage decreased or dose interval lengthened.

Mechanism of Action

Prevents or stops nausea and vomiting by blocking dopamine receptors and emetic impulses at the chemoreceptor trigger zone in the brain.

Contraindications

Children (I.M.); hypersensitivity to trimetho-benzamide, benzocaine, or any of their components

Interaction

DRUGS

apomorphine: Decreased emetic response to apomorphine, increased CNS effects
barbiturates, belladonna alkaloids, phenothiazines: Increased risk of coma, extrapyramidal reactions, opisthotonos, and seizures
CNS depressants: Possibly enhanced effects of both drugs
ototoxic drugs: Possibly masked signs of ototoxicity

Adverse Reactions

CNS: Dizziness, drowsiness, headache
EENT: Blurred vision
GI: Diarrhea
MS: Muscle cramps
Other: Injection-site burning, irritation, pain, redness, or swelling

Nursing Considerations

• Use trimethobenzamide cautiously in dehydrated patients and those with an electrolyte imbalance, encephalitis, encephalopathy, gastroenteritis, or high fever.
• Be aware that trimethobenzamide shouldn't be used in children who have viral illnesses because they're at increased risk for Reye's syndrome, characterized by abrupt onset of irrational behavior; lethargy; persistent, severe vomiting; progressive encephalopathy leading to coma, seizures, and possibly death.
• To minimize injection-site irritation, inject trimethobenzamide deep into a large muscle mass using the Z-track technique, which blocks solution from escaping along the injection route.

PATIENT TEACHING

• Inform patient that drug may cause blurred vision, dizziness, and drowsiness. Advise her to avoid hazardous activities until drug's CNS effects are known.
• Inform patient's parents or caregivers that trimethobenzamide may cause Reye's syndrome, and urge them to notify prescriber immediately if they notice

decreased level of consciousness, irrational behavior, lethargy, or severe vomiting.

trimethoprim
Proloprim, Trimpex

Class and Category
Chemical class: Dihydrofolic acid analogue
Therapeutic class: Antibiotic
Pregnancy category: C

Indications and Dosages
➤ *To treat UTI caused by* Enterobacter species, Escherichia coli, Klebsiella pneumoniae, Proteus mirabilis, *or coagulase-negative staphylococci, including* Staphylococcus saprophyticus

TABLETS
Adults and children age 12 and over. 100 mg every 12 hr or 200 mg daily for 10 days.
DOSAGE ADJUSTMENT For patients with creatinine clearance of 15 to 30 ml/min/1.73 m², dosage usually reduced by 50%.

Mechanism of Action
Inhibits formation of tetrahydrofolic acid, the metabolically active form of folic acid, in susceptible bacteria. This depletes folate, an essential component of bacterial development, thereby disrupting production of bacterial nucleic acid and protein.

Contraindications
Hypersensitivity to trimethoprim or its components, megaloblastic anemia from folate deficiency, severe renal impairment (creatinine clearance less than 15 ml/min/1.73 m²)

Interaction
DRUGS
bone marrow depressants: Increased risk of leukopenia, thrombocytopenia
cyclosporine: Increased risk of nephrotoxicity
dapsone: Increased blood levels and risk of adverse effects (especially methemoglobinemia) of both drugs
folate antagonists: Increased risk of megaloblastic anemia
phenytoin: Decreased phenytoin metabolism, increased risk of phenytoin toxicity

procainamide: Increased blood levels of procainamide and its metabolite, N-acetylprocainamide
rifampin: Increased elimination and decreased effectiveness of trimethoprim
warfarin: Increased anticoagulant activity of warfarin

Adverse Reactions
CNS: Fever, headache
EENT: Glossitis
GI: Abdominal pain, anorexia, diarrhea, elevated liver function test results, epigastric pain, nausea, vomiting
GU: Elevated BUN and serum creatinine levels
HEME: Leukopenia, megaloblastic anemia, methemoglobinemia, neutropenia, thrombocytopenia
SKIN: Exfoliative dermatitis, pruritus, rash

Nursing Considerations
• Obtain urine specimen, as ordered, before trimethoprim therapy starts.
• Give drug on an empty stomach to enhance absorption.
• Evaluate patient's test values for folic acid deficiency and signs of bone marrow depression.
• Monitor serum potassium level and renal function studies, as ordered, in patients with decreased renal function because these patients are at increased risk for hyperkalemia and toxic reactions when receiving trimethoprim.

PATIENT TEACHING
• Instruct patient to complete entire course of trimethoprim therapy, as prescribed, even if she feels better beforehand.
• Advise patient to take drug with food or milk if GI distress occurs.
• Instruct patient to notify prescriber if she experiences rash, severe fatigue, sore throat, or unusual bleeding or bruising.

trimipramine maleate
Apo-Trimip (CAN), Novo-Tripramine (CAN), Rhotrimine (CAN), Surmontil

Class and Category

Chemical class: Dibenzazepine derivative
Therapeutic class: Antidepressant
Pregnancy category: C

Indications and Dosages

➤ *To treat depression*

CAPSULES

Adults in inpatient settings. *Initial:* 100 mg daily in divided doses, increased gradually in a few days to 200 mg daily. *Maximum:* 300 mg daily in 2 to 3 wk.

Adolescents in inpatient settings. *Initial:* 50 mg daily in divided doses, increased, as needed. *Maximum:* 100 mg daily.

Adults in outpatient settings. *Initial:* 75 mg/day in divided doses, increased gradually up to 150 mg daily, as needed. *Maintenance:* 50 to 150 mg daily. *Maximum:* 200 mg daily.

Adolescents in outpatient settings. *Initial:* 50 mg daily in divided doses, increased, as needed. *Maximum:* 100 mg daily.

DOSAGE ADJUSTMENT For elderly patients, initial dosage reduced to 50 mg daily in divided doses, and maximum dosage limited to 100 mg daily.

Route	Onset	Peak	Duration
P.O.	2–3 wk	Unknown	Unknown

Mechanism of Action

Inhibits the reuptake of norepinephrine at presynaptic neurons, thus increasing its concentration in synapses. This action may elevate mood and relieve depression.

Contraindications

Hypersensitivity to trimipramine, other dibenzazepine tricyclic antidepressants, or their components; recovery period after an MI; use within 14 days of an MAO inhibitor, including intravenous methylene blue or linezolid

Interaction

DRUGS

amantadine, anticholinergics, antidyskinetics, antihistamines: Increased anticholinergic effects (confusion, hallucinations, nightmares)
anticonvulsants: Increased CNS depression, lowered seizure threshold (high trimipramine doses), decreased anticonvulsant effect

antithyroid drugs: Risk of agranulocytosis
barbiturates, carbamazepine: Decreased blood level and effects of trimipramine
bupropion, clozapine, cyclobenzaprine, haloperidol, loxapine, maprotiline, molindone, phenothiazines, thioxanthenes: Increased and prolonged sedative and anticholinergic effects of both drugs, increased risk of seizures
cimetidine: Decreased trimipramine metabolism, possibly leading to trimipramine toxicity
clonidine: Decreased hypotensive effect and increased CNS depressant effect of clonidine
CNS depressants: Increased hypotension and CNS and respiratory depression
disulfiram, etchlorvynol: Transient delirium, risk of CNS depression (ethchlorvynol)
fluoxetine: Increased trimipramine level
guanadrel, guanethidine: Decreased hypotensive effect
MAO inhibitors, including intravenous methylene blue or linezolid; serotonergic drugs such as buspirone, fentanyl, lithium, St. John's wort, tramadol, tricyclic antidepressants, triptans: Increased risk of serotonin syndrome, possibly resulting in death, hyperpryrexia, hypertensive crisis, or severe seizures
methylphenidate: Decreased methylphenidate effects, increased blood trimipramine level
metrizamide: Increased risk of seizures
naphazoline (ophthalmic), oxymetazoline (nasal or ophthalmic), phenylephrine (nasal or ophthalmic), xylometazoline (nasal): Increased vasopressor effect of these drugs
oral anticoagulants: Increased anticoagulation
phenothiazines: Increased blood trimipramine level, decreased phenothiazine metabolism
pimozide, probucol: Increased risk of arrhythmias, possibly prolonged QT interval
sympathomimetics: Increased risk of arrhythmias, hyperpyrexia, severe hypertension
thyroid hormones: Increased therapeutic and toxic effects of both drugs

ACTIVITIES

alcohol use: Increased hypotension and CNS and respiratory depression

Adverse Reactions

CNS: Anxiety, ataxia, confusion, delirium, dizziness, drowsiness, excitement, extrapyramidal reactions, hallucinations, headache, insomnia, nervousness, nightmares, parkinsonism, seizures, serotonin syndrome, stroke, suicidal ideation, tremor
CV: Arrhythmias, orthostatic hypotension
EENT: Angle closure glaucoma, blurred vision, dry mouth, increased intraocular pressure, taste perversion, tinnitus, tongue swelling
ENDO: Gynecomastia, syndrome of inappropriate ADH secretion
GI: Constipation, diarrhea, heartburn, ileus, increased appetite, nausea, vomiting
GU: Sexual dysfunction, testicular swelling, urine retention
HEME: Agranulocytosis, bone marrow depression
RESP: Wheezing
SKIN: Alopecia, diaphoresis, jaundice, photosensitivity, pruritus, rash, urticaria
Other: Facial edema, weight gain

Nursing Considerations

• Watch patient closely for suicidal tendencies, especially when therapy starts or dosage changes and particularly if patient is a child, teenager, or young adult.
WARNING Monitor patient closely for serotonin syndrome exhibited by agitation, hallucinations, coma, tachycardia, labile blood pressure, hyperthermia, hyperreflexia, incoordination, nausea, vomiting, or diarrhea. Notify prescriber immediately because serotonin syndrome may be life-threatening, and provide supportive care.
• Expect to reduce trimipramine dosage gradually, as prescribed, before electroconvulsive therapy.

PATIENT TEACHING
• Instruct patient to take the last dose early in the evening to avoid insomnia.
• Advise patient that drug may cause mild pupillary dilation, which may lead to an episode of acute closure glaucoma. Encourage patient to have an eye exam before starting therapy to see if he is at risk.
• Advise patient to avoid hazardous activities until drug's CNS effects are known.

• Urge patient to change position slowly to minimize orthostatic hypotension.
• Urge patient to avoid alcohol during therapy.
• Advise patient to avoid exposure to excessive sunlight and to wear sunscreen when she's outdoors.
• Instruct patient to notify prescriber about the development of unusual bruising and signs of infection.
• Suggest that patient use sugarless gum or hard candy to relieve dry mouth.
• Caution patient to alert all prescribers about trimipramine therapy because of potentially serious drug interactions.
WARNING Urge parents to watch their child or adolescent closely for abnormal behavior, increased aggression or hostility, or suicidal tendencies, especially when therapy starts or dosage is adjusted. Stress need to notify prescriber about changes.

tromethamine

Tham

Class and Category

Chemical class: Organic amine
Therapeutic class: Alkalinizer
Pregnancy category: C

Indications and Dosages

➤ *To treat metabolic acidosis associated with cardiac arrest*

I.V. INFUSION
Adults and children. 3.6 to 10.8 g (111 to 333 ml) of 0.3 M solution.

I.V. INJECTION
Adults and children. If chest is opened, 2 to 6 g injected directly into open ventricular cavity.

➤ *To treat metabolic acidosis during cardiac bypass surgery*

I.V. INFUSION
Adults and children. 9 ml (2.7 mEq or 0.32 g) of 0.3 M solution/kg as a single dose. *Usual:* 500 ml (150 mEq or 18 g) infused over 1 hr. *Maximum:* 500 mg/kg over 1 hr.

Mechanism of Action

Combines with hydrogen ions and their associated acid anions, including lactic, pyruvic, and carbonic acid, to form salts

T

that are excreted in urine. Tromethamine exerts additional alkalinizing effects by acting as an osmotic diuretic, promoting the excretion of alkaline urine that contains increased amounts of carbon dioxide and electrolytes.

Contraindications
Anuria, chronic respiratory acidosis, hypersensitivity to tromethamine or its components, uremia

Interaction
DRUGS
amphetamines, quinidine, other pH-dependent drugs: Altered excretion of these drugs

Adverse Reactions
CNS: Fever
CV: Vasospasm
ENDO: Hypoglycemia
GI: Hepatic necrosis (hemorrhagic)
RESP: Respiratory depression
Other: Hypervolemia; infusion-site infection, phlebitis, or venous thrombosis; metabolic alkalosis

Nursing Considerations
• Evaluate blood pH, blood glucose, and serum bicarbonate and electrolyte levels, and partial pressure of arterial carbon dioxide before, during, and after tromethamine therapy, as ordered.
• Be aware that, except in life-threatening situations, tromethamine therapy is limited to no more than 1 day because of the risk of alkalosis.
WARNING Be aware that exceeding the recommended dosage can cause alkalosis, respiratory depression, and reduced carbon dioxide level.
• Expect I.V. tromethamine administration to increase the risk of hypervolemia and pulmonary edema.
• Assess the infusion site often for infiltration, which may cause inflammation, necrosis, thrombosis, tissue sloughing, and vasospasm.
• Be aware that patients with renal failure have an increased risk of developing hyperkalemia. For such patients, be prepared to monitor ECG continuously and assess serum potassium level frequently.
• Monitor patient's blood glucose level often during and after therapy because rapid

delivery can cause hypoglycemia for several hours.
PATIENT TEACHING
• Inform family members that patient's vital signs and laboratory test results will be measured frequently to monitor her progress.

trospium chloride
Sanctura, Sanctura XR

Class and Category
Chemical class: Quaternary ammonium compound
Therapeutic class: Bladder antispasmodic
Pregnancy category: C

Indications and Dosages
➤ *To treat overactive bladder with symptoms of urge urinary incontinence, urgency, and urinary frequency*
TABLETS
Adults. 20 mg twice daily 1 hr before meals or on empty stomach.
DOSAGE ADJUSTMENT For patients with severe renal insufficiency (creatinine clearance less than 30 ml/min/1.73 m²) and patients age 75 or over, dosage reduced to 20 mg daily at bedtime.
E.R. TABLETS
Adults. 60 mg daily in the morning, 1 hr before a meal or on empty stomach.

Route	Onset	Peak	Duration
P.O.	Unknown	5–6 hr	Unknown

Mechanism of Action
Antagonizes the effect of acetylcholine on muscarinic receptors in the bladder. Trospium's parasympatholytic action reduces the tonus of smooth muscle in the bladder. These actions increase maximum cystometric bladder capacity and volume with the first detrusor contraction, which relieves the sensation of urgency and frequency and enhances bladder control.

Contraindications
Gastric retention, hypersensitivity to trospium or its components, uncontrolled angle-closure glaucoma, urine retention

Interaction

DRUGS

anticholinergics: Increased frequency or severity of adverse effects; possibly reduced absorption of trospium

digoxin, metformin, morphine, pancuronium, procainamide: Possibly increased plasma concentration of trospium, digoxin, metformin, morphine, pancuronium, procainamide

ACTIVITIES

alcohol use: Possibly increased drowsiness

Adverse Reactions

CNS: Confusion, delirium, dizziness, drowsiness, fatigue, fever, hallucinations, headache, insomnia, light-headedness, syncope

CV: Chest pain, hypertensive crisis, palpitations, tachycardia

EENT: Blurred vision; dry eyes, mouth, or throat; visual abnormalities

GI: Abdominal distention or pain, constipation, flatulence, gastritis, indigestion, vomiting

GU: Urine retention

MS: Rhabdomyolysis

SKIN: Decreased sweating, dry skin, flushing, rash, Stevens-Johnson syndrome

Other: Anaphylaxis, angioedema

Nursing Considerations

• Use trospium cautiously in patients with ulcerative colitis, intestinal atony, or myasthenia gravis because drug may decrease GI motility; patients with significant bladder outflow obstruction because drug may cause urine retention; patients with hepatic impairment because drug's effects on the liver are unknown; and patients with renal impairment because drug excretion may be impaired.

• Monitor elderly patients carefully, especially those age 75 or over, for adverse reactions because elderly patients have an increased risk of trospium-induced adverse reactions.

• Monitor patient for anticholinergic central nervous system adverse effects such as dizziness, confusion, hallucinations and somnolence. If present, notify prescriber and expect a dose reduction or drug to be discontinued.

PATIENT TEACHING

• Instruct patient to take trospium on an empty stomach or at least 1 hour before eating because food delays its absorption.

• Caution patient to avoid performing activities in a warm or hot environment because sweating may be delayed, which could cause a sudden increase in body temperature and heatstroke.

• Advise patient to avoid hazardous activities until drug's CNS effects are known.

• Inform patient that alcohol may increase the risk of drowsiness; urge patient to limit or abstain from alcoholic beverages while taking trospium.

• Emphasize importance of reporting allergic reactions, including swelling of her face, lips, throat, or tongue; stopping trospium therapy; and seeking emergency medical care immediately.

• Advise patient to notify prescriber if he develops dizziness, confusion, hallucinations, or somnolence, as dosage may need to be altered or drug discontinued.

tubocurarine chloride

Class and Category

Chemical class: Isoquinoline derivative
Therapeutic class: Anticonvulsant
Pregnancy category: C

Indications and Dosages

➤ *To manage muscle contractions of seizures associated with electroshock therapy*

I.V. INJECTION

Adults. 157 mcg/kg (0.157 mg/kg) over 30 to 90 sec, given just before electroshock therapy. Expect initial dose to be 3 mg less than calculated total dose.

➤ *To produce skeletal muscle paralysis during anesthesia*

I.V. OR I.M. INJECTION

Adults. *Initial:* 6 to 9 mg. *Maintenance:* 3 to 4.5 mg in 3 to 5 min, as needed. For prolonged procedures, 3-mg supplemental doses given.

T

Infants and children. 500 mcg/kg I.V.
Neonates. *Initial:* 250 to 500 mcg/kg I.V.
Maintenance: One-fifth to one-sixth of
initial dose, as needed.
➤ *To facilitate endotracheal intubation
   and aid controlled respiration during
   mechanical ventilation*
I.V. INJECTION
Adults. *Initial:* 16.5 mcg/kg. *Maintenance:*
Dosage individualized based on patient
response.
➤ *To aid in the diagnosis of myasthenia
   gravis*
I.V. INJECTION
Adults. 4 to 33 mcg/kg. After 2 to 3 min,
1.5 mg of neostigmine is given I.V. to
terminate the test.

Route	Onset	Peak	Duration
I.V.	1 min	2–5 min	20–40 min

Incompatibilities
Don't mix tubocurarine with barbiturates,
such as methohexital or thiopental, because
a precipitate may form.

Contraindications
Hypersensitivity to tubocurarine or its
components, in patients for whom
histamine release may be dangerous

Interaction
DRUGS
alfentanil, fentanyl, sufentanil: Prevented or
reversed muscle rigidity from these drugs
*aminoglycosides, anesthetics, capreomycin,
citrate-anticoagulated blood, clindamycin,
lidocaine (I.V.), lincomycin, polymyxins,
procaine (I.V.), trimethaphan:* Additive
neuromuscular blocking effects
beta blockers, calcium salts: Prolonged and
enhanced effects of tubocurarine
magnesium salts, procainamide, quinidine:
Enhanced blockade effects

Mechanism of Action
Tubocurarine reduces the intensity of
skeletal muscle contractions caused
byelectrically induced seizures. Normally,
when a nerve impulse arrives at a
somaticmotor nerve terminal, it triggers
acetylcholine (ACh) stored in synaptic
vesicles to be released into the neuromuscular junction. The released ACh
binds with nicotinic receptors embedded
in the skeletal muscle motor endplate, as
shown below left, triggering muscle cell
depolarization and contraction.

Tubocurarine is a nondepolarizing
neuromuscular blocker that acts as a
competitiveantagonist of ACh. By binding
to the nicotinic receptors, as shown below
right, it prevents transmission of the action
potential at the neuromuscular junction,
thereby sustaining skeletal muscle
relaxation and eliminating the peripheral
muscular manifestations of seizures. The
drug has no effect on the CNS processes
involved with seizures because it doesn't
cross the blood-brain barrier.

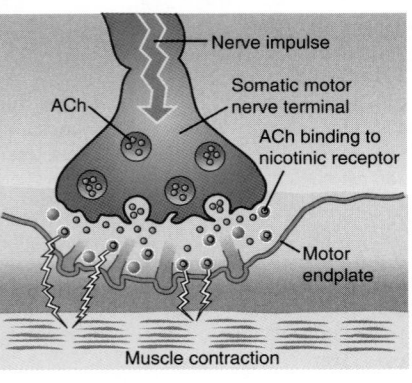

Nerve impulse
Somatic motor
nerve terminal
ACh
ACh binding to
nicotinic receptor
Motor
endplate
Muscle contraction

Tubocurarine
binding to
nicotinic receptor
Muscle relaxation

opioid analgesics: Additive histamine release effects, additive respiratory depressant effects, worsened bradycardia and hypotension

Adverse Reactions

CV: Arrhythmias, bradycardia, edema, hypotension, shock, tachycardia
RESP: Bronchospasm
SKIN: Erythema, flushing, itching, rash
Other: Anaphylaxis

Nursing Considerations

• If patient has a history of CV disease or is hypotensive, monitor her for further decrease in blood pressure.

• Monitor patient for bronchospasm and hypotension because tubocurarine may cause increased histamine release.

• Keep emergency equipment and drugs readily available in case respiratory depression occurs.

PATIENT TEACHING

• Explain the need for frequent hemodynamic monitoring.

U V W

umeclidinium

Incruse Ellipta

Class and Category

Chemical class: Quaternary ammonium bromide compound
Therapeutic class: Bronchodilator
Pregnancy category: C

Indications and Dosages

➤ *To provide long-term maintenance treatment of airflow obstruction in chronic obstructive pulmonary disease (COPD), including chronic bronchitis and/or emphysema*

ORAL INHALATION

Adults. 62.5 mcg (1 inhalation) daily. *Maximum:* 62.5 mcg in a 24-hour period.

Mechanism of Action

Inhibits the muscarinic M_3 receptor in smooth muscle to cause bronchodilation.

Contraindications

Hypersensitivity to umeclidinium or its components, severe hypersensitivity to milk proteins

Interaction

DRUGS

anticholinergics: Possibly additive effects

Adverse Reactions

CNS: Depression, dizziness, headache, vertigo
CV: Atrial fibrillation, idioventricular rhythm, supraventricular extrasystole, tachycardia
EENT: Nasopharyngitis, pharyngitis, rhinitis, worsening of narrow-angle glaucoma
GI: Abdominal pain (upper), diarrhea, dyspepsia, nausea
GU: UTI, worsening of urinary retention
MS: Arthralgia; back, extremity, or neck pain; myalgia
RESP: Cough, paradoxical bronchospasm, respiratory tract infection
SKIN: Rash
Other: Anaphylaxis

Nursing Considerations

• Know that umeclidinium should not be initiated in patients who are experiencing a rapidly deteriorating or potentially life-threatening episode of COPD.
• Do not administer umeclidinium for relief of acute symptoms. Drug is not a rescue inhaler. Instead, acute symptoms should be treated with an inhaled, short-acting $beta_2$-agonist, as ordered.
• Know that patients with a severe milk protein allergy should not receive umeclidinium therapy.
• Use with caution in patients with narrow-angle glaucoma or urinary retention because these conditions may worsen with umeclidinium therapy.

WARNING Monitor patient's respiratory status for paradoxical bronchospasm. Because of its life-threatening nature, notify prescriber immediately, withhold umeclidinium, and prepare to treat patient with an inhaled, short-acting bronchodilator, as ordered. If bronchospasm develops during umeclidinium therapy, expect drug to be permanently discontinued.

PATIENT TEACHING

• Tell patient to take umeclidinium at about the same time every day and not to use more than once in a 24-hour period.
• Teach patient how to use the inhaler.
• Urge patient to notify prescriber if her symptoms worsen, if umeclidinium becomes less effective, or if she needs more inhalations of her prescribed short-acting $beta_2$-agonist than usual. This may indicate that patient's condition is worsening.
• Tell patient to notify prescriber immediately if she develops eye pain or discomfort, blurred vision, visual halos, or colored images in association with red eyes.
• Advise patient to notify prescriber immediately if she develops any difficulty passing urine or painful urination, especially if she has a bladder-neck obstruction or if, in a male patient, prostatic hyperplasia is present.

urea
(carbamide)
Ureaphil

Class and Category
Chemical class: Carbonic acid diamide salt
Therapeutic class: Antiglaucoma, diuretic
Pregnancy category: C

Indications and Dosages
➤ *To reduce cerebral edema and intra-cranial pressure*
I.V. INFUSION
Adults and children age 2 and over.
500 mg to 1.5 g/kg as 30% solution in D$_5$W, D$_{10}$W, or 10% invert sugar solution infused over 30 min to 2 hr at 4 or 6 ml/min, according to manufacturer's instructions. *Maximum:* 2 g/kg daily.
Children under age 2. 100 mg to 1.5 g/kg as 30% solution in D$_5$W, D$_{10}$W, or 10% invert sugar solution infused over 30 min to 2 hr at 4 or 6 ml/min, according to manufacturer's instructions.
➤ *To treat malignant or secondary glaucoma*
I.V. INFUSION
Adults. 500 mg to 1.5 g/kg as 30% solution in D$_5$W, D$_{10}$W, or 10% invert sugar solution infused over 30 min to 2 hr at 4 or 6 ml/min, according to manufacturer's instructions. *Maximum:* 2 g/kg daily.
DOSAGE ADJUSTMENT Dosage reduced or drug withheld for patients with renal impairment if BUN level rises to 75 mg/dl or more or if diuresis fails to occur within 2 hr after administration.

Mechanism of Action
Elevates blood plasma osmolality, creating an osmotic effect that increases movement of water from the brain, CSF, and anterior portion of the eyes into interstitial fluid and plasma. This action reduces cerebral edema, intracranial pressure, CSF volume, and intraocular pressure. Large doses inhibit reabsorption of water and solutes in the renal tubules and induce diuresis by affecting the osmotic pressure gradient of the glomerular filtrate.

Route	Onset	Peak	Duration
I.V.	10 min	1–2 hr	3–10 hr*

Contraindications
Active intracranial bleeding, hepatic failure, hypersensitivity to urea or its components, renal impairment, severe dehydration

Interactions
DRUGS
carbonic anhydrase inhibitors, other diuretics: Additive diuretic and intraocular pressure–reducing effects
lithium: Increased renal excretion of lithium

Adverse Reactions
CNS: Agitation, confusion, fever, headache, hyperthermia, nervousness, subarachnoid hemorrhage, subdural hematoma, syncope
CV: Tachycardia
EENT: Dry mouth, intraocular hemorrhage
GI: Nausea, thirst, vomiting
GU: Elevated BUN level
HEME: Hemolysis
SKIN: Blemishes, extravasation with tissue necrosis and sloughing
Other: Dehydration, hypokalemia, hyponatremia, infusion-site phlebitis or thrombosis

Nursing Considerations
• For maximum reduction of intracranial or intraocular pressure, expect to give urea 60 minutes before ocular or intracranial surgery.
• Don't mix urea with invert sugar solution if patient has fructose intolerance from aldolase deficiency.
• Avoid infusing drug into leg veins to reduce risk of phlebitis and thrombosis.
• Discard unused portion of drug after 24 hours.
• Be aware that rapid administration may cause hemolysis, increased capillary bleeding, and, in patients with glaucoma, intraocular hemorrhage.
• Maintain adequate hydration to minimize adverse reactions. Assess for signs of dehydration, including dry mucous membranes and tenting.

* For diuresis; 5 to 6 hr for reduced intraocular pressure.

• Monitor BUN and serum electrolyte levels as well as fluid intake and output during urea therapy because prolonged use can cause diuresis.

PATIENT TEACHING
• Instruct patient to notify prescriber immediately about difficulty breathing or shortness of breath because drug can cause transient increases in circulatory volume, leading to circulatory overload, worsening of heart failure, or pulmonary edema.
• Tell patient to expect increased urine output.
• Encourage patient to remain on bed rest during therapy.

urokinase
Abbokinase, Abbokinase Open-Cath

Class and Category
Chemical class: Renal enzymatic protein
Therapeutic class: Thrombolytic
Pregnancy category: B

Indications and Dosages
➤ *To treat acute coronary artery thrombosis*
INTRACORONARY INFUSION
Adults. 6,000 international units/min until artery is maximally opened (up to 2 hr may be required). *Usual:* 500,000 international units.
➤ *To treat acute pulmonary thromboembolism including massive events*
I.V. INFUSION
Adults. *Initial:* 4,400 international units/kg over 10 min, followed by 4,400 international units/kg/hr for 12 hr.
➤ *To clear i.v. catheter occlusion*
INSTILLATION
Adults and children. 5,000 international units/ml instilled into occluded line.

Route	Onset	Peak	Duration
I.V.	Unknown	20 min– 2 hr	4 hr
Intra-coronary	Unknown	Unknown	4 hr

Mechanism of Action
Indirectly promotes conversion of plasminogen to plasmin, an enzyme that breaks down fibrin clots, fibrinogen, and other plasma proteins, including procoagulant factors V and VIII.

Incompatibilities
Don't administer I.V. urokinase through same I.V. line as other drugs or add other drugs to urokinase solution.

Contraindications
Arteriovenous malformation, bleeding disorder, hypersensitivity to urokinase or its components, internal bleeding, intracranial aneurysm, intracranial or intraspinal surgery during previous 2 months, intracranial tumor, recent cardiopulmonary resuscitation, recent trauma, severe uncontrolled hypertension (systolic blood pressure 200 mm Hg or higher, or diastolic blood pressure 110 mm Hg or higher), stroke during previous 2 months

Interactions
DRUGS
antifibrinolytics (aminocaproic acid, aprotinin): Mutual antagonism
antihypertensives: Increased risk of severe hypotension
cefamandole, cefoperazone, cefotetan, plicamycin, valproic acid: Increased risk of hypoprothrombinemia and severe hemorrhage
corticosteroids, ethacrynic acid, salicylates (nonacetylated): Increased risk of GI ulceration and bleeding
enoxaparin, heparin, NSAIDs, oral anticoagulants, platelet-aggregation inhibitors: Increased risk of hemorrhage
thiotepa: Increased therapeutic effects of thiotepa

Adverse Reactions
CNS: Chills, CVA, fever, headache
CV: Arrhythmias, including tachycardia; chest pain; cholesterol embolization; hypertension; hypotension
EENT: Orolingual edema
GI: Nausea, vomiting
HEME: Unusual bleeding
MS: Back pain, myalgia
RESP: Bronchospasm, dyspnea, hypoxemia, wheezing

U
V
W

SKIN: Cyanosis, ecchymosis, flushing, pruritus, rash, urticaria
Other: Anaphylaxis, infusion site reactions, metabolic acidosis

Nursing Considerations

• To prevent foaming, don't shake urokinase when reconstituting. Consult pharmacist about giving drug through 0.45-micron or smaller cellulose membrane filter.
• Assess baseline hematocrit, platelet count, thrombin time, APTT, PT, and INR as ordered.
• Monitor heart rate and rhythm by continuous ECG during therapy, especially during rapid lysis of coronary thrombi. Arrhythmias can occur with reperfusion.
• Monitor blood pressure for hypotension. If it occurs, notify prescriber and expect to reduce infusion rate.
• Check for bleeding at puncture sites and in urine and stool. Check for intracranial bleeding by performing frequent neurologic assessments.
• After arterial puncture, apply pressure for at least 30 minutes and then apply pressure dressing. Check often for bleeding during therapy.
• To prevent bleeding and associated complications, avoid venipunctures; use an external blood pressure cuff to measure blood pressure; give acetaminophen (not aspirin), as prescribed, for fever; and handle patient as little as possible.
WARNING If serious bleeding begins and can't be controlled with local pressure, stop infusion immediately and notify prescriber.

PATIENT TEACHING
• Instruct patient to remain on bed rest during urokinase therapy.
• Inform patient that minor bleeding may occur at wounds or puncture sites.

ursodiol
(ursodeoxycholic acid)

Actigall, Urso Forte, URSO 250, Ursofalk (CAN)

Class and Category

Chemical class: Naturally occurring bile acid
Therapeutic class: Bile salt replenisher, cholelitholytic

Pregnancy category: B

Indications and Dosages

➤ *To prevent gallstone formation in obese patients during rapid weight loss*
CAPSULES
Adults and adolescents. 300 mg twice daily. Or, 8 to 10 mg/kg daily in divided doses twice daily or three times a day.
➤ *To dissolve gallstones*
CAPSULES
Adults and adolescents. 8 to 10 mg/kg daily in divided doses twice daily or three times a day.
➤ *To treat primary biliary cirrhosis*
TABLETS
Adults. 13 to 15 mg/kg daily in two to four divided doses.

Mechanism of Action

Suppresses hepatic synthesis, biliary secretion, and intestinal reabsorption of cholesterol. Prolonged use promotes dissolution of gallstones.

Contraindications

Acute cholangiitis; gallstone complications (such as biliary GI fistula; biliary obstruction; calcified, radiopaque, or radiotranslucent bile-pigment gallstones; cholecystitis; pancreatitis); hypersensitivity to ursodiol, other bile acids, or their components

Interactions

DRUGS
aluminum-containing antacids, cholestyramine, colestipol: Decreased absorption and therapeutic effects of ursodiol
clofibrate, estrogens, neomycin, oral contraceptives, progestins: Interference with ursodiol's therapeutic effects; increased risk of gallstone formation
FOODS
any foods: Increased dissolution of drug

Adverse Reactions

CNS: Anxiety, asthenia, depression, dizziness, fatigue, fever, headache, malaise, sleep disturbance
CV: Chest pain, hypertension, peripheral edema
ENDO: Hyperglycemia
EENT: Laryngeal edema, metallic taste, rhinitis, stomatitis
GI: Abdominal discomfort or pain, cholecystitis, constipation, diarrhea,

elevated liver enzymes, esophagitis, flatulence, indigestion, jaundice, nausea, peptic ulcer, vomiting
GU: Elevated creatinine level
HEME: Leukopenia, thrombocytopenia
MS: Arthralgia, back pain, myalgia
RESP: Cough
SKIN: Alopecia, diaphoresis, dry skin, pruritus, rash, urticaria
OTHER: Angioedema

Nursing Considerations
• Administer ursodiol with food to increase drug dissolution.
• Give aluminum-containing antacids, cholestyramine, and colestipol at least 1 hour before or 4 hours after ursodiol because they may decrease drug's effects.
• Monitor patient's liver enzymes every month for 3 months after ursodiol therapy is begun and then every six months thereafter, as ordered. If elevation occurs, notify prescriber as drug may need to be discontinued.
• Expect drug to be discontinued if gall-stones haven't partially dissolved after 12 months of therapy.
• If patient inadvertently takes too much ursodiol, diarrhea will most likely result and may warrant systemic treatment.

PATIENT TEACHING
• Tell patient to take ursodiol with meals.
• Urge patient to take aluminum-containing antacids at least 1 hour before or 4 hours after ursodiol to support absorption.
• Urge patient to notify prescriber immediately if evidence of acute cholecystitis develops, such as acute right-upper-quadrant abdominal pain.
• Inform patient that he may need to take ursodiol for a prolonged period before gallstones dissolve.
• Advise diabetic patient to monitor blood glucose levels during therapy because ursodiol may alter blood glucose control.

ustekinumab
Stelara

Class and Category
Chemical class: Human IgG1k monoclonal antibody

Therapeutic class: Antipsoriatic
Pregnancy category: B

Indications and Dosages
➤ *To treat moderate to severe plaque psoriasis in patients who are candidates for phototherapy or systemic therapy*
SUBCUTANEOUS INJECTION
Adults weighing 100 kg (220 lb) or less:
Initial: 45 mg followed by 45 mg 4 wk later and then 45 mg every 12 wk.
Adults weighing more than 100 kg (220 lb): *Initial:* 90 mg followed by 90 mg 4 wk later and then 90 mg ever 12 wk.
➤ *To treat active psoriatic arthritis as monotherapy or in combination with methotrexate.*
SUBCUTANEOUS INJECTION
Adults. *Initial:* 45 mg, followed by 45 mg 4 wk later, and then 45 mg every 12 wk.
DOSAGE ADJUSTMENT For patients who weigh more than 100 kg (220 lb) and also have coexistent moderate to severe plaque psoriasis in addition to psoriatic arthritis, initial dosage increased to 90 mg followed by 90 mg 4 wk later, and then 90 mg every 12 wk.

Mechanism of Action
Binds to p40 protein subunit used by interleukin (IL)-12 and IL-23 cytokines. These specific cytokines are involved in inflammatory and immune responses, such as natural killer cell activation and CD4+ T-cell differentiation and activation. By disrupting signaling mediated by IL-12 and IL-23, signs and symptoms caused by inflammatory and immune responses in plaque psoriasis are diminished or relieved.

Route	Onset	Peak	Duration
SubQ	Unknown	7–13.5 days	Unknown

Contraindications
Hypersensitivity to ustekinumab or its components

Interactions
DRUGS
cytochrome P-450 substrates such as cyclosporine, theophylline, warfarin: Possibly altered effects or blood levels of these drugs when ustekinumab is started or stopped

live-virus vaccines: Increased risk of adverse vaccine effects

Adverse Reactions

CNS: Depression, dizziness, fatigue, headache, reversible leukoencephalopathy syndrome
ENDO: Nasopharyngitis, pharyngolaryngeal pain
GI: Diarrhea, diverticulitis, gastroenteritis
GU: UTI
MS: Back pain, myalgia, osteomyelitis
RESP: Pneumonia, upper respiratory tract infection
SKIN: Cellulitis, erythrodermic psoriasis, pruritus, pustular psoriasis, rash, urticaria
Other: Anaphylaxis, angioedema, anti-ustekinumab antibodies, injection-site reactions (bruising, erythema, hemorrhage, induration, irritation, pain, pruritus, swelling), malignancies (breast, colorectal, head and neck, kidney, melanoma and nonmelanoma disorders of skin, prostate, or thyroid), serious infection, including bacterial, fungal, and viral infections and reactivation of latent infections

Nursing Considerations

• Make sure patient has a tuberculin skin test before therapy starts. If skin test is positive, treatment of latent tuberculosis should start before ustekinumab therapy starts. Also expect antituberculosis therapy to start if patient has a history of latent or active tuberculosis but adequate therapy can't be confirmed or if patient has a negative test for latent tuberculosis but has risk factors for tuberculosis.
• Make sure patient is current with all immunizations before starting ustekinumab therapy because patient shouldn't receive live vaccines during treatment. BCG vaccines shouldn't be given for 1 year before or after ustekinumab therapy.
• Use caution when administering ustekinumab to a patient undergoing allergen immunotherapy because drug may decrease the protective effect of allergen immunotherapy which in turn may increase the risk of an allergic reaction to a dose of allergen imunotherapy.
• Use ustekinumab cautiously in patients with recurrent infection or increased risk of infection and in patients who live in

regions where tuberculosis and histoplasmosis are endemic.

WARNING Know that if patient has evidence of an active infection when drug is prescribed, therapy shouldn't start until infection has been treated. Monitor all patients for infection during therapy, especially those receiving immunosuppressants. If a serious infection, an opportunistic infection, or sepsis develops, expect prescriber to stop ustekinumab and start appropriate antimicrobial therapy.
• Be aware that patients with a history of cancer or who have genetic deficiencies in IL-12 or IL-23 should be thoroughly evaluated before ustekinumab therapy starts because various cancers have occurred in patients being treated with ustekinumab. Monitor patients throughout therapy for unusual, persistent, or severe signs and symptoms.
• Give ustekinumab using a 27G, half-inch needle into upper arms, gluteal region, thighs, or any quadrant of abdomen. Rotate sites, and avoid areas that are tender, bruised, erythematous, or indurated.
• Note that needle cover on prefilled syringe contains a latex derivative and shouldn't be handled by persons with a latex allergy.
• Know that comparison of the incidence of antibodies to ustekinumab with the incidence of antibodies to other products maybe misleading.
• Monitor patient for hypersensitivity reactions that could become life threatening. At first sign of hypersensitivity, notify prescriber, expect drug to be discontinued, and provide supportive care.
• Monitor patient for headache, seizures, vision disturbances, and confusion, which may signal reversible posterior leukoencephalopathy syndrome, a rare neurologic disorder that may occur with ustekinumab therapy. If present, notify prescriber, discontinue ustekinumab therapy, and provide appropriate treatment, as ordered.
• Inspect patient's skin regularly for evidence of abnormalities because rapid appearance of multiple cutaneous squamous cell carcinoma have occurred in patients who had pre-existing risk factors for non-melanoma skin cancer. Patients

who are over 60 years of age, have a medical history of prolonged immunosuppressant therapy and those with a history of psoralem plus ultraviolet radiation using UVA bands (PUVA) treatment should be closely monitored.

PATIENT TEACHING
• Inform patient that treatment must be supervised by a healthcare professional.
• Teach patient how to administer the drug subcutaneously, if self-administration is ordered by prescriber.
• Inform patient that tuberculosis may occur during ustekinumab therapy. Instruct him to report persistent cough, wasting or weight loss, and low-grade fever to prescriber.
• Teach patient to recognize and report evidence of infection; drug may need to be stopped. Advise patient to avoid people with infections and to have all prescribed laboratory tests performed.
• Inform patient that the risk of developing certain kinds of cancer is higher in patients taking ustekinumab. Emphasize importance of follow-up visits and reporting any unusual, persistent, or sudden-onset signs or symptoms.
• Caution against receiving live-virus vaccines while taking ustekinumab; doing so may adversely affect the immune system.
• Urge patient to inform all healthcare providers about ustekinumab use and to inform prescriber about all OTC medications being taken, including herbal remedies and vitamin and mineral supplements.

---

valproic acid

Alti-Valproic (CAN), Depakene, Depakote ER, Deproic (CAN), Dom-Proic (CAN), Med-Valproic (CAN), Novo-Valproic (CAN), Nu-Valproic (CAN), PMS-Valproic Acid (CAN), Stavzor

valproate sodium

Depacon

divalproex sodium

Depakote, Depakote Sprinkle, Epival (CAN)

Class and Category
Chemical class: Carboxylic acid derivative
Therapeutic class: Anticonvulsant
Pregnancy category: D

Indications and Dosages
➤ *To treat simple or complex absence seizures, complex partial seizures, myoclonic seizures, and generalized tonic-clonic seizures as monotherapy*
CAPSULES, DELAYED-RELEASE SPRINKLE CAPSULES, DELAYED-RELEASE TABLETS, SYRUP, I.V. INFUSION (VALPROIC ACID, VALPROATE SODIUM, DIVALPROEX SODIUM)
Adults and adolescents. *Initial:* 10 to 15 mg/ kg/day in divided doses twice daily or three times a day, increased by 5 to 10 mg/kg daily every wk, as needed. *Maximum:* 60 mg/kg daily.
Children. *Initial:* 15 to 45 mg/kg daily in divided doses twice daily or three times a day, increased by 5 to 10 mg/kg/day every wk, as needed.
➤ *As adjunct to treat simple or complex absence seizures, complex partial seizures, myoclonic seizures, and generalized tonic-clonic seizures*
CAPSULES, DELAYED-RELEASE SPRINKLE CAPSULES, DELAYED-RELEASE TABLETS, SYRUP, I.V. INFUSION (VALPROIC ACID, VALPROATE SODIUM, DIVALPROEX SODIUM)
Adults and adolescents. 10 to 30 mg/ kg/ day in divided doses, increased by 5 to 10 mg/kg/day every wk, as needed.
Children. 30 to 100 mg/kg daily in divided doses.
DOSAGE ADJUSTMENT For adults being converted from immediate-release divalproex tablets to delayed-release tablets, dosage increased to 8% to 20% more than total daily dose of immediate-release tablets and given once daily.
➤ *To treat acute manic phase of bipolar disorder*
DELAYED-RELEASE TABLETS (DIVALPROEX SODIUM), DELAYED-RELEASE CAPSULES (STAVZOR)
Adults. *Initial:* 750 mg daily in divided doses. *Maximum:* 60 mg/kg daily.
➤ *To prevent migraine headache*
TABLETS, TABLETS (DIVALPROEX SODIUM), DELAYED-RELEASE CAPSULES (STAVZOR)
Adults. 250 mg every 12 hr, increased as needed. *Maximum:* 1 g daily.

U
V
W

DELAYED-RELEASE TABLETS (DIVALPROEX SODIUM)
Adults. 500 mg daily, increased, as needed, up to 1 g daily. *Maximum:* 1 g daily.

Mechanism of Action
May decrease seizure activity by blocking reuptake of gamma-aminobutyric acid (GABA), the most common inhibitory neurotransmitter in the brain. GABA suppresses the rapid firing of neurons by inhibiting voltage-sensitive sodium channels.

Contraindications
Children under age 2 suspected of having a POLG-related disorder; hepatic impairment; hypersensitivity to valproic acid, valproate sodium, divalproex sodium, or their components; mitochondrial disease caused by POLG mutations; pregnancy; urea cycle disorders

Interactions
DRUGS
aspirin, heparin, NSAIDs, oral anticoagulants, thrombolytics: Increased inhibition of platelet aggregation and risk of bleeding
barbiturates, primidone: Increased blood levels of both drugs, additive CNS effects
carbamazepine: Possibly decreased valproic acid effectiveness
carbapenem antibiotics (ertapenem, imipenem, meropenem): Reduced serum valproic acid level, causing loss of seizure control
cholestyramine: Decreased bioavailability of valproic acid
clonazepam: Increased risk of absence seizures
CNS depressants: Increased CNS depression
diazepam: Inhibited diazepam metabolism
ethosuximide: Unpredictable blood ethosuximide level
felbamate: Impaired valproic acid metabolism and increased blood drug level
haloperidol, loxapine, MAO inhibitors, maprotiline, phenothiazines, thioxanthenes, tricyclic antidepressants: Increased CNS depression, lowered seizure threshold
lamotrigine: Decreased lamotrigine clearance
mefloquine: Decreased blood levels of valproic acid, divalproex, and valproate sodium; increased risk of seizures
phenytoin: Increased risk of phenytoin toxicity, loss of seizure control

topiramate: Increased risk of hyperammonemia with or without encephalopathy
ACTIVITIES
alcohol use: Additive CNS depression

Adverse Reactions
CNS: Aggression, agitation, behavioral deterioration, ataxia, cerebral pseudoatrophy, confusion, depression, dizziness, drowsiness, euphoria, hallucinations, headache, hostility, hyperactivity, hyperesthesia, hypothermia, lack of coordination, lethargy, loss of seizure control, paresthesia, psychosis, sedation, suicidal ideation, tremor, vertigo, weakness
CV: Bradycardia
EENT: Diplopia, hearing loss, nystagmus, parotid gland swelling, pharyngitis, spots before eyes
ENDO: Breast enlargement, galactorrhea, hyperglycemia, inappropriate ADH secretion
GI: Abdominal pain, anorexia, constipation, diarrhea, elevated liver function test results, hepatotoxicity, increased appetite, indigestion, nausea, pancreatitis, vomiting
GU: Enuresis, menstrual irregularities, UTI
HEME: Agranulocytosis, anemia including aplastic, bone marrow suppression, eosinophilia, hematoma, hypofibrinogenemia, leukopenia, lymphocytosis, macrocytosis, pancytopenia, porphyria (acute, intermittent), prolonged bleeding time, thrombocytopenia
MS: Bone pain, decreased bone mineral density, dysarthria, fractures, osteopenia, osteoporosis
SKIN: Alopecia, cutaneous vasculitis, diaphoresis, erythema multiforme, jaundice, petechiae, photosensitivity, pruritus, rash, Stevens-Johnson syndrome, toxic epidermal necrolysis
Other: Anaphylaxis, decreased carnitine concentration, developmental delay (children), facial edema, hyperammonemia, hyponatremia, injection-site pain, weight gain or loss

Nursing Considerations
• Know that women of childbearing age should not be prescribed valproic acid, valproate, or divalproex unless other treatments have failed or are unacceptable

because drug exposure very early on in pregnancy may cause decreased IQ and major congenital malformations in the fetus.

• Use extreme caution when administering drug to children under the age of 2 because they are at high risk for developing fatal hepatotoxicity.

• Use caution when administering drug to patient with history of hepatic disease, patient receiving multiple anticonvulsants, children of any age, patient with congenital metabolic disorders, patient with severe seizure disorder accompanied by mental retardation, and patient with organic brain disease, because they may be at increased risk for developing hepatotoxicity.

• Give oral valproic acid or divalproex with food to minimize GI irritation, if needed.

• Administer drug at least 2 hours before or 6 hours after cholestyramine.

• Don't mix syrup with carbonated beverages; result may be an unpleasant-tasting mixture and irritate mouth and throat.

• Don't break or let patient chew delayed-release tablets.

• As needed, sprinkle contents of delayed-release sprinkle capsules on small amount of semisolid food just before administration. Instruct patient not to chew contents of delayed-release sprinkle capsules.

• For I.V. administration, dilute prescribed dose with at least 50 ml compatible diluent and infuse over 60 minutes.

• Know that patient should be switched from I.V. to P.O. form of valproic acid as soon as possible.

• Be aware that patient with hypoalbuminemia or another protein-binding deficiency is at increased risk for valproic acid toxicity.

• Watch for evidence of decreased hepatic function, including anorexia, facial edema, jaundice, lethargy, loss of seizure control, malaise, vomiting, and weakness, especially during the first 6 months of treatment.

• Monitor liver function test results, as ordered. Notify prescriber immediately if you suspect hepatotoxicity and, if confirmed, expect drug to be discontinued immediately.

• Monitor platelet count, as ordered, for signs of thrombocytopenia, and notify prescriber if they appear.

WARNING Hyperammonemia may occur even if liver function test results are normal. Monitor ammonia levels, as ordered. If patient develops unexplained lethargy, vomiting, or changes in mental status with an increase in ammonia level; if asymptomatic ammonia elevations are detected and persist; or if patient develops hypothermia even without hyper-ammonemia, expect to discontinue valproic acid.

• Watch patient closely for suicidal tendencies, particularly when therapy starts and dosage changes, because depression may worsen temporarily during these times, possibly leading to suicidal ideation.

• Monitor patient's drug level, as ordered, especially early in therapy and if patient takes other drugs, because interactions can alter the blood level.

• Drug may alter urine ketone test and thyroid function tests.

PATIENT TEACHING

• Instruct patient to swallow capsules whole to prevent irritation to mouth and throat. However, delayed-release sprinkle capsules may be opened and contents mixed with food for easier swallowing. Instruct patient not to chew contents of delayed-release sprinkle capsules.

• Tell patient to notify prescriber immediately and withhold further doses of drug, unless advised otherwise by prescriber, if symptoms such as anorexia, facial edema, lethargy, malaise, weakness, and vomiting occur.

• Advise patient to avoid hazardous activities during therapy because drug may affect mental and motor performance.

• Urge patient to avoid alcohol during therapy.

• Urge woman to notify prescriber at once about suspected or known pregnancy.

• Advise patient to notify prescriber if tremor develops during therapy; it may be dose-related.

U
V
W

- Urge family or caregiver to watch patient closely for suicidal tendencies, especially when therapy starts or dosage changes.
- Instruct women of childbearing age to notify prescriber if pregnancy is suspected or occurs, as valproate exposure in utero can cause adverse effects on the cognitive development of the unborn child. Encourage woman who becomes pregnant while taking valproic acid to enroll in the North American antiepileptic drug pregnancy registry by calling 1-888-233-2334. Explain that the registry is collecting information about the safety of antiepileptic drugs during pregnancy.

valsartan

Diovan

Class and Category

Chemical class: Nonpeptide tetrazole derivative
Therapeutic class: Antihypertensive
Pregnancy category: D

Indications and Dosages

➤ *To manage hypertension, alone or with other antihypertensives*

CAPSULES

Adults. *Initial:* 80 or 160 mg daily, increased as needed and prescribed. *Maximum:* 320 mg/day.

Children ages 6 to 16. 1.3 mg/kg (up to 40 mg total) once daily, increased as needed and prescribed. *Maximum:* 2.7 mg/kg (up to 160 mg) daily.

➤ *To treat New York Heart Association (NYHA) class II to IV heart failure*

CAPSULES

Adults. *Initial:* 40 mg twice daily, increased to 80 mg twice daily and then 160 mg twice daily, as needed. *Maximum:* 320 mg daily.

➤ *To reduce cardiovascular mortality in stable patients with left ventricular failure or dysfunction following an MI*

CAPSULES

Adults. *Initial:* 20 mg twice daily starting as early as 12 hr after MI, increased to 40 mg twice daily within 7 days, followed by subsequent adjustments to 160 mg twice daily as tolerated. *Maintenance:* 160 mg twice daily.

DOSAGE ADJUSTMENT If patient develops symptomatic hypotension or renal dysfunction, dosage decreased.

Route	Onset	Peak	Duration
P.O.	2 hr	6 hr	24 hr

Mechanism of Action

Blocks the hormone angiotensin II from binding to receptor sites in vascular smooth muscle, adrenal glands, and other tissues. This action inhibits vasoconstrictive and aldosterone-secreting effects of angiotensin II, thereby reducing blood pressure.

Contraindications

Concurrent aliskiren therapy in diabetic patients, hypersensitivity to valsartan or its components

Interactions

DRUGS

ACE inhibitors, aliskiren, other angiotensin receptor blockers: Increased risk of hypotension, hyperkalemia, and renal dysfunction
antihypertensives, diuretics: Additive hypotensive effect
cyclosporine, rifampin, ritonavir: Possibly increased blood valsartan level
lithium: Possibly increased serum lithium concentration and toxicity
NSAIDs: Increased risk of renal dysfunction, especially in the elderly and patients with volume depletion or existing renal dysfunction
potassium salts, potassium-sparing diuretics: Possibly hyperkalemia

FOODS

potassium-containing salt substitutes: Possibly hyperkalemia

Adverse Reactions

CNS: Dizziness, fatigue, headache, insomnia, syncope, vertigo
CV: Edema, hypotension including orthostatic hypotension, vasculitis
EENT: Blurred vision, pharyngitis, rhinitis, sinusitis
GI: Abdominal pain, diarrhea, elevated liver enzymes, hepatitis, indigestion, nausea, vomiting
GU: Acute renal failure, increased blood creatinine level
HEME: Thrombocytopenia

MS: Arthralgia, back pain, rhabdomyolysis
RESP: Cough, upper respiratory tract infection
SKIN: Alopecia, bullous dermatitis, rash
Other: Angioedema, hyperkalemia, viral infection

Nursing Considerations
• Know that valsartan shouldn't be given to patients who have hypovolemia or are taking a diuretic, because there is increased risk of severe hypotension from volume depletion. If severe hypotension occurs, place patient in a supine position, notify prescriber, and expect to give an intravenous infusion of normal saline.
• Check patient's blood pressure often during therapy.
• Be aware that maximal blood pressure reduction typically occurs after 4 weeks.
• Monitor serum potassium level because drug may elevate potassium level by blocking aldosterone secretion.
• Obtain a serum creatinine level periodically, as ordered, because changes in renal function can occur during valsartan therapy. Know that patients who are at high risk for renal dysfunction are patients with renal artery stenosis, chronic kidney disease, severe congestive heart failure, or who are volume-depleted. Notify prescriber of an elevated serum creatinine level and changes in voiding patterns because renal dysfunction could lead to acute renal failure.

PATIENT TEACHING
• Instruct patient to take valsartan exactly as prescribed at the same time each day to maintain therapeutic effect.
• Advise patient to avoid hazardous activities until drug's CNS effects are known.
• Advise patient to avoid using potassium-containing salt substitutes without consulting prescriber.
• Instruct female patient of childbearing age to use reliable birth control during therapy and to notify prescriber at once about known or suspected pregnancy, because valsartan will need to be discontinued.
• Urge patient to keep follow-up appointments to monitor progress.

• Tell patients to inform all prescribers of valsartan therapy and any other drug therapy they are taking, including drugs such as ibuprofen and naproxen.

vancomycin hydrochloride
Vancocin

Class and Category
Chemical class: Tricyclic glycopeptide derivative
Therapeutic class: Antibiotic
Pregnancy category: B (oral), C (parenteral)

Indications and Dosages
➤ *To treat pseudomembranous colitis caused by* Clostridium difficile *and enterocolitis caused by staphylococci*
CAPSULES, ORAL SOLUTION
Adults and adolescents. 125 to 500 mg every 6 hr for 7 to 10 days. *Maximum:* 2 g daily.
Children. 10 mg/kg (up to 125 mg) every 6 hr for 7 to 10 days. *Maximum:* 2 g daily.
➤ *To treat bacterial endocarditis caused by methicillin-resistant* Staphylococcus aureus
I.V. INFUSION
Adults. 30 mg/kg daily in equally divided doses twice daily for 4 to 6 wk. *Maximum:* 2 g daily.
➤ *As adjunct to treat bacterial endocarditis caused by methicillin-resistant* S. aureus *in patients with prosthetic heart valve*
I.V. INFUSION
Adults. 30 mg/kg daily in equally divided doses twice daily to four times a day for 6 wk or longer in conjunction with rifampin and gentamicin. *Maximum:* 2 g daily.
➤ *To treat bacterial endocarditis caused by* Streptococcus bovis *or* Streptococcus viridans
I.V. INFUSION
Adults. 30 mg/kg daily in equally divided doses twice daily for 4 wk. *Maximum:* 2 g daily.
➤ *As adjunct to treat bacterial endocarditis caused by enterococci*

I.V. INFUSION
Adults. 30 mg/kg daily in equally divided doses twice daily for 4 to 6 wk in conjunction with gentamicin. *Maximum:* 2 g daily.
➤ *To treat bacterial septicemia, bone and joint infections, pneumonia, and skin and soft-tissue infections caused by staphylococcus, including methicillin-resistant strains, and life-threatening infections*

I.V. INFUSION
Adults and children age 12 and over. 500 mg every 6 hr or 1 g every 12 hr, infused over at least 60 min. *Maximum:* 4 g daily.
Children ages 1 month to 12 years. 10 mg/kg every 6 hr or 20 mg/kg every 12 hr, infused over at least 60 min.
Neonates ages 1 week to 1 month. *Initial:* 15 mg/kg followed by 10 mg/kg every 8 hr, infused over at least 60 min.
Neonates under age 1 week. *Initial:* 15 mg/kg followed by 10 mg/kg every 12 hr, infused over at least 60 min.

Mechanism of Action
Inhibits bacterial RNA and cell wall synthesis; alters permeability of bacterial membranes, causing cell wall lysis and cell death.

Incompatibilities
Don't give I.V. vancomycin through same I.V. line as other drugs. Don't add to albumin-containing solutions, alkaline solutions, aminophylline, amobarbital sodium, aztreonam, cefepime, ceftazidime, chloramphenicol sodium succinate, chlorothiazide sodium, dexamethasone sodium phosphate, foscarnet sodium, heparin sodium, methicillin sodium, penicillin G, pentobarbital sodium, phenobarbital sodium, piperacillin sodium and tazobactam sodium, secobarbital sodium, and sodium bicarbonate. Vancomycin may precipitate with heavy metals.

Contraindications
Hypersensitivity to vancomycin or its components, hypersensitivity to corn or corn products when vancomycin is given with dextrose solutions

Interactions
DRUGS
aminoglycosides (amikacin, gentamicin, tobramycin), amphotericin B, bacitracin (parenteral), bumetanide, capreomycin, carmustine, cidofovir, cisplatin, cyclosporine, ethacrynic acid, furosemide, paromomycin, pentamidine (parenteral), polymyxins, salicylates (parenteral), streptozocin: Additive nephrotoxicity or ototoxicity
antihistamines, buclizine, cyclizine, meclizine, phenothiazines, thioxanthenes, trimethobenzamide: Masked symptoms of ototoxicity
cholestyramine, colestipol: Decreased antibacterial activity of oral vancomycin
dexamethasone: Decreased penetration of vancomycin into CSF
nephrotoxic drugs: Increased risk of nephrotoxicity

Adverse Reactions
CNS: Chills, depression, dizziness, fatigue, fever, headache, insomnia, vertigo
CV: Hypotension, peripheral edema, vasculitis
EENT: Ototoxicity
GI: Abdominal pain, constipation, *Clostridium difficile*-associated diarrhea, diarrhea, flatulence, nausea, vomiting
GU: Nephrotoxicity, UTI
HEME: Anemia, eosinophilia, neutropenia, thrombocytopenia
MS: Back pain
RESP: Dyspnea, wheezing
SKIN: Exfoliative dermatitis; drug rash with eosinophilia and systemic symptoms (DRESS); exfoliative dermatitis; extravasation with pain, tenderness, thrombophlebitis, and tissue necrosis; pruritus; rash; Stevens-Johnson syndrome; toxic epidermal necrolysis; urticaria
Other: Anaphylaxis, drug-induced fever, hypokalemia, injection-site inflammation, superinfection

Nursing Considerations
• To reconstitute 500-mg vial of vancomycin for I.V. use, add 10 ml of sterile water for injection; further dilute with at least 100 ml of compatible I.V. solution. For 1-g vial of dry, sterile powder, add 20 ml of sterile water for injection; further dilute with at least 200 ml of compatible I.V. solution.

WARNING Infuse over at least 1 hour per gram of vancomycin. Rapid delivery may cause hypotension or transient "red man syndrome," characterized by chills; fainting; fever; flushing of face, neck, upper arms, and torso; hypotension; nausea; tachycardia; and vomiting.

• Blood vancomycin concentrations are frequently monitored. Higher trough concentrations of 15-20 mg/L are commonly targeted now, though they are associated with more nephrotoxicity than the lower trough concentrations previously used.

• Monitor serum vancomycin concentration in patients with renal impairment or colitis because significant increases in blood drug level have occurred in such patients taking multiple oral doses of vancomycin.

• If patient has an inflammatory intestinal disorder, assess him often for adverse reactions because vancomycin absorption may be increased in these conditions.

• Check CBC results and serum creatinine and BUN levels during therapy, especially if patient has renal impairment or takes an aminoglycoside.

• Observe I.V. infusion site for evidence of extravasation, including necrosis, pain, tenderness, and thrombophlebitis. If extravasation occurs, discontinue infusion immediately and notify prescriber.

• Assess hearing during therapy. Transient or permanent ototoxicity may occur if patient receives an excessive amount of drug, has an underlying hearing loss, or receives concurrent aminoglycosides.

• Monitor patient closely for diarrhea because it may indicate pseudomembranous colitis caused by *Clostridium difficile*, a risk with many antibiotics. If diarrhea occurs during therapy, notify prescriber and expect to withhold drug. If confirmed, treat with fluids, electrolytes, protein, and an antibiotic effective against *C. difficile*.

• Oral vancomycin is only used for gastrointestinal *C. difficile* and staphylococcal infections, since it is not absorbed. Patients cannot be converted from I.V. to oral vancomycin for other infections.

PATIENT TEACHING

• Instruct patient to use a calibrated measuring device to measure accurate doses of oral solution.

• Advise patient to notify prescriber if no improvement occurs after a few days.

• Instruct patient to complete full course of vancomycin, as prescribed.

• Instruct patient to notify prescriber if she develops severe or persistent diarrhea.

• Instruct patient to keep follow-up appointments during and after treatment.

vardenafil hydrochloride

Levitra, Staxyn

Class and Category

Chemical class: Phosphodiesterase type 5 inhibitor
Therapeutic class: Anti-impotence agent
Pregnancy category: B

Indications and Dosages

➤ *To treat erectile dysfunction*

TABLETS

Adults. 10 mg taken 1 hr before sexual activity; increased to 20 mg or decreased to 5 mg, as needed. *Maximum:* 20 mg and once-daily limit regardless of dosage.

DOSAGE ADJUSTMENT If patient takes ritonavir, vardenafil dosage shouldn't exceed 2.5 mg in 72 hr. If patient takes indinavir, saquinavir, atazanavir, clarithromycin, ketoconazole 400 mg daily, itraconazole 400 mg daily, or another potent CYP3A4 inhibitor, vardenafil dosage shouldn't exceed 2.5 mg in 24 hr. If patient takes ketoconazole 200 mg and itraconazole 200 mg daily, vardenafil dosage shouldn't exceed 5 mg in 24 hr.

ORALLY DISINTEGRATING TABLETS

Adults. 10 mg taken 1 hr before sexual activity. *Maximum:* 10 mg within 24-hr period.

Route	Onset	Peak	Duration
P.O.	30 min	30 min–2 hr	4–5 hr

Mechanism of Action

Enhances effect of nitric oxide (released in the penis by sexual stimulation) and

U
V
W

inhibits phosphodiesterase type 5, which increases cGMP level, relaxes smooth muscle, and increases blood flow into the corpus cavernosum, producing an erection.

Contraindications

Concurrent administration of alpha blockers, concurrent continuous or intermittent nitrate therapy, hypersensitivity to vardenafil or its components

Interactions

DRUGS

alpha blockers, nitrates: Profound hypotension

atazanavir, clarithromycin, erythromycin, indinavir, itraconazole, ketoconazole, ritonavir, saquinavir: Increased vardenafil effects

class IA (procainamide, quinidine) and class III (amiodarone, sotalol) antiarrhythmics: Possibly increased QT-interval prolongation

indinavir, ritonavir: Reduced blood levels of indinavir and ritonavir

FOODS

grapefruit juice: Possibly increased vardenafil effect

Adverse Reactions

CNS: Dizziness, headache, seizures, transient global amnesia

CV: Hypotension

EENT: Decreased vision, hearing loss, loss of vision in one or both eyes, nasal congestion, nonarteritic anterior ischemic optic neuropathy, rhinitis, sinusitis, tinnitus

GI: Indigestion, nausea

GU: Priapism

MS: Back pain

SKIN: Flushing

Other: Flulike symptoms, increased creatine kinase level

Nursing Considerations

• Vardenafil shouldn't be used by men taking class IA (procainamide, quinidine) or class III (amiodarone, sotalol) antiarrhythmics or by men who have congenital prolonged QT interval. Drug may potentiate prolonged QT interval. It should also not be used in men who have unstable angina, hypotension (resting systolic blood pressure of less than 90 mm Hg), uncontrolled hypertension (greater than 170/110 mm Hg), recent history of stroke, presence of life-

threatening arrhythmia, severe cardiac failure, or a myocardial infarction (within last 6 months) because drug use could worsen these conditions.

• Use vardenafil cautiously in men with renal dysfunction (although it should not be used if patient is on dialysis) or mild hepatic impairment (should not be used if patient has moderate to severe hepatic impairment), in elderly men, and in men with penile abnormalities that may predispose them to priapism.

• Also use cautiously in patients with left ventricular outflow obstruction, such as aortic stenosis, and those with severely impaired autonomic control of blood pressure. These conditions increase sensitivity to vasodilators, such as vardenafil.

• Be aware that Levitra tablets are not interchangeable with Staxyn tablets.

• Monitor blood pressure and heart rate before and after giving drug, especially if patient takes an alpha blocker, because of increased risk of symptomatic hypotension.

• Monitor patient's vision, especially if he's over age 50; has diabetes, hypertension, coronary artery disease, or hyperlipidemia; or smokes, because vardenafil rarely leads to nonarteritic ischemic optic neuropathy and decreased vision, possibly permanent.

• Monitor patient's hearing. Sudden decrease or loss, possibly with tinnitus and dizziness, may occur with vardenafil use. Report such changes immediately, and expect drug to be discontinued.

PATIENT TEACHING

• Alert patient that orally disintegrating tablets contain phenylalanine and should not be taken by patients with phenylketonuria. It also contains sorbitol and should not be taken if he has hereditary problems with fructose intolerance.

• For best results, tell patient to take drug 1 hour before anticipated sexual activity.

• Instruct patient to place a prescribed orally disintegrating tablet on his tongue immediately after removing it from the blister package and allow it to dissolve. He should not crush or split the tablet, and tablet should not be taken with any liquid.

WARNING Tell patient not to take vardenafil if he takes an organic nitrate, continuously or intermittently, or within 4 hours of taking an alpha blocker because profound hypotension and death could result.
- Caution patient not to take vardenafil more than once daily or to exceed 20 mg daily for oral tablet or 10 mg for orally disintegrating tablet. Tell him to call his prescriber or go to the emergency department immediately if he accidentally takes more vardenafil than prescribed.
- Tell patient to stop taking vardenafil and notify prescriber if he has a sudden loss of vision in one or both eyes, sudden hearing loss, seizures, or trouble remembering.
- Advise patient to seek sexual counseling to enhance drug's effects.
- Inform patient taking Staxyn that some form of sexual stimulation is needed for an erection to happen.
- To avoid possible penile damage and permanent loss of erectile function, urge patient to notify prescriber at once if erection is painful or lasts longer than 4 hours.

varenicline
Chantix

Class and Category
Chemical class: Tartrate salt
Therapeutic class: Nicotinic blocker
Pregnancy classification: C

Indications and Dosages
➤ *As adjunct to smoking cessation treatment*
TABLETS
Adults. *Initial:* 0.5 mg daily for 3 days; then increased to 0.5 mg twice daily for 4 days, and then increased to 1 mg twice daily for a total of 12 wk of therapy. If effective, an additional 12 wk of therapy may be given.
DOSAGE ADJUSTMENT If patient has severe renal impairment, maximum dosage is 0.5 mg twice daily. If patient is having hemodialysis for end-stage renal disease, maximum dosage is 0.5 mg daily.

Mechanism of Action
Blocks nicotine from activating $alpha_4beta_2$ receptors by binding to them.

This inhibits nicotine stimulation of the central nervous mesolimbic dopamine system, which probably is the area that produces pleasure in and reinforcement of smoking.

Contraindications
Hypersensitivity to varenicline or its components

Interactions
DRUGS
nicotine (transdermal): Increased adverse reactions
ACTIVITIES
alcohol use: Increased intoxicating effects of alcohol

Adverse Reactions
CNS: Abnormal dreams, agitation, anxiety, asthenia, attention difficulties, behavior changes, delusions, depression, dizziness, dysgeusia, fatigue, hallucinations, headache, homicidal ideation, hostility, insomnia, irritability, lethargy, loss of consciousness, malaise, mania, mental impairment, panic, paranoia, psychosis, restlessness, sensory disturbances, seizures, somnolence, stroke, suicidal ideation, thirst
CV: Angina, chest pain, edema, hypertension, MI, peripheral ischemia, thrombosis, ventricular extrasystoles
EENT: Dry mouth, epistaxis, gingivitis, rhinorrhea
ENDO: Hot flashes
GI: Abdominal pain, acute pancreatitis, anorexia, constipation, diarrhea, dyspepsia, flatulence, gastroesophageal reflux disease, GI hemorrhage, increased appetite, liver enzyme abnormalities, nausea, vomiting
GU: Acute renal failure, polyuria, urine retention
HEME: Leukocytosis, lymphadenopathy, splenomegaly, thrombocytopenia
RESP: Asthma, dyspnea, pulmonary embolism
MS: Arthralgia, back pain, muscle cramp, musculoskeletal pain, myalgia
SKIN: Diaphoresis, erythema multiforme, pruritus, rash, Stevens-Johnson syndrome, urticaria
Other: Angioedema, flulike syndrome, hyperkalemia, hypersensitivity, hypokalemia

U
V
W

Nursing Considerations

• Use cautiously in patients with renal disease because varenicline is substantially excreted by the kidneys.

• Review patient's medication history before starting varenicline because dosage adjustments may be needed for such drugs as theophylline, warfarin, and insulin.

WARNING Monitor patient for angioedema, difficult breathing, rash with mucosal lesions, or other signs of hypersensitivity. Report immediately, stop varenicline therapy, and provide supportive emergency care, as prescribed.

• If patient has nausea, the most common adverse reaction to varenicline, notify prescriber. Dosage reduction may help.

• Even with varenicline therapy, nicotine withdrawal symptoms and worsening of underlying psychiatric illness may occur with smoking cessation. Monitor patient for neuropsychiatric symptoms, including changes in behavior, hostility, agitation, depressed mood, and worsening of preexisting psychiatric illness. If present, notify prescriber immediately, institute safety measures, and expect drug to be discontinued.

• Watch patient closely for suicidal tendencies, particularly when therapy starts and dosage changes, because depression may worsen temporarily during these times, possibly leading to suicidal ideation.

• Montior patient for seizures, especially within the first month of therapy, and in patients with a history of seizures or other factors that could lower their seizure threshold.

PATIENT TEACHING

• Explain that using nicotine patches while taking varenicline won't increase its effectiveness and may increase adverse reactions such as dizziness, nausea, and vomiting.

• Instruct patient to set a date to quit smoking and then start taking varenicline 1 week before the quit date. Or, patient can begin therapy and then set a date to quit smoking between days 8 and 35 of treatment.

• Explain how to adjust dose when drug is used for smoking cessation. Tell patient to take drug after eating and with a full glass of water.

• Encourage patient to continue trying to stop smoking even if an early relapse occurs during varenicline therapy.

WARNING Tell patient to seek medical attention immediately if he develops swelling of his face, mouth, limbs, or neck; difficulty breathing; mucosal lesions; rash or other skin reaction; or any other signs of hypersensitivity during therapy.

• Inform patient that the most common adverse reactions to varenicline therapy are nausea and insomnia, usually transient. If they persist, patient should notify prescriber; dosage reduction may help.

• Caution patient to avoid hazardous activities until CNS effects of drug are known. Explain that near miss traffic accidents and other accidental injuries have occurred in patients taking varenicline.

• Explain that vivid, unusual, or strange dreams may occur during therapy.

• Urge family or caregiver to watch patient closely for suicidal tendencies, especially when therapy starts or dosage changes.

• Tell patient that nicotine withdrawal can occur even with varenicline use and that preexisting mental illness may worsen during smoking cessation. Advise patient or family to notify prescriber about abnormal thinking or behavior and to stop taking drug immediately.

• Instruct patient to seek emergency medical care if she experiences a seizure or new or worsening symptoms of cardiovascular disease such as chest pain, shortness of breath, calf pain when walking, or sudden onset of weakness, numbness, or difficulty speaking.

• Advise patient to reduce or avoid alcohol consumption while taking drug until tolerance for alcohol in combination with varenicline therapy is known.

vasopressin
(antidiuretic hormone [ADH])

Pitressin, Pressyn (CAN)

Class and Category
Chemical class: Polypeptide hormone
Therapeutic class: Antidiuretic
Pregnancy category: C

Indications and Dosages
➤ *To prevent or control symptoms of central diabetes insipidus caused by insufficient ADH*

I.M. OR SUBCUTANEOUS INJECTION
Adults. 5 to 10 units twice daily or three times a day, as needed.
Children. 2.5 to 10 units three times a day or four times a day, as needed.
➤ *To prevent or treat abdominal distention*

I.M. INJECTION
Adults. 5 units, increased to 10 units every 3 to 4 hr, as needed.

Route	Onset	Peak	Duration
I.M., SubQ	Unknown	Unknown	2–8 hr

Contraindications
Chronic nephritis with nitrogen retention, hypersensitivity to vasopressin or its components

Interactions
DRUGS
carbamazepine, chlorpropamide, clofibrate, fludrocortisone, tricyclic antidepressants: Increased antidiuretic effect
demeclocycline, lithium, norepinephrine: Decreased antidiuretic effect

Adverse Reactions
CNS: Dizziness, headache, light-headedness, tremor
CV: Angina, MI
EENT: Circumoral pallor
ENDO: Water intoxication
GI: Abdominal cramps, diarrhea, eructation, flatulence, intestinal hypermotility, nausea, vomiting
SKIN: Diaphoresis, pallor
Other: Allergic reaction

Nursing Considerations
• Use vasopressin with extreme caution in patients with coronary artery disease because it may cause angina or MI; in those with hypertension because it may increase blood pressure; and in those with asthma, epilepsy, heart failure, or migraine headache because extracellular fluid may increase rapidly.
• Monitor fluid and electrolyte balance during therapy. Check intake and output at least every 8 hours, and watch for evidence of water intoxication and hyponatremia, including anuria, confusion, drowsiness, headache, listlessness, and weight gain.

PATIENT TEACHING
• Teach patient how to administer vasopressin; stress the need to rotate injection sites.
• Urge patient to notify prescriber immediately if he has evidence of possible water intoxication, including anuria, confusion, drowsiness, headache, listlessness, and unexplained weight gain.
• Inform patient that abdominal cramps, nausea, and skin blanching will subside after a few minutes and can be minimized by drinking one or two glasses of water.

Mechanism of Action
Vasopressin, a synthetic form of antidiuretic hormone, treats diabetes insipidus by decreasing urine output and raising urine osmolality. When vasopressin attaches to vasopressin 2 (V_2) receptors on cell membranes in the nephron's collecting duct, it activates the enzyme adenyl cyclase to convert adenosine triphosphate (ATP) to cyclic adenosine monophosphate (cAMP). This action increases the collecting duct's permeability and enhances water reabsorption into the blood.

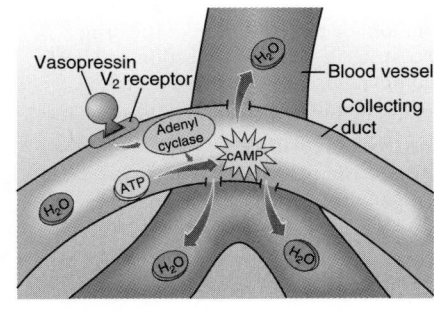

U
V
W

vedolizumab

Entyvio

Class and Category

Chemical class: Humanized IgG$_1$ monoclonal antibody
Therapeutic class: Anti-inflammatory
Pregnancy category: B

Indications and Dosages

➤ *To treat moderate to severe ulcerative colitis or Crohn's disease in patients who have had an inadequate response, lost response, or were intolerant to a tumor necrosis factor blocker or immunomodulator; to treat moderate to severe ulcerative colitis or Crohn's disease in patients who have had an inadequate response, were intolerant to, or demonstrated dependence on corticosteroids*

I.V. INFUSION

Adults. 300 mg infused over 30 min, followed by 300 mg 2 and 6 wk later, and then every 8 wk thereafter.

Mechanism of Action

Binds to a specific integrin and blocks its action with mucosal addressin cell adhesion molecule 1. It also inhibits the migration of memory T lymphocytes across the endothelium into the inflamed gastrointestinal parenchymal tissue. These actions are thought to help relieve the chronic inflammation that occurs with ulcerative colitis and Crohn's disease.

Incompatibilities

Do not mix any other drug with vedolizumab, and do not use any other solution for reconstitution of the drug except sterile water for injection and 0.9% sodium chloride for dilution because incompatibilities are unknown.

Contraindications

Hypersensitivity to vedolizumab or its components

Interaction

DRUGS

natalizumab: Increased risk of progressive multifocal leukoencephalopathy (PML) and other infections

tumor necrosis factor blockers: Increased risk of infections

Adverse Reactions

CNS: Dizziness, fatigue, fever, headache
CV: Hypertension, tachycardia
EENT: Nasopharyngitis, oropharyngeal pain, sinusitis
GI: Elevated bilirubin and liver enzymes, jaundice, hepatic injury (severe), hepatitis, nausea, vomiting
MS: Arthralgia, back or extremity pain
RESP: Bronchitis, bronchospasm, cough, dyspnea, upper respiratory tract infection
SKIN: Flushing, pruritus, rash, urticaria
Other: Anaphylaxis, anti-vedolizumab antibodies, infections, influenza-like symptoms, infusion-related reactions, malignancies, sepsis, septic shock

Nursing Considerations

• Ensure patient is up-to-date with all immunizations prior to initiating vedolizumab therapy.
• Know that vedolizumab is not recommended for use in patients with active, severe infections until the infections are controlled. Ensure that patient has been screened for tuberculosis.
• Use caution when administering vedolizumab to patient with a history of recurring severe infections.
• Reconstitute vedolizumab powder by injecting 4.8 ml of sterile water for injection, using a syringe with a 21- to 25-gauge needle. Gently swirl the vial for at least 15 seconds to dissolve the powder. Do not vigorously shake or invert the vial. Allow solution to sit for up to 20 minutes at room temperature to allow for reconstitution and for any foam to settle; swirl vial, if needed, during this time. If not fully dissolved after 20 minutes, allow another 10 minutes for dissolution. Do not use if the powder is not dissolved after 30 minutes. Solution should be clear or opalescent, colorless to light brownish yellow and free of visible particulates. Prior to withdrawing drug solution from the vial, gently invert vial three times. Withdraw 5 ml (300 mg) of reconstituted solution and add to 250 ml of sterile 0.9% sodium chloride; then gently mix in the infusion bag. Infusion solution may be

stored up to 4 hours in the refrigerator prior to administration.

• Administer as an intravenous infusion over 30 minutes. Never administer as an intravenous push or bolus. Do not add any other drugs to the prepared solution. Flush the intravenous line with 30 ml of sterile 0.9% sodium chloride injection before and after the infusion.

WARNING Monitor patient closely for hypersensitivity reactions during infusion and up to several hours post infusion. Allergic reactions may include bronchospasm, dyspnea, flushing, rash, and urticaria. Blood pressure and heart rate may become elevated. If present, stop infusion, notify prescriber, expect to discontinue drug therapy, as ordered, and provide appropriate treatment according to standard of care.

• Monitor patient for infections because vedolizumab increases risk for infection. Notify prescriber if signs and symptoms occur, as drug may need to be withheld if infection is severe.

WARNING Monitor patient for any new onset or worsening of neurologic signs and symptoms, which may include progressive weakness on one side of the body, clumsiness of extremities, visual disturbances, or changes in thinking, memory, or orientation, because another drug in the same class has been associated with progressive multifocal leukoencephalopathy (PML), a rare and often fatal infection of the central nervous system. If PML is suspected, expect drug to be withheld and patient referred to a neurologist. If PML is confirmed, expect drug to be discontinued.

PATIENT TEACHING

• Stress importance of keeping appointments for vedolizumab administration.

• Instruct patient to notify prescriber immediately if allergic reaction occurs, such as difficulty breathing, rash, or hives.

• Review signs and symptoms of infection and tell patient to notify prescriber immediately if present, as drug may need to be withheld or discontinued.

• Encourage female patients who become pregnant during vedolizumab therapy to register with the pregnancy exposure registry by calling 1-877-825-3327.

venlafaxine hydrochloride
Effexor, Effexor XR

desvenlafaxine fumarate
Desvenlafaxine ER

desvenlafaxine succinate
Khedezla, Pristiq

Class and Category
Chemical class: Phenylethylamine derivative
Therapeutic class: Antidepressant
Pregnancy category: C

Indications and Dosages
➤ *To treat and prevent relapse of major depression*

E.R. CAPSULES (EFFEXOR XR)
Adults. 75 mg daily with a meal at same time each day, morning or evening (for some patients, 37.5 mg daily for 4 to 7 days before increasing to 75 mg daily); then increased by 75 mg daily every 4 days, as prescribed. *Maximum:* 225 mg daily.

DOSAGE ADJUSTMENT Initial daily dose decreased by 25% to 50% for patients with mild to moderate renal impairment and by 50% for patients with hepatic impairment.

E.R. TABLETS (DESVENLAFAXINE ER KHEDEZLA, PRISTIQ)
Adults. 50 mg daily, with a meal, at the same time each day morning or evening
DOSAGE ADJUSTMENT For patients with severe renal impairment and for elderly patients having difficulty tolerating drug, 50 mg every other day.

TABLETS (EFFEXOR)
Adults. 75 mg daily in divided doses twice daily or three times a day, increased by 75 mg daily every 4 days, as needed. *Maximum:* 375 mg daily (225 mg/day for outpatients).

➤ *To treat generalized anxiety disorder or social anxiety disorder*

U
V
W

E.R. CAPSULES (DESVENLAFAXINE ER, EFFEXOR XR)
Adults. 75 mg daily with a meal at same time each day, morning or evening (for some patients, 37.5 mg daily for 4 to 7 days before increasing to 75 mg daily); then increased by 75 mg daily every 4 days, as needed. *Maximum:* 225 mg daily.
DOSAGE ADJUSTMENT Initial daily dose decreased by 25% to 50% for patients with mild to moderate renal impairment and by 50% for patients with hepatic impairment.

Route	Onset	Peak	Duration
P.O.	2 wk	Unknown	Unknown

Mechanism of Action

Inhibits neuronal reuptake of serotonin and norepinephrine, along with its active metabolite, O-desmethylvenlafaxine. These actions raise serotonin and norepinephrine levels at nerve synapses, elevating mood and reducing depression.

Contraindications

Hypersensitivity to desvenlafaxine, venlafaxine, or their components; use of an MAO inhibitor within 14 days, including intravenous methylene blue and linezolid

Interactions

DRUGS
aspirin, NSAIDs, other serotonin-norepinephrine reuptake inhibitors, selective serotonin reuptake inhibitors, warfarin and other anticoagulants: Increased risk of bleeding
cimetidine: Decreased clearance and increased levels of desvenlafaxine and venlafaxine
clozapine: Possibly increased blood clozapine level and serious adverse reactions, including seizures
CYP3A4 inhibitors, ketoconazole: Increased plasma venlafaxine level and risk of adverse reactions
MAO inhibitors: Increased risk of hypertension; hyperthermia; mental status changes, including coma and delirium; muscle rigidity; and severe myoclonus
metoprolol: Increased plasma metoprolol level, but decreased effectiveness in lowering blood pressure
serotonergic drugs such as amitriptyline, clomipramine, desipramine, doxepin,

haloperidol, imipramine, linezolid, lithium, nortriptyline, protriptyline, St. John's wort, tramadol, trazodone, triptans: Possibly serotonin syndrome
warfarin: Possibly increased PT, partial thromboplastin time, and INR

Adverse Reactions

CNS: Abnormal dreams, agitation, amnesia, anxiety, asthenia, attention disturbance, bruxism, cerebral ischemia, chills, confusion, delusions, depersonalization, depression, dizziness, dream disturbances, drowsiness, dyskinesia, extrapyramidal disorder, fatigue, fever, hallucinations, headache, hypesthesia, hypomania, impaired balance and coordination, insomnia, irritability, mania, migraine, mood changes, nervousness, neuroleptic malignant syndrome, paresthesia, seizures, serotonin syndrome, somnolence, suicidal ideation, syncope, tremor, vertigo
CV: Arrhythmias, AV block, chest pain, congestive heart failure, elevated cholesterol and triglyceride levels, edema, extrasystoles, hypertension, hypotension, MI, palpitations, prolonged QT interval, sinus tachycardia, thrombophlebitis, torsades de pointes, vasodilation, worsening of peripheral vascular disease
EENT: Abnormal vision, accommodation abnormality, angle-closure glaucoma, blurred vision, dry mouth, mydriasis, pharyngitis, rhinitis, taste alteration, tinnitus
ENDO: Elevated blood prolactin levels, hot flashes, hyperglycemia, syndrome of inappropriate ADH secretion
GI: Abdominal pain, anorexia, colitis, constipation, diarrhea, elevated liver enzymes, flatulence, GI hemorrhage, indigestion, nausea, vomiting
GU: Anorgasmia (women), decreased libido, ejaculation disorder, impotence, urinary incontinence or urgency, urine hesitancy or retention
HEME: Abnormal bleeding, anemia, leukocytosis, leukopenia, lymphadenopathy, thrombocytopenia
MS: Neck pain, musculoskeletal stiffness, rhabdomyolysis
RESP: Cough, eosinophilic pneumonia, increased dyspnea, interstitial lung disease

SKIN: Diaphoresis, ecchymosis, erythema multiforme, pruritus, rash, Stevens-Johnson syndrome, toxic epidermal necrolysis
Other: Angioedema, hypersensitivity reactions, hyponatremia, weight gain or loss

Nursing Considerations

- Be aware that desvenlafaxine and venlafaxine should not be given to patients with congenital long QT syndrome, bradycardia, hypokalemia or hypo- magnesemia, recent acute myocardial infarction, or uncompensated heart failure because of increased risk of prolonged QT interval and torsades de pointes. It should also not be given to patients who are taking other drugs that prolong the QT interval. Expect hypokalemia and hypomagnesemia to be corrected before drug therapy is begun.
- Use cautiously in patients with a history of mania because desvenlafaxine and venlafaxine therapy may worsen condition. Also use cautiously in patients with a history of seizures, and expect to discontinue drug, as ordered, if seizures occur.
- Use cautiously in patients who have medical conditions that might be made worse by an increased heart rate, as in hyperthyroidism, heart failure, or recent MI.
WARNING Be aware that serotonin syndrome in its most severe form may resemble neuroleptic malignant syndrome, which includes hyperthermia, muscle rigidity, autonomic instability with possibly rapid changes in vital signs, and mental status changes. Notify prescriber, withhold drug immediately, and provide supportive care. Expect drug to be discontinued.
- Monitor blood pressure often during therapy because it may cause dose-related sustained increase in supine diastolic pressure. Expect to reduce or stop drug, as prescribed, if increase develops.
- Assess patient's electrolyte balance, as ordered, because drug can cause hyponatremia, especially in elderly patients and in patients who take diuretics or are volume-depleted. If patient has evidence of hyponatremia (headache, trouble concentrating, confusion, weakness, unsteadiness), notify prescriber.

If imbalance is confirmed, expect to stop drug and give appropriate care.
- Watch patient for suicidal tendencies, especially when therapy starts and dosage changes.
- Be aware that false-positive urine immunoassay screening tests for phencyclidine (PCP) and amphetamine have been found in patients taking desvenlafaxine. Expect different testing to be done to distinguish desvenlafaxine from PCP and amphetamine.
WARNING Drug shouldn't be stopped abruptly, because doing so may cause multiple adverse effects, including asthenia, dizziness, headache, insomnia, nervousness, and flulike symptoms.
- Monitor patient closely for abnormal bleeding that may range from ecchymosis to life-threatening hemorrhage. Know that concomitant use of desvenlafaxine and venlafaxine and drugs known to affect coagulation or bleeding increases the risk of bleeding.

PATIENT TEACHING
- Instruct patient not to crush or chew E.R. capsules or tablets. If she has trouble swallowing capsules, tell her to open capsule, sprinkle contents on a spoonful of applesauce, and swallow immediately without chewing, followed by a glass of water.
- Advise patient that drug may cause mild pupillary dilation, which may lead to an episode of acute closure glaucoma. Encourage patient to have an eye exam before starting therapy to see if he is at risk.
- Advise patient to avoid alcohol during venlafaxine therapy.
- Advise patient not to stop taking desvenlafaxine or venlafaxine abruptly.
- Caution patient to notify prescriber if she becomes pregnant during therapy because she'll need a different antidepressant. Taking desvenlafaxine or venlafaxine during third trimester of pregnancy increases risk of complications in the newborn.
- Advise patient to tell prescriber about all other prescribed drugs or OTC products she takes because of risk of interactions.
- Urge caregivers to monitor patient closely for suicidal tendencies, especially when therapy starts or dosage changes.

U
V
W

- Alert patient that fertility impairment may occur while taking venlafaxine. If this is a concern for the patient, instruct her to discuss with prescriber.
- Caution patient to avoid aspirin and NSAIDs, if possible, while taking desvenlafaxine or venlafaxine.
- Inform patient that urine screening tests for phencyclidine (PCP) and amphetamine may produce a false-positive for several days following discontinuation of desvenlafaxine therapy, but that other tests may be done to distinguish desvenlafaxine from PCP and amphetamine.

WARNING Tell patient to report immediately sudden onset, severe, or persistent symptoms.

verapamil
Apo-Verap (CAN), Calan, Isoptin, Novo-Veramil (CAN), Nu-Verap (CAN)

verapamil hydrochloride
Calan SR, Isoptin SR, Verelan

Class and Category
Chemical class: Phenylalkylamine derivative
Therapeutic class: Antianginal, anti-arrhythmic, antihypertensive
Pregnancy category: C

Indications and Dosages
➤ *To treat chronic angina pectoris*
TABLETS (VERAPAMIL)
Adults and adolescents age 15 and over.
Initial: 80 to 120 mg three times a day, increased every day or wk, as needed.
Maximum: 480 mg daily in divided doses.
Infants and children up to age 15. 4 to 8 mg/kg daily in divided doses.
➤ *To manage hypertension*
E.R. CAPSULES (VERAPAMIL HYDROCHLORIDE)
Adults and adolescents. *Initial:* 240 mg daily, increased every day or wk, as needed.
Maximum: 480 mg daily.
E.R. TABLETS (VERAPAMIL HYDROCHLORIDE)
Adults and adolescents. *Initial:* 180 mg daily, increased every day or wk, as needed,

according to following schedule: 240 mg daily in the morning; 180 mg every 12 hr or 240 mg in the morning and 120 mg in the evening; then 240 mg every 12 hr.
Maximum: 480 mg daily in divided doses.
TABLETS (VERAPAMIL)
Adults and adolescents age 15 and over.
Initial: 80 to 120 mg three times a day, increased every day or wk, as needed.
Maximum: 480 mg daily in divided doses.
Infants and children up to age 15. 4 to 8 mg/kg daily in divided doses.
➤ *To prevent or treat supraventricular tachycardia*
TABLETS (VERAPAMIL)
Adults and adolescents age 15 and over.
Initial: 80 to 120 mg three times a day, increased every day or wk, as needed.
Maximum: 480 mg daily in divided doses.
DOSAGE ADJUSTMENT Initial P.O. dosage, possibly reduced to 40 mg three times a day (120 mg daily for E.R. tablets or capsules) for elderly patients and those with impaired hepatic or left ventricular function. Dosage may need to be reduced in patients with decreased neuromuscular transmission.
I.V. INJECTION (VERAPAMIL HYDROCHLORIDE)
Adults and adolescents age 15 and over.
Initial: 5 to 10 mg slowly over 2 min; then 10 mg, as needed, if response isn't adequate after 30 min.
Children ages 1 to 15. *Initial:* 100 to 300 mcg/kg slowly over 2 min, up to maximum of 5 mg; then 10 mg, as needed, if response isn't adequate after 30 min.
Infants up to age 1. *Initial:* 100 to 200 mcg/ kg slowly over 2 min.
DOSAGE ADJUSTMENT I.V. drug administered over 3 minutes in elderly patients.

Mechanism of Action
Inhibits calcium movement into coronary and vascular smooth-muscle cells by blocking slow calcium channels in cell membranes. The resulting decrease in intracellular calcium level has the following effects:
- inhibits smooth-muscle cell contractions
- decreases myocardial oxygen demand by relaxing coronary and vascular smooth muscle, reducing peripheral vascular resistance, and decreasing systolic and diastolic pressures

• slows AV conduction time and prolongs AV nodal refractoriness
• interrupts reentry circuit in AV nodal reentrant tachycardias.

Route	Onset	Peak	Duration
P.O.	1–2 hr	30–90 min	6–8 hr
P.O. (E.R.)	1–2 hr	30–90 min	Unknown
I.V.	1–5 min	3–5 min	10 min–6 hr

Incompatibilities
Don't mix I.V. verapamil with albumin, amphotericin B injection, hydralazine hydrochloride injection, nafcillin, or sulfamethoxazole and trimethoprim injection. Solutions with pH above 6.0 cause precipitation.

Contraindications
Cardiogenic shock, concomitant use of beta blockers (with I.V. verapamil), hypersensitivity to verapamil or its components, hypotension, severe heart failure unless secondary to supra-ventricular tachycardia that responds to verapamil, severe left ventricular dysfunction, sick sinus syndrome or second- or third-degree heart block unless artificial pacemaker is in place, ventricular tachycardia (with I.V. verapamil)

Interactions
DRUGS
alpha blockers, antihypertensives, general anesthetics (hydrocarbon), prazosin: Hypotensive effects
aspirin: Increased bleeding time
beta blockers: Increased risk of heart failure, hypotension, and severe bradycardia
calcium supplements: Decreased response to verapamil
carbamazepine, cyclosporine, theophylline, valproate: Increased risk of toxicity from these drugs
cimetidine: Decreased metabolism and increased blood level of verapamil
clonidine: Increased risk of severe sinus bradycardia
cyclophosphamide, oncovin, procarbazine, prednisone (COPP) regimen; vindesine, adriamycin, cisplatin (VAC) regimen: Decreased verapamil absorption

dantrolene: Increased risk of hyperkalemia and myocardial depression
digoxin: Increased blood digoxin level and risk of digitalis toxicity
disopyramide, flecainide: Additive negative inotropic effects
doxorubicin: Increased plasma doxorubicin level
erythromycin, ritonavir: Increased blood verapamil level
HMG-CoA reductase inhibitors such as atorvastatin, lovastatin, and simvastatin: Increased risk of myopathy and rhabdo-myolysis
lithium: Increased risk of neurotoxicity
neuromuscular blockers: Prolonged recovery from neuromuscular blockade
NSAIDs, sympathomimetics: Decreased antihypertensive effect of verapamil
paclitaxel: Decreased paclitaxel clearance
phenobarbital: Increased verapamil clearance
procainamide: Increased QT interval, additive negative inotropic effects
protein-bound drugs (hydantoins, salicylates, sulfonamides, sulfonylureas, and warfarin and other oral anticoagulants): Altered blood levels of these drugs
quinidine: Increased risk of quinidine toxicity, increased QT interval, additive negative inotropic effects
rifampin: Decreased bioavailability of oral verapamil
telithromycin: Increased risk of brady-arrhythmias, hypotension, and lactic acidosis
FOODS
grapefruit juice: Increased verapamil level
ACTIVITIES
alcohol use: Increased blood alcohol level and prolonged CNS effects

Adverse Reactions
CNS: Asthenia, confusion, disequilibrium, dizziness, equilibrium disorders, extra-pyramidal reactions, fatigue, headache, insomnia, paresthesia, psychosis, shakiness, somnolence, stroke, syncope
CV: Abnormal ECG, angina, AV conduc-tion disorders, bradycardia, claudication, heart failure, hypertension, hypotension, MI, palpitations, peripheral edema, tachycardia, vasculitis
EENT: Blurred vision, dry mouth, tinnitus

U
V
W

ENDO: Gynecomastia, hyperprolactinemia
GI: Constipation, diarrhea, elevated liver
function test results, GI distress, nausea
GU: Galactorrhea, impotence, increased
urination, menstrual irregularities
MS: Arthralgia, muscle spasms
RESP: Dyspnea, pulmonary edema,
SKIN: Alopecia, diaphoresis, ecchymosis,
erythema multiforme, exanthema, flushing,
hyperkeratosis, rash, Stevens-Johnson
syndrome, urticaria
Other: Allergy aggravated

Nursing Considerations
• Administer I.V. verapamil with compatible
solutions, including Ringer's injection,
D_5W, or normal saline solution.
• Maintain continuous ECG monitoring and
keep emergency resuscitative equipment
and drugs readily available during I.V.
therapy.
• Assess patient with hypertrophic cardiomyopathy or idiopathic hypertrophic
subaortic stenosis for early development
of hypotension and pulmonary edema,
because second-degree AV block and
sinus arrest can result.
• Assess for bradycardia and hypotension,
and notify prescriber if heart rate or blood
pressure declines significantly.
• Disopyramide or flecainide shouldn't be
given within 48 hours before or 24 hours
after verapamil because additive negative
inotropic effects can result.
• Institute measures to prevent constipation,
including a high-fiber diet and a stool
softener, as prescribed.

PATIENT TEACHING
• Instruct patient not to crush or chew
verapamil E.R. tablets or capsules. Inform
her that she may break E.R. tablets in half
if necessary to aid swallowing.
• Direct patient to check her pulse before
taking verapamil and to notify prescriber
if it's below 50 beats/minute or as
instructed by prescriber.
• Caution patient about possible dizziness
and the need to avoid potentially
hazardous activities until drug's CNS
effects are known.
• Inform patient that adverse skin reactions
may subside with continued verapamil
use. Advise her to notify prescriber if rash
persists.

• Encourage patient to increase dietary fiber
intake to help prevent constipation. Advise
her to notify prescriber if problem
becomes persistent or severe.

vigabatrin
Sabril

Class and Category
Chemical class: Amino-hexenoic acid
Therapeutic class: Anticonvulsant
Pregnancy category: C

Indications and Dosages
➤ *As adjunct therapy for refractory*
complex partial seizures in patients with
inadequate response to several alter-
native treatments and for whom
potential benefits outweigh the risk of
vision loss
TABLETS
Adults, adolescents older than 16 years of
age, and children age 10 to 16 weighing
more than 60 kg (132 lbs). *Initial:* 500 mg
twice daily, increased weekly in 500 mg
increments, as needed. *Maximum:* 1.5 g
twice daily.
Children age 10 to 16 years of age
weighing 60 kg (132 lbs) or less. *Initial:*
250 mg twice daily, increased weekly in
250 mg increments, as needed. *Maximum:*
1 gram twice daily.
DOSAGE ADJUSTMENT For patient with
mild renal impairment (creatinine
clearance 51 to 80 ml/min/1.73 m²),
reduce dose by 25%. For patients with
moderate renal impairment (creatinine
clearance 31 to 50 ml/min/1.73 m²),
reduce dose by 50%. For patients with
severe renal impairment (creatinine
clearance 11 to 30 ml/min/
1.73 m²), reduce dose by 75%.
➤ *As monotherapy for pediatric patients*
with infantile spasms for whom poten-
tial benefits outweigh risk of vision
loss
ORAL SOLUTION
Children age 1 month to 2 years. *Initial:*
50 mg/kg/day in 2 divided doses, increased
every 3 days by 25 to 50 mg/kg/day, as
needed. *Maximum:* 150 mg/kg/day.

DOSAGE ADJUSTMENT For patient with mild renal impairment (creatinine clearance 51 to 80 ml/min), reduce dose by 25%. For patients with moderate renal impairment (creatinine clearance 31 to 50 ml/min/1.73 m^2), reduce dose by 50%. For patients with severe renal impairment (creatinine clearance 11 to 30 ml/min/1.73 m^2), reduce dose by 75%.

Route	Onset	Peak	Duration
P.O.	Unknown	1 hr	Unknown

Mechanism of Action
Inhibits the action of gamma aminobutyric acid transaminase (GABA-T), the enzyme responsible for metabolism of the inhibitory neurotransmitter GABA. This increases GABA level in the CNS, which may play a role in suppression of seizure activity.

Contraindications
Hypersensitivity to vigabatrin and its components

Interactions
DRUGS
phenytoin: Decreased serum phenytoin level

Adverse Reactions
CNS: Abnormal magnetic resonance imaging (MRI), abnormal behavior or dreams, acute psychosis, anxiety, apathy, asthenia, attention disturbance, confusion, coordination abnormality, delirium, depression, dizziness, dystonia, encephalopathy, expressive language disorder, fatigue, fever, gait disturbance, headache, hyperreflexia, hypertonia, hypoaesthesia, hyporeflexia, hypomania, hypotonia, insomnia, irritability, lethargy, malaise, malignant hyperthermia, memory loss, myoclonus, nervousness, paresthesia, peripheral neuropathy, postictal state, seizures, sensory disturbance, somnolence, status epilepticus, suicidal ideation, thirst, tremor, vertigo
CV: Chest pain, edema, peripheral edema
EENT: Asthenopia, blurred vision, deafness, diplopia, eye pain, laryngeal edema, nasopharyngitis, nystagmus, optic neuritis, pharyngolaryngeal pain, tinnitus, toothache, vision loss (severe), visual field defect
ENDO: Delayed puberty

GI: Abdominal or stomach pain, cholestasis, constipation, decreased liver enzymes, diarrhea, distention, dyspepsia, esophagitis, GI hemorrhage, nausea, vomiting
GU: Dysmenorrhea, erectile dysfunction, UTI
HEME: Anemia
MS: Arthralgia; back or limb pain; dysarthria; muscle spasticity, spasms or twitching
RESP: Bronchitis, cough, pulmonary edema, respiratory failure, stridor, upper respiratory infection
SKIN: Facial edema, maculopapular rash, pruritus, Stevens-Johnson syndrome, toxic epidermal necrolysis
Other: Angioedema, birth defects, developmental delay, influenza, multi-organ failure, weight gain

Nursing Considerations
• Vigabatrin therapy is only available under a restricted distribution program called the SHARE program (1-888-45-SHARE).

WARNING Monitor patient's vision, and make sure patient has been examined by an ophthalmic professional in which visual fields and retinal examination has been performed no later than 4 weeks after vigabatrin therapy has begun and then periodically thereafter because drug can cause progressive and permanent bilateral concentric visual field constriction and reduce visual acuity. Be aware that while risk increases with total dose and duration of therapy, all patients are at risk for visual abnormalities even after drug has been stopped. Because of the risk of permanent and possibly severe vision loss, drug can be prescribed and obtained only through the SHARE distribution program. Report any visual abnormalities immediately, and expect drug to be discontinued.

• Abnormal MRI results have been noted in some infants receiving vigabatrin.
• Monitor patient for suicidal ideation throughout therapy but especially when therapy starts or dosage changes.
• When discontinuing vigabatrin therapy, expect to do so gradually by decreasing daily dose by 1 gram each week until drug is discontinued, as ordered.
• When discontinuing vigabatrin therapy in children, expect to do so gradually by

U
V
W

decreasing dose by 25 to 50 mg/kg/day every 3 to 4 days.

• Monitor patient for evidence of peripheral neuropathy, such as numbness or tingling in toes or feet, reduced distal lower limb vibration or position sense, or progressive loss of reflexes, starting at the ankles. Alert prescriber if abnormalities are present.

• Assess patient routinely for edema, including peripheral edema.

PATIENT TEACHING

• Explain the risk of possibly permanent vision loss before patient starts vigabatrin.

• Warn patient not to stop taking vigabatrin abruptly; it will need to be weaned off gradually over several weeks.

• Advise female patient of childbearing age to use effective contraception if sexually active and to report suspected or confirmed pregnancy immediately.

• Advise patient or caregiver to notify prescriber if patient has unusual feelings or behaviors, especially if related to suicidal ideation and particularly at the beginning of therapy and during dosage adjustments.

• Caution patient not to perform hazardous activities such as operating equipment until CNS effects of the drug are known.

• Alert patient to monitor his weight because drug may cause weight gain.

vilazodone hydrochloride

Viibryd

Class and Category

Chemical class: Selective serotonin reuptake inhibitor
Therapeutic class: Antidepressant
Pregnancy category: C

Indications and Dosages

➤ *To treat major depressive disorder*

TABLETS

Adults. *Initial:* 10 mg once daily for 7 days, followed by 20 mg once daily for 7 days, then increased to 40 mg once daily.

DOSAGE ADJUSTMENT For patients taking a strong inhibitor of CYP3A4 such as ketoconazole, dosage reduced to 20 mg daily. For patients taking a moderate inhibitor of CYP3A4 such as erythromycin and experiencing intolerable adverse effects, dosage reduced to 20 mg daily. For patients taking a strong CYP3A4 inducer such as carbamazepine for more than 14 days, dosage may be increased up to twofold but not exceeding 80 mg daily.

Mechanism of Action

Exerts antidepressant effects by potentiating serotonin activity in CNS and inhibiting serotonin reuptake at the presynaptic neuronal membrane. Blocked serotonin reuptake increases levels and prolongs activity of serotonin at synaptic receptor sites.

Contraindications

Hypersensitivity to vilazodone or its components, use within 14 days of MAO inhibitor therapy

Interactions

DRUGS

aspirin, NSAIDs, warfarin and other anticoagulants: Increased risk of bleeding

buspirone, MAO inhibitors, serotonin reuptake inhibitors, serotonin norepinephrine reuptake inhibitors, tramadol, triptans, tryptophan: Increased risk of life-threatening adverse effects such as serotonin syndrome

CYP2C8 substrate, highly protein bound drugs: Possibly increased blood concentration of the CYP2C8 substrate or highly protein bound drug

CYP3A4 inhibitors such as erythromycin, ketoconazole: Increased blood vilazodone levels with increased risk of adverse effects

Adverse Reactions

CNS: Abnormal dreams, dizziness, fatigue, feeling jittery, hallucinations, insomnia, irritability, mania, migraine, neuroleptic malignant syndrome-like reactions, panic attack, paresthesia, restlessness, seizures, serotonin syndrome, suicidal ideation, tremor

CV: Palpitations, prolonged QT interval, torsades de pointes, ventricular extrasystoles

EENT: Angle closure glaucoma, blurred vision, cataracts, dry eyes or mouth

GI: Anorexia, diarrhea, dyspepsia, flatulence, gastroenteritis, gastrointestinal

bleeding, increased appetite, nausea, vomiting
GU: Decreased libido, delayed ejaculation, erectile dysfunction, pollakiuria
HEME: Bleeding events
MS: Arthralgia
SKIN: Diaphoresis, night sweats

Nursing Considerations

• Be aware that vilazodine should not be given to patients with congenital long QT syndrome, bradycardia, hypokalemia or hypomagnesemia, recent acute myocardial infarction, or uncompensated heart failure because of increased risk of prolonged QT interval and torsades de pointes. It should also not be given to patients who are taking other drugs that prolong the QT interval. Expect hypokalemia and hypomagnesemia to be corrected before vilazodine therapy is begun.

• •Use vilazodone cautiously in a patient with a seizure disorder because drug effect has not been studied in patients with seizures.

• Expect to taper vilazodone therapy gradually when drug is no longer required; abrupt discontinuation can precipitate withdrawal symptoms.

WARNING Monitor patient closely for serotonin syndrome exhibited by agitation, hallucinations, coma, tachycardia, labile blood pressure, hyper-thermia, hyperreflexia, incoordination, nausea, vomiting or diarrhea. Notify prescriber immediately because serotonin syndrome may be life-threatening; provide supportive care.

WARNING Be aware that serotonin syndrome in its most severe form may resemble neuroleptic malignant syndrome, which includes hyperthermia, muscle rigidity, and autonomic instability with possibly rapid changes in vital signs and mental status. Stop drug immediately, and provide supportive care.

• Watch patient closely for suicidal tenden-cies, particularly when therapy starts and dosage changes, because depression may worsen temporarily during these times, possibly leading to suicidal ideation.

• Watch for mania, which may result from any antidepressant in a susceptible patient.

• Monitor patient closely for evidence of GI bleeding, especially if patient also takes a drug known to cause GI bleeding, such as aspirin, an NSAID, or warfarin.

• Monitor patient's serum sodium level, as ordered, especially in the elderly and patients with volume depletion, because selective serotonin reuptake inhibitors, the class of drugs vilazodone belongs to, have caused hyponatremia. If patient develops a headache, difficulty concentrating, memory impairment, confusion, weakness, and unsteadiness, and sodium level has decreased, notify prescriber and expect drug to be discontinued. Be prepared to provide supportive care.

PATIENT TEACHING

• Instruct patient to take vilazodone with food because drug may not be as effective if taken on an empty stomach.

• Advise patient that drug may cause mild pupillary dilation, which may lead to an episode of acute closure glaucoma. Encourage patient to have an eye exam before starting therapy to see if he is at risk.

• Tell family or caregiver to observe patient closely for suicidal tendencies, especially when therapy starts or dosage changes.

• Tell patient not to take aspirin or NSAIDs during therapy because they increase the risk of bleeding. If patient takes warfarin, tell her to use bleeding precautions and to notify prescriber at once if bleeding occurs.

• Caution patient to alert all prescribers about vilazodone therapy because of potentially serious drug interactions.

vorapaxar

Zontivity

Class and Category

Che*mical class:* Carbamate sulfate
Therapeutic class: Antiplatelet
Pregnancy category: B

Indications and Dosages

➤ *To reduce thrombotic cardiovascular events in patients with a history of myocardial infarction or peripheral arterial disease*

U
V
W

TABLETS
Adults. 2.08 mg once daily.

Mechanism of Action
Inhibits thrombin-induced and thrombin receptor agonist peptide-induced platelet aggregation.

Contraindications
Active pathologic bleeding; history of intracranial hemorrhage, stroke, or transient ischemic attack; hypersensitivity to vorapaxar or its components

Interaction
DRUGS
strong CYP3A inducers such as carbamazepine, phenytoin, rifampin, St. John's wort: Decreased vorapaxar effectiveness
strong CYP3A inhibitors such as boceprevir, clarithromycin, conivaptan, indinavir, itraconazole, ketoconazole, nelfinavir, posaconazole, ritonavir, saquinavir: Increased vorapaxar exposure and adverse reactions

Adverse Reactions
CNS: Depression, intracranial hemorrhage
EENT: Diplopia, oculomotor disturbance, retinal disorder including retinopathy
GI: Gastrointestinal bleeding
HEME: Anemia, bleeding events (mild to severe), iron deficiency
SKIN: Eruptions, exanthema, rash

Nursing Considerations
• Be aware that vorapaxar is usually prescribed along with other antiplatelet agents such as aspirin and/or clopidogrel.
• Know that vorapaxar should not be given to patients with a history of intracranial hemorrhage, stroke, or transient ischemic attack because of an increased risk for intracranial hemorrhage. The drug should be discontinued in a patient who experiences a stroke while taking vorapaxar.
• Assess patient's bleeding risk before beginning vorapaxar therapy, because vorapaxar increases the risk of bleeding in proportion to the patient's underlying bleeding risk. Factors that may increase the patient's risk of bleeding include the use of certain concomitant drugs such as anticoagulants, fibrinolytic therapy, chronic nonsteroidal anti-inflammatory drugs, selective serotonin reuptake inhibitors, or serotonin–norepinephrine reuptake inhibitors; history of bleeding disorders; low body weight; older age; or reduced hepatic or renal function.
• Know that vorapaxar should not be given to patients with severe hepatic impairment because of increased risk for bleeding.

WARNING Monitor patient for bleeding throughout vorapaxar therapy. Suspect bleeding in patient who is hypotensive and has recently undergone coronary angiography, percutaneous coronary intervention, coronary artery bypass graft surgery, or other surgical procedures. Stop vorapaxar therapy and notify prescriber immediately of suspected or known bleeding. Prepare to support patient according to standard of care, as there is no known treatment to reverse the antiplatelet effect of the drug because of its long half-life. Significant inhibition of platelet aggregation has been known to persist for at least 4 weeks after the drug has been discontinued.

PATIENT TEACHING
• Tell patient to take vorapaxar exactly as prescribed and not to discontinue the drug without discussing it with the prescriber.
• Inform patient that he may bleed or bruise more easily. Stress importance of promptly reporting any unanticipated, prolonged, or excessive bleeding, or blood in the stool or urine.
• Review safety precautions to avoid bleeding events, such as using an electric razor and soft toothbrush.
• Remind patient to inform all physicians and dentists of vorapaxar use prior to any surgery or dental procedure. Emphasize that the doctor or dentist performing the procedure should talk to the prescriber before stopping the drug.
• Tell patient to keep prescriber informed of all prescription and over-the-counter drugs and dietary supplements he takes.

voriconazole
Vfend

Class and Category
Chemical class: Triazole

Therapeutic class: Antifungal
Pregnancy category: D

Indications and Dosages

➤ *To treat invasive aspergillosis; to treat serious fungal infections caused by* Scedosporium apiospermum *and* Fusarium *species, including* Fusarium solani, *in patients intolerant of or refractory to other therapy*

I.V. INFUSION

Adults and children age 12 and over.
Initial: 6 mg/kg over 1 to 2 hr at no more than 3 mg/kg/hr every 12 hr for 2 doses. *Maintenance:* 4 mg/kg over 1 to 2 hr at no more than 3 mg/kg/hr every 12 hr.

TABLETS

Adults and children age 12 and over weighing 40 kg (88 lb) or more.
Maintenance: 200 mg every 12 hr, increased to 300 mg every 12 hr, as needed, and taken at least 1 hr before or after a meal.

Adults and children age 12 and over weighing less than 40 kg. *Maintenance:* 100 mg every 12 hr, increased to 150 mg every 12 hr, as needed, and taken at least 1 hr before or after a meal.

➤ *To treat candidemia in nonneutropenic patients and other deep-tissue disseminated* Candida *infections involving the abdomen, kidney, bladder wall, skin, or a wound*

I.V. INFUSION

Adults. *Initial:* 6 mg/kg over 1 to 2 hr at no more than 3 mg/kg/hr every 12 hr for 2 doses. *Maintenance:* 3 to 4 mg/kg over 1 to 2 hr at no more than 3 mg/kg/hr every 12 hr for at least 14 days after symptoms resolve or last positive culture, whichever takes longer.

TABLETS

Adults. *Maintenance:* 200 mg every 12 hr taken at least 1 hr before or after a meal.

➤ *To treat esophageal candidiasis*

TABLETS

Adults. 200 mg every 12 hr taken at least 1 hr before or after a meal for at least 14 days and at least 7 days after signs and symptoms resolve.

DOSAGE ADJUSTMENT If patient can't tolerate drug, I.V. maintenance dose may be reduced to 3 mg/kg every 12 hr and oral maintenance dose by 50-mg decrements to at least 200 mg every 12 hr (100 mg every 12 hr for patients weighing less than 40 kg).

For use with phenytoin, maintenance dose may be increased to 5 mg/kg I.V. every 12 hr or from 200 mg to 400 mg P.O. every 12 hr (100 mg to 200 mg every 12 hr for patients weighing less than 40 kg). For patients with mild to moderate hepatic cirrhosis, standard loading dose should be used but maintenance dose halved for I.V. or P.O. use. For patients with moderate to severe renal insufficiency (creatinine clearance greater than 50 ml/ min/1.73 m^2), only the oral form should be given, if possible.

Mechanism of Action

Prevents fungal ergosterol biosynthesis by inhibiting fungal cytochrome P-450– mediated 14 alpha-lanosterol demethylation. The loss of ergosterol in the fungal cell wall renders the fungal cell inactive.

Incompatibilities

Don't infuse into the same line or cannula with other drugs, including parenteral nutrition, to prevent an increase in subvisible particulate matter. Avoid infusion with blood products and any electrolyte supplements. Don't dilute with 4.2% sodium bicarbonate infusion because the mildly alkaline nature of the diluent causes slight degradation of voriconazole after 24 hours of storage at room temperature.

Contraindications

Coadministration with long-acting barbiturates, carbamazepine, CYP3A4 substrates (astemizole, cisapride, pimozide, quinidine, or terfenadine), efavirenz, ergot alkaloids, rifabutin, rifampin, ritonavir, sirolimus, or St. John's wort; hypersensitivity to voriconazole or its components; galactose intolerance, glucose-galactose malabsorption, or Lapp lactase deficiency (oral form only contains lactose)

Interactions

DRUGS

alfentanil: Increased plasma alfentanil level and increased risk of adverse reactions
benzodiazepines: Possibly prolonged sedative effect of benzodiazepines
calcium channel blockers; HMG-CoA reductase inhibitors, such as lovastatin; omeprazole; sirolimus: Possibly increased plasma levels of these drugs, leading to

increased risk of adverse reactions and toxicity

carbamazepine, long-acting barbiturates, phenytoin, rifampin: Decreased plasma voriconazole concentration

coumarin, warfarin: Possibly increased PTT

cyclosporine, sirolimus, tacrolimus: Increased serum concentrations of these drugs and risk of toxicity, especially nephrotoxicity

CYP3A4 substrates (astemizole, cisapride, pimozide, quinidine, terfenadine): Increased plasma levels of these drugs, which may lead to prolonged QT interval and, rarely, torsades de pointes

ergot alkaloids (ergotamine, dihydro-ergotamine): May increase plasma level of ergot alkaloids, leading to ergotism

fluconazole, oral contraceptives: Increased plasma voriconazole level and risk of toxicity

HIV protease inhibitors (amprenavir, nelfinavir, ritonavir, saquinavir), non-nucleoside reverse transcriptase inhibitors (delavirdine, efavirenz): Possibly inhibited metabolism of these drugs and voriconazole

methadone: Increased plasma level of methadone, possibly leading to toxicity, including QT-interval prolongation

oral contraceptives: Increased plasma voriconazole level and risk of toxicity

rifabutin: Increased rifabutin plasma level; decreased voriconazole plasma level

St. John's wort: Decreased plasma voriconazole level

sulfonylureas: Possibly increased plasma level of sulfonylureas and increased risk of hypoglycemia

vinca alkaloids: Possibly increased risk of neurotoxicity

Adverse Reactions

CNS: Chills, dizziness, fever, hallucinations, headache

CV: Chest pain, hypertension, hypotension, peripheral edema, tachycardia, vasodilation

EENT: Abnormal or blurred vision, altered or enhanced visual perception, change in color perception, chromatopsia, dry mouth, eye hemorrhage, photophobia, visual disturbances

GI: Abdominal pain, diarrhea, elevated liver function test results, nausea, pancreatitis, vomiting

GU: Abnormal kidney function, acute renal failure, elevated serum creatinine level

HEME: Anemia, leukopenia, pancytopenia, thrombocytopenia

MS: Fluorosis, periostitis, skeletal pain

RESP: Respiratory disorders

SKIN: Cholestatic jaundice, erythema multiforme, jaundice, maculopapular rash, photosensitivity, pruritus, rash, Stevens-Johnson syndrome, toxic epidermal necrolysis

Other: Anaphylaxis (I.V. form), elevated alkaline phosphatase, hypokalemia, hypomagnesemia, sepsis

Nursing Considerations

• Use voriconazole cautiously in patients hypersensitive to other azoles and in patients at risk for proarrhythmic events (such as those receiving cardiotoxic chemotherapy or those who have cardiomyopathy or hypokalemia) because some azoles may prolong the QT interval.

• Determine if patient has any problems with galactose intolerance, Lapp lactase deficiency, or glucose-galactose malabsorption before starting therapy because voriconazole tablets contain lactose and shouldn't be given to patients with these conditions.

• Obtain specimens for fungal culture and other relevant laboratory studies (including histopathology), as ordered, before giving first dose. Expect to begin drug before test results are known.

• Assess patient's liver function, including bilirubin, as ordered, at the start of voriconazole therapy and periodically thereafter. Be aware that drug may be discontinued if liver abnormalities occur.

• Check patient's electrolyte levels and correct any imbalances, as ordered, before giving voriconazole because electrolyte imbalances increase the risk of adverse reactions.

• For I.V. infusion, reconstitute powder with 19 ml water for injection to obtain 20 ml of concentrate containing 10 mg/ml voriconazole. To make sure exact amount of water is injected into vial, use a standard 10-ml nonautomated syringe. Shake vial until all powder is dissolved. Further dilute so final concentration is no less than 0.5 mg/ml and no more than 5 mg/ml. This requires withdrawing and discarding at least an equal volume of diluent from infusion bag or bottle before instillation of concentrate.

• Discard partially used vials after mixing. If infusion isn't administered immediately, store at 2° to 8° C (37° to 46° F) for no longer than 24 hours.

• Administer I.V. infusion over 1 to 2 hours at no more than 3 mg/kg/hr.

• Monitor renal function, especially serum creatinine level, when giving I.V. form of voriconazole because drug may accumulate in body when creatinine clearance is less than 50 ml/min/1.73 m^2, increasing the risk of adverse reactions.

WARNING Observe patient receiving I.V. voriconazole closely for anaphylactoid-type reactions—such as flushing, fever, sweating, tachycardia, chest tightness, dyspnea, faintness, nausea, pruritus, and rash—which may occur immediately after starting infusion. Stop infusion if these reactions occur, and notify prescriber immediately.

• Monitor patient closely throughout therapy for rash, which may indicate a serious cutaneous reaction, such as Stevens-Johnson syndrome. If rash occurs, notify prescriber, and expect that voriconazole may be discontinued.

• Monitor cyclosporine, tacrolimus, and warfarin closely for elevated levels when voriconazole is given with any of these drugs.

• Monitor diabetic patients also taking sulfonylureas closely for hypoglycemia, and check blood glucose levels regularly.

• Voriconazole dosage will need to be adjusted when given with phenytoin. Expect to monitor plasma phenytoin level and observe patient closely for phenytoin-related adverse reactions.

• Assess patient's visual function, including visual acuity, visual field, and color perception, if voriconazole therapy continues longer than 28 days.

• Monitor patient closely for pancreatitis, especially if patient is a child or has risk factors for acute pancreatitis, such as recent chemotherapy or hematopoietic stem cell transplantation.

• Report skeletal pain to prescriber and expect skeletal X-rays to be done. If fluoroisis or periostitis is found, anticipate voriconazole therapy to be discontinued.

PATIENT TEACHING

• Instruct patient taking oral voriconazole to take the tablets at least 1 hour before or 1 hour after a meal.

• Inform female patient of possible fetal risk, and emphasize need to avoid pregnancy. Tell her to use effective contraception during therapy and to notify prescriber immediately if pregnancy is suspected.

• Caution patient not to drive at night and to avoid hazardous activities because drug may cause visual disturbances, including blurring or photophobia.

• Advise patient to avoid exposure to direct sunlight or UV light and to wear sunscreen when outdoors.

vortioxetine hydrobromide
Brintellix

Class and Category
Chemical class: Piperazine
Therapeutic class: Antidepressant, Selective Serotonin Reuptake Inhibitor
Pregnancy category: C

Indications and Dosages
➤ *To treat major depressive disorder (MDD)*

TABLETS
Adults. *Initial:* 10 mg once daily, then increased to 20 mg once daily, as tolerated. *Maximum:* 20 mg once daily.
DOSAGE ADJUSTMENT For patients who cannot tolerate higher doses, dosage may be decreased down to 5 mg once daily. For patients taking strong CYP inducers, such as carbamazepine, phenytoin, or rifampin concurrently for longer than 14 days, dosage increased up to 3 times the original dose and when inducer is discontinued, dosage decreased to original level within 14 days. For patients taking strong CYP2D6 inhibitors such as bupropion, fluoxetine, paroxetine or quinidine concurrently, dosage reduced by one half, and when inhibitor is discontinued, dosage increased to original level within 14 days. For patients

U
V
W

who are known CYP2D6 poor metabolizers, maximum dosage is 10 mg once daily.

Mechanism of Action

Enhances serotonergic activity in the central nervous system through inhibiting the reuptake of serotonin. Enhanced serotonergic activity is thought to relieve symptoms of depression.

Contraindications

Hypersensitivity to vortioxetine or its components; use within 14 days of a MAO inhibitor, including intravenous methylene blue and linezolid

Interactions

DRUGS

aspirin, NSAIDs, warfarin and other anticoagulants: Increased risk of bleeding
buspirone, MAO inhibitors, SNRIs, SSRIs, tramadol, triptans, tryptophans: Increased risk of serotonin toxicity
CYP2D6 inhibitors (strong) such as bupropion, fluoxetine, paroxetine, quinidine: Increased plasma vortioxetine levels with increased risk of adverse reactions

Adverse Reactions

CNS: Abnormal dreams, activation of hypomania/mania, dizziness, serotonin syndrome, suicidal ideation, vertigo
EENT: Altered taste, angle-closure glaucoma, dry mouth
GI: Constipation, diarrhea, dyspepsia, flatulence, nausea, vomiting
GU: Decreased libido, sexual performance, or sexual satisfaction
HEME: Abnormal bleeding
RESP: Difficulty breathing
SKIN: Flushing, pruritus, rash, urticaria
Other: Hyponatremia

Nursing Considerations

• Be aware that at least 14 days should elapse between discontinuing a MAO inhibitor used to treat psychiatric disorders and initiation of vortioxetine therapy to avoid risk of patient developing serotonin syndrome. Also, know that at least 21 days should elapse after vortioxetine is discontinued and therapy with a MAO inhibitor used to treat a psychiatric disorder is begun.

• Expect dosage to be decreased to 10 mg once daily for one week before vortioxetine is discontinued to avoid patient experiencing dizziness, headaches, mood swings, including sudden outbursts of anger, muscle tension and runny nose that may occur in the first week of abrupt discontinuation of the drug.

• Watch patient closely for suicidal tendencies, particularly when therapy starts and dosage changes, because depression may worsen temporarily during these times, possibly leading to suicidal ideation.

• Watch for mania, which may result from use of any antidepressant in a susceptible patient.

• Monitor patient closely for evidence of GI bleeding, especially if patient also takes a drug known to cause GI bleeding, such as aspirin, a NSAID, warfarin, or other anticoagulants.

WARNING Monitor patient closely for serotonin syndrome exhibited by agitation, hallucinations, coma, tachycardia, labile blood pressure, hyperthermia, hyperreflexia, incoordination, nausea, vomiting, or diarrhea. Notify prescriber immediately because serotonin syndrome may be life-threatening, and provide supportive care.

• Monitor patient's serum sodium level because hyponatremia has occurred with use of serotonergic drugs, including vortioxetine. Patients at greater risk include the elderly and patients taking diuretics or who are volume-depleted. Report signs and symptoms of hyponatremia, such as confusion, difficulty concentrating, headache, memory impairment, unsteadiness, or weakness. If left untreated, coma, death, hallucinations, seizures, respiratory arrest, or syncope may occur.

PATIENT TEACHING

• Instruct patient to take drug exactly as prescribed and to alert prescriber with concerns.

• Inform patient that nausea is the most common side effect of vortioxetine therapy, and it commonly occurs within the first week of treatment.

• Advise patient that drug may cause mild pupillary dilation, which may lead to an episode of acute closure glaucoma. Encourage patient to have an eye exam before starting therapy to see if he is at risk.

- Tell family or caregiver to observe patient closely for suicidal tendencies, especially when therapy starts or dosage changes.
- Warn patient not to discontinue drug abruptly.
- Advise patient to inform all prescribers of vortioxetine therapy.
- Emphasize importance of reporting any sudden, persistent, or severe symptoms to prescriber.
- Alert patients about risk of bleeding when taking drugs known to increase risk of bleeding, such as aspirin, NSAIDs, or blood thinners.
- Tell patient and caregivers to report any signs of abnormal behavior.
- Inform elderly patient or patient who is taking drugs, such as diuretics, that cause him to be dehydrated of the risk of a low sodium level; tell patient to alert prescriber if he experiences new or sudden onset of symptoms.
- Advise patient to seek emergency medical attention if an allergic reaction such as difficulty breathing, hives, rash, or swelling occurs.
- Instruct female patients of childbearing age to notify prescriber if pregnancy occurs or is suspected.

warfarin sodium

Coumadin

Class and Category

Chemical class: Coumarin derivative
Therapeutic class: Anticoagulant
Pregnancy category: X

Indications and Dosages

➤ *To prevent or treat pulmonary embolism; recurrent MI; thromboembolic complications from atrial fibrillation, heart valve replacement, or MI; and venous thrombosis (and its extension)*

TABLETS

Adults. *Initial:* 2 to 5 mg daily for 2 to 4 days. *Usual:* 2 to 10 mg daily based on

target PT and INR results. *Maximum:* Determined by target PT and INR results, as prescribed.

I.V. INJECTION

Adults. *Initial:* 2 to 5 mg daily infused over 1 to 2 min. *Usual:* 2 to 10 mg daily infused over 1 to 2 min. *Maximum:* Determined by target PT and INR results, as prescribed.

DOSAGE ADJUSTMENT For patients with hepatic dysfunction, dosage reduced to 0.1 mg/kg, as prescribed. For elderly patients, dosage possibly reduced based on PT and INR results.

Route	Onset	Peak	Duration
P.O	24 hr	3–4 days	2–5 days
I.V.	Unknown	3–4 days	2–5 days

Mechanism of Action

Interferes with the liver's ability to synthesize vitamin K–dependent clotting factors, depleting clotting factors II (prothrombin), VII, IX, and X. This action, in turn, interferes with the clotting cascade. By depleting vitamin K–dependent clotting factors and interfering with the clotting cascade, warfarin prevents coagulation.

Incompatibilities

Don't mix warfarin in solution with amikacin sulfate, epinephrine hydrochloride, metaraminol tartrate, oxytocin, promazine hydrochloride, tetracycline hydrochloride, or vancomycin hydrochloride.

Contraindications

Bleeding or bleeding tendencies; blood dyscrasias; cerebral or dissecting aneurysm; cerebrovascular hemorrhage; diverticulitis; eclampsia or preeclampsia; history of warfarin-induced necrosis; hypersensitivity to warfarin or its components; malignant or severe uncontrolled hypertension; malnutrition and emaciation; mental state or condition that leads to lack of patient cooperation; pericardial effusion; pericarditis; polyarthritis; pregnancy; prostatectomy; recent or planned neurosurgery, ophthalmic surgery, or spinal puncture; severe hepatic or renal disease

U
V
W

Interactions

DRUGS

acetaminophen, agrimony, aminoglycosides, amiodarone, androgens, argatroban, beta blockers, bivalirudin, capecitabine, cephalosporins, chloral hydrate, chloramphenicol, chlorpropamide, cimetidine, clofibrate, corticosteroids, cyclophosphamide, dextrothyroxine, diflunisal, disulfiram, erythromycin, ezetimibe, fluconazole, gemfibrozil, glucagon, hydantoins, ifosfamide, influenza virus vaccine, isoniazid, ketoconazole, lepirudin, loop diuretics, lovastatin, metronidazole, miconazole, mineral oil, moricizine, nalidixic acid, NSAIDs, omeprazole, penicillins, phenylbutazones, propafenone, propoxyphene, quinidine, quinine, quinolones, salicylates, streptokinase, sulfamethoxazole-trimethoprim, sulfinpyrazone, sulfonamides, tamoxifen, tetracyclines, thyroid hormones, urokinase, valdecoxib, vitamin E: Increased anticoagulant effect of warfarin, increased risk of bleeding

aminoglutethimide, barbiturates, carbamazepine, cholestyramine, dicloxacillin, estrogens, ethchlorvynol, etretinate, glutethimide, griseofulvin, nafcillin, oral contraceptives, rifampin, spironolactone, sucralfate, thiazide diuretics, trazodone, vitamin C, vitamin K: Decreased anticoagulant effect of warfarin

atorvastatin, pravastatin: Increased or decreased anticoagulant effect of warfarin

herbal remedies (including bromelains, danshen, dong quai, garlic, ginkgo biloba, and ginseng): Increased anticoagulant effect of warfarin, increased risk of bleeding

I.V. lipid emulsion, other medical products that contain soybean oil: Possibly decreased vitamin K absorption and increased anticoagulant effect of warfarin

nicotine patch: Altered response to warfarin

FOODS

certain multivitamins, enteral feedings, vitamin K–rich foods: Decreased warfarin effects

ACTIVITIES

alcohol use: Increased risk of hypoprothrombinemia

smoking, smoking cessation: Altered response to warfarin

Adverse Reactions

CNS: Coma, intracranial hemorrhage, loss of consciousness, syncope, weakness
CV: Angina, chest pain, hypotension
EENT: Epistaxis, intraocular hemorrhage
GI: Abdominal cramps and pain, diarrhea, hepatitis, nausea, vomiting
GU: Hematuria, vaginal bleeding (abnormal)
HEME: Anemia, potentially fatal hemorrhage (from any tissue or organ)
SKIN: Alopecia, ecchymosis, jaundice, petechiae, pruritus, purple-toe syndrome, tissue necrosis
Other: Anaphylaxis

Nursing Considerations

• Reconstitute parenteral warfarin just before administration with 2.7 ml sterile water for injection to yield 2 mg/ml. Then give slowly over 1 to 2 minutes through peripheral I.V.
• Expect to give another parenteral anticoagulant, such as heparin or enoxaparin, with oral warfarin for at least 3 days, or until desired response occurs, before giving warfarin only.
• Avoid I.M. injections during warfarin therapy, if possible, because they can result in bleeding, bruising, and hematoma.
• Monitor INR (daily in acute care setting) and assess for therapeutic effects, as prescribed. Therapeutic INR levels are 2.0 to 3.0 for bioprosthetic heart valve, nonvalvular atrial fibrillation, and venous thromboembolism, and 2.5 to 3.5 after MI and for mechanical heart valve.
• Expect treatment to last up to 12 weeks for bioprosthetic heart valve, 1 to 3 months for nonvalvular atrial fibrillation or venous thromboembolism, and for rest of life after MI and for mechanical heart valve replacement.
WARNING Be aware of the increased risk for intracranial hemorrhage if patient has cerebral ischemia (such as recent transient ischemic attack or minor ischemic stroke) and INR of 3 to 4.5. As prescribed, withhold next warfarin dose and give vitamin K if INR exceeds 4 because of the risk of bleeding.
• Assess for occult bleeding if patient receives I.V. lipid emulsion or other medical product that contains soybean oil.

Such products can decrease vitamin K absorption and increase warfarin's anticoagulant effect.

PATIENT TEACHING

• Explain that warfarin therapy aims to prevent thrombosis by decreasing clotting ability while avoiding the risk of spontaneous bleeding.

• Instruct patient to take drug exactly as prescribed at the same time each evening.

• Urge patient to keep weekly follow-up appointments for blood tests after discharge until PT and INR levels are stabilized.

• Advise patient to avoid alcohol during warfarin therapy.

• Urge patient to take precautions against bleeding, such as using an electric shaver and a soft-bristled toothbrush. Advise him to continue these precautions for 2 to 5 days after therapy stops, as directed, because anticoagulant effect may persist during this time.

• Caution patient to avoid activities that could cause traumatic injury and bleeding.

• Advise patient to eat consistent amounts of vitamin K-rich foods, such as dark green, leafy vegetables.

• Urge patient to notify prescriber immediately about unusual bleeding and any unexplained symptoms, such as abnormal vaginal bleeding; dizziness; easy bruising; gum bleeding; headache; nosebleeds; prolonged bleeding from cuts; red, black, or tarry stool; red or dark brown urine; swelling; and weakness.

• Advise patient to consult prescriber before taking other drugs—including OTC drugs and herbal remedies—during therapy.

• Instruct female patient of childbearing age to stop taking warfarin and notify prescriber immediately if she is or could be pregnant.

• Explain that drug may cause reversible purple-toe syndrome and that this syndrome isn't harmful.

• Urge patient to carry medical identification that reveals he's taking warfarin.

U
V
W

X Y Z

zafirlukast
Accolate

Class and Category
Chemical class: Peptide leukotriene receptor antagonist
Therapeutic class: Antiasthmatic
Pregnancy category: B

Indications and Dosages
➤ *To treat chronic asthma*
TABLETS
Adults and children over age 11. 20 mg twice daily.
Children ages 5 to 11. 10 mg twice daily.

Route	Onset	Peak	Duration
P.O.	1 wk	Unknown	Unknown

Mechanism of Action
Inhibits the selective binding of cysteinyl leukotrienes (arachidonic acid derivatives that usually mediate inflammation in asthma and other inflammatory disorders) by competitively blocking receptor sites. This action causes bronchial relaxation and decreases vascular leakage and edema, mucus secretion, eosinophil movement, and bronchial hyper-responsiveness.

Contraindications
Hepatic impairment including hepatic cirrhosis, hypersensitivity to zafirlukast or its components

Interactions
DRUGS
alprazolam, amitriptyline, calcium channel blockers, carbamazepine, citalopram, corticosteroids, cyclosporine, diazepam, diclofenac, ibuprofen, imipramine, irbesartan, lidocaine, lovastatin, midazolam, phenytoin, quinidine, simvastatin, tolbutamide, tolterodine, triazolam: Inhibited metabolism and, possibly, additive adverse effects of these drugs
aspirin: Increased blood zafirlukast level

erythromycin, terfenadine: Decreased response to zafirlukast
sildenafil: Increased adverse sildenafil effects
theophylline: Decreased zafirlukast level; possibly increased theophylline levels
warfarin: Prolonged PT
FOODS
any food: Possibly decreased bioavailability of zafirlukast

Adverse Reactions
CNS: Asthenia, depression, dizziness, fever, headache, insomnia, malaise
CV: Edema, vasculitis
GI: Abdominal pain, diarrhea, edema, elevated liver function test results, hepatic failure, hepatitis, hyperbilirubinemia, indigestion, nausea, vomiting
HEME: Agranulocytosis, bleeding, systemic eosinophilia
MS: Arthralgia, back pain, myalgia
RESP: Eosinophilic pneumonia
SKIN: Bruising, pruritus, rash, urticaria
Other: Angioedema, generalized pain, hypersensitivity reactions, infections

Nursing Considerations
• Zafirlukast shouldn't be used to treat bronchospasm during an acute asthma attack or status asthmaticus; it can't relieve symptoms quickly enough.
• Assess respiratory rate, depth, and quality, as well as breath sounds, before and during treatment to evaluate response to therapy.
• If patient is being weaned from corticosteroids while taking zafirlukast, monitor her for Churg-Strauss syndrome—a rare allergic reaction characterized by eosinophilia, fever, myalgia, and weight loss—for cardiac complications, neuropathy, and worsening pulmonary symptoms.

PATIENT TEACHING
• Instruct patient to take drug exactly as prescribed, in evenly spaced doses, every day, even during symptom-free periods and acute exacerbations.
• Instruct patient to take drug on an empty stomach at least 1 hour before meals, or 2 hours after.
• Urge patient to continue using prescribed rescue inhalants for acute asthma attacks.

X
Y
Z

- Teach patient how to use peak-flow meter to monitor pulmonary function.
- Tell patient to report immediately any evidence of liver dysfunction, such as right upper-quadrant abdominal pain, nausea, fatigue, lethargy, pruritus, jaundice, flulike symptoms, and anorexia.

zaleplon

Sonata

Class, Category, and Schedule

Chemical class: Imidazopyridine derivative
Therapeutic class: Sedative-hypnotic
Pregnancy category: C
Controlled substance schedule: IV

Indications and Dosages

➤ *Short-term treatment of insomnia*

CAPSULES

Adults up to age 65. 10 mg daily at bedtime, as needed, for up to 35 days. *Usual:* 10 mg daily at bedtime for 7 to 10 days. *Maximum:* 20 mg daily.

DOSAGE ADJUSTMENT For patients who are elderly, have hepatic impairment, or take cimetidine, dosage possibly reduced to 5 mg daily.

Route	Onset	Peak	Duration
P.O.	30 min	Unknown	4 hr

Mechanism of Action

Selectively binds with type 1 benzo-diazepine (BZ1 or omega$_1$) receptors on the gamma-aminobutyric acid-A receptor complex. This binding produces muscle relaxation and sedation as well as antianxiety and anticonvulsant effects.

Contraindications

Hypersensitivity to zaleplon or its components

Interactions

DRUGS

amitriptyline; amoxapine; azatadine; benzodiazepines; brompheniramine; chlorpheniramine; clemastine; clomipramine; clozapine; cyproheptadine; dexchlorpheniramine; diphenhydramine; doxepin; entacapone; haloperidol; hydroxyzine; imipramine; maprotiline; mirtazapine; molindone; nefazodone;

nortriptyline; olanzapine; opioid analgesics; other anxiolytics, sedatives, and hypnotics; phenindamine; phenothiazines; pimozide; pramipexole; promethazine; quetiapine; risperidone; ropinirole; thioridazine; trazodone; trimipramine; tripelennamine: Possibly additive CNS depression
carbamazepine, phenobarbital, phenytoin, rifampin: Reduced zaleplon effects
cimetidine: Increased blood zaleplon level
flumazenil: Reversal of zaleplon's sedation

FOODS

high-fat foods: Prolonged absorption time and reduced effectiveness of zaleplon

ACTIVITIES

alcohol use: Increased CNS depression

Adverse Reactions

CNS: Amnesia, anxiety, complex behaviors (such as sleep driving), depression, dizziness, drowsiness, fever, hallucinations, hypertonia, insomnia, nightmares, paresthesia, seizures, suicidal ideation, tremor, vertigo
EENT: Dry mouth, gingivitis, glossitis, mouth ulcers, stomatitis, throat tightness
GI: Anorexia, colitis, constipation, eructation, esophagitis, flatulence, gastritis, gastroenteritis, increased appetite, indigestion, melena, nausea, rectal bleeding, vomiting
MS: Back pain
RESP: Dyspnea
SKIN: Photosensitivity, pruritus, rash
Other: Anaphylaxis, angioedema, physical and psychological dependence

Nursing Considerations

- Give zaleplon just before bedtime because its onset of action is rapid.
- Avoid giving drug with or after a heavy, high-fat meal because decreased absorption may reduce drug's effects.
- Watch patient closely for suicidal tendencies, particularly when therapy starts and dosage changes, because depression may worsen temporarily during these times, possibly leading to suicidal ideation.
- Monitor patient for signs of drug abuse because zaleplon has an abuse potential similar to that of benzodiazepines and benzodiazepine-like hypnotics.

WARNING Monitor patient closely for hypersensitivity reactions, such as dyspnea, throat tightness, nausea, vomiting, and swelling. If present, discontinue zaleplon immediately, notify prescriber, and provide supportive care.

PATIENT TEACHING
• Explain that zaleplon is intended for short-term use. Advise against using it for any condition other than insomnia.
• Caution patient against exceeding prescribed dosage.
• Instruct patient to take zaleplon immediately before bedtime or right after having trouble falling asleep because of drug's rapid onset of action.
• Teach patient alternative measures for relaxation and sleep induction.
• Advise patient to consult prescriber before taking other CNS depressants.
• Urge patient to avoid alcohol during zaleplon therapy because it increases risk of abnormal behaviors, such as sleep driving.
• Warn patient that zaleplon contains FD & C Yellow No. 5 (tartrazine), which can cause an allergic reaction, especially in those with an aspirin sensitivity. Instruct patient to report allergic reactions, such as rash or difficulty breathing, to prescriber.
• Instruct patient to notify prescriber if inability to sleep continues. Dosage may need to be adjusted.
• Instruct patient to stop taking zaleplon and seek emergency care if she has trouble breathing, throat tightness, nausea, vomiting, or abnormal swelling.
• Explain that drug may cause abnormal behaviors during sleep, such as driving a car, eating, talking on the phone, or having sex without any recall of the event. If family notices any such behavior or patient sees evidence of such behavior upon awakening, prescriber should be notified.
• Urge family or caregiver to watch patient closely for suicidal tendencies, especially when therapy starts or dosage changes.

ziconotide
Prialt

Class and Category
Chemical class: 25 amino acid polybasic peptide

Therapeutic class: Analgesic
Pregnancy category: C

Indications and Dosages
➤ *To manage severe chronic pain in patients intolerant of or refractory to other pain management measures*

INTRATHECAL
Adults. *Initial:* 2.4 mcg daily (0.1 mcg/hr), increased as needed by 2.4 mcg daily but no more than 3 times/wk. *Maximum:* 19.2 mcg/day (0.8 mcg/hr) by day 21.

Contraindications
History of psychosis; hypersensitivity to ziconotide or its components; conditions or treatments that make intrathecal use hazardous (infection at microinfusion site, uncontrolled bleeding diathesis, spinal canal obstruction that impairs CSF circulation).

Interactions
DRUGS
CNS depressants: Increased risk of adverse CNS reactions

Adverse Reactions
CNS: Abnormal gait, agitation, anxiety, aphasia, asthenia, ataxia, chills, confusion, CSF abnormality, decreased reflexes, depression, difficulty concentrating, dizziness, dysesthesia, emotional lability, fever, hallucinations, headache, hostility, hyperesthesia, hypertonia, incoordination, insomnia, malaise, memory loss, meningitis, nervousness, neuralgia, paranoia, paresthesia, psychosis, seizures, somnolence, speech disorder, stroke, stupor, suicidal ideation, syncope, tremor, twitching, unusual dreams, vertigo
CV: Atrial fibrillation, bradycardia, chest pain, edema, hypertension, hypotension, orthostatic hypotension, peripheral edema, tachycardia, T-wave changes on ECG, vasodilation
EENT: Abnormal vision, diplopia, dry mouth, nystagmus, pharyngitis, photophobia, rhinitis, sinusitis, taste perversion, tinnitus
GI: Abdominal pain, anorexia, constipation, diarrhea, indigestion, nausea, vomiting
GU: Acute renal failure, dysuria, urinary hesitancy or incontinence, urine retention, UTI
HEME: Anemia

X
Y
Z

Mechanism of Action

Pain sensations are transmitted by sensory neurons that travel through N-type calcium channels in the dorsal horn of the spinal cord and ascend to the brain, as shown below.

Ziconotide binds to N-type calcium channels on primary nociceptive afferent nerves in superficial layers of the dorsal horn, as shown below. By blocking these channels, the drug prevents excitatory neurotransmitter release in primary afferent nerve terminals and relieves pain.

MS: Arthralgia, arthritis, back pain, leg cramps, muscle spasms or weakness, myalgia, myasthenia, neck pain or rigidity, rhabdomyolysis
RESP: Aspiration pneumonia, bronchitis, cough, dyspnea, lung disorder, pneumonia, respiratory distress
SKIN: Cellulitis, diaphoresis, dry skin, ecchymosis, pruritus, rash
Other: Catheter site infection or pain, dehydration, elevated CK level, flulike

symptoms, generalized pain, hypokalemia, sepsis, viral infection, weight loss

Nursing Considerations

• Determine if patient will receive ziconotide therapy by implanted variable-rate microinfusion device or by external microinfusion device and catheter. Then, follow manufacturer guidelines for programming the microinfusion devise and doing an initial pump fill, including

priming using only undiluted 25-mcg/ml solution and rinsing the internal pump surfaces with 2 ml of drug three times.
• Use strict aseptic technique when preparing ziconotide solution and filling, refilling, or handling the microinfusion device.
• Be aware that initial ziconotide dosage shouldn't exceed 2.4 mcg daily.
• Know that refills can use diluted or undiluted ziconotide solutions. If diluting ziconotide, use only normal saline solution without preservatives, following manufacturer guidelines. Refrigerate solution up to 24 hours if it isn't used immediately. Expect device to need refilling about every 40 days if ziconotide is given diluted or about 60 days if given undiluted.
• Assess patient's response to ziconotide regularly. Notify prescriber if pain relief isn't adequate, and expect to increase dosage.
• Check infusion site regularly, and be aware that meningitis can occur within 24 hours after contamination of delivery system; a disconnected catheter is the most common problem with external devices.
• Monitor patient closely for evidence of meningitis, such as headache, stiff neck, altered mental status, nausea, vomiting, and occasionally seizures caused by inadvertent contamination of micro-infusion device or catheter tract used to deliver ziconotide. Notify prescriber immediately if you suspect meningitis.
• Monitor patient closely for cognitive impairment, hallucinations, or changes in mood or consciousness because ziconotide may cause severe psychiatric symptoms and neurologic impairment. If present, notify prescriber and expect to decrease dosage or stop ziconotide. Provide supportive care, as prescribed, for adverse effects. Tell prescriber again if adverse effects are still present after 2 weeks.
• Expect to stop ziconotide temporarily if patient becomes unresponsive or stuporous during therapy; drug may be continued when patient reverts to previous mental status.
• Ziconotide can be stopped abruptly without causing withdrawal symptoms.

• Monitor patient's serum CK level every other week for first month of therapy and monthly thereafter, as ordered. If levels become elevated, notify prescriber and expect to decrease ziconotide dosage or stop drug until levels return to normal.

PATIENT TEACHING
• Teach caregiver how to care for external device, if present. Emphasize the need for strict aseptic technique with the micro-infusion device and connections and the need to check the site often for problems, such as a disconnected catheter, which increase the risk of meningitis.
• Review evidence of meningitis with caregiver, and tell her to contact prescriber immediately if she suspects meningitis.
• Advise patient to notify prescriber if pain relief isn't adequate.
• Tell patient and caregiver to notify prescriber immediately about muscle pain, soreness, and weakness with or without dark urine or a change in mental status or mood, including depression or suicidal ideation.
• Advise patient to avoid hazardous activities that require mental alertness or motor coordination while receiving ziconotide.
• Caution patient to avoid taking OTC preparations that contain CNS depressants because of the risk of adverse CNS effects.

zileuton
Zyflo CR

Class and Category
Chemical class: Leukotriene inhibitor
Therapeutic class: Antiasthmatic
Pregnancy category: C

Indications and Dosages
➤ *To prevent or treat chronic asthma*
E.R. TABLETS
Adults and adolescents. 600 mg twice daily. *Maximum:* 2,400 mg daily.

Route	Onset	Peak	Duration
P.O.	2 hr	Unknown	Unknown

Mechanism of Action
Inhibits formation of leukotrienes found mainly in neutrophils, eosinophils, monocytes, macrophages, and mast cells.

X
Y
Z

Normally, leukotrienes augment neutrophil and eosinophil migration, neutrophil and monocyte aggregation, leukocyte adhesion, capillary permeability, and smooth-muscle contraction. By inhibiting leukotriene formation, zileuton causes bronchial relaxation and decreases vascular leakage and edema, mucus secretion, eosinophil movement, and bronchial hyperresponsiveness.

Contraindications

Hepatic impairment, hypersensitivity to zileuton or its components

Interactions

DRUGS

propranolol, terfenadine: Increased effects of these drugs
theophylline: Doubled theophylline level
warfarin: Prolonged PT and INR

Adverse Reactions

CNS: Asthenia, dizziness, fever, headache, hypertonia, insomnia, malaise, nervousness, neuropsychiatric events, sleep disorders, somnolence
CV: Chest pain
EENT: Conjunctivitis
GI: Abdominal pain, constipation, flatulence, indigestion, nausea, vomiting
GU: UTI, vaginitis
MS: Arthralgia, myalgia, neck pain or rigidity
SKIN: Pruritus, rash, urticaria
Other: Lymphadenopathy

Nursing Considerations

• Be aware that zileuton should not be used in children under the age of 12 because of the risk of hepatoxicity.
• Know that zileuton shouldn't be used to treat bronchospasm during an acute asthma attack or status asthmaticus; it can't relieve symptoms quickly enough.
• Monitor serum ALT level, as ordered, usually before treatment starts, once a month for 3 months, every 2 to 3 months for remainder of first year, and periodically thereafter during therapy.
• Monitor results of liver and pulmonary function tests and CBC during therapy.
• Monitor patient taking zileuton for neuropsychiatric symptoms including worsening of preexisting psychiatric illness. If present, notify prescriber

immediately, institute safety measures and expect drug to be discontinued.

PATIENT TEACHING

• Advise patient to take drug exactly as prescribed, in evenly spaced doses, every day. Emphasize need to take drug even during symptom-free periods and acute exacerbations.
• Urge patient not to chew, cut, or crush capsule but to swallow it whole.
• Instruct patient to continue using rescue inhalants, as prescribed, for acute attacks.
• Teach patient how to use peak-flow meter to assess and monitor pulmonary function.
• Instruct patient to report any abnormal thoughts or behavior.

zinc acetate

(contains 25 or 50 mg of elemental zinc per capsule)
Galzin

zinc chloride

(contains 1 mg of elemental zinc per ml for I.V. infusion)

zinc gluconate

(contains 1.4 mg of elemental zinc per lozenge; 1.4, 2, 4, 7, 8, 10, 11, 13, 31, 50, or 52 mg of elemental zinc per tablet)
Orazinc

zinc sulfate

(contains 25 or 50 mg of elemental zinc per capsule; 15, 25, 45, or 50 mg of elemental zinc per tablet; 50 mg of elemental zinc per E.R. tablet; and 1 or 5 mg of elemental zinc per ml for I.V. infusion)
Orazinc, Verazinc, Zinc 15, Zinc-220, Zinca-Pak, Zincate

Class and Category

Chemical class: Trace element, mineral
Therapeutic class: Copper absorption inhibitor, nutritional supplement
Pregnancy category: A (oral), C (I.V.)

Indications and Dosages

➤ *To prevent zinc deficiency based on U.S. and Canadian recommended daily allowances*

CAPSULES, E.R. TABLETS, LOZENGES, TABLETS
Men and boys age 11 and over. 15 mg (9 to 12 mg Canadian) elemental zinc daily.
Women and girls age 11 and over. 12 mg (9 mg Canadian) elemental zinc daily.
Pregnant women. 15 mg (15 mg Canadian) elemental zinc daily.
Breastfeeding women. 16 to 19 mg (15 mg Canadian) elemental zinc daily.
Children ages 7 to 10. 10 mg (7 to 9 mg Canadian) elemental zinc daily.
Children ages 4 to 6. 10 mg (5 mg Canadian) elemental zinc daily.
Children from birth to age 3. 5 to 10 mg (2 to 4 mg Canadian) elemental zinc daily.
I.V. INFUSION
Adults and children. 2.5 to 4 mg daily added to total parenteral nutrition (TPN) solution. *Maximum:* 12 mg daily.
Children from birth to age 5. 100 mcg/kg daily added to TPN solution.
Premature infants weighing up to 3 kg. 300 mcg/kg daily added to TPN solution.
➤ *To treat zinc deficiency*
CAPSULES, E.R. TABLETS, LOZENGES, TABLETS
Adults and children. Dosage individualized based on severity of deficiency.
I.V. INFUSION
Adults and adolescents. 2.5 to 4 mg daily added to TPN solution. *Maximum:* 12 mg daily.
Children from birth to age 5. 100 mcg/kg daily added to TPN solution.
Premature infants weighing up to 3 kg. 300 mcg/kg daily added to TPN solution.
➤ *As adjunct maintenance therapy for patients previously treated for Wilson's disease*
CAPSULES
Adults. 50 mg three times a day.
Pregnant women. 25 mg three times a day, increased to 50 mg three times a day if drug effectiveness decreases.
Children age 10 and over. 25 mg three times a day, increased to 50 mg three times a day if drug effectiveness decreases.

Mechanism of Action

Needed for proper function of more than 200 metalloenzymes (those with tightly bound zinc atoms as an integral part of their structure), including carbonic anhydrase, carboxypeptidase A, alcohol dehydrogenase, alkaline phosphatase, and RNA polymerase. Zinc also helps maintain nucleic acid, protein, and cell membrane structure and is essential for certain physiologic functions, including cell growth and division, sexual maturation and reproduction, dark adaptation and night vision, wound healing, host immunity, and taste acuity. This mineral also provides cellular antioxidant protection by scavenging free radicals.

In addition, zinc acetate interferes with intestinal absorption of copper and produces a protein that binds with copper, preventing its transfer to blood. Bound copper is then excreted in stools, thus decreasing copper toxicity in Wilson's disease.

Contraindications

Hypersensitivity to zinc or its components

Interactions

DRUGS
copper supplements: Impaired copper absorption (with large doses of zinc)
oral iron supplements, oral phosphate salts, penicillamine, phosphorus-containing drugs: Decreased zinc absorption
quinolones, tetracyclines: Decreased absorption and possibly decreased effectiveness of these antibiotics
thiazide diuretics: Increased urinary excretion of zinc
zinc-containing preparations: Increased blood zinc level
FOODS
fiber- or phylate-containing foods (such as bran, whole-grain breads, cereal), phosphorus-containing foods (including milk, poultry): Decreased zinc absorption

Nursing Considerations

WARNING Don't give I.V. zinc preparations that contain benzyl alcohol to neonates or premature infants because this preservative may cause a fatal toxic syndrome characterized by metabolic acidosis and CNS, respiratory, circulatory, and renal function impairment.
• Give oral zinc supplements 1 hour before or 2 to 3 hours after meals; at least 2 hours after giving oral iron supplements (to prevent decreased zinc absorption) or copper supplements (to prevent decreased copper absorption); and at least 6 hours before or 2 hours after administering

X
Y
Z

quinolone or tetracycline antibiotics (to prevent decreased absorption of these drugs).
• Monitor patient receiving long-term zinc therapy for sideroblastic anemia, which may result from zinc-induced copper deficiency and is characterized by anemia, leukopenia, neutropenia, granulo-cytopenia, and bone marrow problems. Be aware that these effects are reversible after zinc is discontinued.
• Monitor patient with preexisting copper deficiency for exacerbation of this condition; zinc can decrease serum copper level.
• Assess for signs and symptoms of zinc deficiency, such as growth retardation, hypogonadism, delayed sexual maturation, alopecia, impaired wound healing, skin lesions, immune deficiencies, behavioral disturbances, night blindness, and impaired sense of taste.
• Monitor blood alkaline phosphatase (ALP) level monthly, as ordered; it may increase.
• Be aware that zinc chloride contains aluminum, which may accumulate to the point of toxicity if patient's kidney function is impaired. Assess kidney function regularly.

PATIENT TEACHING
• Explain the need for a zinc supplement.
• Instruct patient to take zinc on an empty stomach, at least 1 hour before or 2 hours after meals. Caution her not to take zinc within 2 hours of iron or copper supplements or phosphorus-containing drugs.
• Instruct patient to let zinc lozenge dissolve in mouth slowly and completely and not to swallow it whole or chew it. Advise her not to take zinc lozenges more often than directed.

ziprasidone hydrochloride

Geodon

ziprasidone mesylate

Geodon for Injection

Class and Category
Chemical class: Benzisoxazole derivative
Therapeutic class: Antipsychotic
Pregnancy category: C

Indications and Dosages
➤ *To treat schizophrenia*
CAPSULES
Adults. *Initial:* 20 mg twice daily. Dosage increased as indicated every 2 or more days. *Usual:* 20 to 80 mg twice daily. *Maximum:* 100 mg twice daily.
I.M. INJECTION
Adults. *Initial:* 10 to 20 mg. 10 mg dose may be given every 2 hr up to maximum dose; 20 mg dose may be given every 4 hr up to maximum dose. *Maximum:* 40 mg daily.
➤ *To treat acute manic or mixed episodes of bipolar disorder*
CAPSULES
Adults. *Initial:* 40 mg twice daily. with food on day 1; then increased to 60 or 80 mg on day 2 with further adjustments as needed.
➤ *As adjunct to lithium or valproate for maintenance treatment of bipolar I disorder*
CAPSULES
Adults. Same dose patient was initially stabilized on that falls within 40 mg to 80 mg twice daily.

Mechanism of Action
Selectively blocks serotonin and dopamine receptors in the mesocortical tract of the CNS, thereby suppressing psychotic symptoms.

Incompatibilities
Don't mix injection form with drugs or solvents other than sterile water for injection.

Contraindications
Concurrent use of other drugs that prolong QT interval, history of arrhythmia, hypersensitivity to ziprasidone or its components, history of prolonged QT interval, recent acute MI, uncompensated heart failure

Interactions
DRUGS
antihypertensives: Additive antihypertensive effects
carbamazepine: Possibly decreased blood ziprasidone level

CNS depressants: Increased CNS depression
dopamine agonists, levodopa: Decreased
therapeutic effects of these drugs
*drugs that prolong QT interval (including
quinidine, dofetilide, pimozide, sotalol,
thioridazine, and sparfloxacin):* Increased
risk of prolonged QT or QTc interval,
torsades de pointes, and sudden death
ketoconazole: Possibly increased blood
ziprasidone level
FOODS
all foods: Increased ziprasidone absorption

Adverse Reactions
CNS: Agitation, akathisia, amnesia, anxiety,
asthenia, CVA, depression, dizziness,
dystonia, extrapyramidal reactions,
headache, hypertonia, hypomania,
insomnia, mania, neuroleptic malignant
syndrome, paresthesia, personality or
speech disorder, serotonin syndrome,
somnolence, syncope, suicidal ideation,
tardive dyskinesia, tremor
CV: Bradycardia, chest pain, hypercholesterolemia, hypertension, orthostatic
hypotension, prolonged QT or QTc
interval, tachycardia, thrombophlebitis,
vasodilation
EENT: Abnormal vision, dry mouth,
increased salivation, rhinitis, tongue
swelling
ENDO: Dysmenorrhea, hyperglycemia,
hyperprolactinemia
GI: Abdominal pain, anorexia, constipation,
diarrhea, dysphagia, indigestion, nausea,
rectal bleeding, vomiting
GU: Priapism, urinary incontinence
HEME: Agranulocytosis, leukopenia,
neutropenia
MS: Arthralgia, back pain, dysarthria,
myalgia
RESP: Cough, pulmonary embolism, upper
respiratory tract infection
SKIN: Allergic dermatitis, diaphoresis,
furunculosis, rash, urticaria
Other: Accidental injury, angioedema, drug
reaction with eosinophilia and systemic
symptoms (DRESS), flulike symptoms,
injection-site pain, weight gain

Nursing Considerations
WARNING Ziprasidone shouldn't be used to
treat elderly patients with dementia-
related psychosis because drug increases
the risk of death in these patients.

• Protect ziprasidone vials from light.
Reconstitute by adding 1.2 ml sterile water
for injection to vial and shaking vigorously until drug is dissolved. Each ml of
reconstituted solution contains 20 mg
ziprasidone. Discard any unused portion.
• Give only by I.M. route.
• Reconstituted drug may be stored 24
hours protected from light or up to 7 days
if refrigerated and protected from light.
• Administer I.M. form cautiously to
patients with impaired renal function.
WARNING Assess cardiac rhythm in patients
with hypokalemia or hypomagnesemia.
Dizziness, palpitations, and syncope may
indicate life-threatening torsades de
pointes. Be prepared to stop ziprasidone if
QTc interval is greater than 500 msec.
• Monitor patient, especially elderly
woman, for involuntary movements,
which may become irreversible tardive
dyskinesia. If symptoms develop, notify
prescriber immediately and be prepared
to stop drug.
• Immediately report evidence of
neuroleptic malignant syndrome, a rare
but potentially fatal adverse reaction
including hyperpyrexia, muscle rigidity,
altered mental status, irregular pulse,
blood pressure changes, tachycardia,
diaphoresis, arrhythmia, myoglobinuria
(rhabdomyolysis), and acute renal failure.
• Monitor patient's blood glucose and lipid
levels routinely, as ordered, because drug
increases risk of hyperglycemia and
hypercholesterolemia.
• Monitor patient's CBC, as ordered,
because serious adverse hematologic
reactions may occur, such as agranulocytosis, leukopenia, and neutropenia.
Monitor more frequently during first
few months of therapy if patient has a
history of drug-induced leukopenia,
neutropenia, or significantly low WBC
count. If abnormalities occur during
ziprasidone therapy, watch for fever and
other evidence of infection, notify
prescriber, and expect to discontinue
drug if severe.
• Monitor patient closely for evidence of
suicidal thinking or behavior, especially
when therapy starts or dosage changes.
• Know that long-standing
hyperprolactinemia caused by ziprasidone

X
Y
Z

therapy may cause decreased bone density if associated with hypogonadism.

PATIENT TEACHING
• Instruct patient to take ziprasidone with food to increase absorption.
• Advise patient to avoid hazardous activities until CNS effects are known.
• Tell family to monitor patient closely for suicidal tendencies; patients with psychotic illness or bipolar disorder are at greater risk.
• Urge patient to rise slowly from seated or lying position to minimize orthostatic hypotension.
• Urge patient to notify prescriber immediately if he develops any sudden onset, unusual, persistent, or servere adverse reactions, especially a rash, fever, or swollen lymph nodes. If present, tell him to stop taking ziprasidone and seek urgent medical care.

zoledronic acid

Reclast, Zometa

Class and Category

Chemical class: Bisphosphonate
Therapeutic class: Antihypercalcemic, bone resorption inhibitor
Pregnancy category: D

Indications and Dosages

➤ *To treat hypercalcemia caused by cancer*
I.V. INFUSION (ZOMETA)
Adults. 4 mg infused over at least 15 min. After 7 days, retreatment with 4 mg if serum calcium level doesn't remain at or return to normal. *Maximum:* 4 mg/dose.
➤ *As adjunct treatment for patients with multiple myeloma or bony metastasis who are receiving standard anti-neoplastic therapy and have a creatinine clearance above 60 ml/min/1.73 m²*
I.V. INFUSION (ZOMETA)
Adults. 4 mg infused over at least 15 min every 3 to 4 wk.
DOSAGE ADJUSTMENT If patient's creatinine clearance is 50 to 60 ml/min/1.73 m², dosage decreased to 3.5 mg; if it's 40 to

49 ml/min/1.73 m², dosage decreased to 3.3 mg; and if it's 30 to 39 ml/min/1.73 m², dosage decreased to 3 mg.
➤ *To treat postmenopausal osteoporosis in women; to treat osteoporosis in men; to treat and prevent glucocorticoid-induced osteoporosis in patients receiving daily prednisone doses of 7.5 mg or greater for at least 12 months*
I.V. INFUSION (RECLAST)
Adults. 5 mg infused over at least 15 min once yearly.
➤ *To treat Paget's disease of the bone*
I.V. INFUSION (RECLAST)
Adults. 5 mg infused over at least 15 min after 2 wk of receiving 1,500 mg elemental calcium daily in divided doses and 800 international units vitamin D daily.
➤ *To prevent osteoporosis in post-menopausal women*
I.V. INFUSION (RECLAST)
Adults. 5 mg infused over at least 15 min every 2 years.

Mechanism of Action

Inhibits resorption of mineralized bone and cartilage by osteoclasts and induces osteoclast breakdown. In cancer-related hypercalcemia, hyperactive osteoclasts cause bone resorption and release of calcium into blood, which causes polyuria, GI disruption, progressive dehydration, and decreasing GFR. This, in turn, increases renal calcium resorption and worsens hypercalcemia. Zoledronic acid interrupts this process.

Incompatibilities

Don't mix zoledronic acid with calcium-containing I.V. solutions, such as lactated Ringer's solution.

Contraindications

Acute renal impairment, creatinine clearance less than 35 ml/min; hyper-sensitivity to zoledronic acid, other bisphosphonates, or their components

Interactions

DRUGS
aminoglycosides: Possibly additive serum calcium–lowering effect
loop diuretics, such as furosemide: Possibly increased risk of hypocalcemia
NSAIDs: Increased risk of nephrotoxicity

Adverse Reactions

CNS: Anxiety, asthenia, chills, confusion, depression, dizziness, fatigue, fever, headache, hyperesthesia, hypoesthesia, insomnia, malaise, paresthesia, tremor, vertigo, weakness
CV: Atrial fibrillation, bradycardia, chest pain, hypertension, hypotension, peripheral edema
EENT: Blurred vision, conjunctivitis, dry mouth, episcleritis, iritis, orbital edema or inflammation, scleritis, sore throat, stomatitis, taste disturbance, uveitis
ENDO: Hypocalcemia
GI: Abdominal pain, anorexia, constipation, diarrhea, dyspepsia, nausea, vomiting
GU: Elevated serum creatinine level, hematuria, proteinuria, renal insufficiency or failure, UTI
HEME: Anemia, neutropenia, thrombocytopenia
MS: Arthralgia; atypical subtrochanteric and diaphyseal femoral fractures; incapacitating bone, joint, or muscle pain; muscle spasms; myalgia; osteonecrosis of the jaw
RESP: Bronchospasm, cough, dyspnea, upper respiratory tract infection
SKIN: Alopecia, dermatitis, diaphoresis, flushing, urticaria
Other: Acute phase reaction-like events (I.V. administration), aggravated malignant neoplasm, anaphylaxis, angioedema, flulike illness, hypersensitivity reaction, hyperkalemia, hypernatremia, hypocalcemia, hypomagnesemia, hypophosphatemia, infusion-site redness and swelling, weight gain

Nursing Considerations

• Be aware that zoledronic acid isn't indicated for hypercalcemia from hyperparathyroidism or other nontumor conditions.
• Use cautiously in patients with aspirin sensitivity because biphosphonates such as zoledronic acid have caused bronchoconstriction in these patients.
• Make sure patient has had a dental checkup before zoledronic acid starts, especially if patient has cancer; is receiving chemotherapy, head or neck radiation, or a corticosteroid; or has poor oral hygiene because risk of osteonecrosis is increased

in these patients, and invasive dental procedures during zoledronic acid therapy may worsen osteonecrosis.
• Expect to aggressively hydrate hypercalcemic patient with I.V. normal saline solution before and during zoledronic acid therapy, as prescribed, to achieve and maintain urine output of about 2 L daily.
WARNING Monitor fluid intake and output often during hydration, and assess patient, especially one with heart failure, for evidence of life-threatening overhydration.
• Know that hypocalcemia and mineral metabolism disorders must be treated before zoledronic acid therapy begins.
• Be aware that Reclast doesn't need reconstitution.
• Reconstitute Zometa by adding 5 ml of sterile water for injection to drug vial to yield solution that contains 4 mg of zoledronic acid. Make sure drug is completely dissolved before withdrawing prescribed dose. Further dilute in 100 ml normal saline solution or 5% dextrose injection, and infuse over no less than 15 minutes.
• Inspect reconstituted and diluted solution before giving drug, and discard it if particles or discoloration are present.
• Expect to give acetaminophen, if not contraindicated, before zoledronic acid to reduce adverse reactions, such as fever, headache, myalgia, and flulike symptoms. These reactions usually occur within first 3 days after zoledronic acid administration and resolve within 3 days (although resolution may take up to 14 days for some patients).
• Refrigerate reconstituted drug at 2° to 8° C (36° to 46° F) and discard after 24 hours.
• Give drug as a single I.V. solution in a separate I.V. line.
WARNING Be aware that a single dose of Zometa shouldn't exceed 4 mg, and that neither Zometa nor Reclast should be infused over less than 15 minutes; exceeding these limits may lead to significant renal function deterioration, which may progress to renal failure.
WARNING Assess patient's renal function, as ordered, before and during zoledronic acid therapy to detect renal deterioration. For patient with a normal serum creatinine

level who develops an increase of 0.5 mg/
dl within 2 weeks of receiving zoledronic
acid, expect to withhold next dose until
serum creatinine level is within 10% of
patient's baseline value. For patient with
an abnormal serum creatinine level who
develops an increase of 1.0 mg/dl within
2 weeks of receiving drug, expect to
withhold next dose until serum creatinine
level is within 10% of baseline value.
• Monitor patient's serum calcium,
magnesium, and phosphate levels, as
ordered, during zoledronic acid therapy. If
hypocalcemia, hypomagnesemia, or
hypophosphatemia occurs, expect to give
short-term supplemental therapy.
• Assess aspirin-sensitive asthma patients
for worsening of respiratory symptoms
during zoledronic acid therapy because
other bisphosphonates have caused
bronchoconstriction in these patients.
• Monitor patient for dehydration. If
present, notify prescriber and expect drug
to be withheld until dehydration has been
corrected.
• Monitor patient for acute phase reaction
(APR) that may occur with intravenous
administration of zoledronic acid. If
patient develops flulike symptoms such as
fever, chills, flushing, bone pain,
arthralgias, and myalgias, notify prescriber.
• Store drug at 25° C (77° F).
• Monitor patient closely for severe and
occasionally incapacitating bone, joint,
and/or muscle pain. If present, notify
prescriber and expect to provide
supportive care, as ordered, for pain relief.

PATIENT TEACHING

• Teach patient the importance of eating a
nutritious diet, including adequate
amounts of calcium and vitamin D.
• Instruct patient to drink at least 2 glasses
of fluid within a few hours before
receiving zoledronic acid intravenously.
• Advise patient to alert prescriber about
muscle or bone pain or new or worsening
thigh or groin pain.
• Instruct patient on proper oral hygiene
and on need to notify prescriber before
undergoing invasive dental procedures.
• Advise women of childbearing age to
notify prescriber immediately if they are
or could be pregnant because drug will
need to be stopped.

zolmitriptan
Zomig, Zomig ZMT

Class and Category
Chemical class: Selective
5-hydroxytryptamine agonist
Therapeutic class: Antimigraine
Pregnancy category: C

Indications and Dosages
➤ *To treat acute migraine headache with
or without aura*
ORAL DISINTEGRATING TABLETS
Adults. *Initial:* 1.25 mg or 2.5 mg, repeated
every 2 hr as needed. *Maximum:* 10 mg in
24 hr or three headaches/mo.
TABLETS
Adults. 2.5 mg or less, repeated in 2 hr.
Maximum: 10 mg in 24 hr or three
headaches/mo.
NASAL SPRAY
Adults. 5 mg, repeated in 2 hr as needed.
Maximum: 10 mg/24 hr.
DOSAGE ADJUSTMENT For patient with
moderate to severe hepatic impairment,
initial dosage should not be higher than
1.25 mg and maximum dose should not
exceed 5 mg in 24 hr. Oral disintegrating
tablets are not recommended for these
patients because the tablet cannot be broken
in half. For patient receiving cimetidine
concurrently, single dosage should not
exceed 2.5 mg and the maximum dosage
should not exceed 5 mg in a 24-hr period.

Mechanism of Action
Constricts inflamed and dilated cranial
blood vessels in the carotid circulation and
inhibits production of proinflammatory
neuropeptides by binding to receptors on
intracranial blood vessels and sensory
nerves in the trigeminal-vascular system to
stimulate negative feedback, which halts the
release of serotonin.

Contraindications
Basilar or hemiplegic migraine, cardiovascular disease, concurrent use of
ergotamine-containing drugs, hypersensitivity to zolmitriptan or its
components, ischemic heart disease,
peripheral vascular disease, Prinzmetal's
angina, symptomatic Wolff-Parkinson-

White syndrome or other accessory pathway conduction disorder, use of another 5-hydroxytryptamine agonist within past 24 hours, use of an MAO inhibitor within 14 days

Interactions

DRUGS

acetaminophen: Delayed peak effect of acetaminophen (by 1 hour)
cimetidine: Prolonged zolmitriptan half-life
ergot alkaloids: Prolonged vasoconstriction effects
fluoxetine, fluvoxamine, paroxetine, sertraline: Hyperreflexia, lack of coordination, and weakness
MAO inhibitors: Increased zolmitriptan effects
naratriptan, rizatriptan, sumatriptan: Prolonged zolmitriptan effects
oral contraceptives, propranolol: Increased blood zolmitriptan level
serotonin and norepinephrine reuptake inhibitors: Increased risk of developing serotonin syndrome

Adverse Reactions

CNS: Asthenia, dizziness, hyperesthesia, paresthesia, somnolence, vertigo
CV: Angina, coronary artery vasospasm, hypertension, MI, palpitations, transient myocardial ischemia, ventricular fibrillation or tachycardia
EENT: Dry mouth, vision disturbance
GI: Abdominal pain, bloody diarrhea, dysphagia, GI or splenic infarction, indigestion, ischemic colitis, nausea, vomiting
MS: Myalgia; myasthenia; pain, pressure, or tightness in jaw, neck, or throat
SKIN: Diaphoresis, flushing
Other: Anaphylaxis, anaphylactoid reaction, angioedema

Nursing Considerations

WARNING Monitor patient for signs and symptoms of vasoconstriction, which may lead to vascular and colonic ischemia with abdominal pain and bloody diarrhea, especially if patient has peripheral vascular disease (including Raynaud's phenomenon) or ischemic bowel disease.

• Monitor elderly patients and those with hepatic impairment for increased blood pressure, and notify prescriber immediately if it occurs.

• Monitor patient closely for signs and symptoms of angina. If patient develops chest pain, notify prescriber.

WARNING Monitor patient closely for signs and symptoms of serotonin syndrome, which may include agitation, hallucinations, coma, tachycardia, labile blood pressure, hyperthermia, hyperreflexia, incoordination, nausea, vomiting, and diarrhea. Notify prescriber immediately because serotonin syndrome may be life-threatening. Be prepared to provide supportive care and discontinue zolmitriptan.

PATIENT TEACHING

• Instruct patient to take zolmitriptan exactly as prescribed. Tell her also not to take more than 10 mg in any 24-hour period, nor should she take drug for 10 or more days a month, because overuse of drug may lead to exacerbation of headache. Tell her to be alert for migraine-like daily headaches developing or marked increase in frequency of migraine headaches that signals overuse may be occurring. Tell her to notify prescriber, as drug may no longer be as effective and drug withdrawal may be needed.

• Advise patient not to remove disintegrating tablet from blister pack until just before taking the tablet. Instruct her to peel open pack, let tablet dissolve on her tongue, and then swallow. Remind her not to break orally disintegrating tablet. However, if she is prescribed the regular 2.5-mg tablet form she may break it in half, if needed for a 1.25-mg dose.

• Urge patient to notify prescriber about unusual or severe adverse reactions.

• Caution patient using nasal spray to avoid spraying drug into her eyes.

• Instruct patient not to take zolmitriptan within 24 hours of other drugs in the same class.

• Tell patient to inform all prescribers of zolmitriptan therapy because serious drug interactions may occur.

zolpidem tartrate

Ambien, Ambien CR, Edluar, Intermezzo, Tovalt, Zolpimist

X
Y
Z

Class, Category, and Schedule
Chemical class: Imidazopyridine derivative
Therapeutic class: Antianxiety, sedative-hypnotic
Pregnancy category: B
Controlled substance schedule: IV

Indications and Dosages
➤ *To provide short-term treatment of insomnia*

TABLETS, ORALLY DISINTEGRATING TABLETS
Adult men. 10 mg at bedtime for 7 to 10 days. *Maximum:* 10 mg daily.
Adult women. 5 mg at bedtime for 7 to 10 days. *Maximum:* 5 mg daily.
DOSAGE ADJUSTMENT For elderly or debilitated patients and those with hepatic impairment, dosage possibly reduced to 5 mg at bedtime, with a maximum of 5 mg daily for nursing facility residents.

E.R. TABLETS
Adult men. 6.25 mg or 12.5 mg immediately before bedtime.
Adult women. 6.25 mg immediately before bedtime.
DOSAGE ADJUSTMENT For elderly or debilitated patients and those with hepatic impairment, dosage reduced to 6.25 mg immediately before bedtime.

➤ *To treat insomnia when a middle-of-the-night awakening occurs and patient cannot get back to sleep and has more than 4 hours of sleep remaining before planned time of waking.*

S.L. TABLETS (INTERMEZZO)
Adult women. 1.75 mg once nightly, as needed.
Adult men. 3.5 mg once nightly, as needed.
DOSAGE ADJUSTMENT For elderly men or male patients with hepatic impairment or who take concomitant CNS depressants, dosage reduced to 1.75 mg once nightly, as needed.

Mechanism of Action
May potentiate the effects of gamma-aminobutyric acid (GABA) and other inhibitory neurotransmitters. By binding to specific benzodiazepine receptors in the limbic and cortical areas of the CNS, zolpidem increases GABA's inhibitory effects, blocks cortical and limbic arousal, and preserves deep sleep (stages 3 and 4).

Contraindications
Hypersensitivity to zolpidem or its components, ritonavir therapy

Interactions
DRUGS
azole antifungals: Increased CNS activity and additive adverse effects of zolpidem
barbiturates, chlorpromazine, general anesthetics, opioid agonists, other CNS depressants, phenothiazines, tramadol, tricyclic antidepressants: Possibly increased CNS depression and reduced psychomotor function
bupropion: Increased blood zolpidem level, possibly visual hallucinations, loss of alertness
desipramine, imipramine: Increased risk of visual hallucinations and reduced alertness
flumazenil: Antagonized sedative effect
haloperidol: Increased CNS depression
nevirapine: Decreased blood zolpidem level
rifabutin, rifampin: Increased zolpidem clearance
selective serotonin-reuptake inhibitors: Increased risk of delusions, disorientation, and hallucinations
FOOD
all foods: Increased time to peak blood zolpidem level, decreased effects of zolpidem
ACTIVITIES
alcohol use: Increased CNS depression

Adverse Reactions
CNS: Abnormal thinking, aggressiveness, amnesia, asthenia, ataxia, behavioral changes, complex behaviors (such as sleep driving), confusion, decreased level of consciousness or inhibition, dizziness, drowsiness, euphoria, hallucinations, headache, insomnia, lethargy, paradoxical CNS stimulation (including agitation, euphoria, hallucinations, hyperactivity, and nightmares), suicidal ideation, vertigo, worsening of depression
EENT: Diplopia, throat tightness, visual abnormality
GI: Constipation, diarrhea, hiccups, indigestion, nausea, vomiting
GU: UTI
MS: Arthralgia, myalgia

RESP: Dyspnea, respiratory depression, upper or lower respiratory infection
Other: Anaphylaxis, angioedema, withdrawal symptoms

Nursing Considerations

• Use zolpidem cautiously in patients with additional disorders because it isn't known if zolpidem therapy might aggravate these conditions, especially conditions with respiratory impairment.
• Administer zolpidem just before patient's bedtime because drug has a rapid onset of action.
• Expect patient to receive no more than a 1-month supply of zolpidem for outpatient therapy.
WARNING If zolpidem is withdrawn abruptly (especially after prolonged therapy), monitor patient for withdrawal symptoms, such as abdominal cramps or discomfort, fatigue, flushing, inconsolable crying, light-headedness, nausea, nervousness, panic attack, rebound insomnia, and vomiting.
• Expect that zolpidem will produce anticonvulsant and muscle relaxant effects at high doses.
• If patient takes other CNS depressants, expect to reduce zolpidem dosage, as prescribed.
• Monitor patient closely for suicidal tendencies, particularly when therapy starts or dosage increases because depression may worsen temporarily during these times, possibly leading to suicide.
WARNING Monitor patient closely for hypersensitivity reactions such as dyspnea, throat tightness, nausea, vomiting, and swelling. If present, discontinue zolpidem immediately, notify prescriber, and provide supportive care.

PATIENT TEACHING
• Caution patient to take drug exactly as prescribed and not to increase dosage unless directed by prescriber.
• Advise patient taking extended-release form to swallow tablet whole and not to break, crush, or chew it.
• Advise patient taking orally disintegrating form to place tablet on tongue, let it dissolve, and then swallow with saliva or, if patient prefers, with water.

• Instruct patient to take zolpidem (except for sublingual tablets) immediately before going to bed, on an empty stomach.
• Tell patient prescribed sublingual tablets to keep tablets at bedside and take only once if awaken during the night but has more than 4 hours of sleep time remaining. Instruct patient to place tablet under his tongue and allow it to dissolve completely before swallowing. Tell him never to swallow the sublingual tablet whole.
• Advise patient to notify prescriber immediately about abdominal cramps or discomfort, fatigue, flushing, inconsolable crying, light-headedness, nausea, nervousness, panic attack, and vomiting.
• Instruct patient to stop taking zolpidem and seek emergency care if she has trouble breathing, throat tightness, nausea, vomiting, or abnormally swelling.
• Advise patient that zolpidem may produce abnormal behaviors during sleep, such as driving a car, eating, talking on the phone, or having sex without any recall of the event. If patient's family notices any such behavior or if patient sees evidence of such behavior upon awakening, prescriber should be notified.
• Tell patient that drug may cause drowsiness or decreased level of consciousness and even next-morning impairment from zolpidem use despite feeling fully awake. Tell her to take precautions against falling and not to perform any hazardous activity such as driving, especially after taking the drug and during the morning hours.
• Tell family or caregiver to observe patient closely for suicidal tendencies, especially when therapy starts or dosage changes.

zonisamide
Zonegran

Class and Category
Chemical class: Benzisoxazole derivative, sulfonamide
Therapeutic class: Anticonvulsant
Pregnancy category: C

X
Y
Z

Indications and Dosages
➤ *As adjunct to treat partial seizures*
CAPSULES
Adults. *Initial:* 100 mg daily. Dosage increased by 100 mg daily every 2 wk, as needed. *Usual:* 200 to 400 mg daily. *Maximum:* 600 mg daily.

Mechanism of Action
May stop seizures and suppress their foci by blocking sodium channels and reducing voltage-dependent, inward currents from calcium channels. This action stabilizes neuronal membranes and suppresses synchronized neuronal hyperactivity.

Contraindications
Hypersensitivity to sulfonamides, zonisamide, or their components

Interactions
DRUGS
carbamazepine, phenobarbital, phenytoin, valproate: Possibly decreased blood zonisamide level
CNS depressants: Additive CNS depressant effects
FOODS
grapefruit juice: Possibly decreased metabolism of zonisamide

Adverse Reactions
CNS: Abnormal gait, agitation, anxiety, asthenia, ataxia, confusion, depression, difficulty concentrating, dizziness, fatigue, headache, incoordination, insomnia, irritability, memory loss, nervousness, paresthesia, schizophrenia, seizures, somnolence, speech abnormalities, suicidal ideation, tremor
CV: Chest pain
EENT: Amblyopia, diplopia, dry mouth, nystagmus, pharyngitis, rhinitis, taste alteration, tinnitus
GI: Abdominal pain, acute pancreatitis, anorexia, constipation, diarrhea, dyspepsia, nausea, vomiting
GU: Renal calculi
HEME: Anemia, leukopenia, thrombocytopenia
MS: Elevated creatine phosphokinase levels, rhabdomyolysis
RESP: Increased cough
SKIN: Ecchymosis, pruritus, rash
Other: Angioedema, flulike symptoms, metabolic acidosis, weight loss

Nursing Considerations
• Obtain a serum bicarbonate level before starting zonisamide and then periodically during therapy, as prescribed because drug may cause metabolic acidosis, especially in patients with predisposing conditions or therapies or who are younger in age.
WARNING Monitor results of patient's CBC and other laboratory tests for signs of blood dyscrasias because zonisamide is a sulfonamide and can be absorbed systemically. Systemic absorption may result in life-threatening reactions, including toxic epidermal necrolysis, Stevens-Johnson syndrome, fulminant hepatic necrosis, agranulocytosis, aplastic anemia, and other blood dyscrasias.
• Be aware that patients receiving doses of 300 mg daily or more are at increased risk for adverse CNS reactions, including decreased concentration, fatigue, drowsiness, and impaired speech.
• Monitor serum creatinine and BUN levels for signs of abnormally decreased glomerular filtration rate (GFR). Expect some decrease in GFR during first 4 weeks of treatment and return to baseline within 2 to 3 weeks after drug is discontinued.
• Monitor patient for signs and symptoms of renal calculi.
• Be aware that zonisamide shouldn't be discontinued abruptly because doing so may increase frequency of seizures.
• Monitor patient closely for evidence of suicidal thinking or behavior, especially when therapy starts or dosage changes.
PATIENT TEACHING
• Inform patient that zonisamide is usually prescribed with other anticonvulsants and that she should continue to take all drugs as prescribed.
• Instruct patient to swallow zonisamide capsules whole and not to chew them or break them open.
• Inform patient that prescriber may have to adjust zonisamide dosage over several weeks or months before stable dose is achieved.
• Advise patient to use caution when driving or performing other activities that are hazardous or require mental alertness because zonisamide commonly causes somnolence, dizziness, and decreased

concentration, particularly during first month of therapy.

• Advise patient to wear a medical identification bracelet or necklace or carry medical identification with information about her seizure disorder.

• Unless contraindicated, encourage patient to drink 6 to 8 glasses of water each day to prevent kidney stones.

• Advise patient to rise slowly from a lying or seated position to reduce the risk of dizziness.

• Urge caregivers to watch closely for evidence of suicidal tendencies, especially when therapy starts or dosage changes, and to report concerns immediately to prescriber.

• Encourage woman who becomes pregnant while taking zonisamide to enroll in the North American antiepileptic drug pregnancy registry by calling 1-888-233-2334. Explain that the registry is collecting information about the safety of antiepileptic drugs during pregnancy.

• Instruct patient to notify prescriber immediately if she develops a skin rash, seizures worsen, signs of kidney stones occur (sudden back pain, abdominal pain, blood in urine), signs of blood abnormalities (fever, sore throat, oral ulcers, easy bruising) are present, or other signs and symptoms such as fast breathing, fatigue, loss of appetite, irregular heart beat, or palpitations develop.

Appendices

Parenteral Insulin Preparations	1267
Oral Allergen Extracts	1270
Antihistamines	1271
Selected Ophthalmic Drugs	1273
Selected Topical Drugs	1283
Selected Antivirals	1299
Selected Antineoplastic Drugs	1308
Selected Antihypertensive Combinations	1326
Selected Obstetrical Drugs	1334
Vitamins	1336
Interferons	1348
Compatible Drugs in a Syringe	1354
Drug Formulas and Calculations	1356
Weights and Equivalents	1361
Equianalgesic Doses for Opioid Agonists	1363
Abbreviations	1364

Parenteral Insulin Preparations

For each category of insulin, the following table lists the species; common trade names; onset, peak, and duration; and key nursing considerations.

CATEGORY, SPECIES, AND TRADE NAMES	KEY NURSING CONSIDERATIONS
Rapid-acting insulin	
Onset: 15 min **Peak:** 30–90 min **Duration:** In 6 hr	
Human • Apidra (insulin glulisine) • Humalog (insulin lispro) • NovoLog (insulin aspart)	• Mix Humalog or NovoLog with other insulin types, but mix Apidra only with NPH insulin, if needed. Administer immediately after mixing. • When mixing rapid-acting insulin with a longer-acting insulin, always draw the rapid-acting insulin into the syringe first to avoid dosage errors. • When giving SubQ, give Humalog up to 15 minutes before a meal; give NovoLog 5 to 10 minutes before a meal; and give Apidra up to 15 to 20 minutes before a meal. When giving rapid-acting insulin via an insulin pump, do not dilute or mix with any other insulin, change the insulin in the reservoir at least every 7days (Apidra at least every 48 hours), and change the infusion sets and insertion site at least every 3 days. • Be aware that 1 unit of rapid-acting insulin has the same glucose-lowering ability as 1 unit of short-acting insulin. • Rapid-acting insulin is available as a cartridge. Make sure to use the correct device for the brand of insulin prescribed, and don't add any other insulin to the cartridge. • Absorption rate of rapid-acting insulin may slow when this type of insulin is mixed in a syringe with human isophane insulin (NPH). Monitor blood glucose level often. • Assess patient taking insulin concurrently with a thiazolidinedione for signs and symptoms of heart failure. If heart failure develops, provide supportive care, as ordered, and expect the thiazolidinedione to be discontinued or dosage reduced.
Short-acting insulin	
Onset: 30 min **Peak:** 2–5 hr **Duration:** 6–8 hr	
Human • Humulin-R • Novolin ge Toronto (CAN) • Novolin R • Novolin R Prefilled • Velosulin BR • Velosulin Human (CAN) **Pork** • Regular (concentrated), Iletin II, U-500	• Don't use short-acting insulin if it's cloudy, discolored, or unusually viscous. • Use the U-500 strength to treat insulin resistance, as prescribed. Be very careful to use conversion chart if U-500 strength is being administered using U-100 syringes. • Mix short-acting insulin with other insulin types, if needed. However, don't mix phosphate-buffered insulin with a zinc-containing insulin because the short-acting insulin's effectiveness may be reduced.

(continued)

Parenteral Insulin Preparations *(continued)*

CATEGORY, SPECIES, AND TRADE NAMES	KEY NURSING CONSIDERATIONS

Short-acting insulin *(continued)*

Onset: 30 min   **Peak:** 2–5 hr   **Duration:** 6–8 hr

- Administer SubQ, I.M., or I.V., as prescribed. Use a continuous SubQ infusion pump, if ordered. For an insulin pump, phosphate-buffered insulin is preferred over nonphosphate-buffered insulin. The catheter tubing and reservoir insulin should be changed every 48 hours or as specified by the pump manufacturer.
- When giving SubQ or I.M. injections, give the short-acting insulin 15 to 30 minutes before a meal or bedtime snack.
- Consider religious restrictions when choosing insulin type.
- Assess patient taking insulin concurrently with a thiazolidinedione for signs and symptoms of heart failure. If heart failure develops, provide supportive care, as ordered, and expect the thiazolidinedione to be discontinued or dosage reduced.

Intermediate-acting insulin

Onset: 1–3 hr   **Peak:** 4–15 hr   **Duration:** 18–24 hr

Human
- Humulin N
- Novolin ge Lente (CAN)
- Novolin ge NPH (CAN)
- Novolin N
- Novolin N Prefilled

- Don't use intermediate-acting insulin if it contains precipitate that is clumped or granular or that clings to the sides of the vial.
- Roll the vial gently between your palms to mix; don't shake it. Also gently turn the prefilled syringe up and down several times before using to achieve a uniform mixture.
- Administer by SubQ injection only, 30 minutes before a meal or bedtime snack.
- Be aware that intermediate-acting insulin rarely produces a blood glucose level that's as close to normal as possible. So expect to mix it with a short-acting insulin, as prescribed, for optimum blood glucose control.
- Consider religious restrictions when choosing insulin.
- Assess patient taking insulin concurrently with a thiazolidinedione for signs and symptoms of heart failure. If heart failure develops, provide supportive care, as ordered, and expect the thiazolidinedione to be discontinued or dosage reduced.

Parenteral Insulin Preparations *(continued)*

CATEGORY, SPECIES, AND TRADE NAMES	KEY NURSING CONSIDERATIONS

Long-acting insulin

Onset: 4–6 hr   **Peak:** 8–20 hr   **Duration:** 24–28 hr

Human
- Humulin-U (CAN)
- Lantus (insulin glargine)
- Levemir (insulin detemir)
- Novolin ge Ultralente (CAN)

- Don't use long-acting insulin if it contains precipitate that is clumped or granular or that clings to the sides of the vial.
- Mix Humulin-U or Novolin ge Ultralente with other insulin types—usually a short-acting insulin—if needed. Do not mix Lantus or Levemir with another insulin or solution.
- Roll the vial gently between your palms to obtain a uniform mixture; don't shake it.
- Administer by the SubQ route only. Inject Humulin-U or Novolin ge Ultralente 30 to 60 minutes before a meal or bedtime snack. Inject Lantus once daily at any time, keeping the daily injection time consistent. Inject Levemir prescribed once daily with the evening meal or at bedtime; inject Levemir prescribed twice daily with the morning meal and with the evening meal, at bedtime, or 12 hours after the morning dose.
- Give Lantus at bedtime, if possible, so that additional insulin can be given while patient is awake if Lantus effects decline before 24 hours pass. If Lantus is given in the morning and its effects don't last 24 hours, hyperglycemia may occur while patient sleeps.
- Assess patient taking insulin concurrently with a thiazolidinedione for signs and symptoms of heart failure. If heart failure develops, provide supportive care, as ordered, and expect the thiazolidinedione to be discontinued or dosage reduced.

Combination insulins

Onset: 30 min   **Peak:** 1–12 hr   **Duration:** 18–24 hr

Human
- Humalog Mix 75/25
- Humalog Mix 50/50
- Humulin 10/90 (CAN)
- Humulin 20/80 (CAN)
- Humulin 30/70 (CAN)
- Humulin 40/60 (CAN)
- Humulin 70/30
- Novolin 70/30
- Novolin ge 10/90 (CAN)
- Novolin ge 20/80 (CAN)
- Novolin ge 30/70 (CAN)
- Novolin ge 40/60 (CAN)
- Novolin ge 50/50 (CAN)
- NovoLog Mix 70/30
- NovoLog Mix 50/50

- Don't use combination insulin if it contains precipitate that is clumped or granular.
- Roll the vial gently between your palms to mix; don't shake it. Also gently turn the prefilled syringe up and down several times before using to achieve a uniform mixture.
- Administer combination insulin by the SubQ route only, 30 minutes before a meal.
- Be aware that Canadian and American products contain the same insulin ratio but express it differently. For example, the Canadian Humulin 30/70 and the American Humulin 70/30 both contain 30 units of a short-acting insulin and 70 units of an intermediate-acting insulin. Canadian products list the short-acting insulin first; American products list it second.
- Assess patient taking insulin concurrently with a thiazolidinedione for signs and symptoms of heart failure. If heart failure develops, provide supportive care, as ordered, and expect the thiazolidinedione to be discontinued or dosage reduced.

Oral Allergen Extracts

Prevention of allergy symptoms in patients diagnosed with an allergy has historically required an extended period of desensitization through the administration of injections given in a healthcare setting. Many patients do not have the time or resources required to undergo such a rigorous desensitization process. A new form of treatment using a sublingual route that the patient can self-administer (after the first dose) is now available for certain types of allergens as summarized in the following chart.

GENERIC AND TRADE NAMES	INDICATIONS	USUAL ADULT DOSAGES	NURSING CONSIDERATIONS FOR ALLERGEN EXTRACTS
grass pollen Grastek	To treat grass pollen–induced allergic rhinitis	2800 Bioequivalent Allergy Unit (1 tablet) sublingual once daily	• Know that allergen extracts are contraindicated in patients with severe, unstable asthma; in patients with a history of any severe systemic allergic reaction, severe local reaction after taking any sublingual allergen immunotherapy, or eosinophilic esophagitis; or in patients with a hypersensitivity to any of the inactive ingredients (gelatin, mannitol, or sodium hydroxide).
mixed pollens allergen extract Oralair	To treat grass pollen–induced allergic rhinitis	300 Index of Reactivity (1 tablet) sublingual once daily	• Monitor patient closely for allergic reactions that could become severe and life threatening, such as anaphylaxis and severe laryngopharyngeal constriction.
ragweed extract Ragwitek	To treat short-term ragweed pollen–induced allergic rhinitis	12 AMB a 1-Unit (1 tablet) sublingual once daily	• First dose must be administered in a healthcare setting and patient observed for at least 30 minutes after administration for signs and symptoms of an allergic reaction.

Antihistamines

Antihistamines are usually used to relieve immediate hypersensitivity reactions. They're also used as sedatives, antiemetics (especially in motion sickness), antitussives, antidyskinetics, and adjuncts to preoperative or postoperative analgesia.

Antihistamines are contraindicated in patients taking drugs that prolong the QT interval (including some macrolide antibiotics, quinidine, itraconazole, ketoconazole, mibefradil, and zileuton). They're also contraindicated in patients hypersensitive to antihistamines or their components.

The table below includes trade names; usual dosages; and onset, peak, and duration for antihistamines your patient is most likely to use daily or intermittently to control symptoms of allergic rhinitis. When caring for a patient who takes an antihistamine, individualize your plan of care but be sure to include these general interventions:
• Use antihistamines cautiously in patients with a history of glaucoma, peptic ulcer, or urine retention because anticholinergic effects may worsen these conditions.
• Before antihistamine therapy, assess the patient for hypokalemia and correct the imbalance, as prescribed, to reduce the risk of arrhythmias.
• Before antihistamine therapy, obtain a detailed medication history to help prevent drug interactions.
• Give antihistamines with food if GI distress occurs.
• Urge patient to avoid alcohol and other CNS depressants during antihistamine use because the combination can cause additive CNS depression.
• Monitor blood pressure because these drugs' anticholinergic effects may cause hypertension.
• Be aware that short- and long-acting antihistamines may be combined and H_2 blockers added to increase antihistamine effects.
• Be aware that products containing pseudoephedrine should be used for less than 7 days.

GENERIC AND TRADE NAMES	USUAL ADULT DOSAGE	ONSET, PEAK, AND DURATION
acrivastine Semprex-D (also include pseudoephedrine)	8 mg P.O. every 4 to 6 hr	**Onset:** 30 min **Peak:** Unknown **Duration:** 6 to 8 hr
azatadine Optimine Trinalin Repetabs (also includes pseudoephedrine)	1 to 2 mg P.O. every 8 to 12 hr 1 tablet P.O. every 12 hr	**Onset:** 15 to 60 min **Peak:** 4 hr **Duration:** 12 hr
azelastine Astelin Astepro 0.1% Astepro 0.15%	2 sprays (137 mcg/spray) in each nostril twice daily 1 to 2 sprays (137 mcg/spray) in each nostril twice daily 1 to 2 sprays (205.5 mcg/ spray) in each nostril twice daily	**Onset:** In 3 hr **Peak:** Unknown **Duration:** 12 hr
carbinoxamine maleate Arbinoxa, Palgic Karbinal ER	4 to 8 mg P.O. three times a day or four times a day (Immediate Release) 6-16 mg P.O. every 12 hrs (Extended Release)	**Onset:** 30 min. **Peak:** Unknown **Duration:** 4 hrs (Arbinoxa, Palgic), 17 hrs (Karbinal ER)

(continued)

Antihistamines *(continued)*

GENERIC AND TRADE NAMES	USUAL ADULT DOSAGE	ONSET, PEAK, AND DURATION
cetirizine Zyrtec Zyrtec D (also includes pseudoephedrine)	5 to 10 mg P.O. daily 5 mg/120 mg twice daily	**Onset:** 30 to 60 min **Peak:** 1 hr **Duration:** Up to 24 hr
desloratadine Clarinex Clarinex Reditabs	5 mg P.O. daily 5 mg P.O. daily	**Onset:** Unknown **Peak:** Unknown (Clarinex); 3 hr (Clarinex Reditabs) **Duration:** Unknown
fexofenadine Allegra Allegra-D (also includes pseudoephedrine)	60 mg P.O. twice daily or 180 mg P.O. daily 1 tablet P.O. every 12 hr	**Onset:** 1 hr **Peak:** 2 to 3 hr **Duration:** 12 hr
levocetirizine Xyzal	2.5 to 5 mg P.O. daily in evening	**Onset:** Less than 1 hr **Peak:** 0.9 hr **Duration:** 24 hr
loratadine Claritin Claritin-D12 (also includes pseudoephedrine) Claritin-D24 (also includes pseudoephedrine)	10 mg P.O. daily 1 tablet P.O. every 12 hr 1 tablet P.O. every 24 hr	**Onset:** 1 to 3 hr **Peak:** 8 to 12 hr **Duration:** At least 24 hr
olopatadine Patanase	2 sprays (665 mcg/spray) in each nostril twice daily	**Onset:** Unknown **Peak:** 15 to 120 minutes **Duration:** Unknown

Selected Ophthalmic Drugs

Although less commonly prescribed than oral drugs, drugs instilled into the eyes are frequently brought into the clinical setting by patients with chronic conditions. In most cases, the patient or a family member has administered these preparations at home. Your patient teaching should include a review of proper administration and storage of these drugs. Have the patient or a family member demonstrate proper use of the drug to make sure it will be administered correctly at home. Use this time to reassess the patient's ability to continue self-medication. Also, instruct him to report any changes in the condition being treated, either negative or positive. A properly educated patient not only ensures safe drug administration, but also is more likely to detect adverse reactions that require a dosage reduction or drug discontinuation, thus preventing the development of more serious health problems.

The following chart lists the generic and trade names, FDA-approved indications, and usual adult dosages for those ophthalmic preparations you're most likely to see in your practice setting. The drugs are divided according to therapeutic use.

GENERIC AND TRADE NAMES	INDICATIONS	USUAL ADULT DOSAGES
Ophthalmic antibiotics		
bacitracin AK-Tracin	To treat surface bacterial infections affecting the conjunctiva and cornea	Small amount of ointment applied to conjunctival sac, as needed
chloramphenicol Diochloram, Dioptic (CAN), Pentamycetin (CAN), Sopamycetin (CAN)	To treat surface bacterial infections affecting the conjunctiva and cornea	Apply small amount of ointment to lower conjunctival sac every 3 to 6 hr and as needed for at least 48 hr after eye resumes normal appearance
ciprofloxacin hydrochloride 0.3% Ciloxan	To treat corneal ulcers due to *Pseudomonas aerugi-nosa, Staphylococcus aureus, Staphylococcus epidermidis, Streptococcus pneumoniae,* and possibly *Serratia marcescens* and *Streptococcus viridans*	2 gtt in affected eye every 15 min for first 6 hr, then 2 gtt every 30 min for rest of first day; on day 2, 2 gtt in affected eye every hr; on days 3 to 14, 2 gtt in affected eye every 4 hr
	To treat bacterial conjunctivitis due to *Haemophilus influenzae, S. aureus, S. epidermidis,* and possibly *S. pneumoniae*	1 or 2 gtt in conjunctival sac of affected eye every 2 hr while awake for first 2 days and then 1 or 2 gtt every 4 hr while awake for next 5 days; or 1/2-inch strip of ointment in affected eye three times a day for 2 days, then twice daily for next 5 days
erythromycin Ilotycin	To treat acute or chronic conjunctivitis and other eye infections	1 cm (0.39 in) of ointment applied in infected eye up to 6 times/day, depending on severity of infection
	To treat chlamydial ophthalmic infections (trachoma)	Small amount applied in each eye twice daily for 2 mo; or twice daily on first 5 days of each month for 6 mo
ganciclovir 0.15% Zirgan	To treat acute herpes keratitis (dendritic ulcers)	1 gtt 5 times daily (about every 3 hr while awake) until corneal ulcer heals; then 1 gtt three times a day for 7 days

(continued)

Selected Ophthalmic Drugs *(continued)*

GENERIC AND TRADE NAMES	INDICATIONS	USUAL ADULT DOSAGES
Ophthalmic antibiotics *(continued)*		
gatifloxacin 0.3% Zymar **gatifloxacin 0.5%** Zymaxid	To treat bacterial conjuncti-vitis due to *Corynebacterium propinquum, Staphylococcus aureus, Staphylococcus epidermidis, Streptococcus mitis, Streptococcus pneumoniae, and Haemophilus influenzae*	1 gtt in affected eye every 2 hr while awake, up to 8 times daily on days 1 and 2; then 1 gtt up to four times daily while awake on days 3 to 7
	To treat bacterial conjuncti-vitis due to Staphylococcus aureus, Staphylococcus epidermidis, Streptococcus mitis, Streptococcus pneumoniae, and Haemophilus influenzae	1 gtt in affected eye every 2 hr while awake, up to 8 times daily on day 1; then 1 gtt twice daily to four times a day while awake on days 2 to 7
gentamicin sulfate Garamycin, Genoptic, Gentacidin, Gentak	To treat blepharitis, blepharo-conjunctivitis, conjunctivitis, corneal ulcers, dacryocystitis, keratoconjunctivitis, or mei-bomianitis due to susceptible organisms	1 or 2 gtt every 4 hr or, for severe infection, up to 2 gtt/hr; alterna-tively, 1 cm (0.39 in) of ointment applied to lower conjunctival sac twice daily or three times daily
levofloxacin 0.5% Quixin	To treat bacterial conjunc-tivitis	On days 1 and 2: 1 or 2 gtt every 2 hr while awake, up to 8 times/ day; on days 3 to 7: 1 or 2 gtt every 4 hr while awake, up to 4 times/day
moxifloxacin 0.5% Vigamox	To treat bacterial conjuncti-vitis due to *Staphylococcus aureus, Staphylococcus epidermidis, Staphylococcus haemolyticus, Staphylococcus hominis, Streptococcus pneu-moniae, Streptococcus* viridans group, *Haemophilus influen-zae, Chlamydia trachomatis*	1 gtt three times a day for 7 days
ofloxacin 0.3% Ocuflox	To treat conjunctivitis due to *Staphylococcus aureus, Staphylococcus epidermidis, Streptococcus pneumoniae, Enterobacter cloacae, Haemophilus influ-enzae, Proteus mirabilis, Pseudomonas aeruginosa, and Propionibacterium acnes*	1 or 2 gtt in conjunctival sac every 2 to 4 hr while awake for first 2 days; then 1 gtt four times a day for up to 5 more days
	To treat bacterial corneal ulcers due to *S. aureus, S. epidermidis, S. pneumoniae, E. cloacae, H. influenzae, P. mirabilis, P. aeruginosa, Serratia marcescens,* and *P. acnes*	1 or 2 gtt every 30 min while awake and 1 or 2 gtt every 4 to 6 hr after retiring for 2 days; then 1 or 2 gtt/hr while awake for up to 7 more days; then 1 gtt four times a day until end of treatment

Selected Ophthalmic Drugs *(continued)*

GENERIC AND TRADE NAMES	INDICATIONS	USUAL ADULT DOSAGES
Ophthalmic antibiotics *(continued)*		
polymyxin B sulfate	To treat superficial eye infections involving the conjunctiva or cornea caused by *Pseudomonas* or other gram-negative organisms	1 to 3 gtt of 0.1% to 0.25% (10,000 to 25,000 units/ml) every hr; or up to 10,000 units in lower conjunctival sac daily
sulfacetamide sodium 10% AK-Sulf, Bleph-10, Ocusulf-10, Sodium Sulamyd 10% (CAN), Sulf-10 **sulfacetamide sodium 15%** Isopto Cetamide	To treat inclusion conjunctivitis, corneal ulcers, and chlamydial infections	1 or 2 gtt solution (10%) in lower conjunctival sac every 2 to 3 hr during day, less often at night; or 1 or 2 gtt (15%) in conjunctival sac every 1 to 2 hr; or 1 gtt (30%) in conjunctival sac every 2 hr; or 1.25 to 2.5 cm ointment (10%) in conjunctival sac four times a day and bedtime
sulfacetamide sodium 30%	To treat trachoma	2 gtt (30%) in lower conjunctival sac every 2 hr in combination with systemic sulfonamide or tetracycline
tobramycin AKTob, Tobrex	To treat superficial ocular infections involving the conjunctiva or cornea	1 to 2 gtt every 1 to 4 hr, depending on severity of infection; or 1 cm (0.39 in) of ointment applied to lower conjunctival sac every 8 to 12 hr for mild to moderate infections or every 3 to 4 hr for severe infections
tobramycin 0.3% (3 mg) and dexamethasone 0.1% (1 mg) TobraDex	To treat steroid-responsive inflammatory ocular conditions for which a corticosteroid is indicated and where superficial bacterial ocular infection or a risk of bacterial ocular infection exists	1 to 2 gtt every 4 to 6 hr; during first 24 to 48 hrs, dosage may be increased to 1 to 2 gtt every 2 hr; or apply 1 cm (0.39 inch) of ointment into the conjunctival sac up to four times a day
Ophthalmic anti-inflammatory drugs		
bromfenac 0.09% Xibrom (0.09%)	To treat postoperative inflammation and reduce ocular pain after cataract extraction	1 gtt in operative eye twice daily starting 24 hr after cataract surgery and continuing through first 2 wk of postoperative period.
Bromday (0.09%) Prolensa (0.07%)	To treat postoperative inflammation and reduce ocular pain after cataract extraction	1 gtt in operative eye once daily, starting 24 hr before cataract surgery and continuing through first 2 wk of postoperative period.

(continued)

Selected Ophthalmic Drugs *(continued)*

GENERIC AND TRADE NAMES	INDICATIONS	USUAL ADULT DOSAGES

Ophthalmic anti-inflammatory drugs *(continued)*

GENERIC AND TRADE NAMES	INDICATIONS	USUAL ADULT DOSAGES
dexamethasone Maxidex **dexamethasone sodium phosphate** AK-Dex, Boldex, R.O. Dexasone (CAN)	To treat allergic conjunctivitis; corneal injury from chemical or thermal burns or from penetration of foreign bodies; inflammatory conditions of the anterior segment of globe, conjunctiva, cornea, or eyelids; iridocyclitis; suppression of graft rejection after keratoplasty; and uveitis	1 or 2 gtt of suspension or solution or 1.25 to 2.5 cm of ointment in conjunctival sac from every hr (in severe disease) to 6 times/day; or ointment may be applied three times a day or four times a day then tapered to twice daily, and then daily.
diclofenac sodium 0.1% Voltaren, Voltaren Ophtha (CAN)	To treat postoperative inflammation after removal of cataract	1 gtt in conjunctival sac four times a day, starting 24 hr after surgery through first 2 postoperative wk
	To treat photophobia in incisional refractive surgery	1 or 2 gtt in operative eye 1 hr before surgery. Then 1 or 2 gtt 15 min after surgery. Then 1 gtt four times a day, starting 4 to 6 hr after surgery for up to 3 days, as needed.
difluprednate Durezol	To treat inflammation and pain associated with ocular surgery	1 gtt in conjunctival sac of affected eye(s) four times a day for 2 wk starting 24 hr after surgery. Then 1 gtt twice daily for 1 wk.
fluoromethalone Fluor-Op, FML Forte, FML Liquifilm, FML S.O.P. **fluoromethalone acetate** Eflone, Flarex	To treat inflammatory and allergic conditions of the anterior uvea, conjunctiva, cornea, or sclera	1 or 2 gtt suspension in conjunctival sac twice daily to four times a day or, in severe conditions, up to every 2 hr during first 1 to 2 days, as needed; or 1 cm (0.39 in) ointment in conjunctival sac once daily to three times a day.
flurbiprofen sodium Ocufen	To inhibit intraoperative miosis	1 gtt in affected eye every 30 min, beginning 2 hr before surgery, up to total of 4 gtt.
ketorolac tromethamine Acular	To relieve ocular itching due to seasonal allergic conjunctivitis	1 gtt in conjunctival sac of each eye four times a day.
	To treat postoperative inflammation in patients who have undergone cataract extraction	1 gtt in operative eye four times a day, starting 24 hr after surgery through first 2 postoperative wk.
Acuvail	To treat postoperative inflammation in patients who have undergone cataract extraction	1 gtt in affected eye twice daily, starting 1 day before surgery, continuing through day of surgery and first 2 wk of postoperative period.

Selected Ophthalmic Drugs *(continued)*

GENERIC AND TRADE NAMES	INDICATIONS	USUAL ADULT DOSAGES
Ophthalmic anti-inflammatory drugs *(continued)*		
loteprednol etabonate Alrex, Lotemax	To relieve seasonal allergic conjunctivitis and to treat steroid-responsive inflammatory conditions of the palpebral and bulbar conjunctiva, cornea, and anterior segment of the globe	1 gtt of 0.2% suspension in affected eyes four times a day; or 1 or 2 gtt of 0.5% suspension in conjunctival sac of affected eye four times a day up to 1 gtt/hr.
	To treat postoperative inflammation following ocular surgery	1 or 2 gtt in conjunctival sac of operated eye four times a day, beginning 24 hr after surgery and continuing through first 2 wk of postoperative period.
medrysone HMS Liquifilm	To treat allergic conjunctivitis, episcleritis, epinephrine sensitivity, and vernal conjunctivitis	1 gtt into conjunctival sac up to every 4 hr.
olopatadine hydrochloride 0.1% Patanol	To treat signs and symptoms of allergic conjunctivitis	1 gtt twice daily at 6- to 8-hr intervals.
prednisolone acetate suspension Econopred Plus, Pred Forte, Pred Mild **prednisolone sodium phosphate solution** AK-Pred, Inflamase Forte, Inflamase Mild	To treat inflammation of the anterior segment of globe, cornea, and palpebral and bulbar conjunctiva	1 or 2 gtt in conjunctival sac twice daily to four times a day (suspension) or up to 6 times/day (solution).
rimexolone Vexol	To treat anterior uveitis	1 or 2 gtt in conjunctival sac every hr while awake in first week; 1 gtt every 2 hr while awake in second week; then tapered until uveitis resolves.
	To treat postoperative inflammation after ocular surgery	1 or 2 gtt in conjunctival sac of affected eye four times a day, starting 24 hr after surgery and continuing through first 2 postoperative wk.
Ophthalmic cycloplegic mydriatics		
atropine sulfate Atropisol, Isopto Atropine, Minims Atropine (CAN)	To treat acute iritis or uveitis	1 gtt up to four times a day; or small strip of ointment applied to conjunctival sac up to twice daily
	To produce dilation for cycloplegic refraction	1 or 2 gtt of 1% solution 1 hr before refraction

(continued)

Selected Ophthalmic Drugs *(continued)*

GENERIC AND TRADE NAMES	INDICATIONS	USUAL ADULT DOSAGES
Ophthalmic cycloplegic mydriatics *(continued)*		
cyclopentolate hydrochloride AK-Pentolate, Cyclogyl, Minims Cyclopentolate (CAN), Pentolair	To produce mydriasis and cycloplegia required in specific diagnostic procedures	1 gtt of 0.5%, 1%, or 2% solution in each eye; then 1 or 2 gtt in 5 to 10 min, as needed
homatropine hydrobromide Isopto Homatropine, Minims Homatropine (CAN)	To dilate pupils for cycloplegic refraction To treat uveitis	1 or 2 gtt in each eye, repeated in 5 to 10 min for 2 or 3 doses, as needed1 or 2 gtt in each eye every 3 to 4 hr
scopolamine hydrobromide Isopto Hyoscine	To dilate pupils for cycloplegic refraction To treat iritis or uveitis	1 or 2 gtt of 0.25% solution 1 hr before refraction 1 or 2 gtt of 0.25% solution once daily to four times a day
tropicamide Mydriacyl, Opticyl, Tropicacyl	To dilate pupils for cycloplegic refraction	1 gtt of 1% solution, repeated in 5 min; additional 1 gtt in 20 to 30 min, as needed
Ophthalmic miotics		
acetylcholine chloride Miochol-E	To produce papillary miosis in anterior segment surgery	0.5 to 2 ml gently into anterior chamber before or after sutures secured
carbachol 0.01% Carbastat, Miostat **carbachol 0.75%, 1.5%, 2.25%, 3%** Carboptic, Isopto Carbachol	To produce papillary miosis in ocular surgery To treat open-angle glaucoma	0.5 ml (solution) into anterior chamber before or after sutures secured 1 or 2 gtt up to three times a day
pilocarpine Ocusert Pilo-20, Ocusert Pilo-40	To treat primary open-angle glaucoma	1 or 2 gtt up to four times a day; or 1-cm (0.39 cm) ribbon of 4% gel at bedtime; or 1 Ocusert Pilo (20 or 40 mcg/hr) every 7 days
pilocarpine hydrochloride Adsorbocarpine, Akarpine, Isopto Carpine, Miocarpine (CAN), Pilocar, Pilopine HS, Pilostat	To treat acute angle-closure glaucoma as emergency therapy	1 gtt of 2% solution every 5 to 10 min for 3 to 6 doses; then 1 gtt every 1 to 3 hr until pressure is controlled
pilocarpine nitrate Pilagan, P.V. Carpine Liquifilm (CAN), Minims Pilocarpine (CAN)	To treat mydriasis due to mydriatic or cycloplegic drug therapy	1 gtt of 1% solution

Selected Ophthalmic Drugs *(continued)*

GENERIC AND TRADE NAMES	INDICATIONS	USUAL ADULT DOSAGES
Ophthalmic miotics *(continued)*		
naphazoline hydrochloride Ak-Con, Albalon Liquifilm, Allerest, Clear Eyes, Comfort Eye Drops, Degest 2, Vasocon Regular	To treat ocular congestion, irritation, or itching	1 gtt of 0.1% solution every 3 to 4 hr; or 1 gtt of 0.012% to 0.03% solution up to four times a day for no more than 72 hr
oxymetazoline hydrochloride OcuClear, Visine L.R.	To provide relief from eye redness due to minor eye irritations	1 or 2 gtt in conjunctival sac twice daily to four times a day (at least 6 hr apart)
phenylephrine hydrochloride Ak-Dilate, Ak-Nefrin, Isopto Frin, Mydfrin, Phenoptic, Relief Eye Drops for Red Eyes	To produce mydriasis without cycloplegia	1 gtt of 2.5% or 10% solution before eye exam, then repeated in 1 hr, as needed
	To produce mydriasis and vasoconstriction	1 gtt of 2.5% or 10% solution as single dose
	To treat chronic mydriasis	1 gtt of 2.5% or 10% solution or three times a day
	To treat posterior adhesion of iris	1 gtt of 2.5% or 10% solution as single dose
proparacaine hydrochloride Alcaine, Ophthaine, Ophthetic	To provide deep anesthesia during cataract extraction	1 gtt every 5 to 10 min for 5 to 7 doses
	To provide anesthesia during removal of eye sutures	1 or 2 gtt 2 to 3 min before procedure
	To provide anesthesia during removal of foreign bodies	1 or 2 gtt in affected eye before surgery
	To provide anesthesia during tonometry	1 or 2 gtt immediately before measurement
tetracaine Pontocaine	To provide eye anesthesia (short term)	1 or 2 gtt, as needed
tetrahydrozoline hydrochloride Collyrium Fresh Eye Drops, Eyesine, Murine Plus, Optigene 3, Tetrasine, Visine Moisturizing, Visine Extra	To treat conjunctival congestion, irritation, and allergic conditions	1 or 2 gtt of 0.05% solution up to four times a day or as directed
Miscellaneous ophthalmic drugs		
alcafiadine 0.25% Lastacaft	To prevent itching associated with allergic conjunctivitis	1 gtt in each eye once daily
apraclonidine hydrochloride Iopidine	To prevent or control elevated intraocular pressure (IOP) before and after ocular laser surgery	1 gtt of 1% solution 1 hr before laser surgery on anterior segment; then 1 drop immediately after surgery

(continued)

Selected Ophthalmic Drugs *(continued)*

GENERIC AND TRADE NAMES	INDICATIONS	USUAL ADULT DOSAGES
Miscellaneous ophthalmic drugs *(continued)*		
azelastine hydrochloride 0.05% Optivar	To treat itching of the eye associated with allergic conjunctivitis	1 gtt in affected eye twice daily
bepotastine besilate 1.5% Bepreve	To treat itching of the eye associated with allergic conjunctivitis	1 gtt in affected eye twice daily
betaxolol hydrochloride Betoptic, Betoptic S	To treat chronic open-angle glaucoma or ocular hypertension	1 or 2 gtt of 0.5% solution or 0.25% suspension twice daily
bimatoprost 0.01%, 0.03% Lumigan	To reduce elevated IOP in patients with open-angle glaucoma or ocular hypertension who can't tolerate or have insufficiently responded to other IOP-lowering medications	1 gtt in affected eye daily in evening
brimonidine tartrate Alphagan, Alphagan P	To reduce IOP in open-angle glaucoma or ocular hypertension	1 gtt in affected eye twice daily, about 8 hr apart
brinzolamide 1% Azopt	To reduce IOP in ocular hypertension or open-angle glaucoma	1 gtt three times a day
brinzolamide 1% and brimonidine tartrate 0.2% Simbrinza	To reduce IOP in open-angle glaucoma or ocular hypertension	1 gtt in affected eye three times a day
carteolol hydrochloride Ocupress	To treat chronic open-angle glaucoma or intraocular hypertension	1 gtt in conjunctival sac of affected eye twice daily
cyclosporine emulsion 0.05% Restasis	To increase tear production in keratoconjunctivitis sicca	1 gtt every 12 hr
cysteamine 0.44% Cystaran	To treat corneal cystine crystal accumulation in patients with cystinosis	1 gtt in each eye, every waking hr
dipivefrin hydrochloride Ophto-Dipivefrin (CAN), Propine	To reduce IOP in chronic open-angle glaucoma	1 gtt of 0.1% solution every 12 hr

Selected Ophthalmic Drugs *(continued)*

GENERIC AND TRADE NAMES	INDICATIONS	USUAL ADULT DOSAGES
Miscellaneous ophthalmic drugs *(continued)*		
dorzolamide hydrochloride Trusopt	To treat increased IOP in ocular hypertension or open-angle glaucoma	1 gtt in conjunctival sac of affected eye three times a day
emedastine difumarate Emadine	To treat allergic conjunctivitis	1 gtt in affected eye up to four times a day
fluorescein sodium AK-Fluor, Fluorescite, Fluor-I-Strip, Fluor-I-Strip-A.T., Ful-Glo, Funduscein-10, Funduscein-25, Ophthifluor	To diagnose corneal abrasions and foreign bodies, fit hard contact lenses, determine lacrimal patency, and assist in fundus photography and applanation tonometry	1 or 2 gtt of 2% solution followed by irrigation; or moisten strip with sterile water, then touch conjunctiva or fornix with moistened tip, and flush with irrigating solution; have patient blink several times after application
ketotifen fumarate Zaditor	To treat allergic conjunctivitis	1 gtt in affected eye twice daily every 8 to 12 hr
latanoprost Xalatan	To reduce IOP in ocular hypertension or open-angle glaucoma	1 gtt in conjunctival sac of affected eye daily in evening
levobunolol hydrochloride AKBeta, Betagan, Novo-Levobunolol (CAN)	To treat chronic open-angle glaucoma or ocular hypertension	1 or 2 gtt of 0.5% solution once daily or 0.25% solution twice daily
levocabastine hydrochloride 0.05% Livostin	To treat signs and symptoms of seasonal allergic conjunctivitis	1 gtt four times a day
metipranolol hydrochloride OptiPranolol	To reduce IOP in ocular hypertension or chronic open-angle glaucoma	1 gtt in affected eye twice daily
nedocromil sodium 2% Alocril	To treat itching associated with both seasonal and perennial allergic conjunctivitis	1 or 2 gtt twice daily
sodium chloride, hypertonic Adsorbonac, AK-NaCl, Muro-128, Muroptic-5	To provide temporary relief from corneal edema	1 or 2 gtt every 3 to 4 hr; or 6 mm (1/4 in) of ointment applied every 3 to 4 hr
tafluprost 0.0015% Zioptan	To reduce IOP in ocular hypertension or open-angle glaucoma	1 gtt in conjunctival sac in affected eye(s) once daily in evening

(continued)

Selected Ophthalmic Drugs *(continued)*

GENERIC AND TRADE NAMES	INDICATIONS	USUAL ADULT DOSAGES
Miscellaneous ophthalmic drugs *(continued)*		
timolol hemihydrate Betimol **timolol maleate** Apo-Timop (CAN), Timoptic **timolol maleateextended-release solution** Timoptic-XE	To reduce IOP in ocular hypertension or open-angle glaucoma	1 gtt of 0.25% solution in affected eye twice daily, then 1 gtt daily; or 1 gtt extended-release solution in affected eye daily
travoprost 0.004% Travatan	To reduce elevated IOP in patients with open-angle glaucoma or ocular hypertension who can't tolerate or have insufficiently responded to other IOP-lowering medication	1 gtt in affected eye daily in evening
unoprostone isopropyl 0.15% Rescula	To reduce elevated IOP in patients with open-angle glaucoma or ocular hypertension who can't tolerate or have insufficiently responded to other IOP-lowering medications	1 gtt in affected eye twice daily

Selected Topical Drugs

Topical drugs consist of an active drug prepared in a specified medium that promotes absorption through the skin. Media commonly are chosen based on drug solubility; rate of drug release; ability to hydrate the outer skin layer; ability to enhance penetration; drug stability; and interactions between the chosen medium, skin, and active ingredient.

Topical media include aerosols, creams, gels, lotions, ointments, powders, tinctures, and wet dressings. Aerosols, gels, lotions, and tinctures are convenient for application to the scalp and other hairy areas. Acutely inflamed areas are best treated with drying preparations, such as lotions, tinctures, and wet dressings. Chronic inflammation does well with applications of lubricating preparations, including creams and ointments.

Because of its physical properties, the skin can act as a holding area for many drugs, allowing slow penetration and prolonged duration of action. (This characteristic makes it important to understand the patient's allergies.) However, when administering topical or transdermal drugs that aren't prescribed for a specific location, keep in mind that penetration properties may vary in different areas of the body. For example, the scrotum, face, axillae, and scalp are more permeable than the limbs, and ventral surfaces typically are more permeable than dorsal surfaces.

Topical Drug Types

Topical drugs are classified as antibacterials, antifungals (the largest group), antivirals, corticosteroids, retinoids, and other miscellaneous preparations.

- *Antibacterials* may be useful in the early treatment of minor skin infections and wounds. Minor skin infections may respond well to topical drugs applied at the infection site. Minor wounds should be treated at the site and in the immediately surrounding area to prevent other pathogens from colonizing the area.
- *Antifungals* usually are used to treat mucocutaneous infections, such as tineas, primarily ringworm and athlete's foot. Systemic use of antifungals is limited by their potentially toxic adverse effects, most commonly renal or hepatic damage. All fungi are completely resistant to conventional antibacterial drugs.
- *Antivirals* are used to inhibit viral replication. They work by targeting any one of the steps involved in viral replication: penetration into

susceptible host cells; uncoating of the viral nucleic acid; synthesis of regulatory proteins, RNA and DNA, and structural proteins; assembly of viral particles; and release of the virus from the cell. Topical antivirals such as penciclovir can shorten the duration of herpetic lesions, lessen lesion pain, and minimize viral shedding.

- *Corticosteroids* reduce the signs and symptoms of inflammation. Topical corticosteroids cause vasoconstriction, probably by suppressing cell degranulation. They also cause decreased cell permeability by reducing histamine release from basal and mast cells.
- *Retinoids,* typically derivatives of vitamin A, are very effective in treating acne vulgaris, although the acne may appear to worsen before it improves. Retinoids are also useful for reducing wrinkles. When applied to the skin, retinoids remain primarily in the dermis; less than 10% of the drug is absorbed into the circulation. Prolonged use of retinoids promotes new dermal growth, new blood vessel formation, and thickening of the epidermis. Because these drugs are absorbed systemically and may have teratogenic effects, they shouldn't be used by pregnant women.
- *Miscellaneous topical drugs* are used to treat a variety of topical skin conditions, including dry skin, ichthyosis, parasitic infestations, psoriasis, and unwanted hair growth.

Administration Tips

Before you apply a topical drug, clean the site and let it dry. Use gloves or a finger cot during application to prevent the drug from being absorbed through your own skin. Inform your patient of any expected discomfort, such as temporary stinging or burning. After application, cover the site only if required; some topical drugs shouldn't be covered with an occlusive dressing.

Be sure to teach the patient and a family member correct administration technique. Also, review possible adverse reactions, highlighting those that should be reported to the prescriber. Stress the importance of complying with the drug regimen because some topical drugs require weeks or months of therapy to eradicate the underlying condition.

The following table includes the generic and trade names of many commonly prescribed topical drugs as well as their FDA-approved indications and usual adult dosages.

Selected Topical Drugs *(continued)*

GENERIC AND TRADE NAMES	INDICATIONS	USUAL ADULT DOSAGES
Antibacterials		
azelaic acid cream Azelex, Finacea, Finevin	To treat mild to moderate inflammatory acne vulgaris	Gently massage thin film into affected area twice daily, morning and evening.
bacitracin	To treat topical infections, abrasions, cuts, and minor burns or wounds	Apply thin film to affected area once daily to three times a day up to 3 wk.
benzoyl peroxide Benzac AC Wash, Clearasil Maximum Strength, Desquam-E 2.5 Gel, Fostex 10 BPO Gel, Triaz	To treat mild to moderate inflammatory acne vulgaris	Apply to affected area once daily, gradually increasing to twice daily or three times a day.
clindamycin phosphate Cleocin, Cleocin T Gel, Cleocin T Lotion, Clinda-Derm, Dalacin, Dalacin T Topical Solution (CAN)	To treat inflammatory acne vulgaris To treat bacterial vaginosis	Apply to affected area twice daily morning and evening. 1 applicatorful (100 mg) intravaginally at bedtime for 7 days.
clindamycin 1% and benzoyl peroxide 5% Benzaclin gel DUAC	To treat acne vulgaris	Apply once or twice daily (morning and/or evening) to affected areas.
clindamycin 1.2% and tretinoin 0.025% Veltin Gel	To treat acne vulgaris	Apply pea-sized amount to affected areas once daily in evening.
erythromycin Akne-Mycin, A/T/S, Erycette, EryDerm, Erygel, Erymax, Ery-Sol (CAN), Erythrogel, ETS (CAN), Sans-Acne (CAN), Staticin, T-Stat (CAN)	To treat inflammatory acne vulgaris	Apply to affected areas twice daily, morning and evening.
erythromycin 3% and benzoyl peroxide 5% Benzamycin	To treat moderate inflammatory acne	Apply to affected areas twice daily, morning and evening.
gentamicin sulfate Garamycin, G-myticin	To prevent or treat superficial skin infections due to susceptible bacteria; to treat superficial burns	Rub small amount gently into skin three times a day or four times a day.
mafenide gel 1% Sulfamylon	As adjunct to treat second- and third-degree burns	Apply 1/16-inch layer aseptically to affected areas once or twice daily.

Selected Topical Drugs *(continued)*

GENERIC AND TRADE NAMES	INDICATIONS	USUAL ADULT DOSAGES
Antibacterials *(continued)*		
metronidazole MetroCream, MetroGel, MetroGel-Vaginal	To treat inflammatory papules and pustules of acne rosacea	Apply thin film to affected area twice daily, morning and evening.
	To treat bacterial vaginosis	1 applicatorful (37.5 mg) intra-vaginally at bedtime or twice daily for 5 days.
mupirocin 2% Bactroban, Bactroban Cream, Bactroban Nasal	To treat impetigo	Apply to affected areas three times a day for 1 to 2 wk.
	To treat secondary infections of traumatic skin lesions due to *Staphylococcus aureus* and *Streptococcus pyogenes*	Apply thin film and cover with an occlusive dressing three times a day for 10 days.
	To eradicate nasal coloniza-tion of methicillin-resistant *S. aureus*	Apply half of the contents of a unit-dose tube to each nostril twice daily for 5 days.
neomycin sulfate Myciguent	To prevent or treat superficial bacterial infections	Rub fingertip-size dose into affected area once daily to three times a day.
nitrofurazone Furacin	As adjunct to treat third-degree burns and to treat infection in skin grafts	Apply aseptically, directly to lesions or on gauze; repeat, as needed.
povidone-iodine Betadine, Betadine Cream, Betadine Spray	To disinfect wounds and burns	Apply or spray to affected area, as needed.
silver sulfadiazine Flamazine (CAN), Silvadene, Thermazine	To prevent and treat bacterial and fungal infection in sec-ond- and third-degree burns	Apply 1/16-inch layer asepti-cally once to twice daily to clean debrided burns; reapply promptly if removed.
sulfacetamide sodium 10% Klaron	To treat acne vulgaris	Apply thin film twice daily.
sulfacetamide sodium 10% and sulfur 5% Sulfacet-R	To treat acne rosacea, acne vulgaris, and seborrheic der-matitis	Apply thin film, and massage into affected area once daily to three times a day.
tetracycline hydrochloride Achromycin, Topicycline	To treat acne vulgaris	Rub solution into affected area twice daily.
	To prevent or treat superficial skin infections due to suscep-tible bacteria	Apply to affected area twice daily. (morning and evening) or three times a day.

(continued)

Selected Topical Drugs *(continued)*

GENERIC AND TRADE NAMES	INDICATIONS	USUAL ADULT DOSAGES
Antifungals		
butenafine hydrochloride 1% Lotrimin Ultra, Mentax	To treat tinea corporis, tinea cruris, or tinea versicolor	Apply to affected surrounding area once daily for 2 wk.
	To treat interdigital tinea pedis due to *Epidermophyton floccosum, Trychophyton mentagrophytes,* or *T. rubrum*	Apply to affected and immediately surrounding area once daily for 4 wk or twice daily for 1 wk.
butoconazole nitrate Femstat, Femstat One, Mycelex 3	To treat vulvovaginal mycotic infections caused by *Candida* species	1 applicatorful (100 mg) intravaginally at bedtime for 3 days; may repeat course for total of 6 days.
Gynazole-1	To treat vulvovaginal infections caused by *Candida albicans*	1 applicatorful (100 mg) intravaginally once anytime day or night.
ciclopirox olamine 1% Loprox 0.77%	To treat candidiasis due to *Candida albicans;* tinea corporis, tinea cruris, and tinea pedis due to *E. floccosum, T. mentagrophytes, T. rubrum,* or *Microsporum canis;* tinea versicolor due to *Malassezia furfur;* onychomycosis due to *T. rubrum;* and seborrheic dermatitis	Massage gently into affected and surrounding area twice daily, morning and evening.
ciclopirox olamine 8% Penlac	To treat onychomycosis of the fingernails and toenails	Apply evenly to entire nail surface and surrounding 5 mm of skin at bedtime for up to 48 wk.
clotrimazole Canesten (CAN), Gyne-Lotrimin, Gyne-Lotrimin 3, Lotrimin, Lotrimin Antifungal, Mycelex, Mycelex-7, Mycelex-G, Mycelex OTC, Trivagizole 3	To treat superficial fungal infections (tinea corporis, tinea cruris, tinea pedis, tinea versicolor, candidiasis)	Apply thin film and massage into affected and surrounding area twice daily, morning and evening, for 2 to 4 wk.
	To treat vulvovaginal candidiasis	Insert 100-mg vaginal tablet at bedtime for 7 days; or 500-mg vaginal tablet at bedtime for 1 day; or 1 applicatorful intravaginally at bedtime for 7 days (or 3 days if using Trivagizole 3).
	To treat oropharyngeal candidiasis	Dissolve oral troche over 15 to 30 min 5 times/day for 14 days.
	To prevent oropharyngeal candidiasis	Dissolve oral troche over 15 to 30 min three times a day for duration of chemotherapy or until corticosteroid dosage is reduced to maintenance levels.

Selected Topical Drugs *(continued)*

GENERIC AND TRADE NAMES	INDICATIONS	USUAL ADULT DOSAGES
Antifungals *(continued)*		
econazole nitrate Ecostatin (CAN), Spectazole	To treat tinea corporis, tinea cruris, tinea pedis, tinea versicolor, cutaneous candidiasis	Rub into affected area once or twice daily for at least 2 wk.
Ecoza	To treat cutaneous candidiasis	Rub into affected area twice daily for 2 wk.
	To treat interdigital tinea pedis	Apply to affected areas once daily for 4 wks.
gentian violet Genapax	To treat candidiasis	Insert 1 intravaginal tampon three times a day to four times a day for 12 days; or apply 1% or 2% solution to affected area once or twice daily for 3 days.
haloprogin Halotex	To treat tinea corporis, tinea cruris, tinea manuum, and tinea pedis due to *E. floccosum, M. canis, T. mentagrophytes, T. rubrum,* or *T. tonsurans;* to treat tinea versicolor due to *M. furfur*	Apply liberally to affected area twice daily for 2 to 3 wk or, for intertriginous lesions, up to 4 wk.
ketoconazole 2% Nizoral	To treat tinea corporis, tinea cruris, and tinea versicolor due to susceptible organisms; to treat cutaneous candidiasis	Apply thin film to affected and immediately surrounding area and cover with occlusive dressing daily for at least 2 wk.
	To treat tinea pedis	Apply to affected and immediately surrounding area daily for 6 wk; or apply shampoo to wet hair, lather, massage for 1 min, leave drug on scalp for 3 min, then rinse and repeat 2 times/wk for 4 weeks (with at least 3 days between shampoos), then intermittently, as needed.
	To treat seborrheic dermatitis	Apply to affected and immediately surrounding area twice daily for 4 wk.
luliconazole 1% cream Luzu	To treat interdigital tinea	Apply to affected area and about 1 inch of the immediate surround area(s) once daily for 2 wks.
	To treat pedis, tinea cruris, and tinca corporis	Apply to affected area and about 1 inch of the immediate surrounding area(s) once daily for 1 wk.

(continued)

Selected Topical Drugs *(continued)*

GENERIC AND TRADE NAMES	INDICATIONS	USUAL ADULT DOSAGES
Antifungals *(continued)*		
miconazole nitrate Femizol-M, Fungoid, M-Zole 3, Micatin, Monistat-Derm, Monistat 3, Monistat 7, Ony-Clear Nail	To treat tinea corporis, tinea cruris, tinea pedis; cutaneous candidiasis; and common dermatophyte infections	Apply cream sparingly (or powder or spray liberally) over affected area twice daily for 2 to 4 wk.
	To treat tinea versicolor	Apply sparingly to affected area daily for 2 wk.
	To treat vulvovaginal candidiasis	1 applicatorful (100 mg) or vaginal suppository (100 mg) at bedtime for 7 days, repeated, as needed; or insert vaginal suppository (200 mg) at bedtime for 3 days.
	To treat onychomycosis	Brush tincture on affected areas of nail surface, beds, and edges and under nail surface twice daily for up to several mo; or spray on clean, dry, affected nails, holding actuator down for 1 or 2 sec.
naftifine hydrochloride Naftin	To treat tinea corporis, tinea cruris, and tinea pedis	Apply cream to affected area daily; or apply gel to affected area twice daily morning and evening.
nystatin Mycostatin, Nadostine (CAN), Nilstat	To treat cutaneous and mucocutaneous infections due to *C. albicans*	Apply cream to affected area twice daily or as indicated; or apply powder twice daily or three times a day; or insert 1 or 2 lozenges (200,000 to 400,000 units) 4 to 5 times/day for up to 48 hr after symptoms have subsided or 14 days; or insert 4 to 6 ml (400,000 to 600,000 units) of oral suspension in mouth four times a day (one-half of dose in each side of mouth) and retain as long as possible before swallowing.
	To treat vulvovaginal candidiasis	Insert 1 intravaginal tablet (100,000 units) or 1 applicatorful (100,000 to 500,000 units) once or twice daily for 14 days.
oxiconazole nitrate Oxistat, Oxizold (CAN)	To treat tinea corporis, tinea cruris, and tinea pedis caused by *E. floccosum*, *T. mentagrophytes*, or *T. rubrum*	Apply to affected and surrounding area once or twice daily for 2 wk (tinea corporis and tinea cruris) or for 4 wk (tinea pedis).
	To treat tinea versicolor caused by *M. furfur*	Apply cream to affected and surrounding area daily for 2 wk.

Selected Topical Drugs *(continued)*

GENERIC AND TRADE NAMES	INDICATIONS	USUAL ADULT DOSAGES
Antifungals *(continued)*		
selenium sulfide SelRX 2.3%, Selsun	To treat tinea versicolor	Apply to scalp, lather with small amount of water, wait 10 min, then rinse, every 7 days.
	To treat dandruff and seborrheic scalp dermatitis	Massage into wet scalp, wait 2 to 3 min, rinse, and repeat 2 times/ wk for 2 wk, then, as needed.
sulconazole nitrate Exelderm	To treat tinea corporis, tinea cruris, and tinea pedis (cream only) caused by *E. floccosum, M. canis, T. mentagrophytes,* or *T. rubrum;* to treat tinea versicolor	Massage small amount gently into affected and surrounding areas once or twice daily (tinea pedis) for up to 6 wk.
terbinafine hydrochloride Lamisil DermGel, Lamisil Solution	To treat tinea versicolor	Apply to affected area twice daily for 1 wk.
Lamisil AT Cream	To treat tinea corporis, tinea cruris, and tinea pedis	Apply thin film to affected area twice daily for 1 wk or 2 wk (plantar tinea pedis).
Lamisil AT Solution	To treat interdigital tinea pedis, tinea corporis, and tinea cruris	Apply between the toes twice daily for 1 wk (interdigital tinea pedis) or to affected area daily for 1 wk (tinea corporis and tinea cruris).
terconazole Terazol 3, Terazol 7	To treat vulvovaginal candidiasis	1 applicatorful (20 mg) intravaginally at bedtime for 3 days (0.4%) or 1 applicatorful (40 mg) for 7 days (0.8%); or insert 80-mg vaginal suppository at bedtime for 3 consecutive days.
tioconazole GyneCure Ovules (CAN), Vagistat-1	To treat vulvovaginal candidiasis	Insert 1 applicatorful (300 mg) or 1 suppository (300 mg) intravaginally at bedtime as a single dose.
tolnaftate Absorbine Footcare, Aftate for Athlete's Foot, Aftate for Jock Itch, Dr. Scholl's Athlete's Foot, Genaspore, NP-27, Pitrex, Quinsana Plus, Tinactin, Ting, Zeasorb-AF	To treat tinea capitis, corporis, cruris, manuum, pedis, and versicolor	Apply 1% aerosol, cream, gel, powder, or solution to affected and surrounding areas twice daily, continue for 2 wk after symptoms subside or up to 6 wk.

(continued)

Selected Topical Drugs *(continued)*

GENERIC AND TRADE NAMES	INDICATIONS	USUAL ADULT DOSAGES
Antivirals		
acyclovir Zovirax	To treat mucocutaneous herpes simplex in immunocompromised patients	Apply cream to affected area 4 to 6 times daily for 10 days. Apply ointment every 3 hr (6 times/day) for 7 days. Use finger cot, rubber glove, or applicator stick for both forms to prevent herpetic whitlow.
docosanol Abreva	To treat recurrent oral-facial herpes simplex	Apply cream gently and completely to affected area 5 times daily, starting with first visible sign of lesion and continuing until lesion is healed.
penciclovir Denavir	To treat recurrent herpes labialis of lips and face	Apply every 2 hr while awake for 4 days.
Corticosteroids		
alclometasone dipropionate Aclovate	To treat corticosteroid-responsive dermatoses	Apply thin film to affected area and massage twice daily to three times a day.
amcinonide Cyclocort	To treat corticosteroid-responsive dermatoses	Apply thin film to affected area and massage twice daily (ointment, lotion) or twice daily to three times a day (cream).
betamethasone benzoate Beben (CAN), Uticort	To treat corticosteroid-responsive dermatoses	Apply thin film or a few drops to affected area once or twice daily up to 45 g/wk (ointment, cream), 50 g/wk (gel), or 50 ml (lotion).
betamethasone dipropionate Diprolene, Diprolene AF, Diprosone, Topilene (CAN)	To treat corticosteroid-responsive dermatoses	Apply thin film or a few drops to affected area once or twice daily up to 45 g/wk (ointment, cream), 50 g/wk (gel), or 50 ml (lotion).
betamethasome valerate Luxiq, Valisone	To treat corticosteroid-responsive dermatoses	Apply foam to scalp, and massage until foam disappears, twice daily. Apply thin film of ointment twice daily.

Selected Topical Drugs *(continued)*

GENERIC AND TRADE NAMES	INDICATIONS	USUAL ADULT DOSAGES
Corticosteroids *(continued)*		
clobetasol propionate Dermovate (CAN), Embeline, Temovate	To treat corticosteroid-responsive dermatoses	Apply thin film to affected area and rub in gently twice daily to three times a day, up to 50 g/wk, for 2 wk.
Olux	To treat corticosteroid-responsive dermatoses of scalp	Apply to affected area of scalp twice daily, once in morning and once at night, for 2 wk.
desonide Desowen, Tridesilon	To treat corticosteroid-responsive dermatoses	Apply thin film to affected area twice daily to four times a day.
desoximetasone 0.25% Topicort	To treat plaque psoriasis	Apply thin film to affected skin areas twice daily.
diflorasone diacetate Florone, Maxiflor, Psorcon	To treat corticosteroid-responsive dermatoses	Apply thin film to affected area once daily to four times a day.
fluocinolone acetonide Bio-Syn, Derma Smooth FS, Fluocet, Fluoderm (CAN), Fluolar (CAN), Fluonid (CAN), Fluonide (CAN), Flurosyn, Synalar, Synalar-HP, Synamol (CAN), Synemol	To treat corticosteroid-responsive dermatoses	Apply thin film to affected area twice daily to four times a day.
fluocinonide Lidemol (CAN), Lidex	To treat corticosteroid-responsive dermatoses	Apply thin film to affected area twice daily to four times a day.
flurandrenolide Cordran, Cordran Tape, Drenison (CAN)	To treat corticosteroid-responsive dermatoses	Apply thin film to affected area and massage twice daily to three times a day; or apply tape every 12 to 24 hr.
fluticasone propionate Cutivate	To treat atopic dermatitis and corticosteroid-responsive dermatoses	Apply thin film daily (atopic dermatitis) or twice daily (dermatoses).
halcinonide Halog	To treat corticosteroid-responsive dermatoses	Apply sparingly and massage once daily to three times a day.
halobetasol propionate Ultravate	To treat corticosteroid-responsive dermatoses	Apply thin film to affected area and rub in gently once or twice daily, up to 50 g/wk, for 2 wk.

(continued)

Selected Topical Drugs *(continued)*

GENERIC AND TRADE NAMES	INDICATIONS	USUAL ADULT DOSAGES

Corticosteroids *(continued)*

GENERIC AND TRADE NAMES	INDICATIONS	USUAL ADULT DOSAGES
hydrocortisone 0.25% Cetacort, Cort-Dome	To treat corticosteroid-responsive dermatoses	Apply thin film (aerosol foam, cream, lotion, ointment, solution) to affected area once daily to four times a day.
hydrocortisone 0.5% Bactine, Cetacort, Cortate (CAN), Cort-Dome, Cortifair, Delacort, DermiCort, Dermtex HC, Emo-Cort (CAN), Hydro-Tex, Hytone, MyCort, Sential (CAN), S-T Cort		
hydrocortisone 1% Ala-Cort, Allercort, Alphaderm, Acticort 100, Barriere-HC (CAN), Beta-HC, Cetacort, Cort-Dome, Cortifair, Cortril, Dermacort, Emo-Cort (CAN), Gly-Cort, Hi-Cor 1.0, Hydro-Tex, Hytone, LactiCare-HC, Lemoderm, Nutracort, Penecort, Prevex-HC (CAN), Rederm, Sarna HC (CAN), Synacort, Unicort (CAN)		
hydrocortisone 2% Ala-Scalp HP		
hydrocortisone 2.5% Allercort, Anusol-HC, Emo- Cort (CAN), Hi-Cor 2.5, Hytone, LactiCare-HC, Lemoderm, Nutracort, Penecort, Synacort		
hydrocortisone acetate 0.1% Corticreme (CAN)		
hydrocortisone acetate 0.5% 9-1-1, Corticaine, Cortacet (CAN), Cortaid, Cortoderm (CAN), FoilleCort, Gynecort, Hyderm (CAN), Lanacort, Novohydrocort (CAN), Pharma-Cort		

Selected Topical Drugs *(continued)*

GENERIC AND TRADE NAMES	INDICATIONS	USUAL ADULT DOSAGES
Corticosteroids *(continued)*		
hydrocortisone acetate 1%, 2%, 2.5% Cortaid, Cortef Feminine Itch, Corticreme (CAN), Cortoderm (CAN), Hyderm (CAN), Maximum Strength Cortaid, Micort HC-Lipocream, Novohydrocort (CAN)	To treat corticosteroid-responsive dermatoses	Apply thin film (aerosol foam, cream, lotion, ointment, solution) to affected area once daily to four times a day.
hydrocortisone acetate topical aerosol foam Epifoam		
hydrocortisone acetate dental paste Orabase-HCA	To treat inflamed oral mucosa	Apply to oral mucosa twice daily to three times a day after meals and at bedtime.
hydrocortisone butyrate Locoid	To treat corticosteroid-responsive dermatoses	Apply to affected area twice daily to three times a day.
hydrocortisone valerate Westcort		
hydrocortisone acetate, polymyxin B sulfate, and neomycin sulfate Cortisporin	To treat corticosteroid-responsive dermatoses (short term) with mild bacterial infection	Apply sparingly and massage twice daily to four times a day.
hydrocortisone and iodoquinol Vytone	To treat corticosteroid-responsive dermatoses with mild bacterial or fungal infection (short term)	Apply to affected area once daily to three times a day.
mometasone furoate Elocom (CAN), Elocon	To treat corticosteroid-responsive dermatoses	Apply thin film or a few drops to affected area daily.
prednicarbate Dermatop	To treat corticosteroid-responsive dermatoses	Apply thin film to affected area twice daily.
triamcinolone acetonide 0.025%, 0.5% Aristocort, Aristocort A, Aristocort D (CAN), Flutex, Kenac, Kenalog, Kenonel, Triacet, Triaderm (CAN), Trianide Mild (CAN)	To treat corticosteroid-responsive dermatoses	Apply thin film (cream) to affected area twice daily to four times a day; 0.025% lotion or ointment once or twice daily; 0.1% lotion or ointment once daily; or 0.5% ointment once daily.

(continued)

Selected Topical Drugs *(continued)*

GENERIC AND TRADE NAMES	INDICATIONS	USUAL ADULT DOSAGES
Corticosteroids *(continued)*		
triamcinolone acetonide 0.1% Aristocort, Aristocort A, Aristocort R (CAN), Delta-Tritex, Flutex, Kenac, Kenalog, Kenalog-H, Kenonel, Triacet, Triaderm (CAN), Trianide Regular (CAN)	To treat corticosteroid-responsive dermatoses	Apply thin film (cream) to affected area twice daily to four times a day; 0.025% lotion or ointment once or twice daily; 0.1% lotion or ointment once daily; or 0.5% ointment once daily.
triamcinolone acetonide 0.5% Aristocort, Aristocort A, Aristocort C (CAN), Flutex, Kenalog, Kenonel, Triacet		
triamcinolone acetonide dental paste Kenalog in Orabase, Oracort, Oralone	To treat inflammatory or ulcerative oral lesions	Apply to oral mucosa twice daily to three times a day after meals and at bedtime.
triamcinolone acetonide topical aerosol Kenalog	To treat corticosteroid-responsive dermatoses	Spray affected area three times a day to four times a day.
Retinoids		
adapalene Differin	To treat acne vulgaris	Apply to affected area at bedtime.
tazarotene 0.05%, 0.1% Avage, Tazorac	To treat plaque psoriasis	Apply thin film to affected area at bedtime.
tazarotene 0.1% Avage, Tazorac	To treat facial acne vulgaris or plaque psoriasis	Apply thin film to affected area at bedtime.
tazarotene 0.1% Fabior	To treat acne vulgaris	Apply thin layer to affected areas of the face and /upper trunk once daily in the evening.
tretinoin Avita, Renova, Retin-A, Retin-A Micro, Stieva-A (CAN)	To treat acne vulgaris	Apply sparingly to clean, dry affected area at bedtime.
Miscellaneous topical drugs		
adapalene 0.1% and benzoyl peroxide 2.5% gel Epiduo	To treat acne vulgaris	Apply sparingly to clean, dry affected area once daily.
ammonium lactate, 12% Lac-Hydrin	To treat dry skin and ichthyosis	Apply to affected area, and rub in twice daily.
anthralin Anthranol 1 (CAN), Drithocreme, Dritho-Scalp	To treat chronic psoriasis To treat chronic scalp psoriasis	Apply sparingly and massage into affected lesions daily. Apply to lesions daily for 1 wk.

Selected Topical Drugs *(continued)*

GENERIC AND TRADE NAMES	INDICATIONS	USUAL ADULT DOSAGES
Miscellaneous topical drugs *(continued)*		
becaplermin Regranex	To treat lower-extremity diabetic neuropathic ulcers that extend into the subcutaneous tissue or beyond and that have an adequate blood supply	Apply to ulcers daily.
brimonidine gel Mirvaso	To treat rosacea	Apply pea-sized amount onto each of the five areas of the face once daily. Do not apply to eyes or lips.
calcipotriene Dovonex	To treat plaque psoriasis	Apply cream or scalp lotion in a thin layer twice daily up to 8 wk. Apply thin layer of ointment once or twice daily up to 8 wk.
calcipotriene hydrate 0.005% and betamethasone dipropionate 0.064% Taclonex, Taclonex Scalp	To treat psoriasis vulgaris	Apply ointment to affected skin; rub in gently and completely once daily for up to 4 wk.
	To treat moderate to severe psoriasis vulgaris of the scalp	Apply suspension to affected scalp areas and rub in gently once daily for 2 to 8 wk or until skin clears.
capsaicin Zostrix Capsin Capzacin-P	To provide temporary pain relief from rheumatoid arthritis and osteoarthritis; to relieve neuralgias from pain following shingles (herpes zoster) infection	Apply to affected area no more than four times a day.
chlorhexidine Hibiclens	To clean skin wounds	Rinse area, apply minimal amount to cover, then wash and rinse thoroughly.
chloroxine Capitrol	To treat dandruff and seborrheic dermatitis	Massage into wet scalp, wait 3 min, rinse, and repeat 2 times/wk.
clotrimazole and betamethasone dipropionate 0.05%, 1% Lotrisone	To treat symptomatic inflammatory tinea corporis, tinea cruris, and tinea pedis	Massage cream gently into affected and surrounding skin areas twice daily for 2 wk (tinea corporis, tinea cruris) or for 4 wk (tinea pedis).
coal tar Zetar, Zetar Shampoo	To treat psoriasis	Add 15 to 20 ml to lukewarm bath, immerse affected area for 15 to 20 min, and rinse thoroughly 3 to 7 times/wk.
	To treat dandruff or scalp seborrhea	Massage into wet scalp, rinse, repeat application and wait 5 min, then rinse again.

(continued)

Selected Topical Drugs *(continued)*

GENERIC AND TRADE NAMES	INDICATIONS	USUAL ADULT DOSAGES
Miscellaneous topical drugs *(continued)*		
crotamiton 10% Eurax	To treat scabies	Massage into cleansed body from chin to soles of feet, and reapply after 24 hr; change bed linens next day, and bathe 48 hr after second dose; repeat in 7 to 10 days if new lesions appear.
desoximetasone Topicort	To relieve inflammatory and pruritic manifestations of corticosteroid-responsive dermatoses, including psoriasis, atopic dermatitis, and eczema	Apply thin film twice daily to affected areas; occlusive dressings may be added for severe dermatoses.
diclofenac sodium 3% Solaraze	To treat actinic keratoses	Massage gel gently onto affected lesion areas twice daily for 60 to 90 days.
doxepin hydrochloride Zonalon	To treat pruritus associated with dermatitis and chronic lichen simplex	Apply thin film to affected area four times a day (every 3 to 4 hr) for up to 8 days.
eflornithine Vaniqa	To retard unwanted hair growth	Apply thin film to affected area of face and chin twice daily (at least 8 hr apart); don't wash treated area for at least 4 hr.
fluocinolone acetonide 0.01%, hydroquinone 4%, tretinoin 0.05% TRI-LUMA Cream	To treat severe facial melasma	Apply a thin film lightly and uniformly to hyperpigmented areas of melasma including about 1/2 in of skin surrounding each lesion daily at least 30 min before bedtime.
fluorouracil cream Carac, Efudex, Fluoroplex	To treat actinic and solar keratoses	Apply to lesions twice daily for 2 to 6 weeks.
hexachlorophene pHisoHex	To treat skin preoperatively	Rinse area, apply minimal amount to cover; then wash and rinse thoroughly.
hydrocortisone acetate, polymyxin B sulfate, and neomycin sulfate Cortisporin	To treat dermatoses associated with secondary bacterial infection	Apply small amount to affected areas twice daily to four times a day.
hydroquinone Alustra, Claripel, Eldopaque, Eldoquin, Glyquin, Melanex	To treat hyperpigmentation and melanin	Apply twice daily to the affected areas for no longer than 2 months.

Selected Topical Drugs *(continued)*

GENERIC AND TRADE NAMES	INDICATIONS	USUAL ADULT DOSAGES
Miscellaneous topical drugs *(continued)*		
imiquimod 3.75% Zyclara	To treat facial or scalp actinic keratoses	Apply to affected area daily for two 2-wk treatment cycles separated by a 2-wk no-treatment period.
imiquinod 5% Aldara	To treat external genital and perianal warts	Apply thin layer to affected area and rub in 3 times/wk at bedtime for up to 16 wk; remove with soap and water after 6 to 10 hr.
ingenol mebutate gel 0.015%, 0.05% Picato	To treat actinic keratosis	Apply 0.015% gel to face and scalp once daily for 3 consecutive days; apply 0.05% gel to trunk and extremities once daily for 2 consecutive days.
ivermectin lotion 0.5% Sklice	To treat head lice	Apply to dry hair in amount sufficient to coat the hair and scalp thoroughly; leave on for 10 minutes, then rinse off with water.
lidocaine and prilocaine EMLA	For local anesthesia	Apply 1 disk or thick layer of 2.5-g cream occlusively for at least 1 hr.
malathion lotion 0.5% Ovide	To treat pediculus humanus capitis	Apply to dry hair in amount just sufficient to wet the hair and scalp thoroughly; then let hair dry naturally. After 8 to 12 hr, shampoo and rinse hair to remove dead lice and eggs. If lice are still present after 7 to 9 days, repeat application.
mequinol 2%, retinol 0.01% Solage	To treat solar lentigines	Apply solution twice daily, morning and evening, at least 8 hours apart. Avoid application to surrounding skin, and do not bathe for 6 hr after application.
minoxidil Rogaine 2% and 5%	To treat alopecia and androgenetica	Apply 1 ml to affected areas twice daily.
monobenzone 20% Benoquin	To treat final depigmentation in extensive vitiligo	Apply twice daily to three times a day for 1 to 4 months, then twice daily weekly for maintenance.
nitroglycerin ointment 0.4% Rectiv	To treat moderate to severe pain associated with chronic anal fissure	Apply 1 inch of ointment intra-anally every 12 hrs for up to 3 wks.

(continued)

Selected Topical Drugs *(continued)*

GENERIC AND TRADE NAMES	INDICATIONS	USUAL ADULT DOSAGES
Miscellaneous topical drugs *(continued)*		
oxybutynin gel 3% Gelnique	To treat overactive bladder with symptoms of urge urinary incontinence, urgency, and frequency	Apply 3 pumps (84 mg) once daily to clean, dry, intact skin on abdomen, upper arms/shoulders, or thighs.
permethrin 1% Nix	To prevent or treat head lice	Wash and dry hair, saturate scalp with 1% cream, leave on hair for 10 min, then rinse; remove nits with provided comb; repeat in 7 days if living mites are still present.
permethrin 5% Acticin, Elimite	To treat scabies	Massage 5% cream into skin from head to soles of feet, and remove after 8 to 10 hr; repeat in 14 days if living mites are still present.
pimecrolimus 1% Elidel	To treat mild-to-moderate atopic dermatitis	Apply to affected areas twice daily.
podofilox Condylox	To treat anogenital warts (gel); to treat external genital warts (gel or solution)	Apply 0.5% gel to anogenital warts for 3 days, then withhold for 4 days; repeat cycle up to 4 times. Apply 0.5% solution or gel to external genital warts every 12 hr in the morning and evening for 3 days, then withhold for 4 days; repeat cycle up to 4 times.
pyrethrum extract and piperonyl butoxide RID, End Lice, Tegrin-LT	To treat head, pubic, and body lice	Apply to dry hair or affected body area. Massage through all hairy areas until hair is wet. Leave on hair for 10 min; then wash with warm water and soap or shampoo. Repeat in 7 to 10 days.
spinosad topical suspension 0.9% Natroba	To treat head lice	Apply to dry scalp and hair using only the amount needed to cover the scalp and hair. Rinse off with warm water after 10 minutes. Repeat in 7 days if live lice are still seen.
tacrolimus ointment 0.03% and 0.1% Protopic	To treat moderate to severe atopic dermatitis in patients unresponsive to other therapies	Apply thin layer to affected areas twice daily, rubbing in gently and completely. Continue for 1 wk after signs and symptoms have disappeared.
urea 41%, 45%	To treat hyperkeratotic conditions	Apply to affected area twice daily and rub in.

Selected Antivirals

Antivirals are used to treat viral infections, such as influenza, human immunodeficiency virus (HIV), herpes simplex virus (HSV) I and II, herpes zoster, and cytomegalovirus (CMV) infections.

The following table lists the generic and trade names, indications, and usual adult dosages for some commonly used antivirals. Although you must individualize your care for a patient who receives an antiviral, be sure to include these general interventions in your plan of care:

• Avoid administering HIV drugs all at once.
• If patient takes an antacid, administer it 1 hour before or 2 hours after an antiviral because antacids may reduce antiviral absorption.

• Monitor hepatic enzyme levels to detect elevations and help prevent hepatotoxicity.
• Monitor BUN and serum creatinine levels to detect signs of impaired renal function.
• Monitor I.V. injection site for pain or phlebitis, which may result from the high pH of reconstituted solutions.
• Assess the immunosuppressed patient for opportunistic infections during antiviral therapy.
• Inform female patient that oral contraceptives may be ineffective when taken with HIV drugs. Suggest alternate contraceptive methods.

GENERIC AND TRADE NAMES	INDICATIONS	USUAL ADULT DOSAGES
Antivirals used for HIV infection		
abacavir sulfate Ziagen	To treat HIV infection	300 mg P.O. twice daily or 600 mg P.O. once daily
abacavir sulfate, dolutegravir, and lamivudine Triumeq	To treat HIV infection	600 mg abacavir, 50 mg dolutegravir, and 300 mg lamivudine (1 tablet) P.O. once daily
abacavir sulfate and lamivudine Epzicom	To treat HIV-1 infection	600 mg abacavir and 300 mg lamivudine (1 tablet) P.O. daily
abacavir sulfate, lamivudine, and zidovudine Trizivir	To treat HIV infection	300 mg abacavir, 150 mg lamivudine, and 300 mg zidovudine (1 tablet) P.O. twice daily
atazanavir sulfate Reyataz	To treat HIV infection in patients not previously treated	400 mg P.O. daily
	To treat HIV infection in patients previously treated	300 mg P.O. daily with ritonavir 100 mg P.O. daily
cobicistat Tybost	As adjunct to treat HIV infection with atazanavir, darunavir, and other antiretroviral agents	150 mg P.O. once daily with atazanavir 300 mg P.O. once daily or darunavir 800 mg P.O. once daily
darunavir Prezista	To treat HIV-1 infection along with ritonavir in patients not previously treated	800 mg P.O. twice daily
	To treat HIV-1 infection along with ritonavir in patients previously treated	600 mg P.O. twice daily

(continued)

Selected Antivirals *(continued)*

GENERIC AND TRADE NAMES	INDICATIONS	USUAL ADULT DOSAGES
Antivirals used for HIV infection *(continued)*		
delavirdine Rescriptor	To treat HIV infection	400 mg P.O. three times a day
dolutegravir Tivicay	To treat HIV infection in treastment naïve or treat-ment-experienced integrase strand transfer inhibitor (INST)-naive	50 mg once daily
	To treat HIV infection along with other antivirals or with suspected INSTI resistance	50 mg twice daily
efavirenz Sustiva	To treat HIV infection	600 mg P.O. daily
elvitegravir Vitekta	As adjunct with an HIV prote-ase inhibitor co-administered with ritonavir and with other antiretroviral drug(s) to treat HIV infection	85 mg P.O. once daily with 100 mg ritonavir P.O. once daily and 300 mg atazanavir P.O. once daily, or with 100 mg ritonavir P.O. twice daily and 400 mg lopinavir P.O. twice daily, or with 100 mg ritonavir P.O. twice daily and 600 mg darunavir P.O. twice daily. Alternatively, 150 mg P.O. once daily with 100 mg ritonavir P.O. twice daily and 700 mg fosamprenavir P.O. twice daily or 200 mg ritonavir P.O. twice daily and 500 mg tipranavir P.O. twice daily.
elvitegravir, cobicistat, emtricitabine, tenofovir Stribild	To treat HIV infection	1 tablet (containing 150 mg elvitegravir, 150 mg cobici-stat, 200 mg emtricitabine, 300 mg tenofovir) P.O. once daily with food
emtricitabine Emtriva	To treat HIV infection	200 mg P.O. daily (capsules) or 240 mg P.O. daily (oral solution)
emtricitabine, rilpivirine, tenofovir Complera	To treat HIV-1 infection	1 tablet (containing 200 mg emtricitabine, 25 mg rilpiv-irine, 300 mg tenofovir) P.O. daily with meal
enfuvirtide Fuzeon	To treat HIV infection	90 mg twice daily SubQ

Selected Antivirals *(continued)*

Antivirals used for HIV infection *(continued)*

GENERIC AND TRADE NAMES	INDICATIONS	USUAL ADULT DOSAGES
etravirine Intelence	To treat HIV-1 infection	200 mg P.O. twice daily
fosamprenavir calcium Lexiva	To treat HIV infection in patients who don't take ritonavir	1,400 mg P.O. twice daily
	To treat HIV infection in patients who take ritonavir but don't take a protease inhibitor	1,400 mg P.O. once daily or 700 mg P.O. twice daily
	To treat HIV infection in patients who take ritonavir and a protease inhibitor	700 mg P.O. twice daily
indinavir Crixivan	To treat HIV infection	800 mg P.O. every 8 hr
lamivudine (3TC, lamivudine triphosphate) Epivir	To treat HIV infection in patients who weigh 50 kg (110 lb) or more	150 mg P.O. twice daily or 300 mg P.O. once daily
	To treat HIV infection in patients who weigh less than 50 kg	2 mg/kg P.O. twice daily
lamivudine and zidovudine (3TC/AZT, 3TC/ZDV) Combivir	To treat HIV infection in patients who weigh 50 kg or more	150 mg of lamivudine and 300 mg of zidovudine P.O. twice daily
lopinavir and ritonavir Kaletra	As adjunct to treat HIV infection in combination with other antiretroviral agents	400 mg lopinavir and 100 mg ritonavir P.O. twice daily
	As adjunct to treat HIV infection in patients who take amprenavir, efavirenz, nelfinavir, or nevirapine	500 mg lopinavir and 125 mg ritonavir P.O. (tablet form) twice daily or 533 mg lopinavir and 133 mg ritonavir P.O. (oral solution) twice daily
	As adjunct to treat HIV infection in patients with fewer than 3 lopinavir resistance associated substitutions and who do not take amprenavir, efavirenz, nelfinavir, or nevirapine	800 mg lopinavir and 200 mg ritonavir P.O. daily
maraviroc Selzentry	To treat HIV infection	150 mg P.O. twice daily with CYP3A inhibitor; 600 mg P.O. twice daily with CYP3A inducers; 300 mg P.O. twice daily with all other drugs

(continued)

Selected Antivirals *(continued)*

GENERIC AND TRADE NAMES	INDICATIONS	USUAL ADULT DOSAGES
Antivirals used for HIV infection *(continued)*		
nelfinavir Viracept	To treat HIV infection	750 mg P.O. three times a day
nelfinavir mesylate Viracept	To treat HIV infection	1,250 mg P.O. twice daily or 750 mg P.O. three times a day
nevirapine Viramune Viramune XR	To treat HIV infection	200 mg P.O. (Viramune) daily. Alternatively, 200 mg P.O. (Viramune) daily for 14 days, followed by 400 mg P.O. (Viramune XR) daily
raltegravir Isentress	To treat HIV-1 infection	400 mg P.O. twice daily or 800 mg P.O. twice daily if given concurrently with rifampin
rilpivirine Edurant	To treat HIV-1 infection	25 mg P.O. daily with meal or 50 mg P.O. once daily if given concurrently with rifabutin
ritonavir Norvir	To treat HIV infection	600 mg P.O. twice daily
saquinavir Fortovase, Invirase	To treat HIV infection	1,200 mg P.O. three times a day (Fortovase) or 1,000 mg (Invirase or Fortovase) and 100 mg ritonavir P.O. twice daily
stavudine Zerit, Zerit XR	To treat HIV infection in patients who weigh 60 kg or more	40 mg P.O. every 12 hr (Zerit) or 100 mg P.O. daily (Zerit XR)
	To treat HIV infection in patients who weigh less than 60 kg	30 mg P.O. every 12 hr (Zerit) or 75 mg P.O. daily (Zerit XR)
tenofovir Viread	To treat HIV infection	300 mg P.O. daily
tenofovir, emtricitabine Truvada	To treat HIV-1 infection Pre-exposure prophylaxis to HIV	300 mg tenofovir and 200 mg emtricitabine (1 tablet) P.O. daily
tipranavir Aptivus	To treat HIV infection	500 mg tipranavir and 200 mg ritonavir P.O. twice daily

Selected Antivirals *(continued)*

GENERIC AND TRADE NAMES	INDICATIONS	USUAL ADULT DOSAGES
Antivirals used for herpes virus infection *(continued)*		
zidovudine (AZT, ZDV) Apo-Zidovudine (CAN), Novo-AZT (CAN), Retrovir	To treat HIV infection	100 mg P.O. every 4 hr while awake, up to 600 mg/day; or 1 to 2 mg/kg I.V. over 1 hr every 4 hr, up to 6 times/day or 6 mg/kg/day.
	To prevent maternal-fetal HIV transmission	100 mg P.O. 5 times daily after 14 wk of pregnancy and continued until labor. During labor and delivery, 2 mg/kg I.V. over 1 hr followed by continuous infusion of 1 mg/kg/hr until umbilical cord clamped. Starting within 12 hr after birth, neonate given 2 mg/kg P.O. every 6 hr for 6 wk.
Antivirals used for CCR5-tropic HIV-1 infection		
maraviroc Selzentry	To treat CCR5-tropic HIV-1 infection	300 mg P.O. twice daily
	To treat CCR5-tropic HIV-1 infection concurrently with potent CYP3A inhibitors (except tipranavir/ritonavir)	150 mg P.O. twice daily
	To treat CCR5-tropic HIV-1 infection concurrently with potent CYP3A inducers	600 mg P.O. twice daily
Antivirals used for herpes virus infection		
acyclovir Zovirax	To treat HSV encephalitis	10 mg/kg I.V. over 1 hr every 8 hr for 21 days.
	To treat HSV genitalis	200 mg P.O. every 4 hr while awake, up to 5 times/day, for 10 days.
	To treat herpes zoster infection	800 mg P.O. every 4 hr while awake, up to 5 times/day, for 7 to 10 days; or 10 mg/kg I.V. over 1 hr every 8 hr for 7 days.
acyclovir Sitavig	To treat recurrent herpes labialis	50 mg applied to upper gum region within 1 hr of symptoms and before appearance of lesions.

(continued)

Selected Antivirals *(continued)*

GENERIC AND TRADE NAMES	INDICATIONS	USUAL ADULT DOSAGES
Antivirals used for herpes virus infection *(continued)*		
famciclovir Famvir	To treat HSV genitalis To treat herpes zoster infection	125 mg P.O. twice daily for 5 days. 500 mg P.O. every 8 hr for 7 days.
foscarnet Foscavir	To treat acyclovir-resistant HSV I and II infections	40 mg/kg I.V. every hr every 8 to 12 hr for 2 to 3 wk or until healed.
idoxuridine Herplex Liquifilm, Stoxil	To treat HSV keratitis	1 cm applied to conjunctiva every 4 hr while awake, up to 5 times/day; or 1 gtt of 0.1% solution every hr during daytime and every 2 hr during nighttime for 7 to 10 days.
penciclovir Denavir	To treat HSV labialis	1% cream applied to lips every 2 hr while awake for 4 days.
valacyclovir Valtrex	To treat HSV genitalis	1 g P.O. twice daily for 10 days for initial episode; 500 mg P.O. twice daily for 3 days for recurrent episodes.
	To suppress recurrent HSV genitalis	1 g P.O. daily; or, 500 mg P.O. daily for patients with a history of nine or fewer recurrences/year or who have HIV.
	To reduce transmission of genital herpes	500 mg P.O. daily for source partner with a history of nine or fewer recurrences/year.
	To treat herpes zoster infection	1 g P.O. three times a day for 7 days.
	To treat herpes labialis (cold sores)	2 g P.O. twice daily for 1 day taken 12 hr apart.
vidarabine Vira-A	To treat acute viral conjunctivitis and recurrent epithelial keratitis caused by HSV infection	1.25 cm applied to conjunctiva every 3 hr until re-epithelialized; then 1.25 cm twice daily for 7 days.

Selected Antivirals *(continued)*

GENERIC AND TRADE NAMES	INDICATIONS	USUAL ADULT DOSAGES
Antivirals used for CMV infection		
cidofovir Vistide	To treat CMV retinitis	5 mg/kg I.V. over 1 hr every wk for 2 wk
foscarnet Foscavir	To treat CMV infection	*Induction:* 90 mg/kg I.V. over 1.5 to 2 hr every 12 hr; or, 60 mg/kg I.V. over 1 hr every 8 hr for 2 to 3 wk *Maintenance:* 90 to 120 mg/kg I.V. over 2 hr every 24 hr
ganciclovir Cytovene	To treat CMV infection	5 mg/kg I.V. over 1 hr every 12 hr for 14 to 21 days *Maintenance:* 1,000 mg P.O. three times a day
valganciclovir hydrochloride Valcyte	To treat CMV retinitis	900 mg P.O. twice daily for 21 days. Then 900 mg P.O. daily
	To prevent CMV infection in high-risk kidney, heart, and kidney-pancreas transplant patients	900 mg P.O. daily, starting within 10 days of transplantation and continuing until 100 days after transplantation
Antivirals used for influenza infection		
oseltamivir phosphate Tamiflu	To treat uncomplicated, acute infections caused by influenza virus A or B in adults who have had symptoms for no more than 2 days	75 mg P.O. twice daily for 5 days, starting within 2 days after symptoms begin *Maximum:* 75 mg twice daily for 5 days
	To prevent influenza following close contact with an infected person	75 mg P.O. daily for 7 days; start within 2 days of exposure
	To prevent influenza during a community outbreak	75 mg P.O. daily during period of potential exposure
peramivir Rapivab	To treat uncomplicated, acute influenza in adults who have had symptoms for no more than 2 days	600 mg I.V. infused over 15 to 30 minutes as a one-time dose
zanamivir Relenza	To treat infections caused by influenza virus A or B	2 inhalations (10 mg) every 12 hr for 5 days

(continued)

Selected Antivirals *(continued)*

GENERIC AND TRADE NAMES	INDICATIONS	USUAL ADULT DOSAGES
Antivirals used for hepatitis B infection		
adefovir dipivoxil Hepsera	To treat chronic hepatitis B	10 mg P.O. daily
		For patients with creatinine clearance of 20 to 49 ml/min/1.73 m^2, dosage interval changed to every 48 hr
		For creatinine clearance of 10 to 19 ml/min/1.73 m^2, dosage interval changed to every 72 hr
		For patients receiving hemodialysis, drug given every 7 days following dialysis
entecavir Baraclude	To treat chronic hepatitis B in patients with compensated liver disease	0.5 mg P.O. once daily
	To treat chronic hepatitis B in patients with decompensated liver disease	1 mg P.O. once daily
lamivudine Epivir HBV	To treat chronic hepatitis B	100 mg P.O. daily
telbivudine Tyzeka	To treat chronic hepatitis B	600 mg P.O. daily
tenofovir Viread	To treat chronic hepatitis B	300 mg P.O. daily
Antivirals used for hepatitis C infection		
boceprevir Victrelisx	To treat chronic hepatitis C in combination with peginterferon alfa and ribavirin in patients with compensated liver disease	800 mg P.O. three times a day with food
ledipasvir and sofosbuvir Harvoni	To treat chronic hepatitis C	90 mg ledipasvir and 400 mg sofosbuvir (1 tablet) P.O. once daily
ombitasvir, paritaprevir, and ritonavir Viekira Pak	To treat chronic hepatitis C in combination with dasabuvir	25 mg ombitasiv, 150 mg paritaprevir, and 100 mg ritonavir (2 tablets) P.O. once daily in morning and 250 mg dasabuvir (1 tablet) P.O. twice daily

Selected Antivirals (continued)

GENERIC AND TRADE NAMES	INDICATIONS	USUAL ADULT DOSAGES
Antivirals used for hepatitis C infection (continued)		
ribavirin Copegus, Rebetol, Ribasphere	To treat chronic hepatitis C in combination with interferon alfa-2b in patients who weigh more than 75 kg (165 lb)	400 mg in the morning and 600 mg P.O. in the evening daily
	To treat chronic hepatitis C in combination with interferon alfa-2b in patients who weigh 75 kg (165 lb) or less	600 mg P.O. twice daily
	To treat chronic hepatitis C in combination with peginterferon alfa-2b	400 mg P.O. twice daily
	To treat chronic hepatitis C in combination with interferon alfa-2a in patients with compensated liver disease who have never received interferon alfa	400 to 600 P.O. mg twice daily
simeprevir Olysio	To treat chronic hepatitis C in combination with peginterferon alfa and ribavirin	150 mg P.O. once daily for 12 weeks
	To treat chronic hepatitis C in combination with sofosbuvir	150 mg P.O. once daily for 12 weeks for patients without cirrhosis and 24 weeks for patients with cirrhosis
sofosbuvir Solvaldi	To treat chronic hepatitis C with ribavirin with or without peginterferon	400 mg P.O. once daily for 12 weeks for patients with genotype 1, 2, or 4; 24 weeks for patients with genotype 3 or for patients with genotype 1 who are ineligible to receive an interferon-based regimen
telaprevir Incivek	To treat chronic hepatitis C in combination with peginterferon alfa and ribavirin in patients with compensated liver disease	1125 mg P.O. twice daily with food (not low-fat)

(continued)

Selected Antineoplastic Drugs

Antineoplastic drugs are the standard of treatment for most types of cancer today. Most of these drugs work by inhibiting cell proliferation, which leads to cell death. They're most effective at killing actively dividing cells.

Cell-specific antineoplastics exert their actions during one or more phases of the cell cycle. S-phase antineoplastics interfere with deoxyribonucleic acid (DNA) synthesis; M-phase drugs interfere with the formation of microtubules and disrupt mitosis.

Most antineoplastics impair DNA in one of the following four ways:
- preventing separation of DNA strands
- inhibiting DNA repair
- mimicking DNA bases
- disrupting the triplicate codons or producing oxygen-free radicals that damage the DNA.

Antineoplastic drugs are cytotoxic, which means that they affect both neoplastic cells and normal cells. As a result, they may cause serious and sometimes life-threatening adverse reactions.

Antineoplastics are most harmful to normal cells that exhibit rapid activity and growth, such as bone marrow tissue, the epithelium of the GI mucosa, and hair follicles. When these drugs suppress bone marrow activity, the patient may develop leukopenia, thrombocytopenia, or anemia. When they affect the GI mucosa, the patient may experience nausea, vomiting, anorexia, bowel dysfunction, and mucosal ulcerations. When antineoplastic drugs affect the hair follicles, the result is hair loss (alopecia), one of the most common adverse reactions. Although not life-threatening, hair loss can be emotionally traumatic for patients, especially women.

Antineoplastic Classification

Antineoplastic drugs are classified according to their mechanism of action.

ALKYLATING DRUGS

The first drugs developed to fight cancer, alkylating drugs are most effective against slow-growing tumors. These agents can damage tissue at the injection site and produce systemic toxicity. They can damage cells during all stages of growth, causing mitotic arrest. Because their actions are not limited to neoplastic cells, they also cause myelosuppression, a predictable adverse reaction. They can also result in secondary tumor development, even years after the initial therapy.

ANTIBIOTICS

Antibiotic antineoplastics originated from a genus of fungus-like bacteria called *Streptomyces*. Their classification is based on their origin, not on mechanism of action, toxicity, pharmacokinetics, or varying clinical indications. Many of these drugs bind to specific bases and block DNA synthesis to interfere with cell replication.

ANTIMETABOLITES

These are cell-cycle-specific drugs that act by preventing synthesis of nucleotides or inhibiting enzymes by mimicking nucleotides. These drugs are often more effective when used in combination.

ANTIMITOTICS

Antimitotic antineoplastics disrupt the formation of microtubule structures in the cell during mitosis. This breakdown of microtubule production stops the formation of the mitotic spindle, inhibiting cellular reproduction.

BIOLOGICAL RESPONSE MODIFIERS

These drugs alter tumor-host metabolic and immunologic relationships.

ANTINEOPLASTIC ENZYMES

Antineoplastic enzymes interfere with the breakdown of extracellular asparagine, an endogenous enzyme that leukemic cells depend on for their survival. The rapid depletion of asparagine eventually kills leukemic cells by fragmenting them into membrane-bound particles that are eliminated by phagocytosis.

HORMONAL DRUGS

These drugs act as agonists to inhibit tumor cell growth or as antagonists to compete with endogenous growth-promoting hormones. Steroid hormones form specific receptor complexes that bind to certain nuclear proteins necessary for DNA transcription.

MISCELLANEOUS ANTINEOPLASTICS

These drugs act in a variety of ways, such as by destroying microtubules that are essential for tumor cell structure before mitosis and by inhibiting topoisomerase, the enzyme that affects the degree of supercoiling in DNA by cutting one or both strands. This inhibition causes DNA strands to break and synthesizes toxic compounds that inhibit DNA strand repair.

The following chart lists the generic and common trade names of common antineoplastic drugs, which are grouped according to mechanism of action. It also includes FDA-approved indications and the usual adult dosage for each drug.

Selected Antineoplastic Drugs *(continued)*

GENERIC AND TRADE NAMES	INDICATIONS	USUAL ADULT DOSAGES
Alkylating drugs		
busulfan Busulfex, Myleran	To provide palliative treatment of chronic myelocytic leukemia (CML)	*Initial:* 0.06 mg/kg P.O. daily until WBC count is below 15,000/mm^3. *Usual:* 4 to 8 mg P.O. daily (but may range from 1 to 12 mg P.O. daily). *Maintenance:* 1 to 3 mg daily. During remission, treatment resumed when WBC count reaches 50,000/mm^3.
	To prepare for hematopoietic progenitor cell transplantation for CML	0.8 mg/kg I.V. over 2 hr every 6 hr for 4 days for a total of 16 doses as an adjunct with cyclophosphamide.
carmustine (BCNU) BiCNU, Gliadel Wafer	To treat primary brain tumors and glioblastoma multiforme	Up to 8 implants per surgical procedure.
	To treat primary brain tumors, Hodgkin's disease, non-Hodgkin's lymphoma, and multiple myeloma	150 to 200 mg/m^2 by slow I.V. infusion as a single dose every 6 to 8 wk; or 75 to 100 mg/m^2 by slow I.V. infusion daily for 2 days every 6 wk.
chlorambucil Leukeran	To provide palliative treatment of chronic lymphocytic leukemia, Hodgkin's disease, malignant lymphomas (including lymphosarcoma and giant follicular lymphoma), and non-Hodgkin's lymphoma	0.1 to 0.2 mg/kg/day as a single dose or in divided doses for 3 to 6 wk. *Usual:* 4 to 10 mg/day as a single dose or in divided doses for 3 to 6 wk.
cyclophosphamide Cytoxan, Neosar, Procytox (CAN)	To treat acute lymphocytic leukemia, acute nonlymphocytic leukemia, chronic lymphocytic leukemia, chronic myelocytic leukemia, breast cancer, epithelial ovarian cancer, Hodgkin's disease, multiple myeloma, neuroblastoma, non-Hodgkin's lymphoma, and retinoblastoma	1 to 5 mg/kg P.O. daily; or 40 to 50 mg/kg I.V. in divided doses over 2 to 5 days; or 10 to 15 mg/kg I.V. every 7 to 10 days; or 3 to 5 mg/kg I.V. 2 times/wk; or 1.5 to 3 mg/kg I.V. daily.
lomustine (CCNU) CeeNU	To treat primary brain tumors and Hodgkin's disease	100 to 130 mg/m^2 P.O. as a single dose every 6 wk.
mechlorethamine hydrochloride (nitrogen mustard) Mustargen	To treat bronchiogenic carcinoma, CML, Hodgkin's disease, lymphosarcoma, and mycosis fungoides	0.4 mg/kg I.V. as a single dose or in divided doses over 2 to 4 days.
	To treat malignant pericardial, peritoneal, or pleural effusions	0.4 mg/kg (peritoneal or pleural effusion); 0.2 mg/kg into affected cavity (pericardial effusion).

(continued)

Selected Antineoplastic Drugs *(continued)*

GENERIC AND TRADE NAMES	INDICATIONS	USUAL ADULT DOSAGES
Alkylating drugs *(continued)*		
melphalan (L-phenylalanine mustard) Alkeran	To treat multiple myeloma	0.15 mg/kg P.O. daily for 7 days; then 0.05 mg/kg daily after 3 wk of no drug. Or, 0.1 to 0.15 mg/kg daily for 2 to 3 wk or 0.25 mg/kg for 4 days; then 2 to 4 mg daily after 2 to 4 wk of no drug.
melphalan hydrochloride Alkeran	To treat epithelial ovarian cancer	16 mg/m^2 I.V. over 15 min every 2 wk for 4 doses, then at 4 wk. 0.2 mg/kg P.O. daily for 5 days, repeated every 4 to 5 wk.
oxaliplatin Eloxatin	To provide adjuvant treatment of stage III colon cancer	85 mg/m^2 I.V. over 2 hr every 2 wk for 12 cycles with 5-fluorouracil.
	To treat advanced colorectal cancer	85 mg/m^2 I.V. over 2 hr every 2 wk with fluorouracil until disease progression or unacceptable toxicity.
streptozocin Zanosar	To treat islet cell or pancreatic carcinoma	500 mg/m^2 I.V. for 5 days every 6 wk, or 1,000 mg/m^2 I.V. every wk for 2 wk.
temozolomide Temodar	To treat astrocytoma	150 mg/m^2 P.O. daily for first 5 days of 28-day cycle, followed by 200 mg/m^2 P.O. daily, if tolerated, for first 5 days of subsequent 28-day cycles.
	To treat glioblastoma multiforme	75 mg/m^2 P.O. or I.V. over 90 min for 42 consecutive days, followed by maintenance dose of 150 mg/m^2 P.O. or I.V. over 90 min daily for first 5 days of every 28 days for 6 cycles as adjunct to radiotherapy.
	To treat refractory anaplastic astrocytoma	150 mg/m^2 P.O. or I.V. over 90 min daily for first 5 days of every 28 days.
thiotepa (TESPA, triethylenethiophosphoramide, TSPA) Thioplex	To treat malignant pericardial or pleural effusions	0.6 to 0.8 mg/kg into affected cavity.
	To treat breast cancer, epithelial ovarian cancer, and Hodgkin's disease	0.3 to 0.4 mg/kg I.V. every 1 to 4 wk, or 0.2 mg/kg for 4 to 5 days every 2 to 3 wk.
	To treat bladder tumors	30 to 60 mg mixed in 30 to 60 ml of normal saline, instilled into bladder every wk for 4 wk.

Selected Antineoplastic Drugs *(continued)*

GENERIC AND TRADE NAMES	INDICATIONS	USUAL ADULT DOSAGES
Antibiotic antineoplastics		
bleomycin sulfate Blenoxane	To treat non-Hodgkin's lymphoma, squamous cell carcinoma, and testicular cancer	0.25 to 0.5 unit/kg or 10 to 20 units/m^2 1 to 2 times/wk I.V., I.M., or SubQ; or 0.25 unit/kg or 15 units/m^2 daily by I.V. infusion over 24 hr
	To treat Hodgkin's disease	0.25 to 0.5 unit/kg I.V., I.M., or SubQ, or 10 to 20 units/m^2 1 to 2 times/wk
	To treat malignant pleural effusions	60 units intrapleural single bolus dissolved in 50–100 ml of normal saline solution
	To treat squamous cell carcinoma of the cervix, head and neck, penis, or vulva	30 to 60 units by arterial infusion over 1 to 24 hr
cisplatin Platinol, Platinol-AQ	To treat bladder cancer	50 to 70 mg/m^2 by I.V. infusion as a single dose every 3 to 4 wk with other agents
	To treat advanced ovarian cancer	75 to 100 mg/m^2 by I.V. infusion as a single dose every 21 days with paclitaxel
	To treat testicular cancer	20 mg/m^2 by I.V. infusion daily for 5 days with bleomycin and etoposide; repeated every 3 wk for two or more cycles
dactinomycin (actinomycin-D) Cosmegen	To treat Ewing's sarcoma, gestational trophoblastic or Wilms' tumors, rhabdomyosarcoma, sarcoma botryoides, and testicular cancer or tumors	0.15 to 500 mcg/kg/day I.V. daily for 5 days; may repeat after 3 wk
	To treat Ewing's sarcoma and sarcoma botryoides	0.05 mg/kg for lower extremity or pelvis; 0.035 mg/kg for upper extremity as an isolation-perfusion
daunorubicin hydrochloride Cerubidine	To treat acute lymphocytic leukemia	45 mg/m^2 daily for first 3 days of a 32-day course of vincristine, prednisone, and asparaginase combination therapy
	To treat acute nonlymphocytic leukemia	45 mg/m^2 daily for first 3 days of first course of cytarabine combination therapy and first 2 days of second course of cytarabine combination therapy

(continued)

Selected Antineoplastic Drugs *(continued)*

GENERIC AND TRADE NAMES	INDICATIONS	USUAL ADULT DOSAGES
Antibiotic antineoplastics *(continued)*		
daunorubicin, liposomal DaunoXome	To treat AIDS-related Kaposi's sarcoma	40 mg/m^2 I.V. over 60 min every 2 wk
doxorubicin hydrochloride Adriamycin PFS, Adriamycin RDF, Rubex	To treat acute lymphocytic leukemia, acute nonlymphocytic leukemia; bladder, breast, gastric, epithelial ovarian, or thyroid cancer; Hodgkin's disease; neuroblastoma or Wilms' tumor; non-Hodgkin's lymphoma; small-cell lung carcinoma; and soft-tissue sarcoma or osteosarcoma	60 to 75 mg/m^2 I.V. as single dose every 21 days; or 25 to 30 mg/m^2 I.V. daily for 2 to 3 days every 3 to 4 wk; or 20 mg/m^2 every wk; or 40 to 60 mg/m^2 every 21 to 28 days in combination with other chemotherapeutic drugs
doxorubicin, liposomal Caelyx (CAN), Doxil	To treat AIDS-related Kaposi's sarcoma	20 mg/m^2 I.V. over 30 min every 3 wk as tolerated
epirubicin hydrochloride Ellence	To treat breast cancer	100 to 120 mg/m^2 by I.V. infusion over 3 to 5 min via a free-flowing I.V. solution as a single dose on day 1 or in divided doses on days 1 and 8, repeated every 3 to 4 wk for 6 cycles in combination with other chemotherapy agents
everolimus Afinitor	To treat advanced hormone receptor-positive, HER2-negative breast cancer, advanced neuroendocrine tumors of pancreatic origin, advanced renal cell carcinoma, and renal angiomyolopoma with tuberous sclerosis complex	10 mg P.O. daily
	To treat subependymal giant cell astrocytomas associated with tuberous sclerosis complex in patients who are not candidates for curative surgical resection	4.5 mg/m^2 as starting dose P.O. once daily, followed by dosage adjustment every 2 wk, as needed
idarubicin hydrochloride Idamycin	To treat acute nonlymphocytic leukemia	12 mg/m^2/day I.V. over 10 to 15 min for 3 days in combination with cytarabine therapy
mitomycin (mitomycin-C) Mutamycin	To treat gastric or pancreatic cancer	20 mg/m^2 as a single dose every 6 to 8 wk

Selected Antineoplastic Drugs *(continued)*

GENERIC AND TRADE NAMES	INDICATIONS	USUAL ADULT DOSAGES
Antibiotic antineoplastics *(continued)*		
plicamycin (mithramycin) Mithracin	To treat testicular cancer	0.025 to 0.03 mg/kg I.V. daily over 4 to 6 hr for 8 to 10 days
	To treat hypercalcemia and hypercalciuria	0.015 to 0.025 mg/kg I.V. daily over 4 to 6 hr for 3 to 4 days; may repeat dose every wk as needed
romidepsin Istodax	To treat cutaneous T-cell lymphoma in patients who have received one previous systemic therapy; to treat peripheral T-cell lymphoma in patients who have received one previous systemic therapy	14 mg/m^2 I.V. over 4 hr on days 1, 8, and 15 of a 28-day cycle, repeated every 28 days
Antimetabolites		
capecitabine Xeloda	To treat locally advanced or metastatic breast cancer or metastatic colorectal cancer	1,250 mg/m^2 P.O. after a meal b.i.d. (morning and evening) for 2 wk, followed by 1-wk rest period; dose repeated in 3-wk cycles
cytarabine (ARA-C, cytosine arabinoside) Cytosar, Cytosar-U	To treat acute nonlymphocytic leukemia	Initially, 100 mg/m^2/day by continuous I.V. infusion for 7 days, alone or with other agents; or 100 mg/m^2 I.V. every 12 hr on days 1 to 7, then consult manufacturer's literature for specific dosing; or high-dose therapy of 2 to 3 g/m^2 I.V. over 1 to 3 hr for 2 to 6 days, then consult manufacturer's literature for specific dosing
	To treat meningeal leukemia	30 mg/m^2 intrathecally as a single dose every 4 days
	To prevent or treat acute lymphocytic leukemia and chronic myelocytic leukemia	Consult manufacturer's literature for specific dosage
floxuridine (fluorodeoxyuridine) FUDR	To treat colorectal or hepatic cancer	0.1 to 0.6 mg/kg/day by continuous intra-arterial infusion for 14 to 21 days, followed by 2 wk of no drug; dose repeated in 5-wk cycles

(continued)

Selected Antineoplastic Drugs *(continued)*

Antimetabolites *(continued)*

GENERIC AND TRADE NAMES	INDICATIONS	USUAL ADULT DOSAGES
fluorouracil **(5-fluorouracil, 5-FU)** Adrucil, Carac, Efudex, Fluoroplex	To treat colorectal, breast, gastric, or pancreatic cancer	7 to 12 mg/kg/day I.V. for 4 days, followed by no drug for 3 days, then 7 to 10 mg/kg every 3 to 4 days for total of 2 wk; or 12 mg/kg/day for 4 days, followed by 1 day of no drug, then 6 mg/kg every other day for 4 or 5 days, for total of 12 days; thereafter, 7 to 12 mg/kg/day I.V. every 7 to 10 days
	To treat multiple actinic (solar) keratoses	0.5% cream (face, anterior scalp), 1% cream (head, neck, chest), or 2% to 5% cream (hands) applied to skin once or twice daily to cover lesions
	To treat superficial basal cell carcinoma	5% cream applied to skin twice daily for up to 12 wk to cover lesions
hydroxyurea Droxia, Hydrea	To treat epithelial ovarian cancer	60 to 80 mg/kg P.O. as a single dose every 3 days alone or with radiation therapy; or 20 to 30 mg/kg P.O. daily
	To treat resistant chronic myelocytic leukemia	20 to 30 mg/kg P.O. once daily or in divided doses twice daily
mercaptopurine **(6-mercaptopurine, 6-MP)** Purinethol, Purixan	For maintenance therapy for acute lymphocytic leukemia	1.5 mg/kg/day to 2.5 mg/kg/day P.O. daily
methotrexate **(amethopterin)** **methotrexate sodium**	To treat chorioadenoma destruens, choriocarcinoma, or hydatidiform mole	15 to 30 mg/day P.O. or I.M. for 5 days; repeat three to five times with 2 to 3 wk between courses

Selected Antineoplastic Drugs *(continued)*

GENERIC AND TRADE NAMES	INDICATIONS	USUAL ADULT DOSAGES
Antimetabolites *(continued)*		
	To treat acute lymphocytic leukemia or meningeal leukemia	Initially, 3.3 mg/m^2/day P.O., I.M., or I.V. in combination with prednisone or other drug; as maintenance dose, 30 mg/m^2/wk P.O. or I.M. in two divided doses or 2.5 mg/kg I.V. every 14 days
	To treat Burkitt's lymphoma (stage I or II)	10 to 25 mg/day P.O. for 4 to 8 days, followed by no drug for 7 to 10 days; course repeated as needed
	To treat Burkitt's lymphoma (stage III)	Same as for stage I or II in combination with other drug
	To treat lymphosarcoma (stage III)	0.625 to 2.5 mg/kg/day P.O.
	To treat mycosis fungoides	2.5 to 10 mg/day P.O. for weeks or months; or 50 mg I.M. every wk or 25 mg I.M. 2 times/wk
	To treat osteosarcoma	12 g/m^2 by I.V. infusion over 12 hr, followed by leucovorin rescue on weeks 4, 5, 6, 7, 11, 12, 15, 16, 29, 30, 44, and 45 after surgery in combination with bleomycin, cisplatin, cyclophosphamide, dactinomycin, and doxorubicin
	To treat breast or head and neck cancer and non–small-cell or small-cell lung carcinoma	Consult manufacturer's literature for specific dosing
pemetrexed disodium Alimta	To treat nonsquamous non–small-cell lung cancer or malignant pleural mesothelioma	500 mg/m^2 I.V. over 10 min on day 1 of each 21-day cycle as adjunct to cisplatin
	To treat nonsquamous non–small-cell lung cancer	500 mg/m^2 I.V. over 10 min on day 1 of each 21-day cycle
thioguanine (6-TG, 6-thioguanine) Lanvis (CAN), Tabloid	To treat acute nonlymphocytic leukemia	2 mg/kg/day P.O. as a single dose; if no improvement after 4 wk, increase to 3 mg/kg/day

Selected Antineoplastic Drugs *(continued)*

GENERIC AND TRADE NAMES	INDICATIONS	USUAL ADULT DOSAGES
Antibiotic antineoplastics		
cabazitaxel Jevtana	To treat hormone-refractory metastatic prostate cancer previously treated with a docetaxel-containing treatment regimen	25 mg/m² I.V. given over 60 min every 3 wk in combination with oral prednisone 10 mg P.O. daily
docetaxel Taxotere	To treat breast cancer	60 to 100 mg/m² by I.V. infusion over 1 hr every 3 wk
	To treat non–small-cell lung carcinoma	75 mg/m² by I.V. infusion over 1 hr every 3 wk
ixabepilone Ixempra	To treat advanced breast cancer	40 mg/m² I.V. over 3 hr every 3 wk, as adjunct to capecitabine, as needed
paclitaxel Taxol Abraxane	To treat ovarian cancer	135 or 175 mg/m² by I.V. infusion over 3 or 24 hr every 21 days
	To treat breast cancer	175 mg/m² by I.V. infusion over 3 or 24 hr every 21 days
	To treat AIDS-related Kaposi's sarcoma	135 mg/m² by I.V. infusion over 3 or 24 hr every 21 days; or 100 mg/m² by I.V. infusion over 3 or 24 hr every 14 days
	To treat non–small-cell lung carcinoma	135 mg/m² by I.V. infusion over 3 or 24 hr, followed by cisplatin 75 mg/m² I.V. every 21 days (Taxol) or 100 mg/m2 I.V. over 30 min on days 1,8, and 15 of each 21 day cycle followed by carboplatin on day 1 of each 21 day cycle immediately after paclitaxel (Abraxane).
	To treat metastatic breast cancer	260 mg/m² I.V. over 30 min. every 3 wks
	To treat non–small-cell lung cancer	100 mg/m² I.V. over 30 min every 3 wks on days 1, 8, and 15 of each 21-day cycle followed immediately by carboplatin 6 mg/min/ml on day 1 of each 21-day cycle
	To treat metastatic adenocarcinoma of the pancreas	125 mg/m² I.V. given over 30 to 40 min on days 1, 8, and 15 of each 28-day cycle, followed immediately by gemcitabine administration

Selected Antineoplastic Drugs *(continued)*

GENERIC AND TRADE NAMES	INDICATIONS	USUAL ADULT DOSAGES
Antibiotic antineoplastics *(continued)*		
vinblastine sulfate (VLB) Velban, Velbe (CAN)	To treat breast cancer, Hodgkin's disease, lymphomas, Kaposi's sarcoma, Letterer-Siwe disease, mycosis fungoides, non-Hodgkin's lymphoma, testicular cancer, and trophoblastic gestational tumors	0.15 to 0.2 mg/kg I.V. every wk
vincristine sulfate (VCR) Oncovin, Vincasar PFS	To treat acute lymphocytic leukemia, Hodgkin's disease, lymphomas, non-Hodgkin's lymphoma, rhabdomyosarcoma, and Wilms' tumor	0.01 to 0.03 mg/kg I.V.; or 0.4 to 1.4 mg/m^2 I.V. every wk as a single dose (maximum of 2 mg)
vinorelbine tartrate Navelbine	To treat non–small-cell lung carcinoma	30 mg/m^2 I.V. over 6 to 10 min every wk alone, or 25 mg/m^2 I.V. over 6 to 10 min every wk with cisplatin 100 mg/m^2 every 4 wk
Antineoplastic enzymes		
asparaginase Elspar, Kidrolase (CAN)	To treat acute lymphoblastic leukemia	6,000 international units/kg I.M. or I.V. three times a week
asparaginase *Erwinia chrysanthemi*	As adjunct to multi-agent chemotherapeutic regimen to treat acute lymphoblastic leukemia in patients who have developed hypersensitivity to *E. coli*–derived asparaginase	*Substitute for dose of pegaspargase:* 25,000 international units/m^2 I.M. or I.V. three times a week for six doses *Substitute for each scheduled dose of native* E. coli *asparaginase:* 25,000 international units I.M. or I.V.
pegaspargase (PEG-L-asparaginase) Oncaspar	To treat acute lymphoblastic leukemia in adults up to age 21	2,500 international units/m^2 I.M. or I.V. every 14 days

(continued)

Selected Antineoplastic Drugs *(continued)*

GENERIC AND TRADE NAMES	INDICATIONS	USUAL ADULT DOSAGES
Biological response modifiers		
bacillus Calmette-Guérin (BCG) live, Connaught strain ImmuCyst (CAN), TheraCys	To treat bladder cancer	81 mg (reconstitute and dilute with 50 ml preservative-free normal saline solution to 53 ml or less) instilled into bladder for 1 to 2 hr every wk for 6 wk, then as a single-dose treatment at 3, 6, 12, 18, and 24 mo
bacillus Calmette-Guérin, Tice strain TICE BCG		50 mg (reconstitute and dilute with 50 ml preservative-free normal saline to 50 ml or less) for 1 to 2 hr every 6 wk; may repeat once, followed by single-dose treatment every mo for 6 to 12 mo
interferon alfa-2a, recombinant Roferon-A	To treat hairy cell leukemia	3 million units/day I.M. or SubQ for 16 to 24 wk, followed by 3 million units 3 times/wk
	To treat AIDS-related Kaposi's sarcoma	36 million units/day I.M. or SubQ for 10 to 12 wk; or 3 million units/day I.M. or SubQ on days 1 to 3, 9 million units/day on days 4 to 6, 18 million units/day on days 7 to 9, and 36 million units/day from day 10 until completion of 10- to 12-wk course; maintenance dose, 36 million units 3 times/wk
interferon alfa-2b, recombinant Intron A	To treat hairy cell leukemia	2 million units/m^2 I.M. or SubQ 3 times/wk
	To treat AIDS-related Kaposi's sarcoma	30 million units/m^2 I.M. or SubQ 3 times/wk
	To treat malignant melanoma	20 million units/m^2 by I.V. infusion on days 1 to 5 every wk for 4 wk, followed by 10 million units/m^2 I.V. 3 times/wk for 48 wk
levamisole hydrochloride Ergamisol	To treat colorectal cancer	Beginning 7 to 30 days after surgery, 50 mg P.O. every 8 hr for 3 days, repeated every 2 wk for 1 yr, with fluorouracil 450 mg/m^2 by rapid I.V. infusion daily for 5 days, starting with first or second course of levamisole

Selected Antineoplastic Drugs *(continued)*

GENERIC AND TRADE NAMES	INDICATIONS	USUAL ADULT DOSAGES
Hormonal antineoplastics		
abiraterone Zytiga	To treat metastatic castration-resistant prostate cancer in combination with prednisone	1,000 mg P.O. once daily
anastrozole Arimidex	To treat breast cancer	1 mg P.O. daily
bicalutamide Casodex	To treat prostate cancer	50 mg P.O. daily in combination with luteinizing hormone-releasing hormone (LHRH) analog or after surgical castration
degarelix Firmagon	To treat advanced prostate cancer	*Initial:* 240 mg SubQ divided into 2 injections; then 80 mg SubQ every 28 days
enzalutamide Xtandi	To treat metastatic castration-resistant prostate cancer in patients who have previously received docetaxel	160 mg P.O. once daily
estramustine phosphate sodium Emcyt	To treat prostate cancer To treat postmenopausal breast cancer	14 mg/kg/day P.O. in three or four divided doses 1 hr before or 2 hr after meals
exemestane Aromasin	To treat prostate cancer	25 mg P.O. daily after a meal
	As adjunct for postmenopausal women with estrogen receptor–positive early breast cancer who have received 2 to 3 yr of tamoxifen therapy	25 mg P.O. daily until completion of 5 years with combined therapy
	To treat advanced breast cancer in postmenopausal women whose disease has progressed after tamoxifen therapy	25 mg P.O. daily
flutamide Euflex (CAN), Eulexin	To treat breast cancer	250 mg P.O. every 8 hr
goserelin acetate Zoladex, Zoladex LA, Zoladex 3-Month	To treat prostate cancer	3.6 mg SubQ into upper abdominal wall every 28 days 3.6 mg SubQ into upper abdominal wall every 28 days; or 10.8 mg SubQ every 12 wk

(continued)

Selected Antineoplastic Drugs *(continued)*

GENERIC AND TRADE NAMES	INDICATIONS	USUAL ADULT DOSAGES
Hormonal antineoplastics *(continued)*		
letrozole Femara	To treat breast cancer	2.5 mg P.O. daily
leuprolide acetate Lupron, Lupron Depot, Lupron Depot-3 Month, Lupron Depot-4 Month, Viadur	To treat prostate cancer	*Regular:* 1 mg SubQ daily; *Depot:* 7.5 mg every mo; or 22.5 mg every 3 mo; or 30 mg every 4 mo; *Implant:* 1 every 12 mo
medroxyprogesterone acetate Depo-Provera	To treat endometrial or renal cancer	400 to 1,000 mg every wk until stable, then 400 mg or more every mo
megestrol acetate Megace	To treat breast cancer	160 mg/day P.O. daily or in divided doses
	To treat endometrial cancer	40 to 320 mg P.O. daily or in divided doses
nilutamide Anandron (CAN), Nilandron	To treat prostate cancer	300 mg P.O. daily up to 30 days, then 150 mg P.O. daily
tamoxifen citrate Apo-Tamox (CAN), Gen-Tamoxifen (CAN), Nolva-dex, Nolvadex-D (CAN), NovoTamoxifen (CAN), Tamofen (CAN), Tamone (CAN)	To prevent breast cancer or reduce the risk of invasive breast cancer in women with ductal carcinoma in situ	20 mg P.O. daily for 5 yr
	To treat breast cancer (node-negative or node-positive)	10 mg P.O. twice daily or, in metastatic disease, 10 to 20 mg P.O. twice daily
testolactone Teslac	To treat breast cancer	250 mg P.O. four times a day
toremifene citrate Fareston	To treat breast cancer	60 mg P.O. daily
triptorelin pamoate Trelstar	To provide palliative treatment of advanced prostate cancer	3.75 mg once every 4 wk, 11.25 mg once every 12 wk, or 22.5 mg once every 24 wk
Miscellaneous antineoplastics		
axitinib Inlyta	To treat advanced renal cell carcinoma after failure of one prior systemic therapy	*Initial:* 5 mg P.O. every 12 hr with dosage adjustment made, as needed.

Selected Antineoplastic Drugs *(continued)*

GENERIC AND TRADE NAMES	INDICATIONS	USUAL ADULT DOSAGES
Miscellaneous antineoplastics *(continued)*		
bevacizumab Avastin	To treat metastatic colorectal cancer	5 or 10 mg/kg I.V. over 90 min every 2 wk as adjunct to I.V. fluorouacil-based chemotherapy.
	To treat nonsquamous, non–small-cell lung cancer	15 mg/kg I.V. over 90 min every 3 wk as adjunct to carboplatin and paclitaxel.
	To treat glioblastoma	10 mg/kg I.V. over 90 min every 2 wk.
	To treat metastatic renal cell cancer	10 mg/kg I.V. over 90 min every 2 wk as adjunct to interferon alfa.
	To treat persistent, recurrent, or metastatic cervical cancer	15 mg/kg I.V. over 90 min every 3 wk as adjunct with I.V. paclitaxel and cisplatin or paclitaxel and topotecan.
Targretin Gel	To treat cutaneous lesions of cutaneous T-cell lymphoma (stages IA and IB)	Apply generously to cover only lesions every other day on 1st wk; then increased as tolerated to once daily on 2nd wk, twice daily on 3rd wk, three times a day on 4th wk and, finally, four times a day on 5th wk.
bortezomib Velcade	To treat multiple myeloma; to treat mantle cell lymphoma	For cycles 1-4:1.3 mg/m^2 I.V. bolus at a concentration of 1 mg/ml or subcutaneous injection at a concentration of 2.5 mg/ml on days 1, 4, 8, 11, 22, 25, 29, and 32 followed by rest period to end of wk 6; then 6-wk cycle repeated 3 more times. For cycles 5-9: 1.3 mg/m^2 I.V. bolus at a concentration of 1 mg/ml or subcutaneous injection at a concentration of 2.5 mg/ml on days 1, 8, 22, and 29 followed by rest period to end of wk 6; then 6-wk cycle repeated 4 more times.

(continued)

Selected Antineoplastic Drugs *(continued)*

GENERIC AND TRADE NAMES	INDICATIONS	USUAL ADULT DOSAGES
Miscellaneous antineoplastics *(continued)*		
dacarbazine DTIC (CAN), DTIC-Dome	To treat Hodgkin's disease	150 mg/m^2 I.V. daily for 5 days in combination with other drugs; may repeat every 28 days; or 375 mg/m^2 every 15 days in combination with other drugs.
	To treat malignant melanoma	2 to 4.5 mg/kg I.V. daily for 10 days and every 28 days thereafter; or 250 mg/m^2 I.V. daily for 5 days and every 21 days thereafter.
eribulin mesylate Halaven	To treat metastatic breast cancer in patients who have previously received at least two chemotherapeutic regimens that included an anthracycline and a taxane	1.4 mg/m^2 I.V. over 2 to 5 min on days 1 and 8 of a 21-day cycle.
erlotinib Tarceva	To treat non-small cell lung cancer	150 mg P.O. once daily.
	To treat pancreatic cancer	100 mg P.O. once daily.
etoposide (VP-16) Toposar, VePesid	To treat germ-cell testicular tumors	50 to 100 mg/m^2/day I.V. on days 1 through 5 up to 100 mg/m^2 I.V. on days 1, 3, and 5; course repeated every 3 to 4 wk.
	To treat small-cell lung carcinoma	35 mg/m^2/day I.V. for 4 days up to 50 mg/m^2/day I.V. for 5 days, repeated every 3 to 4 wk; or 70 mg/m^2/day P.O. for 4 days to 100 mg/m^2/day P.O. for 5 days, repeated every 3 to 4 wk.
etoposide phosphate Etopophos	To treat germ-cell testicular tumors	50 to 100 mg/m^2/day by I.V. infusion on days 1 through 5 to 100 mg/m^2/day by I.V. infusion on days 1, 3, and 5; course repeated every 3 to 4 wk.
	To treat small-cell lung carcinoma	35 mg/m^2/day by I.V. infusion for 4 days to 50 mg/m^2/day by I.V. infusion for 5 days, repeated every 3 to 4 wk.

Selected Antineoplastic Drugs *(continued)*

GENERIC AND TRADE NAMES	INDICATIONS	USUAL ADULT DOSAGES
Miscellaneous antineoplastics *(continued)*		
gemcitabine hydrochloride Gemzar	To treat non–small-cell lung carcinoma	1,000 mg/m^2 by I.V. infusion over 30 min daily on days 1, 8, and 15 every 28 days with cisplatin 100 mg/m^2 on day 28; or 1,250 mg/m^2 I.V. daily on days 1 and 8 every 21 days in combination with cisplatin 100 mg/m^2 I.V. on day 21.
	To treat pancreatic cancer	1,000 mg/m^2 by I.V. infusion over 30 min every wk for 7 wk, followed by 1 wk of no drug; then every wk for 3 wk, followed by 1 wk of no drug; then repeat 4-wk cycle.
imatinib mesylate Gleevec	To treat chronic myeloid leukemia in accelerated phase or blast crisis, or in chronic phase after failure of interferon-alpha therapy	400 mg P.O. daily with food (chronic phase) or 600 mg P.O. daily with food (accelerated phase or blast crisis); after 3 mo, dosage may be increased to 600 mg P.O. daily (chronic phase) or 800 mg P.O. given in 2 divided doses of 400 mg (accelerated phase or blast crisis), as needed.
	To treat GI stromal tumor	400 mg/day P.O. or 600 mg/day P.O.
irinotecan hydrochloride Camptosar	To treat colorectal cancer	125 mg/m^2 I.V. over 90 min every wk for 4 wk, followed by 2 wk of no drug, then repeat 6-wk cycle; or 350 mg/m^2 I.V. over 90 min every 3 wk.
iressa Gefitinib	To treat refractory metastatic non–small-cell lung cancer	250 mg P.O. daily.
ixabepilone Ixempra	To treat metastatic or locally advanced breast cancer in combination with capecitabine after failure with an anthracycline and a taxane; to treat metastatic or locally advanced breast cancer after failure with an anthracycline, a taxane, and capecitabine	40 mg/m^2 I.V. infused over 3 hr every 3 wk.
mitotane (o,p9-DDD) Lysodren	To treat adrenocortical carcinoma	2 to 6 g P.O. daily in divided doses three times a day or four times a day.

(continued)

Selected Antineoplastic Drugs *(continued)*

GENERIC AND TRADE NAMES	INDICATIONS	USUAL ADULT DOSAGES
Miscellaneous antineoplastics *(continued)*		
mitoxantrone hydrochloride Novantrone	To treat hormone-refractory prostate cancer	12 to 14 mg/m^2 I.V. every 21 days.
	To treat acute nonlymphocytic leukemia	12 mg/m^2 by I.V. infusion in free-flowing normal saline solution or D$_5$W over 3 min daily on days 1 to 3, with cytarabine 100 mg/m^2/day by continuous I.V. infusion on days 1 to 7; if response is inadequate, second course at same dosage may be given.
panitumumab Vectibix	To treat wild-type KRAS metastatic colorectal cancer	6 mg/kg I.V. given over 60 min every 14 days.
pazopanib Votrient	To treat advanced renal cell carcinoma	800 mg P.O. once daily, followed by a 400 mg dosage reduction for next dose and then additional increases or decreases in 200 mg steps, as needed. 800 mg P.O. once daily, followed by dosage increases or decreases in 200 mg steps, as needed.
	To treat advanced soft tissue sarcoma in patients who have received prior chemotherapy	
pertuzumab Perjeta	To treat HER2-positive metastatic breast cancer in combination with trastuzumab and docetaxel in patients who have not received prior anti-HER2 therapy or chemotherapy for metastatic disease; or patients with HER2-positive, locally advanced, inflammatory, or early stage breast cancer (either greater than 2 cm in diameter or node-positive)	*Initial:* 840 mg as a 60-min I.V. infusion, followed every 3 wks thereafter with 420 mg as a 30- to 60-min I.V. infusion.
ponatinib Iclusig	To treat T3151-positive chronic myeloid leukemia, T3151-positive Philadelphia chromosome–positive acute lymphoblastic leukemia	45 mg P.O. daily with dosage decreased to as little as 15 mg daily, if needed.
porfimer sodium Photofrin	To treat esophageal cancer and non–small-cell lung carcinoma	2 mg/kg I.V. over 3 to 5 min, followed by laser light illumination and debridement of tumor; may repeat course every 30 days three times.
procarbazine hydrochloride Matulane, Natulan (CAN)	To treat Hodgkin's disease	2 to 4 mg/kg/day (rounded to nearest 50 mg) P.O. as a single dose or in divided doses for 1 wk, followed by 4 to 6 mg/kg/day until leukopenia, thrombocytopenia, or maximal response.

Selected Antineoplastic Drugs *(continued)*

GENERIC AND TRADE NAMES	INDICATIONS	USUAL ADULT DOSAGES
Miscellaneous antineoplastics *(continued)*		
ramucirumab Cyramza	To treat gastric cancer	8 mg/kg I.V. given over 60 min every 2 wk.
	To treat non–small-cell lung cancer	10 mg/kg I.V. given over 60 min on day 1 of each 21-day cycle.
regorafenib Stivarga	To treat metastatic colorectal cancer in patients who have been previously treated with fluoro-pyrimidine-, oxaliplatin-, and irinotecan-based chemotherapy, an anti-VEGF therapy, and, if KRAS wild type, an anti-EGER therapy	160 mg P.O. once daily for the first 21 days of each 28-day cycle.
rituximab Rituxan	To treat non-Hodgkin's lymphomas	375 mg/m^2/day by I.V. infusion every wk for 4 or 8 doses.
	As adjunct to treat CD20-positive chronic lymphocytic leukemia	375 mg/m^2 given on the day prior to the initiation of the first cycle of fludarabine and cyclophosphamide chemotherapy, followed by 500 mg/m^2 given on day 1 of cycles 2 through 6.
romidepsin Istodax	To treat cutaneous or peripheral T-cell lymphoma in patients who have received at least one prior systemic therapy	14 mg/m2 I.V. over 4 hrs on days 1, 8, and 15 of a 28-day cycle. Cycle repeated every 28 days, as needed.
sunitinib malate Sutent	To treat GI stromal tumor progression; to treat advanced renal cell cancer	50 mg P.O. daily for 4 wk, followed by 2 wk off; then cycle repeated as needed.
	To treat progressive, well-differentiated pancreatic neuroendocrine tumors	37.5 mg P.O. daily.
topotecan hydrochloride Hycamtin	To treat ovarian cancer and small-cell lung carcinoma	1.5 mg/m^2 I.V. over 30 min daily for 5 days, repeated every 21 days.
trastuzumab Herceptin	To treat breast cancer	4 mg/kg I.V. over 90 min, followed by 2 mg/kg I.V. over 30 min every 7 days. Alternatively, 8 mg/kg. I.V. over 90 min., followed by 6 mg/kg I.V. over 30 to 90 min every 3 wks.
ziv-aflibercept Zaltrap	To treat metastatic colorectal cancer in combination with 5-fluorouracil, leucovorin, and irinotecan that is resistant to or has progressed following an oxaliplatin-containing regimen	4 mg/kg I.V. infusion over 1 hr every 2 wks.

Selected Antihypertensive Combinations

Antihypertensive drugs are used along with lifestyle changes to manage hypertension. Antihypertensive combinations, which commonly include one or two antihypertensives and a diuretic, are used to simplify patients' drug regimens and, in some cases, to enhance drug actions. The table below lists the generic and trade names; functional classes; usual adult

ANTIHYPERTENSIVE COMBINATION TRADE NAMES	ANTIHYPERTENSIVE GENERIC NAMES	DIURETIC GENERIC NAMES
Aldoril-15	methyldopa 250 mg	hydrochlorothiazide (HCTZ) 15 mg
Aldoril-25	methyldopa 250 mg	HCTZ 25 mg
Aldoril D30	methyldopa 500 mg	HCTZ 30 mg
Aldoril D50	methyldopa 500 mg	HCTZ 50 mg
Amturnide 150/5/12.5	aliskiren 150 mg, amlodipine 5 mg	HCTZ 12.5 mg
Amturnide 300/5/12.5	aliskiren 300 mg, amlodipine 5 mg	HCTZ 12.5 mg
Amturnide 300/5/25	aliskiren 300 mg, amlodipine 5 mg	HCTZ 25 mg
Amturnide 300/10/12.5	aliskiren 300 mg, amlodipine 10 mg	HCTZ 12.5 mg
Amturnide 300/10/25	aliskiren 300 mg, amlodipine 10 mg	HCTZ 25 mg
Apresazide 25/25	hydralazine hydrochloride (HCl4.32 pt) 25 mg	HCTZ 25 mg
Apresazide 50/50	hydralazine HCl 50 mg	HCTZ 50 mg
Apresazide 100/50	hydralazine HCl 100 mg	HCTZ 50 mg
Atacand HCT 16/12.5	candesartan cilexetil 16 mg	HCTZ 12.5 mg
Atacand HCT 32/12.5	candesartan cilexetil 32 mg	HCTZ 12.5 mg
Avalide-150	irbesartan 150 mg	HCTZ 12.5 mg
Avalide-300	irbesartan 300 mg	HCTZ 12.5 mg
Azor 5/20	amlopidine 5 mg, olmesartan 20 mg	None
Azor 5/40	amlodipine 5 mg, olmesartan 40 mg	
Azor 10/20	amlodipine 10 mg, olmesartan 20 mg	
Azor 10/40	amlodipine 10 mg, olmesartan 40 mg	
Benicar HCT 20/12.5	olmesartan medoxomil 20 mg	HCTZ 12.5 mg
Benicar HCT 40/12.5	lmesartan medoxomil 40 mg	HCTZ 12.5 mg
Benicar HCT 40/25	olmesartan medoxomil 40 mg	HCTZ 25 mg
Capozide 25/15	captopril 25 mg	HCTZ 15 mg
Capozide 25/25	captopril 25 mg	HCTZ 25 mg
Capozide 50/15	captopril 50 mg	HCTZ 15 mg
Capozide 50/25	captopril 50 mg	HCTZ 25 mg

dosages; and onset, peak, and duration for commonly used antihypertensive combinations. For information about the mechanisms of action, interactions, adverse reactions, and nursing considerations related to antihypertensive combinations, review the entries for the specific antihypertensives and diuretics that they contain.

FUNCTIONAL CLASSES	USUAL ADULT DOSAGES	ONSET, PEAK, AND DURATION
Centrally acting antiadrenergic and thiazide diuretic	1 tab twice daily or three times daily 1 tab twice daily 1 tab daily 1 tab daily	**Onset:** Unknown **Peak:** 4 to 6 hr **Duration:** 12 to 24 hr
Direct renin inhibitor, calcium channel blocker, and thiazide diuretic	1 tab once daily 1 tab once daily 1 tab once daily 1 tab once daily 1 tab once daily	**Onset:** Unknown **Peak:** 3 to 8 hr **Duration:** Unknown
Peripherally acting arterial dilator and thiazide diuretic	1 cap once or twice daily 1 cap once or twice daily 1 cap once or twice daily	**Onset:** 20 to 30 min **Peak:** 1 to 2 hr **Duration:** 2 to 4 hr
Angiotensin II receptor antagonist and thiazide diuretic	1 tab once or twice daily 1 tab daily	**Onset:** 1 to 2 wk **Peak:** Within 4 wk **Duration:** Unknown
ACE inhibitor and thiazide diuretic	1 tab daily 1 tab daily	**Onset:** Unknown **Peak:** Unknown **Duration:** Unknown
Calcium channel blocker and angiotensin II receptor antagonist	1 tab daily 1 tab daily 1 tab daily 1 tab daily	**Onset:** Unknown **Peak:** 1 to 6 hr **Duration:** 24 hr
Angiotensin II receptor antagonist and thiazide diuretic	1 tab daily 1 tab daily 1 tab daily	**Onset:** Unknown **Peak:** Unknown **Duration:** Unknown
ACE inhibitor and thiazide diuretic	1 tab daily to three times a day 1 tab once or twice daily 1 tab once daily to three times a day 1 tab once or twice daily	**Onset:** 15 to 60 min **Peak:** 60 to 90 min **Duration:** 6 to 12 hr

(continued)

Selected Antihypertensive Combinations *(continued)*

ANTIHYPERTENSIVE COMBINATION TRADE NAMES	ANTIHYPERTENSIVE GENERIC NAMES	DIURETIC GENERIC NAMES
Diovan HCT 80/12.5	valsartan 80 mg	HCTZ 12.5 mg
Diovan HCT 160/12.5	valsartan 160 mg	HCTZ 12.5 mg
Diovan HCT 160/25	valsartan 160 mg	HCTZ 25 mg
Diovan HCT 320/12.5	valsartan 320 mg	HCTZ 12.5 mg
Diovan HCT 320/25	valsartan 320 mg	HCTZ 25 mg
Dyazide	triamterene 37.5 mg	HCTZ 25 mg
Edarbyclor 40/12.5	azilsartan 40 mg	chlorthalidone 12.5 mg
Edarbyclor 40/25	azilsartan 40 mg	chlorthalidone 25 mg
Exforge	amlodipine 5 mg, valsartan 160 mg	None
Exforge HCT 5/160/12.5	amlodipine 5 mg, valsartan 160 mg	HCTZ 12.5 mg
Exforge HCT 10/160/12.5	amlodipine 10 mg, valsartan 160 mg	HCTZ 12.5 mg
Exforge HCT 5/160/25	amlodipine 5 mg, valsartan 160 mg	HCTZ 25 mg
Exforge HCT 10/160/25	amlodipine 10 mg, valsartan 160 mg	HCTZ 25 mg
Exforge HCT 10/320/25	amlodipine 10 mg, valsartan 320 mg	HCTZ 25 mg
Hyzaar 50/12.5	losartan potassium 50 mg	HCTZ 12.5 mg
Hyzaar 100/25	losartan potassium 100 mg	HCTZ 25 mg
Inderide 80/25	propranolol HCl 80 mg	HCTZ 25 mg
Inderide LA 80/50	propranolol HCl 80 mg	HCTZ 50 mg
Inderide LA 120/50	propranolol HCl 120 mg	HCTZ 50 mg
Inderide LA 160/50	propranolol HCl 160 mg	HCTZ 50 mg
Lopressor HCT 50/25	metoprolol tartrate 50 mg	HCTZ 25 mg
Lopressor HCT 100/25	metoprolol tartrate 100 mg	HCTZ 25 mg
Lopressor HCT 100/50	metoprolol tartrate 100 mg	HCTZ 50 mg
Lotensin HCT 5/6.25	benazepril HCl 5 mg	HCTZ 6.25 mg
Lotensin HCT 10/12.5	benazepril HCl 10 mg	HCTZ 12.5 mg
Lotensin HCT 20/12.5	benazepril HCl 20 mg	HCTZ 12.5 mg
Lotensin HCT 20/25	benazepril HCl 20 mg	HCTZ 25 mg

FUNCTIONAL CLASSES	USUAL ADULT DOSAGES	ONSET, PEAK, AND DURATION
ACE inhibitor and thiazide diuretic	1 or 2 tabs daily 1 tab daily 1 tab daily 1 tab daily 1 tab daily	**Onset:** 2 hr **Peak:** 6 hr **Duration:** 24 hr
Potassium-sparing diuretic and thiazide diuretic	1 or 2 caps or tabs daily	**Onset:** 2 to 4 hr **Peak:** 1 day **Duration:** 7 to 9 hr
ACE inhibitor and thiazide-like diuretic	1 tab daily 1 tab daily	**Onset:** Unknown **Peak:** 6 hr **Duration:** 24 hr
Calcium channel blocker and ACE inhibitor	1 or 2 tabs daily	**Onset:** Unknown **Peak:** 6 to 12 hr **Duration:** 24 hr
Calcium channel blocker, ACE inhibitor, and thiazide diuretic	1 tab daily 1 tab daily 1 tab daily 1 tab daily 1 tab daily	**Onset:** Unknown **Peak:** 2 to 6 hr **Duration:** Unknown
ACE inhibitor and thiazide diuretic	1 or 2 tabs daily 1 tab daily	**Onset:** Unknown **Peak:** 6 hr **Duration:** 24 hr or more
Beta blocker and thiazide diuretic	1 or 2 tabs twice daily 1 cap daily 1 cap daily 1 cap daily	**Onset:** Unknown **Peak:** 1 to 1.5 hr **Duration:** Unknown
Beta blocker and thiazide diuretic	1 or 2 tabs daily or 1 tab b.i.d. 1 or 2 tabs daily or 1 tab b.i.d. 1 or 2 tabs daily or 1 tab b.i.d.	**Onset:** 1 hr **Peak:** 1 to 2 hr **Duration:** Unknown
ACE inhibitor and thiazide diuretic	1 tab daily 1 tab daily 1 tab daily 1 tab daily	**Onset:** 1 hr **Peak:** 2 to 4 hr **Duration:** 24 hr

(continued)

Selected Antihypertensive Combinations *(continued)*

ANTIHYPERTENSIVE COMBINATION TRADE NAMES	ANTIHYPERTENSIVE GENERIC NAMES	DIURETIC GENERIC NAMES
Lotrel 2.5/10	amlodipine 2.5 mg, benazepril HCl 10 mg	None
Lotrel 5/10	amlodipine 5 mg, benazepril HCl 10 mg	None
Lotrel 5/20	amlodipine 5 mg, benazepril HCl 10 mg	None
Lotrel 10/20	amlodipine 10 mg, benazepril HCl 20 mg	None
Maxzide 37.5/25	triamterene 37.5 mg	HCTZ 25 mg
Maxzide 75/50	triamterene 75 mg	HCTZ 50 mg
Micardis HCT 40/12.5	telmisartan 40 mg	HCTZ 12.5 mg
Micardis HCT 80/12.5	telmisartan 80 mg	HCTZ 12.5 mg
Moduretic	amiloride 5 mg	HCTZ 50 mg
Prinzide 10/12.5	lisinopril 10 mg	HCTZ 12.5 mg
Prinzide 20/12.5	lisinopril 20 mg	HCTZ 12.5 mg
Prinzide 20/25	lisinopril 20 mg	HCTZ 25 mg
Tekamlo 150/5	aliskiren 150 mg	None
Tekamlo 150/10	amlodipine 5 mg	None
Tekamlo 300/5	aliskiren 150 mg	
Tekamlo 300/10	amlodipine 10 mg	
	aliskiren 300 mg	
	amlodipine 5 mg	
	aliskiren 300 mg	
	amlodipine 10 mg	
Tekturna	aliskiren 150 mg	HCTZ 12.5 mg
Tekturna HCT 150/12.5	aliskiren 150 mga	HCTZ 12.5 mg
Tekturna HCT 150/25	aliskiren 150 mg	HCTZ 25 mg
Tekturna HCT 300/12.5	aliskiren 300 mg	HCTZ 12.5 mg

FUNCTIONAL CLASSES	USUAL ADULT DOSAGES	ONSET, PEAK, AND DURATION
Calcium channel blocker and ACE inhibitor	1 or 2 caps daily 1 cap daily 1 cap daily 1 cap daily	**Onset:** Unknown **Peak:** Unknown **Duration:** 24 hr
Potassium-sparing diuretic and thiazide diuretic	1 tab daily 1 tab daily	**Onset:** 2 to 4 hr **Peak:** 1 day **Duration:** 7 to 9 hr
Angiotensin II receptor antagonist and thiazide diuretic	1 tab once or twice daily 1 tab once or twice daily	**Onset:** Within 3 hr **Peak:** In 4 wk **Duration:** Several days to 1 wk
Potassium-sparing diuretic and thiazide diuretic	1 or 2 tabs daily	**Onset:** 2 hr **Peak:** 6 to 10 hr **Duration:** 24 hr
ACE inhibitor and thiazide diuretic	1 or 2 tabs daily 1 or 2 tabs daily	**Onset:** 1 hr **Peak:** 6 hr **Duration:** 24 hr
Direct renin inhibitor and calcium channel blocker	1 or 2 tabs daily 1 tab daily	**Onset:** Unknown **Peak:** 3–8 hr **Duration:** 24 hr
Direct renin inhibitor and thiazide diuretic	1 tab daily	**Onset:** Unknown **Peak:** 1 to 3 hr **Duration:** Unknown
Direct renin inhibitor and thiazide diuretic	1 tab daily 1 tab daily 1 tab daily	**Onset:** Unknown **Peak:** 1 to 2.5 hr **Duration:** Unknown

(continued)

Selected Antihypertensive Combinations *(continued)*

ANTIHYPERTENSIVE COMBINATION TRADE NAMES	ANTIHYPERTENSIVE GENERIC NAMES	DIURETIC GENERIC NAMES
Timolide 10/25	timolol maleate 10 mg	HCTZ 25 mg
	olmesartan 20 mg	HCTZ 12.5 mg
	amlodipine 5 mg	HCTZ 12.5 mg
	olmesartan 40 mg	HCTZ 25 mg
Tribenzor 20/5/12.5	amlodipine 5 mg	HCTZ 12.5 mg
Tribenzor 40/5/12.5	olmesartan 40 mg	
Tribenzor 40/5/25	amlodipine 5 mg	
Tribenzor 40/10/12.5	olmesartan 40 mg	
	amlodipine 10 mg	
Twynsta 40/5	telmisartan 40 mg, amlodipine 5 mg	None
Twynsta 40/10	telmisartan 40 mg, amlodipine 10 mg	None
Twynsta 80/5	telmisartan 80 mg, amlodipine 5 mg	None
Twynsta 80/10	telmisartan 80 mg, amlodipine 10 mg	None
Uniretic 15/25	moexipril HCl 15 mg	HCTZ 25 mg
Valturna 150/160	aliskiren 150 mg, valsartan 160 mg	None
Valturna 300/320	aliskiren 300 mg, valsartan 320 mg	None
Vaseretic 5/12.5	enalapril maleate 5 mg	HCTZ 12.5 mg
Vaseretic 10/25	enalapril maleate 10 mg	HCTZ 25 mg
Zestoretic 10/12.5	lisinopril 10 mg	HCTZ 12.5 mg
Zestoretic 20/12.5	lisinopril 20 mg	HCTZ 12.5 mg
Zestoretic 20/25	lisinopril 20 mg	HCTZ 25 mg
Ziac 2.5/6.25	bisoprolol fumarate 2.5 mg	HCTZ 6.25 mg
Ziac 5/6.25	bisoprolol fumarate 5 mg	HCTZ 6.25 mg
Ziac 10/6.25	bisoprolol fumarate 10 mg	HCTZ 6.25 mg

FUNCTIONAL CLASSES	USUAL ADULT DOSAGES	ONSET, PEAK, AND DURATION
Beta blocker and thiazide diuretic	1 tab b.i.d. or 2 tabs daily	**Onset:** Unknown **Peak:** 1 to 2 hr **Duration:** Unknown
Angiotensin II receptor antagonist, calcium channel blocker, and thiazide diuretic	1 tab daily	**Onset:** Unknown **Peak:** 1 to 6 hr **Duration:** 24 hr
Angiotensin II receptor antagonist and calcium channel blocker	1 tab daily 1 tab daily 1 tab daily 1 tab daily	**Onset:** Unknown **Peak:** 1 to 6 hr **Duration:** Unknown
Potassium-sparing diuretic and thiazide diuretic	1 or 2 tabs daily	**Onset:** 1 hr **Peak:** 3 to 6 hr **Duration:** 24 hr
Direct renin inhibitor and ACE inhibitor	1 tab daily 1 tab daily	**Onset:** Unknown **Peak:** 1 to 3 hr **Duration:** Unknown
ACE inhibitor and thiazide diuretic	1 tab once or twice daily 1 tab once or twice daily	**Onset:** 1 hr **Peak:** 4 to 6 hr **Duration:** 24 hr
ACE inhibitor and thiazide diuretic	1 or 2 tabs daily 1 or 2 tabs daily 1 or 2 tabs daily	**Onset:** 1 hr **Peak:** 6 hr **Duration:** 24 hr
Beta blocker and thiazide diuretic	1 or 2 tabs daily 1 or 2 tabs daily 1 or 2 tabs daily	**Onset:** Unknown **Peak:** Unknown **Duration:** Unknown

(continued)

Selected Obstetrical Drugs

Obstetrical drugs are used during pregnancy for a variety of reasons, such as control of nausea and vomiting, pain relief, and assistance in the labor and delivery process. Drugs used to control nausea and vomiting throughout pregnancy and analgesics used to provide pain relief, especially during the labor and delivery process, are covered in the main section of the *Nurse Drug Handbook*. While other drugs may be used during pregnancy, not all have FDA approval for such use. For example, misoprostol, a synthetic prostaglandin, is used to treat ulcers. However, it may also be used for indications not approved by the FDA, such as assisting in the termination of a pregnancy, evacuation of the uterine contents in a missed abortion, and dilating the cervix prior to labor. These uses are considered "off-label" uses because they have not been FDA approved. In adherence with the standard of only including FDA-approved indications in the *Nurse Drug Handbook*, following are selected obstetrical drugs that are FDA approved for use with pregnancy issues.

GENERIC NAME AND TRADE NAME	INDICATIONS	ADULT DOSAGES
dinoprostone Cervidil, Prepidil, Prostin E$_2$	Initiation and/or continuation of cervical ripening in patients at or near term in whom there is a medical or obstetrical indication for the induction of labor	10 mg intravaginally designed to release 0.3 mg/hour of the drug over a 12-hour period; removed upon onset of active labor or 12 hours after insertion
hydroxyprogesterone caproate Makena	To reduce risk of preterm birth in women who are carrying only one fetus and who have a history of singleton spontaneous preterm birth	250 mg (1 ml) I.M. once weekly begun between16 weeks, 0 days and 20 weeks, 6 days of gestation and continued weekly until week 37 or delivery, whichever comes first
oxytocin Pitocin	To initiate or improve uterine contractions in situations where there are fetal or maternal concerns, so as to achieve a vaginal delivery	*Initial:* 0.5 mU (milliunits)/min to 1 mU/min I.V., increased in increments of 1 to 2 mU/min every 30 to 60 minutes, as needed; once desired frequency of contractions has been reached and labor has progressed to 5 to 6 cm dilation, dosage may be decreased by 1 mU/min to 2 mU/min every 30 to 60 minutes

GENERIC NAME AND TRADE NAME	INDICATIONS	ADULT DOSAGES
	To produce uterine contractions during the third stage of labor and to control postpartum bleeding or hemorrhage	10 to 40 units added to existing intravenous solution being infused (maximum 40 units to 1,000 ml of solution) and infused at a rate to sustain uterine contraction and control atony
		Alternatively, 10 units (1 ml) I.M. after delivery of placenta
	To treat incomplete, inevitable, or elective abortion	*Initial:* I.V. infusion rate highly individualized (10 units mixed in 500 ml of saline or 5% dextrose-in-water solution)
		Maximum: 30 units in a 12-hour period

Vitamins

As you know, an adequate daily intake of vitamins is essential to vital bodily functions, such as embryonic development (vitamin A), regulation of serum calcium and phosphate (vitamin D), and blood clotting (vitamin K).

Vitamins are classified as one of two types: fat soluble (vitamins A, D, E, and K) and water soluble (vitamin C and all forms of vitamin B). Fat-soluble vitamins can accumulate in body tissue over time; when excessive amounts are ingested through diet or supplementation,

GENERIC AND TRADE NAMES	RECOMMENDED DAILY INTAKE
vitamin A **(retinol)** Aquasol A	***Adult men and boys over age 10.*** 1,000 mcg/day. ***Adult women and girls over age 10.*** 800 mcg/day. ***Pregnant women.*** 800 mcg/day. (900 mcg/day [CAN].) ***Breastfeeding women.*** 1,200 to 1,300 mcg/day. (1,200 mcg/day [CAN].) ***Children ages 7 to 10.*** 700 mcg/day. (700 to 800 mcg/day [CAN].) ***Children ages 4 to 7.*** 500 mcg/day. ***Neonates and children to age 4.*** 375 to 400 mcg/day. (400 mcg/day [CAN].)
vitamin B₁ (thiamine **hydrochloride)** Betaxin (CAN), Bewon (CAN), Biamine	***Adult men and boys over age 10.*** 1.2 to 1.5 mg/day. (0.8 to 1.3 mg/day [CAN].) ***Adult women and girls over age 10.*** 1 to 1.1 mg/day. (0.8 to 0.9 mg/day [CAN].) ***Pregnant women.*** 1.5 mg/day. (0.9 to 1 mg/day. [CAN].) ***Breastfeeding women.*** 1.6 mg/day. (1 to 1.2 mg/day [CAN].)

severe and life-threatening toxicity can develop. Water-soluble vitamins don't accumulate in the body; they are excreted daily so that toxicity is not usually a concern with excessive intake.

The following chart lists the generic and trade names of fat-soluble and water-soluble vitamins, the recommended daily intake to prevent vitamin deficiency, dosages when deficiency occurs, other indications and dosages for vitamin therapy, and guidelines for parenteral administration of vitamins.

OTHER INDICATIONS AND DOSAGES	PARENTERAL ADMINISTRATION GUIDELINES
TO TREAT VITAMIN A DEFICIENCY CAPSULES, ORAL SOLUTION, TABLETS ***Adults and adolescents.*** Dosage individualized based on severity of deficiency, as prescribed. I.M. INJECTION ***Adults and children age 8 and over.*** 15,000 to 30,000 retinol equivalent (RE)/day (50,000 to 100,000 IU/day) for 3 days, followed by 15,000 RE/day (50,000 IU/day) for 2 wk. ***Children ages 1 to 8.*** 1,500 to 4,500 RE/day (5,000 to 15,000 IU/day) for 10 days; for severe deficiency, 5,250 to 10,500 RE/day (17,500 to 35,000 IU/day) for 10 days. ***Infants to age 1 year.*** 1,500 to 3,000 RE/day (5,000 to 10,000 IU/day) for 10 days; for severe deficiency, 2,250 to 4,500 RE/day (7,500 to 15,000 IU/day) for 10 days. I.V. INFUSION ***Adults and children.*** Dosage individualized as part of total parenteral nutrition solution, as prescribed. ***TO TREAT XEROPHTHALMIA*** CAPSULES, ORAL SOLUTION, TABLETS ***Children age 1 and over.*** 60,000 RE (200,000 IU) as a single dose. Dose repeated on day 2 and again in 4 wk. ***Children ages 6 months to 1 year.*** 30,000 RE (100,000 IU) as a single dose. Dose repeated on day 2 and again in 4 wk. ***AS AN ADJUNCT TO TREAT MEASLES*** CAPSULES, ORAL SOLUTION, TABLETS ***Children age 1 and over.*** 60,000 RE (200,000 IU) as a single dose when measles are diagnosed. ***Children ages 6 months to 1 year.*** 30,000 RE (100,000 IU) as a single dose when measles are diagnosed.	• Be aware that anaphylaxis and death have occurred after I.V. administration of vitamin A; I.V. administration is restricted to special solutions, such as in total parenteral nutrition solution. Typically, parenteral administration of vitamin A is by I.M. injection. • Take precautions to protect vitamin A solution from exposure to light because it's light sensitive.
TO TREAT VITAMIN B₁ DEFICIENCY (BERIBERI) ELIXIR, TABLETS ***Adults.*** 5 to 10 mg t.i.d. ***Children and infants.*** 10 mg/day. I.V. OR I.M. INJECTION ***Adults.*** *Initial:* 5 to 100 mg every 8 hr, switched to P.O. vitamin B₁ therapy as soon as possible and continued for total of 1 mo.	• Be aware that I.V. administration of vitamin B₁ has caused severe and life-threatening reactions, especially with repeat administration. Monitor patient closely for angioedema, GI bleeding, respiratory distress, throat tightness, urticaria, vascular collapse, and weakness during and after administration.

(continued)

Vitamins *(continued)*

GENERIC AND TRADE NAMES	RECOMMENDED DAILY INTAKE
vitamin B₁ *(continued)*	***Children ages 7 to 10.*** 1 mg/day. (0.8 to 1 mg/day [CAN].) ***Children ages 4 to 7.*** 0.9 mg/day. (0.7 mg/day [CAN].) ***Children ages 1 to 4.*** 0.3 to 0.7 mg/day. (0.3 to 0.6 mg/day [CAN].)
vitamin B₃ (niacin) Endur-Acin, Nia-Bid, Niac, Niacels, Niacor, Nico-400, Nicobid Tempules, Nicolar, Nicotinex Elixir, Novo-Niacin (CAN), Slo-Niacin	***Adult men and boys age 11 and over.*** 15 to 20 mg/day. (14 to 23 mg/day [CAN].) ***Adult women and girls age 11 and over.*** 13 to 15 mg/day. (14 to 16 mg/day [CAN].) ***Pregnant women.*** 17 mg/day. (14 to 16 mg/day [CAN].) ***Breastfeeding women.*** 20 mg/day. (14 to 16 mg/day [CAN].) ***Children ages 7 to 11.*** 13 mg/day. (14 to 18 mg/day [CAN].) ***Children ages 4 to 7.*** 12 mg/day. (13 mg/day [CAN].) ***Neonates and children to age 4.*** 5 to 9 mg/day. (4 to 9 mg/day [CAN].)
vitamin B₆ (pyridoxine hydrochloride) Beesix, Doxine, Nestrex, Pyri, Rodex, Vita-bee 6	***Adult men and boys age 11 and over.*** 1.7 to 2 mg/day. ***Adult women and girls age 11 and over.*** 1.4 to 1.6 mg/day. ***Pregnant women.*** 2.2 mg/day. ***Breastfeeding women.*** 2.1 mg/day. ***Children ages 7 to 10.*** 1.4 mg/day. ***Children ages 4 to 6.*** 1.1 mg/day. ***Neonates and children to age 3.*** 0.3 to 1 mg/day.

OTHER INDICATIONS AND DOSAGES

PARENTERAL ADMINISTRATION GUIDELINES

TO TREAT WERNICKE'S ENCEPHALOPATHY
I.V. OR I.M. INJECTION
Adults. *Initial:* 100 mg I.V. *Maintenance:* 50 to 100 mg I.V. or I.M. daily until normal recommended daily intake is achieved.

- Rotate sites for I.M. administration of vitamin B_1 to help prevent tenderness and induration that may occur following administration.
- I.M. administration may be painful; use the Z-track method of administration.
- Because of incompatibilities, don't add parenteral vitamin B_1 to alkaline or neutral solutions; also, don't mix it with oxidizing and reducing agents, including barbiturates, carbonates, citrates, and copper.
- Take precautions to protect vitamin B_1 solution from exposure to light because it's light sensitive.

TO TREAT VITAMIN B_3 DEFICIENCY
E.R. CAPSULES, E.R. TABLETS, ORAL SOLUTION, TABLETS
Adults and children age 11 and over. Dosage individualized based on severity of deficiency, as prescribed. *Maximum:* 6 g/day.
I.V. INJECTION
Adults and children age 11 and over. 25 to 100 mg at least twice daily.
Children to age 11. Up to 300 mg daily
I.M. INJECTION
Adults and children age 11 and over. 50 to 100 mg at least 5 times/day.
Children to age 11. Dosage individualized based on severity of deficiency.
TO TREAT HYPERLIPIDEMIA (NIACIN ONLY)
E.R. CAPSULES, E.R. TABLETS, ORAL SOLUTION, TABLETS
Adults. *Initial:* 1,000 mg t.i.d. Dosage increased by 500 mg/day every 2 to 4 wk, as needed. *Maintenance:* 1 to 2 g t.i.d. *Maximum:* 6 g/day.
DOSAGE ADJUSTMENT To reduce or prevent facial flushing, initial dosage reduced to 100 mg/day (tab) or 500 mg/day (E.R. tab), and then gradually increased to 3 to 4 g/day.

- Be aware that I.V. administration of vitamin B_3 may cause CNS or CV adverse reactions, such as arrhythmias, dizziness, headache, peripheral vasodilation, and syncope. Rate of I.V. administration shouldn't exceed 2 mg/min, regardless of method of I.V. administration.
- Vitamin B_3 must be diluted for I.V. use. For direct injection, dilute to 2 mg/ml; for intermittent or continuous infusion, dilute dose in 500 ml of normal saline or other compatible solution.
- Give I.M. injection following routine I.M. administration guidelines. Vitamin B_3 doesn't need to be diluted for I.M. injection.
- Be aware that parenteral administration shouldn't be used to treat hyperlipidemia.

TO TREAT VITAMIN B_6 DEFICIENCY
E.R. CAPSULES, TABLETS
Adults and children. Dosage individualized based on severity of deficiency, as prescribed.
E.R. TABLETS
Adults. Dosage individualized based on severity of deficiency, as prescribed.
I.V. INFUSION
Adults and children. Dosage individualized as part of total parenteral nutrition.

- Be aware that SubQ or I.M. administration of vitamin B_6 may cause injectionsite burning or stinging. Before giving injection, alert patient that this adverse effect may occur.
- Know that I.V. administration is given as part of a multivitamin solution; follow the guidelines for administering an I.V. multivitamin solution as recommended for the product being used.

(continued)

Vitamins *(continued)*

GENERIC AND TRADE NAMES	RECOMMENDED DAILY INTAKE
vitamin B$_6$ *(continued)*	***Children ages 7 to 10.*** 1.4 mg/day. ***Children ages 4 to 6.*** 1.1 mg/day. ***Neonates and children to age 3.*** 0.3 to 1 mg/day. ***Adult men and boys age 11 and over.*** 1.7 to 2 mg/day. ***Adult women and girls age 11 and over.*** 1.4 to 1.6 mg/day. ***Pregnant women.*** 2.2 mg/day. ***Breastfeeding women.*** 2.1 mg/day.
vitamin B$_9$ (folic acid) Apo-Folic (CAN), Folvite, Novo-Folacid (CAN)	***Adult men and boys age 11 and over.*** 150 to 400 mcg/day. (150 to 220 mcg/day [CAN].) ***Adult women and girls age 11 and over.*** 150 to 400 mcg/day. (145 to 190 mcg/day [CAN].) ***Pregnant women.*** 400 to 800 mcg/day. (445 to 475 mcg/day [CAN].) ***Breastfeeding women.*** 260 to 800 mcg/day. (245 to 275 mcg/day [CAN].) ***Children ages 7 to 11.*** 100 to 400 mcg/day. (125 to 180 mcg/day [CAN].) ***Children ages 4 to 7.*** 75 to 400 mcg/day. (90 mcg/day [CAN].) ***Neonates and children to age 4.*** 25 mcg/day. (50 to 80 mcg/day [CAN].)
vitamin B$_{12}$ (cyanocobalamin, hydroxycobalamin)	***Adults age 19 and over.*** 2.4 mcg/day. ***Pregnant women.*** 2.6 mcg/day. ***Breastfeeding women.*** 2.8 mcg/day. ***Adolescents ages 14 to 19.*** 2.4 mcg/day. ***Children ages 9 to 14.*** 1.8 mcg/day. ***Children ages 4 to 9.*** 1.2 mcg/day. ***Children ages 1 to 4.*** 0.9 mcg/day. ***Infants ages 6 to 12 months.*** 0.4 mcg/day. ***Neonates and infants to 6 months.*** 0.5 mcg/day.

OTHER INDICATIONS AND DOSAGES

TO TREAT PYRIDOXINE DEPENDENCY SYNDROME
I.V. OR I.M. INJECTION
Adults and children age 11 and over. 30 to 600 mg daily.
Infants with seizures. *Initial:* 10 to 100 mg, then individualized based on severity of deficiency, as prescribed.
TO TREAT DRUG-INDUCED PYRIDOXINE DEFICIENCY
I.V. OR I.M. INJECTION
Adults and children age 11 and over. 50 to 200 mg/day
for 3 wk, then 25 to 100 mg/day, as needed.

TO TREAT VITAMIN B₉ DEFICIENCY
TABLETS
Adults and children. Dosage individualized based on severity of deficiency, as prescribed.
I.V. INFUSION, I.M. OR SUBCUTANEOUS INJECTION
Adults and children. 0.25 to 1 mg daily until hematologic response occurs.

TO TREAT VITAMIN B₁₂ DEFICIENCY
Caused by nutritional intake imbalance (not for use to treat pernicious anemia) lozenges, tablets
Adults and children. Dosage individualized based on severity of deficiency, as prescribed.
Caused by pernicious anemia; malabsorption disorders (tropical or nontropical sprue, partial or total gastrectomy, regional enteritis, gastroenterostomy, ileal resection); or malignancies, granulomas, strictures, or anastomoses involving the ileum.
SUBCUTANEOUS INJECTION (CYANOCOBALAMIN)
Adults. *Initial:* 30 mcg daily for 5 to 10 days, then switched to I.M. administration for maintenance therapy.

PARENTERAL ADMINISTRATION GUIDELINES

- Vitamin B_6 may increase AST (SGOT) levels. Be aware that at least one manufacturer warns against I.V. administration of vitamin B_6 to patients with heart disease.
- Take precautions to protect vitamin B_6 solution from exposure to light because it's light sensitive.

- Be aware that some vitamin B_9 solutions contain benzyl alcohol. Don't administer these solutions to neonates or immature infants because of a risk of fatal toxic syndrome, which may include CNS, respiratory, circulatory, and renal impairment and metabolic acidosis.
- Unless ordered otherwise, dilute 5 mg/ml of vitamin B_9 with 49 ml of sterile water for injection to provide a solution containing 0.1 mg of vitamin/ml.
- Know that parenteral administration may cause anaphylaxis. Parenteral administration should be used only in patients with severe vitamin deficiency or in those with severely impaired GI absorption.
- Be aware that SubQ administration should be injected deep.
- Take precautions to protect vitamin B_9 solution from exposure to light because it's light sensitive.

- Be aware that parenteral vitamin B_{12} solution is incompatible with many drugs, including ascorbic acid, chlorpromazine hydrochloride, dextrose, heavy metals, phytonadione, prochlorperazine edisylate, warfarin sodium, oxidizing or reducing agents, and alkaline or strongly acidic solutions. Do not administer vitamin with other drugs.
- Know that both cyanocobalamin and hydroxycobalamin may be administered by I.M. injection, but only cyanocobalamin may be administered as a SubQ injection. Be alert to which form is being administered to ensure correct route of administration.

(continued)

Vitamins *(continued)*

GENERIC AND TRADE NAMES	RECOMMENDED DAILY INTAKE
vitamin B₁₂ *(continued)*	**Children ages 7 to 10**. 1 mg/day. (0.8 to 1 mg/day [CAN].) **Children ages 4 to 7**. 0.9 mg/day. (0.7 mg/day [CAN].) **Children ages 1 to 4**. 0.3 to 0.7 mg/day. (0.3 to 0.6 mg/day [CAN].)
vitamin C (ascorbic acid) Ascorbic Acid, Cecon Drops, Cenolate, Cevi-Bid, Vicks Vitamin C Drops	*Adult men.* 90 mg/day. *Adult women.* 75 mg/day. *Pregnant women age 19 and over.* 85 mg/day. *Breastfeeding women age 19 and over.* 120 mg/day. *Adolescent boys ages 14 to 19.* 75 mg/day. *Adolescent girls ages 14 to 19.* 65 mg/day. *Pregnant girls ages 14 to 19.* 80 mg/day. *Breastfeeding girls ages 14 to 19.* 115 mg/day. *Children ages 9 to 14.* 45 mg/day. *Children ages 4 to 9.* 25 mg/day. *Children ages 1 to 4.* 15 mg/day. *Infants ages 7 to 12 months.* 50 mg/day. *Neonates and infants to age 7 months.* 40 mg/day. *Dosage Adjustment* Recommended daily intake for people who smoke is 100 mg/day because of an increased utilization of vitamin C. Recommended daily intake should be increased to promote wound healing and for those with a chronic illness, fever, hemovascular disorder, or infection; the amount of vitamin C increase depends on the severity of the underlying condition.

OTHER INDICATIONS AND DOSAGES

Children. *Initial:* 1,000 to 5,000 mcg given in single daily doses of 100 mcg over 2 or more wk. *Maintenance:* 60 or more mcg/mo.

I.M. INJECTION (CYANOCOBALAMIN OR HYDROXYCOBALAMIN)

Adults. *Initial:* 30 mcg daily for 5 to 10 days. *Maintenance:* 100 to 200 mcg every mo.

Children. *Initial:* 1,000 to 5,000 mcg, given in single daily doses of 100 mcg over 2 or more wk. *Maintenance:* 60 or more mcg/mo.

DOSAGE ADJUSTMENT Dosage adjusted, as needed, to maintain normal hematologic morphology and an erythrocyte count greater than 4.5 million/mm.

Adults. *Initial.* 1 mg/wk for 3 wk. *Maintenance:* 250 mcg/mo.

TO TREAT FAMILIAL SELECTIVE B₁₂ MALABSORPTION

I.M. INJECTION (CYANOCOBALAMIN)

TO TREAT HEREDITARY DEFICIENCY OF TRANSCOBALAMIN II

I.M. INJECTION (CYANOCOBALAMIN)

Adults. 1 to 2 mg/wk.

TO TREAT VITAMIN C DEFICIENCY (SCURVY)

E.R. CAPSULES; LOZENGES; ORAL SOLUTION; E.R. TABLETS; TABLETS; SUBCUTANEOUS, I.M., OR I.V. INJECTION

Adults. 100 to 250 mg once or twice daily until skeletal changes and signs and symptoms of hemorrhagic disorder are reversed (usually within 2 to 21 days).

ORAL SOLUTION; TABLETS; SUBCUTANEOUS, I.M.,OR I.V. INJECTION

Infants and children. 100 to 300 mg/day in divided doses until skeletal changes and signs and symptoms of hemorrhagic disorder are reversed (usually within days).

PARENTERAL ADMINISTRATION GUIDELINES

• Be aware that SubQ administration of cyanocobalamin should be injected deeply.
• Know that vitamin B₁₂ is excreted more rapidly after I.V. injection; I.V. administration isn't recommended.
• Take precautions to protect vitamin B₁₂ solution from exposure to light because it's light sensitive.

• Be aware that I.M. injection is the preferred parenteral route for administering vitamin C, although it may be administered I.V. or SubQ when necessary.
• Rotate sites for I.M. and SubQ administration to help prevent transient mild soreness that may occur following administration. Inform patient that this adverse effect may occur.
• If giving I.V. vitamin C, avoid rapid administration to prevent faintness or dizziness.
• Administer vitamin C solution by itself because it's incompatible with many drugs.
• Be aware that vitamin C solution rapidly oxidizes in air and in alkaline solutions. Take precautions to protect vitamin solution from exposure to air and light.
• Open vitamin C ampules carefully because increased pressure may develop after prolonged storage.

(continued)

Vitamins *(continued)*

GENERIC AND TRADE NAMES	RECOMMENDED DAILY INTAKE
vitamin D₂ (ergocalciferol) Calciferol, Calciferol Drops, Drisdol, Drisdol Drops, Ostoforte (CAN), Radiostol Forte (CAN)	***Adults and children ages 11 and over.*** 200 to 400 IU/day. (100 to 200 IU/day [CAN].) ***Pregnant and breastfeeding women.*** 400 IU/day. (200 to 300 IU/day [CAN].) ***Children ages 7 to 11.*** 400 IU/day. (100 to 200 IU/day [CAN].) ***Children ages 4 to 7.*** 400 IU/day. (200 IU/day [CAN].) ***Neonates and children to age 4.*** 300 to 400 IU/day. (200 to 400 IU/day [CAN].)
vitamin E (alpha tocopherol) Amino-Opti-E, Aquasol E, E-Complex 600, E-Vitamin succinate, Liqui-E, Pheryl E, Vita-Plus E, Webber Vitamin E (CAN)	***Adult men and adolescent boys.*** 16.7 IU/day. (10 to 16.7 IU/day [CAN].) ***Adult women and adolescent girls.*** 13 IU/day. (8.3 to 11.7 IU/day [CAN].) ***Pregnant women.*** 16.7 IU/day. (13 to 15 IU/day [CAN].) ***Breastfeeding women.*** 18 to 20 IU/day. (15 to 16.7 IU/day [CAN].) ***Children ages 7 to 10.*** 11.7 IU/day. (10 to 13 IU/day [CAN].) ***Children ages 4 to 7.*** 11.7 IU/day. (8.3 IU/day [CAN].) ***Infants and children to age 4.*** 5 to 10 IU/day. (5 to 6.7 IU/day [CAN].)

OTHER INDICATIONS AND DOSAGES

PARENTERAL ADMINISTRATION GUIDELINES

TO TREAT VITAMIN D₂ DEFICIENCY
CAPSULES, ORAL SOLUTION, TABLETS
Adults and children. Dosage individualized based on severity of deficiency, as prescribed.
TO TREAT VITAMIN D-RESISTANT RICKETS
CAPSULES, ORAL SOLUTION, TABLETS
Adults. 12,000 to 150,000 IU units daily
TO TREAT VITAMIN D-DEPENDENT RICKETS
CAPSULES, ORAL SOLUTION, TABLETS
Adults. 10,000 to 60,000 IU daily *Maximum:* 150,000 IU daily.
Children. 3,000 to 10,000 IU daily. *Maximum:* 50,000 IU daily.
TO TREAT OSTEOMALACIA CAUSED BY LONG-TERM ANTICONVULSANT USE
CAPSULES, ORAL SOLUTION, TABLETS
Adults. 1,000 to 4,000 IU daily.
Children. 1,000 IU daily.
TO TREAT FAMILIAL HYPOPHOSPHATEMIA
CAPSULES
Adults. 50,000 to 100,000 IU daily.
TO TREAT HYPOPARATHYROIDISM
CAPSULES
Adults. 50,000 to 150,000 IU daily.
Children. 50,000 to 200,000 IU daily.
TO TREAT INTESTINAL MALABSORPTION
I.M. INJECTION
Adults and children. 10,000 IU daily.

- Be aware that vitamin D₂ is usually given orally. However, I.M. injection may be required for patients with GI, liver, or biliary disease associated with malabsorption of vitamin D analogues.
- Take precautions to protect parenteral vitamin D₂ solution from exposure to light because light causes it to decompose.

TO TREAT VITAMIN E DEFICIENCY
CAPSULES (ADULTS ONLY), ORAL SOLUTION, TABLETS
Adults and children. Dosage individualized based on severity of deficiency, as prescribed.

Vitamin E isn't administered parenterally.

(continued)

Vitamins *(continued)*

GENERIC AND TRADE NAMES	RECOMMENDED DAILY INTAKE
vitamin K₁ (phytonadione) AquaMEPHYTON, Mephyton	*Recommended daily intake hasn't been established for vitamin K_1. However, adequate intake is suggested as follows:* ***Adult men age 19 and over.*** 120 mcg/day. ***Adult women age 19 and over, pregnant and breast-feeding women.*** 90 mcg/day. ***Adolescents ages 14 to 19.*** 75 mcg/day. ***Children ages 9 to 14.*** 60 mcg/day. ***Children ages 4 to 9.*** 55 mcg/day. ***Children ages 1 to 4.*** 30 mcg/day. ***Infants ages 7 to 12 months.*** 2.5 mcg/day. ***Neonates and infants to age 7 months.*** 2 mcg/day.

OTHER INDICATIONS AND DOSAGES

TO PREVENT HYPOPROTHROMBINEMIA
DURING PROLONGED USE OF TOTAL PARENTERAL
NUTRITION
I.M. INJECTION
Adults. 5 to 10 mg/wk.
Children. 2 to 5 mg/wk.
TO PREVENT HYPOPROTHROMBINEMIA IN INFANTS WITH
DIETS DEFICIENT IN VITAMIN K (LESS THAN 100 MCG/L)
I.M. INJECTION
Infants. 1 mg/mo.
TO TREAT ANTICOAGULANT-INDUCED
HYPOPROTHROMBINEMIA TABLETS,
I.M. OR SUBCUTANEOUS INJECTION
Adults. 2.5 to 25 mg, repeated 12 to 48 hr after P.O.
dose or 6 to 8 hr after SubQ or I.M. dose, as prescribed.
Maximum: 50 mg/dose.
Children. 2.5 to 10 mg SubQ or I.M., repeated in 6 to 8 hr,
as prescribed.
Infants. 1 to 2 mg SubQ or I.M., repeated in 4 to 8 hr, as
prescribed.
TO TREAT HYPOPROTHROMBINEMIA FROM OTHER CAUSES
TABLETS, I.M. OR SUBCUTANEOUS INJECTION
Adults. 2 to 25 mg. *Usual:* 25 mg.
Maximum: 50 mg/dose.
Children. 5 to 10 mg SubQ or I.M.
Infants. 2 mg SubQ or I.M.
TO PREVENT HEMORRHAGIC DISEASE IN
NEONATES
I.M. OR SUBCUTANEOUS INJECTION
Neonates. 0.5 to 1 mg within 1 hr after birth, repeated in
6 to 8 hr, as prescribed.
TO TREAT HEMORRHAGIC DISEASE IN NEONATES
I.M. OR SUBCUTANEOUS INJECTION
Neonates. 1 mg (or higher dose if mother took an oral
anticoagulant or anticonvulsant during pregnancy).

PARENTERAL ADMINISTRATION GUIDELINES

- Be aware that severe adverse reactions, including anaphylaxis, cardiac and respiratory arrest, hypersensitivity, and shock, may occur during or immediately after I.M. or I.V. administration of vitamin K_1, even if it's diluted to avoid rapid infusion. Administer vitamin by SubQ route whenever possible.
- If vitamin K_1 must be administered I.V., do not exceed rate of 1 mg/min, as prescribed.
- Be aware that some vitamin K_1 solutions contain benzyl alcohol. Don't administer these solutions to neonates or immature infants because of a risk of fatal toxic syndrome, which may include CNS, respiratory, circulatory, and renal impairment and metabolic acidosis.
- Take precautions to protect vitamin K_1 solution from exposure to light because it's light sensitive.

Interferons

Interferons are classified as biological response modifiers or antineoplastics. They fall into three major categories—alpha, beta, and gamma—which are described below.

The table on the following pages lists the trade names, indications, usual adult dosages, adverse reactions, and nursing considerations for these interferons.

Interferon alpha

Highly purified proteins produced by a recombinant DNA process, drugs in this category exhibit antiviral and antitumor activity. Antiviral activity depends on their inhibition of viral protein synthesis. Antitumor activity results from their ability to exert a cytostatic effect, reducing the rate of cell proliferation by delaying RNA and protein production. This delay induces cells to enter a resting stage. These drugs also increase the activity of human natural killer (NK) cells, which have the ability to lyse certain tumor cells and normal targets. They also selectively increase the number of cytotoxic T-cells, thereby affecting tumor growth. Phagocytic activity of macrophages also is increased.

INTERFERON ALFACON

This specific form of interferon is produced by fermentation of genetically engineered *Escherichia coli*. It's structurally and functionally related to interferon beta and has greater biological activity than other interferon alfas.

Interferon beta

Produced by fibroblasts and epithelial cells, drugs in this category neutralize the activity

GENERIC AND TRADE NAMES	INDICATIONS AND USUAL ADULT DOSAGES
Interferon alpha drugs	
interferon alfa-n3 Alferon N	*To treat condyloma acuminatum:* 250,000 units intralesionally at base of wart 2 times/wk for up to 8 wk.
peginterferon alfa-2a PEGASYS	*As monotherapy to treat patients with chronic heptatitis C who have compensated liver disease and have never received an interferon alpha, to treat patients with chronic hepatitis B who have compensated liver disease and evidence of viral replication and liver inflammation:* 180 mcg/wk SubQ for 48 wk.
peginterferon alfa-2b PEG-Intron Sylatron	*As adjunct to treat patients with chronic hepatitis C who have compensated liver disease and have never received an interferon alpha:* 180 mcg/wk SubQ with ribavirin (Copegus) 800 to 1,200 mg/day P.O. in 2 divided doses with food for 48 wk.
	To treat patients with chronic hepatitis C: 1 mcg/kg/wk (PEG-Intron) SubQ every wk on the same day of the wk for 1 year.
	To treat patients with chronic hepatitis C in combination with ribavirin: 1.5 mcg/kg (PEG-Intron) SubQ every wk on the same day of the wk for 48 wk.
	As adjunct treatment of melanoma with microscopic or gross nodal involvement within 84 days of definitive surgical resection: 6 mcg/kg/wk (Sylatron) SubQ for 8 doses followed by 3 mcg/kg/wk (Sylatron) SubQ for up to 5 years.
recombinant interferon alfa-2b Intron A	*To treat hairy cell leukemia:* 2 million units/m^2 I.M. or SubQ 3 times/wk.
	To treat condyloma acuminatum: 1 million units (using only the 10-million units/ml strength) intralesionally at base of wart (up to 5 warts/course) 3 times/wk on alternate days for 3 wk. If response is inadequate 12 to 16 wk after initial treatment, repeat course, as prescribed.

of endogenous interferon gamma (IFNG), the substance believed to be responsible for triggering the autoimmune process that leads to multiple sclerosis. In multiple sclerosis, an initial viral infection may stimulate IFNG production by T cells. Then IFNG induces macrophages to produce proteinases that degrade the myelin sheath around the nerves and spinal cord. Cytotoxic T cells then move to the site of inflammation, recognizing antigens as receptor sites, where they attack the tissue affected by IFNG, resulting in progressive neurologic dysfunction. Interferon beta drugs interfere with IFNG production by lymphocytes and the mRNA transcription caused by IFNG. As a result, cytotoxic T cells can't locate receptor sites and cause further damage in the CNS.

Interferon gamma

Produced from genetically engineered *E. coli*, this type of interferon is chemically and therapeutically distinct from interferon alpha. Drugs in this category have potent phagocyte-activating properties. By enhancing oxidative metabolism, they produce toxic oxygen metabolites in phagocytes, which permits more efficient killing of certain fungi, bacteria, and protozoal microbes. Enhanced antibody-dependent cellular cytotoxicity and NK-cell activity reduce the risk of developing a serious infection in patients with chronic disease. These drugs also stimulate production of cytokines, such as interleukin-1-beta, and regulate the immune system by suppressing the IgE level and inhibiting collagen production.

ADVERSE REACTIONS	NURSING CONSIDERATIONS
CNS: Depression, dizziness, fatigue, headache, homicidal or suicidal ideation, psychosis, seizures, peripheral neuropathy, vertigo **CV:** Hypertriglyceridemia, hypertension, hypotension, palpitations **EENT:** Dry mouth, hearing loss, retinal detachment (with ribavirin) **GI:** Anorexia, diarrhea, hepatotoxicity, nausea, vomiting **GU:** Renal failure **HEME:** Anemia, leukopenia, pure red cell aplasia, thrombocytopenia, thrombotic thrombocytopenic purpura **MS:** Myositis, rhabdomyolysis **SKIN:** Alopecia, rash, Stevens-Johnson syndrome, toxic epidermal necrolysis, urticaria Other: Anaphylaxis, angioedema, bacterial infections, flulike symptoms, liver or renal graft rejection, sepsis, systemic lupus erythematosus	• Use interferon alpha drugs cautiously in patients with renal impairment and in elderly patients. • Be aware that cross-sensitivity may occur among interferon alpha drugs. • Be aware that interferon alpha drugs aren't interchangeable. • Be aware that patients who are sensitive to mouse immunoglobulin also may be sensitive to recombinant interferon alfa-2a. • Unless contraindicated, ensure that patient is well hydrated at the start of and throughout therapy to reduce the risk of hypotension. • Reconstitute by adding 3 ml of diluent provided by manufacturer and swirling gently to dissolve. • Be aware that reconstitution of peginterferon alfa-2a and interferon alfa-n3 is not necessary. • Don't shake vial. • Be aware that cross-sensitivity with interferon alfa-n3 to mouse immunoglobulin, egg protein, or neomycin may occur. ***WARNING*** Because interferon alpha drugs may cause or aggravate fatal or life-threatening autoimmune, ischemic, infectious, or neuropsychiatric disorders, monitor patient periodically with clinical and laboratory evaluations and expect drug to be discontinued if he develops severe or worsening signs and symptoms of these conditions.

(continued)

Interferons *(continued)*

GENERIC AND TRADE NAMES	INDICATIONS AND USUAL ADULT DOSAGES

Interferon alpha drugs *(continued)*

To treat AIDS-related Kaposi's sarcoma: 30 million units/m^2 (using 50 million units/ml) I.M. or SubQ 3 times/wk.

To treat chronic, active hepatitis B and C: 3 million units I.M. or SubQ 3 times/wk.

To treat chronic hepatitis B: 5 million units/day or 10 million units 3 times/wk I.M. or SubQ for 16 wk.

To treat malignant melanoma: 20 million units/m^2 as I.V. infusion for 5 consecutive days/wk for 4 wk, followed by 10 million units/m^2 SubQ 3 times/wk for 48 wk.

Interferon beta drugs

interferon alfacon-1 Infergen	*To treat chronic, active hepatitis C:* 9 mcg SubQ 3 times/wk, at intervals of at least 48 hours, for 24 wk. If inadequate response or relapse occurs, 15 mcg SubQ 3 times/wk, for up to 48 wk. *As adjunct with ribavirin to treat chronic active hepatitis C:* 15 mcg SubQ 3 times/wk at intervals of at least 48 hr, for up to 48 wk.

Interferon beta drugs

interferon beta-1a Avonex	*To treat initial attack or relapsing forms of multiple sclerosis:* 30 mcg I.M. once/wk.
Rebif	*To treat relapsing forms of multiple sclerosis:* 44 mcg SubQ 3 times/wk.
interferon beta-1b Betaseron, Extavia	*To treat relapsing forms of multiple sclerosis:* 63 mcg SubQ on day 1, then 94 mcg SubQ on day 15, and then 125 mcq SubQ on day 29 and every 14 days thereafter.
peginterferon beta-1a Plegridy	*To treat relapsing forms of multiple sclerosis:* 0.25 mg SubQ every other day.

ADVERSE REACTIONS	NURSING CONSIDERATIONS
	• Obtain CBC before and regularly during treatment, as ordered, because interferon alpha drugs may cause bone marrow suppression. Expect drug to be discontinued if patient develops severe decreases in platelet or neutrophil count. • Implement bleeding and infection-control measures, according to facility policy. • Use gamma interferon cautiously in patients previously exposed to cytotoxic drugs or radiation therapy. • Be aware that cross-sensitivity may occur with *Escherichia coli*– derived products. • Discard vial if left at room temperature for more than 12 hours. • Implement bleeding and infection-control measures, according to facility policy. • Administer acetaminophen, as prescribed, to prevent or treat headache and fever.
CNS: Anxiety, confusion, decreased concentration, depression, insomnia, nervousness **EENT:** Abnormal vision **HEME:** Leukopenia, thrombocytopenia	• Be aware that use of interferon alfacon-1 isn't recommended for patients with autoimmune hepatitis or psychiatric disorders. • Be aware that cross-sensitivity may occur with other interferon alfa drugs or *Escherichia coli*–derived products. • Don't shake vial. • Implement bleeding and infection-control measures, according to facility policy. • Monitor patient for signs and symptoms of vision abnormalities.
CNS: Anxiety, confusion, depression, dizziness, emotional lability, fatigue, headache, seizures, suicidal ideation, weakness **CV:** Cardiomyopathy, palpitations, tachycardia, vasodilation **EENT:** Retinal vascular disorders **ENDO:** Thyroid dysfunction **GI:** Autoimmune hepatitis, diarrhea, elevated liver enzyme levels, nausea, pancreatitis, vomiting **HEME:** Anemia, hemolytic uremic syndrome, leukopenia, pancytopenia thrombocytopenia **RESP:** Bronchospasm **SKIN:** Alopecia, pruritus, skin discoloration, urticaria **Other:** Anaphylaxis, flulike symptoms, infection, injection-site reactions (including necrosis), systemic lupus erythematosus, weight changes	• Use beta interferons with extreme caution in patients with depression or seizure disorder. • Be aware that cross-sensitivity may occur with natural or recombinant interferon beta or human albumin. • Reconstitute following manufacturer's directions and refrigerate. Use interferon beta-1a within 6 hours of reconstitution. Use interferon beta-1b within 3 hours of reconstitution. • Implement bleeding and infection-control measures, according to facility policy.

(continued)

Interferons *(continued)*

GENERIC AND TRADE NAMES	INDICATIONS AND USUAL ADULT DOSAGES

Interferon gamma drugs

interferon gamma-1b
Actimmune

To treat chronic granulomatous disease or to delay progression of severe, malignant osteopetrosis in patients with body surface area greater than 0.5 m²: 50 mcg/m² (1 million IU/m²) SubQ 3 times/wk.

To treat chronic granulomatous disease or to delay progression of severe, malignant osteopetrosis in patients with body surface area of 0.5 m² or less: 1.5 mcg/kg/dose SubQ 3 times/wk.

ADVERSE REACTIONS	NURSING CONSIDERATIONS
CNS: Fatigue, headache **GI:** Diarrhea, nausea, vomiting **HEME:** Leukopenia **SKIN:** Rash **Other:** Flulike symptoms	• Use gamma interferon cautiously in patients previously exposed to cytotoxic drugs or radiation therapy. • Be aware that cross-sensitivity may occur with *Escherichia coli*–derived products. • Discard vial if left at room temperature for more than 12 hours. • Implement bleeding and infection-control measures, according to facility policy. • Administer acetaminophen, as prescribed, to prevent or treat headache and fever.

Compatible Drugs in a Syringe

The table below lets you know at a glance whether particular drugs are compatible for at least 15 minutes when mixed together in a syringe for immediate administration. However, keep in mind that drugs listed as compatible when mixed in a syringe may not be compatible when prepared for other routes of adminis-

tration. Drug combinations prepared for immediate administration usually require a more concentrated solution than those prepared for infusion.

Key: C = Compatible; I = Incompatible; n/a = Compatibility information not available, no recommendations can be given.

	atropine	chlorpromazine	dexamethasone	diazepam	diphenhydramine	droperidol	furosemide	glycopyrrolate	haloperidol	
atropine		C	n/a	n/a	C	C	n/a	C	I	
chlorpromazine	C		n/a	n/a	C	C	n/a	C	n/a	
dexamethasone	n/a	n/a		n/a	I	n/a	n/a	n/a	n/a	
diazepam	n/a	n/a	n/a		n/a	n/a	n/a	I	n/a	
diphenhydramine	C	C	I	n/a		C	n/a	C	I	
droperidol	C	C	n/a	n/a	C		I	C	n/a	
furosemide	n/a	n/a	n/a	n/a	n/a	I		n/a	n/a	
glycopyrrolate	C	C	I	C	C	C	n/a		C	
haloperidol	n/a	n/a	n/a	n/a	C	n/a	n/a	n/a		
heparin	C	I	n/a	I	n/a	I	C	n/a	I	
hydromorphone	C	C	n/a	n/a	C	n/a	n/a	C	C	
hydroxyzine	C	C	n/a	n/a	C	C	n/a	C	I	
ketorolac	n/a	n/a	n/a	I	n/a	n/a	n/a	n/a	I	
lidocaine	n/a	n/a	n/a	n/a	n/a	n/a	n/a	C	n/a	
lorazepam	n/a	n/a	n/a	n/a	n/a	n/a	n/a	n/a	n/a	
meperidine	C	C	n/a	C	C	C	n/a	C	n/a	
metoclopramide	C	C	n/a	n/a	C	C	I	n/a	n/a	
midazolam	C	C	n/a	n/a	C	n/a	n/a	C	C	
morphine	C	C	n/a	n/a	C	C	n/a	C	I	
pentobarbital	C	I	n/a	n/a	I	I	n/a	I	n/a	
prochlorperazine	C	n/a	n/a	n/a	C	C	n/a	C	n/a	
ranitidine	C	I	C	n/a	C	n/a	n/a	C	n/a	
scopolamine	C	C	n/a	n/a	C	C	n/a	C	n/a	

heparin	hydromorphone	hydroxyzine	ketorolac	lidocaine	lorazepam	meperidine	metoclopramide	midazolam	morphine	pentobarbital	prochlorperazine	ranitidine	scopolamine
n/a	C	C	n/a	n/a	n/a	C	C	C	C	C	C	C	C
I	C	C	n/a	n/a	n/a	C	C	C	I	I	C	C	C
n/a	C	n/a	n/a	n/a	n/a	n/a	C	n/a	n/a	n/a	n/a	C	n/a
I	n/a	n/a	I	n/a	n/a	n/a	n/a	n/a	n/a	n/a	n/a	I	n/a
n/a	C	C	n/a	n/a	n/a	C	C	C	C	I	C	C	C
I	n/a	C	n/a	n/a	n/a	C	C	C	C	I	C	n/a	C
C	n/a	n/a	n/a	n/a	n/a	n/a	I	n/a	n/a	n/a	n/a	n/a	n/a
n/a	C	C	n/a	C	n/a	C	n/a	C	C	I	C	C	C
I	C	I	I	n/a	n/a	n/a	n/a	n/a	I	n/a	n/a	n/a	n/a
	n/a	n/a	n/a	C	n/a	I	C	n/a	C	n/a	n/a	n/a	n/a
n/a		C	I	n/a	C	n/a	n/a	C	n/a	C	I	C	C
n/a	C		I	C	n/a	C	C	C	C	I	C	C	C
n/a	I	I		n/a	n/a	n/a	n/a	n/a	n/a	n/a	I	n/a	n/a
C	n/a	C	n/a		n/a	n/a	C	n/a	n/a	n/a	n/a	n/a	n/a
n/a	C	n/a	n/a	n/a		n/a	n/a	n/a	n/a	n/a	n/a	I	n/a
I	n/a	C	n/a	n/a	n/a		C	I	I	C	C	C	C
C	C	n/a	n/a	C	n/a	C		C	C	n/a	C	C	C
n/a	C	C	n/a	n/a	n/a	C	C		C	I	I	I	C
C*	n/a	C	n/a	n/a	n/a	n/a	C	C		I	C	C	C
n/a	C	I	n/a	n/a	n/a	I	I	I	I		I	I	C
n/a	I	C	I	n/a	n/a	C	C	I	C	I		C	C
n/a	C	I	n/a	n/a	I	C	C	I	C	I	C		C
n/a	C	C	n/a	n/a	n/a	C	C	C	C	C	C	C	

* Compatible only with morphine doses of 1 mg, 2 mg, and 5 mg.

Drug Formulas and Calculations

When giving drugs, you must be familiar with drug formulas and calculation methods to make sure your patient receives the prescribed drug in the correct dosage, strength, or flow rate. This appendix offers a quick review of ways to calculate the strength of a solution, drug dosages, and I.V. flow rates.

Calculating the Strength of a Solution

Most solutions are prepared in the required strength by the pharmacy or medical supply source. But sometimes only a concentrated form is available, and you'll need to dilute the solution or solid to administer the prescribed strength.

When a solid form of a drug is used to prepare a solution, the drug must be completely dissolved. Solid drug forms, such as tablets, crystals, and powders, are considered 100% strength. (An exception to this is boric acid, which is only 5% at full strength.) The final diluted solution is stated in terms of liquid measurement. To prepare a solution, you'll need to add the prescribed solid or liquid form of the drug (the solute) to the prescribed amount of diluent (the solvent). Two of the most common clinical diluents are normal saline solution and sterile water.

You can use two formulas to calculate the strength of xa solution, as shown in the examples below.

Method 1: Calculating percentage and volume
Use the following formula:

$$\frac{\text{Weaker Solution}}{\text{Stronger Solution}} = \frac{\text{Solute}}{\text{Solvent}}$$

Example: You need to dilute a stock solution of 100% strength to a 5% solution. How much solute will you need to add to obtain 500 ml of the 5% solution?

Calculate as follows:

$$\frac{5\,(\%)\,\text{(weaker solution)}}{100\,(\%)\,\text{(stronger solution)}} = \frac{X\,(g)\,\text{(solute)}}{500\,\text{ml (solvent)}}$$

$$100\,X = (500)(5)\ \text{or}\ 2,500$$

$$X = 25\,g$$

Answer: You'll need to add 25 g of solute to each 500 ml of solvent to prepare a 5% solution.

Method 2: Calculating percentage and volume
Use the following formula:

$$\frac{\text{(Desired Strength)}}{\text{(Available strength)}} \times \frac{\text{Total amount of}}{\text{desired solution}} = X\ \frac{\text{(amount of undiluted drug}}{\text{needed to make solution)}}$$

Example: You need to make 100 ml of a 20% solution, using an 80% solution. How much of the 80% solution must you add to the sterile water to yield a final volume of 100 ml of a 20% solution?

Calculate as follows:

$$\frac{20\,(\%)\text{(Desired Strength)}}{80\,(\%)\text{(Available strength)}} \times \frac{100\,\text{ml (Total amount}}{\text{of desired solution)}} = X$$

$$\frac{0.20}{0.80} = 0.25$$

Drug Formulas and Calculations *(continued)*

$$0.25 \times 100 \ (ml) = X$$

$$x = 25 \ ml \ of \ 80\% \ solution$$

Answer: You'll need to add 25 ml of the 80% solution to the water to make a final volume of 100 ml of a 20% solution.

Calculating Drug Dosages

You may be required to calculate drug dosages when you need to administer a drug that's available only in one measure, but prescribed in another. You should also be prepared to convert various units of measure, such as milligrams (mg) to grains (gr), and dry measurements to liquid. You can use three common methods of ratio and proportion to calculate drug dosages, as shown in the examples below.

CALCULATING ORAL DRUG DOSAGES

Example: You need to give a patient 0.25 mg of digoxin, which comes only in 0.125-mg tablets. How many tablets will you need to give him to attain the proper dosage?

Method 1: Using labeled amount of drug

In this method, true proportions between the drug label and the prescribed dose are used to determine ratio and proportion. The drug label, which states the amount of drug in one unit of measurement—in this case, 0.125 mg in each tablet of digoxin—is the first ratio, expressed as follows:

$$milligrams : tablets = milligrams : tablets$$

$$0.125 \ mg \ (amount \ of \ drug) : 1 \ tablet \ (unit \ of \ measure)$$

The prescribed dose—in this case, 0.25 mg—is the second ratio; it must be stated in the same order and units of measure as the first, as follows:

$$0.125 \ mg : 1 \ tablet = 0.25 \ mg : X \ (tablets)$$

Calculate as follows:

$$0.125 \ X = 0.25$$

$$X = \frac{0.25}{0.125}$$

$$X = 2$$

Answer: You'll need to give the patient 2 tablets of digoxin 0.125 mg.

Be sure to use critical thinking to assess whether your answer is correct. Because the amount of drug prescribed is greater than the amount of drug in one tablet, it's reasonable to expect the required number of tablets to be greater than one.

Method 2: Using an established formula

To determine the correct number of digoxin tablets to give using this method, use the following formula:

$$\frac{Prescribed \ dose}{Dose \ available} \times Quantity \ (unit \ of \ measure) = X \ (unknown \ quantity \ to \ be \ given)$$

(continued)

Drug Formulas and Calculations *(continued)*

Calculate as follows:

$$\frac{0.25 \text{ mg}}{0.125 \text{ mg}} \times 1 \text{ tablet} = X \text{ (number of 0.125-mg tablets)}$$

$$\frac{0.25}{0.125} = 2X$$

$$2 = X$$

Answer: You'll need to give the patient 2 tablets of digoxin 0.125 mg.

Method 3: Calculating according to proportion size

This method uses the same components as method #1, but the ratio is based on proportions according to size. To determine the correct number of digoxin tablets to give using this method, use the following formula:

$$\frac{\text{smaller}}{\text{larger}} = \frac{\text{smaller}}{\text{larger}}$$

Substitute 0.125 into the smaller part and 0.25 into the greater part of the first ratio. Critical thinking leads us to believe that you'll need more than 1 tablet of the weaker 0.125-mg strength to equal the stronger 0.25 mg. Set up the proportion as follows:

$$\frac{0.125 \text{ mg}}{0.25 \text{ mg}} = \frac{1 \text{ (tablet)}}{X \text{ (tablets)}}$$

Calculate as follows:

$$0.125 \, X = 0.25$$

$$X = \frac{0.25}{0.125}$$

$$X = 2 \text{ tablets}$$

Answer: You'll need to give the patient 2 tablets of digoxin 0.125 mg.

CALCULATING PARENTERAL DRUG DOSAGES

The same methods used for calculating oral drugs and solutions can be used for preparing parenteral injections.

Example: You need to administer a prescribed dose of 1 mg morphine sulfate from a unit-dose cartridge containing 4 mg per 2 ml. How many milliliters will you need to give to equal the prescribed dose of 1 mg?

Method 1: Using labeled amount of drug

Using the same ratio as for oral drugs, the drug label—in this case, 4 mg—is the first ratio, and the prescribed dose—in this case, 1 mg—is the second ratio, expressed as follows:

4 mg (the amount of drug) : 2 ml (the unit of measure)

Calculate as follows:

$$4 \text{ mg} : 2 \text{ ml} = 1 \text{ mg} : X \text{ ml}$$

$$4X = 2$$

$$X = \frac{2}{4}$$

$$X = 0.5 \text{ ml}$$

Drug Formulas and Calculations *(continued)*

Answer: You'll need to give 0.5 ml of morphine sulfate
to equal the prescribed dose of 1 mg.

Method 2: Using an established formula
Use this formula:

$$\frac{\text{Prescribed dose}}{\text{Dose available}} \times \text{Quantity (unit of measure)} = \text{X (unknown quantity to be given)}$$

Calculate as follows:

$$\frac{1\ mg}{4\ mg} \times 2\ ml = X\ (\text{number of ml})$$

$$\frac{4}{2} = 0.5$$

Answer: You'll need to give 0.5 ml of morphine sulfate
to equal the prescribed dose of 1 mg.

Method 3: Calculating according to proportion size
To determine the correct amount of morphine sulfate to give using this method, use the
following formula:

$$\text{smaller : greater} = \text{smaller : greater}$$

$$\text{milligrams : milligrams} = \text{milliliters : milliliters}$$

Critical thinking leads us to believe that 1 mg is less than 4 mg and that you'll need less
than 2 ml to give 1 mg of the drug; therefore, 1 mg goes into the smaller part of the first
ratio, and X goes into the smaller part of the second ratio. Set up the proportion as follows:

$$1\ mg : 4\ mg = X\ (ml) : 2\ ml$$

$$4X = 2$$

$$X = \frac{2}{4}$$

$$X = 0.5$$

Answer: You'll need to give 0.5 ml of morphine sulfate
to equal the prescribed dose of 1 mg.

Calculating I.V. Flow Rates
When an I.V. solution is delivered by gravity, you must calculate the number of drops
needed per minute for proper infusion. To calculate I.V. flow rates, you need to know
three things:
- The drip factor—or the number of drops contained in 1 ml for the type of I.V. set you'll be
using. This information is provided on the individual package label.
- The amount and type of fluid that you'll infuse as prescribed on the physician's order sheet
- The infusion duration time in minutes.
    Once you've gathered this information, you can calculate the I.V. flow rate using the
following equation:

$$\frac{\text{Total number of ml}}{\text{Total number of minutes}} \times \text{drip factor (gtt/ml)} = \text{flow rate (gtt/min)}$$

(continued)

Drug Formulas and Calculations *(continued)*

Example 1: If the physician prescribes 1,000 ml of D_5W to infuse over 10 hours, and the drip rate for your administration set is 15 drops (gtt) per ml, calculate as follows:

$$\frac{1,000 \text{ ml}}{10 \text{ hours} \times 60 \text{ minutes}} \times 15 \text{ gtt/ml} = X \text{ gtt/minute}$$

$$\frac{1,000 \text{ ml}}{600 \text{ minutes}} \times 15 \text{ gtt/ml} = X \text{ gtt/minute}$$

$$1.67 \text{ml/minute} \times 15 \text{ gtt/ml} = X \text{ gtt/minute}$$

$$25.05 \text{ gtt/minute} = X$$

Answer: To infuse, round off 25.05 to 25 gtt/minute or according to your institution's policy.

Example 2: If the physician prescribes 500 ml of half-normal (0.45%) saline solution to infuse over 2 hours, and the drip rate for your administration set delivers 10 gtt/ml, calculate as follows:

$$\frac{500 \text{ ml}}{2 \text{ hours} \times 60 \text{ minutes}} \times 10 \text{ gtt/ml} = X \text{ gtt/minute}$$

$$\frac{500 \text{ ml}}{120 \text{ minutes}} \times 10 \text{ gtt/ml} = X \text{ gtt/minute}$$

$$4.17 \text{ml/minute} \times 10 \text{ gtt/ml} = X \text{ gtt/minute}$$

$$4.17 \text{ gtt/minute} = X$$

Answer: To infuse, round off 41.7 to 42 gtt/minute or according to your institution's policy.

Note: When preparing for I.V. administration using a controlled infusion device, the electronic flow-regulator will either count drops using an electronic eye or use a controlled pumping action to deliver the fluid in milliliters. Your final calculation will be based on the unit of measure used by the device: drops per minute, or ml per hour.

Weights and Equivalents

The following three tables show approximate equivalents among systems of measurement.

Table 1 Liquid Equivalents Among Household, Apothecaries', and Metric Systems

HOUSEHOLD	APOTHECARIES'	METRIC
1 teaspoon (tsp)	1 fluid dram	5 milliliters (ml)
1 tablespoon (tbs)	0.5 fluid oz	15 ml
2 tbs (1 ounce [oz])	1 fluid oz	30 ml
1 cupful	8 fluid oz	240 ml
1 pint	16 fluid oz	473 ml
1 quart (qt)	32 fluid oz	946 ml (1 liter)

Table 2 Solid Equivalents Among Apothecaries' and Metric Systems

APOTHECARIES'	METRIC
15 grains (gr)	1 gram (g) (1,000 milligrams [mg])
10 gr	0.6 g (600 mg)
7.5 gr	0.5 g (500 mg)
5 gr	0.3 g (300 mg)
3 gr	0.2 g (200 mg)
1.5 gr	0.1 g (100 mg)
1 gr	0.06 g (60 mg) or 0.065 g (65 mg)
0.75 gr	0.05 g (50 mg)
0.5 gr	0.03 g (30 mg)
0.25 gr	0.015 g (15 mg)
1/60 gr	0.001 g (1 mg)
1/100 gr	0.6 mg
1/120 gr	0.5 mg
1/150 gr	0.4 mg

(continued)

Weights and Equivalents *(continued)*

Table 3 Solid Equivalents Among Avoirdupois, Apothecaries', and Metric Systems

AVOIRDUPOIS	APOTHECARIES'	METRIC
1 gr	1 gr	0.065 g
15.4 gr	15 gr	1 g
1 ounce (oz)	480 gr	28.35 g
437.5 gr	1 oz	31 g
1 pound (lb)	1.33 lb	454 g
0.75 lb	1 lb	373 g
2.2 lb	2.7 lb	1 kg

Equianalgesic Doses for Opioid Agonists

An equianalgesic dose of a synthetic opioid agonist is the dose that produces the same level of analgesia as 10 mg of I.M. or subQ morphine, the prinicipal opioid obtained from opium poppies. If your patient is switched from one opioid to another, expect to use the equi-analgesic dose to decrease the risk of adverse reactions while increasing the likelihood of adequate pain relief. The chart below compares equianalgesic doses (oral and parenteral) for adults and children who weigh 50 kg (110 lb) or more.

OPIOID	ORAL DOSE	PARENTERAL DOSE
codeine	200 mg (not recommended)	120 to 130 mg
hydrocodone	30 mg	Not applicable
hydromorphone	7.5 mg	1.5 mg
levorphanol	4 mg	2 mg
meperidine	300 mg	75 to 100 mg
morphine (around-the-clock dosing)	30 mg	10 mg
morphine (single or intermittent dosing)	60 mg	10 mg
oxycodone	30 mg	Not applicable

Abbreviations

The following abbreviations, which are common to nursing practice, may be used throughout the book.

ABG	arterial blood gas	GABA	gamma aminobutyric acid
ACE	angiotensin-converting enzyme	GFR	glomerular filtration rate
ADH	antidiuretic hormone	GI	gastrointestinal
AIDS	acquired immunodeficiency syndrome	gtt	drop
		GU	genitourinary
ALT	alanine aminotransferase	H_1	histamine$_1$
ANA	antinuclear antibodies	H_2	histamine$_2$
APTT	activated partial thromboplastin time	HDL	high-density lipoprotein
		HEME	hematologic
AST	aspartate aminotransferase	HIV	human immunodeficiency virus
ATP	adenosine triphosphate	HMG-CoA	hydroxymethylglutaryl-
AV	atrioventricular		coenzyme A
BUN	blood urea nitrogen	HPV	human papilloma virus
°C	degrees Celsius	hr	hour
cAMP	cyclic adenosine monophosphate	HSV	herpes simplex virus
(CAN)	Canadian drug trade name	HZV	herpes zoster virus
cap	capsule	ICP	intracranial pressure
CBC	complete blood count	I.D.	intradermal
cGMP	cyclic guanosine monophosphate	IgA	immunoglobulin A
CK	creatine kinase	IgE	immunoglobulin E
Cl	chloride	I.M.	intramuscular
cm	centimeter	INR	international normalized ratio
CMV	cytomegalovirus	I.V.	intravenous
CNS	central nervous system	IVPB	intravenous piggyback
COPD	chronic obstructive pulmonary disease	kg	kilogram
		KIU	kallikrein inactivator units
C.R.	controlled-release	L	liter
CSF	cerebrospinal fluid	LA	long-acting
CV	cardiovascular	lb	pound
CVA	cerebrovascular accident	LD	lactate dehydrogenase
D_5LR	dextrose 5% in lactated Ringer's solution	LDL	low-density lipoprotein
		LOC	level of consciousness
D_5NS	dextrose 5% in normal saline solution	LR	lactated Ringer's solution
		M	molar
$D_5/0.2NS$	dextrose 5% in quarter-normal saline solution	m^2	square meter
		MAO	monoamine oxidase
$D_5/0.45NS$	dextrose 5% in half-normal saline solution	mcg	microgram
		mEq	milliequivalent
D_5W	dextrose 5% in water	mg	milligram
$D_{10}W$	dextrose 10% in water	MI	myocardial infarction
$D_{50}W$	dextrose 50% in water	min	minute
dl	deciliter	ml	milliliter
DNA	deoxyribonucleic acid	mm	millimeter
DS	double-strength	mm^3	cubic millimeter
EC	enteric-coated	mmol	millimole
ECG	electrocardiogram	mo	month
EEG	electroencephalogram	MS	musculoskeletal
EENT	eyes, ears, nose, and throat	msec	millisecond
ENDO	endocrine	Na	sodium
E.R.	extended-release	NaCl	sodium chloride
°F	degrees Fahrenheit	NG	nasogastric
FDA	Food and Drug Administration	ng	nanogram
g	gram	NPH	human isophane insulin

Abbreviations (continued)

NPO	nothing by mouth	RBC	red blood cell
NS	normal saline solution	REM	rapid eye movement
0.225NS	quarter-normal saline (0.225%) solution	RESP	respiratory
		RNA	ribonucleic acid
0.45NS	half-normal saline (0.45%) solution	RSV	respiratory syncytial virus
		SA	sinoatrial
NSAID	nonsteroidal anti-inflammatory drug	sec	second
		S.L.	sublingual
NYHA	New York Heart Association	S.R.	sustained-release
OTC	over the counter	stat	immediately
oz	ounce	SubQ	subcutaneous
PCA	patient-controlled analgesia	supp	suppository
P.O.	by mouth	tab	tablet
P.R.	by rectum	T_3	triiodothyronine
PSVT	paroxysmal supraventricular tachycardia	T_4	thyroxine
		USP	United States Pharmacopeia
PT	prothrombin time	UTI	urinary tract infection
PTCA	percutaneous transluminal - coronary angioplasty	VLDL	very-low-density lipoprotein
		WBC	white blood cell
PTT	partial thromboplastin time	wk	week
PVC	premature ventricular contraction		

Index

Index

- **Generic and alternate names:** lowercase initial
- **letter Trade names:** uppercase initial letter
- **Illustrations:** *i* after page number
- **Tables:** *t* after page number

A

abacavir sulfate, 1299t
abacavir sulfate, lamivudine, and zidovudine, 1299t
abacavir sulfate and lamivudine, 1299t
abatacept, 1–2
Abbokinase, 1213–1214
Abbokinase Open-Cath, 1213–1214
Abbreviations, 1364–1365
abciximab, 3–4
Abelcet, 72–75
Abenol, 8–10
Abilify, 91–94
Abilify Discmelt, 91–94
Abilify Maintena, 91–94
Abitrate, 261–262
Abreva, 1290t
Absorbine Footcare, 1289t
Absorption rates, xxi–xxiii
acamprosate calcium, 4, 5i
acarbose, 6
Accolate, 1247–1248
AccuNeb, 27–29, 28i
Accupril, 1008–1010
Accutane, 618–620
acebutolol hydrochloride, 7–8
Aceon, 923–924
Acephen, 8–10
Acetadote, 14–16
Aceta Elixir, 8–10
acetaminophen, 8–10
Acetaminophen Uniserts, 8–10
Aceta Tablets, 8–10
Acetazolam, 10–12
acetazolamide, 10–12
Acetocot, 1190–1194
acetohexamide, 12–13
acetohydroxamic acid, 13–14
acetylcholine chloride, 1278t
acetylcysteine, 14–16
acetylsalicylic acid, 98–100
Achromycin, 1130–1132, 1285t

Achromycin V, 1130–1132
Acilac, 634–635
AcipHex, 1012–1013
acitretin, 16–18
aclidinium bromide, 18–19
Aclovate, 1290t
Acova, 89–91
acrivastine, 1271t
Act, 460–462, 461i
Actemra, 1165–1167
Acticin, 1298t
Acticort 100, 1292t
Actigall, 1214–1215
Actimmune, 1352t
actinomycin-D, 1311t
Actiprofen Caplets, 575–578
Actiq, 471–477
Activase, 47–48
Activase rt-PA, 47–48
Active diffusion, xxi
Actonel, 1030–1032
Actos, 942–944
Actron, 626–628
Acular, 1276t
Acuvail, 1276t
acyclovir, 1290t, 1303t
Adalat, 837–839
Adalat CC, 837–839
Adalat PA, 837–839
Adalat XL, 837–839
adalimumab, 19–22
adamantanamine hydrochloride, 50–52
adapalene, 1294t
Adcirca, 1108–1110
adefovir dipivoxil, 1306t
Adenocard, 22–24
Adenoscan, 22–24
adenosine, 22–24
ADH, 1226–1227, 1227i
Administration routes, xxi–xxiii, xxviii
Adrenalin, 402–404
Adrenalin Chloride Solution, 402–404
adrenaline, 402–404
Adriamycin PFS, 1312t

Adriamycin RDF, 1312t
Adrucil, 1314t
Adsorbocarpine, 1278t
Adsorbonac, 1281t
Adverse reactions, xv
Advil, 575–578
Aerolate, 1132–1135
Aerolate III, 1132–1135
Aerolate Jr., 1132–1135
Aerolate Sr., 1132–1135
Aerosporin, 950–952
Afko-Lube, 361–362
Afko-Lube Lax, 361–362
Afrezza, 600–602
Aftate for Athlete's Foot, 1289t
Aftate for Jock Itch, 1289t
Aggrastat, 1159–1160
Agonists, xxiv
A-hydroCort, 563–566
Airet, 27–29, 28i
Akarpine, 1278t
AKBeta, 1281t
Ak-Con, 1279t
AK-Dex, 1276t
AK-Dilate, 1279t
AK-Fluor, 1281t
Akineton, 140–141
Akineton Lactate, 140–141
AK-NaCl, 1281t
Ak-Nefrin, 1279t
Akne-Mycin, 1284t
AK-Pentolate, 1278t
AK-Pred, 1277t
AK-Sulf, 1275t
AKTob, 1275t
AK-Tracin, 1273t
Ak-Zol, 10–12
Ala-Cort, 1292t
Ala-Scalp HP, 1292t
alatrofloxacin mesylate, 24–25
Albalon Liquifilm, 1279t
Albert Docusate, 361–362
Albert Glyburide, 538–540
albiglutide, 25–27
albuterol, 27–29, 28i
albuterol sulfate, 27–29, 28i
Alcaine, 1279t
alclometasone dipropionate, 1290t
Alconefrin Nasal Drops 12, 934–936
Alconefrin Nasal Drops 25, 934–936
Alconefrin Nasal Drops 50, 934–936
Alconefrin Nasal Spray 25, 934–936
Aldactone, 1081–1083, 1083i
Aldara, 1297t

Aldomet, 742–743
Aldoril-15, 1326t
Aldoril-25, 1326t
Aldoril D30, 1326t
Aldoril D50, 1326t
alefacept, 29–30
alendronate sodium, 30–32
Aleve, 816–819
Alferon N, 1348t
alfuzosin hydrochloride, 32–33
alglucerase, 33–34
Alimta, 1315t
aliskiren, 34–35, 1326t, 1330t, 1332t
Alkeran, 1310t
Alkylating drugs, 1309–1310t
Allegra, 1272t
Allegra-D, 1272t
Allercort, 1292t
Allerdryl, 353–354
Allerest, 1279t
Allergic reactions, xxiv–xxv
AllerNaze, 1190–1194
Alli, 872–874, 873i
allopurinol, 36–37
allopurinol sodium, 36–37
Almora, 697–700
almotriptan malate, 37–39
Alocril, 1281t
alogliptin, 39–40
Aloprim, 36–37
Alora, 429–435
alosetron hydrochloride, 40–41
Aloxi, 895–898, 897i
Alphacaine, 662–664
Alphaderm, 1292t
alpha-difluoromethyl-ornithine, 389
Alphagan, 1280t
Alphagan P, 1280t
alpha1-proteinase inhibitor (human), 41–42
alpha tocopherol, 1344t
alprazolam, 42–44
alprostadil, 44–47, 45i
Alrex, 1277t
Altace, 1015–1017
alteplase, 47–48
AlternaGEL, 48–49
Alti-Bromocriptine, 146–149, 147i
Alti-Doxycycline, 374–378
Alti-Minocycline, 771–774
Alti-MPA, 984–988
Alti-Sulfasalazine, 1091–1093
Alti-Triazolam, 1195–1197
Alti-Valproic, 1217–1220
Altoprev, 690–692

Alu-Cap, 48–49
Alugel, 48–49
aluminum carbonate, 48–49
aluminum hydroxide, 48–49
Alustra, 1296t
Alu-Tab, 48–49
Alvesco, 242–244
alvimopan, 49–50
amantadine hydrochloride, 50–52
Amaryl, 533–535
Ambien, 1259–1261
Ambien CR, 1259–1261
AmBisome, 72–75
amcinonide, 1290t
Amcort, 1190–1194
Amen, 984–988
Amerge, 819–820
A-methaPred, 748–751
amethopterin, 737–738, 1314t
Amevive, 29–30
Amicar, 54–55
Amigesic, 1049–1050
amikacin sulfate, 52–53
Amikin, 52–53
amiloride hydrochloride, 53–54, 1330t
aminocaproic acid, 54–55
aminoglutethimide, 55–56
Amino-Opti-E, 1344t
aminophylline, 56–58
aminosalicylate sodium, 58
amiodarone hydrochloride, 58–61
Amitiza, 694
amitriptyline hydrochloride, 61–63, 62i
amlodipine besylate, 63–64, 1326t, 1328t, 1330t, 1332t
ammonium chloride, 64–65
ammonium lactate 12%, 1294t
amobarbital sodium, 65–67
amoxapine, 67–68
amoxicillin trihydrate, 68–70
Amoxil, 68–70
amoxycillin, 68–70
amphetamine sulfate, 70–72
Amphocin, 72–75
Amphojel, 48–49
Amphotec, 72–75
amphotericin B, 72–75
amphotericin B cholesteryl sulfate complex, 72–75
amphotericin B lipid complex, 72–75
amphotericin B liposomal complex, 72–75
ampicillin, 75–77
ampicillin sodium, 75–77
ampicillin trihydrate, 75–77

Ampicin, 75–77
amrinone, 590–591
Amturnide 150/5/12.5, 1326t
Amturnide 300/5/12.5, 1326t
Amturnide 300/5/25, 1326t
Amturnide 300/10/12.5, 1326t
Amturnide 300/10/25, 1326t
amyl nitrite, 77–78
Amytal, 65–67
Anadrol-50, 887–889
Anaflex 750, 1049–1050
Anafranil, 262–263
Ana-Guard, 402–404
anakinra, 78–79
Anandron, 1320t
Anaphylactic reactions, xxiv
Anapolon-50, 887–889
Anaprox, 816–819
Anaprox DS, 816–819
Anaspaz, 572–573
Ancalixir, 930–932
Ancasal, 98–100
Ancef, 187–189
Anergan 25, 988–990
Anergan 50, 988–990
Anestacon, 662–664
Anexate, 493–494
Angiomax, 144–145
anidulafungin, 79–80
Aniflex, 874–875
anisindione, 80–82
anisoylated plasminogen-streptokinase activator complex, 82–83
anistreplase, 82–83
Ansaid, 501–503
Antabuse, 358–359
Antagonists, xxiv
anthralin, 1294t
Anthranol I, 1294t
Antibacterial medications, 1284–1285t
Antibiotics, 1273–1275t, 1308, 1311–1313t
antidiuretic hormone, 1226–1227, 1227i
Antifungal medications, 1286–1289t
Antihistamines, 1271–1272t
Antihypertensive drugs, 1326–1333t
Anti-inflammatory ophthalmic drugs, 1275–1277t
Antilirium, 940–941
Antimetabolite medications, 1308, 1313–1314t
Antimitotic medications, 1308, 1313t
Antinaus 50, 988–990
Antineoplastic drugs, 1309–1325t
Antineoplastic enzymes, 1308, 1317t
Anti-Tuss, 545–546

Antivert, 703–704
Antiviral medications, 1290t, 1299–1307t
Anturane, 1093–1094
Anusol-HC, 1292t
Anzemet, 363–364
Apacet Capsules, 8–10
Apacet Elixir, 8–10
Apacet Extra Strength Tablets, 8–10
Apacet Regular Strength Tablets, 8–10
Apidra, 1267t
apixaban, 83–84
Aplenzin, 155–158
Apo-Acetazolamide, 10–12
Apo-Allopurinol, 36–37
Apo-Alpraz, 42–44
Apo-amitriptyline, 61–63, 62i
Apo-Amoxi, 68–70
Apo-Ampi, 75–77
Apo-As, 98–100
Apo-ASEN, 98–100
Apo-Atenol, 100–101
Apo-Benztropine, 132–133
Apo-Bromocriptine, 146–149, 147i
Apo-Cal, 168–170
Apo-Carbamazepine, 176–179, 176i
Apo-Cefaclor, 184–186
Apo-Cephalex, 219–221, 220i
Apo-Chlordiazepoxide, 229–230
Apo-Chlorpropamide, 236–237
Apo-Chlorthalidone, 237–239
Apo-Cimetidine, 245–247
Apo-Clonazepam, 263–264
Apo-Clorazepate, 268–269
Apo-Cloxi, 269–270
Apo-Cromolyn, 285–287, 286i
Apo-Diazepam, 328–331
Apo-Diclo, 334–336
Apo-Diflunisal, 340–342
Apo-Diltiaz, 348–350, 350i
Apo-Dipyridamole FC, 354–355
Apo-Dipyridamole SC, 354–355
Apo-Doxy, 374–378
Apo-Erythro, 416–420
Apo-Erythro-ES, 416–420
Apo-Erythro-S, 416–420
Apo-Famotidine, 460–462, 461i
Apo-Ferrous Gluconate, 478–481
Apo-Ferrous Sulfate, 478–481
Apo-Fluphenazine, 498–500
Apo-Flurazepam, 500–501
Apo-Folic, 1340t
Apo-Furosemide, 522–524
Apo-Gain, 774–776

Apo-Gemfibrozil, 528–529
Apo-Glyburide, 538–540
Apo-Guanethidine, 547–549
Apo-Haloperidol, 551–553
Apo-Hydralazine, 557–558
Apo-Hydroxyzine, 571–572
Apo-Ibuprofen, 575–578
Apo-Imipramine, 582–584
Apo-Indapamide, 593–594
Apo-Indomethacin, 594–597
Apo-Ipravent, 603–606, 604i
Apo-ISDN, 616–618, 617i
Apo-K, 954–958
Apo-Keto, 626–628
Apokyn, 84–86
Apo-Lorazepam, 686–687
Apo-Megestrol, 984–988
Apo-Meprobamate, 716–717
Apo-Methyldopa, 742–743
Apo-Metoclop, 751–753
Apo-Metoprolol, 754–757
Apo-Metronidazole, 757–759
Apo-Minocycline, 771–774
apomorphine hydrochloride, 84–86
Apo-Napro-Na, 816–819
Apo-Naproxen, 816–819
Apo-Nifed, 837–839
Apo-Nitrofurantoin, 841–842
Apo-Nizatidine, 846–847
Apo-Oxazepam, 879–880
Apo-Oxtriphylline, 882–883
Apo-Pen-VK, 915–917
Apo-Perphenazine, 925–927
Apo-Piroxicam, 947–949
Apo-Prednisone, 972–974
Apo-Primidone, 976–977
Apo-Propranolol, 994–997
Apo-Quinidine, 1010–1012
Apo-Ranitidine, 1017–1019
Apo-Selegiline, 1056–1058
Apo-sucralfate, 1086
Apo-Sulfamethoxazole, 1090–1091
Apo-Sulfinpyrazone, 1093–1094
Apo-Sulfisoxazole, 1094–1096
Apo-Sulin, 1096–1098
Apo-Tamox, 1110–1111, 1320t
Apo-Temazepam, 1120–1121
Apo-Tetra, 1130–1132
Apothecary system of measurement, 1361, 1362
Apo-Theo LA, 1132–1135
Apo-Thioridazine, 1138–1140
Apo-Timol, 1154–1155
Apo-Timop, 1282t

Apo-Tolbutamide, 1170–1171
Apo-Triazo, 1195–1197
Apo-Trifluoperazine, 1197–1199
Apo-Trihex, 1201–1202
Apo-Trimip, 1203–1205
Apo-Verap, 1232–1234
Apo-Zidovudine, 1303t
apraclonidine hydrochloride, 1279t
apremilast, 44
aprepitant, 86–88
Apresazide 25/25, 1326t
Apresazide 50/50, 1326t
Apresazide 100/50, 1326t
Apresoline, 557–558
Apriso, 719–720
Aptiom, 422–423
Aptivus, 1302t
Aquachloral Supprettes, 227
AquaMEPHYTON, 1346t
Aquasol A, 1336t
Aquasol E, 1344t
Aqueous diffusion, xxi
ARA-C, 1313t
Aralast NP, 41–42
Aranesp, 305–308
Arava, 643–645
Arcapta Neohaler, 591–592
Aredia, 896–898
arformoterol, 88–89
argatroban, 89–91
Argesic-SA, 1049–1050
Aricept, 365–366
aripiprazole, 91–94
Aristocort, 1190–1194, 1293t, 1294t
Aristocort A, 1293t, 1294t
Aristocort C, 1294t
Aristocort D, 1293t
Aristocort Forte, 1190–1194
Aristocort R, 1294t
Aristopak, 1190–1194
Aristospan, 1190–1194
Arixtra, 509–511
Arm-a-Med Isoetharine, 611–612
Arm-a-Med Metaproterenol, 722–723
Arm and Hammer Pure Baking Soda, 1070–1072
armodafinil, 94–96
Armour Thyroid, 1143–1144
Aromasin, 1319t
Artane, 1201–1202
Arthrinol, 98–100
Arthrisin, 98–100
Arthropan, 241–242
Articulose-50, 969–972

Articulose-LA, 1190–1194
ASA, 98–100
Asacol, 719–720
Ascorbic Acid, 1342t
asenapine, 96–97
Asendin, 67–68
Asmalix, 1132–1135
Asmanex, 789–790
asparaginase, 1317t
A-Spas S/L, 572–573
Aspergum, 98–100
aspirin, 98–100
Aspirin-Free Pain Relief, 8–10
Assessment phase of nursing process, xxxi–xxxiv
Astagraf XL, 1104–1108
Astelin, 113–114, 1271t
Astepro 0.1%, 1271t
Astepro 0.15%, 1271t
Asthmahaler Mist, 402–404
AsthmaNefrin, 402–404
Astramorph PF, 792–796
Atacand, 172–173
Atacand HCT 16/12.5, 1326t
Atacand HCT 32/12.5, 1326t
Atarax, 571–572
atazanavir sulfate, 1299t
Atelvia, 1030–1032
atenolol, 100–101
Ativan, 686–687
Atolone, 1190–1194
atomoxetine hydrochloride, 101–103
atorvastatin calcium, 103–105
atovaquone, 105–106
atracurium besylate, 106–107
Atretol, 176–179, 176i
Atria S.R., 98–100
Atromid-S, 261–262
AtroPen, 107–109
atropine, 107–109, 1354t
atropine sulfate, 107–109, 1277t
Atropisol, 1277t
Atrovent, 603–604, 604i
A/T/S, 1284t
Aubagio, 1126–1128
auranofin, 109–110
Auryxia, 477
Avage, 1294t
Avalide-150, 1326t
Avalide-300, 1326t
avanafil, 110–112
Avandia, 1042–1043
Avapro, 604–606
Avastin, 1321t

Avelox, 796–799
Avelox IV, 796–799
Aventyl, 850–852
Avinza, 792–796
Avita, 1294t
Avodart, 386–387, 387i
Avoirdupois system of measurement, 1362t
Avonex, 1350t
Axert, 37–39
Axid, 846–847
Axid AR, 846–847
axitinib, 1320t
Ayercillin, 915–917
Aygestin, 984–988
Azactam, 117–119
azatadine, 1271t
azathioprine, 112–113
azathioprine sodium, 112–113
azelaic acid cream, 1284t
azelastine hydrochloride, 113–114, 1271t, 1280t
Azelex, 1284t
Azilect, 1020–1022
azilsartan, 1328t
azilsartan medoxomil, 114–115
azithromycin, 115–117
Azopt, 1280t
Azor 5/20, 1326t
Azor 5/40, 1326t
Azor 10/20, 1326t
Azor 10/40, 1326t
Azo-Standard, 927
AZT, 1303t
aztreonam, 117–119
Azulfidine, 1091–1093
Azulfidine EN-Tabs, 1091–1093

B

bacampicillin hydrochloride, 121–122
Baci-IM, 122–123
bacillus Calmette-Guérin, Tice strain, 1318t
bacillus Calmette-Guérin (BCG) live, Connaught
    strain, 1318t
bacitracin, 122–123, 1273t, 1284t
Bactine, 1292t
Bactocill, 875–876
Bactroban, 1285t
Bactroban Cream, 1285t
Bactroban Nasal, 1285t
Balminil Expectorant, 545–546
balsalazide disodium, 123–124
Banflex, 874–875

Banophen, 353–354
Banzel, 1046–1047
Barbita, 930–932
Baridium, 927
Barriere-HC, 1292t
Basaljel, 48–49
Bayer, 98–100
Bayer Select Ibuprofen Pain Relief Formula
    Caplets, 575–578
BayGam, 584–590
BCG live, Connaught strain, 1318t
BCNU, 1309t
B-D Glucose, 327–328
Beben, 1290t
becaplermin, 1295t
Beclodisk, 124–126
beclomethasone dipropionate, 124–126
Beclovent Rotacaps, 124–126
Beconase, 124–126
Beconase AQ, 124–126
Beepen-VK, 915–917
Beesix, 1338t
belimumab, 126–128
belladonna alkaloids, 128–129
Bell/ans, 1070–1072
Belsomra, 1101–1102
Belviq, 687–689
Benadryl, 353–354
Benadryl Allergy, 353–354
benazepril hydrochloride, 129–131, 1328t, 1330t
Benemid, 977–979
Benicar, 859–861, 860i
Benicar HCT 20/12.5, 1326t
Benicar HCT 40/12.5, 1326t
Benicar HCT 40/25, 1326t
Benlysta, 126–128
Benoquin, 1297t
Bentyl, 339–340
Bentylol, 339–340
Benuryl, 977–979
Benylin-E, 545–546
Benzac AC Wash, 1284t
Benzaclin gel DUAC, 1284t
Benzacot, 1202–1203
Benzamycin, 1284t
benzonatate, 131
Benzonatate Softgels, 131
benzoyl peroxide, 1284t
benzquinamide hydrochloride, 131–132
benztropine mesylate, 132–133
bepotastine besilate 1.5%, 1280t
Bepreve, 1280t
bepridil hydrochloride, 133–135
Beta-2, 611–612

Betadine, 1285t
Betadine Cream, 1285t
Betadine Spray, 1285t
Betagan, 1281t
Beta-HC, 1292t
Betaloc, 754–757
Betaloc Durules, 754–757
betamethasone, 135–137
betamethasone acetate-betamethasone sodium
    phosphate, 135–137
betamethasone benzoate, 1290t
betamethasone dipropionate, 1290t, 1295t
betamethasone sodium phosphate, 135–137
betamethasone valerate, 1290t
Betapace, 1077–1079
Betapace AF, 1077–1079
Betapen-VK, 915–917
Betaseron, 1350t
Betaxin, 1336t
betaxolol hydrochloride, 137–139, 1280t
bethanechol chloride, 139–140
Betimol, 1282t
Betnesol, 135–137
Betoptic, 1280t
Betoptic S, 1280t
bevacizumab, 1321t
Bewon, 1336t
Biamine, 1336t
Biaxin, 253–256
Biaxin XL, 253–256
Biaxin XL-PAK, 253–256
bicalutamide, 1319t
Bicillin C-R, 915–917
Bicillin C-R 900/300, 915–917
Bicillin L-A, 915–917
BiCNU, 1309t
Bilax, 361–362
bimatoprost, 1280t
Bioavailability, xxi, xxii
Biological response modifiers, 1308, 1318
Bio-Syn, 1291t
Biotransformation, xxiii
Bio-Well, 667–668
biperiden hydrochloride, 140–141
biperiden lactate, 140–141
bisoprolol fumarate, 141–143, 1332t
bitolterol mesylate, 143–144
bivalirudin, 144–145
Blenoxane, 1311t
bleomycin sulfate, 1311t
Bleph-10, 1275t
Blocadren, 1154–1155
boceprevir, 1306t
Boldex, 1276t

Bonamine, 703–704
Bonine, 703–704
Boniva, 573–574
Bortezomib, 1321t
bosentan, 291, 538, 1062
Brand names of drugs, xx
Breonesin, 545–546
Brethaire, 1125–1126
Brethine, 1125–1126
Bretylate, 145–146
bretylium tosylate, 145–146
Bretylol, 145–146
Brevibloc, 423–425
Bricanyl, 1125–1126
Bricanyl Turbuhaler, 1125–1126
Brilinta, 1147–1148
brimonidine tartrate, 1280t
Brintellix, 1241–1243
brinzolamide 1%, 1280t
Bromday, 1275t
bromfenac 0.09%, 1275t
bromocriptine mesylate, 146–149
Bronalide, 494–495
Bronkaid Mist, 402–404
Bronkaid Mistometer, 402–404
Bronkaid Suspension Mist, 402–404
Bronkometer (0&61%), 611–612
Bronkosol (1%), 611–612
Brovana, 88–89
budesonide, 149–152
bumetanide, 152–153
Bumex, 152–153
Buphenyl, 1073–1074
Buprenex, 153–155
buprenorphine hydrochloride, 153–155
buproion hydrobromide, 155–158
bupropion hydrochloride, 155–158
Busodium, 159–160
BuSpar, 158–159
BuSpar DIVIDOSE, 158–159
buspirone hydrochloride, 158–159
Bustab, 158–159
busulfan, 1309t
Busulfex, 1309t
butabarbital sodium, 159–160
Butalan, 159–160
butenafine hydrochloride, 1286t
Butisol, 159–160
butoconazole nitrate, 1286t
butorphanol tartrate, 160–162
Butrans, 153–155
Bydureon, 455–457, 456i
Byetta, 455–457, 456i
Bystolic, 824–825

C

cabergoline, 163–164
Caelyx, 1312t
Calan, 1232–1234
Calan SR, 1232–1234
calcifediol, 164–165
Calciferol, 1344t
Calciferol Drops, 1344t
Calciject, 168–170
Calcijex, 167–168
Calcilean, 553–555
Calci-Mix, 168–170
Calcionate, 168–170
Calciparine, 553–556
calcipotriene, 1295t
calcipotriene hydrate 0.005% and betamethasone
    dipropionate 0.064%, 1295t
calcitonin, human, 165–167
calcitonin, salmon, 165–167
calcitriol, 167–168
calcium acetate, 168–170
calcium carbonate, 168–170
calcium chloride, 168–170
calcium citrate, 168–170
calcium glubionate, 168–170
calcium gluceptate, 168–170
calcium gluconate, 168–170
calcium lactate, 168–170
Calcium-Sandoz, 168–170
Calcium Stanley, 168–170
Calculations and formulas, 1356–1360
Calderol, 164–165
Caldolor, 575–578
Calmylin Expectorant, 545–546
Calsan, 168–170
Campral, 4–5, 5i
Camptosar, 1323t
canagliflozin, 170–171
Canasa, 719–720
Cancer drugs, 1308–1325t
Cancidas, 182–184, 183i
candesartan cilexetil, 172–173, 1326t
Canesten, 1286t
Capastat, 173–174
capecitabine, 1313t
Capitrol, 1295t
Capoten, 174–175
Capozide 25/15, 1326t
Capozide 25/25, 1326t
Capozide 50/15, 1326t
Capozide 50/25, 1326t
capreomycin sulfate, 173–174

capsaicin, 1295t
Capsin, 1295t
Capsules, xxviii
captopril, 174–175, 1326t
Capzacin-P, 1295t
Carac, 1296t, 1314t
Carafate, 1086
carbachol 0.01%, 1278t
carbachol 0.75%, 1278t
carbachol 1.5%, 1278t
carbachol 2.25%, 1278t
carbachol 3%, 1278t
Carbacot, 736–737
carbamazepine, 176–179, 176i
carbamide, 1212–1213
Carbastat, 1278t
Carbatrol, 176–179, 176i
Carbex, 1056–1058
Carbolith, 679–681
Carboptic, 1278t
Cardene, 832–834
Cardene IV, 832–834
Cardene SR, 832–834
Cardioquin, 1010–1012
Cardizem, 348–350, 350i
Cardizem CD, 348–350, 350i
Cardizem LA, 348–350, 350i
Cardizem SR, 348–350, 350i
Cardura, 370–371
Cardura-1, 370–371
Cardura-2, 370–371
Cardura-4, 370–371
carisoprodol, 179–180
carmustine, 1309t
carteolol hydrochloride, 180, 1280t
Cartrol, 180
carvedilol, 181–182
Casodex, 1319t
caspofungin acetate, 182–184, 183i
Cataflam, 333–336
Catapres, 264–267
Catapres-TTS, 264–267
Caverject, 44–47, 45i
Cayston, 117–119
CCNU, 1309t
Ceclor, 184–186
Ceclor CD, 184–186
Cecon Drops, 1342t
Cedax, 210–211
Cedocard-SR, 616–618, 617i
CeeNU, 1309t
cefaclor, 184–186
cefadroxil, 186–187
Cefadyl, 221–222

cefazolin sodium, 187–189
cefdinir, 189–190
cefditoren pivoxil, 191–192
cefepime hydrochloride, 192–194
cefixime, 194–195
Cefizox, 211–212
cefmetazole sodium, 195–196
Cefobid, 198–199
cefonicid sodium, 196–198
cefoperazone sodium, 198–199
Cefotan, 201–202
cefotaxime sodium, 199–201
cefotetan disodium, 201–202
cefoxitin sodium, 202–204
cefpodoxime proxetil, 204–205
cefprozil, 205–207
ceftaroline fosamil, 207–208
ceftazidime, 208–210
ceftibuten, 210–211
Ceftin, 214–217
ceftizoxime sodium, 211–212
ceftriaxone sodium, 212–214
cefuroxime axetil, 214–217
cefuroxime sodium, 214–217
Cefzil, 205–207
Celebrex, 217–219
celecoxib, 217–219
Celestone, 135–137
Celestone Phosphate, 135–137
Celestone Soluspan, 135–137
Celexa, 251–253
CellCept, 799–802
CellCept Intravenous, 799–802
CellCept Oral Suspension, 799–802
Celontin, 741–742
Cena-K, 954–958
Cenestin, 435–439
Cenocort Forte, 1190–1194
Cenolate, 1342t
cephalexin hydrochloride, 219–221, 220i
cephalexin monohydrate, 219–221, 220i
cephapirin sodium, 221–222
cephradine, 222–223
Cephulac, 634–635
Ceptaz, 208–210
Cerebyx, 516–519
Ceredase, 33–34
certolizumab pegol, 223–226
Cerubidine, 1311t
Cervidil, Prepidil, Prostin E2, 1334
C.E.S., 435–439
Cetacort, 1292t
cetirizine, 1272t
Cevi-Bid, 1342t

cevimeline hydrochloride, 226–227
Chantix, 1225–1226
Chemical names of drugs, xx
Children, xxiii, xxvi
Children's Advil, 575–578
Children's Motrin, 575–578
chloral hydrate, 227
chlorambucil, 1309t
chloramphenicol, 228–230, 1273t
chloramphenicol palmitate, 228–230
chloramphenicol sodium succinate, 228–230
chlordiazepoxide hydrochloride, 229–230
chlorhexidine, 1295t
Chloromag, 697–700
Chloromycetin, 228–230
chlorothiazide, 230–232
chlorothiazide sodium, 230–232
chloroxine, 1295t
chlorphenesin carbamate, 232
Chlorpromanyl, 233–236
chlorpromazine, 233–236, 1354t
chlorpromazine hydrochloride, 233–236
chlorpropamide, 236–237
chlorthalidone, 237–239, 1328t
chlorzoxazone, 239–240
Cholac, 634–635
Choledyl, 882–883
Choledyl SA, 882–883
cholestyramine, 240–241
choline salicylate, 241–242
Chronulac, 634–635
Cialis, 1108–1110
Cibacalcin, 165–167
Cibalith-S, 679–681
ciclesonide, 242–244
ciclopirox olamine, 1286t
cidofovir, 1305t
Cidomycin, 531–533
cilostazol, 244–245
Ciloxan, 1273t
cimetidine, 245–247
cimetidine hydrochloride, 245–247
Cimzia, 223–226
cinacalcet hydrochloride, 247–248
Cinalone 40, 1190–1194
Cipro, 248–251
ciprofloxacin, 248–251
ciprofloxacin hydrochloride 0.3%, 1273t
Cipro I.V., 248–251
Cipro XR, 248–251
cisplatin, 1311t
citalopram hydrobromide, 251–253
Citracal, 168–170
Citracal Liquitabs, 168–170

citrate of magnesia, 697–700
Citrocarbonate, 1070–1072
Citroma, 697–700
Citro-Mag, 697–700
Claforan, 199–201
Claravis, 618–620
Clarinex, 1272t
Clarinex Reditabs, 1272t
Claripel, 1296t
Claripex, 261–262
clarithromycin, 253–256
Claritin, 1272t
Claritin-D12, 1272t
Claritin-D24, 1272t
Classification of drugs, xx–xxi
Clearasil Maximum Strength, 1284t
Clear Eyes, 1279t
Cleocin, 257–259, 1284t
Cleocin Pediatric, 257–259
Cleocin T Gel, 1284t
Cleocin T Lotion, 1284t
clidinium bromide, 256–257
Climara, 429–435
Clinacort, 1190–1194
Clinagen LA 40, 429–435
Clinda-Derm, 1284t
clindamycin 1% and benzoyl peroxide 5%, 1284t
clindamycin 1.2% and tretinoin 0.025%, 1284t
clindamycin hydrochloride, 257–259
clindamycin palmitate hydrochloride, 257–259
clindamycin phosphate, 257–259, 1284t
Clindesse, 257–259
Clinoril, 1096–1098
clobazam, 259–261
clobetasol propionate, 1291t
clofibrate, 261–262
clomipramine hydrochloride, 262–263
Clonapam, 263–264
clonazepam, 263–264
clonidine, 264–267
clonidine hydrochloride, 264–267
clopidogrel bisulfate, 267–268
clorazepate dipotassium, 268–269
clotrimazole, 1295t
clotrimazole and betamethasone dipropionate,
    1295t
cloxacillin sodium, 269–270
Cloxapen, 269–270
clozapine, 270–273
Clozaril, 270–273
CMV medications, 1305
coal tar, 1295t
codeine, 1363t
codeine phosphate, 273–275

codeine sulfate, 273–275
Cogentin, 132–133
Cognex, 1103–1104, 1103i
Colace, 361
Colax, 361
Colazal, 123–124
colchicine, 275–277, 276i
Colcrys, 275–277, 276i
colesevelam hydrochloride, 277–278
Colestid, 278–280
colestipol hydrochloride, 278–280
colistimethate sodium, 280–281
Collyrium Fresh Eye Drops, 1279t
Colprone, 984–988
Coly-Mycin M, 280–281
Combination insulins, 1269t
Combivir, 1301t
Comfort Eye Drops, 1279t
Compatible drugs in syringe, 1354–1355
Compazine, 981–984
Compazine Spansule, 981–984
Competitive antagonists, xxiv
Complera, 1300t
Comtan, 400–402
Concerta, 745–748
Condylox, 1298t
Congest, 435–439
conivaptan hydrochloride, 281–282
Constilac, 634–635
Constulose, 634–635
Copegus, 1307t
Coradur, 616–618, 617i
Cordarone, 58–61
Cordran, 1291t
Cordran Tape, 1291t
Coreg, 181–182
Coreg CR, 181–182
Corgard, 804–806
Corlopam, 468–469
Coronex, 616–618, 617i
Correctol Stool Softener Soft Gels, 361–362
Cortacet, 1292t
Cortaid, 1292t, 1293t
Cortastat, 320–323
Cortastat LA, 320–323
Cortate, 1292t
Cort-Dome, 1292t
Cortef, 563–566
Cortef Feminine Itch, 1293t
Cortenema, 563–566
Corticaine, 1292t
Corticosteroids, 1286t, 1290–1294t
Corticreme, 1292t, 1293t
Cortifair, 1292t

Cortifoam, 563–566
cortisol, 563–566
cortisone acetate, 282–284
Cortisone Acetate-ICN, 282–284
Cortisporin, 1293t, 1296t
Cortoderm, 1292t, 1293t
Cortone, 282–284
Cortone Acetate, 282–284
Cortril, 1292t
Corvert, 578–579
Cosmegen, 1311t
Cotazym, 899–901
Cotazym-S, 899–901
Cotolone, 969–972
Coumadin, 1243–1245
Cozaar, 689–690
Creon, 899–901
Crestor, 1043–1045
Crinone, 984–988
Crixivan, 1301t
crofelemer, 284–285
cromolyn sodium, 285–287, 286i
crotamiton, 287
crotamiton 10%, 1296t
Crysticillin 300 AS, 915–917
Cubicin, 304–305
Cultural considerations, xxv
Cuprimine, 913–915
Curretab, 984–988
Cutivate, 1291t
Cuvposa, 540–542
cyanocobalamin, 1340t
cyclizine hydrochloride, 288–289
cyclizine lactate, 288–289
cyclobenzaprine hydrochloride, 288–289
Cyclocort, 1290t
Cyclogyl, 1278t
Cyklokapron, 1185–1186
cyclopentolate hydrochloride, 1278t
cyclophosphamide, 1309t
Cycloplegic mydriatics, 1277–1278t
cycloserine, 289–290
Cycloset, 146–149, 147i
cyclosporin A, 290–293
cyclosporine, 290–293
cyclosporine emulsion 0.05%, 1280t
Cycrin, 984–988
Cymbalta, 384–386
Cystospaz, 572–573
Cystospaz-M, 572–573
Cytadren, 55–56
cytarabine, 1313t
cytarabine, liposomal, 1313t
Cytomel, 671–673

Cytosar, 1313t
Cytosar-U, 1313t
cytosine arabinoside, 1313t
Cytotec, 780–781
Cytovene, 1305t
Cytoxan, 1309t

D

dabigatran etexilate, 295–297
dacarbazine, 1322t
dactinomycin, 1311t
Dalacin, 1284t
Dalacin C, 257–259
Dalacin C Flavored Granules, 257–259
Dalacin C Phosphate, 257–259
Dalacin T Topical Solution, 1284t
Dalalone, 320–323
Dalalone D.P., 320–323
Dalalone L.A., 320–323
dalbavancin, 297–298
Dalgan, 328
Daliresp, 1039–1040
Dalmane, 500–501
dalteparin sodium, 298–300
Dalvance, 297–298
D-Amp, 75–77
danaparoid sodium, 300–301
Dantrium, 301–302
Dantrium Intravenous, 301–302
dantrolene sodium, 301–302
dapagliflozin, 302–304
daptomycin, 304–305
Daranide, 333
darbepoetin alfa, 305–308
darifenacin, 308–309
darunavir, 1299t
daunorubicin, liposomal, 1312t
daunorubicin hydrochloride, 1311t
DaunoXome, 1312t
Daypro, 877–879
Daytrana, 745–748
Dazamide, 10–12
DC Softgels, 361–362
DDAVP Injection, 318–320
DDAVP Nasal Spray, 318–320
DDAVP Rhinal Tube, 318–320
DDAVP Rhinyle Nasal Solution, 318–320
DDAVP Tablets, 318–320
Decadrol, 320–323
Decadron, 320–323
Decadron Elixir, 320–323

Decadron-LA, 320–323
Decadron Respihaler, 320–323
Decaject, 320–323
Decaject L.A., 320–323
Declomycin, 314–315
deferasirox, 309–311
deferoxamine mesylate, 311–314
degarelix, 1319t
Degest 2, 1279t
Delacort, 1292t
delavirdine, 1300t
Delestrogen, 429–435
Delta-Cortef, 969–972
delta-9-tetrahydrocannabi-nol, 378–379
Deltasone Liquid Pred, 972–974
Delta-Tritex, 1294t
Demadex, 1180–1181
demeclocycline hydrochloride, 314–315
Demerol, 710–711
Demser, 759–760
Denavir, 1290t, 1304t
denosumab, 315–316
Depacon, 1217–1220
Depakene, 1217–1220
Depakote, 1217–1220
Depakote ER, 1217–1220
Depakote Sprinkle, 1217–1220
Depen, 913–915
depGynogen, 429–435
depMedalone, 748–751
DepoDur, 792–796
Depo-Estradiol, 429–435
Depogen, 429–435
Depoject, 748–751
Depo-Medrol, 748–751
Deponit, 842–845
Depopred, 748–751
Depo-Predate, 748–751
Depo-Provera, 984–988, 1320t
Deproic, 1217–1220
Dermacort, 1292t
DermaFlex, 662–664
Derma Smooth FS, 1291t
Dermatop, 1293t
DermiCort, 1292t
Dermovate, 1291t
Dermtex HC, 1292t
Deronil, 320–323
Desferal, 311–314
desipramine hydrochloride, 317–318
Desired effects, xxiv
desloratadine, 1272t
desmopressin acetate, 318–320
desonide, 1291t

Desowen, 1291t
desoximetasone, 1291t
desoximetasone 0.25%, 1291t
Desoxyn, 730–731
Desoxyn Gradumet, 730–731
Desquam-E 2.5 Gel, 1284t
desvenlafaxine succinate, 1229–1232
Detensol, 994–997
Detrol, 1175–1176
Detrol LA, 1175–1176
Dexacen-4, 320–323
Dexacen LA-8, 320–323
Dexacorten, 320–323
Dexacorten-LA, 320–323
Dexacort Turbinaire, 320–323
dexamethasone, 320–323, 1276t, 1354t
dexamethasone acetate, 320–323
Dexamethasone Intensol, 320–323
dexamethasone sodium phosphate, 320–323, 1276t
dexamphetamine sulfate, 70–72
Dexasone, 320–323
Dexasone L.A., 320–323
Dexchlor, 320–323
dexchlorpheniramine maleate, 320–323
DexFerrum, 606–607
Dexilant, 639–642
DexIron, 606–607
dexlansoprazole, 639–642
dexmethylphenidate hydrochloride, 325–326
Dexone, 320–323
Dexone LA, 320–323
dextrose, 327–328
2.5% Dextrose Injection, 327–328
5% Dextrose Injection, 327–328
10% Dextrose Injection, 327–328
20% Dextrose Injection, 327–328
25% Dextrose Injection, 327–328
50% Dextrose Injection, 327–328
60% Dextrose Injection, 327–328
70% Dextrose Injection, 327–328
Dey-Lute Isoetharine, 611–612
Dey-Lute Metaproterenol, 722–723
dezocine, 328
DFMO, 389
d-glucose, 327–328
D.H.E. 45, 346–347
DHT, 347–348
DHT Intensol, 347–348
DiaBeta, 538–540
Diabinese, 236–237
Diagnosis phase of nursing process, xxxii–xxxiii
Dialose, 361
Dialume, 48–49
Diamox, 10–12

Diamox Sequels, 10–12
Diapid, 696
Diastat, 328–331
diazepam, 328–331, 1354t
Diazepam Intensol, 328–331
diazoxide, 331–333
dichlorphenamide, 333
diclofenac potassium, 333–336
diclofenac sodium, 333–336
diclofenac sodium 0.1%, 1276t
diclofenac sodium 3%, 1296t
dicloxacillin sodium, 336–337
dicumarol, 337–339
dicyclomine hydrochloride, 339–340
Didronel, 450–451
Differin, 1294t
Dificid, 483–
diflorasone diacetate, 1291t
Diflucan, 490–492
diflunisal, 340–342
difluprednate, 1276t
Digibind, 344–346
digoxin, 342–344
digoxin immune Fab (ovine), 344–346
dihydroergotamine mesylate, 346–347
Dihydroergotamine-Sandoz, 346–347
dihydrogenated ergot alkaloids, 412–413
dihydromorphinone, 566–568
dihydrotachysterol, 347–348
1,25-dihydroxy-cholecalciferol, 167–168
Dilacor XR, 348–350, 350i
Dilantin, 936–940
Dilantin-30, 936–940
Dilantin-125, 936–940
Dilantin Infatabs, 936–940
Dilantin Kapseals, 936–940
Dilatrate-SR, 616–618, 617i
Dilaudid, 566–568
Dilaudid-5, 566–568
Dilaudid-HP, 566–568
Dilocaine, 662–664
Dilor, 388
diltiazem hydrochloride, 348–350, 350i
Dimelor, 12–13
dimenhydrinate, 350–352
dimethyl fumarate, 352–353
Dinate, 350–352
dinoprostone, 1334
Diochloram, 1273t
Diocto, 361
Diocto-K, 361
dioctyl calcium sulfosuccinate, 361–362
dioctyl potassium sulfosuccinate, 361
dioctyl sodium sulfosuccinate, 361–362

Dioeze, 361
Dioptic, 1273t
Dioval 40, 429–435
Dioval XX, 429–435
Diovan, 1220–1221
Diovan HCT 80/12.5, 1328t
Diovan HCT 160/12.5, 1328t
Diovan HCT 160/25, 1328t
Diovan HCT 320/12.5, 1328t
Diovan HCT 320/25, 1328t
Dipentum, 862–863
Diphenhist CapTabs, 353–354
diphenhydramine hydrochloride, 353–354, 1354t
dipivefrin hydrochloride, 1280t
Diprivan, 993–994
Diprolene, 1290t
Diprolene AF, 1290t
Diprosone, 1290t
dipyridamole, 354–355
dirithromycin, 355–356
Disalcid, 1049–1050
Disipal, 874–875
disodium cromoglycate, 285–287, 286i
disoprofol, 993–994
disopyramide, 356–358
disopyramide phosphate, 356–358
DisperMox, 68–70
Distribution of drugs, xxiii
disulfiram, 358–359
Ditropan, 883–885
Ditropan XL, 883–885
Diulo, 753–754
Diuril, 230–232
divalproex sodium, 1217–1220
Dixarit, 264–267
Dizac, 328–331
Dizmiss, 703–704
dobutamine hydrochloride, 359–361
Dobutrex, 359–361
docetaxel, 1316t
docosanol, 1290t
Dr. Scholl's Athlete's Foot, 1289t
Docucal-P, 361–362
Documentation phase of nursing process, xxxiii–xxxiv
docusate calcium, 361–362
docusate potassium, 361–362
docusate sodium, 361–362
dofetilide, 362–363
DOK, 361–362
Doktors, 934–936
dolasetron mesylate, 363–364
Dolgesic, 575–578
Dolobid, 340–342

Dolophine, 726–730
Dom-Proic, 1217–1220
donepezil hydrochloride, 365–366
Donnamar, 572–573
Donnazyme, 898–899
Dopamet, 742–743
dopamine hydrochloride, 366–368
Dopar, 653–654
Dopram, 369–370
Doral, 1005–1006
Doribax, 368–369
doripenem, 368–369
Doryx, 374–378
dorzolamide hydrochloride, 1281t
D.O.S. Softgels, 361
Dosage calculations, 1356–1360
Dostinex, 163–164
Dovonex, 1295t
doxapram hydrochloride, 369–370
doxazosin mesylate, 370–371
doxepin hydrochloride, 371–373, 1296t
doxercalciferol, 373–374
Doxidan, 361–362
Doxil, 1312t
Doxine, 1338t
doxorubicin, liposomal, 1312t
doxorubicin hydrochloride, 1312t
Doxycin, 374–378
doxycycline calcium, 374–378
doxycycline hyclate, 374–378
doxycycline monohydrate, 375–378
Dramamine II, 703–704
Dramanate, 350–352
Drenison, 1291t
Drisdol, 1344t
Drisdol Drops, 1344t
Drithocreme, 1294t
Dritho-Scalp, 1294t
dronabinol, 378–379
dronedarone, 379–381
droperidol, 381–382, 1354t
Droxia, 1314t
Drug absorption, xxi–xxiii
Drug administration, xxvii–xxx
Drug calculations, 1356–1360
Drug classification, xx–xxi
Drug distribution, xxiii
Drug excretion, xxiii
Drug interactions, xviii
Drug metabolism, xxiii
Drug nomenclature, xx
Drug receptors, xxiii
DTIC, 1322t
DTIC-Dome, 1322t

dulaglutide, 382–383
duloxetine hydrochloride, 384–386
Duphalac, 634–635
Duraclon, 264–267
Dura-Estrin, 429–435
Duragen-20, 429–435
Duragesic, 471–477
Duralith, 679–681
Duramorph, 792–796
Duration, 934–936
Durezol, 1276t
Duricef, 186–187
dutasteride, 386–387, 387i
Duvoid, 139–140
Dyazide, 1328t
Dycill, 336–337
Dymelor, 12–13
Dynabac, 355–356
Dynacin, 771–774
DynaCirc, 620–621
Dynapen, 336–337
dyphylline, 388
Dyrenium, 1194–1195
Dyspep HB, 460–462, 461i

E

Ear medications, xxii, xxx
Easprin, 98–100
EC-Naprosyn, 816–819
E-Complex 600, 1344t
econazole nitrate, 1287t
Econopred Plus, 1t
Ecostatin, 1287t
Ecotrin, 98–100
Ecotrin Maximum Strength, 98–100
E-Cypionate, 429–435
Edarbi, 114–115
Edarbyclor 40/12.5, 1328t
Edarbyclor 40/25, 1328t
Edecrin, 442–444
Edex, 44–47, 45i
ED-SPAZ, 572–573
Edurant, 1302t
E.E.S., 416–420
efavirenz, 1300t, 1301t
Effer-K, 954–958
Effexor, 1229–1232
Effexor XR, 1229–1232
Effient, 966–967
Eflone, 1276t
eflornithine, 1296t

eflornithine hydrochloride, 389
Efudex, 1296t, 1314t
Egrifta, 1129–1130
8-Hour Bayer Time Release, 98–100
8X Pancreatin, 898–899
Eldepryl, 1056–1058
Elderly patients, xxv
Eldopaque, 1296t
Eldoquin, 1296t
eletriptan hydrobromide, 389–390
Elidel, 1298t
Eligard, 645–647
Elimite, 1298t
Eliquis, 83–84
Elixophyllin, 1132–1135
Ellence, 1312t
Elmiron, 920–921
Elocom, 1293t
Elocon, 1293t
Eloxatin, 1310t
Elspar, 1317t
eltrombopag olamine, 391–393
Eltroxin, 660–662
Emadine, 1281t
Embeline, 1291t
Emcyt, 1319t
emedastine difumarate, 1281t
Emend, 86–88
Emend for Injection, 86–88
Emete-Con, 131–132
Eminase, 82–83
EMLA, 1297t
Emo-Cort, 1292t
empagliflozin, 393–394
Epanova, 865–866
Empirin, 98–100
Emsam, 1056–1058
emtricitabine, 1300t, 1302t
Emtriva, 1300t
E-Mycin, 416–420
Enablex, 308–309
enalaprilat, 394–396
enalapril maleate, 394–396, 1322t
Enbrel, 440–442, 441i
Endantadine, 50–52
Endep, 61–63, 62i
End Lice, 1298t
Endur-Acin, 1338t
enfuvirtide, 1300t
Enjuvia, 435–439
enoxacin, 396–398, 397i
enoxaparin sodium, 398–400
entacapone, 400–402
Enteral administration, xxi

Enteral routes of administration, xxviii–xxix
Entereg, 49–50
Entocort EC, 149–152
Entyvio, 1228
Enulose, 634–635
Enzymes, antineoplastic, 1308, 1317t
Epifoam, 1293t
Epimorph, 792–796
epinephrine, 402–404
epinephrine bitartrate, 402–404
EpiPen, 402–404
EpiPen Auto-Injector, 402–404
EpiPen Jr., 402–404
EpiPen Jr. Auto-Injector, 402–404
epirubicin hydrochloride, 1312t
Epitol, 176–179, 176i
Epival, 1217–1220
Epivir, 1301t
Epivir HBV, 1306t
eplerenone, 404–405
EPO, 405–408
epoetin alfa, 405–408
Epogen, 405–408
epoprostenol sodium, 408–410
Eprex, 405–408
eprosartan mesylate, 410–411
eptifibatide, 411–412
Epzicom, 1299t
Equanil, 716–717
Equetro, 176–179, 176i
Equianalgesic doses for opioid agonists, 1363t
Equivalents and weights, 1361–1362t
Eraxis, 79–80
Ergamisol, 1318t
ergocalciferol, 1344t
ergoloid mesylates, 412–413
Ergomar, 413–414
Ergostat, 413–414
ergotamine tartrate, 413–414
eribulin mesylate, 1322t
Eridium, 927
ertapenem sodium, 414–416
Erybid, 416–420
ERYC, 416–420
Erycette, 1284t
EryDerm, 1284t
Erygel, 1284t
Erymax, 1284t
EryPed, 416–420
Ery-Sol, 1284t
Ery-Tab, 416–420
Erythro, 416–420
Erythrocin, 416–420
Erythrocot, 416–420

Erythrogel, 1284t
erythromycin, 416–420, 1273t, 1284t
erythromycin 3% and benzoyl peroxide 5%, 1284t
erythromycin estolate, 416–420
erythromycin ethylsuccinate, 416–420
erythromycin gluceptate, 416–420
erythromycin lactobionate, 416–420
erythromycin stearate, 416–420
erythropoietin alfa, 405–408
escitalopram oxalate, 420–421
Esclim, 429–435
Esidrix, 558–561, 559i
Eskalith, 679–681
Eskalith CR, 679–681
eslicarbazepine acetate, 422–423
esmolol hydrochloride, 423–424
esomeprazole magnesium, 425–428
esomeprazole strontium, 425–428
Esomeprazole strontium, 425–428
estazolam, 428–429
Estinyl, 429–435
Estrace, 429–435
Estraderm, 429–435
estradiol, 429–435
estradiol acetate, 429–435
estradiol cypionate, 429–435
estradiol transdermal system, 429–435
estradiol valerate, 429–435
Estragyn LA 5, 429–435
Estra-L 40, 429–435
estramustine phosphate sodium, 1319t
Estrasorb, 429–435
Estring, 429–435
Estro-Cyp, 429–435
Estrofem, 429–435
Estrogel, 429–435
estrogens (conjugated), 435–439
estrogens (conjugated) and medroxyprogesterone,
    435–439
Estro-L.A., 429–435
Estro-Span, 429–435
eszopiclone, 439–440
etanercept, 440–442, 441i
ethacrynate sodium, 442–443
ethacrynic acid, 442–443
ethambutol hydrochloride, 444–445
ethchlorvynol, 445–446
ethinyl estradiol, 429–435
ethionamide, 446–447
Ethnic considerations, xxv
ethosuximide, 447–448
ethotoin, 448–450
Etibi, 444–445
etidronate disodium, 450–451

etodolac, 451–453
Etopophos, 1322t
etoposide, 1322t
etoposide phosphate, 1322t
etravirine, 1301t
ETS, 1284t
Euflex, 1319t
Euflexxa, 556–557
Euglucon, 572–574
Eulexin, 1319t
Eurax, 287, 1296t
Evalose, 634–635
Evaluation phase of nursing process, xxxiii
Evamist, 429–435
everolimus, 453–454, 1312t
Evista, 1013–1014
E-Vitamin succinate, 1344t
Evoclin, 257–258
Evoxac, 226–227
Exalgo, 566–568
Excedrin IB, 575–578
Excretion of drugs, xxiii
Exdol, 8–10
Exelderm, 1289t
Exelon, 1036–1038
Exelon Patch, 1036–1038
exemestane, 1319t
exenatide, 455–457, 456i
Exforge, 1328t
Exforge HCT 5/160/12.5, 1328t
Exforge HCT 5/160/25, 1328t
Exforge HCT 10/160/12.5, 1328t
Exforge HCT 10/160/25, 1328t
Exforge HCT 10/320/25, 1328t
Exjade, 309–311
Ex-Lax Light Formula, 361
Extavia, 1350t
Extra Strength Bayer Advanced Aspirin, 98–100
Eye medications, xxii, xxx, 1273–1282t
Eyesine, 1279t
EZE-DS, 239
ezetimibe, 457–458, 458i
ezogabine, 459–460

F

Factive, 529–531
famciclovir, 1304t
famotidine, 460–462, 461i
Famvir, 1304t
Fanapt, 580–582
Fareston, 1320t

Farxiga, 302–304
Fat-soluble drugs, xxi
Fazaclo, 270–273
febuxostat, 462–463
felbamate, 464–465
Felbatol, 464–465
Feldene, 947–949
felodipine, 465–466
Femara, 1320t
Femiron, 472–481
Femizol-M, 1288t
Femogex, 429–435
FemPatch, 429–435
Femring, 429–435
Femstat, 1286t
Femstat One, 1286t
Femtrace, 429–435
fenofibrate, 466–468
fenofibric acid, 466–468
fenoldopam mesylate, 468–469
fenoprofen calcium, 469–470
fentanyl citrate, 471–477
fentanyl iontophoretic transdermal, 471–477
fentanyl transdermal system, 471–477
Feosol, 478–481
Feostat, 478–481
Feostat Drops, 478–481
Feraheme, 481–482
Feratab, 478–481
Fer-gen-sol, 478–481
Fergon, 478–481
Fer-In-Sol Capsules, 478–481
Fer-In-Sol Drops, 478–481
Fer-In-Sol Syrup, 478–481
Fer-Iron Drops, 478–481
Fero-Grad, 478–481
Fero-Gradumet, 478–481
Ferospace, 478–481
Ferralet, 478–481
Ferralet Slow Release, 478–481
Ferralyn Lanacaps, 478–481
Ferra-TD, 478–481
Ferretts, 478–481
ferric citrate, 477
Ferrlecit, 1072–1073
ferrous fumarate, 477–481
ferrous gluconate, 478–481
ferrous salts, 478–481
ferrous sulfate, 478–481
Fertinic, 478–481
ferumoxytol, 481–482
fesoterodine fumarate, 481–482
Fetzima, 657–658
Feverall, 8–10

Feverall Sprinkle Caps, 8–10
fexofenadine, 1272t
fidaxomicin, 483
filgrastim, 483–485
Finacea, 1284t
finasteride, 485–486
Finevin, 1284t
fingolimod hydrochloride, 486–488
Firazyr, 579
Firmagon, 1319t
First-pass metabolism, xxii, xxx
Flagyl, 757–759
Flagyl I.V., 757–759
Flagyl I.V. RTU, 757–759
Flamazine, 1285t
Flarex, 1276t
flavoxate hydrochloride, 488
Flebogamma 5% DIF, 584–590
Flebogamma 10% DIF, 584–590
flecainide acetate, 489–490
Flexeril, 288–289
Flexoject, 874–875
Flolan, 408–410
Flomax, 1111–1112
Flonase, 503–504
Flo-Pred, 969–972
Florinef, 492–493
Florone, 1291t
Flovent, 503–505
Flow rate calculations, 1359–1360
Floxin, 855–856
floxuridine, 1313t
fluconazole, 490–492
fludarabine phosphate, 1325t
fludrocortisone acetate, 492–493
Fluid ounces, 1361
flumazenil, 493–494
Flu medications, 1305t
flunisolide, 494–495
Fluocet, 1291t
fluocinolone acetonide, 1291t
fluocinolone acetonide 0.01%, hydroquinone 4%,
    tretinoin 0.05%, 1296t
fluocinonide, 1291t
Fluoderm, 1291t
Fluolar, 1291t
Fluonid, 1291t
Fluonide, 1291t
fluorescein sodium, 1281t
Fluorescite, 1281t
Fluor-I-Strip, 1281t
Fluor-I-Strip-A.T., 1281t
fluorodeoxyuridine, 1313t
fluoromethalone, 1276t

fluoromethalone acetate, 1276t
Fluor-Op, 1276t
Fluoroplex, 1296t, 1314t
fluorouracil, 1314t
5-fluorouracil, 1314t
fluorouracil cream, 1296t
fluoxetine hydrochloride, 495–498
fluphenazine decanoate, 498–500
fluphenazine enanthate, 498–500
fluphenazine hydrochloride, 498–500
flurandrenolide, 1291t
flurazepam hydrochloride, 500–501
flurbiprofen, 501–502
flurbiprofen sodium, 1276t
Flurosyn, 1291t
flutamide, 1319t
Flutex, 1293t, 1294t
fluticasone furoate, 503–505
fluticasone propionate, 503–505, 1291t
fluvastatin sodium, 505–507
fluvoxamine maleate, 507–509
FML Forte, 1276t
FML Liquifilm, 1276t
FML S.O.P., 1276t
Focalin, 325–326
Focalin XR, 325–326
FoilleCort, 1292t
Folex, 737–738
Folex PFS, 737–738
Folvite, 1340t
fondaparinux sodium, 509–511
Foradil Aerolizer, 511–513
formoterol fumarate dihydrate, 511–513
Formulas and calculations, 1356–1360
Formulex, 339–340
Fortamet, 724–726
Fortaz, 208–210
Forteo, 1128–1129, 1129i
Fortovase, 1302t
Fosamax, 30–32
fosamprenavir calcium, 1301t
fosaprepitant dimeglumine, 86–88
foscarnet, 1304t, 1305t
Foscavir, 1304t, 1305t
fosfomycin tromethamine, 513–514
fosinopril sodium, 514–516
fosphenytoin sodium, 516–519
Fosrenol, 642–643, 643i
Fostex 10 BPO Gel, 1284t
4X Pancreatin, 898–899
Fragmin, 298–300
Froben, 501–502
Froben SR, 501–502
Frova, 519–520

frovatriptan succinate, 519–520
5-FU, 1314t
FUDR, 1313t
Ful-Glo, 1281t
Fulyza, 284
Fumasorb, 478–481
Fumerin, 478–481
Funduscein-10, 1281t
Funduscein-25, 1281t
Fungizone Intravenous, 72–75
Fungoid, 1288t
Furacin, 1285t
Furadantin, 841–842
furazolidone, 520–521
furosemide, 522–524, 1354t
Furoside, 522–524
Furoxone, 520–521
Fuzeon, 1300t
Fycompa, 922–923

G

gabapentin, 525–527
gabapentin enacarbil, 525–527
Gabitril, 1146–1147
galantamine hydrobromide, 527–528
Galzin, 1251–1254
Gamimune N 5% S/D, 584–590
Gamimune N 10% S/D, 584–590
Gammagard Liquid, 584–590
Gammagard S/D, 584–590
Gammagard S/D 0.5 g, 584–590
gamma globulin, 584–590
Gammar-P IV, 584–590
Gamunex 10%, 584–590
Gamunex-C, 584–590
ganciclovir, 1273t, 1305t
Gantanol, 109–1091
Gantrisin, 1094–1096
Garamycin, 531–533, 1274t, 1284t
Gastrocrom, 285–287, 286i
Gastrosed, 572–573
gatifloxacin 0.3%, 1274t
gatifloxacin 0.5%, 1274t
GBH, 667–668
Gee-Gee, 545–546
Gefitinib, 1323t
Gelnique, 1298t
Gelnique 10%, 883–884
gemcitabine hydrochloride, 1323t
gemfibrozil, 528–529
gemifloxacin mesylate, 529–531

Gemzar, 1323t
Genahist, 353–354
Gen-Amantadine, 50–52
Genapap Infants' Drops, 8–10
Genapax, 1287t
Genaspore, 1289t
Genatuss, 545–546
Gen-Cimetidine, 245–247
Gen-Clonazepam, 263–264
Genebs Extra Strength, 8–10
Generic names of drugs, xiv
Gen-Fibro, 528–529
Gen-Glybe, 572–574
Gen-Indapamide, 593–594
Gen-K, 954–958
Gen-Medroxy, 984–988
Gen-Metformin, 724–726
Gen-Minocycline, 771–774
Gen-Minoxidil, 774–776
Genoptic, 1274t
Genpril, 575–578
Genprin, 98–100
Gen-Ranitidine, 1017–1019
Gen-Salbutamol, 27–29, 28i
Gen-Selegiline, 1056–1058
Gentacidin, 1274t
Gentak, 1274t
gentamicin sulfate, 531–533, 1274t, 1284t
Gen-Tamoxifen, 1110–1111, 1320t
gentian violet, 1287t
Gen Triazolam, 1195–1197
Geodon, 1254–1256
Geodon for Injection, 1254–1256
Geridium, 927
Gerimal, 412
Gesterol 50, 984–988
Gesterol LA 238, 984–988
GG-CEN, 545–546
Gilenya, 486–488
Glassia, 41–42
Gleevec, 1323t
Gliadel Wafer, 1309t
glibenclamide, 572–574
glimepiride, 533–535
glipizide, 535–536
GlucaGen, 570–571
glucagon, 570–571
Glucagon Diagnostic Kit, 570–572
Glucagon Emergency Kit, 570–572
Glucophage, 724–726
Glucophage XR, 724–726
glucose, 327–328
Glucotrol, 535–536
Glucotrol XL, 535–536

Glu-K, 995–958
Glumetza, 724–726
Glutose, 327–328
glyburide, 572–574
glyceryl trinitrate, 842–845
Glycon, 724–726
glycopyrrolate, 574–576, 1354t
Gly-Cort, 1292t
Glycotuss, 545–546
Glynase PresTab, 572–574
Glyquin, 1296t
Glyset, 767–768
Glytuss, 545–546
G-Mycin, 531–533
G-myticin, 1284t
golimumab, 576–578
goserelin acetate, 1319t
Gralise, 559–561
Grams, 1361
granisetron hydrochloride, 544–545
granulocyte colony-stimulating factor, 483–485
grass pollen, 1334
Grastek, 1270
Gravol, 350–352
guaifenesin, 545–546
Guaituss, 545–46
guanadrel sulfate, 546–547
guanethidine monosulfate, 547–549
guanfacine hydrochloride, 549–550
G-well, 667–668
Gynazole-1, 1286t
Gynecort, 1292t
GyneCure Ovules, 1289t
Gyne-Lotrimin, 1286t
Gyne-Lotrimin 3, 1286
Gynergen, 413–414
Gynogen L.A. 20, 429–435
Gynogen L.A. 40, 429–435

H

Habitrol, 835–837
Halaven, 1322t
halazepam, 550–551
halcinonide, 1291t
Halcion, 1195–1197
Haldol, 551–553
Haldol Concentrate, 551–553
Haldol Decanoate, 551–553
Haldol LA, 551–553
Halenol Children's Junior Strength, 8–10
Half-life, xxiii

halobetasol propionate, 1291t
Halog, 1291t
haloperidol, 551–553, 1354t
haloperidol decanoate, 551–553
haloperidol lactate, 551–553
haloprogin, 1287t
Halotex, 1287t
Halotussin, 545–546
Haltran, 575–578
Hecoria, 1104–1108
Hectorol, 373–374
Hemocyte, 478–481
Hepalean, 553–556
heparin, 1354t
heparin calcium, 553–556
Heparin Leo, 553–556
Heparin Lock Flush, 553–556
heparin sodium, 553–556
Hepatitis B medications, 1306–1307t
Hepatitis C medications, 1307t
Hepsera, 1306t
Heptalac, 634–635
Herceptin, 1325t
Herpes virus medications, 1303–1304t
Herplex Liquifilm, 1304t
hexachlorophene, 1296t
Hexadrol, 320–323
Hexadrol Phosphate, 320–323
Hexit, 667–668
Hibiclens, 1295t
Hi-Cor 1.0, 1292t
Hi-Cor 2.5, 1292t
Hiprex, 732–733
Histantil, 988–990
Hi-Vegi-Lip, 898–899
HIV medications, 1300–1307t
Hizentra 20%, 584–624
HMS Liquifilm, 1277t
homatropine hydrobromide, 1278t
Horizant, 525–527
Hormonal drugs, 1308, 1318–1320t
Household system of measurement, 1361t
Humalog, 1267t
Humalog Mix 50/50, 1269t
Humalog Mix 75/25, 1269t
Humira, 19–22
Humulin 10/90, 1269t
Humulin 20/80, 1269t
Humulin 30/70, 1269t
Humulin 40/60, 1269t
Humulin 70/30, 1269t
Humulin N, 1269t
Humulin-R, 1267t
Humulin-U, 1268t

hyaluronan (high-molecular-weight), 556–557
Hycamtin, 1325t
Hydergine, 412
Hydergine LC, 412
Hyderm, 1292t, 1293t
hydralazine hydrochloride, 557–558, 1326t
Hydrate, 350–352
Hydrea, 1314t
Hydro-chlor, 558–561, 559i
hydrochlorothiazide, 558–561, 559i, 1326t, 1328t,
    1330t, 1332t
hydrocodone, 1363t
hydrocodone bitartrate, 561–563
hydrocortisone, 563–566
hydrocortisone 0.25%, 1292t
hydrocortisone 0.50%, 1292t
hydrocortisone 1%, 1292t
hydrocortisone 2%, 1292t
hydrocortisone 2.5%, 1292t
hydrocortisone acetate, 563–566
hydrocortisone acetate, polymyxin B sulfate, and
    neomycin sulfate, 1293t, 1296t
hydrocortisone acetate 0.1%, 1292t
hydrocortisone acetate 0.5%, 1292t
hydrocortisone acetate 1%, 1293t
hydrocortisone acetate 2%, 1293t
hydrocortisone acetate 2.5%, 1293t
hydrocortisone acetate dental paste, 1293t
hydrocortisone acetate topical aerosol foam, 1293t
hydrocortisone and iodoquinol, 1293t
hydrocortisone butyrate, 1293t
hydrocortisone cypionate, 563–566
hydrocortisone sodium phosphate, 563–566
hydrocortisone sodium succinate, 563–566
hydrocortisone valerate, 1293t
Hydrocortone, 563–566
Hydrocortone Acetate, 563–566
Hydrocortone Phosphate, 563–566
Hydro-D, 558–561, 559i
HydroDIURIL, 558–561, 559i
hydromorphone hydrochloride, 566–568, 1354t,
    1363t
Hydrophilic drugs, xxi
hydroquinone, 1296t
Hydrostat IR, 566–568
Hydro-Tex, 1292t
hydroxychloroquine sulfate, 569–571
hydroxycobalamin, 1340t
hydroxyprogesterone caproate, 984–988, 1334
hydroxyurea, 1314t
hydroxyzine hydrochloride, 571–572, 1354t
hydroxyzine pamoate, 571–572
Hy/Gestrone, 984–988
Hygroton, 237–239

Hylorel, 546–547
Hylutin, 984–988
hyoscyamine sulfate, 572–573
Hypersensitivity reactions, xxv
Hyperstat, 331–332
Hyrexin, 353–354
Hytakerol, 347–348
Hytone, 1292t
Hytrin, 1122–1123
Hytuss, 545–546
Hytuss 2X, 545–546
Hyzaar 50/12.5, 1328t
Hyzaar 100/25, 1328t

I

ibandronate sodium, 573–574
Ibifon 600 Caplets, 575–578
Ibuprin, 575–578
ibuprofen, 575–578
Ibuprohm Caplets, 575–578
Ibu-Tab, 575–578
ibutilide fumarate, 578–579
icatibant, 579
icosapent ethyl, 579–580
I.D. administration, xxii, xxix
Idamycin, 1312t
idarubicin hydrochloride, 1312t
Idiosyncratic responses, xxiv
idoxuridine, 1304t
IFEX, 1309t
ifosfamide, 1309t
IG, 584–590
IGIV, 584–590
IL-2, 1326t
iloperidone, 580–582
Ilosone, 416–420
Ilotycin, 416–420, 1273t
Ilozyme, 899–901
I.M. administration, xxii, xxix
imatinib mesylate, 1323t
IMDUR, 616–618, 617i
imipramine hydrochloride, 582–584
imipramine pamoate, 582–584
imiquimod 3.75%, 1297t
imiquimod 5%, 1297t
Imitrex, 1099–1101
ImmuCyst, 1318t
immune globulin intramuscular (human), 584–590
immune globulin intravenous (human), 584–590
immune globulin subcutaneous (human), 584–590
immune serum globulin, 585–590

Implementation phase of nursing process, xxxiii
Impril, 582–584
Imuran, 112–113
inamrinone (amrinone), 590–591
Inapsine, 381–382
Incivek, 1307t
Incruse Ellipta, 1211
indacaterol maleate, 591–592
Indameth, 594–597
indapamide, 593–594
Inderal, 994–997
Inderal LA, 994–997
Inderide LA 80/25, 1328t
Inderide LA 80/50, 1328t
Inderide LA 120/50, 1328t
Inderide LA 160/50, 1328t
indinavir, 1301t
Indocid, 594–597
Indocid PDA, 595–597
Indocin, 595–597
Indocin I.V., 595–597
Indocin SR, 595–597
indomethacin, 595–597
indomethacin sodium trihydrate, 595–597
InFeD, 606–607
Infergen, 1350t
Inflamase Forte, 1277t
Inflamase Mild, 1327t
infliximab, 597–600
Influenza medications, 1305t
ingenol mebutate gel 0.05%, 1297t
ingenol mebutate gel 0.015%, 1297t
INH, 622–624
Inhalation administration, xxii, xxx
Inlyta, 1320t
Innohep, 1157–1158
InnoPran XL, 994–997
Inocor, 590–591
Inspra, 404–495
Insta-Glucose, 327–328
insulin aspart, 1267t
insulin detemir, 1269t
insulin glargine, 1269t
insulin glulisine, 1267t
insulin, inhaled (rapid-acting), 600–602
insulin lispro, 1267t
Insulin preparations, 1267t–1269t
Insulin Reaction, 327–328
Intal Syncroner, 285–287, 286i
Integrilin, 411–412
Intelence, 1301t
Interactions of drugs, xv
interferon alfa-2a, recombinant, 1307t
interferon alfa-2b, recombinant, 1307t

interferon alfacon-1, 1350t
interferon alfa-n3, 1348t
interferon beta-1a, 1350t
interferon beta-1b, 1350t
interferon gamma-1b, 1352t
Interferons, 1348–1353t
interleukin-2, 1318t
Intermediate-acting insulin, 1268t
Intermezzo, 1259–1261
Intradermal (I.D.) administration, xxii, xxix
Intramuscular (I.M.) administration, xxii, xxix
Intravenous (I.V.) administration, xxii, xxix
Intron A, 1318t, 1348t
Intropin, 366–368
Intuniv, 549–550
Invanz, 414–416
Invega, 893–895
Invega Sustenna, 893–895
Invirase, 1302t
Invokana, 170–171
iodoquinol, 1393t
Ionsys, 471–477
Iopidine, 1279t
ipecac syrup, 602–603
Ipecac Syrup, 602–603
ipratropium bromide, 603–604, 604i
irbesartan, 604–606, 1326t
Ircon, 478–481
iressa, 1323t
irinotecan hydrochloride, 1323t
iron carbonyl, 478–481
iron dextran, 606–607
iron sucrose, 607–609
Irreversible antagonists, xxiv
Isentress, 1302t
ISG, 584–590
Ismelin, 547–549
ISMO, 616–618, 617i
isocarboxazid, 609–611
isoetharine hydrochloride, 611–612
isoetharine mesylate, 611–612
isoniazid, 612–614
isonicotinic acid hydrazide, 612–614
isoprenaline, 614–616
isoproterenol, 614–616
isoproterenol hydrochloride, 614–616
isoproterenol sulfate, 614–616
Isoptin, 1232–1234
Isoptin SR, 1232–1234
Isopto Atropine, 1277t
Isopto Carbachol, 1278t
Isopto Carpine, 1278
Isopto Cetamide, 1275
Isopto Frin, 1279t

Isopto Homatropine, 1278t
Isopto Hyoscine, 1278t
Isordil Tembids, 616–618, 617i
Isordil Titradose, 616–618, 617i
isosorbide dinitrate, 616–618, 617i
isosorbide mononitrate, 616–618, 617
Isotamine, 612–614
isotretinoin, 618–620
isradipine, 620–621
Istodax, 1313t
Isuprel, 614–616
Isuprel Mistometer, 614–616
itraconazole, 621–624
I.V. administration, xxii, xxiv
I.V. flow rate calculations, 1359–1360
Iveegam EN, 584–590
ivermectin lotion 0.5%, 1297t
IVIG, 584–590
ixabepilone, 1316t, 1323t
Ixempra, 1316t, 1323t

J

Januvia, 1069–1079
Jardiance, 393–394
Jenamicin, 531–533
Jenloga, 264–267
Juxtapid, 683–685

K

K-8, 954–958
K-10, 954–958
K+10, 954–958
Kabikinase, 1083–1084
Kadian, 792–796
Kaletra, 1301t
Kalium Durules, 954–958
kanamycin sulfate, 625–626
Kantrex, 625–626
Kaochlor 10%, 954–958
Kaochlor S-F 10%, 954–958
Kaon, 954–958
Kaon-Cl, 954–958
Kapvay, 264–267
Kasof, 361–362
Kato, 954–958
Kay Ciel, 954–958
Kayexalate, 1074–1075
Kaylixir, 955–958
K+Care, 954–958

K+Care ET, 954–958
KCL 5%, 954–958
K-Dur, 954–958
Keflex, 219–220, 220i
Keftab, 219–220, 220i
K-Electrolyte, 954–958
Kenac, 1293t, 1294t
Kenacort, 1190–1194
Kenacort Diacetate, 1190–1194
Kenalog, 1293t, 1294t
Kenalog-10, 1190–1194
Kenalog-40, 1190–1194
Kenalog-H, 1294t
Kenalog in Orabase, 1294t
Kendral-Ipratropium, 603–604, 604i
Ken-Jec-40, 1190–1194
Kenonel, 1293t, 1294t
keoxifene hydrochloride, 1013–1014
Keppra, 649–651
Keppra XR, 649–651
Kerlone, 137–139
Ketek, 1117–1118
ketoconazole 2%, 1287t
ketoprofen, 626–628
ketorolac, 1354t
ketorolac tromethamine, 628–631, 1276t
ketotifen fumarate, 1281t
K-Exit, 1074–1075
Key-Pred, 969–972
K-G Elixir, 955–958
KI, 958–959
K-Ide, 954–958
Kidrolase, 1317t
Kildane, 667–668
Kineret, 78–79
Kionex, 1074–1075
Klaron, 1285t
K-Lease, 954–958
K-Long, 954–958
Klonopin, 263–264
K-Lor, 954–958
Klor-Con 10, 954–958
Klor-Con/25 Powder, 954–958
Klor-Con/EF, 954–958
Klor-Con Powder, 954–958
Klorvess 10% Liquid, 954–958
Klorvess Effervescent Granules, 954–958
Klotrix, 955–958
K-Lyte, 954–958
K-Lyte/Cl, 954–958
K-Lyte/Cl 50, 954–958
K-Lyte/Cl Powder, 955–958
K-Lyte DS, 954–958
K-Med 900, 955–958

K-Norm, 955–958
Kolyum, 955–958
K-Phos M.F., 959–960
K-Phos-Neutral, 959–960
K-Phos No. 2, 959–960
K-Phos Original, 959–960
K-Sol, 955–958
K-Tab, 955–958
Kuvan, 1050–1051
Ku-Zyme HP, 899–901
K-Vescent, 954–958
Kwell, 667–668
Kwellada, 667–668
Kwildane, 667–668
Kynamro, 776–777
Kytril, 544–545

L

labetalol hydrochloride, 631–632
Lac-Hydrin, 1294t
lacosamide, 632–634
LactiCare-HC, 1292t
Lactulax, 634–635
lactulose, 634–635
Lamictal, 635–639
Lamictal XR, 635–639
Lamisil, 1124–1125
Lamisil AT Cream, 1289t
Lamisil AT Solution, 1289t
Lamisil DermGel, 1289t
Lamisil Solution, 1289t
lamivudine, 1299t, 1301t, 1306t
lamivudine triphosphate, 1301t
lamotrigine, 635–639
Lanacort, 1292t
Lanophyllin, 1132–1135
Lanoxicaps, 342–344
Lanoxin, 342–344
Lanoxin Elixir Pediatric, 342–344
Lanoxin Injection, 342–344
Lanoxin Injection Pediatric, 342–344
lansoprazole, 639–642
lanthanum carbonate, 642–643, 643i
Lantus, 1269t
Lanvis, 1315t
Largactil, 233–236
Larodopa, 653–654, 652i
Lasix, 522–524
Lasix Special, 522–524
latanoprost, 1281t
Latuda, 694–694

Laxilose, 634–635
Lazanda, 471–477
L-Caine, 662–664
Ledercillin VK, 915–917
leflunomide, 643–645
Lemoderm, 1292t
Lescol, 505–507
Lescol XL, 505–507
letrozole, 1320t
Leukeran, 1318t
leuprolide acetate, 645–647, 1320t
levalbuterol hydrochloride, 648–649
levamisole hydrochloride, 1318t
Levaquin, 654–657
levarterenol bitartrate, 847–848
Levate, 61–62, 62i
Levatol, 911–913
Levbid, 572–573
Levemir, 1269t
levetiracetam, 649–651
Levitra, 1223–1225
levobunolol hydrochloride, 1281t
levocabastine hydrochloride 0.05%, 1281t
levocetirizine, 651–652, 1272t
levodopa, 653–654, 652i
Levo-Dromoran, 658–660
levofloxacin, 654–657
levofloxacin 0.5%, 1274t
levomilnacipran hydrochloride, 657–658
levonorgestrel, 984–988
Levophed, 847–848
levorphanol tartrate, 658–660, 1363t
Levo-T, 660–662
Levothroid, 660–662
levothyroxine sodium, 660–662
Levoxyl, 660–662
Levsin, 572–573
Levsinex Timecaps, 572–573
Levsin/SL, 572–573
Lexapro, 420–422
Lexiva, 1301t
Lialda, 719–720
Librium, 229–230
Lidemol, 1291t
Lidex, 1291t
lidocaine, 1354t
lidocaine and prilocaine, 1297t
lidocaine hydrochloride, 662–664
Lidoderm, 662–664
lignocaine hydrochloride, 662–664
linaclotide, 664
linagliptin, 664–665
Lincocin, 666–668
lincomycin hydrochloride, 666–667

lindane, 667–668
linezolid, 668–671, 670i
Linzess, 664
liothyronine sodium, 671–673
Lipid diffusion, xxi
Lipitor, 103–105
Lipofen, 466–468
Lipophilic drugs, xxi
Liquadd, 70–71
Liquaemin, 553–556
Liqui-Cal, 168–170
Liquid Cal-600, 168–170
Liquid equivalents, 1361t
Liqui-E, 1344t
Liquiprin Elixir, 8–10
Liquiprin Infants' Drops, 8–10
liraglutide, 673–674
lisdexamfetamine dimesylate, 674–676
lisinopril, 677–679, 1330t, 1332t
Lithane, 679–681
lithium carbonate, 679–681
lithium citrate, 679–681
Lithizine, 679–681
Lithobid, 679–681
Lithonate, 679–681
Lithostat, 13–14
Lithotabs, 679–681
Livalo, 949–950
Livostin, 1281t
Locoid, 1293t
Lodine, 451–453
Lodine XL, 451–453
lomefloxacin hydrochloride, 681–683
lomitapide mesylate, 683–685
lomustine, 1309t
Long-acting insulin, 1269t
Loniten, 774–775
Lopid, 528–529
lopinavir and ritonavir, 1301t
Lopresor, 754–757
Lopresor SR, 754–757
Lopressor, 654–757
Lopressor HCT 50/25, 1328t
Lopressor HCT 100/25, 1328t
Lopressor HCT 100/50, 1328t
Loprox 0.77%, 1286t
Lopurin, 36–37
Lorabid, 685–686
loracarbef, 685–686
loratadine, 1272t
lorazepam, 686–687, 1354t
Lorazepam Intensol, 686–687
lorcaserin hydrochloride, 687–689
losartan potassium, 689–690, 1328t

Losec, 866–868, 867i
Lotemax, 1277t
Lotensin, 129–131
Lotensin HCT 5/6.25, 1328t
Lotensin HCT 10/12.5, 1328t
Lotensin HCT 20/12.5, 1328t
Lotensin HCT 20/25, 1328t
loteprednol etabonate, 1277t
Lotrel 2.5/10, 1330t
Lotrel 5/10, 1330
Lotrel 5/20, 1330
Lotrel 10/20, 1330t
Lotrimin, 1286t
Lotrimin Antifungal, 1286t
Lotrimin Ultra, 1286t
Lotrisone, 1295t
Lotronex, 40–41
lovastatin, 690–692
Lovaza, 864–865
Lovenox, 398–400
Loxapac, 692–693
loxapine hydrochloride, 692–693
loxapine succinate, 692–693
Loxitane, 692–693
Loxitane C, 692–693
Loxitane IM, 692–693
Lozide, 593–594
Lozol, 593–594
L-phenylalanine mustard, 1310t
L-thyroxine sodium, 660–662
L-triiodothyronine, 671–673
L-triiodothyronine sodium, 671–673
lubiprostone, 694–695
Ludiomil, 702–703
Lufyllin, 388
Lumigan, 1280t
Luminal, 930–932
Lunesta, 439–440
Lupron, 645–647, 1320t
Lupron Depot, 645–647, 1320t
Lupron Depot-3 Month, 1320
Lupron Depot-3 Month 11.25 mg, 645–647
Lupron Depot-3 Month 22.5 mg, 645–647
Lupron Depot-4 Month, 1320
Lupron Depot-4 Month 30 mg, 645–647
Lupron Depot-6 Month 45 mg, 645–647
Lupron Depot-Ped-1 Month, 645–647
Lupron Depot-Ped-3 Month, 645–647
lurasidone hydrochloride, 694–695
Luvox, 507–509
Luvox CR, 507–509
Luxiq, 1290t
lypressin, 696
Lyrica, 974–976

Lysodren, 1323t
Lysteda, 1185–1186

M

Macrobid, 841–842
Macrodantin, 841–842
mafenide gel 1%, 1284t
Mag-200, 697–700
Mag-L-100, 697–700
Maglucate, 697–700
magnesium chloride, 697–700
magnesium citrate, 697–700
magnesium gluconate, 697–700
magnesium hydroxide, 697–700
magnesium lactate, 697–700
magnesium oxide, 697–700
magnesium sulfate, 697–700
Magonate, 697–700
Mag-Ox 400, 697–700
Mag-Tab SR Caplets, 697–700
Magtrate, 697–700
Makena, 1334
malathion lotion 0.5%, 1297
Mandelamine, 732–733
mannitol, 700–702
Maolate, 232
Maox, 697–700
maprotiline hydrochloride, 702–703
maraviroc, 1301t, 1303t
Marezine, 287–288
Marinol, 378–379
Marplan, 609–611
Marthritic, 1049–1050
Marzine, 287–288
Matulane, 1324t
Mavik, 1183–1185
Maxair, 946–947
Maxair Autohaler, 946–947
Maxalt, 1038–1039
Maxalt-MLT, 1038–1039
Maxaquin, 681–683
Maxeran, 751–753
Maxidex, 1276t
Maxiflor, 1291t
Maximum Bayer, 98–100
Maximum Strength Cortaid, 1293t
Maxipime, 192–194
Maxzide 37.5/25, 1330t
Maxzide 75/50, 1330t
MB-Tab, 716–717
Measurement systems, 1361–1362t

Mebaral, 715–716
mechlorethamine hydrochloride, 1309
Meclicot, 703–704
meclizine hydrochloride, 703–704
meclofenamate sodium, 704–705
Meclomen, 704–706
meclozine hydrochloride, 703–705
Meda Cap, 8–10
Medi-Glybe, 538–540
Medihaler Ergotamine, 413–414
Medihaler-Iso, 614–616
Medipren, 575–578
Medivert, 703–704
medrogestone, 984–988
Medrol, 748–751
medroxyprogesterone acetate, 987–988, 1320t
medrysone, 1277t
Med-Valproic, 1217–1220
Mefoxin, 202–204
Megace, 984–988, 1320
Megace OS, 984–988
Megacillin, 915–917
megestrol acetate, 984–988, 1320t
Melanex, 1296t
Mellaril, 1138–1140
Mellaril Concentrate, 1138–1140
Mellaril-S, 1138–1140
meloxicam, 706–708
melphalan, 1310
melphalan hydrochloride, 1310
memantine hydrochloride, 708–709, 709i–710i
Menaval-20, 429–435
Meni-D, 703–704
Menostar, 429–435
Mentax, 1286
meperidine hydrochloride, 710–711, 1354t, 1363t
mephentermine sulfate, 712–713
mephenytoin, 713–715
mephobarbital, 715–716
Mephyton, 1346
meprobamate, 716–717
Meprolone, 748–751
Mepron, 105–106
Meprospan, 716–717
mequinol 2% and retinol 0.01%, 1297t
mercaptopurine, 1314
6-mercaptopurine, 1314
meropenem, 717–719
Merrem I.V., 717–719
mesalamine, 719–720
Mesantoin, 713–715
Mesasal, 719–720
M-Eslon, 792–796
mesoridazine besylate, 720–722

Mestinon, 1002–1003
Mestinon-SR, 1002–1003
Mestinon Timespans, 1102–1003
Metabolism of drugs, xxii
Metadate, 745–748
Metadate CD, 745–748
Metadate ER, 745–748
metaproterenol sulfate, 722–723
metaxalone, 723–724
metformin hydrochloride, 724–726
methadone hydrochloride, 726–730
Methadose, 726–730
methamphetamine hydrochloride, 730–731
methazolamide, 731–732
methenamine hippurate, 732–733
methenamine mandelate, 732–733
methicillin sodium, 733–734
methimazole, 734–736
methocarbamol, 736–737
methotrexate, 737–738, 1314t
methotrexate sodium, 737–738, 1314t
methoxypolyethylene glycol-epoetin beta,
    739–741
methscopolamine bromide, 740
methsuximide, 741–742
Methylcotolone, 748–751
methyldopa, 742–743, 1326t
methyldopate hydrochloride, 742–743
Methylin, 745–748
Methylin ER, 745–748
methylnaltrexone bromide, 743–744
methylphenidate hydrochloride, 745–748
methylprednisolone, 748–751
methylprednisolone acetate, 748–751
methylprednisolone sodium succinate, 748–751
Meticorten, 972–974
metipranolol hydrochloride, 1281t
metoclopramide hydrochloride, 751–753, 1354t
Metoclopramide Intensol, 751–753
metolazone, 753–754
metoprolol succinate, 754–757
metoprolol tartrate, 754–757, 1328t
Metric 21, 757–759
Metric system, 1361–1362t
MetroCream, 1285
MetroGel, 757–759, 1285t
MetroGel-Vaginal, 757–759, 1285t
metronidazole, 757–759, 1285t
metronidazole hydrochloride, 757–759
metyrosine, 759–760
Mevacor, 690–692
mevinolin, 690–692
Mexate, 737–738
Mexate-AQ, 737–738

mexiletine hydrochloride, 760–761
Mexitil, 760–761
Mezlin, 761–763
mezlocillin sodium, 761–763
Miacalcin, 165–167
micafungin sodium, 763–764
Micardis, 1118–1119
Micardis HCT 40/12.5, 1330t
Micardis HCT 80/12.5, 1330t
Micatin, 1288t
miconazole nitrate, 1288t
Micort HC-Lipocream, 1293t
Micro-K, 955–958
Micro-K 10, 955–958
Micronase, 538–540
MicroNefrin, 402–404
Microzide, 558–561, 559i
Midamor, 53–54
midazolam hydrochloride, 764–766, 1354t
midodrine hydrochloride, 766–767
Midol IB, 575–578
miglitol, 767–768
Migranal, 346–347
milk of magnesia, 697–700
Milligrams, 1361
Milliliters, 1361
milnacipran hydrochloride, 657–658
milrinone lactate, 770–771, 771i
Miltown, 716–717
Minims Atropine, 1277t
Minims Cyclopentolate, 1278t
Minims Homatropine, 1278t
Minims Pilocarpine, 1278t
Minipress, 968–969
Minitran, 842–845
Minocin, 771–774
minocycline, 771–774
minocycline hydrochloride, 771–774
Minox, 774–776
minoxidil, 1297t
minoxidil (oral), 774–776
minoxidil (topical), 774–776
Minoxigaine, 774–776
Miocarpine, 1278t
Miochol-E, 1278t
Miolin, 874–875
Mio-Rel, 874–875
Miostat, 1278t
Miotics, 1278t
mipomersen sodium, 776–777
mirabegron, 777–778
Miradon, 80–82
Mirapex, 962–964
Mirapex ER, 962–964

Mircera, 739–740
mirtazapine, 778–780
misoprostol, 780–781
Mithracin, 1313t
mithramycin, 1313t
mitomycin, 1312t
mitomycin-C, 1312t
mitotane, 1323t
mitoxantrone hydrochloride, 781–783, 1324t
mixed pollens allergen extract, 1334
Moban Concentrate, 787–789
Mobic, 706–708
modafinil, 783–786
Modane Soft, 361
Modecate, 498–500
Modecate Concentrate, 498–500
Moditen Enanthate, 498–500
Moditen HCl, 498–500
Moduretic, 1330t
moexipril hydrochloride, 785–787, 1332t
molindone hydrochloride, 787–789
Mol-Iron, 478–481
mometasone furoate, 1293t
mometasone furoate monohydrate, 789–790
Monistat 3, 1288t
Monistat 7, 1288t
Monistat-Derm, 1288t
Monitan, 7–8
monobenzone 20%, 1297t
Monocid, 196–198
Monodox, 375–378
Mono-Gesic, 1049–1050
Monoket, 616–618, 617i
Monopril, 514–516
montelukast sodium, 790–792
Monurol, 513–514
Morphine Extra-Forte, 792–796
Morphine Forte, 792–796
Morphine H.P., 792–796
morphine sulfate, 792–796, 1354t, 1363t
Morphitec, 792–796
Motrin, 575–578
Motrin-IB, 575–578
Movantik, 811–812
Moxatag, 68–70
moxifloxacin 0.5%, 1274t
moxifloxacin hydrochloride, 796–799
6-MP, 1314t
MS Contin, 792–796
MSIR, 792–796
MS/L, 792–796
MS/L Concentrate, 792–796
MS/S, 792–796
Mucinex, 545–546

Mucomyst, 14–16
Mucosil, 14–16
Multaq, 379–381
Multipax, 571–572
mupirocin 2%, 1285t
Murine Plus, 1279t
Muro-128, 1281t
Muroptic-5, 1281t
Muse, 44–47, 45i
Mustargen, 1309t
Mutamycin, 1312t
Myambutol, 444–445
Mycamine, 763–764
Mycelex, 1286t
Mycelex 3, 1286t
Mycelex-7, 1286t
Mycelex-G, 1286t
Mycelex OTC, 1286t
Mycifradin, 827
Myciguent, 1285t
mycophenolate mofetil, 799–802
mycophenolate mofetil hydrochloride, 799–802
mycophenolic acid, 799–802
MyCort, 1292t
Mycostatin, 852–853, 1288t
Mydfrin, 1279t
Mydriacyl, 1278t
My-E, 416–420
Myfortic, 799–802
Myidone, 976–977
Mykrox, 753–754
Mylanta-AR, 460–462, 461i
Myleran, 1309t
Myotrol, 874–875
Myrbetriq, 777–778
Myrosemide, 522–524
Mysoline, 976–977
MZM, 731–732
M-Zole 3, 1288t

N

nabumetone, 803–804
nadolol, 804–806
Nadopen-V 200, 915–917
Nadopen-V 400, 915–917
Nadostine, 852–853, 1288t
nafarelin acetate, 806–807
Nafcil, 807–808
nafcillin sodium, 807–808
naftifine hydrochloride, 1288t
Naftin, 1288t

nalbuphine hydrochloride, 809–810
Nalcrom, 285–287, 286i
Nalfon, 469–471
nalidixic acid, 810–811
Nallpen, 807–808
naloxegol, 811–812
naloxone hydrochloride, 812–814
naltrexone hydrochloride, 814–816
Namenda, 708–710, 709i–710i
NANDA (North American Nursing Diagnosis
    Association), xxxiii
naphazoline hydrochloride, 1279t
Naprelan, 816–819
Naprosyn, 816–819
Naprosyn-E, 816–819
Naprosyn-SR, 816–819
naproxen, 816–819
naproxen sodium, 816–819
naratriptan hydrochloride, 819–820
Narcan, 812–814
Nardil, 927–930, 928i
Nasacort, 1190–1194
Nasacort AQ, 1190–1194
Nasacort HFA, 1190–1194
Nasal administration, xxii–xxiii, xxx
Nasalcrom, 285–287, 286i
Nasalide, 494–495
Nasarel, 494–495
Nasogastric administration, xxi, xxviii–xxix
Nasonex, 789–790
natalizumab, 820–822
nateglinide, 822–823, 823i
National Formulary (NF), xx
Natrecor, 830–831
Natroba, 1298t
Natulan, 1324t
Navane, 1141–1143
Navelbine, 1317t
Naxen, 816–819
Nebcin, 1161–1164
nebivolol hydrochloride, 824–825
nedocromil sodium 2%, 1281t
nefazodone hydrochloride, 825–827
NegGram, 810–811
nelfinavir, 1302t
nelfinavir mesylate, 1302t
Nemasol Sodium, 58
Nembutal, 918–920
Neo-Calglucon, 168–170
Neo-Codema, 558–561, 559i
Neo-Fer, 478–481
Neo-Fradin, 827
Neo-K, 954–958
neomycin sulfate, 827, 1285t, 1293t, 1296t

Neopap, 8–10
Neoral, 290–293
Neosar, 1309t
neostigmine bromide, 828–829
neostigmine methylsulfate, 828–829
Neo-Synephrine, 934–936
Neo-Synephrine Nasal Drops, 934–936
Neo-Synephrine Nasal Jelly, 934–936
Neo-Synephrine Nasal Spray, 934–936
Neo-Synephrine Pediatric Nasal Drops, 934–936
Nephro-Fer, 478–481
Nephron, 402–404
Neptazane, 731–732
Nesina, 39–40
nesiritide, 830–831
Nestrex, 1338t
netilmicin sulfate, 831–832
Netromycin, 831–832
Neulasta, 908–909
Neupogen, 483–485
Neuramate, 716–717
Neurontin, 525–527
Neutra-Phos, 959–960
Neutra-Phos-K, 959–960
nevirapine, 1301t
Nexium, 425–428
Nexium I.V., 425–428
Nexterone, 58–61
NF (National Formulary), xx
Nia-Bid, 1338t
Niac, 1338t
Niacels, 1338t
niacin, 1338t
Niacor, 1338t
nicardipine hydrochloride, 832–834
Niclocide, 834–835
niclosamide, 834–835
Nico-400, 1338t
Nicobid Tempules, 1338t
Nicoderm, 835–837
NicoDerm CQ, 835–837
Nicolar, 1338t
Nicorette, 835–837
Nicorette Plus, 835–837
nicotine for inhalation, 835–837
nicotine nasal solution, 835–837
nicotine polacrilex, 835–837
nicotine transdermal system, 835–837
Nicotinex Elixir, 1338t
Nicotrol, 835–837
Nicotrol Inhaler, 835–837
Nicotrol NS, 835–837
Nidagel, 757–759
nifedipine, 837–839

Nilandron, 1320t
Nilstat, 852–853, 1288t
nilutamide, 1320t
9-1-1, 1292t
Nipride, 845–846
Niravam, 42–43
nisoldipine, 840–841
Nitro-Bid, 842–843
Nitrocot, 842–843
Nitro-Dur, 842–843
nitrofurantoin, 841–842
nitrofurazone, 1285t
Nitrogard, 842–843
nitrogen mustard, 1309t
nitroglycerin, 842–843
nitroglycerin ointment 0.4%, 1297t
Nitroglyn E-R, 842–843
Nitroject, 842–843
Nitrol, 842–843
Nitrolingual, 842–843
NitroMist, 842–843
Nitrong SR, 842–843
Nitro-par, 842–843
Nitropress, 845–846
nitroprusside sodium, 845–846
Nitrostat, 842–843
Nitro-time, 842–843
Nix, 1298t
nizatidine, 846–847
Nizoral, 1287t
Nolvadex, 1110–1111
Nolva-dex, 1320t
Nolvadex-D, 1320t
Nomenclature of drugs, xx
Noncompetitive antagonists, xxiv
Nonproprietary names of drugs, xx
norepinephrine bitartrate, 847–848
norethindrone, 984–988
Norflex, 874–875
norfloxacin, 848–850
Norfranil, 582–584
norgestrel, 984–988
Norlutate, 984–988
Normodyne, 631–632
Noroxin, 848–850
Norpace, 356–357
Norpace CR, 356–357
Norplant System, 984–988
Norpramin, 317–318
Nor-Pred T.B.A., 970–972
North American Nursing Diagnosis Association (NANDA), xxxii
nortriptyline hydrochloride, 850–852
Norvasc, 63–64

Norvir, 1302t
Norwich Extra-Strength, 98–100
Nostril Spray Pump, 934–936
Nostril Spray Pump Mild, 934–936
Novamobarb, 65–67
Novamoxin, 68–70
Novantrone, 781–783, 1324t
Nova Rectal, 918–920
Novasen, 98–100
Novo-Alprazol, 42–44
Novo-Ampicillin, 75–77
Novo-Atenol, 100–101
Novo-AZT, 1303t
Novo-Butamide, 1170–1171
Novo-Carbamaz, 176–179, 176i
Novo-Chlorhydrate, 227
Novochlorocap, 228–229
Novo-Chlorpromazine, 233–236
Novo-Cimetine, 245–247
Novo-Clopate, 268–269
Novo-Cloxin, 269–270
Novo-cromolyn, 285–287, 288i
Novo-Difenac, 334–336
Novo-Diflunisal, 340–342
Novo-Digoxin, 342–344
Novo-Diltiazem, 348–350, 350i
Novo-Dipam, 328–331
Novo-Dipiradol, 354–355
Novo-Doxepin, 371–373
Novo-Famotidine, 460–462, 461i
Novoferrogluc, 478–481
Novoferrosulfa, 478–481
Novofibrate, 261–262
Novo-Flupam, 500–501
Novo-Flurprofen, 501–502
Novo-Folacid, 1340t
Novofumar, 478–481
Novo-Furantoin, 841–842
Novo-Gemfibrozil, 528–529
Novo-Glyburide, 538–540
Novo-Hydrazide, 558–561, 559i
Novohydrocort, 1292t, 1293t
Novo-Hydroxyzin, 571–572
Novo-Hylazin, 557–558
Novo-Indapamide, 593–594
Novo-Levobunolol, 1281t
Novo-Lexin, 219–221, 220i
Novolin 70/30, 1269t
Novolin ge 10/90, 1269t
Novolin ge 20/80, 1269t
Novolin ge 30/70, 1269t
Novolin ge 40/60, 1269t
Novolin ge 50/50, 1269t
Novolin ge Lente, 1269t

Novolin ge NPH, 1269t
Novolin ge Toronto, 1267t
Novolin ge Ultralente, 1269t
Novolin N, 1268t
Novolin N Prefilled, 1268t
Novolin R, 1267t
Novolin R Prefilled, 1267t
NovoLog, 1267t
NovoLog Mix 50/50, 1269t
NovoLog Mix 70/30, 1269t
Novo-Lorazem, 686–687
Novo-Medrone, 984–988
Novo-Metformin, 724–726
Novomethacin, 594–597
Novo-Methacin, 594–597
Novometoprol, 754–757
Novo-Minocycline, 771–774
Novo-Naprox, 816–819
Novo-Naprox Sodium, 816–819
Novo-Niacin, 1338t
Novonidazol, 757–759
Novo-Nifedin, 837–839
Novopentobarb, 918–920
Novo-Pen-VK, 915–917
Novo-Peridol, 551–553
NovoPindol, 941–942
Novo-Pirocam, 947–949
Novo-Poxide, 229–230
Novopramine, 582–584
Novopranol, 994–997
Novo-Profen, 575–578
Novo-Propamide, 236–237
Novopyrazone, 1093–1094
Novoquinidin, 1010–1012
Novo-Ranitidine, 1017–1019
Novoreserpine, 1205–1027, 1026i
Novo-Ridazine, 1138–1141
Novo-Rythro, 416–420
Novo-Rythro Encap, 416–420
Novo-Salmol, 27–29, 28i
Novosecobarb, 1054–1055
Novo-Selegiline, 1056–1058
Novosemide, 522–524
Novo-Soxazole, 1094–1096
Novospiroton, 1081–1083, 1083i
Novo-Sundac, 1096–1098
Novo-Tamoxifen, 1110–1111
Novo-Temazepam, 1120–1121
Novo-Tetra, 1130–1132
Novo-Thalidone, 237–239
Novo-Timol, 1154–1155
Novo-Tolmetin, 1173–1175
Novo-Triolam, 1195–1197
Novo-Tripramine, 1203–1205

Novotriptyn, 61–63, 62i
Novo-Valproic, 1217–1220
Novo-Veramil, 1232–1234
Novoxapam, 879–880
Noxafil, 952–954
NP-27, 1289t
Nu-Alpraz, 42–44
Nu-Amoxi, 42–44
Nu-Ampi, 75–77
Nubain, 809–810
Nu-Cephalex, 219–221, 220i
Nu-Cimet, 245–247
Nu-Cloxi, 269–270
Nucynta, 1112–1114
Nucynta ER, 1112–1114
Nu-Diclo, 334–336
Nu-Diltiaz, 348–350, 350i
Nu-Famotidine, 460–462, 461i
Nu-Gemfibrozil, 528–529
Nu-Glyburide, 538–540
Nu-Ibuprofen, 575–578
Nu-Indapamide, 593–594
Nu-Indo, 594–597
Nu-Loraz, 686–687
Nu-Medopa, 742–743
Numorphan, 889–891
Nu-Naprox, 816–819
Nu-Nifed, 837–839
Nu-Pen VK, 915–917
Nu-Pirox, 947–949
Nuprin, 575–578
Nu-Prochlor, 981–984
Nu-Ranit, 1017–1019
Nursing diagnosis, xxxii–xxxiii
Nursing process, xxxi–xxxiv
Nu-Selegiline, 1056–1058
Nu-Tetra, 1130–1132
Nutracort, 1292t
Nu-Valproic, 1217–1220
Nu-Verap, 1232–1234
Nuvigil, 94–96
nystatin, 852–853, 1288t
Nystex, 852–853
Nystop, 852–853
Nytol QuickCaps, 353–354

O

Obstetrical drugs, 1334–1335
Octagam 5%, 584–590
Octamide, 751–753
Octostim, 328–320

octreotide acetate, 853–854
OcuClear, 1279t
Ocufen, 1285t
Ocuflox, 1274t
Ocupress, 1280t
Ocusert Pilo-20, 1278t
Ocusert Pilo-40, 1278t
Ocusulf-10, 1275t
Official names of drugs, xx
Ofirmev, 8–10
ofloxacin, 855–856
ofloxacin 0.3%, 1283t
olanzapine, 857–859
Oleptro, 1188–1190
olmesartan medoxomil, 859–861, 860i, 1326
olodaterol, 861–862
olopatadine, 1272t
olopatadine hydrochloride 0.1%, 1277t
olsalazine sodium, 862–863
Olux, 1291t
omalizumab, 863–864
omega-3-acid ethyl esters, 864–865
omega 3-carboxylic acids, 865–866
omeprazole, 866–868, 867i
Omnaris, 242–244
Omnicef, 189–190
Omnipen, 75–77
Omnipen-N, 75–77
Omontys, 909–911
OMS Concentrate, 792–796
Oncaspar, 1317t
Oncovin, 1317t
ondansetron hydrochloride, 868–871
Onfi, 259–261
Onglyza, 1051–1052
Onsolis, 471–477
Ony-Clear Nail, 1288t
o,p9-DDD, 1323t
Opana, 889–891
Opana ER, 889–891
Ophthaine, 1279t
Ophthalmic administration, xii, xxx
Ophthalmic drugs, 1273–1282t
Ophthetic, 1279t
Ophthifluor, 1281t
Ophto-Dipivefrin, 1280t
Opioid agonists, 1363t
Opticyl, 1278t
Optigene 3, 1279t
Optimine, 1271t
OptiPranolol, 1281t
Optivar, 1280t
Orabase-HCA, 1293t
Oracort, 1294t

Oradexon, 320–323
Oral administration, xxi, xxvii
Oral allergen extracts, 1270
Oral dosage calculations, 1357–1358
Oralair, 1270
Oralone, 1294 t
Oramorph SR, 792–796
Oraphen-PD, 8–10
Orapred ODT, 970–972
Orasone 1, 972–974
Orasone 5, 972–974
Orasone 10, 972–974
Orazinc, 1252–1254
Orbactiv, 871–872
Orbenin, 269–270
Orencia, 1–2
Oretic, 558–561, 559i
oritavancin, 871–872
Orfro, 874–875
Organidin NR, 545–546
Orgaran, 300–301
Orinase, 1170–1171
orlistat, 872–874, 873i
Ornidyl, 389
orphenadrine citrate, 874–875
orphenadrine hydrochloride, 874–875
Orphenate, 874–875
Orthovisc, 556–557
Orudis, 626–628
Orudis KT, 626–628
Orudis-SR, 626–628
Oruvail, 626–628
oseltamivir phosphate, 1305t
Osmitrol, 700–702
Ostoforte, 1344t
Otezla, 44
Otic administration, xxii, xxx
Ovide, 1297t
Ovrette, 984–988
oxacillin sodium, 875–876
oxaliplatin, 1310t
Oxandrin, 876–877
oxandrolone, 877–878
oxaprozin, 877–879
oxazepam, 879–880
oxcarbazepine, 880–882
Oxecta, 885–887
Oxeze Turbuhaler, 511–513
oxiconazole nitrate, 1288 t
Oxistat, 1288 t
Oxizold, 1288 t
oxtriphylline, 882–883
oxybutynin chloride, 883–885
oxybutynin gel 3%, 1298t

oxycodone hydrochloride, 887–887, 1363t
OxyContin, 885–887
oxymetazoline hydrochloride, 1279t
oxymetholone, 887–889
oxymorphone hydrochloride, 889–891
oxytetracycline, 891–892
oxytetracycline hydrochloride, 891–892
oxytocin, 1334
Oxytrol, 883–885

P

Pacerone, 58–61
paclitaxel, 1316t
Palafer, 477–481
paliperidone, 893–895
palonosetron hydrochloride, 895–896
2-PAM chloride, 961–962
Pamelor, 850–852
pamidronate disodium, 896–898
Pamine, 740–741
Pamine Forte, 740–741
Pamprin-IB, 575–578
Panadol, 8–10
Panadol Infants' Drops, 8–10
Pancrease, 899–901
Pancrease MT 4, 899–901
Pancrease MT 10, 899–901
Pancrease MT 16, 899–901
Pancrease MT 20, 899–901
pancreatin, 898–899
Pancreaze MT 4, 899–901
Pancreaze MT 10, 899–901
Pancreaze MT 16, 899–901
Pancreaze MT 20, 899–901
pancrelipase, 899–901
Pancrezyme 4X, 898–899
Panmycin, 1130–1132
Pantoloc, 901–904
pantoprazole sodium, 901–904
para-aminosalicylate, 58
Paraflex, 239–240
Parafon Forte DSC, 239–240
Parenteral dosage calculations, 1358–1360
Parenteral routes of administration, xxii, xxix
paricalcitol, 904–906
Parlodel, 146–149, 147i
Parlodel SnapTabs, 146–159, 147i
Parnate, 1186–1188
paroxetine hydrochloride, 906–908
paroxetine mesylate, 906–908
Partial agonists, xxiv

PAS, 58
Passive diffusion, xxi
Patanase, 1272t
Patanol, 1277t
Pathocil, 336–337
Paxil, 906–908
Paxil CR, 906–908
Paxipam, 550–551
PCE, 416–420
Pediaphen, 8–10
Pediapred, 970–972
Pedi-Dri, 852–853
Peganone, 448–450
pegaspargase, 1317t
PEGASYS, 1348t
pegfilgrastim, 908–909
peginesatide, 909–911
peginterferon alfa-2a, 1348t
peginterferon alfa-2b, 1348t
PEG-Intron, 1348t
PEG-L-asparaginase, 1317t
pemetrexed disodium, 1315t
Penbritin, 75–77
penbutolol sulfate, 911–913
penciclovir, 1290t, 1304t
Penecort, 1292t
Penetrex, 396–398, 396i
Penglobe, 121–122
penicillamine, 913–915
penicillin G benzathine, 915–917
penicillin G potassium, 915–917
penicillin G procaine, 915–917
penicillin G sodium, 915–917
penicillin V potassium, 915–917
Penlac, 1286t
Pentamycetin, 1273t
Pentasa, 719–720
Pentazine, 988–990
pentazocine lactate, 917–918
Pentids, 915–917
pentobarbital sodium, 918–920, 1354t
Pentolair, 1278t
pentosan polysulfate sodium, 920–921
Pentothal, 1136–1138
pentoxifylline, 921–922
Pen Vee, 915–917
Pen Vee K, 915–917
Pepcid, 460–462, 461i
Pepcid AC, 460–462, 461i
Pepcid RPD, 460–462, 461i
perampanel, 922–923
Perforomist, 511–513
Peridol, 551–553
perindopril erbumine, 923–924

Permapen, 915–917
permethrin 1%, 1298 t
permethrin 5%, 1298 t
Permitil, 498–500
Permitil Concentrate, 498–500
perphenazine, 925–927
Persantine, 354–355
Pertofrane, 317–318
pethidine hydrochloride, 710–711
Pexeva, 906–908
Pfizerpen, 915–917
Pfizerpen-AS, 915–917
PGI2, 408–410
PGX, 408–410
Pharmacodynamics, xxiii–xiv
Pharmacognosy, xx
Pharmacokinetics, xxii–xxiii
Pharmacology, xx–xxvi
  classification, xx–xxi
  nomenclature, xx
  pharmacodynamics, xxiii–xxiv
  pharmacokinetics, xxi–xxiii
  pharmacotherapeutics, xxiv–xxv
  special considerations, xxv
Pharma-Cort, 1292t
Pharmacotherapeutics, xxiv–xxv
Phenazine 25, 988–990
Phenazine 50, 908–990
Phenazo, 927
Phenazodine, 927
phenazopyridine hydrochloride, 927
Phencen-50, 988–990
phenelzine sulfate, 927–930, 928i
Phenerzine, 988–990
phenobarbital, 930–932
phenobarbital sodium, 930–932
Phenoject-50, 988–990
Phenoptic, 1279t
phentolamine mesylate, 933–934
phenylephrine hydrochloride, 934–936, 1279t
Phenytex, 936–940
phenytoin, 936–940
phenytoin sodium, 936–940
Pheryl E, 1344t
Phillips' Chewable Tablets, 697–700
Phillips' Magnesia Tablets, 697–700
Phillips' Milk of Magnesia, 797–700
Phillips' Milk of Magnesia Concentrate, 797–700
pHisoHex, 1296t
PhosLo, 168–170
Photofrin, 1324t
Phyllocontin, 56–58
Physicians order sheets, xxvii
physostigmine salicylate, 940–941

phytonadione, 1346t
Picato, 1297 t
Pilagan, 1278t
Pilocar, 1278t
pilocarpine, 1278t
pilocarpine hydrochloride, 1278t
pilocarpine nitrate, 1278t
Pilopine HS, 1278t
Pilostat, 1278t
Pima, 958–959
pimecrolimus 1%, 1298 t
pindolol, 941–942
Pint, 1361
pioglitazone hydrochloride, 942–944
piperacillin sodium, 944–946
piperonyl butoxide and pyrethrum extract, 1298t
Pipracil, 944–946
pirbuterol acetate, 946–947
piroxicam, 947–949
pitavastatin, 949–950
Pitocin, 1334
Pitressin, 1226–1227, 1227i
Pitrex, 1290 t
Placidyl, 445–446
Planning phase of nursing process, xxxiii
Plaquenil, 569–571
Platinol, 1311t
Platinol-AQ, 1311t
Plavix, 267–268
Plendil, 465–466
Pletal, 244–245
plicamycin, 1313t
PMS Benztropine, 132–133
PMS-Bethanechol Chloride, 139–140
PMS-Cephalexin, 219–221, 219i
PMS-Chloral Hydrate, 227
PMS-Cimetidine, 245–247
PMS-Ferrous Sulfate, 478–481
PMS Fluphenazine, 498–500
PMS-Hydromorphone, 556–558
PMS-Hydromorphone Syrup, 566–558
PMS-Isoniazid, 612–614
PMS-Lactulose, 634–635
PMS-Levothyroxine Sodium, 660–662
PMS-Lindane, 667–668
PMS-Methylphenidate, 745–748
PMS-Metoclopramide, 751–753
PMS Perphenazine, 925–927
PMS-Piroxicam, 947–949
PMS Primidone, 763–977
pms Propranolol, 994–997
pms-Pyrazinamide, 1001–1002
PMS-Sodium Polystyrene Sulfonate, 1074–1075

PMS-Sulfasalazine, 1091–1093
PMS-Sulfasalazine E.C., 1091–1093
PMS Theophylline, 1132–1135
PMS Thioridazine, 1138–1140
PMS-Trifluoperazine, 1197–1199
PMS Trihexyphenidyl, 1201–1202
PMS-Valproic Acid, 1217–1220
podofilox, 1298 t
Polaramine, 324–325
Polaramine Repetabs, 324–325
Polycillin, 75–77
Polycillin-N, 75–77
Polygam S/D, 584–590
Polymox, 68–70
polymyxin B sulfate, 950–952, 1275t, 1293t, 1296t
Pontocaine, 1279t
porfimer sodium, 1324t
Portalac, 634–635
posaconazole, 952–954
Potasalan, 955–958
potassium acetate, 954–958
potassium and sodium phosphates, 959–960
potassium bicarbonate, 954–958
potassium bicarbonate and potassium chloride,
    954–958
potassium bicarbonate and potassium citrate,
    954–958
potassium chloride, 954–958
potassium citrate, 954–958
potassium gluconate, 954–958
potassium gluconate and potassium chloride,
    954–958
potassium gluconate and potassium citrate,
    954–958
potassium iodide, 958–959
potassium phosphates, 959–960
Potassium-Rougier, 955–958
Potassium Sandoz, 954–958
Potiga, 459–460
povidone-iodine, 1285t
Pradaxa, 295–297
pralidoxime chloride, 961–962
pramipexole dihydrochloride, 962–964
pramlintide acetate, 964–966
Prandin, 1023–1025
prasugrel, 966–967
Pravachol, 967–968
pravastatin sodium, 967–968
prazosin hydrochloride, 968–969
Precose, 6
Predacort 50, 969–972
Predalone 50, 969–972
Predalone T.B.A., 969–972

Predate 50, 969–972
Predate TBA, 969–972
Predcor-25, 969–972
Predcor-50, 969–972
Predcor-TBA, 969–972
Pred Forte, 1286t
Pred-Ject 50, 969–972
Pred Mild, 1286t
prednicarbate, 1293 t
Prednicen-M, 972–974
Prednicot, 972–974
prednisolone, 969–972
prednisolone acetate, 969–972
prednisolone acetate suspension, 1286t
prednisolone sodium phosphate, 970–972
prednisolone sodium phosphate solution, 1286t
prednisolone tebutate, 970–972
prednisone, 972–974
Prednisone Intensol, 972–974
pregabalin, 974–976
Pregnancy, xvi, xxvi
Prelone, 969–972
Premarin, 435–439
Premarin Vaginal Cream, 435–439
Premphase, 435–439
Prempro, 435–439
Pressyn, 1226–1227, 1227i
Prevacid, 639–642
Prevacid I.V., 639–642
Prevacid SoluTab, 639–642
Prevex-HC, 1292 t
Prezista, 1299t
Prialt, 1248–1251, 1250i
prilocaine, 1297 t
Prilosec, 866–868, 867i
Primacor, 770–771, 771i
Primethasone, 320–323
primidone, 976–977
Principen-250, 75–77
Principen-500, 75–77
Prinivil, 667–669
Prinzide 10/12.5, 1330t
Prinzide 20/12.5, 1330t
Prinzide 20/25, 1130t
Pristiq, 1229–1232
Privigen, 584–590
Pro-50, 988–990
Proair HFA, 27–29, 28i
ProAmatine, 766–767
Probalan, 977–979
Pro-Banthine, 992–993
probenecid, 977–979
procainamide hydrochloride, 979–981

Pro-Cal-Sof, 375–376
Procan SR, 979–981
procarbazine hydrochloride, 1324t
Procardia, 837–839
Procardia XL, 837–839
prochlorperazine, 981–984, 1354t
prochlorperazine edisylate, 981–984
prochlorperazine maleate, 981–984
Procrit, 405–408
Procytox, 1309t
Prodrox, 984–988
Prodrugs, xiii
progesterone, 984–988
progestins, 984–988
Proglycem, 331–333
Prograf, 1104–1108
Prolastin, 41–42
Prolastin-C, 41–42
Prolensa, 1275t
Prolia, 315–316
Prolixin, 498–500
Prolixin Concentrate, 498–500
Prolixin Decanoate, 498–500
Prolixin Enanthate, 498–500
Proloprim, 1203
Promacot, 988–990
Promacta, 391–493
Pro-Med 50, 988–990
Promet, 988–990
promethazine hydrochloride, 988–990
Prometrium, 984–988
Promine, 979–981
Pronestyl, 979–981
Pronestyl-SR, 979–981
propafenone hydrochloride, 991–992
Propanthel, 993–993
propantheline bromide, 992–993
proparacaine hydrochloride, 1279t
Propecia, 485–486
Propine, 1280t
propofol, 993–994
propranolol hydrochloride, 994–997
propylthiouracil, 997–998
Propyl-Thyracil, 997–998
Proquin XR, 248–251
Prorex-25, 988–990
Prorex-50, 988–990
Proscar, 485–486
Pro-Span, 984–988
prostacyclin, 408–410
Prostaphlin, 875–876
ProStep, 835–837
Prostigmin, 828–829

protamine sulfate, 999
Prothazine, 988–990
Protilase, 899–901
Protonix, 901–904
Protopam Chloride, 961–962
Protopic, 1298 t
Protostat, 757–759
protriptyline hydrochloride, 999–1001
Proventil, 26–229, 28i
Proventil HFA, 26–29, 28i
Proventil Repetabs, 26–29, 28i
Proventil Syrup, 26–29, 28i
Provera, 984–988
Provigil, 783–785
Prozac, 495–498
Prozac Weekly, 495–498
Psorcon, 1291 t
PTU, 997–998
Pulmicort Flexhaler, 149–152
Pulmicort Respules, 149–152
Pulmicort Turbuhaler, 149–151
Pulmophylline, 1132–1135
Purinethol, 1314t
Purinol, 36–37
P.V. Carpine Liquifilm, 1278t
pyrazinamide, 1001–1002
pyrethrum extract and piperonyl butoxide, 1298t
Pyri, 1338t
Pyridiate, 927
2-pyridine aldoxime methochloride, 961–962
Pyridium, 927
pyridostigmine bromide, 1002–1003
pyridoxine hydrochloride, 1138t

Q

Q-Profen, 575–578
Quart, 1361
Quarzan, 256–257
quazepam, 1005–1006
Questran, 240–241
Questran Light, 240–241
quetiapine fumarate, 1006–1008
Quibron-T Dividose, 1132–1135
Quibron-T/SR Dividose, 1132–1135
Quinaglute Dura-tabs, 1010–1012
quinapril hydrochloride, 1008–1010
Quinate, 1010–1012
Quinidex Extentabs, 1010–1012
quinidine gluconate, 1010–1012
quinidine polygalacturonate, 1010–1012
quinidine sulfate, 1010–1012

Quin-Release, 1010–1012
Quinsana Plus, 1289t
Quixin, 1283t
QVAR, 124–126

R

rabeprazole sodium, 1012–1013
racepinephrine, 402–404
Radiostol Forte, 1344t
ragweed extract, 1334
Ragwitek, 1270
raloxifene hydrochloride, 1013–1014
raltegravir, 1302t
ramelteon, 1014–1015
ramipril, 1015–1017
Ranexa, 1019–1020
Raniclor, 194–186
ranitidine hydrochloride, 1017–1019, 1354t
ranolazine, 1019–1020
Rapaflo, 1064–1065
Rapamune, 1067–1069
rapamycin, 1067–1069
Rapid-acting insulin, 1267t
rasagiline, 1020–1022
Razadyne, 527–528
Razadyne ER, 527–528
Rebetol, 1307t
Rebif, 1350t
Reclast, 1256–1258
recombinant erythropoietin, 405–408
recombinant interferon alfa-2b, 1348t
Rectal administration, xxii, xxix
Rectiv, 1297 t
Rederm, 1292 t
Redutemp, 8–10
Regitine, 933–936
Reglan, 751–753
Regonol, 1002–1003
Regranex, 1295t
Regular (concentrated) insulin, Iletin II, U-500, 1267t
Regulax SS, 376
Relafen, 803–804
Relaxazone, 239–240
Relenza, 1305t
Relief Eye Drops for Red Eyes, 1279t
Religious considerations, xxv
Relistor, 743–745
Relpax, 389–390
Remeron, 778–780
Remeron SolTab, 778–780

Remicade, 597–600
remifentanil hydrochloride, 1022–1023, 1023i
Remular, 239–240
Remular-S, 239–240
Renagel, 1061–1062
Renedil, 465–466
Renova, 1294 t
Renvela, 1061–1062
ReoPro, 3–4
repaglinide, 1023–1025
Requip, 1040–1042
Rescriptor, 1299 t
Rescudose, 792–796
Rescula, 1282t
Resectisol, 700–702
Reserfia, 1025–1026, 1026i
reserpine, 1025–1026, 1026i
Respbid, 1132–1135
Restasis, 1280t
Restoril, 1120–1121
Resyl, 545–546
Retavase, 1026–1027
reteplase, 1026–1027
Retin-A, 1294 t
Retin-A Micro, 1294 t
Retinoids, 1283t, 1294 t
retinol, 1336t
retinol 0.01% and mequinol 2%, 1297 t
Retrovir, 1303t
Revatio, 1062–1064
ReVia, 814–816
Revimine, 366–368
Rexolate, 1075–1076
Reyataz, 1299 t
rG-CSF, 483–485
Rheumatrex, 737–738
Rhinalar, 494–495
Rhinall, 934–936
Rhinall-10 Children's Flavored Nose Drops,
    934–936
Rhinocort, 149–152
Rhinocort Aqua, 149–152
Rhinocort Turbuhaler, 149–152
Rhodis, 626–628
Rhophylac, 584–590
Rhotrimine, 1203–1205
r-HuEPO, 405–408
Ribasphere, 1307t
ribavirin, 1307t
RID, 1298 t
Ridaura, 109–110
Rifadin, 1027–1029
Rifadin IV, 1027–1029
rifampicin, 1027–1029

rifampin, 1027–1029
rilpivirine, 1300t, 1302t
Rilutek, 1029–1030
riluzole, 1029–1030
Rimactane, 1027–1029
rimexolone, 1277t
Riomet, 724–726
Riphenidate, 745–748
risedronate sodium, 1030–1032
Risperdal, 1032–1034
Risperdal Consta, 1032–1034
risperidone, 1032–1034
Ritalin, 745–748
Ritalin-LA, 745–748
Ritalin-SR, 745–748
ritonavir, 1302t
Rituxan, 1325t
rituximab, 1325t
rivaroxaban, 1034–1036
rivastigmine tartrate, 1036–1038
Rivotril, 263–264
rizatriptan benzoate, 1038–1039
RMS Uniserts, 792–796
R.O. Dexasone, 1279t
Robaxin, 736–737
Robaxin 750, 736–737
Robigesic, 8–10
Robinul, 540–542
Robinul Forte, 540–542
Robitet, 1130–1132
Robitussin, 545–546
Rocaltrol, 167–168
Rocephin, 212–214
Rodex, 1338t
Rofact, 1027–1028
Roferon-A, 1318t
roflumilast, 1039–1040
Rogaine, 774–776
Rogaine 2%, 1297 t
Rogaine 5%, 1297 t
Rogaine ES for Men, 774–776
Rogaine for Men, 774–776
Rogaine for Women, 774–776
Romazicon, 493–494
romidepsin, 1313t, 1325t
ropinirole hydrochloride, 1040–1042
rosiglitazone maleate, 1042–1043
rosuvastatin calcium, 1043–1045
rotigotine, 1045–1046
Routes of administration, xxvii
Rowasa, 719–720
Roxanol, 792–796
Roxanol 100, 792–796
Roxanol UD, 792–796

Roxicodone, 885–887
Roychlor 10%, 955–958
Rozerem, 1014–1015
Rubex, 1312t
Rufen, 575–578
rufinamide, 1046–1047
Rum-K, 955–958
Rybix ODT, 1181–1183
Rythmodan, 356–358
Rythmodan-LA, 356–358
Rythmol, 991–992
Rythmol SR, 991–992

S

Sabril, 1234–1236
St. Joseph Children's, 98–100
St. Joseph Aspirin-Free Infant Drops, 8–10
Sal-Adult, 98–100
Salazopyrin EN-Tabs, 1091–1093
salbutamol, 26–29, 28i
salbutamol sulphate, 26–29, 28i
Salflex, 1049–1050
Sal-Infant, 98–100
salmeterol xinafoate, 1047–1049
Salofalk, 719–720
salsalate, 1049–1050
Salsitab, 1049–1050
Samsca, 1176–1177
Sanctura, 1206–1207
Sanctura XR, 1206–1207
Sancuso, 544–545
Sandimmune, 290–293
Sandoglobulin, 584–590
Sandostatin, 853–854
Sandostatin LAR Depot, 853–854
SangCya, 290–293
Sans-Acne, 1284t
Saphris, 96–97
sapropterin dihydrochloride, 1050–1051
saquinavir, 1302t
Sarafem, 495–498
Sarisol No. 2, 159–160
Sarna HC, 1292 t
S.A.S. Enteric-500, 1091–1093
S.A.S.-500, 1091–1093
Savella, 768–770
saxagliptin monohydrate, 1051–1052
Scabene, 667–668
SCE-A, 435–439
scopolamine, 1354t
scopolamine hydrobromide, 1052–1054, 1278t

scopolamine transdermal system, 1052–1054
Scot-tussin Expectorant, 545–546
SD Deprenyl, 1056–1058
secobarbital sodium, 1054–1056
Seconal, 1054–1056
Sectral, 7–8
Selegiline-5, 1056–1058
selegiline hydrochloride, 1056–1058
selegiline transdermal system, 1056–1058
selenium sulfide, 1289t
Selestoject, 135–137
Selsun, 1289 t
Selzentry, 1302t, 1303t
Semprex-D, 1272t
Sensipar, 247–248
Sential, 1292 t
Serax, 879–880
Serentil, 720–722
Serevent Diskus, 1047–1049
Seromycin, 289–290
Seroquel, 1006–1008
Seroquel XR, 1006–1008
Serpalan, 1025–1026, 1026i
Serpasil, 1025–1026, 1026i
Sertan, 976–977
sertraline hydrochloride, 1058–1061
Serzone, 825–827
sevelamer carbonate, 1061–1062
sevelamer hydrochloride, 1061–1062
Shogan, 988–990
Short-acting insulin, 1267t
Silace, 361–362
Siladryl, 353–354
sildenafil citrate, 1062–1064
Silenor, 371–373
silodosin, 1064–1065
Silvadene, 1285t
silver sulfadiazine, 1285t
Simponi, 542–544
Simron, 478–481
simvastatin, 1065–1067
Sinequan, 371–373
Singulair, 790–792
sirolimus, 1067–1069
sitagliptin, 1069–1070
Sivextro, 1114–1115
Skelaxin, 723–724
Skelex, 736–737
Skelid, 1152–1154
Sklice, 1297 t
Sleep-Eze D Extra Strength, 353–354
Slo-Bid Gyrocaps, 1132–1135
Slo-Niacin, 1338t
Slo-Phyllin, 1132–1135

Slow-Fe, 478–481
Slow-K, 955–958
Slow-Mag, 697–700
Soda Mint, 1070–1072
sodium bicarbonate, 1070–1072
sodium chloride, hypertonic, 1281t
sodium cromoglycate, 285–287, 286i
sodium ferric gluconate, 1072–1073
sodium phenylbutyrate, 1073–1074
sodium phosphates, 959–960
sodium polystyrene sulfonate, 1074–1075
Sodium Sulamyd 10%, 1275t
sodium thiosalicylate, 1075–1076
Solage, 1297 t
Solaraze, 1296 t
Solfoton, 930–932
Solid equivalents, 1361–1362t
solifenacin succinate, 1076–1077
Solodyn, 771–774
Solu-Cortef, 563–566
Solu-Medrol, 748–751
Solurex, 320–323
Solurex LA, 320–323
Solutions, xxx, 1356
Soma, 179–180
Somnol, 500–501
Sonata, 1248–1249
Sopamycetin, 1273t
Sorbitrate, 616–618, 617i
Soriatane, 16–18
Sotacor, 1077–1079
sotalol hydrochloride, 1077–1079
Span-FF, 478–481
sparfloxacin, 1079–1080
Spasmoban, 339–340
Spectazole, 1287t
spectinomycin hydrochloride, 1080–1081
Spectracef, 191–192
Spectrobid, 121–122
spinosad topical suspension 0.9%, 1298 t
Spiriva HandiHaler, 1158–1159
spironolactone, 1081–1083, 1083i
Sporanox, 621–624
SPS Suspension, 1074–1075
SSKI, 958–959
Stadol, 160–162
Stadol NS, 160–162
Staphcillin, 733–734
Starlix, 822–823, 823i
Statex, 792–796
Staticin, 1284t
stavudine, 1302t
Stavzor, 1217–1220
Staxyn, 1223–1225

S-T Cort, 1292 t
Stelara, 1215–1217
Stemetil, 981–984
Stendra, 110–112
Sterapred, 972–974
Sterapred DS, 972–974
Stieva-A, 1294 t
Stimate, 318–320
Stimate Nasal Spray, 318–320
Storzolamide, 10–12
Stoxil, 1304t
Strattera, 101–103
Strength of solution, 1356
Streptase, 1083–1084
streptokinase, 1083–1084
streptomycin sulfate, 1084–1085
streptozocin, 1319t
Strifon Forte DSC, 239–240
Striverdi Respimat, 861–862
Strong agonists, xxiv
Subcutaneous (SubQ) administration, xxiii, xxx
Sublimaze, 471–477
Sublingual administration, xxii, xxx
Subsys, 471–477
Subutex, 153–155
sucralfate, 1086
sucroferric oxyhydroxide, 1086–1087
Sular, 840–841
sulconazole nitrate, 1289 t
Sulcrate, 1086
Sulcrate Suspension Plus, 1086
Sulf-10, 1275t
sulfacetamide sodium 10%, 1275t, 1285t
sulfacetamide sodium 10% and sulfur 5%, 1285t
sulfacetamide sodium 15%, 1275t
sulfacetamide sodium 30%, 1275t
Sulfacet-R, 1285t
sulfadiazine, 1087–1089
sulfamethizole, 1089–1090
sulfamethoxazole, 1090–1091
Sulfamylon, 1284t
sulfasalazine, 1091–1093
sulfinpyrazone, 1093–1094
sulfisoxazole, 1094–1096
sulfisoxazole acetyl, 1094–1096
Sulfizole, 1094–1096
Sulfolax, 361–362
sulindac, 1096–1099
sumatriptan iontophoretic transdermal system, 1099–1101
sumatriptan succinate, 1099–1101
Sumycin, 1130–1132
sunitinib malate, 1325t
Supasa, 98–100

Suprax, 194–195
Surfak, 361–362
Surmontil, 1203–1205
Suspensions, xxviii
Sustiva, 1300 t
Sutent, 1325t
suvorexant, 1101–1102
Sylatron, 1348t
Symax SL, 572–573
Symax SR, 572–573
Symlin, 964–966
Symmetrel, 50–52
Synacort, 1292 t
Synalar, 1291 t
Synalar-HP, 1291 t
Synamol, 1291 t
Synarel, 806–807
Synemol, 1291 t
Syn-Nadolol, 804–806
SynPindol, 941–942
Synthetic Conjugated Estrogens A Vaginal
    Cream, 435–439
synthetic estrogens, A (conjugated), 435–439
synthetic estrogens, B (conjugated), 435–439
Synthroid, 660–662
Syringe, compatible drugs in, 1354–1355t
Systems of measurement, 1361–1362t

T

T3, 671–673
T4, 660–662
Tablespoon, 1361
Tablets, xxvii
Tabloid, 1315t
Taclonex, 1295 t
Taclonex Scalp, 1295 t
tacrine hydrochloride, 1103–1104, 1103i
tacrolimus, 1104–1108
tacrolimus ointment 0.1%, 1298 t
tacrolimus ointment 0.03%, 1298 t
tadalafil, 1108–1110
tafluprost 0.0015%, 1281t
Tagamet, 245–247
Tagamet HB, 245–247
Talwin, 917–918
Tambocor, 489–490
Tamiflu, 1305t
Tamofen, 1110–1111, 1320t
Tamone, 1110–1111, 1320t
tamoxifen citrate, 1110–1111, 1320t

tamsulosin hydrochloride, 1111–1112
Tanzeum, 25–27
Tapanol Extra Strength, 8–10
Tapazole, 734–736
tapentadol, 1112–1114
Targretin Gel, 1321t
Tasmar, 1171–1173
Taxol, 1316t
Taxotere, 1316t
tazarotene 0.1%, 1294 t
tazarotene 0.05%, 1294 t
Tazicef, 208–210
Tazidime, 208–210
Tazorac, 1294 t
Teaspoon, 1361
Tebamide, 1202–1203
Tebrazid, 1001–1002
Tecfidera, 352–353
tedelparin, 298–300
tedizolid, 1114–1115
Teflaro, 207–208
Tegopen, 269–270
Tegretol, 176–179, 176i
Tegretol-XR, 176–179, 176i
Tegrin-LT, 1298 t
Tekamlo 150/5, 1330t
Tekamlo 150/10, 1330t
Tekamlo 300/5, 1330t
Tekamlo 300/10, 1330t
Tekturna, 34–35, 1330t
Tekturna HCT 150/12.5, 1330t
Tekturna HCT 150/25, 1330t
Tekturna HCT 300/12.5, 1330t
telaprevir, 1307t
telavancin, 1115–1117
telbivudine, 1306t
telithromycin, 1117–1119
telmisartan, 1118–1119, 1330t, 1332t
temazepam, 1120–1121
Temodar, 1310t
Temovate, 1291 t
temozolomide, 1310t
Tempra, 8–10
Tempra Drops, 8–10
tenecteplase, 1121–1121
Tenex, 549–550
Ten-K, 955–958
tenofovir, 1300 t, 1302t, 1306t
tenofovir and emtricitabine, 1302t
Tenormin, 100–101
Terazol 3, 1289 t
Terazol 7, 1289 t
terazosin hydrochloride, 1122–1123

terbinafine hydrochloride, 1124–1125, 1289 t
terbutaline sulfate, 1125–1126
terconazole, 1289 t
teriflunomide, 1126–1128
teriparatide, 1128–1129, 1129i
Terramycin, 891–892
Terramycin I.M., 891–892
tesamorelin, 1129–1130
Teslac, 1320t
TESPA, 1310t
Tessalon Perles, 131
testolactone, 1320t
tetracaine, 1279t
Tetracap, 1130–1132
tetracycline hydrochloride, 1130–1132, 1285t
Tetracyn, 1130–1132
Tetracyn 530, 1130–1132
tetrahydroaminoacridine, 1103–1104, 1103 i
tetrahydrozoline hydrochloride, 1279t
Tetrasine, 1279t
Teveten, 410–411
6-TG, 1315t
THA, 1103–1104, 1103 i
Thalitone, 237–239
Tham, 1205–1206
THC, 378–379
Theo-24, 1132–1135
Theobid Duracaps, 1132–1135
Theochron, 1132–1135
Theoclear, 1132–1135
Theoclear LA, 1132–1135
Theo-Dur, 1132–1135
Theolair, 1132–1135
Theolair-SR, 1132–1135
theophylline, 1132–1135
theophylline ethylenediamine, 56–58
Theo-SR, 1132–1135
Theovent Long-Acting, 1132–1135
TheraCys, 1318t
Therapy Bayer, 98–100
Thermazine, 1285t
thiamine hydrochloride, 1336t
thiethylperazine maleate, 1135–1136
thioguanine, 1315t
6-thioguanine, 1315t
Thionex, 667–668
thiopental sodium, 1136–1138
Thioplex, 1310t
thioridazine, 1138–1140
thioridazine hydrochloride, 1138–1140
Thiosulfil Forte, 1089–1090
thiotepa, 1310t
thiothixene, 1141–1143

Thiothixene HCl Intensol, 1141–1143
thiothixene hydrochloride, 1141–1143
Thorazine, 233–236
Thorazine Spansule, 233–236
3TC, 1300 t
3TC/AZT, 1300 t
3TC/ZDV, 1300 t
Thrive, 835–837
Thyrar, 1143–1144
Thyro-Block, 958–959
Thyrogen, 1144–1146
thyroid-stimulating hormone, 1144–1146
Thyroid Strong, 1143–1144
thyroid USP, 1143–1144
thyronine sodium, 671–673
thyrotropin, 1144–1146
thyrotropin alfa, 1144–1146
thyroxine sodium, 660–662
Thytropar, 1144–1146
tiagabine hydrochloride, 1146–1147
TiazacER, 348–350, 350i
ticagrelor, 1147–1148
Ticar, 1148–1149
ticarcillin disodium, 1148–1149
TICE BCG, 1318t
Ticlid, 1149–1151, 1150i
ticlopidine hydrochloride, 1149–1151, 1150i
Tigan, 1202–1203
tigecycline, 1151–1152
Tikosyn, 362–363
Tilone, 1190–1194
tiludronate disodium, 1152–1154
Timolide 10/25, 1332t
timolol hemihydrate, 1282t
timolol maleate, 1154–1155, 1282t, 1332t
timolol maleate extended-release solution, 1282t
Timoptic, 1282t
Timoptic-XE, 1282t
Tinactin, 1289 t
Tindamax, 1155–1156
Ting, 1289 t
tinidazole, 1155–1156
tinzaparin sodium, 1157–1158
tioconazole, 1289 t
tiotropium bromide, 1158–1159
Tipramine, 582–584
tipranavir, 1302t
tirofiban hydrochloride, 1159–1160
tissue plasminogen activator, recombinant, 47–48
Titralac, 168–170
tizanidine hydrochloride, 1160–1161
TNKase, 1121–1122
Tobi, 1161–1164

Tobi Podhaler, 1161–1164
TobraDex, 1275t
Tobramycin, 1161–1164
tobramycin, 1275t
tobramycin 0.3% (3 mg) and dexamethasone 0.1% (1 mg), 1275t
tobramycin sulfate, 1161–1164
Tobrex, 1275t
tocainide hydrochloride, 1164–1165
tocilizumab, 1165–1167
tofacitinib citrate, 1167–1169
Tofranil, 582–584
Tofranil-PM, 582–584
tolazamide, 1169–1170
tolbutamide, 1170–1171
tolcapone, 1171–1173
Tolectin 200, 1173–1175
Tolectin 400, 1173–1175
Tolectin 600, 1173–1175
Tolectin DS, 1173–1175
Tolinase, 1169–1170
tolmetin, 1173–1175
tolnaftate, 1289 t
tolterodine tartrate, 1175–1176
tolvaptan, 1176–1177
Tonocard, 1164–1165
Topamax, 1177–1180
Topical administration, xxii, xxx
Topical drugs, 1284–1298t
Topicort, 1291 t, 1296 t
Topicycline, 1285t
Topilene, 1290 t
topiramate, 1177–1180
Toposar, 1322t
topotecan hydrochloride, 1325t
Toprol-XL, 754–757
Toradol, 628–631
Torecan, 1135–1136
toremifene citrate, 1320t
Tornalate, 143–144
torsemide, 1180–1181
Totacillin, 75–77
Totacillin-N, 75–77
Tovalt, 1259–1261
Toviaz, 482–483
Toxicodynamics, xx
T-Phyl, 1132–1135
Tracrium, 106–107
Trade names of drugs, xiv
Tradjenta, 664–665
Tramacort-D, 1190–1194
tramadol hydrochloride, 1181–1183
Trandate, 631–632

trandolapril, 1183–1185
tranexamic acid, 1185–1186
Transcutaneous routes of administration, xii–xxiii, xxix–xxx
Transderm-Nitro, 842–845
Transderm-Scop, 1052–1054
Transderm-V, 1052–1054
Tranxene, 268–269
Tranxene-SD, 268–269
Tranxene-SD Half Strength, 268–269
tranylcypromine sulfate, 1186–1188
trastuzumab, 1325t
Travatan, 1282t
travoprost 0.004%, 1282t
trazodone hydrochloride, 1188–1190
Trecator-SC, 446–447
Trelstar, 1320t
Trendar, 575–578
Trental, 921–922
tretinoin, 1294 t, 1296 t
Triacet, 1293 t, 1294 t
Triadapin, 371–373
Triaderm, 1293 t, 1294 t
triamcinolone, 1190–1194
triamcinolone acetonide, 1190–1194
triamcinolone acetonide 0.1%, 1294 t
triamcinolone acetonide 0.5%, 1293 t, 1294 t
triamcinolone acetonide 0.025%, 1293 t
triamcinolone acetonide dental paste, 1294 t
triamcinolone acetonide topical aerosol, 1294 t
triamcinolone diacetate, 1190–1194
triamcinolone hexacetonide, 1190–1194
Triam-Forte, 1190–1194
Triamolone 40, 1190–1194
triamterene, 1194–1195, 1328t, 1330t
Trianide Mild, 1293 t
Trianide Regular, 1294 t
Triaz, 1284t
triazolam, 1195–1197
Tribenzagan, 1202–1203
Tribenzor 20/5/12.5, 1332t
Tribenzor 40/5/12.5, 1332t
Tribenzor 40/5/25, 1332t
Tribenzor 40/10/12.5, 1332t
Tricor, 466–468
Tridesilon, 1291 t
Tridil, 842–845
triethylenethiophos-phoramide, 1310t
trifluoperazine hydrochloride, 1197–1199
triflupromazine, 1199–1201
Trihexane, 1201–1202
Trihexy, 1201–1202
trihexyphenidyl hydrochloride, 1201–1202

Tri-K, 955–958
Trikacide, 757–759
trikates, 955–958
Trilafon, 925–927
Trilafon Concentrate, 925–927
Trileptal, 880–882
Trilipix, 466–468
TRI-LUMA Cream, 1296 t
Trimazide, 1202–1203
trimethobenzamide hydrochloride, 1202–1203
trimethoprim, 1203
trimipramine maleate, 1203–1205
Trimox, 68–70
Trimpex, 1203
Trinalin Repetabs, 1272t
Triostat, 671–673
Triptil, 999–1001
triptorelin pamoate, 1320t
Tristoject, 1190–1194
Trivagizole 3, 1286t
Trizivir, 1299 t
Trobicin, 1080–1081
tromethamine, 1205–1206
Tropicacyl, 1278t
tropicamide, 1278t
trospium chloride, 1206–1207
trovafloxacin mesylate, 24–25
Trovan, 24–25
Trovan I.V., 24–25
Trulicity, 382–383
Truphylline, 56–58
Trusopt, 1281t
Truvada, 1302t
Truxophyllin, 1132–1135
TSH, 1144–1146
TSPA, 1310t
T-Stat, 1284t
tubocurarine chloride, 1207–1209, 1208i
Tudorza Pressair, 18–19
Tusal, 1075–1076
Twin-K, 955–958
Twynsta 40/5, 1332t
Twynsta 40/10, 1332t
Twynsta 80/5, 1332t
Twynsta 80/10, 1332t
Tygacil, 1151–1152
Tylenol, 8–10
Tylenol Caplets, 8–10
Tylenol Children's Chewable Tablets, 8–10
Tylenol Extra Strength, 8–10
Tylenol Gelcaps, 8–10
Tylenol Infants' Drops, 8–10
Tysabri, 820–822
Tyzeka, 1306t

U

Uloric, 462–464
Ultiva, 1022–1023, 1023i
Ultram, 1181–1183
Ultram ER, 1181–1183
Ultrase MT 12, 889–901
Ultrase MT 20, 889–901
Ultravate, 1291 t
umeclidinium, 1211
Unicort, 1292 t
Uni-Dur, 1132–1135
Unipen, 807–808
Uniphyl, 1132–1135
Uniretic 15/25, 1332t
Unisom SleepGels Maximum Strength, 353–354
Unithroid, 660–662
Uni-tussin, 545–546
Univasc, 785–787
unoprostone isopropyl 0.15%, 1282t
Urabeth, 139–140
urea, 1212–1213
Ureaphil, 1212–1213
Urecholine, 139–140
Urex, 432–733
Uridon, 237–239
Urispas, 488
Uritol, 522–524
Urobak, 1090–1091
Urocit-K, 955–958
Urodine, 927
Urogesic, 927
urokinase, 1213–1214
Uro-Mag, 797–700
Uroxatral, 32–33
Urozide, 558–560, 559i
URSO 250, 1214–1215
ursodeoxycholic acid, 1214–1215
ursodiol, 1214–1215
Ursofalk, 1214–1215
Urso Forte, 1214–1215
ustekinumab, 1215–1217
Uticort, 1290t

V

Vagifem, 429–435
Vaginal administration, xxiii, xxx
Vagistat-1, 1289 t
valacyclovir, 1304t
Valcyte, 1305t

Valergen 10, 429–435
Valergen 20, 429–435
Valergen 40, 429–435
valganciclovir hydrochloride, 1305t
Valisone, 1290 t
Valium, 328–331
valproate sodium, 1217–1220
valproic acid, 1217–1220
valsartan, 1220–1221, 1328t, 1332t
Valtrex, 1304t
Valturna 150/160, 1332t
Valturna 300/320, 1332t
Vanadom, 179–180
Vancenase, 124–126
Vanceril, 124–126
Vancocin, 1221–1223
vancomycin hydrochloride, 1221–1223
Vaniqa, 1296 t
Vantin, 204–205
Vaponefrin, 402–404
Vaprisol, 281–282
vardenafil hydrochloride, 1223–1225
varenicline, 1225–1226
Vascepa, 580–581
Vascor, 133–135
Vaseretic 5/12.5, 1332t
Vaseretic 10/25, 1332t
Vasocon Regular, 1279t
vasopressin, 1226–1227, 1227i
Vasotec, 394–396
Vasotec I.V., 394–396
V-Cillin K, 915–917
VCR, 1317t
Vectrin, 771–774
vedolizumab, 1228–1229
Veetids, 915–917
Velban, 1317t
Velbe, 1317t
Velcade, 1321t
Veletri, 408–410
Velosef, 222–223
Velosulin BR, 1267t
Velosulin Human, 1267t
Velphoro, 1086–1087
Veltin Gel, 1284t
venlafaxine hydrochloride, 1229–1232
Venofer, 607–609
Venoglobulin-I, 584–590
Venoglobulin-S 5%, 584–590
Venoglobulin-S 10%, 584–590
Ventolin HFA, 26–29, 28i
Ventolin Syrup, 26–29, 28i
VePesid, 1322t

Veramyst, 503–505
verapamil, 1232–1234
verapamil hydrochloride, 1232–1234
Verazinc, 1252–1254
Verelan, 1232–1234
Versed, 764–766
VESIcare, 1076–1077
Vesprin, 1199–1201
Vexol, 1277t
Vfend, 1238–1241
V-Gan-25, 988–990
V-Gan-50, 988–990
Viadur, 1320t
Viagra, 1062–1064
Vibativ, 1115–1117
Vibramycin, 374–378
Vibra-Tabs, 374–378
Vicks Sinex, 934–936
Vicks Vitamin C Drops, 1342t
Victoza, 673–674
Victrelis, 1306t
vidarabine, 1304t
vigabatrin, 1234–1236
Vigamox, 1277t
Viibryd, 1236–1237
vilazodone hydrochloride, 1236–1237
Vimpat, 632–634
vinblastine sulfate, 1317t
Vincasar PFS, 1317t
vincristine sulfate, 1317t
vinorelbine tartrate, 1317t
Viokase Powder, 899–901
Viokase Tablets, 899–901
Vira-A, 1304t
Viracept, 1302t
Viramune, 1302t
Viramune XR, 1302 t
Viread, 1302t, 1306t
Viridium, 927
Visine Extra, 1279t
Visine L.R., 1279t
Visine Moisturizing, 1279t
Visken, 941–942
Vistaril, 571–572
Vistide, 1305t
Vita-bee 6, 1338t
vitamin A, 1336t
vitamin B1, 1336t, 1338t
vitamin B3, 1338t
vitamin B6, 1338t, 1340t
vitamin B9, 1340t
vitamin B12, 1340t, 1342t
vitamin C, 1342t

vitamin D2, 1344t
vitamin E, 1344t
vitamin K1, 1346t
Vitamins, 1336–1346t
Vita-Plus E, 1344t
Vivactil, 999–1001
Vivelle, 429–435
Vivelle-Dot, 429–435
Vivitrol, 814–816
Vivol, 328–331
VLB, 1317t
Volmax, 26–29, 28i
Voltaren, 333–336, 1276t
Voltaren Ophtha, 1276t
Voltaren Rapide, 333–336
Voltaren SR, 333–336
vorapaxar, 1237–1238
voriconazole, 1238–1241
vortioxetine hydrobromide, 1241–1243
VP-16, 1322t
Vytone, 1293 t
Vyvanse, 674–676

W

warfarin sodium, 1243–1245
Water-soluble drugs, xxi
Weak agonists, xxiv
Webber Vitamin E, 1344t
Weights and equivalents, 1361–1362t
Welchol, 277–278
Wellbutrin, 155–158
Wellbutrin SR, 155–158
Wellbutrin XL, 155–158
Westcort, 1293 t
Westhroid, 1143–1144
Winpred, 972–974
WinRho SDF, 584–590
Wintrocin, 416–420
Wyamine, 712–713
Wycillin, 915–917
Wymox, 68–70

X

Xalatan, 1281t
Xanax, 42–44
Xanax XR, 42–44
Xarelto, 1034–1036

Xeloda, 1313t
Xenical, 872–874, 873i
Xibrom, 1275t
Xolair, 863–864
Xopenex, 648–649
Xopenex HFA, 648–649
Xylocaine, 662–664
Xylocard, 662–664
Xyzal, 651–652, 1272t

Z

Zaditor, 1281t
zafirlukast, 1247–1248
Zagam, 1079–1080
zaleplon, 1248–1249
Zanaflex, 1160–1161
zanamivir, 1305t
Zanosar, 1310t
Zantac, 1017–1019
Zantac 150 GELdose, 1017–1019
Zantac 300 GELdose, 1017–1019
Zantac EFFERdose Tablets, 1017–1019
Zarontin, 447–448
Zaroxolyn, 753–754
ZDV, 1303t
Zeasorb-AF, 1289 t
Zebeta, 141–143
Zecuity, 1099–1101
Zefazone, 195–196
Zegerid, 864–868, 867i
Zelapar, 1056–1058
Zemaira, 41–42
Zemplar, 904–906
Zenpep, 899–901
Zerit, 1302t
Zerit XR, 1302 t
Zestoretic 10/12.5, 1332t
Zestoretic 20/12.5, 1332t
Zestoretic 20/25, 1332t
Zestril, 667–669
Zetar, 1295 t
Zetar Shampoo, 1295 t
Zetia, 457–459, 458i
Zetonna, 242–244
Ziac 2.5/6.25, 1332t
Ziac 5/6.25, 1332t
Ziac 10/6.25, 1332t
Ziagen, 1299 t
ziconotide, 1248–1251, 1250 i
zidovudine, 1299 t, 1301t, 1303t

zileuton, 1251–1252
Zinacef, 214–217
Zinc 15, 1252–1254
Zinc-220, 1252–1254
zinc acetate, 1252–1254
Zinca-Pak, 1252–1254
Zincate, 1252–1254
zinc chloride, 1252–1254
zinc gluconate, 1252–1254
zinc sulfate, 1252–1254
Zingo, 662–664
Zioptan, 1281t
ziprasidone hydrochloride, 1254–1256
ziprasidone mesylate, 1254–1256
Zipsor, 333–336
Zirgan, 1273t
Zithromax, 115–117
Zmax, 115–117
Zocor, 1065–1067
Zofran, 868–871
Zofran ODT, 868–871
Zohydro ER, 561–563
Zoladex, 1319t
Zoladex 3-Month, 1319t
Zoladex LA, 1319t
zoledronic acid, 1256–1258
zolmitriptan, 1258–1259

Zoloft, 1058–1061
zolpidem tartrate, 1259–1261
Zometa, 1256–1258
Zomig, 1258–1259
Zomig ZMT, 1258–1259
Zonalon, 1296 t
Zonegran, 1261–1263
zonisamide, 1261–1263
Zontivity, 1237-1238
ZORprin, 98–100
Zortress, 453–455
Zostrix, 1295 t
Zovirax, 1290 t, 1303t
Zuplenz, 868–871
Zyban, 155–158
Zyclara, 1297 t
Zydis, 857–859
Zyflo CR, 1251–1252
Zyloprim, 36–37
Zymar, 1274t
Zymase, 899–901
Zymaxid, 1274t
Zyprexa, 857–859
Zyrtec, 1272t
Zyrtec D, 1272t
Zyvox, 668–671, 670i

Body Mass Index Calculation

Body mass index (BMI) is a formula used to determine obesity; it's calculated by dividing a person's weight in kilograms by height in meters squared (kg/m^2). A BMI of 25 or higher increases your patient's risk of developing hypertension, cardiovascular disease, type 2 diabetes mellitus, and stroke. It also increases the risk that he won't respond effectively to the usual drug dosages. If your patient has an abnormal BMI, be prepared to make dosage adjustments that are individualized based on body weight, as prescribed.

The table below will help you find your patient's BMI easily. The table converts pounds to kilograms and inches to meters, and then it shows the BMI. To use it, simply find the patient's height on either side of the table, then move across the row to the weight that matches your patient's most closely. At the bottom of the column containing the weight, you'll find the BMI for that patient. For example, the BMI for a patient who is 70 inches tall and weighs 208 lb is 30.

WEIGHT (POUNDS)

HEIGHT (INCHES)																		
58	91	96	100	105	110	115	119	124	129	134	138	143	148	153	158	162	167	172
59	94	99	104	109	114	119	124	128	133	138	143	148	153	158	163	168	173	178
60	97	102	107	112	118	123	128	133	138	143	148	153	158	163	168	174	179	184
61	100	106	111	116	122	127	132	137	143	148	153	158	164	169	174	180	185	190
62	104	109	115	120	126	131	136	142	147	153	158	164	169	175	180	186	191	196
63	107	113	118	124	130	135	141	146	152	158	163	169	175	180	186	191	197	203
64	110	116	122	128	134	140	145	151	157	163	169	174	180	186	192	197	204	209
65	114	120	126	132	138	144	150	156	162	168	174	180	186	192	198	204	210	216
66	118	124	130	136	142	148	155	161	167	173	179	186	192	198	204	210	216	223
67	121	127	134	140	146	153	159	166	172	178	185	191	198	204	211	217	223	230
68	125	131	138	144	151	158	164	171	177	184	190	197	203	210	216	223	230	236
69	128	135	142	149	155	162	169	176	182	189	196	203	209	216	223	230	236	243
70	132	139	146	153	160	167	174	181	188	195	202	209	216	222	229	236	243	250
71	136	143	150	157	165	172	179	186	193	200	208	215	222	229	236	243	250	257
72	140	147	154	162	169	177	184	191	199	206	213	221	228	235	242	250	258	265
73	144	151	159	166	174	182	189	197	204	212	219	227	235	242	250	257	265	272
74	148	155	163	171	179	186	194	202	210	218	225	233	241	249	256	264	272	280
75	152	160	168	176	184	192	200	208	216	224	232	240	248	256	264	272	279	287
76	156	164	172	180	189	197	205	213	221	230	238	246	254	263	271	279	287	295
	19	20	21	22	23	24	25	26	27	28	29	30	31	32	33	34	35	36

BODY MASS INDEX